S0-ADO-069

American
DRUG INDEX

29th Edition

American

DRUG INDEX

1985

29th Edition

NORMAN F. BILLUPS, Ph.D., R.Ph.

Dean and Professor of Pharmacy
College of Pharmacy
The University of Toledo

Associate Editor

SHIRLEY M. BILLUPS, R.N.

Oncology Nurse
The Toledo Hospital

J. B. LIPPINCOTT COMPANY
Philadelphia

| London | New York | São Paulo |
| Mexico City | St. Louis | Sydney |

Copyright © 1985, by J. B. Lippincott Company

Copyright © 1956, 1958, 1959, 1960, 1961, 1962, 1963, 1964, 1965, 1966, 1967, 1968, 1969, 1970, 1971, 1972, 1973, 1974, 1975, 1976, 1977, 1978, 1979, 1980, 1981, 1982, 1983, 1984 by J. B. Lippincott Company

2 3 4 5 6 7 8 9

This book is fully protected by copyright and, with the exception of brief excerpts for review, no part of it may be reproduced in any form by print, photoprint, microfilm or any other means, without the written permission of the publishers.

ISBN 0-397-50703-8

Library of Congress Catalog Card Number 55-6286

Printed in the United States of America

Preface

The 29th Edition of the *American Drug Index* (ADI) has been prepared for the identification, explanation, and correlation of the many pharmaceuticals available to the medical, pharmaceutical, and allied health professions. The need for this index has become acute as the variety and number of drugs and drug products have continued to multiply. For this reason the *ADI* should be most useful to pharmacists, nurses, physicians, medical transcriptionists, dentists, sales personnel, students, and teachers in the fields incorporating pharmaceuticals. *Special note to medical transcriptionists:* Although all names in the *ADI* appear in bold capitalized type, trade products are easily identifiable by the manufacturer's name in parentheses immediately following the trade name. The names for official products are preceded by a bullet (•) and should appear in lower case in transcription. The therapeutic and pharmaceutical classes are denoted by a box (■) preceding the name and should be a helpful cross-reference guide.

The organization of the *ADI* falls into the following ten major sections: Monographs of Drug Products, Common Abbreviations Used in Medical Orders, Aproximate Practical Equivalents, Common Systems of Weight and Measure, Glossary, Title Changes For U.S.P. XXI and N.F. XVI Monographs, Container Requirements for U.S.P. XXI Drugs, Container and Storage Requirements for Sterile U.S.P. XXI Drugs, Pharmaceutical Company Labeler Code Index Numbers, and Pharmaceutical Manufacturer and/or Drug Distributor Addresses. The U.S.P. XXI and N.F. XVI Title Changes section has been added to make the *ADI* an even more complete and valuable reference tool.

MONOGRAPHS: The organization of the monograph section of the *ADI* is fundamentally alphabetical with extensive cross-indexing. Names listed are generic (also called non-proprietary, public name, or common name); brand (also called trade-mark, proprietary, or specialty); and chemical. Synonyms that are in general use also are included. All names used for a pharmaceutical appear in alphabetical order with the pertinent data given under the brand name by which it is made available.

The monograph for a typical brand name product consists of the manufacturer, generic and/or chemical names, composition and strength, pharmaceutical forms available, package size, dosage, and use.

Generic names appear in alphabetical order, followed by the corresponding recognition of the drug to the U.S.P. (United States Pharmacopeia), N.F. (National Formulary), and USAN (United States Adopted Names). Each of these officially recognized generic names is preceded by a bullet (•) at the beginning of each entry. The information is in accord with the U.S.P. XXI and N.F. XVI and through Supplement 5, which became official on January 1, 1985; and the USAN-1985.

British Approved Names, indicated by (B.A.N.), are included in this edition with the permission of the Controller of Her Britannic Majesty's Stationery Office.

Because of the multiplicity of specialty names (brand names) used for the same therapeutic agent or the same combination of therapeutic agents, it was apparent that some correlation could be done. As an example of this, please turn to tetracycline HCl. Here under the generic name are listed the various brand names. Following are combinations of tetracycline HCl organized in a manner to point out relationships among the many products. Reference then is made to the specialty name or names having the indicated composition. Under the specialty name are given manufacturer, composition, available forms, sizes, dosage, and use.

The multiplicity of generic names for the same therapeutic agent has complicated the nomenclature of these agents. Examples of multiple generic names for the same chemical substance are (1) parabromdylamine, brompheniramine; (2) acetaminophen, p-hydroxy acetanilid, N-acetyl-p-aminophenol; (3) guaifenesin, glyceryl guaiacolate, glyceryl guaiacol ether, guaianesin, guaifylline, guaiphenesin, guayanesin, methphenoxydiol; (4) methapyrilene HCl, thenylpyramine HCl; and (5) pyrilamine, pyranisamine, pyranilamine, pyraminyl, anisopyradamine.

The cross-indexing feature of the *ADI* permits the finding of drugs or drug combinations when only one major ingredient is known. For example, a combination of aluminum hydroxide gel and magnesium trisilicate is available. This combination can be found by looking under the name of either of the two ingredients, and in each case the specialty names are given. A second form of cross-indexing involves the listing of drugs under various therapeutic and pharmaceutical classes (i.e., antacids, antihistamines, diuretics, laxatives, etc.). Each of these classes is preceded by a box (■) at the beginning of each entry.

ABBREVIATIONS: A listing of Common Abbreviations Used in Medical Orders is included as an aid in interpreting medical orders. The Latin or Greek word and abbreviation are both given with the meaning.

CONVERSION FACTORS: The listing of Approximate Practical Equivalents is added as an aid in calculating and converting dosages among the metric, apothecary, and avoirdupois systems.

WEIGHT AND MEASURE: Tables containing the Common Systems of Weight and Measure are included to aid the practitioner in calculating dosages in the metric, apothecary, and avoirdupois systems.

GLOSSARY: A listing of commonly used terms, with brief definitions, is included as an aid in interpreting the use given for drug monographs listed in the *ADI*.

NEW TITLES AND TITLE CHANGES FOR U.S.P. XXI AND N.F. XVI MONOGRAPHS: 76 official monograph title changes appeared in the

1985 U.S.P. XXI and N.F. XVI, and an additional 535 new monographs have appeared since the 1980 U.S.P. XX and N.F. XV. Since many of these changes apply to commonly used drug products, this section has been added to aid the practitioner in identifying drug products. Among the more significant title changes are diiodohydroxyquin to iodoquinol, dioctyl sodium sulfosuccinate to docusate sodium (and the calcium salt to docusate calcium), gamma benzene hexachloride to lindane, iodochlorhydroxyquin to clioquinol, and levarterenol bitartrate to norepinephrine bitartrate.

CONTAINER AND STORAGE REQUIREMENTS FOR U.S.P. XXI COMPENDIAL DRUGS: This year two new sections have been added on container and storage requirements specified by the U.S.P. XXI for compendial drugs, to aid the practitioner in storing and dispensing.

LABELER CODE INDEX: The Pharmaceutical Labeler Code Index is presented to aid the practitioner in the identification of drug products. In this section, the codes are listed in numerical order followed by the name of the manufacturer.

MANUFACTURER ADDRESSES: The name, address, and zip code of virtually every American Pharmaceutical Manufacturer and/or Drug Distributor are listed in alphabetical order in this section. Additionally, a pharmaceutical labeler code number appears prior to the address of each company as a further aid in the identification of drug products.

A special word of appreciation and acknowledgment is given to my wife, Shirley, who served again this year as my Associate Editor—and helped to compile much of the information that appears in the monograph section of this volume. Special thanks are also extended to the manufacturers who supplied product information and made helpful comments and suggestions for this index, and to Dr. Kenneth S. Alexander, who organized the information on Container and Storage Requirements for U.S.P. XXI Drugs.

Correspondence or communication with reference to a drug or drug products listed in the *American Drug Index* should be directed to Norman F. Billups, Ph.D., Dean, College of Pharmacy; The University of Toledo; Toledo, Ohio 43606, or call 419-537-4235.

Norman F. Billups, Ph.D., R.Ph.

Contents

[•] Denotes official name: Generic name or chemical name approved by
F.D.A. or recognized by the U.S.P., N.F., or USAN.
[■] Denotes therapeutic and pharmaceutical classes.

A

A-200 PYRINATE. (Norcliff Thayer) **Liquid:** Pyrethrins 0.17%, piperonyl butoxide technical 2.00%, petroleum distallate 5.00%. Bot. 2 fl. oz., 4 fl. oz. **Gel:** Pyrethrins 0.33%, piperonyl butoxide technical 4.00%, petroleum distallate 5.33%. Tube 1 oz.
Use: Topically, pediculosis.

A.A.A. OINTMENT. (Jenkins) Ammoniated mercury 2%, acid salicylic 1.25%, acid boric 1%, zinc oxide 15%. Jar 1 oz., 1 lb.
Use: Impetigo, nonspecific eczema & minor skin irritations.

A AND D HAND CREAM. (Schering) Emollients isopropyl myristate & squalane. Tube 2 oz.
Use: Dry skin, sunburn, irritations.

A AND D OINTMENT. (Kenyon) Vits. A & D in lanolin-petrolatum base. Jar 1 lb.

A AND D OINTMENT. (Schering) Petrolatum-lanolin. Tube 1½, 4 oz.; Jar 1 lb.

A & D TABLETS. (Barth's) Vit. A 10,000 I.U., D 400 I.U./Tab. Bot. 100s, 500s.

A AND D VITAMIN CAPSULES. (Lannett) Vit. A 5000 I.U., D 400 I.U./Cap. Bot. 500s, 1000s.
Use: Vit. supplement.

A AND D VITAMIN CREAM. (Eckerd) Bot. 1½ oz., 4 oz.

A & D VITAMIN OINTMENT. (Columbia) Vit. A & D in lanolin-petroleum base Tube 2 oz., Jar 1 lb.
Use: Emollient.

A AND D VITAMIN OINTMENT. (Lannett) In a petrolatum-lanolin base. Jar 1, 5 lb.

A AND D VITAMIN OINTMENT. (Ulmer) Jar 1 lb., 2 oz.

A-A PLUS. (Galen) Al hydroxide gel 400 mg., Mg oxide 175 mg., Na lauryl sulfate 25 mg., Me cellulose 100 mg., hyoscyamine sulfate 0.1037 mg., atropine sulfate 0.0194 mg., hyoscine HBr 0.0065 mg./Tab. Bot. 100s, 1000s. Susp. 1 pt.

AAS INFANTIL TABLETS. (Winthrop Products) Acetylsalicylic acid.
Use: Analgesic, antipyretic.

AAS INFANTIL W/VITAMIN C. (Winthrop Products) Acetylsalicylic acid, Vit. C.
Use: Analgesic, antipyretic.

ABBOCIN. Oxytetracycline, B.A.N.

ABBOKINASE. (Abbott) Urokinase 250,000 I.U./5 ml. Lyophilized powder. Vial 5 ml.
Use: Plasminogen activator.

ABBOKINASE OPEN-CATH. (Abbott) Urokinase for catheter clearance 5,000 I.U./ml. Univial.
Use: Clearance of fibrin occluded catheters.

ABBOTT AFP-EIA. (Abbott) Test Kits 100s.
Use: Enzyme immunoassay for the quantitative measurement of alpha-fetoprotein in human serum to aid in the management of testicular cancer.

ABBOTT CMV TOTAL AB EIA. (Abbott) Test kits 100s.
Use: Enzyme immunoassay for the detection of antibody to cytomegalovirus in human serum, plasma, and whole blood.

ABBOTT-HB$_e$ TEST. (Abbott) Test kits 100s.
Use: Radioimmunoassay or enzyme immunoassay for detection of hepatitis B$_e$ antigen and/or antibody to hepatitis Be antigen.

ABBOTT IgE EIA. (Abbott) Test kits 100s.
Use: Enzyme immunoassay for quantitative determination of IgE in human serum and plasma.

ABC COMPOUND w/CODEINE #3. (Zenith) Aspirin 325 mg., caffeine 40 mg., butalbital 50 mg., codeine phosphate 30 mg./Cap.
Use: Analgesic.

ABCDG VITAMIN CAPSULES. (Lannett) Vit. A 5000 u., D 400 u., B-1 1 mg., B-2 2 mg., C 30 mg./Cap. Bot. 1000s.
Use: Vitamin supplement.

ABDEC BABY VITAMIN DROPS. (Parke-Davis) Vit. A 1500 I.U., D 400 I.U., B-1 0.5 mg., B-2 0.6 mg., B-6 0.4 mg., pantothenic acid 3 mg., niacin 8 mg., C 35 mg./ml. Bot. 1⅔ oz. w/dropper.
Use: Vitamin deficiencies.

ABDEC WITH FLUORIDE BABY VITAMIN DROPS. (Parke-Davis) Vit. A 1500 I.U., D 400 I.U., C 35 mg., B-1 0.5 mg., B-2 0.6 mg., B-6 0.4 mg., niacin 8 mg., pantothenic acid 3 mg./ml. w/fluoride. Bot. 50 ml.
Use: Vitamin therapy with fluoride.

ABDO. (Eastwood) Cap. Bot. 100s.

ABDOL W/MINERALS. (Parke-Davis) Vit. C 50 mg., B-2 2.5 mg., B-12 1 mcg., B-6 0.5 mg., B-1 2.5 mg., niacinamide 20 mg., Vit. A 5000 I.U., D 400 I.U., Ca pantothenate 2.5 mg., folic acid 0.1 mg., iodine 0.15 mg., Mn 1 mg., K 5.0 mg., Fe 15 mg., Cu 1 mg., Zn 0.5 mg., Mg 1 mg., Ca 44 mg., P 34 mg./Cap. Bot. 100s.
Use: Vitamin-mineral deficiency states.

ABSORBABLE CELLULOSE COTTON OR GAUZE. See: Oxidized Cellulose (Various Mfr.)

• **ABSORBABLE DUSTING POWDER,** U.S.P. XXI.

• **ABSORBABLE GELATIN FILM,** U.S.P. XXI. Sterile nonantigenic, absorbable, water-insoluble, gelatin film. See: Gelfilm (Upjohn)

• **ABSORBABLE GELATIN SPONGE,** U.S.P. XXI. Gelatin sponge.
Use: Surgical aid.
See: Gelfoam, Preps. (Upjohn)

• **ABSORBABLE SURGICAL SUTURE,** U.S.P. XXI. (Various Mfr.) Surgical Gut, Surgical Catgut, Catgut suture.
Use: Surgical aid.

• **ABSORBENT GAUZE,** U.S.P. XXI.
Use: Surgical aid.

ABSORBINE ARTHRITIC PAIN LOTION. (W.F. Young) Bot. 2 oz., 4 oz.

ABSORBINE FOOT POWDER. (W.F. Young) Zinc stearate, parachloroxylenol, aluminum chlorhydroxy, allantonate, benzethonium chloride, menthol. Plastic bot. 3 oz. w/shaker top.
Use: Athlete's foot treatment.

ABSORBINE, JR. (W.F. Young) Wormwood, thymol, chloroxylenol, menthol, acetone, zinc stearate, parachloroxylenol, aluminum chlorhydroxy, allantonate, benzethonium chloride, menthol. Liq. Bot. 1 oz., 2 oz., 4 oz., 12 oz. w/applicator.

Use: Muscle soreness, stiffness, treatment of athlete's foot.

ABUSCREEN. (Roche Diagnostics) An immunological and radiochemical assay for morphine and morphine glucuronide in nanogram levels. Utilizes ^3H labeled morphine assayed with liquid scintillation counters using conventional beta counting procedures and ^{125}I labeled morphine requiring gamma scintillation equipment. 100 tests.

ACABEL. Bevonium Methylsulphate, B.A.N.

• **ACACIA**, N.F. XVI. Syrup N.F. XVI. Acacia senegal, gum arabic. (Penick) pow., ¼ lb., 1 lb.; tears, ¼-1 lb.; whole, ¼-1 lb.
Use: Demulcent, emulsifier, suspending agent.

A-CAINE. (A.V.P.) Rectal ointment. Tube 1.25 oz.
Use: Rectal care, anti-hemorrhoidal.

A CAPSULES. (Stanlabs) Natural Vit. A 5,000 I.U., 10,000 I.U., 25,000 I.U., 50,000 I.U./Cap. Bot. 100s. Synthetic or soluble, 10,000 I.U., 25,000 I.U., 50,000 I.U./Cap. Bot. 100s.

A-CAPS. (Drug Industries) Vit. A 50,000 I.U./Cap. Bot. 100s, 500s.
Use: Vitamin A therapy.

• **ACARBOSE.** USAN.
Use: Inhibitor.

ACCELERASE. (Organon) Pancrelipase: Lipase 4000 U., amylase 15,000 U., protease 15,000 U., other pancreatic enzymes mixed with bile salts 65 mg., cellulase 2 mg., calcium carbonate 20 mg./Cap. Bot. 60s.
Use: Functional digestive disorders.

ACCURBRON. (Merrell Dow) Theophylline, anhydrous 10 mg./ml. Bot. pt.
Use: Bronchial asthma treatment.

ACCUSENS T TASTE FUNCTION KIT. (Westport) Test for ability to distinguish among salty, sweet, sour and bitter tastants. Kit contains 15 bottles (60 ml.) tastants and 30 taste record forms.
Use: Diagnostic taste function kit.

ACCUTANE. (Roche) Isotretinoin 10 mg., or 40 mg./Cap. Bot. 100s.
Use: Treatment of severe recalcitrant cystic acne.

A-C-D SOLUTION, U.S.P. Sod. citrate, citric acid & dextrose in sterile pyrogen-free solution.
Baxter-600 cc. bot. with 70, 120 or 300 cc. of sol.; 1000 cc. with 500 cc. of sol.
Cutter-500 cc. bot. with 75 or 120 cc. of sol.; 650 cc. bot. with 80 or 130 cc. of sol.
Diamond-(Abbo-Vac) 250 cc., 500 cc.
Use: Anticoagulant for preparation of plasma or whole blood.

A-C-D SOLUTION MODIFIED. (Squibb) Acid citrate dextrose anticoagulant solution modified.
Use: Anticoagulant for use in radiolabeling red blood cells.

ACDRILE. Methyl Cysteine, B.A.N.

• **ACEBUTOLOL.** USAN. (±)-1-(2-Acetyl-4-butyramido-phenoxy)-3-isopropylaminopropan-2-ol. (Ives) (±)-N-[3-Acetyl-4-[2-hydroxy-3-[(1-methylethyl)amino]pro-poxy]-phenyl] butamide.
Use: Beta adrenergic receptor blocking agent.

• **ACECAINIDE HYDROCHLORIDE.** USAN.
Use: Cardiac depressant.

• **ACECLIDINE.** USAN. 3-Quinuclidinol acetate (ester). Glaucostat. Under study.
Use: Parasympathomimetic.

• **ACEDAPSONE.** USAN. 4',4"-Sulfonylbis (acetanilide).
Use: Antimalarial; antibacterial (leprostatic).

ACEDOVAL. (Vale) Dover's powder 15 mg., ipecac 15 mg., aspirin 162 mg., caffeine anhydrous 8.1 mg., camphor 16.2 mg./Tab. Bot. 100s, 1000s, 5000s.

ACEDYNE. (Vale) Aspirin 64.8 mg., caffeine anhydrous 3.2 mg., atropine sulfate 0.032 mg., magnesium trisilicate 64.8 mg./Tab. Bot. 100s, 1000s, 5000s.

ACEFYLLINE PIPERAZINE. Acepifylline, B.A.N.

• **ACEGLUTAMIDE ALUMINUM.** USAN.

ACELAX. (Marcen) Danthron 100 mg., prune concentrate 64 mg., Chondrus drispus 64 mg./Tab. Bot. 100s, 1000s.
Use: Laxative.

ACENOCOUMAROL. 3-(α-Acetonyl-4-nitrobenzyl)-4-hydroxy-coumarin. Nicoumalone, B.A.N.

A'CENOL. (Kay) Acetaminophen 5 gr./Tab. Bot. 1000s.
Use: Analgesic.

ACEPHEN. (G&W) **Adult:** Acetaminophen 650 mg./Supp. Box 12s, 100s.**Pediatric:** Acetaminophen 120 mg./Supp. Box 12s, 100s.
Use: Analgesic, antipyretic.

ACEPIFYLLINE. B.A.N. Piperazine theophyllin-7-ylacetate. Acefylline Piperazine (I.N.N.). Etophylate.
Use: Spasmolytic.

ACEPROMAZINE. 10(3-Dimethylaminopropyl)-3-acetyl-phenothiazine maleate. Plegicil. (Ayerst) 1-(10-(3-(Dimethylamino)propyl)-10H-phenothiazin-2-yl)ethan-on e(Z)-2-butenedioate.
Use: Tranquilizer.

ACEPROMAZINE. B.A.N. 2-Acetyl-10-(3-di-methylaminopropyl)phenothiazine. Notensil maleate.
Use: Tranquilizer.

• **ACEPROMAZINE MALEATE.** USAN.
Use: Sedative.

ACEROLA C.(Kirkman) Vit. C 100 mg./Wafer. Bot. 100s.

ACEROLA-C. (Barth's) Vit. C 300 mg./Wafer. Bot. 30s, 90s, 180s, 360s.

ACEROLA-PLEX. (Barth's) Vit. C 100 mg., bioflavon-oids 50 mg./Tab. Bot. 100s, 500s.

ACETA. (Century) Acetaminophen. **Elix.** (120 mg./5 cc) Bot. 4 oz., pint, gal. **Tabs.** (5 gr.) Bot. 100s, 1000s, 3000s, 5000s.
Use: Analgesic.

ACETA W/CODEINE. (Century) Acetaminophen 325 mg., codeine phosphate ½ gr./Tab. Bot. 100s.
Use: Analgesic.

ACETAMIDE. N-[5-(Aminosulfonyl)-3-methyl-1,3,4-thi-odiazol-2(3H)-ylidene]-. Methazolamide.

ACETAMIDE, 2,2-DICHLORO-N-[2-HYDROXY-1-(HYDROXYMETHYL)-2-(4-NITROPHENYL)ETHYL]. Chloramphenicol, U.S.P. XXI.

ACETAMIDE, 2-(DIETHYLAMINO)-N-(2,6-DI-METHYLPHENYL)-. Lidocaine, U.S.P. XXI.

ACETAMIDE, N-[5-(AMINOSULFONYL)-1,3,-4-THIADIAZOL-2-YL]-. Acetazolamide, U.S.P. XXI.
ACETAMIDE, N-(4-HYDROXYPHENYL)-. Acetaminophen, U.S.P. XXI.
ACETAMIDE, N-(5,6,7,9-TETRAHYDRO-1,2,3,10-TETRAMETHOXY-9-OXOBENZO[a]-HEPTALEN-7-YL-. Colchicine, U.S.P. XXI.
p-ACETAMIDOBENZOIC ACID SALT of 2-dimethylaminoethanol.
See: Deaner, Tab. (Riker).
5-ACETAMIDO-2,4,6-TRIIODO-N-METHYLISOPHTHALAMIC ACID. Iothalamic Acid, U.S.P. XXI.
5-ACETAMIDO-2,4,6-TRIIODO-N-METHYLISOPHTHALAMIC ACID, SODIUM SALT. Iothalamate Sodium Injection, U.S.P. XXI.
• **ACETAMINOPHEN,** U.S.P. XXI. Elix., for Effervescent Oral Soln., Tabs, Cap. U.S.P. XXI. N-Acetyl-p-amino-phenol. Acetamide, N-(4-hydroxyphenyl)-. 4'-Hydroxyacetanilide.
Use: Analgesic, antipyretic.
See: Acephen, Supp. (G&W)
 Aceta, Tab. Elix., Supp. (Century)
 Acetagesic (Kay)
 Actamin, Tab. (Buffington)
 Acetaminophen Uniserts, Suppos. (Upsher-Smith)
 Aminodyne, Elix. (Bowman)
 Anapap, Tab. (Fellows)
 Anelix, Elix. (Kirkman)
 Anuphen, Supp. (Comatic)
 Apap, Cap., Tab. (Various Mfr.)
 Capital, Tab. (Carnrick)
 Chlor-A-Tyl. (Jenkins)
 Dapa, Tab. (Ferndale)
 Datril 500, Tab. (Bristol-Myers)
 Dimindol, Tab., Elix. (Blue Line)
 Dolanex, Elix. (Lannett)
 Dularin, Syr. (Donner)
 Febridol, Elix., Tab. (Amid)
 Fendon, Tab. (APC)
 G-1 (Hauck)
 Janupap, Tab. (Reid-Provident)
 Lestemp, Elix. (Reid-Provident)
 Liquiprin, Solu. (Norcliff Thayer)
 Lyteca, Syr., Tab. (Westerfield)
 Medigesic (Medics)
 Nebs, Tab., Liq. (Eaton)
 Nilprin 7½, Tab. (AVP)
 Parten, Tab. (Parmed)
 Phenaphen, Cap., Tab. (Robins)
 Proval, Cap., Elix., Drop., Tab. (Reid-Provident)
 SK-Apap, Tab., Elix. (SmithKline)
 Tapar, Tab. (Parke-Davis)
 Temetan, Elix., Tab. (Nevin)
 Tempra, Drop, Syr., (Mead Johnson)
 Tenlap, Elix. (Merrell Dow)
 Tussapap, Tab. (Sutliff & Case)
 Tylenol, Drops, Elix., Liq., Tab., Chew. Tab. (McNeil)
 Tylenol Extra-Strength, Tab., Cap. (McNeil)
 Valadol, Tab., Liq. (Squibb)
 Valorin Tab. (Otis Clapp)

ACETAMINOPHEN W/COMBINATIONS
 Aceta w/Codeine, Tab. (Century)
 Akes-N-Pain, Cap. (Edw. J. Moore)
 Al-Ay Modified, Tab. (Bowman)
 Algecol, Tab. (Winston)
 Allerest Headache Strength, Tab. (Pharmacraft)
 Allylgesic W/Ergotamine, Cap. (Elder)
 Allylvon, Cap. (Elder)
 Alumadrine, Tab. (Fleming)
 Amaphen, Cap. (Trimen)
 Aminodyne, Elix. (Bowman)
 Anaphen, Cap. (Mallard)
 Anodynos-DHC, Tab. (Berlex)
 Anodynos Forte, Tab. (Buffington)
 Apap w/Codeine, Tab. (Central)
 Apapalone, Tab. (Amfre-Grant)
 Arthol Tabs. (Towne)
 Arthralgen, Tab. (Robins)
 Bancaps (Westerfield)
 Bancaps-C (Westerfield)
 Banesin-Forte, Tab. (Westerfield)
 Bexahist, Cap. (Bexar)
 Biophens-S, Tab. (La Crosse)
 Blanex, Cap. (Edwards)
 Bowman Cold Tab. (Bowman)
 B-Pap., Liq. (Wren)
 BQ Cold Tabs (Bristol-Myers)
 Bromo-Seltzer, Gran. (Warner-Lambert)
 Butigetic, Tab. (McNeil)
 Capital w/Codeine, Tab., Susp. (Carnrick)
 Cardui, Tab. (Chattem Labs.)
 Cerose Comp., Cap. (Ives)
 Chexit, Tab. (Dorsey)
 Christodyne-DHC, Tab. (Paddock)
 Clistin-D, Tab. (McNeil)
 Coastaldyne, Tab. (Coastal)
 Coastalgesic, Tab. (Coastal)
 Codalan, Tab. (Lannett)
 Codap (Reid-Provident)
 Codimal, Tab. (Central)
 Colrex Compound, Elix. (Rowell)
 Comtrex, Cap., Liq., Tab. (Bristol-Myers)
 Conar-A, Tab., Susp. (Beecham Labs)
 Conex, Preps. (Westerfield)
 Congesprin, Liq., Tab. (Bristol-Myers)
 Contac Jr., Liq. (Menley & James)
 Coricidin Sinus Headache Tab. (Schering)
 Coryban-D, Syr. (Roerig)
 Corzans, Tab. (Moore Kirk)
 Co-Tylenol, Liq., Tab. (McNeil)
 Dapase, Tab. (Ferndale)
 Darvocet-N, Tab. (Lilly)
 Darvocet-N 100, Tab. (Lilly)
 Daycare, Liq. (Vicks)
 Demerol APAP, Tab. (Winthrop-Breon)
 Dengesic, Tab. (Scott-Alison)
 Desa-Hist AT, Tab. (Pharmics)
 Dolene AP-65, Tab. (Lederle)
 Dolopar, Liq. (O'Neal)
 Drinacet Cap. (Philips Roxane)
 Drinophen, Cap. (Lannett)
 D-Sinus, Cap. (Laser)

Dularin-TH, Tab. (Dooner)
Duoprin, Tab. (Dunhall)
Duo-3X, Tab. (Med. Spec.)
Dynosal, Tab. (Mallard)
Empracet with Codeine, Tab. (Burroughs Wellcome)
Enz-Cold, Cap. (Edw. J. Moore)
Esemgesic, Tab. (Spencer-Mead)
Esgic, Tab. (Gilbert)
Excedrin, Cap., Tab. (Bristol-Myers)
F.C.A.H. Caps. (Scherer)
Femicin, Tab. (Norcliff Thayer)
Fendol, Tab. (Buffington)
Gemnisyn, Tab. (Rorer)
Guaiamine, Cap. (Sutliff & Case)
Histalets, Tab. (Edw. J. Moore)
Histogesic, Tab. (Century)
Histosal #2, Tab. (Ferndale)
Hi-Temp, Tab. (Saron)
Hycomine Comp., Tab. (Du Pont)
Isomel, Cap. (Reid-Provident)
Kiddies Sialco, Tab. (Foy)
Kleer, Syr. (Scrip)
Koryza Tab. (Fellows-Testagar)
Maxigesic, Cap. (W.F. Merchant)
Midran, Tab. (Columbia)
Midrin, Cap. (Carnrick)
Myocalm, Tab. (Parmed)
Myolate, Tab. (Panray)
Naldetuss, Syr. (Bristol)
N-D Gesic, Tab. (Hyrex)
Neo-Pyranistan, Tab. (Standex Labs.)
Nokane, Tab. (Wren)
Novahistine Singlet, Tab. (Merrell Dow)
Novahistine Sinus Tablets, Tab. (Merrell Dow)
Nylorac PB, Tab. (Beard)
Nyquil, Liq. (Vicks)
Opasal, Cap. (Elder)
Ornex, Cap. (Menley & James)
Pamprin, Tab. (Chattem Labs.)
Panitol H.M.B., Tab. (Wesley)
Panritis, Tab. (Pan Amer.)
Parafon Forte, Tab. (McNeil)
Partuss-A, Tab. (Parmed)
Partuss T.D., Tab. (Parmed)
Pavadon Elix. (Coastal)
Pedituss, Liq. (Sutliff & Case)
Pedric, Elix., Wafers (Vale)
Percogesic, Tab. (Du Pont)
Phenahist, Cap., Elix. (Amid)
Phenaphen #2, #3, #4 (Robins)
Phenaphen-650, Tab. (Robins)
Phrenilin, Tab. (Carnrick)
Presalin, Tab. (Mallard)
Prodolor, Tab. (Amfre-Grant)
Proval No. 3, Tab. (Reid-Provident)
Renpap, Tab. (Wren)
Rentuss, Cap., Syr. (Wren)
Repan, Tab. (Everett)
Rhinex, D•Lay, Tab. (Lemmon)
Rhinidrin, Tab. (Central)
Rhinogesic, Tab. (Vale)
Rhinspec, Tab. (Lemmon)

S.A.C. Sinus, Tabs. (Towne)
Salatin w/Codeine, Tab. (Ferndale)
Saleto, Tab. (Mallard)
Saleto-D, Tab. (Mallard)
Salphenyl, Cap., Liq. (Mallard)
Santussin, Prep. (Sandia)
Scotgesic, Cap., Elix. (Scott/Cord)
Scotuss Pediatric Cough Syr. (Scott/Cord)
Sedacane, Cap. (Edw. J. Moore)
Sedalgesic, Tab. (Table Rock)
Sedragesic, Tab. (Lannett)
Sialco, Tab. (Foy)
Sinarest, Tab. (Pharmacraft)
Sine-Aid, Tab. (McNeil)
Sinoze, Tab. (Bowman)
Sinubid, Tab. (Warner Chilcott)
Sinulin, Tab. (Carnrick)
Sinumal, Tab., Liq. (Cook)
Sinus Tab., Tab. (Zenith)
Sinutab, Prods. (Warner-Lambert)
SK-APAP W/codeine, Tab. (SmithKline)
SK-65 APAP, Tab. (SmithKline)
Spantuss, Liq. (Arco)
Spendrisin, Tab. (Spencer-Mead)
Stopain, Tab. (Columbia)
Sunril, Cap. (Emko)
Super-Anahist Tablets (Warner-Lambert)
Symptomax, Liq. (Reid-Provident)
Talacen, Cap. (Winthrop-Breon)
T-Caps, Cap. (Burlington)
Tega-Code, Cap. (Ortega)
Tegapap, Liq., Tab. (Ortega)
Teragen, Tab. (O'Neal)
T-Gesic, Cap. (Tennessee)
Triaminicin, Tab. (Dorsey)
Triaprin, Cap. (Dunhall)
Trind, Syr. (Mead Johnson)
Trind-DM, Syr. (Mead Johnson)
Tussagesic, Tab., Susp. (Dorsey)
Two-Dyne, Tab. (Hyrex)
Tylenol Preps. (McNeil)
Tylenol with Codeine, Elixir, Tab. (McNeil)
Tylox, Cap. (McNeil)
Valihist, Cap. (Clapp)
Vicks Daycare, Liq. (Vicks)
Windolor, Tab. (Winston)
Wygesic, Tab. (Wyeth)
Zenex Comp., Cap. (Zenith)
• **ACETAMINOPHEN AND ASPIRIN TABLETS,**
U.S.P. XXI.
Use: Analgesic.
• **ACETAMINOPHEN ORAL SUSPENSION,** U.S.P.
XXI.
Use: Analgesic.
ACETAMINOPHENOL.
See: Acetaminophen.
ACETAMINOPHEN UNISERTS. (Upsher-Smith)
Acetaminophen 120 mg./Supp. Ctn. 12s; 325
mg./Supp. Ctn. 12s, 50s; 650 mg./Supp. Ctn. 12s,
50s, 500s.
Use: Analgesic, antipyretic.

ACETANILID. (Various Mfr.) (Acetylaminobenzene, acetylaniline, antifebrin) N-phenylacetamide cry.
Use: Antipyretic, analgesic.
ACETARSOL.
See: Acetarsone, Tabs.
ACETARSONE. 3-Acetamido-4-hydroxy-phenylarsonic acid. Acetarsol, Acetphenarsine, Amarsan, Dynarsan, Ehrlich 594, Limarsol, Orarsan, Osarsal, Osvarsan, Paroxyl, Stovarsol.
ACETARSONE SALT OF ARECOLINE.
See: Drocarbil.
ACETAZIDE. Acetazolamide, B.A.N.
• **ACETAZOLAMIDE,** U.S.P. XXI. Tab. U.S.P. XXI. N-(5-Sulfamoyl-1,3,4-thiadiazol-2-yl) acetamide. Acetamide, N-[5-(aminosulfonyl)-1,3,4-thiadiazol-2-yl]-.
Use: Carbonic anhydrase inhibitor.
See: Diamox, Tab., Sequels (Lederle)
Hydrazol, Tab. (Softcon)
ACETAZOLAMIDE. B.A.N. 5-Acetamido-1,3,4-thiadiazole-2-sulfonamide.
Use: Treatment of glaucoma.
See: Acetazide
Diamox
• **ACETAZOLAMIDE SODIUM, STERILE,** U.S.P. XXI.
Use: Carbonic anhydrase inhibitor.
See: Diamox, Inj. (Lederle)
ACET-DIA-MER-SULFONAMIDE. Sulfacetamide, sulfadiazine & sulfamerazine.
See: Buffonamide, Susp., Tab. (Reid-Provident)
Buf-Sul, Tabs. & Susp. (Sheryl)
Cetazine, Tab. (Bowman)
Coco-Diazine, Susp. (Lilly)
Sulfadiazine, sulfamerazine & sulfacetamide, Susp.
ACETEST. (Ames) Sod. nitroprusside, disodium phosphate, aminoacetic acid, lactose. Tab. Bot. 100s, 250s.
Use: Test for acetone or diacetic acid in urine.
• **ACETIC ACID,** U.S.P. XXI, Glacial, Otic soln., U.S.P. XXI. Diluted, N.F. XVI.
Use: Pharmaceutic aid (acidifying agent).
• **ACETIC ACID IRRIGATION,** U.S.P. XXI. 0.25% solution. (Abbott) 250 ml glass cont.; 250 ml.
Use: Irrigating solution
ACETIC ACID, POTASSIUM SALT. Potassium Acetate, U.S.P. XXI.
ACETICYL.
See: Acetylsalicylic Acid.
ACETILUM ACIDULATUM.
See: Acetylsalicylic Acid. (Various Mfr.)
• **ACETOHEXAMIDE,** U.S.P. XXI. Tab. U.S.P. XXI. N-(p-acetylphenylsulfonyl)-N′-cyclo-hexylurea. 1-((p-acetylphenyl)sulfonyl)-3-cyclohexylurea. Benzenesulfonamide, 4-acetyl-N-[[cyclohexylamino]carbonyl].
Use: Blood sugar lowering compound, antidiabetic.
See: Dymelor, Tab. (Lilly)
• **ACETOHYDROXAMIC ACID.** USAN.
ACETOJEN, JR. (Jenkins) Acetylsalicylic acid 1½ gr., phenacetin 1 gr., hyoscyamus ext. 0.0125 gr., (total alkaloids 0.0002 gr.) gelsemium ext. 0.0125 gr./Tab. Bot. 1000s.

ACETOLAX. (Mills) Acetphenylisatin 5 mg., Vit. B-1 1 mg., sod. carboxymethyl cellulose 500 mg./Tab. Bulk Pkg. 1000s.
Use: Laxative.
ACETOL.
See: Acetylsalicylic Acid. (Various Mfr.)
ACETOMEROCTOL. Acetato [2-hydroxy-5-(1,1,-3,3-tetramethylbutyl) phenyl] mercury. Under study.
Use: Topical antiseptic.
• **ACETONE,** N.F. XVI.
ACETONE or DIACETIC ACID TEST.
See: Acetest, Tab. (Ames)
3-(alpha-ACETONYLBENZYL)-4-HYDROXYCOUMARIN SODIUM SALT. Warfarin Sodium.
ACETOPHEN CAPSULE. (Jenkins) Aspirin 3½ gr., phenacetin 2½ gr., caffeine ½ gr./Cap. Bot. 1000s.
ACETOPHEN C.T. GREEN. (Jenkins) Aspirin 3½ gr., phenacetin 2½ gr., caffeine ¼ gr./Tab. Bot. 1000s.
• **ACETOPHENAZINE MALEATE,** U.S.P. XXI. Tab. U.S.P. XXI. 2-Acetyl-10- {3-[4-(-β-hydroxyethyl)-piperazinyl] propyl} phenothiazine dimaleate. 10-[3-[4-(2-Hydroxyethyl)-1-piperazinyl]-propyl)]-phenothiazin-2-yl methyl ketone maleate (1:2).
Use: Tranquilizer.
See: Tindal Maleate, Tab. (Schering)
ACETOPHENETIDIN. Phenacetin, U.S.P. XXI. Ethoxyacetanilide.
Use: Antipyretic, analgesic.
ACETORPHINE. B.A.N. O³-Acetyl-7,8-dihydro-7α[1(R)-hydroxy-1-methylbutyl]-O⁶-methyl-6,-14-endoethenomorphine.
Use: Narcotic analgesic.
ACETOSAL.
See: Acetylsalicylic Acid. (Various Mfr.)
ACETOSALIC ACID.
See: Acetylsalicylic Acid. (Various Mfr.)
ACETOSALIN.
See: Acetylsalicylic Acid. (Various Mfr.)
ACETOSULFONE. 4,4′-Diaminodiphenylsulfone-2-N-acetylsulfonamide sodium. (N¹-acetyl-6-sulfanilylmetanilamido) sodium.
• **ACETOSULFONE SODIUM.** USAN.
Use: Antibacterial.
ACETOXYPHENYLMERCURY.
See: Phenylmercuric acetate.
ACETPHENARSINE.
See: Acetarsone, Tab. (City Chemical)
ACETPHENOLISATIN.
See: Oxyphenisatin Acetate Prep.
W/D-Calcium pantothenate, sodium sulfosuccinate.
See: Peri-Pantyl, Tab. (McGregor)
W/Docusate sodium, sodium carboxymethylcellulose.
See: Scrip-Lax, Tab. (Scrip)
ACETRIZOATE SODIUM. 3-Acetamido-2,4,6,-triiodobenzoate sodium.
W/Polyvinylpyrrolidone.
See: Salpix, Vial (Ortho)
ACETRIZOIC ACID. 3-Acetylamino-2,4,6,-triiodobenzoic acid.
See: Acetrizoate, Sod.

ACET-THEOCIN SODIUM.
See: Theophylline Sod. acetate (Various Mfr.)
ACETYL ADALIN.
See: Acetylcarbromal. (Various Mfr.)
p-ACETYLAMINOBENZALDEHYDE THIOSEMICAR-BAZONE. (Amithiozone, Antib, Berculon A, Benzothiozon, Conteben, Myuizone, Neustab, Tebethion, Thiomicid, Thioparamizone, Thiacetazone).
Use: With streptomycin in the treatment of tuberculosis.
ACETYLAMINOBENZENE.
See: Acetanilid. (Various Mfr.)
N-ACETYL-p-AMINOPHENOL. Acetaminophen, U.S.P. XXI.
ACETYLANILINE.
See: Acetanilid. (Various Mfr.)
ACETYL-BETA-METHYLCHOLINE CHLORIDE.
See: Mecholyl Chloride, Amp. (Baker, J.T.)
ACETYL-BROMO-DIETHYLACETYL-CARBAMIDE.
See: Acetylcarbromal. (Various Mfr.)
ACETYLCARBROMAL. (Meyer) Acetyl adalin, acetylbromodiethylacetyl-carbamide. Pow. for mfg.
Use: Sedative.
See: Paxarel, Tab. (Circle)
W/Bromisovalum, scopolamine aminoxide HBr.
See: Tranquinal, Tab. (Barnes-Hind)
• **ACETYLCHOLINE CHLORIDE,** U.S.P. XXI. For Ophth. Soln., U.S.P. XXI. Ethananinium,2-(acetyloxy)-N, N, N-trimethyl-, chloride. Choline chloride acetate.
Use: S.C., I.M., I.V. Parasympathomimetic agent & vasodilator. Paroxysmal tachycardia.
See: Miochol Ophthalmic (CooperVision)
ACETYLCHOLINE-LIKE THERAPEUTIC AGENTS.
See: Cholinergic agents.
• **ACETYLCYSTEINE,** U.S.P. XXI. Sol. U.S.P. XXI. N-Acetyl-L-cysteine.
Use: Mucolytic agent.
See: Mucomyst, Sol. (Mead Johnson)
• **ACETYLCYSTEINE AND ISOPROTERENOL HYDROCHLORIDE INHALATION SOLUTION,** U.S.P. XXI.
Use: Mucolytic agent.
See: Mucomyst with Isoproterenol, Sol. (Mead Johnson)
ACETYLCYSTEINE. B.A.N. N-Acetyl-L-cysteine. Airbron
Use: Liquefaction of bronchial secretion.
ACETYLDIGITOXIN. α-Digitoxin monoacetate. Acetyl-tridigitoxose. The natural-occurring cardiac glycoside defined as the alpha acetyl ester of digitoxin.
Use: Digitoxin therapy. Cardiotonic.
ACETYLDIHYDROCODEINONE. Thebacon, B.A.N.
ACETYLIN.
See: Acetylsalicylic Acid. (Various Mfr.)
ACETYLMETHADOL, I.N.N. Methadyl acetate, B.A.N.
ACETYLPHENYLISATIN.
See: Oxyphenisatin Acetate.
1-((p-ACETYLPHENYL)SULFONYL)-3-CYCLO-HEXYL-UREA. Acetohexamide.
ACETYLRESORCINOL.
See: Resorcinol Monoacetate. (Various Mfr.)

ACETYLSAL.
See: Acetylsalicylic Acid
ACETYLSALICYLATE ALUMINUM.
See: Aluminum Aspirin
ACETYLSALICYLIC ACID. Aspirin, U.S.P. XXI.
Acidum acetylsalicylicum, 2-acetoxybenzoic acid, Acetilum Acidulatum, Acetophen, Acetol, Acetosal, Acetosalic Acid, Acetosalin, Aceticyl, Acetylsal, Acylpryin, Aspro, Helicon, Rhodine, Salacetin, Salcetogen, Saletin.
See: Aspirin Preps. (Various Mfr.)
ACETYLSALICYLIC ACID, ACETOPHENETIDIN AND CAFFEINE.
See: A.P.C., Prep. (Various Mfr.)
ACETYL SULFAMETHOXYPYRIDAZINE. 3-(N-Acetyl-sulfanilamido)-6-methoxypyridazine.
N¹-ACETYLSULFANILAMIDE. (Albucid; p-Aminoben-zenesulfonacetamide; Sulfacet; Sulfacetamide, N-Sulfanilylacetamide.)
Use: Sulfonamide therapy.
ACETYL SULFISOXAZOLE. Sulfisoxazole Acetyl, U.S.P. XXI.
See: Gantrisin Acetyl, Syr., Susp. (Roche)
Lipo-Gantrisin Acetyl, Liq. (Roche)
ACETYLTANNIC ACID. Tannic acid acetate.
Use: Antiperistaltic.
AC EYE DROPS. (Walgreen) Tetrahydrozoline HCl 0.05%, zinc sulfate 0.25%. Bot. 0.75 oz.
Use: Allergy, colds, eye relief.
ACHLORHYDRIA DETERMINATION.
See: Diagnex Blue, Prep. (Squibb)
ACHLORHYDRIA THERAPY.
See: Acidol. (Various Mfr.)
Glutamic Acid HCl (Various Mfr.)
Muripsin, Tab. (Norgine)
Normacid, Tab. (Stuart)
ACHOL. (Enzyme Process) Vit. A 4000 U., ketocholanic acids 62 mg./Tab. Bot. 100s, 250s.
Use: Vitamin A supplement and therapy.
ACHROMYCIN. (Lederle) Tetracycline HCl.
Intramuscular: (100 mg., 250 mg., buffered w/ascorbic acid) Vial. Box 1s, 100s.
Intravenous: (250 mg., 500 mg., buffered w/ascorbic acid) Vial.
Oint. (3%) Tube 0.5 oz. & 1 oz.
Oint. (Ophth.) 1% Tubes ⅛ oz.
Ophth. Susp. 1%, Plastic dropper bot. 4 ml.
ACHROMYCIN-V. (Lederle) Tetracycline HCl. **Cap.:** 250 mg. Bot. 100s, 1000s, Unit dose 10 × 10s, Unit of use 50 × 40s; 500 mg. Bot. 100s, 1000s; Unit of use 50 × 20s; Unit dose 10 × 10s. **Oral Susp.:** 125 mg./5 cc. w/methylparaben 0.12%, propylparaben 0.03%. Bot. 2 oz., 1 pt.
Use: Treatment of infections caused by both gram-negative and gram-positive bacteria.
ACID ACRIFLAVINE.
See: Acriflavine Hydrochloride (Various Mfr.)
ACID CITRATE DEXTROSE SOLUTION.
See: A.C.D. Sol. (Various Mfr.)
ACID CITRATE DEXTROSE ANTICOAGULANT SOLUTION MODIFIED.
See: A-C-D Solution Modified (Squibb)

ACID HISTAMINE PHOSPHATE.
See: Histamine Phosphate. (Various Mfr.)
ACID MANTLE CREME. (Dorsey) Aluminum acetate in specially prep. water-soluble hydrophilic cream at pH 4.2. Tube 1 oz., Jar 4 oz., 1 lb.
Use: Skin prophylactic agent in restoring normal skin acidity.
ACID MANTLE LOTION. (Dorsey) Aluminum acetate lotion. pH 4.5 Bot. 4 oz.
Use: Dermatitis.
ACIDOL.
See: Betaine Hydrochloride (Various Mfr.)
ACIDOPHILUS W/PECTIN. (Barth's) *Lactobacillus acidophilus* w/natural citrus pectin 100 mg./Cap. Bot. 100s.
Use: Aid to digestion.
ACID TRYPAFLAVINE.
See: Acriflavine Hydrochloride. (Various Mfr.)
ACIDULATED PHOSPHATE FLUORIDE. (Scherer) Flavored soln. containing 0.31% fluoride ion in 0.1 molar phosphate. Bot. 64 oz. Office Product.
Use: Dental caries prevention.
ACIDULIN. (Lilly) Glutamic acid HCl 340 mg./Pulvule. Bot. 100s, 1000s.
Use: Achlorhydria.
ACIGLUMIN.
See: Glutamic Acid Hydrochloride. (Various Mfr.)
ACI-JEL. (Ortho) Glacial acetic acid 0.921%, ricinoleic acid 0.70%, oxyquinoline sulfate 0.025%, glycerine 5%. Tube 85 Gm. w/dose applicator.
Use: Vaginal acidifier.
ACINITRAZOLE. B.A.N. 2-Acetamido-5-nitrothiazole, Aminitrozole (I.N.N.)
Use: Treatment of trichomoniasis.
See: Trichorad
Tritheon
• **ACLARUBICIN.** USAN.
Use: Antineoplastic.
ACLETIN. (Associated Conc.) Lecithin, soya 8 gr. with vitamins/Cap. Bot. 100s, 250s.
Use: Fat metabolism.
ACLOBROM. Propantheline Bromide, B.A.N.
A.C.N. (Person & Covey) Vitamin A palmitate 25M I.U., ascorbic acid 250 mg., niacinamide 25 mg./Tab. Bot. 100s.
Use: Dietary supplement.
ACNAVEEN. (CooperCare)
See: Aveenobar Medicated (CooperCare)
ACNA-VITE. (Cenci) Vit. A 10,000 I.U., C 250 mg., hesperidin 50 mg., niacinamide 25 mg./Cap. Bot. 75s.
Use: Acne vulgaris with Vit. A & C deficiency.
ACNE-AID CLEANSING BAR. (Stiefel) Neutral soap and 6.3 surfactant blend. Non-medicated. Bar 4.0 oz.
Use: Cleanse oily skin.
ACNE-AID CREAM. (Stiefel) Benzoyl peroxide 10% in special cover-up base. Tube, 1.8 oz.
Use: Oily acne treatment.
ACNE-AID LOTION. (Stiefel) Sulfur 10%, alcohol 10% in a washable base. Clear or Tinted Bot. plastic 2 oz.
Use: Treatment of acne.

ACNEDERM. (Lannett) **Lotion:** Dispersable sulfur 5%, zinc sulfate 1%, zinc oxide 10%, alcohol 21%. Bot. 2 oz. **Soap:** Zinc oxide 2%, zinc sulfate 1%, colloidal sulfur 5%. Cake 3.2 oz.
Use: Skin conditions
ACNE-DOME CREAM & LOTION. (Miles Pharm) Regular: sulfur 4%, resorcinol monoacetate 3%, in a vehicle buffered to the pH range of normal skin. **Cream:** Tube 1 oz. **Lotion:** Bot. 2 oz.
Use: Treatment of acne.
ACNE-DOME MEDICATED CLEANSER. (Miles Pharm) Sulfur 2%, salicylic acid 2% in a colloidal soybean complex. Medicated w/sponge 4 oz.
Use: Medicated skin cleanser.
ACNE LOTION. (Weeks & Leo) Benzoyl peroxide 10% in odorless, greaseless, vanishing lotion. Bot. 2 oz.
Use: Treatment for acne.
ACNO CLEANSER. (Baker/Cummins) Isopropyl alcohol 60%. Bot. 8 oz.
Use: Antiseptic astringent for the treatment of acne.
ACNO LOTION. (Baker/Cummins) Micronized sulfur 3%, isopropanol 25%, salicylic acid 2%. Bot. 4 oz.
Use: Acne & related skin conditions.
ACNOMEL. (Menley & James) Resorcinol 2%, sulfur 8%, w/bentonite, propylene glycol, alcohol & titanium dioxide.
Cream: Tube 1 oz.
Use: Acne therapy.
ACNOPHILL. (Torch) Sulfur 5%, Pot. and zinc sulfides and polysulfides 5%, zinc oxide 10% in hydrophilic vehicle. Plain or tinted. Jar 1 lb. and 2 oz.
Use: Acne treatment.
ACNOTEX. (C & M Pharmacal) Sulfur 8%, salicylic acid 2.25%, methylbenzethonium chloride 0.08%, propylene glycol, powder base, acetone, isopropyl alcohol 22%, purified water, color, perfume. Bot. 2 oz., pt., gal.
Use: Anti-acne cover-up lotion.
• **ACODAZOLE HYDROCHLORIDE.** USAN.
Use: Antineoplastic.
ACOTUS. (Whorton) Phenylephrine HCl 5 mg., guaiacol glyceryl ether 100 mg., menthol 1 mg., alcohol, by vol. 10%/5 cc. Bot. 4 oz., 12 oz., gal.
Use: Colds, coughs.
ACR. (Western Research) Ammonium chloride 7.5 gr./Tab. Handicount 28s (36 bags of 28 tab.)
Use: Diuretic.
ACRIFLAVINE. Euflavine, Gonacrine, Neutroflavine Acriflavine neutral; a mixture of 2, 8-diamino-10-methylacridinium chloride & 2,8-diaminoacridine. (Lilly) Tab. 1½ gr. Bot. 100s.
Use: External antiseptic.
ACRIFLAVINE HYDROCHLORIDE. (Various Mfr.) Hydrochloride form of acriflavine. Acid acriflavine, acid trypaflavine, flavine, trypaflavine.
National Aniline—Pow., Bot. (1, 5, 10, 25, & 50 Gm.). Tab. (1½ gr.) Bot. 50s & 100s.
Use: External bacteriostatic.

• **ACRISORCIN,** U.S.P. XXI. Cream U.S.P. XXI. 9-Aminoacridinium 4-hexylresorcinolate.
See: Akrinol Cream (Schering)
Use: Topical, tinea versicolor. Local antifungal.

• **ACRONINE.** USAN. 3, 12-Dihydro-6-methoxy-3,3,12-trimethyl-7H-pyrano[2,3,-c]acridin-7-one. Under study.
Use: Antineoplastic.

A-C TABLET. (Century) Aspirin 6 gr., caffeine 0.5 gr./Tab.
Bot. 100s, 1000s
Use: Analgesic.

ACTACIN-C SYRUP. (Vangard) Codeine phosphate 10 mg., triprolidine HCl 2 mg., pseudoephedrine HCl 20 mg., guaifenesin 100 mg./ 5 ml. Bot. pt., gal.
Use: Antihistamine, decongestant, cough depressant.

ACTACIN SYRUP. (Vangard) Triprolidine HCl 1.25 mg., pseudoephedrine HCl 30 mg./ 5 ml. Bot. pt., gal.
Use: Antihistamine, decongestant.

ACTACIN TABLETS. (Vangard) Triprolidine HCl 2.5 mg., pseudoephedrine HCl 60 mg./Tab. Bot. 100s, 1000s.
Use: Antihistamine/decongestant.

ACTAGEN. (Generix) Triprolidine HCl 2.5 mg., pseudoephedrine HCl 60 mg. Tab. Bot. 100s, 1000s.
Use: Symptomatic treatment of allergic rhinitis.

ACTAL SUSPENSION. (Winthrop Products) Aluminum hydroxide.
Use: Antacid.

ACTAL PLUS TABLETS. (Winthrop Products) Aluminum hydroxide, magnesium hydroxide.
Use: Antacid, demulcent.

ACTAL TABLETS. (Winthrop Products) Aluminum hydroxide.
Use: Antacid.

ACTAMIN. (Buffington) Acetaminophen 325 mg./Tab. Sugar and salt free. Dispens-A-Kit: 500s, Aidpaks 100s. Unit boxes 20s. Medipaks 200s.
Use: Analgesic, anti-pyretic.

ACTAMIN EXTRA. (Buffington) Acetaminophen 500 mg./Tab. Sugar and salt free. Dispens-A-Kit 500s.
Use: Extra strength nonaspirin analgesic and anti-pyretic.

• **ACTAPLANIN.** USAN.
Use: Growth stimulant.

ACTH-ACTEST GEL. (Fellows) Repository corticotropin 40 or 80 u./cc. Vial 5 cc.

ACTH. (Adrenocorticotropic hormone. Adrenocorticotrop(h)in.
See: Corticotropin, U.S.P.
Mallard—(40 u./ml., 5 ml.)
O'Neal, Jones & Feldman—(40 u. or 80 u./ml., 5 ml.)
Parke, Davis—25 units/Vial; 40 units/Vial.
Pharmex—(40 u. or 80 u./ml., 5 ml.)

ACTH GEL, PURIFIED. Arcum.—40 or 80 units/ml., vial 5 ml. Conal.—40 or 80 units/ml., vial 5 ml. Hart Labs.—40 units/ml., vial 5 ml. Bowman—

Adrenocorticotropic hormone 40 u., aqueous gelatin 16%, phenol 0.5%/cc. Vial 5 cc.
Use: Repository corticotropin.
Arcum—(40 u. or 80 u./ml., 5 ml.)
Bell—(40 u. or 80 u./ml., 5 ml.)
Bowman—(40 u./ml., 5 ml.)
Hyrex—(40 u. or 80 u./ml., 5 ml.)
Jenkins—(40 u. or 80 u./ml., 5 ml.)
Vortech—40 units/ml., 80 units/ml., Vial 5 ml.
Rocky Mtn. Pharmacal—40 units/ml., 80 units/ml. Vial 5 ml.
Wesley Pharm.—40 units/ml., vial 5 ml.; 80 units/ml., vial 5 ml.
Wyeth—(40 u. or 80 u./ml. or Tubex)

ACTHAR. (Armour) Corticotropin for Injection. Vial 25, 40 u./Vial. (Lyophilized w/gelatin). Pkg. 10s.
Use: I.M., S.C. or I.V. stimulation of adrenal cortex and diseases related to it.

ACTICORT LOTION 100. (Cummins) Hydrocortisone alcohol 1% in a specially formulated vehicle. Bot. 2 oz.
Use: Anti-inflammatory & antipruritic.

ACTIDIL. (Burroughs Wellcome) Triprolidine HCl **Tab.** 2.5 mg./Tab. Bot. 100s. **Syr.** 1.25 mg./5 ml. Bot. 1 pt.
Use: Antihistamine.

ACTI-DIONE. (Upjohn) Cycloheximide. (3-[2-(3,5-Di-methyl-2-oxocyclohexyl)-2-hydroxyethyl]-glutarimide) 85-100% w/w.
Not for medicinal use. For professional use only. Bot. 4 Gm.

ACTIDOSE. (Paddock) Activated charcoal solution 25 Gm./120 ml. or 50 Gm./240 ml.
Use: Orally or through gastric tube to adsorb toxins in GI tract in drug overdose or poisoning emergency.

ACTIFED. (Burroughs Wellcome) **Tab.:** Triprolidine HCl. 2.5 mg., pseudoephedrine HCl. 60 mg./Tab. Bot. 30s, 100s, 1000s. Boxes 12s, 24s. Unit dose pack 100s. Unit of use 90s. Ctn. 24s. **Syr.:** Triprolidine HCl 1.25 mg., pseudoephedrin HCl 30 mg./5 ml. Bot. 4 oz., 1 pt., gal.
Use: Common cold, allergic rhinitis.

ACTIFED WITH CODEINE COUGH SYRUP. (Burroughs Wellcome) Codeine phosphate 10 mg., triprolidine HCl 2 mg., pseudoephedrine HCl 30 mg., dextromethorphan 100 mg./5 ml. Bot. pt., gal.
Use: Treatment of the common cold.

ACTINOMYCIN. B.A.N. Antimicrobial substances with antitumor activity produced by Streptomyces antibioticus and Streptomyces chrysomallus. Sanamycin is Actinomycin C.

ACTINOMYCIN C. Name previously used for Cactinomycin.

ACTINOMYCIN D. Dactinomycin, U.S.P. XXI.
See: Cosmegen (Merck Sharp & Dohme)

• **ACTINOQUINOL SODIUM.** USAN.
Use: Ultraviolet screen.

ACTINOSPECTOCIN. Name previously used for Spectinomycin.

ACTIVATED ATTAPULGITE.
W/Aluminum hydroxide, magnesium carbonate coprecipitate, compressed gel.
See: Hykasil, Cream (Philips Roxane)
W/Polysorbate 80, colloidal sulfur, salicylic acid, propylene glycol.
See: Sebasorb Lotion (Summers Labs.)

ACTIVATED CHARCOAL TABLETS. (Cowley) 5 gr./Tab. Bot. 1000s.

ACTIVATED 7-DEHYDROCHOLESTEROL.
See: Vitamin D-3 (Various Mfr.)

ACTIVATED ERGOSTEROL.
See: Calciferol.

ACTOL EXPECTORANT. (Beecham Labs) Noscapine 30 mg., guaifenesin 200 mg./5 ml. or Tab. **Syr.** W/alcohol 12.5%. Bot. pt. **Tab.** Bot. 100s.
Use: Treatment of symptoms associated with common cold.

ACTOMOL. Mebanazine, B.A.N.

ACTOQUINOL SODIUM. 8-Ethoxy-5-quinoline-sulfonic acid sodium salt.
Use: Ultraviolet screen.

ACTOS 50. Corticotrophin, B.A.N.

ACTRAPID HUMAN INSULIN. (Squibb Novo) Human insulin 100 Units/ml. Vial 10 ml.
Use: Human insulin (rapid action).

ACTRIOL. Epioestriol, B.A.N.

ACTYLATE. (Kinney) Ammonium salicylate 80 mg., pot. salicylate 80 mg., strontium salicylate 80 mg., pot. para-aminobenzoate 0.32 Gm., ascorbic acid 20 mg./Tab. Bot. 100s.
Use: Rheumatoid arthritis.

ACUCRON. (Seatrace) Acetaminophen 300 mg., salicylamide 200 mg., phenyltoloxamine 20 mg./Tab. Bot. 100s, 1000s, 5000s.
Use: Antihistaminic, analgesic.

ACUTRAN. (Mallinckrodt) Amphecloral.

• **ACYCLOVIR.** USAN.
Use: Antiviral.

ACYCLOVIR. 9-(2-hydroxyethoxymethyl)-guanine.
Use: Management of initial herpes genitalis and mucocutaneous herpes simplex virus infections.
See: Zovirax, Oint. (Burroughs Wellcome)

ACYLPYRIN.
See: Aspirin

ADALAN LANATABS. (Lannett) Amobarbital 50 mg., homatropine methylbromide 7.5 mg., methamphetamine HCl 10 mg./T.D. Tab. Bot. 100s, 1000s.

ADAMANTANAMINE HCl. Amantadine HCl. Anti-flu capsule. This drug is thought to protect cells against entry of the flu virus without actually destroying the virus. Also used in the treatment of Parkinson's disease.
See: Symmetrel, Cap., Syr. (Du Pont)

ADANON. Methadone, B.A.N.

ADAPETTES. (Alcon) Wets contact lens. Pkg. 15 cc.

ADAPIN. (Pennwalt) Doxepin HCl 10 mg., 25 mg. 50 mg., 75 mg., 100 mg./Cap. Bot. 100s, 1000s. 25 mg., 50 mg./Cap. also available in 5000s.
Use: Antianxiety, antidepressant.

ADAPT. (Alcon) Povidone, EDTA 0.1%, thimerosal 0.004%. Wetting sol. Bot. 15 cc.
Use: Contact lens wetting sol.

ADATUSS. (Merchant) Hydrocodone bitartrate 5 mg., guaifenesin 100 mg., alcohol 5%/5 ml. Syr. Bot. pt., gal.
Use: Cough relief.

A.D.C. DROPS. (CMC) Vit. A 3000 I.U., D 400 I.U., C 60 mg./0.6 cc. Bot. 60 cc.

ADCORTYL. Triamcinolone, B.A.N.

ADEECON. (CMC) Vit. A 5000 I.U., D 1000 I.U./Cap. Bot. 1000s.
Use: Supplement.

ADEFLOR CHEWABLE. (Upjohn) Fluoride 1 mg. & 0.5 mg., Vitamin A 4000 I.U., D 400 I.U., C 75 mg., thiamine monitrate (B-1) 2 mg., B-2 2 mg., niacinamide 18 mg., B-6 1 mg., calcium pantothenate 5 mg., B-12 2 mcg./0.5 or 1 mg. Chewable Tab. Bot. 100s, 500s.
Use: Prevention of dental caries.

ADEFLOR DROPS. (Upjohn) Vit. A 2000 I.U., D 400 I.U., C 50 mg., B-6 1 mg., fluoride (as sodium fluoride) 0.5 mg./0.6 ml. Bot. 50 ml. w/dropper.
Use: Prevention of dental caries.

ADEFLOR M TABLETS. (Upjohn) Vit. A 6000 I.U., D 400 I.U., B-1 1.5 mg., B-2 2.5 mg., C 100 mg., niacinamide 20 mg., Vit. B-6 10 mg., calcium pantothenate 10 mg., Vit. B-12 2 mcg., folic acid 0.1 mg., fluoride (as sodium fluoride) 1 mg., calcium (as calcium carbonate) 250 mg., iron 30 mg./Tab. Bot. 100s, 500s.
Use: Dietary supplement.

ADENINE. (Various Mfr.) 6-Aminopurine.

ADENO. (O'Neal, Jones & Feldman) Adenosine monophosphate 25 mg./ml. Vial 10 ml.

ADENO TWELVE GEL INJECTION. (Fellows) Adenosine-5-monophosphate 25 mg., methionine 25 mg., niacin 10 mg./cc. Vial 10 cc.

ADENOCREST. (Nutrition) Adenosine-5-monophosphate sod. 25 mg., nicotinic acid as sod. salt 25 mg., gelatin 100 mg. w/benzyl alcohol 1.5%/cc. Vials 10 cc.
Use: Capillary and arterial vasodilation.

ADENOLIN FORTE. (Lincoln) Adenosine-5-mono-phosphate, 25 mg., methionine 25 mg., niacin 10 mg./cc. Vial 15 cc.
Use: Arthritis, bursitis, tendinitis & other degenerative diseases.

• **ADENOSINE.** F.D.A. 6-Amino-9-beta-D-Ribofurano-syl-9H-purine.

ADENOSINE IN GELATIN. (Fellows) **Forte:** Adenosine-5-monophosphate 50 mg./cc. **Super:** Adenosine-5-monophosphate 100 mg./cc.

ADENOSINE-5-MONOPHOSPHATE AS THE SODIUM SALT.
See: Adenocrest, Amp. (Nutrition)

• **ADENOSINE PHOSPHATE.** USAN. 5-Adenylic acid. B.A.N. Adenosine-5′-(dihydrogen phosphate). Adenosine monophosphate, AMP.
Use: Nutrient.
See: Adenyl
    Cobalasine, Inj. (Keene)
    My-B-Den (Miles Pharm)

ADENYL. Adenosine Phosphate, B.A.N.
ADEPSINE OIL.
See: Petrolatum Liquid (Various Mfr.)
ADICILLIN. B.A.N. 6-[D(+)-5-Amino-5-carboxy-valeramido]penicillanic acid. Penicillin N.
Use: Antibiotic.
• **ADINAZOLAM.** USAN.
Use: Antidepressant, sedative.
ADIPEX-P. CAPSULES. (Lemmon) Phentermine HCl 37.5 mg./Cap. Bot. 100s, 400s.
Use: Anorectic.
ADIPEX-P TABLETS. (Lemmon) Phentermine HCl 37.5 mg./Tab. Bot. 100s, 400s, 1000s.
Use: Anorectic agent.
• **ADIPHENINE HYDROCHLORIDE.** USAN. (2-Diethylaminoethyl diphenylacetate hydrochloride.) Pow. 1 lb. for mfg. use.
Use: Antispasmodic.
ADIPIODONE (I.N.N.). Iodipamide, B.A.N.
3,3'-(ADIPOYLDIIMINO)-BIS[2,4,6-TRI-IODOBEN-ZOIC ACID]. Iodipamide, U.S.P. XXI.
ADIPOST. (Ascher) Phendimetrazine tartrate 105 mg./Slow-rel. Cap. Bot. 100s.
Use: Appetite suppressant.
ADLERIKA. (Last) Magnesium sulfate 4.0 Gm./15 ml. Bot. 12 oz.
Use: Laxative.
ADONIDINE. (City Chem.) Bot. 1 Gm.
Use: Cardiac stimulant.
ADPHEN TABLETS. (Ferndale) Phendimetrazine tartrate 35 mg./Tab. Bot. 100s.
Use: Anorexiant.
A-D-R. (Lincoln) dl-Methionine 250 mg., corn starch lubricant 42 mg./Cap. Bot. 100s, 500s.
Use: Amino acid supplement.
ADRENALIN(E).
See: Epinephrine. (Various Mfr.)
ADRENALIN CHLORIDE SOLUTION. (Parke-Davis) Epinephrine HCl. Principle of the medullary portion of suprarenal glands. **Amp.:** 1:1000-1 ml. Epinephrine 1 mg./ml. with not more than 0.1% sodium bisulfite as preservative. Amps. 10s. **Steri-Vial 1:1000**-1 ml. Epinephrine in isotonic sodium chloride solution with 0.5% chlorobutanol and not more than 0.15% sodium bisulfite as preservative. Vial 30 ml. **Soln. 1:1000-1** ml. Screw cap Bot. 1 oz. (Same desc. as Steri-Vial). **Soln. 1:100.** Each 100 ml. contains 1 Gm. epinephrine HCl dissolved in sodium chloride-citrate buffer solution with Phemerol chloride 0.2 mg./ml. and sodium bisulfite 0.2% as preservative. Bot. ¼ oz.
Use: Sympathomimetic agent.
ADRENALINE HYDROCHLORIDE.
See: Epinephrine Hydrochloride. (Various Mfr.)
• **ADRENALONE.** USAN. 3',4'-Dihydroxy-2-(methylamino)-acetophenone.
Use: Adrenergic (ophthalmic).
ADRENAMINE.
See: Epinephrine (Various Mfr.)
ADRENERGIC AGENTS.
See: Sympathomimetic agents
ADRENERGIC-BLOCKING AGENTS.
See: Sympatholytic agents

ADRENINE.
See: Epinephrine. (Various Mfr.)
ADRENOCHROME.
See: Carbazochrome Salicylate.
ADRENOCHROMAZONE.
See: Carbazochrome Salicylate.
ADRENOCHROME MONOSEMICARBAZONE.
See: Carbazochrome Salicylate
ADRENOCORTICOTROPIC HORMONE. ACTH acts by stimulating the endogenous production of cortisone and the final result is similar whichever substance is administered. The nature of action of each is unknown. Both are necessary in the metabolism of carbohydrates, protein & fat & exert profound effects on neuromuscular metabolism.
See: ACTH gel, Inj. (Bowman)
Corticotropin, U.S.P.
Cortigel (Savage)
ADRENOMIST INHALANT AND NEBULIZERS. (Nephron) Epinephrine 1%, Bot. ½ oz., 1¼ oz.
Use: Inhalant for bronchial asthma.
ADRENOSEM SALICYLATE. (Beecham Labs) Carbazochrome salicylate, benzyl alcohol 2% by volume. **Amp.** (5 mg./ml.) 1 cc., 5s, 100s; (10 mg./2 ml.) 2 ml. 5s, 100s. **Syr.** (2.5 mg./5 ml.) Bot. 4 oz., **Tab.** (2.5 mg.) Bot. 50s.
Use: Orally, I.M.; to increase capillary resistance and suppress bleeding from capillary bed.
ADRENUCLEO. (Enzyme Process) Vit. C 250 mg., d-cal. pantothenate 12.5 mg., bioflavonoids 62.5 mg./Tab. Bot. 100s, 250s.
Use: Vitamin-C supplement therapy.
ADRIAMYCIN. (Adria) Doxorubicin HCl 10 mg., lactose 50 mg./Vial Pkg. 10s. Doxorubicin HCl 50 mg., lactose 250 mg./Vial Ctn. 1s.
Use: Antineoplastic.
ADRUCIL. (Adria) Fluorouracil 500 mg./10 ml. Ampule 10 ml.
Use: Antineoplastic agent.
ADSORBOCARPINE. (Alcon) Pilocarpine HCl 1%, 2%, 4% in adsorbobase, water polymers, & polyvinylpyrrolidone. Vials 15 ml.
Use: Miotic.
ADSORBONAC OPHTH. SOLUTION. (Alcon) Sodium chloride 2% or 5% in vehicle of polyvinylpyrrolidone and BP water soluble polymers. Dropper Vial 15 ml.
Use: Reduction of corneal edema and clearing of the cornea for diagnostic examination.
ADSORBOTEAR. (Alcon) Hydroxyethylcellulose 0.44%, w/polyvinylpyrrolidone, thimerosal 0.002%, EDTA 0.5%. Bot. dropper 15 ml.
Use: Artificial tears.
ADSORMONE. (Herring) Complete set of reagents required. Pow. 100 Gm.
Use: Pregnancy test.
ADVANCE. (Ross) **Ready-to-Feed formula:** (16 cal/fl oz). Each liter contains: Protein 20 g, fat 27 g, carbohydrate 55 g, Ca 0.51 g, P 0.39 g, Na 0.30 g max., Mg 64 mg., Fe 12 mg., Zn 6 mg., Cu 0.9 mg., iodine 60 mcg., Vit. A 2400 IU, D 400 IU, E 18 IU, C 50 mg., B-1 0.75 mg., B-2 0.9 mg., niacin 10

mg. Eq., B-6 0.6 mg., pantothenic acid 4 mg., folic acid 0.1 mg., B-12 2.5 mcg. Bot. 32 fl. oz.
Conc.liquid: (32 Cal/fl oz) 13 fl. oz diluted 1:1 with water to give 16 Cal/fl oz "as feed" beverage see ADVANCE ready-to-feed for composition on "as fed" basis.
Use: A nutritional beverage for older infants.
ADVENT. (Winston) Vit. A 4000 I.U., D 400 I.U., C 200 mg., B-1 2 mg., B-2 1.5 mg., B-6 0.5 mg., B-12 1 mcg., niacinamide 10 mg., Ca. lactate 400 mg., ferrous fumarate 200 mg., iodine 0.01 mg., Pot. 0.835 mg., Cu 0.15 mg., Mn 0.05 mg., Zn 0.085 mg./Tab. Bot. 100s, 1000s.
Use: Pregnancy and lactation.
ADVIL. (Whitehall) Ibuprofen 200 mg. Bot. 8s, 24s, 50s, 100s.
Use: Analgesic.
AERDIL. (Econo Med) Triprolidine HCl 1.25 mg., pseudoephedrine HCl 30 mg./5 ml. Bot. Pts., Gal.
Use: Rhinitis treatment.
AEROCAINE. (Aeroceuticals) Benzyl alcohol 22.7%, benzocaine 13.6%, benzethonium chloride 0.5%. Spray Bot. 0.5 oz., 2.5 oz.
Use: Topical anesthetic, antiseptic, antipruritic.
AEROCELL. (Aeroceuticals) Exfoliative cytology fixative spray. Bot. 2.25 oz.
AERODINE. (Aeroceuticals) Povidone-iodine aerosol. Bot. 3 oz.
Use: Broad range antiseptic germicide.
AEROFREEZE. (Aeroceuticals) Trichloromonofluoromethane & dichlorodifluoromethane. Aerosol containers 8 oz. (12s).
Use: Topical anesthetic.
AEROLATE-III. (Fleming) Theophylline 65 mg./T. D. Cap. Bot. 100s, 1000s.
Use: Bronchodilation.
AEROLATE SR. & JR. (Fleming) **Caps.** Theophylline 4 gr. for Sr. and 2 gr. for Jr./Cap. Bot. 100s, 1000s. **Syrup:** 160 mg./15 ml., Bot. pt., gal.
Use: Bronchodilation.
AEROPURE. (Aeroceuticals) Isopropanol 7.8%, triethylene glycol 3.9%, essential oils 3%, methyldodecyl benzyl trimethyl ammonium chloride 0.12%, methyldodecylxylene bis (trimethyl ammonium chloride) 0.03%, inert ingredients, 85.15%. Bot. 0.8 oz., 4.5 oz.
Use: Concentrated air sanitizer and deodorizer.
AEROSAN. (Ulmer) Air sanitizer, disinfectant & deodorant. Aerosol Spray Can 16.6 oz.
Use: Disinfectant spray.
AEROSEB-DEX. (Herbert) Dexamethasone 0.01%, alcohol 68.5% w/isopropyl myristate and butane propellant. Aerosol 58 Gm.
Use: Corticosteroid-responsive dermatoses.
AEROSEB-HC. (Herbert) Hydrocortisone 0.5%, alcohol 68% w/isopropyl myristate and butane propellant. Aerosol 58 Gm.
Use: Corticosteroid-responsive dematoses.
AEROSEPT. (Dalin) Lidocaine, cetyltrimethylammonium bromide, hexachlorophene. Aerosol Pkg. 6 oz.
Use: Antiseptic, anesthetic.

AEROSIL. (Aeroceuticals) Dimethylpolysiloxane. Bot. 4.5 oz.
Use: Silicone lubricant and protective spray.
AEROAID MERTHIOLATE. (Aeroceuticals) Merthiolate (Lilly) 1:1000 w/alcohol 72%. Spray Bot. 3 oz.
Use: First aid antiseptic spray.
AEROSOL OT.
See: Docusate Sodium, U.S.P.
AEROSOLV. (Aeroceuticals) Isopropyl alcohol, chlorinated solvent, silicone. Aerosol 5.5 oz.
Use: Adhesive tape remover.
AEROSPORIN STERILE POWDER. (Burroughs Wellcome) Polymixin B sulfate 500,000 u./Vial. Multidose Vials 20 ml.
Use: Antibacterial.
AEROSPORIN SULFATE. (Burroughs Wellcome) Polymyxin B sulfate 50 mg., **Sterile Pow.** (500,000 u.) Vial (20 cc.). **Otic Sol.,** sterile. Bot. 10 cc.
Use: Orally for bacillary dysentery, parenteral form for hospital use only.
See: Polymyxin B sulfate, U.S.P.
W/Bacitracin.
See: Polysporin, Oint. (Burroughs Wellcome)
W/Bacitracin & neomycin sulfate.
See: Neosporin, oint. & Ophth. Oint. (Burroughs Wellcome)
W/Bacitracin, neomycin, hydrocortisone.
See: Cortisporin, Prep. (Burroughs Wellcome)
AEROTHERM. (Aeroceuticals) Benzyl alcohol 22.7%, benzocaine 13.6%. Spray Bot. 5 oz.
Use: First aid spray for burns.
AEROTROL. Isoprenaline, B.A.N.
AEROZOIN. (Aeroceuticals) Comp. tr. of benzoin 30%, isopropyl alcohol 44.8%. Spray Bot. 3.5 oz.
Use: Skin conditioner for tape and cast dressing.
AETHYLIS CHLORIDUM.
See: Ethyl Chloride (Various Mfr.)
AFAXIN CAPSULES. (Winthrop Products) Vit. A Palmitate 50,000 I.U., 10,000 I.U./Cap.
Use: Vitamin A deficiency.
A-FIL. (CooperCare) Methyl-anthranilate 5%., titanium dioxide 5% in vanishing cream base. Tube 1.5 oz. Neutral or dark.
Use: Sunscreen.
AFKO-LUBE. (APC) Docusate sodium 100 mg./Cap. Bot. 100s.
Use: Stool softener.
AFKO-LUBE LAX. (APC) Docusate sodium 100 mg., casanthranol 30 mg./Cap. Bot. 100s.
Use: Stool softener.
AFRIKOL. (Citroleum) Suntan lotion w/no cocoa butter or lanolin. Bot. 4 oz.
AFRIN. (Schering) Oxymetazoline HCl 0.5 mg., aminoacetic acid 3.8 mg., sorbitol soln. 57 mg., phenylmercuric acetate 0.02 mg., benzalkonium Cl 0.2 mg./ml. **Nose Drops:** Drop. Bot. 20 ml. **Nasal Spray:** Plastic Spray Bot. 15 ml., 30 ml. **Pediatric Nose Drop:** Oxymetazoline 0.25 mg./ml. Drop. Bot. 20 ml.
Use: Nasal decongestant.

AFRIN MENTHOL NASAL SPRAY. (Schering) Oxymethazoline HCl 0.5 mg./ml. w/menthol. Bot. 15 ml.
Use: Nasal decongestant.

AFRINOL REPETABS. (Schering) Pseudoephedrine sulfate 120 mg./Repeat Action Tab. Box 12s. Bot. 100s.
Use: Nasal decongestant.

AFTATE. (Plough) Tolnaftate 1%. **Gel:** Tube 0.5 oz. **Non-Aerosol Spray:** 1.5 oz. **Spray Liquid:** 4 oz. Aero can; **Spray Powder:** 3.5 oz., 5 oz.; **Sprinkle Powder:** 1.5 oz., 2.25 oz. Can.
Use: Topical antifungal.

• **AGAR,** N.F. XVI. (Various Mfr.) Agar-agar, Bengal Gelatin, Ceylon.
Use: Bulk laxative, suspending aid.
W/Mineral oil.
See: Agoral, Emulsion (Warner-Chilcott)
Petrogalar (Wyeth)

AGGREGATED ALBUMIN.
See: Albumotope-LS (Squibb)

AGOBYL. (C.M.C.) Magnesium sulfate 37.0 Gm., succinic acid 2.0 Gm., peptone (bacteriological) 9.0 Gm., citric acid 4.0 Gm., sod. bicarbonate 6.0 Gm., sucrose (mint flavored) 42.0 Gm./100 Gm. Pkg. 125 Gm.

AGOFOLLIN.
See: Estradiol. (Various Mfr.)

AGORAL. W/Phenolphthalein (Parke-Davis) Phenolphthalein & mineral oil in an emulsion containing agar, tragacanth, egg-albumin, acacia, glycerin and water. Marshmallow flavor. Bot. 8, 16 fl. oz., Raspberry flavored Bot. pint.
Use: Laxative.

AGORAL, PLAIN. (Parke-Davis) Emulsion of mineral oil and an agar-gel. Bot. 16 oz.
Use: Laxative.

A/G-PRO. (Miller) Protein hydrolysate 50 gr. w/essential and nonessential amino acids 45%, l-lysine 50 mg., methionine 12.5 mg. and Fe, Cu, iodine, Mn, K, Zn, Mg./6 Tab. Bot. 180s.
Use: Tissue repair.

AGURIN.
See: Theobromine Sod. Acetate (Various Mfr.)

AHAN. (Eric, Kirk & Gary) Vitamin A acetate 25,000 I.U./Cap. Bot. 100s. 50,000 I.U., 100,000 I.U./Cap. Bot. 100s.

A-HYDROCORT. (Abbott) Hydrocortisone sodium succinate. **Vial:** 100 mg./2 ml. w/diluent. Pkg. 1s, 5s, 25s, 50s, 100s; **Univial:** 100 mg./2 ml. w/diluent. Pkg. 1s, 5s, 25s, 100s; 250 mg./2 ml. Pkg. 1s, 5s, 25s, 100s; 500 mg./4 ml. Pkg. 1s, 5s, 25s, 100s; 1000 mg./8 ml. Pkg. 1s, 5s, 25s.
Use: Anti-inflammatory.

AIR & SURFACE DISINFECTANT. (Aeroceuticals) Dimethylbenzylammonium Cl 0.33%, phenylphenol 0.25%, essential oils 0.10%, ethyl alcohol 44.25%. Aerosol spray.
Use: Air sanitizer, deodorizer..

AIRBRON. Acetylcysteine, B.A.N.

AIR-TABS G.G. (Scrip) Dyphylline 200 mg., guaifenesin 200 mg./Tab. Bot. 100s.
Use: Bronchodilator, expectorant.

AKES-N-PAIN. (Edward J. Moore) Acetaminophen 120 mg., salicylamide 210 mg., caffeine 30 mg., Ca gluconate 60 mg./Cap. Bot. 30s.
Use: Analgesic.

AKES-N-PAIN RUB. (Edward J. Moore) Histamine dihydrochloride, methyl nicotinate, oleoresin capsicum, glycomonosalicylate. Tube 1¼ oz.

AKINETON. (Knoll) Biperiden HCl 2 mg./Tab. Bot. 100s, 1000s.
Use: Anticholinergic and myospasmolytic for Parkinson's disease and drug-induced parkinsonism.

AKINETON LACTATE. (Knoll) Biperiden lactate 5 mg. in aqueous 1.4% sodium lactate solution/cc. Amp 1 cc. Box 10s.
Use: Relief of Parkinson-like dystonic crises.

• **AKLOMIDE.** USAN.
Use: Coccidiostat.

AKNE DRYING LOTION. (Alto) Zinc oxide 12%, urea 10%, sulfur 6%, salicylic acid 2%, benzalkonium chloride 0.2%, isopropyl alcohol 70%, in a base containing menthol, silicon dioxide, iron oxide and perfume. Bot. ¾ oz., 2¼ oz.
Use: Acne vulgaris, acne rosacea, seborrhea.

AKNE SCRUB. (Alto) Povidone iodine with polyethylene granules. Bot. ¾ oz.
Use: Acne cleanser, antiseptic, microbicidal

AKRINOL CREAM. (Schering) Acrisorcin, the hexylresorcinol salt of 9-aminoacridine, 2 mg. in a polyethylene glycol base/Gm. Tube 50 Gm.
Use: Topical treatment of tinea versicolor.

AKSHURN. (Seatrace) Danthron 75 mg./Tab. Bot. 100s, 1000s.
Use: Laxative.

ALA-BATH. (Del-Ray) Bath oil Bot. 8 oz., 12 oz.
Use: Emollient and skin softener.

ALA-CORT. (Del-Ray) Hydrocortisone 1%. **Cream.** Tube 1 oz., 3 oz. **Lotion** 1%, Bot. 4 oz.
Use: Glucocorticoid.

ALA-DERM. (Del-Ray) Emollient lotion. Bot 8 oz., 12 oz.
Use: Emollient lotion.

ALAGEL. (Century) Aluminum hydroxide gel. Bot. 12 oz.
Use: Antacid.

ALA-SEB SHAMPOO. (Del-Ray) Antiseborreic shampoo. Bot. 4 oz., 12 oz.
Use: Antiseborrheic shampoo.

ALA-SEB T SHAMPOO. (Del-Ray) Antiseborreic shampoo. Bot. 4 oz., 12 oz.
Use: Antiseborrheic shampoo.

ALADRINE. (Scherer) Ephedrine sulfate 8.1 mg., secobarbital sod. 16.2 mg./Tab. Bot. 100s. Ephedrine sulfate 8.1 mg., secobarbital sodium 16.2/5 cc. Bot. pt.
Use: Antiasthmatic.

ALAMAG. (Barre) Magnesium-aluminum hydroxide gel. Susp. Bot. pt.
W/Belladonna alkaloid, Susp. Bot. 8 oz.

• **ALAMECIN.** USAN.
Use: Antibacterial.

ALAMINE-C. (Vortech) Codeine phosphate 10 mg., chlorpheniramine maleate 2 mg. phenylpropanol-

amine HCl 18.75 mg./5 ml. W alcohol 5%. Bot. 4 oz., Gal.
Use: Decongestant, antitussive.
ALAMINE EXPECTORANT. (Vortech) Codeine phosphate 10 mg., guaifenesin 100 mg., phenylephrine HCl 10 mg., phenylpropanolamine HCl 18.75 mg./5 ml. W alcohol 7.5% Bot. 4 oz., Gal.
Use: Decongestant, antitussive.
ALAMINE LIQUID. (Vortech) Phenylpropranolamine HCl 18.75 mg., chlorpheniramine maleate 2 mg/5ml. W alcohol 5%. Bot. 4 oz., Gal.
Use: Decongestant.
• **ALANINE,** U.S.P. XXI. $C_3H_7NO_2$. L-Alanine.
β-ALANINE, N-(2,4-DIHYDROXY-3,3-DIMETHYL-1-OXOBUTYL)-, CALCIUM SALT (2:1). Calcium Pantothenate, U.S.P. XXI.
• **ALAPROCLATE.** USAN.
Use: Antidepressant.
ALA-QUIN 0.5%. (Del-Ray) Hydrocortisone, iodochlorhydroxyquin cream. Tube 1 oz.
ALA-SCALP HP 2%. (Del-Ray) Hydrocortisone lotion. Bot. 1 oz.
ALA-TET. (Del-Ray) Tetracycline HCl 250 mg./Cap. Bot. 100s, 1000s.
Use: Antibiotic.
ALAXIN. (Delta) Oxyethlene oxypropylene polymer 240 mg./Cap. Bot. 100s.
Use: Fecal softener, constipation remedy.
AL-AY. (Bowman)**Green Oblong Tube.:** Phenylephrine HCl 5 mg., chlorpheniramine maleate 2 mg., aspirin 162 mg., caffeine 15 mg., aminoacetic acid 162 mg./Tab. Bot. 100s, 1000s.**Dark Green S.C.:** Phenylephrine HCl 5 mg., chlorpheniramine maleate 2 mg., acetaminophen 160 mg., caffeine 15 mg./Tab. Bot. 100s, 1000s.
Use: Nasal decongestant.
AL-AY MODIFIED. (Bowman) Phenylephrine HCl 5 mg., chlorpheniramine maleate 2 mg., acetaminophen 160 mg., caffeine 15 mg./Tab. Bot. 100s, 1000s.
Use: Nasal decongestant.
ALAZANINE TRICHLORPHATE. 3-Ethyl-2-[3-(3-ethyl-2-benzothiazolinylidene) propenyl]-benzothiazolium 2,4,5-trichlorophenoxide salt with two formula weights of 2,4,5[trichlorophenol].
Use: Anthelmintic.
ALBALON-A LIQUIFILM. (Allergan) Naphazoline HCl 0.05%, antazoline phosphate 0.5%, polyvinyl alcohol 1.4%, benzalkonium Cl, edetate disodium, polyvinyl pyrrolidine, sodium Cl., sodium acetate, acetic acid, sodium hydroxide and purified water. Bot. 5 ml., 15 ml.
Use: Ocular antihistamine, decongestant.
ALBALON LIQUIFILM. (Allergan) Naphazoline HCl 0.1%, polyvinyl alcohol 1.4%, benzalkonium Cl, edetate disodium, citric acid, sodium citrate, sodium Cl, sodium hydroxide and purified water. Bot. 5 ml., 15 ml.
Use: Ocular vasoconstrictor.
ALBAMYCIN. (Upjohn) Novobiocin sod. 250 mg./Cap. Bot. 100s.
Use: Wide-range antibiotic therapy.
• **ALBENDAZOLE.** USAN.

Use: Anthelmintic.
ALBOLENE CREAM. (Norcliff Thayer) Unscented: Jar 6 oz., 12 oz. Scented: Jar 6 oz., 12 oz.
ALBUCID.
See: Sulfacetamide
• **ALBUMIN, AGGREGATED.** USAN.
Use: Diagnostic aid.
• **ALBUMIN, AGGREGATED IODINATED 1 131 SERUM,** USAN.
Use: Radioactive agent.
ALBUMINAR 5 AND ALBUMINAR-25. (Armour) Normal serum albumin, Human U.S.P. **5%:** 5% solution with administration set. Bot. 50 ml., 250 ml., 500 ml., 1000 ml. **25%:** 25% solution. Vial 20 ml., 50 ml., 100 ml. with administration set.
• **ALBUMIN, CHROMATED Cr 51 SERUM.** USAN. Radio-Chromated Serum Albumin Human.
See: Chromalbin (Squibb)
• **ALBUMIN HUMAN,** U.S.P. XXI. Normal Human Serum Albumin.
Use: Blood volume supporter
See: Albumisol 5%, 25% conc. (Merck Sharp & Dohme) Proserum 5, Inj. (Merrell Dow)
ALBUMIN HUMAN SALT-POOR.
Use: Shock, hypoproteinemia, renal diseases & cirrhosis.
See: Pro-Bumin, Vial (Lederle)
• **ALBUMIN, IODINATED I-125 SERUM.** USAN. Radio-iodinated (^{125}I) Serum Albumin Human.
Use: Diagnostic aid.
• **ALBUMIN, IODINATED I-131 SERUM,** U.S.P. XXI. Radio-iodinated (^{131}I) Serum Albumin Human. Aggregated Radio-Iodinated (I-131) Albumin Human.
Use: Diagnostic aid.
See: Albumotope-LS (Squibb)
• **ALBUMIN, IODINATED I-131 AGGREGATED INJECTION,** U.S.P. XXI.
Use: Diagnostic aid.
ALBUMIN-SALINE DILUENT. (Hollister-Stier) Pre-measured vials 1.8 ml., 4 ml., 4.5 ml., 9 ml., or 30 ml. Vials 2 ml., 5 ml., 10 ml., 30 ml.
Use: Dilute allergenic extracts & venom products for patient testing and treating.
ALBUMOTOPE I-131. (Squibb) Albumin, Iodinated I-131 Serum (50 uCi).
ALBUSTIX. (Ames) Firm paper reagent strips impregnated with tetrabromphenol blue, citrate buffer and a protein-adsorbing agent. Bot. 100s.
Use: Diagnostic, to indicate the presence of albumin in the urine.
• **ALBUTEROL SULFATE,** USAN.
Use: Bronchodilator.
See: Proventil, Tab. (Schering)
• **ALBUTEROL.** USAN.
Use: Bronchodilator.
• **ALBUTOIN.** USAN. 3-Allyl-5-isobutyl-2-thiohydantoin.
ALCAINE. (Alcon) Proparacaine HCl 0.5%, glycerin, sod. chloride, benzalkonium chloride. Bot. 15 ml.
Use: Ophthalmic topical anesthetic.
ALCLEAR EYE DROPS. (Walgreen) Tetrahydrozoline HCl 0.05%. Bot. 22 ml.
Use: Eye irritation remedy.

ALCLEAR EYE LOTION. (Walgreen) Bot. 8 oz.
Use: Sterile isotonic fluid for eye irritation.
• **ALCLOFENAC.** USAN. 4-Allyloxy-3-chlorophenyla-
cetic acid.
Use: Analgesic; anti-inflammatory.
See: Prinalgin
• **ALCLOMETASONE DIPROPIONATE.** USAN.
Use: Anti-inflammatory.
ALCLOXA. USAN. Tetrahydroxychloro-[(2-
hydroxy-5-oxo-2-imidazolin-4-yl)ureato]-dialuminum.
Use: Astringent, keratolytic.
ALCOBON. Flucytosine, B.A.N.
• **ALCOHOL,** U.S.P. XXI. Ethanol, ethyl alcohol.
Use: Topical anti-infective; pharmaceutic aid (sol-
vent).
• **ALCOHOL, DEHYDRATED,** U.S.P. XXI.
• **ALCOHOL, DEHYDRATED INJECTION,** U.S.P. XXI.
• **ALCOHOL AND DEXTROSE INJECTION,** U.S.P.
XXI.
• **ALCOHOL, DILUTED,** N.F. XVI.
• **ALCOHOL, RUBBING,** U.S.P. XXI. Rubefacient.
ALCOHOL 5% AND DEXTROSE 5%. (Abbott)
Alcohol 5 ml., dextrose 5 Gm./100 ml. Bot. 1000 ml.
ALCOJET. (Alconox) Biodegradable machine washing
detergent and wetting agent. Ctn. 9 × 4 lb., 25 lb.,
50 lb., 100 lb., 300 lb.
Use: Detergent and wetting agent.
ALCOLEC. (American Lecithin) Lecithin w/choline
base, cephalin, lipositol. Caps. 100s. Gran. 8 oz.,
1 lb.
Use: Colloid, emulsifier, antioxidant.
ALCONEFRIN 12 AND 50. (Webcon) Phenylephrine
HCl 0.16% w/benzalkonium chloride. Dropper Bot.
1 oz.
Use: Nasal decongestant.
ALCONEFRIN 25. (Webcon) Phenylephrine HCl
0.25% plus Benzalkonium chloride. Dropper Bot. 30
cc. Spray Pkg. 1 oz.
ALCON LENS CASE. (Alcon) Ctn. of 6s.
Use: Thermal and chemical disinfection regimes of
hard gas permeable and soft contact lenses.
ALCONOX. (Alconox) Biodegradable detergent &
wetting agent. Box 4 lb., Container 25 lb., 50 lb.,
100 lb., 300 lb.
Use: Anionic detergent and wetting agent.
ALCOPAR. Bephenium Hydroxynaphthoate, B.A.N.
ALCOTABS. (Alconox) Tabs., Box 100s, 6s.
Use: Cleaning pipettes and test tubes.
ALCO-VITE. (Galen) Vit. A 6666 I.U., D 333 I.U., B-
1 3.3 mg., B-2 2.66 mg., B-6 3.3 mg., B-12 5 mcg., C
66.6 mg., E 5 I.U., Ca pantothenate 20 mg.,
niacinamide 20 mg., biotin 0.053 mg., folic acid 1.1
mg., PABA 11 mg., inositol 53.3 mg., choline
bitartrate 53.3 mg., desoxycholic acid 1.25
mg./Cap. Bot. 100s, 1000s.
Use: Nutritional supplement—lipotropic therapy.
• **ALCURONIUM CHLORIDE.** USAN.
Diallyldinortoxiferin dichloride.
Use: Muscle relaxant.
See: Alloferin (Roche)
  Toxiferene (Roche)

ALDACTAZIDE TABLETS. (Searle) Spironolactone
and hydrochlorothiazide. **25 mg./25 mg.:** Bot. 100s,
500s, 1000s, 2500s. Unit Dose 100s. **50 mg./50
mg.:** Bot. 100s. Unit Dose 100s.
Use: Antihypertensive, treatment of edema of
cirrhosis & of CHF, nephrotic syndrome.
ALDACTONE TABLETS. (Searle) Spironolactone **25
mg./**Tab. Bot. 100s, 500s, 1000s, 2500s. Unit Dose
100s. **50 mg./**Tab. Bot. 100s. Unit Dose 100s. **100
mg./**Tab. Bot. 100s. Unit Dose 100s.
Use: Antihypertensive; treatment of edema of
cirrhosis & CHF, nephrotic syndrome; in
hypokalemia; primary aldosteronism.
ALDERLIN HYDROCHLORIDE. Pronethalol, B.A.N.
ALDINAMIDE. 2-Carbamoyl pyrazine.
• **ALDIOXA.** USAN. Aluminum dihydroxy allantoinate.
Dihydroxy-[(2-hydroxy-5-oxo-2-imidazolin-4-yl)ureato]
aluminum.
Use: Astringent, keratolytic.
ALDOCLOR-150. (Merck Sharp & Dohme) Methyldopa
250 mg., chlorothiazide 150 mg./Tab. Bot. 100s.
Use: Antihypertensive agent.
ALDOCLOR-250. (Merck Sharp & Dohme) Methyldopa
250 mg., chlorothiazide 250 mg./Tab. Bot. 100s.
Use: Antihypertensive agent.
ALDOCORTEN. Aldosterone, B.A.N.
ALDOMET. (Merck Sharp & Dohme) Methyldopa. 125
mg./Tab. Bot. 100s. 250 mg./Tab. Bot. 100s,
1000s. Single unit pkg. 100s. Unit of use 12 Bot. of
100s. 500 mg./Tab. Bot. 100s, 500s. Single unit
pkg. 100s. Unit of use 12 Bot. of 60s, 100s.
Use: Antihypertensive agent.
W/Chlorothiazide.
See: Aldoclor, Tab. (Merck Sharp & Dohme)
W/Hydrochlorothiazide.
See: Aldoril, Tab. (Merck Sharp & Dohme)
ALDOMET ESTER HCl. (Merck Sharp & Dohme)
Methyldopate HCl 250 mg./5 ml. w/citric acid
anhydrous 25 mg., sodium bisulfite 16 mg.,
disodium edetate 2.5 mg., monothioglycerol 10 mg.
sodium hydroxide to adjust pH, methylparaben
0.15%, propylparaben 0.02% w/water for inj. q.s.
to 5 ml. Vial 5 ml.
Use: Antihypertensive agent.
ALDOMET ORAL SUSPENSION. (Merck Sharp &
Dohme) Methyldopa 250 mg./5 ml. Bot. 473 ml.
Use: Antihypertensive agent.
ALDORIL-15. (Merck Sharp & Dohme) Methyldopa 250
mg., hydrochlorothiazide 15 mg./Tab. Bot. 100s,
1000s. Unit dose pkg. 100s.
Use: Antihypertensive agent.
ALDORIL-25. (Merck Sharp & Dohme) Methyldopa 250
mg., hydrochlorothiazide 25 mg./Tab. Bot. 100s,
1000s. Unit dose pkg. 100s.
Use: Antihypertensive agent.
ALDORIL D30. (Merck Sharp & Dohme) Methyldopa
500 mg., hydrochlorothiazide 30 mg./Tab. Bot. 100s.
Use: Antihypertensive agent.
ALDORIL D50. (Merck Sharp & Dohme) Methyldopa
500 mg., hydrochlorothiazide 50 mg./Tab. Bot.
100s.
Use: Antihypertensive agent.

ALDOSTERONE B.A.N. 11β,21-Dihydroxy-3,-20-di-oxopregn-4-en-18-al. Aldocorten. Electrocortin.
Use: Corticosteroid.

ALDOSTERONE RIA DIAGNOSTIC KIT. (Abbott) Test kit 50s.
Use: Radioimmunoassay for direct measurement of total aldosterone in serum, plasma or urine.

ALERMINE. (Reid-Provident) Chlorpheniramine maleate 4 mg./Tab. Bot. 100s, 500s, 1000s.

ALERMINE T.D. (Reid-Provident) Chlorpheniramine maleate 8 or 12 mg./Granucap. Bot. 1000s.

ALERSULE CAPSULES. (Misemer) Chlorpheniramine maleate 8 mg., phenylephrine HCl 20 mg., methscopolamine nitrate 2.5 mg./Cap. Bot. 100s, 1000s.
Use: Symptoms of common cold and hay fever.

ALERT-PEP. (Approved) Caffeine 200 mg./Cap. Bot. 16s.
Use: General alertness.

• **ALETAMINE HYDROCHLORIDE.** USAN.
Use: Antidepressant.

ALEUDRIN. Isoprenaline, B.A.N.

ALEVAIRE SOLUTION. (Winthrop Products) Superinone.
Use: Mucolytic.

• **ALEXIDINE.** USAN. 1,1'-Hexamethylenebis[5-(2-ethylhexyl) biguanide].
Use: Antibacterial.

• **ALFAPROSTOL.** USAN.
Use: Prostaglandin (veterinary).

ALFENTA. (Janssen) Alfentanil
Use: Analgesic.

• **ALFENTANIL HYDROCHLORIDE.** USAN.
Use: Analgesic, narcotic.

ALFICETYN. Chloramphenicol, B.A.N.

ALFLORONE. Fludrocortisone, B.A.N.

ALGECOL TABLETS. (Winston) Acetaminophen 5 gr., phenylpropanolamine HCl 25 mg., phenylephrine HCl 10 mg., chlorpheniramine maleate 2 mg./Tab. Bot. 100s, 1000s.
Use: Analgesic, decongestant, antihistaminic.

ALGEL. (Faraday) Magnesium trisilicate 0.5 Gm., aluminum hydroxide 0.25 Gm./Tab. Bot. 100s. Susp., Bot. gal.
Use: Antacid.

ALGELDRATE. (Warner-Lambert) Hydrated aluminum hydroxide.
Use: Antacid.

ALGEMIN. (Thurston) Macrocystis pyrifera alga. Powd. Jar 8 oz. Tabs. Bot. 300s.
Use: Dietary aid.

• **ALGESTONE ACETONIDE.** USAN. 16α,-17α-Isopropylidenedioxypregn-4-ene-3,20-dione;
Use: Progestational steroid.

• **ALGESTONE ACETOPHENIDE.** USAN. (R)-16α, 17-Dihydroxypregn-4-ene-3,20-dione cyclic acetal with acetophenone.
Use: Progestin.

ALGETUSS. (Winston) Dextromethorphan HBr 60 mg., ammonium chloride 300 mg., phenylpropanolamine HCl 50 mg., chlorpheniramine maleate 7.5 mg., sodium citrate 720 mg./fl. oz. Bot. pt.

Use: Antitussive, expectorant.

ALGEX LINIMENT. (Approved) Menthol, camphor, methylsalicylate, eucalyptus. Bot. 4 oz.
Use: Heat therapy.

ALGIN.
See: Sodium Alginate, N.F. XVI.

ALGIN-ALL. (Barth's) Sodium alginate from kelp. Tab. Bot. 100s, 500s.

• **ALGINIC ACID,** N.F. XVI.
Use: Pharmaceutic aid (tablet binder; thickening agent).

ALGINIC ACID. W/Aluminum hydroxide dried gel, magnesium trisilicate, and sod. bicarbonate.
See: Gaviscon Foamtabs (Marion)

• **ALGRELDRATE.** USAN.
Use: Antacid.

ALIDINE DIHYDROCHLORIDE OR PHOSPHATE. Anileridine, N.F.

• **ALIFLURANE.** USAN.
Use: Anesthetic.

ALIMEMAZINE (I.N.N.). Trimeprazine, B.A.N.

• **ALIPAMIDE.** USAN. 4-Chloro-3-sulfamoylbenzoic acid 2,2-dimethylhydrazide.
Use: Diuretic, antihypertensive.

ALIPAMIDE. B.A.N. 4-Chloro-2',2'-dimethyl-3-sulfamoylbenzohydrazide.
Use: Diuretic.

ALIPCO. (Drug Products) Strychnine sulfate 0.5 mg., belladonna lvs. ext. 5.4 mg., phenolphthalein 32 mg., aloin 13 mg., podophyllin 4 mg., ipecac 4 mg./Tab. Bot. 1000s.
Use: Adult laxative.

ALISOBUMAL.
See: Butalbital, U.S.P. XXI.

ALKALOL. (Alkalol Co.) Thymol, eucalyptol, menthol, camphor, benzoin, pot. alum, pot. chlorate, sod. bicarb., sod. chloride, sweet birch oil, spearmint oil, pine & cassia oil, alcohol 0.05%. Bot. 1 pt. Nasal douche cup Pkg. 1s.
Use: Eyes, nose, throat & all inflamed mucous membranes.

ALKA-MED LIQUID. (Blue Cross) Aluminum hydroxide 200 mg., magnesium hydroxide 200 mg./ 5 ml. Bot. 8 oz.
Use: Antacid.

ALKA MED TABLETS. (Blue Cross) Magnesium hydroxide, aluminum hydroxide. Bot. 60s.
Use: Antacid.

ALKA-SELTZER. (Miles) Heat treated sodium bicarbonate 1904 mg., citric acid 1000 mg., acetylsalicylic acid 324 mg./Tab. Bot. 8s, 25s; foil 12s, 36s, 72s, 100s.
Use: Effervescent antacid, analgesic.

ALKA-SELTZER PLUS. (Miles) Chlorpheniramine maleate 2 mg., phenylpropanolamine bitartrate 24 mg., aspirin 324 mg./Tab. Foil Pkgs: 20s, 36s.
Use: Relief of cold symptoms.

ALKA-SELTZER SPECIAL EFFERVESCENT ANTACID. (Miles) Heat treated sodium bicarbonate 958 mg., citric acid 832 mg., potassium bicarbonate 312 mg./Tab. Foil Pkgs: 12s, 20s, 36s.
Use: Antacid.

ALKA-2 CHEWABLE ANTACID. (Miles) Calcium carbonate 500 mg./Tab. Rolls 10s, ×3. Bot. 85s.
Use: Antacid.

ALKAVERVIR. Mixture of Veratrum viride alkaloids.

ALKERAN. (Burroughs Wellcome) Melphalan 2 mg./Tab., Bot. 50s.
Use: Treatment of epithial carcinoma of ovary and multiple myeloma.

ALKETS. (Upjohn) Ca carbonate 780 mg., Mg. carbonate 130 mg., Mg. oxide 65 mg./Tab. Bot. 100s.
Use: Antacid.

ALKOHOLA COMPOUND. (Sutliff & Case) Ethyl alcohol 70%. Bot. pt.
Use: Local soothing, cooling and stimulating effect.

ALK-PHOSTEL. (Warner-Lambert) Box 100 test sets.

ALKYLBENZYLDIMETHYLAMMONIUM CHLORIDE.
Benzalkonium Chloride, N.F. XVI.
W/Methylrosaniline chloride,
polyoxyethylenenonylphenol, polyethylene glycol tert-dodecylthioether.
See: Hyva, Tab. (Holland-Rantos)

• **ALLANTOIN.** USAN.
Use: Wounds and resistant ulcers to stimulate the growth of healthy tissue.
See: Cutemol, (Summers)
Sebical Cream Shampoo (Reed & Carnrick)
W/Aminacrine, sulfanilamide.
See: Par Cream (Parmed)
Sufamal, Cream (Milex)
Vagidine, Cream (Elder)
Vagitrol, Cream (Syntex)
W/Balsam, Lano-sil, silicone.
See: Balmex Med. Lot. (Macsil)
W/Camphor, menthol, tinct. benzoin.
See: Siltex, Oint. (Edward J. Moore)
W/Cetyl dimethyl ethyl ammonium Br, pramoxine HCl, pyrilamine maleate.
See: Quad-Creme (Sutliff & Case)
W/p-Chloro-m-xylenol.
See: Cebum, Shampoo (Dermik)
W/Coal tar ext., hexachlorophene, glycerin & lanolin.
See: Pso-Rite, Cream (DePree)
W/Coal tar in cream base.
See: Tegrin Cream (Block Drug)
W/Coal tar solution, isopropyl myristate, psorilan.
See: Psorelief, Sol (Columbia)
W/Dienestrol, sulfanilamide, aminacrine HCl.
See: AVC/Dienestrol Cream, Suppos. (Merrell Dow)
W/Hydrocortisone.
See: Tarcortin, Cream (Reed & Carnrick)
W/Nitrofurazone.
See: Eldezol, Oint. (Elder)
W/Pramoxine HCl, benzalkonium Cl.
See: Perifoam, Aerosol (Rowell Labs.)
W/Resorcinol, hexachlorophene, menthol.
See: Tackle, Gel. (Colgate-Palmolive)
W/Salicylic Acid, sulfur.
See: Neutrogena Disposables (Neutrogena)
W/Sulfanilamide, 9-aminoacridine HCl.
See: Femguard Vaginal, Cream (Reid-Provident)
Nil Vaginal Cream (Century)

Sulfem Vag. Cream (Federal Pharm.)
Triconol Vag. Cream (Coastal)
Vagisan, Creme (Sandia)
Vagisul, Creme (Sheryl)
W/Sulfisoxazole, Aminoacridine.
Use: Topically, aid in the promotion of granulation.
See: Vagilia, Cream, Supp. (Lemmon)
W/Tarbonis.
See: Sebical, Shampoo (Carnrick & Reed)
W/Vit. A, Vit. D.
See: A-D Dressing (LaCrosse)

ALLBEE C-800. (Robins) Vit. E 45 I.U., C 800 mg., B-1 15 mg., B-2 17 mg., niacin 100 mg., B-6 25 mg., B-12 mcg., pantothenic acid 25 mg./Tab. Bot. 60s.
Use: Vitamin supplement.

ALLBEE C-800 PLUS IRON. (Robins) Vit. E 45 I.U., C 800 mg., B-1 15 mg., B-2 17 mg., niacin 100 mg., B-6 25 mg., B-12 12 mcg., pantothenic acid 25 mg., iron 27 mg., folic acid 0.4 mg./Tab. Bot. 60s.
Use: Vitamin supplement with iron.

ALLBEE W/VITAMIN C. (Robins) Vit. B-1 15 mg., B-6 5 mg., B-2 10.2 mg., niacin 50 mg., pantothenic acid 10 mg., Vitamin C 300 mg./Cap. Bot. 30s, 100s, 1000s. Dis-co packs (Caps) 10x100s.
Use: Vitamin supplement.

ALLBEE-T. (Robins) B-1 15.5 mg., B-2 10 mg., B-6 8.2 mg., pantothenic acid 23 mg., niacin 100 mg., Vit. C 500 mg., B-12 5 mcg./Tab. Bot. 100s, 500s.
Use: Vitamin supplement.

ALL BETTER CAPSULES. (Image) Vitamin capsules Bot. 100s.
Use: Supplement.

ALLBEX. (Approved) Vit. B-1 5 mg., B-2 2 mg., B-6 0.25 mg., calcium pantothenate 3 mg., niacinamide 20 mg., ferrous sulfate 194.4 mg., inositol 10 mg., choline 10 mg., Vit. B-12 (conc.) 3 mcg./Cap. Bot. 100s, 1000s.
Use: Vitamin deficiencies.

ALL-DAY B-COMPLEX. (Barth's) Vit. B-12 25 mcg., B-1 7 mg., B-2 14 mg., niacin 4.67 mg., B-6, pantothenic acid, folic acid, choline, aminobenzoic acid, inositol, biotin, Mg, Mn, Cu/Cap. Bot. 30s, 90s, 180s, 360s.

ALL-DAY-C. (Barth's) Vit. C 200 mg./Cap. 500 mg./Tab. with rose hip extract. Bot. 30s, 90s, 180s, 360s.

ALL-DAY IRON YEAST. (Barth's) Iron 20 mg., Vit. B-1 2 mg., B-2 4 mg., niacin 0.57 mg./Cap. Bot. 30s, 90s, 180s.

ALL-DAY-VITES. (Barth's) Vit. A 10,000 I.U., D 400, I.U. B-1 3 mg., B-2 6 mg., niacin 1 mg., C 120 mg., B-12 10 mcg., E 30 I.U./Cap. Bot. 30s, 90s, 180s, 360s.

ALLEGRON. Nortriptyline.

ALLERBEN INJECTION. (Fellows) Diphenhydramine 10 mg./cc. Vial 30 cc.

ALLERCHLOR INJECTION. (Fellows) Chlorpheniramine maleate 10 mg./cc. Vial 30 cc.

ALLERDEC CAPSULES. (Towne) Phenylpropanolamine HCl 25 mg., chlorpheniramine maleate 1 mg., pyrilamine maleate 5 mg./Cap. Bot. 25s, 50s.

ALLEREST. (Pharmacraft) **Tabs:**

Phenylpropanolamine HCl 18.7 mg., chlorpheniramine maleate 2 mg./Tab. Sleeve Pack 24s, 48s. Bot. 75s. **Chewable Tablets for Children:** phenylpropanolamine HCl 9.4 mg., chlorpheniramine maleate 1 mg./Tab. Sleeve Pack 24s. **Timed-Release Caps.:** phenylpropanolamine HCl 50 mg., chlorpheniramine maleate 4 mg./Cap. Bot. 10s. **Nasal Spray:** phenylephrine HCl 0.5%. Bot. 0.5 oz. **Eye Drops:** Naphazoline 0.012%, benzalkonium Cl 0.01%, disodium edetate 0.1% w/boric acid, sodium borate, methylcellulose. Bot. 0.5 oz. **Headache Strength Tabs.:** Acetaminophen 325 mg., phenylpropanolamine HC1 18.7 mg., chlorpheniramine maleate 2 mg./Tab. Sleeve Pack 24s, 48s.
Use: Hay fever, allergy.
ALLERGAN HYDROCARE CLEANING & DISINFECTING SOLUTION. (Allergan) Bot. 4 oz., 8 oz.
Use: Clean, disinfect, & store soft (hydrophilic) contact lenses.
ALLERGAN HYDROCARE PRESERVED SALINE SOLUTION. (Allergan) Bot. 8 oz., 12 oz.
Use: Heat disinfection, rinsing, and storage of soft (hydrophilic) contact lenses.and for rinsing in conjunction with chemical disinfection.
ALLERGAN SORBI-CARE SALINE SOLUTION. (Allergan) Saline solution. Bot. 8 oz.
Use: Rinsing, heat disinfection and storage of soft (hydrophilic) contact lenses.
ALLERGENIC EXT. (Barry) Poison ivy, oak and sumac ext. triple antigen. In hypo-allergenic oil vehicle. Vial 5 cc.
ALLERGENIC EXTRACTS. (Center) Allergenic extracts of pollen, mold, house dust, inhalants, epidermal & insects in saline 0.9% & phenol 0.4% up to 1:10 w/v or 40,000 PNU/ml. in sets or vials up to 30 ml.
Use: Diagnosis & hyposensitization treatment of allergies.
ALLERGENIC EXTRACTS. (Hollister-Stier) Allergenic extracts of pollens, foods, inhalants, epidermals, fungi, insects, miscellaneous antigens, autogenous extracts. Scratch tests, vials.
Use: Diagnosis and treatment of causative factors in allergy.
ALLERGESIC IMPROVED. (Vitarine) Phenylpropanolamine HCl 18.7 mg., chlorpheniramine maleate 2 mg./Tab. Vial 48s.
Use: Relief of upper respiratory allergy symptoms.
ALLERGEX. (Hollister-Stier) Silicones, polyethylene and triethylene glycol, antioxidants, mineral oil with fungicide. Bot. 1 pt. Aerosol Spray, Bot. pt.
Use: Control of house dust allergens.
ALLERGY. (Eckerd) Chlorpheniramine maleate, phenylephrine HCl, ascorbic acid, calcium pantothenate/Tab. Bot. 48s.
ALLERGY II TABLETS. (Eckerd) Chlorpheniramine maleate 4 mg., phenylpropanolamine 37.5 mg./Tab. Bot. 24s., 48s.
Use: Decongestant, antihistamine.

ALLERGY PREPARATIONS.
See: Antihistamine Preparations
ALLERGY TABS. (Weeks & Leo) Phenylpropanolamine HCl 37.5 mg., chlorpheniramine 4 mg./Tab. Vials 30s.
Use: Allergy relief.
ALLERID-D.C. (Trimen) Chlorpheniramine maleate 6 mg., pseudoephedrine HCl 120 mg./Cap. Bot. 100s.
Use: Antihistamine decongestant.
ALLERID-O.D. (Trimen) Chlorpheniramine maleate 8 mg., 12 mg./Cap. Bot. 100s.
ALLERSONE. (Mallard) Hydrocortisone 0.5%, diperodon HCl 0.5%, zinc oxide 5%, sodium lauryl sulfate, propylene glycol, cetyl alcohol, petrolatum, methyl & propyl parabens. Oint. Tube 15 Gm.
Use: Anti-inflammatory, antipruritic & antiallergic.
ALLETORPHINE. B.A.N. N-Allyl-7,8-dihydro-7α-(1(R)-hydroxy-1-methylbutyl)-O⁶-methyl-6,14-endoethenon-ormorphine. N-Allylnoretorphine.
Use: Analgesic.
• **ALLOBARBITAL.** USAN. 5,5-Diallylbarbituric acid.
W/Acetaminophen, salicylamide, caffeine.
See: Allylvon, Cap. (Elder)
W/Aspirin, acetaminophen, aluminum aspirin.
See: Allylgesic, Tab. (Elder)
W/Ergotamine tartrate.
See: Allylgesic w/Ergotamine, Cap. (Elder)
ALLOBARBITONE.
See: Diallylbarbituric Acid (Various Mfr.)
ALLOMETHADIONE. (I.N.N.) Aloxidone, B.A.N.
• **ALLOPURINOL,** U.S.P. XXI. Tablets, U.S.P. XXI. 1 H-Pyrazolo-[3, 4-d] pyrimidin-4-ol.
Use: Antigout, xanthine oxidase inhibitor.
See: Lopurin, Tab. (Boots Pharm)
Zyloprim, Tab. (Burroughs Wellcome)
ALLOPURINOL. B.A.N. 1H-Pyrazolo[3,4-d] pyrimidin-4-ol.
Use: Uricosuric.
ALLPYRAL. (Miles Pharm) Allergenic extracts, alum-precipitated. For subcutaneous inj. pollens, molds, epithelia, house dust, other inhalants, stinging insects.
Use: Allergies.
ALLYLBARBITURIC ACID. Allylisobutyl-barbituric acid, butalbital. Tab. (Various Mfr.)
Use: Sedative.
W/A.P.C.
See: Anti-Ten, Tab. (Century)
Fiorinal, Cap., Tab. (Sandoz)
Marnal, Tab. (Vortech)
Salipral, Tab. (Kenyon)
Tenstan (Standex)
W/Aspirin, acetaminophen, caffeine.
See: Paradol, Tab. (Medics)
W/Acetaminophen, homatropine methylbromide.
See: Panitol H.M.B., Tab. (Wesley)
W/Acetaminophen, salicylamide, caffeine.
See: Renpap, Tab. (Wren)
17-ALLYL-4,5α-EPOXY-3,14-DIHYDROXY-MORPHIN-AN-6-ONE HCl. Naloxone Hydrochloride, U.S.P. XXI.

ALLYLESTRENOL. 17a-Allyl-17b-hydroxy-4-estrene.
**N-ALLYL-14-HYDROXY-NORDIHYDROMORPHI-
NONE HCl.** Naloxone Hydrochloride, U.S.P. XXI.
ALLYL-ISOBUTYLBARBITURIC ACID.
See: Allyl Barbituric Acid.
5-ALLYL-5-ISOPROPYLBARBITURIC ACID.
See: Aprobarbital.
ALLYLISOPROPYLMALONYLUREA.
See: Aprobarbital.
ALLYL ISOTHIOCYANATE, Oil of mustard. (Various Mfr.)
Use: Counterirritant in neuralgia.
4-ALLYL-2-METHOXYPHENOL. Eugenol, U.S.P. XXI.
N-ALLYLNORMORPHINE HCl.
Nalorphine HCl
See: Nalline HCl, Amp. (Merck Sharp & Dohme)
N-ALLYLNOROXYMORPHONE HCl. Naloxone Hydrochloride, U.S.P. XXI.
ALLYLOESTRENOL. B.A.N. 17α-Allyloestr-4-en-17β-ol. Gestanin.
Use: Progestational steroid.
5-ALLYL-5-PHENYLBARBITURIC ACID. Alphenal, Alphenate.
Use: Sedative & hypnotic.
ALLYLPRODINE. B.A.N. 3-Allyl-1-methyl-4-phenyl-4-propionyloxypiperidine.
Use: Analgesic.
5-ALLYL-SEC-BUTYLBARBITURIC ACID.
See: Lotusate, Cap. (Winthrop-Breon)
• **ALMADRATE SULFATE.** USAN. Aluminum magnesium hydroxide-oxide-sulfate-hydrate.
Use: Antacid.
ALMAGUCIN. Antacid mix of gastric mucin, dried aluminum hydroxide gel & mag. trisilicate.
ALMATRI. (Robinson) Aluminum hydroxide gel. 4 gr., Mg trisilicate 7½ gr./Tab. Bot. 100s, 1000s. Bulk Pack 5000s.
Use: Antacid adsorbent.
ALMOCARPINE. (Ayerst) Pilocarpine HCl 1%, 2%, and 4%, Steri-Tainer drop bot. 15 ml. each.
Use: Reduction of intraocular tension.
• **ALMOND OIL,** N.F. XVI. Pharmaceutic aid (emollient and perfume).
ALMORA. (O'Neal, Jones & Feldman) Magnesium gluconate 0.5 Gm./Tab. Pkg. 100s.
Use: Sedative in dysmenorrhea.
ALNYTE. (Mayer) Scopolamine aminoxide HBr. 0.2 mg., salicylamide 250 mg./Tab. Pkg. 16s.
ALOCASS LAXATIVE. (Western Research) Aloin ¼ gr., cascara sagrada ½ gr., rhubarb ½ gr., ginger ¹/₃₂ gr., pow. ext. belladonna ¹/₂₀ gr./Tab. Bot. 1000s. Paks 28.
Use: Laxative.
• **ALOE,** U.S.P. XXI.
Use: See Compound Benzoin Tincture.
ALOE GRANDE CREME. (Gordon) Aloe Vit. E 1500 I.U., A 100,000 u./oz. in cream base. Jar 2 oz.
Use: Skin care cream.
ALOE VERA ACTIVE PRINCIPLE.
See: Alvagel, Oint. (Kenyon)
• **ALOFILCON A.** USAN.
Use: Contact lens material.

ALOIN.. (Baker, J.T.) A mixture of cryst. Pentosides from various aloes. Bot. 1 oz.
Use: Laxative.
W/Ox bile (desiccated), phenolphthalein, cascara sagrada ext., podophyllin.
See: Bilgon (Reid-Provident)
• **ALONIMID.** USAN.
Use: Sedative.
ALOPHEN PILLS. (Parke-Davis) Phenolphthalein 60 mg./Pill Bot. 100s.
Use: Laxative.
ALO-TUSS IMPROVED. (Vortech) Dextromethorphan HBr. 10 mg., phenylephrine HCl 5 mg., chlorpheniramine maleate 2 mg., salicylamide 227 mg., acetophenetidin 100 mg., caffeine 10 mg./Tab. Bot. 100s, 1000s.
Use: Temporary relief of cold symptoms.
ALOXIDONE. B.A.N. 3-Allyl-5-methyloxazolidine-2,4-dione. Allomethadione (I.N.N.) Malidone.
Use: Anticonvulsant.
ALOXIPRIN. B.A.N. Polymeric condensation product of aluminum oxide and O-acetylsalicylic acid. Palaprin.
Use: Antirheumatic.
• **ALPERTINE.** USAN.
Use: Antipsychotic.
• **ALPHA AMYLASE.** USAN. A concentrated form of alpha amylase produced by a strain of nonpathogenic bacteria.
See: Kutrase, Cap. (Kremers-Urban)
Ku-Zyme, Cap. (Kremers-Urban)
ALPHA-AMYLASE W-100. W/Proteinase W-300, cellase W-100, lipase, estrone, testosterone, vitamins, minerals.
See: Geramine, Tab. (Brown)
ALPHA-BEL. (Moore Kirk) Phenobarbital 50 mg., hyoscyamine sulfate 0.3 mg., hyoscine HBr 0.02 mg., atropine sulfate 0.06 mg./timed disintegration Cap. Bot. 100s, 1000s.
Use: Antispasmodic and sedative for pylorospasm, gastritis and colitis, biliary colic.
ALPHACETYLMETHADOL. B.A.N. α-4-Dimethylamino-1-ethyl-2,2-diphenylpentyl acetate.
Use: Analgesic.
ALPHA CHYMAR. (Barnes-Hind) A lyophilized form of crystallized alpha chymotrypsin. Vial 1s. (750 USP units) w/10 ml. diluent for ophthalmic solution.
Use: To dissolve the zonule fibers of the lens of the eye.
ALPHA-CHYMOTRYPSIN.
See: Alpha Chymar, Vial (Armour)
Zolyse, Vial (Alcon)
α-**CYCLOHEXYL-**α-**PHENYL-1-PYRROLIDINEPROP-
ANOL HCl.**
See: Procyclidine HCl (Burroughs Wellcome)
ALPHADERM. (Norwich Eaton) Hydrocortisone 1%, urea 10% in a powder-in-cream base. Tubes 30 Gm, 100 Gm.
Use: Dermatoses treatment.
ALPHADOLONE. B.A.N. 3α,21-Dihydroxy-5α-pregnane-11,20-dione.
Use: Anesthetic component.
ALPHA-E. (Barth's) d-Alpha tocopherol 50 I.U., 100

I.U./Cap. Bot. 100s, 500s, 1000s. 200 I.U./Cap.
Bot. 100s, 250s. 400 I.U./Cap. Bot. 100s, 250s,
500s.
ALPHA E OIL & CREAM. (Towne) 2 oz.
ALPHA-ESTRADIOL. Known to be beta-Estradiol.
See: Estradiol (Various Mfr.)
ALPHA-ESTRADIOL BENZOATE.
See: Estradiol benzoate. (Various Mfr.)
ALPHA FAST. (Eastwood) Bath oil. Bot. 16 oz.
ALPHA-HYPOPHAMINE.
See: Oxytocin Injection
ALPHA-KERI. (Westwood) **Bath Oil:** Mineral oil, lanolin
oil, PEG-4-dilaurate, benzophenone-3, D & C green
#6, fragrance. Bot. 4 oz., 8 oz., 16 oz.; **Spray:** 5
oz. **Cleansing Bar:** bar containing Na tallowate, Na
cocoate, water, mineral oil, fragrance, PEG-75,
glycerin, titanium dioxide, lanolin oil, NaCl, BHT,
EDTA, D&C green # 5, D&C yellow # 10.
Use: Treatment of dry skin.
ALPHAMEPRODINE. B.A.N. α-3-Ethyl-1-methyl-4-pro-
pionyloxypiperidine.
Use: Analgesic.
ALPHAMETHADOL. B.A.N. α-6-Dimethyl-amino-4,4-
diphenylheptan-3-ol.
Use: Analgesic.
ALPHAMIN. (Vortech) Crystalline hydroxocobalamin
1000 mcg./CC. Vial 10 ml., 30 ml.
Use: Pernicious & megaloblastic anemia.
ALPHA-METHYLDOPA. Name previously used for Me-
thyldopa.
ALPHAMUL. (Lannett) Castor oil 60% w/v,
emulsifying agent. Bot. 3 fl. oz., gal.
Use: Laxative.
ALPHA-PHENOXYETHYL PENICILLIN, POTASSIUM.
See: Phenethicillin Potassium.
ALPHAPRODINE. B.A.N. α-1,3-Dimethyl-4-phenyl-4-
propionyloxypiperidine.
Use: Analgesic.
See: Nisentil, Inj. (Roche)
• **ALPHAPRODINE HYDROCHLORIDE,** U.S.P. XXI.
Inj. U.S.P. XXI. dl-Alpha-1,3-Dimethyl-4-phenyl-4-
piperidinol propionate HCl. Inj.
Use: Analgesic.
See: Nisentil HCl, Amp., Vial (Roche)
alphaREDISOL. (Merck Sharp & Dohme)
Hydroxocobalamin 1000 mcg./ml. w/sod. chloride
0.82%, anhydrous sod. acetate 0.02%, acetic acid,
methylparaben 0.15%, propylparaben 0.02%, and
water for injection q.s. Vial 10 ml.
Use: Vitamin B-12 therapy (hematopoietic).
ALPHA-RUVITE. (Savage) Hydroxocobalamin 1000
mcg./cc. Vial 10 cc.
Use: Hematinic.
ALPHASONE ACETOPHENIDE. Name previously
used for Algestone acetonide.
ALPHA-TOCOPHEROL.
See: Dalfatol, Cap. (Reid-Provident)
Tocopherol, Alpha (Various Mfr.)
dl-ALPHA-TOCOPHEROL SUCCINATE.
See: D'Alpha-E, Cap. (Alto)
ALPHA VEE-12. (Schlicksup) Hydroxocobalamin 1000
mcg./ml. Vial 10 ml.

ALPHAXALONE. B.A.N. 3α-Hydroxy-5α-pregnane-11,-
20-dione.
Use: Anesthetic component.
ALPHENAL.
See: 5-Allyl-5-phenylbarbituric acid. (Var. Mfr.)
ALPHOSYL. (Reed & Carnrick) Allantoin 1.7%,
special crude coal tar extracts 5%. Lot.: Bot. 8 fl.
oz. **Cream** 2 oz.
Use: Psoriasis treatment.
• **ALPRAZOLAM.** USAN. 8-Chloro-1-methyl-6-phenyl-
4H-s- triazolo (4,3-α)(1,4)benzodiazepine.
Use: Management of anxiety disorders.
See: Xanax, Tab. (Upjohn)
ALPRENOLOL. B.A.N. 1-(2-Allylphenoxy)-3-
iso-propylaminopropan-2 ol. Betaptin hydro-
chloride.
Use: Beta adrenergic receptor blocking agent.
• **ALPROSTADIL.** USAN. (11α,13E,15S)-11,15 dihy-
droxy-9-oxoprost-13-en-1-oic acid.
Use: Palliative therapy to maintain patency of the
ductus arteriosus in neonates with congenital heart
defects.
See: Prostin VR, Inj. (Upjohn)
• **ALPRENOLOL HYDROCHLORIDE.** USAN.
Use: Anti-adrenergic.
AL-R. (Saron) Chlorpheniramine maleate 6 mg. or 12
mg./S.R. cap.Bot. 100s.
Use: Antihistamine.
• **ALRESTATIN SODIUM.** USAN.
Use: Enzyme inhibitor.
ALSEROXYLON. A fat-soluble alkaloidal fraction ex-
tracted from the root of Rauwolfia serpentina; 1
mg. is equiv. to 0.2 mg. of reserpine.
See: Koglucoid, Tab. (Panray)
Raudolfin, Tabs. (Premo)
Rautensin, Tab. (Dorsey)
Rauwiloid, Tab. (Riker)
Vio-Serpine, Tab. (Rowell)
ALSEROXYLON-ALKAVERVIR. A mixture of partially
purified extracts of Rauwolfia serpentina and
Veratrum viride.
ALSORB GEL. (Standex) Colloidal suspension of
magnesium & aluminum hydroxide.
ALSORB GEL, C.T. (Standex) Calcium carbonate
2 gr., glycine 3 gr., magnesium trisilicate
3 gr./Tab.
ALTACITE. Hydrotalcite, B.A.N.
ALTERNAGEL. (Stuart) Aluminum hydroxide 600
mg./5 ml. Bot. 5 oz., 12 oz.
Use: High-potency, sodium free antacid.
ALTEX. (Cenci) Spironolactone 25 mg./Tab. Bot.
100s, 1000s.
Use: Diuretic, antihypertensive.
ALTEXIDE. (Cenci) Spironolactone 25 mg.,
hydrochlorothiazide 25 mg./Tab. Bot. 100s, 1000s.
Use: Diuretic, antihypertensive.
ALTHIAZIDE. USAN. 3-Allylthiomethyl-3-4-dihydro-6-
chloro-7-sulfamoyl-1,2,4-benzothiadiazine-
1-dioxide.
Use: Hypotensive and diuretic.
ALTILEV. Nortriptyline, B.A.N.
ALTO-PRED LA-100. (Alto) Prednisolone acetate 100
mg./cc. Vial 10 cc.

Use: Repository injectable corticosteroid.
• **ALTRENOGEST.** USAN.
Use: Progestin (veterinary).
ALUCAINE. (Jenkins) Benzocaine 5%, carbolic acid
1.39%, ichthammol 1.39%, balsam peru 0.46%,
alum exsic. 3.7% w/oil cade, oil eucalyptus in oint.
base. Oint. Tube 1 oz., 1 lb.
Use: Relief of pain in burns, scalds, cuts.
ALU-CAP. (Riker) Aluminum hydroxide dried gel 475
mg. w/silicon dioxide and talc/Cap. Bot. 100s.
Use: Antacid.
AL-U-CREME. (MacAllister) Aluminum hydroxide equiv-
alent to 4% aluminum oxide. Susp.: Bot. 1 pt., 1
gal.
Use: Antacid.
ALUDROX. (Wyeth) **Susp.,** Aluminum hydroxide gel
307 mg., w/magnesium hydroxide 103 mg./5 ml.
Bot. 12 fl. oz.: Box 12s. **Tab.** Aluminum hydroxide
233 mg., magnesium hydroxide 83 mg./Tab. Box.
100s.
Use: Antacid.
ALUGAN. Bromocyclen, B.A.N.
ALUKALIN. Activated kaolin.
See: Lusyn, Tab. (Pennwalt)
ALULEX. (Lexington) Magnesium trisilicate 3¼ gr.,
aluminum hydroxide gel 3½ gr., phenobarbital ⅛
gr., homatropine methylbromide ¹⁄₆₀ gr./Tab. Bot.
100s.
Use: Treatment of peptic ulcer.
• **ALUM,** U.S.P. XXI. Sulfuric acid, aluminum
ammonium salt (2:1:1), dodecahydrate. Sulfuric
acid, aluminum potassium salt (2:1:1),
dodecahydrate.
Use: Astringent.
ALUMADRINE. (Fleming) Acetaminophen 500 mg.,
phenylpropanolamine HCl 25 mg., chlorpheniramine
maleate 4 mg./Tab. Bot. 100s, 1000s.
Use: Mild upper respiratory infections.
ALUMATE-HC. (Dermco) Hydrocortisone ⅛% & ¼%,
Cream. ⅛% Pkg. 4 oz., ¼% Pkg. 1 oz., ½% Pkg.
½ oz., 1 oz.; 1% pkg. ½ oz.
Use: Anti-inflammatory agent.
ALUMATE MIXTURE. (Schlicksup) Aluminum hydrox-
ide gel, milk of magnesia/Tsp. Bot. 12 oz., gal.
ALUMID LIQUID. (Vangard) Aluminum hydroxide 225
mg., magnesium hydroxide 200 mg./5 ml. Bot. 12
oz.
Use: Antacid.
ALUMID PLUS LIQUID. (Vangard) Aluminum
hydroxide 100 mg., magnesium hydroxide 200 mg.,
simethicone 20 mg., sodium 0.68 mg./5 ml. Bot. 12
oz.
Use: Antacid, antiflatulent..
ALUMINA HYDRATED POWDER.
W/Activated attapulgite, pectin.
See: Polymagma, Plain, Tabs (Wyeth)
• **ALUMINA AND MAGNESIA ORAL SUSPENSION,**
U.S.P. XXI.
Use: Antacid.
• **ALUMINA AND MAGNESIA TABLETS,** U.S.P. XXI.
Use: Antacid.

• **ALUMINA AND MAGNESIUM TRISILICATE ORAL
SUSPENSION,** U.S.P. XXI.
Use: Antacid.
• **ALUMINA, MAGNESIA, AND CALCIUM CHLORIDE
ORAL SUSPENSION,** U.S.P. XXI.
Use: Antacid.
• **ALUMINA, MAGNESIA, AND CALCIUM
CARBONATE TABLETS.** U.S.P. XXI.
Use: Antacid.
ALUMINETT. (Lannett) Aluminum hydroxide 10
gr./Tab. Bot. 1000s.
Use: Antacid.
ALUMINOSTOMY. (Richards Pharm.) Aluminum pow.
18%, with zinc oxide and zinc stearate in a bland
water repellent ointment. Jars 2 & 6 oz. and 1 lb.
Use: An occlusive dressing for skin protection;
colostomies and ileostomies.
ALUMINUM.
See: Aluminostomy (Richards Pharm.)
ALUMINUM ACETATE.
See: Acid Mantle Creme (Dorsey)
Acid Mantle Lotion (Dorsey)
Buro-Sol, cream & powder (Doak)
W/Phenol, zinc oxide, boric acid, eucalyptol,
ichthammol.
See: Lanaburn, Oint. (Lannett)
W/Salicylic acid, boric acid.
• **ALUMINUM ACETATE TOPICAL SOLUTION,**
U.S.P. XXI. (Various Mfr.). Burow's Solution.
Use: Astringent.
See: Bluboro Powder (Herbert)
Buro-Sol Pow. Conc. (Doak)
Burotor, Emul. (Torch)
Domeboro, Pow. (Miles Pharm)
ALUMINUM AMINOACETATE, DIHYDROXY.
See: Dihydroxy aluminum aminoacetate (Various
Mfr.)
ALUMINUM CARBONATE BASIC.
See: Basaljel, Susp. (Wyeth)
• **ALUMINUM CHLOROHYDRATE.** USAN.
Use: Anhidrotic.
• **ALUMINUM CHLOROHYDREX.** USAN.
Use: Astingent.
ALUMINUM CHLORHYDROXY ALLANTOINATE.
See: Alcloxa (Schuylkill)
• **ALUMINUM CHLORIDE,** U.S.P. XXI. Aluminum
chloride hexahydrate.
Use: Astringent.
W/Oxyquinoline sulfate, benzalkonium chloride.
See: Alochor Stypic (Gordon Labs.)
ALUMINUM CLOFIBRATE. B.A.N. Di-[2-(4-chloro-
phenoxy)-2-methylpropionato]hydroxyaluminum
Use: Treatment of arteriosclerosis.
ALUMINUM DIHYDROXYAMINOACETATE.
See: Dihydroxy Aluminum Aminoacetate, U.S.P.
XXI. (Various Mfr.)
ALUMINUM GLYCINATE, BASIC.
See: Dihydroxy Aluminum Aminoacetate, U.S.P.
XXI.
W/Aspirin, & Mag. carbonate.
See: Bufferin, Tabs. (Bristol-Myers)

• **ALUMINUM HYDROXIDE GEL,** U.S.P. XXI. Aq.
susp. of aluminum hydroxide equiv. to 4%
aluminum oxide.
Use: Antacid.
See: ALterna GEL, Gel (Stuart)
    Al-U-Creme, Susp. (MacAllister)
    Aluminett, Tab. (Lannett)
    Alu-Cap, Cap. (Riker)
    Alu-Tab., Tab. (Riker)
    Amphojel, Susp., Tab. (Wyeth)
    Dialume, Cap. (Armour)
    Hydroxal, Susp. (Blue Line)
    No-Co-Gel, Susp. (Noyes)
    Nutrajel, Bot. (Cenci)
W/Aminoacetic acid, mag. trisilicate.
See: Maracid-2, Tab. (Marin)
W/Aminophylline.
See: Asmadrin, Tab. (Jenkins)
W/Amobarbital, homatropine methylbromide, kaolin
colloidal.
See: Komal, Tab. (O'Neal)
W/Atropine sulfate, mag. trisilicate, phenobarbital.
See: PAMA, Tab. (Vortech)
W/Belladonna ext., magnesium hydroxide.
See: Trialka, Liq., Tab. (Commerce)
W/Calcium carbonate.
See: Alkalade, Susp., Tab. (DePree)
W/Calcium carbonate, magnesium carbonate,
magnesium trisilicate.
See: Marblen, Susp., Tab. (Fleming)
W/Dicyclomine HCl, magnesium hydroxide,
methylcellulose.
See: Triactin Liquid, Tab. (Norwich)
W/Gastric mucin, Mg glycinate.
See: Mucogel, Liq., Tab. (Inwood)
W/Homatropine methylbromide.
See: Aloxed, Susp. (Vortech)
W/Clioquinol, methylcellulose, atropine sulf., hyoscine
HBr, hyoscyamine sulf.
See: Enterex, Tab. (Person & Covey)
W/Kaolin, pectin.
See: Kenpectin, Syr. (Kenwood)
    Metropectin, Liq. (Pennwalt)
W/Magnesium carbonate.
See: Estomul-M Liq., Tabs. (Riker)
W/Magnesium carbonate, calcium carbonate, amino-
acetic acid.
See: Glycogel Tab. or Susp. (Central)
W/Magnesium hydroxide.
See: Alsorb Gel (Standex)
    Aludrox, Susp., Tab. (Wyeth)
    Creamalin, Tab. (Winthrop Products)
    Delcid, Liq. (Merrell Dow)
    Kolantyl, Gel, Wafer (Merrell Dow)
    Maalox, Susp. (Rorer)
    Mylanta, Tab. (Stuart)
    Mylanta II, Tab. (stuart)
    Neutralox, Susp. (Lemmon)
    Nutramag, Liq. (Cenci)
    WinGel, Liq., Tab. (Winthrop Products)
W/Magnesium hydroxide, aspirin.
See: Calciphen, Tab. (Westerfield)

    Cama, Tab. (Dorsey)
    Cama Inlay-Tabs. (Dorsey)
W/Magnesium hydroxide, belladonna ext.
W/Magnesium hydroxide, calcium carbonate.
See: Camalox, Susp. (Rorer)
W/Mag. hydroxide, glycine, magnesium trisilicate,
belladonna ext.
W/Magnesium hydroxide and simethicone.
See: DI-GEL, Liq. (Plough.)
    Maalox Plus, Susp. (Rorer)
    Mylanta, Liq. (Stuart)
    Mylanta-II, Liq. (Stuart)
    Silain-Gel, Lig., Tab. (Robins)
    Simeco, Liq. (Wyeth)
W/Magnesium trisilicate.
See: Antacid G, Tab. (Walgreen)
    Antacid Tablets, Tab. (Panray)
    Arcodex Antiacid, Tab. (Arcum)
    Barosil, Susp. (Barry-Martin)
    Gacid, Tab. (Arcum)
    Malcogel, Susp. (Upjohn)
    Malcotabs (Upjohn)
    Manalum, Tab. (Paddock)
    Neutracomp, Liq., Tab. (C.M.C.)
    Trilox, Susp., Tab. (Blue Line)
    Trisogel, Pulvule, Susp. (Lilly)
W/Magnesium trisilicate, atropine sulf.,
phenobarbital.
See: Pama, Tab. (Vortech)
W/Paregoric, kaolin (colloidal), bismuth subcarbonate,
pectin, aromatics.
See: Kapinal, Tab. (Jenkins)
W/Phenindamine tartrate, phenylephrine HCl, aspirin,
caffeine, magnesium carbonate.
See: Dristan, Tab. (Whitehall)
W/Phenol, zinc oxide, camphor, eucalyptol,
ichthammol.
See: Almophen, Oint. (Bowman)
W/Prednisolone.
See: Fernisolone-B (Ferndale)
    Predoxine, Tab. (Mallard)
W/Sodium salicylate, Acetaminophen, Vit. C.
See: Gaysal-S., Tab. (Geriatric)
• **ALUMINUM HYDROXIDE GEL, DRIED,** U.S.P. XXI.
Tabs. U.S.P. XXI.
Use: Antacid.
See: Amphojel, Tab. (Wyeth)
ALUMINUM HYDROXIDE GEL, DRIED
W/COMBINATIONS
    Alased, Tab. (Norgine)
    Aludrox, Susp., Tab. (Wyeth)
    Alurex, Tab. (Rexall)
    Ascriptin, Tab. (Rorer)
    Ascriptin A/D, Tab. (Rorer)
    Ascriptin W/Codeine, Tab. (Rorer)
    Aspadine, Tab. (Vortech)
    Azolid-A, Cap. (USV Pharm.)
    Banacid, Tab. (Buffington)
    Buffadyne, Tab. (Lemmon)
    Butazolidin Alka, Cap. (Geigy)
    Calciphen, Tab. (Westerfield)
    Camalox, Tab. (Rorer)

Cimadrox, Tab. (Elder)
Coralsone Modif. Tab. (Zemmer)
Creamalin, Tab. (Winthrop-Breon)
Decagesic, Tab. (Merck Sharp and Dohme)
Delcid, Liq. (Merrell Dow)
Estomul, Tab., Liq. (Riker)
Eugel, Tab. (Reid-Provident)
Eulcin, Tab. (Leeds)
Fermalox, Tab. (Rorer)
Gas-Eze, Tab. (Edward J. Moore)
Gaviscon, Foamtabs (Marion)
Gelumina, Tab. (APC)
Gelumina Plus, Liq. (APC)
Gelusil, Preps. (Park-Davis)
Kamadrox, Tab. (Elder)
Kamadrox Jel, Liq. (Elder)
Kao-Lumin, Tab. (Philips Roxane)
Kathmagel, Tab. (Mason)
Kenpectin, Liq. (Kenwood)
Kenpectin-P, Liq. (Kenwood)
Kolantyl, Wafers (Merrell Dow)
Kudrox, Tab., Susp. (Kremers-Urban)
Maalox, Tab. (Rorer)
Maalox Plus, Tab. (Rorer)
Magnatril, Tab., Susp. (Lannett)
Malcotabs, Tab. (Upjohn)
Metropectin, Tab. (Pennwalt)
Mylanta, Tab. and Liq. (Stuart)
Mylanta II, Tab. and Liq. (Stuart)
Neosorb Plus, Tab. (Lemmon)
Neutralox, Tab. (Lemmon)
Pama, Tab. (N. Am. Pharmacal)
Phencaset Improved, Tab. (Elder)
Presalin, Tab. (Mallard)
Silmagel, Tab. (Lannett)
Spasmasorb, Tab. (Hauck)
Syntrogel, Tab. (Block)
Trialatine, Tab. (Bowman)
Trisogel, Pulvules, Liq. (Lilly)
ALUMINUM HYDROXIDE GLYCINE.
See: Dihydroxy aluminum aminoacetate
**ALUMINUM HYDROXIDE MAGNESIUM
CARBONATE.**
See: Aloxine (O'Neal)
DI-GEL, Tab. (Plough)
Magnagel, Susp., Tab. (Mallard)
W/Aminoacetic acid, calcium carbonate.
See: Eugel, Tab., Liq. (Reid-Provident)
W/Dicyclomine HCl, magnesium trisilicate,
methylcellulose.
See: Triactin, Liq., Tab. (Norwich)
W/Magnesium trisilicate.
See: Escot, Cap. (Reid-Provident)
W/Magnesium trisilicate, bismuth aluminate.
See: Escot, Cap. (Reid-Provident)
• **ALUMINUM MONOSTEARATE,** N.F. XVI.
Aluminum, dihydroxy(octadecanoato-O-)-,Dihydroxy
(stearato)aluminum.
ALUMINUM OXIDE.
See: Epi-Clear Scrub Cleanser (Squibb)
ALUMINUM PHENOSULFONATE
See: AR-EX Cream Deodorant (Ar-Ex)

• **ALUMINUM PHOSPHATE GEL,** U.S.P. XXI.
Aluminum phosphate 4.15%.
See: Phosphajel, Susp. (Wyeth)
ALUMINUM SALT OF THE AMINO ACID GLYCINE.
See: Dihydroxy aluminum aminoacetate, Prep.
(Various Mfr.)
• **ALUMINUM SESQUICHLOROHYDRATE.** USAN.
Use: Anhidrotic.
ALUMINUM SODIUM CARBONATE HYDROXIDE.
See: Dihydroxyaluminum Sodium Carbonate
• **ALUMINUM SUBACETATE TOPICAL SOLUTION,**
U.S.P. XXI. (Various Mfr.) Aluminum acetate basic
solution, aluminum subacetate solution.
Use: As an astringent wash.
• **ALUMINUM SULFATE,** U.S.P. XXI.
Use: Pharmaceutic necessity for preparation of
aluminum subacetate solution.
• **ALUMINUM ZIRCONIUM TETRACHLOROHYDREX
GLY.** USAN.
Use: Anhidrotic.
• **ALUMINUM ZIRCONIUM TRICHLOROHYDREX
GLY.** USAN.
Use: Anhidrotic.
ALUPENT. (Boehringer Ingelheim) Metaproterenol
sulfate. Orciprenaline, B.A.N. **Metered dose
inhaler.** 15 cc. **Tab.** 10 mg. or 20 mg. Bot. 100s.
Syr. 10 mg./5 ml., Bot. pt. **Inhalant Sol.** 5%, Bot.
10 ml. Unit Dose 0.9%, 2 ml. vials.
Use: Bronchodilator.
ALURATE. (Roche) Aprobarbital 40 mg./5 ml. Alcohol
20%. Elixir: Red, Bot. 1 pt.
Use: Sedative.
ALUREX. (Rexall) Magnesium-aluminum hydroxide.
Susp. (200 mg.-150 mg./5 cc.) Bot. 12 oz. **Tab.** (400
mg.-300 mg.) Box 50s.
Use: Relief of gastric hyperacidity.
ALU-TAB. (Riker) Aluminum hydroxide gel 600
mg./Tab. Bot. 250s.
Use: Antacid.
ALVAGEL. (Kenyon) 55% Aloe vera active principle
in oint. base. Tube 2 oz., 4 oz.
Use: Topically, for sunburn, eczema, dermatitis, x-
ray & radiation burns.
ALVEDIL CAPS. (Luly-Thomas) Theophylline 4 gr.,
pseudoephedrine HCl 50 mg., butabarbital 15
mg./Cap. Bot. 100s.
Use: Asthma.
• **ALVERINE CITRATE.** USAN. N-ethyl-3,3'-diphenyl
dipropylamine citrate.
Use: Anticholinergic.
See: Spacolin, Tab. (Philips Roxane)
AL-VITE. (Drug Industries) Vit. A 10,000 I.U., D-3 400
I.U., E 25 I.U., C 200 mg., B-1 20 mg., B-2 10 mg.,
B-6 6 mg., Ca. Pantothenate 20 mg., niacinamide 100
mg., B-12 w/intrinsic factor conc. ½ u./Tab. Bot.
100s, 500s.
Use: Vitamin therapy.
AMA. (Wampole-Zeus) Antimitochondrial antibodies
test by IFA. Tests 48s.
Use: Diagnostic aid in the identification of primary
biliary cirrhosis.

• **AMACETAM SULFATE.** USAN.
Use: Cognition Adjuvant.
AMACID. (Kenyon) An acid protein hydrolysate prepared from casein and lactalbumin by special process which retains l-tryptophan and other essential amino acids. Bot. 4 oz., pt., gal.
• **AMADIMONE ACETATE.** USAN.
Use: Progestin.
AMARIL D SPANTAB. (Vortech) Phenlypropanolamine HCl 40 mg., phenylephrine HCl 10 mg., phenyltoloxamine citrate 15 mg., chlorpheniramine maleate 5 mg./Sustained Release Tab. Bot. 1000s.
Use: Antihistamine, decongestant.
AMARIL D SYRUP. (Vortech) Phenylpropanolamine HCl 20 mg., phenylephrine HCl 5 mg., phenyltoloxamine 7.5 mg., chlorpheniramine maleate 2.5 mg./5 ml. Bot. 4 oz., 128 oz.
Use: Antihistamine, decongestant.
AMANOZINE HCl. 2-Amino-4-anilino-s-triazine HCl.
AMANTADINE. B.A.N. 1-Adamantanamine.
Use: Antiviral agent, treatment of Parkinson's disease.
See: Symmetrel, Cap. (Du Pont)
• **AMANTADINE HYDROCHLORIDE,** U.S.P. XXI. Caps, Syr. U.S.P. XXI. 1-Adamantanamine HCl. Tricylo [3.3.1.1³,⁷] decan-1-amine, HCl.
Use: Antiviral agent, treatment of Parkinson's disease.
See: Symmetrel, Caps, Syr. (Du Pont)
AMAPHEN. (Trimen) Butabarbital 50 mg., caffeine 40 mg., acetaminophen 360 mg./Cap. Bot. 100s.
Use: Analgesic.
AMARANTH. 3-Hydroxy-4-[(4-sulfo-1-naphthyl)azo]-2,7-naphthalene-disulfonic acid trisodium salt. F.D. and C. Red No. 2.
Use: Color (Not for internal use).
AMARGYL. Chlorpromazine, B.A.N.
AMARSAN. See: Acetarsone, Tab.
AMATROL LIQUID. (Vortech) Balanced amounts of levulose and dextrose w/orthophosphoric acid, stabilized at optimal pH. Bot. 3 oz., gal.
Use: Antiemetic.
AMAZONE. 1:4-Benzoquinone amidinohydrazone thiosemicarbazone hydrate. Iversal.
AMBAY. (Bay) Codeine sulfate 10 mg., diphenhydramine HCl 8.75 mg., bromodiphenhydramine HCl 3.75 mg., ammonium Cl. 80 mg., potassium guaicolsulfonate 80 mg., menthol 0.5 mg./5 ml. w/alcohol 5%. Bot. 4 oz., pt., gal.
Use: Expectorant.
AMBAZONE. B.A.N. 1,4-Benzoquinone amidinohydrazone thiosemicarbazone.
See: Iversal hydrate
Use: Antiseptic.
AMBENONIUM CHLORIDE. N,N′-bis-(2-Diethyl aminoethyl) oxamide bis-2-chlorobenzyl chloride. [Oxalylbis (iminoethylene)] bis [(o-chlorobenzyl)-diethylammonium] dichloride.
Use: Cholinergic for treatment of myasthenia gravis.
See: Mytelase, Cap. (Winthrop-Breon)

AMBENONIUM CHLORIDE. B.A.N. NN′-Di-[2-(N-2-chlorobenzyldiethylammonio) ethyl] oxamide dichloride.
Use: Cholinesterase inhibitor.
AMBENOXAN. B.A.N. 2-(2-Methoxyethoxyethyl-aminomethyl)-1,4-benzodioxan.
Use: Muscle relaxant.
AMBENYL. (Marion) Codeine phosphate 10 mg., bromodiphendyramine HCl 12.5 mg./5 ml. w/alcohol 5%. Bot. 4 oz. pt., gal.
Use: Relief of upper respiratory symptoms and coughs associated with allergies or common cold.
AMBENYL-D. (Marion) Guaifenesin 200 mg., pseudoephedrine HCl 60 mg., dextromethorphan HBr 30 mg./10 ml. Bot. 1 oz., 4 oz.
Use: Antitussive, expectorant, nasal decongestant.
AMBERLITE, I.R.P.-64. (Rohm and Haas) Polacrilin.
AMBERLITE, I.R.P.-88. (Rohm and Haas) Polacrilin potassium.
AMBILHAR. Niridazole, B.A.N.
• **AMBOMYCIN.** USAN. Isolated from filtrates of *Streptomyces ambofaciens.*
Use: Anti-neoplastic agent.
AMBRAMYCIN. Tetracycline, B.A.N.
AMBROSIACEAE POLLENS.
See: Allergenic Extracts (Ragweed and related pollens) Parke, Davis
• **AMBRUTICIN.** USAN.
Use: Antifungal.
AMBUCAINE. Ambutoxate HCl.
AMBUCETAMIDE. 2-(di-n-Butylamino)-2-(p-methoxyphenyl)acetamide.
AMBUCETAMIDE. B.A.N. α-Dibutylamino-4-methoxyphenylacetamide.
Use: Antispasmodic.
• **AMBUPHYLLINE.** USAN. Theophylline compound with 2-amino-2-methyl-1-propanol. Bufylline
Use: Diuretic, Smooth muscle relaxant.
AMBUSIDE. USAN. 5-Allylsulfamoyl-2-chloro-4-(3-hydroxybut-2-enylideneamino)benzenesulfonamide.
Use: Diuretic.
See: Novohydrin
AMBUTONIUM BROMIDE. Ethyl-dimethylammonium(3-carbamyl-3,3-diphenyl propyl)-ethyl dimethylammonium bromide.
AMBUTONIUM BROMIDE. B.A.N. (3-Carbamoyl-3,3-diphenylpropyl)ethyldimethylammonium bromide.
Use: Antispasmodic.
AMBUTOXATE HYDROCHLORIDE. 2-Diethylaminoethyl-4-amino-2-butoxybenzoate HCl.
AMC. (Schlicksup) Ammonium chloride 7½ gr./Tab. Bot. 1000s.
AMCAP. (Circle) Ampicillin trihydrate equivalent to 250 mg. ampicillin/Cap. Bot. 100s.
Use: Antibiotic.
AMCILL. (Parke-Davis) **Cap:** Ampicillin trihydrate 250 mg. or 500 mg./Cap. Bot. 100s, 500s, unit dose pkg 100s. **Oral Susp.:** 125 mg. or 250 mg./5 ml. Bot. 100 ml., 200 ml. Bot. 100 ml., 200 ml. **Ped. Drops:** 100 mg./ml. w/sod. benzoate 0.1% as preservative. Bot. 20 ml.

Use: Penicillin therapy.
• **AMCINAFAL.** USAN. 9-Fluoro-11β, 16α,17,21-tetrahydroxypregna-1,4-diene-3, 20-dione cyclic 16, 17-acetal with 3-pentanone.
Use: Anti-inflammatory.
• **AMCINAFIDE.** USAN. (R)-9-Fluoro-11β, 16α,17,21-tetrahydroxypregna-1, 4-diene-3,20-dione cyclic 16,-17-acetal with acetophenone.
Use: Anti-inflammatory.
• **AMCINONIDE,** U.S.P. XXI. Cream, Oint., U.S.P. XXI.
Use: Glucocorticoid.
AMCORT. (Keene) Triamcinolone diacetate 40 mg./ml. Vial 5 ml.
Use: Parenteral steroid.
• **AMDINOCILLIN.** USAN.
Use: Antibacterial.
■ **AMEBACIDES.**
See: Acetarsone (Various Mfr.)
Aralen HCl, Inj. (Winthrop-Breon)
Aralen Phosphate, Tab. (Winthrop-Breon)
Carbarsone, Pulvule & Tab. (Lilly)
Chiniofon, Tab. (Various Mfr.)
Diiodohydroxyquin (Various Mfr.)
Diodoquin, Tab. (Searle)
Emetine HCl (Various Mfr.)
Flagyl, Tab. (Searle)
Humatin, Kapseal, Syr. (Parke-Davis)
Yodoxin, Tab. (Glenwood)
AMEBAN.
See: Carbarsone
AMEBAQUIN. (U.S. Products) Iodoquinol 650 mg./Tab.
Bot. 100s.
Use: Amebicidal activity against entamoeba histolytica.
AMECHOL.
See: Methacholine Chloride
• **AMEDALIN HCl.** USAN. 3-Methyl-3-[3-(methylamino)-propyl]-1-phenyl-2-indolinone monohydrochloride.
Use: Antidepressant.
AMEN. (Carnrick) Medroxyprogesterone acetate 10 mg./Tab. Bot. 50s, 1000s.
Use: Progestin.
AMERICAINE AEROSOL. (American Critical Care) Benzocaine 20% in a water-soluble vehicle. Bot. 0.67 oz., 2 oz, 4 oz.
Use: Topical anesthetic.
AMERICAINE ANESTHETIC LUBRICANT. (American Critical Care) Benzocaine 20%, benzethonium chloride 0.1% in a water-sol. polyethylene glycol base. 2.5 Gm. Foil Pack, Pkg. 144s. Tube 1 oz.
Use: Local anesthetic.
AMERICAINE FIRST AID SPRAY. (American Critical Care) Benzocaine 10%, benzethonium chloride 0.1%, alcohol 25%. Pump spray 4 oz.
Use: Topical anesthetic.
AMERICAINE FIRST AID BURN OINTMENT. (American Critical Care) Benzocaine 20%, benzethonium chloride 0.1%, in a water-soluble polyethylene glycol base. Tube 0.75 oz.
Use: Local anesthetic.

AMERICAINE HEMORRHOIDAL OINTMENT. (American Critical Care) Benzocaine 20% and benzethonium chloride 0.1% in a water-soluble polyethylene glycol base. Tube 1 oz. w/rectal applicator.
Use: Hemorrhoidal pain and itching.
AMERICAINE OTIC. (American Critical Care) Benzethonium chloride 0.1%, Benzocaine 20% in a water-soluble base of 1% (w/w) glycerin and polyethylene glycol 300. Bot. 0.5 oz.
Use: Pain and inflammation of otitis media.
AMERTAN. (Lilly) Tannic acid 5%, Merthiolate 1:5000. Tube 1 oz.
Use: Burns.
AMER-TET. (Robinson) Tetracycline HCl 250 mg., 500 mg./Cap. Bot. 100s, 1000s.
Use: Antibiotic.
AMER-TET SUSPENSION. (Robinson) Tetracycline HCl oral suspension 125 mg./5 ml. Bot. pt.
Use: Antibiotic.
AMES ALIQUOT MIXER. (Ames) Formerly Hema-Tek.
Use: Mixer of specimen samples.
• **AMETANTRONE ACETATE.** USAN.
Use: Antineoplastic.
AMETAZOLE. B.A.N. 3-(2-Aminoethyl)pyrazole. Betazole (I.N.N.). Histalog, hydrochloride.
Use: To stimulate gastric secretion in diagnostic tests.
A-METHAPRED UNIVIALS. (Abbott) Methylprednisolone sodium succinate. 40 mg./1 ml. Pkg. 1s, 25s, 50s, 100s; 125 mg./2 ml. Pkg. 1s, 5s, 25s, 50s, 100s; 500 mg./4 ml. Pkg. 1s, 5s, 25s, 100s; 1000 mg./8 ml. Pkg. 1s, 5s, 25s 100s.
Use: Anti-inflammatory.
AMETHOCAINE HYDROCHLORIDE.
See: Pontocaine HCl (Winthrop-Breon)
AMETHOPTERIN.
See: Methotrexate (Lederle)
AMFECLORAL. B.A.N. α-Methyl-N(2,2,2-trichloroethylidene)-phenethylamine.
Use: Appetite suppressant.
• **AMFENAC SODIUM.** USAN.
Use: Anti-inflammatory.
AMFEPRAMONE (I.N.N.). Diethylpropion, B.A.N.
AMFODYNE.
See: Imidecyl Iodine
• **AMFONELIC ACID.** USAN. 7-Benzyl-1-ethyl-4-oxo-1,8-naphthyridine-3-carboxylic acid.
Use: Central nervous system stimulant.
AMFRECIN. (Amfre-Grant) Sodium lauryl sulfate 0.25%, lactose 82%, papain 1%, citric acid 16%, methyl salicylate 0.25%, menthol 0.50%. Bot. 4 oz., 8 oz.
Use: Vaginal douche.
AMIBIARSON.
See: Carbarsone. (Various Mfr.)
AMICAR. (Lederle) 6-Aminocaproic acid. **Syrup** 250 mg./ml. Bot. pt. **Vial** 250 mg./ml. 20 ml. **Tab.** 500 mg./ml. Tab., Bot. 100s.
Use: Antifibrinolytic agent.
AMICARBALIDE. B.A.N. 3,3′-Diamidino-carbanilide. Diampron, isethionate.
Use: Antiprotozoan, veterinary medicine.

• **AMICLORAL.** USAN. 6-0-(2,2,2-Trichloro-1-hydroxye-thyl)-α-D-glucopyranosel-4 polymer with α-D-glucopyranose.
Use: Food additive (veterinary).

• **AMICYCLINE.** USAN.
Use: Antibacterial.

• **AMIDAPSONE.** USAN. p-Sulfanilylphenyl urea.
Use: Antiviral (for poultry).

AMIDATE. (Abbott) Etomidate 2 mg./ml w/propylene glycol 35%. 20 mg./10 ml. single dose Amp.; 40 mg./20 ml. single dose Amp.; 40 mg./20 ml. Abboject syringe.
Use: Anesthesia induction.

AMIDE-VC. (Scrip) Sulfanilamide 15%, 9-aminoacridine HCl 0.2%, allantoin 1.5%. Tube: 4 oz. plus applicator.

AMIDE V/S. (Scrip) Sulfanilamide 500 mg., diiodohydroxyquin 100 mg., diethylstilbestrol 0.1 mg./Insert. Pkg. 12s.
Use: Germicidal; antifungal.

AMIDEPHRINE. B.A.N. 3-(1-Hydroxy-2-methylaminoe-thyl)methanesulfonanilide. Dricol.
Use: Vasoconstrictor; nasal decongestant.

• **AMIDEPHRINE MESYLATE.** USAN.
Use: Adrengergic.

AMIDOFEBRIN.
See: Aminopyrine (Various Mfr.)

AMIDONE HYDROCHLORIDE.
See: Methadone Hydrochloride (Various Mfr.)

AMIDOPYRAZOLINE.
See: Aminopyrine (Various Mfr.)

AMIDOTRIZOIC ACID. Diatrizoic Acid, B.A.N.

AMIDOTRIZOATE, SODIUM.
See: Diatrizoate Sodium

AMID-SAL. (Glenwood) Salicylamide. 3½ gr./Tab. Bot. 100s.
Use: Analgesic, antipyretic.

• **AMIFLUTIZOLE.** USAN.

AMIGEN. (Baxter) Protein hydrolysate 5%. Bot. 500, 1000 ml.; 10% 500, 1000 ml.; 5% w/dextrose 5% Bot. 500 ml., 1000 ml.; 5% w/dextrose 5%, alcohol 5% Bot. 1000 ml.; 5% w/fructose 10% Bot. 1000 ml.; 5% w/fructose 12.5%, alcohol 2.4% Bot. 1000 ml.
Use: Provides amino acids and calories.

• **AMIKACIN,** U.S.P. XXI.
Use: Antibacterial.

• **AMIKACIN SULFATE INJECTION.** U.S.P. XXI. 0-3-Amino-3-deoxy-α-D-glucopyranosyl(1-6)-0-(6-amino-6-deoxy-α-D-glucopyranosyl(1-4)-N-[(S)-4-amino-2-hydroxyl-1-oxobutyl]-2-deoxy-D-streptamine sulfate.
Use: Antibacterial.
See: Amikin, Inj. (Bristol)

AMIKAPRON. Tranexamic Acid, B.A.N.

AMIKIN. (Bristol) Amikacin sulfate injection. 100 mg., 500 mg., 1.0 Gm. vials., 500 mg. Disposable Syringes.
Use: Infections from gram-positive & gram-negative bacteria including pseudomonas species.

AMILORIDE. B.A.N. N-Amidino-3,5-diamino-6-chlo-ropyrazine-2-carboxamide.

Use: Diuretic.
See: Midamor, Tab. (Merck Sharp & Dohme)
W/Hydrochlorthiazide
See: Moduretic, Tab. (Merck Sharp & Dohme)

• **AMILORIDE HYDROCHLORIDE,** U.S.P. XXI. Tab., U.S.P. XXI. Pyrazinecarboxamide,3,5-diamino-N-(ami-noiminomethyl)-6-chloro-,monochloride.
Use: Diuretic.

• **AMILORIDE HYDROCHLORIDE AND HYDROCHLORLTHIAZIDE TABLETS,** U.S.P. XXI.
Use: Diuretic.

• **AMINACRINE.** F.D.A. 9-Aminoacridine.

• **AMINACRINE HYDROCHLORIDE.** USAN. 9-Amino-cridine hydrochloride.
W/Dienestrol, sulfanilamide, allantoin.
See: AVC/Dienestrol Cream, Suppos. (Merrell Dow)
Use: Bacteriostatic agent.
W/Oxyquinoline benzoate.
See: Triva, Vag. Jelly (Boyle)
W/Sulfanilamide, allantoin.
See: AVC, Cream, Suppos. (Merrell Dow)
Femguard Vaginal Cream (Reid-Provident)
Sulfem Vag. Cream (Federal Pharm.)
Triconol Vaginal Cream (Coastal)
Vagidine, Cream (Elder)
Vagitrol, Cream, Suppos. (Lemmon)

AMIN-AID. (American McGaw) Instant drinks & pud-dings.
Use: Dietary aid for renal disease patients.

AMINARSONE.
See: Carbarsone (Various Mfr.)

AMINE RESIN.
See: Polyamine Methylene Resin

AMINESS. (Cutter) Essential aminoacids. 10 Tab. = adult aminoacid MDR. Jar 300s.
Use: Protein restricted diet supplement.

AMINICOTIN.
See: Nicotinamide (Various Mfr.)

AMINITROZOLE. Acinitrazole, B.A.N.

AMINOACETIC ACID. Glycerine U.S.P. XXI. (Various Mfr.) (Glycine, glycocoll) available as elixir, pow. & tab.
Use: Myasthenia gravis, irrigating solution.
W/Aluminum hydroxide, magnesium hydroxide, calcium carbonate.
See: Eugel, Tab. & Liq. (Reid-Provident)
W/Calcium carbonate.
See: Antacid pH, Tab. (Towne)
Eldamint, Tab. (Elder)
W/Calcium carbonate, aluminum hydroxide, magnesium carbonate.
See: Glytabs, Tab. (Pharmics)
W/Calcium carbonate, magnesium carbonate, bismuth subcarbonate, dried aluminum hydroxide gel.
See: Buffer-Tabs (O'Neal)
W/Magnesium trisilicate, aluminum hydroxide.
See: Maracid-2, Tab. (Marin)
W/Phenylephrine HCl, pyrilamine maleate, acetylsalicylic acid, caffeine.
See: Al-Ay, Tabs. (Bowman)
W/Phenylephrine HCl, chlorpheniramine maleate, acetaminophen, caffeine.

See: Codimal, Tab. (Central)
W/Vit. B complex, C and iron.
See: Bironate-B, Cap. (Coastal)
AMINOACETIC ACID & CALCIUM CARBONATE.
W/Lysine.
See: Lycolan, Elix. (Lannett)
AMINO ACID & PROTEIN PREP.
See: Aminoacetic Acid, U.S.P. XXI.
Glutamic Acid
Histidine HCl
Lysine
Phenylalanine
Thyroxine
■ **AMINO ACIDS.**
Use: Amino-acid supplementation.
See: Aminosol, Sol. (Abbott)
Aminosyn, Sol. (Abbott)
Essential-8, Liq. (Medics)
W/Estrone, testosterone, vitamins & minerals.
See: Geramine, Tab. & Inj. (Brown)
W/Vit. B-12.
See: Stuart Amino Acids and B-12, Tab. (Stuart)
AMINOACRIDINE.
Use: Bacteriostatic agent.
See: 9-aminoacridine
9-AMINOACRIDINE HCl. (Various Mfr.)
Aminacrine HCl.
See: Vagisec Plus (J. Schmid)
W/Hydrocortisone acetate, tyrothricin, phenylmercuric
acetate, polysorbate-80, urea, lactose.
See: Aquacort, Vag. Supp. (Webcon)
W/Iodoquinol.
See: Vagitric, Oint. (Elder)
W/Phenylmercuric acetate, tyrothricin, urea, lactose.
See: Trinalis, Vag. Supp. (Webcon)
W/Polyoxyethylene nonyl phenol, sodium edetate,
docusate sodium.
See: Vagisec Plus, Supp. (Schmid)
W/Pramoxine HCl, acetic acid, parachlorometa-
xylenol, methyl-dodecylbenzyltrimethyl ammonium
chloride.
See: Drotic No. 2, Drops (Ascher)
W/Sulfanilamide & allantoin.
See: AVC Cream, Supp. (Merrell Dow)
Nil Vaginal Cream (Century)
Par Cream (Parmed)
Vagisan, Creme (Sandia)
Vagisul, Creme (Sheryl)
W/Sulfisoxazole, allantoin.
See: Vagilia, Cream (Lemmon)
p-AMINOBENZENE-SULFONYLACETYLIMIDE.
See: Sulfacetamide
p-AMINOBENZOATE CALCIUM.
W/Salicylamide, Vit. C, mephenesin.
See: Causalin, Tab. (Amfre-Grant)
• **AMINOBENZOATE POTASSIUM,** U.S.P. XXI. Caps.,
for Oral Soln., Tabs., U.S.P. XXI.
See: Potaba, Pow., Tab. (Glenwood)
W/Hydrocortisone, ammonium salicylate & ascorbic
acid.
See: Neocylate sodium free, Tab. (Central)
W/Potassium salicylate.
See: Pabalate-Sodium Free, Tab. (Robins)

W/Pot. salicylate, ascorbic acid.
See: Pabalan, Tab. (Lannett)
• **AMINOBENZOATE SODIUM,** U.S.P. XXI.
See: PABA Sod., Tab. (Various Mfr.)
W/Phenobarbital, colchicine salicylate, Vit. B-1 & aspi-
rin.
See: Doloral, Tab. (Alamed)
W/Salicylamide, ascorbic acid.
See: Sylapar, Tab. (O'Neal)
W/Sodium salicylate.
See: PABA-C, Tab. (Vortech)
Pabalate, Tab. (Robins)
Salpara, Tab. (Reid-Provident)
W/Salicylamide, sod. salicylate, ascorbic acid,
butabarbital sod.
See: Bisalate, Tab. (Allison Lab.)
• **AMINOBENZOIC ACID,** U.S.P. XXI. Gel., Topical
Soln., U.S.P. XXI. Benzoic acid, 4-amino. PABA. Avail-
able as cap., bot., pow., sol. & tab. Massengill-Sol.
(10%) Bot. 1 pt.
Use: Topical protectant (sun-screening agent).
See: Pabafilm (Owen)
Pabanol, Lot. (Elder)
W/Mephenisin, Salicylamide.
See: Sal-Phenesin, Tab. (Marion)
W/Sod. salicylate & ascorbic acid.
See: Nucorsal, Tab. (Westerfield)
p-AMINOBENZOIC ACID, SALTS.
See: p-Aminobenzoate potassium p-Aminobenzoate
sodium
• **AMINOCAPROIC ACID,** U.S.P. XXI. Syr., Inj., Tab.,
U.S.P. XXI. 6-Aminohexanoic acid.
Use: Antifibrinolytic, hemostatic.
See: Amicar, Syr., Tab., Vial (Lederle)
• **AMINOCAPROIC ACID.** USAN. 6-Aminohexanoic
acid. Amicar. Epsikapron.
Use: Inhibitor of fibrinolytic activity.
AMINOCARDOL.
See: Aminophylline. (Various Mfr.)
AMINO CERV. (Milex) Urea 8.34%, sodium
propionate 0.50%, methionine 0.83%, cystine
0.35%, inositol 0.83%, benzalkonium chloride
0.000004%, buffered to pH 5.5. Tube with
applicator 2¾ oz.
Use: Mild cervicitis, postpartum cervicitis, cervical
tears, post cauterization, post cryosurgery, post
conization.
p-AMINO-N-[2-(DIETHYLAMINO)ETHYL]-BENZAMID-
E MONOHYDROCHLORIDE. Procainamide Hydrochloride, U.S.P. XXI.
AMINODUR DURA-TABS. (Berlex) Aminophylline 300
mg./Tab. Bot. 100s, 250s.
Use: Chronic bronchial asthma and pulmonary
emphysema.
AMINODYNE COMPOUND. (Bowman)
Acetaminophen 2½ gr., aspirin 3½ gr., caffeine ½
gr./Tab. Bot. 100s, 1000s.
2-AMINOETHANOL.
See: Monoethanolamine
(−)-α-(1-AMINOETHYL)-3,4-DIHYDROXYBENZYL
ALCOHOL.
See: Levonordefrin

(−)-α-(AMINOETHYL)-3,4-DIHYDROXYBENZYL AL-
COHOL TARTRATE. Norepinephrine Bitartrate,
U.S.P. XXI.
(±)-α-(1-AMINOETHYL)-2,5-DIMETHOXYBENZYL
ALCOHOL HCl. Methoxamine Hydrochloride, U.S.P.
XXI.
(-)-α-(1-AMINOETHYL)-m-HYDROXYBENZYL ALCO-
HOL TARTRATE. Metaraminol Bitartrate, U.S.P. XXI.
AMINO-ETHYL-PROPANOL.
See: Aminoisobutanol
W/Bromotheophyllin
See: Pamabrom (Various Mfr.)
4-(2-AMINOETHYL)IMIDAZOLE   BIS(DIHYDROGEN
PHOSPHATE). Histamine Phosphate, U.S.P. XXI.
3-AMINO-α-ETHYL-2,4,6-TRIIODOHYDROCINNAMIC
ACID. Iopanoic Acid, U.S.P. XXI.
AMINOFEN. (Dover) Acetaminophen 325 mg./Tab.
Sugar and salt free. Unit Dose 500s.
Use: Analgesic, antipyretic.
AMINOFEN MAX. (Dover) Acetaminophen 500
mg./Tab. Sugar and salt free. Unit Dose 500s.
Use: Extra strength analgesic.
AMINOFORM.
See: Methenamine. (Various Mfr.)
AMINOGEN. (Christina) Vit. B complex & folic acid.
Amp. 2 cc. Box 12s, 24s, 100s.
Vial 10 cc.
Use: Protein hydrolysate therapy.
• AMINOGLUTETHIMIDE, U.S.P. XXI. Tab. U.S.P.
XXI. 2-(p-Aminophenyl)-2-ethylglutarimide.
Use: Treatment of Cushings syndrome.
See: Cytadren, Prods. (Ciba)
6-AMINOHEXANOIC ACID. Aminocaprolic acid
See: Amicar, Syr., Tab., Vial (Lederle)
• AMINOHIPPURATE SODIUM, U.S.P. XXI. Inj.,
U.S.P. XXI. Glycine, N-(4-aminobenzoyl)-, monoso-
dium salt. Monosodium p-aminohippurate. (Merck
Sharp & Dohme) 2 Gm./10 ml. Amp. 10 ml., 50 ml.
Use: I.V., Diagnostic aid for renal plasma flow.
• AMINOHIPPURIC ACID, U.S.P. XXI. Glycine, N-(4-
aminobenzoyl)-.
Use: Diagnostic aid (renal function determination).
N-[p-[[(2-AMINO-4-HYDROXY-6-PTERIDINYL)METH-
YL]AMINO]BENZOYL]- - -GLUTAMIC ACID. Folic
Acid, U.S.P. XXI.
AMINOISOBUTANOL. 2-Amino-2-methylpronanol-1
See: Butaphyllamine
Pamabrom for combinations
AMINOISOMETRADINE.   DL-2-Amino-4-(methylthio)
butyric acid.
See: Methionine
(+)-4-AMINO-3-ISOXAZOLIDINONE.   Cycloserine,
U.S.P. XXI.
8-[(4-AMINO-1-METHYLBUTYL)AMINO]-6-METHOX-
YQUINOLINE PHOSPHATE. Primaquine Phosphate,
U.S.P. XXI.
AMINOMETRADINE. B.A.N.   1-Allyl-6-amino-3-ethyl-
pyrimidine-2,4-dione. Mictine.
Use: Diuretic.
AMINONAT. Protein hydrolysates (oral)
AMINONITROZOLE. N-(5-Nitro-2-thiazolyl) acetamide.
Use: Antitrichomonal.

AMINOPENTAMIDE SULFATE. 4-(Dimethylamino)-2,2-
diphenylvaleramide sulfate.
Use: Anticholinergic.
7-(D-2-AMINO-2-PHENYLACETAMIDO)-3-METHYL-
8-OXO-5-THIA-1-AZABICYCLO-[4.2.0.]OCT-2-ENE
-2-CARBOXYLIC ACID MONOHYDRATE. Ceph-
alexin, U.S.P. XXI.
AMINOPHYLLIN. (Searle) Trademark for
Aminophylline. 100 mg./Tab. Bot. 100s, 1000s.
Unit Dose 100s. 200 mg./Tab. Bot. 100s, 1000s.
Unit Dose 100s.
Use: Bronchodilator.
AMINOPHYLLIN INJECTION. (Searle) Trademark for
Aminophylline. Amp. 250 mg.: 10 ml., 25s, 100s;
500 mg.: 20 ml. 25s, 100s.
Use: Bronchodilator
• AMINOPHYLLINE, U.S.P. XXI. Enema, Inj., Suppos.,
Tabs., U.S.P. XXI. Theophylline compound
w/ethylenediamine (2:1). (Aminocardol,
Ammophyllin, Cardophyllin, Carena, Diophyllin,
Genophyllin, Ionphylline, Metaphyllin, Phyllindon,
Teholamine, Theophyldine.)
Use: Smooth muscle relaxant (bronchodilator).
See: Aminodur, Dura-Tab. (Berlex)
Lixaminol, Elix. (Ferndale)
Panamin, Tab. (Panray)
Phyllocontin, Tab. (Purdue Fredrick)
Rectalad-Aminophylline. (Wallace)
Somophyllin Oral Liquid (Fisons)
Somophyllin Rectal Solution (Fisons)
• AMINOPHYLLINE INJECTION, U.S.P.XXI. (Abbott)
Amp. 250 mg./10 ml., 500 mg./20 ml; Fliptop vial
10 mg./20 ml., 20 mg./50 ml.
Use: Bronchodilator.
AMINOPHYLLINE COMBINATIONS.
Amphedrine Compound, Cap. (Lannett)
Asmacol, Tab. (Vale)
Asmadrin (Jenkins)
Asminorel, Tab. (Reid-Provident)
Asthmacon, Cap. (CMC)
B.M.E., Elix. (Brothers)
Bronchovent, Tab. (Mills)
Dainite, Tab. (Mallinckrodt)
Lixaminol AT/5 cc. (Ferndale)
Mudrane GG-2, Tab. (Poythress)
Orthoxine and Aminophylline, Cap. (Upjohn)
Quinamm, Tab. (Merrell Dow)
Quinite, Tab. (Reid-Provident)
Romaphed, Tab. (Robinson)
Strema, Cap. (Foy)
Theocomp, Cap. (Barry Martin)
Theo-Kaps (Scrip)
AMINOPHYLLINE WITH PHENOBARBITAL
COMBINATIONS.
Amodrine, Tab. (Searle)
Dainite, Tab. (Mallinckrodt)
Mudrane, Tab. (Poythress)
Mudrane GG, Tab. (Poythress)
• AMINOPHYLLINE INJECTION, U.S.P. XXI.
Theophylline ethylenediamine. Amp. 3¾ gr., 7½ gr.
(Various Mfr.).
• AMINOPHYLLINE SUPPOSITORIES, U.S.P. XXI.

7½ gr., 3⅜ gr., (Various Mfr.) Pediatric 0.125 gr. Box 12s (Wyeth).

• **AMINOPHYLLINE TABLETS,** U.S.P. XXI. Plain or enteric coated 1½ gr., 3 gr. (Various Mfr.)

AMINOPHYLLINE-PHENOBARBITAL. (Robinson) Aminophylline 1½ gr., phenobarbital ¼ gr. or ½ gr./Tab. Bot. 100s, 1000s. Bulk Pack 5000s. Aminophylline 3 gr., phenobarbital ¼ gr., or ½ gr./Tab. Bot. 100s, 1000s. Bulk Pack 5000s.

AMINOPHYLLINE-PHENOBARBITAL. (Sutliff & Case) Aminophylline 100 mg., phenobarbital 16 mg., aluminum hydroxide 32 mg./Tab. Bot. 100s, 1000s.

AMINOPHYLLINE-PHENOBARBITAL No. 1. (Sutliff & Case) Aminophylline 1½ gr., Phenobarbital ¼ gr./Tab. Bot. 100s, 1000s.

AMINOPREL. (Pasadena Research) Isolated vegetable protein 4500 mg., 1-lysine monohydrochloride 360 mg., di-methionone 90 mg., all essential amino acids, nonessential amino acids, iron 12 mg., copper 1.5 mg., zinc 12 mg., iodine 0.015 mg., manganese 10 mg., potassium 20 mg., magnesium 240 mg./6 Tab. Bot. 180s.
Use: Dietary supplement.

AMINOPROMAZINE (I.N.N.). Proquamezine, B.A.N.

AMINOPTERIN SODIUM. B.A.N. Sodium N-[4-(2,4-diaminopteridin-6-ylmethyl)aminobenzoyl]-L-glutamate. Sodium N-[p-[[2,4,-(diamino-6-pteridinyl)-methyl]amino]benzoyl]-L-glutamate.
Use: Antineoplastic agent.

4-AMINO-PTEROYLBLUTAMATE SOD. Aminopterin.

2-AMINOPURINE-6-THIOL.
See: Thioguanine

AMINOPYRINE. Amidofebrin, Amidopyrazoline, Anafebrina, Novamidon, Pyradone. Dimethylamino-phenyl-dimethylpyrazolone.
Use: Antipyretic, analgesic.
See: Dipyrone, Vial (Maurry)

AMINOQUIN NAPHTHOATE.
See: Pamaquine Naphthoate

4-AMINOQUINOLINE DERIVATIVES.
See: Aralen HCl (Winthrop-Breon)
Chloroquine Phosphate (Various Mfr.)
Plaquenil Sulfate (Winthrop-Breon)
Primaquine Phosphate (Winthrop-Breon)

8-AMINOQUINOLINE DERIVATIVES.
See: Primaquine Phosphate, U.S.P.

• **AMINOREX.** USAN. 2-Amino-5-phenyl-2-oxazoline.
Use:Appetite suppressant.
See: Apiquel fumarate.

• **AMINOSALICYLATE CALCIUM,** U.S.P. XXI. Cap., Tab., U.S.P. XXI. Calcium 4-Aminosalicylate (1:2) trihydrate. (Dumas-Wilson) 7½ gr., Bot. 1000s.
Use: Tuberculosis therapy.
See: Teebacin Calcium, Tab. (CMC)
Parasal Calcium (Panray)
W/Isoniazid, pyridoxine HCl.
See: Calpas-Inah-6, Tabs. (Amer. Chem. & Drug)

AMINOSALICYLATE POTASSIUM. Monopotassium 4-aminosalicylate.
Use: Antibacterial (tuberculostatic).
See: Parasal Pot., Tab. (Panray)

Paskalium, Tab. & Pow. (Glenwood)
Teebacin Kalium, Tab., Pow. (CMC)

• **AMINOSALICYLATE SODIUM,** U.S.P. XXI. Tab., U.S.P. XXI. Aminosalicyate sodium Benzoic acid, 4-amino-2-hydroxy-, monosodium salt, dihydrate. Monosodium 4-amino-salicylate dihydrate.
Use: Tuberculostatic.
See: Neopasalate, Tab. (Mallincrodt)
Parasal Sodium, Pow., Tab., (Panray)
P.A.S., Pow. (Century)
Pasara Sod., Pow., Tab. (Dorsey)
Pasdium, Tab. (Kasar)
Teebacin, Tab., Pow. (CMC)

• **AMINOSALICYLIC ACID,** U.S.P. XXI. Tablets, U.S.P. XXI. 4-Amino-2-hydroxybenzoic acid. PAS, p-Aminosalicylic acid. (Lilly) 500 mg. Enseal, Bot. 100s.
Use: Adjunct to streptomycin in tuberculosis.
See: Parasal, Tab., Pow. (Panray)
P.A.S. (Lilly)
P.A.S. Acid, Tab. (Kasar)
PASNA (Barnes-Hind)
Teebacin Acid, Tab. (CMC)
W/Isoniazid.
See: Di-Isopacin, Tab. (CMC)
Isopacin, Tab. (CMC)

p-AMINOSALICYLIC ACID SALTS.
See: Aminosalicylate Calcium
Aminosalicylate Potassium
Aminosalicylate Sodium

AMINOSYN. (Abbott) Crystalline amino acid solution. **3.5% M:** 1,000 ml.; **5%:** 250 ml., 500 ml., 1,000 ml. cont.; **7%:** 500 ml.; 7% kit (cs/3); 7% w/Electrolytes, 500 ml.; 7% w/Electrolytes, TPN kit; 10%, 500 ml.; **8.5%:** 1000 ml. w/Electrolytes 1000 ml. Single dose containers.
Use: I.V., nutritional.

AMINOSYN R.F. (Abbott) Single dose containers, 300 ml.
Use: I.V. source of protein.

AMINO-THIOL. (Marcen) Sulfur 10 mg., casein 50 mg., sod. citrate 5 mg., phenol 5 mg., benzyl alcohol 5 mg./cc. Vial 10 cc., 30 cc.
Use: Treatment of arthritis, neuritis.

AMINOTRATE PHOSPHATE. Trolnitrate phosphate.
See: Triethanolamine, preps.

AMINOXYTROPINE TROPATE HCl. Atropine-N-oxide HCl.

AMIPAQUE. (Winthrop-Breon) Metrizamide 3.75 Gm./20 ml. Vial; 6.75 Gm./50 ml. Vial; 2.5 Gm./20 ml. Vial; 13.5 Gm./100 ml. Vial.
Use: Myleography, C.T. cisternography, pediatric angiocardiography, intravenous digital arteriography.

AMIPHENAZOLE. B.A.N. 2,4-Diamino-5-phenyl-thiazole.
Use: Respiratory stimulant.
See: Daptazole

AMIPHENAZOLE HCl. 2,4-Diamino-5-phenylthiazole HCl. Daptazole.

• **AMIQUINSIN HYDROCHLORIDE.** USAN. 4-Amino-6,7-dimethoxyquinoline hydrochloride monohydrate. Under study.

Use: Antihypertensive.

AMIRON HEMATINIC. (Misemer) Ferrous fumarate 275 mg., ascorbic acid 100 mg., folic acid 1 mg., cyanocobalamine 15 mcg., docusate sodium 20 mg./Cap.
Use: Prevention & treatment of iron & folic acid deficiencies.

AMISOMETRADINE. B.A.N. 6-Amino-1,2-methylallyl-3-methylpyrimidine-2,4-dione. Roliction.
Use: Diuretic.

AMITID. (Squibb) Amitriptyline HCl 10 mg., 25 mg., 50 mg./Tab. Bot. 100s, 1000s 75 mg., 100 mg./Tab. Bot. 100s
Use: Antidepressant.

AMITIN. (Thurston) Vit. C 200 mg., lemon bioflavonoid 100 mg., niacinamide 60 mg., methionine 100 mg./Tab. Bot. 100s, 500s.
Use: Dietary supplement and therapy.

AMITONE. (Norcliff Thayer) Calcium carbonate 350 mg./Tab. Bot. 100s.
Use: Antacid.

• **AMITRAZ.** USAN.
Use: Scabicide.
See: Mitaban (Upjohn)

AMITRIL. (Parke-Davis) Amitriptyline HCl 10 mg., 25 mg., 50 mg., 75 mg., 100 mg., 150 mg./Tab. Bot. 100s, 1000s. Unit dose 100s.
Use: Antidepressant.

AMITRIPTYLINE. B.A.N. 3-(3-Dimethylamino-propylidene)dibenzo[a,d]cyclohepta-1,4-diene. Amitriptyline hydrochloride. Laroxyl. Lenitzol. Saroten. Tryptizol.
Use: Antidepressant.
See: Elegen-G, Tab. (Grafton)

• **AMITRIPTYLINE HCl.** U.S.P. XXI. Inj., Tab. U.S.P. XXI. 10,11-dihydro-N, N-dimethyl-5H-dibenzo[a,d]cycloheptene-Δ^5,γ-propylamine hydrochloride.
Use: Antidepressant.
See: Elavil HCl Tabs. & Vials (Merck Sharp & Dohme)
   Endep, Tab. (Roche)
   SK-Amitriptyline, Tab. (SmithKline)
W/Chlordiazepoxide.
See: Limbitrol, Tab. (Roche)
W/Perphenazine.
See: Etrafon, Prod. (Schering)
   Triavil, Tabs. (Merck Sharp & Dohme)

AMLAX TABLETS. (Vortech) Bile salts 1 gr., ext. cascara sagrada ½ gr., phenolphthalein ½ gr., aloin ⅛ gr./Tab. Bot. 100s, 1000s.
Use: Laxative.

AMMENS MEDICATED POWDER. (Bristol-Myers) Boric acid 4.55%, zinc oxide 9.10%, talc and starch. Can. 6.25 oz., 11 oz.
Use: Heat rash, prickly heat or diaper rash.

AMMOIDIN. Methoxsalen.

AMMONIA. Aromatic Ammonia Spirit, U.S.P. XXI. Strong Sol. N.F. XVI. (Lilly) 0.4 ml; pt.; Aspirols 0.4 ml. Pkg. 12s. (Burroughs-Wellcome) Vaporoles 5.41 minims in crushable glass capsule. Box 12s, 100s.
Use: Fainting.

• **AMMONIA SOLUTION, STRONG,** N.F. XVI. (Stanlabs) 28% Bot. pt., gal.

Use: Pharmaceutic aid (source of ammonia).

• **AMMONIATED MERCURY,** U.S.P. XXI. Oint., Ophth. Oint., U.S.P. XXI. (Various Mfr.)
See: Mercuronate 5% Oint. (Bowman)
W/Phenol
See: Pixacreme, Jar (Pixacol)
W/Salicylic acid.
See: Emersal, Liq. (Medco)

AMMONIUM, ALKYLDIMETHYL(PHENYL-METHYL)-, CHLORIDE. Benzalkonium Chloride, U.S.P. XXI.

AMMONIUM BENZOATE.
Use: Urinary antiseptic.

• **AMMONIUM CARBONATE,** N.F. XVI.
Use: Source of ammonia.

• **AMMONIUM CHLORIDE,** U.S.P. XXI. Inj., Tab., U.S.P. XXI. **Tab.** plain or E.C. (5 gr. & 7½ gr.) (Various Mfr.) **Inj.:** (Cutter) 120 mEq./30 ml. Vial.
Use: Diuretic, expectorant, alkalosis.
See: Nodema Tab. (Towne)

AMMONIUM CHLORIDE, ENSEALS. (Lilly) Ammonium chloride. Timed disintegrating tablets. Enseals 7½ gr. Bot. 100s. 15 gr. Bot. 100s.
Use: Acidification of the urine.

AMMONIUM MANDELATE. Ammonium salt of mandelic acid. Syrup, (8 Gm./fl. oz.) Bot pt., gal.
Use: Orally, urinary antiseptic.

• **AMMONIUM MOLYBDATE.** U.S.P. XXI. Inj., U.S.P. XXI.

AMMONIUM NITRATE.
See: Reditemp-C, Cold Pack (Wyeth)

• **AMMONIUM PHOSPHATE,** N.F. XVI. Phosphoric acid diammonium salt. Diammonium phosphate.

AMMONIUM VALERATE.
Use: Sedative.

AMMOPHYLLIN.
See: Aminophylline, U.S.P. XXI. (Various Mfr.)

AMMORID. (Kinney) Benzethonium chloride & zinc oxide in a lanolin absorption base. Tube 2 oz.
Use: Topically, dermatologic ointment.

AMMORID DIAPER RINSE. (Kinney) Methylbenzethonium chloride 5%, plus deionizing & buffering agents in dry powder form, readily soluble in water. Bot. 240 Gm.
Use: Protection against diaper rash.

• **AMOBARBITAL,** U.S.P. XXI. Elixir, Tablets, U.S.P. XXI. (Various Mfr.) 5-Ethyl-5-isoamylbarbituric acid.
Use: Hypnotic of intermediate duration.
See: Amytal, Elix., Pulvule, Tab. (Lilly)

AMOBARBITAL W/COMBINATIONS.
   Amobell, Cap. (Bock)
   Amodex, Cap. (Fellows)
   Amo-Dexules, Cap. (Recsei)
   Amoseco, Cap. (Robinson)
   Amytal & Aspirin, Pulvule (Lilly)
   Aspadine, Tab. (Vortech)
   Asthmacon, Cap. (CMC)
   Barbeloid, Tab. (Vale)
   Bronchovent, Tab. (Mills)
   Buffadyne A-S, Tab. (Lemmon)
   Buffadyne w/Barbiturates, Tab. (Lemmon)
   Butatrax, Cap. (Sutliff & Case)

Dextrobar, Tab. (Lannett)
Ectasule, Cap. (Fleming)
Hydrochol-Plus, Tab. (Elder)
Komal, Tab. (O'Neal)
Milidex, Cap. (Briar)
Monotheamin and Amytal, Pulvule (Lilly)
Obalan Lanatabs, Tab. (Lannett)
Obe-Slim, Tab. (Jenkins)
Penta-E W/Amobarb, Cap. (Recsei)
Phetabar, Cap. (Moore-Kirk)
Scoline-Amobarbital, Tab. (Westerfield)
Spancap No. 2, Cap. (Vortech)
Stim, Prep. (Scrip)
Trimex, Cap. (Mills)
Vasobarb, Cap. (Reid-Provident)
• **AMOBARBITAL SODIUM,** U.S.P. XXI. Capsules, Sterile, XXI. (Various Mfr.) 2,4,6(1H,3H,5H)-Pyrimidi-netrione, 5-ethyl-5-(3-me-thylbutyl)-, monosodium salt. Sodium 5-ethyl-5-isopentylbarbiturate.
Amp.: (1⅞ gr.) 6s, 12s, 25s, 100s; (3¼ gr.) 6s, 12s, 25s, 100s; (7½ gr.) 6s, 12s, 25s, 100s. (Various Mfr.)
Cap.: (3 gr.) Bot. 1000s. (Amer. Drug Prods.)
Pow.: Bot. 4 oz., ½ lb., 1 lb. Pkg. 5 lb. (Various Mfr.)
Vial: (15½ gr.) 10 cc. (Various Mfr.)
Use: Hypnotic of intermediate duration, sedative.
See: Amytal Sod. (Lilly)
W/Ephedrine HCl, theophylline, chlorpheniramine maleate.
See: Theo-Span, Cap. (Scrip)
W/Secobarbital Sod.
See: Amsee, Tab. (Kenyon)
Compobarb, Cap. (Vitarine)
Dusotal, Cap. (Harvey)
Lanabarb, Cap. (Lannett)
AMOBARBITAL-EPHEDRINE CAPSULES. (Lannett) Amobarbital 50 mg., ephedrine sulfate 25 mg./Cap. Bot. 500s, 1000s.
AMOBELL. (Bock) Amobarbital 15 mg., belladonna ext. 10 mg./Cap. Bot. 100s, 1000s.
Use: Sedative & antispasmodic.
AMOCAL JR. (Jenkins) Pyrilamine maleate 3 mg., phenylephrine HCl 1 mg., tartar emetic 1/136 gr., benzoic acid 1/68 gr., ipecac pow. 1/16 gr., amm. chloride ½ gr., iodized Cal. 1/16 gr., licorice ext. 1 gr./Tab. Bot. 1000s.
Use: Expectorant and anodyne.
AMOCILLIN. (Vortech) Crystalline penicillin G potassium, buffered w/sod. citrate, 3,000,000 u./60 cc. Bot. 60 cc.
Use: Antibiotic.
AMO-DERM. (High) Mineral abrasive, lecith. neut. soap base, 3,4,4'-trichlorocarbanilide 1%, allantoin 2%. Pkg. 3½ oz. bars.
Use: Skin cleanser.
AMODEX. (Fellows) Dextroamphetamine HCl 5 mg., amobarbital 20 mg./Tab. Bot. 100s, 1000s.
• **AMODIAQUINE,** U.S.P. XXI. 7-Chloro-4-(3-diethyl-aminomethyl-4-hydroxyanilino)quinoline.
Use: Antimalarial.
• **AMODIAQUINE HYDROCHLORIDE,** U.S.P. XXI.

Tab. U.S.P. XXI. 4-(7-Chloro-4-quinolylamino)-α-(Die-thylamino)-o-cresol-di-HCl.
Use: Antimalarial.
AMODIN. (Vortech) Adenosine-5-monophosphoric acid 25 mg., niacin 10 mg., cyanocobalamin 300 mcg., methionine 25 mg./cc. Vial 10 cc.
AMODRINE. (Searle) Aminophylline 100 mg., racephedrine HCl 25 mg., phenobarbital 8 mg./Tab. Bot. 100s.
Use: Antiasthmatic.
AMOGEL PG. (Vortech) Pow. opium 24 mg., phenobarbital 16.2 mg., kaolin 6 Gm., pectin 142.8 mg., hyoscyamine sulfate 0.1037 mg., atropine sulfate 0.0194 mg., hyoscine HBr 0.0065 mg., sod. benzoate 60 mg. 1 oz. w/alcohol 9.1%. Bot. 4 oz., gal.
Use: Antidiarrheal.
AMOL. Mono-n-amyl-hydroquinone ether.
See: B-F-I, Pow. (Calgon)
AMONIDRIN. (O'Neal, Jones & Feldman) Ammonium chloride 200 mg., guaifenesin 100 mg./Tab. Bot. 100s.
Use: Cough preparation.
AMOPYROQUIN HCl. 4-(7-Chloro-4-quinolylamino)-a-1-pyrrolidyl-o-cresoldihydrochloride.
See: Propoquin.
AMOSAN. (CooperCare) Sodium bitartrate, sodium perborate. Boxes 20, 40 single-dose packets. Liquid Drops 0.5 oz., 2 oz.
Use: Mouth and gum care.
AMOSECO. (Robinson) Secobarbital & amobarbital. Bot. 100s, 1000s.
Use: Sedative.
AMOTRIPHENE. 2,3,3-Tris(p-methoxy-phenyl)-N,N-dimethylallylamine, 3-Dimethylamino-1, 1.2-tris(4-methoxyphenyl)-1-propene HCl.
Use: Coronary vasodilator.
AMOXAL. Pentalamide, B.A.N.
• **AMOXAPINE.** USAN. 2-Chloro-Il-(l-piperazinyl)-dibenz[b,f][1,4]oxazepine.
Use: Antidepressant.
See: Asendin, Tab. (Lederle)
• **AMOXICILLIN.** U.S.P. XXI. Cap., Oral Susp., Tab., U.S.P. XXI. 6-[D-(−)2-Amino-2-(p-hydroxyphe-nyl)acetamido]-3,3-dimethyl-7-oxo-4-thia-1-azabicy-clo[3.2.0]heptane-2-carboxylic acid.
Use: Antibiotic.
See: Amoxil, Preps. (Beecham Labs)
Polymox, Preps. (Bristol)
Sumox, Preps. (Reid-Provident)
AMOXICILLIN TRIHYDRATE.
Use: Antibiotic
See: Amoxil Chewable, Tab. (Beecham Labs)
Polymox, Cap., Susp. (Bristol)
Trimox, Preps. (Squibb)
Utimox, Cap., Susp. (Parke-Davis)
Wymox, Cap, Liq. (Wyeth)
AMOXIL. (Beecham Labs) Amoxicillin, **Cap:** 250 mg. Bot. 100s, 500s. Unit dose 10 × 10. 500 mg. Bot. 50s, 500s. Unit dose 10 × 10. **Oral Suspension:** 125 mg. and 250 mg./5 ml. Bot. 80 ml., 100 ml., 150 ml. Unit dose 5 ml.

AMOXIL CHEWABLE TABLETS. (Beecham Labs) Amoxicillin trihydrate 125 mg./Tab., 250 mg./Tab. Bot. 60s.
Use: Antibiotic.
AMOXIL PEDIATRIC DROPS. (Beecham Labs) Amoxicillin 50 mg./ml. Bot. 15 ml., 30 ml.
AMP. Adenosine Phosphate, B.A.N.
AMPERIL. (Geneva) Ampicillin trihydrate 250 mg., 500 mg./Cap.
Bot. 100s, 500s.
• **AMPHECLORAL.** USAN. α-Methyl-N-(2,2,2-trichloroethylidene) phenethylamine.
Use: Sympathomimetic.
AMPHEDRINE COMPOUND CAPSULES. (Lannett) Aminophylline-ephedrine compound. Bot. 1000s.
AMPHENIDONE. l-(m-Aminophenyl)-2-(1H)-pyridone.
Use: Central stimulant.
AMPHETAMINE, LEVO.
See: Levamphetamine
AMPHETAMINE HYDROCHLORIDE. Rac. amphetamine HCl, methylphenethylamine HCl, dl-1-phenyl-2-aminopropane HCl, dl-methylphenethylamine HCl, rac. desoxynorephedrine HCl. **Amp.** 20 mg./cc 1 cc. (Various Mfr.) **Cap.** (Various Mfr.)
Use: Vasoconstrictor, central nervous system stimulant.
AMPHETAMINE WITH DEXTROAMPHETAMINE AS RESIN COMPLEXES.
See: Biphetamine, Cap. (Pennwalt)
AMPHETAMINE PHOSPHATE. Monobasic dl-a-methylphenethylamine phosphate. Monobasic racemic amphetamine phos.
AMPHETAMINE PHOSPHATE, DIBASIC, Racemic amphetamine phosphate. **Cap.** 5 mg., 10 mg. **Tab.** 5 mg., 10 mg. (Various Mfr.)
• **AMPHETAMINE PHOSPHATE, DEXTRO,** U.S.P. XXI. Tab., U.S.P. XXI. Dextro-amphetamine phosphate. (Various Mfr.).
• **AMPHETAMINE SULFATE,** U.S.P. XXI. Tab., U.S.P. XXI. dl-a-Methylphenethylamine sulfate. (Racemic or dl form). Cap. (5, 10 mg.) (Various Mfr.). Tab. (5, 10 mg.) (Various Mfr.). Vials (20 mg./cc.) (Various Mfr.).
AMPHETAMINE SULFATE, DEXTRO.
See: Dextroamphetamine Sulfate, U.S.P. XXI.
d-AMPHETAMINE CARBOXYMETHYLCELLULOSE SALT.
See: Bontril, T.R. Tab. (Carnrick)
d-AMPHETAMINE HYDROCHLORIDE. (Various Mfr.) Dextroamphetamine HCl. **Cap.** 5 mg., 10 mg. (Various Mfr.) **Tab.** 5 mg., 10 mg. (Various Mfr.)
Use: Vasoconstrictor, central nervous system stimulant.
levo-AMPHETAMINE.
See: Levamphetamine.
AMPHOCAPS. (Blue Cross) Ampicillin 250 mg. or 500 mg./Cap. Bot. 100s
Use: Antibiotic.
AMPHODEX. (Jamieson-McKames) d-Amphetamine sulfate 15 mg., amobarbital 45 mg., Vit. A 6,600 I.U., D 400 I.U., B-1 1.6 mg., B-2 2.5 mg., niacinamide 15.5 mg., C 30 mg., Fe sulfate 20 mg., copper

sulfate 2.8 mg., sod. molybdate 0.45 mg., zinc sulfate 2.8 mg., pot. iodide 0.13 mg./T.R. Cap. Bot. 100s.
Use: Appetite depressant.
AMPHOJEL. (Wyeth) Aq. susp. of aluminum hydroxide, (320 mg./5 ml.) equivalent to 4% aluminum oxide. Bot. 12 fl. oz. Tab. 5 gr. Bot. 100s. Tab. 10 gr. Ctn. 100s. Suspension without flavor. Bot. 12 fl. oz.
Use: Gastric & duodenal ulcer or hyperacidity.
• **AMPHOMYCIN.** F.D.A. An antibiotic produced by *Streptomyces canus*. Amphocortrin.
• **AMPHOMYCIN.** USAN. An antibiotic produced by *Streptomyces canus*.
See: Ecomytrin
AMPHOTERICIN.
See: Fungizone, Prep. (Squibb)
AMPHOTERICIN. B.A.N. Polyene antibiotics isolated from a strain of a Streptomyces species, referred to as *Streptomyces nodosus*. **Amphotericin B.**
See: Fungilin
Fungizone
• **AMPHOTERICIN B,** U.S.P. XXI. Cream, Inj., Lotion, Oint., U.S.P. XXI. A polyene antibiotic substance obtained from cultures of *Streptomyces nodosus*.
Use: Antifungal.
See: Fungizone, Prep. (Squibb)
W/Tetracycline & K metaphosphate.
See: Mysteclin-F, Prep. (Squibb)
• **AMPICILLIN,** U.S.P. XXI. Caps., Oral Susp., Sterile Susp., Tab., U.S.P. XXI. 6[(D)-α-Aminophenylacetamido) penicillanic acid. 6-(D-2-Amino-2-phenylacetamido)-3, 3-dimethyl-7-oxo-4-thia-1-azabicyclo [3.2.0] heptane-2-carboxylic acid.
Use: Antibiotic.
See: Amcill, Prep. (Parke-Davis)
Omnipen, Prep. (Wyeth)
Penbritin, Prep. (Ayerst)
Pfizerpen A, Prep. (Pfipharmecs)
Polycillin, Prep. (Bristol)
Principen, Prep. (Squibb)
Roampicillin, Tab. (Robinson)
Roampicillin Powder, Inj. (Robinson)
Totacillin, Prep. (Beecham Labs)
W/Probenecid
See: Polycillin-PRB, Unit dose (Bristol)
Principen W/Probenecid Cap. (Squibb)
Probampacin (Robinson)
Trojacillin-Plus, Oral Susp. (Young)
• **AMPICILLIN AND PROBENECID CAPSULES,** U.S.P. XXI.
• **AMPICILLIN AND PROBENECID FOR ORAL SUSPENSION,** U.S.P. XXI.
• **AMPICILLIN SODIUM STERILE,** U.S.P. XXI.
Use: Antibiotic.
See: Omnipen-N, Inj. (Wyeth)
Pen A/N, Vial (Pfipharmecs)
Pensyn-N. Sterile (Upjohn)
Polycillin-N (Bristol Labs)
Principen/N, Vial (Squibb)
SK-Ampicillin-N, Vial (SmithKline)
Totacillin-N, Vial (Beecham Labs)

AMPICILLIN TRIHYDRATE. Caps., Oral Susp.
marketed by various manufacturers.
Use: Antibiotic.
AMPICILLIN TRIHYDRATE.
See: Amcap, Cap. (Circle)
Ameril, Cap., Susp. (Geneva)
Ampi-Co, Cap. or Susp. (Coastal)
D-Amp, Cap., Susp. (Dunhall)
Pensyn, Preps. (Upjohn)
Polycillin Prep. (Bristol)
Principen, Cap., Susp. (Squibb)
Principen 250 (Squibb)
SK-Ampicillin, Prep. (SmithKline)
Supen, Cap., Susp. (Reid Provident)
Totacillin, Cap., Susp. (Beecham Labs)
AMPI-CO. (Coastal) Ampicillin trihydrate. **Caps.** 250
mg., 500 mg./Cap. Bot. 100s. **Pow. for oral Susp.**
125 mg./5 cc. Bot. 80 cc. **Susp.** 250 mg./5 cc.,
Bot. 80 cc.
Use: Antibiotic.
AMPROL. (MSD AGVET) Amprolium 25% medicated
feed; 20% soluble powder; 9.6% solution.
Use: Coccidiostat, veterinary medicine.
AMPROL HI-E. (MSD AGVET) Amprolium 25%, ethopa-
bate 8%, medicated feed.
Use: Coccidiostat, veterinary medicine.
AMPROL PLUS. (MSD AGVET) Amprolium 25%,
ethopabate 0.8%., medicated feed.
Use: Coccidiostat, veterinary medicine.
• **AMPROLIUM,** U.S.P. XXI. Oral Powder, Soluble
Powder, U.S.P. XXI. 1-(4-Amino-2-propyl-5-pyrimidi-
nylmethyl)-2-picolinium chloride.
Use: Coccidiostat, veterinary medicine.
See: Amprol (MSD AGVET)
Amprol Hi-E (MSD AGVET)
Amprol Plus (MSD AGVET)
Amprolmix (MSD AGVET)
Amprovine (MSD AGVET)
Corid (MSD AGVET)
Pancoxin hydrochloride (MSD AGVET)
AMPROTROPINE PHOSPHATE. 2-Diethylamino-2,2-
dimethylpropyl tropate.
AMPROVINE. (MSD AGVET) Amprolium Sol. 9.6%,
premix 25%, medicated feed.
Use: Coccidiostat, veterinary medicine, 20% soluble
powder.
• **AMQUINATE.** USAN.
Use: Antimalarial.
• **AMSACRINE.** USAN.
Use: Antineoplastic.
• **AMRINONE.** USAN.
Use: Cardiotonic.
AMSEE. (Kenyon) Amobarbital sod. ¾ gr.,
secobarbital sod. ¾ gr./Cap. Bot. 100s, 1000s.
Use: Sedative.
AMSEE #2. (Kenyon) Amobarbital sod. 1½ gr.,
secobarbital sod. 1½ gr./Cap. Bot. 100s, 1000s.
Use: Sedative.
AM-TUSS ELIXIR. (T.E. Williams) Codeine phosphate
10 mg., phenylephrine HCl 10 mg., phenyl-propanola-
mine HCl 5 mg., prophenpyridamine maleate 12.5
mg., guaifenesin 44 mg., fl. ext. ipecac 0.17 min.,

citric acid 60 mg., sodium citrate 197 mg./5 ml.
w/alcohol 5%. Bot. pt., gal.
Use: Antitussive, vasoconstrictor, antihistaminic
expect.
AMTUSSIN-DM. (American Labs.)
Cough Syrup, Bot. 4 oz.
AM-WAX. (Amlab) Urea, benzocaine, propylene glycol
and glycerin. Bot. 10 cc.
Use: Ear drops.
AMYL. Phenyl phenol, phenyl mercuric nitrate.
See: Lubraseptic Jelly (Guardian)
αAMYLASE.
W/Calcium carbonate, glycine, belladonna ext.
See: Trialka, Tab. (Commerce)
W/Lipase, protease, cellase, hyoscine HBr.
See: Am-Zyme, Tab. (Vortech).
W/Pancreatin, protease, lipase.
See: Dizymes, Caps. (Recsei)
W/Pepsin, homatropine methyl Br, lipase,
protease, bile salts.
See: Digesplen, Tab., Elixir (Med. Prod.
Panamericana)
W/Pepsin, pancreatin, ox bile extract.
See: Gourmase, Cap. (Rowell)
W/Phenobarbital, belladonna, pepsin, amylase,
pancreatin, ox bile extract.
See: Gourmase-PB, Cap. (Rowell)
W/Protease, lipase, simethicone.
See: Tri-Cone, Cap. (Meyer)
• **AMYLENE HYDRATE,** N.F. XVI. Tertiary amyl
alcohol. Tert-pentyl alcohol. 2-Methyl-2-butanol. (Var-
ious Mfr.).
Use: Pharmaceutic aid (solvent).
• **AMYL NITRITE,** U.S.P. XXI. Inhalant, U.S.P. XXI.
Isoamyl nitrite. Isopentyl nitrite. Burroughs
Wellcome—Vaporole (0.18 cc.) (0.3 cc.) Box 12s.
Lilly—Aspirols (0.18 cc., 0.3 cc.) Box 12s.
Use: Inhalation, coronary vasodilator in angina
pectoris.
W/Sodium nitrite, sodium thiosulfate.
See: Cyanide Antidote Pkg. (Lilly)
AMYLOCHROME TEST. (Roche Diagnostics)
Colorimetric test for serum amylase with a built-in
chemical standard. Box 60 tests.
AMYLOLYTIC ENZYME.
W/Butabarbital sod., belladonna ext., cellulolytic
enzyme, proteolytic enzyme, lipolytic enzyme, iron
oxbile.
See: Butibel-Zyme, Tab. (McNeil)
W/Calcium carbonate, glycine, proteolytic and
cellulolytic enzymes.
See: Co-Gel, Tab. (Arco)
W/Cellulolytic, proteolytic and lipolytic enzymes,
hyoscyamine sulfate.
See: Converspaz, Tab. (Ascher)
W/Lipase, proteolytic, cellulolytic enzymes,
phenobarbital, hyoscyamine sulf., atropine sulf.
See: Arco-Lipase Plus, Tab. (Arco)
W/Proteolytic, cellulolytic, lipolytic enzymes, iron, ox
bile.
See: Spaszyme, Tab. (Dooner)
W/Proteolytic enzyme. d-sorbitol.

See: Kuzyme, Cap. (Kremers-Urban)
W/Proteolytic, cellulolytic enzymes.
See: Trienzyme, Tab. (Fellows-Testagar)
W/Proteolytic enzyme, cellulolytic enzyme, lipolytic
enzyme.
See: Arco-Lase, Tab. (Arco)
Zymme, Tab. (Scrip)
W/Proteolytic enzyme (Papain), homatropine
methylbromide, d-sorbitol.
See: Converzyme, Liz. (Ascher)
W/Proteolytic enzyme, lipolytic enzyme, cellulolytic
enzyme, & belladonna ext.
See: Mallenzyme improved, Tab. (Mallard)
AMYLOZINE. Trifluoperazine, B.A.N.
AMYTAL. (Lilly) Amobarbital. **Elixir:** 4 gr./fl. oz.
w/alcohol 34%. Bot. 16 fl. oz.
Tab.:(15 mg.), Bot. 100s, 500s; (30 mg.), Bot. 100s,
1000s; (50 mg.), Bot. 100s, 500s; (100 mg.), Bot.
100s, 500s.
Use: Hypnotic.
W/Aminophylline & ephedrine HCl.
See: Amesec, Cap. (Lilly)
W/Ephedrine.
See: Ephedrine w/Amytal, Cap. (Lilly)
AMYTAL SODIUM. (Lilly) Amobarbital sodium. **Amp.:**
(2 gr.) Pkg. 6s; (4 gr.) Pkg. 6s, 25s; (7½ gr.) Pkg.
6s, 25s; (4 gr., 7½ gr.) w/amp. of water for
injection. **Pulvules:** (1 gr.) Bot. 100s, 500s (3 gr.)
Bot. 100s, 500s. Blister pak 10 × 10s.
Use: Orally, I.M.; I.V., rapid-acting sedative.
W/Seconal sodium.
See: Tuinal, Cap. (Lilly)
AM-ZYME. (Vortech) Pancreatic enzyme concentrate
66 mg., amylase 6666 u., protease 6000 u., lipase
160 u., cellase 1.33 u./inner E.C. Tab.; pancreatic
enzyme concentrate 34 mg., amylase 3334 u.,
protease 3000 u., lipase 80 u., cellase 0.67 mg.,
hyoscine HBr 0.006 mg. outer Tab. Bot. 100s,
1000s.
Use: Digestive aid.
ANA. (Wampole-Zeus) Antinuclear antibodies test by
IFA. Tests 54s.
Use: Aid in the diagnosis of SLE and similar
connective tissue disorders.
ANA HEp-2. (Wampole-Zeus) Antinuclear antibodies
test by IFA. Tests 50s.
Use: Aid in the diagnosis of SLE and similar
connective tissue disorders.
ANABOLEX. Stanolone, B.A.N.
■ **ANABOLIC AGENTS.** These agents stimulate
constructive processes leading to retention of
nitrogen and increasing the body protein.
See: Adroyd, Tab. (Parke-Davis)
Anabolin-IM, Vial (Alto)
Anadrol, Tab. (Syntex)
Anavar, Tab. (Searle)
Android, Tab. (Brown)
Crestabolic, Vial (Nutrition)
Deca-Durabolin, Amp., Vial (Organon)
Dianabol, Tab. (Ciba)
Di Genik, Vial (Savage)
Drolban, Vial (Lilly)

Durabolin, Amp., Vial (Organon)
Halotestin, Tab. (Upjohn)
Maxibolin, Elix., Tab. (Organon)
Ora-Testryl, Tab. (Squibb)
Os-Cal-Mone, Tab. (Marion)
Winstrol, Tab. (Winthrop-Breon)
W/Vitamins and minerals.
See: Dumogran, Tab. (Squibb).
ANABOLIN. (Sig) Methylandrostenediol dipropionate
50 mg., benzyl alcohol 2%, sesame oil q.s./ml. Vial
10 ml. **Aq. susp.:** Methylandrostenediol 50 mg./ml.
in sodium phosphate buffer. Vial 10 ml.
ANABOLIN-IM. (Alto) Nandrolone phenpropionate 50
mg./ml. Vial 2 ml.
Use: Anabolic agent.
ANABOLIN LA-100. (Alto) Nandrolone decanoate
100 mg./ml. Vial 2 ml.
Use: Anabolic, anti-catabolic steroid.
ANACAINE. (Gordon) Benzocaine 10%. Jar. 1 oz., 1 lb.
Use: Anesthetic, antiseptic.
ANACEL. (Softcon) Tetracaine HCl ½%,
w/Methulose (methylcellulose), preservative-ben-
zalkonium chloride 1:10,000, & sod. chloride.
Plastic containers 15 cc.
Use: Topical anesthetic in ophthalmology.
ANACIN-3 CHILDREN'S. (Whitehall) Acetaminophen.
Elixir: 160 mg./5 ml. Bot. 2 oz., 4 oz. **Chewable
Tab.:** 80 mg./Tab. Bot. 30s.
Use: Analgesic.
ANACIN-3 INFANTS. (Whitehall) Acetaminophen 80
mg./0.8 ml. Bot. 0.5 oz.
Use: Analgesic.
ANACIN-3 REGULAR STRENGTH. (Whitehall) Acet-
aminophen 325 mg./Tab. Bot. 24s, 50s, 100s.
Use: Analgesic.
ANACIN-3 WITH CODEINE. (Ayerst) Acetaminophen
and codeine phosphate in 3 strengths:
acetaminophen 325 mg., codeine phosphate 15
mg.; or acetaminophen 300 mg., codeine 30 mg.;
or acetaminophen 300 mg. codeine phosphate 60
mg./Tab. Bot. 100s.
Use: Aspirin-free analgesic, antipyretic, antitussive.
ANACIN CAPSULES. (Whitehall) Aspirin 400 mg.,
caffeine 32 mg./Cap. Bot. 20s, 40s, 75s, 125s.
Use: Analgesic.
ANACIN MAXIMUM STRENGTH. (Whitehall) Aspirin
500 mg., caffeine 32 mg. **Tab.:** Bot. 12s, 20s, 40s,
75s, 150s. **Cap.:** 30s, 60s.
Use: Analgesic.
ANACIN-3 MAXIMUM STRENGTH. (Whitehall)
Acetaminophen 500 mg., **Cap.:** 36s, 72s. **Tab.:** Tins
12s. Bot. 20s, 40s, 75s, 150s.
Use: Analgesic.
ANACIN TABLETS. (Whitehall) Aspirin 400 mg.,
caffeine 32 mg./Tab. Tins 12s. Bot. 30s, 50s, 100s,
200s, 300s.
Use: Analgesic.
ANADROL-50. (Syntex) Oxymetholone 50 mg./Tab.
Bot. 100s.
Use: Anabolic steroid therapy.
ANAFEBRINA.
See: Aminopyrine. (Various Mfr.)

ANAFED. (Everett) **Cap.:** Chlorpheniramine maleate 8 mg., pseudoephedrine HCl 120 mg./T.R. Cap. Bot.100s. **Liq.:** Chlorpheniramine maleate 2 mg., pseudoephedrine HCl 30 mg./5 ml. Bot. pt.
Use: Antihistamine, decongestant.

ANAFER. (British Drug House) Ferrous sulfate 200 mg., Vit. C 10 mg., menadione as diacetyl derivative 1.5 mg./Tab. Bot. 100s, 1000s.
Use: Treatment of iron-deficiency anemia.

ANAFLEX. Polynoxylin, B.A.N.

ANAFRANIL. (Geigy). Under study.
See: Clomipramine HCl

• **ANAGESTONE ACETATE.** USAN. 17-Hydroxy-6α-methylpregn-4-en-20-one acetate.
See: Progestin

• **ANAGRELIDE HYDROCHLORIDE.** USAN.
Use: Antithrombotic.

ANAIDS. (O'Neal, Jones & Feldman) Calcium carbonate 300 mg., sodium phenobarbital 9 mg./Tab. Bot. 100s.
Use: Stomach disorders.

ANA-KIT. (Hollister-Stier) Two dose syringe which allows administration of two measured doses 0.3 ml. each, of epinephrine; four Chol-Amine tablets, each 2 mg. chlorpheniramine maleate; two sterilized swabs, tourniquet, instructions/kit.
Use: For severe potentially anaphylactic insect stings.

ANALATE. (Winston) Magnesium salicylate 600 mg./Tab. Bot. 100s.
Use: Analgesic.

ANALBALM. (Central) Methyl salicylate 5%, menthol 0.55%, camphor 2.75%. Liq. Bot. 4 oz., pt., gal. Green or pink.
Use: Topically, counterirritant to reduce inflammation.

■ **ANALEPTICS.** Usually a term applied to agents with stimulant action particularly on the central nervous system. See also central nervous system stimulants.
See: Amphetamine salts (Various Mfr.)
    Coramine, Amp. Liq. (Ciba)
    Cylert, Tab. (Abbott)
    Deaner, Tab. (Riker)
    Dextroamphetamine salts (Various Mfr.)
    Dopram, Vial (Robins)
    Ephedrine Salts (Various Mfr.)
    Methamphetamine salts (Various Mfr.)
    Metrazol, Amp. (Knoll)
    Nikethamide (Various Mfr.)
    Pentylenetetrazol (Various Mfr.)
    Picrotoxin, Amp. (Various Mfr.)
    Ritalin HCl, Tab. (Ciba)
    Sodium Succinate (Various Mfr.)

ANALGESIC BALM. (Various Mfr.) Menthol w/methyl salicylate in a suitable base.
A.P.C., 1½ oz., 1 lb.
Fougera, 1 oz.
Horton & Converse, 1 oz., 1 lb.
Lilly, 1 oz., 1 lb.
Musterole (Plough)

Stanlabs, 1 oz., pt.
Wisconsin, 1 lb., 5 lb.

ANALGESIC LINIMENT. (C.M.C.) Methyl nicotinate, methyl salicylate, dipropylene glycol salicylate, menthol, camphor, oil of cassia, oleoresins, capsicum, ginger. Plastic Bot. 4 oz.

ANALGESIC LOTION. (Weeks & Leo) Methyl nicotinate 1%, methyl salicylate 10%, camphor 0.1%, menthol 0.1%. Bot. 4 oz.
Use: Relief of symptomatic pain of muscular pain, sprains, & arthritis.

ANALGESIC LIQUID. (Weeks & Leo) Triethanolamine salicylate 10% in an alcohol base. Bot. 4 oz.
Use: Relief for sore aching muscles, neuralgia, arthritis.

ANALGESIC OINTMENT "LANNETT". (Lannett) Camphor, menthol syn., methyl salicylate in lanolin petrolatum base. Tube 1 oz., Jar 1 lb., 5 lb.

ANALGESICS.
See preparations of: Acetanilid-type, Antipyrine-type, Aspirin, Salicylamide.

ANALGESINE.
See: Antipyrine (Various Mfr.)

ANALGETS. (Vale) Aspirin 64.8 mg., magnesium trisilicate 64.8 mg./Tab. Bot. 100s, 1000s, 5000s.
Use: Analgesic.

ANALGIC-C. (Kenyon) Salicylamide 250 mg., acetaminophen 250 mg., ascorbic acid 25 mg./Tab. Bot. 100s, 1000s.
Use: Analgesic.

ANALUCIN. (Lincoln) Pentetrazol 100 mg./cc. Vial 10 cc.
Use: I.M., Subcut. Senile confusion.

ANAMINE T.D. CAPSULES. (Mayrand) Chlorpheniramine maleate 8 mg., pseudoephedrine HCl 20 mg./T.D. Cap. Bot. 100s.

ANAMINE SYRUP. (Mayrand) Chlorpheniramine maleate 2 mg., pseudoephedrine HCl 30 mg./5 cc. Bot. pt.

ANANASE. (Rorer) Bromelains 50,000 u./Tab. Bot. 100s, 500s. 100,000 u./Tab. Bot. 100s, 500s.
Use: Inflammation and edema treatment.

ANAPAP. (Fellows) Acetaminophen 325 mg./Tab. Bot. 100s, 1000s.
Use: Analgesic.

ANAPOLON. Oxymetholone, B.A.N.

ANAPREL. Rescinnamine, B.A.N.

ANAPROTIN. Stanolone, B.A.N.

ANAPROX. (Syntex) Naproxen sodium 275 mg./Tab. Bot. 100s, 500s. Blister pkg. 100s.
Use: Analgesic.

ANAREL. Guanadrel sulfate.

ANAROL. (Kenyon) Acetaminophen 120 mg./5 cc. Bot. 4 oz.
Use: Analgesic, antipyretic.

ANASPAZ. (Ascher) l-Hyoscyamine sulfate 0.125 mg./Tab. Bot. 100s, 500s.
Use: Antispasmodic, anticholinergic therapy for the hyperactive G.I. tract.

ANASPAZ PB. (Ascher) l-Hyoscyamine sulfate 0.125 mg., phenobarbital 15.0 mg./Tab. Bot. 100s, 500s.

Use: Antispasmodic, anticholinergic therapy with sedative for the hyperactive G.I. tract.
ANATUSS SYRUP. (Mayrand) Acetaminophen 130 mg., dextromethorphan HBr 5 mg., phenylephrine HCl 5 mg., phenylpropanolamine HCl 12.5 mg., chlorpheniramine maleate 2 mg., guaifenesin 25 mg./5 cc w/alcohol 12%. Bot. 4 oz., pt.
Use: Decongestant.
ANATUSS TABS. (Mayrand) Guaifenesin 50 mg., acetaminophen 300 mg., dextromethrorphan HBr 10 mg., phenylephrine HCl 5 mg., phenylpropanolamine HCl 25 mg., chlorpheniramine maleate 2 mg./Tab. Bot. 100s, 500s.
Use: Relief of cough.
ANAVAR. (Searle) Oxandrolone. 2.5 mg./Tab. Bot. 100s.
Use: Anabolic agent.
ANAYODIN.
See: Chiniofon
ANAZOLE TABLETS. (Winthrop Products) Stanozolol.
Use: Anabolic steroid.
• **ANAZOLENE SODIUM.** USAN. 4-[(4-Anilino-5-sulfo-1-naphthyl)azo]-5-hydroxy-2,7-naphthalenedisulfonic acid trisodium salt. (2) C.I. acid blue 92 trisodium salt. Sodium Anoxynaphthonate, B.A.N.
Use: Diagnostic aid (blood volume and cardiac output).
See: Coomassie Blue (Ayerst)
ANBESOL GEL. (Whitehall) Benzocaine 6.3%, phenol 0.5%, alcohol 70%. Tube 0.25 oz.
Use: Antiseptic, anesthetic.
ANBESOL LIQUID. (Whitehall) Benzocaine 6.3%, phenol 0.5%, povidone-iodine 0.04%, alcohol 70%. Bot. 0.31 oz., 0.74 oz.
Use: Antiseptic, anesthetic.
ANCARIS. Thenium Closylate, B.A.N.
ANCEF. (SmithKline) Cefazolin sodium. **Vials** equivalent to 250 mg., 500 mg., 1 Gm. of cefazolin; **Multi Packs:** 500 mg., 1 Gm./Pack. 25s.; **Bulk Vials:** 5 Gm., 10 Gm.; **Piggyback Vials:** 500 mg., 1 Gm./100 ml.
Use: Bactericidal.
ANCID TABLET AND SUSPENSION. (Sheryl) Calcium aluminum carbonate, di-amino acetate complex. Tab. 100s, Susp. 1 pt.
Use: Antacid.
ANCOBON. (Roche) Flucytosine 250 mg., 500 mg./Cap. Bot. 100s.
Use: Serious candida and/or Cryptococcus infections.
ANCOLAN DIHYDROCHLORIDE. Meclozine, B.A.N.
ANCOLOXIN. Meclozine, B.A.N.
• **ANCROD.** USAN. An active principle obtained from the venom of the Malayan pitviper Agkistrodon rhodostoma.
Use: Anticoagulant.
See: Arvin
ANDESTERONE SUSPENSION. (Lincoln) Estrone 2 mg., testosterone 6 mg./cc. Vial 15 cc. **Forte:** Estrone 1 mg., Testosterone 20 mg./cc. Inj. vial 15 cc.
Use: I.M. hormone therapy.
ANDOIN. (Ulmer) Allantoin 1% w/vitamin A & D in

ointment base. 1 oz., 1 lb.
Use: Topically, stimulates granulation.
ANDRENEX. (Pasadena Research) Adrenal cortex w/biological activity equiv. to hydrocortisone acetate 100 or 200 mcg./cc. Vial 10 cc., 30 cc.
Use: Hypoadrenal conditions.
ANDREST 90–4. (Seatrace) Testosterone enanthate 90 mg., estradiol valerate 4 mg./ml. Vial 10 cc.
ANDRIOL INJECTION. (Reid-Provident) Methandriol dipropionate 50 mg./cc. Vial 10 cc.
Use: Treatment of senile and postmenopausal osteoporosis.
ANDRO 100. (O'Neal, Jones & Feldman) Testosterone 100 mg./ml. Vial 10 ml.
ANDRO L.A. 200. (O'Neal, Jones & Feldman) Testosterone enanthate 200 mg./ml. Vial 10 ml.
ANDRO-CYP 100. (Keene) Testosterone cypionate 100 mg./ml. Bot. 10 ml.
Use: I.M. long acting androgen therapy.
ANDRO-CYP 200. (Keene) Testosterone cypionate 200 mg./ml. Bot. 10 ml.
Use: I.M. long acting androgen therapy.
ANDRO FEM. (Pasadena Research) Testosterone cypionate 50 mg., estradiol cypionate 2 mg., chlorobutanol 0.5%, cotton seed oil./ml. Vial ml.
Use: Menopause; osteoporosis.
ANDROGEN-860 INJECTION. (Blue Line) Testosterone cypionate 100 mg., benzyl alcohol 0.9% in cottonseed oil/cc. Vial 10 cc.
■ **ANDROGENS.** Substances which possess masculinizing activities.
See: Methyltestosterone
Testosterone
Testosterone cyclopentylpropionate
Testosterone enanthate
Testosterone heptanoate
Testosterone phenylacetate
Testosterone propionate
■ **ANDROGEN-ESTROGEN THERAPY.**
See: Dienestrol with Methyltestosterone
Duomed-P.A., Vial (Medics)
Estradiol Esters with Methyltestosterone
Estradiol Esters with Testosterone
Estrogenic Substance, Conjugated with Methyltestosterone
Estrogenic Substance Mixed with Methyltestosterone
Estrogenic Substance Mixed with Testosterone
Estrone with Testosterone
Gynetone, Tab. (Schering)
ANDROGYN L.A. (O'Neal, Jones & Feldman) Testosterone enanthate 90 mg., estradiol valerate 4 mg./ml. in sesame oil. Vial 10 ml.
ANDROID-5, 10 and 25. (Brown) Methyltestosterone 5 mg./Buccal Tab., 10 mg./Tab. & 25 mg./Tab. Bot. 60s, 250s.
Use: Impotence due to androgenic deficiency.
ANDROID-F. (Brown) Fluoxymeterone 10 mg./Tab. Bot. 60s.
Use: Impotence due to androgenic deficiency, prevention postpartum breast pain and engorgement.

ANDROID HCG. (Brown) Human chorionic gonadotropin 10,000 u. w/diluent. Vial 10 cc.
ANDROID-T. (Brown) Testosterone 50 mg., 100 mg./cc. Aq. susp. Vial 10 cc.
ANDROLAN AQUEOUS. (Lannett) Testosterone 25 mg., 50 mg., 100 mg./cc. susp. Vials 10 cc.
Use: I.M., androgen therapy.
ANDROLAN IN OIL. (Lannett) Testosterone propionate 25 mg., 50 mg., 100 mg./cc. in oil. Vials 10 cc.
Use: I.M. androgen therapy.
ANDROLIN. (Lincoln) Testosterone 100 mg./cc. Vial 10 cc.
Use: I.M., androgen therapy.
ANDROLONE. (Keene) Nandrolone phenpropionate 25 mg./ml. in sesame oil. Vial 5 ml.
Use: Anabolic agent.
ANDROLONE 50. (Keene) Nandrolone phenpropionate 50 mg./ml. in sesame oil. Vial 2 ml.
Use: Prolonged anabolic stimulation.
ANDROLONE-D 50. (Keene) Nandrolone decanoate 50 mg./ml. in sesame oil. Vial 2 ml.
Use: I.M. anabolic maintenance.
ANDROLONE-D 100. (Keene) Nandrolone decanoate 100 mg./ml. in sesame oil. Vial 2 ml.
Use: I.M. anabolic maintenance.
ANDRONAQ-50. (Central) Testosterone 50 mg., sodium carboxymethylcellulose 2 mg., methylcellulose 0.3 mg., povidone 0.3 mg., docusate sodium 0.15 mg., thimerosal 0.08 mg./ml. Vial 10 ml. Box 12s.
Use: I.M., androgen therapy.
ANDRONATE. (Pasadena Research) Testosterone cypionate 100 mg., 200 mg., benzyl alcohol 9 mg./cc. 200 mg. also contains benzyl benzoate 0.2 cc., in cotton seed oil. Multi Dose Vial 10 cc.
Use: Androgen therapy.
ANDRONE. (Rocky Mtn.) Testosterone 25 mg., estrone 2 mg./cc. Vial 10 cc.
ANDRONEX. (Tunex) Methandriol dipropionate 50 mg./ml. Vial 10 cc.
Use: Treatment of senile and post menopausal osteoporosis.
ANDROSTALONE. Mestanolone, B.A.N.
ANDROSTANAZOLE.
See: Stanozolol.
ANDROSTANE-17-(beta)-ol-3one.
See: Stanolone
ANDROSTANOLONE. (I.N.N.) Stanolone.
ANDROST-4-EN-3-ONE, 17-(3-CYCLOPENTYL-1-OXOPROPOXY)-,(17β)-. Testosterone Cypionate, U.S.P. XXI.
ANDROST-4-EN-3-ONE,9-FLUORO-11,17-DIHYDROXY-17-METHYL-,(11β,17β)-. Fluoxymesterone, U.S.P. XXI.
ANDROST-4-EN-3-ONE,17-HYDROXY-17-METHYL-,(17β)-. Methyltesterone, U.S.P. XXI.
ANDROST-4-EN-3-ONE,17-(1-OXOHEPTYL)-OXY-,(17β)-. Testosterone Enanthate, U.S.P. XXI.
ANDROSTENOPYRAZOLE. Anabolic steroid; pending release.

ANDROTEST P.
See: Testosterone Propionate.
ANDRYL. (Keene) Testosterone enanthate, 200 mg./ml. Vial 10 ml.
Use: Androgen.
ANDURACAINE. (Reid-Provident) Procaine base 1.25%, isobutyl-p-aminobenzoate 4.16% in almond oil, benzyl alcohol 4.16%. Vial 5 cc.
Use: Rectal anesthetic.
ANDYLATE FORTE. (Vita Elixir) Acetaminophen 3 gr., salicylamide 3 gr., caffeine ¼ gr./Tab.
Use: Antipyretic, analgesic, circulatory stimulant.
ANDYLATE RUB. (Vita Elixir) Methylnicotinate, methylsalicylate, camphor, dipropyleneglycol salicylate, oil of cassia, oleoresion of capsicum, oleoresin of ginger.
Use: Temporary relief of minor aches and pain.
ANDYLATE TABLETS. (Vita Elixir) Sodium salicylate 10 gr.
Use: Antipyretic, analgesic.
ANECAL CREAM. (Lannett) Benzocaine 3%, calamine 5%, zinc oxide 5%. Jar 1 lb.
ANECTINE. Suxamethonium Chloride, B.A.N.
ANECTINE. (Burroughs Wellcome) Succinylcholine chloride. Sterile Sol. (20 mg./ml.) 10 ml. Vials multiple dose Sterile Pow. Flo-Pak. 500 or 1000 mg. Box 12s.
Use: I.V., short-acting skeletal muscle relaxant.
ANEFRIN NASAL SPRAY. (Walgreen) Phenylephrine HCl 0.5%, pheniramine maleate 0.2%. Bot. 0.5 oz.
Use: Antihistaminic, decongestant.
ANEFRIN NASAL SPRAY, LONG ACTING. (Walgreen) Oxymetazoline 0.05%. Bot. 0.5 oz.
Use: Relief of nasal congestion.
ANELEP-O.D. (Trimen) Phenytoin 250 mg./Cap. Bot. 100s.
Use: Anticonvulsant in epilepsy.
ANERGAN 25. (O'Neal, Jones & Feldman) Promethazine HCl 25 mg./ml. Vial 10 ml.
ANERGAN 50. (O'Neal, Jones & Feldman) Promethazine HCl 50 mg./ml. Vial 10 ml.
ANERTAN.
See: Testosterone Propionate.
ANESTACON. (Webcon) Lidocaine HCl 20 mg./ml. Bot. 15 ml. 12s., 240 ml.
Use: Anesthesia of urethral mucosa.
ANESTHESIN. Ethyl-p-aminobenzoate.
Use: Local anesthetic.
See: Benzocaine, U.S.P. XXI.
ANETHAINE.
See: Pontocaine Hydrochloride (Winthrop-Breon)
• **ANETHOLE,** N.F. XVI. p-Propenylanisole. Benzene, 1-methoxy-4-(1-propenyl)-.
Use: Flavor.
ANEURINE HYDROCHLORIDE.
See: Thiamine HCl, Prep.
(Various Mfr.)
ANEXSIA W/CODEINE. (Beecham Labs) Codeine phosphate 30 mg., aspirin 225 mg., phenacetin 160 mg., caffeine 32 mg./Tab. Bot. 100s, 1000s.
Use: Analgesic.
ANEXSIA-D. (Beecham Labs) Hydrocodone bitartrate 7

37

ANISOTROPINE METHYLBROMIDE

mg., phenacetin 150 mg., aspirin 230 mg., caffeine 30 mg./Tab. Bot. 100s, 1000s.
Use: Analgesic.
ANGEL SWEET. (Garrett) Cosmetic topical aerosol cream of Vitamins A and D-2. 90 Gm.
Use: Protective cream.
ANGEN. (Davis & Sly) Estrone 2 mg., testosterone 25 mg./cc. Aq. susp. Vial 10 cc.
Use: S. C., estrogen and androgen therapy.
ANGERIN. (Kingsbay) Nitroglycerin 1 mg./Cap. Bot. 60s.
Use: Coronary vasodilator.
ANGEX. (Janssen) Lidoflazine.
Use: Coronary vasodilator.
ANGIJEN GREEN. (Jenkins) Pentaerythritol tetranitrate 10 mg., 20 mg./Tab. Bot. 1000s.
Use: Hypertension.
ANGIJEN S.C. SALMON. (Jenkins) Pentaerythritol tetranitrate 10 mg., phenobarbital 8 mg./Tab. Bot. 1000s.
ANGIJEN NO. 1. (Jenkins) Pentaerythritol tetranitrate 20 mg., phenobarbital 15. mg./Tab. Bot. 1000s.
Use: Hypertension.
ANGIL. (Kenyon) Pentaerythritol tetranitrate 10 mg., mephobarbital ¼ gr., phenobarbital ⅛ gr./Tab. Bot. 100s, 1000s.
Use: Vasodilation.
ANGINAR. (Pasadena Research) Erythrityl tetranitrate 10 mg./Tab. Bot. 100s, 1000s. 15 mg./Tab. Bot. 100s. 10 mg. w/Phenobarbital 15 mg./Tab. Bot. 100s.
Use: Prophylaxis and long term treatment of angina pectoris.
ANGIO-CONRAY. (Mallinckrodt) Iothalamate sodium 80% Injection. Vial 50 ml., Pkg. 10s, 50s.
Use: Radiopaque medium.
ANGIOGRAPHIN. Diatrizoic Acid, B.A.N.
ANGIOTENSIN AMIDE. B.A.N. Val⁵-hypertensin II-Asp-β-amide.
Use: Hypertensive.
See: Hypertensin (Ciba)
• **ANGIOTENSIN AMIDE.** USAN. 1-L-asparaginyl-5-L-valyl angiotensin octapeptide. 1L-asparagine-5-L-Valine angiotensin.
ANGIOTENSIN IMMUTOPE KIT I-125. (Squibb) 200 test kits.
Use: Diagnostic-radioimmunoassay.
ANGIOVIST 282. (Berlex) Diatrizoate meglumine 600 mg., edetate calcium 0.1 mg./ml. Vial 50 ml., 100 ml., or 150 ml. Box 10s.
Use: Diagnostic radiopaque medium for parenteral use.
ANGIOVIST 292. (Berlex) Diatrizoate meglumine 520 mg., diatrizoate sodium 80 mg., edetate calcium disodium 0.1 mg./ml. Vial 30 ml., 50 ml., or 100 ml. Box 10s.
Use: Diagnostic radiopaque medium for parenteral use.
ANGIOVIST 370. (Berlex) Diatrizoate meglumine 660 mg., diatrizoate sodium 100 mg., edetate calcium disodium 0.1 mg./ml. Vial 50 ml., 100 ml., 150ml. or 200 ml. Box 10s.

Use: Diagnostic radiopaque medium for parenteral use.
ANGITAB. (Moore Kirk) Pentaerythritol tetranitrate 10 mg., triple-barb (phentobarbital sod., butarbital sod., phenobarbital sod. each 33½%) 8 mg./Tab. Bot. 100s, 1000s.
Use: Coronary vasodilator to prevent attacks of angina pectoris.
ANGITRATE. (Moore Kirk) Pentaerythritol tetranitrate 10 mg., 20 mg./Tab. Bot. 100s, 1000s.
Use: Coronary vasodilator.
ANGOLON HYDROCHLORIDE. Imolamine, B.A.N.
ANG-O-SPAN. (Scrip) Nitroglycerin 2.5 mg./Cap. Bot.: 100s.
ANHYDROHYDROXYPROGESTERONE. Ethisterone.
Use: Corpus luteum hormone deficiency, threatened abortion.
ANHYDRON. (Lilly) Cyclothiazide 2 mg./Tab. Bot. 100s, 1000s.
Use: Diuretic.
• **ANIDOXIME.** USAN. 3-Diethylaminopropiophenone-O-(p-methoxyphenylcarbamoyl)oxime.
Use: Analgesic.
See: Bamoxine (U.S.V. Pharm.)
A-NIL. (Vangard) Codeine phosphate 10 mg., bromodiphenydramine HC1 3.75 mg., diphenhydramine HCl 8.75 mg., ammonium chloride 80 mg., potassium guaiacolsulfonate 80 mg., menthol 0.5 mg./5 ml. w/alcohol 5%. Bot. Pts. Gal.
Use: Antitussive, expectorant.
• **ANILERIDINE,** U.S.P. XXI. Inj., U.S.P. XXI. 4-Piperidinecarboxylic acid, 1-[2-(4-aminophenyl)ethyl]-4-phenyl-ethyl ester. Ethyl 1-(p-amino-phenethyl)-4-phenylisonipecotate. Available as the phosphate salt for injection.
Use: Analgesic.
See: Leritine Injection (Merck Sharp & Dohme)
• **ANILERIDINE HCl,** U.S.P. XXI. Tab., U.S.P. XXI. 1-(4-aminophenethyl)-4-phenylisonipecotic acid ethyl ester.
Use: Analgesic.
See: Leritine HCl, Tab. (Merck Sharp & Dohme).
• **ANILOPAM HYDROCHLORIDE.** USAN.
Use: Analgesic.
ANION EXCHANGE RESINS.
See: Polyamine-Methylene Resin
• **ANIRACETAM.** USAN.
Use: Mental performance enhancer
• **ANISE OIL,** N.F. XVI.
Use: Flavor.
ANISINDIONE. 2-p-Anisyl indandione-1,3,2-(p-methoxyphenyl) indane-1,3-dione.
Use: Anticoagulant.
ANISINDIONE. B.A.N. 2-(4-Methoxyphenyl)-indane-1,3-dione. Miradon.
Use: Anticoagulant.
ANISOPYRADAMINE.
See: Pyrilamine Maleate
• **ANISOTROPINE.** F.D.A. Tropine 2-propylvalerate.
• **ANISOTROPINE METHYLBROMIDE.** USAN. Octatropine Methylbromide, B.A.N. 2-Propyl-pentan-

oyl tropinium methylbromide. 8-Methyltropinium bromide 2 Propylvalerate.
Use: Anticholinergic.
See: Valpin 50, Tab. (Du Pont)
W/Phenobarbital.
See: Valpin 50-PB, Tab. (Du Pont)
2-p-ANISYLINDANDIONE-1,3.
See: Miradon, Tabs. (Schering)
• **ANITRAZAFEN.** USAN.
Use: Anti-inflammatory.
ANOCAINE. (Mallard) Benzocaine, zinc oxide, bismuth subgallate, boric acid, peruvian balsam/Supp. Box 12s.
ANODYNINE. Antipyrine
ANODYNON.
See: Ethyl Chloride
ANODYNOS. (Buffington) Aspirin, salicylamide, acetaminophen, caffeine/Tab. Sugar and salt free. Dispens-A-Kit 500s. Bot. 100s, 500s.
Use: Analgesic, antipyretic, and anti-inflammatory.
ANODYNOS-DHC TABLETS. (Berlex) Hydrocodone bitartrate 5 mg., aspirin 230 mg., acetaminophen 150 mg., caffeine 30 mg./Tab. Bot. 100s.
Use: Narcotic, analgesic, antitussive.
ANODYNOS FORTE. (Buffington) Chlorpheniramine maleate, phenylephrine HCl, salicylamide, acetaminophen, caffeine/Tab. Dispens-A-Kit 500s. Bot. 100s.
Use: Decongestant, antipyretic, antihistaminic and analgesic for treatment of cold, hay fever and sinusitis relief.
ANOQUAN. (Mallard) Butalbital 50 mg., caffeine 40 mg., acetaminophen 325 mg./Cap. Bot. 100s, 1000s.
Use: Analgesic-sedative.
ANOREX. (Dunhall) Phendimetrazine 35 mg./Tab. Bot. 100s.
Use: Anorectic.
■ **ANOREXIGENIC AGENTS.** Appetite depressants.
See: Amphetamine Preps.
Didrex, Tab. (Upjohn)
Plegine, Tab. (Ayerst)
Preludin HCl (Boehringer Ingelheim)
Sanorex, Tab. (Sandoz)
Tenuate (Merrell Dow)
Tepanil, Tab. (Riker)
Wilpo, Tab. (Dorsey)
ANOVLAR. Norethindrone plus ethinylestradiol.
Use: Oral contraceptive.
• **ANOXOMER.** USAN.
Use: Pharmaceutic aid.
ANOXYNAPHTHONATE SODIUM. Anazolene Sodium.
ANQUIL. Benperidol, B.A.N.
ANSPOR. (SmithKline) Cephradine (a semisynthetic cephalosporin) **Caps.** 250 mg./Cap. Bot. 100s. Unit dose 100s. 500 mg./Cap. Bot. 20s, 100s. Unit dose 100s. **Oral Susp.** 125 mg., and 250 mg./5 ml. Bot. 100 ml.
Use: Antibiotic therapy.
ANTABUSE. (Ayerst) Disulfiram 250 mg./Tab. Bot. 100s; 500 mg./Tab. Bot. 50s, 1000s.

Use: Orally, in alcoholism.
ANTACID. (Zenith) Aluminum hydroxide 3¾ gr., Mg trisilicate 7.5 gr./Tab. Bot. 100s.
Use: Antacid.
ANTACID # 2. (Richlyn) Calcium carbonate 5½ gr., magnesium carbonate 2½ gr./Tab. Bot. 100s.
Use: Antacid.
ANTACID NO. 6. (Bowman) Ca carbonate 0.42 Gm., glycine 0.18 Gm./Tab. Bot. 100s.
ANTACID M. (Walgreen) Calcium carbonate 300 mg./Tab. Bot. 100s.
Use: Relief of heartburn, sour stomach and/or acid indigestion.
ANTACID M LIQUID. (Walgreen) Aluminum oxide 0.2 g., magnesium hydroxide 0.1 g/1 Tsp. Bot. 12 oz.
Use: Antacid.
ANTACID PH TABS. (Towne) Calcium carbonate 250 mg., aminoacetic acid 150 mg./Tab. Bot. 100s.
ANTACID POWDER. (DeWitt) Bot. 4 oz.
Use: For heartburn and acid indigestion.
ANTACID RELIEF TABLETS. (Walgreen) Dihydroxyaluminum sodium carbonate 334 mg./Tab. Bot. 75s.
Use: Relief of acid indigestion, heartburn.
ANTACID TABLETS. (Sutliff & Case) Ca carbonate 0.42 Gm., glycine 0.18 Gm./Chewable Tab. Bot. 100s, 1000s.
ANTACID TABLETS. (Reid-Provident) Magnesium trisilicate 3 gr., calcium carbonate 2 gr., glycine 3 gr./Tab.
■ **ANTACIDS.** A drug that neutralizes excess gastric acid.
See: Alka-Seltzer, Tab. (Miles)
Alka-Seltzer Plus, Tab. (Miles)
Alka-Seltzer Special Effervescent Antacid, Tab. (Miles)
Alka-2 Chewable Antacid, Tab. (Miles)
Aluminum Hydroxide Gel (Various Mfr.)
Aluminum Hydroxide Gel W/Combinations (Various Mfr.)
Aluminum Hydroxide Gel Dried (Various Mfr.)
Aluminum Hydroxide Gel Dried W/Combinations (Various Mfr.)
Aluminum Hydroxide Magnesium Carbonate, Tab. (Various Mfr.)
Aluminum Phosphate Gel (Wyeth)
Aluminum Proteinate, Tab. (Rowell)
Amitone, Tab. (Norcliff Thayer)
Calcium Carbonate, Precipitated (Various Mfr.)
Calcium Carbonate Tablets (Various Mfr.)
Carbamine (Key Pharm.)
Ceo-Two, Supp. (Beutlich)
Chooz, Gum Tab. (Plough)
Citrocarbonate, Liq. (Upjohn)
Dicarbosil, Tab. (Arch)
Di-Gel, Liq., Tab. (Plough)
Dihydroxyaluminum Aminoacetate (Various Mfr.)
Dihydroxyaluminum Sodium Carbonate, Tab. (Warner-Lambert)
Magaldrate, Tab., Susp. (Ayerst)
Magnesium Carbonate (Various Mfr.)
Magnesium Glycinate, Tab. (Various Mfr.)

Magnesium Hydroxide (Various Mfr.)
Magnesium Oxide, Tab., Cap. (Various Mfr.)
Magnesium Trisilicate (Various Mfr.)
Neutralox, Susp. (Lemmon)
Oxaine, Susp. (Wyeth)
Ratio, Tab. (Adria)
Rolaids, Tab. (Warner-Lambert)
Romach, Tab. (ROR Pharmacal)
Sodium Bicarbonate, Inj., Tab. (Various Mfr.)
Tums, Tab. (Norcliff Thayer)

ANTACID SPECIAL NO. 1. (Jenkins) Mg carbonate 3 gr., Ca carbonate 2 gr., bismuth subcarbonate 1 gr., cerium oxalate ½ gr./Tab. Bot. 1000s.

ANTACID TABLETS. (Panray) Mg trisilicate 500 mg., aluminum hydroxide gel 250 mg./Tab. Bot. 500s, 1000s.

ANTACID W/PHENOBARBITAL. (Archer-Taylor) Mg hydroxide 0.3 Gm., Ca carbonate 9.3 Gm., atropine 0.2 mg., phenobarbital 8 mg./Tab. Bot. 1000s.
Use: Antacid and sedative.

ANTA GEL. (Blue Cross) Aluminum hydroxide 200 mg., magnesium hydroxide 200 mg., simethicone 20 mg./5 ml. Bot. 12 oz.
Use: Antacid, antiflatulant.

ANTA-GEL II. (Blue Cross) Aluminum hydroxide 400 mg., magnesium hydroxide 400 mg., simethicone 30 mg./5 ml. Bot. 12 oz.
Use: Antiflatulant, antacid.

■ **ANTAGONISTS OF CURARIFORM DRUGS.**
See: Neostigmine Methylsulfate
Tensilon Chloride (Roche)

ANTASTAN.
See: Antazoline Hydrochloride, U.S.P. XXI.

ANTAZOLINE. B.A.N. N-Phenylbenzylamino-methyl-2-imidazoline.
Use: Antihistamine.
See: Antistin
Histostab

ANTAZOLINE HYDROCHLORIDE. Antastan. 2(N-Benzylanilinomethyl)-2-imidazoline HCl.
See: Arithmin, Tab. (Lannett)

• **ANTAZOLINE PHOSPHATE,** U.S.P. XXI. 2-[(N-Benzylanilino)methyl]-2-imidazoline dihydrogen phosphate.
Use: Antihistaminic.
See: Arithmin, Inj. (Lannett)
W/Naphazoline, boric acid, phenylmercuric acetate sod. chloride, sod. carbonate anhydrous.
See: Vasocon-A Ophthalmic, Sol. (Smith, Miller & Patch)
W/Naphazoline HCl, polyvinyl alcohol.
See: Albalon-A Liquifilm, Ophth. Sol. (Allergan)

ANTEPAR. (Burroughs Wellcome) Piperazine citrate. **Syr.** equiv. to 100 mg. of piperazine hexahydrate/ml. Bot. 1 pt. **Tab.** (500 mg.) Bot. 100s.
Use: Orally; anthelmintic, to eradicate pinworms and roundworms.

ANTERIOR PITUITARY.
See: Pituitary, Anterior.

ANTHATEST. (Kay) Testosterone enanthate, oil sol. 200 mg./ml. Vial 10 ml.

Use: Testosterone supplement.

ANTHELMINTIC. A remedy for worms.
See: Alcopara, Granules (Burroughs Wellcome)
Antepar, Preps. (Burroughs Wellcome)
Antiminth, Susp. (Roerig)
Atabrine, Tab. (Winthrop-Breon)
Betanaphthol Benzoate (Various Mfr.)
Carbon Tetrachloride (Various Mfr.)
Gentian Violet
Hetrazan, Tab. (Lederle)
Jayne's PW Vermifuge (Glenbrook)
Jayne's RW, Tab. (Glenbrook)
Mintezol, Preps. (Merck Sharp & Dohme)
Piperazine Prep. (Various Mfr.)
Povan, Tab., Susp. (Parke-Davis)
Terramycin (Various Mfr.)
Tetrachloroethylene

■ **ANTHELMINTICS, VETERINARY USE.** (MSD AGVET)
See: Camvet (MSD AGVET)
Equizole (MSD AGVET)
Equizole A (MSD AGVET)
Equizole B (MSD AGVET)
Omnizole (MSD AGVET)
TBZ (MSD AGVET)
TBZ-2 (MSD AGVET)
TBZ-6 (MSD AGVET)
Thibenzole (MSD AGVET)
Thibenzole 100 (MSD AGVET)
Thibenzole 200 (MSD AGVET)

• **ANTHELMYCIN.** USAN.
Use: Anthelmintic.

ANTHELVET. Tetramisole HCl.

ANTHICAL. Mepyramine, B.A.N.

ANTHIPHEN. Dichlorophen, B.A.N.

ANTHISAN. Mepyramine, B.A.N.
See: Pyrilamine Maleate

ANTHRA-DERM. (Dermik) Anthralin 0.1%, 0.25%,0.-5%, 1.0% in petrolatum ointment base. Tube 1.5 oz.
Use: Psoriasis.

• **ANTHRALIN,** U.S.P. XXI. Ointment. U.S.P. XXI. 1,8,9-Anthracenetriol. Cignolin, Dithranol, Dihydroxy-Anthranol.
Use: Treatment of psoriasis.
See: Anthra-Derm Ointment (Dermik)
Lasan, Cream (Stiefel)
W/Mineral oil
See: Lasan Pomade (Stiefel)

ANTHRALIN PASTE 0.2%. (Durel) Anthralin 0.2%, salicylic acid 0.2%, paraffin 5.0%, Lassar's paste q.s. Jars 1 oz., 1 lb.
Use: Enzyme metabolism inhibition and reduction of mitotic turnover.

ANTHRALIN POMADE 0.4%. (Durel) Anthralin 0.4%, salicylic acid 0.4%, sodium lauryl sulfate, 2.1%, cetyl alcohol 21.9%, mineral oil q.s. Bot. 4 oz., 1 oz.
Use: Enzyme metabolism inhibition and reduction of mitotic turnover.

• **ANTHRAMYCIN.** USAN.
Use: Antineoplastic.

ANTHRAQUINONE OF CASCARA   40

ANTHRAQUINONE OF CASCARA.
See: Cascara Sagrada products

ANTIACID. (Hillcrest North) Aluminum hydroxide, Mg trisilicate, Ca carbonate. Tab. Bot. 100s.

ANTI-ACID NO. 1. (Vortech) Ca carbonate 3½ gr., Mg carbonate 2½ gr., bismuth subnitrate ½ gr., aromatics q.s./Tab. Bot. 100s, 1000s.
Use: Antacid.

ANTI-ALLERGY CAPSULES. (Robinson) Phenylephrine HCl 2.5 mg., phenylpropanolamine HCl 25 mg., pyrilamine maleate 10 mg., chlorpheniramine maleate 2 mg., phenylpyridine HCl 10 mg./Cap. Bot. 100s, 1000s.
Use: Antihistamine.

ANTI-ALLERGY TABLET. (Walgreen) Phenylpropanolamine HCl 18.7 mg., chlorpheniramine maleate 2 mg./Tab. Bot. 24s.
Use: Decongestant, antihistamine.

■ **ANTIARTHRITIC HORMONES.**
Alphadrol, Tab. (Upjohn)
Aristocort, Prep. (Lederle)
Celestone, Prep. (Schering)
Dexamethasone (Various Mfr.)
Fluprednisolone (Various Mfr.)
Haldrone, Tab. (Lilly)
Kenacort, Prep. (Squibb)
Medrol, Prep. (Upjohn)
Methylprednisolone, Prep. (Upjohn)
Prednisolone (Various Mfr.)
Prednisone (Various Mfr.)
Pregnenolone Acetate (Various Mfr.)
Thiodyne, Inj. (Savage)

ANTI-ASTHMA TABLETS. (Panray) Theophylline 130 mg., ephedrine HCl 25 mg., phenobarbital 8 mg./Tab. Bot. 1000s.

■ **ANTIASTHMATIC COMBINATIONS.**
See: Cromolyn Sodium, Cap. (Various Mfr.)
Decadron Respihaler, Aer. (Merck Sharp & Dohme)
Ephedrine HCl (Various Mfr.)
Ephedrine Sulfate (Various Mfr.)
Isoephedrine HCl (Various Mfr.)
Isoetharine (Winthrop-Breon)
Isoetharine HCl (Winthrop-Breon)
Isoetharine Mesylate (Winthrop-Breon)
Isoproterenol HCl (Various Mfr.)
Isoproterenol Sulfate (Various Mfr.)
Methoxyphenamine HCl (Various Mfr.)
Phenylephrine HCl (Various Mfr.)
Phenylpropanolamine HCl (Various Mfr.)
Pseudoephedrine HCl (Various Mfr.)
Racephedrine HCl (Various Mfr.)

ANTIASTHMATIC INHALANT.
See: AsthmaHaler (Norcliff Thayer)
AsthmaNefrin, Sol. (Norcliff Thayer)

ANTI-B. (Eckerd) Phenylephrine HCl 0.5%, pyrilamine maleate 0.5%. **Nasal Spray.** Xylometazoline HCl 0.1%. Bot. 20 cc., 40 cc. **Troches** cetylpyridinium Cl, benzocaine 10 mg., d-methorphan. Bot. 10s, 20s.
Use: Nasal decongestant.

ANTI-B MIST. (Eckerd) Phenylephrine HCl 0.5%, pyrilamine maleate 0.5%, cetalkonium chloride 0.02%, thimerosal 0.002%.

ANTIBACTERIAL SERUMS.
See: Hypertussis Serum
Influenzae Antihaemophilus Type B Serum

ANTIBASON.
See: Methylthiouracil (Various Mfr.)

ANTIBIOPTO. (Softcon) Chloramphenicol 0.5% **Ophthalmic soln.** Bot. 7.5 cc. **Sterile Ophthalmic Oint.** Chloramphenicol 10 mg. (1.0%) in a special base of liquid petrolatum and polyethylene/Gm. Tube 3.5 Gm.
Use: Antibiotic for eye infections.

■ **ANTIBIOTICS**
See: Amoxicillin (Various Mfr.)
Amphotericin B (Squibb)
Ampicillin (Various Mfr.)
Ampicillin Sodium (Various Mfr.)
Ampicillin Trihydrate (Various Mfr.)
Anspor, Cap., Susp. (SmithKline)
Bacitracin (Various Mfr.)
Benzathine Penicillin G (Various Mfr.)
Carbenicillin Disodium, Inj., (Various Mfr.)
Carbenicillin Idanyl Sodium, Tab. (Roerig)
Cefadroxil (Bristol, Mead Johnson)
Cefazolin Sodium, Vial (Various Mfr.)
Cephalexin (Lilly)
Cephalexin Monohydrate, Pulvule, Susp. (Lilly)
Cephaloglycin Dihydrate, Pulvule (Lilly)
Cephaloridine (Lilly)
Cephalothin, Sodium, Vial (Lilly)
Chloramphenicol (Various Mfr.)
Chloramphenicol Sodium Succinate, Inj. (Various Mfr.)
Chlortetracycline HCl (Lederle)
Clindamycin (Upjohn)
Cloxpan, Cap. (Beecham Labs)
Colistimethate Sodium, Inj. (Parke-Davis)
Colistin Sulfate, Ophth., Susp. (Various Mfr.)
Demecycline (Lederle)
Demethylchlortetracycline HCl (Lederle)
Dicloxacillin, Cap., Susp. (Various Mfr.)
Doxycycline (Various Mfr.)
Duricef, Cap. (Mead Johnson)
Erythromycin (Various Mfr.)
Erythromycin Ethylsuccinate (Abbott, Ross)
Erythromycin Lactobionate for Injection (Abbott)
Erythromycin Stearate, Tab. (Various Mfr.)
Flucytosine, Cap. (Roche)
Gentamicin Sulfate (Schering)
Griseofulvin, Tab., Susp. (Various Mfr.)
Griseofulvin Microcry., Tab., Cap. (Various Mfr.)
Hetacillin (Bristol-Myers)
Kanamycin Sulfate, Cap., Inj. (Bristol-Myers)
Ledercillin VK, Prod. (Lederle)
Lincomycin (Upjohn)
Methacycline HCl, Cap., Syr. (Wallace)
Methicillin Sodium, Vial, Pow. (Various Mfr.)
Minocycline, Cap. (Lederle)
Nafcillin, Sodium, Vial, Cap., Pow. (Wyeth)
NegGram, Prod. (Winthrop-Breon)
Nalidixic Acid, N.F.
Neomycin Sulfate, Tab., Sol. (Various Mfr.)
Novobiocin (Various Mfr.)
Novobiocin Calcium (Upjohn)

Novobiocin Sodium, Cap. (Upjohn)
Nystatin (Various Mfr.)
Oxacillin, Sodium (Various Mfr.)
Oxytetracycline (Pfizer)
Paromomycin, Cap., Syr. (Parke-Davis)
Penicillin G, Potassium (Various Mfr.)
Penicillin G, Potassium W/Comb. (Various Mfr.)
Penicillin G, Procaine (Various Mfr.)
Penicillin G, Procaine W/Comb. (Various Mfr.)
Penicillin G, Sodium (Various Mfr.)
Penicillin V Potassium (Various Mfr.)
Phenethicillin Potassium, Tab., Pow., Sol.
  (Various Mfr.)
Phenoxymethyl Penicillin (Various Mfr.)
Polymyxin B Sulfate (Various Mfr.)
Rifampin, Cap. (Various Mfr.)
Rolitetracycline (Various Mfr.)
Seromycin, Pulvule (Lilly)
Sodium Cloxacillin, Cap., Sol. (Bristol-Myers)
Streptomycin Sulfate (Various Mfr.)
Tetracycline (Various Mfr.)
Tetracycline HCl (Various Mfr.)
Tetracycline Phosphate Complex (Various Mfr.)
Triacetyloleandomycin (Various Mfr.)
Troleandomycin, Cap., Susp. (Various Mfr.)
Vancomycin HCl (Lilly)
■ **ANTIBIOTICS, VETERINARY USE.**
  See: Oxytetracycline (Merck Animal Health)
    Penstrep (Merck Animal Health)
    Pro-Penstrep (Merck Animal Health)
    Sulfastrep w/sulfonamides (Merck Animal
      Health)
    Tresaderm w/thiabendazole, dexamethasone &
      neomycin. (Merck Animal Health)
    Vetstrep (Merck Animal Health)
ANTICEPHALGICS. Agents used to prevent or cure a
  headache usually of the recurring type over the
  region of the external carotid artery.
  See: Cafergot, Supp., Tab. (Sandoz)
    DHE-45, Inj. (Sandoz)
    Gynergen, Amp., Tab. (Sandoz)
    Sansert, Tab. (Sandoz)
    Wigraine, Tab., Supp. (Organon)
ANTI-CHLOR. (Galen) Chlorprophenpyridamine male-
  ate 4 mg./Tab. Bot. 100s, 1000s.
  Use: Hay fever, urticaria, allergic eczema, drug
    sensitivity, serum sickness.
■ **ANTICHOLINERGIC AGENTS.** Parasympatholytic
  agents.
  See: Akineton (Knoll)
    Antrenyl Bromide (Ciba)
    Artane HCl (Lederle)
    Atropine preps.
    Banthine Bromide (Searle)
    Belladonna preps.
    Cantil Preps. (Merrell Dow)
    Cogentin (Merck Sharp & Dohme)
    Daricon, Tab. (Beecham Labs)
    Dicyclomine HCl (Various Mfr.)
    Disipal (Riker)
    Donabarb Sr., Cap. (Elder)
    Homatropine methylbromide
    Hybephen, Prods. (Beecham Labs)

Kemadrin, Tab. (Burroughs Wellcome)
Kinesed, Tab. (Stuart)
L-Hyoscyamine, Tab. (Kremers-Urban)
Murel, Amp. (Ayerst)
Norflex, Inj., Tab. (Riker)
Oxyphencyclimine HCl (Various Mfr.)
Pagitane HCl, Tab. (Lilly)
Pamine Bromide, Tab., Sol. (Upjohn)
Panparnit HCl
Parsidol HCl, Tab. (Parke-Davis)
Pathilon (Lederle)
Phenoxene HCl (Merrell Dow)
Prantal Methylsulfate, Tab. (Schering)
Pro-Banthine Bromide, Preps. (Searle)
Robinul, Tab., Inj. (Robins)
Scopolamine methylbromide
Scopolamine methylbromide HBr.
Spasmate, Tab. (Spencer-Mead)
Spasmolin, Tab., Cap. (Spencer-Mead)
Spasmolin TDC, Cap. (Spencer-Mead)
Tral, Preps. (Abbott)
Trihexyphenidyl HCl (Various Mfr.)
Trocinate, Tab. (Polythress)
Valpin 50, Tab. (Du Pont)
Valpin 50-PB, Tab. (Du Pont)
ANTICHOLINESTERASE TOXICITY ANTIDOTE.
  See: Protopam Chloride, vial (Ayerst)
• **ANTICOAGULANT CITRATE DEXTROSE
  SOLUTION,** U.S.P. XXI.
  Use: Anticoagulant for storage of whole blood.
  See: A.C.D. Solution. (Various Mfr.)
• **ANTICOAGULANT CITRATE PHOSPHATE
  DEXTROSE SOLUTION,** U.S.P. XXI.
  Use: Anticoagulant for storage of whole blood.
• **ANTICOAGULANT HEPARIN SOLUTION,** U.S.P.
  XXI.
  Use: Anticoagulant for storage of whole blood.
■ **ANTICOAGULANTS.**
  See: Acenocoumarin
    Anisindione
    Bishydroxycoumarin (Various Mfr.)
    Calciparine, Inj. (American Critical Care)
    Coumadin, Amp., Tab. (Du Pont)
    Depo-Heparin, Sod. (Upjohn)
    Dicumarol (Various Mfr.)
    Dipaxin, Tab. (Upjohn)
    Diphenadione
    Eridione, Tab. (Eric, Kirk & Gary)
    Ethyl Biscoumacetate, Tab.
    Hedulin, Tab. (Merrell Dow)
    Hemostatics
    Heparin, Sod. (Various Mfr.)
    Liquamar, Tab. (Organon)
    Liquaemin Sod., Vial (Organon)
    Miradon, Tab. (Schering)
    Panheprin, Amp., Vial (Abbott)
    Panwarfin, Tab. (Abbott)
    Phenindione, Tab. (Various Mfr.)
    Warfarin (Various Mfr.)
• **ANTICOAGULANT SODIUM CITRATE SOLUTION,**
  U.S.P. XXI. Anticoagulant (plasma and blood,
  fractionation).
■ **ANTICONVULSANTS.** Agents that inhibit muscular

spasms originating in the central nervous system.
See: Amytal Sodium, Ampul (Lilly)
  Celontin, Cap. (Parke-Davis)
  Depakene, Liq., Tab. (Abbott)
  Dilantin, Preps. (Parke-Davis)
  Gemonil, Tabs. (Abbott)
  Glutamic Acid (Various Mfr.)
  Luminal, Ovoids (Winthrop-Breon)
  Magnesium sulf.
  Mephobarbital
  Mesantoin, Tab. (Sandoz)
  Milontin, Cap. (Parke-Davis)
  Paradione, Cap., Sol. (Abbott)
  Peganone, Tab. (Abbott)
  Phenurone, Tab. (Abbott)
  Phenytoin, Susp., Tab. (Various Mfr.)
  Phenytoin Sodium, Cap. (Various Mfr.)
  Phenobarbital (Various Mfr.)
  Tegretol, Tab. (Geigy)
  Tridione, Cap., Dulcet, Sol., Tab. (Abbott)
  Valium, Tab. (Roche)
  Zarontin, Cap., Syrup (Parke-Davis)
■ **ANTIDEPRESSANTS.**
See: Amitid, Tab. (Squibb)
  Amitriptyline HCl (Various Mfr.)
  Aventyl HCl Pulv., Liq. (Lilly)
  Deaner, Tab. (Riker)
  Deprol, Tab., (Wallace)
  Desipramine HCl, Cap., Tab. (Var. Mfr.)
  Elavil Tab., Injection (Merck Sharp & Dohme)
  Imipramine HCl, Amp., Tab. (Var. Mfr.)
  Imipramine Pamoate, Cap. (Geigy)
  Marplan, Tab. (Roche)
  Mono-amine oxidase inhibitors
  Nardil, Tab. (Parke-Davis)
  Niamid, Tab. (Pfizer)
  Norpramin, Preps. (Merrell Dow)
  Pamelor, Cap., Liq. (Sandoz)
  Parnate Sulf., Tab. (SmithKline)
  Pertofrane, Cap. (USV)
  Presamine, Tab. (USV)
  Protriptyline HCl (Merck Sharp & Dohme)
  Ritalin, Tab., Vial (Ciba)
  Sinequan, Caps. (Pfizer)
  Tofranil, Amp., Tab. (Geigy)
  Tofranil-PM, Cap. (Geigy)
  Vivactil, Tab. (Merck Sharp & Dohme)
■ **ANTIDIARRHEICS.**
See: Attapulgite, Activated (Various Mfr.)
  B.K.Z., Elix., Tab. (Sutliff & Case)
  Cantil, Liq., Tab. (Merrell Dow)
  Coly-Mycin S, Oral Susp., (Parke-Davis)
  Corrective Mixture, Liq. (Beecham Labs)
  Corrective Mixture with Paregoric, Liq. (Beecham
    Labs)
  DIA-Quel Liq. (Inter. Pharm. Corp.)
  Diastay, Tab. (Elder)
  Diastop, Liq. (Elder)
  Diatrol, Tab. (Otis-Clapp)
  Donnagel, Susp. (Robins)
  Donnagel-PG (Robins)
  Furoxone Liq., Tab. (Eaton)

Homapin, Preps. (Mission)
Infatol Pink, Liq. (Scherer)
Kaolin (Various Mfr.)
Kaolin Colloidal (Various Mfr.)
Kaomin, Pow. (Lilly)
Kaopectate, Susp. (Upjohn)
Keotin, Susp. (Blue Line)
Lactinex, Tab., Granule (Hynson, Westcott &
  Dunning)
Lactobacillus acidophilus & *bulgaricus* mixed
  culture, Tab. (Hynson, Westcott & Dunning)
Lactobacillus acidophilus, viable culture (Various
  Mfr.)
Lomotil, Liq., Tab., (Searle & Co.)
Milk of Bismuth. (Various Mfr.)
Mycifradin Sulfate, Sol., Tab. (Upjohn)
Palsorb Improved, Liq. (Hauck)
Paocin, Susp. (Massengill)
Paregel, Liq. (Ferndale)
Parelixer, Liq. (Purdue-Fredericks)
Parepectolin, Susp. (Rorer)
Pectocel, Susp. (Lilly)
Pektamalt, Susp. (Warren-Teed)
Pepto-Bismol, Liq. & Tab. (Norwich)
Polymagma, Susp., Tab. (Wyeth)
Sorboquel, Tab. (Schering)
■ **ANTIDIURETICS.**
See: Pitressin, Amp. (Parke-Davis)
  Pitressin Tannate In Oil, Amp. (Parke-Davis)
  Pituitary Post. Inj. (Various Mfr.)
ANTIDOL. Ethosalamide, B.A.N.
ANTIDOTE, NARCOTIC.
See: Nalline Prods (Merck Sharp & Dohme)
■ **ANTIEMETICS.**
See: Antinauseants
ANTIEPILEPTIC AGENT.
See: Anticonvulsants
ANTIFEBRIN.
See: Acetanilid (Various Mfr.)
■ **ANTIFLATULENTS.**
See: Di-Gel, Prods. (Plough)
  Silain, Tab., Gel (Robins)
  Simethicone Prods.
ANTIFOAM A COMPOUND. (Merrell Dow)
Use: Antiflatulent.
See: Simethicone, U.S.P. XXI.
ANTIFOLIC ACID.
See: Methotrexate, Tab. (Lederle)
ANTIFORMIN. Alkaline solution of sod. hypochlorite
in sod. hydroxide 7.5%; available chlorine 5.2%;
may be colored with meta cresol purple.
■ **ANTIFUNGAL AGENTS.**
See: Fungicides
• **ANTIHEMOPHILIC FACTOR,** U.S.P. XXI. Human
antihemophilic factor. (Hyland & Alpha
Therapeutics) Antihemophilic Factor, human.
Method for Syringe Adm. 10 ml. 450 A.H.F. or 300
A.H.F. units/Pkg. W/Syringe 30 ml. or 900 A.H.F.
u/Pkg.
Use: Antihemophilic.
See: Factorate, Vial (Armour)
  Hemofil, Vial (Hyland)

Humafac, Vial (Parke-Davis)
Koate, Vial (Cutter)
ANTIHEPARIN. Protamine Sulfate.
ANTIHISTAMINE CREAM. (Towne) Methapyrilene
HCl 10 mg., pyrilamine maleate 5 mg., allantoin 2
mg., diperodon HCl 2.5 mg., benzocaine 10 mg.,
menthol 2 mg./Gm. Cream. Jar 2 oz.
Use: Skin rashes and itching.
■ **ANTIHISTAMINES.**
See: Actidil, Tab., Syr. (Burroughs Wellcome)
Ambodryl, Kapseal (Parke-Davis)
Benadryl HCl, Preps. (Parke-Davis)
Chlorpheniramine Maleate (Various Mfr.)
Chlorpheniramine Maleate W/Comb. (Various
Mfr.)
Clistin, Elix., Tabs. (McNeil)
Co-Pyronil, Pulvule, Susp. (Lilly)
Diafen, Tab. (Riker)
Dimetane, Preps. (Robins)
Diphenhydramine HCl (Various Mfr.)
Diphenylpyraline HCl (Various Mfr.)
Disophrol, Prod. (Schering)
Doxylamine Succinate (Merrell Dow)
Drixoral, Prod. (Schering)
Forhistal Maleate, Syr., Tab. (Ciba)
Inhiston, Tab. (Plough)
Methapyrilene Salts (Various Mfr.)
Novahistine LP, Tab. (Merrell Dow)
Optimine, Prod. (Schering)
PBZ, Tab. (Geigy)
PPZ-SR, Tab. (Geigy)
Periactin, Syr., Tab. (Merck Sharp & Dohme)
Promethazine HCl (Various Mfr.)
Prophenpyridamine Maleate (Various Mfr.)
Pyrilamine Maleate (Various Mfr.)
Tripelennamine HCl (Various Mfr.)
Triprolidine HCl (Various Mfr.)
■ **ANTIHYPERTENSIVES.**
See: Hypertension Therapy.
ANTI-ITCH CREAM. (Spencer-Mead) Burow's solution
5%, phenol 0.5%, menthol 0.5%, camphor 1% in
washable base. Tube 1 oz.
ANTI-ITCH CREAM. (Towne) Benzocaine 3%, pyrila-
mine maleate 1%, cetyldimethylbenzyl amm.
chloride 0.1%, methylparaben 0.1%, glycerin 5%,
lanolin 1%, greaseless base. Cream. Jar 2 oz.
ANTI-ITCH LOTION. (Towne) Diphenhydramine HCl
1%, pramoxine HCl 0.5%, titanium dioxide 1%, zinc
oxide 4%. Lot. Bot. 4 oz.
ANTILEPROTICS.
See: Hansen's Disease.
ANTILERGE. (Metz) Chlorpheniramine maleate 8 mg.,
phenylephrine HCl 12 mg./Tab. Bot. 30s.
Use: Antihistamine, decongestant.
ANTILEUKEMIA.
See: Antineoplastic Agents
ANTILIRIUM. (O'Neal, Jones & Feldman)
Physostigmine salicylate 2 mg./2 ml. Amp. Box.
12s. Prefilled syringe 1 ml. Box 5s.
Use: Parasympathomimetic.
ANTILUSIN. Pentamethonium Iodide, B.A.N.

■ **ANTIMALARIAL AGENTS.**
See: Amodiaquin HCl
Aralen HCl, Tab. (Winthrop-Breon)
Aralen Phosphate and Aralen Phosphate
W/Primaquine (Winthrop-Breon)
Atabrine Hydrochloride, Tab. (Winthrop-Breon)
Chloroguanide Hydrochloride.
Chloroquine Phosphate (Winthrop-Breon)
Daraprim Tab. (Burroughs Wellcome)
Hydroxychloroquine Sulfate
Paludrine HCl, Tab. (Ayerst)
Pamaquine Naphthoate.
Plaquenil Sulfate, Tab. (Winthrop-Breon)
Plasmochin Naphthoate.
Primaquine Phosphate, Tab. (Winthrop-Breon)
Pyrimethamine
Quinacrine Hydrochloride, Tab.
Quinine Salts (Various Mfr.)
Quinine Sulfate (Various Mfr.)
Totaquine, Pow.
ANTIME. (Rand) Pentaerythritol tetranitrate 30 mg. or
80 mg./Cap. Bot. 60s, 500s.
Use: Smooth muscle relaxant.
ANTIME FORTE. (Rand) Pentaerythritol tetranitrate
30 mg., secobarbital 50 mg./Cap. Bot. 60s,
500s.
Use: Smooth muscle relaxant.
ANTIMINTH. (Pfipharmecs) Pyrantel pamoate 50
mg./5 ml. Bot. 5 ml.
Use: Anthelmintic.
• **ANTIMONY POTASSIUM TARTRATE,** U.S.P. XXI.
Antimonate (2-), bis[u-[2,3-dihydroxybutanedioato (4-
)-0,0:0,0]]-di-, dipotassium, trihydrate, stereoisomer.
Dipotassium bis[u-tar-trato(4-)] diantimonate
(2-) trihydrate. Tartar emetic. (Various Mfr.)
Use: Schistosomiasis, leishmaniasis, expectorant &
emetic.
W/Cocillana, euphorbia pilulifera, squill, senega.
See: Cylana, Syr. (Bowman)
W/Guaifensin, codeine phosphate.
See: Cheracol, Syr. (Upjohn)
W/Guaifenesin, dextromethorphan HBr.
See: Cheracol-D, Syr. (Upjohn)
W/Paregoric, glycyrrhiza fl. ext.
See: Brown Mixture (Lilly)
W/Thenylpyramine HCl, ammonium chloride, sod.
citrate, menthol, aromatics.
See: Histacomp, Syr., Tab. (Approved Pharm.)
■ **ANTIMONY PREPARATIONS.**
See: Antimony Potassium Tartrate (Various Mfr.)
Antimony Sodium Thioglycollate (Various Mfr.)
Tartar Emetic (Various Mfr.)
ANTIMONY SODIUM THIOGLYCOLLATE. (Various
Mfr.)
Use: Schistosomiasis, leishmaniasis & filariasis.
• **ANTIMONY TRISULFIDE COLLOID.** USAN.
Use: Pharmaceutic aid.
ANTIMONYL POTASSIUM TARTRATE.
See: Antimony Potassium Tartrate, U.S.P. XXI.
■ **ANTINAUSEANTS.**
See: Antinauseants Supprettes "WANS" (Webcon)
Atarax, Tab., Syr. (Roerig)

Bendectin, Tab. (Merrell Dow)
Bucladin-S, Softab Tab. (Stuart)
Compazine, Preps. (SmithKline)
Dramamine, and Dramamine-D, Preps. (Searle)
Emesert, Rectal Insert (American Critical Care)
Emetrol, Liq. (Rorer)
Marezine, Preps. (Burroughs Wellcome)
Matropinal, Preps (Comatic)
Meclizine HCl, Tab. (Various Mfr.)
Mepergan, Inj. (Wyeth)
Naus-A-Tories, Supp. (Table Rock)
Nausetrol, Syr. (Medical Chemicals)
Phenergan, Preps. (Wyeth)
Pyridoxine HCl Preparations (Various Mfr.)
Thorazine, Preps. (SmithKline)
Tigan, Preps. (Beecham Labs)
Torecan Amp., Supp., Tab. (Sandoz)
Trilafon, Preps. (Schering)
Vistaril, Cap., Susp., Sol. (Pfizer)

ANTINAUSEA SUPRETTES "WANS." (Webcon)
Child: pyrilamine maleate 25 mg., pentobarbital
sodium 30 mg./Supp. **No. 1:** Pyrilamine maleate 50
mg., pentobarbital sodium 45 mg./Supp. **No. 2:**
Pyrilamine maleate 50 mg., pentobarbital sodium
100 mg./Supp. Box 12s
Use: Nausea, vomiting.

■ **ANTINEOPLASTIC AGENTS.**
See: Adriamycin, Vial (Adria)
Alkeran, Tab. (Burroughs Wellcome)
Blenoxane, Amp. (Bristol)
Cosmegen, Inj. (Merck Sharp & Dohme)
Cytosar, sterile (Upjohn)
Cytoxan, Tab., Vials. (Mead Johnson)
Dicorvin, Tab. (Amfre-Grant)
Drolban, Inj. (Lilly)
Estinyl, Tab. (Schering)
Estradurin, Inj. (Ayerst)
5-Fluorouracil, Amp. (Roche)
FUDR, Vials (Roche)
Hydrea, Cap. (Squibb)
Leukeran, Tab. (Burroughs Wellcome)
Lysodren, Tab. (Calbio)
Matulane, Cap. (Roche)
Medroxyprogesterone Acetate Tab., Vials
(Various Mfr.)
Megace, Tab. (Mead Johnson)
Methosarb, Tab. (Upjohn)
Mercaptopurine, Tab. (Burroughs Wellcome)
Methotrexate, Tab. (Lederle)
Methotrexate Sod., Vial (Lederle)
Meticorten, Tab. (Schering)
Mithracin, Vial (Pfizer)
Mustargen, Inj. (Merck Sharp & Dohme)
Myleran, Tab. (Burroughs Wellcome)
Oncovin, Amp. (Lilly)
Progynon, Pellets, Susp. (Schering)
Purinethol, Tab. (Burroughs Wellcome)
TACE, Cap. (Merrell Dow)
Teslac, Tab., Vial (Squibb)
Thioguanine, Tab. (Burroughs Wellcome)
Thio-Tepa, Vial (Lederle)
Triethylene Melamine, Tab. (Lederle)

Uracil Mustard, Cap. (Upjohn)
Velban, Amp. (Lilly)
Verceyte, Tab. (Abbott)
ANTI 5-NITRO-2-FURALDEHYDE OXIME. Nifuroxime.
■ **ANTI-OBESITY AGENTS.**
See: Thyroid
Amphetamine Preparations (Various Mfr.)
Dextro-amphetamine Preparations (Various Mfr.)
Diethylpropion HCl
Fastin, Cap. (Beecham Labs)
Ionamin, Cap. (Pennwalt)
Levo-Amphetamine
Methamphetamine Preparations (Various Mfr.)
Plegine, Tab. (Ayerst)
Preludin, Tab. (Boehringer Ingelheim)
Sanorex, Tab. (Sandoz)
Statobex, Tab. (Lemmon)
Tenuate (Merrell Dow)
Tepanil, Tab. (Riker)
ANTI-PAK COMPOUND. (Lowitt) Phenylephrine HCl 5
mg., salicylamide 0.23 Gm., acetophenetidin 0.15
gr., caffeine 0.03 Gm., ascorbic acid 50 mg.,
hesperidin complex 50 mg.,
chlorprophenpyridamine maleate 2 mg./Tab. Bot.
30s, 100s.
Use: Cold therapy.
ANTIPARASYMPATHOMIMETICS.
See: Parasympatholytic agents.
ANTI-PELLAGRA VITAMIN.
See: Nicotinic acid.
ANTI-PERNICIOUS ANEMIA PRINCIPLE.
See: Vitamin B-12
ANTIPHEN. Dichlorophen, B.A.N.
ANTIPHLOGISTINE. (Denver) Medicated poultice. Jar
5 oz., 1 lb., Tube 8 oz., Hosp. can 5 lb.
■ **ANTIPROTOZOAN AGENTS.**
See: Antimony Preparations
Arsenic Preparations
Bismuth Preparations
Chiniofon (Various Mfr.)
Diiodohydroxyquinoline
Emetine Hydrochloride (Various Mfr.)
Furazolidone
Iodohydroxyquinoline Sulfonate Sodium
Iodocholohydroxyquinoline
Levofuraltadone
Quinoxyl
Suramin Sodium
• **ANTIPYRINE,** U.S.P. XXI. 2,3-Dimethyl-1-phenyl-3-
pyrazolin-5-one. (Various Mfr.) Analgesine, anody-
nine, dimethyloxyquinazine, oxydimethylquinizine,
parodyne, phenazone, phenylone, pyrazoline,
sedatine.
Use: Analgesic, antipyretic.
W/Benzocaine, glycerin.
See: Aurotis, Liq. (Research Pharmacal Lab.) Ear
Drops, Liq. (Sutliff & Case)
W/Benzocaine, chlorobutanol.
See: G.B.A., Drops (Scrip)
W/Carbamide, benzocaine,
cetyldimethylbenzylammonium HCl.
See: Auralgesic, Liq. (Elder)

W/Phenylephrine HCl, benzocaine.
  See: Tympagesic, Liq. (Adria)
W/Pyrilamine maleate, phenylephrine, benzalkonium.
  See: Prefrin-A Ophthalmic (Allergan)
• ANTIPYRINE AND BENZOCAINE OTIC
  SOLUTION, U.S.P. XXI.
  Use: Local anesthetic.
  See: Auro Ear Drops (Commerce)
      Lanaurine, Drop (Lannett)
      Pyrocaine Eardrop, Liq. (Med. Chem.)
▪ ANTIRHEUMATIC PREPARATIONS.
  See: p-Aminobenzoic Acid and salts (cal., pot., sod.)
      Ammonium Salicylate
      Anti-arthritic Hormones
      Colchicine preps.
      Gentisate Sodium
      Gold Sod. Thiosulfate, Preps. (Various Mfr.)
      Myochrysine, Inj. (Merck Sharp & Dohme)
      Salicylamide preps.
      Sodium Salicylate
      Solganal, Vial (Schering)
▪ ANTIRICKETTSIAL AGENTS.
  See: p-Aminobenzoic Acid (Various Mfr.)
      p-Aminobenzoate, Sod. (Various Mfr.)
      Aureomycin, Preps. (Lederle)
      Chloromycetin, Preps. (Parke-Davis)
      Rocky Mountain Spotted Fever Serum (Rabbit),
        Vial (Lederle)
      Terramycin, Preps. (Pfizer)
ANTI-RUST TABLETS. (Lannett) Not for medicinal use;
  anticorrosive for use with benzalkonium aqueous
  sterilizing solution. Sodium carbonate monohydrate
  1.15 Gm., sodium nitrate 0.50 Gm.for a total of
  1.66 Gm./Tab. Bot. 500s.
ANTI-RUST TABLETS. (Winthrop-Breon) Sodium nitrite
  0.50 Gm., sodium bicarbonate 1.16 Gm. for a total
  of 1.66 Gm./Tab. Bot. 50s, 500s.
  Use: Rust preventive.
ANTISCORBUTIC VITAMIN.
  See: Ascorbic Acid
ANTISEPTIC, CHLORINE, ACTIVE.
  See: Antiseptic, N-Chloro Compounds, Hypochlorite
  Preps.
▪ ANTISEPTIC, DYES.
  See: Acriflavine (Various Mfr.)
      Aminoacridine, HCl
      Bismuth Violet, Prep. (Table Rock)
      Brilliant Green
      Crystal Violet
      Fuchsin
      Gentian Violet (Various Mfr.)
      Methylrosaniline Chloride (Various Mfr.)
      Methyl Violet
      Pyridium, Tab. (Parke-Davis)
      Serenium, Tab. (Squibb)
▪ ANTISEPTIC, MERCURIALS.
  See: Mercresin (Upjohn)
      Mercurochrome, Preps. (Hynson, Wescott &
        Dunning)
      Merthiolate, Preps. (Lilly)
      Phenylmercuric Acetate (Various Mfr.)
      Phenylmercuric Borate (Various Mfr.)

Phenylmercuric Nitrate (Various Mfr.)
Phenylmercuric Picrate (Various Mfr.)
Thimerosal
▪ ANTISEPTIC, N-CHLORO COMPOUNDS.
  See: Chloramine-T (Various Mfr.)
      Chlorazene, Powd., Tab. (Badger)
      Dichloramine-T (Various Mfr.)
      Halazone, Tab. (Abbott)
▪ ANTISEPTIC, PHENOLS.
  See: Anthralin (Various Mfr.)
      Bithionol
      Coal Tar Products (Various Mfr.)
      Creosote (Various Mfr.)
      Cresols (Various Mfr.)
      Guaiacol (Various Mfr.)
      Hexachlorophene (Various Mfr.)
      Hexylresorcinol (Var. Mfr.)
      Methylparaben (Various Mfr.)
      o-Phenylphenol (Various Mfr.)
      Oxyquinoline Salts (Various Mfr.)
      Parachlorometaxylenol (Various Mfr.)
      Phenol (Various Mfr.)
      Picric Acid (Various Mfr.)
      Propylparaben (Various Mfr.)
      Pyrogallol (Various Mfr.)
      Resorcinol (Various Mfr.)
      Resorcinol Monoacetate (Various Mfr.)
      Thymol (Various Mfr.)
      Trinitrophenol (Various Mfr.)
▪ ANTISEPTIC, SURFACE-ACTIVE AGENTS.
  See: Bactine, Preps. (Miles)
      Benzalkonium Chloride (Var. Mfr.)
      Benzethonium Chloride (Var. Mfr.)
      Ceepryn (Merrell Dow)
      Cēpacol Preps. (Merrell Dow)
      Cetylpyridinium Chloride (Var. Mfr.)
      Diaparene Chloride, Preps. (Winthrop-Breon)
      Methylbenzethonium Chloride (Various Mfr.)
      Zephiran Chloride, Preps. (Winthrop-Breon)
▪ ANTISEPTICS.
  See: Furacin, Preps. (Eaton)
      Iodine Products
      Mercurials
      N-Chloro Compounds
      Phenols
      Surface Active Agents
ANTISPAS. (Keene) Dicyclomine HCl 10 mg./ml. Vial
  10 ml.
  Use: Antispasmodic.
▪ ANTISPASMODICS. Usually refers to agents that
  combat the muscarinic effect of liberated
  acetylcholine. The relief of smooth muscle spasms.
  Parasympatholytic agents.
  See: Anticholinergic Agents.
      Spasmolytic Agents
ANTISPASMODIC CAPSULES. (Lemmon)
  Phenobarbital 16.2 mg., hyoscyamine sulfate
  0.1037 mg., atropine sulfate 0.0194 mg.,
  scopolamine HBr 0.0065 mg./Cap. Bot. 1000s.
  Use: Antispasmodic.
ANTISTEREPTOLYSIN-O. Titration procedure.
  See: Aslo (Wampole Labs)

ANTISTERILITY VITAMIN.
See: Vitamin E
ANTISTIN HYDROCHLORIDE OR MESYLATE.
Antazoline, B.A.N.
ANTI-TEN. (Century) Allylisobutylbarbituric acid ¾ gr., aspirin 3 gr., phenacetin 2 gr., caffeine ⅔ gr./Tab. Bot. 100s, 1000s.
Use: Analgesic-sedative.
ANTI-THERM. (Scrip) Sod. chloride 7 gr., dextrose 3 gr., Vit. C 20 mg./Tab. Bot. 1000s.
Use: Sodium chloride deficiency.
■ **ANTITHYROID AGENTS.**
See: Iothiouracil Sodium
Methimazole
Methylthiouracil (Various Mfr.)
Propylthiouracil (Various Mfr.)
Tapazole, Tab. (Lilly)
■ **ANTITOXINS.**
See: Botulism Antitoxin
Diphtheria Antitoxin
Gas Gangrene Antitoxin
Tetanus Antitoxin
■ **ANTITUBERCULOSIS AGENTS.**
See: Aminosalicylates (Na, Ca, K) (Various Mfr.)
Benzapas, Pow., Tab. (Dorsey)
Calcium Benzoylpas (Various Mfr.)
Capastat Sulfate, Amp. (Lilly)
Cycloserine, Pulvule (Lilly)
Diasone Sod., Tab. (Abbott)
Dihydrosteptomycin (Various Mfr.)
Di-Isopacin, Tab. (CMC)
Hyzyd, Tab. (Mallinckrodt)
Isoniazid (Various Mfr.)
Myambutol, Tab. (Lederle)
Natri-Pas, Pow., Tab. (Glenwood)
Niadox, Tab. (Barnes-Hind)
Niconyl, Tab. (Parke-Davis)
Pasara Sod., Pow., Tab. (Dorsey)
Pasdium, Tab. (Kasar)
P.A.S. Acid, Tab. (Kasar)
Pyrazinamide, Tab. (Lederle)
Rifadin, Cap. (Merrell Dow)
Rimactane, Cap. (Ciba)
Seromycin, Pulvule (Lilly)
Streptomycin (Various Mfr.)
Teebacin, Prep. (CMC)
Trecator-SC, Tab. (Ives)
Triniad, Tab. (Kasar)
Uniad, Tab. (Kasar)
Uniad-Plus 5,10, Tab. (Kasar)
ANTI-TUSS. (Century) Guaifenesin 100 mg./5 cc. Bot. 4 oz., pint, gal.
Use: Cough suppressant.
ANTI-TUSS D.M. (Century) Guaifenesin 100 mg., dextromethorphan HBr 15 mg./5 cc. Bot. 4 oz., pint, gal.
Use: Cough suppressant.
ANTI-TUSSIVE. (Canright) Dextromethorphan HBr 10 mg., potassium guaiacol sulfonate 125 mg., terpin hydrate 100 mg., phenylpropanolamine HCl 12.5 mg., pyrilamine maleate 12.5 mg./Tab. Bot. 60's.
Use: Cough suppressor & nasal decongestant.

ANTITUSSIVE COUGH SYRUP. (Weeks & Leo) Chlorpheniramine 2 mg., phenylephrine HCl 5 mg., dextromethorphan 15 mg., ammonium Cl 50 mg./5 ml.
Use: Decongestant, antihistaminic, antitussive, expectorant.
ANTITUSSIVE COUGH SYRUP WITH CODEINE.
(Weeks & Leo) Chlorpheniramine maleate 2 mg., phenylephrine HCl 5 mg., codeine phosphate 10 mg., ammonium Cl 50 mg./5 ml. Bot. 4 oz.
Use: Nasal decongestant, antihistaminic, analgesic, expectorant.
ANTITUSSIVE-DECONGESTANT.
See: St. Joseph Cough Syrup for Children (Plough)
Tussend, Tab., Liq. (Merrell Dow).
• **ANTIVENIN (CROTALIDAE) POLYVALENT,** U.S.P. XXI. Polyvalent crotaline antivenin. Rattlesnake antivenin for four species of pit vipers.
Use: passive immunizing agent for treatment of rattlesnake bite.
• **ANTIVENIN (LATRODECTUS MACTANS),** U.S.P. XXI. (Merck Sharp & Dohme) Black widow spider antivenin. Each vial contains not less than 6000 antivenin units. Thimerosal (mercury derivative) 1:10,000 added as preservative. Vial 2.5 ml.
Use: Treatment of black widow spider bite symptoms.
• **ANTIVENIN (MICRUS FULVIUS),** U.S.P. XXI. (Wyeth) Lyophilized antivenin of animal origin (micrurus fulvius) with phenol 0.25% and thimerosal 0.005% as preservatives. Bacteriostatic water w/phenylmercuric nitrate 1:100,000 as preservative. Combination package. Vial 10 ml.
Use: Bites of North American Coral Snake and Texas Coral Snake.
ANTIVENIN, SNAKE, POLYVALENT. (Wyeth) Antivenin Crotalidae, Polyvalent, U.S.P. XXI. (Crotalidae) Rattlesnake, copperhead & moccasin antitoxic serum. Pkg., Combination w/Phenol 0.25%, thimerosal 1:20,000 as preservatives. One disposable syringe, 10 cc. of bacteriostatic water for inj. w/preservative phenyl mercuric nitrate 1:100,000; one applicator vial iodine tinct. Normal horse serum 1:10, as sensitivity testing material.
Use: Bites by crotalid snakes of the United States.
ANTIVERT. (Roerig) Meclizine HCl 12.5 mg., 25 mg. or 50 mg./Tab. **12.5 mg.:** Bot. 100s, 500s. Unit Dose 100s; **25 mg.:** Bot. 100s, 500s. Chewable 100s, 500s. **50 mg.:** Bot. 100s, 500s.
Use: Vertigo & motion sickness.
ANTIXEROPHTHALMIC VITAMIN.
See: Vitamin A
ANTRENYL. (Ciba) Oxyphenonium bromide 5 mg./Tab. Bot. 100s.
Use: Anticholinergic activity.
ANTROCOL. (Poythress) Atropine sulfate 0.195 mg., phenobarbital 16 mg., bensulfoid 65 mg./Tab. or Cap. Bot. 100s, 500s.
Use: Sedative, antispasmodic.
ANTROCOL ELIXIR. (Poythress) Atropine sulfate 0.039 mg., phenobarbital 3 mg., alcohol 20%. Bot. 1 oz. w/dropper. Bot. pt.

Use: Treatment of a variety of gastro-intestinal disturbances in infants and children.

ANTURAN. Sulphinpyrazone, B.A.N.

ANTURANE. (Ciba) Sulfinpyrazone, U.S.P. 100 mg./Tab. Bot 100s. 200 mg./Cap. Bot. 100s.
Use: Treatment of chronic gout.

ANUCAINE. (Calvin) Procaine 50 mg., butyl-p-aminobenzoate 200 mg., benzyl alcohol 265 mg., in sweet almond oil/5 ml. Amp. 5 ml.
Box 6s, 24s, 100s.
Use: I.M., anesthetic for rectal treatment.

ANUGARD HC. (Vangard) Bismuth subgallate 2.25%, bismuth resorcin compund 1.75%, benzyl benzoate 1.2%, peruvian balsam 1.8%, zinc oxide 11.0%, pramoxine HCl 10 mg./Supp. Bot. 12s.
Use: Hemorrhoid treatment.

ANUJECT. (Hauck) Procaine solution. Vial 5 ml., 10 ml.
Use: Proctologic conditions.

ANULAN SUPPOSITORIES. (Lannett) Bismuth resorcin compound, bismuth subgallate, zinc oxide, boric acid, balsam peru. Box 12s.

ANUPHEN. (Comatic) Acetaminophen 125 mg. 300 mg., 600 mg. In a polyethylene glycol base/Supp. Box 12s.
Use: Analgesic.

ANUSOL. (Parke-Davis) Bismuth subgallate (2.25%), bismuth resorcin compound (1.75%), Peruvian balsam (1.8%), zinc oxide (11.00%), benzyl benzoate (1.2%), dibasic Ca phosphate in hydrogenated vegetable oil. Supp. Boxes 12s, 24s, 48s.
Use: Hemorrhoidal.

ANUSOL-HC. (Parke-Davis) Same as Anusol plus hydrocortisone acetate 10 mg./Supp. Box 12s, 24s.

ANUSOL-HC CREAM. (Parke-Davis) Hydrocortisone acetate 5 mg., bismuth subgallate 22.5 mg., bismuth resorcin compound 17.5 mg., benzyl benzoate 12 mg., propylparaben, methylparaben, polysorbate 60, sorbitan monostearate/Gm. Tube 1 oz.

ANUSOL OINTMENT. (Parke-Davis) Peruvian balsam 18mg., zinc oxide 110mg./Gm. w/bismuth subiodide and pramoxine HCl 1% in a mineral oil glyceryl stearate and water base. Tube 1 oz., 2 oz.
Use: Topically, irritative & inflammatory disorders of the skin.

ANXANIL. (Econo Med) Hydroxyzine HCl 25 mg./Tab. Bot. 100s.
Use: Relief of anxiety and tension.

ANYAGE. (Morton) Vit. A 5000 I.U., D 400 I.U., B-1 3 mg., B-2 3 mg., B-6 1 mg., C 50 mg., niacinamide 20 mg., B-12 2.5 mcg., Ca pantothenate 5 mg./Cap. Bot. 1000s.
Use: Multi-vitamin.

AORACILLIN-B. (Vita Elixir) Penicillin G 200,000 u. and 500,000 u./Tab. Bot. 50s.
Use: Antibiotic.

APAC. (Vortech) Aspirin 325 mg., caffeine 16 mg.,/Tab. Bot 1000s.
Use: Analgesic

APACOMP TABLETS. (Lannett) Bot. 1000s.

APAP. (Stanlabs) Acetaminophen 5 gr./Tab. Bot. 100s, 1000s.

APAP ACETAMINOPHEN TAB. (Towne) 350 mg. Bot. 100s.

APA-SAN. (Bowman) Acetaminophen 324 mg., aspirin 324 mg./Tab. Bot. 100s, 1000s.
Use: Analgesic, antipyretic.

APATATE. (Kenwood) Thiamine HCl 15 mg., Vit. B-12 25 mcg., Vit. B-6 0.5 mg./cc. Bot. Liq. 4 oz., 8 oz.
Use: Orally; nutritional supplement.

• **APAZONE.** USAN. 5-(Dimethylamino)-9-methyl-2-propyl-IH-pyrazolo[1,2,-a][1,2,4] benzotriazine-1,-3(2H)-dione.
Use: Anti-inflammatory.

A.P.C. (Various Mfr.) Aspirin, phenacetin & caffeine. Cap., Tab.
Use: Analgesic.
See: A.S.A. Compound, Preps. (Lilly)
    Aspodyne, Tab. (Blue Line)
    Gelsodyne, Tab. (Blue Line)
    P.A.C. Compound, Cap. or Tab. (Upjohn)
    Pan-APC, Tab. (Panray)
    Phensal, Tab. (Merrell Dow)
W/Aluminum hydroxide gel, magnesium hydroxide.
See: Buffadyne, Tab. (Lemmon)
W/Aluminum hydroxide gel, methapyrilene HCl, magnesium hydroxide.
See: Buffadyne 25, Tab. (Lemmon)
W/Codeine phosphate. (Various Mfr.)
See: Anexsia w/Codeine, Tab. (Beecham Labs)
    Anexsia D, Tab. (Beecham Labs)
    Aspodyne w/Codeine, Tab. (Blue Line)
W/Codeine phosphate, phenolphthalein.
See: Phenodyne, w/Codeine, Cap. (Blue Line)
W/Phenolphthalein.
See: Phenodyne, Tab., Blue Line

APC W/ANTIHISTAMINE TABLET. (Sutliff & Case) Salicylamide 227 mg., acetophenetidin 160 mg., caffeine 32.5 mg., pyrilamine maleate 6.25 mg., methapyriline fumarate 6.25 mg./Tab. Bot 100s, 1000s.

A.P.C. W/GELSEMIUM COMBINATIONS
See: Aidant, Tab. (Noyes)
    Ansemco, No. 2, Tab. (Elder)
    Asphac-G, Tab. (Central)
    Valacet, Tab. (Vale)

APC & GEL #2. (Scrip) Aspirin 3½ gr., acetaminophen 2½ gr., caffeine ¼ gr., tr. gelsemium 3 min./Tab. Bot. 100s.

APCOGESIC. (Apco) Sod. salicylate 5 gr., colchicine 1/320 gr., Ca carbonate 65 mg., dried aluminum hydroxide gel 130 mg., phenobarbital ⅛ gr./Tab. Bot. 100s.
Use: Arthritis, rheumatoid involvement.

APCOHIST. (APC) Phenylpropanolamine HCl 25 mg., chlorpheniramine maleate 1 mg.,/Tab. Bot. 100s.
Use: Antihistaminic; decongestant.

APCORETIC. (APC) Caffeine anhydrous 100 mg., ammonium chloride 325 mg./Tab. Bot. 90s.
Use: Diuretic.

APHCO HEMORRHOIDAL COMBINATION. (APC) Combination package of Aphco Hemorrhoidal

Ointment 1½ oz. tube, Aphco Hemorrhoidal Suppositories, box 12s, 1000s.
Use: Relief of discomfort of piles.
APHONAL TABLETS. (Panray) Isobutyl-allyl-barbituric acid 50 mg., caffeine 40 mg., aspirin 200 mg., acetophenetidin 130 mg./Tab. Bot. 1000s.
Use: Sedative with analgesics.
APICILLIN. D-(-)-α-Aminobenzyl penicillin.
See: Ampicillin
APIQUEL FUMARATE. Aminorex, B.A.N.
APISATE. Diethylpropion, B.A.N.
A.P.L. (Ayerst) Chorionic Gonadotropin for Injection. Dry form, package provides one vial containing 5000 U.S.P. Units, 10,000 U.S.P. Units, or 20,000 U.S.P. Units, and one 10 ml. Amp. w/sterile diluent, w/benzyl alcohol, phenol, lactose, sod. hydroxide or HCl.
Use: Chorionic gonadotropin therapy.
APLISOL. (Parke-Davis) Tuberculin purified protein derivative diluted 5 u./0.1 ml, w/polysorbate 80, pot. & sod phosphates, phenol. Vial 1 ml. (10 tests), 5 ml. (50 tests)
APLITEST. (Parke-Davis) Purified tuberculin protein fraction buffered with pot. & sod. phosphates, phenol 0.5%/Single-use, multipuncture unit. 25s.
APODOL. Anileridine dihydrochloride.
Use: Relief of pain.
APOGEN. (Beecham Labs) Gentamicin sulfate 40 mg./ml. Vial 20 ml.
Use: Antibiotic.
• **APOMORPHINE HYDROCHLORIDE.** U.S.P. XXI. Tablets, U.S.P. XXI. 4H-Dibenzo[de,g] quinoline-10,-11-diol, 5,6,6a,7-tetrahydro-6-methyl HCl hemihydrate. 6α,β-Aporphine-10,11-diol HCl, hemihydrate. Pow., Bot. 5 gr., 15 gr., ⅛ oz., 1 oz. (Various Mfr.) Lilly. H.T. (¹/₁₀ gr.) 100s.
Use: Emetic.
APORPHINE-10, 11-DIOL HYDROCHLORIDE.
See: Apomorphine Hydrochloride
A-POXIDE. (Abbott) Chlordiazepoxide 5 mg., 10 mg., 25 mg./Cap. 5 mg., 10 mg. Bot. 500s; 25 mg. Bot. 100s.
Use: Tranquilizer
APPEDRINE. (Thompson Medical) Phenylpropanolamine HCl 25 mg., multivitamins, caffeine 100 mg./Tab.
Use: Appetite depressant.
APPETITE-DEPRESSANT.
See: Anorexigenic agents
• **APRAMYCIN.** USAN. B.A.N. An antibiotic produced by Streptomyces tenebrarius.
Use: Antibacterial, veterinary medicine.
APRESAZIDE. (Ciba) **25/25 Cap.** Hydralazine HCl 25 mg., hydrochlorothiazide 25 mg. Cap. **50/50 Cap.** Hydralazine HCl 50 mg., hydrochlorothiazide 50 mg./Cap. **100/50 Cap.** Hydralazine 100 mg., hydrochlorothiazide 50 mg./Cap.
Use: Antihypertensive.
APRESOLINE. (Ciba) Hydralazine hydrochloride. **Amp.** 20 mg. w/propylene glycol, methyl- & propylp hydroxy benzoate. 1 ml. Pkg. 5s. **Tab.** 10 mg. Bot.

100s, 1000s, Consumer pack 100s.; 25 mg., 50 mg. Bot. 100s, 500s, 1000s. Consumer pack 100s. Accu-Pak, blister units of 100s.; 100 mg. Bot. 100s. Consumer pack 100s.
Use: Hypertensive disorders.
W/Serpasil.
See: Serpasil Prod., Preps. (Ciba)
APRESOLINE-ESIDRIX. (Ciba) Hydralazine HCl 25 mg., Hydrochlorothiazide 15 mg./Tab. Bot. 100s.
Use: Hypertension.
• **APRINDINE.** USAN. 3-[N-(Indan-2-yl)-N-phenylamino]propyldiethylamine. (Lilly) N-(2,3-Dihydro-1H-inden-2-yl)-N',N'-diethyl-N-phenyl-1,3-propanediamine.
Use: Anti-arrhythmic.
APRINOX. Bendrofluazide, B.A.N.
APROBARBITAL. 5-Allyl-5-isopropylbarbituric acid, Allylisopropylmalonylurea) Pow.
Use: Long acting hypnotic.
See: A.P.B., Tab. (Lemmon)
APROBEE W/C. (Approved) Vit. B-1 15 mg., B-2 10 mg., B-6 5 mg., niacinamide 50 mg., Calc. pantothenate 10 mg., Vit. C 250 mg./Cap. or Tab. **Caps.** Bot. 100s, 1000s. **Tab.** Bot. 50s, 100s, 1000s.
Use: Vitamin deficiencies.
• **APROTININ.** USAN. A polypeptide proteinase inhibitor.
See: Trasylol
A.P.S. Aspirin, phenacetin and salicylamide
APSIN VK. Phenoxymethylpenicillin, B.A.N.
• **APTAZAPINE MALEATE.** USAN.
APTOCAINE. B.A.N. 2-Pyrrolidin-1-ylpropiono-o-toluidide.
Use: Local anesthetic.
See: Pirothesin hydrochloride
APYRON.
See: Magnesium acetylsalicylate
AQ-4B. (Western Research) Trichlormethiazide 4 mg./Tab. Bot. 1000s.
Use: Diuretic.
AQUA-BAN. (Thompson Medical) Caffeine, ammonium chloride/Tab. Bot. 80s.
Use: Pre-menstrual water retention.
AQUA BAN PLUS. (Thompson Medical) Ammonium Cl 650 mg., caffeine 200 mg., bran 6 mg./Tab.
Use: Mild diuretic for pre-menstrual water retention.
AQUABASE. (Vale) Cetyl alcohol, propylene glycol, sodium lauryl sulfate, white wax, purified water. Jar 1 lb.
Use: Hydrophilic ointment base.
AQUACARE. (Herbert) Emollients, moisturizers, urea 2%, benzyl alcohol. **Cream** 2.5 oz. **Lotion** 8 oz.
Use: Dry skin treatment.
AQUACARE/HP. (Herbert) Emollients, moisturizers, urea 10%, benzyl alcohol. **Cream** 2½ oz. **Lotion** 8 oz., 16 oz.
Use: Dry skin treatment.
AQUACHLOR. (Geneva) Chlortetracycline.
Use: Antibiotic.
AQUACHLORAL. (Webcon) Chloral hydrate w/polyethylene glycol and a spreading agent. Supp. (5 gr., 10 gr., 15 gr.) Jar 12s.

Use: (Rectal) sedative.

AQUA-CILLIN 250. (Kenyon) Crystalline penicillin G pot. 3 million u. buffered w/sod. citrate./60 cc. Vial.

AQUACILLIN G. (Geneva) Penicillin G.
Use: Antibiotic.

AQUACORT SUPPRETTES. (Webcon) Hydrocortisone acetate 10 mg., tyrothricin, 2.5 mg., phenylmercuric acetate, 3 mg., 9-aminoacridine HCl 3 mg., polysorbate 80, 10 mg., urea 20 mg., lactose 50 mg./Supprette. Jars 6s, 14s.
Use: Vaginitis.

AQUACYCLINE. (Geneva) Tetracycline HCl.
Use: Antibiotic.

AQUADERM. (C & M Pharmacal) Purified water, glycerin 25%, salicylic acid 0.1%, octoxynol-9 0.03%, 0.0001% FD&C red #40. Bot. 2 oz.
Use: Moisturizer for dry & aging skin.

AQUA-FILM TEARS. (Maurry) Hydroxyethylcellulose 0.-5%, with NaCl, benzalkonium Cl 0.01% as preservative, EDTA and purified water. Bot. 15 cc.
Use: Lubricant.

AQUAFUREN. (Geneva) Nitrofurantoin.
Use: Antibacterial for urinary infections.

AQUA IVY. (Miles Pharm) Poison ivy extract 1:5 dil. Vial 10 cc.
Use: Hyposensitization.

AQUAKAY.
See: Menadione (Var. Mfr.)

AQUA LACTEN LOTION. (Herald Pharmacal) Demineralized water, urea, petrolatum, propylene glycol monostearat sorbitan monosterate, lactic acid. Bot. 8 oz.
Use: Dry Skin.

AQUALIN-PLUS SUPPRETTES. (Webcon) Theop'.yl-line and sod. pentobarbital:-Child: 120 mg. & 24 mg./Cream Supp. 12s; No. 2A: 480 mg. & 48 mg./White Supp. 12s; No. 2: 480 mg. & 100 mg./Light Yellow Supp. Jar 12s.

AQUALOSE. Poloxyl Lanolin, B.A.N.

AQUA MENSE W/IRON. (Stanlabs) Herbal water pill. Bot. 40s.
Use: Diuretic.

AQUAMEPHYTON INJECTION. (Merck Sharp & Dohme) Phytonadione 2 mg. or 10 mg./ml. as an aqueous colloidal solution of Vitamin K-1, w/polyoxyethylated fatty acid derivative 70 mg., dextrose 37.5 mg., benzyl alcohol 0.9%, water for injection q.s. /ml. Available for injection by I.V., I.M., or subcutaneous routes. Amp. 1 mg./0.5 ml. Box 25s; 10 mg./1 ml. 6s, 25s. Vial 10 mg./ml. 2.5 ml. & 5 ml.
Use: Control of hemorrhage, coagulation disorders.

AQUA MIST. (Faraday) Nasal spray. Squeeze Bot. 20 cc.

AQUAMOX. Quinethazone, B.A.N.

AQUAMUCIL. (Cenci) Psyllium hydrophilic mucilloid. Bot. 7 oz., 14 oz.

AQUAMYCIN. (Geneva) Erythromycin.
Use: Antibiotic.

AQUANIL. (Sig) Mersalyl 100 mg., theophylline

(hydrate) 50 mg., methyl paraben 0.18%, propyl paraben 0.02%. Vial 10 cc.

AQUANINE. (Geneva) Quinine HCl.
Use: Antimalarial.

AQUAOXY. (Geneva) Oxytetracycline HCl.
Use: Antibiotic.

AQUAPHENICOL. (Geneva) Chloramphenicol.
Use: Antibiotic.

AQUAPHILIC OINTMENT. (Medco Lab) Hydrated hydrophillic ointment. Jar 16 oz.
Use: Dry skin conditioner and an ointment base.

AQUAPHILIC OINTMENT WITH CARBAMIDE 10% and 20%. (Medco Lab) Stearyl alcohol, white petrolatum, sorbitol, propylene glycol, urea, ionic emulsifier, lactic acid, methylparaben, propylparaben.
Use: Prescription compounding and dry skin.

AQUAPHOR. (Beiersdorf, Germany) Xipamide
Use: Diuretic used to treat edema and hypertension.

AQUAPHOR. Water-miscible ointment base. Jar 1 lb., 5 lb., 45 lb.
Use: Water-miscible ointments.
See: Eucerin, Emulsion (Duke).

AQUAPHYLLIN SYRUP. (Ferndale) Theophylline anhydrous 80 mg./15 ml. Unit dose pks. 15 ml., 30 ml. Bot. 16 oz., gal.
Use: Bronchodilator.

AQUAPOOL CONCENTRATE. (Parker) Additive for whirlpool therapy to control scum formation and foaming. Bot. pt., gal.

AQUAPRES. (Coastal) Benzthiazide 50 mg./Tab. Bot. 100s, 1000s.
Use: Diuretic.

■ **AQUARIUM DRUGS.** (Geneva) Various antibiotic, antifungal, vitamin & antibacterial drugs for aquarium use.

AQUASEC. (Pasadena Research) Benzthiazide 50 mg./Tab. Bot. 100s, 1000s.
Use: Diuretic.

AQUASOL A. (Armour) Water-miscible Vitamin A. **Parenteral** 50,000 I.U./ml. Vial 2 ml. Box 10s. **Caps:** 25,000 I.U./Cap. Bot. 100s. 50,000 I.U./Cap. Bot. 100s, 500s. **Drops:** 5000 I.U./0.1 ml. Bot. 30 ml. w/dropper.
Use: Vitamin A therapy and supplement.

AQUASOL E. (Armour) Vitamin E. **Caps.:** 100 I.U./Cap. Bot. 100s. 400 I.U./Cap. Bot. 30s.**Drops:** 15 I.U./0.3 ml. Bot. 12 ml., 30 ml. w/dropper.
Use: Vitamin E supplement.

AQUASONIC 100. (Parker) Water-soluble contact medium gel for ultrasonic and electrical transmission. Bot. 8 oz., qt., gal.

AQUASONIC 100 STERILE. (Parker) Water-soluble, sterile gel for ultrasonic & electrical transmission. Foil Pouches 15 Gm.
Use: Contact medium gel for medical ultrasound when sterility is indicated.

AQUASULF. (Geneva) Triple sulfa tablet.
Use: Antibacterial.

AQUATAG. (Reid-Provident) Benzthiazide 50 mg./Tab. Bot. 100s.

Use: Antihypertensive, diuretic.
AQUATENSEN. (Wallace) Methyclothiazide 5 mg./Tab. Bot. 100s., 500s.
Use: Diuretic and antihypertensive agent.
AQUAVITE. (Geneva) Soluble multivitamin.
Use: Multivitamin.
AQUAZOL. (Geneva) Sulfisoxazole.
Use: Antibacterial.
AQUEOUS ALLERGENS. (Miles Pharm)
Use: Hyposensitization.
AQUEST. (Dunhall) Estrone (20,000 I.U.) 2 mg./ml. Vial 30 ml.
Use: Estrogen replacement.
AQUEX TABLETS. (Lannett) Trichlormethiazide 4 mg./Tab. Bot. 100s. 1000s.
Use: Diuretic.
AQUINONE.
See: Menadione, U.S.P. XXI.
AQUOL BATH OIL. (Lamond) Vegetable oil, olive oil. Bot. 4 oz., 6 oz., 16 oz., qt., gal.
Use: Dry skin, eczema, pruritic conditions.
1-β-D-ARABINOFURANOSYLCYTOSINE. Cytarabine, U.S.P. XXI.
AR-3. (Stanlabs) Bot. 100s.
Use: Antacid tablets.
ARALEN HYDROCHLORIDE (Winthrop-Breon) Chloroquine HCl 50 mg./ml. 5 ml. Amps. Box 5s.
Use: Malaria; extraintestinal amebiasis.
ARALEN PHOSPHATE. (Winthrop-Breon) Chloroquine phosphate. 500 mg./Tab. Bot. 25s.
Use: Malaria, extraintestinal amebiasis.
ARALEN PHOSPHATE W/PRIMAQUINE PHOSPHATE. (Winthrop-Breon) Aralen phosphate 500 mg., primaquine phosphate 79 mg./Tab. Bot. 100s.
Use: Prophylaxis of malaria.
ARALIS TABLETS. (Winthrop Products) Glycobiarsol, chloroquine phosphate.
Use: Intestinal amebicide.
ARAMINE (Merck Sharp & Dohme) Metaraminol bitartrate (equivalent to metaraminol) 10.0 mg./ml. w/sodium chloride 4.4 mg., water for injection q.s. ad. 1.0 ml., methylparaben 0.15%, propylparaben 0.02%, & sodium bisulfite 0.2%. Vial 1 ml., Box 12s; Vials 10 ml.
Use: Sympathomimetic amine (Vasopressor).
• **ARANOTIN.** USAN.
Use: Antiviral.
• **ARBAPROSTIL.** USAN.
Use: Antisecretory.
ARBOLIC. (Burgin-Arden) Methandriol dipropionate 50 mg./cc. Vial 10 cc.
ARBON INJECTION. (O'Neal, Jones & Feldman) Cyanocobalamine 200 mcg., thiamine HCl 5 mg., riboflavin-5 sodium phosphate 2.86 mg., pyridoxine HCl 10 mg., panthenol 2 mg., niacinamide 50 mg./ml. Vial 30 ml.
Use: multivitamin.
ARBON TABLETS. (O'Neal, Jones & Feldman) Vit. A 5000 I.U., D 400 I.U., C 60 mg., folic acid 0.4 mg., B-1 1.5 mg., B-2 1.7 mg., niacin 20 mg., B-6 2 mg., B-12 6 mcg., iodine 150 mcg., iron 18 mg.,

calcium pantothenate 22 mg., copper 2 mg., zinc 15 mg., magnesium 100 mg., calcium 100 mg., phosphorus 80 mg./Tab. Bot. 100s, 1000s.
ARBON PLUS SC. (O'Neal, Jones & Feldman) Vit. A 5000 I.U., D 400 I.U., E 30 I.U., C 90 mg., folic acid 400 mcg., B-1 2.25 mg., B-2 2.6 mg., niacinamide 20 mg., B-6 3 mg., B-12 9 mcg., pantothenic acid 10 mg., biotin 150 mcg., calcium 162 mg., phosphorus 125 mg., iodine 150 mcg., magnesium 100 mg., copper 3 mg., manganese 7.5 mg., potassium 7.5 mg., zinc 22.5 mg./Tab. Bot. 100s, 1000s.
Use: Vitamin, mineral supplement.
ARBUTAL. (Arcum) Butalbital ¾ gr., phenacetin 2 gr., aspirin 3 gr., caffeine ⅔ gr./Tab. Bot. 100s, 1000s.
Use: Sedative analgesic for tension headache.
ARCOBAN TABLETS. (Arcum) Meprobamate 400 mg./Tab. Bot. 50s, 1000s.
Use: Anxiety and tension states.
ARCOBEX EXTRA STRENGTH CAPS. (Arcum) Vits. B-1 100 mg., B-2 2 mg., B-6 5 mg., niacinamide 125 mg., panthenol 10 mg., B-12 30 mcg., benzyl alcohol 1%, genistic acid ethanolamide 2.5%/cc. Vial 30 cc.
Use: B Vitamin therapy.
ARCOCEE. (Arco) Vit. C 750 mg./Tab. Bot. 30s, 100s, 500s.
Use: Vitamin C deficiency.
ARCOCILLIN. (Arcum) Crystalline penicillin G pot. 400,000 u./Tab. Bot. 100s, 1000s. Powder 400,000 u./5 cc. Bot. 80 cc.
ARCODEX ANTACID TABLETS. (Arcum) Magnesium trisilicate 500 mg., aluminum hydroxide 250 mg./Tab. Bot. 100s, 1000s.
Use: Antiacid.
ARCO-LASE. (Arco) Trizyme 38 mg. (Amylolytic 30 mg., proteolytic 6 mg., celluloytic 2 mg.), lipase 25 mg./Tab. Bot. 50s.
Use: Digestive disorders.
ARCO-LASE PLUS. (Arco) Phenobarbital 8 mg., hyoscyamine sulfate 0.10 mg, atropine sulfate 0.02 mg., trizyme 38 mg., lipase 25 mg./Tab. Bot. 50s.
Use: Treatment of gastrointestinal disturbances.
ARCORET. (Arco) Protease 30 mg., B-12 100 mcg., B-1 30 mg./Tab. Bot. 60s.
Use: Nutritional supplement, protamine appetite, weight gain.
ARCORT W/IRON. (Arco) Elemental iron 150 mg., protease 30 mg., B-12 100 mcg., B-1 30 mg./Tab. Bot. 60s.
Use: Prevention and treatment of iron deficiency anemia.
ARCOSTERONE. (Arcum) Methyltestosterone Oral: 10 mg., 25 mg./Tab. Bot. 100s, 1000s. Subling.: 10 mg./Tab. Bot. 100s, 1000s.
Use: Hormone therapy.
ARCO-THYROID. (Arco) Thyroid 1½ gr./Tab. Bot. 1000s.
ARCOTINIC. (Arco) Ferrous fumarate 5 gr., ferrous sulfate 5 gr., Vit. C 500 mg., desiccated liver 400 mg./Tab. Bot. 100s.
ARCOTINIC LIQUID. (Arco) Ferrous gluconate 9 gr., liver fraction 1 gr., Vit. B-1 4.5 mg., B-2 4.5 mg.,

B-6 1.5 mg., d-panthenol 4 mg., niacinamide 30 mg./Tbsp. Bot. pt.
Use: Iron-deficiency anemia.

ARCOTRATE. (Arcum) Pentaerythritol tetranitrate 10 mg./Tab. **No. 2.** Pentaerythritol tetranitrate 20 mg./Tab. **No. 3.** Pentaerythritol tetranitrate 20 mg., phenobarbital ⅛ gr./Tab. Bot. 100s, 1000s.

ARCOVAL IMPROVED. (Arcum) Vit. A palmitate 10,000 I.U., D 400 I.U., thiamine mononitrate 15 mg., B-2 10 mg., nicotinamide 150 mg., B-6 5 mg., Ca pantothenate 10 mg., Vit. B-12 5 mcg., C 150 mg., E 5 I.U./Cap. Bot. 100s, 1000s.
Use: Dietary supplement.

ARCUM R-S. (Arcum) Reserpine 0.25 mg./Tab. Bot. 100s, 1000s.

ARCUM V-M. (Arcum) Vit. A palmitate 5000 I.U., D 400 I.U., B-1 2.5 mg., B-2 2.5 mg., B-6 0.5 mg., B-12 2 mcg., C 50 mg., niacinamide 20 mg., Ca pantothenate 5 mg., Fe 18 mg./Cap. Bot. 100s, 1000s.
Use: Dietary supplement.

A-R-D. (Birchwood) Anatomically shaped dressing for anorectal wounds, treatment of pruritus ani and other perianal irritations. Dispenser 24s.

ARDEBEN. (Burgin-Arden) Diphenhydramine HCl 10 mg., chlorobutanol 0.5%. Inj. 30 cc. vial.

ARDECAINE 1%. (Burgin-Arden) Lidocaine HCl 1%. Inj. 30 cc. vial.

ARDECAINE 2%. (Burgin-Arden) Lidocaine HCl 2%. Inj. 30 cc. vial.

ARDECAINE 1% W/EPINEPHRINE. (Burgin-Arden) Lidocaine HCl 1% w/epinephrine. Inj. 30 cc. vial.

ARDECAINE 2% W/EPINEPHRINE. (Burgin-Arden) Lidocaine HCl 2% w/Epinephrine. Inj. 30 cc. vial.

ARDEFEM 10. (Burgin-Arden) Estradiol valerate 10 mg./cc. 10 cc. vial.

ARDEFEM 20. (Burgin-Arden) Estradiol valerate 20 mg./cc. 10 cc. vial.

ARDEFEM 40. (Burgin-Arden) Estradiol valerate 40 mg./cc. Vial 10cc.

ARDEPRED SOLUBLE. (Burgin-Arden) Prednisolone 20 mg., niacinamide 25 mg., disodium edetate 0.5 mg., sodium bisulfite 1 mg., phenol 5 mg./cc. Vial 10cc.

ARDERONE 100. (Burgin-Arden) Testosterone enanthate 100 mg./cc. 10 cc. vial.

ANDERONE 200. (Burgin-Arden) Testosterone enanthate 200 mg./cc. 10 cc. vial.

ARDEVILA TABLETS. (Winthrop Products) Inositol hexanicotinate.
Use: Peripheral vasodilator.

ARDIOL 90/4. (Burgin-Arden) Testosterone enanthate 90 mg., estradiol valerate 4 mg./cc. 10 cc. vial.

ARECA. 0.35% of Ether soluble alkaloids, as arecoline.
Use: Anthelmintic (veterinary).

ARECOLINE ACETARSONE SALT.
See: Drocarbil.

ARECOLINE HYDROBROMIDE. (Mallinckrodt) Methyl 1,2,5,-6-tetrahydro-1-methylnicotinate hydrobromide. Hydrobromide of an alkaloid obtained from the dried ripe seed of areca catechu. Tab. (91 to 109% of the labeled amount of arecoline hydrobromide).

Ar-EX BATH OIL. (Ar-Ex) Unscented only. Cholesterol base, mineral oil, isopropyl-myristate, polyethylene glycol 400 dilaurate. Bot. 8 oz.

AR-EX BODY LOTION. (Ar-Ex) Unscented only. Stearic acid, glycerol monostearate, cholesterol base, oil of sesame, sorbitan monooleate, triethanolamine, isopropyl myristate, mineral oil, oxyquinoline benzoate, carbonyl diamide. Bot. 8 oz.

AR-EX BRUSH-ON BROW. (Ar-Ex) Unscented only. Talc, titanium dioxide, microcrystalline wax, butylated hydroxyanisole, cosmetic colors. Tortoise Shell compact with mirror and brush.

Ar-EX BRUSH-ON COMPLEXION COLORING. (Ar-Ex) Unscented only. Talc, colloidal kaolin, zinc stearate, propyl parahydroxybenzoate, mineral oil, titanium dioxide, cosmetic color. Tortoise Shell Compact with mirror and hypo-allergenic nylon brush.

AR-EX BRUSH-ON EYESHADOW. (Ar-Ex) Unscented only. Talc, calcium carbonate, magnesium stearate, isopropyl palmitate, cosmetic colors. Tortoise shell compact with mirror and sponge and brush applicator.

AR-EX CAKE EYELINER. (Ar-Ex) Unscented only. Zinc stearate, calcium carbonate, talc, polyoxyethylene sorbitan monooleate, sorbitan sesquioleate, cetyl alcohol, butylated hydroxyanisole, inorganic pigments. Tortoise shell compact with mirror and brush.

AR-EX CHAP CREAM. (Ar-Ex) Scented or unscented. Diethylene glycol stearate, beeswax, lecithin, cholesterol, carbonyl diamide. Jar. 4 oz., 9 oz., 8 lbs. Tubes 1½ oz.

AR-EX CLEANSING CREAM. (Ar-Ex) Scented or unscented. Liquid petrolatum, beeswax, ozokerite. Scented 4 oz. Unscented 4 oz., 8 oz.

AR-EX COLD CREAM. (Ar-Ex) Scented or unscented. Liquid petrolatum, beeswax, ozokerite. Scented 4 oz. Unscented 4 oz., 8 oz., 7 lbs.

AR-EX COMPACT FACE POWDER. (Ar-Ex) Face powder in compressed cakes, unscented only. Same composition as AR-EX Face Powder, but compressed into cakes. Tortoise Shell Compact with mirror and 7 oz. cake. Refills available.

AR-EX CREAM DEODORANT. (Ar-Ex) Unscented only. Glyceryl monostearate, cholesterol absorption base, spermaceti, glycerine, sorbitol, propylene glycol. Preservatives: methyl and propyl parahydroxybenzoates, aluminum phenolsulfonate. Jar. 1¼ oz. Tube 1 oz.

AR-EX CREAM FOR DRY SKIN. (Ar-Ex) Scented or unscented. Liquid petrolatum, beeswax, ozokerite, cholesterol base. Scented 4 oz., 8 oz. Unscented 4 oz., 8 oz.

AR-EX CREAM FOR OILY SKIN. (Ar-Ex) Unscented only. Ozokerite, cetyl alcohol, petrolatum, petrolatum liquidum. Jar. 3.75 oz.

AR-EX DISAPPEAR-BLEMISH STICK. (Ar-Ex) Unscented only. Carnauba wax, white petrolatum, mineral oil, ozokerite, titanium dioxide, butylated hydroxyanisole, cosmetic colors. Available in combination gold and silver swivel case.

AR-EX EYE CREAM. (Ar-Ex) Unscented only. Cholesterol base, petrolatum, glycerol monostearate, paraffin, oil of sesame, liquid petrolatum, white beeswax. Jar. ½ oz.

AR-EX EYE MAKEUP REMOVER PADS. (Ar-Ex) Unscented only. 100% cotton, specially refined white oil. Jar. 50 Pads.

AR-EX EYE PENCIL. (Ar-Ex) Unscented only, Spermaceti, petrolatum, paraffin wax, japan-wax substitute, zinc stearate, cosmetic grade iron oxide, cosmetic grade carbon black.

AR-EX EYESHADOW STICK. (Ar-Ex) Unscented only. Paraffin wax, petrolatum, liquid petrolatum, cosmetic grade pigments. Swivel container.

Ar-EX FACE POWDER. (Ar-Ex) A hypo-allergenic face powder. Unscented only. Talc, colloidal kaolin, zinc stearate, titanium dioxide, cosmetic colors. Box 2.25 oz.

AR-EX FOUNDATION LOTION. (Ar-Ex) A hypo-allergenic liquid make-up, unscented only. Cetyl alcohol, cholesterol, aluminum magnesium silicate, sodium lauryl sulfate, glycerine, titanium dioxide, triethanolamine stearate, cosmetic iron oxide pigments, Bot. 2 oz.

AR-EX HAIR SPRAY. (Ar-Ex) Unscented only. Polyvinyl plasticizers, polyethoxylated cholesterol, anhydrous alcohol, fluorocarbon propellants. Aerosol cans 7 oz., 14 oz.

AR-EX HAND LOTION. (Ar-Ex) Unscented only. Stearic acid in quince seed extract, glycerin, liquid petrolatum, cholesterol base. Bot. 8 oz.

AR-EX LIP GLOSS & SUN SCREEN STICK. (Ar-Ex) Unscented only. Isopropyl fatty-acid esters, homomenthyl salicylate, mineral oil, candelilla wax, butylated hydroxyanisole. In gold and silver swivel case.

AR-EX A MAN'S HAIR SPRAY. (Ar-Ex) Unscented only. Polyvinyl plasticizers, polyethoxylated cholesterol, anhydrous alcohol, fluorocarbon propellants. Aerosol can 7 oz.

AR-EX MASCARA. (Ar-Ex) Unscented only. Roll-on. Liquid petrolatum, beeswax, carnauba wax, sorbitan sesquioleate, polyoxyethylene sorbitan monostearate, borax, propyl and methyl para-hydroxymenzoate, inorganic cosmetic pigments. Roll-on applicurler Cake in Tortoise shell compact with mirror and spiral brush.

AR-EX MOISTURE CREAM. (Ar-Ex) Unscented only. Glyceryl monostearate, cetyl alcohol, cetyl lactate, depollenized beeswax, isopropyl myristate, sesame oil, glycerine, polyoxyethylene sorbitan monostearate. Jar. 2 oz.

AR-EX MOISTURE LOTION. (Ar-Ex) Scented or unscented. Saturated cholesterol absorption base, stearic acid, glycerol monostearate, oil of sesame, glycerine, triethanolamine. Vial. 2 oz.

AR-EX MULTIBASE. (Ar-Ex) Aliphatic alcohols, polyhydric alcohols, lauric acid esters, petrolatum. Jar 16 oz., 7 lb.

AR-EX NAIL POLISH. (Ar-Ex) Unscented only. Butyl acetate, ethyl acetate, Cellosolve acetate, xylol cellulose acetate, camphor, plasticizer, resin, cosmetic colors. Bot ½ fl. oz. with applicator

AR-EX NAIL POLISH REMOVER. (Ar-Ex) Butyl acetate, ethyl acetate, Cellosolve acetate, xylol. Bot. 2 fl. oz.

AR-EX NIGHT CREAM. (Ar-Ex) Scented or unscented. Cholesterol absorption base, lecithin, beeswax, liquid petrolatum. Jar. Scented or unscented, 2 oz. Unscented only, 4 oz.

AR-EX REGULAR LIPSTICK. (Ar-Ex) Unscented only. Beeswax, castor oil, candelilla wax, butyl stearate, lake colors, certified, tetrabromfluorescein, in brass swivel containers.

AR-EX SAFE-SUDS. (Ar-Ex) Unscented only. A synthetic organic detergent. Alkyl sulfonates. Container 22 oz.

AR-EX SHAMPOO (SOAPLESS). (Ar-Ex) Unscented only. Protein, buffered to a pH of 6.7 approaching the natural pH of the scalp. Bot. 8 oz.

AR-EX SPECIAL FORMULA LIPSTICK. (Ar-Ex) Unscented only. Lipstick without the dye. Composition is the same as AR-EX Indelible Lipstick except contains no Bromofluorescein compounds. Available in silveroid swivel cases.

AR-EX SPRAY DEODORANT. (Ar-Ex) Unscented only. Glycerine, Tween, urea, aluminum phenolsulfonate. Bot. 1½ oz.

AR-EX SUN SCREEN. (Ar-Ex) Unscented only. Glyceryl monostearate, stearic acid, cetyl alcohol, mineral oil, isopropyl myristate, cholesterol absorption base, propylene glycol, homo menthyl salicylate, polyoxyethylene sorbitan monooleate. Bot. 8 oz.

AR-EX SUPERFATTED SOAP. (Ar-Ex) Unscented only. Titanium dioxide, beta methyl umbelliferone, mineral oil, cholesterol absorption base, tallow, coconut oil. Toilet size, Bath size 5.5 oz.

AR-EX TALC. (Ar-Ex) Unscented only. Talc, zinc stearate, boric acid, iron oxide pigment. Shaker can 3 oz.

AR-EX WAVE SET. (Ar-Ex) Unscented only. Quince seed base, plasticized, glycerine, lake color. Bot. 8 fl. oz.

ARFONAD. (Roche) Trimethaphan camsylate 50 mg./ml. w/sod. acetate 0.013%. Amp. 10 ml. Box 10s.
Use: Short-acting vasodilator for control of hypertension.
Note: Refrigerate between 2° and 8° C.

ARGESIC CREAM. (Econo Med) Triethanolamine, methylsalicylate in cream base. Tube 2 oz.
Use: Arthritis, muscular aches and pains.

ARGESIC TABLETS. (Econo Med) Phenyltoloxamine citrate 30 mg., magnesium salicylate 600 mg./Tab. Bot. 100s.
Use: Analgesic, antiinflammatory.

• **ARGININE,** U.S.P. XXI. $C_6H_{14}N_4O_2$. L-Arginine.

• **ARGININE GLUTAMATE.** USAN. L(+)-arginine salt of L(+)-glutamic acid.
Use: Aid in ammonia intoxication due to hepatic failure.

ARGININE GLUTAMATE. B.A.N. L-Arginine salt of L-glutamic acid.
Use: Nutrient.
See: Modumate.

• **ARGININE HYDROCHLORIDE,** U.S.P. XXI. Inj., U.S.P. XXI.
ARGIPRESSIN. B.A.N. 8-Argininevasopressin.
Use: Antidiuretic hormone.
• **ARGIPRESSIN TANNATE.** USAN.
Use: Antidiuretic.
ARGYN.
See: Mild Silver Protein (Various Mfr.)
ARGYROL S.S. 20%. (CooperVision) Mild silver protein 20%. Dropperettes in 1 ml. Box 12s.
Use: Local anti-infective.
ARGYROL STABILIZED SOLUTION 10%. (CooperVision) Mild silver protein 10%. Bot. 0.5 oz., 1 oz.
Use: Local anti-infective.
ARIDOL. (MPL) Pamabrom 52 mg., pyrilamine maleate 30 mg., homatropine methylbromide 1.2 mg., hyoscyamine sulfate 0.10 mg., scopolamine HBr 0.02 mg., methamphetamine HCl 1.5 mg./Tab. Bot. 100s.
Use: Dysmenorrhea, premenstrual tension.
• **ARILDONE.** USAN.
Use: Antiviral.
ARISTOCORT. (Lederle) Triamcinolone. **Tab.** 1 mg. Bot. 50s. 2 mg. 100s. 4 mg. Bot. 30s, 100s, 500s. 8 mg. Bot. 50s. 16 mg. Bot. 30s. **Tab. Aristo-Pk.** 4 mg. Pkg. 16s. **Syr.** (diacetate w/methylparaben 0.08%, propylparaben 0.02%). 2 mg./5 cc. Bot. 4 oz.
Use: Anti-inflammatory steroid.
ARISTOCORT A CREAM. (Lederle) Triamcinolone acetonide w/ethoxylated stearyl alcohol, isopropyl palmitate, glycerin, sorbitol, lactic acid & benzyl alcohol. **0.025% w/Aquatalin.** Tube 15 Gm., 60 Gm. **0.1%.** Tube 15 Gm., 60 Gm. Jar 240 Gm. **0.5%.** Tube 15 Gm. Jar 240 Gm.
Use: Anti-inflammatory steroid.
ARISTOCORT ACETONIDE, SODIUM PHOSPHATE SALT. (Lederle).
Use: Glucosteroid.
See: Aristocort preps.
    Sodium Phosphate Triamcinolone Acetonide
ARISTOCORT CREAM. (Lederle) Triamcinolone acetonide w/stearyl alcohol, polysorbate 80, polysorbate 60, mono and diglycerides, squalane, sorbitol soln., sorbic acid, pot. sorbate. **LP: 0.025%:** Tube 15 Gm. 60 Gm. Jar 240 Gm., 5¼ lb.; **R: 0.1%:** Tube 15 Gm., 60 Gm., Jar 240 Gm., 5¼ lb.; **HP: 0.5%:** Tube 15 Gm. Jar 240 Gm.
Use: Anti-inflammatory steroid.
ARISTOCORT DIACETATE FORTE. (Lederle) Triamcinolone diacetate 40 mg./ml. Vials 1 & 5 ml.
Use: Parenteral steroid, depository.
ARISTOCORT DIACETATE INTRALESIONAL. (Lederle) Triamcinolone diacetate 25 mg./ml. Vial 5 ml.
ARISTOCORT A OINTMENT. (Lederle) Triamcinolone acetonide **0.1%.** Tube 15, 60 Gm. **0.5%.** Tube 15 Gm.
ARISTOCORT OINTMENT. (Lederle) Triamcinolone acetonide. **0.1%:** Tube 15 Gm., 60 Gm. Jar 240 Gm., 5 lb. **0.5%:** Tube 15 Gm. Jar 240 Gm.

Use: Adrenocortical steroid.
ARISTO-PAK. (Lederle) Triamcinolone 4 mg./Tab. 16s.
Use: Glucocorticoid; anti-inflammatory.
ARISTOSPAN INTRALESIONAL. (Lederle) Triamcinolone hexacetonide 5 mg./ml. w/polysorbate 80 0.20% w/v, sorbitol sol. 50% w/v, water q.s., benzyl alcohol 0.90% w/v. Vial 5 ml.
ARISTOSPAN PARENTERAL. (Lederle) Triamcinolone hexacetonide 20 mg./ml. micronized susp. w/polysorbate 80 0.40% w/v, sorbitol sol. 50% w/v, water q.s., benzyl alcohol 0.90% w/v. Vial 1 ml., 5 ml.
Use: Anti-inflammatory.
ARITHMIN INJECTABLE. (Lannett) Antazoline phosphate 100 mg./2 cc. Amp. 12s, 100s.
Use: Antihistaminic.
ARITHMIN TABLETS. (Lannett) Antazoline HCl 100 mg., 200 mg./Tab. Bot. 100s.
Use: Antihistaminic.
ARLACEL 83. (ICI Americas) Sorbitan Sesquioleate.
ARLACEL 165. (ICI Americas) Glyceryl monostearate and PEG-100 stearane nonionic self-emulsifying.
ARLACEL C. (ICI Americas) Sorbitan Sesquioleate. Mixture of oleate esters of sorbitol and its anhydrides.
Use: Surface-active agent.
ARLEF. Flufenamic Acid, B.A.N.
ARLIDIN. (USV Labs.) Nylidrin HCl 6 mg., 12mg./Tab. Bot. 100s, 1000s. Strip dispenser 100s.
Use: Orally, vasodilator, increases peripheral circulation and cardiac output.
ARLIX. (Hoechst) Piretanide HCl.
Use: Diuretic, hypotensive.
ARM-A-CHAR. (Armour) Activated charcoal suspension 30 Gm. in 4 oz. water. Bot. 4 oz.
Use: Adsorbent for use in poisonings or in drug overdosages.
ARMIDEXAN. (Burns) Iron dextran injection.
ARMOUR THYROID. (USV Labs.) Desiccated animal thyroid glands (active thyroid hormones: l-thyroxine, l-triiodothyroxine). ¼, ½, 1, 1½, 2, 3 4, 5 gr./Tab. Most strengths available in several package sizes including: Bot. 100s, 1000s, Handy Hundreds, Carton Strip 100s.
A.R.M. (Menley & James) Chlorpheniramine maleate 4.0 mg., phenylpropanolamine HCl 37.5 mg. Tab. Pkgs. 20s, 40s.
Use: Hay fever, allergy, sinus congestion.
ARMYL. Lymecycline, B.A.N.
ARNE TIMESULES. (Haag) Ferrous fumarate 330 mg., thiamine 5 mg./Cap. Bot. 30s, 100s, 300s, 1000s.
Use: Anemia.
ARNE-C. (Haag) Ferrous fumarate 104 mg., ascorbic acid 60 mg./Tab. Chewable, Bot. 100s, 1000s.
ARNICA TINCTURE. (Lilly) Arnica in alcohol 66%. Bot. 4 fl. oz.
AROMATIC AMMONIA SPIRIT.
See: Ammonia, Aromatic Spirit, U.S.P. XXI.
AROMATIC AMMONIA VAPOROLE. (Burroughs Wellcome) Inhalent. Vial 5 minims.

Use: Inhalent for faintness.
- **AROMATIC ELIXIR,** N.F XVI. (Lilly) Alcohol. 22%. Bot. 16 fl. oz.
Use: Flavored vehicle.
AROXINE. Forminitrazole, B.A.N.
- **ARPRINOCID.** USAN.
Use: Coccidiostat.
ARSAMBIDE.
See: Carbarsone (Various Mfr.)
ARSANILIC ACID. B.A.N. p-Aminophenylarsonic acid.
Use: Treatment of enteritis; growth promotion, veterinary medicine.
See: Maize Pro-Gen
ARSECLOR.
See: Dichlorophenarsine hydrochloride (Var. Mfr.)
- **ARSENIC COMPOUNDS.**
See: Acetarson.
  Arsphenamine
  Carbarsone (Various Mfr.)
  Dichlorophenarsine HCl
  Ferric Cacodylate
  Glycobiarsol
  Neoarsphenamine
  Oxophenarsine HCl
  Sodium Cacodylate (Various Mfr.)
  Tryparsamide
ARSENOBENZENE.
See: Arsphenamine
ARSENPHENOLAMINE.
See: Arsphenamine
ARSTHINOL. Cyclic (hydroxymethyl) ethylene-3-acetamido-4-hydroxydithiobenzenearsonite.
Use: Antiprotozoal.
ARTANE. (Lederle) Trihexyphenidyl HCl. Benzhexol, B.A.N. **Elixir.** Methylparaben 0.08%, propylparaben 0.02% (2 mg./5 ml.), Bot. 1 pt.; **Tab.** (2 mg. & 5 mg.), Bot. 100s, 1000s. Unit dose 10×10 in 10s. **Sequels:** 5 mg., Bot. 60s, 500s.
Use: Parkinsonism.
ARTARAU. (Archer-Taylor) Rauwolfia serpentina 50 mg. or 100 mg./Tab. Bot. 100s, 1000s.
ARTASE. (Jamieson-McKames) Prednisone 0.75 mg., salicylamide 5 gr., C 20 mg., aluminum hydroxide 75 mg./Tab. Bot. 100s.
ARTA-VI-C. (Archer-Taylor) Multivitamins with Vit. C 100 mg./Tab. Bot. 100s.
Use: Supplement.
ARTAZYME. (Archer-Taylor) Autolyzed proteolytic enzyme. Bot. 13 cc.
- **ARTEGRAFT.** USAN. Arterial graft composed of a section of bovine carotid artery that has been subjected to enzymatic digestion with ficin and tanned with dialdehyde starch.
ARTERENOL.
See: Levophed, Amp. (Winthrop-Breon)
ARTERIAL GRAFT. (Johnson & Johnson) Bovine origin.
Use: Arterial grafting.
ARTHOL. (Towne) Acetaminophen 250 mg., salicylamide 250 mg./Tab. Bot. 60s, 100s.
ARTHRALGEN. (Robins) Salicylamide 250 mg., acetaminophen 250 mg./Tab. Bot. 30s, 100s, 500s.

Use: Analgesic.
ARTHRITIC PAIN LOTION. (Walgreen) Triethanolamine salicylate 10%. Bot. 6 oz.
Use: Relief from aches and pains of arthritis and rheumatism.
ARTHRITIS BAYER TIMED RELEASE ASPIRIN. (Glenbrook) Aspirin 650 mg./TR Tab. Bot. 30s, 72s, 125s.
Use: Analgesic, antipyretic, antiinflammatory.
ARTHRITIS PAIN FORMULA. (Whitehall) Aspirin 7½ gr., aluminum hydroxide gel 20 mg., magnesium hydroxide 60 mg./Tab. Bot. 10s, 40s, 100s, 175s.
Use: Analgesic.
ARTHRITIS PAIN FORMULA, ASPIRIN FREE. (Whitehall) Acetaminophen 500 mg./Tab. Bot. 30s., 75s.
Use: analgesic.
ARTHRITIS STRENGTH BUFFERIN. (Bristol-Myers) Aspirin 486 mg./Tab. w/Dialminate (basic aluminum glycinate and magnesium carbonate.) Bot. 40s, 100s.
Use: Analgesic.
ARTHRITIS VACCINES.
See: Streptococcus Vaccine (Lilly)
ARTHROLATE. (Reid-Provident) Sodium thiosalicylate 50 mg., water q.s./cc. Vials 30 cc.
ARTHROPAN LIQUID. (Purdue Frederick) Choline salicylate 870 mg./tsp. Bot. 8, 16 oz.
Use: Analgesic or antipyretic, pain of rheumatoid arthritis and other painful conditions.
ARTICULOSE-50. (Seatrace) Prednisolone acetate 50 mg./ml. Vial 10 cc.
ARTICULOSE L. A. (Seatrace) Triamcinolone diacetate 40 mg./ml. Vial 5 cc.
ARTIFICIAL TANNING AGENT.
See: QT, Prods, (Plough)
  Sudden Tan, Prods. (Plough)
ARTOSIN. Tolbutamide, B.A.N.
ARTRA BEAUTY BAR. (Plough) Triclocarban 1% in soap base. Cake 3.6 oz.
Use: Dermatologic.
ARTRA SKIN TONE CREAM. (Plough) Hydroquinone 2% ointment. Tube ⅓ oz., 1 oz., 2 oz., 4 oz. For normal skin, for dry skin and for oily skin.
Use: Skin lightener.
ARVIN. Ancrod, B.A.N.
ARVYNOL. Ethchlorvynol, B.A.N.
ASA. (Wampole-Zeus) Anti-skin antibodies test by IFA. Tests 48s.
Use: Aid in the diagnosis of pemphigus vulgaris and bullous pemphigoid.
A.S.A.. (Lilly) Aspirin. Acetylsalicylic acid. **Enseals** (5 & 10 gr.) Bot. 100s, 1000s. **Pulvules** (5 gr.) Bot. 100s, 1000s; **Supp.** (5 & 10 gr.) Pkg. 6s; 144s; **Tab.** (5 gr.) Bot. 100s, 1000s. Blisterpak (10 × 10s).
A.S.A. AND CODEINE COMPOUND. (Lilly) Acetylsalicylic acid 380 mg., caffeine 30 mg., codeine phosphate 30 mg./Pulvule or Tab. Bot. 100s.
Use: Analgesic, antipyretic.
ASAFETIDA, EMULSION OF. Milk of Asafetida.

ASALCO NO. 1. (Jenkins) Acetylsalicylic acid 3½ gr., acetophenetidin 2½ gr., caffeine ½ gr./Tab. or Cap. Bot. 1000s.
Use: Colds, neuralgia, muscular soreness.

ASALCO NO. 2. (Jenkins) Dover's powder ¼ gr., acid acetylsalicylic 3½ gr., acetophenetidin 2½ gr., caffeine ½ gr., tinct. gelsemium 2 mg./Tab. or Cap. Bot. 1000s.
Use: Anodyne, analgesic with sedative effects.

ASAPED TABLETS. (Winthrop Products) Acetylsalicylic acid.
Use: Analgesic antipyretic.

ASAWIN TABLETS. (Winthrop Products) Acetylsalicylic acid.
Use: Analgesic, antipyretic.

ASAFEN TABLETS. (Winthrop Products) Paracetamol with other products.
Use: Colds.

A.S.B. (Femco) Calcium carb., magnesium carb., bismuth subcarb., sod. bicarb. & kaolin. Pow., Can 3 oz. Tabs. 50s.
Use: Antacid.

ASBRON G. (Sandoz) Theophylline sodium glycinate 300 mg., guaifenesin 100 mg., alcohol 15% (Elixir only) Tab. Bot. 100s; Elix. Bot. 1 pt.
Use: Relief of acute bronchial asthma & for reversible bronchospasm associated with chronic bronchitis & emphysema.

ASCLEROL. (Spanner) Liver injection crude (2 mcg./cc.) 50%, Vit. B-1 20 mg., B-2 3 mg., B-6 1 mg., B-12 30 mcg., niacinamide 100 mg., panthenol 2.8 mg., choline chloride 20 mg., inositol 10 mg./cc. Multiple dose vial 10 cc.

ASCORVITE. (Vitarine) Vit. C 1000 mg./Gradual Release Tab.
Use: Dietary supplement.

ASCO SOLU-CAPS AND TABLETS. (Sutliff & Case) Aspirin 3 gr., Dover's powder ¼ gr., acetophenetidin 1½ gr., camphor monobromated ¼ gr., atropine sulfate ⅟₅₀₀ gr./Cap. or Tab. Bot. 100s, 1000s.

ASCORBAJEN. (Jenkins) Ascorbic acid and Sodium ascorbate equiv. to 100 mg. of Vit. C/Tab. Bot. 1000s.
Use: Dietary adjuvant.

ASCORBATE SODIUM. Antiscorbutic vitamin.

• **ASCORBIC ACID,** U.S.P. XXI. Injection, Oral Solution, U.S.P. XXI. Tablets, U.S.P. XXI. 3-Oxo-L-gulofuranolactone (enol form). Antiscorbic vitamin; vitamin C.
Cap. (Various Mfr.) 25 mg., 100 mg., 250 mg., 500 mg. **Injection.** (Various Mfr.) Amp. (100 mg./cc.) 1 cc., 2 cc., 5 cc., (200 mg./cc.) 5 cc., (500 mg.) 2 cc., 5 cc., 10 cc., 30 cc. (250 mg./cc.) 10 cc., (1000 mg.) 10 cc. **Tab.** (25 mg., 50 mg., 100 mg., 250 mg., 500 mg.) (Various Mfr.)
Use: Vitamin C therapy
See: Ascorbajen, Tab. (Jenkins)
  Ascorbicap, Cap. (ICN)
  Ascorbineed, Cap. (Hanlon)
  C-Caps 500 (Drug Industries)
  Cecon, Sol. (Abbott)
  Cenolate, Amp. (Abbott)

Cetane, Cap., Vial (Fellows)
Cevalin, Tab., Amp. (Lilly)
Cevi-Bid, Cap. (Geriatric)
Ce-Vi-Sol, Drops (Mead Johnson)
C-Long, Cap., (Reid-Provident)
C-Syrup-500 (Ortega)
Duoscorb, Powd. (Upsher-Smith)
Neo-Vadrin, Preps. (Scherer)
Solucap C, Cap. (Jamieson-McKames)
Synchro-C, Caps. (Carnrick)
Tega-C Tab. (Oretega)

• **ASCORBIC ACID INJECTION,** U.S.P. XXI.
See: Cevalin, Amp, (Lilly)

ASCORBIC ACID SALTS.
See: Bismuth Ascorbate
  Calcium Ascorbate
  Sodium Ascorbate

ASCORBICAP. (ICN) Ascorbic acid 500 mg./Cap. Bot. 50s, 250s.
Use: Treatment of Vit. C deficiency.

ASCORBINEED. (Hanlon) Vit. C 500 mg./T-Cap. Bot. 100s.

ASCORBOCIN POWDER. (Paddock) Vit. C 500 mg., niacin 500 mg., B-1 50 mg., B-6 50 mg., d-αtocopheryl polyethylene glycol 1000 succinate 50 I.U., w/lactose/3 Gm. Bot. 1 lb.
Use: Vitamin supplement.

• **ASCORBYL PALMITATE,** N.F. XVI. L-Ascorbic acid 6-palmitate.
Use: Preservative; antioxidant.

ASCORVITE S.R. (Vitarine) Vit. C 500 mg./Sus. Rel. Cap.
Use: Dietary supplement.

ASCRIPTIN. (Rorer) Aspirin 325 mg., magnesium and aluminum hydroxide (Maalox) 150 mg./Tab. Bot. 50s, 100s, 225s, 500s, also available w/Codeine 15 mg., Bot. 100s. 30 mg. Bot. 100s.
Use: Analgesic, antipyretic, anti-inflammatory.

ASCRIPTIN A/D. (Rorer) Aspirin 325 mg., magnesium and aluminum hydroxides (Maalox) 300 mg./Tab. Bot. 100s, 225s, 500s.
Use: Analgesic, antipyretic, anti-inflammatory.

ASCRIPTIN W/CODEINE No. 2, (Rorer) Codeine phosphate 15 mg., aspirin 325 mg., magnesium and aluminum hydroxides (Maalox) 150 mg./Tab. Bot. 100s.
Use: Orally, analgesic, antipyretic, anti-inflammatory.

ASCRIPTIN W/CODEINE No. 3. (Rorer) Codeine phosphate 30 mg., aspirin 325 mg., magnesium and aluminum hydroxides (Maalox) 150 mg./Tab. Bot. 100s.
Use: Orally, analgesic, antipyretic, anti-inflammatory.

ASELLACRIN. (Serono) Human growth hormone (somatropin) 10 I.U./Vial. plus/vial NaCl diluent; 2 I.U./Vial plus 1 amp. NaCl diluent. Ctn. 1s, 2,s, 4s.
Use: Growth hormone replacement.

ASENDIN. (Lederle) Amoxapine 25 mg., 50 mg., 100 mg., or 150 mg./Tab.
Use: Antidepressant.

ASEPTICHROME.
See: Merbromin (Various Mfr.)
ASLUM. (Drug Products) Carbolic acid 1%, aluminum acetate, ichthammol, zinc oxide, aromatic oils in a petrolatum-stearin base. **Tube** 1 oz. **Jar** 1 lb.
Use: Astringent & soothing dressing.
ASMA. (Wampole-Zeus) Anti-smooth muscle antibody test by IFA. Tests 48.
Use: Diagnostic aid in identifying specific autoimmune disorders.
ASMABAR. (Blue Line) Ephedrine sulfate 25 mg., theophylline 130 mg., butabarbital 20 mg./Tab. Bot. 100s, 1000s.
Use: Treatment of bronchial asthma.
ASMACOL. (Vale) Butabarbital 15 mg., aminophylline 180 mg., phenylpropanolamine HCl 25 mg., chlorpheniramine maleate 2 mg./Tab. w/dihydroxyaluminum aminoacetate as buffer. Bot. 100s, 500s, 1000s.
Use: Bronchospasm due to asthma.
ASMADRIN. (Jenkins) Aminophylline 4 gr., aluminum hydroxide gel, dried, 4 gr., ephedrine HCl ⅜ gr., "trio-bar" ¼ gr. (Representing 33⅓% each of pentobarbital sod., butabarbital sod., and phenobarbital sod)/Tab. Bot. 100s.
ASMA-LIEF. (Columbia) Theophylline 2 gr., ephedrine HCl ⅜ gr., phenobarbital ⅛ gr./Tab. Bot. 50s, 100s, 1000s.
Use: Bronchial asthma and hay fever.
ASMALIX. (Century) Theophylline 80 mg., alcohol 20%, /15 ml. Bot. qt., gal.
Use: Bronchodilator.
ASMASADINA. (Panray) Aminophylline 130 mg., ephedrine HCl 25 mg., amobarbital 25 mg./Cap. Bot. 100s.
ASMA SYRUP. (Coastal) Theophylline 150 mg., guaifenesin 90 mg., alcohol 15%/15 cc. Bot. 16 oz., gal.
ASMATEX. (Kenyon) Chlorpheniremine 1.25 mg., phenylephrine HCl 2.5 mg., acetylsalicylic acid 150 mg. buffered w/aluminum and magnesium hydroxide/Tab. Bot. 100s.
ASMA-TUSS. (Blue Cross) Phenobarbital 4 mg., theophylline 15 mg., ephedrine sulfate 12 mg., guaifenesin 50 mg./5 ml. Bot. 4 oz.
Use: Bronchial asthma treatment.
ASMINOREL. (Reid-Provident) dl-N-Isopropyl arterenol HCl 6 mg., aminophylline 60 mg., ephedrine sulfate 22 mg., Vit. C 10 mg., phenobarbital 8 mg./Tab. Bot. 100s.
Use: Antiasthmatic.
ASMINYL INJECTION. (O'Neal, Jones & Feldman) Dyphylline 250 mg./ml. Vial 10 ml.
ASMINYL TABS. (O'Neal, Jones & Feldman) Phenobarbital sod. 8 mg., ephedrine sulfate 26 mg., theophylline hydrous 130 mg./Tab. Bot. 100s, 500s, 1000s.
Use: Bronchial asthma.
ASMOLIN. (Lincoln) l-Epinephrine 2.5 mg./cc. w/a glycerin solution 25%. Multiple dose vial 10 cc.
Use: For bronchial asthma.
ASOLECTIN. (Associated Conc.) Chemical lecithin 25%, chemical cephalin 22%, inositol phosphatides 16%, soybean oil 2.5%, other miscellaneous sterols and lipids 34.5%.
Use: Hypercholesterolemia, cardiovascular manifestations, and certain skin conditions.
• **ASPARAGINASE.** USAN. L-asparagine amidohydrolase.
Use: Antineoplastic.
I-L-ASPARAGINE-5-L-VALINEANGIOTENSIN II.
See: Angiotensin amide.
• **ASPARTAME,** N.F. XVI. 3-Amino-N-(α-methoxycarbonyl-phenethyl)succinamic acid. L-Aspartyl-L-phenylalanine methyl ester.
Use: Sweetening agent.
• **ASPARTIC ACID.** USAN. Aspartic acid; aminosuccinic acid.
Use: Management of fatigue.
• **ASPARTOCIN.** USAN.
Use: Antibacterial.
A-SPAS. (Hyrex) Dicyclomine HCl 10 mg./ml. Vial 10 ml.
Use: Antispasmodic for I.M. administration.
ASPERBUF. (Bowman) Aspirin 324 gr., aluminum hydroxide dried gel 2 gr./Tab. Bot. 100s, 1000s.
Use: Analgesic.
ASPERCIN. (Otis Clapp) Aspirin 325 mg./Tab. Sugar and salt free. Safety packs 1000s.
Use: Analgesic, antipyretic, anti-inflammatory.
ASPERCIN EXTRA. (Otis Clapp) Aspirin 500 mg./Tab. Sugar and salt free. Safety packs 500s.
Use: Extra strength analgesic, antipyretic, anti-inflammatory.
ASPERCREME. (Stanlabs) Triethanolamine salicylate 10% in a neutral cream base. Bot. 6 oz., Travelettes 5 gm.
ASPERCREME. (Thompson Medical) Triethanolamine salicylate 10% in cream base.
Use: Relief of minor arthritic, rheumatic and muscular aches and pains.
ASPERGILLUS ORYZAE ENZYME. Diastase
See: Taka-Diastase, Preps. (Parke-Davis)
ASPERGUM. (Plough) Aspirin 3.5 gr./1 Gum tablet. Tab. Orange or Cherry flavor. Box 16s, 40s.
Use: Analgesic.
ASPERKINASE. Proteolytic enzyme mixture derived from *aspergillus oryzae.*
• **ASPERLIN.** USAN.
Use: Antibacterial, antineoplastic.
ASPERMIN. (Buffington) Aspirin 325 mg./Tab. Dispens-A-Kits 500s.
Use: Analgesic, antipyretic, anti-inflammatory.
ASPERMIN EXTRA. (Buffington) Aspirin 500 mg./Tab. Dispens-A-Kit 500s.
Use: Analgesic, antipyretic, anti-inflammatory.
ASPIRBAR. (Lannett) Phenobarbital ¼ gr., aspirin 10 gr./Tab. Bot. 1000s.
ASPIR-D COMPOUND CAPSULES. (Lannett) Cap. Bot. 100s.
ASPIR-CODE. (Robinson) Salicylamide 3½ gr., phenacetin 2½ gr., caffeine ½ gr., codeine phosphate 2 mg./Tab. Bot. 36s, 100s.
• **ASPIRIN,** U.S.P. XXI. Caps, Suppos, Tab., U.S.P.

XXI. A.S.A., Acetophen, Acetol, Acetosal,
Acetosalin, Aceticyl, Acetylin, Acetylsal, Empirin,
Saletin. Acetylsalicylic acid, Benzoic acid, 2-(acetylox-
y)-., Salicyclic acid acetate.
Use: Analgesic, antipyretic, & antirheumatic.
   See: A.S.A., Prep. (Lilly)
      Aspergum, Gum, Tab. (Plough)
      Aspirjen Jr., Tab. (Jenkins)
      BC Tablets (Block Drug)
      Buffinol, Tab. (Otis Clapp)
      Ecotrin, Tab. (SmithKline)
      Empirin, Tab. (Burroughs Wellcome)
      Measurin, Tab. (Winthrop-Breon)
      Norwich Aspirin, Tab. (Norwich Eaton)
      St. Joseph, Prods. (Plough)
W/Acetophenetidin & caffeine.
   See: A.P.C. preparations (Various Mfg.)
ASPIRIN-BARBITURATE COMBINATIONS.
   See: Acetabar, Cap., Tab. (Philips Roxane)
      Amytal w/Acetylsal., Cap. (Lilly)
      Anaphen, Cap. (Mallard)
      Aspirbar, Tab. (Lannett)
      Aspirin Uniserts,Suppos. (Upsher-Smith)
      Axotal, Tab. (Warren-Teed)
      Brogesic, Tab. (Brothers)
      Bufabar, Tab. (Philips Roxane)
      Buff-A Comp., Cap., Tabs. (Mayrand)
      Cefinal, Tab. (Alto)
      Doloral, Tab. (Alamed)
      Fiorinal, Cap., Tab. (Sandoz)
      Marnal, Tab., Cap. (Vortech)
      Nipirin, Cap. (Elder)
      Palgesic, Tab., Cap. (Pan Amer.)
      Percobarb, Cap. (Du Pont)
      Rotense, Tab. (Robinson)
      Salibar Jr., Tab. (Jenkins)
      Sedagesic, Tabs. (Kay)
      Sedalgesic, Tab. (Table Rock)
ASPIRIN ENTERIC COATED.
   See: A.S.A., Prep. (Lilly)
      Ecotrin, Tab. (Menley & James)
ASPIRIN PLUS. (Walgreen) Aspirin 400 mg., caffeine
32 mg./Tab. Bot. 100s.
Use: Analgesic.
ASPIRIN SALTS.
   See: Calcium Acetylsalicylate
ASPIRIN W/O.T.C. COMBINATIONS.
   See: A.C.A., Caps., Tabs. (Scrip)
      Alka Seltzer, Tab. (Miles)
      Alka Seltzer Plus, Tab. (Miles)
      Anacin, Tab. (Whitehall)
      Analgestine Forte, Cap. (Mallard)
      Anaphen, Cap. (Mallard)
      Anodynos, Tab. (Buffington)
      A.P.C., Tab. & Cap. (Various Mfr.)
      A.S.A. Comp., Cap., Tab. (Lilly)
      Ascriptin, Tab. (Rorer)
      Ascriptin A/D, Tab. (Rorer)
      Bayer Aspirin Preps. (Glenbrook)
      Bayer Prods. (Glenbrook)
      BC Powder (Block Drug)
      Bexophene, Cap. (Mallard)

Buffaprin, Tab. (Buffington)
Bufferin, Tab. (Bristol-Myers)
Buffinol, Tab. (Otis Clapp)
Cama, Tab. (Dorsey)
Capathyn, Cap. (Scrip)
Capron, Cap. (Vitarine)
Congespirin, Tab. (Bristol-Myers)
Coralsone Modified, Tab. (Zemmer)
Counterpain, Tube (Squibb)
Damason, Prep. (Mason)
Derfort, Cap. (Cole)
Derfule, Cap. (Cole)
Dolor, Tab. (Geriatric Pharm.)
Dynosal, Tab. (Mallard)
Emagrin, Tab. (Otis Clapp)
Emagrin Forte, Tab. (Otis Clapp)
Excedrin, Cap., Tab. (Bristol-Myers)
Excedrin P.M., Tab. (Bristol-Myers)
4-Way, Tab., Spray (Bristol-Myers)
Gemnisyn, Tab. (Rorer)
Liquiprin, Tab. (Mitchum-Thayer)
Midol, Cap., Spray (Glenbrook)
PAC, Cap., Tab. (Upjohn)
Pap, Cap. (Zenith)
Phenacaps, Cap. (Scrip)
Phensal, Tab. (Merrell Dow)
Presalin, Tab. (Mallard)
Saleto, Prep. (Mallard)
Salocol, Tab. (Mallard)
Scrip-Dyne Comp., Cap. (Scrip)
Sine-Off Tablets (Menley & James)
Stanback, Pow., Tab. (Stanback)
St. Joseph Cold Tablets For Children (Plough)
Trigesic, Tab. (Squibb)
Vanquish, Cap. (Glenbrook)
ASPIRIN UNISERTS. (Upsher-Smith) Aspirin 125
mg./Supp. Ctn. 12s, 50s; 300 mg./Supp. Ctn. 12s,
50s, 500s; 600 mg/Supp. Ctn. 12s, 50s, 500s.
Use: Analgesic, antipyretic.
ASPIRJEN Jr. (Jenkins) Aspirin 2½ gr./Tab. Bot.
1000s.
Use: Analgesic.
ASPIR-PHEN. (Robinson) Aspirin 5 gr., phenobarbital ½
gr./Tab. Bot. 100s, 1000s. Bulk Pack 5000s.
Use: Pediatric.
ASPIRTAB. (Dover) Aspirin 325 mg./Tab. Sugar and
salt free. Unit dose 500s.
Use: Analgesic, antipyretic, anti-inflammatory.
ASPIRTAB MAX. (Dover) Aspirin 500 mg./Caplet.
Sugar and salt free. Unit dose 500s.
Use: Extra strength analgesic, antipyretic,
anti-inflammatory.
ASPODYNE. (Blue Line) Aspirin 3½ gr.,
acetophenetidin 2½ gr., caffeine ½ gr./Tab. Bot.
1000s.
W/Codeine phosphate ¼ gr. Bot. 1000s.
Use: Analgesic-antipyretic.
ASPOGEN. Dihydroxyaluminum aminoacetate.
ASPRO.
   See: Acetylsalicylic acid.
ASPROJECT. (Mayrand) Sodium thiosalicylate 50
mg./ml. Vial 30 ml.

Use: Analgesic, antipyretic. **0.5mg.:** Bot. 100s, 500s. Redipak 25s. **1.0 mg.:** Bot. 100s, 500s, 1000s. Redipak 25s. **2 mg.:**
ASTARIL TABLETS. (Winthrop Products) Theophylline anhydrous, ephedrine sulphate.
Use: Antiasthmatic.
• **ASTEMIZOLE.** USAN.
Use: Antihistaminic.
ASTEROL. 6-(2-Diethylaminoethoxy)-2-di-methylaminobenzothiazole dihydrochloride. Diam-thazole Dihydrochloride, B.A.N.
Use: Antifungal drug.
ASTHMACON. (CMC) Aminophylline 130 mg., ephedrine HCl 25 mg., amobarbital 25 mg./Cap. Bot. 100s, 500s, 1000s.
Use: Antiasthmatic.
ASTHMA METER. (Rexall) Epinephrine 0.2 mg./dose. Aerosol nebulizer w/measured dose valve 15 cc. or 300 doses.
ASTHMAHALER. (Norcliff Thayer) Epinephrine bitartrate 7 mg./ml. in an inert propellant. Oral inhaler, 15 ml. with mouthpiece; refills.
Use: Bronchial asthma.
ASTHMANEFRIN SOLUTION & NEBULIZER. (Norcliff Thayer) Racepin (racemic epinephrine) as HCl equivalent to 2.25% epinephrine base, chlorobutanol 0.5%. Bot. ½ fl. oz., 1 fl. oz.
Use: Bronchial asthma.
ASTRING-O-SOL. (Winthrop Products) Alcohol, zinc chloride, methyl salicylate and myrrh extract in a concentrated solution (4 oz. makes 1 gallon). Bot. 4 oz., 8 oz.
Use: Mouthwash.
• **ASTROMICIN SULFATE.** USAN.
Use: Antibacterial.
ASTRO-VITES. (Faraday) Vit. A 3500 I.U., D 400 I.U., C 60 mg., B-1 0.8 mg., B-2 1.3 mg., niacinamide 14 mg., B-6 1 mg., B-12 2.5 mcg., folic acid 0.05 mg., pantothenic acid 5 mg., Fe 12 mg./Tab. Bot. 100s, 250s.
ASUNTOL. Coumaphos, B.A.N.
ASUPIRIN. (Suppositoria) Aspirin 60 mg., 120 mg., 200 mg., 300 mg., 600 mg./1.2 Gm./Suppository. Box 12s, 100s, 1000s.
Use: Alternate route of administration for aspirin.
A.T. 10.
See: Dihydrotachysterol
ATABEE TD. (Defco) Vit. C 500 mg., B-1 15 mg., B-2 10 mg., B-6 2 mg., nicotinamide 50 mg., calcium pantothenate 10 mg./Cap. Bot. 30s, 1000s.
Use: Water-soluble B-complex and ascorbic acid vita-min deficiencies.
ATABRINE HYDROCHLORIDE. (Winthrop-Breon) Quinacrine hydrochloride. **Tab.** (0.1 Gm.) Bot. 100s.
Use: Malaria of all types, giardiasis and tapeworm.
ATARAX. (Roerig) Hydroxyzine HCl **Tab.** (10 mg., 25 mg., 50 mg.) Bot. 100s, 500s, (100 mg.) Bot. 100s. (25 mg., 50 mg., 100 mg.) Unit dose pak 100s. **Syr.** (10 mg./5 cc. w/alcohol 0.5%) Bot. 1 pt.
Use: Treatment of tension, antianxiety & allergic dermatoses.
W/Ephedrine sulfate, theophylline.

See: Marax, Tab., Syr. (Roerig)
W/Penta-erythrityltetranitrate.
See: Cartrax, Tab. (Roerig)
■ **ATARAXIC AGENTS.**
See: Tranquilizers
ATARVET. Acepromazine.
ATEMPOL. Methylpentynol, B.A.N.
ATENOLOL. USAN. 4-(2-Hydroxy-3-isopropylamino-propoxy) phenylacetamide.
Use: Beta adrenergic blocking agent.
See: Tenormin, Tab. (Stuart)
ATENSINE. Diazepam, B.A.N.
AT-EZE. (Faraday) Caps. Vial 30s. Bot. 1000s.
Use: Sleep aid.
ATGAM. (Upjohn) Lymphocyte immune globulin, antithymocyte globulin 250 mg. protein (50 mg./ml.). Amp. 5 ml.
Use: Management of allograft rejection in renal transplant patients.
ATGARD. Dichlorvos, B.A.N.
ATHLETE'S FOOT OINTMENT. (Walgreen) Zinc Undecylenate 20%, undecylenic acid 5%. Tube 1.5 oz.
Use: Antifungal.
ATHROMBIN.
See: Warfarin Sod.
ATHROMBIN-K TABLETS. (Purdue Frederick) Warfarin potassium 5 mg./Tab. Bot. 100s.
Use: Anticoagulant.
ATIVAN INJECTION. (Wyeth) Lorazepam 2 mg., 4 mg./ml. Vials 1 ml., 10 ml. Tubex. Pkg. 10s.
Use: Preanesthesia.
ATIVAN TABLETS. (Wyeth) Lorazepam 0.5 mg., 1 mg. or 2 mg./Tab. **0.5 mg.:** Bot. 100s, 500s. Redipak 25s. **1.0 mg.:** Bot. 100s, 500s, 1000s. Redipak 25s. **2 mg.:** Bot. 100s, 500s, 1000s. Redipak 25s.
Use: Minor tranquilizer for use in treatment of anxiety and tension.
• **ATOLIDE.** USAN. 2-Amino-4'-(diethylamino)-o-benzotoluidide. Under study.
Use: Anticonvulsant.
• **ATRACURIUM BESYLATE.** USAN.
Use: Skeletal muscle relaxant.
ATRIDINE. (Interstate) Tripolidine 2.5 mg., pseudoephedrine HCl 60 mg./Tab. Bot. 100s, 1000s.
Use: Antihistimine, nasal decongestant.
ATROBARB NO. 1 (Jenkins) Phenobarbital sod. ⅛ gr., atropine sulfate ¹⁄₁₀₀₀ gr./Tab. Bot. 1000s.
Use: Sedative.
ATROBARB NO. 2 (Jenkins) Phenobarbital sod. ¼ gr., atropine sulfate ¹⁄₅₀₀ gr./Tab. Bot. 1000s.
Use: Antispasmodic, antiemetic
ATROBARB NO. 3 (Jenkins) Phenobarbital sod. ¼ gr., atropine sulfate ¹⁄₂₅₀ gr./Tab. Bot. 1000s.
Use: Antispasmodic, antiemetic.
ATROCAP. (Freeport) Atropine sulfate 0.06 mg., hyoscyamine sulfate 0.3 mg., hyoscine hydrobromide 0.02 mg., phenobarbital 50 mg./T.R. Cap. Bot. 1000s.
Use: Sedative, anti-spasmodic, anticholinergic.

ATROCHOLIN. (Blue Line) Dehydrocholic acid 2 gr., homatropine methylbromide $^1/_{100}$ gr./Tab. Bot. 100s, 1000s, 5000s.
Use: Antispasmodic & hydrocholeretic.

ATROMID-S. (Ayerst) Clofibrate 500 mg./Cap. Bot. 100s.
Use: Hypercholesterolemia and/or hypertriglyceridemia.

ATROPHYSINE. (Lannett) Physostigmine salicylate 0.6 mg., atropine sulf. 0.6 mg./cc. Vials 30 cc.
Use: I.M., antispasmodic for skeletal muscle.

• **ATROPINE,** U.S.P. XXI. 1αH, 5αH-Tropan-3α-ol dl-Tropate (Ester) (dl-Hyoscyamine)dl-Tropyltropate.
See: Atropine Combinations

ATROPINE AND DEMEROL INJECTION. (Winthrop-Breon) Atropine sulfate 0.4 mg., meperidine HCl 50 mg. or 75 mg./Carpuject.
Use: Preoperative sedation.

ATROPINE BUFOPTO. (Softcon) Atropine sulf. ½%, 1% in methulose w/Benzalkonium chloride. Bot. 15 cc.
Use: Mydriasis and cycloplegia.

■ **ATROPINE-HYOSCINE-HYOSCYAMINE COMBINATIONS. (See also Belladonna Products)**
See: Almezyme, Cap. (Glaxo)
Barbella, Tab., Elix. (Fellows)
Barbeloid, Tab. (Vale)
Barbidonna-CR, Cap. (Mallinckrodt)
Bar-Cy-Amine, Elix. (Sutliff & Case)
Bar-Cy-A-Tab, Tab. (Sutliff & Case)
Bar-Don, Tab., Elix. (Warren-Teed)
Belakoids TT, Tab. (Philips Roxane)
Belbutal No. 2 Kaptabs. (Churchill)
Brobella-P.B., Tab. (Brothers)
Buren, Tab. (Ascher)
Donnacin, Elix., Tab. (Pharmex)
Donnagel, Susp. (Robins)
Donnamine, Elix., Tab. (Tennessee Pharm.)
Donnatal, Cap., Elix., Tab. (Robins)
Donnatal #2, Tab. (Robins)
Donnatal Extentabs, Tab. (Robins)
Donnazyme, Tab. (Robins)
Eldonal, Prep. (Canright)
Haponal, Cap. (Jenkins)
Hyatal, Elix. (Winsale)
Hybephen, Preps. (Beecham Labs)
Hyonal, Prep. (Paddock)
Hyonatol B, Preps. (Bowman)
Hytrona, Tab. (Webcon)
Kinesed, Tab. (Stuart)
Koryza Tab. (Fellows)
Levamine, Tab. (Glaxo)
Maso-Donna, Elix., Tab. (Mason)
Nilspasm, Tab. (Parmed)
Renalgin, Tab. (Meyer)
Sedamine, Tab. (Dunhall)
Sedapar, Tab. (Parmed)
Sedralex, Elix., Tab. (Kay)
Seds, Tab. (Pasadena Research)
Spabelin, Elix. (Arcum)
Spasdel, Cap. (Marlop)
Spasloids, Tab. (G.F. Harvey)
Spasmolin, Tab. (Bell)
Spasquid, Elix. (Geneva)
Spastolate, Elix., Tab. (Barry-Martin)
Uriseptin, Tab. (Blaine)
Urogesic, Tab. (Edwards)
Zemarine Elix., Cap., Tab. (Zemmer)

ATROPINE METHYLNITRATE. (Various Mfr.) dl-Hyoscyamine methylnitrate.
See: Harvatrate, Tab. (O'Neal)
Thitrate W.P., Tab. (Blaine)
W/Hyoscine HBr, hyoscyamine sulfate, amobarbital sodium.
See: Amocine, Tab. (Mallard)
W/Methenamine mandelate & Phenylazodiaminopyridine HCl.
See: Uritral, Cap. (Central)
W/Oxidized bile acids, ox and hog bile ext., phenobarbital.
See: G.B.S., Tab. (O'Neal)
W/Phenobarbital & dihydroxy aluminum aminoacetate.
See: Atromal, Tab. (Blaine)
Harvatrate A, Tab. (O'Neal)
W/Sulfaguanidine, sulfacetamide, neomycin sulf., carob flour.
See: Neogel W/Sulf, Tab. (Vortech)

ATROPINE-N-OXIDE HCl.
See: Atropine Oxide HCl.

• **ATROPINE OXIDE HYDROCHLORIDE.** USAN. Atropine N-oxide hydrochloride.
See: X-Tro. (Xttrium)

• **ATROPINE SULFATE,** U.S.P. XXI. Inj. Ophth. Oint. Ophth. Soln., Tablets, U.S.P. XXI. (Various Mfr.) Benzeneacetic acid, α-(hydroxymethyl-,8-methyl-8-azabicyclo-[3.2.1.]oct-3-yl ester, endo-(+)-, sulfate (2:1) (salt), monohydrate. l-αH, 5-α-H-Tropan-3-α-ol (+)-tropate (ester), sulfate (2:1) (salt) monohydrate. **Pediatric Inj.:** (Abbott) 0.05 mg./ml. 5 ml. Abboject.**Tab-Hypodermic,** $^1/_{500}$, $^1/_{250}$, $^1/_{100}$, $^1/_{50}$, gr./Tab. **Tab-Oral,** $^1/_{500}$, $^1/_{250}$, $^1/_{200}$, $^1/_{150}$, $^1/_{100}$ gr./Tab. **Inj.** (Abbott) 0.1 mg./ml. 10 ml. Abboject syringe. **Lyophilized.** Lyopine (Hyrex)
Use: Anticholinergic, antidote to cholinesterase inhibitors.
See: Isopto-Atropine (Alcon)
Lyopine, Inj. (Hyrex)
Parasympatholytic & antispasmodic agent
W/Chlorpheniramine.
See: Histunex, Inj. (Tunex)
W/Diphenoxylatent
See: Colontil, Tab., Liq. (Mallinckrodt)
W/Ephedrine sulfate.
See: Enuretrol, Tab. (Berlex)

ATROPINE SULFATE W/PHENOBARBITAL.
See: Alised, Tab. (Elder)
Antrocol, Tab., Cap. (Poythress)
Arco-Lase Plus, Tab. (Arco)
Barbeloid, Tab. (Vale)
Bar-Tropin, Tab. (Fellows-Testagar)
Bioxatphen, Tab. (Zemmer)
Briabell, Tab. (Briar)
Briaspaz, Tab. (Briar)
Brobella-P.B., Tab. (Brothers)

Cerebel, Liq. (Xttrium)
Copin, Tab. (Bluco)
Donnatal, Cap., Extentabs, Tab., Elix. (Robins)
Donnatal #2, Tab. (Robins)
Haponal, Cap. (Jenkins)
Histacon, Tab., Syr. (Marsh-Emory)
Hyatal Elix. (Winsale)
Magnased, Tab. (Century)
Magnox, Tabs. (Bowman)
P & A, Tab. (Scrip)
Palbar No. 2, Tab. (Hauck)
PAMA, Tab. (N. Am. Pharm.)
Peece, Cap., Tab. (Scrip)
Ro Trim, Cap. (Rocky Mtn.)
Sedatabs, Tab. (Parkdale)
Seds, Tab. (Pasadena Research)
Spabelin, Elix. (Arcum)
Spasaid, Cap. (Century)
Spasdel, Cap. (Marlop)
Spasidon, Tab. (Haag)
Spasmate, Tab. (Spencer-Mead)
Spasmolin, Tab. (Kenyon)
Spastosed, Tab. (N. Am. Pharm.)
Stannitol (Standex)

ATROPISOL. (CooperVision) Atropine sulfate.
Dropperettes 0.5%, 1%, 2%. 1 ml. 12s. **Sol.** 1%
Dropper Bot. 5 ml, 1% Bot. 15 ml.
Use: Mydriasis, cycloplegia.

ATROSED. (Freeport) Atropine sulfate 0.0195 mg.,
hyoscine HBr 0.0065 mg., hyoscyamine sulfate
0.1040 mg. phenobarbital ¼ gr./Tab. Bot. 1000s,
5000s.
Use: Sedative, anti-spasmodic, anticholinergic.

ATROVENT.
See: Ipratropium bromide, B.A.N.

A/T/S TOPICAL SOLUTION. (Hoechst) Erythromycin
2% topical sol. Bot. 60 ml. W/applicator.
Use: Acne treatment, topical.

ATTAPULGITE, ACTIVATED.
See: Quintess, Susp. (Lilly)
W/Pectin, hydrated alumina powder.
See: Polymagma Plain Tablets (Wyeth)
W/Polysorbate 80, salicylic acid, propylene glycol.
See: Sebasorb Lotion (Summer)

ATTENUVAX. (Merck Sharp & Dohme) Measles virus
vaccine, live, attenuated w/neomycin 25 mcg./Vial.
Single-dose vial w/diluent-containing disposable
syringe; Box of 10 single-dose vials
w/diluent-containing disposable syringes.
Use: Live vaccine for measles.
W/Meruvax.
See: M-R-Vax-II, Vial (Merck Sharp & Dohme)
W/Mumpsvax, Meruvax.
See: M-M-R II, Vial (Merck Sharp & Dohme)

ATURBANE HYDROCHLORIDE. Phenglutarimide,
B.A.N.

ATUSSIN EXPECTORANT. (Amfre-Grant) Chlorpheniramine maleate 2 mg., phenylephrine HCl 5
mg., phenylpropanolamine HCl 5 mg., guaifenesin
100 mg./5 cc Bot. 4 oz., pt., gal.
Use: Coughs

ATUSSIN-D.M. EXPECTORANT. (Amfre-Grant) Chlor-

pheniramine maleate 2 mg., phenylephrine HCl 5
mg., phenylpropanolamine HCl 5 mg., guaifenesin
100 mg., d-methorphan HBr 15 mg./5 cc. Syr. Bot. 4
oz., pt., gal.
Use: Coughs.
W/Pentobarbital sodium, 2-diethylaminoethyl diphenylacetate hydrochloride, aluminum hydroxide.
See: Spasmasorb, Tab. (Hauck)

A.T.V. VAGINAL SUPPOSITORIES. (Amfre-Grant) Estrone 0.2 mg. lactose 50.0 mg./supp. Pkg. 12s with
inserter.
Use: Hormone-estrogen therapy.

AUDINORM. Dioctyl Sodium Sulphosuccinate, B.A.N.

AURA-BELL. (Metro Med) Bot. ½ oz.
Use: Ear solution.

AURAL ACUTE. (Saron) Polymyxin B sulfate 10,000
u., neomycin sulfate 5 mg., hydrocortisone 10
mg./10 cc w/alcohol 0.1%.
Use: Antibiotic ear drops.

AURALGAN OTIC SOLUTION. (Ayerst) Antipyrine 54
mg., benzocaine 14 mg./ml. w/oxyquinoline sulfate
in dehyd. glycerin. (contains not more than 0.6%
moisture). Bot. w/dropper ½ fl. oz.
Use: Treatment otitis media (acute), removal of
cerumen.

AURALGESIC. (Wesley) Carbamide 10%, antipyrine
5%, benzocaine 2.5%, cetyldimethylbenzylammonium HCl 0.2%. Bot. ½ oz.

• **AURANOFIN.** USAN.
Use: Antirheumatic.

AUREOMYCIN PREPARATIONS. (Lederle)
Chlortetracycline HCl.
Oint. Ophth.: 1%. (10 mg./Gm.) Tube ⅛ oz.
Oint. Topical: 3% in white petrolatum, anhydrous
lanolin base. Tube 20 Gm., ½ oz., 1 oz.
Use: Broad spectrum antibiotic.

AUREOQUIN DIAMATE. Name previously used for
Quinetolate.

AURINOL EAR DROPS. (CMC) Benzocaine,
antipyrene, glycerol. Bot. ½ oz., pt., gal.
Use: Removal of wax.

AURISTIL. (Blue Line) Benzocaine 9%,
hexylresorcinol 0.1%, menthol 4%, camphor 2%.
Dropules 50 min., rubber-cap droppers, 12s.
Use: Analgesic for ear-ache.

AURI-TUSS. (Zemmer) Dextromethorphan HBr 15 mg.,
chlorpheniramine maleate 1 mg., guaifenesin 90
mg., phenylephrine HCl 5 mg., alcohol 10%/5 cc.
Syrup. Bot. 3 oz., pt., gal.
Use: Control of cough.

AUROCAINE. (Vita Elixir) Benzocaine 0.15 Gm.,
antipyrine 0.70 Gm., glycerol q.s.
Use: Otic analgesic.

AUROCEIN. (Christina) Gold naphthyl sulfhydryl
derivative. Amp. (5% or 12.5%) 10 cc.
Use: Antirheumatic gold therapy.

AURO-DRI. (Commerce) Boric acid 2.75% in
isopropyl alcohol. Bot. 1 oz.
Use: Relief of swimmer's ear.

AURO EAR DROPS. (Commerce) Carbamide
peroxide 6.5% in a specially prepared base. Tube
0.5 oz.

Use: For softening wax.

AUROLIN.
See: Gold sodium thiosulfate.

AUROMID EARDROPS. (Vangard) Antipyrine 54 mg., benzocaine 14 mg./ml. w/glycerin dehydrated q.s. to 1 ml. Bot. 15 ml.
Use: Decongestant, analgesic.

AUROPIN.
See: Gold sodium thiosulfate.

AUROSAN.
See: Gold sodium thiosulfate.

AUROTHIOBLYCANIDE. 2-Mercaptoacetanilide S-gold (1+) salt.
Use: Antirheumatic.

AUROTHIOGLUCOSE INJECTION.
See: Sterile aurothioglucose suspension.

AUROTHIOMALATE, SODIUM.
See: Gold Sodium Thiomalate, U.S.P. XXI.

AUROTIS. (Research Pharmacal Lab.) Antipyrine 4%, benzocaine 1%, glycerine 95%. 15 cc.
Use: Acute otitis media.

AURTO. (CMC)
Use: Treatment of acute otitis media

AUSAB. (Abbott) Test kit 100s.
Use: Radioimmunoassay or enzyme immunoassay for detection of antibody to hepatitis B surface antigen.

AUSCELL. (Abbott) Test kit 110s, 450s, 1800s.
Use: Reverse passive hemagglutination test for hepatitis B surface antigen.

AUSRIA II-125. (Abbott) Antibody to test for hepatitis B surface antigen. Test kit 100s, 500s, 600s, 700s, 800s, 900s, 1000s.
Use: Radioimmunoassay for detection of hepatitis B antigen.

AUSZYME II. (Abbott) Test kit 100s, 500s.
Use: Enzyme immunoassay for detection of hepatitis B surface antigen.

AUTOANTIBODY SCREEN. (Wampole-Zeus) Autoantibody screening system. Tests 48s.
Use: To screen serum for the presence of a variety of autoantibodies.

AUTOLET KIT. (Ames) Automatic blood letting spring-loaded device.
Use: Obtaining capillary blood samples from fingertips, earlobes or heels.

AUTOPLEX. (Hyland) Anti-inhibitor coagulant complex prepared from pooled human plasma. Vial 30 ml.
Use: Anti-inhibitor coagulant complex.

AUTO SYRINGE INSULIN PUMPS. (Travenol) Insulin infusion pump.

AUTRINIC. Intrinsic factor concentrate.
Use: Increase absorption of Vit. B-12.

AUXOTAB ENTERIC 1 & 2. (Colab) Rapid identification of enteric bacteria and pseudomonas. Test contains capillary units with selective biochemical reagents.

A-VAN. (Stewart-Jackson) Dimenhydrinate 25 mg., niacin 50 mg./Cap. Bot. 100s.
Use: Treatment of vertigo, dizziness, Meniere's syndrome, labyrinthitis.

AVC CREAM. (Merrell Dow) Sulfanilamide 15%, aminacrine HCl 0.2%, allantoin 2% with lactose, in a water-miscible base made from propylene glycol, stearic acid, diglycol stearate to acid pH. Tube 4 oz. w/applicator.
Use: Vulvovaginitis when responsible organism not known *(Trichomonas vaginalis, Candida albicans,* or *Hemophilus vaginitis).*

AVC SUPPOSITORIES. (Merrell Dow) Sulfanilamide 1.05 Gm., aminacrine HCl 0.014 Gm., allantoin 0.14 Gm. with lactose, in a base made from polyethlene glycol 400, polysorbate 80, polyethylene glycol 3350, glycerin, inert glycerin-gelatin covering. Box of 16s w/inserter.
Use: Vulvovaginitis when responsible organism not known *(Trichomonas vaginalis, Candida albicans,* or *Hemophilus vaginalis).*

AVC/DIENESTROL CREAM. (Merrell Dow) Dienestrol 0.01%, sulfanilamide 15%, aminacrine HCl 0.2%, allantoin 2% with lactose, in a water-miscible base made from propylene glycol, stearic acid, diglycol stearate, triethanolamine, butylated hydroxytoluene. Tube 4 oz., w/applicator.
Use: Atrophic vaginitis and kraurosis vulvae associated with menopause and complicated by infection.

AVC/DIENESTROL SUPPOSITORIES. (Merrell Dow) Dienestrol 0.7 mg., sulfanilamide 1.05 Gm., aminacrine HCl 0.014 Gm., allantoin 0.14 Gm. with lactose, in a base made from polyethylene glycol 400, polysorbate 80, polyethylene glycol 3350, glycerin, butylated hydroxytoluene, inert glycerin-gelatin covering. Box of 16s w/inserter.
Use: Atrophic vaginitis and kraurosis vulvae associated with menopause and complicated by infection.

AVEENOBAR MEDICATED. (CooperCare) Aveeno colloidal oatmeal 50%, sulfur 2%, salicylic acid 2%, in soap-free cleansing bar. Formerly Acnaveen. Bar 3.5 oz.
Use: Antipruritic cleanser and shampoo.

AVEENA BATH. (CooperCare) Colloidal oatmeal. Box 1 lb., 4 lb.
Use: Antipruritic bath.

AVEENOBAR OILATED. (CooperCare) Vegetable oils, lanolin derivative, glycerine 29%, Aveeno colloidal oatmeal 30% in soap-free base. Formerly Emulave. Bar. 3 oz.
Use: Lubricates, protects and helps remoisturize dry skin.

AVEENOBAR REGULAR. (CooperCare) A soap-free cleansing bar containing 50% colloidal oatmeal, anionic sulfonate and hypo-allergenic lanolin. Formerly Aveeno Bar. Bar 3.2 oz., 4.4 oz.
Use: Hypoallergenic cleansing agent.

AVEENO COLLOIDAL OATMEAL. (CooperCare) Colloidal oatmeal. Box 1 lb., 4 lb.
Use: Acute, inflammatory "wet" dermatoses.
W/Sulfur, salicylic acid.
See: Acnaveen, Bar (CooperVision)

AVEENO LOTION. (CooperCare) Colloidal oatmeal (A demulcent) in a soothing mildly drying aqueous lotion base. Bot. 6 oz.

Use: Relief of sunburn, poison ivy and oak, diaper rash and other minor skin problems.

AVEENO OILATED. (CooperCare) Aveeno colloidal oatmeal impregnated with a high percentage (35%) of liquid petrolatum and refined olive oil. Box. 8 oz., 2 lb.
Use: Dry skin conditions.

AVENTYL HCl. (Lilly) Nortriptyline HCl equiv. to 10 mg. base/5 ml. **Liq.** Bot. 16 fl. oz. **Pulvule:** equiv. to 10 mg. base or 25 mg. base/Cap. Bot. 100s, 500s. Blisterpak 10 × 10s.
Use: Mental depression and anxiety-tension states.

AVERTIN. Tribromoethanol (Var. Mfr.)

AVICALM HCl. Metoserpate, B.A.N.

AVINAR. Uredepa.
Use: Anti-neoplastic agent.

AVLOCLOR. Chloroquine, B.A.N.

AVLOSULFON. (Ayerst) Dapsone Tab. 100 mg. Bot. 100s.
Use: Treatment of all forms of leprosy.

AVOMINE. Promethazine Theoclate, B.A.N.

AVONIQUE. (Geneva) Vit. A 4000 I.U., D 400 I.U., B-1 1 mg., B-2 1.2 mg., B-6 2 mg., B-12 2 mcg., Ca panothenate 5 mg., B-3 10 mg., C 30 mg., Ca 100 mg., P 76 mg., Fe 10 mg., Mn 1 mg., Mg. 1 mg. Zn 1 mg.
Use: Multiple vitamin.

• **AVOPARCIN.** USAN.
Use: Antibacterial.

A.V.P. CILLIN TABS AND POWDER FOR SYRUP. (A.V.P.) Potassium Penicillin G. **Syr.:** (400,000 u) 250 mg./5 cc. Bot. 80 cc. **Tab.:** 250 mg./Tab. Bot. 100s.
Use: Anti-infective.

A.V.P. NATAL-FA. (A.V.P.) Vitamin A 5000 I.U., iron, elemental from 200 mg., ferrous fumarate 65 mg., calcium 165 mg., phosphorus 75 mg., C 100 mg., B-6 10 mg., folic acid 1 mg./Tab. Bot. 100s.
Use: Dietary supplement during pregnancy or lactation.

• **AVRIDINE.** USAN.

AVR PADS. (Birchwood) Witch hazel-glycerin impregnated flannel pad. 40 pads/Jar.
Use: Personal hygiene.

AXEROPHTHOL.
See: Vitamin A

AXON THROAT SPRAY. (McKesson) Bot. 5.0 gm.
Use: Sore throat remedy.

AXOTAL. (Adria) Butalbital 50 mg., aspirin 650 mg./Tab. Bot. 100s, 500s. Stat-Pak 100s.
Use: Relief of symptomatic complex of tension headaches.

AXSINATE. (Lannett) Styramate 200 mg., salicylamide 210 mg., acetophenetidin 150 mg., caffeine 30 mg./Tab. Bot. 50s.
Use: Analgesic.

AYDS APPETITE SUPPRESSANT CANDY. (Jeffrey Martin) Benzocaine 5 mg. in chewy candy base w/25 cal./Cube candy. Ctn. 12s, 48s, 96s.
Use: Appetite suppressant.

AYGESTIN. (Ayerst) Norethindrone acetate 5 mg./Tab. Bot. 50s. cycle packs 10s.
Use: Progestin hormone therapy.

AYR SALINE NASAL DROPS. (Ascher) Sodium chloride 0.65% adjusted with phosphate buffers to proper tonicity and pH to prevent nasal irritation. Bot. 20 ml.
Use: In babies & children to loosen and remove mucus secretions, etc.

AYR SALINE NASAL MIST. (Ascher) Sodium chloride 0.65% in isotonic spray. Bot. 50 ml.
Use: Dry, congested nasal membranes due to overuse of decongestant nasal sprays and drops.

8-AZABICYCLO[3.2.1.]OCTANE-2-CARBOXYLIC ACID, 3-(BENZOYLOXY)-8-METHYL-, METHYL ESTER, HCl. Cocaine Hydrochloride, U.S.P. XXI.

8-AZABICYCLO[3.2.1]OCTANE, 3-(DIPHENYL-METHOXY)-,endo-, METHANE-SULFONATE. Benztropine Mesylate, U.S.P. XXI.

• **AZABON.** USAN.
Use: Stimulant.

• **AZACITIDINE.** USAN.
Use: Antineoplastic.

• **AZACHLORZINE HYDROCHLORIDE.** USAN.
Use: Vasodilator.

AZACYCLONOL HCl. Alpha, alpha-diphenyl-4-piperidine-methanol HCl.

AZACYCLONOL. B.A.N. α-4-Piperidylbenzhydrol. Frenquel hydrochloride.
Use: Tranquilizer.

AZALOMYCIN. B.A.N. A mixture of related antibiotics produced by Streptomyces hygroscopicus var. azalomyceticus.

AZAMETHONIUM BROMIDE. (Ciba) 3-Methyl-3-azapentamethylenebis (ethyldimethyl-ammonium) dibromide. Pendiomide, Pentamin.
Use: Ganglionic blocking agent.

AZAMETHONIUM BROMIDE. B.A.N. 3-Methyl-3-azapentamethylenedi(ethyldimethylammonium bromide). Pendiomide.
Use: Ganglionic blocking agent.

• **AZANATOR MALEATE.** USAN.
Use: Bronchodilator.

• **AZANIDAZOLE.** USAN.
Use: Antiprotozoal.

• **AZAPERONE.** USAN. 4′-Fluoro-4-[4-(2-pyridyl)-piperazin-l-yl]butyrophenone. Stresnil. Suicalm.
Use: Tranquilizer, veterinary medicine.

AZAPETINE. B.A.N. 6-Allyl-5,7-dihydrodibenz-[c,e]azepine. Ilidar phosphate.
Use: Vasodilator.

AZAPETINE PHOSPHATE. 6-Allyl-6,7-dihydro-5H-dibenz(c,e)azepine, azephine.

AZAPROPAZONE. A fazone.

AZAPROPAZONE. B.A.N. 5-Dimethylamino-9-methyl-2-propyl-1H-pyrazolo[1,2-α][1,2,4]-benzotriazine-1,3 (2H)-dione.
Use: Analgesic; anti-inflammatory.

• **AZARIBINE.** USAN. 2-β-D-Ribofuranosyl-1,2,4-triazine-3,5-(2H,4H)dione2,3′,5′-triacetate. 6-Azauridine 2′,3′,5′-triacetate. Triazure.
Use: Treatment of psoriasis.

• **AZAROLE.** USAN.
Use: Immunoregulator.

- **AZASERINE.** USAN.
  Use: Antifungal.
- **AZATADINE MALEATE,** U.S.P. XXI. 5-H-Benzo (5-6) cyclohepta (1,2-b) pyridine, 6,11-dihydro-11-(1-methyl-4-piperidylidene)-5H-benzo(5,6)-cyclohepta (1,2-b) pyridine maleate (1:2)
  Use: Antihistaminic.
  See: Optimine, Tab. (Schering)
    Trinalin, Tab. (Schering)
- **AZATHIOPRINE,** U.S.P. XXI. Tab., U.S.P. XXI. (Burroughs Wellcome) 6-(1-Methyl-4-nitroimidazol-5-ylthio) purine. IH-Purine, 6-[(l-methyl-4-nitro-IH-imidazol-5-yl)thio]-.6-[(l-Methyl-4-nitroimidazol-5-yl)thio]purine.
  Use: Anti-leukemic compound.
  See: Imuran, Inj., Tab. (Burroughs Wellcome)
AZATHIOPRINE. B.A.N. 6-(1-Methyl-4-nitroimidazol-5-ylthio)purine.
  Use: Antimetabolite.
AZATHIOPRINE SODIUM, U.S.P. XXI.
  Use: Anti-leukemic compound.
- **AZEPINDOLE.** USAN.
  Use: Antidepressant.
- **AZETEPA.** USAN. PP-Diaziridin-1-yl-N-ethyl-1,3,4-thiadiazol-2-ylphosphinamide.
  Use: Antimetabolite.
AZIDOCILLIN. B.A.N. 6-[D(—)-α-Azidophenyl-acetamido]penicillanic acid.
  Use: Antibiotic.
- **AZIPRAMINE HYDROCHLORIDE.** USAN.
  Use: Antidepressant.
AZLIN. (Miles Pharm) Azlocillin sodium. Vials 2 Gm., 3 Gm., or 4 Gm.
  Use: Broad spectrum antibiotic.
- **AZLOCILLIN.** USAN.
  Use: Antibacterial.
  See: Azlin, Inj. (Miles)
- **AZLOCILLIN SODIUM, STERILE,** U.S.P. XXI.
  Use: Antibacterial.
AZLYTAL. (U.S. Ethicals) Phenobarbital 16.2 mg., hyoscyamine sulfate 0.1037 mg., atropine sulfate 0.0194 mg., scopolamine HBr 0.0065 mg./Tab. Bot. 1000s.
  Use: Intestinal anti-spasmodic.
AZMA-AID. (Purepac) Theophylline 2 gr., ephedrine ⅜ gr., phenobarbital ⅛ gr./Tab. Bot. 100s, 250s, 1000s.
  Use: Bronchodilator.
AZMADRINE. (U.S. Ethicals) Aminophylline compound Caps. Bot. 50s, 100s. Tab. 24s.
  Use: Bronchial dilator
AZMADRINE PEDIATRIC SUSPENSION. (U.S. Ethicals) Theophylline 65 mg., ephedrine HCl phenobarbital 4 mg./5 ml.
  Bot. 120 ml., 480 ml.
  Use: Bronchial dilator.
AZMA-EZE. (Eckerd) Theophylline 100 mg., ephedrine HCl 25 mg., guaifenesin 100 mg., chlorpheniramine maleate 2 mg./Tab. Bot. 48s.
  Use: Bronchial asthma.
AZMACORT INHALER. (Rorer) Triamcinolone acetonide 200 mcg. actuation of which

approximately 100 mcg. are delivered from the unit. 20 Gm. canister contains 60 mg. triamcinole acetonide w/oral adapter.
  Use: Treatment of chronic bronchial asthma.
AZO-100. (Scruggs) Phenylazodiaminopyridine HCl 100 mg./Tab. Bot. 100s, 1000s.
  Use: Urinary tract analgesic.
- **AZOCONAZOLE.** USAN.
  Use: Antifungal.
AZO-CYST. (Moore Kirk) Phenylazodiaminopyridine HCl 50 mg., calcium mandelate 120 mg., acid sod. phosphate 120 mg., methenamine 120 mg., hyoscyamine HBr 0.1037 mg., hyoscine HBr 0.0065 mg., atropine sulfate 0.0194 mg./Tab. Bot. 100s, 1000s.
  Use: Urinary tract sterilization.
AZODINE. (Vortech) Phenylazodiaminopyridine HCl 1.5 gr./Tab. Bot. 1000s.
  Use: Urinary anti-infective, analgesic.
AZODYNE.
  W/Sulfadiazine, sulfamethizole
  See: Suladyne, Tab. (Stuart)
AZODYNE HCl
  See: Pyridium, Tab. (Parke-Davis)
AZO GANTANOL. (Roche) Sulfamethoxazole 500 mg., phenazopyridine HCl 100 mg./Tab. Bot. 100s, 500s.
  Use: Treatment of urinary tract infections complicated by pain.
AZO GANTRISIN. (Roche) Sulfisoxazole 500 mg., phenazopyridine HCl 50 mg./Tab. Bot. 100s, 500s.
  Use: Treatment of urinary tract infections complicated by pain.
AZOLID. (USV Labs.) Phenylbutazone 100 mg./Tab. or Caps. Bot. 100s, 1000s.
  Use: Anti-inflammatory.
- **AZOLIMINE.** USAN.
  Use: Diuretic.
AZOMAN. Hexazole, B.A.N.
AZO NEGACIDE TABLETS. (Winthrop Products) Nalidixic acid, phenazopyridine HCl.
  Use: Painful lower urinary tract infection.
- **AZOSEMIDE.** USAN.
  Use: Diuretic.
AZO-SOXAZOLE. (Columbia) Sulfisoxazole 500 mg., phenylazodiaminopyridine HCl 50 mg./Tab. Bot. 100s, 1000s.
AZO-STANDARD. (Webcon) Phenazopyridine HCl 100 mg./Tab. Bot. 30s.
  Use: Urinary tract infections.
AZOSTIX. (Ames) Bromthymol blue, urease, buffers. Bot. 25 strips.
  Use: A colorimetric test for blood urea nitrogen level.
AZO-SULFISOXAZOLE. (Century) Sulfisoxazole 500 mg., phenylazopyridine HCl 50 mg./Tab. Bot. 1000s.
AZO-SULFISOXAZOLE. (Vortech) Sulfisoxazole 500 mg., phenylazodiaminopyridine HCl 50 mg./Tab. Bot. 1000s.
  Use: Urinary tract infections.
AZO-SULFISOXAZOLE. (Richlyn) Sulfisoxazole 500

mg., phenylazopyridine HCl 50 mg./Tab. Bot. 1000s.

AZO-SULFISOXAZOLE. (Fellows) Azo-sulfisoxazole 500 mg., phenylazodiaminopyridine 50 mg./Tab. Bot. 100s, 1000s.

• **AZOTOMYCIN.** USAN. Antibiotic isolated from broth filtrates of *Streptomyces ambofaciens.*
Use: Anti-neoplastic agent.

AZO-URIZOLE. (Jenkins) Sulfisoxazole 0.5 Gm., phenazopyridine HCl 50 mg./Tab. Bot. 1000s.

AZOVAN BLUE. Tetrasodium salt of 4:4′-di-[7-(1-amino-8-hydroxy-2:4-disulpho)-naphthylazo]-3:3′-bitolyl.
See: Evans Blue Dye, Amp. (City Chemical; Harvey)

AZOVAN BLUE. B.A.N. Tetrasodium salt of 4,4′-di-(8-amino-1-hydroxy-5,7-disulfo-2-naphthylazo)-3,3′-bitolyl.
Use: Diagnostic aid.
See: Evans Blue

AZO WINTOMYLON. (Winthrop Products) Nalidixic acid, phenazopyridine HCl.
Use: Painful lower urinary tract infection.

AZPAN. (Zenith) Phenobarbital 8 mg., theophylline 130 mg., ephedrine HCl 24 mg./Tab.
Use: Bronchodilator used in treatment of asthma.

• **AZTREONAM.** USAN.
Use: Antimicrobial.

AZUDIMIDINE. Salazosulphadimidine, B.A.N.

AZULFIDINE ORAL SUSPENSION. (Pharmacia) Sulfasalazine 250 mg./5 ml. Bot. pt.
Use: Mild to moderate ulcerative colitis. Adjunctive therapy in severe ulcerative colitis.

AZULFIDINE TABLETS and EN-TABS. (Pharmacia) Sulfasalazine (salicylazosulfapyridine) 500 mg./En-tab or Tab. Bot. 100s, 500s. Unit dose 100s, 1000s.
Use: Mild to moderate ulcerative colitis and adjunctive therapy in severe ulcerative colitis.

AZURESIN. B.A.N. Prepared from carbacrylic cation exchange resin and azure A dye (3-amino-7-dimethylaminophenazathionium chloride). Diagnex Blue.
Use: Diagnostic aid.

B

B-1. Thiamine hydrochloride.

B-1 50. (Western Research) Vitamin B-1 50 mg./Tab. Bot. 1000s.
Use: Vitamin deficiency supplement.

B-2. Riboflavin.

B-3. Niacinamide.

B-6. Pyridoxine hydrochloride.

B-6 50. (Western Research) Vitamin B-6 50 mg./Tab. Bot. 1000s.
Use: Vitamin deficiency supplement.

B-12. Cyanocobalamin.

B-12 PLEX. (Vortech) Univial 10 ml.
Use: Vitamin B complex.

B & A. (Eastern Research) Sod. bicarbonate, pot.

alum., borax. Hygienic pow. Jar. 8 oz., 5 lb.
Use: Vaginal douche.

B.A. GRADUAL. (Federal) Theophylline 260 mg., pseudo-ephedrine HCl 50 mg., butabarbital 15 mg./Gradual. Bot. 50s, 1000s.

BABY COUGH. (DeWitt) Bot. 3 oz.
Use: Anti-cough for infants and children.

BABY COUGH SYRUP. (Towne) Amm. chloride 300 mg., sod. citrate 600 mg./oz. w/citric acid. Bot. 4 oz.
Use: Antitussive (pediatric).

BABY LIQUID VITAMINS. (Maurry) Vitamin A 3000 I.U., D 400 I.U., C 50 mg., B-1 1 mg., Riboflavin 0.9 mg., Niacinamide 6 mg., B-6 0.5 mg., Panthenol 1 mg./0.6 ml. Bottle: 1 fl. oz., 2 fl. oz.
Use: Pediatric vitamin.

• **BACAMPICILLIN HYDROCHLORIDE,** U.S.P. XXI. for Oral Soln., Tab., U.S.P. XXI.
Use: Antibiotic.

BACARATE. (Reid-Provident) Phendimetrazine tartrate 35 mg./Tab. Bot. 100s, 1000s.
Use: Appetite suppressant.

BACCO-RESIST. (Vita Elixir) Lobeline sulfate 1/64 gr.
Use: Antismoking lozenge.

BACDIP. Quintiofos, B.A.N.

BACID. (Fisons) A specially cultured strain of human *Lactobacillus acidophilus,* sodium carboxymethylcellulose 100 mg./Cap. Bot. 50s, 100s.
Use: Functional diarrhea.

BACIGUENT ANTIBIOTIC OINTMENT. (Upjohn) Bacitracin 500 u./Gm. Oint Tube 0.5 oz., 1 oz., 4 oz.
Use: Topically, pyogenic skin infections.

BACIGUENT OPHTHALMIC OINTMENT. (Upjohn) Bacitracin 500 u./Gm., in a base of white petrolatum, anhydrous lanolin, mineral oil, & chlorobutanol. Tube 3.5 Gm.

• **BACITRACIN,** U.S.P. XXI. Oint., Ophth., Oint., Sterile, U.S.P. XXI. An antibiotic produced by a strain of *Bacillus subtilis.*
Available forms (Various Mfr.)
Diagnostic Tabs.
Ointment
Ophthalmic Oint.
Soluble Tabs.
Systemic Use, Vial.
Topical Use, Vial.
Troches
Vaginal Tabs.
Use: Antibacterial.
See: baciquent, Oint. (Upjohn)
W/Neomycin sulfate.
See: Bacimycin, Oint. (Merrell Dow)
Bacitracin-Neomycin, Oint, Ophth. Oint. (Various Mfr.)
W/Neomycin, polymyxin B sulfate.
See: Baximin, Oint. (Columbia)
BPN Ointment (Norwich Eaton)
Mycitracin, Oint. & Ophth. Oint. (Upjohn)
Neosporin, Oint. & Ophth. Oint., Aerosol, Pwd. (Burroughs Wellcome)
Neo-Thrycex, Oint. (Commerce)

P.B.N., Oint. (Jenkins)
Tigo, Oint. (Burlington)
Tri-Biotic Oint. (Burgin-Arden)
Tri-Biotic, Oint. (Standex)
Tri-Bow Oint. (Bowman)
Triple Antibiotic Oint. (Kenyon, North American Pharmacal, Towne)
W/Neomycin sulf., polymyxin B sulf., hydrocortisone acetate.
  See: Neopolycin-HC, Oint., Ophth. Oint. (Merrell Dow)
W/Neomycin sulfate, polymyxin B sulfate, diperodon HCl.
  See: Epimycin A, Oint. (Delta)
    Mity-Mycin, Oint. (Reid-Provident)
W/Polymyxin B sulfate.
  See: Polysporin, Oint. & Ophth. Oint. (Burroughs Wellcome)
W/Polymyxin B sulfate and neomycin sulfate.
  See: Trimixin, Oint. (Hance)
W/Polymyxin B. sulfate, neomycin sulfate & hydrocortisone free alcohol.
  See: Biotic-Ophth. W/HC, Oint. (Scrip)
    Cortisporin, Preps. (Burroughs Wellcome)
BACITRACIN. B.A.N. An antibiotic produced by a strain of *Bacillus subtilis.*
BACITRACIN-NEOMYCIN OINTMENT. (Various Mfr.) Neomycin sulfate equiv. to 3.5 mg. of base, bacitracin 500 u./Gm. Topical Oint. Tube ½ oz., 1 oz., Ophth. Oint. ⅛ oz.
Use: Treatment of infectious due to gram-positive or gram-negative bacteria.
• **BACITRACIN ZINC,** U.S.P. XXI. Sterile, U.S.P. XXI.(Upjohn) Stevil powder 10,000 u. or 50,000 u./Vial.
Use: Antibiotic.
W/Neomycin sulfate, polymyxin B sulfate.
  See: Neomixin B sulfate.
  See: Neomixin, Oint. (Mallard)
    Neo-polycin, Oint. (Merrell Dow)
    Neosporin, Prods. (Burroughs Wellcome)
    Neotal, Oint. (Mallard)
W/Neomycin sulfate, polymyxin B, benzalkonium chloride.
  See: Biotres, Oint. (Central Pharmacal)
W/Neomycin sulfate, polymyxin B sulfate, hydrocortisone acetate.
  See: Biotres HC, Cream (Central)
    Coracin, Oint. (Mallard)
W/Polymyxin B sulfate, neomycin sulfate.
  See: Ophthel, Ophth. Oint. (Elder)
    Polycin, Oint. (Merrell Dow)
• **BACITRACIN ZINC OINTMENT,** U.S.P. XXI. Bacitracin Zinc in an anhydrous ointment base.
Use: Antibiotic ointment.
• **BACITRACIN ZINC AND POLYMIXIN B SULFATE OINTMENT,** U.S.P. XXI. Ophthalmic Oint., U.S.P. XXI.
Use: Antibiotic.
BACIT-WHITE. (Whiteworth) Bacitracin ointment. Tube 0.5 oz., 1 oz.
Use: Antibiotic ointment.
• **BACLOFEN.** USAN. 4-Amino-3-(4-chlorophenyl)

butyric acid. β-Aminomethyl-p-chlorohydrocinnamic acid.
Use: Muscle relaxant.
See: Lioresal, Tab. (Geigy)
BAC-NEO-POLY OINTMENT. (Burgin-Arden) Bacitracin 400 u., neomycin sulfate 5 mg., polymyxin B sulfate 5000 u./Gm. Tube ½ oz.
BACTAL 1%. (La Crosse) Bar and liquid surgical soap. Bar. 1 doz. Liq. 8 oz., gal.
BACTALIN. (La Crosse) Cetylpyridinium chloride, phosphate buffers. Plastic Bot. 8 oz., 0.5 gal.
Use: Mouth wash.
BACT-CHEK. (Roche)
Escherichia coli, Vial 30 discs.
Enterobacter cloacae, Vial 30 discs.
Proteus vulgaris, Vial 30 discs.
Staphylococcus epidermidis, Vial 30 discs.
Staphylococcus aureus, Vial 30 discs.
Salmonella typhimurium, Vial 30 discs.
Pseudomonas aeruginosa, Vial 30 discs.
Streptococcus pyogenes, Vial 30 discs.
Use: Diagnostic agent.
B.A.C. Gram-Negative: *Pseudomonas aeruginosa, Escherichia coli,* and *Aerobacter aerogenes.* Vial 3½ cc.
B.A.C. Pooled Stock # 1: *Diplococcus pneumoniae* Types I, II, V, VII, and XIV; *Streptococcus pyogenes,* Group A, Types 3, 10, 12, and Granger; *Staphylococcus aureus* and *albus; Streptococcus viridans* strains R1551, R1822, and R353; *Neisseria catarrhalis, Escherichia coli,* and *Haemophilus influenzae* Types a and b. Vial 3½ cc.
B.A.C. Pooled Stock # 2: *Diplococcus pneumoniae* Types III, VI, and XIX; *Klebsiella pneumoniae* Type A, *Streptococcus pyogenes* Types 14, 18, and 19; *Pseudomonas aeruginosa, Escherichia coli,* and *Aerobacter aerogenes.* Vial 3½ cc.
B.A.C. Staphylococcal: *Staphylococcus aureus* and *albus* phage types 42B/52/80/81 obtained from skin lesions, eye, ear, sinus and respiratory tract infections. Vial 3½ cc.
B.A.C. Pooled Skin: *Staphylococcus aureus* and *albus,* and *Proteus vulgaris* isolated from skin lesions in patients with boils, carbuncles, furuncles and acne, Vial 3½ cc.
• **BACTERIOSTATIC WATER FOR INJECTION.** U.S.P. XXI. (Abbott) 30 ml. multiple-dose Fliptop Vial (plastic).
Use: Pharmaceutic acid for diluting and dissolving drugs for injection.
BACTIGEN H. INFLUENZAE. (Wampole) Rapid latex agglutination slide test for the qualitative detection of *Hemophilus influenzae,* type b antigen in cerebrospinal fluid, serum, and urine. Kits 30s, 100s.
Use: Aid in the differential diagnosis of bacterial meningitis.
BACTIGEN N. MENINGITIDIS. (Wampole) Rapid latex agglutination slide test for the qualitative detection of Neisseria meningitidis, serogroups

A,B,C & Y antigens in cerebrospinal fluid, serum & urine. Kits 30s, 100s.
Use: Aid in the differential diagnosis of bacterial meningitis.

BACTIGEN S PNEUMONIAE. (Wampole) Rapitd latex agglutination slide test for the qualitative detection of streptococcus pneumoniae antigens in cerebrospinal fluid, serum and urine. Kits 30s, 100s.
Use: Aid in the differential diagnosis of bacterial meningitis.

BACTINE ANTISEPTIC/ANESTHETIC FIRST AID SPRAY. (Miles) Benzalkonium Cl 0.13%, lidocaine 2.5%. Squeeze Bot. 2 oz., 4 oz., 16 oz. Liquid 3 oz. aerosol.
Use: Antiseptic, anesthetic.

BACTINE HYDROCORTISONE SKIN CREAM. (Miles) Hydrocortisone 0.5% Tube ½ oz.
Use: Antipruritic, antiinflammatory.

BACTOCILL. (Beecham Labs) Oxacillin Sodium **Caps.:** 250 mg. Bot. 100s, Unit dose 10 × 10s. 500 mg. Bot. 100s, Unit dose 10 × 10s. **Vial:** (w/dibasic sod. phosphate 40 mg., methylparaben 3.6 mg., propylparaben 0.4 mg., sodium 3.1 mEq./Gm.) 500 mg., 1 Gm., 2 Gm., 4 Gm./Vial; 10s. Piggyback vial 1 Gm., 2 Gm., 25s. Bulk pharm pkg 10 Gm. Box 25s.
Use: Antibiotic.

BACTRIM. (Roche) Sulfamethoxazole 400 mg., trimethoprim 80 mg./Tab. Bot. 100s, 500s. Teledose 100s. Prescription Paks 40s, 400s.
Use: Urinary infections, otitisimedia, pneumonitis.

BACTRIM ORAL SUSP. (Roche) Sulfamethoxazole 200 mg., trimethoprim 40 mg./5 ml. Bot. pt.
Use: Urinary infections, otitisimedia, pneumonitis.

BACTRIM PEDIATRIC SUSPENSION. (Roche) Trimethorprim 40 mg., sulfamethoxyole 200 mg./5 ml. Bot. 16 oz.
Use: Urinary tract infections.

BACTRIM DS. (Roche) Trimethoprim 160 mg., sulfamethoxazole 800 mg./Tab. Bot. 100s. Teledose 100s. Paks of 20s.
Use: Urinary infections, otitisimedia, pneumonitis.

BACTURCULT. (Wampole) A urinary bacteria culture medium diagnostic urine culture system for urine collection, for bacteriuria screening and presumptive bacterial identification. Kits 10s, 100s.
Use: Diagnosis of bacteria.

BADIONAL. Sulphathiourea, B.A.N.

BAFIL CREAM. (Scruggs) Hydrocortisone ½%, clioquinol 3%, lidocaine 3%, pH adjusted to 6.0 Tube 1 oz.
Use: Broad control of dermatologic disorders.

B.A. GRADUALS. (Amfre-Grant) Theophylline 260 mg., pseudoephedrine HCl 50 mg., butabarbital 15 mg./Tab. Bot. 50s, 1000s.
Use: Bronchial dilators.

BAKERS BEST. (Scherer) Water, alcohol 38%, propylene glycol, ext. capsicum, glycerin, boric acid, Tween 80, diethylphthalate, rose oil, pyrilamine maleate, glacial acetic acid, Uvinul MS 40, hexetidine, benzalkonium chloride 50%, Supercel Hyflo, sodium hydroxide 76%. Bot. 8 oz.
Use: Antipruritic and antiseborrheic.

BAL. (Hynson, Westcott & Dunning) 2,3-Dimercapto-propanol 100 mg., benzyl benzoate 210 mg., peanut oil 680 mg./ml. Amp. 3 ml. Box 10s.
Use: Treatment of arsenic, gold & mercury poisoning, and also acute lead poisoning in combination with edetate calcium disodium injection.

BALANCED SALT SOLUTION. (Alcon) Sod. chloride 0.49%, pot. chloride, 0.075%, cal. chloride 0.036%, mag. chloride 0.03% in sod. acetate-sod. citrate buffer system. Drop-Trainer 15 cc.
Use: Intraocular irrigating solution.

BALMEX BABY POWDER. (Macsil) Specially purified balsam Peru, zinc oxide, talc, starch, calcium carbonate. Shaker top cans. 4 oz.
Use: Adsorbent, emollient, & soothing powder.

BALMEX EMOLLIENT LOTION. (Macsil) Fraction of lanolin, allantoin, specially purified balsam Peru, silicone in a non-mineral oil base. Bot. 6 fl. oz.
Use: Emollient, antibacterial and protective lotion.

BALMEX OINTMENT. (Macsil) Specially purified balsam Peru, Vit. A & D, zinc oxide, & bismuth subnitrate in a base w/silicone. Tubes 1, 2, 4 oz., plastic jars 1 lb.
Use: Emollient, protective, anti-inflammatory, & healing ointment.

BALNEOL. (Rowell) Water, mineral oil, propylene glycol, glyceryl stearate PEG-100 stearate, PEG-40 stearate, laureth-4, PEG-4-dilaurate, lanolin oil, sodium acetate, carbomer-934, triethanolamine, methyl paraben, docusate sodium, acetic acid, fragrance. Bot. 1 oz., 4 oz.
Use: Emollient cleansing of irritated perianal & external vaginal area.

BALNETAR. (Westwood) Tar equivalent to 2.5% Coal Tar, U.S.P. Bot. 8 oz.
Use: Temporary relief of itching & scaling due to psoriasis, eczema and other tar-responsive dermatoses.

BALSAN. Specially purified balsam Peru.
See: Balmex Prod. (Macsil)

BALTRON. (Reid-Provident) Peptonized iron 59 mg., folic acid 2 mg., liver injection USP (equiv. in Vit. B-12 activity to 5 mcg. cyanocobalamin), procaine HCl 1%, phenol 1%, sodium citrate 1%/2 cc., water q.s. Vials 30 cc.

BAMATE. (Century) Meprobamate 400 mg./Tab. Bot. 50s, 100s, 500s, 1000s, 5000s.
Use: Minor tranquilizer.

• **BABMERMYCINS.** USAN.
Use: Antibacterial.

BAMETHAN. B.A.N. 2-Butylamino-1-(4-hydroxyphenyl) ethanol.
Use: Vasodilator.
See: Vasculit sulfate

• **BAMETHAN SULFATE.** USAN. α-[(Butylamino) methyl]-p-hydroxybenzyl alcohol sulfate.
Use: Vasodilator.

BAMIFYLLINE. B.A.N. 8-Benzyl-7-[2-(N-ethyl-2-hydroxy-ethylamino)ethyl]theophylline. Trentadil hydrochloride.
Use: Bronchodilator.

BAMIFYLLINE HYDROCHLORIDE. USAN. 8-Benzyl-7-[2-[ethyl (2-hydroxyethyl) amino]ethyl]-theophylline HCl.
Use: Bronchodilator.

BAMIPINE. B.A.N. 4-(N-Benzylanilino)-1-methyl-piperidine.
Use: Antihistamine.
See: Soventol.

• **BAMNIDAZOLE.** USAN.
Use: Antiprotozoal.

BANACID. (Buffington) Aluminum hydroxide, Mg hydroxide, Mg trisilicate/Tab. Dispens-A-Kit 500s, Medipaks 200s. Unit boxes 8s, 16s.
Use: Antacid.

BANALG. (O'Neal, Jones & Feldman) Menthol, camphor, methyl salicylate & eucalyptus oil in a greaseless base. Regular liniment and hospital strength. Bot. 2 oz., 1 pt., gal.
Use: Topically, a counterirritant.

BANATIL. (Trimen) Butabarbital 32.4 mg., hyoscyamine sulfate 0.25 mg., scopolamine methylnitrate 0.05 mg., atropine sulfate 0.086 mg./D.R. Tab. Bot. 100s. Elix. pt.
Use: G. I. hypermotility & spasm.

BANCAPS. (O'Neal, Jones & Feldman) Acetaminophen 325 mg., butalbital 50 mg./Cap. Bot. 100s, 500s.
Use: Analgesic, muscle relaxant and sedative.

BANCAP HC. (O'Neal, Jones & Feldman) Acetaminophen 500 mg., hydrocodone bitratrate 5 mg./Cap. Bot. 100s, 500s.
Use: Analgesic.

BANCAP W/CODEINE. (O'Neal, Jones & Feldman) Acetaminophen 325 mg., codeine phosphate 30 mg., butalbital 50 mg./Cap. Bot. 100s, 500s.
Use: Analgesic, muscle relaxant and sedative.

• **BANDAGE, ADHESIVE,** U.S.P. XXI.
Use: Surgical aid.

• **BANDAGE, GAUZE,** U.S.P. XXI.
Use: Surgical aid.

BANESIN. (O'Neal, Jones & Feldman) Acetaminophen 500 mg./Tab.
Use: Analgesic.

BANFLEX. (O'Neal, Jones & Feldman) Orphenadrine citrate 30 mg./ml. IM or IV. Vials 10 ml.
Use: Skeletal muscle relaxant.

BANGESIC. (H.L. Moore) Menthol, camphor, methyl salicylate, eucalyptus oil in nongreasy base. Bot. 2 oz., gal.
Use: Local analgesic.

BANOCIDE.
See: Diethylcarbamazine Citrate, U.S.P.

BANTHINE. (Searle) Methantheline bromide 50 mg./Tab. Bot. 100s.
Use: Orally, anticholinergic preparation.

BANTRON BRAND SMOKING DETERRENT TABLETS. (Jeffrey Martin) Magnesium carbonate, 129.6 mg., lobeline sulfate alkaloids 2mg., tribasic calcium phosphate 129.6 mg./Tab. Carton 18s, 36s.
Use: Smoking deterrent.

BARACHLOR TABLETS. (Barry-Martin) Chlorprophenpyridamine maleate 4 mg./Tab. Bot. 1000s.

BARACHLOR T.D. CAPSULES. (Barry-Martin) Chlorpheniramine maleate 8 mg. or 12 mg./Cap. Bot. 100s, 500s, 1000s.

BARACOL EAR DROPS. (Barry-Martin) Antipyrine 1.7 Gm., benzocaine 0.46 Gm., propylene glycol 0.926 fl. oz./fl. oz. Bot. 15 cc., pt., gal.
Use: Ear pain and wax softening.

BARAGESIC SPRAY. (Barry-Martin) Methol, methylsalicylate, camphor, isopropanol, trichloro-fluoromethane, dichlorodifluoromethane, plus essential oils. Can 6 oz.
Use: Relief of aches and pains.

BARAMINE CAPSULES (Barry-Martin) Diphenhydramine HCl 50 mg./Cap. Bot. 100s.

BARAMINE ELIXIR. (Barry-Martin) Diphenhydramine HCl 10 mg./4 cc. Bot., pt., gal.

BARAMINE EXPECTORANT. (Barry-Martin) Diphenhydramine HCl 80 mg., ammonium chloride 12 gr., sod. citrate 5 gr., menthol 0.1 gr./fl. oz. Bot. pt., gal.

BARAZOLE TABLETS. (Barry-Martin) Sulfisoxazole 0.5 Gm./Tab. Bot. 100s, 1000s.

BARAZOLE-AZO TABLETS. (Barry-Martin) Sulfisoxazole 0.5 Gm., phenazopyridine 50 mg./Tab. Bot. 100s, 1000s.

BARBELLA ELIXIR. (Fellows) Phenobarbital ¼ gr., hyoscyamine sulfate 0.1037 mg., atropine sulfate 0.0194 mg., scopolamine HBr 0.0065 mg./alcohol 23%/tsp. Bot. 4 oz., gal.

BARBELLA TABLETS. (Fellows) Phenobarbital 16.2 mg., atropine sulfate 0.0194 mg., hyoscyamine sulfate 0.1037 mg., hyoscine HBr 0.0065 mg./Tab. Bot. 100s, 1000s, 5000s.

BARBELOID. (Vale) Phenobarbital 16.2 mg., hyoscyamine sulfate 0.1037 mg., atropine sulfate 0.0194 mg., scopolamine hydrobromide 0.0065 mg./Tab. Bot. 100s, 500s, 1000s.
Use: Orally, antispasmodic & sedative.

BARBENYL.
See: Phenobarbital.

BARBIDONNA. (Wallace) **Elixir:** phenobarbital 21.6 mg. hyoscyamine sulfate 0.174 mg., atropine sulfate 0.034 mg., scopolamine HBr 0.01 mg., alcohol 15%/5 ml. Bot. 1 pt.; **Tab.:** phenobarbital 16 mg., hyoscyamine sulfate 0.1286 mg., atropine sulfate 0.0250 mg., scopolamine HBr 0.0074 mg./Tab. Bot. 100s, 500s.
Use: Antispasmodic and sedative. Combination for G.I. disorders.

BARBIDONNA NO. 2. (Wallace) Phenobarbital 32 mg., hyoscyamine sulfate 0.1286 mg., atropine sulfate 0.0250 mg., scopolamine HBr 0.0074 mg./Tab. Bot. 100s.
Use: Antispasmodic & sedative combination for G.I. disorders.

BARBINAL CAPSULES. (Fellows) Phenobarbital ½ gr., acetophenetidin 2 gr., aspirin 3 gr., hyoscyamus ¼ gr./Cap. Bot. 100s, 500s.

BARBINAL NO. 3. (Fellows) Phenobarbital ¼ gr., codeine phosphate ½ gr., acetophenetidin 2 mg., aspirin 3 gr., hyoscyamine sulfate .031 mg./Cap. Bot. 100s, 500s.

BARBIPHENYL.
See: Phenobarbital.
BARBITA. (Vortech) Phenobarbital 16 mg./Tab. Bot.
1000s.
Use: Orally, sedative.
BARBITAL. Barbitone, Deba, Dormonal, Hypnogene,
Malonal, Sedeval, Uronal, Veronal, Vesperal,
Diethylbarbituric acid, diethylmalonylurea.
Use: Orally, sedative, hypnotic.
W/Aspirin, caffeine, niacinamide.
See: Mentran, Tab. (Pasadena Research)
BARBITAL SODIUM. Barbitone Sodium,
Diethylbarbiturate Monosodium, Diethylmalonylurea
Sodium, Embinal, Medinal, Veronal Sodium.
Use: Hypnotic, sedative.
BARBITONE.
See: Barbital.
BARBITONE SODIUM.
See: Barbital Sodium.
BARBITURATE-ASPIRIN COMBINATIONS.
See: Aspirin-Barbiturate Combination.
BARBITURATES, INTERMEDIATE DURATION.
See: Butabarbital (Various Mfr.)
Butethal (Various Mfr.)
Diallylbarbituric Acid (Various Mfr.)
Lotusate, Caps. (Winthrop-Breon)
Vinbarbital. (Various Mfr.)
■ **BARBITURATES, LONG DURATION.**
See: Barbital (Various Mfr.)
Mebaral, Tab. (Winthrop-Breon)
Mephobarbital (Var. Mfr.)
Phenobarbital (Various Mfr.)
Phenobarbital Sod. (Various Mfr.)
■ **BARBITURATES, SHORT DURATION.**
See: Amobarbital (Various Mfr.)
Amobarbital Sod. (Various Mfr.)
Butalbital (Var. Mfr.)
Butallylonal (Various Mfr.)
Cyclobarbital (Var. Mfr.)
Cyclopal
Pentobarbital Salts (Var. Mfr.)
Sandoptal
Secobarbital (Various Mfr.)
BARBITURATES, TRIPLE.
See: Butseco, S.C.T., Tab. (Bowman)
Ethobral, Cap. (Wyeth)
BARBITURATES, ULTRASHORT DURATION.
See: Hexobarbital
Neraval
Pentothal Sod., Amp. (Abbott)
Surital Sod., Amp., Vials (Parke-Davis)
Thiopental Sod. (Var. Mfr.)
BARBO COMPOUND LIQUID. (Guild) Bot. 8 oz.
BARBO COMPOUND POWDER. (Guild) Pkg. ¼ oz.
**BARBO COMPOUND INSTANT NO. 1, NO. 2 and
NO. 3.** (Guild) Bot. 1 oz.
BARC GEL. (Commerce) Pyrethrins, piperonyl
butoxide technical and petroleum distillate in gel
base. Tube 1 oz.
Use: Direct application pediculicide. Kills head lice,
crab & egg contact.
BARC LIQUID. (Commerce) Pyrethrins, piperonyl

butoxide technical, petroleum distillate. Bot. 2 oz.
Use: Kills and controls lice, nits and crab lice.
BARC NON-BODY LICE CONTROL SPRAY.
(Commerce) Resmethrin-5-(phenylmethyl)-3-furanyl]
methyl-2, 2-dimethyl-3-(2-methyl-1-propanyl)
cyclopropanecarboxylate. Spray can 5 oz.
Use: Control of lice and louse eggs on inanimate
objects.
BAR-CY-AMINE. (Sutliff & Case) Phenobarbital 16.0
mg., hyoscyamine sulfate 0.0856 mg., atropine
sulfate 0.0171 mg., hyoscine hydrobromide 0.0068
mg., alcohol 20%/5 cc. Bot. 1 pt., 1 gal.
Use: Orally, antispasmodic & sedative.
BAR-CY-A-TAB. (Sutliff & Case) Phenobarbital ¼ gr.,
hyoscyamine sulfate 0.0856 mg., atropine sulfate
0.0171 mg., hyoscine hydrobromide 0.0068
mg./Tab. Bot. 100s, 1000s, 5000s.
Use: Antispasmodic-sedative.
BARHOMA ELIXIR. (Blue Line) Phenobarbital 400
mg., homatropine methylbromide 33.8 mg., alcohol
13.5%/100 cc. Bot. pt., gal.
Use: Sedative.
BARHOMA TABLETS. (Blue Line) Phenobarbital ¼
gr., homatropine methylbromide ¹⁄₄₈ gr./Tab. Bot.
100s, 1000s.
Use: Sedative.
BARIDIUM TABLETS. (Barry-Martin) Phenylazopyridine
HCl 1½ gr./Tab. 24s, 100s, 500s, 1000s.
BARI-STRESS M. (Barre) Vit. B-1 10 mg., B-2 10 mg.,
niacinamide 100 mg., Vit. C 300 mg., B-6 2 mg.,
B-12 4 mcg., folic acid 1.5 mg., cal. pantothenate 20
mg./Cap. or Tab. **Cap:** Bot. 30s, 100s, 1000s. **Tab.**
Bot. 100s, 1000s.
Use: Stress vitamin therapy.
BARITRATE. (Barry-Martin) Pentaerythritol tetranitrate
10 mg. or 20 mg./Tab. Bot. 1000s.
BARITRATE PHENOBARBITAL TABLETS. (Barry-
Martin) Pentaerythritol tetranitrate 10 mg., or 20
mg., phenobarbital 15 mg./Tab. Bot. 1000s.
• **BARIUM HYDROXIDE LIME,** U.S.P. XXI.
Use: Carbon dioxide absorbant.
• **BARIUM SULFATE,** U.S.P. XXI. For Susp., U.S.P.
XXI. (Mallinckrodt) Sulfuric acid, barium salt (1:1).
Barium sulfate U.S.P. for X-ray diagnosis. Canister 1
lb., 5 lb.
Use: Orally or rectally, X-ray diagnostic aid.
See: Esophotrast, cream (Barnes-Hind)
■ **BARIUM SULFATE PREPARATION.**
See: Baroflave, Pow. (Lannett)
Barosperse, Pow. (Mallinckrodt)
Barotrast, Pow., Cream (Barnes-Hind)
Fleet Barobag, Liq. (Fleet)
Raybar, Susp. (Fleet)
Redi-Flow, Susp. (Berlex)
Rugar, Susp. (McKesson)
BARLEVITE. (Barth's) Vit. B-6 0.6 mg., B-12 3 mcg.,
pantothenic acid 0.6 mg., D 3 I.U., l-lysine 20 mg./0.6
ml. 100-Day Supply.
**BARNES-HIND CLEANING AND SOAKING SOLU-
TION.** (Barnes-Hind) Cleaning and buffering agents,
benzalkonium chloride 0.01%, disodium edetate
0.2%. Bot. 4 fl. oz.

Use: Hard contact lens cleaner and disinfectant.

BARNES-HIND GERMICIDAL SOLUTION. (Barnes-Hind) Benzalkonium Cl (1:750) 0.13%, disodium edetate 0.1%. Bot. gal.
Use: Anti-rust disinfectant for medical and dental instruments.

BARNES-HIND WETTING SOLUTION. (Barnes-Hind) Polyvinyl alcohol with disodium edetate 0.02%, benzalkonium chloride 0.004%. Bot. 35 ml., 2 fl. oz.
Use: Hard contact lens wetting solution.

BAROBAG. (Lafayette) Disposable prefilled barium enema bag. 12 oz., 16 oz. w/or w/o retention catheter.
Use: Barium enema.

BARODENSE. (Lafayette) Contains 97% colloidal microbarium sulfate. Drum 100 lb.
Use: Alimentary tract radiography.

BAROFLAVE POWDER. (Lannett) Barium sulfate for diagnostic X-ray use. Bot. 5 lb., Fibre drum 25 lb.

BAROGEL SUSPENSION. (Barry-Martin) Amphoteric aluminum hydroxide gel. Bot. qt., gal.

BAROLOID. (Lafayette) Microbarium sulfate. Drum 100 lbs.
Use: Contrast medium for radiography of the alimentary tract.

BAROPECTIN SUSPENSION. (Barry-Martin) Kaolin 90 gr., pectin 2 gr./fl. oz. Bot. qt., gal.

BAROSIL SUSPENSION. (Barry-Martin) Magnesium trisilicate 0.5 Gm., aluminum hydroxide 0.25 Gm./tsp. Bot. qt., gal.

BAROSMIN.
See: Diosmin.

BAROSPERSE. (Mallinckrodt) Barium sulfate for suspension. Drum 25 lb., 100 lb.; Single dose cups 225 Gm.; Disposable enema units 340 Gm., 454 Gm., 12s; Disposable air contrast colon examination unit 454 Gm., 12s.
Use: For gastrointestinal x-ray diagnosis.

BAROTUSSIN SYRUP. (Barry-Martin) Guaifenesin 100 mg., desoxyephedrine HCl 1 mg./5 cc. Bot. qt., gal.

BAROVITE LIQUID. (Barry-Martin) Vit. B-1 10 mg., B-12 25 mcg./5 cc. Bot. 4 oz., pt., qt.
Use: Appetite stimulant.
W/Iron. Ferric pyrophosphate 250 mg./5 cc. plus Barovite liquid formula.

BARSEB HC SCALP LOTION. (Barnes-Hind) Hydrocortisone 1%, isopropyl alcohol 45%, isopropyl myristate, propylene glycol. Bot. 1.75 oz.
Use: Anti-seborrheic for dermatitis of the scalp.

BARSEB THERA-SPRAY. (Barnes-Hind) Hydrocortisone alcohol 360 mg., salicylic acid 288 mg., benzalkonium chloride 14 mg., propylene glycol, isopropyl myristate, ethanol, butane (propellant). W/plastic applicator 184 Gm.
Use: Anti-seborrheic for dermatitis of the scalp.

BAR-TEST. (Vitarine) Barium sulfate 10 gr./Tab.
Use: Diagnostic agent.

BARTONE. (Rand) Phenobarbital 16.2 mg., scopolamine HBr 0.0065 mg., atropine sulfate 0.0194 mg., hyoscyamine sulfate 0.1037 mg./Tab. or 5 cc. **Tab.** Bot. 100s, 1000s. **Elixir** 1 pt., 1 gal.
Use: Antispasmodic.

BAR-TROPIN. (Fellows) Atropine sulfate $1/200$ gr., phenobarbital $1/4$ gr./Tab. Bot. 100s, 1000s.
Use: Orally, antispasmodic & sedative.

BASA. (Freeport) Acetylsalicylic acid 324 mg./Tab. Bot. 1000s.
Use: Headache and minor aches.

BASALJEL. (Wyeth) Aluminum carbonate gel. **Susp.:** Equiv. to 400 mg./5 cc. Extra strength, aluminum carbonate gel equiv. to 1000 mg. aluminum hydroxide gel. Bot. 12 fl. oz.,**Cap.:** equivalent to 500 mg. aluminum hydroxide. Bot. 100s, 500s. **Tab.:** equivalent to 500 mg. aluminum hydroxide. Bot. 100s.
Use: Orally, prophylaxis of renal stone.

BASELAN. (Metro Med) Jar 1 lb.
Use: Ointment base, emollient.

BASIC ALUMINUM AMINOACETATE.
See: Dihydroxy Aluminum Aminoacetate.

BASIC ALUMINUM CARBONATE.
See: Basaljel, Susp. (Wyeth)

BASIC ALUMINUM GLYCINATE.
See: Dihydroxyaluminum aminoacetate.

BASIC BISMUTH CARBONATE.
See: Bismuth Subcarbonate.

BASIC BISMUTH GALLATE.
See: Bismuth Subgallate (Various Mfr.)

BASIC BISMUTH NITRATE.
See: Bismuth Subnitrate (Various Mfr.)

BASIC BISMUTH SALICYLATE.
See: Bismuth Subsalicylate.

BASIC FUCHSIN.
See: Carbol-Fuchsin Topical Solution, U.S.P. XXI.

BAUMODYNE GEL. (Vortech) Methyl salicylate, menthol, eucalyptus oil, and preservatives in 70% isopropyl alcohol gel.
Use: Relief of joint and muscle pain.

BAMODYNE OINTMENT. (Vortech) Methyl salicylate, menthol, eucalyptus oil, and preservatives in non-greasy base.
Use: Relief of joint and muscle pain.

BAXIMIN OINTMENT. (Columbia) Polymyxin B sulfate 5000 u., bacitracin 400 u., neomycin sulfate 5 mg./Gm. Tube ½ oz.
Use: Antibiotic.

BAYAMINIC EXPECTORANT. (Bay) Phenlypropanolamine HCl 12.5 mg., guaifenesin 100 mg./5 ml. w/alcohol 5%. Bot. 4 oz., pt. gal.
Use: Decongestant, expectorant.

BAYAMINIC SYRUP. (Bay) Phenylpropanolamine HCl 12.5 mg., chlorpheniramine maleate 2 mg./5 ml. Bot. 4 oz., pt., gal.
Use: Decongestant, antihistaminic.

BAYAMINICOL. (Bay) Phenlypropanolamine HCl 12.5 mg., pyrilamine maleate 6.25 mg., pheniramine maleate 6.25 mg. ammonium Cl 90 mg., dextromethorphan HBr 15 mg./5 ml. Bot. 4 oz., pt., gal.
Use: Decongestant, antitussive, antihistaminic.

BAYAPAP. (Bay) Acetaminophen 160 mg./5 ml. w/alcohol 7% Bot. 2 oz., 4 oz., pt., gal.
Use: Pain relief, anti-pyretic.

BAYAPAP DROPS. (Bay) Acetaminophen 80 mg./0.8 ml. w/alcohol 7%. Bot. 15 ml.
Use: Pain relief, anti-pyretic.

BAYAPAP W/CODEINE. (Bay) Codeine phosphate 12 mg., acetaminophen 120 mg./5 ml. w/alcohol 7%. Bot. 4 oz., pt., gal.
Use: Pain relief.

BAY-ASE. (Bay) Phenobarbital gr. ¼, hyoscyamine sulfate 0.1037 mg., atropine sulfate 0.0194 mg., hyosine HBr 0.0065 mg./5 ml. w/alcohol 23%. Bot. 4 oz., pt., gal.
Use: Antispasmodtic, sedative.

BAYCODAN SYRUP. (Bay) Hydrocodone bitartrate 5 mg., homatropine MBr 1.5 mg./5 ml. Bot. 4 oz., pt., gal.
Use: Antitussive.

BAYCOMINE PEDIATRIC. (Bay) Phenylpropanolamine HCl 12.5 mg., hydrocodone bitartrate 2.5 mg./5 ml. Bot. 4 oz., pt., gal.
Use: Antitussive.

BAYCOMINE SYRUP. (Bay) Phenylpropanolamine HCl 25.0 mg., hydrocodone bitartrate 5 mg./5 ml. Bot. 4 oz., pt., gal.
Use: Antitussive.

BAYCOTUSSEND EXPECTORANT. (Bay) Pseudoephedrine HCl 60 mg., hydrocodone bitartrate 5 mg., guaifenesin 200 mg./5 ml. w/alcohol 12.5%. Bot. 4 oz., pt., gal.
Use: Antitussive, expectorant.

BAYCOTUSSEND LIQUID. (Bay) Pseudoephedrine HCl 60 mg., hydrocodone bitartrate 5 mg./5 ml. w/alcohol 5%. Bot. 4 oz., pt., gal.
Use: Antitussive, decongestant.

BAYDEC DM DROPS. (Bay) Pseudoephedrine HCl 25 mg., dextromethorphan HBr 4 mg., carbinoxamine maleate 2 mg./1 ml. Bot. 30 ml.
Use: Decongestant, antitussive, antihistaminic.

BAYDEC DM SYRUP. (Bay) Carbinoxamine maleate 4 mg., pseudoephedrine HCl 60 mg., dextromethorphan HBr 15 mg./5 ml. w/alcohol 0.6%. Bot. 4 oz., pt., gal.
Use: Decongestant, antitussive, antihistaminic.

BAYER ASPIRIN, GENUINE. (Glenbrook) Aspirin 5 gr. (325 mg.)/Tab. Film coated (non-enteric). Bot. 24s, 50s, 100s, 200s, 300s. Plastic 12s.
Use: analgesic, antipyretic, anti-inflammatory.

BAYER ASPIRIN, MAXIMUM. (Glenbrook) Aspirin 500 mg./Tab. Film coated. Bot. 30s, 60s, 100s.
Use: Analgesic, antipyretic, antiinflammatory, antiplatelet.

BAYER CHILDREN'S CHEWABLE ASPIRIN. (Glenbrook) Aspirin 1¼ gr. (81 mg.)/Tab. Bot. 36s.
Use: analgesic, antipyretic, anti-inflammatory.

BAYER CHILDREN'S COLD TABLETS. (Glenbrook) Phenylpropanolamine HCl 3.125 mg., Aspirin 1¼ gr. (81 mg.)/Tab. Bot. 30s.
Use: Analgesic, decongestant.

BAYER COUGH SYRUP FOR CHILDREN. (Glenbrook) Phenylpropanolamine HCl 9 mg., dextromethorphan HBr 7.5 mg./5 ml. w/alcohol 5%. Bot. 3 oz.
Use: Decongestant, antitussive.

BAYER TIMED-RELEASE ASPIRIN, ARTHRITIS. (Glenbrook) Aspirin 10 gr. (650 mg.)/T.R. Tab. Bot. 30s, 72s, 125s.
Use: Analgesic, antipyretic, anti-inflammatory.

BAYER 205.
See: Suramin Sodium. (No Mfr. currently listed.)

BAYFRIN NASAL SPRAY. (Bay) Oxymetazoline HCl 0.05%. Spray Bot. 15 ml.
Use: Decongestant.

BAYHISTINE DH. (Bay) Codeine phosphate 10 mg., chlorpheniramine maleate 2 mg., phenylpropanolamine HCl 18.75 mg./5 ml. w/alcohol 5%. Bot. 4 oz., pt., gal.
Use: Decongestant, antitussive, antihistaminic.

BAYHISTINE ELIXIR. (Bay) Chlorpheniramine maleate 2 mg., phenylpropanolamine HCl 18.75 mg./5 ml. w/alcohol 5%. Bot. 4 oz., pt., gal.
Use: Decongestant, antihistaminic.

BAYHISTINE EXPECTORANT. (Bay) Codeine phosphate 10 mg., guaifenesin 100 mg., phenylpropanolamine HCl 18.75 mg./5 ml. w/alcohol 7.5% Bot. 4 oz., pt., gal.
Use: Expectorant, antitussive, decongestant.

BAYIDYL SYRUP. (Bay) Triprolidine HCl 1.25 mg./5 ml. w/alcohol 4%. Bot. 4 oz., Pt.
Use: Antihistamine.

BAYLOCAINE 2% VISCOUS SOLUTION. (Bay) Lidocaine HCl 2%. Bot. 100 ml.
Use: Local anesthetic.

BAYLOCAINE 4% SOLUTION. (Bay) Lidocaine HCl 4%. Bot. 50 ml. or 100 ml.
Use: Local anesthetic.

BAYLOX. (Bay) Magnesia and alumina oral susp. Bot. 12 oz.
Use: Antacid.

BAYMETHAZINE SYRUP. (Bay) Promethazine HCl 6.25 mg./5 ml. w/alcohol 1.5%. Bot. 4 oz., pt., gal.
Use: Antihistamine

BAYMETHAZINE SYRUP FORTIS. (Bay) Promethazine HCl 25 mg./5 ml. w/alcohol 1.5%. Bot. 4 oz., pt.
Use: Antihistamine.

BAYON ELIXIR. (Bay) Potassium 20 meq./15 ml. Bot. 4 oz., pt., gal.
Use: supplement.

BAYORINADE. (Bay) Phenylpropanolamine HCl 125 mg., caramiphen edisylate 6.7 mg./5 ml. w/alcohol 5%. Bot. 4 oz., pt., gal.
Use: Decongestant, antitussive.

BAYTUSSIN. (Bay) Guaifenesin 100 mg./5 ml. w/alcohol 3.5%. Bot. 4 oz., pt., gal.
Use: Expectorant.

BAYTUSSIN AC. (Bay) Guaifenesin 100 mg., codeine phosphate 10 mg./5 ml. w/alcohol 3.5%. Bot. 4 oz., pt., gal.
Use: Antitussive, expectorant.

BAYTUSSIN DM. (Bay) Guaifenesin 100 mg., dextromethorphan HBr 15 mg./5 ml. w/alcohol 1.4%. Bot. 4 oz., pt., gal.
Use: Antitussive, expectorant.

B-BALM. (Vortech) Phenol 65 mg., zinc oxide 10%, comp. benzoin tr. 0.15 cc., methyl salicylate 20

mg., denatured alcohol 0.45 cc./oz. Jar 1 oz., 2 oz., 1 lb.
Use: Antiseptic.

B-BETTER CAPS. (Image) B-complex 50 mg./Cap. Bot. 100s.
Use: Supplement.

B-BEX T. (Image) Bot. 100s.
Use: Supplement.

BBR. (Western Research) Vit. B-1 10 mg., B-12 25 mcg./Tab. 28 Pack, 1000s.
Use: Vit. B deficiency.

BC-1000. (Reid-Provident) Vit. B-1 50 mg., B-2 5 mg., B-12 1000 mcg., B-6 5 mg., d-panthenol 6 mg., niacinamide 125 mg., ascorbic acid 50 mg., benzyl alcohol 1%/ml. Vial 10 ml.
Use: Vitamin supplement.

B-C-12-1000. (Burgin-Arden) Vit. B-12 1000 mcg., C 50 mg., B-1 50 mg., B-2 5 mg., B-6 5 mg., panthenol 6 mg., niacinamide 75 mg./cc. Vial 10 cc.
Use: B-complex therapy.

B-C-BID CAPSULES. (Geriatric) Vit. B-1 15 mg., B-2 10 mg., B-6 5 mg., niacinamide 50 mg., Ca pantothenate 10 mg., Vit. C 300 mg., B-12 5 mcg./Cap. Bot. 30s, 100s, 500s.

• **BCG VACCINE,** U.S.P. XXI. (Lilly) Prepared from a Glaxo substrain of a Danish strain of BCG bacillus. Vial 1 cc. 10 doses.
Use: Immunization against tuberculosis.

BCNU. 1,3-bis(2-Chloroethyl)-1-nitrosourea.
Use: Antineoplastic agent.
See: BiCNU, Inj. (Bristol)

BCO. (Western Research) Vit. B-1 10 mg., B-2 2 mg., B-6 1.5 mg., B-12 25 mcg., niacinamide 50 mg./Tab. Bot. 1000s.

B-COM. (Century) Vit. B-1 3 mg., B-2 3 mg., B-6 0.5 mg., niacinamide 20 mg., Ca pantothenate 5 mg., B-12 1 mcg., liver desic. (undefatted) 60 mg., debittered brewer's dried yeast 60 mg./Cap. Bot. 100s, 1000s.

B-COMPLEX. (Reid-Provident) Vit. B-1 100 mg., niacinamide 100 mg., B-2 2 mg., B-6 4 mg., calcium pantothenate 10 mg./cc. Vials 30 cc.

B-COMPLEX 2. (Kenyon) Vit. B-1 3 mg., B-2 3 mg., B-6 ½ mg., Ca pantothenate 5 mg., niacinamide 20 mg., dried yeast N.F. 60 mg./Cap. Bot. 100s.

B-COMPLEX NO. 5. (Pharmex) Vit. B-1 100 mg., B-2 2 mg., B-6 4 mg., panthenol 10 mg., niacinamide 100 mg., benzyl alcohol 1%, propylparaben 0.02%, methylparaben 0.18%/cc. Vial 30 cc.

B-COMPLEX 25-25 INJ. (Fellows) Niacinamide 100 mg., B-1 25 mg., B-2 1 mg., B-6 2 mg., pantothenic acid 2 mg./cc. Vial 30 cc.

B COMPLEX 100. (Burgin-Arden) Thiamine HCl 100 mg., riboflavin 5'sodium phosphate 2 mg., pyridoxine HCl 2 mg., panthenol 2 mg., niacinamide 1 ppmg., benzyl alcohol 2%. Vial 30cc.
Use: B complex supplement.

B-COMPLEX 100 (Kenyon) Vit. B-1 100 mg., B-2 2 mg., B-6 4 mg., d-panthenol 4 mg., niacinamide 100 mg./cc. Vial 30 cc.

B COMPLEX #100 (Medical Chem; CMC) B-1 100 mg., Vit. B-2 2 mg., B-6 4 mg., d-panthenol 4 mg., niacinamide 100 mg./cc. Vial 30 cc.

B COMPLEX 100. (Rabin-Winters) Vit. B-1 100 mg., B-2 2 mg., B-6 2 mg., niacinamide 125 mg., panthenol 10 mg./cc. Vial 30 cc.

B-COMPLEX 100/100. (Sandia) Vit. B-1 100 mg., B-2 2 mg., B-6 2 mg., niacinamide 100 mg./cc. Vial 30 cc. Inj.

B COMPLEX CAPSULES. (Arcum) Vit. B-1 1.5 mg., B-2 2 mg., niacinamide 10 mg., B-6 0.1 mg., Ca pantothenate 1.0 mg., liver desic. 70 mg., dried yeast 100 mg./Cap. Bot. 100s, 1000s.

B-COMPLEX CAPSULES. (Vortech) Vit. B-1 1.5 mg., B-2 2 mg., B-6 0.1 mg., Ca pantothenate 1 mg., dried yeast 100 mg., niacinamide 10 mg., desiccated liver 70 mg./Cap. Bot. 100s.

B COMPLEX CAPSULES J.F. (Bryant) Vit. B-1 1 mg., B-2 0.3 mg., nicotinic acid 0.3 mg., B-6 0.25 mg., liver, desic. 0.15 Gm., yeast powder, dried 0.15 Gm./Cap. Bot. 100s, 1000s.

B COMPLEX INJECTION WITH VITAMIN C.
See: Cplex Cap. (Arcum)

B COMPLEX WITH B-12 CAPSULES. (Bryant) Vit. B-1 2 mg., B-2 2 mg., B-6 0.5 mg., niacinamide 10 mg., B-12 2 mcg., biotin 10 mcg., Ca pantothenate 1.5 mg., choline dihydrogen citrate 40 mg., inositol 30 mg., liver, desic. 1 gr., Brewer's yeast 3 gr./Cap. Bot. 100s, 1000s.

B-COMPLEX W/C. (Towne) Vit. C 300 mg., B-1 15 mg., B-2 10 mg., B-6 5 mg., niacinamide 50 mg., calcium pantothenate 10 mg./Cap. Bot. 100s.

B-COMPLEX WITH C. (Sutliff & Case) Vit. B-1 3 mg., B-2 3 mg., C 30 mg., B-6 1.5 mg., pantothenic acid 2 mg., niacin 15 mg., yeast 5 mg./Tab. Bot. 100s, 1000s.
Use: Orally, vitamin B complex w/Vit. C.

B-COMPLEX W/C. (Zenith) Vit. B-1 15 mg., B-2 10 mg., B-6 5 mg., nicotinamide 50 mg., Ca pantothenate 10 mg., Vit. C 300 mg./Cap. Bot. 100s.

B COMPLEX with FOREIGN PROTEIN. (Medical Chem.) Vit. B-1 15 mg., B-2 1 mg., B-6 1 mg., d-panthenol 2 mg., methionine 5 mg., foreign protein 50 mg., niacinamide 50 mg./cc. Vial 30 cc.

B COMPLEX VITAMIN TABLETS. (Squibb) yeast 324 mg., B-1 2 mg., B-2 2 mg., B-6 0.125 mg., cyanocobalamin, niacinamide 10 mg./Tab. Bot. 100s.

B COMPLEX VITAMIN WITH C TABLETS. (Squibb) Vit. C 300mg., B-1 10 mg., B-2 10 mg., B-6 2 mg., B-12 4 mcg., pantothenic acid 20 mg., niacinamide 100 mg./Tab. Box 100s.

BC POWDER. (Block) Aspirin 10 gr., salicylamide 3 gr., caffeine 0.5 gr./Powder. Pkg. 2s, 6s, 24s, 50s, 100s.
Use: Analgesic, antipyretic.

BC TABLETS. (Block) Aspirin 5 gr., Salicylamide 1.5 gr., caffeine 0.25 gr./Tab. Bot. 12s, 50s, 100s.
Use: Analgesic.

BC-VITE. (Drug Industries) Vit. B-1 25 mg., B-2 5 mg., B-6 1 mg., B-12 2 mcg., C 150 mg., pantothenate 10 mg., niacinamide 50 mg./Tab. Bot. 100s, 500s.
Use: Stress therapy.

B-DAY TABLETS. (Barth's) Vit. B-1 7 mg., B-2 14 mg., niacin 4.67 mg., B-12 5 mcg./Tab. Bot. 100s, 500s.

BDEP. Same as Benzathine Penicillin G.

B-DOX. (Lannett) Vit. B-1 100 mg., B-6 100 mg./cc. Vials 10 cc.
Use: I.M. or I.V. nausea and vomiting.

B DOZEN. (Standex) Vit. B-12 25 mcg./Tab. Bot. 1000s.

B-DRAM w/C COMPUTABS. (Dram) Vit. B-2 10 mg., B-6 5 mg.; nicotinamide 50 mg., Ca pantothenate 20 mg., B-1 5 mg./Tab. Bot. 100s.
Use: Vitamin deficiencies.

BEACH GLO. (Eckerd) Ethyl dihydroxypropyl PABA. Bot. 4 oz. Lotion & oil Bot. 4 oz., 8 oz.
Use: Sunscreen.

BEACH GLO ULTRA 21. (Eckerd) Padimate O, oxybenzone. Bot. 4 oz.
Use: Maximum protection sunblock lotion.

BEBATAB NO. 2. (Freeport) Belladonna ⅛ gr., phenobarbital ¼ gr./Tab. Bot. 1000s.
Use: Sedative, anti-spasmodic.

• **BECANTHONE HYDROCHLORIDE.** USAN.
Use: Antischistosomal.

BECEEVITE CAPSULES. (Blue Cross) Vit. C 300 mg., B-1 15 mg., B-2 10 mg., niacin 50 mg., B-6 5 mg., pantothenic acid 10 mg./Tab. Bot. 100s.
Use: Vitamin supplement.

BE-CE FORTE. (Kenyon) B-1 15 mg., B-2 10 mg., niacinamide 80 mg., B-6 20 mg., d-panthenol 23 mg., C 100 mg./2 cc. Vial 20 cc.

BE-CE-PLEX. (CMC) B-6 6 mg., B-1 10 mg., B-2 10 mg., niacinamide 80 mg., panthenol 6 mg., sodium ascorbate 100 mg./2 cc. Vials 30 cc.

BECLAMIDE. B.A.N. N-Benzyl-3-chloropropionamide.
Use: Anticonvulsant.
See: Nydrane

BECLOMETHASONE. B.A.N. 9α-Chloro-11β, 17α, 21-trihydroxy-16β-methylpregna-1, 4-diene-3,20-dione. 9 α-Chloro-16β-methylprednisolone.
Use: Corticosteroid.

• **BECLOMETHASONE DIPROPRIONATE.** USAN.
Use: Corticosteroid.
See: Beclovent Inhaler (Glaxo)
Beconase Nasal Inhaler (Glaxo)
Vancenase Nasal Inhaler (Schering)
Vanceril Inhaler (Schering)

• **BECLOMYCIN DIPROPIONATE,** U.S.P. XXI.
Use: Corticosteroid.

BECLOVENT INHALER. (Glaxo) Beclomethasone diprorionate 42 mcg./dose. Aerosol canister (16.8 Gm.) containing 200 metered inhalations. Canister 16.8 Gm. w/oral adapter. Refill canister 16.8 Gm.
Use: Treatment of chronic bronchial asthma.

BECOMP-C. (Cenci) Vit. C 250 mg., B-1 25 mg., B-2 10 mg., nicotinamide 50 mg., B-6 2 mg., Ca pantothenate 10 mg., hesperidin complex 50 mg./Cap. Bot. 100s, 500s.
Use: Deficiencies of the water-soluble vitamins.

BECONASE NASAL INHALER. (Glaxo) Beclomethasone dipropionate 42 mcg./acuation. Aerosol canister (16.8 Gm.) containing 200 metered inhalations. Canister 16.8 Gm w/nasal adapter.
Use: Corticosteroid.

BECOPLEX. (Blue Line) Vit. B-1 3 mg., B-2 3 mg., B-6 0.25 mg., Ca pantothenate 5 mg., niacinamide 10 mg., dried brewer's yeast 2 gr., liver extract (fraction II) 1 gr./Tab. Bot. 100s.

BECOPLEX FORTIFIED. (Blue Line) Vit. B-1 1 mg., B-2 2 mg., B-12 1 mcg., exc. ferrous sulfate 136 mg., des. liver 200 mg./Cap. Bot. 100s, 1000s.
Use: Orally, vitamin with liver & iron therapy.

BECOTIN. (Dista) Vit. B-1 10 mg., B-2 10 mg., B-6 4.1 mg., niacinamide 50 mg., pantothenic acid 25 mg., Vit. B-12 1 mcg./Pulvule. Bot. 100s.
Use: Orally, vitamin B complex deficiencies.

BECOTIN-T. (Dista) Vit. B-1 15 mg.; B-2 10 mg.; B-6 5 mg., niacinamide 100 mg., pantothenic acid 20 mg.; B-12 4 mcg.; C 300 mg./Tab. Bot. 100s, 1000s. Blister pkg. 10 × 10s.
Use: Vit. B-complex and Vit. C deficiencies.

BECOTIN W/VIT. C. (Dista) Vit. B-1 10 mg., B-2 10 mg., B-6 4.1 mg., niacinamide 50 mg., pantothenic acid 25 mg., Vit. B-12 1 mcg., C 150 mg./Pulvule. Bot. 100s, 500s, 1000s. Blister pkg. 10 × 10s.
Use: Orally, vitamin B complex and vitamin C deficiencies.

BEDOCE. (Lincoln) Crystalline anhydrous B-12 1000 mcg./cc. Vial 10 cc.
Use: I.M., vitamin B-12 therapy.

BEDOCE-GEL. (Lincoln) Vit. B-12 1000 mcg./cc. in 17% gelatin solution. Vial 10 cc.

BEDSORE SPRAY. (Century) Silicone, tincture of benzoin compound. Bot. 7 oz.
Use: Bedsore treatment.

BEECHWOOD CREOSOTE.
See: Creosote, N.F.

BEECOMP. (Vitarine) Vit. B-1 1.5 mg., B-2 2 mg., B-6 1 mg., Ca pantothenate 5 mg., niacinamide 10 mg./Cap. Bot. 50s, 1000s.
Use: Supplement.

BEEF PEPTONES. (Sandia) Water soluble peptones derived from beef 20 mg./2 cc. Vial 30 cc. Inj.

BEEKAPS. (Pharmics) Vit. C 400 mg., lemon bio-flavonoid 200 mg., B-1 25 mg., B-2 10 mg., Ca pantothenate 10 mg., B-6 10 mg., niacinamide 50 mg./Cap. Bot. 100s, 500s, 1000s.
Use: Dietary supplement.

BEELITH. (Beach) Pyridoxine HCl 25 mg., magnesium oxide 600 mg./Tab. Bot. 100s, 500s.
Use: Dietary supplement.

BEEPEN-VK. (Beecham Labs) Penicillin VK. **Tab.:** 250 mg./Tab. Bot. 100s, 1000s; 500 mg./Tab. Bot. 100s, 500s.**Syrup:** 125 mg./5 cc. Bot. 100 cc, 200 cc; 250 mg./5 cc. Bot. 100 cc, 200 cc.
Use: Antibiotics.

BEESIX INJECTION. (Fellows) Pyridoxine HCl 100 mg./cc. Vial 10 cc.

BEE-THI. (Burgin-Arden) Cyanocobalamin 1000 mcg., thiamine HCl 100 mg. in isotonic solution of sodium chloride/cc. Vial 10 cc., 20 cc.

BEE-TWELVE 1000. (Burgin-Arden) Cyanocobalamin 1000 mcg./cc. Vial 10 cc., 30 cc.

BEEZE W/VITAMIN C. (Columbia) Vit. B-1 15 mg., B-2 10 mg., B-6 5 mg., C 300 mg., niacinamide 50 mg., ca pantothenate 10 mg./Cap. Bot. 100s, 1000s.

BEFERRIC. (Kenyon) Ferric ammonium citrate 500

mg., B-1 12 mg., B-2 6 mg., B-6 0.6 mg., folic acid 0.5
mg., Cal. pantothenate 6 mg., niacinamide 15 mg.,
Mg 2 mg., Mg 1 mg., Co 0.1 mg., Zn 2 mg./Fl. oz.
Bot. 4 oz.

BEHEPAN.
See: Vitamin B-12

BEJECTAL. (Abbott) Vit. B-1 100 mg., B-2 20 mg.,
niacinamide 750 mg., B-6 50 mg., sod. pantothenate
50 mg./10 ml. Univial. Box 25s.
Use: I.M. of I.V., vitamin B complex therapy.

BEJECTAL W/ VIT. C. (Abbott) Vit. B-1 20 mg., B-2 3
mg., B-12 2 mcg., niacinamide 75 mg., Vit. B-6 5 mg.,
C 100 mg., sod. pantothenate 5 mg./ml. Univial 10
ml. Box 25s.
Use: I.M. or I.V. Vitamin B complex deficiencies.

BELAP. (Lemmon) Phenobarbital 16.2 mg.,
belladonna extract 10.8 mg./Tab. Bot. 100s, 1000s.
Use: Anticholinergic, sedative.

BELATOL NO. 1; NO. 2. (Cenci) **No. 1:** Belladonna
leaf extract ⅛ gr., phenobarbital ¼ gr./Tab. 100s,
1000s. **No. 2:** Belladonna leaf extract ⅛ gr.,
phenobarbital ½ gr./Tab. Bot. 100s, 1000s.
Use: Antispasmodic and sedative.

BELATOL ELIXIR. (Cenci) Phenobarbital 20 mg.,
belladonna 6.75 min., alcohol 45%/5 cc. Elix. Bot.
pt., gal.
Use: Antispasmodic.

BELBUTAL NO. 2 KAPTABS. (Churchill)
Phenobarbital 32.4 mg., hyoscyamine sulfate
0.1092 mg., atropine sulfate 0.0215 mg., hyoscine
HBr 0.0065 mg./Tab. Bot. 100s.
Use: Antispasmodic sedative.

BELDIN. (Blue Cross) Diphenhydramine HCl 12.5
mg./5 ml. w/alcohol 5%. Bot. gal.
Use: Antitussive.

BELEXAL. (Vale) Vit. B-1 1.5 mg., B-2 2 mg., B-6 0.167
mg., Ca pantothenate 1 mg., niacinamide 10
mg./Tab. w/brewer's yeast. Bot. 100s, 1000s,
5000s.
Use: Vitamin supplement.

BELEXON FORTIFIED IMPROVED. (APC) Liver
fraction No. 2 3 gr., yeast ext. 3 gr., B-1 5 mg., B-2 6
mg., niacinamide 10 mg., Ca pantothenate 2 mg.,
cyanocobalamin 1 mcg., iron 10 mg./Cap. Bot. 100s.

BELFER. (O'Neal, Jones & Feldman) Vit. B-1 2 mg.,
B-2 2 mg., B-12 10 mcg., B-6 2 mg., C 50 mg., iron
gluconate 17 mg., sorbitol 100 mg./Tab. Bot. 100s.
Use: Anemia.

BELIVRON. (Vitarine) Vit. B-1 1 mg., B-2 1 mg., B-12
3 mcg., liver powder 7 gr., iron & ammonium
citrates (green) 3 gr./Cap. Bot. 100s, 250s.
Use: Supplement.

BELIVRON TONIC ELIXIR. (Vitarine) Vit. B-1 6 mg., B-2
3 mg., B-6 2 mg., B-12 6 mcg., niacinamide 30 mg.,
folic acid 0.05 mg., pantothenic acid 6 mg., iron
ammon. citrates 1.3 mg., Mn cit. 130 mg., Cu
sulfate 1.6 mg., Mg sulfate 200 mg., pot. sulfate 20
mg., Zn sulfate 20 mg., liver fraction No. 1 175
mg., beef peptone 175 mg./Fl. oz. Bot. 8 oz., pt.
Use: High-potency tonic.

BELLACHAR. (Wolins) Phenobarbital 20 mg.,
activated charcoal 120 mg., belladonna ext. 5
mg./Tab. Bot. 1000s.

BELLADENAL. (Sandoz) Bellafoline 0.25 mg.,
phenobarbital 50 mg./Tab. Bot. 100s.
Use: Antispasmodic & anticholinergic.

BELLADENAL S. (Sandoz) Bellafoline 0.25 mg.,
phenobarbital 50 mg./Tab. Bot. 100s.
Use: Antispasmodic & anticholinergic.

■ **BELLADONNA ALKALOIDS.**
Use: Intestinal antispasmotic.
W/Combinations.
  See: Accelerase-PB, Cap. (Organon)
    Belladenal, Preps. (Sandoz)
    Bellophen, Tab. (Vortech)
    Belphen, Tab. (Robinson)
    Belphen Elixir (Robinson)
    Belphen Timed Caps. (Robinson)
    Coryztime, Cap. (Elder)
    Decobel, Lanacaps (Lannett)
    Fitacol Stankaps (Standex)
    Kamabel Liq. (Towne)
    Nilspasm, Tab. (Parmed)
    Ultabs, Tab. (Burlington)
    Urilief, Tab. (Mallinckrodt)
    Urised, Tab. (Webcon)
    U-Tract, Tab. (Bowman)
    Wigraine, Tab., Supp. (Organon)
    Woltac, Cap. (Wolins)
    Wyanoids, Supp., Oint. w/applic. (Wyeth)

• **BELLADONNA EXTRACT,** U.S.P. XXI. Tab. U.S.P.
XXI.

■ **BELLADONNA EXTRACT COMBINATIONS.**
  See: Amobell, Cap. (Bock)
    Amsodyne, Tab. (Elder)
    B & O Supprettes (Webcon)
    Belap, Tab. (Lemmon)
    Bellachar, Tab. (Wolins)
    Bellafedrol A-H. Tab. (Lannett)
    Bello-phen, Tab. (Wolins)
    Bellkatal, Tab. (Ferndale)
    Butibel, Tab., Elix. (McNeil)
    Butibel-Zyme, Tab. (McNeil)
    Gelcomul, Liq. (Commerce)
    Hycoff Cold, Caps (Saron)
    Lanothal, Pills (Lannett)
    Phebe (Western Research)
    Rectacort, Supp. (Century)

• **BELLADONNA LEAF,** U.S.P. XXI.
W/Phenobarbital & benzocaine.
Use: Anticholinergic.
  See: Gastrolic, Tab. (Mallard)

■ **BELLADONNA PRODUCTS AND
PHENOBARBITAL COMBINATIONS.**
  See: Accelerase-PB, Cap. (Organon)
    Alised, Tab. (Elder)
    Atrocap, Cap. (Freeport)
    Atrosed, Tab. (Freeport)
    Barbidonna, Elixir and Tab. (Mallinckrodt)
    Bebatab, Tab. (Freeport)
    Belap, Elix., Tab. (Lemmon)
    Belatol, Tab., Elix. (Cenci)
    Belbarb, Tab. (Arnar-Stone)
    Belladenal, Elixir, Spacetab, and Tab. (Sandoz)
    Bellergal, Spacetab., Tab. (Dorsey)
    Bellkatal, Tab. (Ferndale)

Bellophen, Tab. (Richlyn)
B-Sed, Tab. (Scrip)
Chardonna, Tab. (Rorer)
Donabarb, Elix., Tab. (Elder)
Donnafed Jr., Tab. (Jenkins)
Donnatal, Cap., Elixir, Tab., Extentab (Robins)
Donnatal #2, Tab. (Robins)
Donnazyme, Tab. (Robins)
Gastrolic, Tab. (Mallard)
Hypnaldyne, Tab. (North American Pharm.)
Kinesed, Tab. (Stuart)
Mallenzyme, Tab. (Mallard)
Medi-Spas, Elix. (Medical Chemicals)
Phenobarbital and Belladonna Tab. (Lilly)
Phen-o-bel, Tab. (Coastal)
Phen-o-bel-T, T.R. Cap. (Coastal)
Sedapar, Tab. (Parmed)
Sedatromine, Tab. (Sutliff & Case)
Spabelin, Tab. (Arcum)
Spabelin No. 2, Tab. (Arcum)
Spasnil, Tab. (Rhode)
• **BELLADONNA TINCTURE, U.S.P. XXI.**
BELLAFEDROL A-H TABLETS. (Lannett) Pyrilamine maleate 12.5 mg., chlorpheniramine maleate 1 mg., phenylephrine HCl 2.5 mg., ext. belladonna 6 mg./Tab. Bot. 100s, 500s, 1000s.
Use: Antihistamine w/antispasmodic.
BELLAFOLINE. (Sandoz) Levorotatory alkaloids of belladonna as malates. **Amp.** 0.5 mg./cc. SandoPak Pkg. 20s. **Tab.** 0.25 mg./Tab. Bot. 100s.
Use: Antispasmodic for spastic conditions of smooth muscles and excessive secretions.
BELLALPHEN. (CMC) Atropine sulfate 0.0194 mg., hyoscyamine sulfate 0.1037 mg., hyoscine HBr 0.0065 mg., phenobarbital 16.2 mg./Tab. Bot. 100s, 500s, 1000s.
Use: Visceral spasms and hyperirritability.
BELLANEED. (Hanlon) Belladonna & phenobarbital 16 mg./Cap. Bot. 100s.
Use: Antispasmodic.
BELL-ANS. (C.S. Dent) Sodium bicarbonate 264 mg., willow charcoal 38.8 mg., gingerine 0.0003 ml./Tab. Vial 60s, 120s. Also available in double strength. Vial 60s, 120s.
Use: Antacid.
BELLASTAL CAPSULES. (U.S. Ethicals) Phenobarbital 16.2 mg., hyoscyamine sulfate 0.1037 mg., atropine sulfate 0.0194 mg., scopolamine HBr 0.0065 mg./Cap. Bot. 1000s.
Use: Intestinal anti-spasmodic.
BELLASTAL ELIXIR. (U.S. Ethicals) Belladonna alkaloids, phenobarbital 16.2 mg., hyoscyamine sulfate 0.1037 mg., atropine sulfate 0.0194 mg., scopolamine HBr 0.0065 mg./5 ml. Bot. 120 ml., 3840 ml.
Use: Adjunctive therapy in treatment of irritable bowel syndrome.
BELLERGAL. (Sandoz) Bellafoline 0.1 mg., ergotamine tartrate 0.3 mg., phenobarbital 20.0 mg./Tab. Bot. 100s, 1000s.
Use: Orally, sedative w/antispasmodic.
BELLERGAL-S. (Sandoz) Ergotamine Tartrate 0.6 mg.,

Bellafoline 0.2 mg., Phenobarbital 40.0 mg./Spacetab. Bot. 100s.
Use: Menopausal disorders.
BELLKATAL. (Ferndale) Phenobarbital ⅛ gr., Pow. Ext. belladonna leaves ⁴/₂₅ gr., kaolin colloidal 7½ gr./Tab. Bot. 100s, 1000s.
Use: Sedative, antiparasympathomimetic, antispasmodic, absorbent.
BELLOPHEN. (Vortech) Phenobarbital ¼ gr., ext. belladonna ⅛ gr./Tab. Bot. 1000s.
Use: Antispasmodic.
• **BELOXAMIDE.** USAN.
Use: Antihyperlipoproteinemic.
BELPHEN. (Robinson) Belladonna alkaloids, phenobarbital. Bot. Tab. 100s, 1000s.
Use: Antispasmodic, sedative.
BELPHEN ELIXIR. (Robinson) Belladonna alkaloids w/phenobarbital elixir. Bot. pt., gal.
BELPHEN TABLETS. (Stanlabs) #1 Belladonna leaf ext. ⅛ gr., phenobarbital ¼ gr./Tab. #2 Belladonna leaf ext. ⅛ gr., phenobarbital ½ gr./Tab. Bot. 1000s.
Use: Antispasmodic.
BELPHEN TIMED CAPS. (Robinson) Belladonna alkaloids, phenobarbital time disintegration. Bot. 100s, 500s, 1000s.
Use: Antispasmodic, sedative.
BEMEGRIDE. B.A.N. 3-Ethyl-3-methylglutarimide.
See: Megimide
Use: Medullary respiratory stimulant.
BEMINAL 500. (Ayerst) Vit. B-1 25 mg., B-2 12.5 mg., niacinamide 100 mg., B-6 10 mg., calcium pantothenate 20 mg., C 500 mg. cyanocobalamin 5 mcg./Tab. Bot. 100s.
Use: Vitamin B therapy.
BEMINAL FORTE W/VIT. C. (Ayerst) Vit. B-1 25 mg., B-2 12.5 mg., niacinamide 50 mg., B-6 3 mg., calcium pantothenate 10 mg., C 250 mg., B-12 2.5 mcg./Cap. Bot. 100s.
Use: Vitamins B & C therapy.
BEMINAL STRESS PLUS WITH IRON. (Ayerst) Vit. B-1 25 mg., B-2 12.5 mg., B-3 100 mg., B-5 20 mg., B-6 10 mg., B-12 25 mcg., folic acid 400 mcg., C 787 mg., E 45 I.U., iron 27 mg./Tab. Bot. 60s.
Use: Dietary supplement.
BEMINAL STRESS PLUS WITH ZINC. (Ayerst) Vit. B-1 25 mg., B-2 12.5 mg., B-3 100 mg., B-5 20 mg., B-6 10 mg., B-12 25 mcg., C 100 mg., E 45 I.U. Zn 45 mg./Tab. Bot. 60s.
Use: Dietary supplement.
BENACEN. (Cenci) Probenecid 0.5 gm./Tab. Bot. 100s, 1000s.
BENACHLOR. (Jenkins) Diphenhydramine HCl 12.5 mg., ammonium chloride 130 mg., sod. citrate 55 mg., menthol 1.11 mg., alcohol 5%/5 cc. Syr. Bot. 3 oz., 4 oz., gal.
BENACOL. (Cenci) Dicyclomine HCl 20 mg./Tab. Bot. 100s, 1000s.
Use: Smooth muscle spasm.
BENACTYZINE. B.A.N. 2-Diethylaminoethyl benzilate.
Use: Tranquilizer.

See: Suavitil hydrochloride.

BENACTYZINE HYDROCHLORIDE. 2-Diethylamino-
ethyl benzilate HCl.
W/Meprobamate.
　See: Deprol, Tab. (Wallace)
BENA-D-10. (Seatrace) Diphenhydramine HCl 10
mg./ml. Vial 30 cc.
BENA-D-50. (Seatrace) Diphenhydramine HCl 50
mg./ml. Vial 10 cc.
BENADRYL COUGH PREPARATION.
　See: Benylin Cough Syrup (Parke-Davis)
BENADRYL HYDROCHLORIDE. (Parke-Davis)
Diphenhydramine hydrochloride.
　Use: Antihistaminic.
　Amp.: (50 mg./ml.) 1 ml. Box 10s.
　Cap.: (25 mg.) Bot. 100s, 1000s. Unit dose 100s.
　Cream: (2%) Tube 1 & 2 oz.
　Elixir (w/alcohol 14%): (12.5 mg./5 ml.) Bot. 4
　oz., 1 pt., 1 gal. Unit dose 5 ml × 100s.
　Kapseals: (50 mg.) Bot. 100s, 1000s. Unit dose
　100s.
　Steri-Dose: (50 mg./ml., pH adjusted w/HCl or sod.
　hydroxide) Amp. 1 ml. Box 10s. Disposable
　syringes 1 ml. **Steri-Vial:** (10 mg./ml. Phemerol
　benzethonium chloride as germicidal agent. pH
　adjusted w/sod. hydroxide or HCl) 10 ml., 30 ml.
　(50 mg./ml.) 10 ml.
W/Ammonium chloride, sod. citrate, menthol.
　See: Benylin Cough Syrup (Parke-Davis)
W/Ephedrine sulfate. (Parke-Davis) Benadryl
hydrochloride 50 mg., ephedrine sulfate 25
mg./Cap. Bot. 100s.
　Use: Provides the complementary effects of the
　original antihistaminic & the sympathomimetic.
W/Zinc oxide, alcohol.
　See: Ziradryl, Lot. (Parke-Davis)
BENADRYL HCl LOTION OR CREAM.
　See: Caladryl, Cream, Lot. (Parke-Davis)
BENAHIST 10. (Keene) Diphenhydramine 10 mg./ml.
Vial 30 ml.
　Use: Antihistaminic.
BENAHIST 50. (Keene) Diphenhydramine 50 mg./ml.
Vial 10 ml.
　Use: Antihistaminic.
BENANEERIN HCl. 3-(2-Aminoethyl)-1-benzyl-5-me-
thoxy-2-methylindole HCl.
BENANSERIN HYDROCHLORIDE. 3-(2-Aminoethyl)-
1-benzyl-5-methoxy-2-methylindole monohydrochlo-
ride.
　Use: Serotonin antagonist.
BENAPEN.
　See: Benethamine
BENAPRYZINE. B.A.N. 2-(N-Ethylpropylamino)-ethyl
benzilate.
　Use: Treatment of the Parkinsonian syndrome.
• **BENAPRYZINE HYDROCHLORIDE.** USAN.
　Use: Anticholingeric.
BENASE. (Ferndale) Proteolytic enzymes extracted
from Carica papaya 20,000 u. enzyme activity/Tab.
Bot. 1000s.
　Use: Reduction of edema and relief of episiotomy.
BENASEPT. (Blue Line) Benzalkonium chloride

Concentrate 17%. Bot. 4 oz., gal. **Sol.** 1:1000,
stainless. Bot. 1 gal. **Vaginal Jelly** 1:3000, sod.
lactate-lactic acid buffer, tragacanth-pectin-glycerin-
water base, methylparaben, propylparaben,
coloring, perfume, w/applicator, Tube 1½ oz.
　Use: Topically, cationic germicidal.
BENAT-12. (Hauck) Cyanocobalamine 30 mcg., liver injection 0.5 ml., B-1 10 mg., B-2 2 mg., niacinamide 50
mg., d-panthenol 1 mg., B-6 1 mg./ml. w/benzyl alcohol 4%, phenol 0.5%. Vial 10 ml.
　Use: Anti-anemic.
• **BENDAZAC.** USAN. [l-Benzyl-(H-indazol-3yl)oxy]
acetic acid.
　Use: Anti-inflammatory.
BENDECTIN. (Merrell Dow) Doxylamine succinate 10
mg., pyridoxine HCl 10 mg./Tab. 90 tabs. in 3 pkg.
of 30s.
　Use: Nausea and vomiting of pregnancy. **Note:
Manufacturer voluntarily stopped production in
1983.**
BENDROFLUAZIDE. B.A.N. 3-Benzyl-3,4-dihydro-6-
trifluoromethylbenzo-1,2,4-thiadiazine-7-sulfonamide
1,1-dioxide. Bendroflumethiazide (I.N.N.)
　Use: Diuretic.
　See: Aprinox
　　Berkozide
　　Centyl
　　Neo-Naclex
• **BENDROFLUMETHIAZIDE,** U.S.P. XXI. Tab., U.S.P.
XXI. 3-Benzyl-3:4-dihydro-7-sulphamoly-6-tri-
fluoromethylbenzo-1:2:4-thiadiazine 1:1-dioxide. 6-
(Trifluoromethyl)-2H-1,2,4-benzothiadiazine-7-sulfon-
amide 1, 1-dioxide.
　Use: Diuretic; antihypertensive.
　See: Naturetin, Tab. (Squibb)
　　Naturetin-10, Tab. (Squibb)
W/Potassium Chloride.
　See: Naturetin W-K, Tab. (Squibb)
W/Rauwolfia serpentina
　See: Rauzide, Tab.
W/Rauwolfia serpentina, potassium chloride.
　See: Rautrax-N, Tab. (Squibb)
　　Rautrax-N Modified, Tab. (Squibb)
BENDYLATE CAP. (Reid-Provident) Diphenhydramine
HCl 25 mg. & 50 mg./Cap. Bot. 100s, 1000s.
BENDYLATE INJ. (Reid-Provident) Diphenhydramine
HCl 10 mg. in water for inj. w/benzethonium
chloride 1:10,000/cc. Vials 30 cc.
BENEGYN CREAM. (Vortech) Tube. 96 Gm.
w/applicator.
　Use: Trichomoniasis, moniliasis & mixed infections.
BENEMID. (Merck Sharp & Dohme) Probenecid 0.5
Gm./Tab. Bot. 100s, 1000s. Single unit pkg. 100s.
　Use: Uricosuric, adjuvant to antibiotic therapy for
　elevation and prolongation of plasma levels.
W/Colchicine.
　See: Colbenemid, Tab. (Merck Sharp & Dohme)
BENEPHEN ANTISEPTIC MEDICATED POWDER.
(Halsted) Methylbenzethonium chloride 1:1800,
magnesium carbonate, in cornstarch base. Shaker
cans 3.56 oz.
　Use: Deodorant, antiseptic.

BENEPHEN ANTISEPTIC OINTMENT W/COD LIVER OIL. (Halsted) Methylbenzethonium chloride 1:1000, water-repellent base of zinc oxide and cornstarch. Tubes 1½ oz., jars 1 lb.
Use: Antiseptic.

BENEPHEN ANTISEPTIC VITAMIN A & D CREAM. (Halsted) Methylbenzethonium chloride 1:1000, cod liver oil w/vit. A & D in petrolatum & glycerin base. Tubes 2 oz., jars 1 lb.
Use: Antiseptic.

BENETHAMINE PENICILLIN. B.A.N. N-Benzyl-phenethylammonium 6-phenylacetamidopenicillanate. N-Benzylphenethylamine salt of benzylpenicillin. Benapen.
Use: Antibiotic.

BENGAL GELATIN.
See: Agar.

BEN-GAY CHILDREN'S VAPORIZING RUB. (Leeming) Camphor, menthol, w/oils of turpentine, eucalyptus, cedar leaf, nutmeg and thyme in stainless white base. Jar 1.125 oz.
Use: Chest colds.

BEN-GAY EXTRA STRENGTH BALM. (Leeming) Menthol & methylsalicylate. Jars 3.75 oz.
Use: External analgesic.

BEN-GAY GEL. (Leeming) Methyl salicylate, menthol, alcohol 40%. Tube 1.25 oz., 3.0 oz.
Use: External analgesic.

BEN-GAY GREASELESS OINTMENT. (Leeming) Methyl salicylate, menthol. Tube 1.25 oz., 3.0 oz., 5.0 oz.
Use: External analgesic.

BEN-GAY LOTION. (Leeming) Methyl salicylate, menthol in lotion base. Bot. 2 oz., 4 oz.
Use: External analgesic.

BEN-GAY OINTMENT. (Leeming) Methyl salicylate, menthol in ointment base. Tube 1.25 oz., 3 oz., 5 oz.
Use: External analgesic.

BENISONE. (CooperCare) Betamethasone benzoate 0.025% **Cream:** 15 Gm., 60 Gm. **Gel:** 15 Gm., 60 Gm. **Lotion:** 15 ml., 60 ml., **Oint.:** 15 Gm., 60 Gm.
Use: Anti-inflammatory agent.

BENN. (Scrip) Probenecid 500 mg./Tab. Bot. 1000s.
Use: Orally, increase excretion of uric acid.

BENN-C. (Scrip) Probenecid 500 mg., colchicine 0.5 mg./Tab. Bot. 1000s.
Use: Chronic gout and gouty arthritis.

BENOJECT. (Mayrand) Diphenhydramine HCl 50 mg./ml. Vial 10 ml.
Use: Antihistamine, anticholinergic.

BENOQUIN. (Elder) Monobenzone 20% in cream base. Tube 1.25 oz.

BENORAL CAPSULES. (Winthrop Products) Benorylate.
Use: Analgesic, antipyretic.

BENORAL SUSPENSION. (Winthrop Products) Benorylate.
Use: Analgesic, antipyretic.

BENORAL TABLETS. (Winthrop Products) Benorylate.
Use: Analgesic, antipyretic.

• **BENORTERONE.** USAN. 17 β-Hydroxy-17-methyl-β-norandrost-4-en-3-one.
Use: Antiandrogen.

BENORYLATE. B.A.N. 4-Acetamidophenyl O-acetylsalicylate. Benoral.
Use: Analgesic.

• **BENOXAPROFEN.** USAN. 2-(2-p-Chlorophenyl-benzoxazol-5-yl)propionic acid.
Use: Anti-inflammatory; analgesic.

• **BENOXINATE HYDROCHLORIDE,** U.S.P. XXI. Ophth. Soln., U.S.P. XXI. 2-(Diethylaminoethyl)-amino-3-butoxybenzoate HCl.
See: Dorsacaine, Sol. (Dorsey)
W/Fluorescein sod.
See: Flurless, Sol. (Barnes-Hind)

BENOXYL LOTION. (Stiefel) Benzoyl peroxide 5% or 10% in mild lotion base. Bot. 1 oz., 2 oz.
Use: Acne therapy.

• **BENPERIDOL.** USAN. 1-{1-[3-(4-Fluorobenzoyl)-propyl]-4-piperidyl}benzimidazolin-2-one.
Use: Tranquilizer.
See: Anquil

• **BENSALAN.** USAN. 3,5-Dibromo-N-p-bromo-benzyl)-salicylamide. Under study.
Use: Germicide.

• **BENSERAZIDE.** USAN. DL-2-Amino-3-hydroxy-2'-(2,-3,4-trihydroxybenzyl)propionohydrazide.
Use: Treatment of the Parkinsonian syndrome.

BENSULDAZIC ACID. B.A.N. (5-Benzyl-6-thioxo-1,3,5-thiadiazin-3-yl)acetic acid. Defungit sodium salt.
Use: Fungicide, veterinary medicine.

BENSULFOID. (Poythress) 33%**Tabs.** Elemental sulfur 130 mg. by weight, fused on colloidal bentonite. **Pow.:** 1 oz. **Tab.** 2 gr. Bot. 100s.
Use: Prescription compounding.
W/Phenobarbital
See: Solfoton, Tab. or Cap. (Poythress)

BENSULFOID LOTION. (Poythress) Bensulfoid 6%, thymol 0.5%, zinc oxide 6%, alcohol (by vol.) 12%, methyl salicylate 5%, perfume, cosmetic colors, emulsifiers/Lotion Bot. 2 oz.
Use: Topical treatment of acne.

• **BENTAZEPAM.** USAN.
Use: Sedative.

BENTICAL. (Lamond) Bentonite, zinc oxide, zinc carbonate, titanium dioxide. Bot. 4 oz., 6 oz., 8 oz., 16 oz., 32 oz., ½ gal., gal.
Use: Bland lotion.

• **BENTIROMIDE.** USAN.
Use: Diagnostic aid.
See: Chymex, Sol. (Adria)

• **BENTONITE,** N.F. XVI.
Use: Pharm. aid (suspending agent).

• **BENTONITE MAGMA,** N.F. XVI.
Use: Pharmaceutical aid (suspending agent).

BENTONITE PASTE FOR EEG TESTS. (C & M Pharmacal) Jar 32 oz.
Use: Diagnostic aid for EEG test.

BENTRAC 25, 50. (Kenyon) Diphenhydramine HCl 25 mg., 50 mg./Cap. Bot. 100s.

BENTRAC-ELIXIR. (Kenyon) Diphenhydramine HCl 10 mg., alcohol 14%/4 cc. Bot. 4 oz.

BENTRAC EXPECTORANT. (Kenyon)
Diphenhydramine HCl 80 mg., ammonium chloride 12 gr., sod. citrate 5 gr., chloroform 2 gr., menthol 1/10 gr., alcohol 5%/Fl. oz. Bot. 4 oz.
BENTYL. (Merrell Dow) Dicyclomine HCl.**Caps.** 10 mg. Bot. 100s, 500s, 1000s. Unit dose 100s.**Tab.** 20 mg., Bot. 100s, 500s, 1000s. Unit dose 100s. **Syr.** 10 mg./5 ml. Bot. 1 pt. **Inj.** 10 mg./ml. Amp. 2 ml.,syringe 2 ml. (both contain sod. chloride). Vial 10 ml. (also contains sod. chloride, chlorobutanol hydrous).
Use: Antispasmodic for irritable bowel syndrome.
BENTYL WITH PHENOBARBITAL. (Merrell Dow)
Cap. Dicyclomine HCl 10 mg., phenobarbital 15 mg. Bot. 100s. **Syr.** Dicyclomine HCl 10 mg., phenobarbital 15 mg./5 ml. Alcohol 19%. Bot. 1 pt. **Tab.** Dicyclomine HCl 20 mg., phenobarbital 15 mg./Tab. Bot. 100s.
Use: Antispasmodic, for irritable bowel syndrome.
• **BENURESTAT.** USAN.
Use: Enzyme inhibitor.
BENYLIN COUGH SYRUP. (Parke-Davis)
Diphenhydramine HCl 12.5 mg. w/alcohol 5%. Bot. 4 oz., 8 oz., 1 pt., 1 gal. Unit dose 5 ml., 10 ml., Box 100s.
Use: Orally, coughs.
BENYLIN DM COUGH SYRUP. (Parke-Davis)
Dextromethorphan HBr 10 mg./5 ml. w/alcohol 5% Bot. 4 oz., 8 oz.
Use: Cough suppressant.
BENZA. (Century) Benzalkonium chloride 1:5000 and 1:750. Bot. 2 oz., 4 oz.
Use: Antiseptic, germicide.
BENZAC 5 & 10. (Owen) Benzoyl peroxide 5% or 10%w/polyoxyethylene lauryl ether 6%, alcohol 12%, dimethicone, carbomer 940, fragrance & purified water; may contain sodium hydroxide and/or citric acid to adjust pH. Tube 60 Gm.
Use: Acne vulgaris treatment.
BENZAC w 2.5. (Owen) Benzoyl peroxide 2.5%, in gel base of dioctyl sodium sulfosuccinate, edetate disodium, poloxamer 182, carbomer 940, propylene glycol, silicon dioxide, purified water. Tubes 60 Gm., 90 Gm.
Use: Acne vulgaris treatment.
BENZAC w 5 & 10. (Owen) Benzoyl peroxide 5% or 10% w/docusate sodium, edetate disodium, poloxamer 182, carbomer 940, propylene glycol, silicon dioxide purified water and buffer. Tube 60, 90 Gm.
Use: Acne vulgaris treatment.
BENZAC w WASH. (Owen) Benzoyl peroxide 5% in vehicle of sodium C14-16 olefin sulfonate, carbomer 940, purified water. Bot. 4 oz.
Use: Adjunct to primary acne regimens.
BENZAGEL. (Dermik) Benzoyl peroxide 5% or 10% in gel base of water, carbomer 940, alcohol 14%, sodium hydroxide, docusate sodium, fragrance. Tube 1.5 oz., 3 oz.
Use: Treatment of acne.
• **BENZALDEHYDE,** N.F. XVI. Cpd. Elix., N.F. XVI.
Use: Pharm. aid (flavor).

• **BENZALKONIUM CHLORIDE,** N.F. XVI. Sol., N.F. XVI. Alkyldimethylbenzylammonium chloride. Zephirol. Sol. 1:5000. ammonium, alkyldimethyl(phenylmethyl)-, chloride.
Use: Surface antiseptic and antimicrobial preservative.
See: Benasept, Sol. & Tr., Vaginal Jelly (Blue Line)
    Benz-All, Liq. (Xxtrium)
    Econopred, Susp. (Alcon)
    Eye-Stream (Alcon)
    Germicin, Sol. (Consolidated Mid.)
    Hyamine 3500 (Rohm & Haas)
    Otrivin Spray (Geigy)
    Ultra Tears (Alcon)
    Zalkon Conc., Liq. (Gordon)
    Zephiran Chloride Preps. (Winthrop-Breon)
W/Aluminum Cl, oxyquinoline sulfate.
    See: Alochor Styptic, Liq. (Gordon)
W/Bacitracin zinc, polymyxin B, neomycin sulf.
    See: Biotres, Oint. (Central)
W/Benzocaine, benzyl alcohol.
    See: Aerocain, Oint. (Aeroceuticals)
W/Benzocaine, orthohydroxyphenyl-mercuric chloride, parachlorometaxylenol
    See: Unguentine, Aerosol (Norwich)
W/Berberine HCl, sodium borate, phenylephrine HCl, sodium chloride, boric acid.
    See: Ocusol, Eye Lotion, Drops (Norwich)
W/Boric acid, potassium chloride, sodium carbonate anhydrous, disodium edetate.
    See: Swim-Eye, Drops (Savage)
W/Chlorophyll.
    See: Mycomist, Spray Liq. (Gordon)
W/Hydrocortisone.
    See: Barseb Thera-Spray, Sol. (Barnes-Hind)
W/Diperodon HCl, carbolic acid, ichthammol, thymol, camphor, juniper tar.
    See: Boro Oint. (Scrip)
W/Disodium edetate, pot. chloride, isotonic boric acid.
    See: Dacriose (Smith, Miller & Patch)
W/Epinephrine.
    See: Epinal, Sol. (Alcon)
W/Epinephrine bitartrate, pilocarpine HCl, mannitol.
    See: E-Pilo Ophthalmic, Preps. (Smith, Miller & Patch)
W/Ethoxylated lanolin, methylparaben, hamamelis water, & glycerin.
    See: Mediconet, cloth wipes. (Medicone)
W/Gentamicin sulfate, disodium phosphate, monosodium, phosphate, sodium chloride.
    See: Garamycin Ophthalmic Sol., Preps. (Schering)
W/Hydroxypropyl methylcellulose.
    See: Isopto Plain & Tears (Alcon)
W/Hydroxypropyl methylcellulose, disodium edetate
    See: Goniosol (Smith, Miller & Patch)
W/Isopropyl alcohol, methyl salicylate.
    See: Cydonol Massage Lotion (Gordon)
W/Lidocaine, phenol.
    See: Unguentine, spray (Norwich)
W/Methylcellulose.
    See: Tearisol (Smith, Miller & Patch)
W/Methylcellulose, phenylephrine HCl.

See: Efricel ⅛% (Professional Pharmacal)
W/Oxyquinolin sulfate, distilled water.
See: Oxyzal Wet Dressing, Sol. (Gordon)
W/Phenylephrine, pyrilamine maleate, antipyrine.
See: Prefrin-A, Ophthalmic (Allergan)
W/Phenylephrine HCl
See: S.A.C. Nasal Spray (Towne)
W/Pilocarpine HCl, epinephrine bitartrate, mannitol.
See: E-Pilo Ophthalmic, Preps. (Smith, Miller & Patch)
W/Polymyxin B, neomycin sulfate, zinc bacitracin.
See: Biotres, Oint. (Central)
W/Polyoxyethylene ethers.
See: Ionax, Aerosol Can. (Owen)
W/Polyvinyl alcohol.
See: Contique Artificial Tears (Alcon)
W/Potassium alum.
See: Hygefem Douche, Liq., Pwd., Tab. (Blue Line)
W/Pramoxine HCl, allantoin.
See: Perifoam, Aerosol (Rowell)
W/Pramoxine HCl, hydrocortisone.
parachlorometaxylenol, acetic acid.
See: My Cort Otic #2, Ear Drops (Scrip)
Steramine Otic, Drop. (Mayrand)
W/Pramoxine HCl, hydrocortisone.
parachlorometaxylenol, acetic acid, propylene
glycol.
See: Otostan H.C. (Standex)
W/Pyrilamine maleate, pheniramine maleate,
chlorpheniramine maleate, menthol.
See: Trigelamine, Oint. (Edward J. Moore)
W/Sod. borate, sod. bicarbonate, sod. chloride.
See: Zalkon Wet Dressing, Liq. (Gordon)
W/Tripelennamine HCl, methapyrilene.
See: Didelamine, Cream (Commerce Drug)
W/Zinc oxide, urea, sulfur, salicylic acid, isopropyl
alcohol in a base containing menthol, silicon
dioxide, iron oxide and perfume.
See: Akne Drying Lotion, Bot. (Alto)
BENZ-ALL. (Xttrium) Benzalkonium Cl 12.9%. Packets
40 cc., 10 cc. 15s.
Use: Germicidal concentrate with anti-rust factor.
BENZALOIDS. (Jenkins) Benzocaine 5.0 mg., cal.
iodized 12.0 mg., eucalyptol 0.35 mg.,
methenamine 6.5 mg., menthol 0.2 mg./Loz. Bot.
1000s.
**BENZAMIDE, 4-AMINO-N-[2-(DIETHYL-AMINO)-
ETHYL]-,MONOHYDROCHLORIDE.** Procainamide
Hydrochloride, U.S.P. XXI.
**BENZAMIDE, N-(1-METHYLETHYL)-4-[(2-METHYL-
HYDRAZINO)METHYL]-, MONOHYDROCHLO-
RIDE.** Procarbazine Hydrochloride, U.S.P. XXI.
• **BENZATHINE PENICILLIN G,** U.S.P. XXI. Oral Susp.
Sterile, Tab., U.S.P. XXI. N,N′-Dibenzylethylenedia-
mine di(benzylpenicillin) Benzethacil. 3,3-Dimethyl-
7-oxo-6-(2-phenylacetamido)-4-thia-1-azabicyclo [3.
2.0] heptaine-2-carboxylic acid compound with N,N-
Dibenzylethylene-diamine (2:1). Dibencil, Penidural.
Use: Antibiotic.
See: Permapen, Disp. Syr. (Pfipharmecs)
Isoject Permapen, Aq. Susp. (Pfizer)
W/Procaine penicillin G.
See: Bicillin P.A.B., Disp. Syr. (Wyeth)

BENZATHINE PENICILLIN. B.A.N. NN′-Dibenzyle-
thylenedi(ammonium 6-phenylacetamido-penicilla-
nate). NN′-Dibenzylethylenediamine di-(benzylpenicil-
lin).
Use: Antibiotic.
See: Dibencil
Neolin
Penidural
Permapen
BENZAZOLINE HYDROCHLORIDE.
See: Tolazoline HCl
• **BENZBROMARONE.** USAN.
Use: Uricosuric.
BENZCHLORPROPAMID.
Used in Europe under:
Nydrane
Posedrine
BENZ-EASE. (Novocol) Benzocaine, oil of clove, ox-
yquinoline benzoate. Tube ¼ oz., 6s, 36s.
Use: Anesthetic antiseptic adhesive ointment.
BENZEDREX INHALER. (Menley & James)
Propylhexedrine, 250 mg., menthol 12.5 mg. &
aromatics. Single plastic tubes, 12s.
Use: Relieves nasal congestion in colds and hay
fever; ear block and pressure pain during air travel.
BENZEHIST. (Pharmex) Diphenhydramine HCl 10
mg./cc. Vial 30 cc.
Use: Antihistaminic.
**BENZENAMINIUM, 3-[[(DIMETHYLAMINO)-
CARBONYL]OXY]-N,N,N-TRIMETHYL-,** Bromide
or Methyl Sulfate.
See: Neostigmine Bromide, U.S.P. XXI. or Methyl
Sulfate, U.S.P. XXI.
**BENZENE, 1-CHLORO-2-[2,2-DICHLORO-1-(4-CHLO-
ROPHENYL)ETHYL]-.**
See: Mitotane, U.S.P. XXI.
**BENZENEACETIC ACID, α-HYDROXY, 8-METHYL-
8-AZABICYCLO[3.2.1.]-OCT-3-YL ESTER; HYDRO-
BROMIDE, ENDO-(+)-.** Homatropine Hydrobromide,
U.S.P. XXI.
**BENZENECARBOXIMIDAMIDE, 4-[2-[4-(AMINO-
IMINOMETHYL)-PHENYL]ETHENYL]-3-
HYDROXY-, BIS(2-HYDROXYETHANE-
SULFONATE)(SALT).** Hydroxystilbamidine
Isethionate, U.S.P. XXI.
**BENZENEDECANOIC ACID, IODO-t-METHYL-,
ETHYL ESTER.** Iophendylate, U.S.P. XXI.
1,3-BENZENEDIOL. Resorcinol, U.S.P. XXI.
1,4-BENZENEDIOL. Hydroquinone, U.S.P. XXI.
BENZENE HEXACHLORIDE, GAMMA.
See: Lindane, U.S.P. XXI.
**BENZENEMETHANOL, α-(1-AMINOETHYL)-2,5-
DIMETHOXY-, HCl.** Methoxamine Hydrochloride,
U.S.P. XXI.
**BENZENEMETHANOL, α-(1-AMINOETHYL)-3-
HYDROXY-[R-(R*,R*)]-2,3-DIHYDROXY-
BUTANE-DIOATE (1:1) (salt).** Metaraminol
Bitartrate.
**BENZENEMETHANOL, 3-HYDROXY-α-[(METHYL-
AMINO)METHYL]-, HYDROCHLORIDE(S)-.** Pheny-
lephrine Hydrochloride, U.S.P. XXI.

BENZENEPROPANOIC ACID, 3-AMINO-α-ETHYL-2,4,6-TRIIODO-., CALCIUM OR SODIUM SALTS. Iopanoic Acid, Calcium or Sodium, U.S.P. XXI.
BENZENETHANOL, α-[2-(DIMETHYLAMINO)-1-METHYLETHYL]-α-PHENYL-, PROPANOATE (ESTER), HCl. Propoxyphene Hydrochloride, U.S.P. XXI.
BENZESTROL 4,4'-(1,2-Diethyl-3-methyltrimethylene) diphenol.
BENZETHACIL. Dibenzylethylenediamine dipenicillin G DBED.
See: Penicillin G Benzathine, U.S.P. XXI.
BENZETHIDINE. B.A.N. Ethyl 1-(2-benzyloxyethyl)-4-phenylpiperidine-1-carboxylate.
Use: Narcotic analgesic.
• **BENZETHONIUM CHLORIDE, U.S.P. XXI.** Tincture, Topical Sol. U.S.P. XXI. Benzyldimethyl [2-[2-[p-(1,-1,3,3-tetramethylbutyl)phenoxy]ethoxy]ethyl]ammonium chloride.
Use: Surface antiseptic and antimicrobial preservative.
See: Ammorid Diaper Rinse, Oint. (Kinney)
Hyacide, Sol. (Niltig)
Hyamine 1622 (Rohm & Haas)
Phemerol Chloride, Sol. & Tr. (Parke-Davis)
Phemithyn, Liq. (Davis & Sly)
W/Benzocaine.
See: Americaine, Oint., Aerosol (Arnar-Stone)
Dermoplast, Spray (Ayerst)
W/Nonyl phenoxypolyoxyethylene ethanol.
See: Dalkon Foam (Robins)
Emko Pre-Fil, Foam (Emko)
W/Zinc oxide.
See: Ammorid, Oint. (Kinney)
BENZETHONIUM CHLORIDE. B.A.N. Benzyldimethyl-2-[2-[4-(1,1,3,3-tetramethylbutyl)-phenoxy]ethoxy]ethylammonium chloride.
Use: Antibacterial.
See: Phemeride
• **BENZETIMIDE HCl.** USAN. (1)2-(l-Benzyl-4-piperidyl)-2-phenylglutarimide monohydrochloride.
Use: Anticholinergic.
BENZHEXOL. B.A.N. 1-Cyclohexyl-1-phenyl-3-piperidinopropan-1-ol. Trihexyphenidyl (I.N.N.)
Use: Treatment of the Parkinsonian syndrome.
See: Artane
Trinol
N-BENZHYDRYL-N-METHYLPIPERAZINE HCl. Cyclizine Hydrochloride, U.S.P. XXI.
alpha-BENZHYDROL HCl. Diphenylhydroxy-carbinol.
BENZIDE. (Canright) Benzthiazide 50 mg./Tab. Bot. 100s, 1000s.
Use: Diuretic and antihypertensive.
• **BENZILONIUM BROMIDE.** USAN. 1-Ethyl-3-pyrrolidinyl benzilate ethylbromide.
Use: Anticholinergic.
BENZILONIUM BROMIDE. B.A.N. 3-Benziloyloxy-1, 1-diethylpyrrolidinium bromide.
Use: Inhibition of gastric secretion.
See: Portyn
BENZINDAMINE HCl. Benzydamine HCl.
1H-BENZ[E]INDOLIUM, 2-[7-[1,3-dihydro-1,1-dimethyl-

3-(4-sulfobutyl)-2h-benz[e]indol-2-ylidene]-1,3,5-heptatrienyl]-1,1-dimethyl-3-(4-sulfobutyl) hydroxide, inner salt, sodium salt.
See: Indocyanine Green, U.S.P. XXI.
• **BENZINDOPYRINE HYDROCHLORIDE.** USAN. 1-Benzyl-3-[2-(4-pyridyl)-ethyl] indole hydrochloride.
Pyrbenzindole
Use: Tranquilizer.
BENZIODARONE. B.A.N. 2-Ethyl-3-(4-hydroxy-3,5-diiodobenzoyl-benzofuran.
Use: Coronary vasodilator.
See: Cardivix
1,2-BENZISOTHIAZOLIN-3-ONE 1,1-DIOXIDE CALCIUM SALT.
See: Saccharin Calcium, U.S.P. XXI.
1,2-BENZISOTHIAZOLIN-3-ONE 1,1-DIOXIDE SODIUM SALT.
See: Saccharin Sodium, U.S.P. XXI.
BENZO-C. (Freeport) Benzocaine 5 mg., cetalkonium Cl. 5 mg., ascorbic acid 50 mg./Troche. Bot. 1000s, or cello-packed boxes 1000s.
Use: Relief of minor sore throat.
• **BENZOCAINE, U.S.P. XXI.** Cream, Oint., Otic Soln., Topical Aerosol, Topical Soln., U.S.P. XXI. Ethyl-p-aminobenzoate. Anesthesin, orthesin, parathesin.
Use: Local anesthetic.
W/Combinations.
See: Aerotherm, Oint. (Aeroceuticals)
Aerocaine, Oint. (Aeroceuticals)
Americaine, Oint., Aerosol (American Critical Care)
Aminophylline W/Pentobarbital, Tab. (Searle)
Anacaine, Oint. (Gordon)
Anecal, Cream (Lannett)
Aura-Aid, Liq. (Edward J. Moore)
Auralgan, Otic Drops (Ayerst)
Auralgesic, Liq. (Elder)
Auristel, Dropules (Blue Line)
Aurotis, Liq. (Research Pharmacal Lab.)
Benadex, Oint. (Fuller)
Benzo-C, Troche (Freeport)
Benzocol, Oint. (Mallard)
Benzodent, Oint. (Vicks)
Biscolan, Supp. (Lannett)
Boilaid, Oint. (Edward J. Moore)
Bonal Itch Cream, Cream (Edward J. Moore)
Bowman Drawing Paste, Oint. (Bowman)
Boil-Ease Anesthetic Drawing Salve (Commerce)
Burn Gon, Oint. (Edward J. Moore)
20-Cain Burn Relief, Bot. (Alto)
Calamatum, Preps. (Blair)
Caloxide cream W/benzocaine, (Blue Line)
Calsarbain, Tab. (Sutliff & Case)
Cēpacol, Troches (Merrell Dow)
Cetacaine, Preps. (Cetylite)
Chiggerex, Oint. (Scherer)
Chiggertox, Liq. (Scherer)
Chloraseptic Children's Lozenges, (Norwich Eaton)
CPI Hemorrhoidal, Supp. (Century)
Culminal, Cream (Culminal)

D.D.D. Cream (Campana)
Dent's Dental Poultice (C.S. Dent)
Dent's Lotion, Jel (C.S. Dent)
Dent's Toothache Gum (C.S. Dent)
Derma Medicone (Medicone)
Derma Medicone-HC (Medicone)
Dermoplast, Spray (Ayerst)
Diplan, Cap. (Reid-Provident)
Doctient, Supp. (Suppositoria)
Doctient H.C., Supp. (Suppositoria)
Dulzit, Cream (Commerce)
Ear Drops. Liq. (Sutliff & Case)
Epinephricaine, Oint. (Upjohn)
Erase, Supp. (LaCrosse)
E.R.O. Forte, Liq. (Scherer)
Extend, Tab. (Edward J. Moore)
Foille, Preps. (Carbisulphoil)
Formula 44 Cough Control Discs, Loz. (Vicks)
Fung-O-Spray (Scrip)
G.B.A. Drops (Scrip)
Hemocaine, Oint. (Mallard)
Hurricaine, Liq. or Gel (Beutlich)
Isodettes Loz. (Norcliff-Thayer)
Jiffy, Drops (Block Drug)
Kanalka, Tab. (Lannett)
Kankex, Liq. (Edward J. Moore)
Lanaurine, Drop. (Lannett)
Lanazets, Loz. (Lannett)
Listerine Cough Control Lozenges
 (Warner-Lambert)
Medicone Dressing (Medicone)
Meditrating Throat Lozenge, Loz. (Vicks)
My-Cort Drops (Scrip)
Myringacaine, Liq. (Upjohn)
Neo-Cutone, Lot. (Sutliff & Case)
Nilatus, Loz. (Bowman)
Off-Ezy Corn Remover, Liq. (Commerce)
Oracin, Loz. (Vicks)
Oradex-C, Troche (Commerce)
Ora-Jel, Gel. (Commerce)
Otolgesic, Dropules (Blue Line)
Pain-Eze, Oint. (Edward J. Moore)
Pazo, Oint. & Supp. (Bristol-Myers)
Pyrogallic Acid Oint. (Gordon)
Pytosin, Sol. (Blue Line)
Rectal Medicone (Medicone)
Rectal Medicone-HC, Supp. (Medicone)
Rectal Medicone Unguent (Medicone)
Ridupois Capsule (Elder)
Rite-Diet, Cap. (Edward J. Moore)
Robitussets, Troches (Robins)
S.A.C. Throat Lozenges (Towne)
Salicide, Oint. (Gordon)
Scrip, Preps. (Scrip)
Sepo, Loz. (Otis Clapp)
Solarcaine, Lot. (Plough)
Soretts, Loz. (Lannett)
Spec-T Sore Throat-Cough Suppressant Loz.
 (Squibb)
Spec-T Sore Throat-Decongestant Loz. (Squibb)
Sucrets Cold Decongestant Lozenge (Calgon)
Sucrets Cough Control Lozenge (Calgon)

Tanac, Liq. (Commerce)
Thorzetts Lozenges (Towne)
Trocaine Lozenges, Loz. (Vortech)
Tympagesic, Liq. (Adria)
Tyro-Loz, Loz. (Kenyon)
Tyzomint, Loz. (Blue Line)
Unguentine Aerosol (Norwich)
Vicks Cough Silencers, Loz. (Vicks)
Vicks Formula 44 Cough Control Discs, Loz.
 (Vicks)
Vicks Medi-Trating Throat Lozenges, Loz. (Vicks)
Vicks Oracin, Loz. (Vicks)

BENZOCHLOROPHENE SODIUM. The sodium salt of
ortho-benzyl-para-chlorophenol.

BENZOCOL. (Mallard)Benzocaine 5%, Tubes 1 oz.
Use: Surface anesthetic.

BENZOCTAMINE. B.A.N. N-Methyl-9,10-ethanoanthra-
cene-9(10H)-methylamine.
Use: Tranquilizer.
See: Tacitin

• **BENZOCTAMINE HYDROCHLORIDE.** USAN. N-
Methyl-9,10-ethanoanthracene-9(10H)-methylamine
HCl.
Under study.
Use: Muscle relaxant.

BENZODENT. (Vicks Prods) Benzocaine 20%,
eugenol 0.4%, hydroxyquinoline sulfate 0.1%, in an
adhesive ointment base. Tube 0.25 oz., 1 oz.
Use: Analgesic in adjustment to dentures.

BENZODEPA. USAN. Benzyl[bis(aziridinyl)-phosphinyl]
carbamate.
Use: Antineoplastic.

1,4-BENZODIAZEPINE SERIES.
See: Dalmane, Cap. (Roche)
 Librium, Prep. (Roche)
 Serax, Prep. (Wyeth)
 Tranxene, Cap. (Abbott)
 Valium, Preps. (Roche)

BENZODYNE IMPROVED. (Kay) Camphor, menthol,
thymol, propylene glycol, glycerine. Bot. ½ oz.
Use: Softening ear wax.

BENZODYNE-R. (Kay) Ear drops w/dropper. Bot. 15
ml.
Use: Ear drops.

BENZOIC ACID. (Various Mfr.) Pkg. ¼ lb., 1 lb.
Use: Fungistatic & fungicidal.
W/Boric acid, zinc oxide, zinc stearate.
See: Ting, Cream, Pow. (Pharmacraft)
W/Salicylic acid.
See: Whitfield's Oint. (Var. Mfr.)

BENZOIC ACID, 2-HYDROXY. Salicylic Acid, U.S.P.
XXI.

• **BENZOIC AND SALICYLIC ACIDS OINTMENT,**
U.S.P. XXI.
Use: Antifungal (topical).
See: Whitfield's Oint. (Var. Mfr.)

• **BENZOIN,** U.S.P. XXI. Tincture, Compound U.S.P.
XXI.
Use: Topical protectant, expectorant-.
See: Arcum—Bot. 2 oz., 4 oz., pt., gal.
Lilly—Bot. 4 fl. oz., pt.
Rals—Aerosol 12 oz.

Stanlabs—Bot. 2 oz., 4 oz., pt., Cmpnd. Bot. 1 oz., 4 oz., pt.
W/Methyl salicylate, guaiacol.
See: Methagul, Oint. (Gordon)
W/Podophyllum resin.
See: Podoben, Liq. (Maurry)
W/Polyoxyethylene dodecanol, aromatics.
See: Vicks Vaposteam, Liq. (Vicks)
BENZOL. Usually refers to benzene.
• **BENZONATATE.** U.S.P. XXI. Caps., U.S.P. XXI. ω-Meth-oxypoly-(ethyleneoxy)ethyl-p-butylaminobenzoate. 2,5,8,11,14,17,20,23,26-Nonaoxaoctacosan-28-yl p-(butylamino)benzoate. B.A.N.: 3,6,9,12,15,18,21,24,27-non-aoxaoctacosyl 4-N-butylaminobenzoate.
Use: Cough suppressant.
See: Tessalon, Perles (Du Pont)
BENZOPHENONE.
See: Pan Ultra, Lot. & Lipstick (Cummins)
W/Oxybenzone, dioxybenzone.
See: Solbar Lotion (Person & Covey)
BENZOPYRROLATE.
See: Benzopyrronium
BENZOQUINOLIMINE.
See: Emete-Con (Pfizer)
BENZOQUINONIUM CHLORIDE.
Use: Skeletal muscle relaxant (No mfr. listed)
BENZOSULFIMIDE.
See: Saccharin U.S.P. XXI.
BENZOSULPHINIDE SODIUM. Name previously used for Saccharin Sodium.
2H-1,2,4-BENZOTHIADIAZINE-7-SULFONAMIDE, 6-CHLORO-3,4-DIHYDRO-, 1,1,-DIOXIDE. Hydrochlorothiazide, U.S.P. XXI.
2-BENZOTHIAZOLESULFONAMIDE, 6-ETHOXY-. Ethoxzolamide, U.S.P. XXI.
• **BENZOXIQUINE.** USAN.
Use: Disinfectant.
BENZOYL p-AMINOSALICYLIC
See: Benzapas, Pow., Tab. (Dorsey)
BENZOYLPAS CALCIUM Benzoic acid, 4-(benzoylamino)-2-hydroxy-calcium salt (2:1), pentahydrate. Calcium 4-benzamidosalicylate (1:2) pentahydrate.
Use: Antitubercular.
See: Benzapas, Tab., Pow. (Dorsey)
• **BENZOYL PEROXIDE, HYDROUS,** U.S.P. XXI. Gel., Lot., U.S.P. XXI. Peroxide, dibenzoyl.
Use: Keratolytic.
See: Benzagel-5&10, Oint. (Dermik)
Benoxyl, Lot. (Stiefel)
Clearasil Acne Treatment, Cream (Vicks)
Clearasil Antibacterial Acne Lotion (Vicks)
Epi-Clear Antiseptic Lotion, Scrub (Squibb)
Oxy-5 Acne Pimple Medication (Norcliff Thayer)
Oxy-10 Maximum Strength acne-pimple medication (Norcliff Thayer)
Oxy Wash Antibacterial Skin Wash (Norcliff Thayer)
Panoxyl, Bar (Stiefel)
Persadox, Cream, Lot. (Ortho)
Persadox HP Cream, Lot. (Owen)

Persa-Gel, Gel (Ortho)
Topex, Lot. (Vicks)
W/Chlorhydroxyquinoline, hydrocortisone.
See: Loroxide-HC, Lot. (Dermik)
Vanoxide-HC, Lotion (Dermik)
W/Polyoxyethylene lauryl ether
See: Benzac 5&10, Gel (Owen)
Desquam-X, Gels (Westwood)
W/Sulfur.
See: Sulfoxyl Lotion (Stiefel)
N'-BENZOYLSULFANILAMIDE.
See: Sulfabenzamide
W/Sulfacetamide, sulfathiazole, urea.
See: Sultrin, Tab. Cream (Ortho)
BENZPHETAMINE HCl. N-Benzyl-N-α-dimethylphenethylamine HCl, dextro.
Use: Anorexiant.
See: Didrex, Tab. (Upjohn)
BENZPYRINIUM BROMIDE. 1-Benzyl-3-hydroxy-ypyridinium bromide dimethylcarbamate.
• **BENZQUINAMIDE.** USAN. N,N-diethyl-1,3,4,6,7,11b-hexahydro-2-hydroxy-9,10-dimethoxy-2H-benzo[a]quinolizine-3-carboxamide acetate.
Use: Antiemetic agent.
See: Emete-Con, Vial (Roerig)
Quantril (Roerig)
BENZQUINAMIDE. B.A.N. 2-Acetoxy-3-diethylcarbamoyl-1,3,4,6,7,11b-hexahydro-9,10-dimethoxy-2H-benzo[a]quinolizine.
Use: Tranquilizer.
BENZTHIANIDE. 3-Benzylthiomethyl-6-chloro-7-sulfamyl-2H-1,2,4-benzothiadiazine-1,1-di-oxide.   Urese.
• **BENZTHIAZIDE,** U.S.P. XXI. Tabs., U.S.P. XXI. 3-Benzylthiomethyl-6-chloro-7-sulfamyl-1,2,4-benzothiadiazine 1,1-dioxide. 3-((benzylthio)-methyl)-6-chloro-2H-1,2,4,benzothiadiazine-7-sulfonamide 1,1-dioxide. 6-chloro-3[(phenylmethyl) thio] methyl -2H-1,2,4, benzothiadiazine-7-sulfonamide 1,1-dioxide.
Use: Diuretic, antihypertensive.
See: Aquapres, Tab. (Coastal)
Aqua-Scrip, Tab. (Scrip)
Aquasec, Tabs. (Pasadena Research)
Aquatag, Tab. (Reid-Provident)
Diucen, Tab. (Central)
Hy-Drine, Tab. (Zemmer)
Lemazide, Tab. (Lemmon)
Marazide, Tab. (Vortech)
Proaqua, Tab. (Reid-Provident)
Urazide, Tab. (Mallard)
W/Reserpine
See: Exna-R, Tab. (Robins)
BENZTHIAZIDE. B.A.N. 3-Benzylthiomethyl-6-chloro-benzo-1,2,4-thiadiazine-7-sulfonamide 1,1-dioxide.
Use: Diuretic.
See: Fovane.
BENZTROPINE. B.A.N. 3-Benzhydryloxytropane.
Use: Treatment of the Parkinsonian syndrome.
See: Cogentin mesylate.
• **BENZTROPINE MESYLATE,** U.S.P. XXI., Inj., Tab. U.S.P. XXI., Methanesulfonate, 3α-(Diphenylmethoxy)-1αH,5αH-tropane methanesulfonate.
Use: Parasympatholytic; antiparkinsonian.

W/Sodium Chloride.
See: Cogentin, Tab., Amp. (Merck Sharp & Dohme)
BENZTROPINE METHANESULFONATE.
See: Benztropine Mesylate.
BENZYDAMINE. B.A.N. 1-Benzyl-3-(3-dimethyl-amino-propoxy)indazole.
Use: Anti-inflammatory; analgesic.
BENZYDAMINE HCl. USAN. 1-Benzyl-3-[3-(dimethylamino)-propoxyl]-1H-indazole hydro-chloride. Tantum.
Use: Analgesic, anti-inflammatory, antipyretic.
BENZYDROFLUMETHIAZIDE. 3-Benzyl-3,4-dihydro-6-(trifluoromethyl)-1,2,4-benzthiadiazine-7-sulfonami-de, 1,1-dioxide.
See: Bendroflumethiazide
• **BENZYL ALCOHOL,** N.F. XVI. Phenylcarbinol.
Use: Antiseptic, local anesthetic.
See: Topic, Gel (Ingram)
Vicks Blue Mint, Regular & Wild Cherry
Medicated Cough Drops (Vicks)
N-BENZYHYDRYL-N-METHYLPIPERAZINE HCl. Cy-clizine Hydrochloride, U.S.P. XXI.
2-((N-BENZYLANILINO)METHYL)-2-IMIDAZOLINE PHOSPHATE.
See: Antazoline phosphate, U.S.P. XXI.
• **BENZYL BENZOATE,** U.S.P. XXI. Lot., U.S.P. XXI.
Benzoic acid, phenylmethyl ester.
Use: 10 to 30% emuslion in scabies; pharm. necessity.
BENZYL BENZOATE SAPONATED. Triethanolamine 20 Gm., oleic acid 80 Gm., benzyl benzoate q.s. 1000 cc.
BENZYL CARBINOL.
See: Phenylethyl Alcohol, U.S.P. XXI.
BENZYLDIETHYL((2,6-XYLYLCARBAMOYL)METHY-L)AMMONIUM BENZOATE.
See: Denatonium Benzoate
2-[BENZYL[2-(DIMETHYLAMINO)ETHYL]AMINO]-PYRIDINE CITRATE (1:1). Tripelennamine Citrate, U.S.P. XXI.
(+)-N-BENZYL-N,α-DIMETHYLPHENETHYLAMINE HYDROCHLORIDE.
See: Benzphetamine hydrochloride
BENZYLDIMETHYL(2-PHENOXYETHYL)-AMMO-NIUM 3-HYDROXY-2-NAPHTHOATE (1:1). Be-phenium Hydroxynaphthoate, U.S.P. XXI.
p-(BENZYLOXY)PHENOL. Monobenzone, U.S.P. XXI.
BENZYLPENICILLIN-C-14. (Nuclear-Chicago) Carbon-14 labelled penicillin; prepared from phenyl-(acetic acid-1-C-14), 6-aminopenicillanic acid as the potas-sium salt. 23.4 mc/mM (62.9 mc/mg); radiochemical purity is 100%. Vacuum-sealed glass vials 50 microcuries, 0.5 millicuries.
Use: Radioisotope.
BENZYLPENICILLIN 2-DIETHYLAMINO-ETHYL ESTER HI. Neopenil, Estopen. (None listed)
BENZYL PENICILLIN G, POTASSIUM.
See: Penicillin G Potassium.
• **BENZYLPENICILLOYL POLYLYSINE CONCENTRATE,** U.S.P. XXI. Inj., U.S.P. XXI.
Use: Antibiotic.
BENZYL PENICILLIN G, SODIUM.
See: Penicillin G Sodium

BEPANTHEN.
See: Panthenol.
BEPHEDIN. Benzyl ephedrine.
BEPHENIUM BROMIDE. N-Benzyl-N, N-dimethyl-N-(2-phenoxyethyl)ammonium bromide.
• **BEPHENIUM HYDROXYNAPHTHOATE,** U.S.P. XXI. For Oral Susp., U.S.P. XXI. Benzyldimethyl (2-phenoxy-ethyl)ammonium-3-hydroxy-2-naphthoate. Ben-zenemethanaminium,N,N-dimethyl-N-(2-phenox-y-ethyl)-, salt with 3-hydroxy-2-naphthalenecarboxylic acid (1:1).
Use: Anthelmintic (hookworms).
BEPHENIUM HYDROXYNAPHTHOATE. B.A.N. Benzyldimethyl-2-phenoxyethylammonium 3-hydroxy-2-naphthoate.
Use: Treatment of ancylostomiasis and ascariasis.
See: Alcopar.
• **BEPRIDIL HYDROCHLORIDE.** USAN.
Use: Vasodilator.
BERBERINE.
W/Hydrastine, glycerin.
See: Murine, Ophth. Sol.
BERBERINE HYDROCHLORIDE.
W/Borax, sodium chloride, boric acid, camphor water, cherry laurel water, rose water, thimerosol.
See: Lauro, Eye irrigator and drops. (Otis Clapp)
BER-EX. (Dolcin) Cal. succinate 2.8 gr., acetylsalicylic acid 3.7 gr./Tab. Bot. 100s, 500s.
Use: Orally, for treatment of arthritic & rheumatic disorders.
BEROCCA. (Roche) Vit. B-1 15 mg., B-2 15 mg., B-6 5 mg., niacinamide 100 mg., Ca pantothenate 20 mg., B-12 5 mcg., folic acid 0.5 mg., C 500 mg./Tab. Bot. 100s, 500s.
Use: Vitamin B-complex and C.
BEROCCA-C. (Roche) Vit. B-1 10 mg., B-2 10 mg., niacinamide 80 mg., B-6 20 mg., panthenol 20 mg., C 100 mg. & d-Biotin 0.2 mg. benzyl alcohol 1%, sod. hydroxide/2 ml. Amp. 2 ml. Box 10s. Vial 20 ml.
Use: I.V., I.M., water-soluble vitamin therapy.
BEROCCA-C 500. (Roche) In addition to Berocca for-mula, this product contains 400 mg., Vit. C, methyl and propyl parabens 0.2%, sod. bicarb. Amp. 2 ml. Duplex Amps. 2 × 2 ml.
BEROCCA-C PLUS INJECTABLE. (Roche) Vit. B-1 3 mg., biotin 60 mcg., B-2 3.6 mg., niacinamide 40 mg., B-6 4 mg., d-pantethenol 15 mg., C 100 mg./ml. Amp.: Duplex pkg. containing 1 ml. concentrate plus 1 ml. solvent. Box 25s.; Vials: Duplex pkg. containing 20 ml. vial concentrate plus 20 ml. solvent. Box 1s.
Use: I.M. water soluble vitamin therapy.
BEROCCA PLUS TABLETS. (Roche) Vit. A 5000 I.U., E 30 I.U., C 500 mg., B-1 20 mg., B-2 20 mg., niacinamide 100 mg., B-6 25 mg., biotin 0.15 mg., pantothenic acid 25 mg., folic acid 0.8 mg., B-12 50 mcg., iron 27 mg., Cr 0.1 mg., Mg 50 mg., Mn 5 mg., Cu 3 mg., Zn 22.5 mg./Tab. Bot. 100s.
Prescription only.
Use: Multivitamin and mineral supplement for use in physiologic stress.
BEROCCA-WS. (Roche) **Solution No. 1:** Vit. B-1 3 mg., B-2 3.6 mg., biotin 60 mcg., niacinamide 40

mg., B-6 4 mg., C 100 mg., panthenol 15 mg./ml.
Solution No. 2: Vit. B-12 5 mcg., folic acid 400
mg./ml. Multiple dose vials, duplex pckg.
Use: Parenteral dietary supplement of water soluble
vitamins.

BERPLEX-C. (Alton) B & C vitamins. Bot. 100s, 1000s.
Use: Dietary supplement.

BERSOTRIN. (Kenyon) Vit. B-1 15 mg., B-2 10 mg., C
300 mg., Ca pantothenate 10 mg., niacinamide 50
mg., B-6 5 mg./Cap. Bot. 100s.
Use: Dietary supplement.

BERUBIGEN. (Upjohn) Vit. B-12. I.M.; 1000 mcg., benzyl
alcohol 15 mg., NaCl 9 mg. water q.s. to 1 ml. 10
ml. vial 5s.
Use: Hematopoietic.

BERVITE. (Alton) Multiple vitamin. Bot. 100s, 1000s.
Use: Dietary supplement.

• **BERYTHROMYCIN.** USAN. (1) 12-Deoxyery-thromy-
cin; (2) Erythromycin B.
Use: Anti-amebic, antibacterial.

BESAPRIN TABLETS. (Winthrop Products) Aspirin,
chlormezanone.
Use: Analgesic, tranquilizer, muscle relaxant.

BESEROL TABLETS. (Winthrop Products)
Acetaminophen, chlormezanone.
Use: Analgesic, tranquilizer, muscle relaxant.

BESITEX B1. (Mills) Ephedrine ethylenediamine HCl 6
mg./Tab. Bot. 100s.
Use: Appetite depression.

BESITEX B3. (Mills) Ephedrine ethylenediamine HCl 6
mg./Tab. Bot. 100s.
Use: Appetite depression.

BESTA CAPSULES. (Hauck) Vit. B-1 20 mg., B-2 15
mg., niacinamide 100 mg., calcium pantothenate 20
mg., E 50 units, magnesium sulfate 70 mg., zinc
sulfate 80 mg., B-12 4 mcg., B-6 25 mg., Vit. C 300
mg./Tab. Bot. 100s, 1000s.
Use: Vitamin supplement.

BEST C CAPS. (Hauck) Ascorbic acid 500 mg./Cap.
Timed released. Bot. 100s.

BESTRONE INJECTION. (Bluco) Estrone in aqueous
susp. 2 mg. or 5 mg./cc.

BETA-2. (Nephron) Isoetharine HCl 1%. Bot. 10 ml., 30
ml.
Use: Respiratory.

• **BETA CAROTENE,** U.S.P. XXI. Cap., U.S.P. XXI. β,
β-Carotene. All-trans-B-Carotene. (All-E)-1,1-(3,7,-
12,16-Tetramethyl-1,3,5,7,9,11,13,15,17-octadecano-
naene-1,18-diyl) bis (2,6,6-trimethylcyclohexene).

BETACETYLMETHADOL. B.A.N. β-4-Dimethylamino-
1-ethyl-2,2-diphenylpentyl acetate.
Use: Narcotic analgesic.

BETACREST. (Nutrition) Vit. B-1 15 mg., B-2 10 mg., B-6
5 mg., B-12 4 mcg., Ca pantothenate 20 mg., niacinamide 100 mg., Vit. C 600 mg., liver 125
mg./Kapule. Bot. 60s. B-1 100 mg., B-2 2 mg.,
B-6 5 mg., B-12 30 mcg., niacinamide 125 mg., panthenol 10 mg., with benzyl alcohol 1.5%/cc. Vials
30 cc., I.M. or I.V.
Use: Vitamin therapy.

BETACREST KAPULE. (Nutrition) Vit. B-1 30 mg., B-2
20 mg., B-6 10 mg., B-12 8 mcg., Cal. pantothenate
40 mg., niacinamide 200 mg., Vit. C 600 mg., liver

desicc. 250 mg./2 Caps. Bot. 60s.
Use: Therapeutic B-Complex w/Vit. C

BETADINE. (Purdue Frederick) **Povidone-iodine.**
Aerosol Spray, Bot. 3 oz.
Antiseptic Gauze Pads 12s.
Antiseptic Lubricating Gel, Pkg. ⅛ oz. Box 200s.
Disposable Medicated Douche, concentrated
packette w/cannula and 6 oz. water.
Douche, Bot. 1 oz., 8 oz., gal.
Douche Kit w/dispenser 8 oz.
Douche Packette, ½ oz. (6 per carton)
Helafoam Solution Canister 9 oz.
Mouthwash/Gargle, Bot. 6 oz.
Oint., Tube 1 oz., Jar 1 lb., 5 lb.
Oint., packette ¹⁄₃₂ oz., ⅛ oz.
Perineal Wash Conc. Kit, Bot. 8 oz. w/dispenser
Shampoo, Bot. 4 oz.
Skin Cleanser, Bot. 1 oz., 4 oz.
Skin Cleanser Foam, Canister 6 oz.
Solution, ½ oz., 4 oz., 8 oz., 16 oz., 32 oz., gal.
Solution Packette, 1 oz.
Solution Swab Aid, 100s.
Solution Swabsticks, 1s, 3s.
Surgical Scrub, Bot. 1 pt., 1 pt. w/dispenser, 1 qt.,
1 gal., packette ½ oz.
Surgi-prep Sponge-Brush 36s.
Viscous Formula Antiseptic Gauze Pads: 3″ × 9″.
Box 12s. 5″ × 9″ Box 12s.
Whirlpool Concentrate, Bot. gal.
Use: As an antiseptic for uses indicated in product
labeling.

BETA-ESTRADIOL.
See: Estradiol, U.S.P. XXI.

BETAEUCAINE HCl. Name previously used for
Eucaine HCl.

BETAGEN. (Enzyme Process) Vit. B-1 1 mg., B-2 1.2
mg., niacin 15 mg., B-6 18 mg., pantothenic acid 18
mg., choline 1.8 Gm., betaine 96 mg./6 Tab. Bot.
100s, 250s.
Use: Dietary supplement.

BETA-HCG. (Abbott) Test kit 100s.
Use: Enzyme immunoassay for detection of beta
subunit of human chorionic gonadotropin.

• **BETAHISTINE HYDROCHLORIDE.** USAN. 2-(2-Me-
thylaminoethyl) pyridine dihydrochloride.
Use: Meniere's disease. A diamine oxidase
inhibitor. Increase microcirculation.
See: Serc dihydrochloride.

BETA-HYPOPHAMINE.
See: Vasopressin

• **BETAINE HYDROCHLORIDE,** U.S.P. XXI. Acidol
HCl, lycine HCl.
W/Ferrous fumarate, docusate sodium, desic. liver,
vitamins, minerals.
See: Hemaferrin, Tab. (Western Research)
W/Pancreatin, pepsin, and ammonium chloride.
See: Zypan, Tab. (Standard Process)
W/Pepsin.
See: Normacid, Tab. (Stuart)

BETALIN S. (Lilly) Thiamine hydrochloride.
Amp.: (100 mg./ml.) 100s.
Elixir: 2.25 mg./5 ml. w/alcohol 10%. Bot. 1 pt., 1
gal.

Tab.: (25, 50 & 100 mg.) Bot. 100s.
Vial: (100 mg./ml.) 10 ml., 30 ml.
Use: I.M., I.V., orally; Vit. B-1 deficiency.
BETALIN 12 CRYSTALLINE. (Lilly) B-12 100 mcg./ml.
Vial 10 ml. B-12 1000 mcg./1 ml. Also with sod. chloride 0.25%, benzyl alcohol 2%. Vial 5 ml., 10 ml.
Use: B-12 therapy, pernicious anemia.
• **BETAXOLOL HYDROCHLORIDE.** USAN.
BETAMEPRODINE. B.A.N. β-3-Ethyl-1-methyl-4-phenyl-4-propionyloxypiperidine.
Use: Narcotic analgesic.
BETAMETHADOL. B.A.N. β-6-Dimethylamino-4,4-diphenylheptan-3-ol.
Use: Narcotic analgesic.
• **BETAMETHASONE,** U.S.P. XXI. Cream, Syrup, Tabs., U.S.P. XXI. 9-α-Fluoro-11β, 17,21-trihydroxy16 β-methylpregna-1,4-diene-3,20-dione. 9α-Fluoro16β-methylprednisolone. Acetate and sodium phosphate.
Use: Glucocorticoid.
See: Celestone, Cream, Inj., Syr., Tab. (Schering)
• **BETAMETHASONE ACETATE,** U.S.P. XXI. Pregna-1,4-diene-3,20-dione, 9-fluoro-11, 17-dihydroxy-16-methyl-21-(acetyloxy)-, (11β, 16β)-. 9-Fluoro-11β, 17,21-trihydroxy-16β-methylpregna-1,4-diene-3,20-dione 21-acetate.
BETAMETHASONE ACIBUTATE. B.A.N. 21-Acetoxy-9α-fluoro-11β-hydroxy-16β-methyl-17-(2-methylpropionyloxy)pregna-1,4-diene-3,20-dione.
Use: Corticosteroid.
• **BETAMETHASONE BENZOATE,** U.S.P. XXI. Gel, U.S.P. XXI. 9-Fluoro-11β 17,21-trihydroxy-16β-methylpregna-1,4-diene-3,20-dione 17 benzoate.
Use: Glucocorticoid.
See: Benisone. (Warner-Chilcott)
   Flurobate (Texas Pharmacal)
   Uticort, Prods. (Parke-Davis)
• **BETAMETHASONE DIPROPIONATE,** U.S.P. XXI.
Topical Aerosol, Cream, Lotion, Oint., U.S.P. XXI.
See: Diprosone Prods. (Schering) Diprolene, Oint. (Schering)
• **BETAMETHASONE SODIUM PHOSPHATE,** U.S.P. XXI. Pregna-1,4-diene-3,20-dione, 9-fluoro-11,17-dihydroxy-16-methyl-21-(phosphonoxy)-, disodium salt, (11β, 16β). 9-Fluoro-11β,17,21-trihydroxy-16β-methylpregna-1,4-diene-3,20-dione   21-(disodium phosphate).
See: Celestone Phosphate Inj. (Schering)
• **BETAMETHASONE SODIUM PHOSPHATE AND BETAMETHASONE ACETATE SUSPENSION, STERILE,** U.S.P. XXI.
See: Celestone Soluspan (Schering)
• **BETAMETHASONE VALERATE,** U.S.P. XXI.
Topical Aerosol, Cream, Lotion, Oint. U.S.P. XXI.
Pregna-1,4-diene-3,20-dione,9-fluoro-11,21-dihydroxy-16-methyl-17-[(1-oxopentyl)oxy]-,(11β,16β)-.   9-Fluoro-11β,17,21-trihydroxy-16β-methylpregna-1,4-diene-3,20-dione 17-valerate.
See: Betatrex Prods. (Savage)
• **BETAMICIN SULFATE.** USAN.
Use: Antibacterial.
BETANAPHTHOL. 2-Naphthol.

Use: Parasiticide.
BETANAPHTHOL BENZOATE. (Amend) Pow. 1 oz., ¼ lb., 1 lb. Merck-Pow. 1 oz., ¼ lb., 1 lb.
Use: Antiseptic & parasiticide.
BETAPEN-VK. (Bristol) Penicillin V potassium.
Oral Solution: 125 mg., 250 mg./5 ml. Bot. 100 ml., 200 ml. **Tab:** 250 mg./Tab. Bot. 100s, 1000s; 500 mg./Tab. Bot. 100s.
Use: Treatment of infections where penicillin is effective.
BETAPRODINE. B.A.N. β-1,3-Dimethyl-4-phenyl-4-propionyloxypiperidine.
Use: Narcotic analgesic.
BETAPRONE. (O'Neal, Jones & Feldman) Beta-propiolactone. Pkg. 100 cc. Amp. 5 cc., 12s.
Use: Sterilization of vaccines and tissue grafts.
BETA-PROPIOLACTONE.
See: Betaprone, Vial (O'Neal, Jones & Feldman)
BETA-PYRIDYL-CARBINOL. Nicotinyl alcohol. Alcohol corresponding to nicotinic acid.
See: Roniacol, Elixir & Tab. (Roche Lab.)
BETA-TEC. (Wampole) Double antibody radioimmunoassay for the qualitative detection and quantitative determination of B-hCG/hCG in serum. Kits 125s.
Use: Aid in the diagnosis of pregnancy.
BETA-TEC QUALITATIVE. (Wampole) Double antibody radio-immunoassay for the qalitative detection of B-hCG/hCG in serum. Kits 125s.
Use: Aid in the diagnosis of pregnancy.
BETATREX. (Savage) Betamethasone valerate 0.1%. Cream and Ointment. Tubes 15 Gm., 45 Gm.; Lotion Bot. 60 cc.
Use: Relief of inflammatory and provitic manifestations.
BETA-VAL CREAM. (Columbia) Betamethasone valerate 0.1% in cream base. Tube 15 Gm., 45 Gm.
Use: Anti-inflammatory.
BETA-VAL CREAM. (Lemmon) Betamethasone valerate 0.1% in cream base. Tube 15 Gm., 45 Gm.
Use: Topical anti-inflammatory, anti-pruritic.
BETA-VITE LIQUID ELIXIR. (Vortech) Vit. B-1 10 mg., B-12 25 mcg./5 cc. Bot. 4 oz., gal.
Use: Appetite stimulant.
BETA-VAL OINTMENT. (Columbia) Beta-methasone valerate 0.1% in ointment base. Tube 15 Gm., 45 Gm.
Use: Anti-inflammatory.
BETA-VITE W/IRON LIQUID. (Vortech) Vit. B-12 25 mcg., B-1 10 mg., ferric pyrophosphate 250 mg./5 cc. Bot. 4 oz., gal.
Use: Appetite stimulant.
• **BETAXOLOL HYDROCHLORIDE.** USAN.
Use: Anti-anginal, antihypertensive.
BETAZOLE HCl. XXI. 1H-Pyrazole-3-ethanamine, dihydrochloride. 3-(2-Aminoethyl)pyrazole diHCl.
Use: Diagnostic aid (gastric secretion indicator).
See: Histalog, Amp. (Lilly).
BETAZYME. (Inwood) Vit. B-1 2.5 mg., B-1 (Cocarboxylase from yeast) 2.5 mg., B-2 10 mg., niacinamide 50 mg., calcium pantothenate 25 mg., B-6 2.5 mg., menadione (2 methyl-1-4-naphthoquinone) 2 mg.,

choline HCl 10 mg., high potency yeast concentrate 200 mg., Brewer's type yeast 200 mg., yeast protein hydrolysate 1 Gm., sodium nucleate 100 mg., glutamic acid 50 mg., glycine 50 mg., cysteine HCl 25 mg., iron 50 mg., manganese 50 mg., magnesium 50 mg., zinc 5 mg./3 Tabs. Bot. 100s, 1000s.
Use: Vitamin, mineral, enzyme supplement.
• **BETHANECHOL CHLORIDE,** U.S.P. XXI. Inj., Tabs., U.S.P. XXI. (2-Hydroxypropyl) trimethylammonium Chloride Carbamate. Carbamylmethylcholine chloride.
Use: Parasympathomimetic.
See: Duvoid, Tab. (Norwich Eaton)
Myotonachol, Tab., Amp. (Glenwood)
Urecholine, Amp. & Tab. (Merck Sharp & Dohme)
Vesicholine, Tab. (Star)
• **BETHANIDINE.** USAN. 2-Benzyl-1,3-dimethylguanidine.
Use: Hypotensive.
See: Bethanid
Esbatal sulfate.
BETTER GEN M. (Image) multiple vitamin. Bot. 100s. 250s.
Use: Supplement.
• **BEVANTOLOL HYDROCHLORIDE.** USAN.
Use: Antianginal, antihypertensive, cardiac depressant.
BEVONIUM METHYLSULFATE. B.A.N. 2-Benziloyloxy-methyl-1,1-dimethylpiperidinium methylsulfate.
Use: Antispasmodic.
See: Acabel
BEXIBEE. (Vortech) Vit. B-1 100 mg., cyanocobalamin 1000 mcg., benzyl alcohol 1.5%/ml. Vial 10 ml.
Use: Vitamin B therapy.
• **BEZAFIBRATE.** USAN.
Use: Antihyperlipoproteinemic.
BEZITRAMIDE. B.A.N. 4-[4-(2-Oxo-3-propionylben-zimidazolin-1-yl)piperidino]-2,2-diphenylbutyronitrile.
Use: Narcotic analgesic.
BEZON. (Whittier) Vits. B-1 5 mg., B-2 3 mg., niacinamide 20 mg., pantothenic acid 3 mg., B-6 0.5 mg., C 50 mg., B-12 1 mcg./Cap.
Bot. 30s, 100s.
BEZON FORTE. (Whittier) Vits. B-1 25 mg., B-2 12.5 mg., niacinamide 50 mg., pantothenic acid 10 mg., B-6 5 mg., C 250 mg./Cap. Bot. 30s, 100s.
B-F-I POWDER. (Beecham Products) Bismuth-formic-iodide zinc phenolsulfonate, bismuth subgallate, amol, pot. alum, boric acid, menthol, eucalyptol, thymol & inert diluents. Can ¼ oz., 1¼ oz., 8 oz.
Use: Antiseptic first-aid powder.
B-GEN WITH C. (Image) Vitamin B and C Bot. 100s, 250s.
Use: Supplement.
B.G.O. (Calotabs) Iodoform, salicylic acid, sulfur, zinc oxide, phenol (liquefied) 1%, calamine, menthol, petrolatum, lanolin and mineral oil, undecylenic acid 1%. Jar ⅞ oz., Tube 1⅛ oz.
Use: Antiseptic, antifungal.

B-HCG. (Roche) Rapid RIA assay for Beta-human chorionic gonadotropin. 100 test kit.
• **BIALAMICOL.** F.D.A. 5,5'-Diallyl-alpha,alpha'-bis-(die-thylamino) m,m'-bitolyl-4,4'-diol.
BIALAMICOL. 6,6'-Dially-α,α'-bisdiethylaminomethyl-4,4'-dihydroxydiphenyl, dihydrochloride. Biallylamicol
Use: Antiamebic.
BIALAMICOL. B.A.N. 3,3'-Diallyl-5,5'-bisdiethyl-aminomethyl-4,4'-dihydroxybiphenyl.
Use: Treatment of amebiasis.
See: Camoform dihydrochloride
• **BIALAMICOL HCl.** USAN. 5,5'-Diallyl-α,α'-bis-(die-thylamino)-m,m'-bitolyl-4,4'-diol HCl.
Use: Antiamebic.
BIAMINE. (O'Neal, Jones & Feldman) Thiamine HCl 100 mg./ml. Vial 30 cc.
BI-AMINE. (Ulmer) n-alkyl dimethyl benzyl ammonium chloride 4.5%, n-alkyl dimethyl ethylbenzyl ammonium chloride 4.5%, tetrasodium ethylenediamine tetraacetate 2%, Na carbonate 4%. Bot. gal.
Use: Quaternary germicide, detergent, deodorant solution.
BIAPHASIC INSULIN INJECTION. A suspension of insulin crystals in a solution of insulin buffered at pH 7. Insulin Novo Rapitard.
BIAVAX-II. (Merck Sharp & Dohme) Rubella & mumps virus vaccine, live. See details under Meruvax-II and Mumpsvax. Single-dose vial w/diluent-containing disposable syringe. Box of 10 single-dose vials; Box of 10 single-dose vials w/diluent-containing disposable syringes.
BIBENZONIUM BROMIDE. B.A.N. 2-(1,2-Diphenyle-thoxy)ethyltrimethylammonium bromide.
Use: Cough suppressant.
See: Thoragol
BICALPHO IN-A-TAB. (Blue Line) Vitamin A acetate 1000 I.U., D-2 100 I.U., B-1 0.25 mg., B-2 0.33 mg., C 16.67 mg., niacinamide 3.33 mg., calcium 250 mg., iron 2.5 mg./Tab. Bot. 100s, 175s, 1000s.
BICHLORACETIC ACID. (Kahlenberg) Dichloroacetic acid full strength. Treatment kit. ½ oz. ea. 10 ml.
Use: Escharotic.
BICHOLAN. (Galen) Ox bile extract 1.5 gr., cascara ext. 5 gr., phenolphthalein 5 gr., oleoresin capsicum 0.05 gr./Tab. Bot. 100s, 1000s.
Use: Choleretic-Laxative.
BICHOLATE. (Blue Line) Desic. ox gall 2¼ gr., phenophthalein ½ gr., cascarin ½ gr./Tab. Bot. 100s, 1000s.
Use: Orally, choleretic & cholagogue.
BICILLIN. (Wyeth) Penicillin G benzathine 200,000 u./Tab. Bot. 36s.
Use: Antibiotic.
BICILLIN C-R. (Wyeth) Penicillin G benzathine 150,000 u., procaine penicillin G 150,000 u./cc. w/sod. citrate, lecithin, povidone, C.M.C., sorbitan monopalmitate, polyoxyethylene sorbitan monopalmitate, methyl- and propylparaben. Vial 10 cc. Bicillin 300,000 u., procaine penicillin G 300,000 u./1 cc. w/sod. citrate, lecithin, C.M.C. povidone, methyl- and propylparaben. Tubex cartridge. Pkg.

10s, 50s. Bicillin 600,000 u., procaine penicillin G 600,000 u./2 cc. Tubex cartridge. Pkg. 10s, 50s, and 2 cc. single dose syringe, 10s. Bicillin 1,200,000 u., procaine penicillin G 1,200,000 u./4 cc. single-dose syringe, 2,400,000 u./single-dose disp. syringe, 10s, 4 cc.
Use: Antibiotic.

BICILLIN C-R 900/300 INJECTION. (Wyeth) Penicillin G benzathine 900,000 u., penicillin G procaine 300,000 u./2 ml. Tubex. Pkg. 10s.
Use: Antibiotic.

BICILLIN LONG-ACTING. (Wyeth) Penicillin G benzathine 300,000 U./cc. w/sod. citrate, lecithin, povidone, C.M.C., sorbitan monopalmitate, polyoxyethylene sorbitan monopalmitate, methyl- and propylparaben. 300,000 U/ml. Vial 10 cc. 600,000 u./Tubex., 900,000 u./Tubex. Pkg. 10s. Tubex w/sod. citrate, lecithin, C.M.C. povidone, methyl- and propylparaben. 10s.
1,200,000 u./2 cc. Tubex 10s. Single dose disp. syringe, 10s. 2,400,000 U./4 cc. single dose disp. syringe, 10s.

BICITRA. (Willen) Sodium citrate dihydrate 500 mg., citric acid monohydrate 334 mg., 5 mEq sodium ion/5 ml. Shohl's Solution. Bot. 4 oz., 1 pt., 1 gal.
Use: Systemic alkalizer potassium free and sugar free.

BiCNU. (Bristol) Carmustine (BCNU) 100 mg., sterile diluent (absolute ethanol) 3 ml./Vial.
Use: Antineoplastic injection.

BICOZENE CREAM. (Creighton) Benzocaine 6%, resorcinol 1.66% in cream base. Tube 1 oz.
Use: External itching or irritation of vaginal and rectal areas.

BICYCLINE. (Knight) Tetracycline HCl 250 mg./Cap. Bot. 100s.
Use: Broad-spectrum antibiotic.

BICYCLO[2.2.1]HEPTANE-2-ONE, 1,7,7-TRI-METH-YL-. Camphor, U.S.P. XXI.

[BICYCLOHEXYL]-1-CARBOXYLIC ACID, 2-(DIE-THYLAMINO)-ETHYL ESTER HCl. Dicyclomine Hydrochloride, U.S.P. XXI.

BIDIMAZIUM IODIDE. B.A.N. 4-(Biphenyl-4-yl)-2-(4-dimethylaminostyryl)-3-methylthiazolium iodide.
Use: Anthelmintic.

BIDROLAR. (Forrest) Docusate sodium ⅔ gr., ox bile 1 gr./Tab. Bot. 30s, 100s.
Use: Treatment of constipation.

BIFE. (Jenkins) Thiamine HCl 1 mg., ferrous sulfate, exsic. 3 gr./Tab. Bot. 1000s.
Use: Iron deficiency anemias and B-1 avitaminosis.

BIFLURANOL. B.A.N. erythro-4,4′-(1-Ethyl-2-methyle-thylene)di-(2-fluorophenol).
Use: Benign hypertrophy of the prostate.

• **BIFONAZOLE.** USAN.
Use: Antifungal.

BIG LEAGUE RUB. (Eckerd) Bot. pt.

BIHISTOL. (Sutliff & Case) Pyrilamine maleate 25 mg./Tab. Bot. 100s, 1000s.
Use: Antihistaminic.

BI-K. (USV Labs.) Liquid potassium supplement. Bot. 16 oz.

Use: Treatment of hypokalemia.

BILAMIDE. (Norgine) Ox bile 200 mg., homatropine methylbromide 1.4 mg., phenobarbital 8 mg./Tab. Bot. 50s, 250s.
Use: Management of symptoms in hypermotility of the GI tract. Management of symptoms in hypermotility of the GI tract.

BILAX. (Drug Industries) Dehydrocholic acid 50 mg., docusate sodium 100 mg./Cap. Bot. 100s, 500s.
Use: Fecal softener.

BILE ACIDS, OXIDIZED. Note also dehydrocholic acid.
W/Atropine methyl nitrate, ox & hog bile ext., phenobarbital.
See: G.B.S., Tab. (O'Neal)
W/Bile whole (desiccated), dessicated whole pancreas, homatropine methylbromide.
See: Pancobile, Tab. (Reid-Provident)
W/Ox bile, steapsin, phenobarbital & homatropine methylbromide.
See: Oxacholin, Tab. (Philips Roxane)

BILECHOL. (Manne) Atropine sulfate 0.12 mg., nitroglycerin 0.12 mg., magnesium sulfate 0.3 Gm., ext. ox bile/Tab.
Bot. 1000s.
Use: Biliary stimulant & laxative.

BILE EXTRACT. (Various Mfr.) Pow. ¼ lb., 1 lb.
W/Cascara sagrada, dandelion root, podophyllin, tr. nux vomica.
See: Oxachol, Liq. (Philips Roxane)
W/Dehydrocholic acid, homatropine methylbromide, phenobarbital.
See: Neocholan, Tab. (Merrell Dow)
W/Pancreatic substance, dl-methionine, choline bitartrate.
See: Licoplex, Tab. (Mills)

BILE EXTRACT, OX. Purified oxgall.
Lilly—Enseal 5 gr., Bot. 100s, 500s, 1000s.
C. D. Smith—Tab. 5 gr., Bot. 1000s.
Stoddard—Tab. 3 gr., Bot. 100s, 500s, 1000s.
W/Cellulase, pepsin, glutamic acid HCl, pancreatin
See: Kanulase, Tab. (Dorsey)
W/Cellulase, pepsin, glutamic acid HCl, pancreatin, methscopolamine nitrate, & pentobarbital.
See: Kanumodic, Tab. (Dorsey)
W/Colcynth comp. ext., cascara sagrada ext., podophyllin & hyoscyamus ext.
See: Bileo-Secrin Compound Tablets (First Texas)
W/Dehydrocholic acid, homatropine methylbromide, phenobarbital.
See: Bilamide, Tab. (Norgine)
W/Dehydrocholic acid, pepsin, & homatropine methylbromide.
See: Biloric, Cap. (Arcum)
W/Desoxycholic acid, oxidized bile acids, pancreatin.
See: Bilogen, Tab. (Organon)
W/Enzyme conc., pepsin & dehydrocholic acid, belladonna ext.
See: Ro-Bile, Tab. (Rowell)
W/Oxidized bile acids, steapsin, phenobarbital & homatropine methylbromide.
See: Oxacholin, Tab. (Philips Roxane)
W/Pepsin, pancreatic enzyme concentrate.

See: Konzyme, Tab. (Brunswick)
Nu'Leven, Tab. (Lemmon)
Nu'Leven Plus, Tab. (Lemmon)
W/Phenolphthalein, cascarin.
See: Bicholate, Tab. (Blue Line)
W/Sod. salicylate, phenolphthalein, chionanthus ext.,
cascara sagrada ext., sod. glycocholate, sod.
taurocholate.
See: Glycols, Tab. (Bowman)
BILEIN. Bile salts obtained from ox bile.
BILE-LIKE PRODUCTS.
See: Zanchol, Tab. (Searle)
■ **BILE PRODUCTS.**
See: Bile Salts
Dehydrocholic Acid
Desoxycholic Acid
Ketocholanic Acid
■ **BILE SALTS.** Sod. glycocholate & taurocholate.
Note also Bile Ext., Ox, and oxidized bile acids.
Lilly—Enseal 5 gr., Bot. 100s.
See: Bilein
Bisol, Tab. (Paddock)
Chobile, Tab. (Mallinckrodt)
Ox Bile Extract
Oxidized Bile Acids
W/Belladonna & nux vomica comp. Bile salts 60 mg.,
belladonna leaf ext. 5 mg., nux vomica ext. 2 mg.,
phenolphthalein 30 mg. Sod. salicylate 15 mg.,
aloin 15 mg./Tab. Bot. 1000s.
Use: Orally, laxative w/antispasmodic.
W/Cascara, phenophthalein, aloin.
See: Amlax, Tab. (Vortech)
W/Cascara ext., phenolphthalein, oleoresin capsicum.
See: Bilocomp, Tab. (Lannett)
W/Cascara sagrada, phenolphthalein, capsicum
oleoresin & peppermint oil.
See: Torocol, Tab. (Plessner)
W/Cellulase, calcium carbonate & pancrelipase.
See: Accelerase, Cap. (Organon)
W/Cellulase, pancrelipase, cal. carbonate, belladonna
alkaloids, phenobarbital.
See: Accelerase-PB, Cap. (Organon)
W/Dehydrocholic acid & pancreatic substance.
See: Depancol, Tab. (Parke-Davis)
W/Dehydrocholic acid, pepsin, pancreatin.
See: Progestive, Tab. (NCP)
W/Iron.
See: Bilron, Pulvule (Lilly)
W/Pancreatin, pepsin, dehydrocholic acid,
desoxycholic acid.
See: Enzylax, Tab. (Kay)
Pepsatal, Tab. (Kenyon)
W/Pancrelipase, cellulase.
See: Cotazym-B, Tab. (Organon)
W/Papain, cascara sagrada ext., phenolphthalein &
capsicum oleoresin.
See: Torocol Compound, Tab. (Plessner)
W/Pepsin, homatropine, methylBr, amylase, lipase,
protease.
See: Digesplen, Tab., Elixir, Drops (Med. Prod.
Panamericana)
W/Phenophthalein, ext. chionanthus.
See: Bile Anthus Comp., Cap. (Scrip)

W/Sod. salicylate, phenolphthalein, chionanthus ext.,
bile ext., cascara sagrada ext.
See: Glycols, Tab. (Bowman)
BILE, WHOLE DESICCATED.
W/Pancreatin, mycozyme diastase, pepsin, ext. nux
vomica.
See: Enzobile, Tab. (Mallard)
BILEZYME. (Geriatric) Amylolytic enzyme 30 mg.,
proteolytic enzyme 6 mg., dehydrocholic acid 200
mg., desoxycholic acid 50 mg./Tab. Bot. 42s, 100s,
500s.
Use: Digestive aid.
BILEZYME PLUS. (Geriatric) Phenobarbital 8 mg.,
homatropine methylbromide 2.5 mg., gerilase 30
mg., geriprotase 6 mg., dehydrocholic acid 200 mg.,
desoxycholic acid 50 mg./Tab. Bot. 42s, 100s,
500s.
Use: Constipation, liver, gall bladder disease, colic.
BILI-LABSTIX. (Ames) Reagent strips. Bot. 100s.
Use: Diagnostic test for pH, protein, glucose,
ketones, bilirubin and blood in urine.
BILIVIST. (Berlex) Ipodate sodium 500 mg./Cap.
Catch cover Box 6s, 20s.
Use: Oral radiopaque medium for cholecystography
and cholangiography.
BILOCOMP TABLETS. (Lannett) Bile salts 1½ gr.,
ext. cascara ½ gr., phenolphthalein ½ gr.,
oleoresin capsicum 1/20 min./Tab. Bot. 1000s.
Use: Laxative.
BILOGEN. (Organon) Ox bile ext. 120 mg., oxidized
mixed ox bile acids 75 mg. (equiv. to 75 mg.
dehydrocholic acid), desoxycholic acid 30 mg.,
pancreatin 250 mg./Tab. Bot. 100s.
Use: Orally, choleretic & digestant.
BILOGEST. (Mills) Mixed oxidized bile acids 65 mg.,
desoxycholic acid 60 mg., ext. ox bile 40 mg.,
pepsin 100 mg., pancreatin 100 mg., inositol 40
mg., dimethionine 120 mg., betaine HCl 75 mg.,
choline bitartrate 100 mg., diazyme 10 mg./Tab.
Bot. 100s.
Use: Gallbladder disorders, indigestion, cirrhosis,
obesity.
BILOPAQUE. (Winthrop-Breon) Tyropanoate sodium
750 mg./Cap. Envelopes of 4 caps. Box 25s.
Use: Cholecystography.
BILORIC. (Arcum) Pepsin 9.0 mg., ox bile 160
mg./Cap. Bot. 100s, 1000s.
Use: Antispasmodic.
BILRON. (Lilly) Iron bile salts. Pulvule 150mg./Cap.
Bot. 100s. 300 mg./Cap Bot. 100s,
500s.
Use: Orally, physiologic laxative.
BILSTAN. (Standex) Bile salts ½ gr., cascara
sagrada pow. ext. ½ gr., phenolphthalein ½ gr.,
aloin ⅛ gr., podophyllin 1/20 gr./Tab. Bot. 100s.
BILTRICIDE. (Miles) Praziquantel 600 mg./Tab. Bot.
6s.
Use: Trematodicide.
BIMETHOXYCAINE LACTATE. Bis-[b-(o-methoxy-phe-
nyl) isopropyl] amine lactate. Isocaine Lactate.
BI-NATE. (Tunex) Testosterone enanthate 90 mg.,
estradiol valerate 4 mg./ml. in sesame oil. Vial
10 cc.

Use: Androgen & estrogen therapy.

BINAZINE. Todrazoline, B.A.N.

BINDAZAC. B.A.N. 1-Benzylindazol-3-yloxyacetic acid. Bendazac (I.N.N.)
Use: Anti-inflammatory.

BINEX-C. (Scruggs) B complex formula with C vitamins. Tab. Bot. 100s, 1000s.

• **BINIRAMYCIN.** USAN.
Use: Antibiotic.

BINTRON TABLETS. (Madland) Liver fraction 4.6 gr., ferrous sulfate 5 gr., Vit. B-1 3 mg., B-2 0.5 mg., B-6 0.15 mg., C 20.0 mg., Ca pantothenate 0.3 mg., niacinamide 10 mg./Tab. Bot. 100s, 1000s.
Use: Hematinic.

BIOCAL 250. (Miles) Calcium 250 mg./Chewable Tab. Bot. 60s.
Use: Calcium supplement.

BIOCAL 500. (Miles) Calcium 500 mg./Tab. Bot. 60s.
Use: Calcium supplement.

BIOCEPT-G. (Wampole) Radioreceptor assay for the qualitative detection of hCG in serum. Kits 30s, 150s.
Use: Aid in the diagnosis of pregnancy.

BIO-CREST. (Nutrition) Citrus bioflavonoid complex 200 mg., Vit. C 250 mg., rutin 50 mg./Tabseal. Bot. 100s.
Use: Abnormal capillary permeability, fragility, & bleeding.

BIO/DOPA. (DDR Pharm.) Levodopa 125 mg., 250 mg., 500 mg./Cap. Bot. 100s.
Use: Parkinsonism.

BIO-FLAVONOID COMPOUNDS. Vit. P.

BIO-FLAVONOID COMPOUND, CITRUS.
W/Vit. C.
See: C.V.P. Syr. & Cap. (USV Pharm.)
Mevanin-C, Cap. (Beutlich)
Mevatinic-C, Tab. (Beutlich)
Peridin-C, Tab. (Beutlich)
Pregent, Tab. (Beutlich)

BIOGASTRONE:
See: Carbenoxolone.

• **BIOLOGICAL INDICATOR FOR DRY-HEAT STERI-LIZATION, PAPER STRIP,** U.S.P. XXI.
Use: Indicator.

• **BIOLOGICAL INDICATOR FOR ETHYLENE OXIDE STERILIZATION, PAPER STRIP,** U.S.P. XXI.
Use: Indicator.

• **BIOLOGICAL INDICATOR FOR STEAM STERILIZATION,** U.S.P. XXI.
Use: Indicator.

BIO-MEDI-PEC. (Medi-Rx) Neomycin sulfate 300 mg., kaolin 6 Gm., pectin 0.13 Gm./Fl. oz. Bot. pt., gal.
Use: Diarrhea therapy.

BIONATE 50-2. (Seatrace) Testosterone cypionate 50 mg., estradiol cypionate 2 mg./ml. Vial 10 ml.

BIOPAR, FORTE. (USV Labs.) Vit. B-12 w/intrinsic factor concentrate 0.5u., Cobalamin 25 mcg./Tab. Bot. 30s.

BIORAL.
See: Carbenoxolone.

BIOS I.
See: Inositol.

BIOSONE. (Kay) Hydrocortisone acetate 50 mg.,

methylparaben, propylparaben, sodium chloride 9 mg./cc. Vial 5 cc.
Use: Hydrocortisone therapy.

BIO-SORB ABSORBABLE DUSTING POWDER. (Arbrook) Corn starch & magnesium oxide 2%. Packet 1.6 Gm., Bag 10 lb.
Use: Glove lubricant.

BIO-STIK. (Commerce) Benzocaine, allantoin, octyl dimethyl PABA, camphor, menthol in special base and core. Swivel stick 0.1 oz.
Use: Relief of chapped, dry lips.

BIOTEXIN.
See: Novobiocin.

BIOTIC-OPH. (Scrip) Bacitracin 400 u., polymyxin B sulfate 5000 u., neomycin sulfate 5 mg., in a petroleum and mineral oil base 3 mg. ophthalmic/Gm. Tube ⅛ oz.

BIOTIC-T-400. (Scrip) Penicillin G (buffered w/calcium carb.)400,000 u./Tab. Bot. 100s.

BIOTRES. (Central) Zinc bacitracin 500 u., polymyxin B sulfate 10,000 u./Gm. Tube ½ oz.
Use: Antibiotic.

BIOTRUM. (Vitarine) Vitamin and mineral replacement.
Use: Dietary supplement.

BIO-TYTRA. (Approved) Neomycin sulfate 2.5 mg., gramicidin 0.25 mg., benzocaine 10 mg./Troche. Box 10s.
Use: Antibiotic.

BIOXATPHEN. (Zemmer) Phenobarbital ⅛ gr., atropine sulfate 1/1000 gr., bismuth subnitrate 2 gr., cerium oxalate 2 gr./Tab.
Bot. 100s, 1000s.
Use: Orally, antispasmodic & sedative.

BIOZYME-C. (Armour) Collagenase 250 units/Gm. in white petrolatum base.
Use: Debriding chronic dermal ulcers and severely burned areas.

• **BIPERIDEN,** U.S.P. XXI. 1-Piperidinepropanol,α-bicyclo[2.2.1]hept-5-en-2-yl-α-phenyl-.α-5-Norbornen-2-yl-α-phenyl-1-piperidinepropanol.
Use: Anticholinergic.

BIPERIDEN. B.A.N. 1-(Bicyclo[2.2.1]hept-5-en-2-yl)-1-phenyl-3-piperidinopropan-1-ol.
Use: Treatment of the Parkinsonian syndrome.
See: Akineton (hydrochloride or lactate)

• **BIPERIDEN HYDROCHLORIDE,** U.S.P. XXI. Tabs., U.S.P. XXI. 1-Piperidinepropanol, -α-bicyclo[2.2.1]-hept-5-en-2-yl-α-phenyl-, hydrochloride. α-5-Norbornen-2-yl-α-phenyl-1-piperidinepropanol hydrochloride.

• **BIPERIDEN LACTATE INJECTION,** U.S.P. XXI. 1-Piperidinepropanol, α-bicyclo[2.2.1]hept-5-en-2-yl-α-phenol, compound with 2-hydroxypropanoic acid (1:1). α-5-Norbornen-2-yl-α-phenyl-1-piperidine-propanol lactate (salt).

BIPERIDEN HCI and LACTATE.
(Alpha-(Bicyclo[2,2,1] hept-5-en-2-yl)-alpha-phenyl-1-piperidine propanol.
See: Akineton, Amp., Tab. (Knoll)

BIPHASIC INSULIN INJECTION. B.A.N. A suspension of insulin crystals in a solution of insulin buffered at pH 7.
Use: Hypoglycemic agent.

See: Insulin Novo Rapitard
• **BIPHENAMINE HYDROCHLORIDE.** USAN. 2-Diethylaminoethyl-3-phenylsalicylate hydrochloride.
BIPHETAMINE 12½. (Pennwalt) Dextroamphetamine (as resin complex) 6.25 mg., amphetamine (as resin complex) 6.25 mg./Cap. Bot. 100s
Use: Appetite suppressant.
BIPHETAMINE 20. (Pennwalt) Dextroamphetamine (as resin complex) 10 mg., amphetamine (as resin complex) 10 mg./Cap. Bot. 100s.
Use: Appetite suppressant.
BIPOLE-S. (Spanner) Testosterone 25 mg., estrone 2 mg./cc. Vial 10 cc.
BIRONATE-B. (Coastal) Fe sulfate exs. 100 mg., aminoacetic acid (glycine) 175 mg., Vit. B-1 5 mg., B-2 1 mg., desiccated liver 150 mg., B-12 0.85 mcg., folic acid 0.25 mg., niacinamide 5 mg., Vit. C 120 mg./Cap. Bot. 100s.
Use: Dietary supplement.
■ **BIRTH CONTROL.**
See: Oral Contraceptive.
BIS (ACETOXYPHENYL) OXINDOL.
See: Oxyphenisatin.
• **BISACODYL,** U.S.P. XXI. Suppos., Tabs.: U.S.P. XXI. Phenol, 4,4′-(2-pyridinylmethylene)bis-,diacetate (ester). Di-(p-acetoxyphenyl)-2-pyridylmethane. 4-4′-(2-pyridylmethylene) diphenol diacetate (ester).
Use: Cathartic.
See: Bisacodyl Uniserts, Suppos. (Upsher-Smith)
Deficol, Tab., Supp. (Vangard)
Delco-Lax, Tab. (Delco)
Dulcolax, Tab., Supp. (Boehringer Ingelheim)
Theralax, Tab. & Supp. (Beecham Labs)
BISACODYL. B.A.N. Di-(4-acetoxyphenyl)-2-pyridylmethane.
Use: Laxative.
BISACODYL PATIENT PACK. (Roxane) Each pack contains: 1 bisacodyl 10 mg. supp., 3 bisacodyl 5 mg. Tab., 1 tube lubricant, 1 disposable glove, detailed instructions. 50s.
Use: Preparation for GI series.
• **BISACODYL TANNEX.** USAN. Water-soluble complex of bisacodyl and tannic acid.
Use: Contact laxative.
See: Clysodrast, packet (Barnes-Hind)
BISACODYL UNISERTS. (Upsher-Smith) Bisacodyl 10 mg./Suppos. Carton 12s, 50s, 500s.
Use: Laxative.
BISALATE. (Allison) Sod. salicylate 5 gr., salicylamide 2½ gr., Sod. paraminobenzoate 5 gr., ascorbic acid 50 mg., butabarbital sod. ⅛ gr./Tab. Bot. 100s, 1000s.
Use: Rheumatic disorders.
• **BISANTRENE HYDROCHLORIDE.** USAN.
Use: Antineoplastic.
BISARSONATE. (Marcen) Arsenic 3 mg., bismuth 7 mg., benzyl alcohol 5 mg., phenol 5 mg., sod. citrate 5 mg./cc. Vial 30 cc.
Use: Syphilis.
BISATIN.
See: Oxyphenisatin.

1,4-BIS(3-BROMOPROPIONYL)PIPERAZINE.
See: Pipobroman
2-[BIS(2-CHLOROETHYL)AMINO]TETRAHYDRO-2H-1,3,2-OXAZAPHOSPHORINE 2-OXIDE MONOHYDRATE. Cyclophosphamide, U.S.P. XXI.
BISCOLAN SUPPOSITORIES. (Lannett) Bismuth subgallate, benzocaine, resorcin, cod liver oil, lanolin, zinc oxide/Supp. Box 12s.
BISCOLAN HC SUPPOSITORIES. (Lannett) Same as Biscolan Supp. w/hydrocortisone acetate 10 mg./Supp. Box 12s.
N,N′-BIS(p-ETHOXYPHENYL)ACETAMIDINE MONOHYDROCHLORIDE.
See: Phenacaine Hydrochloride, U.S.P. XXI.
1,4-BIS(2-ETHYLHEXYL)SULFOSUCCINATE, CALCIUM SALT. Docusate Sodium, U.S.P. XXI.
BIS 5-[3-(DIMETHYLAMINO)PROPYL]-10,11-DIHYDRO-5H-DIBENZ[b,f] AZEPINE COMPOUND (2:1) WITH 4,4-METHYLENE-BIS-[3-HYDROXY-2-NAPHTHOIC ACID].
See: Imipramine Pamoate (Geigy)
BISHYDROXYCOUMARIN.
See: Dicumarol, U.S.P. XXI.
3,3-BIS(p-HDROXYPHENYL)PHTHALIDE. Phenolphthalein, U.S.P. XXI.
BISMOSALICATE COMPOUND. (Blue Line) Cal. carb. 48 gr., mag. trisilicate 40 gr., bismuth subcarb. 8 gr., zinc phenolsulphonate 4 gr. Bot. 14 oz., 1 gal.
Use: Orally, antacid.
BISMU-KINO. (Denver) Bismuth oxycarb. 10 gr., eucalyptus gum 6 gr., phenyl salicylate, camphor, menthol & carminative oils of nutmeg & clove in soothing, demulcent base, w/alcohol 2%/fl. oz. Bot. 4 oz., 1 pt.
Use: Stomach and intestinal upset.
BISMUTH ALUMINATEW/Magnesium trisilicate, aluminum hydroxide and magnesium carbonate coprecipitate.
See: Escot, Cap. (Reid-Provident)
BISMUTH BETANAPHTHOL. (Amend) Bi-$_2$O$_3$ 75%, betanaphthol 18%. Bot. 1 oz., ¼ lb.
Use: Intestinal astringent.
BISMUTH GLYCOLLYLARSANILATE. B.A.N. Bismuthyl N-glycoloylarsanilate. Glycobiarsol (I.N.N.)
Use: Treatment of amebiasis.
BISMUTH GLYCOLYLARSANILATE. Bismuthyl N-glycollylarsanilate.
Use: Antiamebic.
See: Glycobiarsol, N.F. XVI.
BISMUTH HYDROXIDE.
See: Milk of Bismuth, U.S.P. XXI.
BISMUTH, INSOLUBLE PRODUCTS.
See: Bismuth Oxyiodide (Mallinckrodt)
Bismuth Subgallate (Various Mfr.)
Bismuth Subsalicylate (Various Mfr.)
Bismuth Tribromophenate (N.Y. Quinine)
BISMUTH, MAGMA. Name previously used for Milk of Bismuth.
• **BISMUTH, MILK OF,** N.F. XVI.
Use: Astringent, antacid.
BISMUTH OXYCARBONATE.
See: Bismuth Subcarbonate

BISMUTH OXYIODIDE. (Mallinckrodt) Bismuth subiodide.
Use: Local antiseptic.
W/Ephedrine sulfate, ext. belladonna, zinc oxide, boric acid, bismuth subcarbonate, peruvian balsam.
See: Wyanoids, Preps. (Wyeth)
BISMUTH POTASSIUM TARTRATE. Basic bismuth pot. bismuthotartrate.
Brewer—25 mg./cc. Amp. 2 cc.
Miller—Amp. (0.016 Gm./cc.) 2 cc., Box 12s, 100s; Bot. 30 cc., 60 cc.
Raymer—(2½%) Amp. 2 cc., Box 12s, 100s.
Use: I.M.; syphilis.
BISMUTH RESORCIN COMPOUND.
W/Bismuth subgallate, balsam peru, benzocaine, Zn oxide, boric acid.
See: Bonate, Supp. (Suppositoria)
W/Bismuth subgallate, balsam peru, Zn oxide, boric acid.
See: Versal, Supp. (Suppositoria)
W/Bismuth subgallate, zinc oxide, boric acid, balsam peru.
See: Anulan, Supp. (Lannett)
BISMUTH SODIUM TARTRATE.
Use: I.M.; syphilis.
BISMUTH SUBBENZOATE. (N.Y. Quinine)
Use: Dusting powder for wounds.
BISMUTH SUBCARBONATE.
Use: Gastroenteritis, diarrhea.
W/Benzocaine, cod liver oil, lanolin, zinc oxide, resorcin, balsam Peru.
See: Doctient, Supp. (Suppositoria)
W/Benzocaine, zinc oxide, boric acid.
See: Aracain Rectal Supp. (Commerce)
W/Calcium carbonate, magnesium carbonate.
See: Dimacid, Tab. (Otis Clapp)
W/Calcium carbonate, magnesium carbonate, aminoacetic acid, dried aluminum hydroxide gel.
See: Buffertabs, Tab. (O'Neal)
W/Charcoal and ginger.
See: Harv-a-carbs, Tab. (O'Neal)
W/Hydrocortisone acetate, belladonna extract, ephedrine sulfate, zinc oxide, boric acid, balsam peru, cocoa butter.
See: Rectacort, Supp. (Century)
W/Kaolin, pectin.
See: B-K-P Mixture, Liq. (Sutliff & Case) K-C, Liq. (Century)
W/Paregoric, Kaolin (colloidal), aluminum hydroxide, Pectin.
See: Kapinal, Tab. (Jenkins)
W/Paregoric, phenyl salicylate, zinc phenolsulfonate, pepsin.
See: Bismuth, salol, zinc and paregoric. (Bowman)
W/Pectin, kaolin, opium pow.
See: KBP/O, Cap. (Cole)
W/Phenyl salicylate, zinc phenolsulfonate, pepsin.
See: Bismuth, salol, zinc compound (Bowman)
W/Phenyl salicylate, chloroform, eucalyptus gum, camphor.
See: Bismu-Kino, Liq. (Denver Chem.)

W/Ephedrine sulfate, ext. belladonna, zinc oxide, boric acid, bismuth oxyiodide, peruvian balsam.
See: Wyanoids, Preps. (Wyeth)
W/Sodium salicylate, phenolphthalein, bismuth subgallate.
See: Laxogen, Tab. (Vortech)
BISMUTH SUBGALLATE. (Various Mfr.) Dermatol.
Use: Topically for skin conditions; Orally as an antidiarrheal.
W/Balsam of peru, Zn oxide, cod liver oil.
See: Pile-Gon, Oint. (Edward J. Moore)
W/Benzocaine, resorcin, cod liver oil, lanolin, zinc oxide.
See: Biscolan, Supp. (Lannett)
W/Benzocaine, zinc oxide, boric acid, peruvian balsam.
See: Anocaine, Supp. (Mallard)
W/Bismuth oxyiodide, bismuth resorcin comp, benzocaine, boric acid.
See: Bonate, Supp. (Suppositoria)
W/Bismuth resorcin comp., balsam peru, benzocaine, Zn oxide, boric acid.
See: Bonate, Supp. (Suppositoria)
W/Bismuth resorcin compound, zinc oxide, boric acid, balsam peru.
See: Anulan, Supp. (Lannett)
Versal, Supp. (Suppositoria)
W/Cod liver oil, benzocaine, lanolin, zinc oxide, resorcin, balsam Peru, hydrocortisone.
See: Doctient HC, Supp. (Suppositoria)
W/Hydrocortisone acetate, bismuth resorcin comp., zinc oxide, peruvian balsam, benzyl benzoate.
See: Anusol-HC, Cream, Supp. (Parke-Davis)
W/Diethylaminoacet-2, 6-xylidide, zinc oxide, aluminum subacetate, & peruvian balsam.
See: Xylocaine Suppositories (Astra)
W/Kaolin, colloidal.
See: Diastop, Liq. (Elder)
W/Kaolin colloidal, calcium carbonate, magnesium trisilicate, papain, atropine sulphate.
See: Kaocasil, Tab. (Jenkins)
W/Kaolin, opium, zinc phenolsulfonate, pectin.
See: Cholactabs, Tab. (Philips Roxane)
W/Kaolin, pectin, zinc phenolsulfonate, opium pow.
See: Diastay, Tab. (Elder)
W/Kaolin, zinc phenolsulfonate, opium pow.
See: B-K-Z, Tab. (Sutliff & Case)
W/Nux vomica, activated charcoal, pepsin, berberis, diastase, pancreatin, hydrastis, papain.
See: Digestalin, Tab. (Vortech)
W/Opium pow., pectin, kaolin, and zinc phenolsulfonate.
See: Amogel, Tab. (Vortech)
Bismuth, Pectin & Paregoric (Lemmon)
B.K.Z., Tab. (Sutliff & Case)
W/Sodium salicylate, bismuth subcarbonate, phenolphthalein.
See: Laxogen, Tab. (Vortech)
W/Zinc oxide, bis. resorcin comp., peruvian bal., benzyl benzoate.
See: Anugesic, Supp., Oint. (Parke-Davis)
Anusol, Supp., Oint. (Parke-Davis)

BISMUTH SUBIODIDE.
See: Bismuth oxyiodide.
• **BISMUTH SUBNITRATE,** U.S.P. XXI.
Use: Gastroenteritis, amebic dysentery & locally for wounds.
W/Atropine sulfate, phenobarbital & cerium oxalate.
See: Bioxatphen, Tab. (Zemmer)
W/Calcium carbonate, magnesium carbonate.
See: Antacid No. 2, Tab. (Bowman)
Maygel, Tab. (Century)
W/Sodium bicarbonate, Mg carbonate.
See: Bismatesia, Can (Noyes)
W/Sod. bicarbonate, magnesium carbonate, diastase, papain.
Panacarb, Tab. (Lannett)
BISMUTH SUBSALICYLATE. Basic bismuth salicylate
Use: I.M., to treat syphilis.
W/Calcium carbonate, glycocoll
See: Pepto-Bismol, Tab. (Norwich)
W/Calcium carbonate, Ca phenolsulfonate.
See: Pan-Bis-Cal, Liq. (Noyes)
W/Pectin, salol, kaolin, zinc sulfocarbolate, aluminum hydroxide.
See: Wescola Antidiarrheal-Stomach Upset (Western Research)
W/Phenylsalicylate, zinc phenolsulfonate, methylcellulose, magnesium aluminum silicate.
See: Pepto-Bismol, Liq. (Norwich)
BISMUTH TANNATE. (Various Mfr.) Tanbismuth.
Use: Astringent & protective in G.I. disorders.
BISMUTH TRIBROMOPHENATE. (N.Y. Quinine).
Use: Intestinal antiseptic.
BISMUTH VIOLET. (Table Rock) Bismuth Violet.
Oint. 1%, Jar 1 oz., 1 lb. **Sol.** ½%, Bot. ½ oz., 6 oz., pt., gal. **Tr.** ½%, Bot. 6 oz., 1 pt., also 1% w/benzoic and salicylic acid Bot. ½ oz., 6 oz., 1 pt.
Use: Bactericidal & fungicidal.
BISMUTH, WATER-SOLUBLE PRODUCTS.
See: Bismuth Potassium Tartrate (Various Mfr.)
• **BISOBRIN LACTATE.** USAN. Meso-1,1'-tetramethlenebis[1,2,3,4-tetrahydro-6,7-dimethoxyisoquinoline]-dilactate.
Use: Fibrinolytic.
BISODOL POWDER. (Whitehall) Sodium bicarbonate 644 mg., magnesium carbonate 475 mg./Tsp. Bot. 3 oz., 5 oz.
Use: Antacid.
BISODOL TABLETS. (Whitehall) Calcium carbonate 194 mg., magnesium hydroxide 178 mg./Tab. Bot. 30s, 100s.
Use: Antacid.
BISOXATIN. B.A.N. 2,3-Dihydro-2,2-di(4-hydroxyphenyl)-1,4-benzoxazin-3-one.
Use: Laxative.
See: Laxonalin diacetate
• **BISOXATIN ACETATE.** USAN.
Use: Cathartic.
BISQUADINE. (Sterwin) Alexidine.
BIS(2,2,2-TRIFLUOROETHYL) ETHER.
See: Fluorthyl.
BIS-TROPAMIDE, Tropicamide.
See: Mydriacyl, Sol. (Alcon)

BITE & ITCH LOTION. (Weeks & Leo) Pramoxine HCl 1%, pyrilamine maleate 2%, pheniramine maleate 0.2%, chlorpheniramine maleate 0.2%. Bot. 4 oz.
Use: First aid lotion for sunburn, minor burns, cuts, insect bites & irritations.
BITHIONOL. 2,2'-Thiobis(4,6-dichlorophenol)
Use: Local anti-infective.
See: Actamer (Monsanto Chem.)
W/Allantoin salicylic acid.
See: Domerine, Shampoo (Miles Pharm)
W/Resorcinol monoacetate, sulfur.
See: Acne-Dome, Preps. (Miles Pharm)
BITHIONOL. B.A.N. 2,2'-Thiobis-(4,6-dichlorophenol).
Use: Antiseptic.
• **BITHIONOLATE SODIUM.** USAN. Disodium 2,2'-thiobis-(4,6-dichlorophenoxide).
• **BITOLTEROL MESYLATE.** USAN.
Use: Bronchodilator.
BITRATE. (Arco) Phenobarbital 15 mg., pentaerythritol tetranitrate 20 mg./Tab. Bot. 100s.
Use: Angina pectoris.
B-K-P MIXTURE. (Sutliff & Case) Kaolin 40 gr., bismuth subcarbonate 20 gr., pectin 10 gr./fl. oz. Bot. 1 pt., 1 gal.
B-K-Z TABLETS, CHEWABLE. (Sutliff and Case) Kaolin 370 mg., bismuth subgallate 60 mg., Zn phenolsulfonate 16 mg., powd. opium 5 mg./Tab. Bot. 100s, 1000s.
Use: Diarrhea.
BLACK AND WHITE BLEACHING CREAM. (Plough) Hydroquinone 2%. 0.75 oz., Tube 1.5 oz.
Use: Skin lightener.
BLACK AND WHITE OINTMENT. (Plough) Phenol 0.5%, resorcinol 5%. Tube 0.75 oz., 2.25 oz.
Use: Antiseptic-antipruritic dressing.
BLACK DRAUGHT SYRUP. (Chattem Labs.) Casanthrol 90 mg./Tablespoonful. Bot. 2 oz., 4 oz.
Use: Laxative.
BLACK DRAUGHT TABLETS. (Chattem Labs.) Casanthrol 30 mg./Tab. Bot. 30s.
Use: Laxative
BLACK WIDOW SPIDER, ANTIVENIN.
See: Antivenin, Inj. (Merck Sharp & Dohme)
BLAINE P.N.F. (Blaine) Tab. 100s.
Use: Vitamin mineral prenatal.
BLANEX. (Edwards) Chlorzoxazone 250 mg., acetaminophen 300 mg./Cap. Bot. 100s.
Use: Relief of pain and muscle spasm.
BLAUD STRUBEL. (Strubel) Ferrous sulfate 190 mg./Cap. Bot. 100s.
Use: Treatment of iron deficiency anemia.
BLASTOMYCIN.
Use: Diagnostic aid (dermal reactivity).
BLEFCON. (Madland) Sod. sulfacetamide 30% ointment, ophthalmic. Tube ⅛ oz.
BLENOXANE. (Bristol) Bleomycin sulfate 15 u./Vial. in 10s; Single units in 1s.
Use: Antineoplastic injection.
BLEOMYCIN. (B.A.N.) Antibiotic obtained from cultures of Streptomyces verticillus.
Use: Antineoplastic.

• **BLEOMYCIN SULFATE, STERILE,** U.S.P. XXI.
See: Blenoxane, Inj., (Bristol)

BLEPH-10 LIQUIFILM. (Allergan) Sulfacetamide
sodium 10%, polyvinyl alcohol 1.4%, thimerosal
0.005%, polysorbate 80, sod. thiosulfate, pot.
phosphate monobasic, edetate disodium, sod.
phosphate dibasic (anhydrous), hydrochloric acid
and purified water. Plastic dropper bot. 5 ml., 15
ml. Unit Dose 2.5 ml.
Use: Topical anti-infective agent for ophthalmic
use.

BLEPH-10 S.O.P. STERILE OPHTHALMIC OINTMENT
. (Allergan) Sulfacetamide sodium 10%, phenylmercuric acetate 0.0008% w/white petrolatum, mineral
oil, lanolin derivatives. Tube 3.5 Gm.
Use: Topical anti-infective agent for opthalmic use.

BLEPHAMIDE LIQUIFILM. (Allergan) Sulfacetamide
sodium 10%, prednisolone acetate 0.2%, polyvinyl
alcohol 1.4%. Dropper Bot. 5 ml. & 10 ml. Unit
Dose 2.5 ml.
Use: Treatment of blepharitis.

BLEPHAMIDE S.O.P. OPHTH. OINTMENT. (Allergan)
Prednisolone acetate 0.2%, sulfacetamide sodium
10%. Tube 3.5 Gm.
Use: Eye anti-infective.

BLINK-N-CLEAN. (Allergan) Polyoxyl 40 stearate and
polyethylene glycol 300 with 0.5% chlorobutanol.
Bot. 7.5 ml., 15 ml. Unit dose 1 ml.
Use: Hard contact lens cleaning and rewetting
solution.

BLINX. (Barnes-Hind) Sterile, isotonic, alkaline borate
buffer containing boric acid and sodium borate,
phenylmercuric acetate 0.004%. Bot. 1 oz. & 4 oz.
Use: Ophthalmic Irrigation and eye wash.

BLIS. (Commerce) Bot. 7 oz.
Use: Foot bath.

BLIST-AWAY CREAME. (Towne) Thymol and undecylenic acid. **Liq.** Bot. 1 & 2 oz.
Powder: Benzoic acid, salicylic acid, thymol, &
boric acid. Can. 2 oz. **Aerosol** 6 oz.

BLIS-TO-SOL. (Chattem Labs.) **Liquid:** Salicylic acid,
undecylenic acid. Bot. 1 oz., 2 oz. **Powder:**
Benzoic acid, salicylic acid. Bot. 2 oz.
Use: Topical anti-fungal.

BLOCADREN. (Merck Sharp & Dohme) Timolol
maleate 10 mg. or 20 mg./Tab. Bot. 100s.
Use: Antihypertensive, prevention of recurrent
myocardial infarction.

BLOOD, ANTICOAGULANTS.
See: Anticoagulants.

• **BLOOD CELLS, RED,** U.S.P. XXI.
Use: Blood replenisher.

BLOOD COAGULATION.
See: Hemostatics

BLOOD CULTURE PREP KIT. (Marion) Isopropyl
alcohol 70%, acetone sol. 10%, povidone iodine
sol. 10%, SEPP, Isopropyl alcohol wipe. Ctn. 20s.
Use: Skin prep kit.

BLOOD FRACTIONS.
See: Albumin (Human) Salt-Poor (Armour; Hyland)

BLOOD GLUCOSE CONCENTRATOR.
See: Glucagon (Lilly)

• **BLOOD GROUPING SERUMS,** U.S.P. XXI. Anti-Rh.

(Anti-D) 85%-Tubes, 10 tests; Vial, with pipette, 5 cc.
Anti-Rh. (Anti C plus D) 17%-Tube, 10 tests; Vial, with
pipette, 5 cc.
Use: Diagnostic aid in the determination of Rh. (D)
and Rh. (C plus D) factors in red blood cells.

• **BLOOD GROUPING SERUM, ANTI-A,** U.S.P. XXI.
Use: Diagnostic aid (in vitro, blood).

• **BLOOD GROUPING SERUM, ANTI-B,** U.S.P. XXI.
Use: Diagnostic aid (invitro, blood).

• **BLOOD GROUP SPECIFIC SUBSTANCES A, B
AND AB,** U.S.P. XXI. Blood neutralizer
(isoagglutinins, group O blood).

BLOOD PLASMA.
See: Normal Human Plasma

BLOOD PLASMA SUBSTITUTES.
See: Dextran (Cutter; Pharmachem)

BLOOD VOLUME DETERMINATION.
See: Evans Blue, dye (Harvey; City)

• **BLOOD, WHOLE HUMAN,** U.S.P. XXI.
Use: Blood replenisher.

BLU-6. (Bluco) Pyridoxine HCl 100 mg./ml. Vial 10 ml.
Use: Vitamin B-6 supplement.

BLU-12 100. (Bluco) Cyanocobalamin 100 mcg./ml. Vial
30 ml.
Use: Vitamin B-12 injectable.

BLU-12 1000. (Bluco) Cyanocobalamin 1000 mcg./ml.
Vial 30 ml.
Use: Vitamin B-12 injectable.

BLUDEX. (Burlington) Methenamine 40.8 mg.,
methylene blue 5.4 mg., phenyl salicylate 18.1 mg.,
atropine sulfate 0.03 mg. hysocyamine 0.03 mg.,
benzoic acid 4.5 mg./Tab. Bot. 100s, 1000s.
Use: Urinary antiseptic and antispasmodic.

BLUE-GRAY (HEMORRHOIDAL) SUPPOSITORIES.
(Columbia) Bismuth subiodide, bismuth
subcarbonate, zinc oxide, boric acid, benzocaine.
Boxes 12s.
Use: Treatment of hemorrhoids.

BLUTENE CHLORIDE. Tolonium chloride, Toluidine
blue O chloride, 3-amino-7-dimethylamino-2-methyl-
phenazathonium salt.

B-MAJOR. (Barth's) Vit. B-1 7 mg., B-2 14 mg., niacin
2.35 mg., B-12 7.5 mcg., B-6 0.15 mg., pantothenic
acid 0.37 mg., choline 85 mg., inositol 6 mg., biotin,
folic acid, aminobenzoic acid./Cap. Bot. 1s, 3s, 6s,
12s.

B.M.E. (Brothers) Aminophylline 32 mg., ephedrine
sulfate 8 mg., phenobarbital 8 mg.,
chlorpheniramine maleate 2 mg., alcohol 15%/5
cc. Bot. pt.

B-N. (Eric, Kirk & Gary) Bacitracin 500 units; neomycin
sulfate, 5 mg./Oint. ½ oz.
Use: Dermatitis, impetigo, burns.

B-NUTRON TABLETS. (Nion) Vit. B-1 2 mg., niacinamide 18 mg., B-6 2.2 mg., cyanocobalamine 3
mcg., folic acid 0.4 mg., iron 6 mg., pantothenic
acid 3.3 mg., plus vit. B complex as provided by
150 mg. Brewer's yeast/Tab. Bot. 100s, 500s.
Use: Dietary supplement.

B and O SUPPRETTES NO. 15A & NO. 16A.
(Webcon) Opium 30 mg. or 60 mg., belladonna ext.
15 mg./Supp. Jars 12s.
Use: Analgesic, antispasmodic, sedative.

BOBID. (Boyd) Phenylpropanolamine HCl 50 mg., chlorpheniramine maleate 8 mg., methscopolamine bromide 2.5 mg./Cap. Bot. 100s.

BODY ALL. (Lehn & Fink) With or w/or talc. Spray can 5 oz., 8 oz., 16 oz.
Use: Body deodorant.

BOILAID. (Edward J. Moore) Benzocaine, tetracaine, ichtchammol, resin cerate, thymol iodide. Jar 1 oz.
Use: Anesthetic drawing salve.

BOIL-EASE ANESTHETIC DRAWING SALVE. (Commerce) Benzocaine, ichthammol, sulfur, camphor, juniper tar. Tube. 1 oz.
Use: Boils.

BOILnSOAK. (Alcon) Sodium chloride 0.7%, thimerosal 0.001%, disodium edetate 0.1%. Plastic dropper vial ¼ oz., Bot. 12 oz., 8 oz.
Use: Soft contact lenses care.

• **BOLANDIOL DIPROPIONATE.** USAN.
Use: Anabolic.

• **BOLASTERONE.** USAN.
Use: Anabolic.

BOLAX. (Boyd) Docusate sodium 240 mg., phenolphthalein 30 mg., dihydrocholic acid ¾ gr./Cap. Bot. 100s.

BOLDENONE. B.A.N. 17β-Hydroxyandrosta-1,4-dien-3-one.
Use: Anabolic steroid.

• **BOLDENONE UNDECYLENATE.** USAN. 17β Hydroxyandrosta-1,4-dien-3-one 10 undecenoate. Parenabol. Under study.
Use: Anabolic.

• **BOLENOL.** USAN. 19-Nor-17-α-pregn-5-en-17-ol. 17 α-ethyl-5-estren-17-ol. Under study.
Use: Anabolic.

BOLINE HOUDE, BOLDINE. (C.M.C.) Bot. 40s.

• **BOLMANTALATE.** USAN. 17β-Hydroxyestr-4-en-3-one adamantane-1-carboxylate.
Use: Anabolic steroid.

BON-A-DAY, IMPROVED. (Inwood) Vit. A 5000 I.U., D 400 I.U., B-1 1.5 mg., B-2 1.7 mg., niacinamide 20 mg., C 60 mg., B-6 2 mg., folic acid 0.1 mg., pantothenic acid 10 mg., B-12 5 mcg./Tab. Bot. 100s, 250s, 365s.

BON-A-DAY w/IRON, IMPROVED. (Inwood) Same formula as above with iron 18 mg./Tab. Bot. 100s, 250s, 365s.

BONAL ITCH CREAM. (Edward J. Moore) Benzocaine, dibucaine, tetracaine in water-washable base. Tube 1 oz.
Use: Itching; anesthetic.

BON-A-LETS. (Inwood) Vit. A 10,000 I.U., D 1000 I.U., B-1 5 mg., B-2 5 mg., nicotinamide 25 mg., B-6 2 mg., B-12 2 mcg., Ca pantothenate 5 mg., C 100 mg.,/Tab. Bot. 100s, 250s.

BON-A.M. (Inwood) Vit. A 5000 I.U., D 500 I.U., C 75 mg., B-1 3 mg., B-2 3 mg., B-6 2 mg., Ca pantothenate 5 mg., B-12 1 mcg., E 3 I.U., niacinamide 20 mg., iron 10 mg./Tab. Bot. 100s.

BONATE. (Suppositoria) Bismuth subgallate, Peru balsam, benzocaine, zinc oxide/Suppository. Box 12s, 100s, 1000s.
Use: Antihemorrhoidal.

BON-BEE W/C CAPSULES. (Inwood) Vit. B-1 15 mg., B-2 10 mg., B-6 5 mg., nicotinamide 50 mg., Ca pantothenate 10 mg., C 300 mg./Cap. Bot. 100s.

BON-BEE FORTE W/C CAPSULES. (Inwood) Vit. B-1 25 mg., B-2 12.5 mg., nicotinamide 50 mg., B-6 3 mg., Ca pantothenate 10 mg., C 250 mg., B-12 2.5 mcg./Cap. Bot. 100s, 250s.

BONINE. (Roerig) Meclizine HCl 25 mg./Chewable Tab. Bot. 100s, 500s.
Use: Motion sickness.

BONINE OTC. (Pfipharmecs) Meclizine HCl 25 mg./Chewable Tab. Pkg. 8 tabs.
Use: Motion sickness.

BON-O-TIN W/C CAPSULES. (Inwood) Vit. B-1 10 mg., B-12 10 mg., B-6 5 mg., niacinamide 50 mg., Ca pantothenate 25 mg., liver des. & def. 350 mg., B-12 1 mcg., C 150 mg./Cap. Bot. 100s, 250s.

BONTRIL PDM. (Carnrick) Phendimetrazine tartrate 35 mg./3 layer Tab. Bot. 100s, 1000s.
Use: Anorexiant.

BONTRIL SLOW RELEASE CAPSULES. (Carnrick) Phendimetrazine tartrate 105 mg./Cap. Bot. 100s, 1000s.
Use: Anorexiant.

BOPEN-VK. (Boyd) Pot. phenoxymethyl penicillin 400,000 u./Tab. Bot. 100s.

BORAX. Sodium Borate, N.F. XVI.

BORGHESE LA RIVIERA SUN PRODUCTS. (Revlon) Padimate O, Oxybenzone in cream & gel bases giving sun protection factors of 2, 4, 6, and 8..
Use: Sunburn prevention.

• **BORIC ACID,** N.F. XVI. Cryst. or Pow.
Use: Mild antiseptic.
See: Borofax, Oint. (Burroughs Wellcome)
W/Combinations.
See: Saratoga Ointment (Blair)

BORIC ACID OINTMENT. (Various Mfr.) 5% to 10%.

2-BORNANONE. Camphor, U.S.P. XXI.

BORNAPRINE. B.A.N. 3-Diethylaminopropyl 2-phenyl-bicyclo[2.2.1]-heptane-2-carboxylate.
Use: Spasmolytic.
See: Sormodren

• **BORNELONE.** USAN.
Use: Ultraviolet screen.

BOROFAX OINTMENT. (Burroughs Wellcome) Boric acid 5%. Tube 1.75 oz.
Use: Topically, for chafed and chapped skin.

BOROGLYCERIN. Glycerol borate. (Emerson) Bot. pt.

BOROGLYCERIN GLYCERITE. Boric acid 31 parts & glycerin 96 parts.
Use: Externally, in dermatitis.

BOROTANNIC COMPLEX. Boric Acid 31 mg., Tannic acid 50 mg.
W/Salicylic acid, ethyl alcohol.
See: Onycho-Phytex, Liq. (Unimed)

• **BOTULISM ANTITOXIN,** U.S.P. XXI.
Use: Prophylaxis & treatment of the toxins of C. botulinum, Types A or B; passive immunizing agent.

BOURBONAL.
See: Ethyl Vanillin, N.F. XVI.

BOWMAN COLD TABS. (Bowman) Acetaminophen 324 mg., phenylpropanolamine HCl 24.3 mg., caffeine 16.2 mg./Tab. Bot. 100s, 1000s, 5000s.
Use: Decongestant, analgesic.
BOWMAN'S POISON ANTIDOTE KIT. (Bowman) Syrup ipecac 1 oz., 1 Bottle; activated charcoal liquid 2 oz., 3 Bottles.
Use: First aid for accidental poisoning.
BOWTUSSIN D.M. (Bowman) Guaifenesin 100 mg., dextromethorphan HBr. 15 mg./5 ml. w/alcohol 15%.
Use: Antitussive, expectorant.
BOWSTERAL. (Bowman) Isopropanol 60%. Bot. pt., gal.
Use: Anti-rust disinfectant for surgical instruments.
BOWTUSSIN D.M.. (Bowman) Guaifenesin 100 mg., dextromethorphan HBr 15 mg./ 5 ml. w/alcohol 15%. Bot. 3 oz., pt., gal.
Use: Coughs.
• **BOXIDINE.** USAN. 1-[2-[[4′-(Trifluoromethyl)-4-biphenylyl]-oxy]ethyl]pyrrolidine.
Use: Adrenal steroid blocker.
BOYLEX. (Approved) Diperodon, hexachlorophene, rosin cerate, ichthammol, carbolic acid, thymol, camphor, juniper tar. Tube 1 oz.
Use: Drawing salve.
B-PAP. (Wren) Acetaminophen 120 mg., sod. butabarbital 15 mg./5 cc. Bot. pt., gal.
B-PAS.
See: Calcium Benzoylpas
B-PLEX 100, INJECTABLE. (Jenkins) Vit. B-1 100 mg., B-2 2 mg., B-6 2 mg., panthenol 10 mg., niacinamide 125 mg., ethanolamide of gentisic acid 2.5%/cc. Vial 30 cc.
Use: Vitamin B therapy.
B-PLEX 100 W/B-12. (Jenkins) Vit. B-1 100 mg., B-2 2 mg., B-6 5 mg., niacinamide 125 mg., panthenol 10 mg., B-12 30 mcg., ethanolamide of gentisic acid 2.5%/cc. Vial 30 cc. 12s.
Use: Dietary supplement.
B-PLUS. (Enzyme Process) Vit. B-1 5 mg., B-2 mg., niacin 20 mg., B-6 4 mg., pantothenic acid 15 mg., B-12 15 mcg./4 Tab. Bot. 100s, 250s.
Use: Dietary supplement.
B-P-M CREAM. (Durel) Burow's solution 5%, phenol 0.5%, menthol 0.5%, camphor 1% in Duromantel cream. Jars 1 oz., lb., 6 lb.
Use: Generalized, widespread eczematous eruptions.
BPP LEMMON. (Lemmon) Powd. opium 1.2 mg. (Equiv. to 0.3 ml. paregoric), bismuth subgallate 120 mg., pectin 15 mg., kaolin 120 mg., zinc phenolsulfonate 15 mg./Tab. Bot. 1000s.
Use: Antidiarrheal.
BP-PAPAVERINE. (Burlington) Papaverine HCl 150 mg./Sus. Rel. Cap. Bot. 50s.
Use: For relief of cerebral & peripheral ischemia associated with arterial spasm & myocardial ischemia complicated by arrhythmias.
BQ COLD TABLETS. (Bristol-Myers) Acetaminophen 325 mg., phenylpropanolamine HCl 12.5 mg., chlorpheniramine maleate 2.0 mg./Tab. Card 16s; Bot. 30s, 50s.

Use: Cold treatment.
B.Q.R. (Calotabs) Fl. extract Cascara sagrada aromatic, sodium salicylate, syrup of ipecac, menthol, balsam peru in elix. lactated pepsin base w/Alcohol 8½%. Bot. 2 fl. oz.
Use: Cold discomforts.
BRACE. (Norcliff Thayer) Denture adhesive. Tube 1.4 oz., 2.4 oz.
BRADOSOL BROMIDE. (Ciba) Domiphen bromide.
BRAN FIBER WAFERS. (Nion) Unprocessed wheat bran 1000 mg., celery, parsley, watercress, lecithin. Six wafers daily with a glass of water at mealtime. Bot. 180s.
Use: Dietary supplement.
BRASIVOL FINE, MEDIUM AND ROUGH. (Stiefel) Aluminum oxide scrub particles in a surfactant cleansing base. **Fine**—Jar 5.1 oz. **Medium**—Jar 6 oz. **Rough**—Jar 6½ oz.
Use: Scrub cleanser.
BRASIVOL BASE. (Stiefel) Cleansing paste containing polyoxyethylene lauryl ether and a surfactant cleanser. Jar 4.1 oz.
Use: Degreasing skin cleanser.
BREACOL DECONGESTANT COUGH MEDICATION. (Glenbrook) Dextromethorphan HBr 10 mg., phenylpropanolamine HCl 37.5 mg., alcohol 10%, chlorpheniramine maleate 4 mg./Tsp. Bot. 3 oz., 6 oz.
Use: Antitussive, decongestant antihistaminic.
BREATHEASY. (Pascal Co.) Racemic epinephrine HCl sol. 2.2% inhaled by use of nebulizer. Bot. ¼ oz., ½ oz., 1 oz.
Use: Relief of bronchial congestion due to asthma or related respiratory allergies.
BREEZEE MIST. (Pedinol) Aluminum chlorohydroxide complex, undecylenic acid, zinc undecylenate, menthol. Bot. 4 oz.
Use: Foot powder.
BREONESIN. (Winthrop-Breon) Guaifenesin 200 mg./Cap. Bot. 100s.
Use: Expectorant.
BRETHINE. (Geigy) Terbutaline sulfate. **Tab.:** 2.5 mg./Tab. Bot. 100s, 1000s, unit dose 100s; 5 mg./Tab. Bot. 100s, 1000s, unit dose 100s; Gy-Pak 100s. **Amp.:** 1 mg./ml. Box 10s, 100s.
Use: Bronchodilator.
• **BRETYLIUM TOSYLATE.** USAN. 2-Bromobenzyl-ethyldimethylammonium toluene-p-sulfonate.
Use: Hypotensive.
See: Bretylate
  Bretylol, Inj. (American Critical Care)
  Darenthin
BRETYLOL. (American Critical Care) Bretylium tosylate 50 mg./ml. Amp. 10 ml.
Use: Anti-arrythmic, antifibrillatory agent.
BREVICON. (Syntex) Norethindrone 0.5 mg., ethinyl estradiol 0.035 mg./Tab. 21 & 28 day (7 inert tabs) Wallette.
Use: Oral contraceptive.
BREVITAL SODIUM. (Lilly) Methohexital sodium. **Powder:** (anhydrous Na carbonate) 500 mg., 50 ml.

Vial: 1s, 25s, w/diluent 50 ml. 1s, 2.5 Gm. 1s, 25s. 250 ml. 1s, 25s. 5.0 Gm. 1s, 500 ml. 1s, 25s.
Use: (1%) Ultrashort-acting intravenous anesthetic.

BREWER'S YEAST. (Various Mfr.) Pow., Tab. 6 gr., 7½ gr., 1 lb.
W/Docusate sodium.
See: Doss or Super Doss, Tab., Cap. (Ferndale)
W/Psyllium seed, plantago ovata, karaya gum.
See: Plantamucin Granules, (Elder)

BREXIN. (Savage) Pseudoephedrine HCl 60 mg., carbinoxamine maleate 4 mg., guaifenesin 100 mg./Cap. Bot. 100s, 500s.
Use: Decongestant.

BREXIN L.A. (Savage) Chlorpheniramine maleate 8 mg., pseudoephedrine HCl 120 mg./L.A. Bot. 100s.
Use: Temporary relief of cold symptoms.

BREXIN LIQUID. (Savage) Pseudoephedrine HCl 30 mg., carbinoxamine maleate 2 mg., guaifenesin 100 mg./5 ml. Bot. Pts.
Use: Temporary relief of cough, cold symptoms.

BRIABELL. (Vortech) Phenobarbital 16.2 mg., hyoscyamine sulfate 0.104 mg., atropine sulfate 0.0195 mg., scopolamine hydrobromide 0.0065 mg./Tab. Bot. 1000s.
Use: Antispasmodic & sedative.

BRICANYL INJECTION. (Merrell Dow) Terbutaline sulfate 1 mg., sod. chloride 8.9 mg., hydrochloric acid to adjust pH to 3.0-5.0/Amp. 1 ml. 10s.
Use: Bronchodilator.

BRICANYL TABLETS. (Merrell Dow) Terbutaline sulfate 2.5 or 5 mg./Tab. **2.5 mg.** Bot. 100s, 1000s, unit dose 100s; **5 mg.** Bot. 100s, 1000s, unit dose 100s.
Use: Bronchodilator.

BRIGEN-G. (Grafton) Chlordiazepoxide 5 mg., 10 mg., or 25 mg./Tab. Bot. 500s.
Uses: Emotional disturbances, sedative.

BRIJ-721. (ICI Americas) Polyoxyethylene 21 stearyl ether (100% active).
Use: Surface active agent.

BRILLIANT GREEN.
W/Benzocaine and Mag. Sulf.
See: Osmopak, Oint. (Mallinckrodt)

• **BRINOLASE.** USAN. Fibrinolytic enzyme produced by *Aspergillus oryzae.*
Use: Fibrinolytic.

BRIREL W/SUPERINONE. (Winthrop Products) Hexahydropyrazine, hexahydrate.
Use: Anthelmintic.

BRISTAMYCIN. (Bristol) Erythromycin stearate 250 mg./Tab. Bot. 100s, 500s.
Use: Antibiotic therapy, antibacterial.

BRISTOJECT. (Bristol) Prefilled disposable syringes w/needle.
Atropine Sulf: 5 mg./5 ml. or 1 mg./ml. 10s.
Ca Chloride: 10%. 10 ml. 10s.
Dexamethasone 20 mg./5 ml.
Dextrose: 50%. 50 ml. 10s.
Diphenhydramine 50 mg./5 ml.
Ephedrine 50 mg./10 ml.
Epinephrine: 1:10,000 10 ml. 10s.

Lidocaine HCl. 1%: 5 ml., 10 ml.; 2%: 5 ml.; 4%: 25 ml., 50 ml.; 20%: 5 ml., 10 ml.
Magnesium Sulf: 5 Gm./10 ml. 10s.
Metaraminol: 1%, 10 ml.
Sod. Bicarbonate: 7.5% 50 ml., 8.4% 50 ml. 10s.

BRITISH ANTI-LEWISITE. Dimercaprol
See: BAL

BROBELLA-P.B. (Brothers) Atropine sulfate 0.0195 mg., hyoscine HBr 0.0065 mg., hyoscyamine sulfate 0.1040 mg., phenobarbital ¼ gr./Tab. Bot. 100s, 1000s.

BROCILLIN. (Brothers) Pot. penicillin G 400,000 u./Tab. or 5 cc. Bot. 100s. Bot. 80 cc.

BROCON C.R. (Forest) Brompheniramine maleate 12 mg., phenylephrine HCl 15 mg., phenylpropanolamine HCl 15 mg./Tab. Bot. 100s.
Use: Antihistamine, decongestant.

• **BROCRESINE.** USAN. 0-(4-Bromo-3-hydroxybenzyl)-hydroxylamine. Alpha(amino-oxy)-6-bromo-m-cresol.
Use: Histidine decarboxylase inhibitor.
See: Contramine phosphate

BROCYCLINE. (Brothers) Tetracycline HCl 250 mg./Cap. Bot. 100s, 1000s.

BROFEZIL. B.A.N. 2-(4-p-Bromophenylthiazol-2-yl)propionic acid.
Use: Anti-inflammatory.

• **BROFOXINE.** USAN.
Use: Antipsychotic.

BROGESIC. (Brothers) Isobutylalkylbarbituric acid ¾ gr., aspirin 5 gr., caffeine ¾ gr., phenacetin 3.75 gr./Tab. Bot. 100s, 500s. W/Codeine/Tab. Bot. 100s.

BROHEMBIONE. (Brown) Vit. B-12 100 mcg., liver inj. USP (10 mcg. B-12/cc.), B-1 25 mg., B-2 2 mg., B-6 10 mg., w/benzyl alcohol 1.5% & procaine HCl 1%/cc. Vial 10 cc.
Use: Liver plus Vit. B complex.

BROLADE. (Brothers) Chlorpheniramine maleate 8 mg., phenylephrine HCl 20 mg., methscopolamine nitrate 2.5 mg./Cap. Bot. 50s, 500s.

BROMACRYLIDE. N-(acrylamidomethyl)-3-bromopropionamide.

• **BROMADOLINE MALEATE.** USAN.
Use: Analgesic.

BROMALATE. (Webber) Magnesium glutamate HBr 300 mg./Cap. Bot. 50s, 100s, 500s. Liq.: 150 mg./5 cc. Bot. 6 oz.
Use: Sedative-tranquilizer.

BROMALEATE. A mixture of 2-amino-2-methyl-1-propanol and 8-bromotheophylline.
See: Pamabrom.

BROMALIX. (Century) Bromphenramine maleate 4 mg., phnylephrine HCl 5 mg., phenylpropanolamine HCl 5 mg., alcohol 2.3%/5 ml. Bot. 4 oz., pt., gal.
Use: Antihistaminic, decongestant.

BROMAPAPP. (Zenith) Brompheniramine maleate 4 mg., phenylephrine HCl 5 mg., phenylpropanolamine HCl 5 mg./Tab. Bot. 100s.
Use: Antihistamine.

BROMAURIC ACID. Hydrogen tetrabromoaurate.

• **BROMAZEPAM.** USAN. 7-Bromo-1,3-dihydro-5-(2-Pyridyl)-2H-1,4-benzodiazepin-2-one.

Use: Minor tranquilizer.
BROMAZINE.
See: Ambodryl HCl, Elix., Kapseal (Parke-Davis)
BROMBAY ELIXIR. (Bay) Brompheniramine maleate
2 mg./5 ml. w/alcohol 3%. Bot. 4 oz., pt., gal.
Use: Antihistamine.
• **BROMCHLORENONE.** USAN. 6-Bromo-5-chloro-2-
benzoxazolinone. (Maumee) Vinyzene.
Use: Local anti-infective.
BROMEBRIC ACID. B.A.N. cis-3-Bromo-3-p-anisoyla-
crylic acid.
Use: Cytotoxic agent.
See: Cytembena sodium salt
• **BROMELAINS.** USAN. A concentrate of proteolytic
enzymes derived from pineapple plant, *Ananas
comosus.*
Use: Oral depolymerizing enzyme; anti-inflammatory,
antiedema.
See: Ananase, Tab. (Rorer)
BROMENZYME. (Barth's) Bromelain 40 mg./Tab. Bot.
100s, 250s, 500s.
Use: Digestive aid.
BROMEPAPH ELIXIR. (Columbia) Brompheniramine
maleate 4 mg., phenylephrine HCl 5 mg.,
phenylpropanolamine HCl 5 mg., alcohol 2.3%/5
cc. Bot. pt., gal.
BROMEPAPH EXTENDED-ACTION TABLETS. (Co-
lumbia) Brompheniramine maleate 12 mg.,
phenylephrine HCl 15 mg., phenylpropanolamine
HCl 15 mg./Tab. Bot. 100s, 1000s.
BROMETHOL.
See: Avertin
BROMEZYME. (Barth's) Bromelain 40 mg., papaya
fruit, papain enzyme/Tab. Bot. 100s, 250s, 500s.
BROMFED. (Muro) Brompheniramine maleate 12 mg.,
psuedoephedrine HCl 120 mg./TR Cap. Bot. 100s,
500s.
Use: Antihistamine, decongestant.
BROMFED-PD. (Muro) Brompheniramine maleate 6
mg., pseudoephedrine HCl 60 mg./TR Cap. Bot.
100s.
Use: Allergy therapy.
BROMHEXINE. B.A.N. N-(2-Amino-3,5-dibromobenzyl)-
N-cyclohexylmethylamine.
Use: Bronchial mucolytic.
See: Bisolvon hydrochloride.
• **BROMHEXINE HCl.** USAN. (1) 3,5-Dibromo-Nα-cy-
clohexyl-Nα-methyltoluene-α,2-diamine monohydro-
chloride. (2) N-cyclohexyl-N-methyl-(2-amino-3,-5-
dibromobenzyl) ammonium chloride.
Use: Expectorant; mucolytic.
See: Bisolvon (Boehringer Ingelheim)
BROMIDES.
See: Lanabrom, Elix. (Lannett)
Neurosine, Liq., Tab. (Dios)
Peacocks Bromides, Liq. (Natcon)
■ **BROMIDE SALTS.**
See: Calcium Bromide
Ferrous Bromide
Potassium Bromide
Sodium Bromide
Strontium Bromide

BROMI-LOTION. (Gordon) Aluminum hydroxychloride
20%. in emollient base. Bot. 1.5 oz., 4 oz.
Use: Antiperspirant.
• **BROMINDIONE.** USAN. 2-(4-Bromophenyl)(2)2-(p-
Bromophenyl)-1,3-indandione.
Use: Anticoagulant.
See: Circladin
BROMISOVALUM. α-Bromoisovaleryl urea. (Premo)
Pow. Bot. 1 oz., ¼ & 1 lb. Tab. (5 gr.) Bot. 100s,
1000s.
W/Acetaminophen, salicylamide.
See: Sedalgesic Tablets (Table Rock)
W/Acetylcarbromal, acetaminophen.
See: Isomel, Cap. (Reid-Provident)
Vannor, Cap. (Vortech)
W/Acetylcarbromal, scopolamine aminoxide HBr.
See: Tranquinal, Tab. (Barnes-Hind)
W/Carbromal.
See: Bro-T's, Tab. (Brothers)
BROMI-TALC. (Gordon) Pot. alum, bentonite, talc.
Shaker can 3.5 oz., 1 lb., 15 lb.
Use: Bromidrosis, hyperhidrosis.
2-BROMO-2-CHLORO-1,1,1-TRIFLUOROETHANE.
See: Halothane, U.S.P. XXI.
• **BROMOCRIPTINE.** USAN. 2-Bromo-α-ergocryptine.
Use: Prolactin inhibitor.
See: Parlodel, Tab. (Sandoz)
• **BROMOCRIPTINE MESYLATE.** USAN.
Use: Enzyme inhibitor.
• **BROMOCRIPTINE MESYLATE,** U.S.P. XXI. Tab.,
U.S.P. XXI.
Use: Prolactin inhibitor.
BROMOCYCLEN. B.A.N. 5-Bromomethyl-1,2,3,4,7,7-
hexachloronorborn-2-ene.
Use: Insecticide; acaricide, veterinary medicine.
See: Alugan.
BROMODIETHYLACETYLUREA.
See: Carbromal.
**2-(p-BROMO-α-(2-(DIMETHYLAMINO)-ETHYL BEN-
ZYL)PYRIDINE MALEATE (1:1)**
See: Brompheniramine Maleate, U.S.P. XXI.
Dexbrompheniramine Maleate, U.S.P. XXI.
BROMODIPHENHYDRAMINE. B.A.N. N-2-(4-Bromo-
benzhydryloxy)ethyldimethylamine. Bromazine
(I.N.N.)
Use: Antihistamine.
• **BROMODIPHENHYDRAMINE HCl,** U.S.P. XXI.
Caps., Elix., U.S.P. XXI. 2-[(4-Bromophenyl)phenyl-
methoxy]-N,N-dimethyl-, hydrochloride. 2-(p-Bromo-
α-phenylbenzyl)oxy)-N,N-dimethylethylamine hydro-
chloride. Ethanamine.
W/Combinations.
See: Ambenyl Prods. (Marion)
BROMOFROM. Tribromomethane.
BROMOISOVALERYL UREA. Alpha, bromoisovaleryl
urea.
See: Bromisovalum
**2-((p-BROMO-α-PHENYLBENZYL)OXY)-N,N-
DIMETHYLETHYLAMINE HYDROCHLORIDE.**
Bromodiphenhydramine hydrochloride, U.S.P. XXI.
BROMOPHIN.
See: Apomorphine HCl (Various Mfr.)

BROMO QUININE COLD TABLETS.
See: BQ Cold Tablets (Bristol-Myers)
BROMO-SELTZER. (Warner-Lambert) Acetaminophen 325 mg., sodium bicarbonate 2.78 Gm. and citric acid 2.22 Gm. which when dissolved, forms sodium citrate 2.85 Gm./Dose. Lg. (2⅝ oz.), King (4¼ oz.), Giant (9 oz.), Foil pack, single dose 48s.
Use: Effervescent antacid, analgesic.
8-BROMOTHEOPHYLLINE W/2-amino-2-methyl-1-propanol.
See: Pamabrom
BROMOTHEOPHYLLINATE AMINOISOBUTANOL.
See: Pamabrom
BROMOTHEOPHYLLINATE PYRILAMINE.
See: Pyrabrom
BROMOTHEOPHYLLINATE PYRANISAMINE.
See: Pyrabrom
• **BROMOXANIDE.** USAN.
Use: Anthelmintic.
• **BROMPERIDOL.** USAN.
Use: Antipsychotic.
BROMPHENIRAMINE. B.A.N. 3-(4-Bromophenyl)-3-(2-pyridyl)propyldimethylamine.
Use: Antihistamine.
See: Dimotane hydrogen maleate
BROMPHENIRAMINE EXPECTORANT. (Columbia) Brompheniramine maleate 2 mg., guaifenesin 100 mg., phenylephrine HCl 5 mg., phenylpropanolamine HCl 5 mg., alcohol 3.5%/5 ml. Syr. Bot. pint, gal.
Use: Expectorant.
• **BROMPHENIRAMINE MALEATE,** U.S.P. XXI. Elix., Inj., Tabs., U.S.P. XXI. 2-{p-Bromo-α-[2-di-methylamino)ethyl]-benzyl}}-pyridine maleate.
Use: Antihistaminic.
See: Dimetane, Tab., Elixir, Inj. (Robins)
  Histapp Prods. (Upsher-Smith)
  Rolabromophen, Tab. (Robinson)
  Rolabromophen Decongestant Elixir (Robinson)
  Rolabromophen Elixir (Robinson)
  Rolabromophen Expectorant (Robinson)
  Rolabromophen Forte, Tab. (Robinson)
  Rolabromophen Injection (Robinson)
  Rolabromophen Timed, Tab. (Robinson)
  Symptom 3, Liq. (Parke-Davis)
  Veltane (Lannett)
BROMPHENIRAMINE MALEATE W/COMBINATIONS.
See: Bro-Expectorant W/Codeine, Liq. (Reid-Provident)
  Bromapapp, Cap. (Zenith)
  Bromepaph, Preps. (Columbia)
  Brompheniramine Expect. Syr. (Columbia)
  Bro-Tane, Liq. (Scrip)
  Bro-Tapp, Liq. (Scrip)
  Cortane, Preps. (Standex)
  Cortapp, Elix. (Standex)
  Dimetane Decongestant, Tab., Elix. (Robins)
  Dimetane Expectorant, Liq. (Robins)
  Dimetane Expectorant-DC, Liq. (Robins)
  Dimetapp Extentabs, Elix. (Robins)
  Eldatapp, Tab., Liq. (Elder)

BROMTAPP. (Blue Cross) Brompheniramine maleate 4 mg., phenylephrine HCl 5 mg., phenylpropanolamine HCl 5 mg./5 ml. Bot. 16 oz., gal.
Use: Antihistaminic, decongestant.
BRONCAJEN. (Jenkins) Pyrilamine maleate 10 mg., phenylephrine HCl 2 mg., potassium guaiacol sulfonate 2 gr., ammonium chloride 2 gr., ipecac ⅛ gr./Tab. Bot. 1000s.
BRONCHIAL SYRUP. (Eckerd) Potassium guaiacolsulfonate 200 mg., alcohol 5%./5 cc. **DM:** Potassium guaiacol sulfonate 200 mg., dextro-methorphan HBr 15 mg./5 cc. Bot. pt. Bot. 8 oz.
BRONCHIAL SYRUP DM. (Eckerd) Guaifenesin 150 mg., dextromethorphan H Br 15 mg./Dose. Bot. 4 oz., 8 oz.
Use: Expectorant, cough syrup.
BRONCHOHIST. (Sutliff & Case) Guaifenesin 250 mg., phenylephrine HCl 25 mg., chlorpheniramine maleate 6 mg., Sod. citrate 280 mg./Fl. Oz. Bot. 1 pt., 1 gal.
Use: Orally, non-narcotic antihistamine expectorant.
BRONCHOLATE SYRUP. (Bock) Ephedrine HC1 6.25 mg., potassium quaiacolsulfonate 100 mg./15 cc.
Use: Bronchodilator.
BRONCHOVENT. (Mills) Aminophylline 90 mg., guaifenesin 50 mg., amobarbital 16 mg./coated Tab. Bot. 100s.
Use: Bronchodilator, expectorant, sedative.
BRONCOL. (Pasadena Research) Guaiacol 0.1 Gm., iodoform 0.02 Gm. camphor 0.05 Gm., eucalyptol 0.08 Gm., benzyl alcohol 2%/ 2 cc. Vial 30 cc.
Use: Liquefacient expectorant for intramuscular injection.
BRONDECON. (Parke-Davis) **Tab.:** Oxtriphylline 200 mg., guaifenesin 100 mg./Tab. Bot. 100s. **Elix.** Oxtriphylline 100 mg., guaifenesin 50 mg./5 ml., w/alcohol 20%. Bot. 8 oz., 16 oz.
Use: Expectorant-bronchodilator.
BRONICOF. (Jenkins) Ethylmorphine HCl 2.5 mg., syrup hydriodic acid 50%, pot. citrate 438 mg., sod. benzoate 10 mg., aromatics/5 cc. Bot. 3 oz., 4 oz., gal.
Use: Cough sedative and expectorant.
BRONITIN. (Whitehall) Theophylline hydrous 130 mg., guaifenesin 100 mg., ephedrine HCl 24.3 mg., pyrilamine maleate 16.6 mg./Tab. Bot. 18s, 50s.
Use: Bronchodilator.
BRONKAID MIST. (Winthrop Products) Epinephrine 0.5%. Each spray releases 0.25 mg. epinephrine. Bot. ½ oz., ¾ oz.
Use: Treatment of bronchial asthma.
BRONKAID MIST SUSPENSION. (Winthrop Products) Epinephrine bitartrate 0.7%. Each spray releases 0.3 mg. epinephrine bitartrate equiv. to 0.16 mg. epinephrine base. Bot. 10cc.
Use: Treatment of bronchial asthma.
BRONKAID TABLETS. (Winthrop Products) Ephedrine sulfate 24 mg., guaifenesin 100 mg., theophylline 100 mg./Tab. Box 24s, 60s.
Use: Bronchial congestion and bronchial asthma.

BRONKASMA TABLETS. (Winthrop Products) Theophylline anhydrous, ephedrine sulphate, thenyldiamine.
Use: Antiasthmatic.

BRONKEPHRINE. (Winthrop-Breon) Ethylnorepinephrine HCl 2 mg./ml. in a sterile isotonic sol. sod. chloride 0.7% w/sod. acetone bisulfite 0.2% and sod. hydroxide or HCl to adjust pH to 2.9-4.5. Amp., 1 ml., 5s, 25s.
Use: S.C., I.M., bronchodilator in bronchial asthma.

BRONKODYL. (Winthrop-Breon) Theophylline 100 mg., 200 mg./Cap. Bot. 100s. Elix. 80 mg./15 ml. Bot. Pints.
Use: Bronchodilator.

BRONKODYL S-R. (Winthrop-Breon) Theophylline 300 mg./Cap. Sust. Release. Bot. 100s.
Use: Bronchodilator.

BRONKOLATE "G". (Parmed) Dyphylline 200 mg., guaifenesin 200 mg./Tab. Bot. 100s, 1000s.
Use: Bronkodilator, expectorant.

BRONKOLIXIR. (Winthrop-Breon) Guaifenesin 50 mg., ephedrine sulfate 12 mg., theophylline 15 mg., phenobarbital 4 mg./5 cc. Bot. pt.
Use: Bronchodilater.

BRONKOMETER. (Winthrop-Breon) Isoetharine mesylate 0.61% w/ saccharin, menthol and alcohol 30%. Metered dose in fluoro hydrocarbon propellant. Bot. w/nebulizer 10 ml., 20 ml. Refill 10 ml. 20 ml.
Use: Bronchodilator.

BRONKOSOL. (Winthrop-Breon) Isoetharine HCl 1% in aqueous glycerin sol. for oral inhalation. Bot. 10 ml., 30 ml.
Use: Bronchodilator.

BRONKOSOL UNIJET. (Winthrop-Breon) Isoetharine HCl inhalation 0.25% in sterile aqueous sol. for oral inhalation w/sodium Cl., citric acid, sodium hydroxide, acetone sodium bisulfite. Unijet 2 ml. Box 10s.
Use: Bronchodilator.

BRONKOTABS. (Winthrop-Breon) Ephedrine sulf. 24 mg., theophylline 100 mg., guaifenesin 100 mg., phenobarb. 8 mg./Tab. Bot. 100s, 1000s.
Use: Bronchodilator.

BRONKOTUSS. (Hyrex.) Chlorpheniramine maleate 4 mg., guaifenesin 100 mg., ephedrine sulfate 8.216 mg., hydriodic acid syrup 1.67 mg./5 ml. W/alcohol 5% Bot. 16 oz., 128 oz.
Use: Expectorant.

BRONOPOL. B.A.N. 2-Bromo-2-nitropropane-1,3-diol.
Use: Antiseptic; preservative.

BRON-SED. (Southern Pharm.) Ephedrine HCl 20 mg., pyrilamine maleate 12.5 mg., pot. iodide 15 mg., fl. ext. Ipecac 0.25 min., phenobarbital 1/8 gr./5 cc. Elixir. Bot. pt.
Use: Bronchodilator.

• **BROPERAMOLE.** USAN.
Use: Anti-inflammatory.

BROSERPINE. (Brothers) Reserpine 0.25 mg./Tab. Bot. 250s, 1000s.

BRO-T'S. (Brothers) Bromisovalum 0.12 Gm., carbromal 0.2 Gm./Tab. Bot. 100s, 1000s.

Use: Sedative, tranquilizer.

BROTANE EXPECTORANT. (Blue Cross) Guaifenesin 100 mg., brompheniramine maleate 2 mg., phenylephrine HCl 5 mg., phenylpropanolamine HCl 5 mg./5 ml. w/alcohol 3.5% Bot. 16 oz.
Use: Expectorant, antihistaminic, decongestant.

BRO-TANE EXPECTORANT. (Scrip) Brompheniramine maleate 2 mg., guaifenesin 100 mg., phenylephrine HCl 5 mg., phenylpropanolamine HCl 5 mg./5 ml. Bot. 4 oz.

BRO-TAPP ELIXIR. (Scrip) Brompheniramine maleate 4 mg., phenylephrine HCl 5 mg., phenylpropanolamine 5 mg./5 ml. Bot. 4 oz.

BROTIANIDE. B.A.N. 2-Bromo-4-chloro-6-(4-bromophenylthiocarbamoyl)phenyl acetate.
Use: Anthelmintic, veterinary medicine.

• **BROTIZOLAM.** USAN.
Use: Hypnotic.

BRO-TUSS. (Brothers) Dextromethorphan HBr 15 mg., chlorpheniramine maleate 2 mg., phenylephrine HCl 5 mg., ammonium Cl 100 mg., sod. citrate 150 mg., Vit. C 30 mg./10 cc. Bot. 4 oz., pt., gal.

BRO-TUSS A.C. (Brothers) Acetaminophen 120 mg., codeine phosphate 10 mg., phenylephrine HCl 5 mg., chlorpheniramine maleate 2 mg., menthol 1 mg., alcohol 10%/5 cc. Bot. pt., gal.

BRUCELLA VACCINE. Undulant fever vaccine.
Use: I.M., S.C., undulant fever.

BRYREL SYRUP. (Winthrop Products) Piperazine citrate anhydrous 110 mg./ml. Bot. 1 oz.
Use: Anthelmintic.

B-SCORBIC. (Pharmics) Vit. C 400 mg., B-1 25 mg., B-2 10 mg., B-12 2 mcg., calcium pantothenate 10 mg., nicotinamide 50 mg., hesperidin 200 mg./Tab. Bot. 100s, 1000s.
Use: Vitamin supplement.

BSS PLUS. (Alcon) Balanced salt solution with bicarbonate dextrose, glutathione. Two part solution: Part I contains 480 ml., Part II (20 ml. Vial) mixed within 6 hrs. of surgery.
Use: Intraocular irrigating solution

BSS SOLUTION. (Alcon) Balanced salt solution of sodium, potassium and calcium chloride, magnesium chloride hexahydrate, sodium acetate, sodium citrate dihydrate. Bot. 15 ml., 250 ml., 500 ml.
Use: Eye irrigating solution.

B-TRIM. (Amlab) Pectin cellulose 45 gr., choline bitartrate 450 mg., lecithin 45 mg., dextrose 450 mg., niacinamide 90 mg., Vit. A 1500 I.U., D 150 I.U., E 1 I.U., B-1 1 mg., B-2 2 mg., C 30 mg., B-6 0.05 mg., B-12 0.5 mcg., Ca pantothenate 1 mg., Fe 6 mg., iodine 0.05 mg., Ca phosphate 225 mg./Cap. Caps. 24s, 90s.
Use: Appetite control.

• **BUCAINIDE MALEATE.** USAN.
Use: Cardiac depressant.

BUCETIN. B.A.N. N-3-Hydroxybutyryl-p-phenetidine.
Use: Analgesic.

BUCHU.
See: Barosmin
BUCINDOLOL HYDROCHLORIDE. (Mead Johnson) (USAN)
Use: Investigative: antihypertensive.
BUCLADIN-S. (Stuart) Buclizine HCl 50 mg., Softab. Tab. Bot. 100s.
Use: Prevention and treatment of nausea, vomiting and dizziness associated with motion sickness.
BUCLIZINE. B.A.N. 1-(4-t-Butylbenzyl)-4-(4-chlorobenz-hydryl)piperazine.
Longifene and Vibazine dihydrochloride.
Use: Antiemetic.
• **BUCLIZINE HYDROCHLORIDE.** USAN. 1-(p-tert Butylbenzyl)-4-(p-chloro-alpha-phenylbenzyl) pipera-zine dihydrochloride.
See: Bucladin-S, Tab. (Stuart)
BUCLOSAMIDE. B.A.N. N-Butyl-4-chlorosalicyl-amide.
Use: Antimycotic.
• **BUCRYLATE.** USAN.
Use: Surgical aid.
• **BUDESONIDE.** USAN.
Use: Anti-inflammatory.
BUF ACNE CLEANSING BAR. (3M Products)
Salicylic acid 1%, sulfur 1%, in detergent cleansing bar, 3½ oz.
Use: Acne treatment.
BUF BODY SCRUB. (3M Products) Round cleansing sponge on plastic handles.
Use: Cleansing hard to reach parts of the body.
BUFFASAL. (Dover) Aspirin 325 mg./Tab. buffered w/Mg oxide. Unit dose boxes 500s.
Use: Buffered analgesic, antipyretic, anti-inflamma-tory.
BUFFASAL MAX. (Dover) Aspirin 500 mg./Tab. buffered w/Mg. oxide. Unit dose boxes 500s.
Use: Extra strength buffered analgesic, antipyretic, anti-inflammatory.
BUF FOOT CARE KIT. (3M Products) Cleansing system for the feet.
Use: Cleansing and moisturizing feet.
BUF FOOT CARE LOTION. (3M Products)
Moisturizing lotion for feet.
Use: Foot moisturizer.
BUF FOOT CARE SOAP. (3M Products) Bar 3.5 oz.
Use: Foot cleanser.
• **BUFILCON A.** USAN.
Use: Contact lens material.
BUF KIT FOR ACNE. (3M Products) Cleansing sponge, cleansing bar 3.5 oz. w/booklet, holding tray.
Use: Cleansing system for acne.
BUF LOTION. (3M Products) Moisturizing lotion.
Use: Moisturizer.
BUF-OXAL. (3M Products) Benzoyl peroxide 5% or 10%. Tube 2 oz.
Use: Topical treatment of acne, pimples, blemishes.
BUF-PED NON MEDICATED CLEANSING SPONGE.
(3M Products) Abrasive cleansing sponge.
Use: Cleansing skin on feet.
BUF PUF BODYMATE. (3M Products) Oval two-sided cleansing sponge. Abrasive/gentle.

Use: Cleansing all areas of the body.
BUF-PUF NON MEDICATED CLEANSING SPONGE.
(3M Products) Abrasive cleansing sponge.
Use: Skin cleansing.
BUFACET. (Jenkins) Acetylsalicylic acid 3½ gr., acetophenetidin 2½ gr., caffeine alkaloid ½ gr., aromatics and buffered w/alum. hydroxide gel./Tab. Bot. 1000s.
Use: Analgesic.
BUFEXAMAC. B.A.N. 4-Butoxyphenylacetohydroxamic acid.
Use: Anti-inflammatory.
See: Droxaryl.
BUFF, Full Strength. (Travenol) Sod. carbonate 69 mg., sod. phosphate 83 mg./liter. Also available in Half Strength. Pkg. single dose incert vial, 100s.
Use: Admixture parenteral solution.
BUFF-A. (Mayrand) Aspirin acid 5 gr./Tab. buffered w. mixture of magnesium hydroxide and aluminum hydroxide dried gel. Bot. 100s, 1000s.
Use: Analgesic.
BUFFACETIN. (Kay) Aspirin 3½ gr., phenacetin 2½ gr., caffeine ½ gr./Tab. Bot. 100s, 500s, 1000s.
Use: Analgesic.
BUFF-A-COMP. (Mayrand) **Tab.:** Aspirin 648 mg., caffeine 40 mg., butalbital 50 mg./Tab. **Cap.:** Butalbital 50 mg., aspirin 325 mg., caffeine 40 mg./Cap. Bot. 100s.
Use: Analgesic, antipyretic.
BUFF-A-COMP NO. 3. (Mayrand) Butalbital 50 mg., aspirin 325 mg., caffeine 40 mg., codeine phosphate 30 mg./Tab. Bot. 100s.
Use: Analgesic.
BUFFAPRIN. (Buffington) Aspirin 325 mg./Tab. and buffered with magnesium oxide. Dispens-A-Kit 500s.
Use: Buffered analgesic, antipyretic, anti-inflamma-tory.
BUFFAPRIN EXTRA. (Buffington) Aspirin 500 mg./Tab. buffered with magnesium oxide. Dispens-A-Kits 500s.
Use: Extra strength buffered aspirin analgesic, antipyretic, anti-inflammatory.
BUFFASAL. (Dover) Aspirin 325 mg./Tab. w/ magnesium oxide. Sugar and salt free.
Use: Buffered aspirin.
BUFFASAL MAX. (Dover) Aspirin 500 mg./Tab. w/ magnesium oxide. Sugar and salt free.
Use: Extra strength buffered aspirin.
BUFFERIN CAPSULES. (Bristol-Myers) Aspirin 325 mg./Cap. buffered with magnesium carbonate, magnesium oxide, calcium carbonate. Bot 30s, 50s, 75s.
Use: Analgesic.
BUFFERIN EXTRA STRENGTH CAPSULES.
(Bristol-Myers) Aspirin 500 mg./Cap buffered with magnesium carbonate, magnesium oxide, calcium carbonate. Bot. 24s.,50s., 75s.
Use: Analgesic.
BUFFERIN EXTRA STRENGTH TABLETS.
(Bristol-Myers) Aspirin 500 mg./Tab. buffered with magnesium carbonate, aluminum glycinate. Bot. 30s, 60s, 100s.

Use: Analgesic.

BUFFERIN TABLETS. (Bristol-Myers) Aspirin 325 mg./Tab. buffered with aluminum glycinate, magnesium carbonate. Bot. 12s, 36s, 60s, 100s, 165s, 225s, 375s. Industrial 200 × 2s, 1000s.
Use: Mild analgesic.

BUFFERIN WITH CODEINE. (Bristol) Codeine phosphate 30 mg., aspirin 325 mg., aluminum glycinate 48.6 mg., magnesium carbonate 97.2 mg./Tab. Bot. 100s.
Use: Analgesic.

BUFFETS II. (Bowman) Aspirin 226 mg., acetaminophen 162 mg., caffeine 32.4 mg./Tab. Bot. 100s, 1000s.
Use: Analgesic, antipyretic.

BUFFINOL. (Otis Clapp) Aspirin 325 mg./Tab. buffered with magnesium oxide. Sugar and salt free. Safety packs 1000s. Bot. 100s. Aidpaks 100s. Unit boxes 20s. Medipaks 200s.
Use: Buffered analgesic, antipyretic.

BUFFINOL EXTRA. (Otis Clapp) Aspirin 500 mg./Tab. Sugar and salt free. Safety packs 500s.
Use: Extra strength buffered analgesic, anti-pyretic, anti-inflammatory agent.

BUFOPTO ATROPINE. (Softcon) Atropine 0.5%, 1% in a vehicle (Methulose) methylcellulose, benzalkonium chloride 1:10,000 as preservative, w/monobasic sod. phosphate, dibasic sod. phosphate, & sod. chloride. Dropper Bot. 15 ml.

BUFOPTO ZINC SULFATE. (Softcon) Zinc sulfate 0.25% in benzalkonium chloride solution, 1:25,000 as preservative. Dropper Bot. ½ oz., 1 oz.
Use: Eye anti-infective.

• **BUFORMIN.** USAN. 1-Butylbiguanide. Silubin.
Use: Oral hypoglycemic agent.

BUFOSAL. (Table Rock) Sod. salicylate 15 gr./Dr. w/cal. carb. & sod. bicarb. as granulated effer. Bot. 4 oz.
Use: Orally, analgesic & antipyretic.

BUFROLIN. B.A.N. 6-Butyl-1,4,7,10-tetrahydro-4,10-dioxo-1,7-phenanthroline-2,8-dicarboxylic acid.
Use: Treatment of allergic airway obstruction.

BUFS. (Moore Kirk) Acetylsalicylic acid 3½ gr., phenacetin 2½ gr., caffeine ½ gr./Tab. Bot. 100s, 1000s.
Use: Relief of pain in simple headache, neuralgia, and common cold.

BUF-SUL TABLETS AND SUSPENSION. (Sheryl) 167 mg. of each sulfacetamide, sulfadiazine & sulfamerazine. Tab. 100s, Susp. pt.
Use: Antibacterial.

BUF-TABS. (Blue Cross) Aspirin 5 gr./Tab. w/aluminum hydroxide, glycine magnesium carbonate. Bot. 100s.
Use: Analgesic.

BUFURALOL. B.A.N. 2-tert-Butylamino-1-(7-ethylben-zofuran-2-yl)ethanol.
Use: Beta adrenergic blocking agent.

BUFYLLINE. B.A.N. Theophylline compound with 2-amino-2-methylpropan-1-ol (1:1).
Use: Bronchodilator.
See: Ambuphylline

BUGS BUNNY. (Miles) Vit. A 2500 I.U., E 15 I.U., C 60 mg., folic acid 0.3 mg., B-1 1.05 mg., B-2 1.2 mg., niacin 13.5 mg., B-6 1.05 mg., B-12 4.5 mcg., D 400 I.U./Tab. Bot. 60s, 100s.
Use: Multivitamin supplement.

BUGS BUNNY PLUS IRON. (Miles) Vit. A 2500 I.U., E 15 I.U., C 60 mg., folic acid 0.3 mg., B-1 1.05 mg., B-2 1.2 mg., niacin 13.5 mg., B-6 1.05 mg., B-12 4.5 mcg., D 400 I.U., iron 15 mg./Tab. Bot. 60s, 100s.
Use: Multivitamin supplement with iron.

BUGS BUNNY WITH EXTRA C. (Miles) Vit. A 2500 I.U., D 400 I.U., E 15 I.U., C 250 mg., folic acid 0.3 mg., B-1 1.05 mg., B-2 1.20 mg., niacin 13.50 mg., B-6 1.05 mg., B-12 4.5 mcg./Tab. Bot. 60s.
Use: Chewable multivitamin supplement with extra vitamin C.

BU-LAX-100 AND -250. (Ulmer) Docusate sodium 100 mg. or 250 mg./Cap. Bot. 100s, 1000s.
Use: Stool softener.

BU-LAX-PLUS. (Ulmer) Docusate sodium 100 mg., casanthranol 30 mg./Cap. Bot. 100s, 1000s.
Use: Stool softener, laxative.

BULBORO POWDER. (Herbert) Aluminum sulfate, calcium acetate 1.9 Gm./Pkt. Ctn. 12s, 100s.
Use: Astrigent soaking solution.

BULKOGEN. A mucin extracted from the seeds of *Cyanopsis tetragonaloba.*

• **BUMETANIDE.** USAN. 3-Butylamino-4-phenoxy-5-sulfamoylbenzoic acid.
Use: Diuretic.
See: Bumex, Tab. (Roche)

• **BUMETRIZOLE.** USAN.
Use: Ultraviolet screen.

BUMEX. (Roche) Bumetanide 0.5 mg. or 0.1 mg./Tab. Bot. 100s, 500s. Tel-E-Dose 30s. Ampuls 2 ml., 0.25 mg./ml. Box 10s.
Use: Potent diuretic.

BUMINATE. (Hyland) Normal serum Albumin (Human) **25%** solution in 20 ml. w/o administration set, 50 ml. and 100 ml. w/administration set; **5%** sol in 250 ml. and 500 ml. with administration set.

BUMINTEST. (Ames) Sulfosalicylic acid in effer. tab. Tab., Bot. 100s.
Use: Test for albumin in urine.

BUNAMIDINE. B.A.N. NN-Dibutyl-4-hexyloxy-1-naphthamidine
Use: Anthelmintic, veterinary medicine.
See: Buban hydroxynaphthoate
  Scolaban hydrochloride

• **BUNAMIDE HYDROCHLORIDE.** USAN.
Use: Anthelmintic.

BUNAMIODYL SODIUM. Sodium 3-butyramido-α-ethyl-2,4,6-triiodocinnamate.
Use: Diagnostic aid (radiopaque medium).

BUNIODYL. B.A.N. 3-(3-Butyramido-2,4,6-triiodophenyl)-2-ethylacrylic acid. Bunamiodyl (I.N.N.)
Use: Radio-opaque substance.
See: Orabilix sodium salt

• **BUNOLOL HCl.** USAN. (±)-5-[3-(tert)-butylamino)-2-hydroxypropoxy]-3,4-dihydro-1-(2H)-naphthalenone hydrochloride.

Use: Antiadrenergic (β-receptors).

BUPHENINE. B.A.N. 1-(4-Hydroxyphenyl)-2-(1-methyl-3-phenylpropylamino)propan-1-ol.
Use: Peripheral vasodilator.
See: Perdilatal hydrochloride

• **BUPICOMIDE.** USAN.
Use: Antihypertensive.

BUPIVACAINE. B.A.N. 1-Butyl-2-(2,6-xylylcarbamoyl)-piperidide. 1-Butyl-2′,6′-pipecoloxylidide. (Abbott) 0.5% Soln. Amp 20 ml.
Use: Local anesthetic.

• **BUPIVACAINE AND EPINEPHRINE INJECTION,** U.S.P. XXI.
See: Marcaine w/Epinephrine, Inj. (Winthrop-Breon)

• **BUPIVACAINE HYDROCHLORIDE,** U.S.P. XXI. Inj. U.S.P. XXI. 2-piperidinecarboxamide, 1-butyl-N-(2, 6-dimethylphenyl)-, monohydrochloride, monohydrate.
Use: Local anesthetic.
See: Marcaine, Injectable (Winthrop-Breon)
    Sensorcaine, Inj. (Astra)

BUPRENORPHINE. B.A.N. N-Cyclopropylmethyl-7,8-dihydro-7α-(1-(S)-hydroxy-1,2,2-trimethylpropyl)-O⁶-methyl-6,14-endoethanonormorphine.
Use: Analgesic.

• **BUPRENORPHINE HYDROCHLORIDE.** USAN.
Use: Analgesic.

• **BUPROPION HYDROCHLORIDE.** USAN.
Use: Antidepressant.

• **BUQUINOLATE.** USAN. Ethyl 4-hydroxy-6,7-diisobutoxy-3-quinolinecarboxylate.
Use: Coccidostat for poultry.

• **BURAMATE.** USAN. 2-Hydroxyethyl benzylcarbamate. Hyamate.
Use: Anti-convulsant, tranquilizer.
See: Hyamate (Xttrium)

BURDEO. (Hill) Aluminum subacetate 100 mg., boric acid 300 mg./Oz. Bot. 3 oz. Roll-on 8 oz.
Use: Deodorant.

BURLESON RECTAL OINTMENT. (Burleson) Phenol, zinc oxide, zinc stearate, boric acid, eucalyptol, lanolin, white petrolatum. Tube 2 oz.
Use: Temporary relief of itching and discomfort due to hemorrhoids and rectal problems.

BURNATE. (Burlington) Vit. A 4000 I.U., D-2 400 I.U., thiamine HCl 3 mg., riboflavin 2 mg., niacinamide 10 mg., pyridine HCl 2 mg., cyanocobalamin 5 mcg., calcium pantothenate 0.5 mg., folic acid 0.4 mg., ascorbic acid 50 mg., ferrous fumarate 300 mg., calcium 200 mg., iodine 0.15 mg., copper 1 mg., magnesium 5 mg., zinc 1.5 mg. Tab. Bot. 100s.
Use: Prenatal Vitamin.

BURN GON. (Edward J. Moore) Benzocaine, cod liver oil, boric acid, lanolin. Tube 1¼ oz.
Use: Burn and first aid ointment.

■ **BURN THERAPY.**
See: Americaine, Prep. (Arnar-Stone)
    Amertan, Jelly (Lilly)
    Burn-A-Lay, Cream (Ken-Gate)
    Burnicin, Oint. (Columbia)
    Burn-Quel, Aerosol (Halperin)

Butesin Picrate Oint. (Abbott)
Foille, Prep. (Carbisulphoil)
Kip, Prep. (Youngs Drug Prod.)
Nupercainal, Oint. (Ciba)
Silvadene, Cream (Marion)
Solarcaine, Prep. (Plough)
Sulfamylon, Cream (Winthrop-Breon)
Unguentine, Prep. (Norwich)

BURN-A-LAY. (Ken-Gate) Chlorobutanol 0.75%, oxyquinoline benzoate 0.025%, zinc oxide 2%, thymol 0.5%. Cream. Tube 1 oz.
Use: Burn remedy.

BURN-QUEL. Halperin Aerosol dispenser. 1 oz., 2 oz.
Use: Burn therapy.

BURNTAME SPRAY. (Otis Clapp) Benzocaine 8-hydroxyquinoline. Aerosol can 2.5 oz.
Use: Anethetic/antiseptic burn spray.

BUR-OIL-ZINC. (Durel) Zinc oxide, talcum, lanolin, olive oil, Burow's solution. Bot. 4 oz., pt., gal.
Use: Generalized and widespread eczematous eruptions, acute and subacute inflammatory processes, exfoliative dermatitis.

BUR-OIL-ZINC LOTION PLUS. (Durel) Menthol 0.25%, phenol 0.5% added to Bur-oil-zinc comp. Bot. 4 oz., pt., gal.
Use: Antipruritic.

BURO-SOL ANTISEPTIC POWDER. (Doak) Contents make a dilute Burow's Sol.—aluminum acetate topical sol. plus benzethonium chloride. Pkg. (2.36 Gm.) 12s, 100s. Bot. Pow. 4 oz., 1 & 5 lb.

BUROTOR. (Torch) W/O emulsion of aluminum acetate basic 5%. Bot. 4 oz., 8 oz.
Use: Dilute 1:20 with water as bland, soothing, astringent lotion for dermatoses.

BUROW'S SOLUTION. Aluminum Acetate Topical Solution, U.S.P. XXI.
See: Buro-Sol, Cream, Pow. (Doak)
    Domeboro, Pow., Tab. (Miles Pharm)
W/Boric acid, acetic acid.
See: Star-Otic, Drops (Star)

BURSUL. (Burlington) Sulfamethiazole 500 mg./Tab. Bot. 100s.
Use: Sulfa-specific urinary inf.

BUR-TUSS. (Burlington) Chlorpheniramine maleate 2 mg., phenylepherine HCl 5 mg., phenylpropanolamine HCl 5 mg., guaifenesin 100 mg., alcohol 2.5%/5 cc. Bot. Pt., Gal.
Use: Expectorant.

BUR-ZIN. (Lamond) Aluminum acetate solution 2%, zinc oxide 10%. Bot. 4 oz., 8 oz., pt., qt., gal. Also w/o lanolin.
Use: Treatment of exzema, pruritic conditions, irritated skin.

• **BUSERELIN ACETATE.** USAN.
Use: Gonad-stimulating principle.

• **BUSPIRONE HYDROCHLORIDE.** USAN. (Mead Johnson)
Use: Investigative: antianxiety.

• **BUSULFAN,** U.S.P. XXI. Tabs. U.S.P. XXI. Tetramethylene dimethanesulfonate. 1-4-Dime-

thanesulphonyloxybutane. 1,4-Butanediol dimethane-
sulfonate.
Use: Chronic myeloid leukemia.
See: Myleran, Tab. (Burroughs Wellcome)
BUSULPHAN. B.A.N. Tetramethylene
di(methanesulphonate).
Use: Antineoplastic agent.
See: Myleran
• **BUTABARBITAL,** U.S.P. XXI 5-sec-Butyl-5-ethylbar-
bituric acid.
Use: Sedative, hypnotic.
See: BBS, Tab. (Reid-Provident)
   Butisol, Prods. (McNeil)
   Da-Sed, Tab. (Sheryl)
   Expansatol, Caps. (Merit)
   Medarsed, Elixir, Tab. (Medar)
W/Acetaminophen.
See: Coastalgesic, Tab. (Coastal)
   G-3, Tab. (Hauck)
   Sedapap, Elixir (Mayrand)
   Sedapap-10, Tab. (Mayrand)
W/Acetaminophen, & codeine phosphate.
See: Coastaldyne, Tab. (Coastal)
   G-3, Cap. (Hauck)
W/Acetaminophen, mephenesin.
See: T-Caps, Cap. (Burlington)
W/Acetaminophen, phenacetin, caffeine.
See: Windolor, Tab. (Winston)
W/Acetaminophen, salicylamide, phenyltoloxamine
citrate.
See: Dengesic, Tab. (Scott-Alison)
   Scotgesic, Cap., Elixir (Scott/Cord)
W/Acetysalicylic acid, phenacetin, caffeine,
hyoscyamine sulfate, codeine phosphate.
See: Butadeine, Cap. (Sutliff & Case)
W/Ambutonium bromide, aluminum hydroxide, mag.
hydroxide.
See: Aludrox, Susp., Tab. (Wyeth)
W/Aminophylline, phenylpropanolamine HCl,
chlorpheniramine maleate, aluminum hydroxide,
magnesium trisilicate.
See: Asmacol, Tabs. (Vale)
W/Amobarbital.
See: Butatrax, Caps. (Sutliff & Case)
W/Carboxyphen.
See: Bontril Timed No. 2, Tab. (G. W. Carnrick)
W/Chlorpheniramine maleate, hyoscine hydrobromide.
See: Pedo-Sol, Tab., Elixir (Warren Pharmacal)
W/Dihydroxypropyl theophylline, ephedrine HCl.
See: Airet R, Tabs. (Baylor Labs.)
W/Ephedrine sulfate, theophylline.
See: Asmabar, Tabs. (Bluline)
W/Ephedrine sulfate, theophylline.
See: Airet Y, Tab., Elix. (Baylor)
W/Ephedrine HCl, theophylline, guaifenesin.
See: Quibron Plus, Cap., Elix. (Mead Johnson)
W/Ephedrine HCl, theophylline, isoproterenol.
W/Ephedrine sulfate, theophylline, guaifenesin.
See: Broncholate, Cap., Elix. (Bock)
W/I-Hyoscyamine.
See: Cystospaz-SR, Caps. (Webcon)
   Levamine, Tabs., Caps. (Meyer)

W/Hyoscyamine sulfate, atropine sulfate, hyoscine
HBr, homatropine methylbromide.
See: Butabell HMB, Tabs., Elix. (Saron)
W/Hyoscyamine sulfate, scopolamine methylnitrate,
atropine sulfate.
See: Banatil, Cap., Elixir (Trimen)
W/Nitroglycerin.
See: Nitrodyl-B, Cap. (Bock)
W/Pentaerythritol tetranitrate.
See: Petn Plus (Saron)
W/Pentobarbital & phenobarbital.
See: Quiess, Tab. (O'Neal)
   Triple Barbiturate Elixir (CMC)
W/Phenazopyridine & hyoscyamine HBr.
See: Pyridium Plus, Tab. (Parke-Davis)
W/Phenazopyridine, scopolamine HBr, atropine
sulfate, hyoscyamine sulfate.
See: Buren, Tab. (Ascher)
W/Phenobarbital, pentobarbital, hyoscyamine sulfate,
hyoscine hydrobromide, atropine sulfate.
See: Neoquess, Tab. (O'Neal)
W/Salicylamide.
See: Dapco, Tab. (Mericon)
W/Secobarbital.
See: Monosyl, Tab. (Arcum)
W/Secobarbital, pentobarbital phenobarbital.
See: Quad-Set, Tab. (Kenyon)
W/Theophylline.
See: Theobid, Cap. (Meyer)
W/Theophylline, pseudoephedrine HCl.
See: Asmadil, Cap. (Reid-Provident)
   Ayr, Liq. (Ascher)
   Ayrcap, Cap. (Ascher)
   Az-Kap, Cap. (Keene)
   B. A., Prods. (Federal)
   Bronchobid, Duracap (Meyer)
• **BUTABARBITAL SODIUM.** U.S.P. XXI. Caps., Elix.,
Tabs., U.S.P. XXI. Sod. 5-sec-butyl-5-ethylbarbiturate.
Use: Sedative & hypnotic.
See: BBS, Tab. (Reid-Provident)
   Butalan, Elix. (Lannett)
   Butazem, Tab., Elix. (Zemmer)
   Buticaps, Cap. (McNeil)
   Butisol Sodium, Elixir, Tab. (McNeil)
   Expansatol, Cap. (Merit)
   Quiebar, Spantab, Tab (Nevin)
   Renbu, Tab. (Wren)
   Soduben Tab., Elxr. (Arcum)
W/Acetaminophen.
See: Amino-Bar, Tab. (Bowman)
   Minotal, Tabs. (Carnrick)
W/Acetaminophen, aspirin, caffeine.
See: Dolor Plus, Tab. (Geriatric)
W/Acetaminophen, caffeine.
See: Dularin-TH, Tab. (Donner)
   Phrenilin, Tab. (Carnrick)
W/Acetaminophen, mephenesin, codeine phosphate.
See: Bancaps-C, Cap. (Westerfield)
W/Acetaminophen, phenacetin, caffeine anydrous
See: Butigetic, Tab. (McNeil)
W/Acetaminophen, salicylamide.

See: Banesin Forte, Tab. (Westerfield)
Indogesic, Tab. (Century)
W/Acetaminophen, salicylamide, d-amphetamine
sulfate, hexobarbital, secobarbital sod., pheno-
barbital.
See: Sedragesic, Tab. (Lannett)
W/Aluminum hydroxide dried gel, Mg glycinate, Powd.
ext. belladonna leaf.
See: Bellabarbital Buffered, Cap. (Consol.-Midland)
W/d-Amphetamine sulfate.
See: Bontril, Tab. (Carnrick)
W/Ascorbic acid, Sod. p-aminobenzoate, salicylamide,
Sod. salicylate.
See: Bisalate, Tab. (Allison)
W/Atropine sulfate, hyoscyamine HBr, alcohol,
hyoscine HBr.
See: Hyonatol Tab., Hyonatol B Elixir, Hexett, Tab.
(Bowman)
W/Belladonna ext.
See: Butibel, Tab., Elix. (McNeil)
Quiebel, Elixir, Cap. (Nevin)
W/Belladonna ext., enzymes, & iron oxbile.
See: Butibel-zyme, Tab. (McNeil)
W/Dehydrocholic acid, belladonna extract.
See: Decholin-BB, Tabs. (Miles Pharm)
W/Hyoscine HBr, hyoscyamine sulfate, atropine
sulfate.
See: Zemarine, Elix., Tab., Cap. (Zemmer)
W/Methscopolamine bromide, aluminum hydroxide gel
dried & Mag. trisilicate.
See: Eulcin, Tab. (Leeds)
W/Pentaerythritol tetranitrate.
See: Covap, Tab. (Blue Line)
Perbuzem, Tab. (Zemmer)
W/Pentobarbital sod., phenobarbital sod.
See: Trio-Bar, Tab. (Jenkins)
W/Phenobarbital sod. acetaminophen, phenacetin,
caffeine.
See: Two-Dyne, Tab. (Key)
W/Salicylamide, mephenesin.
See: Metrogesic, Tab. (Metro)
W/Secobarbital sodium.
See: Monosyl, Tab. (Arcum)
W/Secobarbital sod., pentobarbital sod. &
phenobarbital.
See: Nidar, Tab. (Armour)
Quadrabarb, Tab. (Vortech)
W/Secobarbital Sodium & phenobarbital.
See: S.B.P., Tab. (Lemmon)
W/Simethicone, hyoscyamine sulfate, atropine sulfate,
hyoscine HBr.
See: Sidonna, Tab. (Reed & Carnrick)
W/Theophylline, pseudoephedrine HCl.
See: Dilorbron, Cap. (Hauck)
BUTABELL HMB. (Saron) Butabarbital 15 mg.,
hyoscyamine sulfate 0.1037 mg., atropine sulfate
0.0194 mg., hyoscine HBr 0.0065 mg./Tab. Bot.
100s, 1000s.
BUTACAINE.
Use: Surface anesthetic.
See: Butyn Dental Oint. (Abbott).
BUTACAINE SULFATE. 1-Propanol,3-(dibutyl-

amino)-,4-aminobenzoate (ester), sulfate (salt) (2:1).
3-(Dibutylamino)-1-propanol, p-aminobenzoate (ester)
sulfate (2:1). Various manufacturers.
Use: Surface anesthetic.
• **BUTACETIN.** USAN. 4′-Tert-butoxyacetanilide.
Use: Analgesic.
• **BUTACLAMOL HYDROCHLORIDE.** USAN.
Use: Antipsychotic.
BUTALAMINE. B.A.N. 5-(2-Dibutylaminoethyl)-amino-
3-phenyl-1,2,4-oxadiazole.
Use: Vasodilator.
BUTALBITAL, U.S.P. XXI. 5-Allyl-5-isobutyl-barbituric
acid. Allylbarbituric Acid.
Use: Sedative.
See: Buff-A-Comp #3 (Mayrand)
Lotusate, Cap. (Winthrop-Breon)
Sandoptal, Prep. (Sandoz)
W/Acetaminophen, caffeine.
See: Esgic, Tab. (Gilbert)
W/Acetaminophen, phenacetin, caffeine.
See: Arbutal, Tab. (Arcum)
Buff-A-Comp, Tab.-Cap. (Mayrand)
Cefinal, Tab. (Alto)
Protension, Tab. (Blaine)
Repan, Tab. (Everett)
W/Aspirin, phenacetin, caffeine.
See: Duogesic, Cap. (Western Research)
Fiorinal, Cap., Tab. (Sandoz)
W/Aspirin, phenacetin, caffeine, codeine phosphate.
See: Buff-A-Comp, Tab w/Codeine. (Mayrand)
Fiorinal With Codeine, Cap. (Sandoz)
W/Caffeine, aspirin, acetaminophen.
See: Anaphen, Cap. (Mallard)
W/Caffeine, aspirin, aluminum hydroxide.
See: Kengesin, Tab. (Kenwood)
W/Phenacetin, aspirin, caffeine.
See: Arbutal, Tab. (Arcum)
BUTALGIN.
See: Methadone HCl (Various Mfr.)
BUTALAN ELIXIR. (Lannett) Sodium butabarbital 0.2
Gm./30 cc. Bot. pt., gal.
Use: Sedative.
BUTALIX. (Vale) Alcohol 10%, sod. butabarbital 200
mg./Fl. oz. Bot. pt., gal.
BUTALLYLONAL. 5-(2-Bromoallyl)-5-sec-butylbarbitu-
ric acid. (Pernocton)
Use: Hypnotic.
• **BUTAMBEN,** U.S.P. XXI. Benzoic acid, 4-amino-,butyl
ester. Butyl p-aminobenzoate.
Use: Anesthetic, local.
• **BUTAMBEN PICRATE.** USAN.
Use: Topical anesthetic.
See: Butesin Picrate, Oint. (Abbott)
• **BUTAMIRATE CITRATE.** USAN.
Use: Antitussive.
• **BUTAMISOLE HYDROCHLORIDE.** USAN.
Use: Anthelmintic.
BUTAMYRATE. B.A.N. 2-(2-Diethylaminoethoxy)-ethyl
2-phenylbutyrate.
Use: Cough suppressant.
See: Sinecod citrate

- **BUTANE,** N.F. XVI.
BUTANEDIOIC ACID, MONO[2-[(2,2-DICHLORO-ACETYL) AMINO]-3-HYDROXY-3-(4-NITRO-PHENYL)PROPYL]ESTER, MONOSODIUM SALT. Chloramphenicol Sodium Succinate, U.S.P. XXI.
BUTANEDIOIC ACID,SULFO-, 1-4-BIS(2-ETHYLHEX-YL)ESTER, SODIUM SALT. Docusate Sodium, U.S.P. XXI.
1,4-BUTANEDIOL DIMETHANESULFONATE. Busulfan, U.S.P. XXI.
BUTANILICAINE. B.A.N. 2-Butylamino-6'-chloroacet-o-toluidide.
  Use: Local anesthetic.
BUTANISAMIDE. 1-Butyl-1-(o-methoxyphenyl) urea.
1-BUTANONE,4-[4-(4-CHLOROPHENYL-4-HYDROX-YL-1-PIPERIDINYL]-1-(4-FLUOROPHENYL)-. Haloperidol, U.S.P. XXI.
- **BUTAPERAZINE.** USAN. 1-{ 10-[3-(4-Methyl-1-piperazinyl)propyl]phenothiazin-2-yl }-1-butanone.
  Use: Psychotropic agent.
  See: Repoise (Robins)
- **BUTAPERAZINE MALEATE.** USAN.
  Use: Antipsychotic.
BUTAPHYLLAMINE. Ambuphylline. Theophylline aminoisobutanol. Theophylline with 2-amino-2-meth-yl-1-propanol.
BUTAPRO ELIXIR. (Approved) Butabarbital sod. 0.2 Gm./30 cc. Bot. pt., gal.
BUTATRAN. (Hauck) Butabarbital 0.5 gr./Tab. Bot. 100s.
  Use: Sedative.
BUTATRAX. (Sutliff & Case) Amobarbital 20 mg., butabarbital 30 mg./Cap. Bot. 100s, 1000s.
  Use: Sedative.
BUTAZEM. (Zemmer) Butabarbital sodium **Tab.:** 15 mg., 30 mg. 0.1 Gm./Tab. Bot. 100s, 1000s.
  Elix.: Bot. 3 oz., pt. gal.
  Use: Sedative.
BUTAZOLIDIN. (Geigy) Phenylbutazone 100 mg./Tab. or Cap. Bot. 100s, 1000s. Unit Dose 100s.
  Use: Analgesic, anti-inflammatory, antiarthritic and antipyretic.
BUTAZOLIDIN. (Geigy) Phenylbutazone 100 mg./Cap. Bot. 100s, 1000s, Unit Dose 100s. Gy-Pak 100s.
  Use: Anti-inflammatory, analgesic, antipyretic and an-tiarthritic.
BUTELLINE.
  See: Butacaine Sulfate (Various Mfr.)
2-BUTENEDIOIC ACID,(E)-,IRON(2+)-SALT. Ferrous Fumarate, U.S.P. XXI.
- **BUTERIZINE.** USAN.
  Use: Vasodilator.
BUTESIN PICRATE. n-Butyl-p-aminobenzoate. Bu-tamben picrate.
BUTESIN PICRATE OINTMENT. (Abbott) Contains 1% butamben picrate. Tube 1 oz.
  Use: Minor burns of various kinds—electrical, steam, hot metal & scalds.
BUTETHAL. (Various Mfr.) 5-Ethyl-5-butylbarbituric acid.
  Use: Sedative & hypnotic.

BUTETHAMATE. B.A.N. 2-Diethylaminoethyl 2-phenyl-butyrate.
  Use: Antispasmodic.
BUTETHAMINE FORMATE. 2-Isobutyl aminoethyl-p-aminobenzoate formate.
BUTETHAMINE HYDROCHLORIDE. 2-(Isobutylamino) ethyl-p-amino benzoate HCl.
  See: Dentocaine (Amer. Chem. & Drug)
BUTETHANOL.
  See: Pontocaine Phydrochloride, Preps. (Winthrop-Breon)
BUTHALITONE SODIUM. B.A.N. A mixture of 100 parts by weight of the monosodium derivative of 5-allyl-5-isobutyl-2-thiobarbituric acid and 6 parts by weight of dried sodium carbonate.
  Use: Hypnotic; sedative.
  See: Transithal
    Ulbreval
- **BUTHIAZIDE.** USAN. 6-Chloro-3, 4-dihydro-3-isobu-tyl-2H-1,2,4-benzothiadiazine-7-sulfonamide 1,1-di-oxide.
  Use: Diuretic, antihypertensive
BUTIBEL Tab. and Elixir. (Wallace) Butabarbital sod. 15 mg., belladonna ext. 15 mg./Tab. or 5 cc. **Tab.** Bot. 100s. **Elixir** (alcohol 7%), Bot. pt.
  Use: Antispasmodic and sedative combination for G.I. disorders.
BUTIBEL-ZYME. (McNeil Pharm) Butabarbital Sod. 15 mg., belladonna ext. 15 mg., proteolytic enzyme 10 mg., amylolytic enzyme 20 mg., cellulolytic enzyme 5 mg., lipolytic enzyme 100 mg., iron ox bile 30 mg./Tab. Bot. 100s.
  Use: Digestive aid.
BUTICAPS. (Wallace) Butabarbital sodium 15 mg., 30 mg./Cap. Bot. 100s.
  Use: Sedative and hypnotic.
- **BUTIKACIN.** USAN.
  Use: Antibacterial.
- **BUTIFENIN.** USAN.
  Use: Diagnostic aid.
- **BUTIROSIN SULFATE.** USAN. A mixture of the sulfates of the A and B forms of an antibiotic produced by *Bacillus circularis*.
  Use: Antibacterial.
BUTISOL SODIUM. (Wallace) Butabarbital sodium. **Elixir:** 30 mg/5cc. Bot pt., gal. **Tab:** 15 mg., 30 mg., 50mg. or 100mg. Bot. 100s, 1000s.
  Use: Intermediate sedative & hypnotic.
  See: Buticaps, Cap. (McNeil)
W/Belladonna ext.
  See: Butibel, Tab. and Elixir. (McNeil)
W/Belladonna ext., digestive enzymes & iron oxbile.
  See: Butibel-Zyme, Tab. (McNeil)
- **BUTIXIRATE.** USAN.
  Use: Analgesic, antirheumatic.
- **BUTOCONAZOLE NITRATE.** USAN.
  Use: Antifungal.
BUTOLAN. Benzylphenyl carbamate.
- **BUTONATE.** USAN.
  Use: Anthelmintic.
- **BUTOPAMINE.** USAN.
  Use: Cardiotonic.

BUTOPYRONOXYL. (Indalone) Butyl mesityl oxide.
   Use: Insect repellant, used in Comp. Dimethyl
   Phthalate Solution.
• **BUTORPHANOL.** USAN.
   Use: Analgesic, antitussive.
• **BUTORPHANOL TARTRATE,** U.S.P. XXI. Inj.,
   U.S.P. XXI.
   Use: Analgesic.
   See: Stadol, Inj., (Bristol)
BUTOXAMINE. B.A.N. ($\pm$)-erythro-1-(2,5-Dimethoxy-
   phenyl)-2-t-butylaminopropan-1-ol.
   Use: Inhibitor of fatty acid mobilization.
• **BUTOXAMINE HCl.** USAN. α-[1-(Tertbutylamino)e-
   thyl]-2,5-dimethoxybenzyl alcohol HCl.
   Use: Oral hypoglycemic; antilipemic.
**2-BUTOXY-N-(2-(DIETHYLAMINO)ETHYL)-CINCHON-
INAMIDE.** Dibucaine, U.S.P. XXI.
BUTRIPTYLINE. B.A.N.DL-3-(10,11-Dihydro-5H-diben-
   zo[a,d]cycloheptene-5-yl)-2-methyl-propyldimethyla-
   mine.
   Use: Antidepressant.
• **BUTRIPTYLINE HYDROCHLORIDE.** USAN. dl-10,
   11-Dihydro-N, N, β-trimethyl-5H-dibenzo (a,d)cy-
   cloheptene-5-propylamine hydrochloride.
   Use: Antidepressant.
• **BUTYL ALCOHOL,** N.F. XVI. Butyl alcohol is *n*-butyl
   alcohol.
BUTYL AMINOBENZOATE. n-Butyl
   p-Aminobenzoate. Scuroforme.
   Use: Surface anesthetic.
W/Benzocaine, tetracaine HCl.
   See: Cetacaine, Preps. (Cetylite)
W/Benzyl alcohol, phenylmercuric borate, benzocaine.
   See: Dermathyn, Oint. (Davis & Sly)
W/Procaine, benzyl alcohol, in sweet almond oil
   See: Anucaine, Amp. (Calvin)
W/Tetracaine
   See: Pontocaine, Oint. (Winthrop-Breon)
• **BUTYLATED HYDROXYANISOLE,** N.F. XVI. tert-
   Butyl-4-methoxyphenol.
   Use: Pharmaceutic aid (antioxidant).
BUTYLATED HYDROXYANISOLE. B.A.N. 2-t-Butyl-
   4-methoxyphenol.
   Use: Antioxidant.
• **BUTYLATED HYDROXYTOLUENE,** N.F. XVI. 2.6-
   Di-tert-butyl-P-cresol.
   Use: Pharmaceutic aid (antioxidant).
BUTYLATED HYDROXYTOLUENE. B.A.N. 2,6-Di-t-
   butyl-p-cresol.
   Use: Antioxidant.
4-BUTYL-1,2-DIPHENYLPYRAZOLIDINE-3,5-DIONE.
   Phenylbutazone, U.S.P. XXI.
BUTYL p-HYDROXYBENZOATE. Butylparaben, N.F.
   XVI.
• **BUTYLPARABEN,** N.F. XVI. Butyl p-Hydroxy-benzo-
   ate.
   Use: Pharmaceutical aid (antifungal preservative).
BUTYLPHENAMIDE. N-n-butyl-3-phenyl-salicylamide.
BUTYLPHENYLSALICYLAMIDE.
   See: Butylphenamide
1-BUTYL-3-(p-TOLYLSULFONYL)UREA. Tolbut-
   amide, U.S.P. XXI.

BUTYN DENTAL OINTMENT. (Abbott) Butacaine 4%
   oint. Tube 0.25 oz., 1 oz.
   Use: Relief of pain due to dentures.
B-VITE. (Bluco) B-1 100 mg., B-2 2 mg., B-6 4 mg.,
   niacinamide 100 mg., d-penthenol 4 mg./cc. Vial 30
   cc.
   Use: B vitamin deficiency.
BVU.
   See: Bromisovalum.
BYLA'S. (C.M.C.) Musculosine. Bot. 4¾ oz.

C

CABADON-M. (Reid-Provident) Cyanocobalamin 1000
   mcg./cc. Vials 10 cc, 30 cc. I.M. or S.C
• **CABUFOCON B.** USAN.
   Use: Contact lens material.
CACODYLIC ACID SALTS.
   Ferric Salt
   Iron Salt
   Sodium Salt
• **CACTINOMYCIN.** USAN. Dactinomycin 10%;
   actinomycin C_2 45% and actinomycin C_3 45%.
   Actinomycin C.
   Use: Antineoplastic agent.
   See: Sanamycin (FBA Pharm.)
CADE OIL.
   See: Juniper Tar
CADE OIL CREAM NO. 26. (Durel) Cade oil 3%,
   ammoniated mercury 2%, in Duromantel cream.
   Jars 1 oz., lb., 6 lb.
   Use: Psoriasis vulgaris.
CADE OIL CREAM NO. 27. (Durel) Cade oil 5%,
   sulfur 5%, salicylic acid 3%, added to Duromantel
   cream. Jars 1 oz., lb., 6 lb.
   Use: Psoriasis vulgaris, hyperkeratotic eczemas of
   the palms and soles.
CAD-O-BATH. (Durel) Oil of cade 35%, polysorbate
   "20" 35%. Bot. 8 oz., pt., gal.
   Use: Generalized pruritus, pruritic dermatoses,
   psoriasis.
CAFEDRINE. B.A.N. L-7-[2-(β-Hydroxy-
   α-methylphenethylamino)ethyl]-
   theophylline.
   Use: Analeptic.
CAFENOL. (Winthrop Products) Aspirin, caffeine.
   Use: Analgesic.
CAFERGOT P-B SUPPOSITORIES. (Sandoz) Ergotamine tartrate 2 mg., caffeine 100 mg., bellafoline
   0.25 mg., pentobarbital 60 mg./Suppos. Box 12s.
   Use: Treatment of migraine with tension &
   gastrointestinal disturbances.
CAFERGOT P-B TABLETS. (Sandoz) Ergotamine
   tartrate 1 mg., caffeine 100 mg., bellafoline 0.125
   mg., pentobarbital sodium 30 mg./Tab. SigPak
   dispensing pkg. of 90s, 250s.
   Use: Migraine with tension & gastrointestinal
   disturbances.
CAFERGOT SUPPOSITORIES. (Sandoz) Ergotamine
   tartrate 2 mg., caffeine 100 mg. in cocoa butter
   base. Box 12s.

Use: Treatment of migraine.

CAFERGOT TABLETS. (Sandoz) Ergotamine tartrate 1 mg., caffeine 100 mg./S.C. Tab. Bot. 250s. SigPak dispensing pkg. of 90s.
Use: Treatment of migraine.

• **CAFFEINE,** U.S.P. XXI. 1H-Purine-2,6-dione, 3,-7-dihydro-1,3,7-trimethyl-xanthine. (Various Mfr.) Guaranine; Methyltheobromine; Thein.
Use: Cardiac, respiratory & psychic stimulant.
See: Enerjets, Loz. (Chilton)
   Femicin, Tab. (Norcliff Thayer)
   Nodoz, Tabs. (Bristol-Myers)
   Stim 250, Cap. (Scrip)
   Tirend (Norcliff-Thayer)
   Vivarin, Tab. (J.B. Williams)

CAFFEINE CITRATED.
Use: Central nervous system stimulant.

CAFFEINE SODIO-BENZOATE.
See: Caffeine sod. benzoate

• **CAFFEINE SODIUM BENZOATE INJECTION,** U.S.P. XXI. Approximately equal parts of caffeine and sod. benzoate. (Various Mfr.) Amp. (3¾ & 7½ gr.) 2 cc., Box 12s, 100s. Hypo Tab. (1 gr.) Tube 20s, 100s & Pow.
Use: Orally & I.M. Central nervous system stimulant.

CAFFEINE SODIUM SALICYLATE. (Various Mfr.) Bot. 1 oz.; Pkg. ¼ lb., 1 lb.
Use: See caffeine.

CAFFEINE-THEOPHYLLINE COMPOUND, w/Nux Vomica Ext.
See: Xanthinux, Tab. (Cole)

CAFFIN-T.D. (Kenyon) Caffeine 250 mg./Cap. Bot. 100s.

CAG. (Western Research) Calcium gluconate 1004 mg./Tab. Bot. 1000s.
Use: Supplement.

CAGOL. (Harvey) Guaiacol 0.1 Gm., eucalyptol 0.08 Gm., iodoform 0.2 Gm., camphor 0.05 Gm./2 cc. in olive oil. Vial 30 ml.
Use: I.M., expectorant.

20-CAIN BURN RELIEF. (Alto) Benzocaine 20%, benzyl alcohol 2.3%, urea 5.38%, p-chloro-m-xylenol 0.51%, propylene glycol 71.81%. Spray Bot. 6 oz.
Use: Relief from sunburn, minor burns, nonvenomous insect bites, and itching from minor skin irritations.

CALADRYL. (Parke-Davis) 1% Benadryl HCl in specially prepared calamine base. **Cream;** tube, 1½ oz., Bot. 6 oz. Plastic Squeeze Bot. 2½ oz.
Use: Antihistaminic & antipruritic.

CALAFORMULA. (Eric, Kirk & Gary) Ferrous gluconate 130 mg., calcium lactate 130 mg., Vit. A 1000 I.U., D 400 I.U., B-1 2 mg., B-2 2 mg., niacinamide 5 mg., ascorbic acid 20 mg., folic acid 0.130 mg., Mg 0.250 mg., Cu 0.250 mg., Zn 0.250 mg., Mn 0.250 mg., K 0.075 mg./Cap. Bot. 50s, 100s, 500s, 1000s, 5000s.
Use: Prenatal dietary supplement.

CALAFORMULA WITH AMPHETAMINE. (Eric, Kirk & Gary) Calaformula with amphetamine sulfate 5 mg./Cap. Bot. 100s.

Use: Control appetite.

CALAFORMULA F. (Eric, Kirk & Gary) Calaformula plus fluorine 0.333 mg./Tab. Bot. 100s.
Use: Protect against decay of teeth.

CALAHIST LOTION. (Walgreen) Diphenhydramine HCl 1% in calamine. Bot. 6 oz.
Use: Antihistamine & antipruritic.

CALAMATUM. (Blair) **Lotion** Zinc oxide, calamine, benzocaine 3%. Bot. 3¾ oz. **Oint.** Zinc oxide, calamine, phenol, camphor, benzocaine. Tube 1.5 oz.
Use: Relief of minor skin irritations.

CALAMATUM AEROSOL SPRAY. (Blair) Benzocaine 3% w/zinc oxide, calamine, phenol, camphor. Spray Can 3 oz.
Use: Relief of minor skin irritations.

• **CALAMINE,** U.S.P. XXI. Lotion, Phenolated Lotion, U.S.P. XXI. (Various Mfr.) Iron oxide mixture with zinc oxide.
Use: Astringent and mild antiseptic.

CALAN. (Searle) Verapamil HCl 80 mg. or 120 mg./Tab. Bot. 100s, Unit Dose 100s. mg./Tab. Bot. 100s, 500s, 1000s. Unit Dose 100s.
Use: Calcium antagonist, antianginal, antiarrhythmic.

CALAN I.V. (Searle) Verapamil HCl. **Amp.:** 5 mg./2 ml. Ctn. 10s. **Vial:** 5 mg./2 ml. 10 mg./4 ml. Ctn. 5s, 10s. **Syringe:** 5 mg./2 ml. 10 mg./4 ml. Ctn. 5s, 10s.
Use: Antiarrhythmic.

CALBRODEX. (Pasadena Research) Calcium gluconate 0.5 Gm., strontium Br 0.5 Gm., dextrose 1 Gm./10 cc. Amp. for IV use. 25s, 100s.

CAL-C-BATE. (Kay) Calcium gluconate 700 mg., calcium lactate 300 mg., dextrose 500 mg., Vit. C 1 gm./10 cc. 25/10 ml. ampules. I.V.
Use: Calcium deficiencies.

CALCEE. (Pasadena Research) Calcium gluconate 350 mg., calcium lactate 150 mg., dextrose 250 mg., ascorbic acid 500 mg./5 cc. amp. 25s, 100s. Amp. 10 cc. 25s, 100s.

CALCET. (Mission) Calcium lactate 240 mg. calcium gluconate 240 mg., calcium carbonate 240 mg., calcium 152.8 mg., Vit. D-2 100 u./Tab. Bot. 100s.
Use: Dietary supplement.

CALCIBIND. (Mission) Sodium cellulose phosphate 2.5 Gm./Packet. Box 90s.
Use: Absorptive hypercalciuria.

CALCICAPS. (Nion) Calcium 750 mg., phosphorus 360 mg., Vit. D 300 I.U./6 Tab. Bot. 100s, 500s.
Use: Dietary supplement.

CALCICAPS-FOUR. (Nion) Sugar free. Calcium 800 mg., Vit D 400 I.U./4 Tab. Bot. 100s.
Use: Dietary supplement.

CALCICAPS WITH IRON. (Nion) Calcium 750 mg., phosphorus 360 mg., Vit. D 400 I.U., ferrous gluconate 384 mg./6 Tab. Bot. 100s, 500s.
Use: Dietary supplement.

CALCICAPS, SUPER. (Nion) Calcium 334 mg., phosphorus 41.7 mg., Vit. D 133 I.U./Tab. Bot. 100s.
Use: Dietary supplement.

CALCIDE. (Blue Line) Available iodine in combination with lime and starch 0.2 gr./Tab. Bot. 1000s.

CALCIDRINE SYRUP. (Abbott) Codeine 8.4 mg., cal. iodide anh. 152 mg. alcohol 6%/5 ml. Bot. 4 oz., pt., gal.
Use: Treatment of cough due to colds.

• **CALCIFEDIOL,** U.S.P. XXI. Caps., U.S.P. XXI.
Use: Calcium regulator.

CALCIFEROL. Ergocalciferol, U.S.P. XXI. Vitamin D-2, viosterol, synthetic vitamin D, irradiated ergosterol, activated ergosterol.
Use: Vitamin D (Antirachitic).
See: Calciferol, Tab., Inj. (Kremers-Urban)
Calderol, Tab. (Upjohn)
Deltalin, Gelseal (Lilly)
Drisdol, Cap., Sol. (Winthrop-Breon)

CALCIFEROL DROPS. (Rorer) Ergocalciferol 8000 U (0.2 mg.)/ml. Bot. 60 ml. w/dropper.
Use: Prevention Vit. D deficiency in infants, children & adults.

CALCIFEROL INJECTION. (Rorer) Ergocalciferol 500,000 U (12.5 mg.)/cc. Amp. 1cc. Box 5s.
Use: Hypoparathyroidism & refractory rickets.

CALCIFEROL TABLETS. (Rorer) Ergocalciferol 50,000 U/Tab. Bot. 100s.
Use: Hypoparathyroidism and refractory rickets.

CALCIGARDS. (Eckerd) Bot. 300s.

CALCIMAR SOLUTION. (USV Labs.) A calcitonin solution (Salmon origin) containing 200 I.U. (MCR)/ml. Vial 2 ml.
Use: To lower bone reabsorption of calcium, symptomatic treatment of Paget's Disease.

CALCIPARINE. (American Critical Care) Heparin Calcium Injection. **5000** u/0.2 ml. prefilled syringe. Box 10s. **12500** u/0.5 ml. Amp w/disposable syringe & needle. Box 10s. **20000** u/0.8 ml. Amp w/disposable syringe & needle. Box 10s.
Use: IM, IV, or SC anticoagulant.

• **CALCITONIN.** USAN. Hormone from thyroid gland.
Use: Plasma hypocalcemic hormone.

CALCITONIN SALMON.
See: Calcimar, Inj. (Armour)

• **CALCITRIOL.** USAN. 9, 10-seco (5Z, 7E)-5, 7, 10 (19)-cholestatriene-1a, 3b, 25-triol.
Use: Management of hypocalcemia in chronic renal dialysis patients.
See: Rocaltrol, Cap. (Roche)

CALCIUM ACETYLSALICYLATE. Kalmopyrin, kalsetal, soluble aspirin, tylcalsin.
Use: As aspirin.

CALCIUM ALUMINUM CARBONATE.
W/Dl-Amino Acetate Complex.
See: Ancid Tablet and Suspension (Sheryl)

CALCIUM AMINOSALICYLATE. Aminosalicylate Calcium, N.F. XVI.

CALCIUM AMPHOMYCIN.
See: Amphomycin.

• **CALCIUM AND MAGNESIUM CARBONATES TABLETS,** U.S.P. XXI.
Use: Antacid.

CALCIUM 4-BENZAMIDOSALICYLATE. Calcium Aminacyl B-PAS. Benzoylpas Calcium.

See: Benzapas, Pow., Tab. (Dorsey)

CALCIUM BENZAMIDOSALICYLATE. B.A.N. Calcium 4-benzamido-2-hydroxybenzoate.
Use: Treatment of tuberculosis.

CALCIUM BENZOYL-p-AMINOSALICYLATE.
See: Benzoylpas calcium

CALCIUM BENZOYLPAS.
See: Benzoylpas Calcium

CALCIUM BIS-DIOCTYL SULFOSUCCINATE.
See: Dioctyl Calcium Sulfosuccinate

CALCIUM CARBASPIRIN. F.D.A. Calcium salicylate diacetate compound with urea.
W/Triaminic.
See: Ursinus, Tab. (Dorsey)

• **CALCIUM CARBONATE AND MAGNESIA TABLETS,** U.S.P. XXI.
Use: Antacid.

CALCIUM CARBONATE, AROMATIC. (Lilly) Calcium carbonate 10 gr./Tab. Bot. 100s, 1000s.

• **CALCIUM CARBONATE, PRECIPITATED,** U.S.P. XXI. (Various Mfr.) Precipitated chalk; carbonic acid, calcium salt (1:1).
Use: Antacid.
See: Amitone, Tab. (Norcliff Thayer)
Biocal Prods. (Miles)
Cal-Sup, Tab. (Riker)
Dicarbosil, Tab. (Arch)
Mallamint, Tab. (Mallard)
Tums, Tab. (Norcliff Thayer)

CALCIUM CARBONATE W/COMB.
See: Accelerase, Cap. (Organon)
Alised, Tab. (Elder)
Alka-2, Tab. (Miles)
Alkalade, Susp., Tab. (DePree)
Alkets, Tab. (Upjohn)
Anti-Acid No. 1, Tab. (N. Amer. Pharm.)
Antacid pH, Tab. (Towne)
Antacin, Tab. (Reid-Provident)
Calsarbain, Tab. (Sutliff & Case)
Camalox, Tab., Susp. (Rorer)
Ca-Plus, Tab. (Miller)
Carbonates No. 3, Tab. (Noyes)
Co-Gel, Tab. (Arco)
Diatrol, Tab. (Otis Clapp)
Dimacid, Tab. (Otis Clapp)
Equilets, Tab. (Mission Pharm.)
Eugel, Susp., Tab. (Reid-Provident)
Gas-Eze, Tab. (Edward J. Moore)
Glytabs, Chew. Tab. (Pharmics)
Hycidol, Pow. (Mallard)
Iodized Lime, Tab. (Elder)
Kanalka, Tab. (Lannett)
Kaocasil, Tab. (Jenkins)
Lactocal, Tab. (Laser)
Marbien, Susp., Tab. (Fleming)
Maygel, Tab. (Century)
Natabec, Prep. (Parke-Davis)
Os-Cal 500, Tab. (Marion)
Os-Cal-Mone, Tab. (Marion)
Pan-Bis-Cal, Susp. (Noyes)
P.H. Tablets, Chewable (Scrip)
Pregent, Tab. (Beutlich)

Ratio, Tab. (Adria)
Spastosed, Tab. (N. Amer. Pharm.)
Titralac, Liq., Tab. (Riker)
• **CALCIUM CARBONATE TABLETS,** U.S.P. XXI.
Use: Antacid.
CALCIUM CARBIMIDE. Calcium cyanamide.
CALCIUM CASEINATE.
See: Casec, Pow. (Mead Johnson)
CALCIUM CHEL 330. (Geigy).
Use: Heavy metal antagonist.
See: Calcium Trisodium Pentetate.
• **CALCIUM CHLORIDE,** U.S.P. XXI. Inj., U.S.P. XXI.
Use: Calcium replenisher.
• **CALCIUM CHLORIDE CA 45.** USAN.
Use: Radioactive agent.
• **CALCIUM CHLORIDE CA 47.** USAN.
Use: Radioactive agent.
• **CALCIUM CHLORIDE INJECTION.** U.S.P. XXI.
(Upjohn) 1 Gm. Amp. 10 ml., 25s. (Torigian)1 Gm.
Amp. 10 ml. 12s, 25s, 100s. (Trent) 10% Amp. 10
ml. (Cutter) 13.6 mEq./10 ml. Vial.
Use: I.V., hypocalcemic tetany.
CALCIUM CYCLAMATE. Calcium
cyclohexanesulfamate.
CALCIUM CYCLOBARBITAL. Calcium 5-(l-cyclohex-
en-l-yl)-5-ethylbarbiturate.
Use: Central depressant.
CALCIUM CYCLOHEXANESULFAMATE.
See: Calcium Cyclamate
CALCIUM DL-PANTOTHENATE. Calcium Pantothe-
nate, Racemic, U.S.P. XXI.
CALCIUM 3-((DIMETHYLAMINO)METHYLENE)-
AMINO)-2,4,6-TRIIODOHYDROCINNAMATE,
See: Calcium Ipodate.
CALCIUM DIOCTYL SULFOSUCCINATE. Docusate
Calcium, U.S.P. XXI.
See: Surfak (Hoechst)
CALCIUM DISODIUM EDATHAMIL.
See: Edetate Calcium Disodium, U.S.P. XXI.
CALCIUM DISODIUM EDETATE. Edetate Calcium
Disodium, U.S.P. XXI.
CALCIUM DISODIUM VERSENATE. (Riker) Calcium
Disodium Edetate U.S.P. Amp. 1 gm./5 ml. in water
for injection. Box 6s.
Use: I.V.; lead poisoning.
CALCIUM EDETATE SODIUM. Edetate Calcium
Disodium, U.S.P. XXI.
CALCIUM EDTA.
See: Calcium Disod. Versenate, Amp., Tab. (Riker)
CALCIUM FOLINATE. B.A.N. Calcium N-[4-(2-amino-
5-formyl-5,6,7,8-tetrahydro-4-hydroxy-pteridin-6-
ylmethyl-aminobenzoyl]-L-glutamate.
Use: Antidote to folic acid antagonists.
See: Leucovorin Calcium
• **CALCIUM GLUBIONATE.** USAN. (1) (D-Gluconato)
(lactobionato) calcium monohydrate; (2) Calcium D-
gluconate lactobionate monohydrate.
Use: Calcium replenisher.
• **CALCIUM GLUCEPTATE,** U.S.P. XXI. (Lilly) Calcium
salt of d-glucoheptonic acid represents 0.09 Gm. cal-
cium (4.5 mEq.)/5 cc. Amp. 5 cc. 25s.
Use: Treatment of hypocalcemia.

• **CALCIUM GLUCEPTATE INJECTION,** U.S.P. XXI.
(Abbott) Calcium gluceptate 1.1 Gm. containing 90
mg. Ca/5 ml. Abboject Syringe (22G × 1½") 5 ml.,
Ampul 5 ml.
Use: Calcium therapy.
CALCIUM GLUCOHEPTONATE. (Various Mfr.) Cal.
D-glucoheptonate O.
Use: Uncontrolled muscular spasms due to lack of
calcium in blood.
• **CALCIUM GLUCONATE,** U.S.P. XXI. Injection, Tab.,
U.S.P. XXI. D-Gluconic acid, calcium salt.(2:1) **Inj.:**
(Upjohn) Each 10 ml. provides 94.68 mg. (4.72
mEq.) of Ca. **Amp.** 10 ml.; **Tab.** 5 gr., 7.5 gr., 10 gr.
or 15 gr.; **Wafers** 15 gr. (Various Mfr.)
W/Calcium ascorbate, benzyl alcohol, sodium bisulfite.
See: Cal-C-Bate, Amps. (Kay)
W/Vit. D (Lilly) Vit. D 660 u., cal. gluconate 1
Gm./Tab., Cal. gluconate 5 gr., Vit. D 330
u./Pulvule. Bot. 100s.
Use: Calcium and vitamin-D supplement.
CALCIUM GLYCEROPHOSPHATE. Neurosin.
(Various Mfr.)
• **CALCIUM HYDROXIDE,** U.S.P. XXI. Topical
Solution U.S.P. XXI.
Use: Astringent; pharm. necessity for calamine
lotion.
CALCIUM HYPOPHOSPHITE. (N.Y. Quinine & Chem.
Works)
CALCIUM IODIDE.
W/Codeine phosphate.
See: Calcidrine Syrup (Abbott)
W/Chloral hydrate, ephedrine HCl.
See: Iophed, Syr. (Marsh-Emory)
CALCIUM IODIZED.
Cal-Lime #1, Tab. (Scrie)
W/Calcium creosotate.
See: Niocrese, Tab. (Noyes)
W/Ipecac, ext. hyoscyamus, ext. licorice.
See: Kaldifane, Tab. (Noyes)
CALCIUM IODOBEHENATE. Calioben. (Various Mfr.)
CALCIUM IPODATE, Ipodate Calcium, U.S.P. XXI.
See: Oragrafin Calcium, Granules (Squibb)
CALCIUM KINATE GLUCONATE. Kinate is
hexahydrotetrahydroxybenzoate. Calcium Quinate
• **CALCIUM LACTATE,** U.S.P. XXI. Tab., U.S.P. XXI.
Propanoic acid, 2-hydroxy-, calcium salt (2:1), hy-
drate. Tab. (Upjohn) 650 mg. (4.2 mEq.) Ca/Tab.
Bot. 100s.
Use: Calcium deficiency and prophylaxis.
W/Calcium glycerophosphate.
See: Calphosan, Amp., Vial (Carlton)
W/Ca glycerophosphate, phenol, sod. chloride
solution.
See: Calpholac, Vial (Century)
Calphosan, Inj. (Brown)
W/Niacinamide, folic acid, ferrous gluconate,
vitamins.
See: Pergrava No. 2, Cap. (Arcum)
W/Phenobarbital, ext. hyoscyamus, terpin hydrate,
guaifenesin.
See: Gylanphen, Tab. (Lannett)
W/Theobromine sodium salicylate, phenobarbital.

See: Theolaphen, Tab. (Elder)
W/Thiamine HCl.
See: Nycralan, Tab. (Lannett)
W/Zinc sulfate.
See: Zinc-220, Cap. (Alto)
CALCIUM LACTOPHOSPHATE. Lactic acid hydrogen phosphate calcium salt.
CALCIUM LEUCOVORIN. Leucovorin Calcium, U.S.P. XXI.
Use: Overdosage folic acid antagonists.
• **CALCIUM LEVULINATE,** U.S.P. XXI. Inj., U.S.P. XXI. Pentanoic acid, 4-oxo-,calcium salt (2:1), dihydrate. Amp. 10%.
Use: Calcium replenisher.
See: Calcium Levulinate, Pow. (City Chemical)
Levucal, Amp. (Kay)
CALCIUM MANDELATE. (Various Mfr.). Urisept (Grail)
Use: Orally, urinary antiseptic & acidifier.
CALCIUM NOVOBIOCIN. Calcium salt of an antibacterial substance produced by *Streptomyces niveus.*
Use: Antibiotic.
CALCIUM OROTATE.
See: Calora, Tab. (Miller)
CALCIUM OXYTETRACYCLINE. Oxytetracycline Calcium, N.F. XIV.
• **CALCIUM PANTOTHENATE,** U.S.P. XXI. Tab., U.S.P. XXI. β-Alanine, N-(2,4-dihydroxy-3,3-dimethyl-1-oxobutyl)-,calcium salt (2:1). Vit. B-5. D(+)-N-(alpha, gamma dihydroxy-beta,beta-dimethyl-butyryl)-beta aminopropionic acid, calcium salt, dextro form.
Use: Vitamin B (enzyme co-factor).
See: Liver-Iron B Complex With Vitamin B-12, inj. (Maurry)
Pantholin, Tab. (Lilly)
W/Ascorbic acid, niacinamide, Vits. B-1, B-2, B-6, B-12, A, D, E.
See: Tota-Vi-Caps Gelatin Capsule, Cap. (Elder)
W/Calcium carbonate.
See: Ilomel, Pow. (Warren-Teed)
W/Calcium carbonate, ferrous fumarate, niacinamide.
See: Prenatag, Tab. (Reid-Provident)
W/Danthron.
See: Modane, Tab., Liq. (Warren-Teed)
Parlax, Tab. (Parmed)
W/Docusate sodium.
See: Pantyl, Tab. (McGregor)
W/Docusate sodium, acetphenolisatin.
See: Android-Plus, Tab. (Brown)
Peri-Pantyl, Tab. (McGregor)
W/Methoscopolamine nitrate, mephobarbital.
See: Ilocalm, Tabs. (Warren-Teed)
W/Niacin, vitamins.
See: Hi-Bee, Cap. (Vortech)
W/Niacinamide and vitamins.
See: Allbee C-800, Prods. (Robins)
Allbee T, Caps. (Robins)
Allbee with C, Caps. (Robins)
Ferrovite, Tab. (Laser)
Fumatinic, Tab. (Laser)
Maintenance Vitamin Formula, Tab. (Burgin-Arden)

Mulvidren, Tab. (Stuart)
OB-Tabs, Tab. (Laser)
Probec, Tab. (Stuart)
Probec-T, Tab. (Stuart)
Stuart Hematinic, Tab. (Stuart)
Stuart Therapeutic Multivitamin, Tab. (Stuart)
Therapeutic Vitamin Tablets, Tab. (Vortech)
Vita Cebus, Tab. (Cenci)
W/Niacinamide, B-1, B-2, B-6.
See: Noviplex Capsules, Cap. (Elder)
W/B-1, niacinamide, B-2, B-6, B-12, Vit. B-12, choline chloride, inositol, dl-methionine, testosterone, estrone, procaine.
See: Gerihorm, Inj. (Burgin-Arden)
W/Vitamin complex, ferrous fumarate, folic acid, calcium lactate, niacinamide.
See: Vitanate, Tab. (Century)
W/Vit. A, D, B-1, B-2, C, niacinamide, calcium. phosphorus, iron, Vit. B-6, B-12, E, magnesium, manganese, potassium, zinc, choline bitartrate, inositol.
See: Geriatric Vitamin Formula, Tab. (Burgin-Arden)
W/Vitamin C, niacin zinc sulf., Vit. E, B-1, B-2, B-6, B-12.
See: Z-Bec, Tab. (Robins)
W/Vitamin complex and iron.
See: Vita-iron, Tab. (Century)
W/Vitamins and minerals, niacinamide.
See: Arcum-VM, Cap. (Arcum)
Capre, Tab. (Marion)
Orovimin, Tab. (Reid-Provident)
Os-Cal Forte, Tab. (Marion)
Os-Vim, Tab. (Marion)
Stuartinic, Tab. (Stuart)
Theramin, Tab. (Arcum)
Theron, Tab. (Stuart)
Uplex, Cap. (Arcum)
Vit-Min-I-Fact, Tab. (Sutliff & Case)
W/Vitamins, minerals, methyl testosterone, ethinyl estradiol, niacinamide.
See: Geritag, Cap. (Reid-Provident)
W/Vitamin complex, yeast, niacinamide, desiccated liver.
See: B-Complex, Cap. (Vortech)
W/Vit. C, niacinamide, zinc sulf., magnesium sulf., Vit. B-1, B-2, B-6.
See: Vicon-C, Cap. (Meyer)
W/Zinc sulf., niacinamide, magnesium sulf., manganese Cl, Vitamin complex.
See: Vicon Plus, Cap. (Meyer)
• **CALCIUM PANTOTHENATE, RACEMIC,** U.S.P. XXI. β-Alanine, N-(2,4-dihydroxy-3,3-dimethyl-1-oxobutyl)-, calcium salt (2:1), (+-Calcium DL-pantothenate (1:2).
Use: Vitamin B (enzyme co-factor).
See: Pantholin (Lilly)
• **CALCIUM PHOSPHATE, DIBASIC,** U.S.P. XXI. Tab., U.S.P. XXI.
See: Dicalcium Phosphate
Diostate D, Tab. (Upjohn)
CALCIUM PHOSPHATE, MONOCALCIUM.
See: Dicalcium Phosphate

• **CALCIUM PHOSPHATE, TRIBASIC,** N.F. XVI.
(Various Mfr.)
CALCIUM-PHOSPHORUS-FREE.
See: Fosfree, Tab. (Mission)
• **CALCIUM POLYCARBOPHOL,** U.S.P. XXI.
Use: Cathartic.
CALCIUM PROPIONATE.
See: Propionate-caprylate mixtures.
CALCIUM QUINATE.
See: Calcium Kinate Gluconate
• **CALCIUM SACCHARATE,** U.S.P. XXI.
Use: Sweetening agent.
CALCIUM SACCHARIN. Saccharin Calcium, U.S.P.
XXI.
Use: Sweetening agent.
CALCIUM SALICYLATE, THEOBROMINE.
See: Theocalcin, Tab., Pow. (Knoll)
CALCIUM SALTS OF SUGAR ACIDS.
See: Gluco-Calcium, Vial (Lilly)
• **CALCIUM SILICATE,** N.F. XVI. A compound of
calcium oxide and silicon dioxide.
• **CALCIUM STEARATE,** N.F. XVI.
Use: Pharmaceutic aid (tablet lubricant).
CALCIUM SUCCINATE.
W/Aspirin.
See: Ber-Ex, Tab. (Dolcin)
Dolcin, Tab. (Dolcin)
W/Phenobarbital, salicylamide, Vit. C.
See: Calsuxaphen, Cap., Tab. (Lannett)
• **CALCIUM SULFATE,** N.F. XVI.
Use: Pharmaceutic aid (tablet diluent).
CALCIUM TRISODIUM PENTETATE. Calcium
trisodium   (carboxymethylimino)-bis(ethyl-enenitrilo)
tetra-acetic acid.
Use: Heavy metal antagonist.
See: Calcium Chel 330 (Geigy)
CALCIUM TRISODIUM PENTETATE. B.A.N. Calcium
chelate of the trisodium salt of diethylenetriamine-
NNN'N″N″-penta-acetic acid.
Use: Chelating agent.
CALCIUM UNDECYLENATE.
See: Caldesene, Pow. (Pharmacraft)
Cruex, Aerosol, Squeeze Pow., Cream
(Pharmacraft)
W/Hydrocortisone.
See: Caldecort, Oint. (Pennwalt)
CALCIWAFERS. (Nion) Calcium 165 mg., Vit. D. 66.7
I.U./Wafer. Bot. 96s.
Use: Dietary supplement.
CALDECORT CREAM. (Pharmacraft) Hydrocortisone
acetate equivalent to hydrocortisone 0.5% in cream
base. Tube 0.5 oz., 1 oz.
Use: Temporary relief from itching.
CALDECORT SPRAY. (Pharmacraft) Hydrocortisone
acetate 0.5%. Aerosol can 1.5 oz.
Use: Relief from itching.
CALDEE. (Jenkins) Ascorbic acid (sodium ascorbate
equiv. to 10 mg. Vit. C) 10 mg., Vit. D 200 I.U.,
dicalcium phosphate 7½ gr., irradiated yeast/Tab.
Bot. 1000s.
Use: Calcium deficiencies.

CALDEROL. (Upjohn) Calcifediol 20 mcg. or 50
mcg./Tab. Bot. 60s.
Use: Treatment of metabolic bone disease or
hypercalcemia associated with chronic renal failure
in renal dialysis patients.
CALDESENE. (Pharmacraft) **Oint:** Cod liver oil,
lanolin, petrolatum, talc, zinc oxide. Tube 1¼ oz.
Pow.: calcium undecylenate 10% pkg. 2 oz.,
5 oz.
Use: Diaper rash, burns, chafing.
CAL-D-MINT. (Enzyme Process) Calcium 800 mg., magnesium 150 mg., iron 18 mg., iodine 0.10 mg.,
copper 2 mg., Vit. D 200 I.U./2 Tab. Bot. 100s,
250s.
Use: Dietary mineral supplement.
CAL-D-PHOS. (Archer-Taylor) Dicalcium phosp. 4.5 gr.,
cal. gluconate 3 gr. w/D/Tab. Bot. 1000s.
CALFER-VITE. (Drug Industries) Ca 250 mg., iron 30
mg., Mn 2 mg., Cu 0.2 mg., Zn 1 mg., iodine 0.15
mg., niacinamide 20 mg., lemon bioflavonoid
complex 25 mg., A 5000 I.U., D 400 I.U., C 75 mg.,
B-1 3 mg., B-2 3 mg., B-6 2 mg., B-12 2 mcg., Ca
pantothenate 5 mg./Tab. Bot. 100s, 500s, 1000s.
Use: Prenatal vitamin and mineral supplement.
CALICARB. (Jenkins) Calcium carbonate 0.25 Gm.,
magnesium carbonate 0.15 Gm., bismuth subnitrate
60 mg., powd. ipecac 0.25 mg., aromatics/Tab.
Bot. 1000s.
Use: Gastric hyperacidity.
CALICYLIC CREME. (Gordon) Salicylic acid 10% in
cream base. Jar. 2 oz.
Use: Removal of heavy callus.
CAL-IM. (Standex; Kenyon) Calcium glycerophosphate
1%, calcium levulinate 1½%. Vial 30 cc.
CALINATE-FA. (Reid-Provident) Calcium 250 mg., Vit. A
4000 I.U., D 400 I.U., B-1 3 mg., B-2 3 mg., B-6 5 mg.,
B-12 1 mcg., folic acid 1 mg., C 50 mg., niacinamide
20 mg., d-panthenol 1 mg., iron 60 mg., iodine 0.02
mg., manganese 0.2 mg., magnesium 0.2 mg., zinc
0.1 mg., copper 0.15 mg./Tab. Bot. 100s, 1000s.
Use: Prenatal dietary supplement.
CALIOBEN.
See: Calcium Iodobehenate
CALIVITE. (Apco) Ca carbonate 885 mg., Fe sulfate
199 mg., Vit. A 3600 I.U., D 400 I.U., C 75 mg., B-1
1.5 mg., B-2 1.95 mg., B-6 0.75 mg., nicotinic acid 15
mg., Vit. B-12 activity 0.025 mcg., choline 1500 mcg.,
inositol 2500 mcg., pantothenic acid 75 mcg., folic
acid 25 mcg., p-aminobenzoic acid 12 mcg., K 10 mg.,
Mg 1.0 mg., Zn 0.075 mg., Mn 0.02 mg., Cu 0.01
mg., Co 0.02 mcg./Tab. Bot. 100s.
Use: Dietary supplement and prenatal vitamin.
CAL-LIME-1. (Scrip) Calcium iodized 1 gr./Tab. Bot.
1000s.
CALMOL 4-SUPPOSITORIES. (Mentholatum) Zinc
oxide in a cocoa butter-lanolin alcohol base. Box 12s,
24s.
Use: Rectal suppository that protects against
irritation and trauma.
CALMOSIN. (Spanner) Cal. gluconate, strontium
bromide. Ampul 10 cc. 100s.
CALOMEL. Mercurous chloride.

Use: Cathartic.

CALORA. (Miller) Calcium (as calcium orotate) 65 mg./3 Tab. Bot. 100s.

CALOR-AID. (American McGaw) Instant drink, high calorie, protein-free dietetic aid.
Use: Dietary supplement.

CALOTABS, Reformulated. (Calotabs) Docusate sodium 100 mg., casanthranol 30 mg./Tab. Box 10s.
Use: Laxative.

CALOXIDE CREAM W/BENZOCAINE. (Blue Line) Calamine 10%, zinc oxide 10%, ethyl aminobenzoate (benzocaine) 3% in a water miscible base. Tube 1½ oz.
Use: Topically, protective & antiseptic.

CALOXIDINE (IODIZED CALCIUM).
See: Calcium Iodized

CAL-NOR. (Vortech) Ca glycerophosphate 1%, Ca levulinate 1.5%. Vial 100 ml.
Use: Calcium deficiency.

CALPHOSAN. (Brown) Cal. lactate 50 mg. & cal. glycerophosphate 50 mg., phenol 0.25% (preservative), physiological solution of sodium chloride q.s./10 cc. Amp. 10 cc. Box 10s, 100s; Vial 60 cc.
Use: Therapy for calcium deficiency.

CALPHOSAN-B-12. (Brown) Calphosan plus Vit. B-12 300 mcg./10 cc. Vials 60 cc.
Use: Therapy for calcium deficiency.

CALSA. (Amlab) Aspirin 2 gr., sodium salicylate 3 gr., calcium carbonate 1 gr., calcium ascorbate 10 mg., para-aminobenzoic acid 10 mg./Tab. Bot. 60s, 100s.
Use: Analgesic, anodyne.

CALSAN. (Burgin-Arden) Calcium glycerophosphate 10 mg., calcium levulinate 15 mg., chlorobutanol 0.5%/cc. Inj. Vial, 100 cc.
Use: Calcium therapy.

CALSARBAIN TABLETS. (Sutliff & Case) Phenobarbital ¼ gr., Ca carbonate 3 gr., sod. bicarbonate 3 gr., papain 1 gr., pancreatin 1 gr., benzocaine ¼ gr./Tab. Bot. 100s, 1000s.

CALSCORBATE. (O'Neal, Jones & Feldman) Vit. D 50 I.U., C 89.5 mg., calcium 262 mg., phosphorus 194 mg./Tab. Bot. 100s.
Use: Multivitamin.

CAL-SUP. (Riker) Calcium carbonate 750 mg./Tab. Bot. 100s.
Use: Calcium supplement.

CALSUXAPHEN. (Lannett) Calcium succinate 2½ gr., salicylamide 4 gr., phenobarbital ⅛ gr., Vitamin C 30 mg./Cap., Tab. Bot. 250s, 500s, 1000s.
Use: Sedative.

CALTRATE 600. (Lederle) Calcium carbonate 600 mg./Tab. Bot. 60s.
Use: High potency calcium supplement.

• **CALUSTERONE.** USAN. (1) 17β-Hydroxy-7β, 17-dimethylandrost-4-ene-3-one; (2) 7β, 17α-dimethyl testosterone.
Use: Antineoplastic.

CAMA ARTHRITIS PAIN RELIEVER. (Dorsey) Aspirin 500 mg., magnesium oxide 150 mg., aluminum hydroxide gel 150 mg./Tab. Bot. 36s, 50s, 100 200s.
Use: Temporary relief of minor arthritic pain.

CAMALOX. (Rorer) Suspension of aluminum hydroxide 225 mg., magnesium hydroxide 200 mg., calcium carbonate 250 mg./5 ml. Bot. 12 oz.
Use: Antacid.

CAMALOX TABLETS. (Rorer) Magnesium hydroxide 200 mg., aluminum hydroxide 225 mg., calcium carbonate 250 mg./Tab. Bot. 50s.
Use: Antacid.

• **CAMBENDAZOLE.** USAN. Isopropyl 2-(4-thiazolyl)-5-benzi-midazolecarbamate.
Use: Anthelmintic, veterinary medicine.
See: Camvet (MSD AGVET)

CAMELLIA LOTION. (O'Leary) Moisturizer lotion for face, hands and body. Bot. 4 oz.

CAMEO OIL. (Medco Lab) Mineral oil base, synthetic spreading oil, de-waxed oil-soluble principle of lanolin, and proper surfactants. Pl. bot. 8 oz., 16 oz., 32 oz.
Use: Emollient, antipruritic and cleansing agent as bath oil.

CAMPHO-PHENIQUE. (Winthrop Products) **Liq.:** Phenol 4.7%, camphor 10.8%. Bot. 0.75 oz., 1.5 oz., 4 oz. **Gel.:** 0.23 oz., 0.5 oz.
Use: Topical antiseptic.

CAMPHO-PHENIQUE LIP BALM. (Winthrop Products) Padimate O, hydrogenated vegetable oil, microcrystalline wax, mineral oil, cetyl esters, wax, lanolin oil, camphor, phenol. Stick 0.15 oz.
Use: Antiseptic.

• **CAMPHOR,** U.S.P. XXI. Spirit U.S.P. XXI. Bicyclo-[2.2.1.]heptane-2-one, 1,7,7-trimethyl. 2-Bornanone.
Use: Topical antipruritic; anti-infective; pharm. necessity for camphorated phenol, paregoric and flexible collodion, antitussive, expectorant, local counterirritant, nasal decongestant.
See: Vicks Inhaler (Vicks)
    Vicks Regular and Wild Cherry Medicated Cough Drops (Vicks)
    Vicks Medi-Trating Throat Lozenges (Vicks)
    Vicks Sinex, Nasal Spray (Vicks)
    Vicks Vaporub, Oint. (Vicks)
    Vicks Vaposteam, Liq. (Vicks)
    Vicks Va-Tro-Nol, Nose Drops (Vicks)

CAMPHOR, MONOBROMATED. 3-Bromo-2-borna-none.

• **CAMPHORATED, PARACHLOROPHENOL,** U.S.P. XXI.
Use: Anti-infective (dental).

CAMPHORIC ACID. 1,2,2-Trimethyl-1,3-cyclopentanedicarboxylic acid.

CAMPHORIC ACID ESTER. Ester of p-Tolylmethylcarbinal as Diethanolamine Salt.

CAMPTROPIN. (Jenkins) Caffeine alkaloid 5 mg., camphor 12 mg., atropine sulfate 0.1 mg./Tab. Bot. 1000s.
Use: Common cold and hay fever.

CAMVET. (MSD AGVET) Cambendazole
Paste: 45% cambendazole;
Pellets: 5.3% cambendazole;
Susp.: 3%.

Use: Anthelmintic, veterinary medicine.

CANDEX. (Miles Pharm) **Lotion:** Nystatin 100,000 u./ml. Bot. 30 ml.
Use: Treatment moniliasis.

• **CANDICIDIN,** U.S.P. XXI. Oint., Vag. Tab., U.S.P. XXI. An antifungal antibiotic derived from *Strep. griseus.*
Use: Local antifungal.
See: Candeptin, Vag. Tabs, Oint. (Julius Schmid) Vanobid, Oint. & Vag. Tab. (Merrell Dow)

CANDICIDIN. B.A.N. One or more of a mixture of heptanes with antifungal activity produced by *Streptomyces griseus* and other *Streptomyces* species.

C & T. (Hyrex) Vit B-12 1000 mg., thiamine 100 mg./ml. Vial 10 ml.
Use: Vitamin B deficiencies.

CANDYCON. (Allison) Chlorprophenpyridamine maleate 2 mg., phenylephrine HCl 5 mg./Tab. Bot. 50s.
Use: Antihistamine-Decongestant.

CANNABINOL. B.A.N. 6,6,9-Trimethyl-3-pentyl-benzo[c]chromen-l-ol.

CANOPAR. (Burroughs Wellcome).
See: Thenium closylate

• **CANRENOATE POTASSIUM.** USAN.
Use: Aldosterone antagonist.

• **CANRENONE.** USAN.
Use: Aldosterone antagonist.

CANTHARIDIN.
Use: Treatment for removal of warts.
See: Cantharone, Liq. (Ingram)

CANTIL. (Merrell Dow) Mepenzolate bromide. 25 mg./Tab. Bot. 100s.
Use: Adjunctive treatment of peptic ulcer.

CANTIL W/PHENOBARBITAL. (Merrell Dow) Mepenzolate bromide 25 mg., phenobarbital 16 mg./Tab. Bot. 100s.
Use: Adjunctive treatment of peptic ulcer and irritable bowel.

CANTRI. (Hauck) Sulfisoxazole 10%, aminacrine HCl 0.2%, allantoin 2%/Tube. Tube 90 Gm.
Use: Treatment of vaginitis and cervicitis.

CANZ. (O'Neal, Jones & Feldman) Pepsin 260 mg., pancreatin 260 mg., dehydrocholic acid 40 mg./Tab. Bot. 100s, 500s, 1000s.
Use: Digestive aid.

C-A-P. (Eastman) Cellulose acetate phthalate.

CAPA. (U.S. Ethicals) Acetaminophen 432 mg./Tab. Bot. 20s, 100s, 500s.
Use: Antipyretic, analgesic.

CAPAHIST-DMH. (Freeport) Chlorpheniramine maleate 8 mg., phenylpropanolamine HCl 50 mg., atropine sulfate ¹/₁₈₀ gr., dextromethorphan HBr 20 mg./T.R. Cap.
Use: Relief from coughing and URI congestion.

CAPASTAT SULFATE. (Lilly) Capreomycin sulfate 1 Gm./10 ml. Vial 10 ml. Box 10s.
Use: Antituberculostatic.

CAPILLARIS X OINTMENT. (Guild) Pkg. 1 oz., 3½ oz.
CAPILLARIS X SHAMPOO. (Guild) Pkg. 6 oz.
CAPITAL W/CODEINE. (Carnrick) Codeine

phosphate 30 mg., acetaminophen 325 mg./Tab. Bot. 100s.
Use: Analgesic.

CAPITAL WITH CODEINE SUSPENSION. (Carnrick) Acetaminophen 120 mg., codeine phosphate 12 mg./5 ml. Bot. 16 oz.
Use: Analgesic.

CAPITROL CREAM SHAMPOO. (Westwood) 5,7-dichloro-8-hydroxyquinoline. Chloroxine 2% in a shampoo base containing: Sodium octoxynol-3 sulfonate, PEG-6 lauramide, dextrin, stearyl alcohol/ceteareth-20, sodium lauryl sulfoacetate, docusate sodium, magnesium aluminum silicate, PEG-14M, EDTA, benzyl alcohol 1%, citric acid, water, color, fragrance. Tube 85 Gm.
Use: Treatment of dandruff & mild to moderately severe seborrheic dermatitis of the scalp.

Ca-PLUS. (Miller) Calcium (as contained in a calcium-protein complex made with specially isolated soy protein and torula yeast) 280 mg./Tab. Bot. 100s.
Use: Calcium deficiency.

CAPNITRO. (Freeport) Nitroglycerin 6.5 mg./T.R. Cap. Bot. 100s.
Use: Peripheral vasodilator.

• **CAPOBENATE SODIUM.** USAN. Sodium 6-(3,4,5-trimethoxybenzamido) Hexanoate.
Use: Cardiac depressant (antiarrhythmic).

• **CAPOBENIC ACID.** USAN. 6-(3,4,5-Trimethoxybenzamido)-hexanoic acid.
Use: Cardiac depressant (antiarrhythmic).

CAPOTEN. (Squibb) Captopril 25 mg., 50 mg., or 100 mg./Tab. Bot 100s.
Use: Antihypertensive agent.

CAPREOMYCIN. B.A.N. An antibiotic produced by *Streptomyces capreolus.*
See: Capastat sulfate

• **CAPREOMYCIN SULFATE STERILE,** U.S.P. XXI. An antibiotic derived from *Streptomyces capreolus.* Caprocin.
Use: Antibiotic (tuberculostatic).
See: Capastat Sulfate, Amp. (Lilly)

CAPROCHLORONE. Levo-gamma-(o-chlorobenzyl)-delta-oxo-gamma-phenylcaproic acid.

CAPRON. (Vitarine) Acetaminophen 227 mg., aspirin 227 mg., caffeine anh., 32.4 mg./Cap. Bot. 18s, 1000s.
Use: Analgesic.

CAPROXAMINE. B.A.N. (E)-3′-Amino-4′-methyl-hexanophenone O-(2-aminoethyl)oxime.
Use: Antidepressant.

CAPRYLATE-PROPIONATE MIXTURES.
See: Sopronol, Preps. (Wyeth)

CAPRYLATE, SALTS.
See: Sodium Caprylate
Zinc Caprylate

CAPRYLATE SODIUM, INJECTION.
Ingram—Amp. 33%, 1 cc. Pkg. 12s, 25s, 100s.
Use: Fungus infections of skin.
See: Sodium Caprylate Preps.

CAPSICUM OLEORESIN.
W/Alcohol, benzocaine, oxyquinoline, thymol, capsicum oleoresin.

See: Dent's Dental Poultice (C. S. Dent)
W/Alcohol, chlorobutanol hydrous (chloroform
derivative), phenol, eugenol, cresol.
See: Dent's Toothache Drops Treatment (C. S.
Dent)
W/Benzocaine, phenol.
See: Dent's Toothache Gum (C. S. Dent)
W/Camphor, corn oil, cajuput oil and turpentine oil.
See: Capsolin, Oint. (Parke-Davis)
W/Methyl salicylate, oil of camphor, oil of pine,
turpentine oil.
See: Sloan's Liniment, Liq. (Warner-Lambert)
CAPSULES, EMPTY GELATIN. (Lilly) Lilly markets
clear empty gelatin capsules in sizes
000,00,0,1,2,3,4,5.
* **CAPTAMINE HYDROCHLORIDE.** USAN. N-(2-mer-
captoethyl)dimethylamine hydrochloride.
Use: Cutaneous depigmenting activity.
CAPTODIAME. B.A.N. 4-Butylthiobenzhydryl 2-dime-
thylaminoethyl sulfide.
Use: Tranquilizer.
See: Covatin hydrochloride.
CAPTODIAME HCl. 4-Butylthio-a-phenylbenzyl 2-dime-
thylaminoethyl sulfide. Covatin hydrochloride.
* **CAPTOPRIL.** USAN. Angiotensin I converting
enzyme inhibitor.
Use: Antihypertensive agent.
See: Capoten, Tab. (Squibb)
CAPULETS. (Vitarine) Vit. A 5000 I.U., D 400 I.U.,
B-1 2.5 mg., B-2 2.5 mg., B-6 0.5 mg., C 50 mg., cal.
pantothenate 5 mg., niacinamide 20 mg., cobalamin
2 mcg./Cap. Bot. 100s, 250s, 1000s.
CAPULETS M CAPTABS. (Vitarine) Vit. A 5000 I.U.,
D 400 I.U., B-1 2.5 mg., B-2 2.5 mg., C 50 mg., niacina-
mide 20 mg., B-6 0.5 mg., Ca. pantothenate 5 mg.,
B-12 2 mcg., Fe 10 mg., iodine 0.05 mg., Cu 0.5 mg.,
Mn 0.5 mg., Mg 6 mg., Zn 0.5 mg., Ca 50 mg./Tab. Bot.
100s.
* **CAPURIDE.** USAN.
Use: Hypnotic.
CAQUIN. (O'Neal, Jones & Feldman) Hydrocortisone
1%, clioquinol 3%. Cream. Tube 20 Gm.
Use: Derma-steroid.
* **CARACEMIDE.** USAN.
Use: Antineoplastic.
CARAFATE. (Marion) Sucralfate 1 Gm./Tab. Bot.
100s. Unit dose, Ctn. 500s.
Use: Treatment of duodenal ulcers.
* **CARAMEL,** N.F. XVI.
Use: Pharm. aid (Color).
CARAMIPHEN. B.A.N. 2-Diethylaminoethyl 1-phenylcy-
clopentane-1-carboxylate.
Use: Treatment of the Parkinsonian syndrome.
See: Parpanit hydrochloride
Taoryi edisylate
CARAMIPHEN EDISYLATE.
W/Phenylpropanolamine.
See: Tuss-Ornade, Prods. (SmithKline)
CARAMIPHEN ETHANEDISULFONATE.
W/Phenylephrine hydrochloride, phenindamine
tartrate.
See: Dondril, Tab. (Whitehall)

CARAMIPHEN HYDROCHLORIDE. 1-Phenylcyclo-
pentanecarboxylic acid 2-diethyl-aminoethyl ester hy-
drochloride.
Use: Proposed for muscular spasm & tremor in
Parkinson's disease.
* **CARAWAY,** N.F. XVI. Oil, N.F. XVI.
Use: Flavor.
CARBACEL. (Softcon) Sterile buffered aqueous
methulose solution containing carbachol U.S.P. in
¾%, 1½%, 3% strengths, with benzalkonium
chloride. 15 cc. plastic direct-application bots.
Use: Glaucoma.
* **CARBACHOL,** U.S.P. XXI. Intraocular Sol., Ophth.
Soln., U.S.P. XXI. Ethanaminium, 2-(aminocarbonyl-
)oxy-N,N,N-trimethyl-, chloride. Carbamycholine chlo-
ride. Choline chloride carbamate, Lentin, Carbolin.
Use: Parasympathomimetic agent; cholinergic.
See: Carbacel, Sol. (Softcon)
Miostat Intraocular, Solution (Alcon)
Murocarb, Soln. (Muro)
W/Methylcellulose.
See: Isopto Carbachol, Soln. (Alcon)
CARBACRYLAMINE RESINS.
Use: Cation-exchange resin.
* **CARBADOX.** USAN. Methyl 3-quinoxalin-2-yl-
methylenecarbazate N¹N⁴-dioxide.
Use: Antibacterial, veterinary medicine.
See: Mecadox.
CARBAMATE.
See: Valmid, Tab. (Lilly)
CARBAMAZEPINE. B.A.N. Dibenz[b,f]azepine-5-
carboxamide.
Use: Treatment of trigeminal neuralgia.
See: Tegretol
* **CARBAMAZEPINE,** U.S.P. XXI. Tab., U.S.P. XXI.
5H-dibenz[b,f]azepine-5-carboxamide.
Use: Treatment epilepsy & trigeminal neuralgia.
See: Tegretol, Tab. (Geigy)
CARBAMIDE.
See: Urea U.S.P. XXI. (Various Mfr.)
CARBAMIDE COMPOUNDS.
See: Acetylcarbromal (Various Mfr.)
Bromisovalum (Various Mfr.)
Bromural, Tab. (Knoll)
Carbrital, Elix. & Kap. (Parke-Davis)
Carbromal (Various Mfr.)
Carbropent, Tab. (Blue Line)
Iotis, Liq. (Research Pharmacal Lab.)
Sedamyl, Tab. (Riker)
* **CARBAMIDE PEROXIDE TOPICAL SOLUTION,**
U.S.P. XXI. Urea compound w/hydrogen peroxide
(1:1).
Use: Local anti-infective (dental).
See: Clear Drops. (Internat. Pharm.)
Urea-Peroxide (Various Mfr.)
CARBAMIDE PEROXIDE, 6.5% IN GLYCERIN.
Use: Softening hardened ear wax
See: Murine Ear Drops (Abbott)
Murine Ear Wax Removal System (Abbott)
N-CARBAMOYLARSANILIC ACID.
See: Carbarsone, U.S.P. XXI. (Var. Mfr.)

CARBAMINO PHENYL-ARSONIC ACID.
See: Carbarsone (Various Mfr.)
**(3-CARBAMOYL-3,3-DIPHENYLPROPYL)-DIISOPRO-
PYLMETHYLAMMONIUM IODIDE.**
See: Isopropamide Iodide
CARBAMYLCHOLINE CHLORIDE.
See: Carbachol
CARBAMYLMETHYLCHOLINE CHLORIDE.
See: Urecholine, Tab., Inj. (Merck Sharp & Dohme)
• **CARBANTEL LAURYL SULFATE.** USAN.
Use: Anthelmintic.
• **CARBARSONE,** U.S.P. XXI. Caps., U.S.P. XXI. (Var.
Mfr.) N-carbamoylarsanilic acid. Amabevan, ameban,
amibiarson, arsambide, fenarsone, leucarsone,
aminarsone, amebarsone. p-Ureidobenzenearsonic
acid.
Pulvule (Lilly) (250 mg.) Bot. 20s.
Use: Acute & chronic amebiasis & trichomoniasis.
CARBARYL. B.A.N. 1-Naphthyl methylcarbamate.
Use: Insecticide, veterinary medicine.
See: Sevin
• **CARBASPIRIN CALCIUM.** USAN.
Use: Analgesic.
• **CARBAZERAN.** USAN.
Use: Cardiotonic.
CARBAZOCHROME SALICYLATE. Adrenochrome
Monosemicarbazone Sod. Salicylate Complex.
See: Adrenosem Salicylate, Amp, Syr., Tab.
(Beecham-Massengill)
CARBAZOCINE. (Warner-Lambert) cis-14-(Cyclo-
propylmethyl)-1,2,3,4,4a,5,6,11-octa-hydro-5-11b-imi-
noethano-11bH-benzo(a)carbazole.
Use: Analgesic.
CARBENICILLIN. B.A.N. 6-(α-Carboxyphenyl-acetami-
do)penicillanic acid.
Use: Antibiotic.
See: Pyopen.
• **CARBENICILLIN DISODIUM, STERILE,** U.S.P. XXI.
Sterile, U.S.P. XXI. 4-Thia-1-azabicyclo[3.2.0]-hep-
tane-2-carboxylic acid, 6-[(carboxyphenylacetyl)-ami-
no]-3,3-dimethyl-7-oxo-, disodium salt. N-(2-Carboxy-
3,3-dimethyl-7-oxo-4-thia-1-azabicyclo-[3.2.0]-hept-
6-yl)-2-phenylmalonamic acid disodium salt.
Use: Antibacterial.
See: Geopen disodium, Vial (Roerig)
Pyopen, Inj. (Beecham Labs)
• **CARBENICILLIN INDANYL SODIUM,** U.S.P. XXI.
Tabs., U.S.P. XXI.
See: Geocillin, Tab. (Roerig)
• **CARBENICILLIN PHENYL SODIUM.** USAN.
Use: Antibacterial.
• **CARBENICILLIN POTASSIUM.** USAN.
Use: Antibacterial
CARBENOXOLONE. B.A.N. 3β-(3-Carboxypropionylox-
y)-11-oxo-olean-12-en-30-oic acid.
Use: Treatment of peptic ulcer.
See: Biogastrone
Bioral
Duogastrone disodium salt
• **CARBENOXOLONE SODIUM.** USAN.
Use: Glucocorticoid.
CARBENZIDE. (Warner-Lambert) Ethyl 3-(a-methylbe-
nyl) carbazate. Under study.

Use: Anti-depressant, monoamine oxidase inhibitor.
CARBETAPENTANE CITRATE. 2-[2-(Diethylamino)e-
thoxy] ethyl 1-phenyl-cyclopentyl-1-carboxylate dihy-
drogen citrate.
Use: Antitussive.
W/Codeine phosphate, chlorpheniramine maleate,
guaifenesin.
See: Tussar-2, Syr. (Armour)
W/Terpin hydrate, menthol, alcohol, sod. citrate, citric
acid, glycerin.
See: Toclonol Expectorant, Liq. (Cenci)
W/Terpin hydrate, sod. citrate, citric acid, menthol
glycerin, alcohol, codeine.
See: Toclonol W/Codeine, Liq. (Cenci)
CARBETAPENTANE TANNATE
W/Chlorpheniramine tannate, ephedrine tannate,
phenylephrine tannate.
See: Rynatuss Tabules, Susp., Tab. (Mallinckrodt)
CARBETHOXYSYRINGOYL METHYLRESERPATE.
See: Singoserp, Tab. (Ciba)
CARBETHYL SALICYLATE.
See: Sal-Ethyl Carbonate, Tab. (Parke-Davis)
• **CARBETIMER.** USAN.
• **CARBIDOPA,** U.S.P. XXI. 2-(3,4-Dihydroxybenzyl)-
2-hydrazinopropionic acid; (-)-Lα-hydrazino-α-
methyl-β-(3,4-dihydroxybenzene) propanoic acid
monohydrate.
Use: Decarboxylase inhibitor.
W/Levodopa
See: Sinemet, Tab. (Merck Sharp & Dohme)
• **CARBIDOPA AND LEVODOPA TABLETS,** U.S.P.
XXI.
Use: Treatment of Parkinsonian syndrome.
CARBIMAZOLE. B.A.N. Ethyl 3-methyl-2-thioimidazo-
line-1-carboxylate.
Use: Antithyroid substance.
See: Bimazol
Neo-Mercazole.
CARBIMAZOLE. 1-Ethoxycarbonyl-2:3-di-hydro-3-
methyl-2-thioimidazole. Neo-Mercazole.
CARBINOXAMINE. B.A.N. 2-(4-Chloro-α-2-pyridylben-
zyloxy-ethyldimethylamine. Davenol. Extil hydrogen
maleate.
Use: Antihistamine.
See: Clistin, Tab. (McNeil)
CARBINOXAMINE HCl.
W/acetaminophen, phenylephrine HCl.
• **CARBINOXAMINE MALEATE,** U.S.P. XXI. Tabs.,
U.S.P. XXI. 2-[p-Chloro-alpha-[(2-(dimethyl-amino-
ethoxy)]benzyl]pyridine bimaleate.
Use: Antihistaminic.
See: Clistin Elix., Tab. (McNeil)
W/Acetaminophen.
See: Clistin-D, Tab. (McNeil)
W/Ammonium chloride, pot. guaiacol sulfonate, sod.
citrate.
See: Clistin Expectorant (McNeil)
W/Pseudoephedrine HCl.
See: Rondec Prods. (Ross)
W/Pseudoephedrine HCl, dextromethorphan HBr.
See: Rondec DM, Drops and Syrup (Ross)
CARBIPHENE. B.A.N. α-Ethoxy-N-methyl-N—

[2-(N-methylphenethylamino)ethyl]diphenyl-
acetamide.
See: Jubalon hydrochloride.
Use: Analgesic.

CARBIPHENE HCl. USAN. 2-Ethoxy-N-methyl-n-[2-
(methylphenethylamino)ethyl]-2, 2-diphenyl-aceta-
mide HCl.
Use: Analgesic.

CARBOCAINE. (Cook-Waite) Mepivacaine HCl 30 mg.,
NaCl 3 mg./1.8 ml. Cartridge. Mepivacaine HCl 20
mg., levonordefrin 0.05 mg., NaCl 4 mg., acetone
sodium bisulfite not more than 2 mg./1.8 ml.
Cartrige.
Use: Local anesthetic (dental).

CARBOCAINE HCl. (Winthrop-Breon) Mepivacaine
HCl. **1%**: Single Dose Vial 30 ml. Multiple Dose
Vial 50 ml.; **1.5%**: Single Dose Vial 30 ml.; **2%**:
Single Dose Vial 20 ml. Multiple Dose Vial 50 ml.
Use: Nerve block, caudal, epidural, and infiltration.

CARBOCLORAL. USAN. Ethyl (2,2,2,-trichloro-1-hy-
droxyethyl)carbamate.
Use: Hypnotic.
See: Chloralurethane.
   Prodorm (Parke-Davis)

CARBOCYSTEINE. USAN.
Use: Mucolytic.

CARBOL-FUCHSIN PAINT. Original fuchsin formula
known as Castellani's Paint. Fuchsin 0.3%, boric
acid 1%, phenol 4.5%, resorcinol 10%, acetone
5%, alcohol 10%, water q.s. 1 oz., 4 oz., 1 pt.
Use: Local antifungal.
See: Carfusin, Sol. (Rorer)
   Castaderm, Lot. (Lannett)
   Castellani's Paint (Various Mfr.)

CARBOL-FUCHSIN TOPICAL SOLUTION, U.S.P.
XXI.
Use: Topical antifungal.

CARBOLONIUM BROMIDE. B.A.N.
Hexamethylenedi(carbamoylcholine bromide).
Hexcarbacholine Bromide (I.N.N.)
Use: Muscle relaxant.
See: Imbretil.

CARBOMER, N.F. XVI. A polymer of acrylic acid,
crosslinked with a polyfunctional agent.
Use: Pharmaceutic aid (suspending agent);
emulsifying agent.
See: Carbopol 934 P (Goodrich)

CARBOMER. B.A.N. A polymer of acrylic acid
crosslinked with allyl sucrose.
Use: Pharmaceutical aid.
See: Carbopol 934.

CARBOMER 910. USAN.
Use: Pharmaceutic aid.

CARBOMER 934. USAN.
Use: Pharmaceutic aid.

CARBOMER 934P. USAN.
Use: Pharmaceutic aid.

CARBOMER 940. USAN.
Use: Pharmaceutic aid.

CARBOMER 941. USAN.
Use: Pharmaceutic aid.

CARBOMYCIN. An antibiotic from *Streptomyces
halstedii.*

CARBON DIOXIDE, U.S.P. XXI.
Use: Inhalation, respiratory stimulant.
See: Ceo-Two, Supp. (Beutlich)

CARBON TETRACHLORIDE, N.F. XVI.
Benzinoform. (Var. Mfr.)
Use: Pharm. aid (solvent).

CARBONATES NO. 3. (Noyes) Calcium carbonate
3½ gr., Mg carbonate 2½ gr., bismuth
subcarbonate ½ gr./Tab. Bot. 100s, 1000s.

CARBONIC ACID, DILITHIUM SALT. Lithium
Carbonate, U.S.P. XXI.

CARBONIC ACID, DISODIUM SALT. Sodium
carbonate, N.F. XVI.

CARBONIC ACID, MONOSODIUM SALT. Sodium
Bicarbonate, U.S.P. XXI.

CARBONIC ANHYDRASE INHIBITOR.
See: Daranide, Tab. (Merck Sharp & Dohme)
   Diamox, Tab., Sequel, Vial (Lederle)
   Hydrazol, Tab. (Softcon)
   Neptazane, Tab. (Lederle)

CARBONIS DETERGENS, LIQUOR.
See: Coal Tar Solution.

CARBONYL DIAMIDE.
See: Chap Cream (Ar-Ex)

CARBOPHENOTHION. B.A.N. S-(4)Chlorophenylthi-
omethyl)00)diethyl phosphorodithioate.
Use: Insecticide, veterinary medicine.
See: Garrathion
   Trithion

CARBOPLATIN. USAN.
Use: Antineoplastic.

CARBOPOL 934 P. (Goodrich) Carbomer.

CARBOPROST. USAN.
Use: Oxytocic.

CARBOPROST TROMETHAMINE, U.S.P. XXI. Inj.,
U.S.P. XXI.
Use: Oxytocic.
See: Prostin, Amp. (Upjohn)

CARBOSE D.
See: Carboxymethylcellulose sodium, Prep. (Various
Mfr.)

CARBOTABS. (Jenkins) Sodium bicarbonate 3⅓ gr.,
magnesium carbonate 1 gr., calcium carbonate ¾
gr., papain ¹/₃₂ gr., pancreatin ¹/₃₂ gr./Tab. Bot.
1000s.
Use: Effervescent antacid.

CARBOWAX, 300, 400, 1540, 4000. Polyethylene
glycol 300, 400, 1540, 4000.

CARBOXIN. (Kay) Methocarbamol 500 mg., or 750
mg./Tab. Bot. 100s, 500s.
Use: Musculo-skeletal conditions.

**CARBOXYMETHYLCELLULOSE SALT OF
DEXTROAMPHETAMINE.** Carboxyphen.
See: Bontril Timed Tab. (Carnrick)

CARBOXYMETHYLCELLULOSE SODIUM, U.S.P.
XXI. Paste, Tab., U.S.P. XXI. Cellulose,
carboxymethyl ester, sod. salt. Carbose D, C.M.C.
(Hercules Pow. Co.)
Use: Pharm. aid (suspending agent; tablet
excipient; viscosity-increasing agent); cathartic.
W/Acetphenolisatin, docusate sodium.
See: Scrip-Lax, Tab. (Scrip)
W/Alginic acid, sodium bicarbonate.

See: Pretts, Tabs. (Marion)
W/Belladonna ext., kaolin, pectin, zinc
phenosulfonate.
See: Gelcomul, Liq. (Commerce)
W/Danthron, Vit. B-1, oxyethylene oxpropylene
polymer.
See: Evactol, Cap. (Delta)
W/Digitoxin.
See: Foxalin, Cap. (Standex)
Thegitoxin (Standex)
W/Docusate sodium.
See: Dialose, Cap. (Stuart)
W/Docusate sodium, casanthranol.
See: Dialose Plus, Cap. (Stuart)
Disolan Forte, Cap. (Lannett)
Tri-Vac, Cap. (Rhode)
W/Docusate sodium, oxyphenisatin acetate.
See: Dialose Plus, Cap. (Stuart)
W/Methylcellulose.
See: Ex-Caloric, Wafer (Eastern Research)
W/Testosterone, estrone, sod. chloride.
See: Tostestro, Inj. (Bowman)
• **CARBOXYCELLULOSE SODIUM 12,** N.F. XVI.
CARBOXYMETHYLCYSTEINE. B.A.N. S-Carboxyme-
thylcysteine.
Use: Mucolytic agent.
See: Mucodyne
Thiodril
3,3-CARBOXYMETHYLENE Bis-(4-Hydroxycouma-
rin)ethyl ester. Tromexan.
CARBOXYPHEN
W/Butabarbital.
See: Bontril, Timed Tab. (G. W. Carnrick)
CARBROMAL. (Various Mfr.) Bromodiethylacetylurea,
bromadel, nyctal, planadalin, uradal.
Use: Sedative & mild hypnotic.
W/Bromisovalum (Bromural).
See: Bro-T's, Tab. (Brothers)
W/Pentobarbital sod.
See: Carbropent, Tab. (Blue Line)
CARBROPENT. (Blue Line) Pentobarbital sod. 1½
gr., carbromal 4 gr./Tab. Bot. 100s, 1000s.
Use: Sedative & hypnotic.
CARBUTAMIDE. B.A.N. 1-Butyl-3-sulphanilylurea.
Use: Hypoglycemic agent.
See: Bucrol
Invenol
Nadisan
CARBUTAMIDE. N-Butyl-N'-sulfanilyl-urea. Burcol;
BZ. 55; Invenol; Nadisan.
Use: Oral hypoglycemic agent.
• **CARBUTEROL HYDROCHLORIDE.** USAN.
Use: Bronchodilator.
CARDABID. (Saron) Nitroglycerine 2.5 mg./S.R.Tab.
Bot. 60s, 100s.
Use: Antianginal.
• **CARDAMON** N.F. XVI. Oil, seed, Cpd. Tincture; N.F.
XVI.
Use: Flavor.
CARDENZ. (Miller) Vit. C 25 mg., E 5 mg., inositol 30
mg., p-aminobenzoic acid 9 mg., A 2000 I.U., B-6 1.5
mg., B-12 1 mcg., D 100 I.U., niacinamide 20 mg., Mg

23 mg., I 0.05 mg. Pot. 8 mg., lemon bioflavonoid
complex 10 mg./Tab. Bot. 100s.
Use: Adults dietary supplement.
CARDIAMID.
See: Nikethamide. (Various Mfr.)
CARDIAZOL.
See: Metrazol, Preps. (Knoll)
CARDILATE. (Burroughs Wellcome) Erythrityl
tetranitrate. **Tab.** 5 mg. 100s, 10 mg. 100s, 1000s.
Chewable Tab. 10 mg., Bot. 100s.
Use: Prophylaxis and long-term treatment of patients
with recurrent anginal pain.
CARDIOGRAFIN. (Squibb) Diatrizoate
methylglucamine 85% in a sterile, aqueous
solution. Vial 50 cc.
Use: Diagnostic agent.
CARDIO-GREEN. (Hynson, Westcott & Dunning) Sterile
Indocyanine Green. Vials 25 mg. and 50 mg.
Use: For indicator dilution, hepatic function and
ophthalmic angiography studies.
CARDIO-GREEN DISPOSABLE UNIT. (Hynson, West-
cott & Dunning) Vial Cardio-green, ampule aqueous
solvent & calibrated syringe. 10 mg., 40 mg.
Use: For indicator dilution, hepatic function and
ophthalmic angiography studies.
CARDIOQUIN TABLETS. (Purdue Frederick)
Quinidine polygalacturonate 275 mg. equivalent to
quinidine sulfate 200 mg./Tab. Bot. 100s, 500s.
Use: Cardiac arrhythmias.
CARDIOTROL-CK. (Roche) Lyophilized human serum
containing three CK isoenzymes from human tissue
source. Suitable for use as a quality control for
immunochemical or electrophoretic assays.
CARDIOTROL-LD. (Roche) Lyophilized human serum
containing all LD isoenzymes from human tissue
source. 10x1ml.
CARDIZEM. (Marion) Diltiazem HCl 30 mg. or 60
mg./Tab. Bot. 100s. Unit Dose 100s.
Use: Treatment of angina.
CARDOPHYLLIN.
See: Aminophylline. (Various Mfr.)
CARDOXIN. (Vita Elixir) Digoxin 0.25 mg./Tab.
Use: Cardiotonic.
CARENA.
See: Aminophylline (Various Mfr.)
CARFECILLIN. B.A.N. 6-(α-Phenoxycarbonyl-
phenylacetamido) penicillanic acid.
Use: Antibiotic.
• **CARFENTANIL CITRATE.** USAN.
Use: Analgesic, narcotic.
CARGENTOS.
See: Silver Protein, Mild
CARGESIC. (Rand) Bot. 2 oz.
Use: Analgesic, counterirritant.
CARICA PAPAYA ENZYME.
See: Caroid, Preps. (Winthrop-Breon)
Papain (Various Mfr.)
W/Diastase.
See: Caripeptic, Liq. (Upjohn)
CARINDACILLIN. B.A.N. 6-(α-Indan-5-yloxycarbonyl-
phenylacetamido)penicillanic acid.
Use: Antibiotic.

CARISOPRODOL. B.A.N. 2-Carbamoyloxymethyl-2-N-isopropylcarbamoyloxymethylpentane.
Use: Muscle relaxant.
See: Carisoma

CARISOPRODOL. N-isopropyl meprobamate. Isomeprobamate, N-isopropyl-2-methyl-2-propyl-1, 3 propanediol dicarbamate.
See: Rela, Tab. (Schering)
Soma, Tab. (Wallace)
W-Acetophenetidin, caffeine.
See: Soma Compound, Tabs. (Wallace)
W/Acetophenetidin, caffeine, codeine phosphate.
See: Soma Compound w/codeine, Tab. (Wallace)
W/Phenacetin.
See: Soma Compound Tabs. (Wallace)

CARI-TAB. (T.E. Williams) Fluoride 0.5 mg., Vitamin A 2000 U., D 200 U., C 75 mg./Softab. Bot. 100s.
Use: Aid in development of caries-resistant teeth and prophylaxis of vitamin A, D & C deficiencies.

• **CARMANTADINE.** USAN.
Use: Antiparkinsonian.

CARMOL 10. (Syntex) Urea (carbamide) 10% in hypoallergenic water-washable lotion base. Bot. fl. 6 oz.
Use: Dry skin.

CARMOL 20. (Syntex) Urea (carbamide) 20% in hypoallergenic vanishing cream base. Tube 3 oz., Jar 1 lb.
Use: Dry & Hyperkeratotic skin.

CARMOL-HC CREAM 1%. (Syntex) Micronized hydrocortisone acetate 1%, in water-washable base containing urea. Tube 1 oz. Jar 4 oz.
Use: Topical corticosteroid.

• **CARMUSTINE.** USAN. 1, 3-Bis-(2-chloroethyl)-1-nitrosourea.
Use: Antineoplastic.
See: Bicnu, Inj. (Bristol)

CARNATION INSTANT BREAKFAST. (Carnation) Non-fat instant breakfast containing 280 K cal. w/15 Gm. protein and 8 oz. whole milk. Pkt. 35 Gm. Ctn. 6s. Six flavors.
Use: Nutritionally complete enteral meal supplement.

• **CARNIDAZOLE.** USAN. Methyl-nitro-imidazole.
Use: Antiparasitic, antiprotozoal.

CAROID LAXATIVE. (Winthrop Products) Phenolphthalein 32.4 mg., Cascara Sagrada extract 50 mg./Tab. Bot. 20s, 50s, 100s.
Use: Laxative.

CAROID TOOTH POWDER. (Winthrop Products) Calcium carbonate, magnesium carbonate, sodium bicarbonate, saccharin. Cans 2.0 oz., 4.1 oz.
Use: Dentrifice, tooth polish.

• **CAROXAZONE.** USAN.
Use: Antidepressant.

CARPERIDINE. B.A.N. Ethyl 1-(2-carbamoylethyl)-4-phenylpiperidine-4-carboxylate.

CARPHENAZINE. B.A.N. 10-{3-[4-(2-Hydroxyethyl)piperazin-1-yl]propyl}-2-propionylphenothiazine.
Use: Tranquilizer.

• **CARPHENAZINE MALEATE,** U.S.P. XXI. Oral Sol., U.S.P. XXI. 1-{10-(3-[4-(2-Hydroxyethyl)-1-piperazi-nyl]-propyl)   phenothiazin-2-yl}-1-propanone   bis (maleate).
Use: Chronic psychosis.
See: Proketazine, Tab., Liq. (Wyeth)

• **CARRAGEENAN,** N.F. XVI.

CARSALAM. B.A.N. 1,3-Benzoxazine-2,4-dione. O-Carbamoylsalicylic acid lactam
Use: Analgesic.

• **CARTAZOLATE.** USAN.
Use: Antidepressant.

• **CARTEOLOL HYDROCHLORIDE.** USAN.
Use: Anti-adrenergic.

CARTER'S LITTLE PILLS. (Carter Products) Bisacodyl 5 mg./Pill. Vial 30s, 85s.
Use: Laxative.

CARTICAINE. B.A.N. Methyl 4-methyl-3-(2-propylaminopropionamido)thiophene-2-carboxylate.
See: Ultracain hydrochloride.
Use: Local anesthetic.

CARTRAX 10. (Roerig) Atarax 10 mg. & pentaerythritoltetranitrate 10 mg./Tab. yellow. Bot. 100s.
Use: Angina pectoris & decubitus.

CARTRAX 20. (Roerig) Atarax 10 mg., pentaerythritoltetranitrate 20 mg./Tab. pink. Bot. 100s.
Use: Angina pectoris & decubitus.

CARTUCHO COOK WITH RAVOCAINE. (Winthrop Products) Ravocaine, novocain and levophed or neo-cobefrin.
Use: Dental anesthetic.

• **CARUBICIN.** USAN.
Use: Antineoplastic.

CAR-VIT. (Mericon) Ascorbic acid 60 mg., vitamin A acetate 4000 I.U., D-2 400 I.U., ferrous fumarate 90 mg. (iron 30 mg.), oyster shell 600 mg. (calcium 230 mg.)/Cap. Bot. 90s, 1000s.

CARZENIDE. p-Sulfoamoylbenzoic acid.
Use: Carbonic anhydrase inhibitor.

CASA-DICOLE. (Blue Cross) Docusate sodium 100 mg., casanthrol 30 mg./Cap. Bot. 100s.
Use: Laxative, stool softeners.

CASAFRU. (Key) Extract of dried senna fruit. Bot. 2 oz., 4 oz., 8 oz.
Use: Laxative.

• **CASANTHRANOL.** USAN. A purified mixture of the anthranol glycosides derived from Cascara sagrada.
Use: Cathartic.
See: Black Draught, Prods. (Chattem Labs.)
W/Bile of ox, phenolphthalein.
See: Bicholate, Tab., (Blue Line)
W/Docusate sodium
See: Bu-Lax-Plus, Cap. (Ulmer)
Calotabs, Tabs. (Calotabs)
Comflax-Plus, Cap. (Rorer)
Comfolax-Plus, Cap. (Searle)
Comfula-Plus (Searle)
Constiban, Cap. (Columbia)
Diolax, Cap. (Century)
Dio-Soft (Standex)
Diothron, Cap. (Vortech)
Disanthrol, Cap. (Lannett)
Disulans, Cap. (Noyes)

D-S-S W/Casanthranol, Cap. (Wolins)
Easy-Lax Plus, Cap. (Walgreen)
Genericace, Cap. (Fellows-Testagar)
Neo-Vardin D-S-S-C, Cap. (Scherer)
Nuvac, Cap. (LaCrosse)
Peri-Colace, Cap., Syr. (Mead Johnson)
Sodex, Cap. (Mallard)
Sofflax, Cap. (Medics)
Stimulax, Cap. (Geriatric)
Syncelax, Cap. (Blue Line)
Tonelax Plus, Cap. (A.V.P.)
W/Docusate sodium, sod. carboxymethylcellulose.
  See: Dialose Plus, Cap. (Stuart)
      Disolan Forte, Cap. (Lannett)
      Tri-Vac, Cap. (Rhode)
W/Mineral oil and irish moss.
  See: Neo-Kondremul, Liq. (Fisons)
CASCARA. (Lilly) Cascara 150 mg./Tab. Bot. 100s.
  Use: Cathartic.
CASCARA, AROMATIC (Lilly) Alcohol 19%. Bot. 16
fl. oz.
  Use: Cathartic.
CASCARA COMPOUND (Lilly) Ext. cascara sagrada
  16 mg., aloin 16 mg., podophyllum resin 10 mg.,
  ext. belladonna 8 mg., oleoresin ginger 4 mg./Tab.
  Bot. 100s.
  Use: Cathartic.
• **CASCARA FLUIDEXTRACT, AROMATIC,** U.S.P.
XXI.
  Use: Cathartic.
W/Psyllium husk pow. & prune pow.
  See: Casyllium, Pow. (Upjohn)
CASCARA GLYCOSIDES.
  Use: Cathartic.
• **CASCARA SAGRADA,** U.S.P. XXI. Extract,
  Fluidextract, U.S.P. XXI. (Various Mfr.)
  Use: Pharmaceutical necessity for Aromatic
  Cascara Fluidextract.
• **CASCARA SAGRADA EXTRACT,** U.S.P. XXI.
  Use: Cathartic.
W/Bile salts, phenolphthalein, aloin.
  See: Amlax, Tab. (Vortech)
W/Bile salts, phenolphthalein, aloin, papain, ext. nux
vomica.
  See: Taurocolate, Tab. (Vortech)
W/Bile salts, papain, phenolphthalein, capsicum
oleoresin.
  See: Torocol Compound, Tab. (Plessner)
W/Bile salts, phenolphthalein, capsicum oleoresin &
peppermint oil.
  See: Torocol, Tab. (Plessner)
W/Capsicum, ginger.
  See: Flatulence, Tab. (Wolins)
W/Docusate sodium.
  See: Dioctyl-Zem, Tab. (Zemmer)
W/Ox bile (desiccated), phenolphthalein, aloin,
podophyllin.
  See: Bilgon, Tab. (Reid-Provident)
W/Oxgall, dandelion root, podophyllin, tr. nux vomica.
  See: Oxachol, Liq. (Philips Roxane)
W/Pancreatin, pepsin, sod. salicylate.
  See: Bocresin, Liq. (Scrip)

W/Phenolphthalein, sodium glycocholate, sodium
taurocholate, aloin.
  See: Bicholax, Tab. (Elder)
      Oxiphen, Tab. (Webcon)
W/Sod. salicylate, phenoiphthalein, chionanthus ext.,
bile ext., sod. glycocholate, sod. taurocholate.
  See: Glycols, Tab. (Bowman)
• **CASCARA SAGRADA FLUID EXTRACT,** U.S.P.
  XXI. (Parke-Davis) Alcohol 18% Bot. 1 pt., 1 gal.,
  Unit dose 5 ml..
  Use: Cathartic.
  See: Cas-Evac, Liq. (Parke-Davis)
      Bilstan (Standex)
CASCARA SAGRADA FLUID EXTRACT AROMATIC
. Aromatic Cascara Fluidextract, U.S.P. XXI.
W/Psyllium husk pow., prune pow.
  See: Casyllium, Granules (Upjohn)
• **CASCARA TABLETS,** U.S.P. XXI.
  Use: Cathartic.
CASCARIN.
  See: Casanthranol (Various Mfr.)
CASEC. (Mead Johnson) Calcium caseinate (derived
from skim milk curd and calcium carbonate). Pow.
Can 3⅓ oz.
  Use: Provides extra protein for infants, children or
adults.
CASOATE-A. (Marcen) Hydrolyzed casein 100 mg., his-
tidine monohydrochloride 4 mg., benzyl alcohol 5
mg., phenol 5 mg./cc. Vial 10 cc.
  Use: Gastro-duodenal ulcer therapy.
CASTADERM. (Lannett) A lotion of boric acid,
resorcinol, acetone & soln. of carbol fuchsin. Bot.
1, 4 & 16 oz.
  Use: Eczematoid conditions of epidermatophytic
origin.
CASTEL-MINUS. (Syosset) Resorcinl 8%, alcohol
8.5% w/acetone, fuchsin. Bot. 1 oz.
  Use: Antifungal.
CASTELLANI PAINT. (Pedinol) Fuchsin, phenol
resorcinol, acetone, alcohol. Bot. 1 oz., 16 oz./w
color; colorless 1 oz., 16 oz.
  Use: Local antifungal drying agent.
CASTELLANI'SPAINT. (Archer-Taylor) Bot. 4 oz., 16
oz.
  Use: Fungicide solution.
CASTELLANI'S PAINT. (Penta) Carbol-fuchsin sol.
Fuchsin 0.3%, phenol 4.5%, resorcinol 10.0%,
acetone 1.5%, alcohol 13%. Bot. 1 oz., 4 oz., pt.
  Use: Dermatological formulation, for external use
only under direct supervision of a physician.
• **CASTOR OIL,** U.S.P. XXI. Aromatic, Caps., U.S.P.
  XXI. (Squibb) Bot. 2 oz., 4 oz.
  Use: Cathartic; pharmaceutic aid (plasticizer).
  See: Neoloid (Lederle)
CASTOR OIL ELASTIC FILLED CAPSULES (Lilly)
Castor oil 10 min./Cap. Bot 100s.
  Use: Cathartic.
• **CASTOR OIL EMULSION,** U.S.P. XXI.
  Use: Cathartic.
• **CASTOR OIL, HYDROGENATED,** N.F. XVI.
  Use: Cathartic.
CATAPRES. (Boehringer Ingelheim) Clonidine HCl 0.1

mg., 0.2 mg. or 0.3 mg./Tab. **0.1mg.:** Bot. 100s, 1000s. Unit Dose 100s. **0.2 mg.:** Bot. 100s, 1000s. Unit Dose 100s. **0.3 mg.:** Bot. 100s, 1000s.
Use: Antihypertensive.

CATARASE. (CooperVision) Chymotrypsin 1:5,000 (300 units) in a 2 chamber vial with 2 ml. sterile diluent; Chymotrypsin 1:10,000 (150 units) in a 2 chamber vial with 2 ml. sterile diluent.
Use: Intracapsular lens extraction.

CATARRHALIS, KILLED NEISSERIA.
W/Klebsiella pneumoniae, Diplococcus pneumoniae, Streptococci, staphylococci.
See: Combined Vaccine No. 4 W/Catarrhalis, Inj. (Lilly)

CATHOMYCIN CALCIUM. Calcium novobiocin.

CATHOMYCIN SODIUM. Novobiocin sod.

■ CATIONIC RESINS.
See: Resins, Sodium Removing

CAUSALIN. (Amfre-Grant) Magnesium salicylate 600 mg./Tab. Bot. 100s 1000s.
Use: Analgesic, antiinflammatory.

CAVACAINE. (Graham) Mepivacaine HCl 3%. Vial 20 ml.
Use: Anesthetic.

C-BIO. (Barth's) Vit. C. 150 mg., citrus bioflavonoid complex 100 mg., rutin 50 mg./Tab. Bot. 100s, 500s, 1000s.

C-B-PLEX CAPSULES. (Barry-Martin) Vit. B-1 15 mg., B-2 10 mg., niacinamide 50 mg., Ca pantothenate 10 mg., C 250 mg., B-6 5 mg./Cap. Bot. 100s, 500s.
Use: Vitamin supplement.

C-B TIME. (Arco) Ascorbic acid 200 mg., Vit. B-1 10 mg., B-2 10 mg., B-6 5 mg., B-12 10 mcg., niacinamide 50 mg., calcium pantothenate 10 mg./Cap. Vit. C 300 mg., B-1 15 mg., B-2 10 mg., B-6 5 mg., cobalamin concentrate 5 mcg., niacinamide 100 mg., D-panthenol 20 mg./5 cc. **Caps.** Bot. 40s, 120s, 500s.
Liq., Bot. 4 oz.
Use: Vitamin supplements.

C-B TIME 500. (Arco) Vit. C 500 mg., B-1 10 mg., B-2 10 mg., B-6 5 mg., cyanocobalamin 10 mg., niacinamide 50 mg., Ca pantothenate 10 mg./Tab. Bot. 30s, 100s, 500s.

C-B VONE CAPSULES. (Armour) Vitamin B Complex and C supplement. Bot. 100s.
Use: Vitamins B and C supplement.

C-CAPS 500. (Drug Industries) Vitamin C 500 mg./Cap. Bot. 100s.
Use: Vitamin C supplement.

CCNU. Lomustine.
See: CeeNu, Tab. (Bristol)

C.D.M. EXPECTORANT. (Lannett) Dextromethorphan HBr 10 mg., chlorpheniramine maleate 1 mg., phenylephrine HCl 5 mg., sodium citrate 15 mg., guaifenesin 25 mg./5 cc. Bot. pt., gal.
Use: Antihistaminic, antitussive cough expectorant.

CEA. (Abbott) Test kits 100s.
Use: Radioimmunoassay or enzyme immunoassay for quantitative measurement of carcinoembryonic antigen in human serum or plasma.

CEA-ROCHE. (Roche) Radioimmunoassay capable of

detecting and measuring plasma levels of CEA in the nanogram range. Sensitivity-0.5 ng./ml. of CEA.

CEA-ROCHE TEST KIT. (Roche) Carcinoembryonic antigen, a glycoprotein which is a constituent of the glycocalyx of embryonic entodermal epithelium. Test Kit.
Use: Diagnostic agent.

CEB NUGGETS. (Scott/Cord) Vit. B-1 15 mg., B-2 15 mg., B-6 5 mg., B-12 5 mcg., C 600 mg., niacinamide 100 mg., E 40 I.U., calcium pantothenate 20 mg., folic acid 0.1 mg./Nugget. Bot. 60s.

CEBEFORTIS. (Upjohn) Vit. B-1 5 mg., B-2 5 mg., B-6 1 mg., cal. pantothenate 10 mg., niacinamide 50 mg., ascorbic acid 150 mg., Vit. B-12 activity 2 mcg./Tab. Bot. 100s.
Use: Vitamin B-complex therapy.

CEBENASE. (Upjohn) Intrinase 0.167 N.F. unit (oral), Sod. ascorbate 150 mg., B-1 10 mg., B-2 10 mg., B-6 2.5 mg., Cal. pantothenate 10 mg., niacinamide 75 mg./Tab. Bot. 50s.
Use: Hematinic.

CEBO-CAPS. (O'Neal, Jones & Feldman) Placebo timed capsules.

CEBRAL. (Kenwood) Ethaverine HCl 100 mg./Blue, green, or orange. Bot. 100s, 1000s. B-2 5 mg., B-6 2 mg., pantothenic acid 10 mg.,

CEBRALAN-M TABLETS. (Lannett) B-1 10 mg., Cap. Bot. 50s, 500s.
Use: Relief of cerebral and peripheral ischemia. niacinamide 30 mg., B-12 3 mcg., C 100 mg., E 5 I.U., A 10,000 I.U., D 1000 I.U., Fe 15 mg., Cu 1 mg., iodine 0.15 mg., Mn 1 mg., Mg 5 mg., Zn 1.5 mg./Tab. Bot. 100s, 1000s.
Use: Mineral-vitamin supplement.

CEBRALAN M.T. TABLETS. (Lannett) Vit. B-1 15 mg., B-2 10 mg., B-6 2 mg., pantothenic acid 10 mg., niacinamide 100 mg., B-12 7.5 mcg., C 150 mg., E 5 I.U., A 25,000 I.U., Cu 1 mg., Fe 15 mg., iodine 0.15 mg., Mn 1 mg., Mg 5 mg., Zn 1.5 mg./Tab. Bot. 100s, 1000s.
Use: High potency mineral-vitamin tablet.

CECLOR. (Lilly) **Pulvules:** Cefaclor 250 or 500 mg./Pulvule. Bot. 15s,100s. Blister pkg. 10 × 10s. **Oral Susp.:** Cefaclor 125 or 250 mg./5 ml. Bot. 75 ml., 150 ml.
Use: Antibiotic.

CECON SOLUTION. (Abbott) Ascorbic acid 10% in propylene glycol. Each drop from enclosed dropper supplies 2.5 mg. ascorbic acid; each ml. contains 100 mg. Bot. w/dropper 50 ml.
Use: Vitamin-C therapy.

CEDILANID-D. (Sandoz) Deslanoside, desacetyllanatoside C. 0.4 mg./2 ml. w/citric acid, sodium phosphate, alcohol 9.8%, glycerin 15%, Water for injection qs 2 ml./Amp. SandoPak Pkg. 20s.
Use: Parenterally, digitalization.

CEEAMIDE. (Image) Vitamin Tab. Bot. 100s. Liquid Bot. 16 oz.
Use: Supplement.

CEEBATE. (Mallard) Ascorbic acid 250 mg./ml. Vial 30 ml.
Use: Scurvy treatment and prevention.

CeeNU. (Bristol) Lomustine (CCNU) 10 mg., 40 mg., 100 mg./Cap. Bot. 20s. Dose pk. of two cap. each of three strengths.
Use: Antineoplastic agent.

CEEPA. (Geneva) Theophylline 130 mg., ephedrine HCl 24 mg., phenobarbital 8 mg./Tab. Bot. 100s, 1000s.

CEEPRYN. Cetylpyridinium chloride.
Use: Antiseptic.
See: Cēpacol Lozenges, Sol., Troches (Merrell Dow)

CEETOLAN CONCENTRATE. (Lannett) Cetyldimethylbenzyl ammonium chloride 1:5500/2 oz. Bot. diluted w/1 gal. water. Bot. 2 oz.
Use: Mouth wash.

• **CEFACLOR,** U.S.P. XXI. Capsules, For Oral Susp., For Oral Susp., U.S.P. XXI.
Use: Antibacterial.
See: Ceclor, Cap. (Lilly)

• **CEFACTOR.** USAN.
Use: Antibacterial.

• **CEFADROXIL,** U.S.P. XXI. Caps., Tabs., Oral Susp., U.S.P. XXI. 7-[[D-2-amino-2-(4 hydroxyphenyl) acetyl] amino]-3-methyl-8-oxo-5-thia-1-azabicyclo [4.2.0] Oct-2-ene-2-carboxylic acid monohydrate.
Use: Antibiotic
See: Duricef, Cap., Tab., Susp. (Mead Johnson) Ultracef, Cap. (Bristol)

CEFADYL. (Bristol) Cephapirin sodium 500 mg., 1 Gm., 2 Gm./Vial.; Piggyback vials 1 Gm., 2 Gm., 4 Gm.; Bulk vial 20 Gm.
Use: Antibiotic, IM & IV.

• **CEFAMANDOLE.** USAN.
Use: Antibacterial.

• **CEFAMANDOLE NAFATE, STERILE,** U.S.P. XXI. For Inj. U.S.P. XXI. 5-Thia-1-azabicyco (4.2.0) oct-2-ene-2-carboxylic acid, 7-(((formyloxy,) phenylacetyl) amino) -3- (((1-methyl-1H-tetrazol -5-yl)thio)methyl) -8- oxo-, monosodium salt, (6R-(6 α, 7 β (R)))—.
Use: Antibiotic
See: Mandol, Amp. (Lilly)

• **CEFAMANDOLE SODIUM,** U.S.P. XXI. For Inj., U.S.P., Sterile, U.S.P. XXI.
Use: Antibiotic.

• **CEFAPAROLE.** USAN.
Use: Antibacterial.

CEFAPIRIN. B.A.N. 7-[α-(4-Pyridylthioacetamido)]-cephalosporanic acid.
Use: Antibiotic.
See: Cefatrex Cefatrexyl sodium salt.

• **CEFATRIZINE.** USAN.
Use: Antibacterial.

• **CEFAZAFLUR SODIUM.** USAN.
Use: Antibacterial.

• **CEFAZOLIN,** U.S.P. XXI.
Use: Antibiotic.

• **CEFAZOLIN SODIUM, STERILE,** U.S.P. XXI. Inj., U.S.P. XXI. Sodium salt of 3-[(5-methyl-1, 3, 4-thiadia-zol-2-yl) thio]-methyl -8-oxo 7-[2-(1H-tetrazol-1-yl)acetanido]-5-thia-1-azabicyclo[4-2.0]oct-2-ene-2-carboxylic acid.

Use: Antibiotic.
See: Ancef, Vial (SmithKline) Kefzol, Amp. (Lilly)

CEFERA. (Haag) Ferrous fumarate 200 mg. (equiv. to 60 mg. Iron), ascorbic acid 100 mg./Tab. Bot. 100s, 1000s.
Use: Treatment of iron deficiency.

CEFERA PLUS. (Haag) Ferrous fumarate 194 mg., Vit. C 50 mg., B-1 2 mg., B-2 2 mg., niacinamide 15 mg., B-6 0.5 mg., B-12 5 mcg./Tab. Bot. 100s, 500s, 1000s.
Use: Iron and vitamin deficiency.

• **CEFETAMET.** USAN.

CEFINAL II. (Alto) Salicymide 150 mg., acetaminophen 250 mg., doxylamine succinate 25 mg./Tab. Bot. 100s.
Use: Nighttime analgesic.

CEFIZOX. (SmithKline) Semisynthetic cephalosporin equivalent to 1 Gm. or 2 Gm. of ceftizoxime/Vial.
Use: Bactericidal.

• **CEFMENOXINE HYDROCHLORIDE.** USAN.
Use: Antibacterial.
See: Takeda (Abbott)

CEFOBID. (Roerig) Cefoperazone sodium 2 Gm. or 4 Gm./Vial
Use: Antibiotic for I.V. or I.M. administration.

CEFOL FILMTAB. (Abbott) Vit. B-1 15 mg., B-2 10 mg., B-6 5 mg., B-12 6 mcg., C 750 mg., E 30 I.U., Ca pantothenate 20 mg., niacinamide 100 mg., folic acid 500 mcg./Tab. Bot. 100s.

• **CEFONICID MONOSODIUM.** USAN.
Use: Antibacterial.

• **CEFONICID SODIUM.** USAN.
Use: Antibacterial.

• **CEFOPERAZONE SODIUM, STERILE,** U.S.P. XXI.
Use: Antibacterial.
See: Cefobid, Inj. (Roerig)

• **CEFORANIDE.** USAN.
Use: Antibacterial.

• **CEFOTAXIME SODIUM.** USAN.
Use: Antibacterial.
See: Claforan, Inj. (Hoechst)

• **CEFOTETAN.** USAN.

• **CEFOTETAN DISODIUM.** USAN.

• **CEFOTIAM HYDROCHLORIDE.** USAN.
Use: Antibacterial.

• **CEFOXITIN.** USAN.
Use: Antibacterial.

• **CEFOXITIN SODIUM, STERILE,** U.S.P. XXI. 5-Thia-1-azabicyclo (4.2.0) oct-2-ene-2-carboxylic acid, 3-((aminocarbonyl) oxy) methyl)-7-methoxy-8-oxo-7-((2-thienylacetyl)-amino)-, sodium salt (6R-cis)-.
Use: Antibiotic.

• **CEFROXADINE.** USAN.
Use: Antibacterial.

• **CEFSULODIN SODIUM, STERILE,** U.S.P. XX1.
Use: Antibacterial.

• **CEFTAZIDIME.** USAN.
Use: Antibacterial.

• **CEFTIZOXIME SODIUM.** USAN.
Use: Antibacterial.

• **CEFTRIAXONE SODIUM.** USAN.
Use: Antibacterial.

• **CEFUROXIME.** USAN (6R, 7R)-3-Carbamoyloxymeth-
yl-7-[(2Z)-2-(2-furyl)-2-methoxyiminoacetamido]-ceph
-3-em-1-carboxylic acid.
Use: Antibiotic.

• **CEFUROXIME AXETIL.** USAN.
Use: Antibiotic.

CELESTONE. (Schering) Betamethasone 0.6 mg./
Tab. Bot. 100s, 500s. Tab-Pack 21s. **Syr.:** 0.6 mg./5
cc. Alcohol < 1%. Bot. 4 oz.
Use: Anti-inflammatory steroid.

CELESTONE CREAM. (Schering) Betamethasone
(0.2%) 2 mg./Gm. Tubes 15 Gm.
Use: Dermatoses.

CELESTONE PHOSPHATE INJECTION. (Schering)
Betamethasone sodium phosphate 4 mg./ml.
equivalent to betamethasone alcohol 3 mg./ml.
Ampules 1 ml. Multidose vials, 5 ml.
Use: Anti-inflammatory.

CELESTONE SOLUSPAN. (Schering) Betamethasone
sodium phosphate 3 mg., betamethasone acetate 3
mg., dibasic sod. phosphate 7.1 mg., monobasic
sod. phosphate 3.4 mg., edetate disodium 0.1 mg.,
benzalkonium chloride 0.2 mg./ml. Vial 5 ml.
Use: Anti-inflammatory.

CELLABURATE. (Eastman) Cellulose acetate
butyrate.
Use: Pharmaceutic aid (plastic filming agent).

• **CELIPROLOL HYDROCHLORIDE.** USAN.
Use: Anti-adrenergic.

CELLACEPHATE. B.A.N. A partial mixed acetate and
hydrogen phthalate ester of cellulose.
Use: Enteric coating.

CELLASE W-100. W/Alpha-amylase W-100, proteinase
W-300, lipase, estrone, testosterone, vitamins, miner-
als.
See: Geramine, Tab. (Brown)
W/Amylase, protease, lipase, hyoscine HBr.
See: Am-Zyme, Tab. (Vortech)

CELLEPACBIN. (Arthrins) Vit. A 1200 I.U., B-1 1.5 mg.,
B-2 1.5 mg., B-6 0.75 mg., niacinamide 7.5 mg., panthenol 3 mg., C 20 mg., B-12 2 mcg., E 1 I.U./Cap. Bot.
180s.
Use: Dietary supplement.

CELLOTHYL. (C-D Consumer Products)
Methylcellulose 0.05 Gm./Tab. 100s, 1000s.
Use: Bulk laxative.

• **CELLULASE.** USAN. A concentrate of cellulose-split-
ting enzymes derived from *Aspergillus niger* and
other sources.
Use: Digestive Aid.
W/Bile salts, mixed conjugated, pancrelipase.
See: Cotazym-B, Tab. (Organon)
W/Mylase, prolase, calcium carbonate, magnesium
glycinate.
See: Zylase, Tabs. (Vitarine)
W/Mylase, prolase & lipase.
See: Ku-Zyme, Cap. (Kremers-Urban)
W/Pepsin, glutamic acid, pancreatin, ox bile ext.
See: Kanulase, Tab. (Dorsey)
W/Pepsin, pancreatin enz. conc., dehydrocholic acid.
See: Gastroenterase, Tabs. (Wallace)

CELLULOSE.
W/Hexachlorophene.

See: ZeaSorb, Pow. (Stiefel)

• **CELLULOSE, ACETATE,** N.F. XVI.

**CELLULOSE, ACETATE, 1,2-BENZENEDICARBOXY-
LATE.** Cellulose Acetate Phthalate, N.F. XVI.

• **CELLULOSE ACETATE PHTHALATE,** N.F. XVI.
Cellulose, acetate, 1,2-benzenedicarboxylate.
Use: Pharm. aid (tablet-coating agent).

CELLULOSE, CARBOXYMETHYL, SODIUM SALT.
Carboxymethylcellulose Sodium, U.S.P. XXI.

CELLULOSE, HYDROXYPROPYL METHYL ETHER.
Hydroxypropyl Methylcellulose, U.S.P. XXI.

CELLULOSE METHYL ETHER.
See: Methylcellulose, Prep. (Various Mfr.)

• **CELLULOSE MICROCRYSTALLINE,** N.F. XVI.
Use: Tablet diluent.

CELLULOSE, NITRATE. Pyroxylin, U.S.P. XXI.

CELLULOSE, OXIDIZED. Oxidized Cellulose, U.S.P.
XXI.
Use: Local hemostatic.

CELLULOSE, OXIDIZED REGENERATED, U.S.P.
XXI.

• **CELLULOSE, POWDERED,** N.F. XVI.

CELLULOSIC ACID.
See: Oxidized Cellulose. (Various Mfr.)

CELLULOLYTIC.
W/Amylolytic, proteolytic.
See: Trienzyme, Tabs. (Fellows-Testagar)

CELLULOLYTIC ENZYME.
See: Cellulase (Various Mfr.)
W/Amylolytic, proteolytic enzymes, lipase,
phenobarbital, hyoscyamine sulf., atropine sulf.
See: Arco-Lipase Plus, Tab. (Arco)
W/Amylolytic enzyme, proteolytic enzyme, lipolytic
enzyme, butisol sodium, belladonna.
See: Butibel-zyme Tabs (McNeil)
W/Calcium carbonate, glycine, amylolytic and
proteolytic enzymes.
See: Co-Gel, Tab. (Arco)
W/Proteolytic enzyme, amylolytic enzyme, lipolytic
enzyme.
See: Ku-Zyme, Cap. (Kremers-Urban)
Zymme, Cap. (Scrip)
W/Proteolytic, amylolytic, lipolytic enzymes, iron, ox
bile.
See: Spaszyme., Tab. (Dooner)

CELOID. (Xttrium) Lemon bioflavonoid complex 100
mg., ascorbic acid 100 mg./Cap. Bot. 100s, 1000s.

CELONTIN. (Parke-Davis) Methsuximide. Kapseal 150
mg., 300 mg. Bot. 100s.
Use: Petit mal and psychomotor attacks.

CENAFED. (Century) Pseudoephedrine HCl 60
mg./Tab. Bot. 100s, 1000s.
Use: Bronchodilator.

CENAFED SYRUP. (Century) Pseudoephedrine HCl
30 mg./5 cc. Bot. 4 oz., pint, gal.
Use: Bronchodilator.

CENAHIST. (Century) Chlorpheniramine maleate 8
mg., phenylephrine HCl 20 mg., methscopolamine
nitrate 2.5 mg./Cap. Bot. 100s, 500s, 1000s.
Use: Relief from allergic conditions.

CENAID. (Century) Salicylamide 227 mg., phenacetin
100 mg., caffeine 10 mg., ascorbic acid 20 mg.,

phenylephrine HCl 5 mg., chlorpheniramine maleate 2 mg./Tab. Bot. 100s, 1000s.
Use: Analgesic.
CENA-K. (Century) Potassium chloride 20%. Bot. pt., gal.
CENALAX. (Century) Bisacodyl. **Tab.:** 5 mg./Tab. Bot. 100s, 1000s. **Supp.:** 10 mg./Supp. Pkgs. 12s, 1000s.
Use: Laxative.
CENALONE. (Kay) Triamcinolone acetonide 40 mg./ml. Vial 5 ml.
Use: Glucocorticoid.
CENALONE INJECTION. (Century) Prednisolone sod. phosphate 20 mg./cc. Vial 10 cc.
CENALONE L.A. (Century) Prednisone sodium phosphate and prednisolone acetate 80 mg.
CEN-E. (Century) Vitamin E 100 I.U./Cap., 200 I.U./Cap., 400 I.U./Cap. Bot. 100s, 1000s.
CENOCORT A-40. (Central) Triamcinolone acetate 40 mg./ml. Vials 5 ml. Box 12s.
Use: Glucocorticoid.
CENOCORT FORTE. (Central) Triamcinolone diacetate 40 mg./ml. Vials 5 ml. Box 12s.
Use: Glucocorticoid.
CENOLATE. (Abbott)
Use: Treatment of Vitamin C deficiency.
CENTER-AL. (Center) Allergenic extracts, alum precipitated 10,000 PNU/ml. or 20,000 PNU/ml. Vials 10 ml.
Use: Treatment of allergy due to pollens or house dust.
■ **CENTRAL NERVOUS SYSTEM DEPRESSANTS.**
See: Sedatives
■ **CENTRAL NERVOUS SYSTEM STIMULANTS.**
See: Amphetamine (Various Mfr.)
D-Amphetamine (Various Mfr.)
Anorexigenic agents
Benzedrine, Cap., Tab. (SmithKline)
Caffeine (Various Mfr.)
Coramine, Liq., Inj. (Ciba)
Deaner, Tab. (Riker)
Desoxyephedrine HCl, Tab. (Various Mfr.)
Desoxyn HCl, Tab. Gradumet. (Abbott)
Dexedrine, Preps. (SmithKline)
Methamphetamine HCl (Various Mfr.)
Metrazol, Preps. (Knoll)
Nikethamide (Various Mfr.)
Pentylenetetrazol (Various Mfr.)
Picrotoxin
Ritalin HCl, Tab., Inj. (Ciba)
CENTRAX. (Parke-Davis) Prazepam. **Cap.:** 5 mg., 10 mg., or 20 mg./Cap. Bot. 100s, 500s. **Tab.** 10 mg./Tab. Bot. 100s. Unit dose 100s.
Use: Symptomatic relief of anxiety and tension associated with anxiety disorders, transient situational disorders, functional or organic disorders.
CENTRUM. (Lederle) Vit A 5000 I.U., E 30 I.U., C 90 mg., folic acid 400 mcg., B-1 2.25 mg., B-2 2.6 mg., B-6 3 mg., niacinamide 20 mg., B-12 9 mcg., D 400 I.U., biotin 150 mcg., pantothenic acid 10 mg., Ca 162 mg., phosphorus 125 mg., iodine 150 mcg.,

iron 27 mg., Mg. 100 mg., K 7.7 mg., Mn 7.5 mg., Cr 15 mcg., Se 15 mcg., molybdenum 15 mcg., zinc 22.5 mg./Tab.
Use: Vitamin & Mineral supplement.
CENTRUM JR. (Lederle) Vit. A 5000 I.U., D 400 I.U., E 15 I.U., C 60 mg., folic acid 400 mcg., B-1 1.5 mg., B-6 2 mg., B-12 6 mcg., riboflavin 1.7 mg., niacinamide 20 mg., iron 18 mg., magnesium 25 mg., copper 2 mg., zinc 10 mg., manganese 1 mg., potassium 1.6 mg., chloride 1.4 mg./Tab. Bot.60s.
Use: Vitamin, mineral, iron supplement for children.
CENTURY HOSPITAL RUB. (Century) Lanolins, menthol, allantoin in soothing base. Bot. 8 oz.
Use: Emollient lotion.
CENTUSS. (Century) Dextromethorphan HBr 10 mg., salicylamide 227 mg., phenacetin 100 mg., caffeine 10 mg., ascorbic acid 20 mg., phenylephrine HCl 5 mg., chlorpheniramine maleate 2 mg./MLT Tab. Bot. 100s, 1000s.
Use: Antitussive and analgesic.
CEO-TWO. (Beutlich) Potassium bitartrate and sod. bicarbonate in polyethylene glycol base. Supp. 10s.
Use: Laxative.
CEPACOL. (Merrell Dow) Ceepryn (brand of cetylpyridinium chloride) 1:2000, alcohol 14%, phosphate buffers and aromatics.Bot. 12 oz., 18 oz., 24 oz., 32oz., 4 × 2 qt.
Use: Mouthwash and gargle for oral hygiene.
CEPACOL ANESTHETIC LOZENGES. (Merrell Dow) Benzocaine,cetylpyridinium chloride 1:1500, aromatics in citrus flavored hard candy base. Pkg. 18s, 324s.
Use: Temporary relief of minor throat & mouth pain.
CEPACOL THROAT LOZENGES. (Merrell Dow) Cetylpyridinium chloride 1:1500, benzyl alcohol 0.3%, aromatics in mint flavored hard candy base. Pkg. 18s, 648s.
Use: Temporary relief of dryness and minor mouth & throat irritations.
CEPASTAT. (Merrell Dow) Mouthwash/gargle/spray w/phenol 1.4%. Spray Bot. 3 oz.
Use: Temporary relief of sore throat.
CEPASTAT LOZENGES. (Merrell Dow) Phenol 1.45%, menthol 0.12%/Lozenge w/sorbitol, eucalyptus oil. Pkg. 18s, 300s, 648s.
Use: Temporary relief of minor sore throat pain.
CEPASTAT CHERRY FLAVOR LOZENGES. (Merrell Dow) Phenol 0.73%, menthol 0.12% in sorbitol base. Box 18s.
Use: Temporary relief of sore throats in children 6 and older.
CEPHACETRILE SODIUM. Sodium 7-(2-cyanoacetamido)-3-(hydroxy-methyl)-8-oxo-5-thia-1-aza-bicyclo [4.3.0]oct-2-ene-2-carboxylate acetate (ester).
Use: Antibacterial.
• **CEPHADRINE TABLETS,** U.S.P. XXI.
• **CEPHALEXIN,** U.S.P. XXI. Caps., Oral Susp., Tabs. U.S.P. XXI. 7-(D-2-Amino-2-phenyl-acetamido)-3-methyl-8-oxo-5-thia-1-azabicyclo-[4.2.0]oct-2-3n3-2-carboxylic acid. 5-Thia-1-azabicyclo[4.2.0].oct-2-ene-2-carboxylic acid,7-[(aminophenylacetyl)amino]-3-methyl-8oxo-, monohydrate.

Use: Antibiotic.
CEPHALEXIN. B.A.N. 7-(D-α-Aminophenylacetamido)-3-cephem-4-carboxylic acid.
Use: Antibiotic.
See: Ceporex
  Keflex
CEPHALEXIN MONOHYDRATE.
See: Keflex, Pulvule & Susp. (Lilly)
CEPHALIN.
W/Lechithin with choline base, lipositol.
See: Alcolec, Cap., Granules (American Lecithin)
CEPHALOGLYCIN. 7-(D-2-Amino-2-phenyl-acetamido)-3-(hydroxymethyl)-8-oxo-5-thia-1-azabicyclo[4.2.0]oct-t-2-ene-2-carboxylic acid, acetate(ester) dihydrate.
Use: Antibiotic.
CEPHALOGLYCIN. B.A.N. 7-[(—)-α-Amino-phenylacetamido]cephalosporanic acid.
Use: Antibiotic.
See: Kefglycin
CEPHALOGLYCIN DIHYDRATE.
See: Kafocin, Pulvule (Lilly)
CEPHALONIUM. B.A.N. 3-(4-Carbamoyl-1-pyridiniomethyl)-7-(2-thienylacetamido)-3-cephem-4-carboxylate.
Use: Antibiotic.
CEPHALORAM. B.A.N. 7-Phenylacetamidocephalosporanic acid.
Use: Antibiotic.
CEPHALORIDINE. B.A.N. 7-[(2-Thienyl)acetamido]-3-(1-pyridylmethyl)-3-cephem-4-carboxylic acid betaine.
Use: Antibiotic.
See: Ceporin
CEPHALORIDINE, STERILE. 1-[[2-Carboxy-8-oxo-7-[2-(2-thienyl)acetamido]-5-thia-1-azabicyclo[4.2.0]oct-2-en-3-yl]methyl]pyridinium hydroxide inner salt.
Use: Antibacterial.
See: Loridine, Amp. (Lilly)
CEPHALOSPORIN C. B.A.N. 7-(5-Amino-5-carboxyvaleramido)cephalosporanic acid.
Use: Antibiotic.
CEPHALOTHIN. B.A.N. 7-(2-Thienylacetamido) cephalosporanic acid. A semisynthetic antibiotic using the fungus Cephalosporium. Not inactivated by penicillinase.
Use: Antibiotic.
See: Keflin Prods (Lilly)
• **CEPHALOTHIN SODIUM, STERILE,** U.S.P. XXI. Inj., Sterile, For Inj., U.S.P. XXI. (Lilly) 7-(2-Thienyl acetamido) cephalosporanic acid sod. salt. 5-Thia-1-azabicyclo[4.2.0]oct-2-ene-2-carboxylic acid,3-[(acetyloxy)methyl]-8-oxo-7-[(2-thienylacetyl)-amino]-,monosodium salt.
Use: Antibacterial, antibiotic.
See: Keflin, Vial (Lilly)
CEPHAMANDOLE. B.A.N. 7-D-Mandelamido-3-[(1-methyltetrazol-5-yl)thiomethyl]-3-cephem-4-carboxylic acid.
Use: Antibiotic.
• **CEPHAPIRIN SODIUM, STERILE,** U.S.P. XXI.
Sodium 3-(hydroxymethyl)-8-oxo-7-[2-(4-pyridylthio)

acetamido]-5-thia-1-azabicyclo[4.2.0]oct-2-ene-2-carboxylate acetate (ester).
Use: Antibiotic.
See: Cefadyl, Vial (Bristol)
CEPHAZOLIN. B.A.N. 3-[(5-Methyl-1,3,4-thiadiazol-2-yl)thiomethyl]-7-(tetrazol-1-ylacetamido)-3-cephem-4-carboxylic acid.
Use: Antibiotic.
CEPHAZOLIN SODIUM.
See: Ancef (SmithKline)
  Kefzol (Lilly)
CEPHOXAZOLE. B.A.N. 7-(3-o-Chlorophenyl-5-methylisoxazole-4-carboxamido)-cephalosporanic acid.
Use: Antibiotic.
• **CEPHRADINE,** U.S.P. XXI. Cap., Inj., Oral Susp., Sterile U.S.P. XXI. 7-[D-2-Amino-2-(1,4-cyclohexadien-1-yl-acetamido)-3-methyl-8-oxo-5-thia-1-azabicyclo[4.2.0]oct-2-ene-2-carboxylic acid monohydrate.
Use: Antibiotic.
See: Anspor, Cap., Susp. (SmithKline)
  Eskacef
  Velosef, Cap., Inj., Susp. (Squibb)
CEPHULAC. (Merrell Dow) Lactulose syrup 10 G./15 ml. Bot. pt., 2 qt. Unit dose 30 ml. Box 100s.
Use: Prevention & treatment of portal-systemic encephalopathy.
CERABEX-T. (Vitarine) Vit. C 500 mg., with high potency vitamins.
Use: Dietary supplement.
CERAPON. Triethanolamine Polypeptide Oleate-Condensate. (Purdue-Frederick)
See: Cerumenex, Drops (Purdue-Frederick)
CEREBEL. (Xttrium) Phenobarbital elix. 2.02 ml., milk of bismuth 2.5 ml., cerium oxalate 300 mg., hyoscyamine sulfate 5.2 mcg., atropine sulfate 0.01 mg., hyoscine HBr 3 mcg., alcohol 6%/5 cc. Bot. pt.
Use: Antidiarrheal.
CEREBID-150. (Saron) Papaverine HCl 150 mg./Sus. Rel. Cap. Bot. 100s, 1000s.
Use: Cerebral and peripheral ischemia.
CEREBID-200. (Saron) Papaverine HCl 200 mg./Sus. Rel. Tab. Bot. 100s, 1000s.
Use: Cerebal and peripheral ischemia.
CERELOSE.
See: Glucose (Various Mfr.)
CERESPAN. (USV Labs.) Papaverine HCl 150 mg./Sustained release cap. Bot. 100s, 1000s.
Use: Cerebral and peripheral ischemia.
CERETEX. (Enzyme Process) iron 15 mg., B-12 10 mcg., B-1 2 mg., B-6 1 mg., niacinamide 1 mg., pantothenic acid 0.15 mg., B-2 2 mg., iodine 15mg./2 cc. Bot. 60 cc., 8 Oz.
Use: Supplement.
CEROSE COMPOUND. (Ives) Chlorpheniramine maleate 4 mg., phenylephrine HCl 10 mg., acetaminophen 325 mg./Cap. Bot. 100s.
Use: Relief of allergy, common cold, pain, fever, sinusitis, nasal congestion.
CEROSE, DM. (Ives) Dextromethorphan HBr 10 mg., phenindamine tartrate 5 mg., phenylephrine HCl 5 mg., fl. ex. ipecac 0.17 min., glycerin 40 min., pot.

guaiacolsulfonate 86 mg., sod. citrate 3 gr., citric acid 1 gr. & alcohol 2½%/5 cc. Sugar free. Bot. 4 oz., 1 pt.
Use: Symptomatic relief of coughs due to colds, nasal congestion, sinusitis.

CERTANE. (Ladco) Vaginal cones 6s. Vaginal jelly tube 12s.
Use: Contraceptive.

CERTANE DOUCHE POWDER. (Ladco) Oxyquinoline sulfate, boric acid, sod. chloride & sod. sulfo-dioctyl succinate. Can 4 oz., 12 oz. Packettes 9s, 18s.
Use: Vaginal cleanser.

CERTANE JELLY. (Ladco) Phenylmercuric acetate 0.02%, w/oxyquinoline sulfate, boric acid, sod. sulfo-dioctyl succinate. Tube 2¼ oz., 4¼ oz.
Use: Contraceptive jelly.

CERUBIDINE. (Ives) Daunorubicin HCl 5 mg./ml. once reconstituted w/4 ml. water for injection. Vial 20 mg.
Use: Antineoplastic.

• **CERULETIDE.** USAN.
Use: Stimulant.

CERUMENEX DROPS. (Purdue Frederick) Triethanolamine polypeptide oleate-condensate. Dropper bot. 6 cc., 12 cc.
Use: Removal of cerumen (ear wax).

CERVO. (Sutliff & Case) Sod. citrate 560 mg., ammonium chloride 520 mg., pot. guaiacol sulfonate 520 mg., antimony pot. tartrate 5.4 mg./Fl. oz. Bot. pt., gal.
Use: Cough due to sore throat or colds.

CES. (I.C.N.) Conjugated estrogens, 0.625 mg., 1.25 mg., 2.5 mg./Tab.
Use: Hormone.

• **CESIUM CHLORIDE.** USAN.
Use: Myocardial scanning.

• **CETABEN SODIUM.** USAN.
Use: Antihyperlipoproteinemic.

CETACAINE. (Cetylite) Benzocaine 14%, butyl aminobenzoate 2%, tetracaine HCl 2%, benzalkonium Cl 0.5%, cetyl dimethyl ethyl ammonium bromide 0.005%, **Aerosol Spray** 56 Gm. 50 cc. **Liquid:** 56 Gm.**Oint.:** Jar 37 Gm., flavored. **Hosp. Gel:** 29 Gm.
Use: Topical anesthetic.

CETACIN. (Jenkins) Cetylpyridinium Cl 4 mg., sodium propionate 10 mg., benzocaine 6 mg./Tab. Bot. 1000s.
Use: Anesthetic throat lozenge.

CETACORT LOTION. (Owen) Hydrocortisone in concentrations of 0.25%, 0.5%, or 1% w/cetyl alcohol, propylene glycol, stearyl alcohol, sodium lauryl sulfate, butylparaben, methylparaben, propylparaben and purified water. Bot. 2 oz., 4 oz.
Use: Relief of inflammatory manifestations of corticosteroid-responsive dermatoses.

• **CETALKONIUM.** F.D.A.
Benzylhexadecyldimethylammonium ion.

• **CETALKONIUM CHLORIDE.** USAN.
Cetyldimethylbenzyl ammonium chloride.
Use: Antibacterial agent.
W/Phenylephrine, pyrilamine maleate, thimerosal.
See: Anti-B Mist (DePree)

CETALKONIUM CHLORIDE. B.A.N.
Benzylhexadecyldimethylammonium chloride.
Use: Anti-infective.

CETAMIDE. (Alcon) Sulfacetamide sod. 10%. Sterile ophthalmic oint. Tube 3.5 Gm.

• **CETAMOLOL HYDROCHLORIDE.** USAN.
Use: Anti-adrenergic

CETANE. (O'Neal, Jones & Feldman) **Cap.:** Ascorbic acid 500 mg./Cap. Bot. 100s, 1000s. **Inj.:** Sodium ascorbate 250 mg. or 500 mg./ml. Vial 30 ml.
Use: Vit. C deficiency.

CETAPHIL CREAM. (Owen) Purified water, cetyl alcohol, propylene glycol, sodium lauryl sulfate, stearyl alcohol, methylparaben, propylparaben, butylparaben. Jar 1 lb.
Use: Skin cleanser for soap intolerant people.

CETAPHIL LOTION. (Owen) Cetyl alcohol, stearyl alcohol, propylene glycol, sod. lauryl sulfate, methylparaben, propylparaben, butylparaben, purified water. Bot. 8 fl. oz., 16 fl. oz.
Use: Lipid-free skin cleanser.

CETAPRED. (Alcon) Sulfacetamide sodium 10%, prednisolone 0.25% in a methylcellulose vehicle. Soln. Ophth. Oint. Tube 3.5 Gm.
Use: Inflammatory and infectious conditions of the eye.

CETAZOL. (Professional Pharmacal) Acetazolamide 250 mg./Tab. Bot. 100s.
Use: Glaucoma treatment, carbonic anhydrase inhibitor.

• **CETIEDIL CITRATE.** USAN.
Use: Vasodilator.

• **CETOCYCLINE HYDROCHLORIDE.** USAN.
Use: Antibacterial.

CETOMACROGOL 1000. B.A.N. Polyethylene glycol 1000 monocetyl ether. Polyoxyethylene glycol 1000 monocetyl ether.
Use: Pharmaceutical aid.

• **CETOPHENICOL.** USAN. D-threo-N- {p-[acetyl-β-hydroxy-α-(hydroxymethyl)-phenethyl]}-2,2-dichloroacetamide.
Use: Antibacterial agent.

• **CETOSTEARYL ALCOHOL,** N.F. XVI.
Use: Pharmaceutic aid (emulsifying agent).

CETOXIME. B.A.N. N-Benzylanilinoacetamidoxime.
Use: Antihistamine.
See: Febramine

• **CETRAXATE HYDROCHLORIDE.** USAN.
Use: Anti-ulcerative.

CETRIMONIUM CHLORIDE. B.A.N.
Hexadecyltrimethylammonium chloride.
Use: Antiseptic detergent.

CETRO-CIROSE. (Ives) Codeine phosphate 30 mg., potassium guaiacolsulfonate 8 gr., glycerin 240 minims, ipecac flext. 1 min., sod. citrate 18 gr., citric acid 6 gr./5 cc w/alcohol 1.5% Bot. 1 pt., 1 gal.
Use: Narcotic cough preparation.

CETYBEN TROCHES. (Sutliff & Case) Cetylpyridinium chloride (1:1000) 1 mg., diperodon HCl 1 mg./Troche. Box 100s, 1000s.
Use: Throat irritations.

• **CETYL ALCOHOL,** N.F. XVI. 1-Hexadecanol.

Use: Emulsifying & stiffening agent.
• **CETYL ESTERS WAX**, N.F. XVI.
CETYLCIDE SOLUTION. (Cetylite) Cetyldimethylethyl
ammonium Br 6.5%, benzalkonium Cl 6.5%,
isopropyl alcohol 13%. Inert ingredients 74%,
including sodium nitrite. Amp. 10 cc., Bot. 32 oz.,
16 oz.
Use: Disinfectant.
CETYLDIMETHYL BENZYL AMMONIUM CHLORIDE.
See: Ceetolan Concentrate, Liq. (Lannett)
W/Benzocaine, ascorbic acid.
See: Locane, Troches (Reid-Provident)
Trocaine Lozenges (Vortech)
W/Phenylephrine HCl, pyrilamine maleate.
See: Dalihist, Nasal Spray (Dalin)
• **CETYLPYRIDINIUM CHLORIDE**, U.S.P. XXI.
Topical Soln., Loz., U.S.P. XXI. 1-Hexadecyl-
pyridinium chloride.
Use: Local anti-infective.
See: Bactalin, Bot. (LaCrosse)
W/Benzocaine.
See: Axon Throat Loz. (McKesson)
Cēpacol, Throat Lozenges, (Merrell Dow)
Coirex, Preps. (Rowell)
Lanazets, Loz. (Lannett)
Oradex-C, Troches (Commerce)
Semets, Troches (Beecham Labs)
Spec-T Sore Throat Loz. (Squibb)
Tyro-Loz. (Kenyon)
Vicks Medi-Trating Throat Lozenges (Vicks)
W/Benzocaine.
See: Cepacol Anticeptic Lozenges (Merrell Dow)
W/Benzocaine, Menthol, camphor, eucalyptus oil.
See: Vicks Medi-Trating Throat Lozenges (Vicks)
W/Dextromethorphan HBr, benzocaine.
See: Thorzettes Logenes (Towne)
W/Methapyrilene HCl, naphazoline.
See: Korizol, Spray (Sutliff & Case)
W/d-Methorphan HBr, phenyltoloxamine dihydrogen ci-
trate, and sodium citrate.
See: Exo-Kol, Cough Syrup, Spray, Tab. (Inwood)
W/Phenylephrine HCl, methapyrilene HCl, menthol,
eucalyptol, camphor, methyl salicylate.
See: Vicks Sinex Nasal Spray (Vicks)
W/Phenylpropanolamide HCl, benzocaine, terpin
hydrate.
See: S.A.C. Throat Lozenges (Towne)
CETYLPYRIDINIUM CHLORIDE. B.A.N. 1-Hexadecyl-
pyridinium chloride.
Use: Antiseptic detergent.
See: Ceepryn
Merocet
CETYLTRIMETHYL AMMONIUM BROMIDE. (Bio
Labs.) Cetrimide B.P., Cetavlon, CTAB.
Use: Antiseptic, Surface-active agent.
W/Hydrocortisone, phenylephrine, methapyrilene,
chlorobutanol.
See: T-Spray (Saron)
W/Lidocaine, hexachlorophene.
See: Aerosept, Aerosol (Dalin)
CEVALIN. (Lilly) Ascorbic acid. **Amp.:** (100 mg.) 2
cc. pkg. 6s, 100s. (500 mg.) 1 cc. Pkg. 25s. (1

Gm.) 10 cc. Pkg. 25s. **Tab.:** (100 mg.) Bot. 100s,
(250 mg.) Bot. 100s. (500 mg.) Bot. 100s, 500s.
Use: I.M., I.V., S.C. & orally, Vitamin C deficiency.
CEVI-BID. (Geriatric) Ascorbic acid 500 mg./Cap. Bot.
30s, 100s, 500s.
Use: Vitamin C therapy.
CEVI-FER. (Geriatric) Ascorbic acid 300 mg., ferrous
fumarate 60 mg., folic acid 1 mg./Cap. Bot. 30s.
Use: Treatment secondary anemias.
CE-VI-SOL. (Mead Johnson) Ascorbic acid 35 mg./0.6
ml. Bot. w/dropper 50 ml.
Use: Vitamin C supplementation.
CEVITA. (Kay) **Chewable Tabs.** Ascorbic acid 100
mg. or 250 mg./Chewable Tab. Bot. 100s, 1000s.
Tabs. 500 mg. 100s, 1000s. Kaykaps T.D. 500 mg.,
Bot. 60s, 250s, 500s, 1000s.
Use: Vitamin supplement.
CEVITA INJECTION. (Kay) Sodium ascorbate 250
mg./ml. Vial 30 ml.; 10 Gm./50 ml. Vial 50 ml.; 200
mg./ml. Amp. 5 ml.
Use: Vitamin C supplement.
CEVITAMIC ACID.
See: Ascorbic acid.
CEVITAN.
See: Ascorbic acid.
CEWIN TABLETS. (Winthrop Products) Ascorbic acid.
Use: Vitamin C supplement.
CEYLON GELATIN.
See: Agar.
CEZ. (Dattel) Vit. A 2,000 I.U., C 250 mg., E 100 I.U.,
zinc sulfate 25 mg./Cap. Bot. 60s.
Use: Vitamin supplement.
C.G. (Sig) Choronic gonadotropin (lyophilized) 10,000
u., mannitol 100 mg., supplied with diluent. Univial
10 ml.
CG DISPOSABLE UNIT.
See: Cardio Green, Vial (Hynson, Westcott &
Dunning)
CG RIA. (Abbott) Test kit 100s.
Use: Diagnostic kit for cholyglycine.
CHAP CREAM. (Ar-Ex) Carbonyl diamide. Tubes 1½
oz., 3¼ oz. Jar 4 oz., 9 oz., 18 oz.
Use: Hypoallergenic hand cream.
CHAPOLINE CREAM LOTION. (Wade) Glycerine,
boric acid, chlorobutanol ½%, alcohol 10%. Bot. 4
oz., pt., gal.
Use: Skin irritation.
CHARCOAID. (Requa) Activated charcoal in sorbital
slurry. Bot. 6 oz.
Use: Antidote for acute toxic injestion.
CHARCOAL.
See: Requa's Charcoal, Prods. (Requa)
• **CHARCOAL, ACTIVATED**, U.S.P. XXI.
Use: Antidote: pharmaceutic aid (Adsorbent).
See: Charcodote, Pow. (Panray)
W/Nux vomica, bismuth subgallate, pepsin, berberis,
diastase, pancreatin, hydrastis, papain.
See: Charcocaps, Cap. (Requa)
Charcotabs, Tab. (Requa)
Digestalin, Tab. (Vortech)
CHARCOAL ANTIDOTE. (U.S. Products) Activated
charcoal 15 Gm., 30 Gm. Box 12s.

Use: Poison antidote.

CHARCOCAPS. (Requa) Activated charcoal 260 mg./Cap. Bot. 36s, 300s.
Use: G.I. Detoxicant, antiflatulent, antidiarrheal, indigestion.

CHARCODOTE. (Panray) Activated charcoal. 15 Gm., 30 Gm./unit dose.
Use: Antidote, poison control.

CHARDONNA-2. (Rorer) Phenobarbital 15 mg., belladonna extract 15 mg./Tab. Bot. 100s.
Use: Antispasmodic, antisecretory, sedative.

CHARDOSE POWDER. (Upsher-Smith) Activated charcoal USP 20 gm. or 30 gm./Unit Dose Bottle.
Use: Oral adsorbent.

CHARGERS. (Eckerd) Caffeine 100 mg.
Use: CNS stimulant. Tab. Bot. 40s.

CHARO SCATTER-PAKS. (Requa) Activated charcoal 5 Gm./Packet.
Use: Odor absorber.

CHAZ SCALP TREATMENT DANDRUFF SHAMPOO. (Revlon) Zinc pyrithione 1% in liquid shampoo.
Use: Anti-Dandruff shampoo

CHECKMATE. (CooperCare) Acidulated phosphate fluoride 1.23%. Bot. 2 oz., 16 oz.
Use: Topical application to aid in dental caries prevention.

CHEK-STIX REAGENT STRIPS. (Ames) Bot. 25s.
Use: Control strips for visual urinalysis.

CHELAFRIN.
See: Epinephrine.

CHELAMIDE INJECTION. (Vortech) Disodium edetate 150 mg./ml. Vial 20 ml.
Use: Chelating agent.

CHELATING AGENT.
See: Bal, Amp. (Hynson, Westcott & Dunning)
  Calcium Disodium Versenate, Amp., Tab. (Riker)
  Desferal, Amp. (Ciba)
  Endrate Disodium, Amp. (Abbott)
  Magora, Tab. (Miller)

CHELEN.
See: Ethyl Chloride.

CHEL-IRON. (Kinney) Ferrocholinate, Iron choline citrate complex 0.33 Gm. equiv. to 40 mg. of elemental iron/Tab. Bot. 100s.
Use: Iron deficiency anemias.

CHEL-IRON LIQUID. (Kinney) 0.417 Gm. ferrocholinate equiv. to 50 mg. of elemental iron per teaspoonful. Bot. 8 fl. oz.
Use: Pediatric oral iron therapy.

CHEL-IRON PEDIATRIC DROPS. (Kinney) 0.208 Gm. Ferrocholinate, equiv. to 25 mg. of elemental iron/cc. Bot. 60 cc. with calibrated dropper.
Use: Pediatric oral iron therapy.

CHEL-IRON PLUS. (Kinney) Ferrocholinate 200 mg. (equiv. to 24 mg. elemental iron) Vit. B-12 with intrinsic factor concentrate ⅓ u., Vit. C 50 mg., B-1 2 mg., B-2 2 mg., B-6 HCl 2 mg., niacin 25 mg./Tab. Bot. 100s.
Use: Iron deficiency anemias.

CHEMIPEN. Pot. phenethicillin.
Use: Infections amenable to therapy with oral penicillin.

CHEMOVAG SUPPS. (Fellows) Sulfisoxazole 0.5 Gm./Supp. Bot. 12s w/applicators.
Use: Cervicitis, vaginitis, vulvitis and related gynecologic disorders.

CHEMOZINE. (Tennessee Pharm.) Sulfadiazine, 0.167 Gm., sulfamerazine, 0.167 Gm., sulfamethazine, 0.167 Gm./Tab. Bot. 100s, 1000s. Susp. Bot. 1 pt., 1 gal.

CHENATAL. (Miller) Ca 580 mg., phosphorus 450 mg., dl-methionine 20 mg., Mg 27 mg., Vit. C 100 mg., l-lysine 25 mg., lemon bioflavonoid complex 30 mg., folic acid 0.075 mg., A 5000 I.U., D 400 I.U., B-1 3 mg., B-2 3 mg., B-6 5 mg., B-12 9 mcg., niacinamide 30 mg., Ca pantothenate 5 mg., tocopherols (mixed) 10 mg., Fe 20 mg., Cu 1 mg., Mn 2 mg., K 10 mg., Zn 2 mg., iodine 0.1 mg./3 Tabs. Bot. 100s.
Use: Prenatal vitamin-mineral combination.

CHENIX. (Rowell) Chenodiol 250 mg./Tab. Bot. 100s.
Use: Cholesterol gallstone disolution.

• **CHENODIOL.** USAN.
Use: Anticholelithogenic.
See: Chenix, Tab. (Rowell)

CHERACOL D. (Upjohn) Dextromethorphan HBr 10 mg., guaifenesin 100 mg./ 5 ml. w/alcohol 4.75%. Bot. 2 oz., 4 oz., 6 oz. Bilingual Label Bot. 4 oz.
Use: Coughs due to colds.

CHERACOL. (Upjohn) Codeine phosphate 10 mg., guaifenesin 100 mg./5 ml. w/alcohol 4.75%. Bot. 2 oz., 4 oz., pt.
Use: Narcotic-containing cough mixture.

CHERACOL PLUS. (Upjohn) Phenylpropanolamine HCl 25 mg., dextromethorphan HBr 20 mg., chlorpheniramine maleate 4 mg./15 ml. Bot. 4 oz., 6 oz.
Use: Treatment of head cold symptoms.

CHERALIN SYRUP. (Lannett) Pot. guaiacol sulfonate 8 gr., ammonium chloride 8 gr., antimony and pot. tartrate 1/12 gr. in white pine & wild cherry/Fl. oz. Bot. pt., gal.; also with codeine 1 gr./Oz. Bot. pt., gal.
Use: Cough preparation.

CHERAPAS. (Kay) Hydrochlorothiazide 15 mg., reserpine 0.1 mg., hydralazine 25 mg./Tab. Bot. 1000s.
Use: Treat hypertension.

CHERASULFA PEDIATRIC. (Cenci) Triple sulfa. (5 gr.): Sulfadiazine, 1.67 gr., sulfamethazine, 1.67 gr., sulfamerazine 1.67 gr., sodium citrate 6 gr./5 cc. Bot. 16 oz. **F.S. Liq.:** (7.5 gr.) Bot. 16 oz. **Tab.:** 7.5 gr. Bot. 100s, 1000s, 5000s.
Use: Infections caused by sulfonamide-susceptible organisms.

CHERASULFA SUSPENSION. (Sutliff & Case) Sulfadiazine 167 mg., sulfamethazine 167 mg., sulfamerazine 167 mg., sod. citrate 51 mg./5 cc. Susp. Bot. pt., gal.
Use: Triple sulfonamide therapy.

CHERATUSSIN COUGH SYRUP. (Towne) Dextromethorphan HBr 45 mg., ammon. chloride 575 mg., citrate sodium 280 mg./Fl. oz. Bot. 4 oz.

CHERI-APRO. (Approved) Codeine phos. 1 gr., pot.

GUAIACOLSULFONATE 8 gr., tartar emetic $\frac{1}{12}$ gr./fl. oz. Bot. 4 oz., gal.

CHERIJEN MORPHINE SULFATE. (Jenkins) Alcohol 7%, morphine sulfate 2.5 mg., ammonium chloride 88 mg., potassium guaiacolsulfonate 88 mg., tartar emetic 0.9 mg./5 cc. Syr. 4 oz., gal.

CHERO-TRISULFA-V. (Vita Elixir) Sulfadiazine 0.166 Gm., sulfacetamide 0.166 Gm., sulfamerazine 0.166 Gm., sodium citrate 0.500 Gm./5 cc. Susp. Bot. pt.
Use: Multiple sulfonamide therapy.

CHERRALEX. (Barre) Pot. guiacolsulfonate 8 gr., ammonium chloride 3 gr., tartar emetic $\frac{1}{12}$ gr., alcohol 3%/Fl. oz. Also w/codeine phosphate 1 gr. Bot. pt., gal.
Use: Coughs due to colds.

CHERRY-B. (Vortech) Nicotinamide 10 mg., Vit. B-1 2.5 mg., B-2 0.5 mg., B-6 0.15 mg., d-pantothenyl alcohol 0.20 mg./cc. Bot. 1 oz., pt., Gal.
Use: B-complex therapy.

• **CHERRY JUICE,** N.F. XVI.
Use: Flavor.

• **CHERRY SYRUP,** N.F. XVI.
Use: Pharmaceutic aid (Vehicle)

CHESTAMINE. (Leeds) Chlorpheniramine maleate 8 or 12 mg./Cap. Bot. 50s.
Use: Allergic states responsive to antihistamines.

CHEW HIST. (Kenyon) Phenylephrine HCl 7½ mg., chlorpheniramine maleate 2 mg., C 50 mg./Wafer. Bot. 100s.

CHEWIES TABLETS. (Barry-Martin) Vit. A 5000 I.U., D 500 I.U., B-1 3 mg., B-2 2.5 mg., B-6 1 mg., B-12 1 mcg., C 50 mg., niacinamide 20 mg./Tab. Bot. 100s, 250s. Also available w. minerals.
Use: Multivitamin.
W/Fluoride. Chewies Tab. formula plus fluoride 0.5 mg./Tab.
Use: Vitamin supplement

CHEW-VIMS.(Barth's)Vit.A5000I.U.,D400I.U.,B-13mcg., B-2 6 mg., niacin 1.71 mg., C 100 mg., B-12 5 mcg., E 5 I.U./Tab. Bot. 30s, 90s, 180s, 360s.
Use: Multivitamin.

CHEW-VI-TAB. (Blue Cross) Vit A 2,500 I.U., D 400 I.U. E 15 I.U., C 60 mg., folic acid 0.3 mg., B-1 1.05 mg., B-2 1.2 mg., niacin 13.5 mg., B-6 1.05 mg., B-12 4.5 mcg./Tab. Bot. 100s.
Use: Vitamin supplement.

CHEW-VI-TAB WITH IRON. (Blue Cross) Vit. A 5,000 I.U., C 60 mg., E 15 I.U., folic acid 0.4 mg., B-1 1.5 mg., B-2 1.7 mg., niacin 20 mg., B-6 2 mg., B-12 6 mcg., D 400 I.U., iron 18 mg./Tab. Bot. 100s.
Use: Vitamin and iron supplement.

CHEW-VITE. (Vortech) Vit. A. 5000 I.U., D 500 I.U., C 50 mg., B-1 3 mg., B-2 2.5 mg., B-6 1 mg., Niacinamide 20 mg., B-12 1 mcg./Tab. Bot. 100s, 1000s
Use: Multiple vitamin.

CHEWVITES. (Zenith) Vit. A 3,500 I.U., D 400 I.U., B-1 1.1 mg., B-2 1.2 mg., niacinamide 15 mg., C 40 mg., B-6 1.2 mg., B-12 5 mcg., folic acid 0.1 mg., pantothenic acid 5 mg./Tab. Bot. 100s.
Use: Chewable vitamins.

CHEW VITES. (Kenyon) Vit. A 5000 I.U., D 500 I.U., B-1 2 mg., B-2 2 mg., B-6 1 mg., B-12 2 mcg. Ca pantothenate 2 mg., C 50 mg., niacinamide 10 mg., fluoride 0.05 mg./Tab. Bot. 100s.

CHEXIT. (Dorsey) Pheniramine maleate 12.5 mg., pyrilamine maleate 12.5 mg., phenylpropanolamine 25 mg., dextromethorphan HBr 30 mg., terpin hydrate 180 mg., acetaminophen 325 mg./Tab. Dispenser 12s. Industrial Pak 100-1s.
Use: Decongestant & antitussive.

CHIGGEREX. (Scherer) Benzocaine 0.02% w/camphor, menthol, peppermint oil, olive oil, clove oils, pegosperse, methylparaben, distilled water. Oint. Jar 50 Gm.
Use: Chigger bites.

CHIGGERTOX. (Scherer) Benzocaine 2.1%, benzyl benzoate 21.4%, soft soap, isopropyl alcohol. Liq. Bot. 1 oz.
Use: Chigger, tick, and mosquito bites.

CHILDREN'S COLD TABLETS. (Towne) Chlorpheniramine maleate 0.75 mg., phenylephrine HCl 1 mg., salicylamide 100 mg., caffeine 16.25 mg./Tab. Bot. 36s.

CHILDREN'S CONGEST-AFED DM SYRUP. (Eckerd) Pseudoephedrine HCl 30 mg., guaifenesin 100 mg., dextromethorphan HBr 10 mg./5 ml. w/alcohol 10%. Bot. 4 oz.
Use: Decongestant, expectorant, antitussive.

CHILDREN'S COUGH SYRUP. (Eckerd) Phenylpropanolamine HCl 6.25 mg., guaifenesin 75 mg., dextromethorphan 5 mg.,/5 ml. w/alcohol 5%. Bot. 4 oz.
Use: Expectorant, decongestant, antitussive.

CHILDREN'S HOLD 4-HOUR COUGH SUPPRESSANT & DECONGESTANT. (Beecham Products) d-Methorphan HBr, phenylpropanolamine HCl. Loz. 10s.
Use: Antitussive & decongestant.

CHILDREN'S NO ASPIRIN ELIXIR. (Walgreen) Acetaminophen 80 mg./2.5 ml. Bot. 4 oz.
Use: Analgesic.

CHINESE GELATIN.
See: Agar

CHINESE ISINGLASS. 7-Iodo-8-hydroxyquinoline-5-sulfonic acid sodium salt. Yatren.
Use: Amebic dysentery.

CHINIOFON. 7-Iodo-8-hydroxyquinoline-5-sulfonic acid, anayodin, yatren, quinoxyl. (CMC) Chiniofon 250 mg., 8-hydroxy-7-iodoquinoline-5-sulfonic acid 80%, sod. bicarbonate 20%/Tab. Bot. 100s, 1000s.
Use: Intestinal amebiasis.

CHINOSOL. (Vernon) 8-Hydroxyquinoline sulfate. Tab. 7½ gr. Vial 6s. Trit. Tabs. ($\frac{3}{5}$ gr.) Bot. 50s. Vial 110s. Pow. 1 oz.
Use: Antiseptic sol.

CHLAMYDIAZYME. (Abbott) Test kits 100s.
Use: Enzyme immunoassay for detection of chlamydin trachomatis from urethral or urogenital swabs.

CHLO-AMINE. (Hollister-Stier) Chlorpheniramine maleate 2 mg./Chewable Tab. Box 24x4 mg. Tab. Packages.
Use: Allergy therapy.

- **CHLOPHEDIANOL.** F.D.A. 2-Chloro-alpha-[2-(dimethylamino)ethyl] benzhydrol.
CHLOPHEDIANOL. B.A.N. 2-Chloro-α-(2-dimethylaminoethyl)benzhydrol.
Use: Cough suppressant.
See: Detigon Hydrochloride
- **CHLOPHEDIANOL HCl.** USAN. a-(2-Dimethylaminoethyl)-o-chlorobenzyhydrol HCl.
See: Ulo, Syr. (Riker)
W/Diphenylpyraline HCl, phenylephrine HCl, gualifenesin, alcohol.
See: Acutuss Expectorant (Philips Roxane)
CHLOR-4. (Mills) Chlorpheniramine maleate 4 mg./Tab. Bot. 100s.
CHLOR-100. (Vortech) Chlorpheniramine maleate 100 mg./ml. Vial 10 ml.
Use: Antihistaminic.
CHLORACET CAP. (Jenkins) Chlorpheniramine maleate 4 mg., salicylamide 3 gr., phenacetin 2 gr., caffein ½ gr., ascorbic acid 50 mg./Cap. Bot. 1000s.
CHLORAFED. (Hauck) Chlorpheniramine maleate 2 mg., pseudoephedrine HCl 30 mg./5 ml. Alcohol, dye, sugar and corn free. Bot. Pts.
Use: Allergy and common cold treatment.
CHLORAFED TIMECELLES. (Hauck) Chlorpheniramine maleate 8 mg., pseudoephedrine HCl 120 mg./Sustained action timeceles. Bot. 100s, 500s. Unit dose 100s.
Use: Allergy and common cold treatment.
CHLORAFED H.S. TIMECELLES. (Hauck) Chlorpheniramine maleate 4 mg., pseudoephedrine HCl 60 mg./S.R. Cap. Bot. 100s, 500s.
Use: Allergy & common cold treatment.
CHLORAFED INJECTION. (Hauck) Chlorpheniramine maleate 5mg.,atropinesulfate0.2mg./ml.Vial10ml.
Use: Allergy & common cold treatment.
CHLORAHIST. (Evron) Chlorpheniramine maleate 4 mg./Tab. Bot. 100s, 1000s. Chlorpheniramine maleate 8 or 12 mg./Cap. Bot. 250s, 1000s. Syr. 2 mg./4 cc. Bot. qt.
Use: Symptomatic relief of allergic manifestations.
- **CHLORAL BETAINE.** USAN.
Use: Sedative.
CHLORALFORMAMIDE. N-(2,2,2-trichloro-l-hydroxyethyl) formamide.
- **CHLORAL HYDRATE,** U.S.P. XXI. Caps., Syr. U.S.P. XXI. 1,1-Ethanediol, 2,2,2-trichloro-ethanol. Chloral.
Use: Hypnotic and sedative.
See: Aquachloral Supprettes, Supp. (Webcon)
Cohidrate, Cap. (Coastal)
Felsules, Cap. (Fellows-Testagar)
H.S. Need, Cap. (Hanlon)
Maso-Chloral, Cap. (Mason)
Noctec, Cap. & Syr. (Squibb)
Oradrate, Cap. (Coast Labs.)
Rectules, Supp. (Fellows-Testagar)
SK-Chloral Hydrate, Cap. (SmithKline)
Somnos, Elixir. (Merck Sharp & Dohme)
Generic Products:
Fellows-Cap. (3¾ gr.) Bot. 100s, 500s, 1000s.

Columbia- (7½ gr.) Bot. 100s.
G.F. Harvey-Cap. (3¾ gr.) Bot. 100s; (7½ gr.) Bot. 100s.
Lederle-Cap. 500 mg. 100s.
Pacific Pharm. Corp.-Cap. (7½ gr.) Bot. 100s, 1000s.
Parke, Davis—Cap. (500 mg.) Bot. 100s, unit dose 100s.
Stayner-Cap. (250 mg. and 500 mg.) Bot. 100s, 500 mg. Bot. 1000s, Crystals Bot. 1 lb. and 5 lbs.
West-Ward-Cap. (3¾ gr., 7½ gr.) Bot. 100s.
CHLORAL HYDRATE BETAINE (1:1) COMPOUND. Chloral Betaine.
CHLORAL-METHYLOL OINTMENT. (Ulmer) Methyl salicylate, methol. Jar. 1 oz., 1 lb.
Use: Analgesic ointment.
CHLORALPYRINE DICHLORALPYRINE.
See: Dichloralantipyrine
CHLORALURETHANE. Name used for Carbochloral.
CHLORAMAN. (Rasman) Chlorpheniramine maleate 12 mg./Tab. Bot. 100s, 500s, 1000s.
Use: Antihistaminic.
- **CHLORAMBUCIL,** U.S.P. XXI. Tab. U.S.P. XXI. 4-{p-[Bis(2-chlorethyl)-amino]-phenyl} butyric acid. Benzenebutanoic acid. 4-[bis(2-chloroethyl)-amino]-.
Use: Antineoplastic.
See: Leukeran, Tab. (Burroughs-Wellcome)
CHLORAMBUCIL. B.A.N. 4-[4-Di-(2-chloroethyl) aminophenyl]butyric acid.
Use: Antineoplastic agent.
See: Leukeran
CHLORAMINE-T. Sod. paratoluenesulfan chloramide, chloramine & chlorozone.
Lilly-Tab. (0.3 Gm.), Bot. 100s, 1000s.
Mallinckrodt, Pow., 1 lb.
Robinson, Pow., 1 oz.
Use: Antiseptic, deodorant.
See: Chlorazene, Prep. (Badger)
- **CHLORAMPHENICOL.** U.S.P. XXI. Caps., Cream, Oral Soln., Tab., Otic Soln., Sterile, Ophth. Sol., Ophth. Oint., for Ophth. Sol. Inj., U.S.P. XXI. D(-)-threo-2, 2-Dichloro-N[Beta-hydroxy-alpha-(hydroxymethyl)-p-nitrophenethyl]acetamide.
Use: Antibacterial, antirickettsial.
See: Antibiopto, Soln. Oint. (Softcon)
Chlorcetin
Chloromycetin, Prep. (Parke-Davis)
Chloroptic Ophth. Oint. (Allergan)
Chloroptic S.O.P. Ophth. Oint. (Allergan)
Econochlor, Soln., Oint. (Alcon)
Kemicetine
Mychel, Cap. (Rachelle)
Ophthochlor, Sol. (Parke-Davis)
Paraxin
W/Polymixin B.
Use: Treatment of superficial ocular infections involving the conjuctivia and/or cornia caused by susceptible organisms.
See: Chloromyxin Ophthalmic Oint. (Parke-Davis)
W/Polymyxin B, Hydrocortisone.
See: Ophthocort, Oint. (Parke-Davis)

W/Prednisolone alcohol.
See: Chloroptic-P S.O.P. Ophth. Oint. (Allergan)
CHLORAMPHENICOL. B.A.N. D-threo-2-Di-
chloroacetamido-1-(4-nitrophenyl)propane-1,
3-diol.
Use: Antiseptic; antibiotic.
• **CHLORAMPHENICOL AND HYDROCORTISONE
ACETATE FOR OPHTHALMIC SUSPENSION,**
U.S.P. XXI.
Use: Antibiotic, anti-inflammatory.
See: Chloromycetin, Prods. (Parke-Davis)
• **CHLORAMPHENICOL AND POLYMYXIN B
SULFATE OPHTHALMIC OINTMENT,** U.S.P. XXI.
Use: Antibiotic.
• **CHLORAMPHENICOL, POLYMIXIN B SULFATE,
AND HYDROCORTISONE ACETATE
OPHTHALMIC OINTMENT,** U.S.P. XXI.
Use: Antibiotic, anti-inflammatory.
See: Chloromycetin, Prods. (Parke-Davis).
• **CHLORAMPHENICOL AND PREDNISOLONE
OPHTHALMIC OINTMENT,** U.S.P. XXI.
Use: Antibiotic, steroid combination.
See: Chloromycetin, Prods. (Parke-Davis)
• **CHLORAMPHENICOL PALMITATE,** U.S.P. XXI.
Oral Susp. U.S.P. XXI.
Use: Antibacterial, antirickettsial.
See: Chloromycetin Palmitate, Oral Susp.
(Parke-Davis)
• **CHLORAMPHENICOL PANTOTHENATE
COMPLEX.** USAN. A complex consisting of 4 parts
of chloramphenicol to one part of calcium
pantothenate. Pantofenicol
Use: Antibiotic.
• **CHLORAMPHENICOL SODIUM SUCCINATE,
STERILE,** U.S.P. XXI.
Use: Antibacterial, antirickettsial.
See: Chloromycetin Succinate, Inj., (Parke-Davis)
Mychel-S, IV. (Rachelle)
CHLORANIL. 2,3,5,6-Tetrachloro-1,4-benzoquinone.
CHLORASEPTIC CHILDREN'S LOZENGES. (Procter
& Gamble) Benzocaine 5 mg./Loz. Pkg. 18s.
Use: Anesthetic for temporary relief of minor sore
throat pain.
CHLORASEPTIC LIQUID. (Procter & Gamble) Total
phenol 1.4% as phenol and sodium phenolate.
Menthol and cherry flavors. Pkg. 6 oz. w/sprayer, 8
& 12 oz. Spray 1.5 oz. Spray also contains
compressed nitrogen.
Use: Antiseptic and anesthetic mouthwash and
gargle for temporary relief of sore throat pain.
CHLORASEPTIC LOZENGE. (Procter & Gamble)
Total phenol 32.5 mg./lozenge as phenol and
sodium phenolate, sugar, corn syr. solids. Menthol
and cherry flavors. Pkg.: 18s, 45s.
Use: Anesthetic and antiseptic lozenge for
temporary relief of minor sore throat pain.
CHLOR-A-TYL. (Jenkins) Acetyl-p-aminophenol 160
mg., chlorpheniramine maleate 1 mg.,
phenylephrine HCl 7½ mg., ascorbic acid 15
mg./Tab. Bot. 1000s.
CHLORAZANIL HCl. 2-Amino-4-(p-chloroanilino)-s-tria-
zine HCl. Daquim

CHLORAZENE. (Badger) Chloramine-T, sod. p-toluene-
sulfonchloramide. Pow., Pkg. No. 1 & No. 2; Bot. 1 lb.,
5 lb. Aromatic Pow. (5%), Bot. 1 lb., 5 lb. Tab. (0.3
Gm.), Bot. 20s, 100s, 1000s, 5000s.
Use: Topically; antiseptic, deodorant.
CHLORAZEPATE DIPOTASSIUM.
Use: Minor tranquilizer.
See: Tranxene Prods. (Abbott)
CHLORAZEPTATE MONOPOTASSIUM.
Use: Minor tranquilizer
CHLORAZONE.
See: Chloramine-T
CHLOR BENZO MOR, A AND D OINTMENT. (Wade)
Vitamins A and D fortified, chlorobutanol 3%,
benzocaine 2%, benzyl alcohol 3%, actamer 1%,
in lanolin and petrolatum base. Tube 1 oz., Jar 1
oz., lb.
Use: Antiseptic, anesthetic.
CHLOR BENZO MOR SPRAY. (Wade) Vitamin A and
D fortified, chlorabutanol 3%, benzocaine 2%,
benzyl alcohol 3%, and actamer 1%, in lanolin and
mineral oil base. Bot. 2 oz., 11 oz.
Use: Antiseptic, anesthetic.
CHLORBETAMIDE. B.A.N. Dichloro-N-(2,4-di-
chlorobenzyl)-N-(2-hydroxyethyl)acetamide.
Use: Treatment of amebiasis.
See: Mantomide
Pontalin
CHLORBUTANOL.
See: Chlorobutanol, N.F. XVI.
CHLORBUTOL.
See: Chlorobutanol, N.F. XVI.
CHLORCYCLIZINE. B.A.N. 1-(4-Chlorobenzhydryl)-4-
methylpiperazine.
Use: Antihistamine.
See: Di-paralene Histantin hydrochloride
• **CHLORCYCLIZINE HYDROCHLORIDE,** N.F. XVI. 1-
(p-Chloro-α-phenylbenzyl)-4-methylpiperazine HCl. 1-
(p-Chlorobenzhydryl)-4-methylpiperazine HCl. Histan-
tin.
Use: Antihistaminic.
W/Hydrocortisone acetate.
See: Mantadil, Cream (Burroughs Wellcome)
W/Pseudoephedrine HCl.
See: Fedrazil, Tab. (Burroughs Wellcome)
• **CHLORDANTOIN.** F.D.A. 5-(1-Ethylpentyl)-3-[(tri-
chloromethyl) thio] hydantoin.
• **CHLORDANTOIN.** USAN. 5-(1-Ethylamyl)-3-trichloro-
methyl thiohydantoin.
Use: Antifungal.
See: Sporostacin Cr. (Ortho)
CHLORDIAZACHEL. (Rachelle) Chlordiazepoxide HCl
5 mg., 10 mg., 25 mg./Cap. Bot. 100s, 500s.
Use: Tranquilizer.
• **CHLORDIAZEPOXIDE,** U.S.P. XXI. Tab., U.S.P. XXI.
3H-1, 4-Benzodiazepin-2-amine, 7-chloro-N-methyl-
5-phenyl-, 4-oxide; 7-chloro-2-(methylamino)-5-phe-
nyl-3H-1, 4-benzodiazepine 4-oxide.
Use: Tranquilizer.
See: A-poxide, Cap. (Abbott)
Brigen-G, Tab. (Grafton)

Libritabs, Tab. (Roche)
Menrium, Tab. (Roche)
W/Amitriptyline
  See: Limbitrol, Tab. (Roche)
• **CHLORDIAZEPOXIDE HCI,** U.S.P. XXI., Caps,
  Sterile U.S.P. XXI. 7-Chloro-2-methylamino-5-phenyl-
  3H-1, 4-benzodiazepine-4-oxide HCI. Metha-
  minodiazepine HCI.
  Use: Emotional disturbance, sedative.
  See: A-poxide, Cap. (Abbott)
    Chlordiazachel, Cap. (Rachelle)
    Librium, Cap., Inj. (Roche)
    Screen, Cap. (Foy)
    SK-Lygen, Cap. (SmithKline)
    Zetran, Cap. (Hauck)
W/Clidinium bromide
  See: Chlordinium Sealets, Cap. (Lemmon)
    Librax, Cap. (Roche)
• **CHLORDIAZEPOXIDE AND AMITRIPTPTYLINE
  HCL TABLETS,** U.S.P. XXI.
  Use: Tranquilizer.
  See: Limbitrol, Tab. (Roche)
CHLORDIMORPHINE HCI. γ-Morpholino-propyl-2-chlo-
  ro-4-phenylphenyl ether HCI.
CHLORDINIUM SEALETS. (Lemmon)
  Chlordiazepoxide HCI 5 mg., clidinium Br 2.5
  mg./Cap. Bot. 100s, 500s, 1000s.
  Use: Gastrointestinal disorders.
CHLOREN 4. (Wren) Chlorpheniramine maleate 4
  mg./Tab. Bot. 100s, 1000s.
CHLOREN 8 T.D. (Wren) Chlorpheniramine maleate 8
  mg./Tab. Bot. 100s, 1000s.
CHLOREN 12 T.D. (Wren) Chlorpheniramine maleate
  12 mg./Tab. Bot. 100s, 1000s.
CHLORESIUM DENTAL OINT. (Rystan) Water-soluble
  chlorophyll 0.5% in hydrophilic base. Tube 0.5 oz.
  Use: Tissue repair.
CHLORESIUM OINTMENT. (Rystan) Water soluble
  chlorophyll "a" (0.5%) in specially prepared water-
  soluble base. Tube 1 oz., 4 oz. Jar 1 lb.
  Use: Promote tissue growth and deodorize.
CHLORESIUM SOLUTION. (Rystan) Water-soluble
  chlorophyll "a" (0.2%) in isotonic saline solution.
  Bot. 2 oz., 8 oz., 32 oz.
  Use: Cleansing and deodorization of purulent
  wounds.
CHLORESIUM TOOTH PASTE. (Rystan) Purified
  chlorophyllin (water-soluble). Tube 3.25 oz.
CHLORETHYL.
  See: Ethyl Chloride
CHLORFENVINPHOS. B.A.N. 2-Chloro-1-(2,4-dichloro-
  phenyl)vinyl diethyl phosphate.
  Use: Insecticide, veterinary medicine.
  See: Birlane
CHLORGUANIDE HYDROCHLORIDE.
  See: Chloroguanide HCI (Various Mfr.)
CHLORHEXADOL. 2-Methyl-4-(2',2',2',-trichlor-1'-hy-
  droxyethoxy)-2-pentanol. Lora
CHLORHEXADOL. B.A.N. 2-Methyl-4-(2,2,2-trichloro-
  1-hydroxyethoxy)pentan-2-ol.
  Use: Hypnotic; sedative.
  See: Chloralodol (I.N.N.)
    Medodorm

• **CHLORHEXIDINE.** F.D.A. 1,1'-Hexamethylenebis-
  [5-(ρ-chlorophenyl) biguanide]
  Use: Antiseptic.
  See: Hibiclens
    Hibiscrub
    Hibitane
    Lisium
    Rotersept
• **CHLORHEXIDINE GLUCONATE.** USAN. 1,1'-Hex-
  amethylenebis[5-(ρ-chlorophenyl)biguanide] dihydro-
  chloride.
  Use: Antimicrobial skin cleanser.
  See: Hibiclens, Liq. (Stuart)
    Hibistat, Liq. (Stuart)
• **CHLORHEXIDINE HYDROCHLORIDE.** USAN.
  Use: Anti-infective, topical.
CHLOR-HYDRO CREAM. (Vortech) Tube. 15 Gm.
  Use: Antipruritic, anti-inflammatory, anesthetic.
CHLORHYDROXYQUINOLIN.
  See: Quinolor Comp., Oint. (Squibb)
CHLORINATED AND IODIZED PEANUT OIL.
  Chloriodized Oil.
• **CHLORINDANOL.** USAN. 7-Chloro-4-indanol.
  Use: Antiseptic, spermaticide.
CHLORINE COMPOUND, ANTISEPTIC. Antiseptics,
  Chlorine.
CHLORIODIZED OIL. Chlorinated and iodized peanut
  oil.
CHLORISONDAMINE CHLORIDE. 4,5,6,7-Tetra-
  chloro-2-(2-dimethylaminoethyl)-isoindoline dimetho-
  chloride.
CHLORISONDAMINE CHLORIDE. B.A.N. 4,5,6,7-Tet-
  rachloro-2-(2-trimethylammonioethyl)-isoindolinium
  dichloride.
  Use: Hypotensive.
  See: Ecolid
CHLORMADINONE. B.A.N. 6-Chloro-17α-hydroxypreg-
  na-4,6-diene-3,20-dione.
  Use: Progestational steroid.
  See: Clordion
    Normenon
    Verton
• **CHLORMADINONE ACETATE.** USAN. 6-Chloro-6-
  dehydro-17α-acetoxyprogesterone. 6-Chloro-17-hy-
  droxypregna-4,6-diene-3,20 dione Acetate.
CHLOR MAL w/SAL + APAP S.C. (Richlyn)
  Chlorpheneramine maleate 2 mg., acetaminophen
  150 mg., salicylamide 175 mg./Tab. Bot. 1000s.
  Use: Antihistamine, analgesic.
CHLORMENE. (Robinson) Chlorpheniramine maleate
  4 mg./Tab.
  Bot. 100s, 1000s.
  Use: Antihistamine.
CHLORMENE INJECTION. (Robinson)
  Chlorpheniramine maleate injection. 10 mg., 30 cc.
  Vial; 100 mg. 10 cc. Vial.
CHLORMENE REPEAT ACTION. (Robinson)
  Chlorpheniramine 8 mg., 12 mg./Tab. Bot. 100s,
  1000s.
CHLORMENE TIMECAPS. (Robinson)
  Chlorpheniramine maleate time disintegration 8
  mg., 12 mg./Tab. Bot. 100s, 500s, 1000s.
CHLORMERODRIN. 3-Chloro-mercuri-2-methoxy-

propylurea. Chloro (2-methoxy-3-ureidopropyl) mercury. Mercloran.
Use: Diuretic.

CHLORMERODRIN Hg 197 INJECTION. Mercury-197HG, [3-[(aminocarbonyl)amino]-2-methoxypropyl]-chloro-. Chloro(2-methoxy-3-ureidopropyl)mercury-197Hg.
Use: Diagnostic aid (renal scanning).

CHLORMERODRIN Hg 203 INJECTION. Mercury-203Hg,[3-[(aminocarbonyl)amino]-ureidopropyl)mercury-203Hg.
Use: Diagnostic aid (tumor localization).

CHLORMETHIAZOLE. B.A.N. 5-(2-Chloroethyl)-4-methylthiazole.
Use: Hypnotic; sedative.
See: Heminevrin (base or the edisylate)

CHLORMEZANONE. Chlormethazanone. 2-(4-Chlorophenyl)-3-methyl-4-methathiazanone-1-2-dioxide
Use: Tranquilizer.
See: Trancopal, Cap. (Winthrop-Breon)

CHLORMIDAZOLE. B.A.N. 1-(4-Chlorobenzyl)-2-methylbenzimidazole.
Use: Antifungal agent.

CHLOR-NIRAMINE ALLERGY TABS. (Whiteworth) Chlorpheniramine maleate 4 mg./Tab. Bot. 24s, 100s.
Use: Antihistaminic.

CHLOROAZODIN. Alpha, alpha, Azobis-(chloroformamidine).

6-CHLORO-H-1,2,4-BENZOTHIADIAZINE-7-SULFONAMIDE 1,1-DIOXIDE.
See: Chlorothiazide

1-(γ-(p-CHLOROBENZYL) CINNAMYL) PYRROLIDINE PHOSPHATE (1:2).
See: Pyrrobutamine Phosphate

• **CHLOROBUTANOL**, N.F. XVI. 1,1,1-Trichloro-2-methyl-2-propanol. Sedaform. (Various Mfr.)
Use: Anesthetic, antiseptic & hypnotic; pharmaceutic aid (antimicrobial preservative).
See: Cerumenex, Drops. (Purdue-Frederick)
Pre-Sert(Allergan)
W/Atropine sulfate, chlorpheniramine maleate, phenylpropanolamine HCl.
See: Decongestant, Inj. (Century)
W/Benzocaine and camphor.
See: Eardro, Liq. (Jenkins)
W/Calcium glycerophosphate, calcium levulinate.
See: Cal San, Inj. (Burgin-Arden)
W/Cetyltrimethylammonium Br, methapyrilene HCl, phenylephrine HCl, hydrocortisone.
See: T-Spray, Liq. (Saron)
W/Diphenhydramine HCl.
See: Ardeben, Inj. (Burgin-Arden)
W/Ephedrine hydrochloride, sodium chloride.
See: Efedron HCl Nasal Jelly (Hart)
W/Estradiol cypionate, testosterone cypionate.
See: Depo-Testadiol, Vial (Upjohn)
Depotestogen, Vial (Hyrex)
Testadiate-Depo, Vial (Kay)
W/Glycerin, anhydrous.
See: Ophthalgan, Liq. (Ayerst)
W/Liquifilm.

See: Liquifilm Tears (Allergan)
W/Methylcellulose.
See: Lacril (Allergan)
W/Myristyl-gamma-picolinium chloride.
See: Wet Tone, Soln. (Riker)
W/Nonionic lanolin derivative.
See: Lacri-Lube, Ophthalmic Ointment (Allergan)
W/Polyethylene glycol, polyoxyl 40 stearate.
See: Blink-N-Clean (Allergan)
W/Sod. chloride.
See: Ocean, Liq. (Fleming)
W/Tannic acid, isopropyl alcohol.
See: Outgro, Sol. (Whitehall)
W/Testosterone enanthate.
See: Anthatest, Vial (Kay)
W/Vit. B-1, B-2, B-6, niacinamide, calcium pantothenate, benzyl alcohol.
See: Lanoplex, Inj. (Lannett)

CHLOROCON. (CMC) Chloroquine phosphate 250 mg./Tab. Bot. 100s, 500s, 1000s.
Use: Antimalarial.

• **CHLOROCRESOL.** USAN.
Use: Antiseptic, disinfectant.

7-CHLORO-6-DEMETHYLTETRACYCLINE HYDROCHLORIDE.
See: Demeclocycline Hydrochloride

7-CHLORO-1,3-DIHYDRO-3-HYDROXY-5-PHENYL-2H-1,4-BENZODIAZEPIN-2-ONE.
See: Oxazepam

7-CHLORO-1,3-DIHYDRO-1-METHYL-5-PHENYL-2H-1,4-BENZODIAZEPIN-2-ONE.
See: Diazepam

7-CHLORO-4,6-DIMETHOXYCOUMARAN-3-ONE-2-SPIRO-1'-(2'-METHOXY-6'-METHYLCYCLOHEX-2'-EN-4'-ONE). Griseofulvin.

2-(p-CHLORO-α-(2-(DIMETHYLAMINO)-ETHOXY)BENZYL)PYRIDINE MALEATE (1:1).
See: Carbinoxamine Maleate

(+)-2-(p-CHLORO-α-(2-(DIMETHYLAMINO)-ETHYL)BENZYL) PYRIDINE MALEATE (1:1).
See: Dexchlorpheniramine Maleate

2-CHLORO-10-[3-(DIMETHYLAMINO)-PROPYL]PHENOTHIAZINE. Chlorpromazine, U.S.P. XXI.

(E)-2-CHLORO-N,N-DIMETHYLTHIOZANTHENE-Δ-9 γ-PROPYLAMINE.
See: Chlorprothixene

CHLOROETHANE.
See: Ethyl Chloride

CHLORODRI. (Kenyon) Chlorpheniramine maleate 5 mg., phenylpropanolamine HCl 12.5 mg., atropine sulfate 0.2 mg./cc. Vial 10 cc.

1-CHLORO-3-ETHYL-1-PENTEN-4-YN-3-OL.
See: Ethchlorvynol, U.S.P. XXI.

• **CHLOROFORM**, N.F. XVI. Bot. 1 lb., 5 lb.
Use: Inhalation anesthetic: solvent.

4-CHLORO-N-FURFURYL-5-SULFAMOYL-ANTHRANILIC ACID. Furosemide, U.S.P. XXI.

CHLOROGUANIDE HYDROCHLORIDE. (Various Mfr.) (Proguanil HCl) 1-(p-Chlorophenyl)-5-isopropyl-biguanidine HCl. Guanatol HCl.
Use: Antimalarial.

CHLOROHYDRATES. Same as Hydrochloride.

6-CHLORO-17-HYDROXYPREGNA-4,6-DIENE-3, 20-DIONE ACETATE.
See: Chlormadinone Acetate

CHLORO-IODOHYDROXYQUINOLINE.
See: Clioquinol, U.S.P. XXI.

5-CHLORO-7-IODO-8-QUINOLINOL.
See: Clioquinol, U.S.P. XXI.

p-CHLOROMETAXYLENOL.
W/Benzocaine, benzyl alcohol, propylene glycol.
See: 20-Cain Burn Relief, Bot. (Alto)
W/Hydrocortisone, pramoxine HCl.
See: Orlex HC, Otic (Baylor)

CHLOROMETHAPYRILENE CITRATE.
See: Chlorothen Citrate.

CHLORO(2-METHOXY-3-UREIDOPROPYL)-MERCURY.
See: Chlormerodin

7-CHLORO-2-(METHYLAMINO)-5-PHENYL-3H-1,4-BENZODIAZEPINE 4-OXIDE.
See: Chlordiazepoxide, U.S.P. XXI.

2-CHLORO-10-(3-(4-METHYL-1-PIPER-AZINYL)-PRO-PYL)PHENOTHIAZINE.
See: Prochlorperazine, U.S.P. XXI.

CHLOROMYCETIN. (Parke-Davis) Chloramphenicol.
Cream: (1%) w/cetyl alcohol, sod. lauryl sulfate, liq. petrolatum, buffered with sod. phosphate, and propylparaben. Tube 1 oz.
Kapseal: (250 mg.) Bot. 16s, 100s. Unit dose 100s.
Ophth. Oint.: (1%) in base of petrolatum and polyethylene. Tube 3.5 Gm.
Ophth. Sol.: (25 mg.) Bot. w/dropper 15 cc. (dry). Sol. 5 mg./ml. Plastic dropper Bot. 5 ml.
Otic Drops: (0.5%) 5 mg./ml. w/propylene glycol Bot. 15 ml.
Palmitate, Oral Susp. (150 mg./5 ml.) w/Sodium benzoate 0.5% Bottles 60 ml.
Use: Antibiotic.

CHLOROMYCETIN-CORTISOL OPHTHALMIC.
(Parke-Davis) Chloromycetin 12.5 mg., hydrocortisone acetate 25 mg., borate buffer, phemerol. Vial 5 ml. Stable at room temperature for 10 days after reconstitution with water.
Use: Inflammatory infections.

CHLOROMYCETIN SODIUM SUCCINATE I.V.
(Parke-Davis) Chloramphenicol sodium succinate dried powder which when reconstituted contains chloromycetin 100 mg./ml. Steri-vials 1 Gm. 10s.
Use: I.V. treatment of salmonella typhi infections.

CHLOROMYXIN. (Parke-Davis) Chloramphenicol 10 mg., polymixin B 5000 units/Gm. in base of liquid petrolatum & polyethylene. Tube 3.5 Gm.
Use: Treatment of occular infections.

CHORON 10. (O'Neal, Jones & Feldman) Chorionic gonadotropin 1000 units. Vial 10 ml.

CHLOROPHEN. (C.M.C.) Chlorpheniramine maleate 20 mg./cc. Vial 10 cc. 100 mg./cc. Vial 10 cc.
Use: Antihistamine therapy.

CHLOROPHEN. (Robinson) Chlorphentermine HCl 65 mg./Tab. Bot. 100s, 1000s.

p-CHLOROPHENOL.
See: Parachlorophenol

CHLOROPHENOTHANE.   1,1,1-Trichloro-2,2-bis(p-

chlorophenyl) ethane. Gesarol, Neocid, Dicophane
Use: Pediculicide.

4-(3-(2-CHLOROPHENOTHIAZIN-1-yl)-PROPYL)-1-PIPERAZINEETHANOL.
See: Perphenazine, U.S.P. XXI.

1-(p-CHLORO-α-PHENYLBENZYL)-4-METHYL-PIPE-RAZINE MONOHYDROCHLORIDE.
See: Chlorcyclizine Hydrochloride, U.S.P. XXI.

4-(4-(p-CHLOROPHENYL)-4-HYDROXYPIPERIDINO)-4-FLUOROBUTYROPHENONE.
See: Haloperidol, U.S.P. XXI.

CHLOROPHYLL. W/Formalin, benzalkonium chloride.
See: Mycomist, Spray Liq. (Gordon)

CHLOROPHYLL "a" OINTMENT.
See: Chloresium Oint. (Rystan)

CHLOROPHYLL "a" SOLUTION (Chlorophyllin).
See: Chloresium Sol. (Rystan)

CHLOROPHYLL COMPLEX PERLES. (Standard Process) Natural chlorophyll extracted from alfalfa and tillandsia. Vit. K 3.3 mg./6 Perles. Bot. 60s, 350s. Oint. Tube 1½ oz., Jar 3 oz.

CHLOROPHYLL TABLETS.
See: Derifil, Tab. (Rystan)
Nullo, Tab. (Depree)

CHLOROPHYLL, WATER-SOLUBLE. (Various Mfr.) Chlorophyllin.
See: Chloresium Prep. (Rystan)
Derifil, Pow. (Rystan)

CHLOROPHYLLIN.
Use: Healing agent & deodorizer.

• **CHLOROPHYLLIN COPPER COMPLEX.** USAN.
Use: Deodorant.

• **CHLOROPROCAINE HCl,** U.S.P. XXI. Inj., U.S.P. XXI. beta, Diethylamino-ethyl 2-chloro-4-amino-benzoate HCl. 4-amino-2-chloro-, 2-(diethylamino) ethyl ester, HCl. 2-(Diethylamino) ethyl 4-amino-2-chloro-benzoate HCl. (Abbott) 2% or 3%. Concentration in Abboject Syringe, Ampul or Vial.
See: Nesacaine, Vial (Pennwalt)
Nescaine-CE, Vial (Pennwalt)

CHLOROPTIC. (Allergan) Chloramphenicol 0.5%, chlorobutanol 0.5%. Dropper bot. 7.5 ml. Unit dose 2.5 ml. Sterile Ophth. Oint. 1.0%, Tube 3.5 ml.
Use: Bacterial conjunctivitis.

CHLOROPTIC-P S.O.P. STERILE OPHTHALMIC OINTMENT. (Allergan) Chloramphenicol 1%, prednisolone alcohol 0.5%. Ophth. Oint. Tube 3.5 Gm.
Use: Eye infections.

• **CHLOROQUINE,** U.S.P. XXI. 7-Chloro-4-[[4-(diethylamino)-1-methyl butyl]amino]quinoline.
Use: Pharmaceutic necessity for chloroquine HCl.
See: Aralen HCl Prods. (Winthrop-Breon)

CHLOROQUINE. B.A.N. 7-Chloro-4-(4-diethyl-amino-1-methylbutylamino)-quinoline.
Use: Antimalarial.
See: Aralen
Avloclor
Bemasulph
Nivaquine
Resochin
Roquine, Tab. (Robinson)

• **CHLOROQUINE HYDROCHLORIDE, INJ.,** U.S.P. XXI.
  Use: Antiamebic, antimalarial.
• **CHLOROQUINE PHOSPHATE,** U.S.P. XXI. Tab. U.S.P. XXI. Nivaquine.
  Use: Febrile attacks of malaria; antiamebic; lupus erythematosus suppressant.
  See: Aralen Phosphate, Tab. (Winthrop-Breon)
      Chlorocon, Tab. (C.M.C.)
4-((7-CHLORO-4-QUINOLYL)AMINO)-α-(DIETHYLA- MINO)-0-CRESOL DIHYDROCHLORIDE. Amodiaquine Hydrochloride U.S.P. XXI.
5-CHLORO-SALICYLANILIDE.
7-CHLOROTETRACYCLINE HYDROCHLORIDE.
  Use: Antibacterial, antiprotozoan.
  See: Chlortetracycline Hydrochloride, U.S.P. XXI.
CHLOROTHEN. 2-[(5-Chloro-2-thenyl)(2-dimethylaminoethyl)amino]pyridine hydrochloride & citrate salts (Chlorothenylpyramine, chloromethapyrilene, Pyrithen).
  Use: Symptomatic relief in allergic disorders.
CHLOROTHEN CITRATE. (Whittier) 2-[-(5-Chloro-2-thenyl)]2-dimethylamino)-ethyl]amino]pyridine dihydrogen citrate. Chloromethapyrilene, Chlorothenylpyramine, pyrithen. Tab., Bot. 100s.
  Use: (Oral 25 to 50 mg.) Antihistaminic in relief of allergic disorders.
W/Pyrilamine, thenylpyramine.
  See: Derma-Pax, Liq. (Recsei)
2-((5-CHLORO-2-THENYL)(2-DIMETHYLAMINO)ETH- YL)AMINO)PYRIDINE CITRATE (1:1).
  See: Chlorothen Citrate
CHLOROTHENYLPYRAMINE. Chlorothen, Prep.
CHLOROTHEOPHYLLINATE W/BENADRYL.
  See: Dramamine, Prep. (Searle)
• **CHLOROTHIAZIDE,** U.S.P. XXI. Oral Susp., Tabs., U.S.P. XXI. 6-Chloro-2H-1,2,4-benzothiadiazine-7-sulfonamide 1,1-dioxide.
  Use: Diuretic.
  See: Diuril, Tab., Susp. (Merck Sharp & Dohme)
W/Methyldopa
  See: Aldoclor, Tab. (Merck Sharp & Dohme)
W/Reserpine
  See: Diupres, Tab. (Merck Sharp & Dohme)
CHLOROTHIAZIDE. B.A.N. 6-Chlorobenzo-1,2,4-thiadiazine-7-sulphonamide 1,1-dioxide.
  Use: Diuretic.
  See: Chlotride
      Diuril, Prods. (Merck Sharp & Dohme)
      Saluric
• **CHLOROTHIAZIDE SODIUM FOR INJECTION,** U.S.P. XXI.
  See: Sodium Diuril, Vial (Merck Sharp & Dohme)
CHLOROTHYMOL. 6-Chlorothymol.
  Use: Antibacterial.
• **CHLOROTRIANISENE,** U.S.P. XXI. Cap., U.S.P. XXI. Chlorotris (p-methoxyphenyl)ethylene.
  Use: Estrogen.
  See: TACE, Cap. (Merrell Dow)
CHLOROTRIANISENE. B.A.N. Chlorotri-(4-methoxy-phenyl)ethylene.
  Use: Estrogen.

See: TACE, Cap. (Merrell Dow)
CHLOROTRIS(p-METHOXYPHENYL)ETHYLENE,
  See: Chlorotrianisene, U.S.P. XXI.
β-CHLOROVINYL ETHYNYL CARBINOL.
  See: Placidyl, Cap. (Abbott)
• **CHLOROXINE.** USAN.
  Use: Antiseborrheic.
• **CHLOROXYLENOL.** USAN. 4-Chloro-3,5-xylenol. p-Chloro-m-xylenol; parachloro-metaxylenol; benzytol.
  Use: Antiseptic.
W/Benzocaine, menthol, lanolin.
  See: Unburn, Spray, Cream, Lot. (Leeming-Pacquin)
W/Hexachlorophene.
  See: Desitin, Preps. (Leeming-Pacquin)
W/Methyl salicylate, menthol, camphor, thymol, eucalyptus oil, isopropyl alcohol.
  See: Gordobalm, Balm (Gordon)
CHLORPHEN. (Wolins) Chlorpheniramine maleate 0.75 mg., salicylamide 80 mg., phenacetin 16 mg./Tab. Bot. 1000s.
CHLORPHENADE. (Wolins) Atropine sulfate 1/180 gr., chlorpheniramine maleate 8 mg., phenylpropanolamine HCl 50 mg./T.D. Cap. Bot. 100s, 1000s.
• **CHLORPHENESIN.** F.D.A. 3-(p-Chlorophenoxy)-1,2-propanediol.
CHLORPHENESIN. B.A.N. 3-(4-Chlorophenoxyl)-propane-1,2-diol.
  Use: Antifungal agent.
  See: Mycil
• **CHLORPHENESIN CARBAMATE.** USAN. 3-(p-Chlorophenoxy)-2-hydroxypropyl carbamate.
  Use: Muscle relaxant.
  See: Maolate, Tab. (Upjohn)
CHLORPHENEX CAPS. (Wolins) Acetaminophen 325 mg., phenylpropanolamine HCl 18 mg./Cap. Bot. 100s, 1000s.
CHLORPHENIRAMINE. B.A.N. 1-(4-Chlorophenyl)-3-dimethylamino-1-(2-pyridyl)propane. 3-(4-Chlorophenyl)-3-(2-pyridyl)propyldimethylamine.
  Use: Antihistamine.
  See: Chlorphenamine (I.N.N.)
      Chlorprophenpyridamine
      Haynon
W/Atropine sulfate.
  See: Histunex, Inj. (Tunex)
W/Phenylephrine HCl, phenylpropanolamine HCl, phenyltoloxamine citrate.
  See: Naldecon, Tab., Drops, Syr.
      (Bristol-Myers)
W/Phenylephrine, analgesics, and Vitamin C.
  See: Corico, Caps. (Haag)
• **CHLORPHENIRAMINE MALEATE,** U.S.P. XXI. Inj., Syr., Tab., U.S.P. XXI. 2-[p-Chloro-alpha(2-dimethylaminoethyl)benzyl]pyridine maleate, chlorprophenpyridamine maleate. 2-Pyridinepropanamine, gamma-(4-chlorophenyl)-N,N-dimethyl-,(Z)-2-butenedioate(1:1).
  Use: Antihistaminic.
  See: Alermine, Tab. (Reid-Provident)
      Barachlor T.D., Cap., Tab. (Barry Martin)
      Chestamine, Cap. (Leeds)

Chlo-Amine, Tab. (Hollister-Stier)
Chloraman, Tab. (Rasman)
Chloren, Preps. (Wren)
Chlor-4, Tab. (Mills)
Chlormene, Tab. (Robinson)
Chlormene Injection (Robinson)
Chlormene Repeat Action, Tab. (Robinson)
Chlormene Timecaps, Tab. (Robinson)
Chlor-Niramine, Tab. (Whiteworth)
Chlorophen, Vial (Medical Chem.)
Chlor-pen, Vial, Tab. (Amer. Chem. & Drug)
Chlor-Span, Cap. (Burlington)
Chlortab, Tab., Cap., Inj. (North American Pharmacal)
Chlor-Trimeton Maleate, Prep. (Schering)
Cosea, Preps. (Center)
Histacon, Tab., Syr. (Marsh-Emory)
Histaspan, Cap. (USV Labs.)
Histex, Cap. (Mallard)
Nasahist (Keene)
Panahist, Tab. (Panray)
Phenetron, Preps. (Lannett)
Polaramine, Tab., Syr. (Schering)
Pyranistan Tab. (Standex)
Rhinihist, Elix. (Central)
Teldrin, Spansule, Cap. (Menley & James)
Trymegen (Medco)

CHLORPHENIRAMINE MALEATE W/COMBINATIONS

See: Al-Ay, Preps (Bowman)
Alclear Anti-allergy, Tab. (Walgreen)
Alcon Decongestant, Tab., Liq. (Webcon)
Algetuss, Syr. (Winston)
Alka-Seltzer Plus, Tab. (Miles)
Allercomp, Tab. (Wolins)
Allerdec, Cap. (Towne)
Allerest Prods. (Pharmacraft)
Allergesic, Tab. (Vitarine)
Allergy (Eckerd)
Alo-Tuss, Tab. (North Amer. Pharm.)
Alumadrine, Tab. (Fleming)
Amohist, Tab. (Vortech)
A.R.M., Tab. (Menley & James)
Atussin Expectorant, Liq. (Federal)
Atussin-D.M. Expectorant, Liq. (Federal)
Bayer Prods. (Glenbrook)
Bellafedrol A-H, Tab. (Lannett)
B.M.E., Liq. (Brothers)
Bobid, Cap. (Boyd)
Breacol Cough Medication, Liq. (Glenbrook)
Brolade, Cap. (Brothers)
Bronchohist, Syr. (Sutliff & Case)
Bur-Tuss Expectorant (Burlington)
CDM, Expect. (Lannett)
Cenahist, Caps. (Century)
Cenaid, Tabs. (Century)
Centuss, Tab. (Century)
Cerose Comp., Liq. (Ives)
Chew-Hist, Wafer (Kenyon)
Children's Cold Tab. (Towne)
Chlorodri, Vial (Kenyon)
Chlorpel, Caps. (Santa)

Chlorphen, Vial (Kenyon)
Chlorphen, Tab. (Wolins)
Chlorphenade, T.D. Cap. (Wolins)
Chlorphenwol, Cap. (Wolins)
Chlor-Trimeton, Preps. (Schering)
Chlor-Trimeton Expect. (Schering)
Codimal, Tab. (Central)
Co-Histine DH, Elix. (Kay)
Col-Decon, Tab. (Columbia)
Colrex Compound, Preps. (Rowell)
Comhist, Tabs., Elix. (Baylor)
Comtrex, Cap., Liq., Tab. (Bristol-Myers)
Conalsyn Croncap, Cap. (Cenci)
Conhist, Cap. (Mallard)
Conjec, Inj., (Mallard)
Contac, Cap. (Menley & James)
Cophene No. 2, Cap. (Dunhall)
Cophene-S, Syr. (Dunhall)
Coricidin, Prep. (Schering)
Coriforte, Cap. (Schering)
Corilin, Liq. (Schering)
Corizahist, Preps. (Mason)
Coryban-D, Cap., Syrup (Roerig)
Coryzaid, Tab. (Elder)
Coryztime, Cap., Vial (Elder)
Corzone, Syr. (Xttrium)
Co-Sansprin, Tab. (Wolins)
Cotrol-D, Tab. (Beecham Labs)
Co-Tylenol, Preps. (McNeil)
Covanamine, Liq., Tab. (Mallinckrodt)
Covangesic, Liq., Tab. (Mallinckrodt)
C3 Capsules (Menley & James)
Dallergy, Cap., Tab., Syr. (Laser)
Dasikon, Cap. (Beecham Labs)
Decobel, Cap. (Lannett)
Decojen, Tab., Vial (Jenkins)
Deconamine, Cap., Tab., Elxr., Syrup (Berlex)
Decongestant, Tab. (Panray)
Decongestant, Vial (Century)
Dehist, Cap. (O'Neal, Jones & Feldman)
Demazin, Tab., Syr. (Schering)
Derma-Pax, Lot. (Recsei)
Desa-Hist AT, Tab., Syr. (Pharmics)
Desa-Hist PF Elixir, PF-8, Cap. (Pharmics)
Dextromal, Liq. (Mallard)
Dezest, Cap. (Geneva Drugs)
Dodamin, Tab. (Reid-Provident)
Donatussin, Liq., Syr. (Laser)
Dri-Drip, Cap., Liq. (Coastal)
Dri-Hist Meta-Kaps, Cap. (Sutliff & Case)
Drinus, Syr., Cap., (Amfre-Grant)
Drinus-M, Cap. (Amfre-Grant)
Dristan, Preps. (Whitehall)
Drucon, Elix. (Standard Drug)
Drynal (Blaine)
Efricon Expectorant, (Lannett)
Expectico, Syr. (Coastal)
Expecto Hist, Tab. (Wolins)
Extendryl, Cap., Syr., Tab. (Fleming)
F.C.A.H., Caps (Scherer)
Fedahist, Prods. (Donner)
Fitacol (Standex)

Forcold, Syr. (Lemmon)
Formadrin, Liq. (Kenyon)
Gomahist, Liq. (Burgin-Arden)
Guahist (Hickam)
Guaiamine, Cap. (Sutliff & Case)
Guaiodol-Plus, Vial (Kenyon)
Guistrey Fortis, Tab. (Bowman)
Hista-Compound #5, Tab. (Vortech)
Histacon, Syr., Tab. (Marsh-Emory)
Histapco, Tabs. (Apco)
Hista-Vadrin, Cap., Syrup, Tab. (Scherer)
Histine Prods. (Freeport)
Histogesic, Tab. (Century)
Histone, Tab. (Blaine)
Historal, Cap., Liq. (W.F. Merchant)
Histussinol, Syr. (Bock)
Hycoff, Cap., Syr. (Saron)
Hycoff-X, Expect. (Saron)
Hycomine Comp., Tab. (Du Pont)
Infantuss, Liq. (Scott/Cord)
Kiddi-Koff, Liq. (Reid-Provident)
Kiddisan, Tab. (O'Neal)
Koldeze, Cap. (Scrip)
Koryza, Tabs. (Fellows-Testagar)
Kronofed-A, Cap. (Ferndale)
Lanatuss, Expect. (Lannett)
Marhist (Marlop)
Medcohist, Tabs. (Hauck)
Midran, Tab. (Columbia)
Naldecon, Preps. (Bristol)
Napril, Cap. (Marion)
Narine, T.R. Cap. (Dooner)
Narspan, Cap. (Coast Labs.)
Naso-Dex, Cap. (Commerce)
Neo-Pyranistan, Tab. (Standex)
Nilcol, Tabs. and Elix. (Parke-Davis)
Nolamine, Tab. (Carnrick)
Novafed A, Cap., Liq. (Merrell Dow)
Novahistine, Preps. (Merrell Dow)
Oraminic, Prep. (Vortech)
Oriphan, Tab. (Panray)
Ornade, Prods. (SmithKline)
Para-Hist, Cap., Syr. (Pharmics)
Partuss, Liq. (Parmed)
Partuss T.D., Tab. (Parmed)
Pectorine, Liq. (Scrip)
Pedo-Sol, Elix., Tab. (Warren)
Pertussin Plus Night-Time Cold Medicine, Syr.
   (Chesebrough-Pond's)
Phenahist, Preps (Amid)
Phenchlor Prods. (Freeport)
Phenetron Comp., Tab. (Lannett)
Phenylin, Cap. (Mallard)
Polytuss-DM, Liq. (Rhode)
P.R. Syrup, Liq. (Fleming)
Pyma, Cap., Vial (Fellows-Testagar)
Pyristan, Cap., Elix. (Arcum)
Pyranistan (Standex)
Quartets, Cap. (DePree)
Quelidrine, Syr. (Abbott)
Rentuss, Cap., Syr. (Wren)
Resclor, Tab. (Dunhall)

Rhinex D M, Syr., Tab. (Lemmon)
Rhinogesic, Tab. (Vale)
Rhinosyn, Cap, Liq. (Comatic)
Rid-A-Col, Tab. (Panray)
Rid-A-Col D, Tab. (Panray)
Rinocidin, Cap., Liq. (Cenci)
Rohist-D, Cap. (Rocky Mtn.)
Rolanade, Cap. (Robinson)
Romilar CF, Syr. (Block)
Ryna, Liq. (Mallinckrodt)
Ryna-tussadine, Tab., Liq. (Mallinckrodt)
Salphenyl, Cap. (Mallard)
Scotcof, Liq. (Scott/Cord)
Scotuss Liq. (Scott/Cord)
Scotnord (Scott/Cord)
Shertus, Liq. (Sheryl)
Sialco, Tab. (Foy)
Sinaprel, Cap. (Pasadena Research)
Sinarest, Tab., (Pharmacraft)
Sine-Off, Tab. (Menley & James)
Sino-Comp., Tab. (Bio-Factor)
Sinodec, Cap. (Primedics)
Sinovan Timed, Cap. (Drug Ind.)
Sinucol, Cap., Vial (Tennessee)
Sinulin, Tab. (Carnrick)
Sinutab Extra Strength, Cap. (Warner-Lambert)
Spantuss, Liq., Tab. (Arco)
Spectab, Tab. (Reid-Provident)
Statomin Maleate CC, Tab. (Bowman)
Sudafed Plus, Tab., Syr. (Burroughs Wellcome)
Supercitin, Syr. & Sugar-Free, Cap. (Vitarine)
Symptrol, Cap. (Saron)
T.A.C. Cap. (Towne)
Tercol, Liq. (Commerce)
Thor, Cap. (Towne)
Tonecol, Syr., Tab. (A.V.P.)
Triamincin Chewables, (Dorsey)
Trigelamine, Oint. (Edward J. Moore)
Trisohist, Cap. (Riker)
Turbilixir, Liq. (Burlington)
Turbispan Leisurecaps, Cap. (Burlington)
Tusquelin, Syr. (Circle)
Tussar-2, Syr. (Armour)
Tusscaps, Cap. (Martin-Phillips)
Tussi-Organidin, Liq. (Wallace)
U-R-D, Prods. (Hickam)
Valihist, Cap. (Otis Clapp)
Vernate, Inj. (Reid-Provident)
Wesade, Cap. (Western Research)

d-CHLORPHENIRAMINE MALEATE.
   See: Polarmine Expect., Syr., Tab. (Schering)
CHLORPHENIRAMINE RESIN W/COMBINATIONS.
   See: Omni-Tuss, Liq. (Pennwalt)
CHLORPHENIRAMINE TANNATE.
W/Carbetapentane tannate, ephedrine tannate,
   phenylephrine tannate.
   See: Rynatuss Tabules, Susp. (Mallinckrodt)
W/Phenylephrine tannate, pyrilamine tannate.
   See: Rynatan, Tab., Susp. (Mallinckrodt)
CHLORPHENOCTIUM AMSONATE. B.A.N. 2,4-Di-
chlorophenoxymethyldimethyloctylammonium 4,4'-
diaminostilbene-2,2'-disulfonate.

Use: Antifungal agent.
CHLORPHENOXAMINE. B.A.N. N-2-(4-Chloro-α-methylbenzhydryloxy)ethyldimethylamine.
Use: Treatment of the Parkinsonian syndrome.
See: Clorevan
• **CHLORPHENOXAMINE HCl,** U.S.P. XXI. Tab.,
U.S.P. XXI. beta-Dimethylaminoethyl (p-chlor-alpha-methyl-benzhydryl-ether HCl.
• **CHLORPHENTERMINE.** F.D.A. 4-Chloro-alpha, alpha-dimethylphenethylamine.
CHLORPHENTERMINE. B.A.N. 4-Chloro-αα-dimethyl-phenethylamine.
Use: Appetite suppressant.
See: Lucofen
• **CHLORPHENTERMINE HCl.** USAN.
p-Chloro-α, α-dimethylphenethylamine HCl.
Use: Anorexic.
See: Chlorophen, Tab. (Robinson)
CHLORPHTHALIDONE. 1-Oxo-3-(3′-sulfanyl-4′-chlorphenyl)-3-hydroxy-isoindoline.
See: Chlorthalidone
CHLORPROGUANIL. B.A.N. 1-(3,4-Dichlorophenyl)-5-isopropylbiguanide.
Use: Antimalarial.
See: Lapudrine
• **CHLORPROMAZINE,** U.S.P. XXI. Supp. U.S.P. XXI.
2-Chloro-10-[3-(dimethylamino)propyl]-phenothiazine. 10H-Phenothiazine-10-propanamine,2-chloro-N,N-dimethyl-
Use: Anti-emetic; tranquilizer.
See: Chloractil
    Largactil
• **CHLORPROMAZINE HCl,** U.S.P. XXI. Inj., Syr., Tab.
U.S.P. XXI.
Use: Anti-emetic; tranquilizer.
See:
    Chlorzine, Inj. (Mallard)
    Promachlor, Tab. (Geneva)
    Promapar, Tab. (Parke-Davis)
    Promaz, Inj. (Keene)
    Sonazine, Tab. (Reid-Provident)
    Terpium, Tab. (Scrip)
    Thorazine, Amp., Supp., Syr., Tab., Cap., Liq.
    (SmithKline)
• **CHLORPROPAMIDE,** U.S.P. XXI. Tabs. U.S.P. XXI.
1-[(p-Chlorophenyl)-sulfonyl]-3-propylurea. Benzene-sulfonamide, 4-chloro-N-[(propylamino)carbonyl]-.
Use: Hypoglycemic agent.
See: Diabinese, Tab. (Pfizer Laboratories)
CHLORPROPAMIDE. B.A.N. 1-(4-Chlorobenzenesulphonyl)-3-propylurea.
Use: Oral hypoglycemic agent.
See: Diabinese
CHLORPROPHENPYRIDAMINE MALEATE.
See: Chlorpheniramine Maleate, U.S.P. XXI.
• **CHLORPROTHIXENE,** U.S.P. XXI. Inj., Oral Susp.,
Tab., U.S.P. XXI. 1-Propanamine, 3-(2-chloro-9H-thioxanthene-9-ylidene)-N,N-dimethyl-,(Z)-; (Z)-2-Chloro-N,N-dimethylthioxanthene-Δ⁹γ-propylamine.
Use: Tranquilizer; antiemetic.
See: Taractan, Tab., Conc., Inj. (Roche)

CHLORQUINALDOL. 5,7-Dichloro-8-hydroxyquinaldine.
CHLORQUINALDOL. B.A.N. 5,7-Dichloro-8-hydroxy-2-methylquinoline.
Use: Antiseptic; fungicide.
See: Steroxin
CHLORQUINOL. A mixture of the chlorinated products of 8-hydroxyquinoline containing about 65 per cent of 5,7-dichloro-8-hydroxyquinoline. Quixalin.
CHLOR-SPAN. (Burlington) Chlorpheniramine maleate 8 mg./Sus. Rel. Cap. Bot. 60s.
Use: Antihistaminic.
CHLORSPAN-12. (Vortech) Chlorpheniramine maleate 12 mg./Cap. Bot. 1000s.
Use: Antihistaminic.
CHLORTAB. (Vortech) Chlorpheniramine maleate 4 mg. or 8 mg./Tab.
Bot. 30s, 1000s.
Vial 100 mg./cc., 10 cc.; Spancap: 12 mg./Cap.
Use: Antihistaminic.
• **CHLORTETRACYCLINE HCl,** U.S.P. XXI. Caps.,
Oint., Ophth. Oint., Sterile. U.S.P. XXI. 7-Chlorotetracycline hydrochloride.
Use: Antibiotic.
See: Aureomycin, Prep. (Lederle)
• **CHLORTHALIDONE,** U.S.P. XXI. Tabs. U.S.P. XXI.
2-Chloro-5-(1-hydroxy-3-oxo-1-isoindolinyl)benzenesulfonamide. Benzenesulfonamide, 2-chloro-5-(2,3-dihydro-1-hydroxy-3-oxo-1H-isoindol-1-yl)-.
Use: Diuretic, antihypertensive.
See: Combipres, Tab. (Boehringer-Ingelheim)
    Hygroton, Tab. (USV Labs.)
W/Reserpine.
See: Demi-Regroton, Tab. (USV Labs.)
    Regroton, Tab. (USV Labs.)
CHLORTHENOXAZIR. B.A.N. 2-(2-Chloroethyl)-2,3-dihydro-1,3-benzoxazin-4-one.
Use: Anti-inflammatory; analgesic.
CHLOR-TRIMETON. (Schering) Chlorpheniramine maleate **Inj.** 10 mg./ml. Amp. 1 ml. 100s. **Allergy Tab.** 4 mg./Tab. Box 24s. Bot. 100s, 1000s, 5000s.
Long Acting Allergy Repetabs: 8 mg./Tab. Box 24s., 48s. Bot. 100s, 1000s, 5000s; (12 mg.) Bot. 100s, 1000s. **Syr.** 2 mg./5 ml. Bot. 4 oz., gal.
Use: Antihistaminic.
CHLOR-TRIMETON W/COMBINATIONS. (Schering) Chlorpheniramine maleate.
W/Aspirin
See: Coricidin, Tab., Medilets (Schering)
    Coricidin Medilets, Tab. (Schering)
W/Aspirin, phenylpropanolamine.
See: Coricidin "D", Prods. (Schering)
W/Aspirin, phenylephrine.
See: Coricidin Demilets (Schering)
W/Aspirin, chlorpheniramine maleate, phenylephrine HCl.
See: Coricidin Demilets, Tab. (Schering)
W/Phenylephrine HCl.
See: Demazin, Prods. (Schering)
W/Pseudoephedrine sulfate.
See: Chlor-Trimeton Long-Acting Decongestant Repetabs (Schering)

W/Salicylamide, phenacetin, caffeine, Vit. C.
    See: Coriforte, Cap. (Schering)
W/Sod. salicylate, amino acetic acid.
    See: Corilin, Liq. (Schering)
CHLOR-TRIMETON DECONGESTANT TABLETS.
    (Schering) Chlorpheniramine maleate 4 mg.,
    pseudoephedrine sulfate 60 mg./Tab. Box 24s,
    48s.
    Use: Decongestant, antihistaminic.
CHLOR-TRIMETON EXPECTORANT. (Schering)
    Chlorpheniramine maleate 2 mg., phenylephrine HCl
    10 mg., ammonium chloride 100 mg., sod. citrate
    50 mg., guaifenesin 50 mg./5 ml. Alcohol < 1%.
    Bot. 16 oz.
    Use: Antihistaminic, antitussive, decongestant.
**CHLOR-TRIMETON LONG-ACTING
    DECONGESTANT REPETABS.** (Schering)
    Chlorpheniramine maleate 8 mg., pseudoephedrine
    sulfate 120 mg./S.R. Tab. Box 12s.
    Use: Antihistamine, nasal decongestant.
CHLORTRON. (Pharmex) Chlorpheniramine maleate
    10 mg./Vial. Vial 30 cc.
CHLORULAN TABLETS "500" (Lannett) 500 mg.
    Bot. 100s, 1000s.
CHLORZIDE. (Foy) Hydrochlorothyazide 50 mg./Tab.
    Bot. 1000s.
    Use: Diuretic.
• **CHLORZOXAZONE,** U.S.P. XXI. Tab., U.S.P. XXI. 5-
    Chlorobenzoxazolin-2-one. 5-Chlorobenzoxazoli-
    none.
    Use: Muscle relaxant.
    See: Paraflex, Tab. (McNeil)
W/Acetaminophen.
    See: Blanex, Cap. (Edwards)
        Parafon Forte, Tab. (McNeil)
• **CHLORZOXAZONE AND ACETAMINOPHEN
    CAPSULES,** U.S.P. XXI.
    Use: Muscle relaxant, analgesic.
• **CHLORZOXAZONE AND ACETAMINOPHEN
    TABLETS,** U.S.P. XXI.
    Use: Muscle relaxant, analgesic.
CHOICE 10. (Whiteworth) Potassium Cl 10% solution,
    unflavored. Bot. Gal.
    Use: Replacement therapy for potassium deficiency
    states.
CHOICE 20. (Whiteworth) Potassium Cl 20% solution,
    unflavored. Bot. Gal.
    Use: Replacement therapy for potassium deficiency
    states.
CHOLACRYLAMINE RESIN. An anion exchange
    resin consisting of a water soluble polymer having
    a molecular weight equivalent between 350 and
    360 in which aliphatic quaternary amine groups
    are attached to an acrylic backbone by ester
    linkages.
CHOLAJEN. (Jenkins) Ox bile ext. 3½ gr.,
    desoxycholic acid ⅛ gr., dehydrocholic acid ⅛ gr.,
    pancreatin 1.0 gr., betaine HCl 1.0 gr. Bot. 1000s.
    Use: Cholagogue laxative.
CHOLALIC ACID.
    See: Cholic Acid

CHOLAN-DH. (Pennwalt) Dehydrocholic acid 250
    mg./Tab. Bot. 100s.
    Use: Stimulate bile flow.
CHOLAN-HMB. (Pennwalt) Phenobarbital 8 mg., dehy-
    drocholic acid 250 mg., homatropine methylbromide
    2.5 mg./Tab. Bot. 100s, 1000s.
    Use: Nonobstructive biliary disease.
CHOLANIC ACID. Dehydrodesoxycholic acid.
CHOLA-ZEM. (Zemmer) Atropine sulfate 1/500 gr., sod.
    glycocholate 1 gr., taurocholate 1 gr., nitroglycerin
    1/500 gr., mag. sulfate 5 gr./Tab. Bot. 100s, 1000s.
    Use: Choleretic & cholagogue with antispasmodic.
CHOLEBRINE. (Mallinckrodt) Iocetamic acid 750
    mg./Tab. Box 20s, 30s, 100s, 150s, Bot. 100s.
    Use: Diagnostic aid.
• **CHOLECALCIFEROL,** U.S.P. XXI. Vit. D-3, Activated
    5,7-Cholestadien-3β-ol. 9,10-Secocholesta-5,7,-
    10(19)-trien-3-ol.
    Use: Antirachitic vitamin.
    See: Decavitamin Cap. & Tab.
CHOLECALCIFEROL. B.A.N. 9,10-Secocholesta-5,7,-
    10(19)-trien-3β-ol.
    Use: Treatment of vitamin D deficiency.
    See: Vitamin D-3
▪ **CHOLECYSTOGRAPHY AGENTS.**
    See: Bilopaque, Cap., (Winthrop-Breon)
        Iodized Oil (Various Mfr.)
        Iophendylate Inj.
        Pantopaque, Amp. (LaFayette)
        Telepaque, Tab. (Winthrop-Breon)
CHOLEDYL. (Parke-Davis) Oxtriphylline. **Tab.** (100
    mg.) Bot. 100s, (200 mg.) Bot. 100s, 1000s. Unit
    dose 100s. **Elix.** 100 mg./5 ml., alcohol 20%. Bot.
    pt. **Pediatric Syrup:** 50 mg./5 ml. Bot. pt.
    Use: Theophylline therapy.
CHOLEDYL SA. (Parke-Davis) Oxtriphylline 400 mg.
    or 600 mg./Tab. Bot. 100s. Unit dose 100s.
    Use: Relief of acute and chronic bronchial asthma.
• **CHOLERA VACCINE,** U.S.P. XXI. (Lederle) India
    Strains, Vials 1.5 cc. (Lilly) Vials 1.5 cc. (Wyeth)
    Vials 1.5 cc., 20 cc.
    Use: Active immunizing agent.
CHOLERETIC.
    See: Bile Preps. and Forms
        Dehydrocholic Acid
        Desoxycholic Acid
        Tocamphyl, Tab. (Various Mfr.)
CHOLESTERIN.
    See: Cholesterol.
• **CHOLESTEROL,** N.F. XVI. Cholest-5-en-3β-ol. 5,6-
    Cholesten-3-Ol(Cholesterin). (Various Mfr.)
    Use: Pharmaceutic aid (emulsifying agent).
• **CHOLESTYRAMINE RESIN,** U.S.P. XXI. A styryl-divi-
    nyl-benzene copolymer (about 2% divinylbenzene)
    containing quaternary ammonium groups.
    Use: Resin producing insoluble bile acid
    complexes.
    See: Questran (Mead Johnson)
• **CHOLESTYRAMINE FOR ORAL SUSPENSION,**
    U.S.P. XXI.
CHOLIC ACID. 3,7,12-Trihydroxycholanic acid. Cholalic
    acid. Dehydrocholic Acid.

CHOLIC ACID SALTS.
W/Ketocholanic acids.
  See: Chobile, Tab. (Mallinckrodt)
CHOLINATE. (Cenci) Choline dihydrogen citrate 1
  Gm./4 cc. Bot. 16 oz., gal.
  Use: Liver disorders.
CHOLINE BITARTRATE.
W/Bile extract, pancreatic substance, dl-methionine.
  See: Licoplex, Tab. (Mills)
W/Hesperidin, niacinamide, protein hydrolysate,
  methionine, inositol, vitamins, minerals.
  See: Norimex-Plus, Cap. (Vortech)
W/Inositol, B-Vitamins.
  See: Lipotriad Cap., (Smith, Miller & Patch)
W/Lemon bioflavonoid complex, inositol, Vit. C,
  B-Vitamins.
  See: Lipoflavonoid, Cap. (Smith, Miller & Patch)
W/Methionine, inositol, liver desiccated, Vitamin B-12.
  See: Limvic, Tab. (Briar)
W/Mucopolysaccharide, epinephrine neutralizing
  factor, pancreatic lipotropic fraction, dl-methionine,
  inositol, bile ext.
  See: Lipo-K, Cap. (Marcen)
W/d-Pantothenyl alcohol.
  See: Ilopan-Choline, Tab. (Adria)
W/Pentylenetetrazol, nicotinic acid, methyl-testoster-
  one, ethinyl estradiol, Vit. B-1, B-2, B-6, B-12, C, pan-
  thenol, inositol.
  See: Benizol Plus, Elixir, Tab. (ICN)
W/Safflower oil, whole liver, soybean, lecithin, inositol,
  methionine, natural tocopherols, B-6, B-12, pan-
  thenol.
  See: Nutricol, Cap., Vial (Nutrition Control)
CHOLINE CHLORIDE. (Various Mfr.)
  Use: Liver disorders.
W/Inositol, methionine, Vit. B-12.
  See: Cho-Meth, Vial (Kenyon)
    Lychol-B, Inj. (Burgin-Arden)
W/Methionine, vitamins, niacinamide, panthenol.
  See: Minoplex, Vial (Savage)
W/Panthenol, inositol, vitamins, minerals, estrone,
  testosterone.
  See: Geramine, Inj. (Brown)
W/Panthenol, inositol, vitamins, minerals, estrone,
  testosterone, polydigestase.
  See: Geramine, Tab. (Brown)
W/B-1, niacinamide, B-2, B-6, calcium pantothenate,
  cyanocobalamin, Vit. B-12, inositol, dl-methionine,
  testosterone, estrone, procaine.
  See: Gerihorm, Inj. (Burgin-Arden)
CHOLINE CHLORIDE, CARBAMATE. Carbachol,
  U.S.P. XXI.
CHOLINE CHLORIDE SUCCINATE.
  See: Succinylcholine Chloride, U.S.P. XXI.
CHOLINE CITRATE, TRICHOLINE CITRATE.
W/Inositol, methionine, Vit. B-12.
  See: Cholimeth Tab. (Central)
CHOLINE DIHYDROGEN CITRATE. 2-Hydroxy-ethyl
  trimethylammonium citrate-U.S. Vit. 0.5 Gm. Bot.
  100s, 500s.
  Use: Liver disorders.
  See: Cholinate, Liq. (Cenci)

CHOLINE SALICYLATE.
  See: Arthropan, Liq. (Purdue Frederick)
CHOLINE MAGNESIUM TRISALICYLATE.
  Use: Anti-inflammatory agent.
  See: Trilisate, Tab. (Purdue Fredrick)
CHOLINE SALICYLATE. B.A.N. Choline salt of
  salicylic acid.
  Use: Analgesic; antipyretic.
CHOLINE THEOPHYLLINATE.
  See: Oxtriphylline.
CHOLINE THEOPHYLLINATE. B.A.N. Choline salt of
  theophylline.
  Use: Bronchodilator.
  See: Choledyl
■**CHOLINERGIC AGENTS,**
  (Parasympathomimetic Agents).
  See: Mecholyl Chloride, Inj. (Baker)
    Mestinon, Tab., Amp., Syr. (Roche)
    Mytelase, Cap. (Winthrop-Breon)
    Pilocarpine Nitrate (Var. Mfr.)
    Prostigmin Bromide, Tab. (Roche)
    Prostigmin Methylsulfate, Inj. (Roche)
    Tensilon, Inj. (Roche)
    Urecholine, Inj., Tab. (Merck Sharp & Dohme)
■**CHOLINERGIC BLOCKING AGENTS.**
  See: Parasympatholytic agents
CHO-LIV-12. (Jenkins) Choline 100 mg., cyanocoba-
  lamin 200 mcg., liver equal to Vit. B-12 10 mcg./cc.
  Vial 10 cc., 12s.
CHOL METH IN B. (Esco) Choline bitartrate 235 mg.,
  inositol 112 mg., methionine 70 mg., betaine
  anhydrous 50 mg., Vit. B-12 6 mcg., Vit. B-1 6 mg., Vit.
  B-6 3 mg., niacin 10 mg./Cap. Bot. 500s, 1000s.
  Use: Vitamin supplement.
CHOLOGRAFIN MEGLUMINE. (Squibb) Iodipamide
  methylglucamine (52%) 0.52 Gm./10 ml. Amp.
  10.3% 100 ml.
  Use: I.V., Cholangiography and cholecystography.
CHOLOGRAFIN SODIUM. Disodium salt of N,N'-adipyl
  bis-(3-amino-2:4:6 triodobenzoic acid).
CHOLOXIN. (Flint) Sodium dextrothyroxine 1 mg., 2
  mg., 4mg., 6 mg./Tab. 2 mg., 4 mg. Bot. 100s,
  250s; 1 mg., 6 mg. Bot. 100s.
  Use: Hypocholesterolemic.
CHOLYGLYCINE.
  See: CG RIA, Kit (Abbott)
CHO-METH. (Kenyon) Methionine 30 mg., choline chlo-
  ride 200 mg., inositol 100 mg., Vit. B-12, 12 mcg./2 cc.
  Vial 30 cc.
CHONDODENDRON TOMENTOSUM.
  See: Curare
CHONDRUS. Irish Moss
W/Petrolatum, Liq.
  See: Kondremul, Liq. (Fisons)
CHOO E PLUS C. (Stayner) Vit. E 100 I.U., Vit. C 250
  mg./Tab. Bot. 100s.
CHOOZ. (Plough) Calcium carbonate 360 mg./Gum
  tablet. Pkg. 10s, 20s.
  Use: Antacid.
CHOREX 5. (Hyrex) Chorionic gonadotropin 5,000
  I.U., urea 100 mg., thimerosal 1.0 mg., sodium
  phosphate buffer/Vial. Vial 10 ml.

Use: Hormone therapy.
CHOREX 10. (Hyrex) Chorionic gonadotropin 10,000
I.U., urea 100 mg., thimerosal 1.0 mg., sodium
phosphate buffer/Vial 10 cc.
Use: Hormone therapy.
CHORIGON. (Dunhall) Chorionic gonadotropin (dried)
1000 I.U./ml. Vial 10 ml.
Use: Cryptorchidism, functional uterine bleeding.
CHORION-PLUS. (Pharmex) Chorionic gonadotropin
10,000 u./Vial. Diluent: Glutamic acid 52 mcg., B-1
25 mg., procaine 1%/cc. Vial 10 cc.
• **CHORIONIC GONADOTROPIN,** U.S.P. XXI. Inj.
U.S.P. XXI. 5,000 I.U./Vial w/diluent 10 cc., 10,000
I.U./Vial w/diluent 10 cc. (Serono) 10,000 I.U. of
hCG, mannitol 100 mg., benzyl alcohol 0.9%/10
ml. vial.
Use: Prepubertal cryptorchidism, hypogonadotropic
hypogonadism, & induction of ovulation &
pregnancy in anovulatory women.
See: Antuitrin-S (Parke-Davis)
    A.P.L., Inj. (Ayerst)
    C-G-10, Vial. (Scrip)
    Chorigon, Amp. (Dunhall)
    Chorex 5, Vial. (Hyrex)
    Chorex 10, Vial. (Hyrex)
    Chorion-Plus, Vial (Pharmex)
    Follutein, Vial (Squibb)
    Gonadex (Continental Dist.)
    Khorion (Hickam)
    Neovital-Diluent, Inj. (Pasadena Research)
    Pre-Ine, Inj. (Kay)
    Rochoric, Inj. (Rocky Mtn.)
CHRISTODYNE-DHC. (Paddock) Acetyl-p-amino-phe-
nol 150 mg., aspirin 230 mg., caff. 30 mg.,
dihydrocodeinone bitartrate 5 mg./Tab. Bot. 100s,
500s.
Use: Analgesic, antitussive.
CHROMAGEN. (Savage) **Cap:** Ferrous fumarate 200
mg., Vit. C 250 mg., B-12 activity 10 mcg., desiccated
stomach substances 100 mg./soft gelatin cap. Bot.
100s, 500s. **Injectable:** Iron peptonized 100 mg.,
B-12 5 mcg., cyanocobalamin 25 mcg. lidocaine HCl
1%/2 cc. Vials 10 cc., 30 cc.
Use: Hematinic.
CHROMALBIN. (Squibb) 100 uCi containing
chromium CR 51 and human albumin.
CHROMARGYRE.
See: Merbromin (Var. Mfr.)
• **CHROMATE Cr-51, SODIUM FOR INJECTION,**
U.S.P. XXI.
CHROMATED (Cr-51) SERUM ALBUMIN (HUMAN).
CHROMATED SOLUTION (51Cr).
See: Chromitope sodium (Squibb)
CHROMELIN COMPLEXION BLENDER. (Summers)
Dihydroxyacetone 5%, alcohol 50%. Bot. 1 oz.
Use: Cosmetic darkening of whitened skin areas.
CHROMIC ACID, DISODIUM SALT. Sodium
Chromate Cr 51 Injection, U.S.P. XXI.
• **CHROMIC CHLORIDE,** U.S.P. XXI. Inj., U.S.P. XXI.
Chromium chloride (CrCl3) hexahydrate. Chromium
(3+) chloride hexahydrate.

Use: Chromium deficiency treatment.
See: Chrometrace, Inj. (Armour)
• **CHROMIC CHLORIDE Cr 51.** USAN.
Use: Radioactive agent.
See: Chromitope Chloride (Squibb)
• **CHROMIC PHOSPHATE Cr 51.** USAN.
Use: Radioactive agent.
• **CHROMIC PHOSPHATE P 32 SUSPENSION,**
U.S.P.XXI.
Use: Radioactive agent.
CHROMETRACE. (Armour) Chromic chloride injection
containing Chromium 4 mcg./ml. Vial 10 ml. Box
25s.
Use: Supplement to I.V. Solutions for chromium
deficiency.
CHROMITOPE SODIUM. (Squibb) Chromate Cr 51,
Sodium for Injection 0.25 mCi.
• **CHROMONAR HCl.** USAN. Ethyl[[3-[-2-(di-
ethylamino)-ethyl]-4-methyl-2-oxo-2H-1-benzopyran-
7-yl]oxy]acetate HCl. Intensain
Use: Recommended as coronary vasodilator, upon
release.
CHRONULAC. (Merrell Dow) Lactulose 10 Gm./15
ml. Bot. 8 oz., 32 oz. Unit dose 30 ml. Box 100s.
Use: Treatment of constipation.
CHRYSAZIN.
See: Danthron, N.F. XVI.
CHUR-HIST. (Churchill) Chlorpheniramine 4 mg./Kap-
tab. Bot. 100s.
Use: Antihistamine.
CHYMEX. (Adria) Bentiromide 500 mg./7.5 ml.
w/propylene glycol 40%.
Use: Screening test for pancreatic exocrine
insufficiency. Monitoring the adequacy of
supplemental pancreatic activity.
CHYMODIACTIN. (Smith) Chymodiactin 10,000 units,
sodium L-cysteinate HCl. Vial 10,000 units.
Use: Treatment of herniated lumbar intervertebral
discs.
• **CHYMOPAPAIN.** USAN. Proteolytic enzyme isolated
from papaya latex, differing from papain in
electrophoretic mobility, solubility, and substrate
specificity.
Use: Proteolytic enzyme.
See: Discase (Travenol)
CHYMORAL. (USV Labs.) Trypsin and chymotrypsin,
50,000 Armour units (activity in ratio of
approximately 6 to 1)/Tab. Bot. 48s.
Use: Oral anti-inflammatory.
CHYMORAL-100. (USV Labs.) Trypsin and chymotrypsin 100,000 Armour units/Tab. (Activity ratio
approximately 6 to 1). Bot. 48s, 250s.
Use: Oral enzymes for treatment of inflammation.
• **CHYMOTRYPSIN,** U.S.P. XXI. Ophth. Sol. U.S.P.
XXI. An enzyme, α-Chymotrypsin obtained in crystal-
line form from mammalian pancreas by aqueous
acid extraction of its proenzyme, chymotrypsinogen,
and subsequent conversion with trypsin to chymotryp-
sin.
Use: Proteolytic enzyme.
See: Avazyme, Tab. (Wallace)
    Catarase, Sol. (CooperVision)

W/Trypsin.
  Chymoral, Tab. (Armour)
  Orenzyme, Tab. (Merrell Dow)
W/Trypsin, neomycin palmitate.
  See: Biozyme, Oint. (Armour)
CHYMOTRYPSIN. B.A.N. An enzyme obtained from
  chymotrypsinogen by activation with trypsin.
  Use: Proteolytic enzyme.
  See: α-Chymotrypsin
    Chymar
    Chymar-Zon
CIBALITH-S. (Ciba) Lithium 8 mEq./5 ml. in
  sugar-free, raspberry-flavored syrup. Bot. 480
  ml.
  Use: Manic-depressive states.
C.I. BASIC VIOLET 3. Gentian Violet, U.S.P. XXI.
• **CIBENZOLINE.** USAN.
  Use: Cardiac depressant (anti-arrhythmic).
• **CICLAFRINE HYDROCHLORIDE.** USAN.
  Use: Antihypotensive.
CICLAZINDOL. B.A.N. 10-m-Chlorophenyl-2,3,4,-10-
  tetrahydropyrimido[1,2-α]-indol-10-ol.
  Use: Antidepressant.
CICLOPIROX. B.A.N. 6-Cyclohexyl-1-hydroxy-4-methyl-
  2-pyridone.
  Use: Fungicide.
  See: Batrafen (ethanolamine salt).
• **CICLOPIROX OLAMINE,** U.S.P. XXI. Cream, U.S.P.
  XXI.
  Use: Antifungal.
  See: Loprox, Cream (Hoechst)
• **CICLOPROFEN.** USAN. 2-(2-Fluorenyl)propionic acid.
  Use: Anti-inflammatory.
CICLOXOLONE. B.A.N. 3β-(cis-2-Carboxycyclo-hexyl-
  carbonyloxy)-11-oxo-olean-12-en-30-oic acid.
  Use: Treatment of gastric ulcers.
CIDEX. (Arbrook) Activated dialdehyde solution. Bot.
  qt., gal., 5 gal.
  Use: Sterilizing & disinfecting solution.
C.I. DIRECT BLUE 53 TETRASODIUM SALT. Evans
  Blue, U.S.P. XXI.
• **CIDOXIEPIN HCl.** USAN.
  Use: Psychotherapeutic.
• **CIGLITAZONE.** USAN.
CIGNOLIN.
  See: Anthralin (Var. Mfr.)
• **CILASTATIN SODIUM.** USAN.
CILFOMIDE TABLETS. (Winthrop Products) Inositol
  hexanicotinate.
  Use: Hypolipedemic, peripheral vasodilator.
• **CIMETIDINE.** USAN. 1-Methyl-3-[2-(5-methylimidazol-
  4-ylmethylthio)ethyl]guanidine-2-carbonitrile.
  Use: H-2-receptor histamine antagonist.
  See: Tagamet, Tab., Inj. (SmithKline)
CINACORT SPAN. (Foy) Triamcinolone acetonide 40
  mg./ml. Vial 5 ml.
  Use: Adrenocortical steroid replacement therapy.
• **CINANSERIN HYDROCHLORIDE.** USAN.
  2′-[[3-(Dimethylamino)-propyl]thio]cinnamanilide
  HCl.
  Use: Serotonin antagonist.

CINCHONA BARK. (Various Mfr.)
  Use: Antimalarial & tonic.
W/Anhydrous quinine, cinchonidine, cinchonine,
  quinidine & quinine.
  See: Totaquine, Pow. (Various Mfr.)
W/Iron oxide, nux vomica, Vitamin B-1, alcohol.
  See: Briatonic, Liq. (Briar)
**CINCHONAN-9-OL, 6′-METHOXY-, (9S)-,
  MONO-D-GLUCONATE (SALT), OR SULFATE
  (SALT).** Quinidine Gluconate, Sulfate.
CINCHONIDINE SULFATE.
CINCHONINE SALTS. (Various Mfr.)
  Use: As quinine dihydrochloride.
CINCHOPHEN. 2-Phenylcinchoninic acid.
  Use: Analgesic.
CINEPAZATE. B.A.N. Ethyl 4-(3,4,5-trimethoxy-cin-
  namoyl)piperazin-1-ylacetate.
  Vascoril hydrogen maleate.
  Use: Treatment of angina.
• **CINEPAZET MALEATE.** USAN.
  Use: Anti-anginal.
CINEPAZIDE. B.A.N. 1-Pyrrolidin-1-ylcarbonyl-methyl-
  4-(3,4,5-trimethoxycinnamoyl)-piperazine.
  Use: Peripheral vasodilator.
  See: Vasodistal hydrogen maleate.
CINEX-40. (Tunex) Triamcinolone diacetate 40
  mg./ml. Vial 5cc.
  Use: Parenteral steroid, depository.
• **CINGESTOL.** USAN. 19-Nor-17α-pregn-5-en-20-yn-
  17-ol.
  Use: Progestogen.
CINNAMALDEHYDE.
• **CINNAMEDRINE.** USAN. a-[1-(Cinnamyl-me-
  thylamine)-ethyl] benzyl alcohol.
  Use: Uterine antispasmodic.
  See: Midol, Tab. (Glenbrook)
CINNAMIC ALDEHYDE. Name previously used for
  Cinnamaldehyde.
• **CINNAMON,** N.F. XVI.
  Use: Flavoring agent.
• **CINNAMON OIL,** N.F. XVI. (Various Mfr.)
  Use: Pharmaceutic aid. (flavor)
CINNAMYL EPHEDRINE HCl.
W/Acetaminophen, homatropine methylbromide.
  See: Periodic, Cap. (Towne)
• **CINNARIZINE.** USAN. 1-Diphenylmethyl-4-trans-cin-
  namylpiperazine; 1-Benzhydryl-4-cinnamylpiperazine;
  F.D.A. 1-Cinnamyl-4-diphenyl-methylpiperazine.
  See: Mitronal
    Stugeron
CINNASIL. (Amfre-Grant) Rescinnamine Tab. 0.5 mg.
  Graduals 0.5 mg. Bot. 100s.
  Use: Treatment of hypertension.
CINNOPENTAZONE. INN for Cintazone.
CINO-40. (Reid-Provident) Triamcinolone diacetate 40
  mg./ml. Vial. 5 ml.
  Use: Glucocorticoid.
CINOBAC. (Dista) Cinoxacin. 250 mg./Pulvule. Bot.
  40s. 500 mg./Pulvule. Bot. 50s.
  Use: Treatment of urinary tract infections.
• **CINODINE HYDROCHLORIDE.** USAN.
  Use: Antibacterial.

• **CINOXACIN,** U.S.P. XXI. Caps. U.S.P. XXI. 1-Ethyl-4-oxo[1,3]dioxolo-[4,5-g]cinnoline-3-carboxylic acid.
Use: Antibacterial.
See: Cinobac, Cap. (Dista).

• **CINOXATE.,** U.S.P. XXI. Lotion, U.S.P. XXI. 2-Ethoxyethyl p-methoxycinnamate.
Use: Ultraviolet screen.
See: Sundare Prods. (Cooper).
W/Methyl anthranilate.
See: Maxafil Cream (Cooper).

CINOXOLONE. B.A.N. Cinnamyl 3β-acetoxy-11-oxo-olean-12-en-30-oate.
Use: Treatment of gastric ulcers.

• **CINPERENE.** USAN. 1-Cinnamyl-4-(2,6-dioxo-3-phenyl-3-piperidyl)piperidine.
Use: Tranquilizer.

CIN-QUIN. (Rowell) Quinidine sulfate. **Tab:** 100 mg., 200 mg., 300 mg./Tab. Bot. 100s, 1000s, Unit dose 100s. **Cap.:** 200 mg./Cap. Bot. 100s, 1000s; 300 mg./Cap. Bot. 100s, 500s. Unit dose 100s.
Use: Cardiac depressant.

• **CINTAZONE.** USAN. 2-Pentyl-6-phenyl-1H-pyrazolo [1,2-a] cinnoline-1,3(2H)-dione.
Use: Anti-inflammatory.

• **CINTRIAMIDE.** USAN.
Use: Antipyschotic.

• **CIPREFADOL SUCCINATE.** USAN.
Use: Analgesic.

• **CINROMIDE.** USAN.
Use: Anticonvulsant.

• **CIPROCINONIDE.** USAN.
Use: Adrenocortical steroid.

• **CIPROFIBRATE.** USAN.
Use: Antihyperlipoproteinemic.

• **CIRAMADOL.** USAN.
Use: Analgesic.

CIRAMINE. (Zemmer) Chlorpheniramine maleate. **Elixir:** 3 oz., pt., gal. **Parenteral:** (100 mg./cc.) Vial 10 cc. **Tab.:** 4 mg., Bot. 100s, 1000s. **Tab. T.R.:** 8 mg., Bot. 100s, 1000s, 12 mg. Bot. 100s, 1000s.
Use: Antihistaminic.

CIRBED. (Boyd) Papaverine HCl 150 mg./Cap. Bot. 100s.
Use: Antispasmodic effect on smooth muscle.

CIRCANOL. (Riker) **0.5 mg. Sublingual Tab.:** Dihydroergocornine 0.167 mg., dihydroergocristine 0.167 mg., dihydroergocryptine 0.167 mg. (alpha-beta ratio 2:1) mesylates/0.5 mg. Tab.; **1.0 mg. Tab:** dihydroergocornine 0.333 mg., dihydroergocristine 0.333 mg., dihydroergocryptine (alkpha-beta ratio 2:1) mesylates/1 mg. Tab. Bot. 100s, 1000s.
Use: To improve performance of self-care in elderly, mood elevator.

CIRCAVITE T. (Circle) Vit. A acetate 25,000 I.U, D-2 400 I.U., B-1 15 mg., B-2 10 mg., B-6 5 mg., C 300 mg., B-12 10 mcg., E 5 I.U., niacinamide 100 mg., pantothenic acid 20 mg., ferrous sulfate 15 mg., calcium 110 mg./Tab. w/KI, Cu, Mg, Zn Bot. 100s.
Use: Vitamin and mineral supplement.

CIRCUBID. (Merchant) Ethaverine HCl 150 mg./Cap. Bot. 100s, 1000s.
Use: Peripheral and cerebral vascular insufficiency.

CIRIN. (Zemmer) Aspirin 300 mg., ascorbic acid 50 mg./Tab. Bot. 100s, 1000s.
Use: Analgesic.

• **CIROLEMYCIN.** USAN.
Use: Antibacterial, antineoplastic.

• **CISAPRIDE.** USAN.

CISPLATIN. USAN.
Use: Antineoplastic agent.
See: Platinol, Inj. (Bristol)

CITANEST. (Astra) Prilocaine HCl w/sod. chloride, sod. hydroxide. Vial 30 cc., 1%, 2%. Ampul 1% 30 cc.; 2% 30 cc.; 3% 20 cc.
Use: Local anesthetic.

• **CITENAMIDE.** USAN.
Use: Anticonvulsant.

CITHAL CAPSULES. (Table Rock) Ext. watermelon seed 2 gr., theobromine 4 gr., phenobarbital ¼ gr./Cap. Bot. 100s, 500s.
Use: Hypertension.

CITRA CAPSULES. (Boyle) Phenylephrine HCl 10 mg., ascorbic acid 50 mg., pheniramine maleate 6.25 mg., pyrilamine maleate 8.33 mg., salicylamide 227 mg., phenacetin 120 mg., caffeine alk. 30 mg. chlorpheniramine maleate 1 mg./Cap. Bot. 16s, 100s.
Use: Antihistamine, decongestant, analgesic.

CITRA FORTE CAPSULES. (Boyle) Dihydrocodeinone bitartrate 5 mg., Vit. C 50 mg., pheniramine maleate 6.25 mg., pyrilamine maleate 8.33 mg., phenylephrine HCl 10 mg., salicylamide 227 mg., caffeine 30 mg., phenacetin 120 mg./Cap. Bot. 50s, 500s.
Use: Antitussive, antihistaminic, decongestant, analgesic.

CITRA FORTE SYRUP. (Boyle) Dihydrocodeinone bitartrate 5 mg., ascorbic acid 30 mg., pheniramine maleate 2.25 mg., pyrilamine maleate 3.33 mg., potassium citrate 150 mg., 5 cc. alcohol 2%. Bot. pt., gal.
Use: Antitussive, antihistaminic and expectorant.

CITRAMIN-500. (Thurston) Vit. C 500 mg., rose hips, acerola with mixed bioflavonoids/Loz. Bot. 100s, 250s, 1000s.
Use: Trauma, corticotropin therapy, pregnancy and lactation.

CITRASAN B. (Sandia) Lemon bioflavonoid complex 300 mg., Vit. C 300 mg., B-1 30 mg., B-2 10 mg., B-6 5 mg., B-12 4 mcg., cal. pantothenate 10 mg., niacinamide 50 mg./Tab. Bot. 100s, 1000s.

CITRASAN K LIQUID. (Sandia) Vit. C 125 mg., Vit. K 0.66 mg., lemon bioflavonoid complex 125 mg./5 cc. Bot. pt., gal.

CITRASAN K-250. (Sandia) Vit. C 250 mg., Vit. K 1 mg., lemon bioflavonoid 250 mg./Tab. Bot. 100s, 1000s.

CITRATED CAFFEINE.
See: Caffeine Citrate

CITRATED NORMAL HUMAN PLASMA.
See: Plasma, Normal Human.

CITRESCO-K. (Esco) Vit. C 100 mg., citrus bioflavonoid

complex 100 mg., vit. K 0.7 mg./Cap. Bot. 100s, 500s, 1000s.
Use: Treatment of vit. K deficiencies.

• **CITRIC ACID,** U.S.P. XXI. 1,2,3-Propanetricarboxylic acid, 2-hydroxy-.

CITRIN.
See: Vitamin P

CITRIN CAPSULES. (Table Rock) Ext. watermelon seed 4 gr./Cap. Bot. 100s, 500s.
Use: Hypertension.

CITROBIC. (Blue Line) Hesperidin 100 mg., ascorbic acid 100 mg./Tab. Bot. 100s, 1000s.
Use: Fragile capillaries.

CITRO-C CAPSULES. (Barry-Martin) Bioflavonoids 100 mg., Vit. C 100 mg./Cap. Bot. 100s, 500s.

CITROCARBONATE. (Upjohn) Sod. bicarbonate 0.78 Gm., sod. citrate anhydrous 1.82 Gm./teaspoon. Bot. 4 oz., 8 oz.
Use: Increase alkali reserve.

CITROHIST. (Robinson) Prophenpyridamine 6.75 mg., pyrilamine maleate 8.33 mg., hesperidin 50 mg., C 50 mg., ephedrine sulfate 16.2 mg., salicylamide 3½ gr., phenacetin 2 gr., caffeine alkaloid ½ gr., atropine sulfate ¹/₆₀₀ gr./Cap. Bot. 100s, 1000s. Bulk Pack 5000s. Vial 20s.
Use: Cold symptoms.

CITROLEUM SUNBURN CREME. (Citroleum) Bot. 4 oz.

CITROLITH. (Beach) Potassium citrate 50 mg., sodium citrate 950 mg./Tab. Bot. 100s.
Use: Urinary alkalizer.

CITROPAM. (Jenkins) No. 1 Ammonium chloride 0.5 Gm., citric acid 0.5 Gm., potassium quaiacolsulfonate 0.5 Gm./fl. oz. Bot. 3 oz., 4 oz., gal. Also Citropam No. 2 w./codeine phosphate 30 mg./fl., oz.
Bot. 3 oz., 4 oz., gal.
Use: Cough syrup.

CITROTEIN. (Doyle) Orange Flavor: Sucrose, pasteurized egg white solids, maltodextrin, citric acid, natural & artificial flavors, mono & diglycerides, partially hydrogenated soybean oil, vitamins & minerals, FD&C yellow No. 5 and No. 6. Powder 1.57 oz./packet, Cans 14.16 oz. Orange, grape and punch flavors.
Use: Supplementary oral feeding.

CITROVORUM FACTOR. Leucovorin Calcium, U.S.P. XXI.
See: Leucovorin Calcium (Lederle) Folinic Acid.

CITRUS BIOFLAVONOID COMPOUND.
See: Bioflavonoid Cpds. (Various Mfr.)
     C.V.P., Syr. (USV Pharm.)
     Vitamin P
W/Ascorbic acid, phenyltoloxamine dihydrogen citrate, salicylamide, acetyl p-aminophenol, caffeine, racemic amphetamine sulf.
See: Euphenex, Tab. (Westerfield)

C-JECT. (Lincoln) Ascorbic acid 2,000 mg., sodium bisulfite 0.1%, disodium sequestrene 0.01%, 10 cc. Ampule 10 cc. "Score-Break" Box 25s.

C-JECT WITH B. (Lincoln) When mixed with 10 cc. of Diluent each vial contains: Vit. C 2,000 mg., B-1 50

mg., B-2 5 mg., B-6 10 mg., nicotinamide 100 mg., with methylparaben 0.89 mg., propyparaben 0.22 mg., sodium bisulfite 10 mg., disodium sequestrene 1 mg. Box of 6 lyophilized plugs and 6 10-cc. vials of Sterile Diluent.

CKA CANKER AID. (Pannett Prod.) Benzocaine, aluminum hydrate, mag. trisilicate, sod. acid carbonate. Pow.
Use: Cold-canker sore.

CLAFORAN. (Hoechst) Cefotaxime sodium 1.0 Gm., 2.0, and 10 Gm./Vial. Infusion Bottles 1.0 Gm. and 2.0 Gm.
Use: Broad spectrum antibiotic.

CLAMIDOXIC ACID. B.A.N. [2-(3,4-Dichlorobenz-amido)phenoxy]acetic acid.
Use: Antirheumatic.

CLAMOXYQUIN. B.A.N. 5-Chloro-7-(3-diethylamino-propylaminomethyl)-8-hydroxyquinoline.
Use: Treatment of amebiasis.

• **CLAMOXYQUIN HYDROCHLORIDE.** USAN. 5-Chlo-ro-7-(((3-(diethylamino)propyl)-amino)methyl)-8-quino-linol dihydrochloride.
Use: Amebicide.

CLARETIN-12.
See: Vitamin B-12

• **CLAZOLAM.** USAN.
Use: Tranquilizer.

• **CLAZOLIMINE.** USAN.
Use: Diuretic.

CLEANING & SOAKING SOLUTION. (Barnes-Hind) Benzalkonium chloride 0.01%, EDTA 0.2%. Bot. 4 oz.
Use: Hard contact lens cleaner and disinfectant.

CLEAN-N-SOAK. (Allergan) Hard contact lens cleaning & soaking solution. Bot. 4 oz.

CLEARASIL ACNE TREATMENT CREAM. (Vicks Prods) Benzoyl peroxide 10% in tinted or vanishing base. Tube 0.65 oz., 1.0 oz.
Use: Topical acne medication.

CLEARASIL ANTIBACTERIAL ACNE LOTION. (Vicks Prods) Benzoyl peroxide 5%, Bot. 1 oz.
Use: Topical acne medication.

CLEARASIL ANTIBACTERIAL SOAP. (Vicks Prods) Triclosan 0.75% in soap cake 3.25 oz.
Use: Skin cleanser.

CLEARASIL PORE DEEP CLEANSER. (Vicks Prods) Salicylic acid 0.5%, alcohol 43%. Bot. 4 oz., 8 oz.
Use: Medicated skin cleanser.

CLEARASIL STICK. (Vicks Prods) Sulfur 8%, resorcinol 1%. Stick. ⅛ oz.
Use: Topical acne medication.

CLEAR BY DESIGN. (Herbert) Benzoyl peroxide 2.5% in cream base. Tubes, 1.5 oz., 3 oz.
Use: Acne skin medication.

CLEAR EYES. (Abbott Products) Naphazoline HCl 0.012%, benzalkonium chloride 0.01%, disodium edetate 0.1%, boric acid, sodium borate. Bot. 0.5 oz.,1.5 oz.
Use: Ophthalmic decongestant.

CLEAREX ACNE CREAM. (Approved) Allantoin, sulfur, resorcinol, d-panthenol, isopropanol. Tube 1½ oz.

CLEFAMIDE. B.A.N. αα-Dichloro-N-(2-hydroxy-ethyl)-N-[4-(4-nitrophenoxy)benzyl]acetamide.
Use: Treatment of amebiasis.
See: Mebinol

CLEMASTINE. USAN. (+)-2-[2-(4-Chloro-α-methyl-benzhydryloxy)ethyl]-1-methylpyrrolidine.
Use: Antihistamine.
See: Tavegil hydrogen fumarate
Tavist, Tab. (Dorsey)

CLEMASTINE FUAMARATE. USAN.
Use: Antihistaminic.

CLEMASTINE FUMARATE TABLETS, U.S.P. XXI.
Use: Antihistaminic.

CLEMIZOLE. B.A.N. 1-(4-chlorobenzyl)-2-pyrrolidin-1-ylmethylbenzimidazole.
Use: Antipruritic.

CLEMIZOLE HCl. 1-p-Chlorobenzyl-2-pyrrolidyl-methyl benzimidazole. Reactrol.

CLEMIZOLE PENICILLIN. B.A.N. Benzylpenicillin combined with 1-(4-chlorobenzyl)-2-pyrrolidin-1-ylmethylbenzimidazole. Neopenyl.
Use: Antibiotic.

CLENPYRIN. B.A.N. 1-Butyl-2-(3,4-dichloro-phenylimino)pyrrolidine.
Use: Insecticide, veterinary medicine.

CLEOCIN HCl. (Upjohn) Clindamycin HCl equiv. to clindamycin base 75 mg./Cap. Bot. 100s; 150 mg./Cap. Bot. 16s, 100s. Unit-Dose 100s.
Use: Antibiotic.

CLEOCIN PEDIATRIC, (Upjohn) Clindamycin palmitate HCl equivalent to 75 mg., clindamycin/5 ml. when reconstituted as directed. Bot. 100 ml.
Use: Antibiotic.

CLEOCIN PHOSPHATE. (Upjohn) Clindamycin phosphate equivalent to 150 mg. clindamycin/ml. **300 mg.:** Amp. 2 ml. w/disodium edetate 1 mg., benzyl alcohol 18.9 mg. Box 25s, 100s. **600 mg.:** Amp. 4 ml. w/disodium edetate 2 mg., benzyl alcohol 37.8 mg. Box 25s, 100s.
Use: Antibiotic.

CLEOCIN T. (Upjohn) Clindamycin phosphate 1%. Bot. 30 ml., 60 ml.; pt.
Use: Antibiotic.

CLERA. (Alcon) Naphazoline HCl 0.05% Bot. 15 cc.
Use: Ocular vasoconstrictor decongestant.

CLERZ. (CooperVision) A neutral hypertonic balanced salt soln. Lubricating and rewetting eye drops. Bot. 25 ml. w/dropper.
Use: For hard and soft contact lenses.

CLERZ 2. (CooperVision) Lubricating/rewetting eye drops. A neutral balanced salt sol. Bot. 15 ml. w/Dropper.
Use: For hard and soft contact lenses.

C-LEST. (Tunex) Betamethasone sodium phosphate equivalent to betamethasone 3 mg., sodium phosphate 10 mg./ml. Vial 5 cc.
Use: Anti-inflammatory.

CLETOQUINE. B.A.N. 7-Chloro-4-[4-(2-hydroxy-ethylamino)-1-methylbutyl]aminoquinoline.
Use: Anti-inflammatory.

CLIDINIUM BROMIDE, U.S.P. XXI. Caps., U.S.P. XXI. 1-Methyl-3-benzil-oyloxy-quinuclidinium bromide.

3-Hydroxy-1-methyl-quinuclidinium bromide benzilate.
Use: Anticholinergic.
See: Quarzan, Cap. (Roche)
W/Chlordiazepoxide.
See: Chloridinium Sealets, Cap. (Lemmon)
Librax, Cap. (Roche)

CLIMESCO. (Esco) Methyl testosterone 5 mg., yohimbine HCl 5 mg., ext. nux vomica 5 mg., thiamine HCl 25 mg./Cap. Bot. 100s, 500s, 1000s.
Use: Male climacteric and hypogonadal impotence; neurasthenia.

CLINDAMYCIN. USAN. Methyl 7-chloro-6,7,8-tri-deoxy-6-(trans-1-methyl-4-propyl-L-2-pyrrolidine-carboxamido)-1-thio-L-threo-α-D-galactooctopy-ranoside.
Use: Antibiotic.
See: Dalacin C

CLINDAMYCIN HYDROCHLORIDE, U.S.P. XXI. Caps. U.S.P. XXI.
Use: Antibacterial.
See: Cleocin HCl A.D.T., Cap. (Upjohn)

CLINDAMYCIN PALMITATE HYDROCHLORIDE, U.S.P. XXI. Oral Soln., U.S.P. XXI.
Use: Antibacterial.
See: Cleocin Pediatric (Upjohn)
Cleocin T, Liq. (Upjohn)

CLINDAMYCIN PHOSPHATE, U.S.P. XXI. Inj., Topical Sol., Sterile, U.S.P. XXI.
Use: Antibacterial.
See: Cleocin phosphate, Inj. (Upjohn)

CLINISTIX. (Ames) Glucose oxidase, peroxidase and orthotolidine. Diagnostic test for glucose in urine. Bot. 50s.
Use: Diagnostic agent: glucosuria.

CLINITEST. (Ames) Reagent tablets containing copper sulfate, sod. hydroxide & heat-producing agents. Patient's plastic set; Tab. refills, **Bot.** 36s, 100s, 250s, **Box** 100s, 500s, sealed in foil. **Child-resistant Bot.** 36s, 100s.
Use: For urine-sugar determination.

CLINITEST DROPPERS. (Ames) Pkgs. 3s.
Use: Droppers for use with Clinitest reagent tablets.

CLINITEST REAGENT TABLETS 2-DROP METHOD. (Ames) Bot. 36s, 100s. Pt. plastic set.
Use: Test for urine sugar.

CLINITEST SET. (Ames) Urine-sugar analysis set with bottle of 36 tablets and 2 foil wrapped tablets.

CLINITEST TEST TUBES. (Ames) Carton 6s.

CLINOCAINE HCl.
See: Procaine HCl

CLINORIL. (Merck Sharp & Dohme) Sulindac 150 mg. and 200 mg./Tab. Bot. 100s. Unit dose 100s. Unit of use 60s, 100s.
Use: Nonsteroidal anti-inflammatory and analgesic for treatment of osteoarthritis, rheumatoid arthritis, ankylosing spondylitis, acute painful shoulder, and acute gouty arthritis

CLIOQUINOL, U.S.P. XXI. Comp. Pow., Cream, Oint., U.S.P. XXI. 5-Chloro-7-iodo-8-quinolinol. Quinambicide, Rometin. Iodohydroxyquin.
Use: Antiamebic; local anti-infective.

See: HCV Creame (Saron)
   Quin III, Cream (Lemmon)
   Quinoform, Oint., Cream, Lot. (C & M Pharmacal)
   Torofor, Cream, Oint. (Torch)
   Vioform, Prep. (Ciba)
W/Aluminum acetate solution, hydrocortisone.
See: Hydrelt, Cream, Oint. (Elder)
W/Hydrocortisone.
See: Bafil, Cream (Skruggs)
   Caquin Cream (O'Neal, Jones, Feldman)
   Coidocort Cream (Coast)
   Corticoid, Cream (Jenkins)
   Cort Nib V, Cream (Cenci)
   Domeform-HC, Cream (Miles Pharm)
   Durel-Cort 'V,' Cream, Oint., Lot. (Durel)
   Hi-Form Cream (Blaine)
   Hydrelt, Cream (Elder)
   Hysone, Cream, Oint. (Mallard)
   Ido-Cortistan Ointment (Standex)
   Iodocort, Cream (Ulmer)
   Iohydro, Cream (Freeport)
   Kencort, Cream (Kenyon)
   Lanvisone, Cream (Lannett)
   Maso-Form, Cream (Mason)
   Mity-Quin Cream (Reid-Provident)
   Racet, Cream (Lemmon)
   Racet Forte, Cream (Lemmon)
   Vioform-Hydrocortisone, Cream, Oint., Lotion (Ciba)
   Vio-Hydrocort, Cr. and Oint. (Columbia)
W/Hydrocortisone acetate.
See: Quinsone, Oint. (Sutliff & Case)
   Viotag Cream (Reid-Provident)
W/Hydrocortisone acetate, lidocaine.
See: Lidaform-HC, Creme, Lot. (Miles Pharm)
W/Hydrocortisone, coal tar solution.
See: Tar-Quin-HC, Oint. (Jenkins)
W/Hydrocortisone, lidocaine.
See: Bafil Lotion (Scruggs)
   HIL-20 Lotion (Reid-Provident)
W/Hydrocortisone, chlorobutanol.
See: Hc-Form, Jelly (Recsei)
W/Hydrocortisone, coal tar extract.
See: Racet LCD, Cream (Lemmon)
W/Hydrocortisone and pramoxine HCl.
See: Dermarex Cream (Hyrex)
   Quinsone, Cream (Sutliff & Case)
   Sherform-HC, Oint. (Sheryl)
   Stera-Form Creme (Mayrand)
   V-Cort, Cream (Scrip)
   Vio-Hydrosone, Cream (Vortech)
W/Methylcellulose, aluminum hydroxide, atropine sulf., hyoscine HBr, hyoscyamine sulf.
See: Enterex, Tab. (Person & Covey)
W/Nystatin.
See: Nystaform, Oint. (Miles Pharm)
• **CLIOXANIDE.** USAN. 2-(4-Chlorophenylcarbamoyl)-4,6-di-iodophenylacetate.
Use: Anthelmintic, veterinary medicine.
See: Tremerad
• **CLIPROFEN.** USAN.
Use: Anti-inflammatory.

CLISTIN. (McNeil Pharm) Carbinoxamine maleate 4 mg./Tab. Bot. 100s.
Use: Antihistamine.
CLISTIN-D. (McNeil Pharm) Carbinoxamine maleate 2 mg., Acetaminophen 300 mg., phenylephrine HCl 10 mg./Tab. Bot. 100s.
Use: Common cold.
• **CLOBAMINE MESYLATE.** USAN.
Use: Antidepressant.
• **CLOBAZAM.** USAN. 7-Chloro-1-methyl-5-phenyl-1,5-benzodiazepine-2,4-dione.
Use: Tranquilizer.
CLOBENZTROPINE. 3-(p-Chloro-a-phenylbenzyl-oxy) tropane.
CLOBETASOL. B.A.N. 21-Chloro-9α-fluoro-11β, 17α-dihydroxy-16β-methylpregna-1,4-diene-3,20-dione.
Use: Corticosteroid.
• **CLOBETASOL PROPIONATE.** USAN.
Use: Corticosteroid.
CLOBETASONE. B.A.N. 21-Chloro-9α-fluoro-17α-hydroxy-16β-methylpregna-1,4-diene-3,11,20-trione.
Use: Corticosteroid.
• **CLOBETASONE BUTYRATE.** USAN.
Use: Corticosteroid.
CLOCIGUANIL. B.A.N. 4,6-Diamino-1-(3,4-dichloroben-zyloxy)-1,2-dihydro-2,2-dimethyl-1,3,5-triazine.
Use: Antimalarial.
• **CLOCORTOLONE ACETATE.** USAN.
Use: Glucocorticoid.
• **CLOCORTOLONE PIVALATE,** U.S.P. XXI. Cream, U.S.P. XXI.
Use: Glucocorticoid.
CLOCREAM. (Upjohn) Vit. A & D in vanishing base. Tube 1 oz.
Use: Relief of minor skin irritations.
• **CLODANOLENE.** USAN.
Use: Relaxant.
• **CLODAZON HYDROCHLORIDE.** USAN.
Use: Antidepressant.
CLODERM. (Ortho) Clocortolone pivalate cream 0.1%. Tube 15 Gm., 45 Gm.
Use: Steroid responsive dermatoses.
• **CLODRONIC ACID.** USAN.
Use: Regulator.
• **CLOFAZIMINE.** USAN. 3-(p-Chloroanilino) 10-(p-chlorophenyl)-2,10-dihydro-2-(isopropylimino)-phenazine.
Use: Tuberculostatic; leprostatic.
CLOFAZIMINE. B.A.N. 3-(4-Chloroanilino)-10-(4-chlorophenyl)-2,10-dihydro-2-isopropylimino-phenazine.
Use: Treatment of leprosy.
See: Lamprene
• **CLOFIBRATE,** U.S.P. XXI. Caps., U.S.P. XXI. Ethyl 2-(p-chlorophenoxy-2-methyl-propionate. Propanoic acid, 2-(4-chlorophenoxy)-2-methyl-, methyl ester.
Use: Cardiovascular disorders; antihyperlipidemic.
See: Atromid S., Caps. (Ayerst)
• **CLOFILIUM PHOSPHATE.** USAN.
Use: Cardiac depressant.
• **CLOFLUCARBAN.** USAN. 4,4'-Dichloro-3-(trifluoromethyl)-carbanilide. Irgasan, CF3.

Use: Recommended as antiseptic, on release.

CLOFLUPEROL. B.A.N. 4-(4-Chloro-3-trifluoro-methyl-phenyl)-1-[3-(4-fluorobenzoyl)propyl]piperidin-4-ol.
Use: Neuroleptic.

CLOGESTONE. B.A.N. 6-Chloro-3β, 17-dihydroxypreg-na-4,6-diene-20-one.
Use: Progestational steroid.

CLOGESTONE ACETATE. USAN. 6-Chloro-3β, 17-dihydroxypregna-4,6-dien-20-one diacetate. Under study.
Use: Progestogen.

CLOGUANAMILE. B.A.N. 1-Amidino-3-(3-chloro-4-cyanophenyl)urea.
Use: Antimalarial.

CLOMACRAN. B.A.N. NN-Dimethyl-3-(2-chloro-9, 10-dihydroacridin-9-yl)propylamine.
Use: Tranquilizer.

CLOMACRAN PHOSPHATE. USAN. 2-Chloro-9-[3-dimethyl-amino)propyl] acridan phosphate (1:1). Under study.
Use: Tranquilizer.

CLOMEGESTONE ACETATE. USAN. 6-Chloro-17-acetoxy-1,6α-methyl-4,6-pregnadiene-3,20-dione. Under study.
Use: Progestogen.

CLOMETHERONE. USAN. 6α-Chloro-16α-methyl-pregn-4-ene-3,20-dione.
Use: Anti-estrogen.

CLOMID. (Merrell Dow) Clomiphene citrate 50 mg./Tab. Carton 30s.
Use: Ovulatory failure (dysfunction) in patient desiring pregnancy.

CLOMINOREX. USAN.
Use: Anorexic.

CLOMIPHENE CITRATE. U.S.P. XXI. Tabs., U.S.P. XXI. 2-[p-(2-Chloro-1,2-diphenyl-vinyl)phenoxy]ure-thylamine dihydrogen citrate. Ethanamine, 2-[4-(2-chloro-1,2-diphenylethenyl)-phenoxy]-N,N-diethyl-, 2-hydroxy-1,2,3-propanetricarboxylate(1:1).
Use: Fertility agent.
See: Clomid, Tab. (Merrell Dow)
    Serophene, Tab. (Serono)

CLOMIPRAMINE. B.A.N. 3-Chloro-5-(3-dimethylamino-propyl-10,11-dihydrodibenz[b,f]azepine.
Use: Antidepressant.
See: Anafranil hydrochloride

CLOMIPRAMINE HCl. USAN. 3-Chloro-5-[3-(dimethyl-amino)propyl]-10, 11-dihydro-5H-dibenz-[b,f] azepine monohydrochloride.
Use: Antidepressant.

CLOMOCYCLINE. B.A.N. N²-(Hydroxymethyl)-chlortet-racycline.
Use: Antibiotic.
See: Chlormethylencycline Megaclor

CLONAZEPAM, U.S.P. XXI. Tab. U.S.P. XXI. 5-(o-Chlorophenyl)-1,3-dihydro-7-nitro-2H-1,4-benzodiaze-pin-2-one. B.A.N. 5-(2-Chlorophenyl)-1,3-dihydro-7-nitro-2H-1,4-benzodiazepin-2-one. Rivotril.
Use: Anticonvulsant.
See: Clonopin, Tab. (Roche)

C-LONG. (Reid-Provident) Ascorbic acid 500 mg./long-acting Cap. Bot. 100s.

CLONIDINE. USAN. 2-(2,6-Dichloroanilino)-2-imida-zoline.
Use: Hypotensive.
See: Catapres
    Dixarit

CLONIDINE HYDROCHLORIDE, U.S.P. XXI. Tabs., U.S.P. XXI. Benzamine, 2,6-dichloro-N-2-imidazolidi-nyl-idene-, monochloride. (1)2-(2,6-Dichloranilino)-2-imidazoline monohydrochloride. (2)2-(2,6-Dichloro-phenylamino)-2-imidazoline HCl.
Use: Antihypertensive.
See: Catapres, Tab. (Boehringer Ingelheim)

CLONIDINE HYDROCHLORIDE AND CHLORTHALIDONE TABLETS, U.S.P. XXI.
Use: Antihypertensive, diuretic.
See: Combipres, Tab. (Boehringer Ingelheim)

CLONITAZENE. B.A.N. 2-(4-Chlorobenzyl)-1-(2-die-thylaminoethyl)-5-nitrobenzimidazole.
Use: Narcotic analgesic.

CLONITRATE. USAN. 3-Chloro-1,2-propanediol dini-trate. Dylate
Use: Coronary vasodilator.

CLONIXERIL. USAN.
Use: Analgesic.

CLONIXIN. USAN.
Use: Analgesic.

CLONOPIN. (Roche) Clonazepam 0.5 mg., 1 mg., 2.0 mg./Tab. Pkg. 100s.
Use: Anticonvulsant (petit mal).

CLOPAMIDE. USAN. (1) 4-Chloro-N-(2,6-dimethyl-piperidino)-3-sulfamoylbenzamide; (2)4-chloro-3-sul-famoylbenzoic acid 1,5-dimethylpentamethylenehy-drazide.
Use: Antihypertensive; diuretic.
See: Aquex, Tab. (Lannett)
    Brinaldix

CLOPENTHIXOL. USAN. 4-[3-(2-Chlorothioxanthen-9-ylidene)propyl]-1-piperazine-ethanol.
Use: Antipsychotic.
See: Sordinol (Ayerst)

CLOPERIDONE HYDROCHLORIDE. USAN. 3-[3-[4-(m-Chlorophenyl)-1-piperazinyl] propyl]-2,-4-(IH, 3H)-quinazolinedione HCl.
Use: Sedative; tranquilizer.

CLOPHEDIANOL HCl.
See: Acutuss, Tab., Expect. (Philips Roxane)

CLOPHENOXATE HCl. 2-Dimethylamino-ethyl p-chlor-phenoxyacetate HCl.
Use: Cerebral stimulant.

CLOPENTHIXOL. B.A.N. 2-Chloro-9- 3-[4-(2-hydroxye-thyl)piperazin-1-yl]-propylidene thiaxanthene.
Use: Psychotropic.
See: Sordinol dihydrochloride

CLOPIDOL. USAN. 3,5-Dichloro-4-hydroxy-2,6-dime-thylpyridine.
Use: Antiprotozoan, veterinary medicine.
See: Coyden 25

CLOPIMOZIDE. USAN.
Use: Antipyschotic.

CLOPIPAZAN MESYLATE. USAN.
Use: Antipsychotic.

CLOPIRAC. USAN. 1-p-Chlorophenyl-2,5-dimethylpyr-rol-3-ylacetic acid.
Use: Anti-inflammatory.
CLOPONONE. B.A.N. β,4-Dichloro-α-dichloro-acetamidopropiophenone.
Use: Antiseptic.
• **CLOPREDNOL.** USAN.
Use: Glucocorticoid.
CLOPROSTENOL. B.A.N. ($\pm$)-7- (1R,2R,3R,5S)-2-[(3R)-4-(3-Chlorophenoxy)-3-hydroxybut-1-(E)-enyl]-3,5-dihydroxycyclopent-1-yl hept-5-(Z) enoic acid.
Use: Synchronization of estrus; infertility, veterinary medicine.
• **CLOPROSTENOL SODIUM.** USAN.
Use: Prostaglandin.
CLOQUINATE. B.A.N. Chloroquine di-(8-hydroxy-7-iodoquinoline-5-sulfonate).
Use: Treatment of amebiasis.
See: Resotren
• **CLORAZEPATE DIPOTASSIUM.** USAN. 7-Chloro-2,3-dihydro-2,2-dihydroxy-5-phenyl-IH-1,4-benzodiaz-epine-3-carboxylic acid dipotassium salt.
Use: Minor tranquilizer.
See: Tranxene, Cap. (Abbott)
• **CLORAZEPATE MONOPOTASSIUM.** USAN.
Use: Minor tranquilizer.
CLORAZEPIC ACID. B.A.N. 7-Chloro-2,3-dihydro-2,2-dihydroxy-5-phenyl-1H-1,4-benzodiazepine-3-carbox-ylic acid.
Use: Sedative.
See: Azene, monopotassiuim salt (Du Pont)
Tranxene dipotassium salt (Abbott)
• **CLORETHATE.** USAN.
Use: Sedative, hypnotic.
CLOREXOLONE. USAN. 5-Chloro-2-cyclohexyl-6-sul-famoylisoindolin-1-one.
Use: Diuretic.
See: Nefrolan
CLORFED II. (Stewart-Jackson) Chlorpheniramine 4 mg., pseudoephedrine 60 mg./Tab. Bot. 100s.
Use: Decongestant, antihistamine.
CLORFED CAPSULES. (Stewart-Jackson) Chlorpheniramine 8 mg., pseudoephedrine 120 mg./Cap. Bot. 100s.
Use: Antihistamine, decongestant.
CLORFED EXPECTORANT. (Stewart-Jackson) Pseudoephedrine 30 mg., guaifensen 100 mg., codeine 10 mg. Bot. pt.
Use: Decongestant, antihistamine, expectorant, antitussive.
CLORFED LIQUID. (Stewart-Jackson) Chlorpheniramine 2 mg., pseudoephedrine 30 mg. w/alcohol by volume 5%. Bot. pt.
Use: Decongestant, antihistamine.
CLORGYLINE. B.A.N. N-3-(2,4-Dichlorophenoxy) pro-pyl-N-methylprop-2-ynylamine.
Use: Monoamine oxidase inhibitor; antidepressant.
CLORINDIONE. B.A.N. 2-(4-Chlorophenyl)indane-1,3-dione.
Use: Anticoagulant.
See: Indalitan
• **CLOROPERONE HYDROCHLORIDE.** USAN.
Use: Antipsychotic.

CLORPACTIN WCS-90. (Guardian) Sodium oxychloro-sene. Bot. 2 Gm. 5s.
Use: Topical antiseptic for irrigation of infected areas.
• **CLOROPHENE.** USAN. 4-Chloro-alpha-phenyl-o-cre-sol.
Use: Disinfectant.
See: Santophen 1 (Monsanto)
CLORPRENALINE. B.A.N. 1-(2-Chlorophenyl)-2-iso propylaminoethanol.
Use: Sympathomimetic.
• **CLORPRENALINE HYDROCHLORIDE.** USAN. (formerly Isoprophenamine HCl) 1-(α-Chlorophenyl)-2-isopropyl-aminoethanol hydrochloride hydrate. Vor-tel
Use: Bronchodilator.
• **CLORSULON.** USAN.
Use: Antiparasitic, fasciolicide.
• **CLORTERMINE HCl.** USAN. o-Chloro-α,α-dimethyl-phenethylamine HCl.
Use: Anorexic.
See: Voranil (USV Labs.)
• **CLOSANTEL.** USAN.
Use: Anthelmintic.
• **CLOSIRAMINE ACETURATE.** USAN.
Use: Antihistaminic.
CLOSTEBOL ACETATE. B.A.N. 17β-Acetoxy-4-chlo-roandrost-4-en-3-one.
Use: Anabolic steroid.
• **CLOTHIAPINE.** USAN. 2-Chloro-11-(4-methyl-pipera-zin-1-yl)dibenzo[b,f][1,4]thiazepine.
Use: Tranquilizer.
• **CLOTHIXAMIDE MALEATE.** USAN. 4-[3-(2-Chloro-thioxanthen-9-ylidene)propyl]-N-methyl-1-piperazine-propionamide dimaleate.
Use: Tranquilizer.
• **CLOTRIMAZOLE,** U.S.P. XXI. Cream, Topical Soln., Vaginal Tabs., U.S.P. XXI. I-(o-Chloro-α,α-diphenyl-benzyl)-imidazole.
Use: Antifungal.
See: Gyne-Lotrimin, Cream, Vaginal Tab. (Schering)
Lotrimin, Cream, Sol. (Schering)
Myclex, Cream, Sol. (Miles Pharm)
Myclex-G, Vag. Suppos. (Miles Pharm)
• **CLOVE OIL,** N.F. XVI.
Use: Pharmaceutic aid (flavor).
CLOVERINE. (Medtech) White salve. Tin 1 oz.
Use: Temporary relief of minor skin irritations & burns.
CLOVOCAIN. (Vita Elixir) Benzocaine, oil of cloves.
Use: Dental medicine, surface anesthetic.
CLOXACILLIN. B.A.N. 6-[3-(2-Chlorophenyl)-5-methylisoxazole-4-carboxamido]penicillanic acid. 3-(2-Chlorophenyl)-5-methylisoxazol-4-ylpenicillin.
Use: Antibiotic.
See: Orbenin sodium salt
• **CLOXACILLIN SODIUM,** U.S.P. XXI., Caps., For Oral Soln., U.S.P. XXI. 4-Thia-1-azabicyclo[3.2.0]hep-tane-2-carboxylic acid,6-[[[3-(2-chlorophenyl)-5-methyl-4-isoxazoly]carbonyl]amino]-3,3-dimethyl-7-oxo-,monosodium salt, monohydrate. Monosodium 6-[3-(o-chlorophenyl)-5-methyl-4-isoxazolecarboxami-

do]-3,3-dimethyl-7-oxo-4-thia-1-azabicyclo[3.2.0]hept-ane-2-carboxylate monohydrate.
Use: Antibiotic for resistant staph infections.
See: Cloxapen, Cap. (Beecham Labs)
   Tegopen, Cap., Granules (Bristol)

CLOXAPEN. (Beecham Labs) Cloxacillin sodium 250 mg. & 500 mg./Cap. Bot. 100s.
Use: Antibiotic.

• **CLOXYQUIN.** USAN.
Use: Antibacterial.

• **CLOZAPINE.** USAN. 8-Chloro-11-(4-methylpiperazin-1-yl)-5H-dibenzo[b,e][1,4]-diazepine.
Use: Sedative.

CLUSIVOL CAPSULES. (Ayerst) Vit. A 10,000 U.S.P. Units, D-2 400 U.S.P. Units, C 150 mg., B-1 10 mg., B-2 5 mg., B-6 0.5 mg., d-panthenol 1 mg., B-12 2.5 mcg., niacinamide 50 mg., E 0.5 I.U., Fe 15 mg., Ca 120 mg., Mn 0.5 mg., Zn 0.6 mg., Mg 3 mg./Cap. 100s.
Use: Nutritional supplement.

CLUSIVOL SYRUP. (Ayerst) Vit. A 2500 U.S.P. Units, D-2 400 U.S.P. Units, C 15 mg., B-12 2 mcg., B-1 1 mg., B-2 1 mg., niacinamide 5 mg., d-panthenol 3 mg., B-6 0.6 mg., manganese, 0.5 mg., zinc. 0.5 mg., magnesium, 3 mg./5 ml. Bot. 8, 16 fl. oz.
Use: Nutritional supplement.

CLUSIVOL TABLETS. (Ayerst) Vit. A 10,000 U.S.P. Units, D-2 400 U.S.P. Units, C 150 mg., B-1 10 mg., B-2 5 mg., B-6 0.5 mg., d-panthenol 1 mg., B-12 2.5 mcg., niacinamide 50 mg., E 0.5 I.U., Fe 15 mg., Ca 120 mg., Mn 0.5 mg., Zn 0.6 mg., Mg 3 mg./Tab. Bot. 130s.
Use: Nutritional supplement.

CLYSODRAST. (Barnes-Hind) Bisacodyl 1.5 mg., tannic acid 2.5 Gm./packet. 25s, 50s.
Use: Stimulant laxative.

C.M.C. CELLULOSE GUM.
See: Carboxymethylcellulose Sodium, Preps.

CMV. (Wampole-Zeus) Cytomegalovirus antibody test system. Tests 100s.
Use: For the qualitative and semi-quantitative detection of CMV antibody in human serum.

COAGULANTS.
See: Hemostatics

• **COAL TAR,** U.S.P. XXI. Oint., Sol., U.S.P. XXI.
Use: Topical antieczematic; antipsoriatic.
See: Balnetar, Liq. (Westwood)
   Estar, Gel (Westwood)
   L.C.D. Comp., Oint., Sol. (Almay)
   Polytar Bath, Liq. (Stiefel)
   Tarbonis, Cream (Reed & Carnrick)
   Zetar, Preps. (Dermik)
W/Allantoin, hydrocortisone.
See: Alphosyl-HC, Lot., Cream (Reed & Carnrick)
W/Hydrocortisone.
See: Doak Oil Forte, Liq. (Doak)
   Tarcortin, Cream (Reed & Carnrick)
W/Iodoquinol, hydrocortisone.
See: ZeTar-Quin, Cream (Dermik)
W/Mercury oleate, salicylic acid, phenol, p-nitrophenol.
See: Prosol, Emulsion (Torch)
W/Zinc oxide.
See: Tarpaste, Paste (Doak)

COAL TAR BATH. (Durel) Coal tar solution 20%, polysorbate "20" 5%, isopropanol 75%. Bot. 8 oz., pt., gal.
Use: Generalized pruritus, pruritic dermatoses, psoriasis.

COAL TAR CREAM COTASOL. (Durel) Coal tar solution 5% in Duromantel cream. Jars 1 oz., 1 lb., 6 lb.
Use: Atopic dermatitis, mild forms of contact dermatitis, seborrheic dermatitis.

COAL TAR, DISTILLATE.
See: Lavatar, Liq. (Doak)
   Syntar, Cream (Elder)
W/Sulfur & salicylic acid.
See: Pragmatar, Oint. (Menley & James)

COAL TAR EXTRACT
W/Allantoin, hexachlorophene.
See: Sebical Cream (Reed & Carnrick)
W/Allantoin, hexachlorophene, glycerin, lanolin.
See: Pso-Rite, Cream (DePree)
W/Allantoin, salicylic acid & perhydrosqualine.
See: Skaylos Cream (Ambix)
   Skaylos Lotion (Ambix)
W/Salicylic acid, resorcinol, benzoic acid.
See: Mazon Cream (Norcliff-Thayer)

COAL TAR PASTE.
W/Zinc paste.
See: Tarpaste, Paste (Doak)

• **COAL TAR TOPICAL SOLUTION,** U.S.P. XXI.
Liquor Carbonis Detergens. L.C.D.
See: Balnetar, Liq. (Westwood)
   Estar, Gel (Westwood)
   L.C.D. Compound Oint., Sol. (Almay)
   Psorigel, Gel (Owen)
   Wright's Soln. (Fougera)
   Zetar, Emuls., Shampoo (Dermik)
W/Allantoin, psorilan, myristate.
See: Iocon, Shampoo (Owen)
   Psorelief, Cream (Columbia)
W/Hydrocortisone, iodoquinol.
See: Cor-Tar-Quin, Cream, Lotion (Miles Pharm)
W/Hydrocortisone alcohol, clioquinololine and diperodon HCl, Vit. A, D.
See: Pentarcort, Cream (Dalin)
W/Robane (perhydrosqualene).
See: Skaylos Shampoo (Ambix)
W/Salicylic acid.
See: Epidol, Sol. (Spirt)
   Ionil T, Shampoo (Owen)
W/Salicylic acid, sulfur, protein.
See: Vanseb-T Tar Shampoo (Herbert)

COASTALDYNE. (Coastal) Codeine phosphate 30 mg., acetaminophen 500 mg./Tab. Bot. 100s, 1000s.
Use: Analgesic.

COASTALGESIC. (Coastal) Acetaminophen 7½ gr., caffeine ½ gr., butabarbital ¼ gr./Tab. Bot. 100s, 1000s.
Use: Analgesic.

• **COBALAMINE CONCENTRATE,** U.S.P. XXI.
Use: Hematopoetic vitamin.
See: Vitamin B-12 (Var. Mfr.)

COBALASINE. (Keene) Adenosine phosphate Inj. 25 mg./ml. Vial 10 ml.

COBALIN. (Ulmer) Thiamine HCl 100 mg., cyanocobalamin 500 mcg./cc. Vial 10 cc.
Use: Treatment of vit. B-12 and thiamine deficiency.

COBALT CHLORIDE.
W/Ferrous gluconate, Vit. B-12, duodenum whole desic.
See: Bitrinsic-E, Cap. (Elder)

COBALT GLUCONATE.
W/Ferrous gluconate, B-12 activity, desiccated stomach substance, folic acid.
See: Chromagen, Cap., Inj. (Savage)

COBALT-LABELED VITAMIN B-12.
See: Rubratope-57 (Squibb)

• **COBALTOUS CHLORIDE Co 57.** USAN.
Use: Radioactive agent.

• **COBALTOUS CHLORIDE Co 60.** USAN.
Use: Radioactive agent.

COBALT STANDARDS FOR VITAMIN B-12.
See: Cobatope-57, and Cobatope-60 (Squibb)

COBAN SODIUM SALT.
See: Monensin, B.A.N.

COBATOPE-57. (Squibb) Cobaltous Chloride Co 57.

COBEX 100. (Standex) Vit. B-12 100 mcg.

COBEX 1000. (Standex) Vit. B-12 1000 mcg./10 cc. Vial 30 cc.

CO-BILE. (Western Research) Hog bile 64.8 mg., pancreas sub. 64.8 mg., papain-pepsin complex 97.2 mg., diatase malt 16.2 mg., papain 48.6 mg., pepsin 48.6 mg./Tab. Bot. 1000s.
Use: Digestant.

COBIONE.
See: Vit. B-12

COBIRON. (Pharmex) Cyanocobalamin 100 mcg., hydroxycobalamine 50 mcg., ferrous gluconate 60 mg., liver injection 5 mcg./2 cc.; procaine HCl 2%, phenol 0.5%. Vial 30 cc.

COBRA VENOM.
See: Cobroxin, Amp. (Hynson, Westcott & Dunning)
Nyloxin, Inj. (Hynson, Westcott & Dunning)

• **COCAINE,** U.S.P. XXI. Methyl 3β-Hydroxy-1αH,-5αH-tropane-2β-carboxylate Benzoate (Ester) Alkaloid, Pow. (Mallinckrodt) Hydrochloride, Pow. (Mallinckrodt).

• **COCAINE HYDROCHLORIDE,** U.S.P. XXI. Tab., for Topical Sol., U.S.P. XXI. 8-Azabicyclo[3.2.1]octane-2-carboxylic acid, 3-(benzoyloxy)-8-methyl-, methyl ester, hydrochloride. Methyl 3β-hydroxy-1αH,5αH-tropan-2β-carboxylate, benzoate (ester) hydrochloride.

CO-CARBOXYLASE. B.A.N. Pyrophosphoric ester of aneurine.
Use: Co-enzyme.

■ **COCCIDIOSTATS, VETERINARY USE.**
See: Amprol (MSD AGVET)
Amprol Hi-E (MSD AGVET)
Amprol Plus (MSD AGVET)
Amprovine (MSD AGVET)
Corid (MSD AGVET)
Nicarb (MSD AGVET)
S.Q. (MSD AGVET)

COCCULIN.
See: Picrotoxin, Inj. (Various Mfr.)

COCILAN SYRUP. (Approved) Euphorbia, wild lettuce, cocillana, squill, senega and cascarin (bitterless). Bot. gal. Available w/codeine. Bot. gal.

COCILLANA.
W/Euphorbia pilulifera, squill, antimony potassium tartrate, senega.
See: Cylana Syr. (Bowman)

COCILLIN V-K. (Coastal) Pot. phenoxymethyl penicillin 250 mg. (400,000 u.)/Tab. Bot. 100s, 1000s.

• **COCOA,** N.F. XVI. Syr., N.F. XVI.
Use: Pharm. Aid (Flavor; flavored vehicle).

• **COCOA BUTTER,** N.F. XVI.
Use: Pharm. Aid (Suppository base).

CODACTIDE. B.A.N. D-Ser[1]-Lys[17,18]-β[1-18]-corticotrophin amide.
Use: Corticotrophic peptide.

CODAHIST SYRUP. (Towne) Codeine phosphate 8.7 mg., pyrilamine maleate 5 mg., pot. guaiacol sulfonate, ammonium chloride, menthol & raspberry/4 cc. Bot. 4 oz., 1 pt.
Use: Cough due to colds.

CODAHIST THROAT LOZENGES. (Towne) Bot. 12s

CODALAN NO. 1. (Lannett) Codeine phosphate 8 mg., salicylamide 230 mg., acetaminophen 150 mg., caffeine 30 mg./Tab. Bot. 100s, 500s, 1000s. **Codalan No. 2** contains codeine phosphate 15 mg./Tab; Bot. 100s, 500s, 1000s. **Codalan No. 3** contains codeine phosphate 30 mg./Tab. Bot. 100s, 500s, 1000s.

CODAMINE PEDIATRIC. (Columbia) Hydrocodone bitartrate 2.5 mg., phenylpropanolamine HCl 12.5 mg./5 ml. Bot. pt., gal.
Use: Antitussive, antihistaminic.

CODAMINE SYRUP. (Columbia) Hydrocodone bitartrate 5.0 mg., phenylpropanolamine HCl 25 mg./5 ml. Bot. pt., gal.
Use: Antitussive, Antihistaminic.

CODANOL OINTMENT. (A.P.C.) Vit. A, Vit. D, hexachlorophene, zinc oxide.
Tube 1½ oz., 4 oz.
Jar 1 lb.
Use: Diaper rash, minor burns, skin irritations.

CODAP. (Reid-Provident) Codeine phosphate 32 mg., acetaminophen 325 mg./Tab. Bot. 500s.
Use: Analgesic.

CODAPRIN. (Cenci) APC w/codeine **No. 2:** (¼ gr.), **No. 3:** (½ gr.), **No. 4:** (1 gr.). Bot. 100s, 1000s.

CODASA I. (Stayner) Codeine phosphate ¼ gr., aspirin 5 gr./Cap. Bot. 100s, 500s.
Use: Analgesic.

CODASA II. (Stayner) Codeine phosphate ½ gr., aspirin 5 gr./Cap. Bot. 100s, 500s.

CODASA FORTE. (Stayner) Codeine phosphate ½ gr., aspirin 10 gr./Cap. Bot. 100s, 500s.

CODASA TABS. (Stayner) Codeine phosphate ½ gr. or ¼ gr., aspirin 5 gr./Tab. Bot. 100s, 1000s.

CODASPRO No. 1 & No. 2. (Mallinckrodt) New name for Bellaspro, Tab. W/Codeine.

• **CODEINE,** U.S.P. XXI. 7,8-Didehydro-4,5α-epoxy-3-

methoxy-17-methylmorphinan-6α-ol   monohydrate.
Cryst. or Pow. Bot. ⅛ oz., & 1 oz.
Use: analgesic (Narcotic); antitussive.
CODEINE COMBINATIONS.
See: Actifed-C, Exp., Syr. (Burroughs-Wellcome)
  Anexsia w/Cod., Tab. (Beecham Labs)
  APAP w/Codeine, Tab. (Central)
  A.P.C. w/Cod., Tab. (Various Mfr.)
  Ascriptin W/Codeine No. 2, Tab. (Rorer)
  Ascriptin W/Codeine No. 3, Tab. (Rorer)
  Asphac-G w/Codeine, Tab. (Central)
  Aspodyne w/Cod., Tab. (Blue Line)
  Bancap w/Codeine, Cap. (Westerfield)
  Bri-Stan, Liq. (Briar)
  Buff-A-Comp., Tab. (Mayrand)
  Butadeine, Cap. (Sutliff & Case)
  Calcidrine Syr. (Abbott)
  Capital w/Codeine, Tab., Susp. (Carnrick)
  Cerose, Liq. (Ives)
  Cetro-Cirose, Liq. (Ives)
  Cheracol, Syr. (Upjohn)
  Chlor-Trimeton Expect. (Schering)
  Coastaldyne, Tab. (Coastal)
  Codalan, Tab. (Lannett)
  Codap, Tab. (Reid-Provident)
  Codasa I & II, Cap. (Stayner)
  Codel, Exp., Syr. (Elder)
  Colrex Compound, Cap., Elix. (Rowell)
  Cosanyl Cough Syrup (Health Care Ind.)
  Co-Xan, Liq. (Central)
  Drucon w/Codeine, Liq. (Standard Drug)
  Empirin, No. 1, No. 2, No. 3, No. 4, Tab.
    (Burroughs-Wellcome)
  Fedahist-C, Expect. (Dooner)
  Fiorinal w/Codeine, Cap. (Sandoz)
  G-3, Cap. (Hauck)
  Golacol, Syr. (Arcum)
  Guialyn W/Codeine, Liq. (Scrip)
  Histussinol W/C, Syr. (Bock)
  Isoclor, Expect. (Arnar-Stone)
  Kiddi-Koff, Liq. (Republic)
  Mallergan, Liq. (Mallard)
  Maxigesic, Cap. (W.F. Merchant)
  Novahistine, Expect. (Merrell Dow)
  Nucofed, Liq. (Beecham)
  Partuss AC (Parmed)
  Pavadon Elix. (Coastal)
  Pediacof, Syr. (Winthrop-Breon)
  Percogesic-C, Tab. (Du Pont)
  Phenaphen, #2, #3, #4 Cap. (Robins)
  Phenaphen-650, Tab. (Robins)
  Phenatuss, Liq. (Dalin)
  Phenergan Expectorant w/Codeine, Troches
    (Wyeth)
  Phenodyne w/Codeine Phos., Cap. (Blue Line)
  Poly-histine Expectorant, Liq. (Bock)
  Proval No. 3, Tab. (Reid-Provident)
  Prunicodeine, Syr. (Lilly)
  Respi-Sed, Liq. (Vortch)
  Robitussin A-C, DAC (Robins)
  Ryna-Cx, Liq. (Mallinckrodt)
  SK-APAP W/Codeine, Tab. (SmithKline)

  Syrcodate, Syr. (Blue Line)
  Tega-Code, Cap. (Ortega)
  Tolu-Sed, Elix. (Scherer)
  TSG Croup Liquid, Liq. (Elder)
  Tussar-2, Syr. (Armour)
  Tussi-Organidin, Liq. (Wallace)
  Tylenol w/Codeine, No. 1, No. 2, No. 3, No. 4
    Tab. (McNeil)
  Tylenol w/Codeine Elixir (McNeil)
  Vasotus, Liq. (Sheryl)
CODEINE RESIN COMPLEX COMBINATIONS.
  See: Omni-Tuss, Liq. (Pennwalt)
CODEINE METHYLBROMIDE. Eucodin.
  Use: Narcotic cough depressant.
• **CODEINE PHOSPHATE,** U.S.P. XXI. Inj., Tablets,
  U.S.P. XXI. (Various Mfr.) Pow. Bot. ⅛ oz., ¼ oz.,
  ½ oz. & 1 oz.
  Use: Narcotic analgesic antitussive.
• **CODEINE SULFATE,** U.S.P. XXI. Tab., U.S.P. XXI.
  7,8-Didehydro-4,5α-epoxy-3-methoxy-17-methyl-mor-
  phinan-6α-ol sulfate.
CODELCORTONE.
  See: Prednisolone.
CODICLEAR DH SYRUP. (Central) Hydrocodone
  bitartrate 5 mg., potassium guaiaco/sulfonate 300
  mg./5 ml. Bot. 4 oz., pts.
  Use: Antitussive-expectorant.
CODIMAL-A. (Central) Brompheniramine maleate 10
  mg./ml. w/methylparaben 0.18%, propylparaben
  0.02%. I.M. Vial 10 ml.
  Use: Antihistaminic.
CODIMAL CAPSULES (Central) Chlorpheniramine
  maleate 2 mg., pseudoephedrine HCl 30 mg.,
  acetaminophen 325 mg./Cap. Bot. 24s, 100s,
  1000s.
  Use: Temporary relief of cold symptoms.
CODIMAL DH SYRUP. (Central) Hydrocodone
  bitartrate 1.66 mg., phenylephrine HCl 5 mg.,
  pyrilamine maleate 8.33 mg./5 ml. Bot. 4 oz., pt.,
  gal.
  Use: Antihistaminic expectorant.
CODIMAL DM. (Central) Dextromethorphan HBr 10
  mg., phenylephrine HCl 5 mg., pyrilamine maleate
  8.33 mg./5 ml. w/ alcohol 4%. Sugar Free. Bot. 4
  oz., pt., gal.
CODIMAL EXPECTORANT. (Central)
  Phenylpropanolamine HCl 25 mg., guaifenesin 100
  mg./5 ml. Bot. 4 oz., Pt.
  Use: Temporary relief of coughs due to common
  cold.
CODIMAL-L.A. (Central) Chlorpheniramine maleate 8
  mg., pseudoephedrine HCl 120 mg./Cap. Bot.
  100s, 1000s.
  Use: Antihistamine, decongestant.
CODIMAL PH SYRUP. (Central) Codeine phosphate
  10 mg., phenylephrine HCl 5 mg., pyrilamine
  maleate 8.33 mg./5 ml. Bot. 4 oz., pt., gal.
  Use: Sedative expectorant for coughs due to
  colds.
CODIMAL TABLETS. (Central) Chlorpheniramine
  maleate 2 mg., pseudoephedrine HCl 30 mg.,

acetaminophen 325 mg./Tab. Bot. 24s, 100s, 1000s.
Use: Relief symptoms of common cold.

CODISTAN. (Vortech) Codeine sulf. 64 mg., pyranisamine maleate 200 mg., guaifenesin 100 mg., alcohol 8%/oz. Syr. Bot. 4 oz., Gal.
Use: Treatment of coughs and colds.

• **COD LIVER OIL,** U.S.P. XXI. Emulsion, emulsion w/malt.
Use: Vitamin A & D therapy.

W/Anesthesin, zinc oxide, hydroxyquinoline.
See: Medicone Dressing. (Medicone)

W/Benzocaine.
See: Morusan, Oint. (Beecham Labs)

W/Creosote. (Bryant) Cod liver oil 9 min., creosote 1 min./Cap. Bot. 100s.

W/Malt ext. (Burroughs Wellcome) Vit. A 6450 I.U., Vit. D 645 I.U. Bot. 10 fl. oz., 20 fl. oz.

W/Methylbenzethonium Cl.
See: Benephen, Prods. (Halsted)

W/Viosterol.
Abbott-Vit. A 2800 I.U., Vit. D 255 I.U./Gm. Bot. 12 fl. oz.
Squibb-Vit. A 2000 I.U., Vit. D 440 I.U./Gm. Bot. 4 & 12 fl. oz.

W/Zinc oxide.
See: Caldesene, Oint. (Pharmacraft)
Desitin, Prep. (Leeming)

COD LIVER OIL CONCENTRATE. (Schering) Concentrate of cod liver oil with vitamins A and D added. **Cap.** Bot. 40s, 100s. **Tab.** Bot. 100s, 240s. Also W/Vit. C. Bot. 100s.

COD LIVER OIL OINTMENT.
See: Moruguent, Oint. (Beecham Labs)

• **CODORPHONE HYDROCHLORIDE.** USAN.
Use: Analgesic.

• **CODOXIME.** USAN.
Use: Antitussive.

• **CODOXY.** (Halsey) Oxycodone HCl 4.50 mg., oxycodone terephthalate 0.38 mg., aspirin 325 mg./Tab. Bot. 100s.
Use: Pain relief.

CODROXOMIN INJECTION. (Fellows) Crystalline hydroxocobalamin 1000 mcg./cc. Vial 10 cc.

COENZYME-B. (Inwood) Diphosphothiamin (Co-carboxylase) 25 mg./Cap. Bot. 50s. Amp. (50 mg./2 cc.). Bot. 12s, 25s, 50s, 100s.
Use: Coenzyme for Vitamin B-1.

CO-ESTRO. (Robinson) Conjugated estrogen 0.625 mg., 1.25 mg., 2.5 mg./Tab. Bot. 100s, 500s, 1000s.
Use: Estrogen therapy.

COFFEE BREAK. (O'Connor) Phenylpropanolamine HCl 37.5 mg./cube. Bot. 42s.
Use: Appetite suppressant.

CO-GEL. (Arco) Calcium carbonate 300 mg., glycine 85 mg., Trizyme (amylolytic enzyme 3 mg., proteolytic enzyme 0.6 mg., cellulolytic enzyme 0.2 mg.) 3.8 mg./Tab. Bot. 100s.
Use: Hyperacidity.

COGENTIN. (Merck Sharp & Dohme) Benztropine Mesylate **Tab.:** 0.5 mg. Bot. 100s; 1 mg. Bot. 100s,

Unit dose pkg. 100s; 2 mg. Bot. 100s, 1000s, Unit dose pkg. 100s. **Inj.:** benztropine mesylate 1 mg./1 ml. w/sodium chloride 9 mg. and water for injection q.s. to 1 ml. Amp. 2 ml., Box 6s.
Use: Parkinsonism, extrapyramidal disorders due to neuroleptic drugs.

CO-GESIC. (Central) Hydrocodone bitartrate 5 mg., acetaminophen 500 mg./Tab. Bot. 100s.
Use: Analgesic.

COHEMA. (Sutliff & Case) Manganese 5 mg., copper 0.2 mg., molybdenum 0.2 mg., cobalt 0.5 mg., zinc 1 mg., Vit. B-1 1 mg., niacinamide 10 mg., Vit. B-12 1 mcg. Vit. C 60 mg., ferrous fumarate 325 mg./Tab. Bot. 100s, 1000s.
Use: Hematinic

CO-HEP-TRAL. (Davis & Sly) Folic acid 10 mg., B-12 100 mcg., liver injection, q.s./cc. Vial 10 cc.
Use: Anemias and sprue.

COHIDRATE. (Coastal) Chloral hydrate 500 mg./Cap. Bot. 100s, 1000s.
Use: Sedative.

CO-HISTINE DH. (Kay) Codeine phosphate 10 mg., phenylpropanolamine HCl 18.75 mg., chlorpheniramine maleate 2 mg./5 ml. w/alcohol 5%. Bot. 1 Gal.
Use: Decongestant, antitussive, antihistamine.

CO-HISTINE EXPECTORANT. (Kay) Codeine phosphate 10 mg., phenylpropanolamine HCl 18.75 mg., guaifenesin 100 mg./5 ml w/alcohol 7.5%. Bot. Gal.
Use: Relief of cough and nasal congestion.

COIDOCORT CREAM. (Coast) Hydrocortisone free alcohol 1%, clioquinol 3% in aqueous emulsion. Tubes, 20 Gm.
Use: Dermatitis, eczema, & pruritis.

COLACE. (Mead Johnson) Docusate sodium. **Cap.** (50 mg. or 100 mg.) Bot. 30s, 60s, 250s, 1000s. Single unit pack 10s, (100 mg. only), 100s. **Liq.** 1%, Bot. 30 cc., pt. Syr. (20 mg./5 cc.) Bot. 8 oz., 1 pt.
Use: Orally, fecal softener.

W/Casanthrol.
See: Peri-Colace, Cap., Syr. (Mead Johnson)

COLAGYN. (Smith) Zinc sulfocarbolate, pot, oxyquinoline sulfate, lactic acid and boric acid, Jelly. Tube w/applicator & refill 6 oz. Douche Pow. 3 oz., 7 oz., 14 oz.
Use: Contraceptive.

COLANA SYRUP. (Hance) Tinct. euphorbia pilulifera 8 cc., syr. wild lettuce 8 cc., tinct. cocillana 2.5 cc., syr. squill cmpd. 1.5 cc., cascara 0.25 Gm., menthol 4.8 mg./fl. oz. Bot. 4 fl. oz., gal. Also w. Dionin 15 mg./fl. oz. Bot. gal.
Use: Cough preparation.

COLASPASE B.A.N. L-Asparagine amidohydrolase obtained from cultures of Escherichia coli.
See: Crasnitin

COLBENEMID. (Merck Sharp & Dohme) Probenecid 0.5 Gm., colchicine 0.5 mg./Tab. Bot. 100s.
Use: Uricosuric for chronic gouty arthritis.

COLBENI-MOR. (H.L. Moore) Probenecid 0.5 mg./Tab. Bot. 100s, 1000s.
Use: Chronic gouty arthritis.

COLCHICINE, U.S.P. XXI. Tab., Inj. U.S.P. XXI.
Acetamide, N-(5,6,7,9-tetrahydro-1,2,3,10-tetrame-thoxy-9-oxobenzo[a]heptalen-7-yl)-.
(Various Mfr.)
Use: Gout suppressant.
W/Benemid.
  See: Colbenemid, Tab. (Merck Sharp & Dohme)
W/Methyl salicylate. (Parke-Davis) Colchicine 1/250 gr.,
methyl salicylate 3 min./Cap. Bot. 100s, 500s,
1000s.
  Use: Orally, gout therapy.
W/Probenecid
  See: Benn-C, Tab. (Scrip)
    Colbenemid, Tab. (Merck Sharp & Dohme)
    Robenecid with colchicine, Tab. (Robinson)
W/Sod. salicylate.
  See: Salcoce, Tab. (Cole)
W/Sod. salicylate, calcium carbonate, dried aluminum
hydroxide gel, phenobarbital.
  See: Apcogesic, Tabs. (Apco)
W/Sod. salicylate & pot. iodide.
  See: Bricolide, Tab. (Briar)
    Colsalide, Tab. (Vortech)
COLCHICINE SALICYLATE.
W/Phenobarbital, Sod. p-aminobenzoate, Vit. B-1 & as-
pirin.
  See: Doloral, Tab. (Alamed)
COLD-CAPS TIMED RELEASE. (Stayner) Replaces
Super-Polyhist Cold Capsules. Pack of 12.
• **COLD CREAM,** U.S.P. XXI.
  Use: Emollient; water-in-oil emulsion ointment base.
COLD CREAM FOR COMPOUNDING
PRESCRIPTIONS. (Lilly) Ointment (Not U.S.P.) Bot.
16 oz.
COL-DECON. (Columbia) Chlorpheniramine maleate 5
mg., phenylephrine HCl 10 mg., phenylpropanola-
mine HCl 40 mg., phenyltoloxamine citrate 15
mg./Tab. Bot. 100s, 1000s.
  Use: Decongestant.
COLDONYL. (Dover) Acetaminophen, phenylephrine
HCl 5 mg., atropine sulfate 0.08 mg./Tab. Sugar
and salt free.
  Use: Antihistiminic and decongestant for cold &
allergy relief.
COLDRAN. (Blue Cross) Phenelephrine HCl 5 mg.,
chlorpheniramine maleate 2 mg., salisylamide
1½ gr., acetaminophen ½ gr., caffeine/ Tab.
Bot. 30s.
  Use: Colds, allergies, sinus congestion.
COLDRINE. (Mallard) Acetaminophen 200 mg.,
pseudoephedrine HCl 30 mg./Tab. Bot. 1000s.
Sani-Pak 1000s.
  Use: Analgesic, decongestant.
COLD SORE LOTION. (DeWitt) Camphor 3.7%, Tr.
benzoin 4.1%, phenol 0.3%, menthol 0.3%
w/alcohol 90%. Bot. 0.5 oz.
  Use: Cold sore, fever blister and cracked lip
relief.
COLD SORE LOTION. (Purepac) Camphor, benzoin,
aluminum chloride. Bot. 0.5 oz.
  Use: Astringent, analgesic, protectant for cold
sores and fever blisters.

COLD TABLETS. (Walgreen) Phenylephrine HCl 5
mg., chlorpheniramine maleate 2 mg., aspirin 325
mg., caffeine 16.2 mg./Tab.
Bot. 50s.
  Use: Decongestant, antihistamine, analgesic.
COLD TABLETS MULTIPLE SYMPTOM. (Walgreen)
Acetaminophen 325 mg., phenylpropanolamine HCl
12.5 mg., chlorpheniramine maleate 1 mg.,
dextromethorphan HBr 10 mg./Tab. Bot. 50s.
  Use: Symptomatic relief of colds;
decongestant.
COLD VACCINES, ORAL. Sherman—Oral Tabs.
  See: Entoral, Pulvule (Lilly)
COLESTID. (Upjohn) Colestipol HCl 5 Gm./pkt. Box
30s, Bot. 500 Gm.
  Use: Adjunctive therapy to diet for reduction of
elevated serum cholesterol in hypercholesterolemic
patients.
• **COLESTIPOL HYDROCHLORIDE.** USAN.
  Use: Antihyperlipoproteinemic.
COL-EVAC. (Fellows) Pot. bitartrate, bicarbonate of
soda and a blended base of polyethylene glycols.
Supps. 2s, 12s.
COLEXUSS. (Jenkins) White pine 56.7 mg., wild
cherry 56.7 mg., American spikenard 6 mg., poplar
bud 6 mg., sanguinaria 5 mg., menthol 0.5 mg./fldr.
Bot. 3 oz., 4 oz., gal.
  Use: Cough syrup.
COLFANT. (Jenkins) Paregoric 2 min. (pow. opium
1/125 gr.), sod. bicarbonate 1 gr., Mg trisilicate 5/8 gr.,
ext. catnip 1/50 gr., ext. chamomile 1/100 gr.
(Matricaria), oil fennel q.s./Tab. Bot. 1000s.
  Use: Antacid, analgesic.
COLICELL. (Sutliff & Case) Whole bile ext. 227 mg.,
ketocholanic acids 97 mg., methyl cellulose 130
mg., homatropine methylbromide 2.5 mg./Tab. Bot.
100s, 1000s.
  Use: Laxative w/antispasmatic.
COLIMYCIN SODIUM METHANESULFONATE.
(Parke-Davis)
  See: Colistimethate Sod.
COLIMYCIN SULFATE. (Parke-Davis)
  See: Coly-Mycin, Preps. (Parke-Davis)
• **COLISTIMETHATE SODIUM, STERILE,** U.S.P. XXI.
  Sod. Colistin Methanesulfonate.
  Colistinmethanesulfonic acid, pentasodium salt.
  Pentasodium colistinmethanesulfonate.
  Use: Antibiotic.
  See: Coly-Mycin-M, Injectable (Parke-Davis)
COLISTIN. B.A.N. A mixture of polypeptides produced
by strains of Bacillus polymyxa var. colistinus.
  Use: Antibiotic.
  See: Colomycin sulfate
COLISTIN BASE.
W/Neomycin base, hydrocortisone acetate,
thonzonium bromide, polysorbate 80, acetic acid,
sodium acetate.
  See: Coly-Mycin Otic W/Neomycin and Hydrocorti-
sone, Liq. (Parke-Davis)
COLISTIN AND NEOMYCIN SULFATES AND
HYDROCORTISONE ACETATE OTIC
SUSPENSION, U.S.P. XXI.

Use: Antibiotic, anti-inflammatory.

COLISTIN METHANESULFONATE.
See: Colistimethate Sodium

• **COLISTIN SULFATE,** U.S.P. XXI. Oral Susp., U.S.P. XXI. The sulfate salt of an antibiotic substance elaborated by Aerobacillus colistinus.
Use: Antibacterial.
See: Colymycin-S Ophthalmic (Softcon)
Coly-Mycin S Susp. (Parke-Davis)

COLISTIN SULFOMETHATE. B.A.N. An antibiotic obtained from colistin sulfate by sulfomethylation with formaldehyde and sodium bisulfite.

COLITUSSIN. (Dalin) Bot. 4 oz. Pediatric. Bot. 4 oz.

CO-LIVER. (Standex) Folic acid 1 mg., Vit. B-12 100 mcg., liver 10 mcg./cc. Vial 10 cc.

COLLADERM. (C & M Pharmacal) Purified water, glycerin, soluble collagen, hydrolysed elastin, allantoin, ethylhydroxycellulose, sorbic, octoxynol-9. Bot. 2.3 oz.
Use: Moisturizer & protein replenisher for dry & aging skin.

COLLAGENASE.
See: Santyl (Knoll)

COLLAGENASE ABC OINTMENT. (Advance Biofactures) Collagenase 250 u./Gm. in white petrolatum. 25 Gm., 50 Gm.
Use: Debridement of dermal ulcers and burned areas.

• **COLLODION,** U.S.P. XXI. Flexible, U.S.P. XXI.
Use: Topical protectant.

COLLOIDAL ALUMINUM HYDROXIDE.
See: Aluminum Hydroxide Gel, U.S.P. XXI.

COLLOIDAL GOLD.
See: Aureotope (Squibb)

COLLOIDAL SILVER IODIDE.
See: Neo-Silvol, Sol. (Parke-Davis)

COLLYRIUM. (Wyeth) Neutral borate sol. with boric acid, sodium borate, thimerosal 0.002% and water. Bot. 6 fl. oz. with eyecup.
Use: Eye lotion.

COLLYRIUM, WITH EPHEDRINE. (Wyeth) Neutral isotonic sol. of boric-acid & borax, containing 0.4% antipyrine & 0.1% ephedrine, thimerosal 0.002%. Bot. 0.5 fl. oz. w/dropper.
Use: Eye lotion.

COLOCTYL. (Vitarine) Docusate sodium 100 mg./Cap. Bot. 100s, 1000s. Unit dose 1000s.
Use: Stool softener.

COLOGEL. (Lilly) Methylcellulose 9 Gm./100 ml. w/alcohol 5% Bot. 16 fl. oz.
Use: Constipation.

COLODNYL. (Dover) Acetaminophen, phenylephrine HCl atropine sulfate/Tab. Unit dose boxes 500s.
Use: Antihistamine-free remedy for colds, hay fever, sinusitis.

COLREX. (Rowell) Chlorpheniramine maleate 2 mg., phenylephrine HCl 5 mg., acetaminophen 325 mg./Cap. Bot. 24s, 100s.

COLREX COMPOUND. (Rowell) Codeine phosphate 16 mg., acetaminophen 325 mg., phenylephrine

HCl 10 mg., chlorpheniramine maleate 2 mg./Cap. Bot. 100s, 1000s.
Use: Relief of symptoms from common cold.

COLREX COMPOUND ELIXIR. (Rowell) Codeine phosphate 8 mg., acetaminophen 120 mg., chlorpheniramine maleate 1 mg., phenylephrine HCl 5 mg./5 ml. Alcohol 9.5%. Sugar free elixer. Bot. 60 ml., 480 ml., gal.
Use: Relief of cough, congestion.

COLREX DECONGESTANT. (Rowell) Chlorpheniramine maleate 4 mg., tripelennamine HCl 50 mg., phenylpropanolamine HCl 25 mg., phenylephrine HCl 10 mg./Tab. Bot. 100s.
Use: Decongestant.

COLREX EXPECTORANT. (Rowell) Guaifenesin 100 mg./5 cc. w/alcohol 4.7%. Bot. 120 ml., 480 ml. Sugar free base
Use: Bronchial secretions.

COLREX SYRUP. (Rowell) Dextromethorphan HBr 10 mg., phenylephrine HCl 5 mg., chlorpheniramine maleate 2 mg./5 cc. w/alcohol 4.5% Bot. Sugar free base. 120 ml.
Use: Relief of cough.

COLREX TROCHES. (Rowell) Benzocaine 10 mg., cetylpyridinium chloride 2.5 mg./Troche. 20s.
Use: Relief of sore throat due to the common cold.

COLSALIDE. (Vortech) Colchicine 0.65 mg./Tab. Bot. 1000s.
Use: Gout & gouty arthritis & neuritis.

COLSPAN. (Zenith) Chlorpheniramine maleate 1 mg., phenylpropanolamine HCl 50 mg., belladonna alkaloids 0.16 mg., pheniramine maleate 12.5 mg./Cap. Bot. 10s, 100s.

• **COLTEROL MESYLATE.** USAN.
Use: Bronchodilator.

COLY-MYCIN M PARENTERAL. (Parke-Davis) Colistimethate sodium equivalent 150 mg. colistin base per vial.
Use: Urinary tract infections.

COLY-MYCIN S OTIC DROPS W/NEOMYCIN AND HYDROCORTISONE. (Parke-Davis) Colistin base as the sulfate 3 mg., neoymycin base as the sulfate 3.3 mg., hydrocortisone acetate 10 mg., thonzonium bromide, polysorbate 80, acetic acid, sodium acetate/cc. 5 ml. w/dropper. 10 ml. Bot. 5 cc.
Use: Acute and chronic external otitis.

COLY-MYCIN S. (Parke-Davis) Colistin sulfate 300 mg./60 ml. For oral susp. Bot. 300 mg.
Use: Acute bacterial diarrhea.

COMBICAL D. (Mills) Calcium 375 mg., Vit. D 400 I.U., phosphorus 180 mg., magnesium 144 mg./3 Tab. Bot. 1000s.
Use: Vitamin, nutrition therapy.

COMBICHOLE. (Trout) Dehydrocholic acid 2 gr., desoxycholic acid 1 gr./Tab. Bot. 100s, 1000s.
Use: Stimulate bile flow.

COMBID. (SmithKline) 'Darbid' (isopropamide) as the iodide 5 mg., 'Compazine' (prochlorperazine) as the maleate 10 mg./Spansule. Bot. 50s, 500s. Unit pkg. 100s.

Use: Gastro-intestinal disorders.

COMBIPRES TABLETS. (Boehringer Ingelheim) Clonidine HCl 0.1 or 0.2 mg., chlorthalidone 15 mg./Tab. Bot. 100s, 1000s.
Use: Antihypertensive.

COMBISTIX. (Ames) Protein test-tetrabromphenol blue, citrate buffer, protein-absorbing agent; glucose test area-glucose oxidase, orthotolidin and a catalyst; pH test area methyl red and bromthymol blue. Box, strips, 100s.
Use: Diagnostic agent. Proteinuria, glucosuria, pH.

COMFORT DROPS. (Barnes-Hind) A nonionic cleaning and wetting system in a mildly alkaline, isotonic vehicle preserved with disodium edetate 0.02% and benzalkonium chloride 0.005%. Plastic dropper bot. 15 ml.
Use: Cushion, rewet, & clean hard contact lenses while they are being worn.

COMFORT FORMULA. (Ex-Lax) Docusate sodium 100 mg./Tab. Pkg. 30s.
Use: Stool softener.

COMFORT GEL LIQUID. (Walgreen) Aluminum hydroxide compressed gel 200 mg., hydro-magma paste 200 mg., simethicone 25 mg./5 ml. Bot. 12 oz.
Use: Antacid-antiflatulent.

COMFORT GEL TABLETS. (Walgreen) Magnesium hydroxide 85 mg., simethicone 25 mg., aluminum hydroxide-magnesium carbonate codried gel 282 mg./Tab. Bot. 100s.
Use: Antacid-antiflatulent.

COMFORTINE. (Dermik) Zinc oxide 12%, Vit. A & D, lanolin in protective base. Oint. Tube 1½ oz. 4 oz.
Use: Antiseptic & protective ointment.

COMHIST LIQUID. (Norwich Eaton) Chlorpheniramine maleate 2 mg., phenylephrine HCl 5 mg./5 cc. Bot. pt.
Use: Relief of allergies and congestion.

COMHIST L.A. CAPSULES. (Norwich Eaton) Phenylephrine HCl 20 mg., chlorpheniramine maleate 4 mg., phenyltoloxamine citrate 50 mg./Cap. Bot. 100s.
Use: Relief of allergies and congestion.

COMHIST TABLETS. (Norwich Eaton) Phenylephrine HCl 10 mg., chlorpheniramine maleate 2 mg., phenyltoloxamine citrate 25 mg./Tab. Bot. 100s.
Use: For the relief of allergies and congestion.

COMPAL. (Reid-Provident) Dihydrocodeine 16 mg., promethazine HCl 6.25 mg., acetaminophen 356.4 mg., Caffeine 30 mg./Cap. Bot. 100s.
Use: Analgesic.

COMPAZINE. (SmithKline) Prochlorperazine as the maleate. **Tab.:** 5 mg., 10 mg., 25 mg., Bot. 100s, 1000s. Unit dose 100s. **Inj.,** Edisylate salt 2 ml. (5 mg./ml.) Boxes 10s, 100s, 500s. Multiple-dose vials-Edisylate salt 10 ml. (5 mg./ml.) 1s, 20s, 100s.; Disposable Syringe 5 mg./ml. Syringe 2 ml. Box 10s, 100s. **Spansule** Maleate Salt 10 mg., 15 mg., 30 mg., Bot. 50s, 500s. Unit dose 100s. **Supp.:** 2.5 mg., 5 mg., 25 mg., Box 12s. **Syrup:** Edisylate salt 5 mg./5 ml. Bot. 4 fl. oz.

Use: Treatment of mental & emotional disturbances; also nausea & vomiting.

COMPLEAT-B. (Doyle) Deionized water, beef puree, hydrolyzed cereal solids, green bean puree, pea puree, nonfat milk, corn oil, maltodextrin, peach puree, orange juice, mono & diglycerides, carrageenan, vitamins & minerals. Bot. 250 ml. Cans 250 ml.
Use: Tube feeding.

COMPLEAT-MODIFIED FORMULA. (Doyle) Deionized water, hydrolyzed cereal solids, beef puree, pea puree, green bean puree, corn oil, peach puree, mono and diglycerides, orange juice, carrageenan, vitamins & minerals. Cans 250 ml.
Use: Lactose free, low sodium, isotonic blenderized tube feeding.

COMPLETONE ELIXIR FORT. (Winthrop Products) Ferrous gluconate.
Use: Hematinic.

COMPLEX 15 CREAM. (Baker/Cummins) Bot. 4 oz.
Use: Moisturizing cream.

COMPLEX 15 LOTION. (Baker/Cummins) Bot. 8 oz.
Use: Moisturizing lotion.

COMPOUND 42.
See: Warfarin (Various Mfr.)

COMPOUND B.
See: Corticosterone (Various Mfr.)

COMPOUND CB3025.
See: Alkeran, Tabs. (Burroughs Wellcome)

COMPOUND E. (Kendall)
See: Cortisone Acetate. (Various Mfr.)

COMPOUND F.
See: Hydrocortisone (Various Mfr.)

COMPOUND W. (Whitehall) Salicylic acid 17% w/w in flexible collodion vehicle W/ether 63.5%. Bot. 0.31 oz.
Use: Wart remover.

COMPOZ. (Jeffrey Martin) Diphenhydramine HCl 50 mg./Tab. Ctn. 24s.
Use: Night-time sleep aid.

COMPRELETS. (Columbia) Vit. A 10,000 I.U., B-1 25 mg., B-2 12 mg., B-3 75 mg., B-5 3 mg., B-6 1.2 mg., B-12 mcg., C 150 mg., D 400 I.U., E 3.3 I.U., biotin 2 mcg., Ca 40 mg., iron 3 mg., K 0.5 mg., Cu 1.25 mcg., Mn 1.0 mg., Mg 0.8 mg., Zn 1.25 mg., & amino acid factors/Tab. Bot. 100s, 1000s.
Use: Vitamin, mineral, amino acid therapy.

COM-PRO-SPAN. (Columbia) Prochlorperazine 10 mg., isopropamide 5 mg./Cap. Bot. 100s, 500s.
Use: Gasto-intestinal disorders.

COMTREX CAPSULES MULTI-SYMPTOM COLD RELIEVER. (Bristol-Myers) Acetaminophen 325 mg., phenylpropanolamine HCl 12.5 mg., chlorpheniramine maleate 1.0 mg., dextromethorphan HBr 10 mg./Cap. Bot. 16s, 36s.
Use: Analgesic, decongestant, antihistamine, cough reliever.

COMTREX LIQUID MULTI-SYMPTOM COLD RELIEVER. (Bristol-Myers) Acetaminiophen 650 mg.,

phenylpropanolamine HCl 25 mg., chlorpheniramine maleate 2 mg., dextromethorphan HBr 20 mg./30 ml. w/alcohol 20%. Bot. 6 oz., 10 oz.
Use: Analgesic, decongestant, antihistamine, cough reliever.

COMTREX NIGHTIME. (Bristol-Myers) Acetaminophen 1000 mg., pseudoephedrine HCl 60 mg., chlorpheniramine maleate 4 mg., dextromethorphan HBr 30 mg./30 ml. w/alcohol 25%. Bot. 6 oz., 10 oz.
Use: Analgesic, decongestant, antihistamine, cough reliever.

COMTREX TABLETS MULTI-SYMPTOM COLD RELIEVER. (Bristol-Myers) Acetaminophen 325 mg., phenylpropanolamine HCl 12.5 mg., chlorphemiramine maleate 1.0 mg., dextromethorphan HBr 10 mg./Tab. w/F D and C Yellow #5. Bot. 24s, 50s, 100s.
Use: Analgesic, decongestant antihistamine, cough reliever.

CONACETOL. (CMC) Acetaminophen 5 gr./Tab. **Tabs.** Bot. 50s, 100s, 1000s. **Elix:** 120 mg., Bot. pt., gal.
Use: Analgesic antipyretic.

CONACETON ELIXIR. (CMC) Acetaminophen elixir.
Use: Analgesic.

CONALSYN. (Cenci) Chlorpheniramine maleate 8 mg., phenylephrine HCl 20 mg., methscopolamine nitrate 2.5 mg./T.R. Cap. Bot. 30s, 250s, 500s.
Use: Hay fever and similar allergies.

CONAR. (Beecham Labs) Noscapine 15 mg., phenylephrine HCl 10 mg./5 ml. Bot. pt.

CONAR-A SUSPENSION. (Beecham Labs) Noscapine 7.5 mg., phenylephrine HCl 5.0 mg., acetaminophen 150.0 mg., guaifenesin 50.0 mg./cc. Bot. pt.

CONAR-A TAB. (Beecham Labs) Noscapine 15 mg., phenylephrine HCl 10 mg., acetaminophen 300 mg., guaifenesin 100 mg./Tab. Bot. 100s. Unit dose 20s.

CONAR EXPECTORANT. (Beecham Labs) Noscapine 15 mg., phenylephrine HCl 10 mg., guaifenesin 100 mg.,/5 cc. Bot. 4 oz. in 12s, pt.

CONCENTRATED OLEOVITAMIN A & D. See: Oleovitamin A & D, Concentrated, Cap. (Various Mfr.)

CONCENTRATED TUBERCULIN.

CONCEPTROL CONTRACEPTIVE GEL. (Ortho) Nonoxynol-9 in 4% concentration. Tube 70 Gm. w/applicator.
Use: Contraceptive jelly.

CONCEPTROL CREAM. (Ortho) Nonoxynol-9 5%, in an oil-in-water emulsion at pH 4.5. Tube 70 Gm. with applicator.
Use: Contraceptive cream.

CONCEPTROL DISPOSABLE CONTRACEPTIVE GEL. (Ortho) Nonoxynol-9 in 4% concentration. Pkg. 6 or 10 disposable applicators.
Use: Contraceptive jelly.

CONDOL SUSPENSION. (Winthrop Products) Dipyrone, chlormezanone.
Use: Analgesic, muscle relaxant.

CONDOL TABLETS. (Winthrop Products) Dipyrone, Chlormezanone.
Use: Analgesic, muscle relaxant.

CONEST. (Grafton) Conjugated estrogens 0.625 mg., 1.25 mg., or 2.5 mg./Tab. Bot. 100s, 1000s.
Use: Female hormone supplement.

CONESTORAL. (Galen) Sodium estrone sulfate 0.625 mg./Tab. Bot. 100s, 1000s.
Use: Treatment of menopausal syndrome, hypogenitalism, functional uterine bleeding.

CONEX-DA. (O'Neal, Jones & Feldman) Phenyl-propanolamine HCl 50 mg., chlorpheniramine maleate 8 mg./Dual action Tab. Bot. 100s, 1000s.
Use: Orally, relief of nasal congestion.

CONEX LOZENGE CT. (O'Neal, Jones & Feldman) Benzocaine 5 mg., methylparaben 2 mg., propylparaben 0.5 mg., cetylpyridinium chloride 0.5 mg./Bot. 1000s.
Use: Topical anesthetic, antibacterial.

CONEX PLUS. (O'Neal, Jones & Feldman) Phenylpropanolamine HCl 12.5 mg., chlorpheniramine maleate 4 mg., acetaminophen 325 mg./Tab. Bot. 100s, 1000s.
Use: Orally, analgesic and relief of nasal congestion.

CONEX SYRUP. (O'Neal, Jones & Feldman) Phenylpropanolamine HCl 12 mg., guaifenesin 100 mg./10 cc. Bot. 4 oz., 1 pt.
Use: Treatment of cough due to colds.

CONEX WITH CODEINE. (O'Neal, Jones & Feldman) Codeine phate 10 mg., guaifenesin 100 mg., phenylpropanolamine HCl 12.5 mg./5 ml. Bot. 4 oz.

CONFIDENT. (Block) Carboxymethylcellulose gum, ethylene oxide polymer, petrolatum/mineral oil base. Tube 0.7 oz., 1.4 oz., 2.4 oz.
Use: Denture adhesive cream.

CONGESPIRIN COUGH SYRUP. (Bristol-Myers) Dextromethorphan hydrobromide 5 mg./5 ml. Bot. 3 oz.
Use: Children's antitussive.

CONGESPIRIN FOR CHILDREN, ASPIRIN FREE. (Bristol-Myers) Acetaminophen 81 mg., phenyleph-rine HCl 1.25 mg./Tab. Bot. 24s.
Use: Analgesic, nasal decongestant, antipyretic.

CONGESPIRIN LIQUID COLD MEDICINE. (Bristol-Myers) Acetaminophen 130 mg., phenylpropanolamine HCl 6.25 mg., alcohol 10%/5 ml. Bot. 3 oz.
Use: Children's analgesic, decongestant.

CONGESPIRIN TABLETS. (Bristol-Myers) Aspirin 81 mg., phenylephrine HCl 1.25 mg./Tab. Bot. 36s.
Use: Children's analgesic decongestant.

CONGEST-AFED DM SYRUP. (Eckerd) Pseudoephe-drine HCl 30 mg., guaifenesin 150 mg., dextromethorphan HBr 10 mg./ 5 ml. w/alcohol 20%. Bot. 4 oz.
Use: Decongestant, expectorant, antitussive.

CONGESTERONE. (Kenyon) Conjugated estrogens 0.625 mg., 1.25 mg., or 2.5 mg./tab. Bot. 100s.

CONGO RED. Injection.
Use: Hemostatic in hemorrhagic disorders.

CONGESS. (Fleming) **Sr.:** Guaifenesin 250 mg., pseudoephedrine HCl 120 mg./Cap. **Jr.:**

Guaifenesin 125 mg., pseudoephedrine HCl 60 mg./Cap. Bot. 100s, 1000s.
Use: Expectorant/bronchodilator.

CO-NIB OINTMENT. (Guild) ¼ oz.

CONJEC. (Mallard) Atropine sulfate 0.2 mg., chlorpheniramine maleate 5 mg./cc. Vial 10 ml.

CONJUGATED ESTROGENS.
See: Estrogens, Conjugated (Various Mfr.)

CONJUGENS. (Coastal) Conjugated estrogens 1.25 mg./Tab. Bot. 100s.

CONJUTABS. (Rand) Conjutabs 62: estrogens, 0.625 mg./Tab. Conjutabs 125: estrogens, 1.25 mg./Tab. Conjutabs 250: estrogens, 2.50 mg./Tab. (Enteric coated) Bot. 100s, 500s.
Use: Estrogen therapy and supplementation.

CONMEN. (Winthrop Products) Dipyrone as drops, syrup, suppositories (adult and child strength), injection and tablets.
Use: Analgesic, antipyretic, anti-inflammatory.

CONRAY. (Mallinckrodt) lothalamate meglumine Inj. 60%. Vials 20, 30, 50 ml. Pkg. 25s, 50s, 100s; 100 ml. Pkg. 6s.
Use: Radiopaque medium.

CONRAY-30. (Mallinckrodt) lothalamate meglumine Inj. 30%. Bot. 300 ml. Pkg. 6s.
Use: Radiopaque medium.

CONRAY-400. (Mallinckrodt) lothalamate sodium inj. 66.8%. Vial 25 ml., 50 ml. Pkg. 25s, 50s, 100s.
Use: Radiopaque medium.

CONSIN COUMOUND SALVE. (Wisconsin) Carbolic acid ointment. Jar 2 oz., 1 lb.
Use: Minor cuts, burns, skin irritations.

CONSIN WHITE IODINE. (Wisconsin) Decolorized iodine Bot. ½ oz, 16 oz.
Use: Antiseptic, nail hardner.

CONSOTUSS ANTITUSSIVE SYRUP. (Merrell Dow) Dextromethorphan HBr 15 mg., doxylamine succinate 3.75 mg./5 ml. w/alcohol 10%. Bot. 6 oz.
Use: Antitussive, antihistaminic.

CONSTAB-100. (Kenyon) Docusate sodium 100 mg./Tab. Bot. 100s, 1000s.

CONSTANT-T. (Geigy) Theophylline anhydrous 200 mg., or 300 mg./Sus. Rel. Tab. Bot. 100s.
Use: Asthma and reversible bronchospasm.

CONSTIBAN. (Columbia) Casanthranol 30 mg., docusate sodium 100 mg./Cap. Bot. 30s, 100s, 1000s.
Use: Constipation.

CONSTONATE 60. Docusate sodium 100 mg., 250 mg./Cap. Bot. 100s, 1000s.
Use: Fecal softener.

CONTAC. (Menley & James) Phenylpropanolamine HCl 75 mg.; chlorpheniramine maleate 8 mg./Continuous action capsule. Pkg. 10s, 20s, 30s, 40s.
Use: Treatment of nasal congestion due to common cold, hay fever and sinusitis.

CONTAC JR. (Menley & James)
Phenylpropanolamine HCl 9.375 mg., acetaminophen 162.5 mg., dextromethorphan HBr 5.0 mg./5cc w/alcohol 10%. Bot. 4 oz.
Use: Congestion, aches, fever & cough due to colds.

CONTAC SEVERE COLD FORMULA. (Menley & James) Pseudoephedrine HCl 30 mg., acetaminophen 500 mg., dextromethorphan HBr. 15 mg., chlorpheniramine maleate 2 mg./Cap. Bot. 10s, 20s.
Use: Colds with flu-like symptoms.

CONTACTISOL. (CooperVision) Sterile buffered isotonic soln. preserved with benzalkonium chloride 0.01%, edetate disodium 0.01%. Bot. 1.9 oz.
Use: Cleaning and wetting solution for hard contact lenses.

CONTIQUE. (Alcon) Artificial Tears w/polyvinyl alcohol 2%, benzalkonium chloride & salts. ½ oz.
Wetting Solution 2 oz.
Soaking Solution 4 oz.
Cleaning Solution 1 oz.
Flow-Thru Contact Lens Case
Swirl Clean Hard Lens Cleaner

■ **CONTRACEPTIVES.**
See: Oral Contraceptives (Var. Mfr.)
Foams, Vaginal.
See: Delfen, Vaginal Foam (Ortho Pharm.)
Emko, Vaginal Foam (Emko)
Jellies & Creams, Vaginal.
See: Colagyn, Jel (Smith)
Colagyn, Jel (Smith)
Conceptrol, Cream, Gel (Ortho)
Gynol II, Gel (Ortho)
Immolin, Cream-Jel (Schmid)
Koromex-A, Jelly (Holland-Rantos)
Koromex, Cream or Jelly (Holland-Rantos)
Ortho-Creme (Ortho)
Ortho-Gynol, Jelly (Ortho)
Suppositories, Vaginal.
See: Intercept, Inserts (Ortho)
Lorophyn, Supp., Jelly (Eaton)

CONTRAPAR. (Wellcome; Gloxazone. (B.A.N.)

CONTROLYTE. (Doyle) Polysaccharides obtained by deionization of a partial hydrolysate of corn starch, partially hydrogenated soybean oil with BHA, hydroxylated lecithin and polyglycerol esters of fatty acids. Powder. Cans, 14 oz.
Use: Calorie supplement.

CONVERSPAZ. (Ascher) Cellulase 5 mg., protease 10 mg., amylase 30 mg., lipase 13 mg., l-hyoscyamine sulfate 0.0625 mg./Cap. Bot. 100s.
Use: To aid digestion of food.

CONVERZYME CAPS. (Ascher) Cellulase 5 mg., protease 10 mg., amylase 30 mg., lipase 13 mg./Cap. Bot. 100s.
Use: Aid for digestion of food.

COOPERVISION BALANCED SALT SOLUTION.
(CooperVision) Sterile intraocular irrigation sol. Bot. 15 ml., 500 ml.
Use: Intraocular irrigating solution during intraocular surgical procedures.

COPAVIN. (Lilly) Caps. Bot. 100s.

COPE. (Glenbrook) Aspirin 421.2 mg., magnesium hydroxide 50 mg., dried aluminum hydroxide gel 25

mg., caffeine 32 mg./Tab. Bot. 15s, 36s, 60s.
Use: Tension headaches, muscular aches, neuritic pain, fevers.

COPENE. (Kenyon) Chlorphentermine HCl 65 mg./Tab. Bot. 100s.

COPHENE #2. (Dunhall) Chlorpheniramine maleate 12 mg., phenylpropanolamine HCl 50 mg., phenylephrine HCl 25 mg./Time Cap. Bot. 100s, 500s.
Use: Decongestant, antihistaminic.

COPHENE INJECTABLE. (Dunhall) Atropine sulf. 0.2 mg., phenylpropanolamine HCl 12.5 mg., chlorpheniramine maleate 5 mg./ml. Pkg. 10 ml.
Use: Decongestant, antihistaminic.

COPHENE-PL. (Dunhall) Phenylephrine HCl 20 mg., phenylpropanolamine HCl 20 mg., chlorpheniramine maleate 5 mg./5 cc. Bot. 16 oz.
Use: Cough due to colds and allergy.

COPHENE-S. (Dunhall) Dihydrocodone bitartrate 3 mg., phenylephrine HCl 20 mg., phenylpropanolamine HCl 20 mg., chlorpheniramine maleate 5 mg./5 cc. Bot. pt.
Use: Antitussive.

COPHENE-X. (Dunhall) Carbetapentane citrate 20 mg., phenylephrine HCl 10 mg., phenylpropanolamine HCl 20 mg., chlorpheniramine maleate 2.5 mg., potassium guaiacolsulfonate 45 mg./Cap. Bot. 100s, 500s.
Use: Antihistamine, decongestant, expectorant, antitussive.

COPHENE-XP SYRUP. (Dunhall) Carbetapentane citrate 20 mg., phenylephrine HCl 10 mg., phenylpropanolamine HCl 20 mg., chlorpheniramine maleate 2.5 mg. potassium guaiacolsulfonate 45 mg./5 ml. Bot. pt.
Use: Antihistamine, decongestant, antitussive.

COPPERHEAD BITE THERAPY.
See: Antivenin, Snake Polyvalent Inj. (Wyeth)

COPPERIN. (Vernon) Iron ammonium citrate w/copper (6 gr.). "A" adult dose, "B" children dose. Bot. 30s, 100s, 500s.
Use: Treatment of secondary anemias.

COPPERTONE. (Plough) A series of products marketed under the coppertone name including: Dark Tanning Butter, (SPF 2), Dark Tanning Oil, (SPF 2), For Faces Only (SPF 2, 4, 6, 15), Lite Formula Oil (SPF 2), Lite Lotion (SPF 4), Noskote, (SPF 8), QT Quick Tanning Lotion, (SPF 2), Shade Sunscreen Lotion, (SPF 6), Shade Plus, Sudden Tan, Suntan Lotion, (SPF 4), Super Shade Sunblocking Lotion, (SPF 15), Tan Care, Sunger Products and Tropical Blend Products. Most contain one or more of the following ingredients in various oil and lotion bases: homosalate, oxybenzone, padimate O.
Use: Ultraviolet sunscreen.

COPPERTONE NOSKOTE. (Plough) Homosalate 7% and Oxybenzone 3% sunscreen ointment. (SPF 8). Jar. 1 oz. Tube 7/16 oz.
Use: Ultraviolet sunscreen.

COPPERTRACE. (Armour) Cupric chloride injection containing copper 0.4 mg./ml. Vial 10 ml. Box 25s.
Use: Supplement to I.V. solutions for copper deficiency.

COPPER UNDECYLENATE.
W/Sod. propionate, Sod. caprylate, propionic acid, undecylenic acid, salicylic acid.

COPROBATE. (Coastal) Meprobamate 400 mg./Tab. Bot. 100s, 1000s.
Use: Muscle relaxant and tranquilizer.

CO-PYRONIL 2. (Dista) Chlorpheniramine maleate 4 mg., pseudoephedrine HCl 60 mg./Pulvule. Bot. 100s, 1000s.
Use: Allergic symptoms, antihistaminic.

CO-PYRONIL 2 PEDIATRIC. (Dista) Chlorpheniramine maleate 2 mg., pseudoephedrine HCl 30 mg./Pulvule. Bot. 100s. Liquid 16 fl. oz.
Use: Allergic symptoms, antihistaminic.

CORAB. (Abbott) Test kit 100s.
Use: Radioimmunoassay for detection of antibody to hepatitis B core antigen.

CORACE INJECTION. (Fellows) Cortisone acetate 50 mg./cc. Vial 10 cc.

CORAL. (Lorvic) Fluroide ion 1.23%, 0.1 molar phosphate. Jar 250 Gm., Coral II: 180 disposable cup units/carton.
Use: Phosphate/fluoride prophylaxis paste.

CORAL/PLUS. (Lorvic) Free fluoride ion 2.2%, recrystallized kaolinite. Tube 250 Gm.

CORALSONE MODIFIED. (Zemmer) Aspirin 300 mg., ascorbic acid 50 mg., aluminum hydroxide 35 mg./Tab. Bot. 100s, 1000s.

CORAMINE. (Ciba) Nikethamide, Liq. 25%. Bot. 3 oz. Amp. 25% 1½ cc. Pkg. 20s.
Use: Respiratory stimulant.

CORANE CAPSULES. (Fellows) Pyrilamine maleate 25 mg., pheniramine maleate 10 mg., phenylpropanolamine HCl 25 mg., phenylephrine HCl 10 mg./Cap. Bot. 100s, 500s, 1000s.

CORBICIN-125. (Arthrins) Vit. C 125 mg./Cap. Bot. 100s.
Use: Vitamin C supplement.

CORDRAN LOTION. (Dista) Flurandrenolide 0.05% w/cetyl alcohol, benzyl alcohol, stearic acid, glyceryl monostearate, polyoxyl 40 stearate, glycerin, mineral oil, menthol and purified water. Squeeze bot. 15 ml. and 60 ml.
Use: Dermatologic steroid.

CORDRAN OINTMENT. (Dista) Flurandrenolide 0.025%, 0.05%; emulsified petrolatum base/Gm. 0.05% Tube 15 Gm., 30 Gm., 60 Gm. Jar 225 Gm. 0.025%. Tube 30 Gm., 60 Gm. Jar 225 Gm.
Use: Dermatologic steroid.

CORDRAN-N CREAM & OINTMENT. (Dista) Flurandrenolide 0.5 mg.; neomycin sulfate 5 mg./Gm. Tube 15 Gm., 30 Gm., 60 Gm.
Use: Dermatologic steroid.

CORDRAN SP. (Dista) Flurandrenolide 0.025% and 0.05%, in emulsified base w/cetyl alcohol, stearic acid, polyoxyl 40 stearate, mineral oil, propylene glycol, sodium citrate, citric acid, purified water. 0.05%, Tube 15 Gm., 30 Gm., 60 Gm., Jar 225 Gm.; 0.025%, Tube 30 Gm., 60 Gm. Jar 225 Gm.
Use: Dermatologic steroid.

CORDRAN TAPE. (Dista) Flurandrenolide 4 mcg./sq. cm. Roll 7.5 cm. × 60 cm., 7.5 cm. × 200 cm.

CORDROL. (Vita Elixir) Prednisolone 5 mg. or 20 mg./Tab. Bot. 100s
Use: Treatment of inflammatory conditions.

COREGA POWDER. (Block) Denture adhesive containing polyethyleneoxide polymer w/peppermint oil, karaya gum. Pkg.: pocket 0.7 oz.; medium 1.15 oz.; economy 3.55 oz.
Use: Denture adhesive powder.

CORGARD. (Squibb) Nadolol 40 mg., 80 mg., 120 mg. or 160 mg./Tab. Bot 100s, 1000s. Unit Dose 100s.
Use: Antihypertensive and antiangina beta-blocker.

CORGONJECT-5. (Mayrand) Human chorionic gonadotropin 500 u./ml. Vial 10 ml.

• CORIANDER OIL, N.F. XVI.
Use: Pharm. Aid (flavor).

CORIBAN. Diamphenethide, B.A.N.

CORICIDIN. (Schering) Chlorpheniramine maleate 2 mg., aspirin 325 mg./Tab. Bot. 12s, 24s, 60s, 100s, 1000s. Box 100 x 4 Tab. packets.
Use: Common cold.

CORICIDIN COUGH SYRUP. (Schering) Guaifenesin 100 mg., phenylpropanolamine HCl 12.5 mg., dextromethorphan HBr. 10 mg./5 ml. w/alcohol < 0.5%. Bot. 4 oz.
Use: Antitussive.

CORICIDIN 'D' DECONGESTANT TABLETS. (Schering) Chlorpheniramine maleate 2 mg., aspirin 325 mg., phenylpropanolamine HCl 12.5 mg./Tab. Bot. 12s, 24s, 50s, 100s. Box 100 x 4 Tab packets.
Use: Nasal decongestant & treatment of common cold.

CORICIDIN DEMILETS. (Schering) Aspirin 80 mg. (1¼ gr.), chlorpheniramine maleate 1.0 mg., phenylpropanolamine HCl 6.25 mg./Chewable Tab. Box 24s, 36s.
Use: Decongestant.

CORICIDIN EXTRA STRENGTH SINUS HEADACHE TABLETS. (Schering) Acetaminophen 500 mg., phenylpropanolamine HCl 12.5 mg., chlorpheniramine maleate 2 mg/Tab. Box 24s.
Use: Antihistaminic, decongestant and analgesic.

CORICIDIN MEDILETS. (Schering) Chlorpheniramine maleate 0.5 mg., aspirin 80 mg. (1¼ gr.)/Chewable tab. Box 24s, 36s.
Use: Antihistaminic with analgesic.

CORICIDIN NASAL MIST. (Schering) Phenylephrine HCl 5 mg./ml. Bot. 20 ml.
Use: Decongestant.

CORICO. (Haag) Phenylephrine, chlorpheniramine, analgesics and Vitamin C. Capsules, Bot. 100s, 500, 1000s.
Use: Common cold treatment.

CORID. (MSD AGVET) Amprolium: 20% sol. powder; 9.6% solution, 1.25% crumbles.
Use: Coccidiostat, veterinary medicine.

CORIFORTE. (Schering) Chlorpheniramine maleate 4 mg., salicylamide 190 mg., phenacetin 130 mg., caffeine 30 mg., ascorbic acid 50 mg./Cap. Bot. 100s.
Use: Antihistaminic, analgesic, antipyretic.

CORILIN INFANT LIQUID. (Schering) Chlorpheniramine maleate 0.75 mg., sod. salicylate 80 mg., aminoacetic acid 25 mg./ml. w/alcohol < 1% Bot. 30 ml.
Use: Antihistamine, analgesic, antipyretic.

CORMED.
See: Nikethamide (Various Mfr.)

• CORMETHASONE ACETATE. USAN.
Use: Anti-infammatory.

CORN FIX. (Last) Turpentine oil 2.4%, liquefied phenol 2.25%. Bot. 0.3 oz.
Use: Corn remedy.

CORN HUSKERS LOTION. (Warner-Lambert) Glycerin 6.7%, alcohol 5.7%. Bot. 4 oz., 7 oz.
Use: Moisturizing skin lotion.

• CORN OIL, N.F. XVI.
Use: Pharm. Aid (solvent: oleaginous vehicle).
See: G. B. Prep Emulsion (Gray)
Lipomul-Oral, Liq. (Upjohn)

CORNS-O-POPPIN. (Ries-Hamly) Salicylic acid 6.5%, benzoic acid 12%.
Use: Treatment of corns

CORON IRON TABLETS. (Jamieson-McKames) Cobalt gluconate 25 mg., ferrous gluconate 200 mg./Tab. Bot. 100s.

COR-OTICIN. (Maurry) Hydrocortisone acetate 15 mg., neomycin sulf. 5 mg., sod. cit., polysorbate 80, carboxymethylcellulose, sod. metabisulf., sodium chloride, chlorobutanol 0.5%, sod. hydr./cc. Aq. susp. 5 cc.
Use: Anti-inflammatory, antibiotic.

COROVAS TYMCAPS. (Amfre-Grant) Pentaerythritol tetranitrate 30 mg., secobarbituric acid 50 mg./Cap. Bot. 60s, 120s, 500s, 1000s.
Use: Prolonged action coronary vasodilator.

CORPUS LUTEUM, EXTRACT (WATER SOLUBLE).
See: Progesterone, Preps. (Var. Mfr.)

CORRECTIVE MIXTURE W/PAREGORIC. (Beecham Labs) Zinc sulfocarbolate 10 mg., phenyl salicylate 22 mg., bismuth subsalicylate 85 mg., pepsin 45 mg., paregoric 0.6 ml./5cc. w/alcohol 2%. Bot. Gal.
Use: Antidiarrheal.

CORRECTOL LIQUID. (Plough) Yellow phenolphthalein 65 mg./15 ml. Bot. 2 oz., 8 oz., 16 oz.
Use: Laxative.

CORRECTOL TABLETS. (Plough) Docusate sodium 100 mg., yellow phenolphthalein 65 mg./Tab. Box 4s, 15s, 30s, 60s, 90s.
Use: Stool softener and laxative.

CORSALONE MODIFIED. (Zemmer) Aspirin 300 mg., ascorbic acid 50 mg., aluminum hydroxide 35 mg./E.C. Tab., Bot. 100s.

CORTAID. (Upjohn) Hydrocortisone acetate equivalent to hydrocortisone 5 mg./Gm.**Cream:** 0.5 oz., 1 oz. tube. **Lotion:** 1 oz., 2 oz. Bot. **Ointment:** 0.5 oz., 1 oz. tube. **Spray:** 1.5 fl. oz.
Use: Anti-inflammatory, antipruritic.

CORTAN. (Blue Cross) Presnisone 5 mg./Tab. Bot. 1000s.
Use: Anti-inflammatory.

CORTANE D.C. EXPECTORANT. (Standex)
Brompheniramine maleate 2 mg., guaifenesin 100
mg., phenylephrine HCl 5 mg.,
phenylpropanolamine HCl 5 mg., codeine
phosphate 10 mg., alcohol 3.5%/5 cc. Bot. pt.

CORTANE EXPECTORANT. (Standex)
Brompheniramine maleate 2 mg., guaifenesin 100
mg., phenylephrine 5 mg., phenylpropanolamine
HCl 5 mg., alcohol 3.5%/5 ml. Bot. pt.

CORTAPP ELIXIR. (Standex) Brompheniramine
maleate 5 mg., phenylephrine HCl 5 mg.,
phenylpropanolamine HCl 5 mg., alcohol 2.3%/5
cc. Bot. pt.

CORT-DOME. (Miles Pharm) Hydrocortisone alcohol;
Cream: ⅛%—1 oz., 4 oz. ¼%, 1 oz., 4 oz., 1 lb.
½%—½ oz., 1 oz. Jar 4 oz., 1 lb.; 1%—½ oz., 1
oz. **Lotion:** ⅛%, 6 oz.; ¼%,-4 oz.; ½%—½ oz., 1 oz.,
4 oz., 1%—½ oz., 1 oz. **Supp.** (25 mg., 15 mg.)
Box 12s.
Use: Topically; dermatitis.

CORTEF ACETATE OINTMENT. (Upjohn)
Hydrocortisone acetate 10 and 25 mg./Gm.
w/lanolin (anhydrous), white petrolatum, and
mineral oil. Tube 5 Gm. (25 mg./Gm.) and 20 Gm.
(10 mg./Gm.)
Use: Anti-inflammatory corticosteroid for topical application.

CORTEF ACETATE STERILE SUSPENSION.
(Upjohn) Hydrocortisone acetate 50 mg., sodium
carboxymethylcellulose 4.8 mg., polysorbate 80 3.9
mg. sod. chloride 8.7 mg., benzyl alcohol 8.83
mg./ml. Vial 5 ml.
Use: Anti-inflammatory corticosteriod for local
injection.

CORTEF FEMININE ITCH CREAM. (Upjohn)
Hydrocortisone acetate equivalent to
hydrocortisone 5 mg./Gm. Tube 0.5 oz.
Use: Anti-inflammatory, antipruritic.

CORTEF ORAL SUSPENSION. (Upjohn)
Hydrocortisone 10 mg./5 ml. (as 13.4 mg.
hydrocortisone cypionate). Oral susp. Bot. 4 oz.
Use: Anti-inflammatory corticosteriod for oral administration.

CORTEF RECTAL ITCH OINTMENT. (Upjohn)
Hydrocortisone acetate equivalent to
hydrocortisone 5 mg./Gm. Tube 0.5 oz.
Use: Anti-infammatory, antipruritic.

CORTEF STERILE SUSPENSION IM. (Upjohn)
Hydrocortisone 50 mg., sodium
carboxymethylcellulose 4.8 mg., sod. chloride 8.7
mg., benzyl alcohol 8.83 mg., polysorbate 80 3.85
mg., water q.s./ml. Vial 5 ml.
Use: Anti-inflammatory corticosteroid for I.M. injection.

CORTEF TABLETS. (Upjohn) Hydrocortisone. Tab. 5
mg., Bot. 50s; 10 mg. & 20 mg., Bot. 100s.
Use: Anti-inflammatory corticosteriod.

CORTENEMA. (Rowell) Hydrocortisone 100 mg., in
aqueous solution w/carboxypolymethylene,
polysorbate 80, & methylparaben 0.18%/60 ml.
Bot. w/applicator. Pkg. 7s. Unit dose 1s.
Use: Idiopathic nonspecific ulcerative colitis.

CORTENIL.
See: Desoxycorticosterone Acetate, Preps. (Various
Mfr.)

■ **CORTICAL HORMONE PRODUCTS.**
See: Adrenal Cortex Ext. (Various Mfr.)
Aristocort, Preps. (Lederle)
Corticotropin, Preps. (Var. Mfr.)
Hydrocortisone, Preps. (Var. Mfr.)
Cortisone Acetate, Preps. (Var. Mfr.)
Desoxycorticosterone Acetate, Preps. (Var. Mfr.)
Dexamethasone, Tab. (Var. Mfr.)
Fludrocortisone (Var. Mfr.)
Kenacort, Prep. (Squibb)
Lipo-Adrenal Cortex, Inj. (Upjohn)
Medrol, Preps. (Upjohn)
Methylprednisolone, Tab. (Var. Mfr.)
Prednisolone, Tab. (Var. Mfr.)
Prednisone, Tab. (Var. Mfr.)
Triamcinolone, Tab. (Var. Mfr.)

CORTICAL OINT. (Jenkins) Hydrocortisone 0.33%,
calamine 5.0%, pyrilamine maleate 0.25%,
petrolatum, stearyl alcohol, mineral oil, propylene
glycol, polyoxyl 40 stearate, methyl and propyl
parabens (preservatives), purified water.
Tube ½ oz.

CORTICOID. (Jenkins) Hydrocortisone alcohol 10
mg., clioquinol 30 mg., methyl paraben 0.5 mg.,
propyl paraben 0.5 mg./Gm. Tube 20 Gm.

CORTICOSTERONE. Kendall's Compound B (Various
Mfr.)

CORTICOTROPHIN. B.A.N. Adrenocorticotrophic
hormone.
Use: Adrenocorticotrophin; ACTH
See: Acthar
Actos 50
Cortic-Gel
Cortrophin ZN

CORTICOTROPIN-GEL PURIFIED. (Wilson) Corticotropin in gelatin menstruum, Vial (40 u./cc. & 80
u./cc.) 5 cc.
Use: I.M., S.C.; corticotropin therapy.

CORTICOTROPIN HIGHLY PURIFIED.
See: H. P. Acthar Gel. Vial. (Armour)

• **CORTICOTROPIN INJECTION,** U.S.P. XXI. ACTH.
Adrenocorticotropic hormone or
adrenocorticotrop(h)in or corticotropin.
Use: Adrenocorticotropic hormone; adrenocortical
steroid (anti-inflammatory): diagnostic aid (adrenocortical insufficiency).
See: Cortrophin Gel, Vial, Amp. (Organon)

• **CORTICOTROPIN FOR INJECTION,** U.S.P. XXI.
Use: Adrenocorticotropic hormone; adrenocortical
steroid (anti-inflammatory); diagnostic aid (adrenocortical insufficiency).

• **CORTICOTROPIN INJECTION, REPOSITORY,**
U.S.P. XXI. (Various Mfr.)
Use: I.M. anterior pituitary hormone therapy:
adrenocortical steroid (anti-inflammatory); diagnostic
aid (adrenocortical insufficiency).
See: Acthar Gel, Vial (Armour)
ACTH Gel. Purified (Var. Mfr.)
Cortigel, Vial (Savage)

Cortrophin Gel Amp., Vial (Organon)
H.P. Acthar Gel, Vial (Armour)

CORTICOTROPIN ZINC.
See: Cortrophin-Zinc, Vials (Organon)

• **CORTICOTROPIN-ZINC HYDROXIDE SUSPEN-SION, STERILE,** U.S.P. XXI. Absorbed on zinc hydroxide.
Use: Adrenocorticotropic hormone; adrenocortical steroid (anti-inflammatory); diagnostic aid (adrenocortical insufficiency).

CORTIFOAM. (Reed & Carnrick) Hydrocortisone acetate 10% in an aerosol foam w/propylene glycol, emulsifying wax, steareth 10, cetyl alcohol, methylparaben propylparaben, trolamine, water and inert propellants. Container 20 Gm. w/rectal applicator for 14 applicatorfuls.
Use: Rectal foam, glucocorticoid therapy.

CORTIGEL. (Savage) Purified corticotropin 40 or 80 u./cc. in 16% gelatin solution. Vial 5 cc.
Use: Adrenocorticosteroid.

CORTIGESTIC OTIC DROPS. (Century) Bot. 10 cc.
Use: Ear drops.

CORTIKAY CREAM. (Kay) Dubicaine w/hydrocortisone 0.5% in cream base Bot. 1 oz.
Use: Topical anti-inflammatory, anesthetic.

CORTIN 1% CREAM. (C & M Pharmacal) Hydrocortisone 1%, clioquinol 3%. Tube 20 Gm.
Use: Allergic & atopic eczemas.

CORTINAL. (Kenyon) Micronized hydrocortisone alcohol in a nonallergenic water washable base 5 mg./Gm. Tube 1 oz.

CORTIPREL CREAM. (Pasadena Research) Hydrocortisone acetate 0.5%, 1% in special base. 0.5% Tube 1 oz., 1% Tube 0.5 oz.

CORTISOL.
See: Hydrocortisone, U.S.P.XXI.
Note: Cortisol was the official published name for hydrocortisone in U.S.P.XXI. The name was changed back to Hydrocortisone, U.S.P. in Supplement 1 to the U.S.P.XXI.

CORTISOL CYCLOPENTYLPROPIONATE.
See: Cortef Fluid, Susp., Tab. (Upjohn)

CORTISONE. B.A.N. 17α,21-Dihydroxypregn-4-ene-3,11,20-trione. 17-Hydroxy-11-dehydrocorticosterone.
Adreson, Cortelan, Cortistab, and Cortisyl are the 21-acetate
Use: Corticosteroid.

• **CORTISONE ACETATE,** U.S.P. XXI. Sterile Susp., Tab., U.S.P. XXI. 17,21-Dihydroxypregn-4-ene 3,11,-20-trione 21 acetate. (Kendall's Comp. E) Tab. (Upjohn) 5 mg., 10 mg., or 25 mg./Tab. Bot. 50s, 100s, 500s.
Use: Adrenocortical steroid (anti-inflammatory).
See: Cortistan (Standex)
Cortone Acetate, Tab., Inj. (Merck Sharp & Dohme)
Pantisone, Tab. (Panray)

CORTISPORIN CREAM. (Burroughs Wellcome) Polymyxin B sulfate 10,000 u., neomycin sulfate 5 mg., gramicidin 0.25 mg., hydrocortisone acetate 5 mg./Gm. w/methylparaben 0.25%. Tube 7.5 Gm.

Use: Anti-inflammatory.

CORTISPORIN OINTMENT. (Burroughs Wellcome) Polymyxin B sulfate 5,000 u., bacitracin zinc 400 u., neomycin sulfate 5 mg., hydrocortisone (1%) 10 mg./Gm. in petrolatum base. Tube 0.5 oz.
Use: Anti-inflammatory and antibacterial.

CORTISPORIN OPHTHALMIC OINTMENT. (Burroughs Wellcome) Polymyxin B sulfate 10,000 u., bacitracin 400 u., neomycin sulfate 5 mg., hydrocortisone (1%) 10 mg./Gm. in petrolatum base. Tube ⅛ oz. Sterile.
Use: Anti-inflammatory & antibacterial.

CORTISPORIN OPHTHALMIC SUSPENSION. (Burroughs Wellcome) Polymyxin B sulfate 10,000 u., neomycin sulfate 5 mg., hydrocortisone (1%) 10 mg., in sterile, saline, isotonic/ml. W/thimerosal, cetyl alcohol, glyceryl monostearate, liq. petrolatum, polyoxyl 40 stearate, propylene glycol. Drop bot. 5 ml. Sterile.
Use: Optic, inflammation.

CORTISPORIN OTIC SOLUTION STERILE. (Burroughs Wellcome) Polymixin B sulf. 10,000 u., neomycin sulf. 5 mg., hydrocortisone 10 mg./ml. w/glycerin, HCl, propylene glycol, & K metabisulfite 0.1%. Bot. W/dropper 10 ml. Sterile.
Use: External ear infections.

CORTISPORIN OTIC SUSPENSION. (Burroughs Wellcome) Polymyxin B sulf. 10,000 u., neomycin sulf. 5 mg., hydrocortisone free alcohol 10 mg./ml. W/cetyl alcohol, propylene glycol, polysorbate 80, thimerosal. Bot. w/dropper 10 ml. Sterile.
Use: Ear infections.

CORTISTAN. (Standex) Cortisone 25 mg./10 cc.

• **CORTIVAZOL.** USAN. 11B,17,21-trihydroxy-6, 16α-dimethyl-2′-phenyl-2′H-pregna-2,4,6-trieno[3,2-c]-pyrazol-20-one 21-acetate.
Use: Anti-inflammatory.

CORTIZONE-S, MAXIMUM STRENGTH. (Thompson Medical) Hydrocortisone 0.5%. Tubes.
Use: Relief of dermatitis, itch, rash.

CORT-NIB CREAM. (Cenci) Hydrocortisone alcohol, 0.-25%, 0.5%, 1.0%. **Cream:** Tube 1 oz. Jar 1 lb.
Use: Anti-inflammatory agent.

CORT-NIB V CREAM. (Cenci) Hydrocortisone alcohol ½%, clioquinol 3%. Tube 1 oz.
Use: Anti-inflammatory agent.

• **CORTODOXONE.** USAN. 17,21-Dihydroxy-pregn-4-ene-3,20-dione. Cortexolone.
Use: Anti-inflammatory.

CORTOGEN ACETATE. Cortisone acetate.

CORTONE ACETATE. (Merck Sharp & Dohme) Cortisone acetate. **Tab.** 25 mg., Bot. 100s. **Saline Susp.,** 25 mg./ml. and 50 mg./ml. W/sod. chloride 9 mg., polysorbate 80-4 mg., sodium carboxymethyl-cellulose 5 mg., benzyl alcohol 9 mg./ml., water for injection q.s. 1 ml. **25 mg./**ml. Vial, 20 ml.; **50 mg./**ml. Vial, 10 ml.
Use: Anti-inflammatory corticosteroid.

CORTOXIDE GEL. (Syosset) Hydrocortisone 0.5% or 1% in gel base. Bot. 1.5 oz.
Use: treatment of dermatoses.

CORT-QUIN. (Miles Pharm) Hydrocortisone alcohol

¼%, iodoquinol 1% in vehicle buffered to the pH range of normal skin. Hydrocortisone alcohol ½%, iodoquinol 1% in Acid Mantle vehicle of cetyl alcohol, stearyl alcohol, sod. lauryl sulfate, beeswax, white petrolatum, liquid petrolatum glycerin methylparaben. Tube ½ oz., 1 oz.
Use: Antibacterial, antiprotozoal, antifungal.

CORTRIL TOPICAL OINTMENT 1%. (Pfipharmecs) Hydrocortisone 1% W/cetyl and stearyl alcohol, propylene glycol, sod. lauryl sulfate, petrolatum, cholesterol, mineral oil, methyl and propyl parabens in ointment base. Tube ½ oz.
Use: Anti-inflammatory.

CORTROPHIN GEL. (Organon) Corticotropin, Gel. **40 U/cc.** Vial 5 ml. **80 U./cc.** Vial 5 ml. Box 1s.
Use: Hormone (ACTH).

CORTROPHIN-ZINC. (Organon) Corticotropin zinc 40 u./ml. Vial 5 cc.
Use: Hormone (ACTH).

CORTROSYN INJECTION. (Organon) Cosyntropin 0.25 mg., mannitol 10 mg., lyophilized pow./1 ml. Vial. Pkg. w/1 ml. amp. diluent. Box 10s. Vial.
Use: Hormone (ACTH).

CORT-TOP OINTMENT. (Standex) Topical hydrocortisone 1%. Tube 20 Gm.

CORUBEEN. (Spanner) B-12 crystalline 1000 mcg./cc. Vial 10 cc.

CORYBAN-D. (Pfipharmecs) Phenylpropanolamine 25 mg., chlorpheniramine maleate 2 mg., caffeine 30 mg./Cap. Bot. 24s.
Use: Common cold.

CORYBAN-D SYRUP. (Pfipharmecs) Phenylephrine HCl 5 mg., acetaminophen 120 mg., guaifenesin 50 mg., d-methorphan HBr 7.5 mg., and alcohol 7.5%/5 cc. tsp. Bot. 4 oz. 12s
Use: Common cold, allergies.

CORYZEX. (Vitarine) Acetaminophen 325 mg., phenylpropanolamine HCl 12.5 mg., chlorpheniramine maleate 1 mg., dextromethorphan HBr. 10 mg./Cap.
Use: Symptomatic relief of discomforts of cold.

CORZANS. (Moore Kirk) Acetaminophen 160 mg., chlorpheniramine maleate 1 mg., phenylephrine HCl 7½ mg., ascorbic acid 15 mg./Tab. Bot. 100s, 1000s.
Use: Treatment of common cold and hay fever.

CORZIDE. (Squibb) Nadolol 40 mg., Bendrolumethiazide 5 mg./Tab or Nadolol 80 mg., bendroflumethiazide 5 mg./Tab. Bot. 100s.
Use: Antihypertensive, B-blocker diuretic combination.

CORZONE. (Xttrium) Dextromethorphan HBr 15 mg., chlorpheniramine maleate 1.8 mg., phenyltoloxamine dihydrogen citrate 8 mg., phenylpropanolamine HCl 12.5 mg., ammonium Cl 90 mg./5 cc. Bot. pt., gal.
Use: Relief of coughs due to colds.

CORZYME. (Abbott) Test kit 100s.
Use: Enzyme immunoassay for detection of antibody to hepatitis B core antigen.

CORZYME-M. (Abbott) Test kits 100s.
Use: Enzyme immunoassay for the detection of IgM antibody to hepatitis B core antigen.

COSALDON. Pentifylline, B.A.N.

CO-SANSPRIN. (Wolins) Acetaminophen 325 mg., chlorpheniramine maleate 1 mg., phenylephrine HCl 5 mg./Tab. Bot. 1000s.

COSANYL. (Health Care Industries) Codeine sulfate 10 mg., d-pseudoephedrine HCl 30 mg./5 ml. w/alcohol 6% in peach flavored base. Bot. 4 oz., 1 pt., 1 gal.

COSANYL-DM. (Health Care Industries) Dextromethorphan HBr 15 mg., d-pseudoephedrine HCl 30 mg./5 ml. w/alcohol 6% in a peach flavored base. Bot. 4 oz., gal.
Use: Sedative, expectorant.

COSMEGEN. (Merck Sharp & Dohme) Actinomycin D (dactinomycin) 0.5 mg. (lyophilized powder), mannitol 20 mg./Vial.
Use: Antineoplastic.

COSMOLINE.
See: Petrolatum

COSPRIN. (Glenbrook) Aspirin 325 mg. or 650 mg./Tab. **650 mg.**/Tab. Bot. 36s, 72s; **325 mg** ./Tab. Bot. 60s, 125s.
Use: Analgesic, anti-inflammatory.

COSULID. (Ciba) Sulfachloropyridazine.

• COSYNTROPIN. USAN.
Use: Adrenocorticotropic hormone.
See: Cortrosyn, Vial (Organon)

COTARNINE CHLORIDE. Cotarnine hydrochloride.

COTARNINE HYDROCHLORIDE.
See: Cotarnine Chloride

COTAZYM. (Organon) Pancrelipase, Lipase 8,000 u., protease 30,000 u., amylase 30,000 u. having digestive power for 17 Gm. dietary fat, trypsin, having digestive power for 34 Gm. dietary protein; amylase, having digestive power for 40 Gm. dietary starch, plus other enzymes from whole hog pancreas/Cap. Bot. 100s, 500s. Cherry flavored. Cap. Bot. 100s.
Use: Pancreatic enzyme deficiency.

COTAZYM-B. (Organon) Mixed conjugated bile salts 65 mg., pancrelipase 165 mg., cellulase 2 mg./Tab. Bot. 60s.
Use: Enzyme digestant.

CORTAZYM-S. (Organon) Pancrelipase spheres, lipase 5,000 U., protease 20,000 U., amylase 20,000 U./Tab.
Use: Pancreatic enzyme deficiency.

COTIN. (Pasadena Research) Pepsin 250 mg., pancreatin 300 mg., bile salts 150 mg., dehydrocholic acid 25 mg./Tab. Bot. 100s, 1000s.

CO-TINIC INJECTION. (Vortech) Iron peptonized 59 mg., folic acid 5 mg., liver injection equiv. to B-12 5 mcg., procaine HCl 1%, sod. citrate 1%, pheno 1.5%/2 cc. Vial 30 ml.
Use: Hematinic.

COTININE FUMARATE. (-)-1-Methyl-5-(3-pyridyl)-2 pyrrolidinone compound (2:1) with fumaric acid.
Use: Psychomotor stimulant.

COTRIM. (Lemmon) Sulfamethoxazole 400 mg., trimethoprim 80 mg./Tab. Bot. 100s, 500s. Unit Dose 100s.
Use: Antibacterial.

COTRIM D.S. (Lemmon) Sulfamethoxazole 800 mg., trimethoprim 160 mg./Tab. Bot. 100s, 500s. Unit Dose 100s.
Use: Anti-infective.

COTRIM PREDIATRIC. (Lemmon) Sulfamethoxazole 200 mg., trimethoprim 40 mg./5 ml. Bot. pt.
Use: Anti-infective.

COTRIM S.S.. (Lemmon) Sulfamethoxazole 400 mg., trimethoprim 800 mg./Tab. Bot. 100s.
Use: Anti-infective.

CO-TRIMOXAZOLE. B.A.N. Compounded preparations of trimethoprim and sulfamethoxazole in the proportions of 1 part to 5 parts.
Use: Antibacterial.
See: Bactrim Prods (Roche)
Septra (Burroughs Wellcome)
Septrin

COTROL-D. (Beecham Labs) Pseudoephedrine HCl 60 mg., chlorpheniramine maleate 4 mg./Tab. Bot. 100s.
Use: Relief of upper respiratory and bronchial congestion.

• **COTTON, PURIFIED,** U.S.P. XXI.
Use: Surgical aid.

• **COTTONSEED OIL,** N.F. XVI.
Use: Pharm. aid, solvent, oleaginous vehicle.

COTYLENOL CHILDREN'S LIQUID COLD FORMULA. (McNeil Prods) Acetaminophen 160 mg., chlorpheniramine maleate 1 mg., phenylpropanolamine HCl 6.25 mg./5 ml. w/Alcohol 7%. Bot. 4 oz.
Use: Analgesic, antipyretic, decongestant.

COTYLENOL COLD FORMULA CAPSULES. (McNeil Prods) Acetaminophen 325 mg., chlorpheniramine maleate 2 mg., pseudoephedrine HCl 30 mg., dextromethorphan HBr 15 mg./Cap. Bot. 20s. Bot. 40s.
Use: Multisymptom cold and cough formula.

COTYLENOL LIQUID COLD FORMULA. (McNeil Prods) Acetaminophen 650 mg., chlorpheniramine maleate 4 mg., pseudoephedrine HCl 60 mg., dextromethorphan HCl 30 mg./30 ml. w/alcohol 7.5% Bot. 2 oz., 5 oz., 10 oz.
Use: Multisymptom cough and cold formula.

COTYLENOL TABLETS. (McNeil Prods) Chlorpheniramine maleate 2 mg., dextromethorphan HBr 15 mg., pseudoephedrine HCl 30 mg., acetaminophen 325 mg./Tab. Vial 10s; Box 24s; Bot. 50s, 100s.
Use: Multisymptom cough and cold formula.

COUGH EEZ. (Kay) Dextromethorphan 15 mg., benzocaine 3 mg./Cap. Bot.
Use: Cough & minor sore throat.

COUGH WAFERS. (Wolins) Benzocaine ⅛ gr., plant ext. licorice ¹⁄₁₆ gr., anise oil q.s., eucalyptol q.s., menthol q.s./Tab. Bot. 1000s.

COUMADIN. (Du Pont) Warfarin sodium crystalline. 2 mg., 2½ mg., 5 mg., 7½ mg., 10 mg./Tab. Bot. 1000s. Hospital pack Box. 100s. **Inj.** 50 mg./Vial w/diluent sod. chloride, thimerosal, and sod. hydroxide to adjust pH. Box 6s.
Use: Anticoagulant.

COUMAPHOS. B.A.N. 0-3-Chloro-4-methylcoumarin-7-y100-diethylphosphorothioate.
Use: Insecticide, veterinary medicine.
See: Asuntol

COUMARIN.
Use: Pharmaceutic aid.

• **COUMERMYCIN,** USAN. Antibiotic derived from *Streptomyces rishiriensis.*
Use: Antibiotic.

COUNTERPAIN RUB. (Squibb) Methyl salicylate, eugenol, menthol. Oint. Tube 1 oz.
Use: External analgesic.

COVAP. (Blue Line) Pentaerythritol tetranitrate 15 mg., sod. butabarbital 20 mg./Tab. Bot. 100s, 1000s.
Use: Angina pectoris.

COVERMARK. (O'Leary) Neutral cream, hypoallergenic, opaque, greaseless. Jars 1 oz., 3¼ oz., avail. in eight shades.
Use: Conceals birthmarks and skin discolorations.

COVERMARK CREAM ROUGE. (O'Leary) Same basic formulation as Covermark: Regular and waterproof formulas. Shades: Blonde, medium and brunette. Bot. Waterproof ¾ oz., 2¾ oz. Regular 1.24 oz., 4 oz.
Use: To conceal birthmarks and skin discolorations.

COVICONE CREAM. (Abbott) Silicone, nitrocellulose, castor oil suspended in vanishing cream base. Tube 1 oz.
Use: Topically for protecting skin from irritation.

CO-XAN SYRUP. (Central) Theophylline sod. glycinate 165 mg., ephedrine HCl 25 mg., Guaifenesin 100 mg., codeine phosphate 15 mg., alcohol 10%/15 ml. Bot. 1 pt.
Use: Bronchial spasms.

COYDEN 25. Clopidol, B.A.N.

COZ OINTMENT. (Sentinel) Zinc oxide, cod liver oil, menthol, phenol. Jar 2 oz., 1 lb.
Use: Skin irritation.

CP. (Western Research) Phenylpropanolamine 75 mg., caffeine 140 mg./Cap. Bot. 1000s.
Use: Anorectic-decongestant.

CP-2. (Century) Aspirin 4 gr., phenacetin 2 gr., caffeine ¼ gr./Tab. Bot. 100s, 1000s, 5000s.

C.P.C. PLUS. (Coastal) Phenylephrine HCl 5 mg., phenylpropanolamine HC1 25 mg., chlorpheniramine maleate 2 mg., vit. C 60 mg./Tab. Bot. 50s, 100s, 500s.
Use: Antihistaminic and decongestant.

CPI HEMORRHOIDAL SUPPS. (Century) Bismuth subgallate, bismuth oxyiodide, bismuth resorcin comp., balsam Peru, benzocaine, Zn oxide, boric acid. 12s.
Use: Antihemorrhoidal.

CPLEX. (Arcum) Vit. B-1 10 mg., B-2 10 mg., B-6 5 mg., B-12 10 mcg., niacinamide 100 mg., calcium pantothenate 25 mg., Vit. C 150 mg., liver 50 mg., dried yeast 50 mg./Cap. Bot. 100s, 1000s.
Use: Dietary supplement.

CREAMALIN. (Winthrop Products) Aluminum hydroxide 248 mg., magnesium hydroxide 75 mg./Tab. Bot. 50s, 100s, 200s.

Use: Antacid.

CREMACOAT 1. (Vicks) Dextromethorphan HBr 30 mg./15 ml. Bot. 3 oz., 6 oz.
Use: Cough suppressant.

CREMACOAT 2. (Vicks) Guaifenesin 200 mg./15 ml. Bot. 3 oz., 6 oz.
Use: Expectorant.

CREMACOAT 3. (Vicks) Dextromethorphan HBr 20 mg., phenylpropanolamine HCl 37.5 mg., guaifenesin 200 mg./15 ml. Bot. 3 oz., 6 oz.
Use: Cough suppressant, nasal decongestant, expectorant.

CREMACOAT 4. (Vicks) Dextromethorphan HBr 20 mg., phenylpropanolamine HCl 37/5 mg., doxylamine succinate 7.5 mg./15 ml. Bot. 3 oz, 6 oz.
Use: Cough suppressant, nasal decongestant, antihistaminic.

CREMAGOL. (Cremagol) Emulsion of liq. petrolatum, agar agar, acacia, glycerin. Bot. 14 oz. Also w/cascara 11 gr./oz. Bot. 14 oz., also w/phenolphthalein 2 gr./oz. Bot. 14 oz.
Use: Laxative.

CREMESONE. (Dalin) Hydrocortisone alcohol 5 mg./Gm. Tube 1 oz.
Use: Inflammatory skin diseases or allergic dermatitis.

CREOMULSION COUGH MEDICINE. (Creomulsion) Beechwood creosote, cascara, ipecac, menthol, white pine, wild cherry w/alcohol. For Adults. Bot. 4 & 8 fl. oz.
Use: Coughs and bronchial irritations due to colds.

CREOMULSIN FOR CHILDREN. (Creomulsion) Beechwood creosote, cascara, ipecac, menthol, white pine, wild cherry w/alcohol. For Children. Bot. 4 fl. oz., 8 fl. oz.
Use: Coughs and bronchial irritations due to colds.

CREOSANT COUGH SYRUP. (DeWitt) Ammonium chloride, beechwood creosote, menthol, w/alcohol 3%. Bot. 4 oz.
Use: Cough relief.

CREOSOTE. Wood creosote, creosote, beechwood creosote.
W/Ipecac, menthol, licorice, white pine, wild cherry, cascara, Vitamin C.
See: Creozets, Loz. (Creomulsion)

CREOSOTE CARBONATE.

CREOTERP. (Jenkins) Terpin hydrate 2 gr., potassium iodide 1/8 gr., creosote 1/10 min., eucalyptol 1/10 min. Tab. Bot. 1000s.
Use: Antitussive.

CREO-TERPIN. (Denver) Creosote 0.12 ml., sod. glycerophosphate 259 mg., terpin hydrate 130 mg., chloroform 0.06 ml., alcohol 25%/30 ml. Bot. 3 oz., 6 oz.
Use: Antitussive.

■ **CRESCORMON.** (Kabi) Somatropin 4 I.U./Vial. I.M. administration.
Use: Long-term therapy for children who have growth failure secondary to somatropin deficiency.
Note: Crescormon will be available only for patients who qualify for treatment; full

documentation for prospective patients to be submitted to Kabi Group Inc. for approval.

CRESCORMON. (Pharmacia) Somatropin 4 I.U./Vial + 2 ml. NaCl injection.
Use: Long term treatment of children with growth failure secondary to somatropin deficiency.

• **CRESOL,** N.F. XVI. Mixture of 3 isomeric cresols. Phenol, methyl cresol.
Use: Antiseptic & disinfectant.

CRESOL PREPARATIONS.
Use: Antibacterial (inanimate objects).
See: Cresol, Sol. (Various Mfr.)
Cresylone, Liq. (Parke-Davis)
Saponated Cresol Sol.

CRESTABOLIC. (Nutrition) Protein anabolic steroid, methandriol dipropionate 50 mg./ml. w/benzyl alcohol 5% in sesame oil. Vial 10 cc.
Use: Treatment of conditions where tissue building action is desired.

m-CRESYL-ACETATE.
See: Cresylate, Liq. (Recsei)

CRESYLATE. (Recsei) M-cresyl-acetate. Otic sol. 1/2 oz. dropper bot., Pts.
Use: Otomycosis due to aspergillus niger & furunculosis.

CRESYLIC ACID. Same as Cresol.

CRITICARE HN. (Mead Johnson) High nitrogen elemental diet. Protein 14%, fat 3%, carbohydrate 83%. Bot. 8 oz.
Use: Complete, high-quality elemental nutrition.

CROFERRIN. (Fellows) Iron peptonate 50 mg., liver inj. 2.5 mcg., Vit. B-12 12.5 mcg., lidocaine HCl 1%, phenol 0.5%, Na citrate 0.125%, Na bisulfite 0.009%/ml. Vial 10 ml., 30 ml.
Use: Iron deficiency anemia.

• **CROFILCON A.** USAN
Use: Contact lens material.

• **CROMITRILE SODIUM.** USAN.
Use: Antihistaminic.

CROMOGLYCIC ACID. B.A.N. 1,3-Di-(2-car-boxy-4-oxochromen-5-yloxy)propan-2-ol.
Use: Treatment of allergic airway obstruction.

• **CROMOLYN SODIUM,** U.S.P. XXI. For Inhalation, U.S.P. XXI. Disodium 5,5'-[(2-hydroxytrimethylene)dioxy]bis[4-oxo-4H-1-benzopyran-2-carboxylate].
Use: Treatment of allergic airway obstruction.
See: Intal, Cap. (Fisons)

C-RON. (Rowell) Ascorbic acid 100 mg., ferrous fumarate 200 mg./Tab. Bot. 100s, 1000s.
Use: Anemias.

C-RON F.A. (Rowell) Ferrous fumarate 200 mg., Vit. C 600 mg., folic acid 0.5 mg./Tab. Bot. 100s.
Use: Iron-deficiency and megaloblastic anemias of pregnancy.

C-RON FORTE. (Rowell) Ferrous fumarate 200 mg., ascorbic acid 600 mg./Tab. Bot. 100s, 1000s.
Use: Iron deficiency anemia.

C-RON FRECKLES. (Rowell) Vitamin C 50 mg., ferrous fumarate 100 mg./Chewable Tab. Bot. 100s,
Use: Iron deficiency in children.

CRONETAL.
See: Disulfiram

CROPROPAMIDE. B.A.N. NN-Dimethyl-2-(N-propyl-crotonamido)butyramide.
Use: Respiratory stimulant.
C ROSE HIPS. (Robinson) 100 mg., 250 mg., 500 mg./Tab. Bot. 100s, 250s, 1000s.
• **CROSCARMELLOSE SODIUM,** N.F. XVI.
Use: Tablet disintegrant.
• **CROSPOVIDONE,** N.F. XVI.
Use: Pharmaceutic aid (tablet excipient).
CROSS ASPIRIN. (Cross) Aspirin 325 mg./Tab. Bot. 100s, 1000s
Use: Analgesic, antipyretic, anti-inflammatory.
CROTALINE ANTIVENIN, POLYVALENT. Antivenin Crotalidae Polyvalent, U.S.P. XXI. North and South American Antisnakebite serum.
Use: Passive immunizing agent.
• **CROTAMITON,** U.S.P. XXI. Cream, U.S.P. XXI. N-Crotonyl-N-ethyl-o-toluidine.
Use: Antipruritic.
See: Eurax, Cream, Lot. (Geigy)
CROTETHAMIDE. B.A.N. 2-(N-Ethylcrotonamido)-NN-dimethylbutyramide.
Use: Respiratory stimulant.
CRPA, CRPA LATEX TEST. (Laboratory Diagnostics) CRPA, 1 ml.—CRP Positest Control, 0.5 ml. CRPA Latex Test Kit.
Use: Rapid latex agglutination test for the qualitative determination of C reactive protein.
CRUDE TUBERCULIN.
See: Tuberculin, Old, Vial (Parke-Davis)
CRUEX AEROSOL POWDER. (Pharmacraft) Hydrocarbon propellant w/zinc undecylenate 20%, undecylenic acid 2% in talc base. Aerosol 5.5 oz.
Use: Jock itch (Tinea cruris) treatment.
CRUEX CREAM. (Pharmacraft) Zinc undecylenate 20%, undecylenic acid 3%. Tube 15 Gm.
Use: Jock itch (Tinea cruris) treatment.
CRUEX SQUEEZE POWDER. (Pharmacraft) Calcium undecylenate 10%. Bot. 1.5 oz., 3.0 oz. squeeze container.
Use: Jock itch (Tinea cruris).
• **CRUFOMATE.** USAN. 4-tert-Butyl-2-chlorophenyl methyl methylphosphoramidate.
Use: Insecticide; anthelmintic, veterinary medicine.
See: Ruelene.
CRYPTENAMINE ACETATE & TANNATE. Esters of alkaloids of veratrum viride.
See: Unitensen, Preps. (Mallinckrodt)
CRYPTENAMINE.
W/Methyclothiazide.
See: Diutensen, Tabs. (Mallinckrodt)
W/Methyclothiazide, reserpine.
See: Diutensen-R, Tab. (Mallinckrodt)
CRYPTOLIN. (Hoechst) Gonadorelin in nasal spray.
Use: Cryptorchism treatment.
CRYSPEN-400. (Knight) Buffered penicillin G potassium 400,000 u./Tab. Bot. 100s.
Use: Anti-infective.
CRYSTALLINE TRYPSIN. Highly purified prep. of enzyme as derived from mammalian pancreas glands.

See: Tryptar, Inj. (Armour)
CRYSTALLOSE. (Jamieson-McKames) Saccharin sodium. Crystals, Box ¼ oz., ¾ oz. Liquid, plas. squeeze bot. ¾ oz., 2 oz.
Use: Sweetening agent.
CRYSTAL VIOLET.
See: Methylrosaniline Chloride, U.S.P.
CRYSTAMINE. (Dunhall) Cyanocobalamin 1,000 mcg./ml. Vial 10 ml, or 30 ml.
Use: Vitamin B-12 deficiency.
CRYSTI-12. (Hauck) Vitamin B-12 1000 mcg./ml. Vial 10 ml., 30 ml.
Use: B-12 parenteral.
CRYSTICILLIN 300 A.S. (Squibb) Sterile procaine penicillin G suspension U.S.P. 300,000 u./ml. w/lecithin, povidone, sod. citrate, sod. formaldehyde sulfoxylate, sod. carboxymethylcellulose, methylparaben & propylparaben. Vial 10 cc.
Use: Bactericidal agent against penicillin-sensitive microorganisms during the stage of active multiplication.
CRYSTICILLIN 600 A.S. (Squibb) Sterile procaine penicillin G suspension 600,000 u./1.2 cc. w/lecithin, phenol, povidone, sod. citrate, sod. carboxymethylcellulose, sod. formaldehyde sufoxylate, methylparaben, & propylparaben. Vial 12 ml.
Use: Bactericidal agent against penicillin-sensitive microorganisms during the stage of active multiplication.
CRYSTODIGIN TABLETS. (Lilly) Crystalline digitoxin 0.05 mg./Tab. Bot. 100s, 500s; 0.1 mg./Tab. Bot. 100s, 500s, 5000s. Blister pkg. 10 × 10s; 0.15 mg./Tab. Bot. 100s, 500s; 0.2 mg./Tab. Bot. 100s, 500s.
Use: Congestive heart failure.
CRYSTOGRAFIN. Meglumine diatrizoate.
Use: Contrast medium.
C-SPAN. (Edwards) Ascorbic acid 500 mg./Timed Release Cap. Bot. 100s.
Use: Treatment of Vit. C deficiency.
C SPERIDIN. (Marlyn) Bioflavanoids with Vitamin C. Bot. 100s, 1000s.
C.S.R. UNIT. Unit represents the amount of veratrum viride extract per Kg. of body weight which will just abolish the pressor response to the carotid sinus reflex resulting from occlusion of the carotid arteries in dogs.
See: Cryptenamine
C-SYRUP-500. (Ortega) Ascorbic acid 500 mg./5 ml. Bot. pt., gal.
CTAB.
See: Cetyl Trimethyl Ammonium Bromide
CTD COMPLEX TABLETS. (Image) Vitamin C. Bot. 100s.
Use: Supplement.
C-TUSSIN. (Century) Codeine phosphate 10 mg., phenylpropanolamine HCl 18.72 mg., guaifenesin 100 mg./5 ml. w/alcohol 7.5%. Bot. 10 cc., gal.
Use: Expectorant.
CULMINAL. (Culminal) Benzocaine 3% in water

miscible ointment base. Tube 1 oz.
Use: Prevention of premature ejaculation.
CUMETHAROL. B.A.N. 4,4'-Dihydroxy-3,3'-(2-methoxy-ethylidene)dicoumarin.
Use: Anticoagulant.
See: Dicumoxane
CUPREX. (Beecham Products)
Tetrahydronaphthalene, copper oleate. Bot. 3 oz., 1 pt.
Use: Topically, pediculocide.
• **CUPRIC ACETATE Cu 64.** USAN.
Use: Radioactive agent.
• **CUPRIC CHLORIDE,** U.S.P. XXI., Inj., U.S.P. XXI.
Use: Copper deficiency treatment.
See: Coppertrace, Inj. (Armour)
• **CUPRIC SULFATE,** U.S.P. XXI. Inj., U.S.P. XXI.
Use: Antidote to phosphorus.
W/Zinc sulfate & camphor.
See: Dalibour, Pow. (Doak)
CUPRIMINE. (Merck Sharp & Dohme) Penicillamine 125 mg., 250 mg./Cap. Bot. 100s.
Use: Wilson's disease, cystinuria, rheumatoid arthritis.
• **CUPRIMYXIN.** USAN.
Use: Antibacterial.
CURARE.
Use: Muscle relaxant.
See: d-Tubocurarine Salts (Various Mfr.)
CURARE ANTAGONIST.
See: Neostigmine Methylsulfate Inj. (Various Mfr.)
Tensilon, Amp. (Roche)
CURBAN. (Pasadena Research) Dextroamphetamine sulfate 10, 15 mg./Tab. Bot. 100s, 1000s.
Use: Central stimulant.
CURRAL.
See: Diallyl Barbituric Acid, Tab. (Various Mfr.)
CURRETAB. (Reid-Provident) Medroxyprogesterone acetate 10 mg./Tab. Bot. 50s.
Use: Progestin.
CUTAR. (Summers) Coal tar solution 7½% w/Liquid petrolatum, isopropyl myristate, acetylated lanolin, lanolin alcohols extract. Bot. 6 oz.
Use: Bath oil emulsion.
CUTEMOL EMOLLIENT CREAM. (Summers)
Allantoin 0.2%, hypoallergenic lanolin fractions, with additional emollient agents and a nonionic emulsifier in a high-aqueous content water-in-oil cream base. Tube 2 oz., Bath Oil 6 oz.
Use: Dermatologic.
CUTICURA ACNE CREAM. (Jeffrey Martin) Benzoyl peroxide 5%, allantoin, phenoxyethanol, alcohol 1%.
Use: Dermatologic, acne.
CUTICURA ANTIBACTERIAL MEDICATED SOAP.
(Jeffrey Martin) Triclocarban 1%. Bars 3.25 oz., 5 oz.
Use: Cleaning combination for the skin.
CUTICURA MEDICATED SHAMPOO. (Jeffrey Martin)
Sodium lauryl sulfate, sodium stearate, salicylic acid, protein, sulfur. Tube 3 oz.
Use: Antidandruff shampoo.
CUTICURA MEDICATED SOAP. (Jeffrey Martin)

Triclocarban 1%, petrolatum, emollients. Bars 3½ oz. 5½ oz.
Use: Antibacterial skin care.
CUTICURA OINTMENT. (Jeffrey Martin) Beeswax synthetic, isopropyl palmitate, mineral wax, mineral oil, oxyquinoline, pine oil phenol, petrolatum, precipitated sulfur, rose geranium oil. Tin ¾ oz., 1¾ oz. Jar. 4¼ oz.
Use: Skin care.
CUTTER INSECT REPELLENT. (Miles) N,N-Diethyl-meta-toluamide 28.5%, other isomers 1.5% Vial 1 oz. Foam, Can 2 oz.; Spray 7 oz., 14 oz. aerosol can; Assortment Pack; First Aid Kits, Trial Pack, 6s; Marine Pack, 3s; Camp Pack, 4s. Pocket Pack, Travel Pack.
Use: Insect repellent.
C VITAMIN.
See: Ascorbic Acid, Prep.
C.V.P. CAPSULES. (Armour) Bioflavonoids 100 mg./Cap Bot. 100s.
Use: Vitamin supplement.
CYACETAZIDE. B.A.N. Cyanoacetohydrazide.
Use: Anthelmintic, veterinary medicine.
CYADE-GEL. (Kenyon) Adenosine-5-monophosphate 100 mg., Vit. B-12 100 mcg./cc. Vial 10 cc.
CYANIDE ANTIDOTE PACKAGE. (Lilly) 2 Amp. (300 mg./10 ml.) sodium nitrite; 2 Amp. (12.5 Gm./50 ml.) w/sodium thiosulfate; 12 aspirols amyl nitrite 5 min./Pkg. Check exact dosage before administration.
Use: Treatment of cyanide poisoning.
CYANOCOB. (Paddock) Vit. B-12 1000 mcg./cc. Bot. 1000 cc. Vials 10 cc.
Use: Vitamin B-12 deficiency.
CYANOCOBALAMIN. B.A.N. α-(5,6-Dimethyl-benzimidazol-1-yl)cobamide cyanide.
Vitamin B-12.
Use: Treatment of megaloblastic anemia.
See: Cobastab
Cytacon
Cytamen
• **CYANOCOBALAMIN,** U.S.P. XXI. Inj. U.S.P. XXI.
Use: Vitamin B-12 (hematopoietic).
See: Vitamin B-12, Preps.
• **CYANOCOBALAMIN CO 57,** USP XXI. Cap., Oral Soln., U.S.P. XXI.
Use: Diagnostic aid (pernicious anemia)
• **CYANOCOBALAMIN CO 60,** U.S.P. XXI. Cap., Oral Soln., U.S.P. XXI.
Use: Diagnostic aid (pernicious anemia).
CYANOJECT 10 AND 30. (Mayrand) Vit. B-12 1000 mcg./ml. Vial 10 ml.
CYANOVER. (Research Supplies) Cyanocobalamin 100 mcg., liver inj. 10 mcg., folic acid 10 mg./cc. Lyo-layer vials 10 cc. with 10 cc. vials of diluent.
Use: Treatment of pernicious anemia.
• **CYCLACILLIN,** U.S.P. XXI. For Oral Susp., Tab., U.S.P. XXI. 6-(1-Aminocyclohexanecarbox-amide)-3,3-dimethyl-7-oxo-4-thia-1-azabicyclo-[3.2.0] heptane-2-carboxylic acid.
Use: Antibacterial.
See: Cyclapen-W, Liq., Tab. (Wyeth)

CYCLAINE. (Merck Sharp & Dohme) Hexylcaine HCl 50 mg., methylparaben 1.5 mg., propylparaben 0.2 mg./ml., water. 60 ml. Bot. 60 ml.
Use: Local topical anesthetic.

CYCLAMATE SODIUM. Cyclohexanesulfamate dihydrate salt.

• **CYCLAMIC ACID,** USAN. N-Cyclohexylsulfamic acid. Hexamic Acid. Cyclohexanesulfamic acid. Currently banned in U.S.
Use: Sweetening agent.

CYCLANDELATE. 3,3,5-Trimethylcyclohexyl mandelate.
See: Cyclospasmol, Tab., Cap. (Ives)

CYCLANDELATE. B.A.N. 3,3,5-Trimethylcyclohexyl mandelate.
Use: Treatment of vascular disorders.
See: Cyclospasmol

CYCLAPEN-W. (Wyeth) Cyclacillin 250 mg. or 500 mg./Tab. Bot. 100s.
Use: Antibiotic.

CYCLAPEN-W FOR ORAL SUSPENSION. (Wyeth) Cyclacillin 125 mg./5 ml. or 250 mg./5 ml. Bot. to make 100 ml., 150 ml., 200 ml.
Use: Antibiotic.

CYCLARBAMATE. B.A.N. 1,1-Di(phenylcarbamoyl-oxymethyl)cyclopentane.
Use: Muscle relaxant; tranquilizer.
See: Casmalon

• **CYCLAZOCINE.** USAN. 3-(Cyclopropylmethyl)-1,2,3,-4,5,6-hexahydro-6, 11-dimethyl-2,6-methano-3-benzazocin-8-ol. This product is under study.
Use: Analgesic.

• **CYCLINDOLE.** USAN.
Use: Antidepressant.

• **CYCLIRAMINE MALEATE.** USAN.
Use: Antihistaminic.

• **CYCLIZINE,** U.S.P. XXI. Piperazine, 1-(diphenylme-thyl)-4-methyl-1-(Diphenylmethyl)-4-methyl pipera-zine.
Use: Antihistamine.
See: Marzine (hydrochloride)
Valoid (hydrochloride or lactate)

• **CYCLIZINE HYDROCHLORIDE,** U.S.P. XXI. Tab. U.S.P. XXI. 1-Diphenylmethyl-4-methylpiperazine. N-Benzhydryl-N-methyl piperazine.
Piperazine, 1-(diphenylmethyl)-4-methyl-,monohydrochloride.
Use: Antiemetic.
See: Marezine Hydrochloride and lactate, Preps. (Burroughs Wellcome)
W/Ergotamine tartrate, caffeine.
See: Migral, Tab. (Burroughs Wellcome)

• **CYCLIZINE LACTATE INJECTION,** U.S.P. XXI. A sterile soln. of cyclizine lactate in water for injection.
Use: Antihistamine, antiemetic.

CYCLOBARBITAL. 5-(1-Cyclohexen-1-yl)-5-ethylbar-bituric acid.
Use: Central depressant.

CYCLOBARBITAL CALCIUM. Cyclobarbitone, namuron, palinum, cyclobarbital Cal. 5-(1-Cyclohex-enyl)-5-Ethylbarbituric Acid.

Use: Hypnotic & sedative w/intermediate action.

CYCLOBARBITONE. B.A.N. 5-(Cyclohex-1-enyl)-5-ethylbarbituric acid.
Use: Hypnotic; sedative.
See: Phanodorm
Rapidal (calcium salt)

CYCLO-BELL. (Moore Kirk) Scopolamine HBr 0.0065 mg., hyoscyamine HBr 0.1037 mg., atropine sulfate 0.0194 mg., Triple Barb 5.4 mg., each of phenobarbital sodium, butabarbital sodium, pentobarbital sodium, 16.2 mg./Tab. Bot. 100s, 1000s.
Use: Antispasmodic and sedative.

• **CYCLOBENDAZOLE.** USAN.
Use: Anthelmintic.

CYCLOBENZAPRINE HCl. U.S.P. XXI. Tab., U.S.P. XXI. 5-(3-Dimethylamino-propylidene)-dibenzo(a.e.)-cycloheptatriene HCl.
Use: Relief of muscle spasm associated with acute, painful musculoskeletal conditions.
See: Flexeril, Tab. (Merck Sharp & Dohme)

CYCLOCORT. (Lederle) Amcinonide in Aquatain hydrophilic base 0.1%. Tubes 15 Gm., 30 Gm., 60 Gm.
Use: Topical corticosteroid.

CYCLOCUMAROL. 3,4-Dihydro-2-methoxy-2-methyl-4-phenyl-2H,5H-pyrano[3,2c][1]benzopyran-5-one.
Use: Anticoagulant.

CYCLOCOUMAROL. B.A.N. 3,4-Dihydro-2-methoxy-2-methyl-4-phenylpyrano[3,2-c]coumarin.
Use: Anticoagulant.
See: Cumopyran

CYCLOFENIL. B.A.N. 4,4′-Diacetoxybenz-hydrylidenecyclohexane.
Use: Treatment of infertility.
See: Ondonid
Sexovid

• **CYCLOFILCON A.** USAN.
Use: Contact lens material.

CYCLOGUANIL EMBONATE. B.A.N. 4,6-Diamino-1-(4-chlorophenyl)-1,2-dihydro-2,2-dimethyl-1,3,5-tria-zine compound with 4,4′-methylenedi-(3-hydroxy-2-naphthoic acid) (2:1).
Use: Antimalarial.

• **CYCLOGUANIL PAMOATE.** USAN. 4,6-Diamino-1-(p-chlorophenyl)-1,2-dihydro-2,2-dimethyl-s-triazine compound (2:1) with 4,4′-methylenebis-[3-hydroxy-2-naphthoic acid].
Use: Antimalarial.

CYCLOGYL. (Alcon) Cyclopentolate HCl. Sol. ½%, 1% & 2%. Droptainer 2 ml., 5 ml., 15 ml.
Use: Cycloplegic & mydriatic.

CYCLOHEPTENYLETHYL BARBITURIC ACID. Heptabarbital.

CYCLOHEXANE, 1,2,3,4,6,6-HEXACHLORO-. Benzene Hexachloride, Gamma.

• **CYCLOHEXIMIDE.** USAN.
Use: Antipsoriatic.

1-(CYCLOHEXYLAMINO)-2-PROPANOL BENZOATE (ESTER) HYDROCHLORIDE.
See: Hexylcaine Hydrochloride, U.S.P. XXI.

(3-CYCLOHEXYL-3-HYDROXY-3-PHENYLPROPYL)-TRIETHYLAMMONIUM CHLORIDE.
See: Tridihexethyl Chloride, U.S.P. XXI.

α-CYCLOHEXYL-α-PHENYL-1-PIPERIDINEPROPAN-OL HYDROCHLORIDE. Trihexyphenidyl
Hydrochloride, U.S.P. XXI.

CYCLOMETHYCAINE. B.A.N. 3-(2-Methylpiperidino)-propyl 4-cyclohexyloxybenzoate.
Use: Local anesthetic.
See: Surfathesin sulfate

CYCLOMETHYCAINE AND METHAPYRILENE.
See: Surfadil Cream, Lot. (Lilly)

• **CYCLOMETHYCAINE SULFATE,** U.S.P. XXI.
Creme, Jelly, Oint., Supp., U.S.P. XXI. 3-(2-Methyl-piperidino) propyl p-(cyclohexyloxy) benzoate sulfate.
Use: Topical anesthesia.
See: Surfacaine, Prep. (Lilly)
W/Methapyrilene.
See: Surfadil, Cream, Lot. (Lilly)

CYCLOMETHYCAINE AND THENYLPYRAMINE.
See: Surfadil Cream, Lot. (Lilly)

CYCLOMINE. (Tunex) Dicyclomine HCl 10 mg./ml.
Vial 10 cc.
Use: Antispasmodic.

CYCLOMYDRIL. (Alcon) Phenylephrine HCl 1%,
cyclopentolate HCl 0.2% in a sterile ophthalmic
solution. Bot. 7.5 ml. Droptainer 2 ml. & 5 ml.
Use: Mydriatic.

CYCLONIL. (Seatrace) Dicyclomine HCl 10 mg./ml.
Vial 10 cc.

CYCLOPAL. 5-Allyl-5(2-cyclopenten-1-yl)-barbituric
acid. Cyclopentenyl allylbarbituric acid.

CYCLOPAR. (Parke-Davis) Tetracycline HCl
250 mg. Cap. Bot. 100s, 1000s.
500 mg. Cap. Bot. 100s.
Use: Antibiotic.

CYCLOPENTAMINE. B.A.N. 1-Cyclopentyl-2-methylaminopropane.
Use: Vasoconstrictor.
See: Clopane (hydrochloride)

• **CYCLOPENTAMINE HYDROCHLORIDE,** U.S.P.
XXI. Nasal Soln., U.S.P. XXI. N-a-Dimethylcyclopen-taneethylamine HCl.
Use: Adrenergic (vasoconstrictor).
See: Clopane hydrochloride, nasal sol. (Dista)
W/Aludrine.
See: Aerolone Compound, Sol. (Lilly)
W/Chlorpheniramine.
See: Hista-Clopane, Pulvule (Lilly)

CYCLOPENTENYL - ALLYL - BARBITURIC ACID.
See: Cyclopal

• **CYCLOPENTHIAZIDE.** USAN. 6-Chloro-3-(cyclo-pen-tylmethyl)-3,4-dihydro-2H-1,2,4-benzothiadiazine-7-sulfonamide 1,1-dioxide.
Use: Diuretic, anti-hypertensive.
See: Navidrex

CYCLOPENTOLATE. B.A.N. 2-Dimethylaminoethyl 2-(1-hydrocyclopentyl)-2-phenylacetate.
Use: Mydriatic.
See: Cyclogyl
Mydrilate (hydrochloride)

• **CYCLOPENTOLATE HYDROCHLORIDE,** U.S.P.
XXI. Ophth. Soln., U.S.P. XXI. β-Di-methyl-aminoethyl

(1-hydroxycyclopentyl) phenylacetate HCl. 2-(Dime-thylamino)ethyl 1-Hydroxy-α-phenylcyclopentane-acetate HCl. Benzeneacetic acid, α-(1-hydroxy-cyclopentyl)-,2-(dimethylamino)ethyl ester,
hydrochloride.
Use: Anticholinergic (ophthalmic).
See: Cyclogyl, Sol. (Alcon)
W/Phenylephrine HCl.
See: Cyclomydril, Sol. (Alcon)

α-CYCLOPENTYL-α-PHENYL-1-PIPERIDINEPROPA-NOL HYDROCHLORIDE.
See: Cycrimine Hydrochloride, U.S.P. XXI.

CYCLOPENTYLPROPIONATE.
See: Depo-Testosterone, Vial (Upjohn)

• **CYCLOPHENAZINE HYDROCHLORIDE.** USAN.
Use: Antipsychotic.

CYCLOPHOSPHAMIDE. B.A.N. 2-[Di-(2-chloroethyl)-amino]-1-oxa-3-aza-2-phosphacyclohexane 2-oxide.
Use: Antineoplastic agent.
See: Cytoxan
Endoxana

• **CYCLOPHOSPHAMIDE,** U.S.P. XXI. Inj., Tabs.,
U.S.P. XXI. N,N-bis(2-Chloroethyl)-tetrahydro-,2-oxide, monodydrate. 2 H-1,3,2-Oxazaphosphorin-2-amine. phordiamidic acid cyclic ester monohydrate.
2-[bis(2-Chloroethyl) amino] tetrahydro-2H-1,3,2-ox-azaphosphorine-2-Oxide.
Use: Antineoplastic; Immunosuppressive.
See: Cytoxan, Tab., Vial (Mead Johnson)

• **CYCLOPROPANE,** U.S.P. XXI. Trimethylene.
Use: Inhalation anesthetic.

CYCLOPYRRONIUM BROMIDE. (Robins) 1-Ethyl-3-pyrrolidyl a-phenylcyclo-pentane-acetate metho-bromide.
Use: Anticholinergic.

CYCLORPHAN. (Roche) On trial.
Use: Morphine antagonist.

CYCLOSERINE. B.A.N. D-4-Aminoisoxazolid-3-one.
Use: Antibiotic.
See: Seromycin

• **CYCLOSERINE,** U.S.P. XXI. Caps., U.S.P. XXI. D-(+)-4-Amino-3-isoxazolidinone. 3-Isoxazolidinone, 4-amino-, (R)-. An antibiotic produced by *Streptomycin orchidaceus.* Oxamycin.
Use: Antibacterial (tuberculostatic).
See: Seromycin, Cap. (Lilly)

CYCLOSPASMOL CAPSULES. (Ives) Cyclandelate.
200 mg. or 400 mg./Cap. **200 mg.:** Bot. 100s,
500s, 1000s. Clinipak. **400 mg.:** Bot. 100s, 500s.
Clinipak.
Use: Vasodilator.

CYCLOSPASMOL TABLETS. (Ives) Cyclandelate 100
mg./Tab. Bot. 100s, 500s.
Use: Vasodilator.

• **CYCLOSPORINE.** USAN.
Use: Immunosuppressive.
See: Sandimmune, Inj., Oral Soln. (Sandoz)

CYCLO-TAB. (Jenkins) Butabarbital sod. 5.4 mg., pen-tobarbital sod. 5.4 mg., phenobarbital sod. 5.4 mg.,
hyoscyamine HBr 0.1037 mg., scopolamine HBr
0.0065 mg., atropine sulfate 0.0194 mg./Tab. Bot.
1000s.

• **CYCLOTHIAZIDE,** U.S.P. XXI. Tabs., U.S.P. XXI. 6-

Chloro-3-(2-norbornenyl-5)-7-sulfamyl-3,4-dihydro-
1,2,4-benzothiadiazine-1,   1-dioxide,-6-Chloro-3,4-
dihydro-3-(5-norbornen-2-yl)-2H-1,2,4-benzothiadiazi-
ne-7-sulfonamide-1,-1-Dioxide. Bot. 100s, 1000s.
Use: Diuretic.
See: Anhydron, Tab. (Lilly)
    Fluidil, Tab. (Adria)
CYCOSTAT HCl. Robenidine, B.A.N.
CYCRIMINE. B.A.N. 1-Cyclopentyl-1-phenyl-3-
piperidinopropan-1-ol.
Use: Treatment of the Parkinsonian syndrome.
CYCRIMINE HYDROCHLORIDE. a-Cyclopentyl-a-phe-
nyl-1-piperidine propanol HCl.
See: Pagitane Hydrochloride, Tab. (Lilly)
CYDEL. (Hauck) Cyclandelate 200 mg./Cap. Bot.
100s, 1000s.
Use: Vasodilator.
CYDONOL MASSAGE LOTION. (Gordon) Isopropyl
alcohol 14%, methyl salicylate, benzalkonium
chloride. Bot. 4 oz., gal.
Use: Massage lotion for feet.
• CYHEPTAMIDE. USAN.
Use: Anticonvulsant.
CYLERT CHEWABLE TABLETS. (Abbott) Pemoline
37.5 mg./Tab. Bot. 100s.
Use: Childhood attention-defect syndrome
(hyperkinetic syndrome).
CYLERT TABLETS. (Abbott) Pemoline 18.75, 37.5,
75 mg./Tab. Bot. 100s.
Use: Childhood attention-defect syndrome
(hyperkinetic syndrome).
p-CYMEN-3-OL. Thymol, N.F. XVI.
CYNOBAL. (Arcum) Cyanocobalamin injection Vial
100 mcg./cc. 30 cc. 1000/mcg./cc. 10 cc. 30 cc.
CYOMIN. (O'Neal, Jones & Feldman)
Cyanocobalamin 1000 mcg./ml. Vial 30 ml.
• CYPENAMINE HCL. USAN. 2-Phenylcyclopentyla-
mine Hydrochloride.
Use: Antidepressant.
• CYPOTHRIN. USAN.
Use: Insecticide.
• CYPRAZEPAM. USAN.
Use: Sedative.
CYPRENORPHINE. B.A.N. N-Cyclopropylmethyl-7,8-
dihydro-7α-(1-hydroxy-1-methylethyl)-O⁶-methyl-6,
14-endoethenonormorphine.
Use: Narcotic antagonist.
CYPROHEPTADINE. B.A.N. 4-(1,2:5,6-Dibenzo-
cycloheptatrienylidene)-1-methylpiperidine.
Use: Antihistamine.
See: Periactin
• CYPROHEPTADINE HYDROCHLORIDE, U.S.P.
XXI. Syrup, Tabs., U.S.P. XXI. 4-(5H-Dibenzo-
[a,d]cyclohepten-5-ylidene)-1-methylpiperidene
Hydrochloride. 1-Methyl-4-(5-dibenzo-[a,e]cyclo-
heptatrienylidene) piperidine HCl monohydrate.
Use: Antihistaminic; antipruritic.
See: Periactin, Tab., Syr. (Merck Sharp & Dohme)
• CYPROLIDOL HYDROCHLORIDE. USAN. Diphenyl
(2-(4-pyridyl)cyclo-propyl)-methanol hydrochloride.
Use: Psychotherapeutic drug.
• CYPROQUINATE. USAN.
Use: Coccidiostat (for poultry)

CYPROTERONE. B.A.N. 6-Chloro-17α-hydroxy-1α,2α-
methylenepregna-4,6-diene-3,20-dione.
Use: Antiandrogen.
• CYPROTERONE ACETATE. USAN. 6-Chloro-17-hy-
droxy-1α-2α-methylenepregna-4,6-diene-3, 20-dione
acetate.
Use: Anti-androgen.
• CYPROXIMIDE. USAN.
Use: Antidepressant.
CYREN A.
See: Diethylstilbestrol Prep. (Various Mfr.)
CYRIMINE HCl. 1-Phenyl-1-cyclopentyl-3-piperidino-
1-propanol HCl.
Use: Antispasmodic.
See: Pagitane HCl, Tab. (Lilly)
CYSTAMIN.
See: Methenamine, Tab. (Various Mfr.)
CYSTAMINE. (Tennessee) Methenamine 2 gr., phenyl
salicylate ½ gr., phenazopyridine HCl 10 mg.,
benzoic acid ⅛ gr., hyoscyamine sulfate ¹/₂₀₀₀ gr.,
atropine sulfate ¹/₂₀₀₀ gr./S.C. Tab. Bot. 100s,
1000s.
Use: Urinary tract infections.
CYSTEX. (CooperVision) Methenamine, salicylamide,
sodium salicylate, benzoic acid/Tab. Bot. 40s,
100s.
Use: Antibacterial and analgesic for relief of
symptoms of bladder and kidney irritation.
• CYSTINE. USAN. An essential amino acid. Delta—
Bot. 100 Gm.; Mann—Bot. 25 Gm.; Abbott—50
mg./ml. HCl salt solution.
Use: Amino acid replacement therapy, an additive
for infants on TPN.
• CYSTEINE HCL, U.S.P. XXI. Lotion, U.S.P. XXI.
L-Cysteine hydrochloride monohydrate.
Use: Amino acid for replacement therapy.
CYSTISED (IMPROVED). (Jenkins) Atropine sulfate
0.03 mg., hyoscyamine 0.03 mg., gelsemium 6.1
mg., methenamine 40.8 mg., salol 18.1 mg.,
benzoic acid 4.5 mg., methylene blue 5.4 mg./Tab.
Bot. 1000s.
CYSTITOL. (Vortech) Atropine sulfate 0.03 mg.,
hyoscyamine 0.03 mg., gelsemium 6.1 mg.,
methenamine 40.8 mg., salol 18.1 mg., benzoic
acid 4.5 mg./Tab. Bot. 1000s.
CYSTO. (Freeport) Methenamine 40.8 mg., methylene
blue 5.4 mg., phenyl salicylate 18.1 mg., atropine
sulfate 0.03 mg., hyoscyamine 0.03 mg., benzoic
acid 4.5 mg./Tab. Bot. 1000s.
Use: Cystitis, pyelitis, trigonitis in pregnancy,
urethritis.
CYSTO-CONRAY. (Mallinckrodt) Iothalamate meglumin
43%. Vial 50 ml., Pkg. 10s, 50s; 100 ml. Pkg. 6s.
Bot. 250 ml., Pkg. 6s. Dilution unit, 250 ml. 500 ml.
Bot. 6s.
Use: Radiopaque medium.
CYSTOGRAFIN. (Squibb) Meglumine diatrizoate 30%,
bound iodine 14%, EDTA 0.04%. Bot. 100 cc. Box
10s. 300 cc. Box 10s.
Use: Retrograde cystourethrography.
CYSTOGRAFIN-DILUTE. (Squibb) Diatrizoate, meglu-
mine 18% organically-bound iodine 85 mg./ml. Vial
300 ml, 500 ml.

Use: Contrast agent, retrograde cystourethrography.

CYSTOSOL. (Travenol) **Pre-diluted:** sorbitol 2.5 Gm., mannitol 0.5 Gm., hexitols 3%/100 ml. Bot. 1500 ml. **Conc.:** sorbitol 50 Gm., mannitol 10 Gm., hexitols 60%/100 ml. Bot. 150 ml., 500 ml.

CYSTO-SPAZ. (Webcon) l-Hyoscyamine 0.15 mg./Tab. Bot. 100s.
Use: Antispasmodic.

CYSTO-SPAZ-M. (Webcon) Hyoscyamine sulfate 375 mcg./Cap. Bot. 100s.

CYSTREA. (Moore Kirk) Methenamine 2 gr., phenyl salicylate ½ gr., methylene blue ⅛ gr., benzoic acid ¹⁄₁₀ gr., hyoscyamine alkaloid ¹⁄₂₀₀₀ gr., atropine sulfate ¹⁄₂₀₀₀ gr./Tab. Bot. 100s, 1000s.
Use: Urinary antiseptic.

CYTADREN. (Ciba) Aminoglutethimide 250 mg./Tab. Bot. 100s.
Use: Cushing's syndrome.

CYTAL, PRE-DILUTED. (Cutter) Sorbitol 2-7 Gm., mannitol 0.54 Gm./100 ml. Bot. 1500 ml.
Use: Urological irrigant.

• **CYTARABINE,** U.S.P. XXI. Sterile, U.S.P. XXI. 2(1H)-Pyrimidihone, 4-amino-1-β- -arabinofuranosyl- . 1-β- -Arabinofuranosylcytosine.
Use: Antineoplastic.
See: Cytosar, Inj. (Upjohn)

• **CYTARABINE HYDROCHLORIDE.** USAN. 1-Arabinoluranosylcytosine hydrochloride.
Use: Management of acute leukemias.
See: Cytosar-U, Vial (Upjohn)

CYTOMEL. (SmithKline) Liothyronine sod. L-triiodothyronine sod. Tab. 5 mcg., 25 mcg., 50 mcg. Bot. 100s. 25 mcg. Bot. 1000s.
Use: Treatment of inadequate endogenous thyroid production.

CYTOSAR-U. (Upjohn) Cytarabine (**20 mg./ml.**) 100 mg./5 ml. Vial 5 ml. w/5 ml. amp. diluent; (**50 mg./ml.**) 500 mg./10 ml. w/10 ml. amp. diluent.
Use: Management of acute granulocytic leukemias.

CYTOSINE ARABINOSIDE HCl. Cytarabine HCl.

CYTOSINE, 5-FLUORO-. Flucytosine, U.S.P. XIX.

CYTOX. (MPL) Cyanocobalamin 500 mcg., B-6 20 mg., B-1 100 mg., benzyl alcohol 2% in isotonic solution of sod. chloride./ml. Inj. Vial 10 cc.
Use: Treatment of polyneuritis, osteoarthritis, alcohol neuritis, migraine headache.

CYTOXAN. (Mead Johnson) Cyclophosphamide. **Vial.** 100 mg., 10 cc., 200 mg., 20 cc., 500 mg., 25 cc., 12s., 1 Gm., 2 Gm. **Tab.** 25 mg. or 50 mg. Bot. 100s, single unit pack 100s and Bot. 1000s 50 mg. only.
Use: Certain forms of cancer.

D

DAA.
See: Dihydroxy Aluminum Aminoacetate

• **DACARBAZINE,** U.S.P. XXI. For Inj., U.S.P. XXI. 5-(3,3-Dimethyltriazeno)-imidazole-4-carboxamide.
Use: Antineoplastic.
See: Dtic-Dome, Inj. (Miles Pharm)

DACRIOSE. (CooperVision) Isotonic, buffered solution

of purified water, sodium chloride, potassium chloride, sodium hydroxide, sodium phosphate, and preserved with benzalkonium chloride 0.01% and edetate disodium 0.03%. Bot. 0.5 oz., 1 oz., 4 oz.
Use: Ophthalmic irrigating solution.

• **DACTINOMYCIN,** U.S.P. XXI. Inj., U.S.P. XXI. Actinomycin D.
Use: Antineoplastic.
See: Cosmegen, Vial (Merck Sharp & Dohme)

DACURONIUM BROMIDE. B.A.N. 3α-Acetoxy-17β-hydroxy-5α-androstan-2β,16β-di-(1-methyl-1-piperidinium) dibromide.
Use: Neuromuscular blocking agent.

DAILY/JET. (Kirkman) Multiple vitamins. Bot. 100s.

DAILY VITAMIN LIQUID. (Bay) Vit. A 2500 I.U., D 400 I.U., E 15 I.U., C 60 mg., B-1 1.2 mg., B-2 1.2 mg., B-6 1.05 mg., B-12 4.5 mcg., nicainamide 13.5 mg./5 ml. Bot. 8 oz., pt., gal.
Use: Multivitamins.

DAILY VITAMINS. (Kirkman) Vit. A 5,000 I.U., D 400 I.U., C 50 mg., B-1 3 mg., B-2 2.5 mg., B-6 1 mg., B-12 1 mcg., niacinamide 20 mg., d-calcium pantothenate 1 mg./Tab. Bot. 100s.
Use: Multivitamins.

DAILY VITAMINS W/IRON. (Kirkman) Vit. A 5,000 I.U., D 400 I.U., B-1 2 mg., B-2 2.5 mg., B-6 1 mg., B-12 1 mcg., niacinamide 20 mg., d-calcium pantothenate 1 mg., iron 18 mg./Tab. Bot. 100s.
Use: Multivitamins with iron.

DAILY VITES. (Image) Multiple vitamin. Bot. 100s, 365s.
Use: Supplement.

DAINITE TABLETS. (Wallace) Aminophylline 200 mg., pentobarbital sodium 16 mg., ephedrine HCl 16 mg., dried aluminum hydroxide gel 160 mg., benzocaine 16 mg./Tab. Bot. 100s.
Use: Bronchodilator for treatment of bronchial asthma.

DAINITE-KI. (Wallace) Aminophylline 200 mg., phenobarbital 16 mg., ephedrine HCl 16 mg., potassium iodide 325 mg., dried aluminum hydroxide gel 160 mg., benzocaine 16 mg./Tab. Bot. 100s.
Use: Bronchodilator and expectorant combination for treatment of bronchial asthma.

DAISY 2 PREGNANCY TEST KIT. (Ortho) 2 tests per kit.
Use: Accurate pregnancy test result in 45 minutes, for use as 3 days after a missed period.

DAKIN'S SOLUTION.
See: Sodium Hypochlorite Solution Diluted.

DALALONE. (O'Neal, Jones & Feldman) Dexamethasone sodium phosphate 4 mg./ml. Vial 5 ml.

DALALONE I.L. (O'Neal, Jones & Feldman) Dexamethasone acetate 2 mg./ml. Vial 5 ml.

DALALONE L.A. (O'Neal, Jones & Feldman) Dexamethasone 8 mg./ml. Vial 5 cc.
Use: Adrenocortical steroid therapy.

DALALONE D.P. (O'Neal, Jones & Feldman) Dexamethasone acetate 16 mg./ml. Vial 1 ml. Box 5s; 2 ml. Box 10s.

DALCA. (Ascher) Phenylpropanolamine HCl 12.5 mg.,

magnesium salicylate 325 mg./Tab. Pkgs. 24s, 48s. Bot. 100s.
Use: Temporary relief of nasal congestion & headache.

DALCAINE. (O'Neal, Jones & Feldman) Lidocaine HCl 2%. Vial 2 ml. Box 10s.

DALEDALIN TOSYLATE. USAN. 3-Methyl-3-[3-(methylamino)propyl]-1-phenylindoline mono-p-toluene sulfonate.
Use: Antidepressant.

DALEX. (Dalin) Dextromethorphan HBr 45 mg., phenylephrine HCl 15 mg., chlorpheniramine maleate 6 mg., guaifenesin 180 mg., ammonium chloride 600 mg./Fl. oz. Syr., Bot. 4 oz., pt. Throat lozenge 10s, 18s. Cap. 20s. Pediatric, Bot. 4 oz. T.R. 15s.
Use: Coughs and colds.

DALICOTE. (Dalin) Hexachlorophene, pyrilamine maleate, diperodon HCl, 0.25%, dimethyl polysiloxane, silicone, zinc oxide, camphor. Lot. Bot. 4 fl. oz.
Use: Antihistaminic, antipruritic, anesthetic for chickenpox, pityriasis rosea, and allergic pruritus.

DALICREME. (Dalin) Vit. A 750 I.U., D 75 I.U., diperodon HCl 0.25%, quaternary ammonium cpd. Tubes: 1½ and 4 oz. Jar, 16 oz.
Use: Vit. A & D therapy.

DALIDERM LIQUID. (Dalin) Night applic. Ethyl alc, 66%, quat. ammonium cpd., carbolic acid, benzoic acid, salicylic acid, resorcin, camphor, tannic acid, soln. coal tar and chlorthymol. Bot. ½ oz., 1 oz.
Use: Antipruritic, fungicidal, deodorant liq.

DALIDERM POWDER. (Dalin) Zinc undecylenate, sod. propionate, quat. ammonium cpd., salicylic acid, boric acid, aluminum acetate, alum. Can 2 oz., 3½ oz.
Use: Antipruritic, fungicidal, deodorant pwdr.

DALIDYNE. (Dalin) Methylbenzethonium chloride, tannic acid, benzocaine, ethyl alcohol, benzyl alcohol, camphor, menthol, & chlorothymol. Lot. Bot. ¼, ½, 1 fl. oz.
Use: Cancrum, stomatitis, thrush, painful gums.

DALIDYNE JEL. (Dalin) Benzocaine, cherry-flavored base. Tube 10 Gm.

DALIDYNE THROAT SPRAY. (Dalin) Lidocaine, cetyldimethylbenzyl ammonium chloride, ethyl alcohol. Aerosol ⅓ oz.
Use: Anesthetic, antiseptic.

DALIFORT. (Dalin) Vit. A 25,000 I.U., D 400 I.U., C 500 mg., B-1 10 mg., B-2 5 mg., B-6 5 mg., B-12 5 mcg., niacinamide 100 mg., d-calcium pantothenate 20 mg., iron 10 mg., magnesium oxide 5 mg., zinc sulfate 1.5 mg., copper sulfate 1 mg./Tab. Bot. 30s, 100s.
Use: Vitamin-mineral dietary supplement.

DALIHIST. (Dalin) Phenylephrine HCl 0.5%, pyrilamine maleate 0.15%, cetyl benzyldimethyl ammon. chloride 0.04% in aq. isotonic sol. Nasal Spray 20 cc
Use: Decongestant, antihistaminic.

DALIMYCIN. (Dalin) Oxytetracycline HCl 250 mg./Cap. Bot. 24s, 100s.
Use: Broad spectrum antibiotic.

DALISEPT. (Dalin) Vit. A 750 I.U., D 75 I.U., diperodon HCl 1%, methylbenzethonium Cl 0.1%. Tubes, 2 & 4 oz. Jar, 16 oz.
Use: Antiseptic, anesthetic, Vit. A & D ointment.

DALIVIM FORTE. (Dalin) Iron ammonium citrate 18 gr., liver fraction 3 gr., Vit. B-12 60 mcg., A palmitate 10,000 I.U., D 1000 I.U., B-1 12 mg., B-2 4 mg., niacinamide 20 mg., Vit. B-6 2 mg., Ca pantothenate 12 mg., mixed tocopherols 30 mg., Ca glycerophosphate 65 mg., manganese glycerophosphate 17.5 mg./Oz. Bot. 4 oz., 8 oz., 16 oz.
Use: Hematinic and dietary supplement.

DALIVIM FORTE TABLETS. (Dalin) Fe fumarate 100 mg., liver desic. 150 mg., B-12 10 mcg., Vit. A palmitate 1667, D 167 I.U., C 50 mg., B-1 3 mg., B2 3 mg., niacinamide 10 mg., B-6 0.5 mg., cal. pantothenate 2 mg., cal. glycerophosphate 11 mg., manganese glycerophosphate 3 mg./Tab. Bot. 50s, 100s.
Use: Vitamin and mineral supplement.

DALLERGY CAPSULES. (Laser) Chlorpheniramine maleate 8 mg., phenylephrine HCl 20 mg., methscopolamine nitrate 2.5 mg./Cap. Bot. 100s, 1000s.
Use: Antihistaminic, decongestant, antisecretory.

DALLERGY SYRUP. (Laser) Chlorpheniramine maleate 2 mg., phenylephrine HCl 10 mg., methscopolamine nitrate 0.625 mg./5 ml. Bot. pt., gal.
Use: Antihistaminic, decongestant, antisecretory.

DALLERGY TABLETS. (Laser) Chlorpheniramine maleate 4 mg., phenylephrine HCl 10 mg., methscopolamine nitrate 1.25 mg./Tab. Bot. 100s, 1000s.
Use: Antihistiminic, decongestant, antisecretory.

DALMANE. (Roche) Flurazepam HCl 15 mg., 30 mg./Cap. Bot. 100s, 500s. Tel-E-Dose pkg. 100s. Prescription Pak 30s, 300s. Teledose 100s (4 rolls x 25 Caps.), RNP (Reverse Numbered Packages).
Use: Hypnotic agent.

D-ALPHA-E CAP. (Alto) di-Alpha-tocopherol acetate 100 mg. I.U./Cap. Bot. 100s.
Use: Vit. E therapy.

DAMASON-P. (Mason) Hydrocodone bitartrate 5 mg., aspirin 224 mg., caffeine 32 mg./Tab. Bot. 100s, 500s.
Use: Analgesic, antitussive.

DAMBOSE.
See: Inositol, Tabs.

D-AMP. (Dunhall) Ampicillin trihydrate 500 mg./Cap. Bot. 100s. **Susp.** 250 mg./5 cc. Bot. 200 cc.
Use: Antibiotic.

DANATROL CAPSULES. (Winthrop Products) Danazol.
Use: Gonadotropin inhibitor.

• **DANAZOL,** U.S.P. XXI. Caps., U.S.P. XXI. 17α-Pregna-2,4-dien-20-yno-[2,3-d]isoxazol-17-ol.
Use: Pituitary gonadotropin suppressant.
See: Danocrine, Cap. (Winthrop-Breon)

DANDRUFF SHAMPOO. (Walgreen) Zinc pyrithione. Bot. 11 oz. Tube 7 oz.
Use: Dandruff control.

DANEX PROTEIN ENRICHED DANDRUFF SHAMPOO. (Herbert) Pyrithione zinc 1%. Bot. 4 oz.
Use: Antidandruff.

DANIVAC. (Fellows) 1, 8-Dihydroxyanthraquinone (Danthron) 75 mg./Tab. Bot. 1000s.
Use: Constipation.

DANOCRINE. (Winthrop-Breon) Danazol 50 mg., 100 mg., or 200 mg./Cap. Bot. 100s.
Use: Treatment of endometriosis, fibrocystic breast disease, hereditary angioedema.

DANOGAR TABLETS. (Winthrop Products) Danazol.
Use: Gonadotropin inhibitor.

DANOL CAPSULES. (Winthrop Products) Danazol.
Use: Gonadotropin inhibitor.

DANTHANE. (Western Research) Danthron 75 mg./Tab. Handicount 28 (36 bags of 28s)
Use: Cathartic

• **DANTHRON,** U.S.P. XXI. Tabs., U.S.P. XXI. 1,8-Dihydroxy-anthraquinone, dioxyanthraquinone, Chrysazin.
Use: Cathartic.
See: Danivac, Tab. (Fellows-Testagar)
  Danthane, Tab. (Western Research)
  Dorbane, Tab. (Riker)
  Modane, Prod. (Adria)
W/d-Calcium pantothenate.
See: Dantrolax, Tab. (Wolins)
  Danvac, Tab. (Kenyon)
  Parlax, Tab. (Parmed)
  Weslax, Tab. (Western Research)
W/Calcium docusate.
See: Doxidan, Cap. (Hoechst)
W/Chondrus drispus, prune concentrate.
See: Acelax, Tab. (Marcen)
W/Docusate sodium.
See: Doctate-P, Cap. (Glaxo)
  Dorbantyl, Cap. (Riker)
  Dorbantyl Forte, Cap., (Riker)
  Doxan, Tab. (Hoechst)
  Doxate-D, Tab. (Dunhall)
  Guarsol, Tab. (Western Research)
W/Oxyethylene oxpropylene polymer, B-1, carboxymethyl cellulose.
See: Evactol, Cap. (Delta)
W/Sod. lauryl sulfate.

DANTRIUM. (Norwich Eaton) Dantrolene sodium 25 mg./Cap. Bot. 100s, 500s, & Unit dose 100s; 50 mg./Cap. Bot. 100s; 100 mg./Cap. Bot. 100s, unit dose 100s.
Use: Skeletal muscle relaxant, prophylaxis of malignant hyperthermia.

DANTRIUM I.V. (Norwich Eaton) Dantrolene sodium 20 mg./Vial.
Use: Treatment of malignant hyperthermia.

DANTROLAX. (Wolins) Danthron 75 mg., D-calcium pantothenate 25 mg./Tab. Bot. 1000s.

• **DANTROLENE.** USAN. 1(((5-(4-nitrophenyl) -2-furanyl) methylene) amino)-2, 4- nidazolidinedione.
Use: Skeletal muscle relaxant.

• **DANTROLENE SODIUM.** USAN.
See: Dantrium, Cap. (Norwich Eaton)

DANVAC. (Kenyon) Danthron 37.5 mg., 75 mg., d-calcium pantothenate 12.5 mg., 25 mg./Tab. Bot. 100s.
Use: Laxative.

DAPA TABLETS. (Ferndale) Acetaminophen 324 mg./Tab. Bot. 100s.
Use: Analgesic.

DAPCO. (Schlicksup) Salicylamide 300 mg., butabarbital 15 mg./Tab. Bot. 100s, 1000s.
Use: Analgesic w/sedative.

DAPEX. (Ferndale) Phentermine HCl 37.5 mg./Cap. Bot. 100s.
Use: Anorectic.

• **DAPSONE,** U.S.P. XXI. Tabs., U.S.P. XXI. Benzenamine, 4,4′-sulfonyl-bis-. Diaminodiphenylsulfone. 4,4′-Sulfonyldianiline.
Use: Treatment of leprosy; dermatitis herpetiformis suppressant.
See: Avlosulfon, Tab. (Ayerst)

DAPTAZOLE. Amiphenazole, B.A.N.

DARAGEN. (Owen) Collagen polypeptide and benzalkonium chloride in a mild amphoteric base. Bot. 8 oz.
Use: Hair repair shampoo.

DARA SOAPLESS SHAMPOO. (Owen) Purified water, potassium coco hydrolyzed protein, sulfated castor oil, pentasodium triphosphate, sodium benzoate, sodium lauryl sulfate, fragrance. Bot. 8 oz., 16 oz.
Use: For people with sensitive scalp.

DARANIDE. (Merck Sharp & Dohme) Dichlorphenamide. Tab. 50 mg. Bot. 100s.
Use: Carbonic anhydrase inhibitor for reduction of intraocular pressure in glaucoma.

DARAPRIM. (Burroughs Wellcome) Pyrimethamine 25 mg./Tab. Bot. 100s.
Use: Orally, antimalarial.

DARBID. (SmithKline) Isopropamide Iodide 5 mg./Tab. Bot. 50s.
Use: Anticholinergic.
W/Compazine.
See: Combid, Cap. (SmithKline)

DARENTHIN. Bretylium Tosylate, B.A.N.

DARICON. (Beecham Labs) Oxyphencyclimine HCl 10 mg./Tab. Bot. 60s, 500s.
Use: G-I & G-U disorders.

DARICON-PB. (Beecham Labs) Oxyphencyclimine HCl 5 mg., phenobarbital 15 mg./Tab. Bot. 100s.
Use: Anticholinergic with sedative.

DARO TABLETS-C.T. (Fellows) Dextroamphetamine HCl 5 mg./Tri-tab. Bot. 100s, 1000s, 5000s.

DARO TIMED CAPSULES. (Fellows) d-Amphetamine HCl 15 mg./Cap. Bot. 100s, 1000s.

DARVISIL. Diaveridine, B.A.N.

DARVOCET-N 50. (Lilly) Propoxyphene napsylate 50 mg., acetaminophen 325 mg./Tab. Bot. 100s (Rx Pak), 500s; Blister pkg. 10 × 10s; Rx Pak 20 × 50s.
Use: Analgesic.

DARVOCET-N 100. (Lilly) Propoxyphene napsylate 100 mg., acetaminophen 650 mg./Tab. Bot. 100s (Rx Pak), 500s; Blister pkg. 10 × 10s; 500 single cut

blisters; Unit dose rolls 20 × 25s; Rx Pak 25 × 30s.
Use: Relief of mild to moderate pain.
DARVON. (Lilly) Propoxyphene HCl **32** mg./Pulvule. Bot. 100s (Rx Pak), 500s; Blister pkg. 10 × 10s. **65 mg.**/Pulvule. Bot. 100s (Rx Pak), 500s; Blister pkg. 10 × 10s; 500 single-cut individually labeled blisters; Unit dose 20 rolls × 25s; Rx Pak 25 × 30s, 20 × 50s.
Use: Analgesic.
DARVON COMPOUND. (Lilly) Propoxyphene HCl 32 mg., aspirin 389 mg., caffeine 32.4 mg./Pulvule. Bot. 100s (Rx Pak), 500s.
Use: Antipyretic and analgesic.
DARVON COMPOUND-65. (Lilly) Propoxyphene HCl 65 mg., aspirin 389 mg., caffeine 32.4 mg./Pulvule Bot. 100s (Rx Pak), 500s; Blister pkg. 10 × 10s; Unit dose 20 rolls × 25s.
Use: Acute, chronic or recurrent pain.
DARVON-N. (Lilly) Propoxyphene napsylate **Tabs.**: 100 mg./Tab. Bot. 100s (Rx Pak), 500s; Blister pkg. 10 × 10s; Rx Pak 20 × 50s. **Susp.** 50 mg./5 ml. Bot. 16 fl oz.
W/A.S.A. Propoxyphene napsylate 100 mg., aspirin 325 mg./Tab. Bot. 100s (Rx Pak), 500s; 500 single-cut individually labeled blisters.
Use: Analgesic.
DARVON WITH A.S.A. (Lilly) Darvon 65 mg., A.S.A. 325 mg./Pulvule. Bot. 100s (Rx Pak), 500s.
Use: Analgesic without caffeine.
DA-SED TABLET. (Sheryl) Butabarbital ½ gr./Tab. Tab. 100s.
Use: For mild, prolonged "daytime" sedation.
DASIKON. (Beecham Labs) Chlorpheniramine maleate 2 mg., caffeine 32 mg., acetylsalicylic acid 195 mg., phenacetin 130 mg., atropine sulfate 0.065 mg./Cap. Bot. 1000s.
Use: Colds.
DASIN. (Beecham Labs) Ipecac 3 mg., acetylsalicylic acid 130 mg., phenacetin 100 mg., camphor 15 mg., caffeine 8 mg., atropine sulfate 0.13 mg./Cap. Bot. 100s, 1000s.
Use: Analgesic, antipyretic, diaphoretic.
D-ASMA-S. (Dunhall) Secobarbital sodium 16.2 mg., ephedrine sulfate 8.1 mg./5 ml. w/alcohol 9%. Bot. Pt.
Use: Anti-asthmatic.
DATRIL EXTRA STRENGTH CAPSULES. (Bristol-Myers) Acetaminophen 500 mg./Cap. Bot. 24s, 50s.
Use: Analgesic.
DATRIL EXTRA STRENGTH TABLETS. (Bristol-Myers) Acetaminophen 500 mg./Tab. Bot. 30s, 60s, 100s.
Use: Analgesic.
DATURINE HBr.
See: Hyoscyamine Salts (Var. Mfr.)
DAUNORUBICIN. B.A.N.
Use: Antineoplastic.
• **DAUNORUBICIN HCL,** U.S.P. XXI. For Inj., U.S.P. XXI. An antibiotic produced by *Streptomyeces ceruleorubidus.* 3-Acetyl-1,2,3,-4,6,11-hexahydro-3,5,

12-trihydroxy-10-methoxy-6,11-dioxonaphthacen-1-yl-3-amino-2,3,6-trideoxy-β-D-galactopyranoside.
Use: Antineoplastic.
See: Cerubidin, Inj. (Ives)
• **DAUNORUBICIN HYDROCHLORIDE.** USAN.
Use: Antineoplastic.
DAVITAMON K.
See: Menadione Inj., Tab. (Various Mfr.)
DAVOSIL. (Hoyt) Silicon carbide in glycerin base. Jar 8 oz., 10 oz.
Use: Clean and polish teeth.
DAYALETS. (Abbott) Vit. B-1 1.5 mg., B-2 1.7 mg., A 5000 I.U., C 60 mg., D 400 I.U. niacinamide 20 mg., B-6 2 mg., B-12 6 mcg., E 30 I.U., folic acid 0.4 mg./Filmtab. Bot. 100s. Abbo-Pac 100s.
Use: Vitamin.
DAYALETS PLUS IRON. (Abbott) Vit. B-1 1.5 mg., B-2 1.7 mg., niacinamide 20 mg., B-6 2 mg., C 60 mg., A 5000 I.U., D 400 I.U., E 30 I.U., B-12 6 mcg., iron 18 mg., folic acid 0.4 mg./Filmtab. Bot. 100s.
Use: Dietary supplement.
DAY CAPS. (Towne) Vit. A 5,500 I.U., D 400 I.U., B-1 3 mg., B-2 3 mg., B-6 0.5 mg., B-12 4 mcg., C 50 mg., Ca pantothenate 5 mg., niacinamide 20 mg./Cap. Bot. 120s, 300s.
DAY CAP TABS-M. (Towne) Vit. A 5,500 I.U., D 400 I.U., B-1 3 mg., B-2 3 mg., B-6 0.5 mg., B-12 4 mcg., C 50 mg., niacinamide 20 mg., Ca pantothenate 5 mg., l-Lysine HCl 15 mg., Fe 10 mg., Zn 1.5 mg., Mn 1 mg., iodine 0.1 mg., Cu 1 mg., K 5 mg., Mg 6 mg./Captab Bot. 100s, 250s.
DAY SWEET. (Towne) Vit. A 5000 I.U., D 400 I.U., E 30 I.U., C 60 mg., folic acid 0.4 mg., B-1 1.5 mg., B-2 1.7 mg., niacin 20 mg., B-6 2 mg., B-12 6 mcg./Tab. Bot. 100s.
DAY-TABS. (Towne) Vit. A 5000 I.U., D 400 I.U., B-1 1.5 mg., B-2 1.7 mg., C 60 mg., niacinamide 20 mg., B-6 2 mg., folic acid 0.1 mg., pantothenic acid 10 mg., B-12 5 mcg./Tab. Bot. 100s, 200s.
DAY-TABS PLUS IRON. (Towne) Iron 18 mg., Vit. A 5000 I.U., D 400 I.U., B-1 1.5 mg., B-2 1.7 mg., niacinamide 20 mg., C 60 mg., B-6 2 mg., pantothenic acid 10 mg., B-12 5mcg., folic acid 0.1 mg./Tab. Bot. 100s.
DAY-VITE. (Drug Industries) Vit. A 10,000 I.U., D-3 1000 I.U., E 10 I.U., C 100 mg., B-1 5 mg., B-2 5 mg., B-6 2 mg., B-12 2 mcg., niacinamide 25 mg., Ca pantothenate 10 mg./Tab. Bot. 100s, 500s.
Use: Dietary supplement.
• **DAZANDROL MALEATE.** USAN.
Use: Antidepressant.
• **DAZOPRIDE FUMARATE.** USAN.
• **DAZOXIBEN HYDROCHLORIDE.** USAN.
Use: Antithrombotic.
DB ELECTRODE PASTE. (Day-Baldwin) Tube 5%.
DBED. Dibenzylethylenediamine dipenicillin G.
See: Benzathine penicillin G Susp.
DCA
See: Desoxycorticosterone acetate Preps. (Various Mfr.)
D-CAINE. (Century) Dibucaine 1%, with rectal tube. 1 oz.

Use: Local anesthetic.
DDAVP. (Centerchem) Desmopressin acetate 0.1 mg./ml. Vial 2.5 ml. w/applicator tubes.
Use: Antidiuretic therapy.
DDAVP. (USV Labs.) Desmopressin acetate 0.1 mg., chlorobutanol 5.0 mg., sodium chloride 9.0 mg./ml. Vial 2.5 ml. w/applicator tubes.
Use: Antidiuretic therapy in central diabetes insipidus.
D-DIOL. (Burgin-Arden) Testosterone cypionate 50 mg., estradiol cypionate 2 mg./cc. Vial 10 cc.
DDS.
See: Dapsone Tab., U.S.P. XXI.
DDT.
See: Chlorophenothane.
DEACETYLLANATOSIDE C.
See: Deslanoside, U.S.P. XXI.
DEADLY NIGHTSHADE LEAF, U.S.P.
See: Belladonna Leaf, U.S.P. XXI.
DEANOL. B.A.N. 2-Dimethylaminoethanol.
Use: Central nervous system stimulant.
See: Deaner, Tab. (Riker)
DEANOL ACETAMIDOBENZOATE. (2-Di-methylaminoethanol as the p-acetamido-benzoic acid salt).
See: Deaner, Tab. (Riker)
DEAPRIL-ST. (Mead Johnson) Dihydrogenated ergot alkaloids (ergoloid mesylates): dihydroergocornine, dihydroergocristine, & dihydroergokryptine as the mesylates, 1:1:1 ratio. Bot. 100s 1 mg. sublingual Tab.
Use: Selected symptoms in elderly patients.
DEBA.
See: Barbital (Various Mfr.)
DEBRIDING (enzymatic) AGENT, VETERINARY USE.
See: Dornavac Prods. (Merck, Sharp & Dohme)
DEBRISAN. Dextranomer, B.A.N.
DEBRISAN. (Pharmacia) Spherical hydrophilic beads, 0.1-0.3 mm diameter. Bot. 60 Gm., 120 Gm. Pks. 7 × 4g, 14 × 14g. U.S. distributor Johnson & Johnson Products.
Use: Cleansing exuding lesions such as venous stasis ulcers, decubitus ulcers, infected traumatic and surgical wounds, and infected burns.
• **DEBRISOQUIN SULFATE.** USAN. 3,4-Dihydro-2(1H)-isoquinolinecarboxamidine sulfate. Formerly Isocaramidine Sulfate
Use: Hypotensive agent.
DEBRISOQUINE. B.A.N. 2-Amidino-1,2,3,4-tetra-hydroisoquinoline.
Use: Hypotensive.
See: Declinax (sulfate)
DEBROX. (Marion) Carbamide peroxide 6.5% in anhydrous glycerol. Plastic Squeeze Bot. 0.5 oz., 1 oz.
Use: Excess ear wax.
DECA-BON. (Barrows) Vit. A 3000 I.U., D 400 I.U., C 60 mg., B-1 1 mg., B-2 1.2 mg., niacinamide 8 mg., B-6 1 mg., panthenol 3 mg., B-12 1 mcg., biotin 30 mcg./0.6 cc. Drops Bot. 50 cc. Chewable Tabs. Bot. 100s, 250s.
Use: Vitamin supplement.

DECADERM IN ESTERGEL. (Merck Sharp & Dohme) Dexamethasone 0.1% w/isopropyl myristate gel, wood alcohols, refined lanolin alcohol, micro-crystalline wax, anhydrous citric acid, anhydrous sod. phosphate dibasic. Tube 30 Gm.
Use: Corticosteroid (glucocorticoid).
DECADROL. (Paddock) Dexamethasone sodium phosphate 4 mg./cc. Vial 5 cc.
Use: Corticosteroid.
DECADRON. (Merck Sharp & Dohme) Dexamethasone. **Tabs.** 0.25 mg., Bot. 100s; 0.5 mg., Bot. 100s, 1000s. Single unit pkg. 100s; 0.75 mg., 5-12 Pak, 12s, Bot. 100s, 1000s. Single unit pkg. 100s; 1.5 mg. Bot. 50s. Single unit pkg. 100s; 4 mg. Bot. 50s. Single unit pkg. 100s.
Elixir 0.5 mg./5 ml., benzoic acid 0.1%, alcohol 5% Bot. w/dropper 100 ml., Bot. w/out dropper 237 ml.
W/Neomycin sulfate.
See: NeoDecadron, Ophth. Soln., Ophth. Oint., Cream (Merck Sharp & Dohme)
NeoDecaspray topical aerosol. (Merck Sharp & Dohme)
DECADRON-LA SUSPENSION. (Merck Sharp & Dohme) Dexamethasone acetate equiv. to 8 mg. dexamethasone/1ml. w/sod. chloride 6.67 mg., creatinine 5 mg., disodium edetate 0.5 mg., sodium carboxymethylcellulose 5 mg., polysorbate 80 0.75 mg., sod. hydroxide, benzyl alcohol 9 mg., water for injection, sod. bisulfite 1 mg./1 ml. Vials 1 ml., 5 ml.
Use: Corticosteroid (glucocorticoid).
DECADRON PHOSPHATE. (Merck Sharp & Dohme) Dexamethasone sod. phosphate.
Ophth. Sol. 0.1% w/creatinine, sod. citrate, sod. borate, polysorbate 80, sodium hydroxide (hydrochloric acid for Ocumeter disodium edetate, water for inj., Sod. Bisulfite 0.32% (0.1% for Ocumeter), phenylethanol 0.25%, benzalkonium Cl 0.02%. Dropper Bot. 2.5 ml., 5 ml.
Use: Corticosteroid responsive inflammatory conditions of the eye and ear.
Ophth. Oint. 0.05% w/white petrolatum and mineral oil. Tube 3.5 gm.
Use: Corticosteroid responsive inflammatory conditions of the eye or ear.
Ocumeter Ophth. Sol. 0.1%, 5 ml. plastic dispenser with controlled dropper tip.
Topical Cream 0.1% w/stearyl alcohol, cetyl alcohol, mineral oil, polyoxyl 40 stearate, sorbitol sol., methyl polysilicone emul., creatinine, purified water, sod. citrate, disod. edetate, sod. hydroxide, methylparaben 0.15%, sorbic acid 0.1%. Tube 15 Gm., 30 Gm.
Use: Corticosteroid responsive dermatoses.
Turbinaire Each metered spray dispenses 0.1 mg. dexamethasone sodium phosphate equivalent to 0.084 mg. dexamethasone w/fluorochlorohydrocarbons as propellants and alcohol 2%. Aerosol container 170 sprays w/nasal applicator; refill package without nasal applicator.
Use: Allergic or inflammatory nasal conditions.

W/Neomycin
  Use: Corticosteroid, antibiotic.
  See: NeoDecadron, Ophth. Soln., Ophth. Oint.,
  Cream (Merck Sharp & Dohme)
    Neo-Decaspray, topical aerosol (Merck Sharp &
    Dohme)
W/Xylocaine **Inj.** Dexamethasone phosphate 4 mg.,
  lidocaine HCl 10 mg., citric acid 10 mg., creatinine
  8 mg., sodium bisulfite 0.5 mg., disodium edetate
  0.5 mg., sod. hydroxide, water, methylparaben 1.5
  mg., propylparaben 0.2 mg./ml. Vial 5 ml.
  Use: Corticosteriod (glucocorticoid).
DECADRON PHOSPHATE INJECTION. (Merck Sharp
  & Dohme) Dexamethasone sod. phosphate 4
  mg./ml. and 24 mg./ml., with creatinine 8 mg., sod.
  citrate 10 mg., disodium edetate 0.5 mg. (24
  mg./ml, only), sod. hydroxide, sod. bisulfite 1 mg.,
  methylparaben 1.5 mg., propylparaben 0.2 mg./ml.
  4 mg./ml.: Disposable syringe 1 ml., 2.5 ml., 1s.;
  Vial 1 ml., 25s.; Vial 5 ml. 1s.; Vial 25 ml. 1s. **24
  mg./ml.** (for I.V. use only): Vial 5 ml., 1s; 10 ml.,
  1s.
  Use: Corticosteroid (glucocorticoid).
DECADRON PHOSPHATE RESPIHALER. (Merck
  Sharp & Dohme) Each metered spray dispenses
  dexamethasone sodium phosphate equivalent to
  0.1 mg. dexamethasone phosphate or 0.084 mg.
  dexamethasone, w/fluorochlorohydrocarbons as
  propellants, alcohol 2%. Aerosol for oral inhalation,
  170 sprays in pressurized container. Refill package.
  Use: Bronchial asthma treatment.
DECA-DURABOLIN. (Organon) Nandrolone decanoate
  injection w/benzyl alcohol 10%. **50 mg./ml.** Amp.
  1 ml. Box 4s; Multidose Vial 2 ml. **100 mg./ml.**
  Multidose Vial 2 ml. Box 1s, 25s. 200 mg./ml.
  Multidose vial 1 ml. Box 1s, 25s.
  Use: I.M. depot-anabolic.
DECA-DURABOLIN REDIJECT SYRINGES. (Organon)
  Nandrolone decanoate. 200 mg./ml., 100 mg./ml.,
  50 mg./ml. Syringes 1 ml. Box 25s.
  Use: Depot-anabolic.
**DECAHYDRO-4α,7,9-TRIHYDROXY-2-METHYL-6,8-
  BIS(METHYLAMINO)-4H-PYRANO 2,3-β[1,4]BEN-
  ZODIOXIN-4-ONE DIHYDROCHLORIDE PEN-
  TAHYDRATE.** Sterile Spectinomycin Hydrochloride,
  U.S.P. XXI.
DECAJECT 5 AND 10. (Mayrand) Dexamethasone
  sod. phosphate 4 mg./ml. Vial 10 ml.
  Use: Anti-inflammatory corticosteroid.
DECAJEST LA. (Mayrand) Dexamethasone acetate 8
  mg./ml. Vial 5 ml.
  Use: Anti-inflammatory corticosteroid.
DE-CAL. (Vortech) Calcium 250 mg., Vit. D 1.25 u./Tab.
  Bot. 100s, 1000s.
  Use: Calcium and Vitamin D therapy.
DECALIX. (Pharmed) Dexamethasone 0.5 mg./5 ml.
  Bot. 100 ml.
  Use: Adrenocortical steroid therapy.
DECAMETH. (Foy) Dexamethasone sodium
  phosphate inj. 4 mg./5cc vial.
  Use: Adrenocortical steroid therapy.
DECAMETH L.A. (Foy) Dexamethasone sodium

phosphate injection. 8 mg./ml.; 5 ml. vials.
  Use: Steroid therapy.
DECAMETH TABLETS. (Foy) Dexamethasone 0.75
  mg./Tab. Bot. 1000s.
  Use: Steroid therapy.
DECAMETHONIUM BROMIDE.
  Use: Muscle relaxant.
  See: Syncurine, Vial (Burroughs Wellcome)
DECAMETHONIUM IODIDE. B.A.N.
  Decamethylenedi(trimethylammonium iodide).
  Use: Muscle relaxant.
  See: Eulissin
DECAPRYN. (Merrell Dow) Doxylamine succinate.
  12.5 mg./Tab. Bot. 100s.
  Use: Antihistamine.
W/Pyridoxine HCl.
  See: Bendectin, Tab. (Merrell Dow)
DECASONE INJECTION. (Fellows) Dexamethasone
  sod. phosphate equiv. to dexamethasone
  phosphate 4 mg./cc. Vial 5 cc.
DECASPRAY. (Merck Sharp & Dohme) Topical
  dexamethasone aerosol. Every second of spray
  dispenses approximately 0.075 mg. of dexametha-
  sone. Dexamethasone 10 mg., isopropyl myristate,
  isobutane in pressurized container 25 Gm.
  Use: Corticosteroid responsive dermatoses.
• **DECAVITAMIN CAPSULES AND TABLETS,** U.S.P.
  XXI. Vit. A 4000 I.U., D 400 I.U., C 70 mg., calcium
  pantothenate 10 mg., B-12 5 mcg., folic acid 100
  mcg., nicotinamide 20 mg., B-6 2 mg., B-2 2 mg.,
  B-1 2 mg./Cap. or Tab.
  Use: Vitamin therapy.
DECCASOL-T. (Kenyon) Vit. B-1 10 mg., B-2 5 mg.,
  B-6 2 mg., pantothenic acid 10 mg., niacinamide 30
  mg., B-12 3 mcg., C 100 mg., E 5 I.U., A 10,000 I.U.,
  D 1000 I.U., Fe 15 mg., Cu 1 mg., Mn 1 mg., Mg 5
  mg., Zn 1.5 mg./Tab. Bot. 100s.
DECCOX. Decoquinate, B.A.N.
DECHOLIN. (Miles Pharm) Dehydrocholic acid 250
  mg./Tab. Bot. 100s, 500s, 1000s.
  Use: Laxative.
DECHOLIN SODIUM. (Miles Pharm) Sodium
  dehydrocholate 20% aqueous sol. Amp. 5cc, Boxes
  20 amps.
  Use: Diagnostic.
DECHLORISON ACETATE. 9-alpha, 11-beta, di-chloro-
  1,4-pregnadiene-17-alpha, 21-diol-3,20-dione-21 ac-
  etate. Diloderm.
DECICAIN. Tetracaine HCl.
• **DECLENPERONE.** USAN.
  Use: Sedative.
DECLOFEN SR CAPSULES. (U.S. Ethicals)
  Theophylline 250 mg./S.R. Cap. Bot. 100s.
  Use: Prolonged relief and/or prevention of
  symptoms of asthma and reversible bronchospasm.
DECLOMYCIN HCl. (Lederle) **Cap.** Demeclocycline
  HCl 150 mg./Cap. Bot. 100s. **Tab.** 150 mg./Tab.,
  Bot. 100s; 300 mg./Tab. Bot. 12s, 48s
  Use: Broad spectrum antibiotic.
DECOBEL LANACAPS. (Lannett) Belladonna
  alkaloids 0.128 mg., phenylpropanolamine HCl 50

mg., chlorpheniramine maleate 1 mg., pheniramine maleate 12.5 mg./Cap. Bot. 100s, 1000s.
Use: Decongestant.

DECOHIST CAPSULES. (Towne) Chlorpheniramine maleate 1 mg., phenylpropanolamine HCl 12.5 mg., salicylamide 180 mg., caffeine 15 mg./Cap. Bot. 18s.
Use: Antihistaminic.

DECOJEN. (Jenkins) Aspirin 2.5 gr., chlorpheniramine maleate 1.25 mg., phenylephrine HCl 2.5 mg./Tab. Bot. 1000s.
Use: Nasal decongestant.

DECOJEN INJECTION. (Jenkins) Atropine sulfate 0.2 mg., phenylpropanolamine HCl 12.5 mg., chlorpheniramine maleate 5 mg., water for injection q.s./cc. Vials 10 cc. 12s.

DECOLONE-50. (Kay) Nandrolone decanoate 50 mg., or 100 mg./ml. Vial 2 ml.
Use: anabolic.

DECONAMINE ELIXIR. (Berlex) Chlorpheniramine maleate 2 mg., d-pseudoephedrine HCl 30 mg., alcohol 15%/5 ml. Bot. 473 ml.
Use: Antihistaminic, decongestant.

DECONAMINE SR CAPSULES. (Berlex) Chlorpheniramine maleate 8 mg., d-pseudoephedrine HCl 120 mg./Cap. Bot. 100s, 500s.
Use: Antihistaminic-decongestant.

DECONAMINE SYRUP. (Berlex) Chlorpheniramine maleate 2 mg., d-pseudoephedrine HCl 30 mg./ 5 ml. Bot. 473 ml.
Use: Antihistaminic-decongestant.

DECONAMINE TABLETS, DYE-FREE. (Berlex) Chlorpheniramine maleate 4 mg., d-pseudoephedrine HCl 60 mg./Tab. Bot. 100s, 500s.
Use: Antihistaminic, decongestant.

DECONGESTANT. (Century) Atropine sulfate 0.2 mg., chlorpheniramine maleate 5 mg., phenylpropanolamine HCl 12.5 mg., chlorobutanol 0.5%, water for inj./cc. Inj. Vial 10 cc.

DECONGESTANT NA. (Vitarine) Acetaminophen 325 mg., phenylpropanolamine HCl 18 mg./Cap.
Use: Decongestant.

DECONGESTANT TABLETS. (Panray) Chlorpheniramine maleate 2 mg., aspirin 388.8 mg., caffeine 32.4 mg., phenylephrine 10 mg./Tab. Bot. 1000s.

DECONTABS. (Zenith) Phenylpropanolamine HCl 40 mg., phenlephrine HCl 10 mg., phenylteoloxamine citrate 15 mg., chlorpheniramine maleate 5 mg./SR Tab.
Use: Decongestant, antihistaminic.

• **DECOQUINATE.** USAN. Ethyl 6-decyloxy-7-ethoxy-4-hydroxyquinoline-3-carboxylate.
Use: Antiprotozoan, veterinary medicine.
See: Deccox.

• **DECTAFLUR.** USAN.
Use: Dental caries prophylactic.

DECUBITEX. (Merchant) Scarlet red modified 1%, peruvian balsam, castor oil, zinc oxide in an ointment base containing starch, white petrolatum, liquid petrolatum & plasticized hydrocarbon gel. Jars 4 oz., 16 oz.
Use: Decubitus care.

DECURITIS. (Sween) Cream, Jar 2 oz. Pads, Jar 80s.
Use: Bed sores treatment.

DEEP DOWN PAIN RELIEF RUB. (Beecham Products) Methyl salicylate 15%, menthol 5%, methyl nicotinate 0.7%, camphor 0.5%. Tubes 1.25 oz., 3 oz.
Use: Relieve pain of minor arthritis, sore joints, muscle aches, sprains, backaches, lumbago.

DEEP STRENGTH MUSTEROLE. (Plough) Methyl salicylate 30%, menthol 3%, methyl nicotinate 0.5% Tube 1.25 oz., 3 oz.
Use: Analgesic rub.

• **DEFEROXAMINE.** USAN.
Use: Chelating agent for iron.

• **DEFEROXAMINE HYDROCHLORIDE.** USAN.
Use: Chelating agent for iron.

• **DEFEROXAMINE MESYLATE,** U.S.P. XXI. Sterile, U.S.P. XXI. N-[5-[3-[(5-aminopentyl)-hydroxycarbamoyl]propionamido]-pentyl]-3-[[5-(N-hydroxyacetamido)pentyl]-carbamoyl]-propionohydroxamic acid.
Use: Iron depleter.
See: Desferal, Amp. (Ciba)

DEFICOL. (Vangard) **Tab.:** Bisacodyl 5 mg./Tab. Bot. 100s, 1000s. **Supp.:** Bisacodyl 10 mg./supp. Box 12s.
Use: Laxative.

DEFINATE. (Fellows) Docusate sodium 100 mg./Tab. Bot. 1000s.

DEFUNGIT SODIUM SALT. Bensuldazic acid, B.A.N.

DEGEST-2. (Barnes-Hind) Naphazoline HCl 0.012%, benzalkonium chloride 0.0067%, disodium edetate 0.02% Bot. 15 ml.
Use: Ophthalmic decongestant for eye irritations.

DEHIST CAPSULES. (O'Neal, Jones & Feldman) Phenylpropanolamine HCl 75 mg., chlorpheniramine maleate 12 mg./Cap. S.R. Bot. 100s.
Use: Decongestant, antihistaminic.

• **DEHYDROACETIC ACID.** N.F. XVI.
Use: Pharmaceutic aid (preservative).

• **DEHYDROCHOLATE SODIUM INJ.,** U.S.P. XXI. Sodium 3,7,12-trioxo-5B-Cholan-24-oate.
Use: Relief of liver congestion; diagnosis of cardiac failure.
See: Decholine Sodium, Inj. (Miles Pharm)

7-DEHYDROCHOLESTEROL, ACTIVATED. (Various Mfr.) Vitamin D-3.

DEHYDROCHOLIC ACID. B.A.N. 3,7,12-Trioxo-5β-cholanic acid.
Use: Laxative.
See: Bilostat
  Decholin, Tab. (Miles Pharm)
  Dehydrocholin

• **DEHYDROCHOLIC ACID,** U.S.P. XXI. Tabs., U.S.P. XXI. 3,7,12-Trioxo-5β-cholan-24-oic acid. Ketocholanic acid, oxidized cholic acid, bile acids oxidized.
Use: Orally, hydrocholeretic & choleretic.
See: Cholan-DH, Tab. (Pennwalt)
  Ketocholanic acid
  Neocholan, Tab. (Merrell Dow)
W/Amyloytic and proteolytic enzymes, desoxycholic acid.
See: Bilezyme, Tab. (Geriatric)

W/Bile, homatropine methylbromide, pepsin.
  See: Biloric, Caps. (Arcum)
W/Bile, homatropine methylbromide, phenobarbital.
  See: Bilamide, Tab. (Norgine)
W/Bile ext., methyl cellulose, homatropine
  methylbromide.
  See: Colicell, Tab. (Sutliff & Case)
W/Bile ext., pepsin, pancreatin.
  See: Progestive, Tab. (NCP)
W/Cholic acid.
  See: Chobile, Tab. (Mallinckrodt)
W/Desoxycholic acid.
  See: Combichole, Tab. (F. Trout)
    Ketosox, Tab. (Ascher)
W/Docusate sodium.
  See: Dubbalax-B, Cap. (Redford)
    Dubbalax-N, Cap. (Redford)
    Neolax, Tab. (Central)
W/Docusate sodium, phenolphthalein.
  See: Bolax, Cap. (Boyd)
    Sarolax (Saron)
    Tripalax, Cap. (Redford)
W/Homatropine methylbromide.
  See: Atrocholin. Tab. (Blue Line)
    Cholan V, Tab. (Pennwalt)
    Dranochol, Tab. (Marin)
    Hepahydrin, Tab. (Comatic)
W/Homatropine methylbromide, sod. pentobarbital.
  See: Homachol, Tab. (Lemmon)
W/Methscopolamine, ox bile, amobarbital.
  See: Hydrochol Plus, Tab. (Elder)
W/Ox bile, homatropine methylbromide,
  phenobarbital.
  See: Bilamide, Tab. (Norgine)
W/Pancreatin, pepsin, bile salts, desoxycholic
  acid.
  See: Enzylax, Tab. (Kay)
    Pepsatal, Tab. (Kenyon)
W/Pancreatin, pepsin, ox bile, belladonna ext.
  See: Ro-Bile, Tab. (Rowell)
W/Pepsin, pancreatin.
  See: Digestozyme, Tab. (Wolins)
W/Pepsin, pancreatin, ox bile ext. papain.
  See: Canz, Tab. (Cole)
W/Pepsin, pancreatin enz. conc., cellulase.
  See: Gastroenterase, Tab (Wallace)
W/Phenobarbital & homatropine methylbromide.
  See: Cholan-HMB, Tab. (Pennwalt)
W/Phenobarbital, homatropine methylbromide,
  gerilase, geriprotase, desoxycholic acid.
  See: Bilezyme Plus, Tabs. (Geriatric)
W/Phenolphthalein, docusate sodium.
  See: Sarolax, Cap. (Saron)
W/Prolase-300, Mylase-100, hyoscine HBr, atropine sulfate.
  See: Almezyme, Cap. (Meyer)
DEHYDROCHOLIN.
  See: Dehydrocholic acid.
11-DEHYDRO-17-HYDROXYCORTICOSTERONE.
  See: Cortisone.
DEHYDRODESOXYCHOLIC ACID.
  See: Cholanic acid
DEHYDROEMETINE. B.A.N. 3-Ethyl-1,6,7,11b-tetrahy-

dro-9,10-dimethoxy-2-(1,2,3,4-tetrahydro-6,7-dimeth-
oxy-1-isoquinolylmethyl)-4H-benzo[a]-quinolizine.
2,3-Dehydroemetine.
  Use: Treatment of amebiasis.
  See: Mebadin
DEKA. (Winthrop Products) Codeine alkaloid, alcohol,
  wild cherry fluid extract, tolu balsam tincture, squill
  extract.
  Use: Expectorant, antitussive.
DEKASOL. (Seatrace) Dexamethasone phosphate 4
  mg./ml. Vial 5 cc or 10 cc.
DEKASOL L.A. (Seatrace) Dexamethasone acetate 8
  mg./ml. Vial 5 cc.
DEKA-VITES TABLETS. (Barry-Martin) Vit. A 5000 I.U.,
  D 1000 I.U., B-1 2.5 mg., B-2 2.5 mg., B-6 0.5 mg.,
  B-12 2 mcg., niacinamide 20 mg., Ca pantothenate 5
  mg., C 50 mg., dicalcium phosphate 69.45
  mg., ferrous sulfate, dried 51 mg., potassium
  iodide 0.2 mg., manganese sulfate 3.2 mg., cop-
  per sulfate monohydrate 2.8 mg., zinc sulfate, dried
  2.77 mg., magnesium sulfate 21.58 mg., potassium
  sulfate 1.2 mg./Tab.Bot. 100s, 250s.
  Use: Vitamin supplement w. minerals.
DEKEN'S OINTMENT. (Guild) Bot. 4 oz.
DE-KOFF. (Whiteworth) Terpin hydrate w/dextrome-
  thorphan elixir. Bot 4 oz.
  Use: Antitussive.
DELACORT LOTION. (Mericon) Hydrocortisone
  0.5%. Bot. 1 oz., 4 oz.
DELADIOL-40. (Dunhall) Estradiol valerate 40
  mg./ml. Vial 10 ml.
  Use: Long-acting estrogen.
DELADUMONE. (Squibb) Testosterone enanthate 90
  mg., estradiol valerate 4 mg. in sesame oil/ml.,
  chlorobutanol 0.5%. Vial 5 ml., 1 dose (1 cc.).
  Use: Androgen and estrogen therapy.
DELADUMONE OB. (Squibb) Testosterone enanthate
  180 mg., estradiol valerate 8 mg. in sesame oil/cc.
  Vial w/benzyl alcohol 2%. 2 cc./dose. Unimatic
  disp. syringe w/needle. (2 cc.) Pkg. 1s, 10s.
DELALUTIN. (Squibb) 17-α-Hydroxyprogesterone caproate 125 mg./cc., in sesame oil, benzyl benzoate
  30%, benzyl alcohol 2%; 250 mg./cc., in castor oil,
  benzyl benzoate 46%, benzyl alcohol 2%. 125
  mg./cc. Vial 2 cc. 10 cc. 250 mg./cc. Vial 5 cc.
  Unimatic 1-dose syringe 1 cc.
  Use: I.M., long-acting progestational agent.
DELANEX. (Tunex) Hydroxyprogestrone caproate 250
  mg./ml. w/benzyl benzoate 46%, benzyl alcohol
  2% as preservative. Vial 5 cc.
  Use: Long-acting progestional agent.
DEL-ANTHRA OINTMENT. (Del-Ray) Anthralin 0.03%
  Jar 4 oz.
  Use: Treatment of psoriasis.
DELAPAV. (Dunhall) Papaverine HCl 150 mg./Time
  Cap. Bot. 100s, 1000s.
  Use: Vasodilator.
DEL-AQUA-5. (Del-Ray) Benzoyl peroxide 5%. Tube
  1.5 oz.
  Use: Topical aid for acne vulgaria.
DEL-AQUA-10. (Del-Ray) Benzoyl peroxide 10%. Tube
  1.5 oz.
  Use: Topical aid for acne vulgaria.

DELAQUIN LOTION. (Schlicksup) Hydrocortisone 0.5%, Iodoquin 3%. Bot. 3 oz.
DELATEST. (Dunhall) Testosterone enanthate 100 mg./ml. Amp. 10 ml.
Use: Androgen therapy.
DELATESTADIOL. (Dunhall) Testosterone enanthate 90 mg., estradiol valerate 4 mg./ml. Amp. 10 ml.
Use: Androgen and estrogen therapy.
DELATESTRYL. (Squibb) Testosterone enanthate 200 mg./cc. in sesame oil, chlorobutanol 0.5%. Vial 5 cc. 1-dose Unimatic syringe (1 cc.) 1s, 10s.
Use: I.M., androgen therapy.
DELAXIN. (Ferndale) Methocarbamol 500 mg./Tab. Bot. 100s, 500s.
Use: Musculoskeletal conditions.
DELCID. (Merrell Dow) Aluminum hydroxide 600 mg., magnesium hydroxide 665 mg./5 ml. Bot. plastic 8 oz.
Use: Antacid.
DEL-CLENS, (Del-Ray) Soapless cleanser. Bot. 8 oz.
DELCOBESE. (Delco) d-Amphetamine sulfate 25%, d-amphetamine adipate 25%, amphetamine adipate 25%, amphetamine sulfate 25%, Cap., Time Cap. 5, 10, 15, 20 mg. Bot. 1000s. Tab.,
Use: Anorexiant, CNS stimulant.
DELCO-LAX. (Delco) Bisacodyl 5 mg./Tab. Bot. 1000s.
Use: Laxative.
DELCOPLEX. (Delco) Multivitamin & multimineral Tab. Bot 1000s, 5000s, 10,000s.
Use: Sugar free vit. & mineral replacement.
DELCO-RETIC. (Delco) Hydrochlorothiazide 25 mg., 50 mg./Tab. Bot. 1000s.
Use: Diuretic and antihypertensive.
DELCOZINE. (Delco) Phendimetrazine tartrate. 70 mg./Tab. Bot. 1000s, 5000s.
Use: Anorexiant, CNS stimulant.
DELESTREC. Estradiol 17-undecanoate.
Use: Estrogen.
DELESTROGEN. (Squibb) Estradiol valerate 10 mg./cc., in sesame oil, chlorobutanol 0.5%. Vial 1 cc. 20 mg./cc., in castor oil, benzyl benzoate 20%, benzyl alcohol 2%. Vial 5 cc. 40 mg./cc., in castor oil, benzyl benzoate 40%, benzyl alcohol 2%. Vial 5 cc. Unimatic single dose syringe: 20 mg., 1 cc. 1s, 10s.
Use: I.M., amenorrhea, menopausal syndrome.
DELFEN CONTRACEPTIVE FOAM. (Ortho) Nonoxynol-9 12.5% in an oil-in-water emulsion at pH 4.5 to 5.0. Can with applicator 20 Gm. Can only 20 Gm. 50 Gm.
Use: Contraceptive foam.
DELINAL. Propenzolate Hydrochloride.
DELMADINONE. B.A.N. 6-Chloro-17α-hydroxypregna-1,4,6-triene-3,20-dione.
Use: Progestational steroid.
• **DELMADINONE ACETATE.** USAN. 6-Chloro-17-hydroxypregna-1, 4, 6-triene-3, 20-dione acetate.
Use: Progestin.
See: Delmate (Syntex)
DELNAV. Dioxathion, B.A.N.
DELSYM. (Pennwalt) Dextromethorphan resin

complex equivalent to dextromethorphan HBr 30 mg./5 ml. Bot. 3 oz.
Use: Antitussive.
DELTA-CORTEF. (Upjohn) Prednisolone 5 mg./Tab. Bot. 100s, 500s.
Use: Orally, rheumatoid arthritis & intractable bronchial asthma.
DELTA-CORTRIL.
Prednisolone.
DELTA-1-CORTISONE.
See: Deltasone, Tab. (Upjohn)
DELTACORTONE.
Prednisone.
• **DELTAFILCON A.** USAN.
Use: Contact lens material.
DELTA-1-HYDROCORTISONE.
See: Prednisolone (Var. Mfr.)
DELTA¹, 6-METHYL-HYDROCORTISONE.
See: Medrol, Preps. (Upjohn)
DELTAPEN. (Trimen) Potassium penicillin G, U.S.P. 400,000 u./5 cc. Oral Susp. Bot. "16 dose." Tab. Bot. 100s.
Use: Antibiotic.
DELTASONE. (Upjohn) Prednisone. **2.5 mg.**/Tab. Bot. 100s, **5 mg.**/Tab. Bot. 100s, 500s. Unit-Dose 100s. Dosepak 21s. **10 mg., 20 mg.**/Tab. Bot. 100s, 500s. Unit-Dose 100s. **50 mg.**/Tab. 100s, Unit Dose 100s.
Use: Orally, rheumatoid arthritis & intractable bronchial asthma.
DEL-TRAC. (Del-Ray) Acne lotion. Bot. 2 oz.
Use: Topical aid for acne.
DELTRA-STAB.
See: Prednisolone (Var. Mfr.)
DEL-STAT. (Del-Ray) Abradent cleaner. Jar 2 oz.
Use: Topical aid for acne.
DELYSID. Lysergic acid diethylamide.
Use: Potent psychotogenic.
DEMAZIN. (Schering) **Syr.:** Chlorpheniramine maleate 1 mg., phenylphrine HCl 2.5 mg./5 ml., alcohol 7.5%. Bot. 4 oz. **Repetab:** Outer and inner layers: chlorpheniramine maleate 2 mg./layer, phenylephrine 10 mg./layer. Box 24s. Bot. 100s, 1000s.
Use: Antihistamine, decongestant.
• **DEMECARIUM BROMIDE,** U.S.P. XXI. Ophth. Sol. U.S.P. XXI.
Use: Cholinergic (ophthalmic).
See: Humorsol, Sol. (Merck Sharp & Dohme)
• **DEMECLOCYCLINE,** U.S.P. XXI. Oral Susp., U.S.P. XXI. 7-Chloro-4-(dimethylamino)-1,4,4α,5,5α,6,11,12 α-octahydro-3,6,10,-12,12α-pentahydroxy-1,11-dioxo -2-naphthacene-carboxamide.
Use: Antibacterial.
See: Declomycin Prods (Lederle)
Ledermycin Prods (Lederle)
• **DEMECLOCYCLINE HYDROCHLORIDE,** U.S.P. XXI. Caps., Tabs., U.S.P. XXI.
Use: Antibacterial.
See: Declomycin, HCl, Preps. (Lederle)
• **DEMECLOCYCLINE HYDROCHLORIDE AND NYSTATIN CAPSULES,** U.S.P. XXI.

Use: Antibacterial.
See: Declostatin, Cap.(Lederle)
DEMECLOCYCLINE HYDROCHLORIDE AND NYSTATIN TABLETS, U.S.P. XXI.
Use: Antibacterial
See: Declostatin, Tab. (Lederle)
DEMECOLCINE. B.A.N. N-Methyl-N-deacetyl-colchicine.
Use: Antimitotic, leukemia therapy.
See: Colcemid
• **DEMECYCLINE.** USAN.
Use: Antibacterial.
DEMEROL APAP. (Winthrop-Breon) Meperidine HCl 50 mg., acetaminophen 300 mg./Tab. Bot. 100s.
Use: Analgesic.
DEMEROL HYDROCHLORIDE. (Winthrop-Breon) Meperidine HCL. **Syrup:** (50 mg./tsp.) Bot. 16 fl. oz. **Inj.: Detecto-Seal, Carpuject, Sterile Cartridge-Needle Units, Uni-Amp. 2.5%:** (25 mg./ml.), **5%:** (50 mg./ml.), **7.5%:** (75 mg./ml.), **10%:** (100 mg./ml.), Boxes 10s. **Uni-Amp. 5%:** 0.5 ml (25 mg.)/Amp., 1 ml. (50 mg.)/Amp., 1.5 ml. (75 mg.)/Amp., and 2 ml (100 mg.)/Amp. Box 25s; **10%:** 1 ml. (100 mg.)/Amp. Box 25s. **Uni-Nest 5%:** 0.5 ml (25 mg.)/Amp., 1 ml. (50 mg.)/Amp., 1.5 ml (75 mg.)/Amp. and 2 ml (100 mg.)/Amp. Box 25s; **10%:** 1 ml./Amp. Box 25s. **Vials: 5%** multiple-dose vials/30 ml. Box 1s; **10%** multiple dose vials/20 ml. Box 1s.**Tab.:** (50 mg.) Bot. 100s, 500s. (100 mg.) Bot. 100s, 500s.
Use: Analgesic.
DEMETHYL CHLORTETRACYCLINE HCI.
See: Demeclocycline HCl, U.S.P. XXI.
DEMI-REGROTON. (USV Labs.) Chlorthalidone 25 mg., reserpine 0.125 mg./Tab. Bot. 100s., 1000s.
Use: Antihypertensive.
• **DEMOXEPAM.** USAN. 7-Chloro-1, 3-dihydro-5-phenyl-2H-1, 4-benzodiazepin-2-one-4-oxide.
Use: Minor tranquilizer.
DEMSER. (Merck Sharp & Dohme) Metyrosine 250 mg./Cap. Bot. 100s.
Use: Treatment of patients with pheochromocytoma.
DEMULEN 1/50-21. (Searle) Ethynodiol diacetate 1 mg., ethinyl estradiol 50 mcg./Tab. Compack Disp. 21s, 6×21., 24 × 21. Refills 21s, 12×21.
Use: Oral contraceptive.
DEMULEN 1/35-21. (Searle) Ethynodiol diacetate 1 mg., ethinyl estradiol 35 mcg./Tab. Compack disp. 21s, 6 ×21s, 24 × 21. Refill 21s, 12 × 21.
Use: Low estrogen oral contraceptives.
DEMULEN 1/35-28. (Searle) Ethynodiol diacetate 1 mg., ethinyl estradiol 35 mcg./Tab. Compack 28s: 21 active tabs, 7 placebo tabs. Compack 6×28, 24 × 28. Refills 28s, 12 × 28.
Use: Low-estrogen oral contraceptive.
DEMULEN 1/50-28. (Searle) Ethynodiol diacetate 1 mg., ethinyl estradiol 50 mcg./Tab. Compack 28s: 21 active tabs, 7 placebo tabs. Compack Disp. of 28, 6×28, 24×28. Refills 28s, 12×28.
Use: Oral contraceptive.

DENALAN DENTURE CLEANSER. (Whitehall) Sodium percarbonate 30%. Bot. 7 oz., 13 oz.
Use: Denture cleanser.
• **DENATONIUM BENZOATE,** N.F. XVI. Bitrex (MacFarlan Smith, Ltd. Scotland) Benzyldiethyl [(2, 6-xylylcarbamoyl) methyl] ammonium benzoate.
Use: Denaturant for ethyl alcohol.
See: Bitrex
DENCORUB. (Last) Methyl salicylate 20%, menthol 0.75%, camphor 1%, oil eucalyptus 0.5%. Tube 1.25 oz., 2.75 oz.
Use: Greaseless analgesic rub.
DENDRID. (Alcon) 2-Deoxy-5-iodouridine Ophth. Sol. 0.1% sol. w/benzalkonium chloride, phenylmercuric nitrate, boric acid, purified water. Bot. w/dropper 15 cc.; Isotonic sol. idoxuridine 0.1% Vials 15 cc.
Use: Ocular herpes simplex.
DENGESIC. (Scott-Alison) Salicylamide 100 mg., acetaminophen 240 mg., phenyltoloxamine dihydrogen citrate 30 mg., butabarbital ⅛ gr./Tab. Bot. 60s, 500s.
Use: Analgesic w/sedative.
• **DENOFUNGIN.** USAN.
Use: Antifungal, antibacterial.
DENOREX. (Whitehall) Coal tar solution 9.0%, menthol 1.5%. Bot. 4 oz., 8 oz.
Use: Medicated shampoo.
DENOREX GEL. (Whitehall) Coal tar solution 9%, menthol 1.5%. Tube 2 oz., 4 oz.
Use: Medicated shampoo.
DENOREX MOUNTAIN FRESH. (Whitehall) Coal tar sol. 9%, menthol 1.5%. Bot. 4 oz., 8 oz.
Use: Medicated shampoo.
DENOREX WITH CONDITIONERS. (Whitehall) Coal tar sol. 9%, menthol 1.5%. Bot 4 oz., 8 oz.
Use: Medicated shampoo.
DENQUEL. (Vicks Prods) Potassium nitrate 5%. Tube 1.6 oz., 3 oz., 4.5 oz.
Use: Sensitive teeth toothpaste.
DENTAL CARIES PREVENTIVE. (Hoyt) Fluoride ion 1.2%, alumina abrasive. 2 Gm. Box 200s, Jars 9 oz.
Use: Clean and polish teeth.
DENTAVITE CHEWABLE TABLETS. (Reid-Provident) Vit. A 3000 I.U., D 400 I.U., C 60 mg., B-1 1 mg., B-2 1.2 mg., B-6 1 mg., niacinamide 8 mg., calcium pantothenate 3 mg., fluoride 1 mg./Tab. Bot. 100s.
Use: Fluoride with vitamin supplement.
DENTROL. (Block) Carboxymethylcellulose, polyethylene oxide homopolymer, peppermint & spearmint in mineral oil base. Bot. 0.9 oz., 1.8 oz.
Use: Liquid denture adhesive.
DENT'S DENTAL POULTICE. (C.S. Dent) Alcohol 64%, benzocaine, oxyquinoline, thymol, capsicum oleoresin. Box 6s, 12s.
DENT'S EAR WAX DROPS. (C.S. Dent) Glycerine, propylene glycol, mineral oil, chloroform 1%, polyoxyethylene sorbitan monooleate. Bot. ⅛, ¼ oz.
DENT'S LOTION-JEL. (C.S. Dent) Benzocaine in special base. Tube ³⁄₁₆ oz.
Use: Toothache, teething pain, denture irritation.

DENT'S TOOTHACHE DROPS TREATMENT. (C.S. Dent) Alcohol 60%, chlorobutanol hydrous (chloroform derivative) 0.09%, phenol, eugenol, cresol and capsicum oleoresin. Bot. ⅛ fl. oz.

DENT'S TOOTHACHE GUM. (C.S. Dent) Benzocaine, phenol, capsicum oleoresin in base of cotton and wax. Box 21 grs.

DENYL SODIUM.
See: Diphenylhydantoin Sodium, Cap (Various Mfr.)

DEOXYCHOLIC ACID.
See: Desoxycholic Acid, Tab. (Various Mfr.)

11-DEOXYCORTICOSTERONE ACETATE. Desoxycorticosterone Acetate, U.S.P XXI.

DEOXYCORTICOSTERONE ACETATE.
See: Desoxycorticosterone acetate, U.S.P. XXI.

2-DEOXY-5-FLUOROURIDINE.
See: FUDR, Vial (Roche)

2-DEOXY-5-IODOURIDINE. Idoxuridine, U.S.P. XXI.

1-DEOXY-1-(METHYLAMINO)-d-GLUCITOL. Meglumine, U.S.P. XXI.

1-DEOXY-1-(METHYLAMINO)-D-GLUCITOL ⅝ — ACETAMIDO-2,4,6,-TRIIODO-N-METHYLISOPHTH-ALAMATE (SALT). Iothalamate Meglumine Injection, U.S.P. XXI.

1-DEOXY-1-(METHYLAMINO)-D-GLUCITOL 3,3'-(ADIPOYLDIIMINO) BIS[2,4,6-TRI-IODOBEN-ZOATE] (2:1) (SALT). Iodipamide Meglumine Injection, U.S.P. XXI.

1-DEOXY-1-(METHYLAMINO)-D-GLUCITOL 3, 5-DIACETAMIDO-2,4,6-TRIIODOBENZOATE (SALT). Diatrizoate Meglumine, U.S.P. XXI.

D.E.P.-75. (Merchant) Diethylpropion HCl 75 mg./Cap. Bot. 100s.
Use: Anorexant.

DEPAKENE. (Abbott) Valproic acid **Cap.:** 250 mg./Cap. Bot. 100s. Unit dose 100s. **Syrup:** 250 mg./5 ml. Bot. pt.
Use: Anticonvulsant.

DEPAKOTE. (Abbott) Divalproex sodium 250 mg. or 500 mg./Enteric Coated Tab. Bot. 100s. Unit dose 100s.
Use: Antiepileptic agent.

dep ANDRO 100. (O'Neal, Jones & Feldman) Testosterone cypionate in cottonseed oil 100 mg./ml. Vial 10 ml.

dep ANDROGYN. (O'Neal, Jones & Feldman) Testosterone cypionate 50 mg., estradiol cypionate 2 mg./ml. Vial 10 ml.

dep ANDRO 200. (O'Neal, Jones & Feldman) Testosterone cypionate in cottonseed oil 200 mg./ml. Vial 10 ml.

DEPEN TITRATABLE TABLETS. (Wallace) Penicillamine 250 mg./Tab. Bot. 100s.
Use: Disease modifying anti-rheumatoid agent for severe active rheumatoid arthritis unresponsive to conventional therapy.

DEPEPSEN. Amylosulfate sodium.
Use: Peptic ulcer therapy.

DEP-ESTRADIOL. (Rocky Mtn.) Estradiol cypionate 5 mg./cc. Vial 10 cc.
Use: Female hormone therapy.

DEPESTRO. (Kay) Estradiol cypionate 5 mg./ml. Vial 10 ml.
Use: Hormone supplement.

dep GYNOGEN. (O'Neal, Jones & Feldman) Estradiol cypionate in cottonseed oil 5 mg./ml. Vial 10 ml.

dep MEDALONE 40. (O'Neal, Jones & Feldman) Methylprednisolone acetate in aqueous suspension 40 mg./ml. Vial 5 ml.

dep MEDALONE 80. (O'Neal, Jones & Feldman) Methylprednisolone acetate 80 mg./ml. Vial 5 ml.

DEPOESTRA. (Tennessee Pharm.) Estradiol cypionate 5 mg./cc. Vial 10 cc.
Use: Estrogen therapy.

DEPO-ESTRADIOL. (Upjohn) Estradiol cypionate 1 mg., 5 mg./ml. chlorobutanol anhydrous 5.4 mg./ml. w/cottonseed oil. Estradiol cypionate **1 mg./ml.** Vial 10 ml. **5 mg./ml.** Vial 5 ml.

DEPOGEN. (Sig) Estradiol valerate 10 mg., 20 mg./ml. in oil. Vial 10 ml.
Use: Estrogen therapy.

DEPOGEN. (Hyrex) Estradiol cypionate 5 mg., Vial 10 cc.
Use: Long acting estrogen.

DEPO-MED 40. (Tunex) Methylprednisolone acetate 40 mg./ml. Vial 5 cc.
Use: Anti-inflammatory.

DEPO-MED 80. (Tunex) Methylprednisolone acetate 80 mg./ml. Vial 5 cc.
Use: Anti-inflammatory.

DEPO-MEDROL. (Upjohn) Methylprednisolone acetate 20 mg., 40 mg., or 80 mg./ml. suspended in polyethylene glycol 3350 (29.6 mg., 29 mg., or 28 mg./ml), sod. chloride (8.9 mg., 8.7 mg. or 8.5 mg./ml.), myristyl-gamma-picolinium chloride 0.19 mg. **20 mg./ml.:** Vials 5 ml. Box 1s, 5s, 25s, 50s, 100s. **40 mg./ml.:** Vials 1 ml., 5 ml., 10 ml. Box 1s, 5s, 25s, 50s, 100s. **80 mg./ml.:** Vials 1 ml., 5 ml. 1s, 5s, 25s, 50s, 100s. Unit-Dose 1 ml. U-Ject. 5s, 25s, 50s, 100s.
Use: Anti-inflammatory.

DEPO-PRED. (Hyrex) Methylprednisolone acetate suspension 40 mg./ml. Vial 5 ml. 80 mg./ml. Vial 5 ml.
Use: Steroid-anti-inflammatory.

DEPO-PRED 100. (Vortech) Prednisolone acetate 100 mg., sodium chloride 0.65%, pectin 0.2%, niacinamide 25 mg./ml. w/preservative and buffer. Vial 10 ml.
Use: Adrenocortical steroid.

DEPO-PROVERA. (Upjohn) Medroxyprogesterone acetate 100 mg. and 400 mg./ml. **100 mg./ml.:** suspended in polyethylene glycol 3350, 27.6 mg., polysorbate 80, 1.84 mg., sod. chloride, 8.3 mg., methylparaben, 1.75 mg., propylparaben 0.194 mg./ml. Vial 5 ml. 1s, 5s, 25s. **400 mg./ml.:** suspended in polyethylene glycol 3350, 20.3 mg. sod. sulfate (anhydrous), 11 mg., myristyl-gamma-picolinium chloride, 1.69 mg./ml. Vial 2.5 ml., 10ml. 1 ml. U-Ject. 1s, 5s, 25s.
Use: Long-acting (16da.) progestational agent.

DEPOTEST. (Hyrex) Testosterone cypionate 100 mg. and 200 mg. Vial 10 cc.
Use: Male hormone, long acting.

DEPOTEST. (Kay) Testosterone cypionate 100 mg. or 200 mg./ml. Vial 10 ml.
Use: Androgen.

DEPO-TESTADIOL. (Upjohn) Sterile sol. testosterone cypionate 50 mg., estradiol cypionate 2 mg., chlorobutanol 5.4 mg./ml. w/cottonseed oil 874 mg./ml. Vial 1 ml., 10 ml. Box 1s, 5s, 25s.
Use: Androgen-estrogen therapy.

DEPOTESTOGEN. (Hyrex) Testosterone cypionate 50 mg., estradiol cypionate 2 mg., chlorobutanol 5 mg., in cottonseed oil/cc. Vial 10 cc.
Use: Androgen-estrogen therapy, long acting.

DEPO-TESTOSTERONE. (Upjohn) Testosterone cypionate 50 mg., 100 mg., or 200 mg./ml. **50 mg./ml.:** testosterone cypionate in chlorobutanol (anhydrous), 5.4 mg. cottonseed oil, 874 mg./ml. Vial 10 ml. 1s, 5s, 25s. **100 mg./ml.:** testosterone cypionate in benzyl alcohol 9.45 mg., cottonseed oil, 736 mg./ml. Vial 1 ml., 10 ml. 1s, 5s, 25s. **200 mg./ml.:** testosterone cypionate in benzyl benzoate, 0.2 ml., benzyl alcohol, 9.45 mg., cottonseed oil, 560 mg./ml. Vial 1 ml., 10 ml. 1s, 5s, 25s.
Use: I.M., long-acting androgen therapy.

DEPRODONE. B.A.N. 11 β 17α-Dihydroxypregna-1, 4-diene-3,20-dione.
Use: Corticosteroid.

DEPROL TABLETS. (Wallace) Meprobamate 400 mg., benactyzine HCl 1 mg./Tab. Bot. 100s, 500s. Unit dose 500s, 1000s.
Use: Antidepressant.

• **DEPROSTIL.** USAN.
Use: Antisecretory.

DEP-TEST. (Sig) Testosterone cypionate 100 mg./ml. Vial 10 ml.
Use: Androgenic.

DEP-TESTOSTERONE. (Rocky Mtn.) Testosterone cypionate 200 mg. /cc. Vial 10 cc. 100 mg./cc. 1 cc.
Use: Male hormone therapy.

DEP-TESTRADIOL. (Rocky Mtn.) Estradiol cypionate 2 mg., testosterone cypionate 50 mg./cc. Vial 10 cc.

DEPTROPINE. B.A.N. 3-(10, 11-Dihydrodibenzo-[a, d]cycloheptadien-5-yloxy)tropane.
Use: Bronchodilator.
See: Brontina (dihydrogen citrate)

DEQUALINIUM CHLORIDE. B.A.N. Decamethylenedi-(4-aminoquinaldinium chloride).
Use: Antiseptic.
See: Dequadin

DEQUIBOLIN-100. (Vortech) Nandrolone decandate 100 mg./ml. Vial 2 ml.
Use: I.M. androgen, anabolic, anti-catabolic steroid.

DERIFIL. (Rystan) Water-soluble derivatives of chlorophyll 100 mg./Tab. or 5 ml. of prepared sol. Bot. 30s, 100s, 1000s. Pow. 1 oz., 10 oz.
Use: Designed to control colostomy or ileostomy odors; odor of incontinent patients.

DERISOL. (Wolins) Amobarbital ½ gr., aspirin 2½ gr., N-acety-p-aminophenol 2½ gr./Tab. Bot. 1000s.
Use: Analgesic.

DERMACARE. (Jenkins) Hexachlorophene, camphor, menthol, lanolin. Bot. 2 oz. , 6 oz., pt., gal.

Use: Antiseptic skin lotion.

DERMACOAT AEROSOL SPRAY. (Century) Benzocaine 4.5%. Bot. 7 oz.
Use: Topical anesthetic.

DERMACON. (Paddock) Dermal contact ionogenic catalytic emulsoid. Bot. gal.

DERMACORT CREAM. (Rowell) Hydrocortisone 1% in a water soluble cream of stearyl alcohol, cetyl alcohol, isopropyl palmitate, citric acid, polyoxethylene 40 stearate, sod. phosphate, propylene glycol, water, benzyl alcohol & buffered to pH 5.0. Jar 1 lb.
Use: Inflammatory skin disorders.

DERMACORT LOTION. (Rowell) Hydrocortisone 0.5% or 1% in lotion base, buffered to pH 5.0 Paraben free. Bot. 120 ml.
Use: Topical corticosteroid cream.

DERMA-COVER. (Scrip) Sulfur, salicylic acid, hyamine 10x, isopropyl alcohol 22%, in powder film forming base. Bot. 2 oz.

DERMA-GUARD. (Greer) Protective adhesive pow. Can w/sifter top, 4 oz. Spray top Bot. 4 oz., pkg. 1 lb. Rings. Pkg. 5s, 10s.
Use: Protective powder for skin.

DERMAL-RUB. (Mallard) Menthol racemic 7%, camphor 1%, methyl salicylate 1%, cajuput oil 1%. Cream. Jar 1 oz., 1 lb.
Use: Analgesic.

DERMA-MEDICONE. (Medicone) Benzocaine 20 mg., oxyquinoline sulfate 10.5 mg., menthol 4.8 mg., ichthammol 10 mg., zinc oxide 137 mg./Gm. w/petrolatum, lanolin, perfume, certified color. Oint., Tube 1 oz.; Jar 1 lb.
Use: Antipruritic & vasoconstrictor.

DERMA MEDICONE-HC. (Medicone) Hydrocortisone acetate 10 mg., benzocaine 20 mg., oxyquinoline sulfate 10.5 mg., ephedrine HCl 1.1 mg., menthol 4.8 mg., ichthammol 10 mg., zinc oxide 137 mg./Gm. w/petrolatum, lanolin, perfume. Oint., Tube 7 Gm. & 20 Gm.
Use: Dermatoses.

DERMANEED. (Hanlon) Zirconium oxide 4.5%, calamine 6%, zinc oxide 4%, actamer 0.1% in bland lotionized base. Bot. 4 oz.
Use: Poison ivy.

DERMA-PAX. (Recsei) Methapyrilene HCl 0.22%, chlorothenylpyramine maleate 0.06%, pyrilamine maleate 0.22%, benzyl alcohol 1%, chlorobutanol 1%, isopropyl alcohol 40%. Liq. 4 oz., pt.
Use: Topically, antipruritic w/antihistamine.

DERMAPHILL. (Torch) Aluminum acetate 1%, phenol 1%, menthol ½%, camphor 3%, in hydrophilic vehicle. Jar 1 lb., 2 oz.
Use: General soothing and cooling applications.

DERMA-pH SKIN LOTION. (Day-Baldwin) pH 4.6 to 4.9. Mentholated or plain. Plastic Squeeze Bot. 4 oz., 8 oz. Plastic Bot. gal.

DERMAREX. (Hyrex) Hydrocortisone 1%, clioquinol 3%, pramoxine HCl 0.5%. Cream Tubes, ½ oz.
Use: Antifungal and antibacterial agent.

DERMA-SMOOTHE/FS OIL. (Hill) Fluocinolone acetonide 0.01% topical oil. Bot. 4 oz.

Use: Psoriasis, seborrheic dermatitis & atopic dermatitis.

DERMA+SOFT CREAM. (Creighton) salicylic acid 2.5%, in a cream base. Tube 1 oz.
Use: Removal of corns & callouses.

DERMA-SMOOTHE OIL. (Hill) Refined peanut oil, mineral oil in lipophilic base.
Use: Relieves itching, softens skin.

DERMA-SONE 1%. (Hill) Hydrocortisone 1%, pramoxine HCl 1%, cetyl alcohol, glyceryl monosterate, isopropyl myristate, potassium sorbate, furcelleran.
Use: Relief of the inflammatory manifestations of corticosteroid responsive dermatoses.

DERMASSAGE. (Colgate) Mineral oil, TEA-stearate, propylene glycol, stearic acid, menthol, diammonium phosphate, methylparaben, lanolin, oxyquinoline sulfate, urea, propylparaben. Lot. 6, 12, 16 oz., Cream 3.5 oz.

DERMA SOAP. (Ferndale) Dowicil 0.1%. 4 oz. w/dispenser.

DERMA-SOFT. (Vogarell) Medicated cream. Salicylic acid, castor oil, triethanolamine. Tube ¾ oz.
Use: Removal of corns, calluses, warts.

DERMASORCIN. (Lamond) Resorcin 2%, sulfur 5%. Bot. 1 oz., 2 oz., 4 oz., 8 oz., pt., 32 oz., ½ gal.
Use: Treatment of acne and seborrhea.

DERMASTRINGE. (Lamond) Bot. 4 oz., 6 oz., 8 oz., pt., 32 oz., gal.
Use: Skin cleansing solution.

DERMASUL. (Lamond) Sulfur 5%. Bot. 1 oz., 2 oz., 4 oz., 8 oz., pt., 32 oz., ½ gal., gal.
Use: Treatment of acne and seborrhea.

DERMATHYN. (Davis & Sly) Benzyl alcohol 3%, benzocaine 3.5%, butyl-p-aminobenzoate 1% & phenylmercuric borate. Tube 1 oz.
Use: Topical local anesthetic.

DERMATIC BASE. (Whorton) Compounding cream base. Bot. 16 oz.
Use: Preparing creams and lotions with water-based materials.

DERMATOL.
See: Bismuth subgallate, Preps. (Various Mfr.)

DERMAX. (Dermco) Methphenoxydiol 100 mg., (3-(2-methosyphenoxy)-1, 2-propanediol) Bot. 100s, 1000s.
Use: Tension states.

DERMEZE. (Premo) Thenylpyramine HCl 2%, benzocaine 2%, tyrothricin 0.25 mg./Gm. Massage Lotion 5¾ oz.
Use: Topically; antihistaminic, antibiotic & anesthetic.

DERMIDON ANTI-ITCH CREAM. (Republic) Pyrilamine maleate 0.5%, phenyltoloxamine dihydrogen citrate 0.5%, diperidon HCl 0.25%, benzalkonium chloride 0.1%, menthol, camphor, water washable cream. Tube 1¼ oz.
Use: Relief of itching.

DERMOLATE ANTI-ITCH CREAM. (Schering) Hydrocortisone 0.5% in a greaseless, vanishing cream. Tube 15 gm., 30 gm.
Use: Antipruritic.

DERMOLATE ANTI-ITCH SPRAY. (Schering) Hy-

drocortisone 0.5%, alcohol 24%. Pump spray bot. 45 ml.
Use: Antipruritic.

DERMOLATE ANAL-ITCH OINTMENT. (Schering) Hydrocortisone 0.5%. Tube 30 gm.
Use: Antipruritic.

DERMOLATE SCALP-ITCH LOTION. (Schering) Hydrocortisone 0.5%, alcohol 47%. Squeeze Bot. 30 ml.
Use: Antipruritic.

DERMOLIN. (Mallard) Menthol racemic, methyl salicylate, camphor, mustard oil, isopropyl alcohol 8%. Liniment. Bot. 3 oz., pt., gal.
Use: Topically, for pain.

DERMO PEDIC ELBOW LOTION. (CMC) Bot. 4 oz.
Use: Soothing elbow lotion.

DERMO PEDIC FOOT LOTION. (CMC) Bot. 4 oz.
Use: Soothing foot lotion.

DERMOPLAST AEROSOL SPRAY. (Ayerst) Benzocaine 20%, menthol 0.5%, in water-dispersible base of Tween 85, PEG 400 monolaurate, methylparaben as preservative, and propellants. Spray 2.75 oz., 6 oz.
Use: Topically as anesthetic, antipruritic.

DERMOVAN. (Owen) Glyceryl stearate, spermaceti, mineral oil, glycerin, cetyl alcohol, butylparaben, methylparaben, propylparaben, & purified water. Vanishing-type base, Jar 1 lb.
Use: Cream base (lanolin free).

DESACCHROMIN. A nonprotein bacterial colloidal dispersion of polysaccharide.

DESA-HIST AT. (Pharmics) Phenylpropanolamine HCl 50 mg., chlorpheniramine maleate 6 mg., dextromethorphan HBr 30 mg., terpin hydrate 180 mg., acetaminophen 325 mg./Tab. Tabs. Bot. 100s. Syr. Bot. pt., gal.
Use: Decongestant, antihistamine, antitussive, expectorant and analgesic.

DESA-HIST PF CAPSULES. (Pharmics) Chlorpheniramine maleate 8 mg., phenylpropanolamine HCl 50 mg./Cap. Bot. 100s, 500s.
Use: Decongestant, antihistaminic combination for nasal congestion due to allergies.

DESA-HIST PF ELIXIR. (Pharmics) Chlorprophenpyridamine maleate 2 mg., 1-phenylephrine HCl 3 mg., alcohol 7.5% in a syrup base/5 cc. Bot. pts., gal.
Use: Systemic nasal decongestant.

DESAMYCIN. (Pharmics) Tetracycline HCl 250 mg./Cap. Bot. 100s.
Use: Tetracycline therapy.

• **DESCINOLONE ACETONIDE.** USAN.
Use: Glucocorticoid.

DESENEX. (Pharmacraft) Oint. Undecylenic acid 5%, zinc undecylenate 20%. Tube 0.9 oz., 1.8 oz. Jar 1 lb. Pow. Undecylenic acid 2%, zinc undecylenate 20%. Can 1.5 oz., 3 oz. Carton 1 lb. Soap: Undecylenic acid 2%. Cake 3.25 oz. Liquid: Undecylenic acid 10%, isopropyl alcohol 47.1%. Pump Spray Bot. 1.5 oz. Aerosol Powder (hydrocarbon): Undecylenic acid 2%, Zn undecylenate 20%. Can 2.7 oz., 5.5 oz. Foam:

Undecylenic acid 10% isopropyl alcohol 35.2%. Can 1.5 oz.
Use: Fungus infections.

DESENEX FOOT & SNEAKER SPRAY. (Pharmacraft) Aluminum chlorhydrate complex, alcohol 89.3% v/v, menthol Bot. Aerosol 2.7 oz.
Use: Foot deodorant, antiperspirant.

DE SERPA. (de Leon) Reserpine, Tab. 0.25, 0.5 mg., Bot. 100s, 500s. Tab. 0.25 mg. Bot. 1000s.
Use: Tranquilizer and hypotensor.

DESERPIDINE. B.A.N. 11-Demethoxyreserpine.
Use: Tranquilizer.

DESERPIDINE. An alkaloid derived from *Rauwolfia canescens.* 11-Desmethoxyreserpine (Raunormine)
Use: Treatment of hypertension.
See: Harmonyl, Tab. (Abbott)
W/Hydrochlorothiazide
See: Oreticyl, Tab. (Abbott)
W/Methyclothiazide
See: Enduronyl and Enduronyl Forte, Tabs. (Abbott)

DESFERAL. (Ciba) Deferoxamine mesylate 500 mg./5 ml. Amp. 4s.
Use: Iron salt poisoning.

DESFERRIOXAMINE. B.A.N. 30-Amino-3,14,25-tri-hydroxy-3,9,14,20,25-penta-azatriacontane-2,10,-13,21,24-pentaone. Deferoxamine (I.N.N.)
Use: Chelating agent.
See: Desferal, Amp. (Ciba)

• **DESIPRAMINE HYDROCHLORIDE,** U.S.P. XXI. Caps., Tab., U.S.P. XXI. 10, 11-Dihydro-5-[3-(methylamino)propyl]-5H-dibenz[b,f]azepine hydrochloride.
Use: Antidepressant.
See: Norpramin, Tab. (Merrell Dow)
Pertofrane, Cap. (USV Labs.)

DESITIN. (Leeming) Pow. Talc. Can 3 oz., 7 oz., 10 oz. **Oint.** Cod liver oil, zinc oxide, talc, petrolatum, lanolin. Tube 1.25 oz., 2.25 oz., 4.25 oz., 8 oz. Jar 1 lb.
Use: Diaper rash remedy.

• **DESLANOSIDE,** U.S.P. XXI. Inj., U.S.P. XXI. Deacetyllanatoside C.
Use: Cardiotonic.
See: Cedilanid-D, Amp. (Sandoz)

DESMA. (Tablicaps) Diethylstilbesterol 25 mg./Tab. Patient dispensers 10s.
Use: Estrogen therapy.

11-DESMETHOXY RESERPINE. Deserpidine.
See: Harmonyl, Tab. (Abbott)

DESMOPRESSIN. B.A.N. 1-Desamino-8-D-arginine-vasopressin.
Use: Treatment of diabetes insipidus.

• **DESMOPRESSIN ACETATE.** USAN.
Use: Treatment of diabetes insipidus.
See: DDVAP, Liq. (Centerchem)

DESO-CREME. (Columbia) Zinc undecylenate 20%, caprylic acid 5%, sod. propionate 2%. Tubes 1 oz.
Use: Athlete's foot, ringworm and fungus infections.

DESOMORPHINE. B.A.N. 7,8-Dihydro-6-deoxy-morphine.
Use: Narcotic analgesic.

• **DESONIDE.** USAN. 16-alpha-Hydroxyprednisolone-16, 17 acetonide. B.A.N. 11 β,21-Dihydroxy-16α, 17 α-isopropylidenedioxypregna-1,4-diene-3,20-dione.
Use: Anti-inflammatory.
See: Tridesilon, Cream (Miles Pharm)

• **DESOXIMETASONE GEL,** U.S.P. XXI.

DESOXYCHOLIC ACID. (Various Mfr.) Deoxycholic acid, 3,12-Dihydroxycholanic acid. Tab. 1½ gr.
Use: Choleretic.
See: Droxolan, Tab. (O'Neal)
W/Dehydrocholic acid.
See: Combichole, Tab. (Trout)
Foydox, Tab. (Foy)
Ketosox, Tab. (Ascher)
W/Dehydrocholic acid, ox bile extract, phenobarbital.
See: Oxsorbil PB, Cap. (Ives)
W/Dehydrocholic acid, bile ext., sorbitan mono-oleate, oleic acid.
See: Oxsorbil, Cap. (Ives)
W/Dehydrocholic acid, choline methionine tartrate, & adiphenine HCl.
See: Desacholine, Tab. (Mallard)
W/Ox bile ext., mixed ox bile acids, pancreatin.
See: Bilogen Tabs. (Organon)
W/Pancreatin, pepsin, bile salts, dehydrocholic acid.
See: Enzylax, Tab. (Kay)
Pepsatal, Tab. (Kenyon)
W/Phenobarbital, homatropine methylbromide, gerilase, geriprotase, dehydrocholic acid.
See: Bilezyme Plus, Tabs. (Geriatric)

• **DESOXIMETASONE,** U.S.P. XXI. Cream, U.S.P. XXI.
Use: Adrenocortical steroid.

• **DESOXYCORTICOSTERONE ACETATE,** U.S.P. XXI. Inj., Pellets, U.S.P. XXI. Pregn-4-ene-3,20-dione, 21-(acetyloxy)-. 11-Deoxycorticosterone acetate. (Various Mfr.) (DCA, Deoxycostone acetate, Cortate, Cortiron, Cortenil, Cortigen, Syncort, Syncortyl.) Aq. susp., 5 mg./cc. Vial 10 cc.; in sesame oil, 5 mg./cc. Vial 10 cc.
Uses: I.M. or S.C. (2-5 mg.) adrenal cortical insufficiency; (salt-regulating).
See: Doca Acetate, Inj. (Organon)
Percorten, Amp., Pellet & Vial (Ciba)

• **DESOXYCORTICOSTERONE PIVALATE,** U.S.P. XXI. Sterile Susp. U.S.P. XXI. Pregn-4-ene-3,20-dione, 21-(2,2-dimethyl-1-oxopropoxy)-11-deoxycorticosterone pivalate.
Use: Salt-regulator; adrenocortical steroid.
See: Percorten Privalate, Vial (Ciba)

• **DESOXYCORTICOSTERONE TRIMETHYL-ACETATE.** 11-Deoxycorticosterone pivalate.
Use: Adrenocortical steroid (salt-regulating).

DESOXYCORTONE ACETATE.
See: Desoxycorticosterone Acetate, Prep. (Various Mfr.)

DESOXYEPHEDRINE HYDROCHLORIDE. (Various Mfr.) Dextro-l-phenyl-2-methylaminopropane, d-phenylisopropylmethylamine, d-N-methylamphetamine.
See: Methamphetamine HCl, Prep.

dl-DESOXYEPHEDRINE HYDROCHLORIDE.
See: dl-Methamphetamine HCl

DESOXYMETHASONE. B.A.N. 9α-Fluoro-11β,-21-dihy-droxy-16α-methylpregna-1,4-diene-3,20-dione.
Use: Topical corticosteroid.
See: Esperson
DESOXYN. (Abbott) Methamphetamine HCl.
Tab.: 5 mg., Bot. 100s, 1000s.
Gradumets: 5 mg., Bot. 100s, 10 & 15 mg. Bot. 100s, 500s.
Use: Central nervous system stimulant.
DESOXY NOREPHEDRINE.
Use: Central nervous system stimulant.
See: Amphetamine HCl, Preps. (Various Mfr.)
DESOXYRIBONUCLEASE.
W/Fibrinolysin.
See: Elase, prep. (Parke-Davis)
DESQUAM-X 5% or 10% GEL. (Westwood) Benzoyl peroxide 5% or 10%, laureth-4 6% in a gel base w/water, carbomer 940, diisopropanolamine, disodium edetate. Tube. 1.5 oz., 3 oz.
Use: Antibacterial and drying lotion for control of acne.
DESQUAM-X 4% or 10% WASH. (Westwood) Benzoyl peroxide 4% or 10% in a lathering base of sodium oxtoxynol-3 sulfonate, docusate sodium, magnesium aluminum silicate, methylcellulose, EDTA. Bot. 5 oz.
Use: Topical antibacterial and skin cleanser for the control of acne vulgaris.
D-EST. (Burgin-Arden) Estradiol cypionate 5 mg./cc. 10 cc. vial.
DESYREL. (Mead Johnson) Trazodone HCl 50 mg., 100 mg./Tab. Unit dose 100s.
Use: Antidepressant.
DETACHOL. (Ferndale) Bland, nonirritating liquid for removing adhesive tape. Pkg. 4 oz.
DE TAL. (de Leon) Phenobarbital ¼ gr., hyosciamine sulfate 0.1037 mg., atropine sulfate 0.0194 mg., hyoscine HBr 0.0065 mg./Tab. or 5 cc. **Tab.** Bot. 100s; **Elix.** alcohol 20%, Bot. pt.
DETANE. (Commerce) Tube 0.5 oz.
Use: Desensitizing lubricant.
• **DETERENOL HYDROCHLORIDE.** USAN.
Use: Adrenergic.
DETERGENTS, Surface-Active.
See: pHisoDerm, Liq. (Winthrop Products)
pHisoHex, Liq. (Winthrop-Breon)
Zephiran, Prods. (Winthrop-Breon)
DETIGON HYDROCHLORIDE.
See: Chlophedianol HCl. (Var. Mfr.)
• **DEUTIERIUM OXIDE.** USAN.
Use: Radioactive agent.
DETUSS. (Zenith) Caramiphen edisylate 40 mg., phenylpropanolamine HCl 75 mg., isopropamide iodide equiv. to 2.5 mg. of isopropamide/S.R. Cap.
Use: Allergy, cold treatment.
DETUSSIN EXPECTORANT. (Columbia)
Pseudoephedrine HCl 60 mg., hydrocodone bitartrate 5 mg., guaifenesin 200 mg./5 ml. Bot. pt., gal.
Use: Antitussive, decongestant, expectorant.
DETUSSIN LIQUID. (Columbia) Hydrocodone bitartrate 5 mg., pseudoephedrine HCl 60 mg./5 ml. w/alcohol 57. Bot. pt., gal.

Use: Antitussive, decongestant.
DeWITT'S COUGH CONTROL MEDICINE. (DeWitt) Dextromethorphan HBr 8 mg., ammonium chloride 80 mg., pot. guaiacolsulfonate 75 mg., glycerin, alcohol 3%/5 ml. Bot. 4 oz.
Use: Antitussive.
DeWITT'S PILLS. (DeWitt) Analgesic and mild diuretic pills. Blister Packs 20s, 40s, 80s.
Use: Backache and joint pain relief.
DEXACEN-4. (Central) Dexamethasone phosphate (furnished as dexamethasone sodium phosphate) 4 mg./ml. w/sodium citrate 10 mg., sodium bisulfite 1 mg., methylparaben 1.5 mg., propylparaben 0.2 mg., creatinine 8 mg./ml. and sodium hydroxide to adjust pH. Vial 10 ml. Box 12s.
Use: Corticosteroid therapy by I.M. and soft tissue injection.
DEXACEN-LA-8. (Central) Dexamethasone acetate equivalant to dexamethasone 8 mg./ml. w/sodium Cl 6.67 mg., creatinine 5 mg., disodium edetate 0.5 mg., sodium carboxymethylcellulose 5 mg., polysorbate-80 0.75 mg., benzyl alcohol 9 mg., sodium bisulfite 1 mg./ml. Vial 5 ml. Box 12s.
Use: Corticosteroid therapy by I. M. and soft tissue injection.
DEXACILLIN. Epicillin, B.A.N.
DEX-A-DIET ORIGINAL FORMULA. (O'Connor) Phenylpropanolamine HCL 75 mg., caffeine 200 mg./Cap. Pkg. 3s, 6s, 10s, 24s, 48s.
Use: Appetite suppressant/diuretic.
DEX-A-DIET CAFFEINE FREE. (O'Connor) Phenylpropanolamine HCl 75 mg./Cap. Pkg. 3s, 6s, 20s, 40s.
Use: Appetite suppressant.
• **DEXAMETHASONE,** U.S.P. XXI. Tab., Elix., Gel, Ophth. Susp., Topical Aerosol, U.S.P. XXI. Pregna-1,4-diene-3,20-dione,9-fluoro-11,17,21-trihydroxy-16-methyl-, (11β,16α). 9-fluoro-11β, 17,21-trihydroxy-16α-methyl-, pregna-1,4-diene-3,20-dione.
Use: Adrenocortical steroid (anti-inflammatory); Same as for prednisone or prednisolone; Dose: Individualized according to disease, 0.75 mg. is equivalent to 4 mg. triacinolone, 5 mg. prednisone/prednisolone, 20 mg. hydrocortisone or 25 mg. cortisone.
See: Aeroseb-Dex, Aerosol (Herbert)
Decaderm in Estergel (Merck Sharp & Dohme)
Decadron, Tab., Elxr. (Merck Sharp & Dohme)
Decameth, Inj. (Foy)
Decameth L.A., Inj. (Foy)
Decaspray, Aerosol (Merck Sharp & Dohme)
Dexaport, Tab. (Freeport)
Dezone, Tab. (Reid-Provident)
Dexone TM, Tab. (Rowell)
Hexadrol, Tab. Elxr., Cream. (Organon)
Maxidex Ophth. liq. (Alcon)
SK-Dexamethasone, Tab. (SmithKline)
W/Neomycin Sulf.
See: NeoDecadron, Prep. (Merck Sharp & Dohme)
NeoDecaspray, Aerosol (Merck Sharp & Dohme)
W/Neomycin sulf., polymyxin B sulf.
See: Maxitrol Ophth. Susp., Oint. (Alcon)

• **DEXAMETHASONE ACETATE,** U.S.P. XXI. Sterile Susp.., U.S.P. XXI.
Use: Adrenocortical steroid (anti-inflammatory)
See: Dexzone LA, Ind. (Tunex)
   Tendron, Inj. (Amfre-Grant)
• **DEXAMETHASONE SODIUM PHOSPHATE.** U.S.P. XXI. Inhalation Aerosol, Cream, Ophth. Oint., Ophth. Soln., Inj., U.S.P. XXI. Pregn-4-ene-3,20-dione, 9-fluoro-11, 17-dihydroxy-16-methyl-21-(phosphonooxy)-disodium salt, (11β, 16α)-9-Fluoro-11β, 17,21-trihydroxy-16α-methylpregna-1,4-diene-3,20-dione-21-(dihydrogen phosphate) disodium salt.
Use: Adrenocortical steroid (anti-inflammatory).
See: Dexzone, Inj. (Tunex)
   Decadron Phosphate, Preps. (Merck Sharp & Dohme)
   Decadron Phosphate Respihaler (Merck Sharp & Dohme)
   Decaject, Vial (Mayrand)
   Decameth, Inj. (Foy)
   Dexone, Inj. (Keene, Mallard)
   Dezone, Inj. (Reid-Provident)
   Hexadrol Phosphate, Inj. (Organon)
   Savacort D, Inj. (Savage)
   Solurex, Inj. (Hyrex)
   Tendron, Inj. (Amfre-Grant)
W/Lidocaine (Xylocaine)
See: Decadron Phos w/Xylocaine, Inj. (Merck Sharp & Dohme)
W/Neomycin sulfate.
See: NeoDecadron, Prep. (Merck Sharp & Dohme)
• **DEXAMISOLE.** USAN.
Use: Antidepressant.
DEXAMPEX. (Lemmon) Dextroamphetamine sulfate. **Tab.:** 5 mg./Tab. Bot. 1000s, 5000s,. 10 mg./Tab. 1000s, 5000s. **Cap.:** 15mg./Cap. Bot. 1000s, 5000s.
Use: Central stimulant, narcolepsy treatment.
DEXAMPHETAMINE. B.A.N. (+)-α-Methyl-phenethylamine. (+)-Amphetamine.
Use: Central nervous system stimulant; appetite suprassant.
See: Dexamed
   Dexedrine
DEXAMPHETAMINE.
See: Dextroamphetamine (Var. Mfr.)
DEXA-PED CHEWABLE VITAMINS. (Xttrium) Vit. A 5000 I.U., D 400 I.U., B-1 2 mg., B-2 2 mg., B-6 1.5 mg., B-12 5 mcg., C 75 mg., niacinamide 10 mg., Ca pantothenate 2 mg., E 1 I.U./Tab. Bot. 150s, 250s.
DEXA-PED VITAMIN DROPS. (Xttrium) Vit. A 3000 I.U., D 400 I.U., C 60 mg., B-1 1 mg., B-2 1.2 mg., niacinamide 8 mg., B-6 1 mg., panthenol 3 mg., B-12 1 mcg., biotin 30 mcg./0.6 cc. Bot. 60 cc.
DEXAPORT. (Freeport) Dexamethasone 0.75 mg.,/Tab. Bot. 1000s.
Use: Anti-inflammatory.
DEXASONE. (Ferndale) Dexamethasone sodium phosphate 4 mg./ml. Vial 10 cc.
Use: Adrenocortical steroid therapy.
DEXASONE INJECTION. (Hauck) Dexamethasone sodium phosphate 4 mg./ml. Vial 5 ml.

Use: Advenocortical steroid.
DEXASONE-L.A. INJECTION. (Hauck) Dexamethasone acetate 8 mg./ml. Vial 5 ml., 30 ml.
Use: Adrenocortical steroid.
DEXASPORIN OPHTHALMIC SUSPENSION. (Columbia) Dexamethasone 0.1%, neomycin 3.5 mg., polymyxin B sulfate 10,000 u./ml. Bot. 5 ml.
Use: Anti-inflammatory, antibiotic.
DEXATRIM. (Thompson Medical) Phenylpropanolamine HCl, caffeine. Available in Regular, Extra Strength, Caffeine Free and Caffeine Free plus Vitamins.
Use: Appetite suppressant.
DEXBROM. (Zenith) Dexbrompheniramine maleate 6 mg., pseudoephedrine sulfate 120 mg./Time Release Tab.
Use: Antihistaminic, decongestant.
• **DEXBROMPHENIRAMINE MALEATE,** U.S.P. XXI. (+)-2-[p-Bromo-α-[2-(dimethylamino) ethyl]-[benzyl]-pyridine maleate. Dextro form of brompheniramine. Dextroparabromdylamine 1-(p-bromophenyl-1-(2-pyridyl)-3-dimethylamino propane maleate. (+)-2-(p-Bromo-α-(2-(dimethylamino)ethyl)benzyl)-pyridine-Maleate (1:1)
Use: Antihistaminic.
W/Pseudoephedrine sulfate.
See: Disophrol Chronotab, Tab. (Schering)
   Drixoral S.A., Tab. (Schering)
• **DEXCHLORPHENIRAMINE MALEATE,** U.S.P. XXI. Syrup, Tabs., U.S.P. XXI. d-2-[p-Chloroalpha(2-dimethyl-amino-ethyl)benzyl] pyridine bimaleate. (+)-2-(p-Chloro-α-(2-dimethylamino)-ethyl)benzyl)pyridin-e-Maleate (1:1) Dextro-Chlorpheniramine Maleate.
Use: Antihistaminic.
See: Polaramine, Repetabs Tab., Tab., Syr. (Schering)
W/Pseudoephedrine sulfate, guaifenesin, alcohol.
See: Polaramine Expect. (Schering)
• **DEXCLAMOL HYDROCHLORIDE.** USAN.
Use: Sedative.
DEXEDRINE. (SmithKline) Dextroamphetamine sulfate. **Elixir:** 5 mg./5 ml. (Alcohol 10%.) Bot. 16 oz. **Tab.:** (5 mg.) Bot. 100s, 1000s. **Spansule:** 5 mg. Bot. 50s; 10 mg., 15 mg. Bot. 50s, 500s.
Use: Central nervous system stimulant.
• **DEXETIMIDE.** USAN. (+)-3-(1-Benzyl-4-piperidyl)-3-phenylpiperidine-2,6-dione.
Use: Treatment of the Parkinsonian syndrome.
• **DEXIMAFEN.** USAN.
Use: Antidepressant.
• **DEXIVACAINE.** USAN.
Use: Anethetic.
DEXO-LA. (Mallard) Dexamethasone 8 mg./ml. Vial 5 ml.
Use: Adrenocortical steroid.
DEXON. (Kay) Dexamethasone sodium phosphate 4 mg./ml. Vial 10 ml.
Use: Anti-inflammatory.
DEXON. (Pasadena Research) Desoxycorticosterone acetate 5 mg./ml. Vial 10 cc. (In sesame oil).
DEXON L.A. (Kay) Dexamethasone acetate 8 mg./ml. Vial 5 ml.

Use: Anti-inflammatory.

DEXONE. (Mallard) Dexamethasone sodium phosphate. 4 mg./ml. Amp. 5 ml.
Use: Anti--inflammatory.

DEXONE. (Keene) Dexamethasone sodium phosphate 4 mg./ml. Vial 5 ml., 10 ml.
Use: Anti-inflammatory.

DEXONE L.A.. (Keene) Dexamethasone acetate suspension equiv. to 8 mg. dexamethasone. Vial 5 ml.

DEXONE TM. (Rowell) Dexamethasone 0.5 mg., 0.75 mg., 1.5 mg., 4 mg. Tab. Bot. 100s. Unit dose 100s.

• **DEXOXADROL HYDROCHLORIDE.** USAN. d-2-(2,2-Diphenyl-1,3-dioxolan-4-yl) piperidine hydrochloride. Dextro form of dioxadrol HCl.
Use: Antidepressant.

• **DEXPANTHENOL,** U.S.P. XXI. Preparation, U.S.P. XXI. (+)-2,4-Dihydroxy-N-(3-hydroxypropyl)-3,3-dimethylbutyramide.
Use: Treatment of paralytic ileus and postoperative distention
See: Bepanthen
  Ilopan, Inj. (Adria)
  Intrapan, Vial (Intra; Arcum)
  Panthoderm Lotion, Cream (USV Labs.)
  Tonestat, Inj. (A.V.P.)

DEXPROPRANOLOL. B.A.N. (+)-1-Isopropylamino-3-(1-naphthyloxy)propan-2-ol.
Use: Antiarrhythmic.

• **DEXPROPANOLOL HCl.** USAN. (+)-l-(Iso-propylamino)-3-(l-naphthyloxy)-2-propanol HCl.
Use: Cardiac depressant (antiarrhythmic).

DEX-SALT. (Columbia) Sodium chloride 7 gr., vit. B-1 1 mg., dextrose 3 gr./Tab. Bot. 100s, 1000s.

DEXSONE INJECTION (Vortech) Dexamethasone sod. phosphate equiv. to dexmethasone phos. 4 mg., creatinine 8 mg., sod. citrate 10 mg., sod. bisulfite 1 mg., methyl paraben 1.5 mg., propyl paraben 0.2 mg./cc. Vial 5 cc.
Use: Adrenocortical steroid (Anti-inflammatory).

DEXTRAN. B.A.N. Polyanhydroglucose.
Use: Restoration of blood volume.
See: Dextraven
  Intradex

DEXTRAN.
Use: Blood volume expander.
See: LMWD-Dextran 40 (Pharmchem)
  Macrodex, Sol. (Pharmacia)

DEXTRAN 6%. (Abbott)
See: Dextran 75, I.V. (Abbott)

• **DEXTRAN 40.** USAN. Polysaccharide (m.w. 40,000) produced by the action of Leuconostoc mesenteroides on saccharose.
Use: Blood suspension stabilizer.
See: LMD 10% (Abbott)
  Rheomacrodex, Sol. (Pharmacia)

DEXTRAN 45, 75. Polysaccharide (m.w. 45,000 & 75,000) produced by the action of Leuconostoc mesenteroides on saccharose. Rheotran (45).
Use: Blood plasma volume extender, antithrombogenic agent.

• **DEXTRAN 70.** USAN. A polysaccharide.
  Macrodex, Sol. (Pharmacia)
Use: Blood volume expander.

• **DEXTRAN 75.** USAN. Dextran 75 6% in 0.9% saline. Flask 500 ml.; Dextran 75 6% in 5% dextrose. Flask 500 ml.
Use: Blood plasma expander.

DEXTRANOMER. B.A.N. Dextran cross-linked with epichlorohydrin.
Use: Promoter of wound-healing.
See: Debrisan.

• **DEXTRATES,** N.F. XVI. Mixture of sugars (approximately 92% dextrose monohydrate and 8% higher saccharides; dextrose equivalent is 95 to 97%) resulting from the controlled enzymatic hydrolysis of starch.
Use: Pharmaceutic aid (tablet binder and diluent).

DEXTRIFERRON. B.A.N. A colloidal solution of ferric hydroxide in complex with partially hydrolyzed dextrin.
Use: Treatment of iron-deficiency anemia.
See: Astrafer

DEXTRIFERRON. The hematinic preparation of a colloidal solution of ferric hydroxide in complex with partially hydrolyzed dextrin.
See: Imferon, Amps. (Merrell Dow)

• **DEXTROAMPHETAMINE.** USAN.
Use: Stimulant.

DEXTROAMPHETAMINE WITH AMPHETAMINE AS RESIN COMPLEX.
See: Biphetamine 12½, 20, Cap. (Pennwalt)

DEXTROAMPHETAMINE HYDROCHLORIDE. (Various Mfr.) d-Amphetamine HCl. (+)-2-Aminopropylbenzene.
See: Daro, Preps. (Fellows- Testagar)

DEXTROAMPHETAMINE PHOSPHATE. Monobasic d-a-methylphenethlyamine phosphate. (+)-α-Methylphenethylamine phosphate.
Use: Central stimulant.
See: d-Amphetamine Phos. for combinations

• **DEXTROAMPHETAMINE SULFATE,** U.S.P. XXI. Caps., Elix., Tabs, U.S.P. XXI. Benzeneethanamine, α-methyl-, sulfate (2:1). (+)-α-Methylphenethylamine sulfate (2:1). d-Amphetamine sulfate, d-Methylphenylamine sulfate.
Use: Central stimulant.
See: Amphedex, Cap. (Paddock)
  Dexampex, Cap., Tab. (Lemmon)
  Dexedrine, Prep. (SmithKline)
  Diphylets, Granucaps (Reid-Provident)
  Oxydess, Tab. (Vortech)
  Robese P., Tab., Vial (Rocky Mtn.)
  Spancap #1, #4. (Vortech)
  Tidex Tabs. (Allison)

DEXTROAMPHETAMINE SULFATE W/COMBINATIONS.
See: Amphedex, Cap. (Jamieson-McKames)
  Delcobese (Delco)
  Dextrobar, Tab. (Lannett)
  Min-Gera, Tab. (Scrip)
  Ro Trim, Cap. (Rocky Mtn.)
  Trimex, Trimex #2, Cap. (Mills)

DEXTROAMPHETAMINE TANNATE.
See: Obotan & Obotan Forte, Tab. (Mallinckrodt)
DEXTROBAR. (Lannett) Dextroamphetamine sulfate 5
mg., amobarbital 32 mg./Tab. Bot. 500s, 1000s.
Use: Central stimulant.
DEXTROCAINE. (Wolins) Dextromethorphan HBr 5
mg., benzocaine 1 mg./Loz. Bot. 1000s.
DEXTROCELL. (Jones) Dextroamphetamine sulfate
2.5 mg., methylcellulose 5 gr./Tab. Bot. 100s,
1000s.
DEXTRO-CHEK. (Ames) Solution containing 0.1% glu-
cose. Vials 5 ml. Ctn. 2s.
Use: With Dextrostix and Visidex reagent strips to
quality control test.
DEXTRO-CHEK CALIBRATOS. (Ames) Clear liquid sol.
containing measured amounts of glucose. Low
calibrator contains 0.05% w/v glucose. High
calibrator contains 0.30% w/v glucose.
Use: Dextrostix to perform calibration procedure
with glucometer reflectance photometer.
DEXTRO-CHLORPHENIRAMINE MALEATE.
See: Polaramine, Repetab, Tab., Expect., Syr.
(Schering)
DEXTRO DESOXYEPHEDRINE HCl.
See: Dee-10, Tab. (Scrip)
• **DEXTROMETHORPHAN,** U.S.P. XXI. (+)-3-Methoxy-
N-methylmorphinan.
Use: Cough suppressant.
See: Benylin DM Cough Syrup (Parke-Davis)
Delsym, Lig. (Pennwalt)
Extend-12, Liq. (Robins)
Romilar (hydrobromide)
W/Benzocain, menthol, peppermint oil.
See: Vicks Formula 44 Cough Control Discs, Loz.
(Vicks)
• **DEXTROMETHORPHAN HYDROBROMIDE,** U.S.P.
XXI. Syrup, U.S.P. XXI. d-3-Methoxy-N-methylmorphi-
nan. (+)-3-Methoxy-17-methyl-9α, 13α,-14α-morphi-
nan HBr. Dormethan. d-Methorphan.
Use: Antitussive.
See: Benylin DM Cough Syrup, Syr.
(Parke-Davis)
Dicodethal, Elix. (Lannett)
Maxefed, Tab. (Noyes)
Mediquell, Tab (Warner-Lambert)
Romilar, Loz., Syr., Cap., Tab. (Block)
St. Joseph Cough Syrup (Plough)
Symptom 1, Liq. (Parke-Davis)
Tus-F, Liq. (Orbit)
Tussade Tab. (Westerfield)
DEXTROMETHORPHAN HBr W/COMBINATIONS
See: Algetuss, Syr. (Winston)
Alo-Tuss, Tab. (Vortech)
Ambenyl-D, Liq. (Marion)
Anti-Tuss D.M., Liq. (Century)
Anti-Tussive, Tab. (Canright)
Bayer Prods. (Glenbrook)
Breacol cough Medication, Liq. (Glenbrook)
Capahist-DMH, Cap. (Freeport)
C.D.M., Expect. (Lannett)
Centuss, MLT, Tabs. (Century)
Cerose Compound, Cap. (Ives)

Cerose DM, Liq. (Ives)
Cheracol-D, Cough Syr. (Upjohn)
Cheratussin, Cough Syr. (Towne)
Chexit, Tab. (Dorsey)
Children's Hold 4-Hour Cough Suppressant &
Decongestant, Loz. (Calgon)
Chloraseptic DM Cough Control Lozenges
(Eaton)
Codimal DM, Liq. (Central)
Colchek, Tab. (Creomulsion)
Colrex, Syr. (Rowell)
Combi-Tuss, Syr. (Table Rock)
Comtrex, Cap., Liq. Tab. (Bristol-Myers)
Congespirin Cough Syrup (Bristol-Myers)
Consin-DM, Syr. (Wisconsin)
Consotuss Antitussive, Syr. (Merrell Dow)
Contac Jr., Liq. (Menley & James)
Coricidin Childrens Cough Syrup (Schering)
Corzone, Syr. (Xttrium)
C3 Capsules (Menley & James
Daycare, Liq. (Vicks)
Dextrocaine, Loz. (Wolins)
Dextro-Tuss GG, Liq. (Ulmer)
Dextro-Tussin, Liq. (Ulmer)
Dimacol, Cap. (Robins)
Donatussin, Syr. (Laser)
Dorcol Ped. Cough Syr. (Dorsey)
Dristan Cough Formula, Syr. (Whitehall)
End-A-Koff, Jr. Syr. (Columbia)
Endotussin-N N, Syr. (Du Pont)
Formula 44 Prods. (Vicks)
G-100/DM, Syr. (Bock)
Halls Mentho-Lyptus Decongestant Cough For-
mula, Liq. (Warner-Lambert)
Histalets, DM, Syr. (Reid Provident)
Histivite-D, Syr. (Vitarine)
Hold 4-Hour Cough Suppressant, Loz. (Calgon)
Hycoff, Prep. (Seton)
Infantuss, Liq. (Scott/Cord)
Ipsatol, Syr. (Lakeside)
Listerine Cough Control Lozenges
(Warner-Lambert)
Naldetuss, Syr. (Bristol)
Niltuss, Syr. (Minn. Pharm.)
N-N Cough Syrup (Vitarine)
Nyquil, Liq. (Vicks)
Ornacol, Cap., Liq. (Menley & James)
Orthoxicol, Syr. (Upjohn)
Para-Hist DM, Tab. (Pharmics)
Partuss, Liq. (Parmed)
Phenergan, Pediatric, Liq. (Wyeth)
Propahist-DM, Syr. (Blue Line)
Pyraldine, Syr. (Mallinckrodt)
Polytuss-DM, Liq. (Rhode)
Quartets, Cap. (DePree)
Quelidrine, Syr. (Abbott)
Queltuss, Syr., Tab. (Westerfield)
Rentuss, Tab., Syr. (Wren)
Rentuss, Tab. (Wren)
Rhinex DM, Liq., Tab. (Lemmon)
Robitussin-DM, Syr., Loz. (Robins)
Robitussin-CF (Robins)

Romilar Prods. (Block)
Rondec DM, Drops and Syrup (Ross)
S.A.C. Cough Formula (Towne)
Scotcof Liq. (Scott/Cord)
Scotuss, Pediatric Cough Syr. (Scott/Cord)
Shertus, Liq. (Sheryl)
Silence Is Golden Children's Cough Lozenges (Bristol-Myers)
Silence Is Golden Cough Lozenges (Bristol-Myers)
Silexin, Syr. (Clapp)
Sorbase Cough Syr. (Fort David)
Spantuss, Liq., Tab. (Arco)
Spec-T Sore Throat-Cough Suppressant Lozenges (Squibb)
Sucrets Cough Control Lozenge (Calgon)
Sudafed Cough Syrup (Burroughs Wellcome)
Synatuss-One, Liq. (Freeport)
Tercol, Liq. (Commerce)
Thor, Cough Syr. (Towne)
Thor Capsules (Towne)
Thorzettes Lozenges (Towne)
Tolu-Sed DM, Liq. (Scherer)
Tonecol, Syr., Tab. (A.V.P.)
Triaminic-DM Cough Formula (Dorsey)
Triaminicol, Syr. (Dorsey)
Trihista-Cod, Tab. (Recsei)
Tri-Medicol, Syr. (Medical Chemical)
Trind-DM, Syr. (Mead Johnson)
Tusquelin, Syr. (Circle)
Tussagesic, Tab., Susp. (Dorsey)
Tusscaps, Cap. (Martin-Phillips)
Tuss-Chlorphenade, Cap. (Wolins)
Tusscidin Expectorant D, Liq. (Cenci)
Unproco, Cap. (Reid-Provident)
Vicks Cough Prods. (Vicks)
Vicks Daycare, Liq. (Vicks)
Vicks Formula 44 Prods. (Vicks)
Vicks Nyquil, Liq. (Vicks)
Wal-Tussin DM, Syr. (Walgreen)

DEXTROMORAMIDE. B.A.N. (+)-1-(3-Methyl-4-morpholino-2, 2-diphenylbutyryl) pyrrolidine.
Use: Narcotic analgesic.
See: Jetrium
    Palfium [hydrogen tartrate]

DEXTROMORAMIDE TARTRATE. dl-(3-Methyl-4-morpholino-2, 2-d-phenyl-butyryl) pyrrolidine.

DEXTRO-PANTOTHENYL ALCOHOL.
See: Panthenol (Var. Mfr.)

DEXTROPROPOXYPHENE. B.A.N. α-(+)-4-Dimethylamino-3-methyl-1, 2-diphenyl-2-propionyl-oxybutane. α-(+)-1-Benzyl-3-dimethylamino-2-methyl-1-phenylpropyl propionate.
Use: Analgesic.
See: Darvon Prods. (Lilly)
    Depronal SA [hydrochloride]
    Doxolene [napsylate]

DEXTRO PROPOXYPHENE HCl.
See: Propoxyphene HCl, Caps. (Var. Mfr.)
W/Acetylsalicylic acid, phenaglycodol.
See: Darvo-Tran, Pulvule (Lilly)

DEXTRORPHAN. B.A.N. (+)-3-Hydroxy-N-methylmorphinan.
Use: Narcotic analgesic.
See: Dextromethorphan HBr (Var. Mfr.)

• **DEXTROSE,** U.S.P. XXI. Inj., U.S.P. XXI. d-Glucose. -Glucose, monohydrate.
Use: Fluid and nutrient replenisher.
W/Cal. ascorbate & benzyl alcohol inj.
See: Calscorbate, Amp. (Cole)
W/Psyllium mucilloid.
See: V-lax, Pow. (Century)

• **DEXTROSE EXCIPIENT,** N.F. XVI.
Use: Pharmaceutic aid (tablet excipient)

• **DEXTROSE & SODIUM CHLORIDE INJECTION,** U.S.P. XXI. (Abbott) 10% Dextrose and 0.225% Sodium Chloride Injection. Single dose container 500 ml.
Use: Fluid and electrolyte replenisher.

DEXTROSE LARGE VOLUME PARENTERALS. (Abbott)
Dextrose 2 ½% in Water-1000 ml.
Dextrose 2 ½% in ½ Str. Lact. Ringer's or in ½ Str. Saline-1000 ml.
Dextrose 5% in Water-150, 250, 500, 1000 ml. in Abbo-Vac glass or LifeCare flexible plastic cont.; partial-fill glass: 50 in 200 ml., 50 in 300 ml., 100 in 300 ml., 400 in 500 ml.; partial-fill plastic: 50 in 150 ml., 100 in 150 ml.
Dextrose 5% in Lact. Ringer's-250, 1000 ml. glass; 1000 ml. plastic cont.
Dextrose 5% in Ringer's-500, 1000 ml.
Dextrose 5% in Saline 0.9% or in ¼, ⅓ or ½ Str. Saline-250, 500, 1000 ml. glass or plastic cont.
Dextrose 10% in Water-250, 500, 1000 ml. cont.
Dextrose 20% in Water-500 ml.
Dextrose 50% in Water-500 ml.
Dextrose 20%, 30%, 40%, 50%, 60% and 70% Injections, U.S.P. in partial-fill cont., 500 ml. in 1000 ml.
Dextrose Injection 50%. Bot. 1000 ml
Dextrose 50% and Injection w/Electrolytes in partial-fill cont., 500 ml. in 1000 ml.
Dextrose Injection 70%. Bot. 1000 ml.
Use: Fluid, calorie and electrolyte source.

DEXTROSE SMALL VOLUME PARENTERALS. (Abbott) Dextrose 10%, 5 ml. ampul; Dextrose 50%, 50 ml. Abboject Syr. (18 G × 1½")
Use: Caloric source.

DEXTROSTIX. (Ames) A cellulose strip containing glucose oxidase and indicator system. Bot. 25s, 100s. Box 10s foil wrapped.
Use: Blood-glucose test.

DEXTROTHYROXINE. B.A.N. 3-[4-(4-Hydroxy-3,5-diiodophenoxy)-3, 5-di-iodophenyl]-D-alanine.
Use: Treatment of hypercholesterolemia.
See: Choloxin [sodium derivative]

DEXTROTHYROXINE SODIUM, U.S.P. XXI.
Tab., U.S.P. XXI. D-Tyrosine, 0-(4-hydroxy-3, 5-diiodophenyl)- 3, 5-diiod-, monosodium salt hydrate.
Use: Anticholesteremic.
See: Choloxin, Tab. (Flint)

DEXTRO-TUSS GG. (Ulmer) Guaifenesin 100 mg., dextromethorphan HBr 15 mg./5 ml. W/alcohol 1.4%. Bot. 16 oz.
Use: Expectorant, cough suppressant.

DEXULE. (Approved) Vit. A 1333 I.U., D 133 I.U., B-1 0.33 mg., B-2 0.4 mg., C 10 mg., niacinamide 3.3 mg., Fe 3.3 mg., Ca 29 mg., P 15 mg., methylcellulose 100 mg., benzocaine 3 mg./Cap. Bot. 21s, 90s.
Use: Reducing aid.

DEXYL. (Pinex) Dextromethorphan HBr 15 mg., Vit. C 20 mg./Tab. Box 20s.
Use: Cough due to cold.

• **DEZAQUANINE.** USAN.

• **DEZAQUANINE MESYLATE.** USAN.

DEXZONE. (Tunex) Dexamethasone sod. phosphate equiv. to 4 mg./ml. Vial 5 cc.
Use: Corticosteroid.

DEXZONE LA. (Tunex) Dexamethasone acetate equiv. to 8 mg./ml. Vial 5 cc.
Use: Corticosteroid.

DEZEST. (Geneva) Atropine sulfate, phenylpropanolamine HCl, chlorphenaramine maleate. Bot. 100s.
Use: Decongestant.

• **DEZOCINE.** USAN.
Use: Analgesic.

DEZONE. (Reid-Provident) Dexamethasone 0.75 mg./Tab. Bot. 100s **Inj.,** Dexamethasone sodium phosphate 4 mg./ml. Vial 5 ml.
Use: Synthetic adrenocortical steroid.

D-FILM. (CooperVision) Cleaning gel. Poloxamer 407, benzalkonium chloride 0.025%, edetate trisodium 0.25%. 25 Gm.
Use: Cleaning gel for hard contact lenses.

DFP. Diisopropyl fluorophosphate (Var. Mfr.)

D.H.E. 45. (Sandoz) Dihydroergotamine mesylate. Amp. 1 mg./ml., methanesulfonic acid/sod. hydroxide, alcohol 6.1%, glycerin 15%, Water for Injection U.S.P., q.s. to 1 ml. SandoPak Pkg. 20s.
Use: Parenterally, treatment of migraine.

DHS CONDITIONING RINSE. (Person & Covey) Conditioning ingredients. Bot. 8 oz.
Use: Dermatalogical hair care.

D.H.S. SHAMPOO. (Person & Covey) Blend of cleansing surfactants and emulsifiers. Plastic Bot. w/dispenser 8 oz., 16 oz.
Use: Dermatological hair and scalp shampoo.

DHS TAR SHAMPOO. (Person & Covey) Coal tar 0.5% in DHS shampoo. Bot. 4 oz., 8 oz.
Use: Seborrhea and psoriasis of the scalp.

DHS ZINC SHAMPOO. (Person & Covey) Zinc pyrithione 2% in DHS shampoo. Bot. 6 oz., 12 oz.
Use: Anti-dandruff shampoo.

DHT. (Roxane) Dihydrotachysterol. **Tab.:** 0.125, 0.2 or 0.4 mg./Tab. **Oral Sol.:** 0.2 mg./5 ml. Bot. 500 ml. **Intensol:** Dihydrotachysterol 0.2 mg./ml. w/alcohol 20%. Bot. 30 ml. w/dropper
Use: Calcium regulator.

DIABETA. (Hoechst) Glyburide. 1.25 mg., 2.5 mg. or 5.0 mg./Tab.
Use: Oral antidiabetic agent.

DIABETUSSIN EXPECTORANT. (Research Pharmacal Lab.) Guaifenesin 100 mg., pot. citrate, glycerine, citric acid, menthol/5 cc. sugar free. Bot. 4 oz., pt., gal.
Use: Expectorant.

DIABINESE. (Pfizer Laboratories) Chlorpropamide 100 mg./Tab. Bot. 100s, 500s. Unit dose 100s; 250 mg./Tab. 100s, 250s, 1000s. Unit dose 100s.
Use: Hypoglycemic agent.

DIABISMUL LIQUID. (O'Neal, Jones & Feldman) Opium 7 mg., pectin 80 mg., kaolin 2500 mg./15 ml. Bot. 8 oz.
Use: Anidiarrheal.

DIABISMUL TABLETS. (O'Neal, Jones & Feldman) Bismuth subcarbonate 125 mg., powdered opium 1.23 mg., calcium carbonate 125 mg./Tab. Bot. 1000s.
Use: Antidiarrheal.

DIACETAMATE. B.A.N. 4-Acetamidophenyl acetate.
Use: Analgesic.

3, 5-DIACETAMIDO-2, 4, 6-TRIIODOBENZOIC ACID. Diatrizoic Acid, U.S.P. XXI.

DIACETIC ACID TEST.
See: Acetest, Tab. (Ames)

DIACETO. (Archer-Taylor) Aspirin 3½ gr., acetophenetidin 2½ gr., caffeine ½ gr./Tab. Bot. 100s, 1000s.

DIACETO W/CODEINE. (Archer-Taylor) Codeine ¼ gr. or ½ gr./Tab. or Cap. Bot. 500s, 1000s.

DIACETO W/GELSEMIUM. (Archer-Taylor) Phenobarbital ½ gr. gelsemium 3 min./Tab. Bot. 1000s.

• **DIACETOLOL HYDROCHLORIDE.** USAN.
Use: Anti-adrenergic.

DIACETRIZOATE, SODIUM.
See: Diatrizoate (Var. Mfr.)

• **DIACETYLATED MONOGLYCERIDES,** N.F. XVI. Glycerin esterfied with edible fat-forming fatty acids and acetic acid.

DIACETYLCHOLINE CHLORIDE. Succinyl-choline Chloride.
See: Anectine Chloride, Inj., Pow. (Burroughs-Wellcome)

DIACETYL-DIHYDROXYDIPHENYLISATIN.
See: Oxyphenisatin acetate (Var. Mfr.)

DIACETYLDIOXYPHENYLISATIN.
See: Oxyphenisatin acetate (Var. Mfr.)

DIACETYLMORPHINE SALTS. Heroin. Forbidden in U.S.A. by Federal statute because of its addiction-causing nature.

DIACETYLNALORPHINE. B.A.N. O³O⁶-Diacetyl-N-allylnormorphine.
Use: Narcotic analgesic.

DIACTION. (Boots) Diphenoxylate HCl 2.5 mg., atropine sulfate 0.025 mg./Tab. Bot. 100s, 500s.
Use: Antidiarrheal.

DIADAX CAPSULES. (O'Connor) Phenylpropanolamine HCl 50 mg./Cap. Bot. 14s, 30s, 40s.
Use: Appetite suppressant.

DIADAX TABLETS. (O'Connor) Phenylpropanolamine HCl 25 mg./Tab. Bot. 21s, 100s.
Use: Appetite suppressant.

DI-ADEMIL.
　See: Hydroflumethiazide, Tab. (Var. Mfr.)
DIA-EAZ. (Central) Bismuth subgallate 0.15 Gm., kaolin
　5.5 Gm./15 ml. w/preservatives and aromatics.
　Bot. 8 oz.
　Use: Antidiarrheal.
DIAGARD. (Vitarine) Cassanthranol 30 mg., docusate
　sodium 100 mg./Cap.
　Use: Fecal softener.
DIAGNIOL.
　See: Sodium Acetrizoate
DIAGNOSTIC 50+. (Barry) Allergenic extracts
　scratch test kit 3% (1:30 dilution w/v). Vial 1.5
　cc/w dropper.
　Use: Testing for common allergies to dust, molds;
　and various tree, grass and weed pollens.
■ **DIAGNOSTIC AGENTS.**
　See: Acholest, Kit. (Fougera)
　　Baroflave, Pow. (Lannett)
　　Cardio-Green, Vial (Hynson Westcott & Dunning)
　　Cardiografin, Vial (Squibb)
　　Cea-Roche, Kit (Roche)
　　Cholografin, Prep. (Squibb)
　　Coccidioidin, Vial (Cutter)
　　Dextrostix, Strips (Ames)
　　Diptheria Toxin for Schick Test (Var. Mfr.)
　　Evans Blue, Amp. (Harvey)
　　Fertility Tape (Weston Labs.)
　　Fluorescein Sodium Ophth. Sol. (Various Mfr.)
　　Fluor-I-Strip (Ayerst)
　　Fluor-I-Strip A.T. (Ayerst)
　　Fluress, Ophth. Sol. (Barnes-Hind)
　　Glucola, Sol. (Ames)
　　Hema-Combistix Strips (Ames)
　　Hemastix Strips (Ames)
　　Histalog, Amp. (Lilly)
　　Histoplasmin, Vial (Parke-Davis)
　　Indigo Carmine (Var. Mfr.)
　　Mannitol Sol., Inj. (Merck Sharp & Dohme)
　　Phenolsulfonphthalein (Var. Mfr.)
　　Phentolamine Methanesulfonate, Inj. (Var. Mfr.)
　　Regitine, Amp. & Tab. (Ciba)
　　Rheumanosticon Slide Test (Organon)
　　Rocky Mountain Spotted Fever Antigen, Vial
　　　(Lederle)
　　Sodium Dehydrocholate, Inj. (Var. Mfr.)
　　Tes-Tape (Lilly)
　See also: Cholecystography Agents
　　Kidney Function Agents
　　Liver Function Agents
　　Urography Agents
■ **DIAGNOSTIC AGENTS FOR URINE.**
　See: Acetest, Tab. (Ames)
　　Albustix, Strips (Ames)
　　Bumintest, Tab. (Ames)
　　Clinistix, Strips (Ames)
　　Clinitest, Tab. (Ames)
　　Hema-Combistix, Strip (Ames)
　　Hemastix, Strip (Ames)
　　Hematest, Tab. (Ames)
　　Icotest, Tab. (Ames)

　　Ketostix, Strips (Ames)
　　Pheniplate, Preps. (Ames)
　　Phenistix, Strips (Ames)
　　Uristix, Strips (Ames)
DIAGNOSTIC '10' KIT. (Panray) 10-2 cc. A.T.V. vials.
　Mxd molds Vial 2 cc., mxd inhalants-D Vial 2 cc., mxd
　insects Vial 2 cc., mxd epidermals Vial 2 cc., house
　dust Vial 2 cc., mxd ragweed Vial 2 cc., mxd trees
　Vial 2 cc., mxd grasses Vial 2 cc., mxd weeds Vial
　2 cc., control vial Vial 2 cc.
DIAHIST ELIXIR. (Century) Diphenhydramine HCl
　12.5 mg./ml. Bot. gal.
　Use: Antihistaminic.
DIALLYLAMICOL. Diallyl-diethylaminoethyl phenol di
　HCl.
DIALLYBARBITURIC ACID. Allobarbital,
　Allobarbitone, Curral.
　W/Acetaminophen, aluminum aspirin, aspirin.
　　See: Allylgesic, Tab. (Elder)
　W/Atropine sulfate, Mag. carb., Cal. carb. precipitated
　　& bismuth subcarb.
　　See: Dia-Tropine, Tab. (O'Neal)
DIALLYLNORTOXIFERINE.
　See: Alloferin (Roche)
DIALMINATE. Mixture mag. carb. and (alminate)
　dihydroxyaluminum glycinate.
　W/Aspirin.
　　See: Bufferin, Preps. (Bristol-Myers)
DIALOSE. (Stuart) Docusate potassium 100 mg./Cap.
　Bot. 36s, 100s, 500s,
　Unit Dose 100s.
　Use: Stool softener for treatment of constipation
　due to lack of moisture in stool.
DIALOSE PLUS. (Stuart) Docusate potassium 100
　mg., casanthranol 30 mg./Cap.
　Bot. 36s, 100s, 500s,
　Unit Dose 100s.
　Use: Stool softener with peristaltic activator for
　constipation caused by decreased intestinal motility.
DIALUME. (Armour) Aluminum hydroxide gel 500
　mg./Cap. Bot. 100s, 500s.
　Use: Antacid.
DIA-MER-SULFONAMIDES. Sulfadiazine, Sulfamera-
　zine.
　　See: Aldiazol-M, Susp. (Beecham-Massengill)
　　　Sulfonamide Duplex, Susp. (Lilly)
　W/Alkaline agents.
　　See: Aldiazol-M, Susp. (Beecham-Massengill)
DIAMETHINE.
　See: Dimethyl tubocurarine (Var. Mfr.)
DIAMINE DIPENICILLIN G.
　See: Benzethacil (Var. Mfr.)
**DI-AMINO ACETATE COMPLEX W/Calcium Alumi-
　num Carbonate.**
　See: Ancid Tab. & Susp. (Sheryl)
**4,6-DIAMINO-1(P-CHLOROPHENYL)-1,2-DIHYDRO-
　2,2-DIMETHYL-S-TRIAZINE COMPOUND (2:1)
　WITH 4,4'-METHYLENEBIS-[3-HYDROXY-2-
　NAPHTHOIC ACID].** Camolar
**2,4-DIAMINO-5-(p-CHLOROPHENYL)-6-ETHYLPYRI-
　MIDINE.** Pyrimethamine, U.S.P. XXI.

DIAMINODIPHENYLSULFONE. Dapsone, U.S.P. XXI.
Use: Treatment of malaria.
See: Avlosulfon, Tab. (Ayerst)
Diasone Sod., Tab. (Abbott)
Glucosulfone Sod., Inj. (Var. Mfr.)
2,6-DIAMINO-3-PHENYLAZOPYRIDINE HYDRO-CHLORIDE.
Use: Urogenital antiseptic.
See: Phenazopyridine HCl (Var. Mfr.)
Phenylazo-diaminopyridine hydrochloride
DIAMINOPROPYL TETRAMETHYLENE.
See: Spermine
L-(+)-N-[p][2,4-DIAMINO-6-PYERIDINYL)METHYL] METHYLAMINO[BENZOYL]-GLUTAMIC ACID. Methotrexate, U.S.P. XXI.
DIAMOCAINE. B.A.N. 1-(2-Anilinoethyl)-4-(2-diethylaminoethoxy)-4-phenylpiperidine.
Use: Local anesthetic.
• **DIAMOCAINE CYCLAMATE.** USAN. (1) 1-(2-Anilinoethyl)-4-[2-(diethylamino)-ethoxy]-4-phenylpiperidine bis(cyclohexanesulfamate); (2) Cyclohexanesulfamic acid compound with 1-(2-anilinoethyl)-4-[2-(diethylamino)ethoxy]-4-phenylpiperidine (2:1).
Use: Local anesthetic.
DIAMOX. (Lederle) Acetazolamide (2-acetylamino-1,-3,4-thiadiazole-5-sulfonamide). **Tab.** 125 mg., Bot. 100s; 250 mg. Bot. 100s, 1000s. **Parenteral Vial** sod. salt 500 mg., (sod. hydroxide to adjust pH).
Use: Diuretic. Carbonic anhydrase inhibitor, glaucoma therapy.
DIAMOX SEQUELS. (Lederle) Acetazolamide 500 mg./Cap. Bot. 30s, 100s.
Use: Diuretic, glaucoma therapy.
DIAMPHENETHIDE. B.A.N. ββ'-Oxydi(aceto-p-phenetidide).
Use: Anthelminitic, veterinary medicine.
See: Coriban
DIAMPROMIDE. B.A.N. N-[2-(N-Methylphenethylamino)propyl]propionanilide.
Use: Analgesic.
DIAMPRON ISETHIONATE. Amicarbalide, B.A.N.
DIAMTHAZOLE. B.A.N. 6-(2-Diethylaminoethoxy)-2-dimethylaminobenzothiazole.
Dimazole (I.N.N.)
Use: Antifungal agent.
See: Asterol (dihydrochloride)
DIAMTHAZOLE DIHYDROCHLORIDE. Asterol.
DIANEAL. (Travenol) Na 141 mEq, Ca 3.5 mEq, Mg 1.5 mEq, Cl 101 mEq, lactate 45 mEq/Liter. w/Dextrose 1.5% or 4.25%. Bot. 1000 ml., 2000 ml.
DIANEAL 137. (Travenol) Na 132 mEq, Ca 3.5 mEq, Mg 1.5 mEq, Cl 102 mEq, lactate 35 mEq/Liter W/Dextrose 1.5% or 4.25%. Bot. 2000 ml.
DIANEAL K. (Travenol) Dextrose (Hydrous) U.S.P. 15 Gm., sodium 141 mEq, chloride 101 mEq, calcium 3.5 mEq, magnesium 1.5 mEq, lactate 45 mEq, potassium 4mEq./L. Bot. 1.5% dextrose solution. 1000 ml., 2000 ml.
Use: Peritoneal dialysis.
DIANEAL K-141. (Travenol) Na 132 mEq, Ca 3.5 mEq,

Mg 1.5 mEq, Cl 106 mEq, lactate 35 mEq, K 4 mEq/Liter. W/Dextrose 1.5% or 4.25%. Bot. 2000 ml.
1,4:3,6-DIANHYDRO-D-GLUCITOL DINITRATE.
Diluted Isosorbide Dinitrate, U.S.P. XXI.
1,4:3,6-DIANHYDRO-SORBITOL-2,5-DINITRATE.
Diluted Isosorbide Dinitrate, U.S.P. XXI.
DIAPAKARE. (Paddock) Antibacterial agent. Cans 9 oz. (Powd.)
Use: Diaper rash, prickly heat.
DIAPAKARE ANTIBACTERIAL POWDER. (Paddock) Diaphene, corn starch, sod. bicarbonate.
• **DIAPAMIDE.** USAN.
Use: Diuretic, antihypertensive.
DIAPANTIN. (Janssen) Isoprofamide bromide.
Use: Anticholinergic.
DIAPARENE. (Glenbrook) Methylbenzethonium chloride. **Pow.** 1:1000, Bot. 4 oz., 9 oz., 12½ oz. **Oint.,** 1:1000, Tube 1 oz., 2 oz., 4 oz.
Use: Surface-active disinfectant.
DIAPARENE CRADOL EMULS. (Glenbrook) Methylbenzethonium chloride in pet. and lanolin Base. Plast. Bot. 3 oz.
Use: Seborrhea capitis.
DIAPARENE OINTMENT. (Glenbrook) Methylbenzethonium Cl. 0.1% w/petrolatum & glycerin. Tubes 1 oz., 2 oz., 4 oz.
Use: Soothe, soften, protect irritated areas.
DIAPARENE PERI-ANAL CREAM. (Glenbrook) Methylbenzethonium chloride 1:1000, zinc oxide, starch, cod liver oil & casein. Cream, Tube 1 oz., 2 oz., 4 oz.
Use: Rectally, dermatitis.
DIAPER RASH CREAM. (Eckerd) Bot. 4 oz.
Use: Protective and emollient.
DIAPHENYLSULFONE. Dapsone, U.S.P. XXI.
DIAPID. (Sandoz) Lypressin synthetic lysine-8-vasopressin. Equiv. to 50 U.S.P. units posterior pituitary/cc. (0.185 mg./cc.). Nasal spray. Bot. Plastic squeeze 8 ml.
Use: Diabetes insipidus.
DIAPARESS. (Jenkins) Cod liver oil, diperodon HCl 0.25%, Zinc oxide, starch, aluminum acetate, Peruvian balsam. Tubes 1.5 oz.
Use: Minor skin irritations.
DI-AP-TROL. (Foy) Phendimetrazine tartrate 35 mg./Tab. Bot. 100s, 1000s.
DIAQUA. (Hauck) Hydrochlorthiazide 50 mg./Tab. Bot. 100s, 1000s. Unit dose 100s.
Use: Diuretic.
DIAR AID. (Thompson Medical) Activated attapulgate and pectin.
Use: Antidiarrheal.
DIARREST. (Dover) Calcium carbonate, pectin/Tab. Sugar and salt free. Unit dose boxes 500s.
Use: Antidiarrheal.
DIARRHEA RELIEF WITH PAREGORIC. (Weeks & Leo) Bismuth subsalicylate 63 mg., kaolin 675 mg., pectin 27 mg. paregoric 0.6 ml./5 ml. Bot. 4 oz.
Use: Relief of diarrhea and nausea.
DIARRHEA THERAPY.
See: Antidiarrheics

DIASPORAL. (Doak) Formerly Sulfur Salicyl
Diasporal. Sulfur 3%, salicylic acid 2%, isopropyl
alcohol in diasporal base. Cream: Jar 3¾ oz.
Use: Topical antiseptic.

DIASTASE.
See: Aspergillus oryzae enzyme
W/Bismuth subnitrate, sod. bicarb., magnesium
carbonate, papain.
See: Panacarb, Tab. (Lannett)
W/Carica papaya enzyme.
See: Caripeptic, Liq. (Upjohn)
W/Sod. bicarbonate, magnesium carbonate, bismuth
subnitrate, papain.

DIASTIX. (Ames) Broad range test for glucose in
urine. Containing glucose oxidase, peroxidase,
potassium iodide/w blue background dye. Tab. Pkg.
50s, 100s.
Use: Dip-and-Read test for urine glucose.

DIATRIC. (Pasadena Research) Methyl testosterone
5 mg., ethinyl estradiol 0.02 mg./Tab. Bot. 100s,
1000s.
Use: Anabolic.

DIATRIZOATE.   3,5-diacetamido-2,4,6-triiodobenzoic
acid.

• **DIATRIZOATE MEGLUMINE,** U.S.P. XXI. Inj., U.S.P.
XXI. Benzoic acid, 3,5-bis(acetylamino)-2,4,6-tri-
iodo-, compound with 1-deoxy-1-(methylamino)-
-glucitol (1:1).
Use: Diagnostic aid (radiopaque medium).
See: Angiovist 282, Inj. (Berlex)
Cardiografin, Vial (Squibb)
Cystographin, Inj. (Squibb)
Gastrografin, Liq. (Squibb)
Hypaque-Cysto, Liq. (Winthrop-Breon)
Hypaque Melgumide, Liq. (Winthrop-Breon)
Hypaque Meglumine (Winthrop-Breon)
Renografin, Inj. (Squibb)
Reno-M-DIP, Inj. (Squibb)
Reno-M-30, Inj. (Squibb)
Reno-M-60, Inj. (Squibb)
Urovist, Prods. (Berlex)
W/Iodipamide methylglucamine.
See: Sinografin, Vial (Squibb)
W/Sod. Diatrizoate.
See: Renovist, Inj. (Squibb)

• **DIATRIZOATE MEGLUMINE AND DIATRIZOATE
SODIUM INJECTION,** U.S.P. XXI.
Use: Diagnostic aid (radiopaque medium).
See: Angiorist 292, Inj. (Berlex)
Angiovist 370, Inj. (Berlex)
Gastrovist, Sol. (Berlex)
Hypaque-M Prods. (Winthrop-Breon)

• **DIATRIZOATE MEGLUMINE AND DIATRIZOATE
SODIUM SOLUTION,** U.S.P. XXI.
See: Gastrografini Sol. (Squibb)
Renografin-60, Sol. (Squibb)
Renografin-76, Sol. (Squibb)
Renovist, Sol. (Squibb)

DIATRIZOATE METHYLGLUCAMINE.
See: Diatrizoate Meglumine, U.S.P. XXI.

DIATRIZOATE METHYLGLUCAMINE SODIUM. Sod.
salt of N-methylglucamine salt of 3,5-diacetamido-
2,4,6-triiodobenzoate.

• **DIATRIZOATE SODIUM,** U.S.P. XXI. Inj., Sol.,
U.S.P. XXI. Benzoic acid, 3,5-bis(acetylamino)-2,4,6-
triiodo-, monosodium salt.
Use: Diagnostic aid (radiopaque medium).
See: Hypaque Prods. (Winthrop-Breon)
Urovist Sodium, Inj. (Berlex)
W/Meglumine diatrizoate.
See: Gastrografin, Liq. (Squibb)
Renografin-60, -76, Vial (Squibb)
Renovist II, Vial (Squibb)
W/Methylglucamine diatrizoate, sodium citrate,
disodium ethylenediamine tetra-acetate dihydrate,
methylparaben, propylparaben.
See: Renovist, Vial (Squibb)

• **DIATRIZOATE SODIUM I-125.** USAN.
Use: Radioactive agent.

• **DIATRIZOATE SODIUM I-131.** USAN.
Use: Radioactive agent.

• **DIATRIZOIC ACID.** USAN. 3,5-Diacetamido-2,4,6-
tri-iodobenzoic acid.
Use: Radio-opaque substance.
See: Amidotrizoic Acid
Hypaque sodium salt

• **DIATRIZOIC ACID,** U.S.P. XXI. Benzoic acid, 3,5-
bis(acetylamino)-2,4,6-triiodo-.   3,5-Diacetamido-2,-
4,6-triiodobenzoic acid.
Use: Radiopaque medium (urographic).

DIATRO. (Whiteworth) Diphenoxylate w/atropine
sulfate. 2.500/ 0.25 mg. Tab. 100s, 500s,
1000s.
Use: Antidiarrheal.

DIATROL. (Otis Clapp) Pectin, calcium
carbonate/Tab. Safety Pack 500s; Bot. 100s.
Aidpaks 100s. Unit boxes 20s.
Use: Antidiarrheal.

• **DIAVERIDINE.** USAN. 2,4-Diamino-5-(3,4-dimethox-
ybenzyl)pyrimidine. Present in Darvisul
Use: Antiprotozoan, veterinary medicine.

• **DIAZEPAM,** U.S.P. XXI. Cap., Extended-Release Cap.,
Inj., Tabs: U.S.P. XXI. 2H-1,4-Benzodiazepin-2-one, 7-
chloro-1,3-dihydro-1-methyl-5-phenyl-. 7-Chloro-1,3-
dihydro-1-methyl-5-phenyl-2H-1,4-benzodiazepin-2-
one. B.A.N. 7-Chloro-1,3-dihydro-1-methyl-5-phenyl-
2H-1,4-benzodiazepin-2-one.
Use: Agent for control of emotional disturbances;
sedative; tranquilizer.
See: Valcaps, Cap. (Roche)
Valium, Tab. (Roche)
Valrelease, S.R. Cap. (Roche)

DIAZINON.
See: Dimpylate, B.A.N.

• **DIAZIQUONE.** USAN.
Use: Antineoplastic.

DIAZMA. (Pharmex) Diphylline 250 mg./cc. Vial 10
cc.

DI-AZO. (Kay) Phenazopyridine HC1 100 mg./Tab.
Bot. 50s, 100s, 1000s.
Use: Urinary analgesic.

DIAZOMYCINS A, B, & C. Antibiotic obtained from
Streptomyces ambofaciens. Under study.

6-DIAZO-5-OXO-L-NORLEUCINE.

DIAZO-TEL TEST SYSTEM. (Warner-Lambert) A bilirubin test system.

Use: Aid in the diagnosis of red blood cell break-down, liver disease or blockage of the bile duct.
• **DIAZOXIDE,** U.S.P. XXI. Cap., Oral Susp., Inj., U.S.P. XXI. 7-Chloro-3-methyl-2H-1,-2, 4-benzothiadiazine-1, 1-dioxide.
Use: Antihypertensive.
See: Hyperstat, Inj. (Schering)
Proglycem Capsules (Schering)
Proglycem Suspension (Schering)
• **DIBASIC CALCIUM PHOSPHATE,** U.S.P. XXI.
See: D.C.P. 340, Tabs. (Parke-Davis)
Diostate D, Tab. (Upjohn)
DIBASIC CALCIUM PHOSPHATE w/VITAMIN D.
(Lilly) Dibasic calcium phosphate, anhydrous, equiv. to 500 mg. of dibasic calcium phosphate dihydrate, Vit. D synthetic 33 I.U. (0.825 mcg.)/Pulvule. Bot. 100s.
DIBENCIL.
See: Benzathine Penicillin G. (Var Mfr.)
DIBENT. (Hauck) **Tab.:** Dicyclomine HCl 20 mg./Tab. Bot. 100s. **Injection:** Dicyclomine HCl 10 mg., sodium Cl 9 mg./ml. Vial 10 ml.
Use: Smooth muscle relaxant of G.I. tract.
DIBENT-PB. (Hauck) Dicyclomine HCl 20 mg., phenobarbital 15 mg./Tab. Bot. 100s.
Use: Adjunct therapy in treatment of peptic ulcer.
DIBENZEPIN. B.A.N. 10-(2-Dimethylaminoethyl)-5-methyldibenzo[b,e][1,4]diazepin-11-one.
Use: Antidepressant.
See: Noveril hydrochloride
5H-DIBENZ[b,f]AZEPINE-5-CARBOXAMIDE. Carbamazepine, U.S.P. XXI.
5H-DIBENZ[b,f]AZEPINE-5-PROPANAMINE, 10,11-DIHYDRO-N,N-DIMETHYL-, HCl. Imipramine HCl, U.S.P. XXI.
• **DIBENZEPIN HCl.** USAN. 10-[2-Dimethylamino)ethyl]-5,10-dihydro-5-methyl-IlH-dibenzo-[b,e][1,4]diazepin-11-one monohydrochloride.
Use: Antidepressant.
4-(5H-DIBENZO(a,d)CYCLOHEPTEN-5-YLIDENE)-1-METHYLPIPERIDENE HYDROCHLORIDE.
See: Cyproheptadine Hydrochloride, Syr., Tab. (Merck Sharp & Dohme)
• **DIBENZOTHIOPHENE.** USAN.
Use: Keratolytic.
(+)-1,3-DIBENZYLDECAHYDRO-2-OXOIMIDAZO[4,5-c]THIENO[1,2-a]-THIOLIUM 2-OXO-10-BORNANESULFONATE (1:1). Trimethaphan Camsylate, U.S.P. XXI.
DIBENZYLETHYLENEDIAMINE DIPENICILLIN G, U.S.P.
See: Benzethacil
DIBENZYLINE. (SmithKline) Phenoxybenzamine HCl 10 mg./Cap. Bot. 100s.
Use: Long-acting adrenergic blocking agent.
• **DIBROMSALAN.** USAN. 4′, 5-Dibromosalicylanilide. Diaphene
Use: Germicide.
• **DIBUCAINE,** U.S.P. XXI. Cream, Oint., U.S.P. XXI. 2-Butoxy-N-[2-(diethylamino)ethyl]-cinchoninamide.
Use: Local anesthetic.
See: D-caine, Oint. (Century)

Dulzit, Cream (Commerce)
Nupercainal, Oint. (Ciba)
W/Benzocaine.
See: Extend, Tab. (Edward J. Moore)
W/Benzocaine, tetracaine.
See: Bonal Itch Cream, Cream (Edward J. Moore)
W/Hydrocortisone.
See: Corticaine Cream (Blue Line)
W/Dextrose.
See: Nupercaine Heavy Soln. (Ciba)
W/Sod. bisulfite.
See: Nupercainal, Cream, Oint. (Ciba)
W/Zinc oxide, bismuth subgallate, acetone sod. bisulfite.
See: Nupercainal, Oint., Supp (Ciba)
• **DIBUCAINE HYDROCHLORIDE,** U.S.P. XXI. Inj., U.S.P. XXI. 2-Butoxy-N-(2-diethylamino-ethyl) cinchoninamide HCl. (Cinchocaine, Percaine)
Use: Surface & spinal anesthesia.
See: Nupercaine HCl, Sol., (Ciba)
W/Antipyrine, hydrocortisone, polymyxin B sulfate. neomycin sulfate.
See: Otocort, Liq. (Lemmon)
W/Colistin sodium methanesulfonate, citric acid, sodium citrate.
See: Coly-Mycin M, Injectable (Warner-Chilcott)
W/Hydrocortisone.
See: Cortacaine, Cream (Meyer)
DIBUPYRONE. B.A.N. Sodium N-(2,3-dimethyl-1-phenyl-5-oxopyrazolin-4-yl)-N-isobutylamino-methanesulfonate.
Use: Analgesic.
DIBUTOLINE SULFATE. Ethyl(2-hydroxy-ethyl)-dimethylammonium sulfate (2:1) bis(dibutyl-carbamate).
Use: Anticholinergic.
DI-CAL. (Kenyon) Dibasic calcium phosphate 261.9 mg., calcium gluconate 162 mg., Vit. D 333 I.U./Cap. Bot. 100s, 1000s.
DICALCIUM PHOSPHATE. Dibasic Calcium Phosphate, U.S.P., Monocalcium Phosphate. (Various Mfr.) **Cap.** 7½ gr., 10 gr. **Tab.** 7½ gr., 10 gr., 15 gr. Wafers 15 gr.
Use: Calcium supplement.
See: Irophos-D, Cap. (Lannett)
W/Cal. gluconate & Vit. D. (Various Mfr.) Cap., Tab. & Wafer.
See: Calcicaps, Tab. (Nion)
Di-Cal, Cap. (Kenyon)
W/Iron & Vit. D. (Various Mfr.)
Lilly—Pulvule, Bot. 100s.
Premo-Cap. Bot. 100s, 1000s.
W/Liver protein, vitamins, minerals.
See: Pet-A-Vite, Prep. (Vortech)
W/Methyl testosterone, ethinyl estradiol, linoleic acid, cobalt sulf, niacin, desic. liver, Mg sulf., Mn sulf., Cu sulf., Fe peptonate, pot. iodide
See: Gera-Pet, Tab. (North. Amer. Pharm.)
W/Vitamin D. (Squibb) Ca 85 mg., phosphorous 60 mg., Vit.-D. 41 I.U.
DICAL-D. (Abbott) Dibasic calcium phosphate containing calcium 116.7 mg., phosphorous 90 mg., Vit. D 133 I.U./Cap. Bot. 100s, 500s.

Use: Increase oral intake of calcium & phosphorus.

DICAL-D WITH IRON. (Abbott) Dibasic calcium phosphate containing calcium 116.7 mg., phosphorus 90 mg., Vit. D 133 I.U., iron pyrophosphate soluble 87 mg./Cap. Bot. 100s.
Use: Calcium, phosphorus & iron supplement.

DICAL-D WITH VITAMIN C. (Abbott) Dibasic calcium phosphate containing calcium 116.7 mg., phosphorus 90 mg., Vit. D 133 I.U., ascorbic acid 15 mg./Cap. Bot. 100s.
Use: Calcium, phosphorus & Vitamin C supplement.

DICAL-D WAFERS. (Abbott) Dibasic calcium phosphate containing calcium 232 mg., phosphorus 180 mg., Vit. D 200 I.U./Wafer. Box of 51s.
Use: Calcium & phosphorus supplement.

DICAL-DEE. (Barre) Vit. D 350 I.U., dibasic calcium phosphate 4½ gr., Cal. gluconate 3 gr./Cap. Bot. 100s, 1000s.
Use: Calcium supplement.

DICALDEL. (Faraday) Dibasic calcium phosphate 300 mg., calcium gluconate 200 mg., Vit. D 33 I.U./Cap. Bot. 100s, 250s, 500s, 1000s.
Use: Calcium supplement.

DICALTABS. (Faraday) Dibasic calcium phosphate 108 mg., Ca gluconate 140 mg., Vit. D 35 I.U./Tab. Bot. 100s, 250s, 1000s.
Use: Calcium supplement.

DICARBOSIL. (Arch) Calcium carbonate 500 mg./Tab. 12 Rolls 12s.
Use: Antacid.

DICEN. (Mallard) Dicyclomine HCl 10 mg., sodium chloride 9 mg., chlorobutanol hydrate 5 mg./ml. Vial 10 ml.
Use: Anticholinergic.

DI-CET. (Sanford & Son) Methylbenzethonium chloride 24.4 Gm., Sod. carb. monohydrate 48.8 Gm., Sod. nitrite 24.4 Gm., trisodium ethylenediamine tetra-acetate monohydrate 2.4 Gm. Pow. Pkg. 2.4 Gm., Box 24s.
Use: Disinfection of dental instruments.

DICHLORALANTIPYRINE. Dichloralphenazone. Chloralpyrine. A complex of 2 mol. chloral hydrate with 1 mol. antipyrine. Sominat.
W/Isometheptene mucate, N-acetyl-p-amino-phenol.
See: Midrin, Caps. (Carnrick)

DICHLORALPHENAZONE. B.A.N. A complex of chloral hydrate and phenazone. Dichloralantipyrine (Various Mfr.)
Use: Hypnotic.
See: Fenzol
    Welldorm
W/Isometheptine mucate, acetaminophen.
See: Midrin, Cap. (Carnrick)

DICHLORAMINE   T. P-Toluenesulfone-dichloramine (Var. Mfr.)
Use: (1 to 5% in chlorinated paraffin) Antiseptic.

DICHLOREN.
See: Mechlorethamine HCl, Sterile Inj. (Var. Mfr.)

DICHLORISONE ACETATE. 9a, 11b-dichloro-dl,-4-pregnadiene-17a,21-diol-3,20-dione-21-acetate.

DICHLORMETHAZANONE. 2-(3,4-dichlorophenyl)-3-methyl-4-metathiazanone-1-dioxide.

4,5-DICHLORO-m-BENZENEDISULFONAMIDE. Dichlorphenamide, U.S.P. XXI.

1,1-DICHLORO-2-(o-CHLOROPHENYL)-2-(p-CHLOROPHENYL)-ETHANE. Mitotane, U.S.P. XXI.

2-DICHLORO-1,1-DIFLUOROETHYL METHYL ETHER. Methoxyflurane, U.S.P. XXI.

• **DICHLORODIFLUOROMETHANE,** N.F. XVI.
Use: Aerosol propellant.

DICHLORODIPHENYL TRICHLOROETHANE.
See: Chlorophenothane (Var. Mfr.)

5-7-DICHLORO-8-HYDROXYQUINALDINE. Sterosan.

5, 7-DICHLORO-8-HYDROXYQUINOLINE.
See: Capitrol, Liq. (Westwood)

[2, 3-DICHLORO-4-(2-METHYLENEBUTYRYL)-PHENOXY] ACETIC ACID.
See: Ethacrynic Acid, U.S.P. XXI.

2, 2'-DICHLORO-n-METHYL-DIETHYLAMI-NE HCl.
See: Mechlorethamine HCl, U.S.P. XXI.

DICHLOROPHEN. B.A.N. Di(5-chloro-2-hydroxy-phenyl) methane.
Use: Anthelminitic.
See: Antiphen

DICHLOROPHENARSINE. B.A.N. 3-Amino-4-hydroxy-phenyldichloroarsine.
Use: Antifungal agent.

DICHLOROPHENARSINE HYDROCHLORIDE, (Chlorarsen, Clorarsen, Fontarsol, Halarsol.)

DICHLOROPHENE. Didroxane. G-4, bis(5-Chloro-2-hydroxyphenyl) methane. Related to hexachlorophene.
W/Parachlorometaxylenol, propylparaaminobenzoate, hexachlorophene, benzocaine.
See: Triguent, Oint. (Commerce)
W/Undecylenic acid.
See: Fungicidal Talc. (Gordon)
    Onychomycetin, Liq. (Gordon)
W/Undecylenic acid, salicylic acid, hexachlorophene.
See: Podiaspray, aerosol pow. (Dalin)

• **DICHLOROTETRAFLUOROETHANE,** N.F. XVI.
1, 2-Dichlorotetrafluoroethane.
Use: Aerosol propellant.

4, 4'-DICHLORO-3-(TRIFLUOROMETHYL)-CARBANI-LIDE. Cloflucarban

DICHLOROXYLENOL. B.A.N. 2,4-Dichloro-3,5-xylenol.
Use: Bactericide.

• **DICHLORPHENAMIDE.** U.S.P. XXI. Tab. U.S.P. XXI. 1,3-Benzenedisulfonamide, 4,5-dichloro-. 1,3-Disulfamyl-4-5-dichloro-benzene. B.A.N. 4,5-Dichlorobenzene-1,3-disulfonamide.
Use: Treatment of glaucoma.
See: Daranide, Tab. (Merck Sharp & Dohme)

N,N-DICHLOR SULFAMIDOBENZOIC ACID.
See: Halazone, Tab. (Abbott)

• **DICHLORVOS.** USAN. 2, 2-Dichlorovinyl dimethyl phosphate.
Use: Anthelmintic; insecticide, veterinary medicine.
See: Atgard
    Canogard
    Equigard
    Vapona

DICHOLIN. (Kenyon) Ox bile ext. ⅜ gr., iron lactate

¾ gr., calumba ¾ gr., chamomile flowers 1⅝ gr., rhubarb 1⅝ gr./Cap. Bot. 100s, 1000s.

DICHROMIUM TRIOXIDE. B.A.N. Chromium sesquioxide.
Use: Diagnostic aid.

• **DICIRENONE.** USAN.

DICKEY'S OLD RELIABLE EYE WASH. (Dickey Drug) Berberine sulfate, boric acid, propyl parasept, methyl parasept. Plastic dropper bot. 8 cc., 12 cc., 1 oz.
Use: Minor eye irritations.

DICLOFENAC. B.A.N. [2-(2,6-Dichloroanilino) phenyl]-acetic acid.
Use: Anti-inflammatory.
See: Voltarol (sodium salt)

• **DICLOFENAC SODIUM.** USAN.
Use: Anti-inflammatory.

• **DICLORALUREA.** USAN.
Use: Food additive.

• **DICLOXACILLIN.** USAN. 6-[3-[2,6-Dichlorophenyl)-5-methyl-4-isoxazolecarboxamido]-3,3-dimethyl-7-oxo-4-thia-1-azabicyclo[3.2.0]-heptane-2-carboxylic acid.
Use: Antibiotic.
See: Dynapen, Cap., Susp. (Bristol)
  Pathocil, Cap., Susp. (Wyeth)
  Veracillin, Cap., Inj. (Ayerst)

• **DICLOXACILLIN SODIUM,** U.S.P. XXI. Capsules, Sterile, For Oral Suspension U.S.P. XXI.
Use: Antibiotic.
See: Dycill, Cap. (Beecham)
  Dynapen, Cap., Sol. (Bristol)

DICODETHAL ELIXIR. (Lannett) D-methorphan HBr 10 mg./5 cc. in el. terpin hydrate. Bot. 1 pt., 1 gal.
Use: Cough preparation.

DICOLE. (Blue Cross) Docusate sodium 100 mg./Cap. Bot. 100s.
Use: Stool softener.

DICOPHANE.
See: Chlorophenothane (Var. Mfr.); DDT.

DICOUMARIN.
See: Dicumarol, Preps. (Var. Mfr.)

DICOUMAROL.
See: Dicumarol, U.S.P. XXI.

• **DICUMAROL,** U.S.P. XXI. Caps., Tab., U.S.P. XXI. 2H-1-Benzopyran-2-one 3,3'-methylenebis 4-hydroxy-3,3'-methylenebis(4-hydroxycoumarin). Dicoumarol. Dicoumarin. Bishydroxycoumarin. Melitoxin. (Abbott) Tab. 25 mg., 50 mg. Bot. 100s, 1000s; 100 mg. Bot. 1000s. (Columbia) Tab. 25 mg., 50 mg., Bot. 100s. (Lilly) Pulvule. 25 mg. Bot. 100s, 1000s; 50 mg. Bot. 100s.
Use: Blood anticoagulant.

DICYCLOMINE. B.A.N. 2-Diethylaminoethyl bicyclohexyl-1-carboxylate. Dicycloverine (I.N.N.)
Use: Antispasmodic.
See: Merbentyl
  Wyovin [hydrochloride]

• **DICYCLOMINE HYDROCHLORIDE,** U.S.P. XXI. Caps., Inj., Syrup, Tabs., U.S.P. XXI. Bicyclohexyl-1-carboxylic acid, 2-(diethylamino) ethyl 3w534 HCl.

2-(Diethylamino)ethyl (Bicyclohexyl)-1-carboxylate hydrochloride.
Use: Antispasmodic.
See: Antispas, Inj. (Keene)
  Benacol, Tab. (Cenci)
  Bentyl, Amp. Syringe, Cap., Tab. & Syr. (Merrell Dow)
  Cyclomine, Inj. (Tunex)
  Dysaps, Tab., Liq., Inj. (Savage)
  Nospaz, Vial (Reid-Provident)
  Rocyclo Preps. (Robinson)
  Rotyl HCl, Vial (Rocky Mtn.)
  Stannitol (Standex)
W/Aluminum hydroxide, magnesium hydroxide, methylcellulose.
See: Triactin Liquid & Tab. (Norwich)
W/Phenobarbital.
See: Bentyl with Phenobarbital, Prods. (Merrell Dow)

DI-CYCLONEX. (Pasadena Research) Dicyclomine HCl 10 mg./ml. Injectable vial. Vial 10 cc.

DICYCLON-M. (Kenyon) Dicyclomine HCl 10 mg., pyrilamine maleate 10 mg., pyridoxine HCl 10 mg./Tab. Bot. 100s, 1000s.
Use: Antinauseant.

DICYCLON NO. 1. (Kenyon) Dicyclomine HCl 10 mg./Tab. Bot. 100s, 1000s.
Use: Antispasmodic.

DICYCLON NO. 2. (Kenyon) Dicyclomine HCl 10 mg., phenobarbital 15 mg./Tab. Bot. 100s, 1000s.

DICYCLON NO. 3. (Kenyon) Dicyclomine HCl 20 mg., phenobarbital 15 mg./Tab. Bot. 100s, 1000s.

DICYNENE. (Baxter)
Use: Hemostatic agent.
See: Ethamsylate

DICYSTEINE.
See: Cystine, Pow. (Various Mfr.)

7,8-DIDEHYDRO-4,5-EPOXY-3-ETHOXY-17-METHYL-MORPHINAN-6-ol HYDRO-CHLORIDE.
See: Ethylmorphine Hydrochloride. (Mallinckrodt)

7,8-DIDEHYDRO-4,5α-EPOXY-3-METHOXY-17-METHYLMORPHINAN-6α-OL.
See: Codeine, U.S.P. XXI. Cryst., Pow. (Var. Mfr.)

7,8-DIDEHYDRO-4,5α-EPOXY-3-METHOXY-17-METHYLMORPHINAN-6α-OL PHOSPHATE (1:1) (Salt).
Codeine Phosphate, U.S.P. XXI.

7,8-DIDEHYDRO-4,5-EPOXY-3-METHOXY-17-METHYL-MORPHINAN-6α-OL SULFATE (2:1).
See: Codeine Sulfate, U.S.P. XXI. Tab., Pow. (Var. Mfr.)

7,8-DIDEHYDRO-4,5α-EPOXY-17-METHYL-MORPHINAN-3,6α-DIOL SULFATE (2:1) (SALT) PENTAHYDRATE. Morphine Sulfate, U.S.P. XXI.

(+)-9,10-DIDEHYDRO-N-(1-(HYDROXY-METHYL)-PROPYL)-1,6-DIMETHYLERGO-LINE-8β-CARBOX-AMIDE MALEATE (1:1)
See: Methysergide Maleate, U.S.P. XXI. (Sandoz)

9,10-DIDEHYDRO-n-[(S)-2-HYDROXY-1-METHYLETHYL]-6-METHYLERGOLINE-8β-CARBOXAMIDE MALEATE. Ergonovine Maleate.

9,10-DIDEHYDRO-N-[(S)-1-(HYDROXY-METHYL)PROPYL]-6-METHYLERGOLINE-8β-CARBOXAMIDE

MALEATE (1:1). Methylergonovine Maleate, U.S.P. XXI.

DI-DELAMINE GEL. (Commerce) Tripelennamine HCl, diphenhydramine HCl, benzalkonium chloride, menthol in a special clear gel. Gel. Tube 1.25 oz.
Use: Relief of itching.

DI-DELAMINE SPRAY. (Commerce) Tripelennamine HCl, diphenhydramine HCl, menthol Spray pump 4 oz.
Use: Relief of itching due to allergies, hives, non-poisonous insect bites.

3[(O-2,6-DIDEOXY-β-D-ribo-HEXOPYRANOSYL-(14) -0-2,6-DIDEOXY-β-D-ribo-HEXOPYRANOSYL-(14) -2,6-DIDEOXY-β-D-ribo-HEXOPYRANOSYL)OXY]- 12, 14-DIHYDROXY-5β-CARD-20(22)-ENOLIDE. Digoxin, U.S.P. XXI.

DIDREX. (Upjohn) Benzphetamine HCl 25 mg./Tab. Bot. 100s; 50 mg./Tab. Bot. 100s, 500s.
Use: Appetite depressant.

DIDRONEL. (Norwich Eaton) Etidronate disodium 200 mg./Tab. Bot. 60s.
Use: Treatment of symptomatic Paget's disease of bone and prevention and treatment of heterotopic ossification due to spinal cord injury and prevention and treatment of heterotropic ossification following total hip replacement.

DIELDRIN. B.A.N. Product containing 85 per cent of 1,2,3,4,10, 10-hexachloro-6,7-epoxy-1,4,4a,5,6,7,-8,8a-octahydro-exo-1,4-endo-5,8-dimethanona-phthalene.
Use: Treatment of arthropod infestation.

• **DIENESTROL,** U.S.P. XXI. Cream, U.S.P. XXI. Non-steroid, synthetic estrogen. Dienoestrol. 4,4'-(Diethylideneethylene)diphenol. **Cream:** (Ortho) Dienestrol 0.01%. Tube 78 Gm. w/applicator.
Use: Estrogen therapy, atropic vaginitis.
See: D V Cream (Merrell Dow)
   D V Suppositories (Merrell Dow)
   Ortho Dienestrol Cream (Ortho)
W/Sulfanilamide, aminacrine HCl, allantoin.
See: AVC/Dienestrol Cream, Supp. (Merrell Dow)

DIETAC MAXIMUM STRENGTH ONCE-A-DAY DIET AID CAPSULES. (Menley & James) Phenylpropanolamine HCl 75 mg. Pkg. 20s, 40s.
Use: Appetite suppressant.

DIETAC ONCE-A-DAY DIET AID CAPSULES. (Menley & James) Phenylpropanolamine HCl 50 mg., caffeine 200 mg./Cap. Pkg. 14s, 28s.
Use: Appetite suppressant.

DIETETIC COUGH SYRUP. (Eckerd) Bot. 8 oz.

DIETHADIONE. B.A.N. 5,5-Diethyloxazine-2,4-dione.
Use: Analeptic agent.
See: Dietroxine (I.N.N.)
   Toce

• **DIETHANOLAMINE,** N.F. XVI.
Use: Pharmaceutic acid (alkalizing agent).

DIETHAZINE. B.A.N. 10-(2-Diethylaminoethyl)-Phenothiazine.
Use: Treatment of the Parkinsonian syndrome.
See: Diparcol (hydrochloride)

DIETHAZINE HCl. 10-(β-Diethylaminoethyl)-phenothiazine HCl. Diparcol.

DIETHANOLAMINE.
See: Diolamine

DIETHOXIN. Intracaine HCl

2-(DIETHYLAMINO)-2′, 6′-ACETOXYLIDIDE. Lidocaine, U.S.P. XXI.

2-(DIETHYLAMINO)-2′, 6′-ACETOXYLIDIDE HCl.
See: Lidocaine HCl, U.S.P. XXI.

2-(2-(DIETHYLAMINO)ETHOXY)ETHYL 1-PHENYL-CYCLOPENTANECARBOXYLATE CITRATE (1:1).
See: Carbetapentane Citrate.

2-(DIETHYLAMINO)ETHYL p-AMINOBENZOATE HCl.
See: Procaine HCl, U.S.P. XXI.

2-(DIETHYLAMINO)ETHYL 4-AMINO-2-CHLORO-BENZOATE MONOHYDROCHLORIDE.
See: Chloroprocaine Hydrochloride, U.S.P. XXI. (Var. Mfr.)

2-(DIETHYLAMINO)ETHYL 4-AMINO-2-PROPOXY-BENZOATE MONOHYDROCHLORIDE.
See: Chloroprocaine Hydrochloride, U.S.P. XXI. (Var. Mfr.)

2-(DIETHYLAMINO)ETHYL 4-AMINO-2-PROPOXY-BENZOATE MONOHYDROCHLORIDE.
See: Propoxycaine Hydrochloride, U.S.P. XXI. (Var. Mfr.)

2-(DIETHYLAMINO)ETHYL 3-AMINO-4-PROPOXY-BENZOATE MONOHYDROCHLORIDE. Proparacaine Hydrochloride, U.S.P. XXI.

2-(DIETHYLAMINO)ETHYL(BICYCLOHEXYL)-1-CARBOXYLATE HYDROCHLORIDE.
See: Dicyclomine Hydrochloride U.S.P. XXI. (Var. Mfr.)

2-(DIETHYLAMINO)PROPIOPHENONE HYDROCHLORIDE.
See: Diethylpropion Hydrochloride, Tab. (Var. Mfr.)

10-[2-(DIETHYLAMINO)PROPYL]PHENOTHIAZINE MONOHYDROCHLORIDE. Ethopropazine Hydrochloride, U.S.P. XXI.

DIETHYLCARBAMAZINE. B.A.N. 1-Diethyl-carbamoyl-4-methylpiperazine.
Use: Treatment of filariasis.
See: Banocide
   Ethodryl
   Hetrazan dihydrogen citrate

• **DIETHYLCARBAMAZINE CITRATE,** U.S.P. XXI. Tab., U.S.P. XXI. Diethylcarbamazine Dihydrogen Citrate. N, N-Diethyl-4-methyl-1-piperazine-carboxamide dihydrogen citrate. 1-Piperazinecarboxamide, N,N-diethyl-4-methyl-, 2-hydroxy-1,2,3-propanetricarboxylate. Banocide, Ethodryl.
Use: Antifilarial.

DIETHYLENEDIAMINE CITRATE. Piperazine Citrate, Piperazine Hexahydrate.
See: Antepar, Syr., Tab., Wafer (Burroughs Wellcome)

13,17alpha-DIETHYL-17-HYDROGEN-4-EN-3-ONE. Genabol.

DIETHYL(2-HYDROXYETHYL)METHYL-AMMONIUM BROMIDE α-CYCLOPENTYL-2-THIOPHENE-GLYCOLATE.
See: Penthienate Bromide, Tab. (Var. Mfr.)

DIETHYL(2-HYDROXYETHYL)METHYL-AMMONIUM BROMIDE XANTHENE-9-CARBOXYLATE.
See: Methantheline Bromide, Tab. (Var. Mfr.)

4,4'-(DIETHYLIDENEETHYLENE)DIPHENOL.
See: Dienestrol, Cream, Tab. (Var. Mfr.)
DIETHYLMALONYLUREA.
See: Barbital, Tab. (Var. Mfr.)
5,5-DIETHYL-1-METHYLBARBITURIC ACID.
See: Metharbital, Tabs. (Var. Mfr.)
3, 3-DIETHYL-5-METHYL-2,4-PIPERIDINE-DIONE.
See: Methyprylon, Preps. (Var. Mfr.)
4, 4'-(1, 2-DIETHYL-3-METHYLTRIMETHYLENE) DI-PHENOL.
See: Benzestrol, Tabs. (Var. Mfr.)
N, N-DIETHYLNICOTINAMIDE.
See: Nikethamide. (Var. Mfr.)
N-N-DIETHYL-M-TOLUAMIDE. W/N-Octyl Bicyclohep-tene Dicarboximide, 2,3,4,5-bis(delta-2-butylene)tet-rahydrofurfural, Di-n-propyl isocincho-meronate, iso-propanol and other isomers.
See: Bansum, Bot. (Summers)
• **DIETHYL PHTHALATE,** N.F. XVI.
Use: Plasticizer.
DIETHYLPROPION. B.A.N. α-Diethylaminopropiophe-none.
Use: Appetite suppressant.
See: Amfepramone (I.N.N.)
• **DIETHYLPROPION HCl,** U.S.P. XXI. Tab., U.S.P.
XXI. 1-Phenyl-2-diethylaminopropanone-1 HCl. 2-(Di-ethylamino)propiophenone HCl.
Use: Anorexic.
See: D.E.P.-75
Nu-Dispoz, Tab. (Coastal)
Ro-Diet, Tab. (Robinson)
Ro-Diet Timed (Robinson)
Tenuate, Tab. (Merrell Dow)
Tepanil, Tab. (Riker)
Tepanil Ten-Tab, Tab. (Riker)
α,α'-**DIETHYL-4,4'-STILBENEDIOL.** Diethylstilbestrol,
U.S.P. XXI.
(E)-$\alpha\alpha'$-**DIETHYL-4,4'-STILBENEDIOL DIPROPIONATE.**
See: Diethylstilbestrol Dipropionate, Preps. (Var. Mfr.)
• **DIETHYLSTILBESTROL,** U.S.P. XXI. Inj. Supp.,
Tab., U.S.P. XXI. Phenol 4,4'-(1,2-diethyl-1,2-ethenediyl)bis-. (Cyren A, Domestrol, Estrobene, Fonatol, New-Oestranol 1, Oestrogenine, Oestromie-nin, Palestrol, Synthoestrin, Stiboestroform, Stilbestrol, Synestrin) alpha, alpha'-Diethyl-4,4'-stil-benediol.
Use: Estrogen.
See: Acnestrol, Lot. (Dermik)
Mase-Bestrol, Tab. (Mason)
W/Clioquinol, sulfanilamide.
See: D.I.T.I. Creme (Dunhall)
W/Nitrofurazone, diperodon HCl.
See: Furacin-E Urethral Inserts (Eaton)
W/Sulfadiazine, clioquinol.
See: Benegyn, Vag. Insert, Cream (Vortech)
• **DIETHYLSTILBESTROL DIPHOSPHATE,** U.S.P.
XXI. Inj., U.S.P. XXI.
Use: Estrogen.
See: Stilphostrol, Inj., Tab. (Miles Pharm)
DIETHYLSTILBESTROL DIPROPIONATE, a,a'-Dieth-yl-4, 4' stilbenediol dipropionate. Cyren B, Estilben,

Estroben DP, New-Oestranol 11, Orestol, Pabestrol D, Stilbestronate, Stilboestrol DP, Stilronate, Synestrin Amp. (Various Mfr.) Amp. in oil, 0.5 mg., 1 mg., 5 mg./cc. Tab. 0.5 mg., 1 mg., 5 mg.
Use: Estrogen.
DIETHYLTHIAMBUTENE. B.A.N. 3-Diethyl-amino-1, 1-di(2-thienyl)but-1-ene.
Use: Narcotic analgesic.
See: Themalon
• **DIETHYLTOLUAMIDE,** U.S.P. XXI. Topical Soln., U.S.P. XXI. Benzamide, N, N-diethyl-3-methyl-N, N-Diethyl-m-toluamide.
Use: Repellent (arthropod).
See: RV Pellent, Oint. (Elder)
N, N-DIETHYLVANILLAMIDE.
See: Ethamivan, Inj. (Var. Mfr.)
DIET PLAN CAPSULES. (Towne) Vit. A palmitate 1333 I.U., D 133 I.U., B-1 0.33 mg., B-2 0.40 mg., C 10 mg., niacinamide 3.33 mg., iron 3.33 mg., benzocaine 3.0 mg., sodium carboxymethylcellulose 167 mg./Cap. Bot. 24s, 90s.
DIET-TRIM. (Pharmex) Phenylpropanolamine, carboxy-methylcellulose, benzocaine/Tab. Bot. 21s, 90s.
DIETTS. (Image) 75 mg. timed tablet.
Use: Weight control.
DIET-TUSS. (Approved) d-Methorphan 30 mg., thenyl-pyramine HCl and pyrilamine maleate 80 mg., sod. salicylate 200 mg., sod. citrate 600 mg., ammonium chloride 100 mg./Fl. Oz. Bot. 4 oz.
Use: Sugar-free antihistaminic.
DI-FACTOR. (Sutliff & Case) Vit. D 133 I.U., cal. carb. 200 mg., ferrous gluconate 15 mg., Vit. B-1 2 mg., B-2 2 mg., C 30 mg., magnesium carb. 5 mg., mang. sulf. 1 mg., copper sulf. 1 mg./Tab. Bot. 100s, 1000s.
Use: Prenatal dietary supplement.
• **DIFENOXIMIDE HYDROCHLORIDE.** USAN.
Use: Antiperistaltic.
• **DIFENOXIN.** USAN. 1-(3-Cyano-3, 3-diphenyl-propyl)-4-phenylpiperidine-4-carboxylic acid.
Use: Antidiarrheal.
DIFETARSONE. B.A.N. NN'-Ethylene-1, 2-diarsanilic acid.
Use: Arsenical.
See: Bemarsal disodium salt
• **DIFLORASONE DIACETATE.** USAN. 6α, 9α-difluoro 11β, 17, 21 trihydroxy-16β methyl-pregna-1, 4-diene-3, 20-dione 17, 21 diacetate.
Use: Anti-inflammatory, antipruritic.
See: Florone, Cream, Oint. (Upjohn)
Maxiflor, Cream, Oint. (Herbert)
• **DIFLUANINE HCl.** USAN. (McNeil) 1-(2-Anilinoethyl)-4-[4, 4-bis(p-fluorophenyl)butyl]-piperazine trihydro-chloride.
Use: CNS stimulant.
• **DIFLUCORTOLONE.** USAN. 6α,9-Difluoro-11β, 21-dihydroxy-16α-methylpregna-1, 4-diene-3, 20-dione.
Use: Glucocorticoid.
• **DIFLUCORTOLONE PIVALATE.** USAN.
Use: Glucocorticoid.
DIFLUMIDONE. B.A.N. 3'-Benzoyldifluorometha-nesulfonanilide.

Use: Anti-inflammatory.
- **DIFLUMIDONE SODIUM.** USAN.
  Use: Anti-inflammatory.
- **DIFLUNISAL,** U.S.P. XXI. Tab., U.S.P. XXI.
  Use: Analgesic, anti-inflammatory.
  See: Dolobid, Tab. (Merck Sharp & Dohme)
- **DIFTALONE.** USAN.
  Use: Anti-inflammatory.

6α, 9-DIFLUORO-11β, 16 α, 17, 21-TETRAHY-DROXY-PREGNA-1,4-DIENE-3, 20-DIONE, CYCLIC 16, 17-ACETAL WITH ACETONE. Fluocinolone Acetonide, U.S.P. XXI.

6α, 9-DIFLUORO-11β, 17, 21-TRIHYDROXY-16α-METHYL-PREGNA-1, 4-DIENE-3,20-DIONE 21 PIVALATE. Flumethazone Pivalate, U.S.P. XXI.

- **DIFLUPREDNATE.** USAN. 6α, 9-difluoro-11β, 17, 21-trihydroxypregna-1, 4-diene-3, 20-dione 21-acetate-17-butyrate.
  Use: Anti-inflammatory.

DI-GEL LIQUID. (Plough) Aluminum hydroxide 282 mg., mag. hydroxide 87 mg., simethicone 20 mg./5 ml. Bot. 6 oz., 12 oz. Mint or lemon-orange.
  Use: Antacid, antiflatulent.

DI-GEL TABLETS. (Plough) Aluminum hydroxide, mag. carb. 282 mg., mag. hydroxide 85 mg., simethicone 25 mg./Tab. Box 30s, 60s, 90s.
  Use: Antacid, antiflatulent.

DIGENZYMES. (Maurry) Ox bile ext. 130 mg., pancreatin 130 mg., papain 65 mg., duodenal substances desiccated defatted 65 mg./Tab. Bot. 100s, 1000s.
  Use: Colitis, faulty protein, carbohydrate, and fat digestion, gall bladder stasis.

DI-GESIC. (Central) Hydrocodone bitartrate 5 mg., acetaminophen 150 mg., aspirin 230 mg., caffeine 30 mg./Tab. Bot. 100s, 1000s.
  Use: Analgesic.

DIGESTALIN. (Vortech) Activated charcoal 5.3 mg., bismuth subgallate 3.8 mg., pepsin 2.0 mg., berberis 1.2 mg., papain 1.2 mg., pancreatin 0.40 mg., hydrastis 0.08 mg./Tab. Bot. 100s, 1000s.
  Use: Digestive aid.

DIGESTAMIC. (Metro Med) **Tabs.** #1. Bot. 50s, 500s. #2. Bot. 50s, 500s. **Liq.** Bot. 8 oz., gal.
  Use: Flatulence and bloating.

DIGESTANT. (Canright) Pancreatin 5¼ gr., ox bile ext. 2 gr., pepsin 5 gr., betaine HCl 1 gr./Tab. Bot. 100s, 1000s.
  Use: Digestant formula.

DIGESTEX. (Pasadena Research) Pancreatin 130 mg., iron oxbile 130 mg., prolase 3 mg., mylase 15 mg., celase 1 mg./Tab. Bot. 100s, 1000s.
  Use: Digestive enzymes.

DIGESTIVE COMPOUND. (Thurston) Betaine HCl 3.25 gr., pepsin 1 gr., papain 2 gr., mycozyme 2 gr., ox bile 2 gr./2 Tabs. Bot. 100s, 500s.
  Use: Hypochlorhydria, achlorhydria, impaired digestive ability.

DIGESTOZYME. (Wolins) Pepsin 250 mg., pancreatin 300 mg., dehydrocholic acid 25 mg./Tab. Bot. 1000s.

DIGIGLUSIN. (Lilly) Digitalis glucosides **Tab.** 1 u. (sugar-coated) Bot. 100s.
  Use: Digitalis therapy.
- **DIGITALIS,** U.S.P. XXI. Cap., Pow., Tab., U.S.P. XXI.
  Use: Digitalis therapy, cardiotonic.
  See: Digitora, Tab. (Upjohn)
- **DIGITALIS GLYCOSIDES.**
  Use: Digitalis therapy.
  See: Acylanid, Tab. (Sandoz)
    Cedilanid, Tab. (Sandoz)
    Cedilanid-D, Amp. (Sandoz)
    Crystodigin, Tab., Amp., Vial (Lilly)
    Deslanoside, Inj. (Var. Mfr.)
    Digiglusin, Tab. (Lilly)
    Digitaline Nativelle, Sol., Tab., Elxr. (Savage)
    Digitoxin, Preps. (Var. Mfr.)
    Digoxin, Preps. (Var. Mfr.)
    Gitaligin, Tab. (Schering)
    Gitalin, Tab. (Var. Mfr.)
    Lanatoside C, Inj., Tab. (Var. Mfr.)
    Lanoxin, Tab., Inj., Elix. (Burroughs Wellcome)
    Purodigin, Tab., (Wyeth)

DIGITALIS LEAF, POWDERED.
  Use: Digitalis therapy.
  See: Pil-Digis, Pill (Key)

DIGITALIS TINCTURE.
  Use: Digitalis therapy.
- **DIGITOXIN,** U.S.P. XXI. Inj., Tab., U.S.P. XXI. (Various Mfr.) Amp. (0.2 mg./cc.) 1 cc., Cap. in oil, 0.1 mg., 0.2 mg., Tab. 0.1 mg., 0.2 mg.
  Use: Digitalis therapy; cardiotonic.
  See: Crystodigin, Tab. (Lilly)
    De-Tone 0.1, 0.2, Tab. (Scrip)
    Digitaline Nativelle, Prep. (Savage)
    Maso-Toxin, Tab. (Mason)
    Purodigin, Tab. (Wyeth)
  W/Carboxymethylcellulose & Sod.
  See: Foxalin, Cap. (Standex)

DIGITOXIN, ACETYL.
  Use: Digitalis therapy.
  See: Acylanid, Tab. (Sandox)

α-DIGITOXIN MONOACETATE.
  Use: Digitalis therapy.
  See: Acetyldigitoxin, Tab. (Var. Mfr.)

DIGOLASE. (Boyle) Pancreatin 80 mg., aspergillus oryzae 15 mg., papain 3 mg., polysorbate-80 20 mg./Cap. Bot. 100s.
  Use: Orally, digestive enzyme deficiencies.
- **DIGOXIN,** U.S.P. XXI. Elix., Inj., Tab. U.S.P. XXI. Cryst. glycoside isolated from lvs. of digitalis lanata. 0.25 mg./Tab. Bot. 1000s. Unit dose 100s.
  Use: Digitalization; cardiotonic.
  See: Lanoxin, Prep. (Burroughs Wellcome)
    Masoxin, Tab. (Mason)

DIGOXIN I-125 IMUSAY. (Abbott) Digoxin diagnostic kit. 100s, 300s.
  Use: Quantitative determination of serum digoxin.

DIGOXIN CLASP RIA KIT. (Squibb) Solid phase I-125 digoxigenin assay. 200 tests/kit.
  Use: Radio assay.

DIGOXIN RIABEAD. (Abbott) Test kit 100s, 300s.

Use: Solid-phase radioimmunoassay for quantitative measurement of serum digoxin.

• **DIHEXYVERINE HYDROCHLORIDE.** USAN.
  Use: Anticholinergic.

DIHYDAN SOLUBLE.
  See: Phenytoin Sodium (Various Mfr.)

DIHYDRALLAZINE. B.A.N. 1,4-Dihydrazinophthalazine.
  Use: Hypotensive.
  See: Nepresol [mesylate or sulfate]

DIHYDREX CAPSULES. (Kay) Dipehnhydramine HCl 12.5 mg./5 ml. w/alcohol 14% Bot. 4 oz., 16 oz., gal.
  Use: Antihistaminic.

DIHYDREX EXPECTORANT. (Kay) Diphenhydramine HCl 80 mg., ammonium chloride 12 gr., sod. citrate 5 gr., menthol 1 mg./5 ml. w/alcohol 5%. Bot. pt.
  Use: Cough control.

DIHYDREX INJECTION. (Kay) Diphenhydramine HCl 10 mg./ml., or 50 mg./ml. Vial 30 ml.
  Use: Antihistaminic.

DIHYDROCODEINE. Paracodin. Drocode.
  Use: Antitussive & analgesic.

DIHYDROCODEINONE BITARTRATE.
  Use: Narcotic.
  See: Hydrocodone Bitartrate, U.S.P. XXI.
W/Caffeine, phenacetin, aspirin.
  See: Drocogesic #3, Tab. (Rand)
       Duradyne DHC, Liq. (O'Neal, Jones, & Feldman)
W/Caffeine, phenacetin, aspirin, promethazine HCl.
  See: Synalgos-DC, Cap. (Ives)

DIHYDROCODEINONE RESIN COMPLEX.
W/Phenyltoloxamine resin complex.
  See: Tussionex, Prep. (Pennwalt)

10, 11-DIHYDRO-N,N-DIMETHYL-5H-DIBENZO-[a,d]CYCLOHEPTENE-PROPYLAMINE HCl.
  Amitriptyline Hydrochloride, U.S.P. XXI.

DIHYDRO-DIETHYLSTILBESTROL.
  See: Hexestrol, Tab. & Vial (Various Mfr.)

DIHYDROERGOCORNINE. Ergot Alk. component of Hydergine.
  See: Circanol, Tab. (Riker)
       Deapril-ST, Tab. (Mead Johnson)

DIHYDROERGOCRISTINE. Ergot Alk. component of Hydergine.
  See: Circanol, Tab. (Riker)
       Deapril-ST, Tab. (Mead Johnson)

DIHYDROERGOCRYPTINE. Ergot Alk. component of Hydergine.
  See: Circanol, Tab. (Riker)
       Deapril-ST, Tab. (Mead Johnson)

DIHYDROERGOTAMINE. (D.H.E. 45) (Sandoz) Dihydroergotamine mesylate. Amp.

• **DIHYDROERGOTAMINE MESYLATE,** U.S.P. XXI.
  Inj., U.S.P. XXI. Dihydroergotamine methanesulfonate.
  Use: Treatment of migraine; antiadrenergic.
  See: DHE 45, Amp. (Sandoz)
W/Scopolamine HBr, phenobarbital Sod., barbital Sod. & Sandoptal.
  See: Plexonal, Tab. (Sandoz)

DIHYDROFOLLICULAR HORMONE.
  See: Estradiol (Various Mfr.)

DIHYDROFOLLICULINE.
  See: Estradiol (Various Mfr.)

DIHYDROHYDROXYCODEINONE. Oxycodone.
  (Ducodal, Eukodal, Eucodal)
  Use: Narcotic, analgesic.

DIHYDROHYDROXYCODEINONE HCl or BITARTRATE. Oxycodone HCl or Bitartrate.
W/Combinations.
  See: Cophene-S, Syr. (Dunhall)
       Corizahist-D, Syr. (Mason)
       Damason-P, Tab. (Mason)
       Percobarb, Cap. (Du Pont)
       Percodan, Tab. (Du Pont)
       Triaprin-DC, Cap. (Dunhall)

10,11-DIHYDRO-5-(3-(METHYLAMINO)-PROPYL)-5H-DIBENZ(b,f) AZAPINE MONOHYDROCHLORIDE.
  See: Desipramine Hydrochloride, U.S.P. XXI.

10,11-DIHYDRO-N-METHYL-5H-DIBENZO-(a,d)CYCLOHEPTENE-Δ^{5v}PROPYLAMINE HYDROCHLORIDE.
  See: Nortriptyline Hydrochloride, U.S.P. XXI.

DIHYDROMORPHINONE HCl.
  See: Dilaudid, Prep. (Knoll)

• **DIHYDROTACHYSTEROL,** U.S.P. XXI. Caps., Oral Soln., Tabs., U.S.P. XXI. 9, 10-Seco-5,7,22-ergostartien-3-β-ol
  See: Hytakerol, Cap. Sol. (Winthrop-Breon)

DIHYDROTACHYSTEROL. B.A.N. 9, 10-Secoergosta-5,7,22-trien-3β-ol.
  Use: Treatment of hypocalcemia.

DIHYDROTACHYSTEROL. (Philips Roxane) Dihydrotachysterol 0.2 mg./Tab. Bot. 100s. Unit dose 100s.
  Use: Calcium replacement.

DIHYDROTESTOSTERONE. Androstane-17-beta-ol-3-one.
  See: Stanolone.

DIHYDROTHEELIN.
  See: Estradiol (Var. Mfr.)

DIHYDROXYACETONE.
  See: Chromelin, Liq. (Summers)
       QT, Liq. (Plough)
       Sudden Tan, Liq. (Plough)

• **DIHYDROXYALUMINUM AMINOACETATE,** U.S.P. XXI. Magma, Tab., U.S.P. XXI. Aluminum, (glycinato-N,O)dihydroxy-,hydrate. (Glycinato)-dihydroxyaluminum hydrate. Aluminum dihydroxyaminoacetate; basic aluminum aminoacetate. (Glycinato)dihydroxyaluminum.
  Use: Antacid.
  See: Hyperacid, Tab. (Wolins)
W/Methscopolamine bromide, sod. lauryl sulfate & magnesium hydroxide.
  See: Alu-Scop, Cap., Susp. (Westerfield)
W/Phenobarbital & atropine methyl nitrate.
  See: Harvatrate A, Tab. (O'Neal)
W/Salicylsalicylic acid, aspirin.
  See: Salsprin, Tab. (Seatrace)

• **DIHYDROXYALUMINUM SODIUM CARBONATE,** U.S.P. XXI. Tab., U.S.P. XXI. Aluminum sodium

carbonate hydroxide. Sodium (carbonato)-dihydroxyaluminate(1-)hydrate.
Use: Antacid.
See: Rolaids, Tab. (Warner-Lambert)
1,8-DIHYDROXYANTHRANOL. Anthrolin.
1,8-DIHYDROXYANTHRAQUINONE. Dioxyanthraquinone.
See: Danthron, U.S.P. XXI.
2,5-DIHYDROXYBENZOATE SODIUM. Gentisic acid.
See: Gentisate Sodium. (Various Mfr.)
3,12-DIHYDROXYCHOLANIC ACID.
See: Desoxycholic acid. (Var. Mfr.)
DIHYDROXYESTRIN.
See: Estradiol (Various Mfr.)
DIHYDROXYFLUORANE. Fluorescein.
3,4-DIHYDROXY-α-[)ISOPROPYLAMINO)METHYL]-BENZYL ALCOHOL HCl. Isoproterenol Hydrochloride, U.S.P. XXI.
(−)-3,4-DIHYDROXY-α-[(METHYLAMINO)-METHYL]-BENZYL ALCOHOL. Epinephrine, U.S.P. XXI.
DIHYDROXYPHENYLISATIN.
See: Oxyphenisatin (Var. Mfr.)
(−)-3-(3,4-DIHYDROXYPHENYL)-L-ALA-NINE.
See: Levodopa, U.S.P. XXI.
2,2'-DIHYDROXY-4-METHOXYBENZOPHEN-ONE. Dioxybenzone, U.S.P. XXI.
L-3-(3,4-DIHYDROXYPHENYL)-2-METHYLALANINE SESQUIHYDRATE. Methyldopa, U.S.P. XXI.
DIHYDROXYPHENYLOXINDOL.
See: Oxyphenisatin (Var. Mfr.)
17,21-DIHYDROXYPREGNA-1,4-DIENE-3,11,-20-TRI-ONE. Prednisone, U.S.P. XXI.
DIHYDROXYPROPYLTHEOPHYLLINE. Dyphylline.
See: Airet, Preps. (Norwich Eaton)
Neothylline, Tab., Elix., Inj. (Lemmon)
W/Ephedrine HCl, butabarbital.
See: Airet R, Tabs. (Baylor Labs.)
W/Guaifenesin.
See: Airet G. G., Caps. & Elix. (Baylor Labs.)
DIHYDROXY(STEARATO)ALUMINUM. Aluminum Monostearate, N.F. XVI.
DIIODOHYDROXYQUIN.
See: Iodoquinol, U.S.P. XXI.
DI-IODOHYDROXYQUINOLINE. B.A.N. 8-Hydroxy-5,7-di-iodoquinoline.
Use: Treatment of amebiasis.
See: Diodoquin
Embequin
Floraquin
DIIODOHYDROXYQUINOLINE.
See: Iodoquinol, U.S.P. XXI.
5,7-DIIODO-8-QUINOLINOL.
See: Iodoquinol, U.S.P. XXI.
3,5-DI-IODO-THYROACETIC ACID. Diac.
DIISOPROMINE HCl. N,N-diisopropyl-3,3-diphenyl-propylamine HCl. (Lab. for Pharmaceutical Development, Inc.)
See: Desquam-X (Westwood)
• **DIISOPROPANOLAMINE,** N.F. XVI.
Use: Pharmaceutic aid (alkalizing agent).
DIISOPROPYL PHOSPHOROFLUORIDATE.
See: Isofluorophate, U.S.P. XXI.
Floropryl, Oint. (Merck Sharp & Dohme)

DIISOPROPYL SEBACATE.
See: Delavan, Cream (Miles Pharm)
DILACAP. (Coastal) Dyphylline 100 mg., guaifenesin 100 mg., ephedrine HCl 16 mg., phenobarbital 16 mg./Cap. Bot. 100s, 1000s.
DILAMINATE. Mixture of mag. carb. and dihydroxy aluminum glycinate.
DILANTIN. (Parke-Davis) Phenytoin. **30′ Suspension:** 30 mg./5 ml. Bot. 8 oz. Unit dose 5 ml.**125′ Suspension:** 125 mg./5 ml. Bot. 8 oz. Unit dose 5 ml. **Infatabs:** 50 mg./Tab. Bot. 100s. Unit dose 100s.
DILANTIN SODIUM. (Parke-Davis) Extended phenytoin sodium **Kapseal** 30 mg., 100 mg. Bot. 100s, 1000s. Unit dose 100s. **Amp.:** (w/propylene glycol 40%, alcohol 10%, sod. hydroxide) 100 mg./2 ml. Unit dose 10s; 250 mg./5 ml. Amp. 10s. Unit dose 10s.
Use: Anticonvulsant.
DILANTIN SODIUM W/PHENOBARBITAL KAPSEAL. (Parke-Davis) Phenytoin sod. 100 mg., phenobarbital ¼ gr. or ½ gr./Cap. Bot. 100s, 1000s. ½ gr. Unit dose 100s.
Use: Anticonvulsant w/sedative.
DILATRATE SR. (Reed & Carnrick) Isosorbide dinitrate 40 mg./Sustained Release Cap. Bot. 100s.
Use: Control of angina pectoris and coronary insufficiency.
DILAUDID COUGH SYRUP. (Knoll) Hydromorphone HCl 1 mg., guaifenesin 100 mg., alcohol 5%/5 cc. Bot. pts.
Use: Harassing and nonproductive coughs.
DILAUDID-HP. (Knoll) Hydromorphone 10 mg./ml. Amp. 1 × 10s.
Use: Analgesic for narcotic tolerant patients.
DILAUDID HYDROCHLORIDE. (Knoll) Hydromorphone HCl. **Amp.:** (w/sod. citrate 0.2%, citric acid sol. 0.2%): 1mg., 2mg., or 4mg./ml. Box 10s. 2 mg., Box 25s. **Tab.:** 1 mg., 3 mg. Bot. 100s. 2 mg., 4 mg. Bot. 100s, 500s. Hospital Pack 100s. **Pow.:** Vial, 15 gr. Multiple dose vial 10 ml., 20 ml. 2 mg./ml. **Rectal Supp.:** (in cocoa butter base, w/colloidal silica 1%): 3 mg. Box 6s.
Use: Analgesic.
W/Guaifenesin.
See: Dilaudid Cough Syrup. (Knoll)
DILAX. (Mission) Docusate sodium 100 mg. or 250 mg./Cap. Bot. 100s.
Use: Stool softener.
• **DILEVALOL HYDROCHLORIDE.** USAN.
DILIN. (Hauck) Dyphylline 250 mg./ml. Vials 10 ml.
Use: Smooth muscle relaxant.
DILITHIUM CARBONATE. Lithium Carbonate, U.S.P. XXI.
DILOCAINE. (Hauck) Lidocaine HCl 1% or 2%. Bot. 50 ml.
Use: Anesthetic.
DILOCOL. (Bell Pharmacal) Hydromorphone HCl ⅒ gr., sod. citrate 20 gr., antimony pot. tartrate ⅒ gr./fl. oz. Bot. 1 pt., 1 gal.
Use: Cough depressant.

DILOMINE. (Kay) Dicyclomine HCl 10 mg./ml. Vial 10 ml.
Use: Antispasmodic.

DILOR. (Savage) **Injectable:** Dyphylline 500 mg./2 cc. Amp. Box 6s, 50s. 250 mg./cc. Vial 10 cc. **Tab.:** Dyphylline 200 mg./Tab. Bot. 100s, 1000s. Unit dose 100s. **Elixir:** Dyphylline 160 mg./15 cc. Bot. Pt., gal.
Use: Vasodilator; bronchodilator.

DILOR 400. (Savage) Dyphylline 400 mg. Bot. 100s, 1000s. Unit dose 100s.
Use: Vasodilator, bronchodilator.

DILOREX. (Tunex) Dyphylline 250 mg./ml. Vial 10cc.
Use: Vasodilator, bronchodilator.

DILOR G LIQUID. (Savage) Dyphylline 300 mg., Guaifenesin 300 mg./15 ml. Bot. pts., gals.

DILOR G TABLETS. (Savage) Dyphylline 200 mg., guaifenesin 200 mg., 400 mg./Tab. Bot. 100s, 1000s. Unit dose 100s.

DILOXANIDE. B.A.N. 4-(N-Methyldichloroacetamido) phenol.
Use: Treatment of amebiasis.
See: Entamide
    Furamide [2-furoate]

• **DILTIAZEM HYDROCHLORIDE.** USAN.
Use: Vasodilator.

DIMACID. (Otis Clapp) Mg carbonate, Ca carbonate/Tab. Sugar and salt free. Bot. 100s. Safety packs 1000s.
Use: Antacid.

DIMACOL. (Robins) Pseudoephedrine HCl 30 mg., dextromethorphan HBr 15 mg., guaifenesin 100 mg./Cap. or 5 cc. Alcohol content of liquid 4.75% **Caps.** Bot. 100s, 500s; Pre-Pack 12s, 24s. **Liq.** Bot. pt.
Use: Expectorant, decongestant, cough suppressant.

DIMAZOLE (I.N.N.). Diamthazole, B.A.N.

• **DIMEFADANE.** USAN. N, N-Dimethyl-3-phenyl-1-in-danamine.
Use: Non-narcotic analgesic.

DIMEFLINE. B.A.N. 8-Dimethylaminomethyl-7-methoxy-3-methylflavone.
Use: Respiratory stimulant.
See: Remeflin hydrochloride. (Wallace)

• **DIMEFLINE HYDROCHLORIDE.** USAN.
Use: Stimulant.

• **DIMEFOLCON A.** USAN.
Use: Contact lens material.

DIMELOR. Acetohexamide, B.A.N.

DIMENATE. (Tunex) Dimenhydrinate 50 mg./ml. Vial 10cc.
Use: Motion sickness.

DIMENEST. (Fellows) Dimenhydrinate 50 mg./cc. Vials 10 cc.
Use: Antivertigo and antiemetic agent.

• **DIMENHYDRINATE,** U.S.P. XXI. Syr., Tab., Inj., U.S.P. XXI. Beta-dimethylaminoethyl benzohydryl ether-8-chlorotheophyllinate. 8-Chlorotheophylline 2-(Diphenylmethoxy)-N, N-dimethylethylamine compound (1:1). IH-Purine-2,6-dione,8-chloro-3,7-dihydro-1,3-dimethyl-, compound with 2-(diphenylmethoxy)-N,N-dimethylethanamine (1:1). Gravol.
Use: Anti-emetic, antihistamine.

See: Dimenate, Inj. (Tunex)
    Dimenest, Inj. (Fellows-Testagar)
    Dimentabs, Tab. (Bowman)
    Dipendrate, Tab. (Kenyon)
    Dramaject, Vial (Mayrand)
    Dramamine, Prep. (Searle)
    Dramocen, Inj. (Central)
    Dymenate, Inj. (Keene)
    Eldadryl, Preps. (Elder)
    Eldodram, Tab. (Elder)
    Hydrate, Vial (Hyrex)
    Marmine, Inj., Tab. (Vortech)
    Reidamine, Inj. (Reid-Provident)
    Signate, Inj. (Sig)
    Trav-Arex, Cap. (Columbia)
    Traveltabs, Tab. (Geneva Drugs)

DIMENOXADOLE. B.A.N. 2-Dimethylaminoethyl 2-ethoxy-2, 2-diphenylacetate.
Use: Narcotic analgesic.

DIMENSYN. (Ortho) Acetaminophen 500 mg., pamabrom 25 mg., pyrilamine maleate 15 mg./Cap. Bot. 24s, 48s.
Use: Maximum strength menstrual discomfort relief.

DIMENTABS. (Bowman) Dimenhydrinate 50 mg./Tab. Bot. 100s, 1000s
Use: Antinauseant.

DIMEPHEPTANOL. B.A.N. 6-Dimethylamino-4, 4-di-phenylheptan-3-ol.
Use: Narcotic analgesic.
See: Methadol

DIMEPREGNEN. B.A.N. 3β-Hydroxy-6α, 16α-dimethyl-pregn-4-en-20-one.
Use: Anti-estrogen.

DIMEPROPION. B.A.N. α-Dimethylaminopropio-phenone. Metamfepramone (I.N.N.)
Use: Anorexigenic.

• **DIMERCAPROL,** U.S.P. XXI. Inj. U.S.P. XXI. 2, 3-Dimercaptol-1-propanol.
Use: Antidote to gold, arsenic, mercury poisoning; metal complexing agent.
See: BAL Amp. (Hynson, Wescott & Dunning)

2, 3-DIMERCAPTOPROPANOL.
See: Dimercaprol, U.S.P. XXI.

DIMESONE. B.A.N. 9α-Fluoro- 11β, 21-dihydroxy-16α, 17-dimethylpregna-1, 4-diene-3, 20-dione.
Use: Anti-inflammatory steroid.

DIMETANE. (Robins) Brompheniramine maleate. **Tabs.** (4 mg.) Bot. 100s, 500s. Pre-Pack 24s. **Extentabs:** (8 mg., 12 mg.) Bot. 100s, 500s. **Elixir:** (2 mg./5 cc.) Bot. 4 oz., 1 pt., 1 gal. **Amps.:** pH adjusted with sod. hydroxide. (10 mg./cc.) 1 cc. Box 25s.
Use: Antihistamine.
W/Phenylephrine hydrochloride, phenylpropanolamine hydrochloride.
See: Dimetapp Elix., Extentabs (Robins)

DIMETANE DECONGESTANT ELIXIR. (Robins) Brompheniramine maleate 2 mg., phenylephrine HCl 5 mg./5 ml. w/2.3% alcohol. Bot. 4 oz.
Use: Relief of nasal congestion due to colds and allergies.

DIMETANE DECONGESTANT TABLETS. (Robins)

Brompheniramine maleate 4 mg., phenylephrine HCl 10 mg./Tab. Ctn. 24s, 48s.
Use: Nasal decongestant, antihistaminic.

DIMETANE EXPECTORANT. (Robins)
Brompheniramine maleate 2 mg., guaifenesin 100 mg., phenylephrine HCl 5 mg.,
phenylpropanolamine HCl 5 mg./5 ml. w/alcohol 3.5%. Bot. pt., gal.
Use: Antihistaminic, decongestant, expectorant.

DIMETANE EXPECTORANT-DC. (Robins) Same as Dimetane Expectorant plus codeine phosphate 10 mg./5 cc. Bot. pt., gal.
Use: Antihistaminic, antitussive, decongestant, expectorant.

DIMETAPP ELIXIR. (Robins) Brompheniramine maleate 4 mg., phenylephrine HCl 5 mg., phenylpropanolamine HCl 5 mg./5 cc. alcohol 2.3% Bot., 4 fl. oz., pt., gal. Dis-Co Pack 5 ml. 10 × 10s.
Use: Antihistaminic, nasal decongestant.

DIMETAPP EXTENTABS. (Robins) Brompheniramine maleate 12 mg., phenylephrine HCl 15 mg., phenylpropanolamine HCl 15 mg./Tab. Bot. 100s, 500s. Dis-Co Pack 100s.
Use: Antihistaminic, nasal decongestant.

• **DIMETHADIONE.** USAN. 5, 5-Dimethyl-2, 4-oxazolidine-dione. Eupractone (Travenol).
Use: Anticonvulsant.

DIMETHAZAN. 1, 3-Dimethyl-7-(2-dimethylamino-ethyl) xanthine.

• **DIMETHICONE.** N.F. XVI. Dimethylsiloxane polymers. dimethyl polysiloxane.
Use: Prosthetic aid, component of barrier creams.
See: Covicone, Cream (Abbott)
Silicone, Oint. (Various Mfr.)
Silicote, Prep. (Arnar-Stone)

• **DIMETHICONE 350.** USAN.
Use: Prosthetic aid for soft tissue.

DIMETHINDENE. B.A.N. 2- 1-[2-(2-Dimethylaminoethyl) inden-3-yl]ethyl pyridine.
Use: Antihistamine.
See: Fenostil [hydrogen maleate]

DIMETHINDENE MALEATE. Dimethpyridene. 2- 1-[2-(2-dimethyl-amino-ethyl)inden-3-yl] ethyl-pyridine maleate.
Use: Antihistamine.
See: Forhistal Maleate, Tab., Syr. (Ciba)

DIMETHISOQUIN. B.A.N. 3-Butyl-1-(2-dimethyla-mino-ethoxy)isoquinoline. Quinisocaine (I.N.N.)
Use: Antipruritic.
See: Quotane [hydrochloride]

DIMETHISOQUIN HYDROCHLORIDE. 3-Butyl-1-2-(di-methyl-amino)-ethoxy isoquinoline HCl.
Use: Local anesthetic.
See: Quotane Hydrochloride, Oint. Lot. (Menley & James)

• **DIMETHISTERONE.** USAN.
Use: Preogestin.

DIMETHOLIZINE PHOSPHATE. 1-(2-Methoxy-phenyl)-4-(3-methoxypropyl)piperazine phosphate. Ansiv.

DIMETHOTHIAZINE. B.A.N. 10-(2-Dimethylamino-propyl)-2-dimethysulfamoylphenothiazine.
Use: Treatment of migraine.

See: Fonazine
Banistyl [mesylate]

DIMETHOXANATE. B.A.N. 2-(2-Dimethylamino-ethoxy) ethyl phenothiazine-10-carboxylate.
Use: Cough suppressant.

DIMETHOXYPHENYL PENICILLIN SODIUM.
See: Methicillin Sod. (Var. Mfr.)

N1-(2, 6-DIMETHOXY-4-PYRIMIDINYL)SULFANIL-AMIDE.
See: Sulfadimethoxine.

6, 7-DIMETHOXY-1-VERATRYLISOQUINOLINE HY-DROCHLORIDE.
See: Papaverine Hydrochloride, U.S.P. XXI.

DIMETHPYRIDENE MALEATE. Dimethindene Maleate, U.S.P. XXI.
See: Dimethindene Maleate, U.S.P. XXI.

6-(DIMETHYLAMINO)-4, 4-DIPHENYL-3-HEPTA-NONE HYDROCHLORIDE. Methadone Hydrochloride, U.S.P. XXI.

2-(DIMETHYLAMINO)ETHYL p-(BUTYLAMINO) BEN-ZOATE.
See: Tetracaine (Var. Mfr.)

β-DIMETHYLAMINOETHYL (1-HYDROXY-CY-CLOPENTYL)PHENYLACETATE HYDROCHLO-RIDE. Cyclopentolate Hydrochloride, U.S.P. XXI.

2-(DIMETHYLAMINO)ETHYL 1-HYDROXY-α-PHE-NYLCYCLOPENTANE-ACETATE HYDROCHLO-RIDE. Cyclopentolate Hydrochloride, U.S.P. XXI.

2(1-(2-(2-(DIMETHYLAMINO)ETHYL)-INDEN-3-yl)ET-HYL)PYRIDINE MALEATE (1:1).
See: Dimethindene Maleate, U.S.P. XXI.

2-((2-(DIMETHYLAMINO)ETHYL) (p-METHOXYBEN-ZYL)AMINO)PYRIDINE MALEATE (1:1).
See: Pyrilamine Maleate, U.S.P. XXI.

2-((2-(DIMETHYLAMINO)ETHYL)-2-THENYLAMINO)-PYRIDINE MONOHYDROCHLORIDE.
See: Methapyrilene Hydrochloride, U.S.P. XXI.

(+)-4-(DIMETHYLAMINO)-3-METHYL-1, 2-DI-PHENYL-2-BUTANOL PROPIONATE (ESTER) HYDROCHLORIDE. Propoxyphene Hydrochloride, U.S.P. XXI.

(-)-α-4-(DIMETHYLAMINO)-3-METHYL-1, 2-DI-PHENYL-2-BUTANOL PROPIONATE (ESTER) 2-NAPHTHALENE-SULFONATE (SALT).
See: Levopropoxyphene Napsylate (Var. Mfr.)

(−)-10-(3-(DIMETHYLAMINO)-2-METHYLPROPYL)-2-METHOXYPHENOTHIAZINE.
See: Methotrimeprazine, U.S.P. XXI.

10-3-(DIMETHYLAMINO)-2-METHYLPROPYL PHENOTHIAZINE TARTRATE (2:1). Trimeprazine Tartrate, U.S.P. XXI.

DIMETHYLAMINOPHENAZONE.
See: Aminopyrine (Various Mfr.)

4, 7-BIS(DIMETHYLAMINO)-1, 4, 4a, 5, 5a, 6, 11,-12a-OCTAHYDRO-3, 10, 12, 12a-TETRAHYDRO-1, 11-DIOXO-2-NAPHTHACENE-CARBOXAMIDE MONOHYDROCHLORIDE. Minocycline Hydrochloride, U.S.P. XXI.

[4-[BIS[p-(DIMETHYLAMINO)PHENYL]-METHYL-ENE]-2, 5-CYCLOHEXADIEN-1-YLIDENE]DI-METHYLAMMONIUM CHLORIDE. Gentian Violet, U.S.P. XXI.

-[3-(DIMETHYLAMINO)PROPYL]-10, 11-DIHYDRO-
5H-DIBENZ[b,f]AZEPINE MONOHYDRO-
CHLORIDE. Imipramine Hydrochloride, U.S.P. XXI.
10-(3-(DIMETHYLAMINO)PROPYL)PHENO-
THIAZINE. Promethazine HCl, U.S.P. XXI.
10-(3-(DIMETHYLAMINO)PROPYL)-2-(TRIFLUORO-
METHYL)PHENOTHIAZINE MONOHYDRO-
CHLORIDE.
　See: Triflupromazine Hydrochloride (Var. Mfr.)
DIMETHYLAMINO PYRAZINE SULFATE.
　See: Ampyzine Sulfate
DIMETHYLCARBAMATE of
3-Hydroxy-1-Methylpyridinium Bromide.
　See: Mestinon, Tab. (Roche)
I, α-DIMETHYLCYCLOHEXANEETHYLAMINE.
　See: Propylhexedrine, U.S.P. XXI.
I,-DIMETHYLCYCLOPENTANEETHYLAMINE HY-
DROCHLORIDE.
　See: Cyclopentamine Hydrochloride, U.S.P. XXI.
N, N-DIMETHYLDIBENZ [b, e] OXEPIN-Δ$^{11(6m)}$,-
γ-PROPYLAMINE HYDROCHLORIDE. Curatin.
DIMETHYLHEXESTROL DIPROPIONATE.
　Promethestrol Dipropionate.
　See: Meprane Dipropionate, Tab. (Reed & Carnrick)
N11-(3, 4-DIMETHYL-5-ISOXAZOLYL)SULFANIL-
AMIDE. Sulfisoxazole, U.S.P. XXI.
N-(3,4-DIMETHYL-5-ISOXAZOLYL)-N-SULFANIL-
YLACETAMIDE, Sulfisoxazole, Acetyl, U.S.P. XXI.
N,N-DIMETHYL-2-((o-METHYL-α-PHENYLBENZYL)-
OXY)ETHYCAMINE CITRATE (1:1).
　See: Orphenadrine Citrate, U.S.P. XXI.
3, 3-DIMETHYL-7-OXO-6-(2-PHENOXYL-ACETAMI-
DO-4-THIA 1-AZABICYCLO[3.2.0.] HEPTANE-2-
CARBOXYLIC ACID. Penicillin V, U.S.P. XXI.
(+)-1, 3-DIMETHYL-4-PHENYL-4-PIPERIDINOL PRO-
PIONATE HYDROCHLORIDE.
　See: Alphaprodine Hydrochloride, U.S.P. XXI.
2, 3-DIMETHYL-1-PHENYL-3-PYRAZOLIN-5-ONE.
　See: Antipyrine, U.S.P. XXI.
N, 2-DIMETHYL-2-PHENYLSUCCINIMIDE.
　See: Methsuximide, U.S.P. XXI.
DIMETHYL POLYSILOXANE.
　See: Dimethicone (Var. Mfr.)
W/Benzocaine, bismuth subcarbonate, carbamide,
hexachlorophene, phenylephrine HCl, pyrilamine
maleate, zinc oxide.
W/Hexachlorophene, zinc oxide, pyrilamine maleate,
tetracaine HCl, methyl salicylate, zirconium oxide.
N^1-(4, 6-DIMETHYL-2-PYRIMIDINYL)-SULFANIL-
AMIDE. Sulfamethazine, U.S.P. XXI.
• DIMETHYL SULFOXIDE, U.S.P. XXI. Irrigation,
U.S.P. XXI. Methyl sulfoxide. DMSO
　Use: Topical anti-inflammatory agent.
　See: Demasorb (Squibb)
　　　Demeso (Merck Sharp & Dohme)
　　　Domoso (Syntex)
　　　Dromisol (Merck Sharp & Dohme)
DIMETHYLTHIAMBUTENE. B.A.N. 3-Dimethylamino-
1, 1-di-(2-thienyl)but-1-ene
　Use: Narcotic analgesic.
(+)-0,0'-DIMETHYLTUBOCURARINE DIIODIDE.
　See: Dimethyl Tubocurarine Iodide.

DIMETHYLTUBOCURARINE. B.A.N. Dimethyl ether
of (+)-tubocurarine.
　Use: Neuromuscular blocking agent.
　See: Diamethine [bromide]
DIMETHYL-TUBOCURARINE IODIDE.
　Use: Skeletal muscle relaxant.
　See: Metocurine Iodide, U.S.P. XXI.
DIMETHYLURETHIMINE.
　See: Meturedepa (Armour)
1, 3-DIMETHYLXANTHINE.
　See: Theophylline, U.S.P. XXI.
3, 7-DIMETHYLXANTHINE.
　See: Theobromine, Prep. (Various Mfr.)
DIMETRIDAZOLE. B.A.N. 1, 2-Dimethyl-5-
nitroimidazole. Emtryl.
　Use: Antiprotozoan, veterinary medicine.
DIMINAZENE. B.A.N. pp'-Diamidinodiazoamino-ben-
zene.
　Use: Antiprotozoan; bactericide, veterinary
medicine.
DIMINDOL. (Blue Line) Acetaminophen 325 mg./Tab.
Bot. 100s, 1000s.
DIMINDOL ELIXIR. (Blue Line) Acetaminophen 120
mg., alcohol 9%/5 ml. Bot. 4 fl. oz., pt., gal.
　Use: Analgesic.
DIMOTANE HYDROGEN MALEATE.
　Brampheniramine, B.A.N.
• DIMOXAMINE HYDROCHLORIDE. USAN.
　Use: Memory adjuvant.
DIMPYLATE. B.A.N. 00-Diethyl 0-(2-isopropyl-6-methyl-
pyrimidin-4-yl) phosphorothioate.
　Use: Insecticide, veterinary medicine.
　See: Diazinon
DIMYCOR. (Standard Drug) Pentaerythritol tetranitrate
10 mg., phenobarbital 15 mg./Tab. Bot. 1000s.
　Use: Management of coronary insufficiency.
DINACRIN. (Winthrop Products) Isonicotinic acid,
hydrazide.
　Use: Antitubercular agent.
DINATE. (Seatrace) Dimenhydrinate 50 mg./ml. Vial
10 cc.
DINDEVAN.
　See: Phenindione (Var. Mfr.)
DINITOLMIDE. B.A.N. 3, 5-Dinitro-o-toluamide.
　Use: Antiprotozoan, veterinary medicine.
　See: Zoalene
DINOL. (Seatrace) Salicylamide 200 mg.,
acetaminophen 300 mg./Tab. Bot. 100s, 1000s.
　Use: Analgesic, antipyretic.
• DINOPROST. USAN. 7-[3α, 5α-Dihydroxy-2β-[3S-)
hydroxy-trans-oct-1-enyl]cyclopent-1-yl]cis-hept-5-
enoic acid.
　Use: Smooth muscle activator.
　See Prostaglandin F-$_{2α}$
• DINOPROST TROMETHAMINE. USAN.
　Use: Oxytocic (prostaglandin)
　See: Prostin F2 Alpha, Amp. (Upjohn)
• DINOPROSTONE. USAN. 7-[3α-Hydroxy-2β-[(3S)-
hydroxy-trans-oct-1-enyl]-5-oxocyclopent-1-yl]-cis-
hept-5-enoic acid.
　Use: Smooth muscle activator.
　See: Prostaglandin E-2

18, 19-DINORPREGN-4-EN-20-YN-3-ONE, 13-ETHYL-17-HYDROXY-, (17α)-(+)-. Norgestrel, U.S.P. XXI.

DI-N-PROPYL ISOCINCHOMERONATE W/N-N-diethyl-m-toluamide, N-Octyl Bicycloheptene Dicarboximide, 2, 3, 4, 5-bis (delta-2-butylene) Tetrehydrofurfural other isomers, isopropanol.
See: Bansum, Bot. (Summers)

• **DINSED.** USAN. N,N′-Ethylenebis (3-nitrobenzenesulfonamide)
Use: Coccidiostat.

DIOCTIN. (Janssen) Difenoxin HCl.
Use: Antiperistalic.

DIOCTO. (Purepac) Docusate sodium 100 mg. or 200 mg./Cap. Bot. 100s.
Use: Stool softener.

DIOCTYL CALCIUM SULFOSUCCINATE. Docusate Calcium, U.S.P. XXI.

DIOCTYL POTASSIUM SULFOSUCCINATE.
W/Glycerin, pot. oleate and stearate.
See: Rectalad, Liq. (Wallace)

DIOCTYL SODIUM SULFOSUCCINATE. B.A.N. Docusate Sodium, U.S.P. XXI.
Use: Non-laxative fecal softener.

DIOCTYL-ZEM. (Zemmer) Docusate sodium 60 mg., ext. cascara sagrada 4 mg./Tab. Bot. 100s, 1000s.
Use: Fecal softener and peristaltic stimulant.

DIODONE INJECTION.
See: Iodopyracet injection.

DIOEZE. (Century) Dioctyl sodium sulfosuccinate 250 mg./Cap. Bot. 100s, 1000s.
Use: Laxative.

• **DIOHIPPURIC ACID I-125.** USAN.
Use: Radioactive agent.

• **DIOHIPPURIC ACID I-131.** USAN.
Use: Radioactive agent.

DIO-HIST. (Approved) d-Methorphan 30 mg., thenylpyramine HCl 80 mg., phenylephrine HCl 20 mg., pot. tartrate 1/24 gr./oz. Bot. 4 oz.
Use: Antihistamine.

DIOLAMINE. Diethanolamine.

DIOLAX. (Century) Docusate sodium 100 mg., casanthranol 50 mg./Cap. Bot. 30s, 100s, 1000s.
Use: Stool softener and laxative.

DIOLOSTENE.
See: Methandriol

DIO-MEDICONE. (Medicone) Docusate sodium 50 mg./Tab. Vials 50s.
Use: Fecal softener.

DIONEX. (Interstate) Docusate sodium 100 mg. or 250 mg./Cap. Bot. 100s, 250s, 1000s.
Use: Laxative.

DIONIN. Ethylmorphine HCl.
Use: Orally; cough depressant, ocular lymphagogue.

DIONOSIL OILY. (Picker) Propyliodone 60% in peanut oil. Inj.
Use: Bronchographic contrast medium.

DIOPHYLLIN.
See: Aminophylline, Prep. (Various Mfr.)

DIOPTERIN. Pteroyldiglutamic acid, PDGA, Pteroyl-alpha-glutamylglutamic acid.
Use: Treatment of neoplastic diseases.

DIORAPIN. (Standex) Estrogenic conjugate 0.625 mg., methyl testosterone 5 mg./Tab. Bot. 100s.
Inj. Estrone 2 mg., testosterone 25 mg./cc. Vial 10 cc.
Use: Hormone therapy to promote anabolism.

DIOSATE. (Towne) Docusate sodium Caps. 100 mg., 250 mg./Tab. Bot. 100s.

DIO-SOFT. (Standex) Docusate sodium 100 mg., casanthranol 30 mg./Cap. Bot. 100s.

DIOSMIN. Buchu resin obtained from lvs. of barosma serratifolia & allied rutaceae.

DIOSTATE D. (Upjohn) Vit. D 400 I.U., calcium 343 mg., phosphorus 265 mg./3 Tabs. Bot. 100s.
Use: Calcium w/ Vit. D and mineral therapy.

DIOSUCCIN. (CMC) Docusate sodium. Cap. 100 mg., 250 mg., Bot. 100s. **Syr.** Bot. pt., gal.
Use: Fecal softener.

DIO-SUL. (Vortech) Docusate sodium 100 mg./Tab. or Cap. Bot. 1000s.
Use: Orally, fecal softener.

DIOSUX CAPSULES. (Jenkins) Docusate sodium 100 mg./Cap. Bot. 1000s.
Use: Laxative.

DIOSUX TABS. (Jenkins) Docusate sodium 60 mg., danthron 40 mg./Tab. Bot. 1000s.

DIOTHRON. (Vortech) Casanthranol 30 mg., docusate sodium 100 mg./Cap. Bot. 1000s.
Use: Fecal softener, laxative.

DIOTHYL. Pyrimithate, B.A.N.

• **DIOTYROSINE I-125.** USAN.
Use: Radioactive agent.

DIOVAL. (Keene) Estradiol valerate, 10 mg./ml. Vial 10 ml.

DIOVAL XX. (Keene) Estradiol valerate, 20 mg./ml. Vial 10 ml.

DIOVAL 40. (Keene) Estradiol valerate, 40 mg./ml. Vial 10 ml.

DIOVOCYLIN. (Ciba)
See: Estradiol, Prep. (Various Mfr.)

• **DIOXADROL HYDROCHLORIDE.** USAN.
Use: Antidepressant.

DIOXAMATE. B.A.N. 4-Carbamoyloxymethyl-2-methyl-2-nonyl-1,3-dioxolan.
Use: Treatment of the Parkinsonian syndrome.

DIOXAPHETYL BUTYRATE. B.A.N. Ethyl 4-morpholino-2,2-diphenylbutyrate.
Use: Narcotic analgesic.

DIOXATHION. B.A.N. A mixture consisting essentially of cis- and trans-SS′-1,4-dioxan-2,3-diyl bis (00-diethyl phosphorodithioate).
Use: Insecticide; acaricide, veterinary medicine.
See: Delnav.

DIOXINDOL. Diacetylhydroxyphenylisatin.

DIOXYANTHRANOL.
See: Anthralin, N.F. (Various Mfr.)

DIOXYANTHRAQUINONE. 1,8-Dihydroxy-anthra-quinone.
See: Danthron, U.S.P. XXI.

• **DIOXYBENZONE,** U.S.P. XXI. Dioxybenzone and Oxybenzone Cream, U.S.P. XXI. Methanone, (2-hydroxy-4-methoxyphenyl)(2-hydroxyphenyl)1.
W/Oxybenzone, benzophene.

Use: Sunscreen agent.
See: Solbar, Lot. (Person & Covey)

DIOXYLINE. (Laboratoires Franca, Canada)
Benzoxiquine.

DIOXYLINE PHOSPHATE. 6,7-Dimethoxy-1-(4'-
ethoxy-3'-methoxybenzyl))-3-methylisoquinoline.
Use: Smooth muscle relaxant.
See: Paveril Phosphate, Tab. (Lilly)

DI-PARALENE. Chlorcyclizine, B.A.N.

DIPARCOL HYDROCHLORIDE. Diethazine.

DIPEGYL.
See: Nicotinamide, Prep. (Various Mfr.)

DIPENDRATE. (Kenyon) Dimenhydrinate 50 mg./Tab.
Bot. 100s, 1000s.

DIPENICILLIN G.
See: Benzethacil

DIPENINE BROMIDE. B.A.N. 2-Dicyclopentyl-acetoxy-
ethyltriethylammonium bromide.
Use: Antispasmodic.
See: Diponium Bromide (I.N.N.)

DIPERODON. B.A.N. 3-Piperidinopropane-1,2-diol
di(phenylcarbamate).
Use. Local anesthetic.

DIPERODON, U.S.P. XXI. Oint., U.S.P. XXI. 3-Piperidino-
1,2-propanediol dicarbanilate (ester) monohydrate.
Use: Local anesthetic.

DIPERODON HYDROCHLORIDE.
Use: Anesthetic.
See: Diothane Ointment (Merrell Dow)
Proctodon, Cream (Rowell)
W/Bacitracin, neomycin sulfate, polymyxin.
See: Epimycin A, Oint. (Delta)
W/Benzalkonium chloride, ichthammol, thymol,
camphor, juniper tar.
See: Boro Oint. (Scrip)
W/Cetylpyridinium chloride.
See: Cetyben, Troches (Sutliff & Case)
W/Furacin (nitrofurazone)
See: Furacin E Urethral Inserts (Eaton)
Furacin H.C. Urethral Inserts (Eaton)
W/Furacin (nitorfurazone) & Microfur (nituroxime).
See: Furacin Otic, Drops. (Eaton)
W/Hydrocortisone, polymyxin B sulfate, neomycin.
See: My Cort Otic # 1, Ear Drops (Scrip)
W/Hydroxyquinoline Benzoate.
See: Diothane, Oint. (Merrell Dow)
W/Methapyrilene HCl, pyrilamine maleate, allantoin,
benzocaine, menthol.
See: Antihistamine Cream (Towne)
W/Neomycin sulfate, polymyxin B sulfate.
See: Aural Acute (Saron)
W/Thimerosal, isopropyl alcohol.
See: Earobex, Ear Drops (Mallard)

DIPHEMANIL METHYLSULFATE. B.A.N. 4-Benzhy-
drylidene-1, 1-dimethylpiperidinium methyl-sulfate.
Use: Parasympatholytic.
See: Diphenatil

• **DIPHEMANIL METHYLSULFATE,** U.S.P. XXI. Tab.,
U.S.P. XXI. 4-(Diphenylmethylene)-1,1-dimethyl-
piperidinium methylsulfate. Diphenmethanil methylsulfate.
Use: Anticholinergic.

See: Prantal, Tab. (Schering)

DI-PHEN. (Vortech) Diphenylhydantoin sod.   1.5
gr./Cap. Bot. 1000s.
Use: Anticonvulsant in epilepsy.

DIPHENACEN-10. (Central) Diphenhydramine HCl 10
mg./ml. w/chlorobutanol 0.5%. Vial 30 ml.
Use: Antihistaminic.

DIPHENACEN-50. (Central) Diphenhydramine HCl 50
mg./ml. w/chlorobutanol 0.5%. Vial 10 mg.
Use: Antihistaminic.

DIPHENADIONE. B.A.N. 2-Diphenylacetylinedane-1,3-
dione.
Use: Anticoagulant.
See: Didandin
Oragulant

DIPHENADIONE. 2-(Diphenylacetyl)-1-3, indandione.
Use: Anticoagulant.
See: Dipaxin, Tab. (Upjohn)

DIPHENADRIL. (Vitarine) Diphenhydramine HCl 75
mg., alcohol 5%/oz. Bot. 4 oz., gal.
Use: Expectorant.

DIPHENATIL.
See: Diphemanil methylsulfate

DIPHEN COUGH SYRUP. (Bay) Diphenhydramine HCl
12.5 mg./5 ml. w/alcohol 5%. Bot. 4 oz., pt., gal.
Use: Antihistaminic.

DIPHEN ELIXIR. (Bay) Diphenhydramine HCl 12.5
mg./5 ml. w/alcohol 14%. Bot. 4 oz., pt., gal.
Use: Antihistaminic.

DIPHEN-EX SYRUP. (Columbia) Diphenhydramine HCl
12.5 mg., alcohol 5%/5 ml. Bot. pt., gal.
Use: Cough relief.

DIPHENHYDRAMINE. B.A.N. 2-Benzhydryloxyethyl-
dimethylamine.
Use: Antihistamine.
See: Benadryl
Histex hydrochloride

DIPHENHYDRAMINE COMPOUND EXPECTORANT.
(Kay) Diphenhydramine HCl 80 mg., ammonium
chloride 12 gr., sod. citrate 5 gr., menthol ¹/₁₀ gr.,
alcohol 5%/fl. oz. Bot. 4 oz., pt., gal.
Use: Antitussive.

DIPHENHYDRAMINE EXPECTORANT. (CMC)
Diphenhydramine HCl 80 mg., ammonium chloride
12 gr./oz. w/menthol alcohol 5%, sod. citrate. Bot.
pt., gal.

• **DIPHENHYDRAMINE HYDROCHLORIDE.** U.S.P.
XXI. Cap., Elix., Inj., U.S.P. XXI. Ethanamine, 2-(di-
phenylmethoxy)-N,N-dimethyl-,HCl. 2-Diphenyl-
methoxy)-N,N-dimethylethylamine HCl.
Use: Antihistaminic.
See: Baramine, Prod. (Barry Martin)
Baramine Expectorant (Barry Martin)
Bax, Cap., Elix., Expect., (McKesson)
Benachior, Syr. (Jenkins)
Benadryl Hydrochloride, Prep. (Parke-Davis)
Benahist, Preps. (Keene)
Bentrac, Cap. (Kenyon)
Benylin Cough Syrup (Warner-Lambert)
Diphen-Ex, Syr. (Columbia)
Fenylhist, Cap. (Mallard)
Histine Prods. (Freeport)

Hyrexin, Inj. (Hyrex)
Nordryl, Prep. (North. Amer. Pharm.)
Rodryl, Inj. (Rocky Mtn.)
Rodryl-50, Inj. (Rocky Mtn.)
Rohydra, Elix. (Robinson)
SK-Diphenhydramine, Tabs., Cap. Elix. (Smith-Kline)
Span-Lanin, Cap. (Scrip)
T-Dryl 10, Inj. (Tunex)
T-Dryl 50, Inj. (Tunex)
Tusstat, Expect. (Century)
W/Ammonium chloride, menthol.
  See: Bentrac Expectorant, Liq. (Kenyon)
    Eldadryl Expectorant, Liq. (Elder)
    Fenylex, Exp. (Mallard)
    Tusstat Expectorant (Century)
W/Antihistamines.
  See: Symptrol, Syr., Cap., Inj. (Saron)
W/Benzethonium Cl.
  See: Bendylate, Inj. (Reid-Provident)
W/Chlorobutanol.
  See: Ardeben, Inj. (Burgin-Arden)
W/Pheniramine maleate pyrilamine maleate,
  phenylephrine HCl, phenylpropanolamine HCl.
  See: Symptrol, Syr. (Saron)
W/Phenylephrine HCl, phenylpropanolamine HCl,
  potassium guaiacolsulfonate, menthol, codeine
  phosphate.
  See: Para-Hist Antitussive, Syr., Cap. (Pharmics)
W/Pramoxine HCl, titanium dioxide, zinc oxide.
  See: Anti-Itch, Lot. (Towne)
W/Zinc oxide.
  See: Ziradryl, Lot. (Parke-Davis)
DIPHENIDOL. B.A.N. 1,1-Diphenyl-4-piperidino-butan-1-ol
  Use: Anti-emetic.
• DIPHENIDOL. USAN. α,α-Diphenyl-1-piperidinebutanol.
  See: Vontrol, Prep. (SmithKline)
• DIPHENIDOL HCl. USAN. $\alpha\alpha$-Diphenyl-1-piperidinebutanol HCl.
  Use: Anti-emetic.
• DIPHENIDOL PAMOATE. USAN. α,α-Diphenyl-1-piperidinebutanol compound with 4,4'-methylenebis
  [3-hydroxy-2-naphthoic acid](2:1).
  Use: Anti-emetic.
DIPHENMETHANIL METHYLSULFATE. 4-Diphenyl-methylene-1,1-dimethylpiperidinium methylsulfate.
  See: Diphemanil Methylsulfate (Var. Mfr.)
DIPHENOXYLATE. B.A.N. Ethyl 1-(3-cyano-3,3-di-phenylpropyl)-4-phenylpiperidine-4-carboxylate.
  Use: Antidiarrheal.
• DIPHENOXYLATE HCl, U.S.P. XXI. 4-Piperidinecar-boxylic acid, 1-(3-cyano-3,3-diphenylpropyl-4-phenyl-,
  ethyl ester, HCl, 2,2-Diphenyl-4-(4-carbethoxy-4-phe-nyl-1-pyeridino)butyronitrite ethyl ester HCl. Ethyl 1-
  (3-Cyano-3,3 diphenyl-propyl)-4-phenylisonipecotate
  Hydrochloride.
  Use: Antiperistaltic to treat diarrhea.
W/Atropine.
  See: Diaction, Tab. (Boots Pharm.)

Lomotil, Tab., Liq. (Searle)
SK-Diphenoxylate, Tab. (SmithKline)
• DIPHENOXYLATE HYDROCHLORIDE AND
  ATROPINE SULFATE, U.S.P. XXI. Oral Sol., Tabs.,
  U.S.P. XXI.
  Use: Antiperistaltic.
DIPHENYLAN SODIUM. (Lannett) Diphenyl-hydantoin
  sodium ½ gr. & 1½ gr./Cap. Bot. 500s, 1000s.
  Use: Epilepsy.
2,2-DIPHENYL-4-(4-CARBETHOXY-4-PHENYL-1-PY-
  ERIDINO)-BUTYRONITRITE ESTHYL ESTER HY-
  DROCHLORIDE. Diphenoxylate Hydrochloride,
  U.S.P. XXI.
DIPHENYLHYDROXYCARBINOL. Benzhydrol HCl.
5,5-DIPHENYLHYDANTOIN. Phenytoin, U.S.P. XXI.
DIPHENYLHYDANTOIN. Phenytoin, U.S.P. XXI.
  Use: Anticonvulsant.
5,5-DIPHENYLHYDANTOIN SODIUM. Phenytoin, So-dium, U.S.P. XXI.
DIPHENYLHYDANTOIN SODIUM. Phenytoin Sodium,
  U.S.P. XXI.
  Use: Anticonvulsant.
DIPHENYLISATIN.
  See: Oxyphenisatin (Var. Mfr.)
2-(DIPHENYLMETHOXY)-N,N-DIMETHYLETHYLAMI-
  NE HYDROCHLORIDE. Diphenhydramine Hydrochlo-ride, U.S.P. XXI.
3-DIPHENYLMETHOXYTROPANE METHANESUL-
  FONATE. Benztropine Mesylate, U.S.P. XXI.
1-(DIPHENYLMETHYL)-4-METHYLPIPERAZINE
  MONOHYDROCHLORIDE. Cyclizine Hydrochloride,
  U.S.P. XXI.
1,2-DIPHENYL-4-2-(PHENYLSULFINYL)-ETHYL-3,5-
  PYRAZOLIDINEDIONE. Sulfinpyrazone, U.S.P. XXI.
alpha, alpha-DIPHENYL-1-PIPERIDINEBUTANOL.
  See: Vontrol, Prods.
DIPHENYLPYRALINE. B.A.N. 4-Benzhydryloxy-1-methylpiperidine.
  Use: Antihistamine.
  See: Histryl
    Lergoban (hydrochloride)
• DIPHENYLPYRALINE HCl, U.S.P. XXI. Tab., U.S.P.
  XXI. 4-Diphenyl-methoxy-1-methypiperidine HCl.
  See: Diafen, Tab. (Riker)
    Hispril, Cap. (SmithKline)
W/Chlorphedianol HCl, phenylephrine HCl,
  guaifenesin, alcohol.
  See: Acutuss Expectorant (Philips Roxane)
DIPHOSPHONIC ACID.
  See: Etidronic acid
DIPHOSPHOPYRIDINE (DPN). Treating alcoholism.
  Under study.
DIPHOSPHOTHIAMIN. Cocarboxylase.
  See: Coenzyme-B, Cap. & Inj. (Inwood)
DIPHOXAZIDE. N^1-(b-hydroxy-b,b-diphenylpropionyl)-N^2-acetylhdrazine. Inductin.
• DIPHTHERIA ANTITOXIN, U.S.P. XXI. (Squibb-Con-naught) 20,000 units/Vial.
  Use: I.M., S.C.; protection & treatment of diphtheria.
  See: Diphtheria Toxoid, U.S.P. XXI.
• DIPHTHERIA & TETANUS TOXOIDS, U.S.P. XXI.

• **DIPHTHERIA & TETANUS TOXOIDS ABSORBED,** U.S.P. XXI. (Dow; Lilly) Vial 5 ml.
Use: Active immunizing agent.

DIPHTHERIA & TETANUS TOXOIDS ADSORBED, ALUMINUM PHOSPHATE ADSORBED. (Wyeth) Vial 5 cc. Tubex 0.5 cc. Pkg. 10s. Available in pediatric and adult strengths.

DIPHTHERIA AND TETANUS TOXOIDS, COMBINED PUROGENATED. (Lederle) Vial 5 ml. Lederject disposable syringe 10 × 0.5 ml.

DIPHTHERIA & TETANUS TOXOIDS, ALUMINUM PHOSPHATE ADSORBED, PUROGENATED. (Lederle) Adult, pediatric. Vial 5 ml.

• **DIPHTHERIA & TETANUS TOXOIDS & PERTUSSIS VACCINE,** U.S.P. XXI. (Squibb-Connaught) Vial 7.5 ml. for pediatric use.
Use: Prevention against diphtheria, tetanus and pertussis.
See: Tri-immunol, Vial (Lederle)
Tri-Solgen Vial, Hyporet (Lilly)

DIPHTHERIA & TETANUS TOXOIDS & PERTUSSIS VACCINE COMBINED, ALUMINUM HYDROXIDE ADSORBED.
See: Triogen, Vial (Parke-Davis)

DIPHTHERIA & TETANUS TOXOIDS & PERTUSSIS VACCINE COMBINED, ALUMINUM PHOSPHATE-ADSORBED.
See: Tri-Immunol, Vial (Lederle)

DIPHTHERIA & TETANUS TOXOIDS & PERTUSSIS VACCINE COMBINED, ALUM PRECIPITATED.
See: Triple Antigen, Vial (Wyeth)

DIPHTHERIA TOXIN, DIAGNOSTIC. Schick Test.

DIPHTHERIA TOXIN, INACTIVATED DIAGNOSTIC. Schick test control.

• **DIPHTHERIA TOXIN FOR SCHICK TEST,** U.S.P. XXI.
Use: Diagnostic aid (dermal reactivity indicator).
See: Diphtheria Toxin, Diagnostic

• **DIPHTHERIA TOXOID,** U.S.P. XXI.
Use: Active immunizing agent.

• **DIPHTHERIA TOXOID ADSORBED,** U.S.P. XXI. Alum. Precipitated (Antoxin-Ramon, Diphtheria Ana-toxin).
Use: Active immunizing agent.

DIPHTHERIA TOXOID & PERTUSSIS VACCINE. Lilly —Vial 10 tests.

DIPHYLLINE.
See: Diazma, Vial (Pharmex)

DIPIPANONE. B.A.N.4,4-Diphenyl-6-piperidino-heptan-3-one.
Use: Narcotic analgesic.
See: Pipadone (hydrochloride)

• **DIPIVEFRIN.** USAN.
Use: Adrenergic.

DIPIVEFRIN HYDROCHLORIDE. (+)-3,4-dihydroxy-a-(methylamino) methyl benzyl alcohol 3,4-dipivalate HCl.
Use: Treatment of chronic open-angle glaucoma.
See: Propine, Sol. (Allergan))

DIPONIUM BROMIDE (I.N.N.). Dipenine Bromide, B.A.N.

DIPRENORPHINE. B.A.N. N-Cyclopropylmethyl-7,8-

dihydro-7 α-(1-hydroxy-1-methylethyl)-O⁶-methyl-6,14 endoethanonormorphine.
Use: Narcotic antagonist.

DIPRIDAMOLE. (Foy) Dipyridamole 25 mg./Tab. Bot. 1000s.
Use: Coronary vasodilator.

DIPROLENE OINTMENT 0.05%. (Schering) Betamethasone dipropionate 0.64 mg., in ointment base. Tubes 15 Gm., 45 Gm.
Use: Topical anti-inflammatory, anti-pruritic agent.

DIPROPHYLLINE. B.A.N. 7-(2,3-Dihydroxypropyl)-theophylline.
Use: Bronchodilator.
See: Isophylline
Neutraphylline
Silbephylline

DIPROSONE AEROSOL 0.1%. (Schering) Betamethasone dipropionate 6.4 mg. (equiv. to 5 mg. bethamethasone) in vehicle of mineral oil, caprylic-capric triglyceride w/isopropyl alcohol 10%, inert hydrocarbon propellants. (propane & isobutane). Pkg. 85 Gm.
Use: Topical anti-inflammatory

DIPROSONE CREAM 0.05%. (Schering) Betamethasone dipropionate 0.64 mg. (equiv. to 0.5 mg. betamethasone) w/mineral oil, white petrolatum, polyethylene glycol 1000 monocetyl ether, cetostearyl alcohol, phosphoric acid and monobasic sod. phosphate with 4-chloro-m-cresol as preservative. Tube 15 Gm., 45 Gm.
Use: Anti-inflammatory dermatological.

DIPROSONE LOTION 0.05%. (Schering) Betamethasone dipropionate 0.64 mg. (equiv. to 0.5 mg. betamethasone) W/isopropyl alcohol (46.8%) & purified water. Bot. 20 ml., 60 ml.
Use: Topical anti-inflammatory.

DIPROSONE OINTMENT 0.05%. (Schering) Betamethasone dipropionate 0.64 mg. (eqiv. to 0.5 mg. betamethasone) in white petrolatum & mineral oil base. Tubes 15 Gm., 45 Gm.
Use: Topical anti-inflammatory agent.

DIPTEREX. Metriphonate, B.A.N.

• **DIPYRIDAMOLE,** U.S.P. XXI. Tab., U.S.P. XXI. 2,6-Di [di-(2-hydroxy-ethyl)-amino]-4,8-dipiperidinopyrimido [5,4-d]-pyrimidine.
Use: Coronary vasodilator.
See: Persantin

• **DIPYRIDAMOLE.** USAN. 2,2′,2″-2‴,-[4,8-Dipiperidinopyrimido[5,4-d]pyrimidine-2,6-diyl)-dinitril-o]tetraethanol.
Use: Coronary dilator.
See: Persantine, Tabs. (Boehringer-Ingelheim)

• **DIPYRITHIONE.** USAN.
Use: Antibacterial, antifungal.

• **DIPYRONE.** USAN. Sodium N-(2,3-dimethyl-1-phenyl-5-oxopyrazolin-4-yl)-N-methylamino-methanesulfonat-e. Sodium noramidopyrine methanesulfonate. Sodium phenyldimethylpyrazolon-methylamino-me-thane sulfonate, sodium (anti-pyrinylmethylamino)-methane sulfonate hydrate; novalgin, methylmelubrin, methampyrone, 4-Sod. methanesulfonate methylamine-antipyrine.

Use: Analgesic, antipyretic & antirheumatic.
Note: Product removed from the market.
DIRIDONE. (Premo) Phenylazo-diamino-pyridine HCl.
100 mg./Tab. Bot. 100s, 1000s.
Use: Urinary anesthetic and antiseptic.
DIROX TABLETS. (Winthrop Products) Paracetamol.
Use: Analgesic, antipyretic,
DISALCID. (Riker) Salsalate. **Tab.:** 500 mg., 750
mg./Tab. Bot. 100s, 500s.**Cap.:** 500 mg./Cap. Bot.
100s.
Use: Anti-inflammatory, analgesic in arthritis.
DISAMIDE. Disulfamide, B.A.N.
DISANTHROL CAPSULES. (Lannett) Docusate
sodium 100 mg., casanthranol 30 mg./Cap. Bot.
100s, 1000s.
Use: Laxative.
DISIPAL. (Riker) N,N-dimethyl-2-(0-methyl-α-phenyl-
benzyloxy) ethylamine. Orphenadrine HCl. Tab. (50
mg.) Bot. 100s.
Use: Parkinsonism.
DISMISS DOUCHE. (Schering) Sodium chloride,
sodium citrate, citric acid, cetaryl octoate,
ceteareth-27 & fragrance. Powder for dilution. Pkg. 1s,
2s, 3s.
Use: Vaginal cleanser.
• **DISOBUTAMIDE.** USAN.
Use: Cardiac depressant.
DISODIUM CARBONATE. Sodium Carbonate, N.F.
XVI.
DISODIUM CHROMATE. Sodium Chromate Cr 51
Injection, U.S.P. XXI.
**DISODIUM 3,3′-DIOXO[Δ^2,$^{2′}$-BINDOLINE]-5,5′-DI-
SULFONATE.** Indigotindisulfonate Sodium, U.S.P.
XXI.
DISODIUM EDATHAMIL.
See: Edathamil Disodium (Var. Mfr.)
DISODIUM EDETATE. B.A.N. Disodium dihydrogen
ethylenediamine-NNN′N′-tetra-acetate.
Use: Chelating agent.
DISODIUM EDETATE. Disodium
ethylenediaminetetraacetate.
See: Edetate Disodium, U.S.P. XXI.
**DISODIUM (ETHYLENEDINITRILO)TETRA-ACETO
CALCIATE(2-)HYDRATE.** Edetate Calcium
**DISODIUM (ETHYLENEDINITRILO)TETRA-ACETO
DIHYDRATE.** Edetate Disodium, U.S.P. XXI.
DISODIUM PHOSPHATE.
See: Sodium Phosphate, U.S.P. XXI.
DISODIUM PHOSPHATE HEPTAHYDRATE. Sodium
Phosphate, U.S.P. XXI.
**DISODIUM SALT OF N-(3-CARBOXY-METHYL-THIO-
MERCURI-2-METHOXY-PROPYL) CAM-
PHORAMIC ACID.** Mercaptomerin Sodium, U.S.P.
XXI.
DISODIUM THIOSULFATE PENTAHYDRATE.
Sodium Thiosulfate, U.S.P. XXI.
DI-SODIUM VERSENATE.
See: Edathamil Disodium (Var. Mfr.)
• **DISOFENIN.** USAN.
Use: Diagnostic aid.
DISOLAN. (Lannett) Docusate sodium 100 mg.,

phenolphthalein 65 mg./Cap. Bot. 100s, 500s,
1000s.
Use: Constipation therapy.
DISOLAN FORTE CAPSULES. (Lannett)
Casanthranol 30 mg., sod. carboxymethylcellulose
400 mg., Docusate sodium 100 mg./Cap. Bot.
100s, 500s, 1000s.
Use: Laxative.
DISONATE. (Lannett) Docusate sodium 60 mg., 100
mg., 240 mg./Cap. **Caps.** Bot. 100s, 500s, 1000s.
Tab. 100 mg., Bot. 1000s **Liq.** 10 mg./ml. Bot. pt.
Syr. 20 mg./5 ml. Bot. pt., gal.
Use: Fecal softener.
DISOPHROL CHRONOTABS. (Schering)
Dexbrompheniramine maleate 6 mg., pseudo-
ephedrine sulf. 120 mg./S.A. Tab. Bot. 100s.
Use: Antihistamine-decongestant.
• **DISOPYRAMIDE.** USAN. 4-Di-isopropylamino-2-phe-
nyl-2-(2-pyridyl)butyramide.
Use: Anti-arrhythmic.
See: Rythmodan
• **DISOPYRAMIDE PHOSPHATE,** U.S.P. XXI. Caps.,
U.S.P. XXI.
DI-SOSUL. (Drug Industries) Docusate sodium 50
mg./Tab. Bot. 100s, 500s.
Use: Stool softener.
DI-SOSUL FORTE. (Drug Industries) Docusate sodium
100 mg., casanthranol 30 mg./Tab. Bot. 100s,
500s.
Use: Stool softener and laxative.
DISOTATE. (O'Neal, Jones & Feldman) Disodium
edetate 150 mg./cc. Vial 20 cc.
DI-SPAZ. (Vortech) Dicyclomine HCl **Cap.** 10 mg./Cap.
Bot. 100s, 1000s; **Inj.:** w/sod. chloride 0.9%,
chlorobutanol 0.5%/cc. Vial 10 cc.
Use: Antispasmodic.
DISTAQUAINE.
See: Penicillin V.
DISTIGMINE BROMIDE. B.A.N. NN′-Hexamethyl-
enedi-[1-methyl-3-(methylcarbamoyloxy)-pyridinium
bromide].
Use: Anticholinesterase.
See: Ubretid
DISTIGMINE BROMIDE. Hexamarium bromide.
DISULANS-PLUS. (Noyes) Docusate sodium 100 mg.,
casanthrol 30 mg./Cap. Bot. 100s, 1000s.
Use: Stool softener with laxative.
• **DISULFIRAM,** U.S.P. XXI. Tab., U.S.P. XXI. Bis-(die-
thylthiocarbamoyl)disulfide. Tetraethylthiuram
Disulfide.
Use: Treatment of alcoholism
See: Antabuse, Tab. (Ayerst)
DISULFONAMIDE.
See: Dia-Mer-Sulfonamides (Var. Mfr.)
DISULFAMIDE. B.A.N. 5-Chlorotoluene-2,4-disulfona-
mide.
Use: Diuretic.
See: Disamide
DITAN. (Mallard) Phenytoin sodium 100 mg./Cap.
Bot. 1000s.
Use: Anticonvulsant.

DITATE. (Savage) Estradiol valerate 4 mg., testosterone enanthate 90 mg./ml. Vial 10 ml.

DITATE-DS. (Savage) Estradiol valerate 8 mg., testosterone enanthate 180 mg./ml. Vial 2 ml., syringe 2 ml., 10s.

DITHIAZANINE. B.A.N. 3-Ethyl-2-[5-(3-ethyl-benzothiazolin-2-ylidene)penta-1,3-dienyl]benzothiazolium.
Use: Anthelmintic.
See: Delvex
   Telmid (iodide)

DITHRANOL.
See: Anthralin, U.S.P. XXI. (Var. Mfr.)

D.I.T.I. CREME. (Dunhall) Iodoquinol 100 mg., sulfanilamide 500 mg., diethylstilbestrol 0.1 mg./Gm. Jar. 4 oz.
Use: Intra-vaginal infections.

D.I.T.I.-2 CREME. (Dunhall) Sulfanilamide 15.0%, aminacrine HCl 0.2%, allantoin 2.0%. Tube 5 oz.
Use: Intra-vaginal creme.

DITOPHAL. B.A.N. SS'-Diethyl dithioisophthalate.
See: Etisul
Use: Antileprotic.

DITROPAN. (Marion) Oxybutynin chloride 5 mg./Tab. Bot. 100s, 1000s. Unit dose identification paks of 100s.
Use: Relief of symptoms in voiding with neurogenic bladder.

DITROPAN SYRUP. (Marion) Oxybutynin Cl. 5 mg./5 ml. Bot. 16 oz.
Use: Relief of symptoms in voiding with neurogenic bladder.

DIUCARDIN. (Ayerst) Hydroflumethiazide 50 mg./Tab. Bot. 100s.
Use: Diuretic, antihypertensive.

DIULO. (Searle) Metolazone. 2½ mg./Tab. Bot. 100s. 5 mg./Tab. Bot. 100s, 500s. 10 mg./Tab. Bot. 100s.
Use: Diuretic, antihypertensive.

DIUPRES. (Merck Sharp & Dohme) Chlorothiazide 250 mg. or 500 mg., reserpine 0.125 mg./Tab. Bot. 100s, 1000s.
Use: Antihypertensive.

DIURESE. (Key) Trichlormethiazide 4 mg./Tab. Bot. 100s, 1000s.
Use: Diuretic.

DIURETANE #1. (Wolins) Uva ursi pow. ext. 32.4 mg., buchu leaves pow. ext. 32.4 mg., corn silk pow. ext. 32.4 mg., juniper pow. ext. 16.2 mg., caffeine 16.2 mg./Tab. Bot. 100s, 1000s.

DIURETANE #2. (Wolins) Buchu pow. ext. 65 mg., couch grass 65 mg., corn silk pow. ext. 32.5 mg., hydrangea pow. ext. 32.5 mg./Tab. Bot. 100s, 1000s.

■ **DIURETICS.**
See: Aldactazide, Tab. (Searle)
   Aldactone, Tab. (Searle)
   Aminophylline (Var. Mfr.)
   Aquazide, Tab. (Western Research)
   Benzthiazide (Var. Mfr.)
   Carbamide
   Carbonic Anhydrase Inhibitors
   Diamox (Lederle)

   Diamox, Sequels (Lederle)
   Dicurin Procaine, Inj. (Lilly)
   Diuril, Tab., Oral Susp. (Merck Sharp & Dohme)
   Dyazide, Cap. (SmithKline)
   Dyrenium, Caps. (SmithKline)
   Edecrin, Tab. (Merck Sharp & Dohme)
   Esidrix, Tab. (Ciba)
   Exna, Tab. (Robins)
   Fleet Theophylline Rectal Unit, Sol. (Fleet)
   Flumethiazide
   Glycerin, Liq. (Var. Mfr.)
   Hydrochlorothiazide, Tab. (Var. Mfr.)
   Hydroflumethiazide, Tab. (Bristol)
   Hydromox, Tab. (Lederle)
   Hygroton, Tab. (USV)
   Lasix, Tab., Inj. (Hoechst)
   Mannitol (Var. Mfr.)
   Mercurial diuretics
   Mersalyl and Theophylline (Var. Mfr.)
   Metahydrin, Tab. (Merrell Dow)
   Methazolamide (Var. Mfr.)
   Methyclothiazide, Tab. (Var. Mfr.)
   Naqua, Tab. (Schering)
   Naquival, Tab. (Schering)
   Naturetin, Tab. (Squibb)
   Neothylline, Amp., Elix., Tab. (Lemmon)
   Proaqua, Tab. (Reid-Provident)
   Renese, Tab. (Pfizer)
   Sodium Diuril, I.V. Inj., Vial (Merck Sharp & Dohme)
   Sodium Edecrin, I.V. Inj., Vial (Merck Sharp & Dohme)
   Theocalcin, Pow., Tab. (Knoll)
   Trichlormethiazide, Tab. (Var. Mfr.)
   Triticoll, Tab. (Western Research)
   Urea (Var. Mfr.)
   Zaroxolyn, Tab. (Pennwalt)

DIURETIC TABLETS. (Faraday) Buchu leaves 150 mg., uva ursi leaves 150 mg., juniper berries 120 mg., bone meal, parsley, asparagus/Tab. Bot. 100s.

DIURETTE INJECTION. (Ortega) Mersalyl, USP, 100 mg.; theophylline USP, 50 mg./cc. Vial 10 cc.
Use: Diuresis, especially in cardiac edema.

DIURETTS. (Faraday) Tab. Bot. 84s.
Use: Diuretic.

DIURIL. (Merck Sharp & Dohme) Chlorothiazide, U.S.P. **Tabs.:** 250 mg. Bot. 100s, 1000s. Single unit pkg. 100s; 500 mg. Bot. 100s, 1000s, 5000s. Single unit pkg. 100s. **Oral Susp.:** 250 Gm./5ml. w/methylparaben 0.12%, propylparaben 0.02%, benzoic acid 0.1%, alcohol 0.5%. Bot. 237 ml. **I.V. Inj.:** 0.5 Gm./Vial w/0.25 Gm. mannitol, sodium hydroxide & 0.4 mg. thimerosal.
Use: Diuretic therapy for edema.
W/Reserpine.
See: Diupres, Tab. (Merck Sharp & Dohme)

DIURIL. (MSD AGVET) Chlorothiazide 2 Gm. bolus, 0.25 Gm/Tab.
Use: Diuretic, veterinary medicine.

DIURSAL. (Harvey) Mersalyl 100 mg., theophylline 50 mg./cc. Amp. 2 cc., Box 25s, 100s.

Use: Diuretic.

DIU-SCRIP. (Scrip) Hydrochlorothiazide 25 mg., 50 mg./Tab. Bot. 1000s.

DIU-TABS. (Wisconsin) Bot. 35s, 100s.
Use: Elimination of excess water.

DIUTENSEN. (Wallace) Cryptenamine (as the tannate salts) 2 mg., methyclothiazide 2.5 mg./Tab. Bot. 100s, 500s.
Use: Hypertension.

DIUTENSEN-R. (Wallace) Methyclothiazide 2.5 mg., reserpine 0.1 mg./Tab. Bot. 100s, 500s.
Use: Hypertension.

• **DIVALPROEX SODIUM.** USAN.
Use: Anticonvulsant.

DIVINYL OXIDE. Vinyl Ether, Divinyl Ether.
Use: Inhalation anesthetic.

DIXARIT HYDROCHLORIDE. Clonidine, B.A.N.

DIZYMES. (Recsei) Protease and amylase equiv. to 250 mg. "Lipase 3,000"/Cap. Cap. 250 mg. Bot. 100s, 500s.
Use: Digestive enzymes.

DIZMISS. (Bowman) Meclizine HCl 25 mg/Tab. Bot. 100s, 1000s.
Use: Antinauseant for motion sickness.

DMCT. (Lederle) Demethylchlortetracycline.
See: Declomycin HCl, Prep. (Lederle)

DM 4 CHILDREN'S COUGH CONTROL. (DeWitt) d-Methorphan. Bot. 3 oz.

DM 8 COUGH CONTROL MEDICINE. (DeWitt) d-Methorphan. Bot. 4 oz.

DM COUGH SYRUP. (Bay) Dextromethorphan HBr 10 mg./5 ml. w/alcohol 5%. Bot. 4 oz. pt., gal.
Use: Antitussive.

D-MED. (Ortega) Methylprednisolone acetate 40 or 80 mg./ml. Vials 5 ml.
Use: Adrenocortical steroid.

DMSO. (Crown Zellerbach; Syntex)
See: Dimethyl sulfoxide.

DOAK-OIL. (Doak) Tar distillate 2%, in a lanolin, mineral oil suspension. Pl. Bot. 8 oz.
Use: Dermatologic.

DOAK OIL FORTE. (Doak) Tar distillate 5%, Bot. 4 oz.
Use: Dermatologic.

DOAK TAR LOTION. (Doak) Tar distillate 5%. Bot. 4 oz.
Use: Dermatological lotion.

DOAK TAR SHAMPOO. (Doak) Tar distillate 3% in shampoo base. Bot. 4 oz.
Use: Dermatological shampoo.

DOAK TERSASEPTIC. (Doak) A liquid cleanser, pH 6.8. Bot. 4 oz., pt., gal.
Use: Liquid detergent.

DOAN'S BACKACHE SPRAY. (Jeffrey Martin) Methyl salicylate 15%, menthol 8.4%, methyl nicotinate 0.6%. Aerosol can 4 oz.
Use: External analgesic.

DOAN'S PILLS. (Jeffrey Martin) Magnesium salicylate 325 mg./Tab. Ctn. 24s, 48s.
Use: Analgesic.

DOB BATH OIL. (Person & Covey) Bot. 8 oz.
Use: Bath & shower for dry skin.

DOBELL'S SOLUTION. Sodium Borate Solution Compound.
(Emerson) Bot. 4 oz., pt.
(Stanlabs) Bot. pt.

• **DOBUTAMINE.** USAN. (±)-4-[2-(3-p-Hydroxy-phenyl-1-methylpropylamino)ethyl]pyrocatechol.
Use: Cardiac stimulant.

• **DOBUTAMINE HYDROCHLORIDE.** U.S.P. XXI. For Inj., U.S.P. XXI.
Use: Cardiac stimulant.
See: Dobutrex, Inj. (Lilly)
Inotrex (Lilly)

DOBUTREX. (Lilly) Dobutamine HCl 250 mg./vial. Vial 20 ml.
Use: Inotropic agent.

DOCA ACETATE. (Organon) Desoxycorticosterone acetate 5 mg./ml. in oil. Vial 10 ml.
Use: Adrenocortical insufficiency.

• **DOCONAZOLE.** USAN.
Use: Antifungal.

DOCTASE. (Purepac) Docusate sodium 100 mg., casanthranol 30 mg./Cap. Bot. 100s.
Use: Stool softener.

DOCTIENT HC. (Suppositoria) Cod liver oil, hydrocortisone acetate 10 mg., lanolin, zinc oxide, bismuth subgallate, benzocaine, /Supp. Box 12s, 100s, 1000s.
Use: Antihemorrhoidal.

DOCTYL. (Approved) Docusate sodium 100 mg./Tab. Bot. 40s, 100s, 1000s.
Use: Constipation.

DOCTYLAX. (Approved) Docusate sodium 100 mg., acetophenolisatin 2 mg., prune conc. ¾ mg./Tab. Bot. 40s, 100s, 1000s.
Use: Corrective laxative.

• **DOCUSATE CALCIUM,** U.S.P. XXI. Cap. U.S.P. XXI. 1, 4-Bis(2-ethylhexyl)sulfosuccinate, cal. salt. Calcium bis-dioctyl-sulfosuccinate.
Use: Fecal softener.
See: Surfak, Cap. (Hoechst)
Doxidan, Cap. (Hoechst)

• **DOCUSATE POTASSIUM,** U.S.P.XXI. Cap., U.S.P. XXI.
Use: Stool softener
See: Dialose, Cap. (Stuart)
Dialose Plus, Cap. (Stuart)
Kasof, Cap. (Stuart)

• **DOCUSATE SODIUM,** U.S.P. XXI. Cap., Soln., Syr., Tab., U.S.P. XXI. Aerosol OT. (Am. Cyanamid). Bis-(2-ethoxy)-S-sodium sulfosuccinate. Sodium 1, 4-Bis (2-ethylhexyl) sulfosuccinate.
Use: Pharm. aid (surfactant); stool softener.
See: Bu-Lax, Cap. (Ulmer)
Colace, Cap., Liq., Syr. (Mead Johnson)
Coloctyl, Cap. (Vitarine)
Comfolax, Cap. (Searle)
Constab-100, Tab. (Kenyon)
Dilax, Cap. (Mission)
Diomedicone, Tab (Medicone)
Diosate Caps. (Towne)
Diosuccin, Cap., Syr. (CMC)
Dio-Sul, Cap. (Vortech)

Diosux, Cap. (Jenkins)
Disonate, Cap., Tab. Syr., Liq. (Lannett)
Doss, Super Doss, Tab. (Ferndale)
Doxinate, Cap., Liq. (Hoechst)
DSS (Parke-Davis)
Duosol, Cap. (Kirkman)
Dynoctol, Cap. (Reid-Provident)
Easy-Lax, Cap. (Walgreen)
Konsto, Cap. (Freeport)
Laxatab, Tab. (Freeport)
Liqui-Doss, Liq. (Ferndale)
Modane Soft, Cap. (Adria)
Neo-Vadrin, Cap. (Scherer)
Peri-Doss, Cap. (Ferndale)
Regul-Aid, Syr. (Columbia)
Regutol, Tab. (Plough)
Revac Supprettes, Supp. (Webcon)
Rodox, Caps. (Rocky Mtn.)
Softon, Cap. (Stanlabs)
Stulex, Tab. (Bowman)
Surfak, Cap. (Hoechst)
W/Ascorbic acid, ferrous fumarate.
See: Hemaspan Cap. (Bock)
W/Betaine HCl, zinc, manganese, molybdenum.
See: Hemaferrin (Western Research)
W/Bisacodyl
See: Laxadan, Supp.(Lemmon)
W/Brewer's yeast.
See: Doss or Super Doss, Tab. (Ferndale)
W/Casanthranol.
See: Bu-Lax-Plus, Cap. (Ulmer)
Calotabs, Tabs. (Calotabs)
Constiban (Columbia)
Diolax, Caps. (Century)
Dio-Soft (Standex)
Diothron, Cap. (Vortech)
Disanthrol, Cap. (Lannett)
Di-Sosul Forte, Tab. (Drug)
D-S-S W/Casanthranol, Cap. (Wolins)
Disulans-Plus, Cap. (Noyes)
Easy-Lax Plus, Cap. (Walgreen)
Genericace, Cap. (Fellows-Testagar)
Neo-Vadrin D-D-S, Cap. (Scherer)
Nuvac, Cap. (LaCrosse)
Peri-Colace, Cap., Syr. (Mead Johnson)
Rodox, Cap. (Rocky Mtn.)
Sodex, Cap. (Mallard)
Sofflax, Cap. (Medics)
Stimulax, Cap. (Geriatric)
Syncelax, Cap. (Blue Line)
W/Casanthranol, sodium carboxymethylcellulose.
See: Dialose Plus, Cap. (Stuart)
Disolan Forte, Cap. (Lannett)
Tri-Vac, Cap. (Rhode)
W/Cascara sagrada extract.
See: Dioctyl-Zem, Tab. (Zemmer)
W/Danthron.
See: Danthross, Cap. (Elder)
Doctate-P, Cap. (Glaxo)
Doxate-D, Tab. (Dunhall)
W/Danthron, guar gum.
See: Guarsol, Tab. (Western Research)

W/Dehydrocholic acid.
See: Dubbalax-B, Cap. (Redford)
Dubbalax-N, Cap. (Redford)
Neolax, Tab. (Central)
W/D-calcium pantothenate and acetphenolisatin.
See: Peri-Pantyl, Tab. (McGregor)
W/Cascara sagrada extract.
See: Dioctyl-Zem, Tab. (Zemmer)
W/Dorbane.
See: Dorbantyl, Cap. (Riker)
Dorbantyl Forte, Cap. (Riker)
W/Ferrous fumarate, Vit. C.
See: Hemaspan, Cap. (Bock)
Recoup, Tab. (Lederle)
W/Ferrous fumarate, vitamins.
See: Bevitone, Tab. (Lemmon)
W/Ferrous fumarate, betaine HCl, desic. liver,
vitamins, minerals.
See: Hemaferrin, Tab. (Western Research)
W/Guar gum, prune concentrate.
See: D-S-S Compound, Cap. (Wolins)
W/Glycerin.
See: Rectalad Enema, Liq. (Wampole)
W/Isobornyl thiocyanoacetate.
See: Barc, Cream, Liq. (Commerce)
W/Petrolatum.
See: Milkinol, Liquid, Emulsion (Kremers-Urban)
W/Phenolphthalein.
See: Correctol, Tab. (Plough)
Disolan, Cap. (Lannett)
Feen-A-Mint, Pills (Plough)
Novalax, Cap. (Coastal)
W/Phenolphthalein, dehydrocholic acid.
See: Bolax, Cap. (Boyd)
Sarolax, Caps. (Saron)
Tripalax, Cap. (Redford)
W/Polyoxyethylene nonyl phenol, sodium edetate,
and 9-aminoacridine HCl.
See: Vagisec Plus Suppositories (Schmid)
W/Psyllium.
See: Sof-Cil, Pow. (Zemmer)
W/Senna concentrate.
See: Gentlax S, Tab. (Blair)
Sarolax (Saron)
Senokap-DDS, Cap. (Purdue Frederick)
Senokot S, Tab. (Purdue Frederick)
W/Sod. propionate, propionic acid, salicylic
acid.
See: Prosal, Liq. (Gordon)
W/Vitamin-mineral combination.
See: Geriplex-FS, Kapseal (Parke-Davis)
Materna 1.60., Tab. (Lederle)
DODERLEIN BACILLI.
See: Redoderlein, Vial (Fellows-Testagar)
DODICIN. B.A.N. 3,6,9-Triazaheneicosanoic acid.
Dodecyldi(aminoethyl)glycine.
Use: Surface active agent.
DOFAMIUM CHLORIDE. B.A.N. 2-(N-Dodecanoyl-N-
methylamino)ethyldimethyl-(phenylcarbamoyl-
methyl)ammonium chloride.
Use: Antiseptic.
See: Desogen.

DoFUS. (Miller) Freeze dried *Lactobacillus acidophilus* minimum of 200,000 I.U./Tab. Bot. 100s.
Use: To restore intestinal flora.

DOGMATYL. (Laboratories Delagrange, France) Sulpiride.

DOKTORS NOSE DROPS AND SPRAY. (Scherer) Phenylephrine HCl 0.25%. Spray Bot. 0.5 oz., 1 oz. Drops Bot. 1 oz.
Use: Nasal decongestant.

DOLACET C-3. (Hauck) Propoxyphene HCl 65 mg., acetaminophen 650 mg./Tab. Bot. 100s, 500s.
Use: Analgesic.

DOLAMIN. (Harvey) Ammonium sulf. 0.75% with sod. chlor. and benzyl alc. Amp. 10 cc.
Use: Various neuralgias. 12s, 25s, 100s.

DOLANEX ELIXIR. (Lannett) Acetaminophen 325 mg./5 mg., alcohol 23%. Bot. 4 oz., 16 oz.
Use: Analgesic.

DOLANTIN.
See: Meperidine Hydrochloride, U.S.P. XXI.

DOLCIN. (Dolcin) Aspirin 3.7 gr., cal. succinate 2.8 gr./Tab. Bot. 100s, 200s.
Use: Analgesic, antipyretic.

DOLDRAM. (Dram) Salicylamide 7½ gr./Tab. Bot. 100s.
Use: Analgesic.

DOLEAR. (Eastwood) Ear drops. Bot. ½ oz.

DOLENE AP-65. (Lederle) Propoxyphene HCl 65 mg., acetaminophen 650 mg./Tab. Bot. 100s, 500s.
Use: Analgesic.

DOLENE COMPOUND-65. (Lederle) Propoxyphene HCl 65 mg., aspirin 389 mg., caffeine 32.4 mg./Cap. Bot. 100s, 500s.
Use: Analgesic.

DOLENE PLAIN. (Lederle) Propoxyphene HCl 65 mg./Caps. Bot. 100s, 500s.
Use: Analgesic.

DOLICAINE. (Reid-Provident) Lidocaine HCl 2%/cc. Vials 50cc.

DOLOBID. (Merck Sharp & Dohme) Diflunisal 250 mg. or 500 mg./Tab. Unit of use 60s. Unit dose 100s.
Use: Analgesic, anti-inflammatory.

DOLOMITE. (Barth's) Magnesium 297 mg., calcium 474.9 mg./Tab. Bot. 100s, 500s, 1000s.

DOLOMITE PLUS CAPSULES. (Barth's) Magnesium 37 mg., Ca 187 mg., P 50 mg., iodine 0.25 mg./Cap. Bot. 100s, 500s, 1000s.

DOLOMITE TABLETS. (Columbia) Magnesium 396 mg., calcium 633 mg./4 Tab. Bot. 250s, 500s.

DOLOMITE. (Blue Cross) Calcium 426 mg., magnesium 246 mg./3 Tabs. w/guar and acacia gum. Bot. 250s.
Use: Calcium and magnesium deficiency.

DOLOMITE TABLETS. (Faraday) Calcium 150 mg., magnesium 90 mg./Tab. Bot. 250s.

DOLONIL. (Parke-Davis)
See: Pyridium Plus, Tab. (Parke-Davis)

DOLOPHINE HYDROCHLORIDE. (Lilly) Methadone HCl. **Amp.:** (10 mg./ml.; sod. chloride 0.9%) 1 ml. 12s, 100s. **Vial:** (10 mg./ml.) 20 ml. (Sod. chloride 0.9%, chlorobutanol 0.5%). 1s, 25s. **Tab.:** 5 mg. Bot. 100s. 10 mg. Bot. 100s.

Use: Narcotic, analgesic & antitussive.

DOLOPIRONA TABLETS. (Winthrop Products) Dipyrone with chlormezanone.
Use: Analgesic, muscle relaxant.

DOLORAL. (Progressive Enterprises) Colchicine salicylate 0.1 mg., phenobarbital 8 mg., sod. p-aminobenzoate 15 mg., Vit. B-1 25 mg., aspirin 325 mg./Tab. Bot. 100s, 1000s.
Use: Treatment of gout, arthritis & rheumatism.

DOLORGON. (Kenyon) Mephenesin 200 mg., salicylamide 75 mg., acetyl-p-aminophenol 75 mg., ascorbic acid 50 mg./Tab. Bot. 100s, 1000s.
Use: Analgesic.

DOLOSAL.
See: Meperidine Hydrochloride (Var. Mfr.)
Demerol HCl, Prods. (Winthrop-Breon)

DOLVANOL.
See: Meperidine Hydrochloride (Var. Mfr.)
Demerol HCl, Prod. (Winthrop-Breon)

• **DOMAZOLINE FUMARATE.** USAN.
Use: Anticholinergic.

DOMEBORO. (Miles Pharm) Aluminum sulfate & cal. acetate when added to water gives therapeutic effect of Burow's. One pkg. or Tab./Pt. water approx. equiv. to 1:40 dilution. **Pkg.:** 2.2 Gm., 12s, 100s. **Tab.:** effer. Box 12s, 100s, 1000s.
Use: Externally; in inflammatory skin conditions.

DOMEBORO OTIC. (Miles Pharm) Acetic acid 2%, in an aluminum acetate solution buffered to pH of 5.0 Plas. Bot. w/otic tip 2 oz.
Use: Otitis externa.

DOMEFORM-HC. (Miles Pharm) Hydrocortisone alcohol ½%, clioquinol 3%, in vehicle buffered to the pH range of normal skin w/cetyl alcohol, stearyl alcohol, sod. lauryl sulfate, beeswax, glycerin, petrolatum, & methylparaben. Cream: Tube ½ oz.
Use: Treatment of skin infections.

DOME-PASTE BANDAGE. (Miles Pharm) Zinc oxide, calamine, glycerine & gelatin bandage. Pkg. flesh-colored 4″ × 10 yd. and 3″ × 10 yd. impregnated gauze bandage.
Use: Treatment of leg ulcers.

DOMERINE MEDICATED SHAMPOO. (Miles Pharm) Salicylic acid 2%, allantoin 0.2%, in vehicle combining surface-active wetting agents with protein condensate (pH 5.3). Bot. 4 oz.
Use: Seborrheic conditions of the scalp.

DOMESTROL.
See: Diethylstilbestrol, Prep. (Various Mfr.)

D.O.M.F.
See: Merbromin (Mercurochrome) (City Chem.)

• **DOMIODOL.** USAN.
Use: Mucolytic.

• **DOMIPHEN BROMIDE.** USAN. Dodecyldimethyl-2-phenoxyethylammonium bromide. Phenododecinium Bromide (I.N.N.).
Use: Antiseptic.
See: Bradosol
Domibrom

DOMMANATE. (O'Neal, Jones & Feldman) Dimenhydrinate 50 mg./ml. Vial 10 ml.

DOMPERIDONE. USAN.
Use: Anti-emetic.

DONATUSSIN. (Laser) **Pediatric Drops:** Guaifenesin 20 mg., chlorpheniramine maleate 1 mg., phenylephrine HCl 2 mg./ml. Drop. bot. 30 ml. **Syr.:** Dextromethorphan HBr 7.5 mg., phenylephrine HCl 10 mg., chlorpheniramine maleate 2 mg., guaifenesin 100 mg./5 ml. Bot. pt., gal.
Use: Antitussive, antihistamine, decongestant.

DONATUSSIN DC SYRUP. (Laser) Hydrocodone bitartrate 2.5 mg., phenylephrine HCl 7.5 mg., guaifenesin 50 mg./5 ml. Bot. 4 oz., pt.
Use: Cough and nasal congestion.

DONDRIL. (Whitehall) Dextromethorphan HBr 10 mg., phenylephrine HCl 5 mg., chlorpheniramine maleate 1 mg./Cap. Bot. 24s.

DONNA. (Arcum) Menthol, thymol, eucalyptol, alum exsiccated, boric acid. 4 oz., 14 oz.
Use: Antiseptic douche.

DONNACIN. (Pharmex) Phenobarbital 16.20 mg., hyoscyamine sulfate 0.1037 mg., atropine sulfate 0.194 mg., hyoscine HBr 0.0065 mg./5 cc. or Tab. **Elixir:** Bot. pt., gal. **Tab.:** Bot. 1000s.
Use: Antispasmodic.

DONNAFED Jr. (Jenkins) Ephedrine HCl 1/16 gr., belladonna ext. 1/20 gr. (total alkaloids, 0.0006 gr.), salicylamide 1 1/4 gr./Tab. Bot. 1000s.
Use: Coryza, rhinitis, asthmatic conditions.

DONNAGEL. (Robins) Hyoscyamine sulfate 0.1037 mg., atropine sulfate 0.0194 mg., hyoscine HBr 0.0065 mg., sod. benzoate (preservative), 60 mg., kaolin 6 Gm., pectin 142.8 mg., 30 ml. alcohol 3.8%/oz. Susp., Bot. 4 oz., 1 pt.
Use: Antidiarrheal

DONNAGEL-PG. (Robins) Po. opium 24 mg., Kaolin 6 Gm., pectin 142.8 mg., hyoscyamine sulfate 0.1037 mg., atropine sulfate 0.0194 mg., hyoscine HBr 0.0065 mg., sodium benzoate 60 mg./30 cc. alcohol 5%. Bot. 6 oz., 1 pt.
Use: Control diarrhea.

DONNAMINE. (Tennessee) Hyoscyamine HBr 0.1280 mg., hyoscine HBr 0.0072 mg., atropine sulfate 0.0240 mg., phenobarbital 1/4 gr./Tab. Bot. 100s, 1000s.
Use: Antispasmodic.

DONNAMINE ELIXIR. (Tennessee) Alcohol 23%, phenobarbital 16 mg., hyoscyamine sulfate 0.1037 mg., atropine sulfate 0.0194 mg., hyoscine HBr 0.0065 mg./5 cc. Bot. pt.
Use: Antispasmodic.

DONNA-PHENAL ELIXIR. (Columbia) Atropine sulfate 0.0194 mg., hyoscyamine sulfate 0.1037 mg., hyoscine HBr 0.0065 mg., phenobarbital 16.2 mg. alcohol 23%. Bot. pt., gal.
Use: Antispasmodic and sedative.

DONNAPHEN ELIXIR. (Approved) Phenobarbital 16.2 mg., hyoscyamine sulfate 0.1037 mg., atropine sulfate 0.0194 mg., hyoscine HBr 0.0065 mg./5 cc. Bot. pt., gal.
Use: Antispasmodic and sedative.

DONNA-SED LIQUID. (Vortech) Phenobarbital 16.2 mg., hyoscyamine HBr 0.1037 mg., atropine sulfate

0.0194 mg., hyoscine HBr 0.0065 mg./5 cc. Bot. 4 oz., Gal.
Use: Sedative, antispasmodic.

DONNATAL. (Robins) Tab., Cap. or 5 cc. of Elixir contains hyoscyamine sulfate 0.1037 mg., atropine sulfate 0.0194 mg., hyoscine HBr 0.0065 mg., phenobarbital 16.2 mg.,**Cap. & Tab.:** Bot. 100s, 1000s. **Elixir:** w/alcohol 23%. Bot. 4 oz., 1 pt., 1 gal. Dis-Co packs 5 ml., 100s.
Use: Sedative & antispasmodic.

DONNATAL DIS-CO UNIT DOSE PACK. (Robins) Hyoscyamine sulfate 0.1037 mg., atropine sulfate 0.0194 mg., hyoscine HBr 0.0065 mg., phenobarbital 16.2 mg. (1/4 gr.)/Tab., 5 cc. **Tab.:** Unit dose pack 100s. **Elixir:** Unit dose pack (5 cc.) 25s.
Use: Antispasmodic and sedative.

DONNATAL EXTENTABS. (Robins) Hyoscyamine sulfate 0.3111 mg., atropine sulfate 0.0582 mg., hyoscine HBr 0.0195 mg., phenobarbital 48.6 mg. (3/4 gr.)/Tab. Bot. 100s, 500s. Dis-Co pack 100s.
Use: Long-acting antispasmodic & sedative.

DONNATAL #2. (Robins) Phenobarbital 32.4 mg. (0.5 gr.), hyoscyamine sulfate 0.1037 mg., atropine sulfate 0.0194 mg., hyoscine HBr 0.0065 mg./Tab. Bot. 100s, 1000s.
Use: Antispasmodic & sedative.

DONNAZYME. (Robins) Hyoscyamine sulf. 0.0518 mg., atropine sulf. 0.0097 mg., hyoscine HBr 0.0033 mg., phenobarbital 8.1 mg. (1/8 gr.), pepsin 150 mg./Tab. in outer layer, and pancreatin 300 mg., bile salts 150 mg./Tab. in core. Bot. 100s, 500s.
Use: Functional G.I. disorders.

DONPHEN. (Lemmon) Phenobarbital 15 mg., hyoscyamine sulfate 0.1 mg., atropine sulfate 0.02 mg., scopolamine HBr 6 mcg./Tab. Bot. 100s, 1000s.
Use: Antispasmotic.

DON'T. (Commerce) Sucrose octa acetate isopropyl alcohol. Bot. 0.45 oz.
Use: Discourage nail biting and thumb sucking.

DOPAMANTINE. USAN.
Use: Antiparkinsonian

DOPAMINE. (Astra) Dopamine. **Amp.:** 200 mg./5 ml. Amp. Box 10s; 400 mg./10 ml. Amp. Box 5s. **Additive Syringe:** 200 mg./5 ml. Syr. Box 1s; 400 mg./10 ml Syr. Box 1s.
Use: Shock treatment.

• **DOPAMINE HYDROCHLORIDE,** U.S.P. XXI. Inj., U.S.P. XXI. 4-(2-Aminoethyl)pyrocatechol HCl.
Use: Adrenergic.
   Intropin, Amp. (American Critical Care)

• **DOPAMINE HYDROCHLORIDE AND DEXTROSE INJECTION,** U.S.P. XXI.
Use: Adrenergic, emergency treatment of low blood pressure.

DOPAMINE HCL. (Abbott) Dopamine 40 mg./ml. or 80 mg./ml. Amp. 5 ml., 10 ml.
Use: Emergency treatment of low blood pressure.

DOPAR. (Norwich Eaton) Levodopa 100 mg., 250

mg./Cap. Bot. 100s. 500 mg./Cap. Bot. 100s, 1000s.
Use: For treatment of Parkinson's disease.
DOPASTAT. (Parke-Davis) Dopamine HCl 40 mg./ml. Vial 5 ml.
Use: Adrenergic.
DOPHENCO. (Blue Line) Opium pow. 1/20 gr., ipecac pow. 1/20 gr., acetophenetidin 1½ gr., atropine sulf. 1/500 gr., acetylsalicylic acid 3 gr., camphor monobromated ½ gr., caffeine ⅛ gr./Cap. Bot. 100s, 1000s.
Use: Analgesic antipyretic.
DOPRAM. (Robins) Doxapram HCl 20 mg./ml. w/chlorobutanol (preservative) 0.5%. Vial 20 ml.
Use: Respiratory stimulant.
DORAPHEN COMPOUND 65. (Cenci) Propoxyphene HCl 65 mg., aspirin 227 mg., phenacetin 162 mg., caffeine 32.4 mg./Cap. Bot. 100s, 500s, 1000s.
Use: Analgesic.
DORAPHEN HCL. (Cenci) Propoxyphrene HCl 65 mg./Cap. Bot. 100s, 1000s.
Use: Analgesic.
DORBANE. (3M Products) Danthron. 75 mg./Tab. Bot. 100s, 500s, 1000s.
Use: Constipation.
DORBANTYL. (3M Products) Docusate sodium 50 mg., danthron 25 mg./Cap. Bot. 30s, 100s, 250s.
Use: Fecal softener and laxative.
DORBANTYL FORTE. (3M Products) Docusate sodium 100 mg., Danthron 50 mg./Cap. Bot. 30s, 100s, 250s.
Use: Fecal softener and laxative.
DORCOL CHILDREN'S COUGH SYRUP. (Dorsey) Dextromethorphan HBr 5 mg., pseudoephedrine HCL 15 mg., guaifenesin 50 mg./5 ml. w/alcohol 5%. Bot. 4 oz., 8 oz.
Use: Cough prep.
DORICO DROPS (Winthrop Products) Paracetamol.
Use: Analgesic, antipyretic.
DORICO TABLETS. (Winthrop Products) Paracetamol.
Use: Analgesic, antipyretic.
DORIDEN. (USV Labs.) Glutethimide. 250 mg./Tab. Bot. 100s; 500 mg./Tab. Bot. 100s, 500s, 1000s. Strip Pkg. 100s.
Use: Nonbarbiturate hypnotic.
DORIMIDE. (Cenci) Gluthethimide 0.5 gm./Tab. Bot. 100s, 1000s.
Use: Sedative, hypnotic.
DORME. (A.V.P.) Promethazine HCl 12.5 mg., 25 mg., 50 mg./Cap. Bot. 100s.
Use: Antihistaminic.
DORMEER. (Pasadena Research) Scopolamine aminoxide HBr 0.2 mg./Cap. Bot. 100s, 1000s.
DORMETHAN.
See: Dextromethorphan HBr. (Var. Mfr.)
DORMIN SLEEPING CAPSULES. (Randob) **25 mg.** /Cap. #4 pink Cap. Bot. 12s, 36s, 72/Bot. **50 mg.** /Cap. 14 caps./carton.
Use: Assist in restful sleep.
DORMIRAL.
See: Phenobarbital, Prep. (Various Mfr.)

DORMONAL.
See: Barbital, Prep. (Various Mfr.)
DORMUTOL. (Approved) Scopolamine aminoxide HBr 0.2 mg./Cap. Bot. 24s, 60s.
Use: OTC sedative
• **DORSATINE HYDROCHLORIDE.** USAN.
Use: Antihistaminic.
DOSS SYRUP. (Bay) Docusate sodium 20 mg./5 ml. Bot. pt., gal.
Use: Stool softener.
DOSS W/CASANTHRANOL. (Bay) Casanthranol 30 mg., docusate sodium 60 mg./15 ml. w/alcohol 10%, cc. Bot. pt., gal.
Use: Stool softener, laxative.
• **DOTHIEPIN HCL.** USAN. 11-(3-Dimethylamino-propylidene)-6H-dibenzo[b,e]thiepin hydrochloride. Dosulepin (I.N.N.)
Use: Antidepressant.
See: Prothiaden (hydrochloride)
DOTIROL. (Winthrop Products) Ampicillin trihydrate available in Cap, Suspension, Inj. (IV, IM.).
Use: Antibiotic.
DOUBLE-A. (Edwards) Acetaminophen 325 mg., aspirin 325 mg./Tab. Bot. 100s.
Use: Arthritic conditions.
DOUBLE DANDERINE. (Medtech) Benzalkonium chloride 10%. Bot. 10 oz.
Use: Treatment of dandruff.
DOUCHE. (Jenkins) Acid boric, borax, acid tannic, sodium salicylate, zinc sulfate, pow. alum, hydrastine HCl, thymol, w/sod. bicarbonate and acid tartaric/Tab. Bot. 1000s.
DOVAPHEN CAP. (Jenkins) Dover's powder 16.2 mg. (opium 1.62 mg.), ipecac 1.62 mg., aspirin 2½ gr., phenacetin 1½ gr., caffeine ⅛ gr., camphor ¼ gr., atropine sulfate 1/1000 gr./Cap. Bot. 1000s.
DOVAPHEN JR. (Jenkins) Dover's pow. 8.1 mg., acetophenetidin ½ gr., atropine sulfate 1/4000 gr., salicylamide ½ gr., caffeine 1/10 gr./Tab. Bot. 1000s.
Use: Analgesic.
DOVER'S POWDER. Ipecac 1 part, opium 1 part, lactose 8 parts.
Use: Analgesic sedative & diaphoretic.
W/Acetophenetidin, atropine sulfate, aspirin, camphor, caffeine, sod. sulfate dried.
See: Dovium, Cap. (Hance)
W/Acetophenetidin, atropine sulfate, salicylamide, caffeine.
See: Dovaphen Jr., Tab. (Jenkins)
W/Acetophenetidin, camphor, aspirin, caffeine, atropine sulfate.
See: Analgestine, Cap. (Mallard)
W/Acetophenetidin, sodium citrate, potassium guaiacolsulfonate.
See: Doverlyn, Cap., Tab. (Davis & Sly)
W/A.P.C., & camphor monobromated.
See: Coldate, Tab. (Elder)
W/Aspirin, acetophenetidin, camphor monobromated, caffeine, atropine sulfate.
See: Asco, Cap., Tab. (Sutliff & Case)
W/Aspirin, phenacetin, camphor monobromated, caffeine.

See: Coldate, Tab. (Elder)
Doveram, Prep. (Vortech)
W/Atropine sulf., A.P.C., camphor.
See: Dasin, Cap. (Beecham-Massengill)
W/Phenacetin, aspirin, camphor, caffeine alkaloid,
atropine sulfate.
See: Analgestine Forte, Cap. (Mallard)
Dovernon, Cap. (Reid-Provident)
Phenacaps, Cap. (Scrip)
W/Pheneacetin, camphor, caffeine.
See: Doverlyn Adult, Tab. (Scrip)
W/Pyrilamine maleate, racephedrine HCl,
salicylamide, phenacetin.
See: Asphamal-D, Tab. (Central)
W/Sodium salicylate, potassium iodide, camphor,
gelsemium tincture.
See: Ricor, Tab. (Vortech)
DOVIUM. (Hance) Dover pow. ½ gr., acetophenetidin
1½ gr., atropine sulfate 1/500 gr., aspirin 2 gr.,
camphor ¼ gr., caffeine ⅛ gr., sod. sulfate dried
7½ gr./Cap. Bot. 100s, 1000s.
Use: Analgesic & antipyretic.
DOWICIL 200.
See: Derma Soap (Ferndale)
DOW-ISONIAZID. (Merrell Dow) Isoniazid 300 mg./Tab.
Bot. 30s.
Use: Tuberculosis treatment.
DOXAMIN. (Fellows) Thiamine HCl 100 mg., Vit.
B-6 100 mg./cc. Vial 10 cc.
• DOXAPRAM HYDROCHLORIDE, U.S.P. XXI. Inj.,
U.S.P. XXI. 1-Ethyl-4-(2-morpholinoethyl)-3,3-
diphenyl-2-pyrrolidinone HCl.
Use: Respiratory & CNS stimulant.
See: Dopram, Vial (Robins)
• DOXAPROST. USAN.
Use: Bronchodilator.
• DOXAPROST. USAN.
Use: Bronchodilator.
DOXATE. Docusate sodium.
Use: Stool softener.
• DOXAZOSIN MESYLATE. USAN.
Use: Antihypertensive.
DOXEPIN. B.A.N. 11-(3-Dimethylaminopropylidene)-
6H-ibenz[b,e]oxepin.
Use: Antidepressant.
See: Sinequan [hydrochloride]
• DOXEPIN HYDROCHLORIDE, U.S.P. XXI. Caps.,
Oral Soln., U.S.P. XXI. N,N-Dimethyldibenz[b,e] oxe-
pin-Δ¹¹(⁶ᴴ), y-propylamine hydrochloride.
Use: Psychotherapeutic drug.
See: Adapin, Cap. (Pennwalt)
Sinequan, Cap. (Roerig)
DOXIDAN. (Hoechst) Danthron 50 mg., docusate
sodium 60 mg./Cap. Bot. 30s, 100s, 1000s. Unit
dose 100s. Display Packs 10s.
Use: Laxative.
DOXINATE. (Hoechst) Docusate sodium. Cap.: 60
mg. or 240 mg./Cap. Bot. 100s. Soln.: 5% pediatric
solution. Bot. 60 ml., gal.
Use: Orally, a wetting agent that keeps the stool soft.
DOXOLENE NAPSYLATE. Dextropropoxyphene,
B.A.N.

• DOXORUBICIN. USAN.
Use: Antineoplastic.
DOXORUBICIN HYDROCHLORIDE, U.S.P. XXI. Inj.,
U.S.P. XXI. 14-Hydroxydaunorubicin. An antibiotic
produced by Streptomyces peuceticus var. caesius.
See: Adriamycin (Adria)
• DOXPICOMINE HYDROCHLORIDE. USAN.
Use: Analgesic.
DOXYBETASOL. B.A.N. 9α-Fluoro-11β, 17α-dihydroxy-
16β-methylpregna-1,4-diene-3,20-dione.
Use: Corticosteroid.
DOXY-C. (Century) Doxycycline hyclate 100 mg./Cap.
Bot. 50s.
Use: Antibiotic.
DOXY-CAPS. (Edwards) Doxycycline hyclate 100
mg./Cap. Bot. 50s.
Use: Broad spectrum antibiotic.
DOXYCHEL CAPSULES. (Rachelle) Doxycycline
hyclate 50 mg. or 100 mg./Cap. Bot. 50s, 500s.
Unit dose 100s.
Use: Antibiotic.
• DOXYCYCLINE. U.S.P. XXI. For Oral Susp. U.S.P.
XXI. 4-(Dimethylamino)-1,4,4a,5,5a,6,11,12a-octahy-
dro-3,5,10,12,12a-pentahydroxy-6-methyl-1,11-dioxo
-2-naphthacenecarboxamide.
Use: Antibiotic.
See: Vibramycin for Oral Suspension (Pfizer
Laboratories)
• DOXYCYCLINE CALCIUM ORAL SUSPENSION,
U.S.P. XXI.
• DOXYCYCLINE HYCLATE, U.S.P. XXI. Caps., Inj.,
Sterile, Tab., U.S.P. XXI. 2-Naphthacenecarboxa-
mide, 4-(dimethyl-amino)-1,4,4a,5,5a,6,11,12a-oc-
tahydro-3,5,10,12-12a-pentahydroxy-6-methyl-1,11-
dioxo-, HCl compound with ethanol monohydrate.
Use: Antibacterial.
See: Doxy-Caps, Cap. (Edwards)
Vibra-Tabs, Tab. (Pfizer Laboratories)
Vibramycin, Cap., Tab., Vial (Pfizer Laboratories)
• DOXYLAMINE SUCCINATE, U.S.P. XXI. Syr., Tab.,
U.S.P. XXI. 2-[α(2-Dimethylamino-ethoxy)-α-methyl-
benzyl]pyridine bisuccinate.
Use: Antihistamine.
See: Decapryn, Prep. (Merrell Dow)
Unisom, Tab. (Leeming Pacquin)
W/Acetominophen, ephedrine sulfate,
dextromethorphan HBr, alcohol.
See: Nyquil, Liq. (Vick)
W/Dextromethorphan HBr, alcohol.
See: Consotuss Antitussive, Syr. (Merrell Dow)
W/Dextromethorphan HBr, sodium citrate, alcohol.
See: Vicks Formula 44 Cough Mixture, Syr. (Vicks)
W/Mercodol.
See: Mercodol w/Decapryn, Syr. (Merrell Dow)
W/Pyridoxine HCl,
See: Bendectin, Tab. (Merrell Dow)
DOXY-LEMMON CAPSULES. (Lemmon) Doxycycline
hyclate equiv. to 100 mg./Cap. of doxycycline
base. Bot. 50s, 500s. Unit dose 100s.
Use: Anti-Infective.
DOXY-LEMMON TABLETS. (Lemmon) Doxycycline hy-

clate equiv. to 100 mg./Tab. of doxycycline base.
Bot. 50s.
Use: Anti-infective.

DOXY-TABS. (Rachelle) Doxycycline hyclate 100 mg./Film Coated Tab. Bot. 50s, 500s.
Use: Antibiotic.

DOXY-TABS-50. (Rachelle) 50 mg./Tab. Bot. 50s.
Use: Antibiotic

DRAMABAN. (Mallard) Dimenhydrinate 50 mg./Tab. Bot. 1000s.
Use: Prevention and treatment of nausea & vomiting.

DRAMAJECT. (Mayrand) Dimenhydrinate 50 mg./ml. Vial 10 ml.

DRAMAL. (Galen) Phenyltoloxamine dihydrogen citrate 50 mg./Tab. Bot. 100s, 1000s.
Use: Antihistamine.

DRAMAMINE. (Searle) Dimenhydrinate.**Liq.** 12.5 mg./4cc. Bot. 3 oz., 1 pt. **Tab.:** 50 mg. Bot. 36s, 100s, 1000s. Unit Dose 100s. Ciba Strip 12s, 4 × 12.
Use: Motion sickness.

DRAMAMINE INJECTION. (Searle) Dimenhydrinate. **Amp.** 50 mg., 1cc., Carton 5s, 25s, 100s. **Vial:** 250 mg./5cc. Carton 5s, 25s, 100s.
Use: Antinauseant.

DRAMARIN.
See: Dramamine, Prep. (Searle)

DRAMILIN. (Kay) Dimenhydrinate 50 mg./ml. Vial 10 ml.
Use: Antihistamine.

DRAMOCEN. Central Dimenhydrinate 50 mg./ml. Vial 10 ml. Box 12s.
Use: Anti-emetic, antihistaminic.

DRAMYL.
See: Dramamine, Prep. (Searle)

DRANOCHOL. (Marin) Dehydrocholic acid 200 mg., homatropine methylbromide 5 mg./Tab. Bot. 60s, 500s, 1000s.
Use: Hydrocholeretic, antispasmodic.

DRAPOLENE. Benzalkonium Chloride, B.A.N.

DRAWING SALVE. (Eckerd) Resorcinol, salicilic acid, zinc oxide, kaolin, phenol 0.25%. Tube 1½ oz.
Use: Drawing poultice.

DRAWING SALVE. (Towne) Tube 1 oz.

DRAWING SALVE with TRIQUINODIN. (Towne) Tube 2 oz.

DR. CALDWELL SENNA LAXATIVE. (Glenbrook) Senna 7.0%, Alcohol 4.5%. bot. 5 oz., 12 oz.
Use: Laxative.

DRC PERI-ANAL CREAM. (Xttrium) Lassar's paste 37.5%, anhydrous lanolin USP 37.5%, cold cream 25%. Tube 5 oz.
Use: Diaper rash.

DR. DRAKE'S COUGH MEDICINE. (Last) Dextromethorphan HBr 10 mg./5 ml. Bot. 2 oz.
Use: Antitussive cough remedy.

DREST. (Dermik) Polyvinylpyrrolidone, benzalkonium chloride 0.125%, alkylisoquinolinium bromides 0.15%, in gel base. Tubes 3.5 oz.
Use: Antiseptic hair dressing.

• **DRIBENDAZOLE,** USAN.

DRICOL MESYLATE. Amidephrine, B.A.N.

DRI-DRIP. (Coastal) Chlorpheniramine maleate 8 mg., phenylpropanolamine HC1 50 mg., atropine sulfate ¹⁄₈₀ gr./Cap. Bot. 100s, 500s.
Use: Treatment of cold symptoms.

DRI-DRIP LIQUID. (Coastal) Phenylephrine HC1 5 mg., phenylpropanolamine 8 mg., chlorpheniramine maleate 2 mg., alcohol 3%/5 cc. Bot. 4 oz., 16 oz.
Use: Treatment of cold symptoms.

DRI-A CAPS. (Barth's) Vit. A 10,000 I.U./Cap. Bot. 100s, 500s.

DRI A&D CAPS. (Barth's) Vit. A 10,000 I.U., D 400 I.U./Cap. Bot. 100s, 500s.

DRI-E. (Barth's) Vit. E 100 I.U./Cap. Bot. 100s, 500s, 1000s. 200 I.U./Cap. Bot. 100s, 250s, 500s. 400 I.U./Cap. Bot. 100s, 250s.

• **DRIED ALUMINUM HYDROXIDE GEL,** U.S.P. XXI.
See: Aluminum Hydroxide Gel, Dried

DRIED YEAST.
See: Yeast, dried

DRI-HIST META-KAPS. (Sutliff & Case) Chlorpheniramine maleate 8 mg., phenylpropanolamine 50 mg., atropine sulfate 0.36 mg./S.A. Cap. Bot. 100s, 1000s.
Use: Antihistaminic and sympathomimetic.

DRI-HIST NO. 2 META-KAPS. (Sutliff & Case) Pyrilamine maleate 25 mg., pheniramine maleate 10 mg., phenylpropanolamine HCl 25 mg., phenylephrine HCl 10 mg./Cap. Bot. 100s, 1000s.

DRINOPHEN CAPSULES. (Lannett) Phenyl-propanolamine HCl 15 mg., acetylsalicylic acid 230 mg., acetaminophen 200 mg., caffeine 15 mg./Cap. Bot. 1000s.
Use: Analgesic.

DRINUS GRADUALS. (Amfre-Grant) Chlorpheniramine maleate 8 mg., phenylephrine HCl 20 mg., methscopolamine nitrate 2.5 mg./Cap. Bot. 30s, 250s, 1000s.
Use: Antihistamine & decongestant.

DRINUS-M GRADUALS. (Amfre-Grant) Chlorpheniramine maleate 8 mg., phenylephrine HCl 20 mg./Cap. Bot. 50s, 250s, 1000s.
Use: Antihistamine, decongestant.

DRINUS SYRUP. (Amfre-Grant) Chlorpheniramine maleate 2 mg., phenylpropanolamine 12.5 mg./5 cc. Bot. 4 oz. pt., gal.
Use: Antihistamine, decongestant.

DRISDOL. (Winthrop-Breon) Ergocalciferol (Vitamin D) 200 I.U./drop in propylene glycol solvent. Bot. 60 ml.
Use: Prevention of Vitamin D deficiency.

DRISDOL 50,000 UNIT CAPSULES. (Winthrop-Breon) Vit. D-2, 50,000 I.U./Cap. Bot. 50s.
Use: Treatment of refractory rickets, hypoparathyroidism, familial hypophosphatemia.

DRISTAN 12 HOUR. (Whitehall) Chlorpheniramine maleate 4 mg., phenylephrine HCl 20 mg./Cap. Bot. 6s, 10s, 15s.
Use: Decongestant, analgesic.

DRISTAN-AF. (Whitehall) Phenylephrine HCl 5 mg., chlorpheniramine maleate 2 mg., acetaminophen

325 mg., caffeine 16.2 mg./Tab. Tins 12s, Bot. 24s, 50s, 100s.
Use: Antihistamine, nasal decongestant, analgesic.

DRISTAN CAPSULES. (Whitehall)
Phenylpropanolamine HCl 12.5 mg.,
chlorpheniramine maleate 2 mg., acetaminophen
325 mg./Cap. Bot. 16s, 36s, 75s.
Use: Decongestant, analgesic.

DRISTAN COUGH FORMULA. (Whitehall)
Dextromethorphan HBr 7.5 mg., phenylephrine HCl
5 mg., chlorpheniramine maleate 1 mg.,
guaifenesin, 30 mg./5ml. w/alcohol 12%. Bot. 3 oz.
Use: Antitussive.

DRISTAN LONG LASTING NASAL MIST. (Whitehall)
Oxymetazoline HCl 0.05%. Bot. ½ oz., 1 oz.
Use: Nasal decongestant.

DRISTAN MENTHOL NASAL MIST. (Whitehall)
Phenylephrine HCl 0.5%, pheniramine maleate
0.2% Bot. ½ oz., 1 oz.
Use: Nasal decongestant.

DRISTAN NASAL MIST. (Whitehall) Phenylephrine
HCl 0.5%, pheniramine maleate 0.2%/ml. Bot. ½
oz., 1 oz.
Use: Nasal decongestant

DRISTAN TABLETS. (Whitehall) Phenylephrine HCl 5
mg., chlorpheniramine maleate 2 mg.,
acetaminophen 325 mg./Tab. Bot. 24s, 50s, 100s.
Use: Antihistamine, oral nasal decongestant,
analgesic.

DRISTAN ULTRA COLD FORMULA. (Whitehall)
Acetaminophen 500 mg., pseudoephedrine HCl 30
mg., chlorpheniramine maleate 2 mg.,
dextromethorphan 15 mg./Tab. or Cap. Tab. Bot.
20s, 48's; Cap. Pkg. 16s, 36s; Liq. Bot. 6 oz.
Use: Relief of cold symptoms.

DRITHOCREME. (American Dermal) Anthralin 0.1%,
0.25% or 0.5%. Tube 50 gm.
Use: Psoriasis treatment.

DRITHOCREME HP 1.0%. (American Dermal)
Anthralin 1.0%. Tube 50 Gm.
Use: Psoriasis treatment.

DRIXORAL. (Schering) Dexbrompheniramine maleate
6 mg., pseudoephedrine sulfate 120 mg./S.A. Tab.
Box 10s, 20s, 40s. Bot. 100s.
Use: Nasal decongestant, antihistamine.

DRIZE. (Ascher) Phenylpropanolamine HCl 75 mg.,
chlorpheniramine maleate 12 mg./S.R. Cap. Bot.
100s.
Use: Allergic rhinitis, common cold.

• **DROBULINE.** USAN.
Use: Cardiac depressant.

DROCARBIL. Acetarsone salt of arecoline. Arecoline
n-acetyl-4-hydroxy-m-arsanilate.
Use: Anthelmintic in animals.

• **DROCINONIDE.** USAN.
Use: Anti-inflammatory.

DROCODE.
See: Dihydrocodeine.

DROLBAN INJECTION. (Lilly) Dromostanolone
propionate 50 mg./ml. in sesame oil q.s., phenol
0.5%. Vial 10 ml. Ctn. 10s.
Use: Metastatic carcinoma of the breast.

DROMORAN, LEVO. Levorphanol, Levorphan.
See: Levo-Dromoran, Vial, Amp., Tab. (Roche)

DROMOSTANOLONE PROPIONATE. 2α-Methyland-
rostan-17-(β)-0l-3-one propionate. 17 β-Hydroxy-2α-
methyl-5α-androstan-3-one propionate.
Use: Antineoplastic.
See: Drolban, Inj. (Lilly)

DROP CHALK. (Various Mfr.) Cal. carb., prepared.

• **DROPERIDOL,** U.S.P. XXI. Inj., U.S.P. XXI. 1-{1-[3-
(p-Fluorobenzoyl)propyl-1,2,3,6-tetrahydro-4-pyridyl]
}-2-benzimidazolinone.
Use: Tranquilizer.
See: Inapsine, Inj. (Janssen)

W/Fentanyl citrate.
Use: Tranquilizer.
See: Innovar, Inj. (Janssen)

• **DROPRENILAMINE.** USAN.
Use: Vasodilator

DROPROPIZINE. B.A.N. 1-(2,3-Dihydroxypropyl)-4-phe-
nylpiperazine.
Use: Antitussive.
See: Katril
    Catabex
    Tussilex

DROSTANOLONE. B.A.N. 17β-Hydroxy-2α-methyl-5α-
androstan-3-one.
Use: Anabolic steroid.
See: Dromostanolone
    Methalone
    Masteril (propionate)

DROTEBANOL. B.A.N. 3,4-Dimethoxy-17-methyl-mor-
phinan-6β, 14-diol.
Use: Analgesic; antitussive.

DROTIC. (Ascher) Hydrocortisone 1%, acetic acid
2%, citric acid 0.2%, in propylene glycol vehicle
containing propylene glycol diacetate 3%,
benzethonium Cl 0.02%, sodium acetate 0.015%.
Dropper Bot. 10 ml.
Use: Otitis externa.

• **DROXACIN SODIUM.** USAN.
Use: Antibacterial.

DROXARYL. Bufexamac, B.A.N.

• **DROXIFILCON A.** USAN.
Use: Contact lens material.

DROXINE L.A. (Shear-Kershman) Dyphylline 400
mg./Tab. (long acting). Bot. 100s.
Use: Smooth muscle relaxant.

DROXOVITE. (Kay) Hydroxocobalamin, 1000
mcg./cc. Vehicle; Sodium chloride 0.82%, sodium
acetate 0.10%, methylparaben 0.15%,
propylparaben 0.02%, acetic acid/cc. Vial 10
cc.
Use: Pernicious anemia, megaloblastic anemia.

DROXYPROPINE. B.A.N. 1-[2-(2-Hydroxyethoxy)-
ethyl]-4-phenyl-4-propionylpiperidine.
Use: Cough suppressant.

DR. PIERCE'S GOLDEN MEDICAL DISCOVERY.
(Medtech) Gentian root, oregan root, blood root.
Tab. Bot. 100s. Liq. Bot. 8 oz.
Use: Aids digestion.

DR. SCHOLL'S ATHLETE'S FOOT GEL. (Scholl)
Tolnaftate 1%. Tube 0.5 oz.

Use: Anti-fungal.

DR. SCHOLL'S ATHLETE'S FOOT POWDER.
(Scholl) Tolnaftate 1%. Shaker: Plastic bottle 2.5oz.
Spray: Aerosal can 3.5 oz.
Use: Anti-fungal.

DR. SCHOLL'S ATHLETE'S FOOT SPRAY. (Scholl)
Tolnafatate 1%. Aerosol Can 3.5 oz.
Use: Anti-fungal.

DR. SCHOLL'S CALLOUS SALVE. (Scholl) Salicylic
acid 15%. Tube 0.4 oz.
Use: Callous remover.

DR. SCHOLL'S CORN SALVE. (Scholl) Salicylic acid
15.0%. Jar 0.4 oz.
Use: Corn remover.

**DR. SCHOLL'S "2" DROP CORN/CALLOUS
REMOVER.** (Scholl) Salicylic acid 12.6%. Bot.0.33
oz.
Use: Corn and callous remover.

DR. SCHOLL'S ONIXOL. (Scholl) Sodium sulfide 1%.
Bot. 0.33 oz.
Use: Treatment of in-grown toenail

**DR. SCHOLL'S PRO COMFORT ATHLETE'S FOOT
SPRAY.** (Scholl) Tolnaftate 1%. Aerosol Can 4 oz.
Use: Anti-fungal.

**DR. SCHOLL'S PRO COMFORT JOCK ITCH
SPRAY.**(Scholl)Tolnaftate1%.Aerosolcan3.5oz.
Use: Anti-fungal.

DR. SCHOLL'S WART REMOVER KIT. (Scholl)
Salicylic acid 17%. Bot. 3.25 oz.
Use: Wart Removal.

**DR. SCHOLL'S ZINO PADS/WITH MEDICATED
DISKS.** (Scholl) Salicylic acid 40% or 20%.
Protective pads designed for use with & without
salicylic acid-impregnated disks.
Use: For removal of soft and hard corns, callouses.

DRUCON. (Standard Drug) Phenylephrine HCl 5 mg.,
chlorpheniramine maleate 2 mg., menthol 1 mg.,
alcohol 5%/5 ml. Elixir Bot. pt., gal.
Use: Relief of respiratory congestion in infants and
children.

DRUCON C R. (Standard Drug) Phenylephrine HCl 25
mg., chlorpheniramine maleate 4 mg./Tab. Bot.
100s.
Use: Relief of nasal congestion of colds or allergy.

DRUCON WITH CODEINE. (Standard Drug) Codeine
phosphate 10 mg., phenylephrine HCl 10 mg.,
chlorpheniramine maleate 2 mg., menthol 1 mg.,
alcohol 5%/5 ml. Bot. pt.
Use: Relief of respiratory congestion.

DRY & CLEAR ACNE MEDICATION. (Whitehall)
Benzoyl peroxide 5%. Bot. 1 oz., 2 oz.
Use: Acne medication.

DRY & CLEAR CLEANSER. (Whitehall) Alcohol 50%,
salicylic acid 0.5%, benzoic acid 0.5%,
benzethonium Cl. 0.1%. Bot. 4 oz., 8 oz.
Use: Acne medication.

DRY & CLEAR DOUBLE STRENGTH CREAM.
(Whitehall) Benzoyl peroxide 10%. Tube 1 oz.
Use: Acne medication.

DRY SKIN CREME. (Gordon) Cetyl alcohol,
lubricating oils in a water soluble base. Jar 2 oz., 1
lb., 5 lb.

Use: Dry skin, moisturizer, vehicle.

DRYSOL. (Person & Covey) Aluminum C1 20% in
anhydrous ethyl alcohol. Bot. 37.5 cc. Dab-O-Matic
Rx in 35 ml. plastic bottle w/applicator head.
Use: Hyperhidrosis.

DRYSUM. (Summers) Two soapless, lathering
detergents, alcohol, acetone, perfume. Plastic Bot.
4 oz.
Use: Shampoo.

DRYTERGENT. (C & M Pharmacal) TEA-dodecylben-
zenesulfonate, boric acid, lauramide DEA,
propylene glycol, purified water, color, fragrance.
Bot. 8 oz., 16 oz., 1 Gal.
Use: Cleanser for acne therapy.

DRYTEX. (C & M Pharmacal) Salicylic acid 2%,
methylbenzethonium chloride 0.1% non-ionic wetting
agent, acetone, isopropyl alcohol 40%, purified
water, color and perfume. Lot. Bot. 8 fl. oz., pt., gal.
Use: Cleanser for acne and seborrhea.

d-SEB. (CooperCare) Blend of 2 synthetic detergents,
parachlorometaxylenol 2%, isopropanol 7.6%. Tube
60 Gm.
Use: For cleansing of excessive skin oil or as an
aid in the control of acne and pimples.

D-SINUS. (Laser) Phenylpropanolamine HC1 18 mg.,
acetaminophen 325 mg./Cap. Bot. 24s, 100s, 1000s.
Use: Decongestant, analgesic.

D-S-S CAPSULES. (Parke-Davis) Docusate sodium 100
mg./Cap. Bot. 100s, 1000s. Unit dose 100s.

D-S-S COMPOUND. (Wolins) Docusate sodium 100
mg., guar gum 200 mg., prune concentrate 50
mg./Cap. Bot. 100s.

D-S-S W/CASANTHRANOL. (Wolins) Docusate sodium 100 mg., casanthranol 30 mg./Cap. Bot.
100s, 1000s.

D-S-S PLUS CAPSULES. (Parke-Davis) Docusate sodium 100 mg., casanthranol 30 mg./Cap. Bot.
100s, 1000s. Unit dose 100s.

DST. Dihydrostreptomycin.
See: Dihydrostreptomycin, Prep. (Various Mfr.)

D-TEST 200. (Burgin-Arden) Testosterone cypionate
200 mg./cc. 10 cc. vial.

D-TEST 100. (Burgin-Arden) Testosterone cypionate
100 mg./cc. 10 cc. vial.

DTIC-DOME. (Miles Pharm) Dacarbazine 100 mg., 200
mg./Vial. Vial 10 ml., 20 ml.
Use: Metastatic malignant melanoma.

DUADACIN. (Hoechst) Phenylpropanolamine HCl 12.5
mg., chlorpheniramine maleate 2.0 mg.,
acetaminophen 325.0 mg./Cap. Bot. 100s, 1000s.
Carton 5000s. 8 paks 1000s.
Use: Cold syndrome.

DUALEX-E ELIXIR. (Scruggs) Bot. pt., gal.

DUAL FORMULA FEEN-A-MINT PILLS. (Plough) Yellow phenolphthalein 65 mg., docusate sodium 100
mg./Tab. Box. 15, 30, 60.
Use: Stool softener, laxative.

DUAL-PRED. (Tunex) Prednisolone acetate 80 mg.,
prednisolone sodium phosphate 20 mg., sodium Cl.
6.5 mg., pectin 2 mg./ml. w/sodium acetate 0.8%,
benzalkonium Cl. 0.01%.
Use: Anti inflammatory agent.

DUAL-WET. (Alcon) Polyvinyl alcohol & duasorb water soluble polymetric system, benzalkonium chloride 0.01%, disodium edetate 0.05%. Bot. 2 oz.
Use: Wetting sol. for hard contact lens.

• DUAZOMYCIN. USAN. Antibiotic isolated from broth filtrates of *Streptomyces ambofaciens.*
Use: Anti-neoplastic agent.

DUAZOMYCIN A. Name used for Duazomycin.

DUAZOMYCIN B. Name used for Azotomycin.

DUAZOMYCIN C. Name used for Ambomycin.

DUBILE. (Kenyon) Ox bile ext. 1.5 gr., mixed oxidized bile acids 1.5 gr., homatropine MeBr ¹⁄₁₂₀ gr./Tab. Bot. 100s, 1000s.

DULCETS. (Wolins) Cetylpyridium chloride 2.5 mg., benzocaine 10 mg./oz. Bot. 10s.

DULCOLAX. (Boehringer Ingelheim) Bisacodyl. **Tab.** E.C. 5 mg. Box 4s, 24s. Bot. 100s, 1000s. Unit dose 100s. **Supp.** 10 mg. Box 2s, 4s, 8s, 50s, 500s. **Bowel Prep Kit.** 4 tablets and 1 suppository/Kit. 5 Kits/box
Use: Laxative.

DU-MIN 4. (Scrip) Chlorpheniramine maleate 4 mg., caffeine 15 mg./Tab. Bot. 100s.

DUO. (Norcliff Thayer) Surgical adhesive. Tube ½ oz.

DUOBARBITAL.(Wolins)Amobarbitalsodiumsecobarbital sodium 1.5 gr. or 3 gr. Cap. Bot. 1000s.
Use: Sedative-hypnotic.

DUO-C.V.P. CAPSULES. (Armour) Bioflavonoids 200 mg./Cap. Bot. 100s, 500s.
Use: Vitamin supplement.

DUO-CYP. (Keene) Testosterone cypionate 50 mg., estradiol cypionate, 2 mg./ml. Vial 10 ml.

DUODENAL SUBSTANCE.
W/Ox bile extract, pancreatin, papain.
See: Digenzyme, Tab. (Burgin-Arden)

DUODENUM WHOLE, DESICCATED & DEFATTED.
See: Viodenum, Tab., Pow. (VioBin)
W/Ferrous gluconate, Vit. B-12, cobalt chloride.
See: Bitrinsic-E, Cap. (Elder)

DUOFILM. (Stiefel) Salicylic acid 16.7%, lactic acid 16.7% in flexible collodion. Bot. 0.5 oz.
Use: Warts, keratolytic agent.

DUO-FLOW. (CooperVision) Bot. 4 oz.
Use: Cleaning and soaking solution for hard contact lenses.

DUOGASTRONE DISODIUM SALT. Carbenoxolone, B.A.N.

DUO-IONATE. (Tunex) Testosterone cypionate 50 mg., estradiol cypionate 2 mg./ml. w/chlorobutanol 0.5% in cottonseed oil. Vial 10cc.
Use: Androgen-estrogen therapy.

DUOJECT. (Mallard) Cyanocobalamin 1000 mcg., thiamine HCl 100 mg./cc.

DUOLUBE. (Muro) Petrolatum, sterile. Tube 3.5 Gm.
Use: Corneal Lubricant.

DUO-MEDIHALER. (Riker) Isoproterenol HCl 4.0 mg., phenylephrine bitartrate 6.0 mg./ml. in an inert propellant. Oral adapter w/15 ml. Vial; Oral adapter w/22.5 ml Vial. Refill vials 15 ml. and 22.5 ml.
Use: Treatment of asthma.

DUOMINE. (Kenyon) Dextromethorphan HBr 7.5 mg., chlorpheniramine maleate 10 mg., ammonium Cl 80 mg., pot. guaiacolate 80 mg., tartar emetic 0.8 mg./5 cc. Bot. 4 oz., pt., gal.

DUOMYCIN.
See: Aureomycin, Prep. (Lederle)

DUOPRIN. (Dunhall) Acetaminophen 250 mg., salicylamide 250 mg./Tab. Bot. 30s, 100s, 250s. **Cap.** Bot. 30s, 100s, 500s.
Use: Non-salicylate analgesic.

DUOPRIN-S. (Dunhall) Acetaminophen 90 mg., salicylamide 90 mg., menthol 1 mg./5 ml. Bot. pt.
Use: Analgesic.

DUOSOL. (Kirkman) Ducosate sodium 100 mg./Cap. Bot. 100s, 1000s.
Use: Fecal softener.

DUOSCORB. (Upsher-Smith) Ascorbic acid 2 Gms./Pkt. Pkt. 50s.
Use: Renal dialysis use.

DUOTAL. (Approved) 1½ gr.: Secobarbital sod. ¾ gr., amobarbital ¾ gr./Cap. 3 gr.: Secobarbital sod. 1½ gr., amobarbital 1½ gr./Cap. Bot. 100s, 500s, 1000s.

DUOTAL.
See: Guaiacol Carbonate (Various Mfr.)

DUOTRATE. (Marion) Pentaerythritol tetranitrate 30 mg./Time release Cap. Bot. 100s.
Use: Coronary vasodilation.

DUOTRATE-45. (Marion) Pentaerythritol tetranitrate 45 mg./Time release Cap. Bot. 100s.
Use: Coronary vasodilation.

DUOTRONE. (Arnar-Stone; Dunhall) Estrone 2 mg., testosterone 25 mg./cc. Vial 10 cc.

DUOVAL-P.A. (Reid-Provident) Testosterone enanthate 90 mg., estradiol valerate 4 mg./cc. Vials 10 cc. 1s, 6s, 12s.

DUOVIN-S. (Spanner) Estrone 2.5 mg., progesterone 25 mg./1 cc. Vial 10 cc.

DUO-WR, No. 1 & No. 2. (Whorton) **No. 1:** Salicylic acid, compound tincture benzoin. **No. 2:** Compound tincture benzoin, formaldehyde. Bot. ¼ oz.
Use: Topical application in the removal of warts.

DUPHRENE. (Vale) Phenylephrine HCl 5 mg., chlorpheniramine maleate 1 mg., pyrilamine maleate 12.5 mg./Tab. Bot. 100s, 500s, 1000s.
Use: Antihistaminic.

DUPLAST. (Beiersdorf) Adhesive coated elastic cloth 8"×4", Box 10 strips. 10"×5", Box 8 & 10 strips.

DUPLEX SHAMPOO. (C & M Pharmacal) Sodium lauryl sulfate, lauramide DEA, purified water. Bot. pt., gal.
Use: Shampoo.

DUPLEX T SHAMPOO. (C & M Pharmacal) Sodium lauryl sulfate, purified water, lauramide DEA, solution of coal tar, alcohol 8.3%. Bot. pt., gal.
Use: Anti-dandruff shampoo.

DUPONOL.
See: Gardinol-type Detergents (Sod. Lauryl Sulfate) (Various Mfr.)

DURABOLIN-25. (Organon) Nandrolone phenpropionate 25 mg./ml. in sesame oil, w/ Benzyl alcohol 5%. Amp. 1 ml. Box 3s; Vial 5 ml.
Use: Anabolic agent.
See: Deca-Durabolin, Inj. (Organon)

DURABOLIN-50. (Organon) Nandrolone phenpropionate 50 mg./ml. in sterile sesame oil w/ 10%
benzyl-alcohol. Vials 2 cc.
Use: Anabolic agent.

DURA-C 500. (Amfre-Grant) Vit. C 500 mg./Timed Release Cap. Bot. 100s, 500s.
Use: Vit. C deficiency.

DURA-CHORION PLUS. (Pharmex) Estradiol valerate
10 mg./cc. Vial 10 cc.

DURACID. (Fielding) Antacid. Bot 100s.
Use: Antacid.

DURACILLIN A.S. (Lilly) Penicillin G procaine
300,000 u./ml. w/lecithin 1%, sod. citrate 4%,
povidone 0.1%, w/methylparaben 0.15%,
propylparaben 0.02%, benzylalcohol 1% as
preservatives. Vial 10 ml. Box 1s. Traypak
100s.
Use: Antibiotic.

DURADYNE. (O'Neal, Jones & Feldman) Aspirin 230
mg., acetaminophen 180 mg., caffeine 15 mg./Tab.
Bot. 100s. **Forte:** Bot. 100s. **No. 2:** Bot. 100s.

DURADYNE DHC. (O'Neal, Jones & Feldman)
Dihydrocodeinone bitartrate 5 mg., acetaminophen
500 mg./Tab. Bot. 50s.
Use: Analgesic.

DURA-ESTRIN. (Hauck) Estradiol cypionate 5 mg./ml.
Vial 10 ml.
Use: Estrogen deficiency.

DURAGEN. (Hauck) Estradiol valerate 10 mg., 20
mg., or 40 mg./ml. Vial 10 ml.
Use: Estrogen therapy.

DURA-KELLIN. (Pharmex) Estrone 2 mg., potassium
estrone sulfate 1 mg., sod. phosphate buffer, sod.
carboxymethylcellulose 0.2%, thimerosal 1:20,000,
benzyl alcohol 1.5%/cc. Vial 10 cc.
Use: Deficiency of estrogens.

DURALEX. (American Urologicals) Pseudoephedrine
HCl 120 mg., chlorpheniramine maleate 8 mg./Cap.
Bot. 100s.
Use: Nasal decongestant, antihistaminic.

DURALONE. (Hauck) Methylprednisolone acetate 40
mg., or 80 mg./ml. Vial 5 ml., 10 ml.
Use: Steroid therapy.

DURA-METH. (Foy) Methylprednisolone 40 mg./ml.
Vials 5 ml., 10 ml.
Use: Replacement therapy in adrenocortical
deficiency states.

DURANDROL. (Pharmex) Methandriol dipropionate 50
mg./cc. Vial 10 cc.

DURANEST BASE AND HCl. Etidocaine, B.A.N.
Use: Local anesthetic.
See: Duranest HCl (Astra)

DURANEST HCl. (Astra) Etidocaine 1%
w/epinephrine 1:200,000. Vial 30 ml.
Use: Local anesthetic.

• **DURAPATITE.** USAN.
Use: Prosthetic aid.

DURAPHYL. (McNeil Pharm) Anhydrous theophylline
controlled released 100 mg., 200 mg., or 300
mg./Tab. Bot. 100s.
Use: Bronchodilator.

DURAPRED. (Amfre-Grant) Prednisolone acetate 100
mg./ml. Vial 10 mg.

Use: Hormone.

DURAPRED T.B.A. (Amfre-Grant) Prednisolone T-buty-
lacetate 20 mg./ml. Vial 10 ml.
Use: Hormone.

DURAQUIN. (Parke-Davis) Quinidine gluconate 330
mg./Tab. (Sustained release). Bot. 100s. Unit dose
100s.
Use: Cardiac depressant.

DURASAL. (Seatrace) Magnesium salicylate 600
mg./Tab. Bot. 100s, 500s.
Use: Anti-arthritic, analgesic, anti-pyretic.

DURASIL. (Seatrace) Aluminum hydroxide dried gel
200 mg., magnesium trisilicate 200 mg., D-calcium
pantothenate 10 mg./Tab. Bot. 100s.
Use: Dietary supplement.

DURATEARS OINTMENT. (Alcon) Tube 3.5 Gm.
Use: Ocular lubricant.

DURATEST. (Hauck) Testosterone cypionate 100 mg.
or 200 mg./ml. Vial 10 ml.
Use: Androgen therapy.

DURA-TESTOSTERONE. (Pharmex) Testosterone enthanate 200 mg./cc. Vial 10 cc.

DURA-TESTRONE. (Pharmex) Testosterone enthanate
90 mg., estradiol valerate 4 mg./cc.
Use: Androgen therapy.

DURA-TESTERONE FORTE. (Pharmex) Testosterone
enthanate 180 mg., estradiol valerate 8 mg./cc.
Vial 10 cc.
Use: Androgen therapy.

DURATHESIA. (Vortech) Procaine base 15 mg.,
propyl p-aminobenzoate 60 mg., benzyl alcohol 5C
mg./cc. Vial 10 cc.
Use: Local anesthetic for proctologic use only.

DURATION MENTHOLATED VAPOR SPRAY.
(Plough) Oxymetazoline HCl 0.05%, aromatics.
Squeeze Bot. 0.5 oz.
Use: Nasal decongestant.

DURATION MILD 4-HOUR NASAL SPRAY. (Plough)
Phenylephrine HCl 0.5% Bot. 0.5 oz.
Use: Nasal decongestant.

DURATION NASAL SPRAY. (Plough)
Oxymethazoline HCl 0.05%. Aqueous sol. Squeeze
Bot. 0.5 oz., 1 oz.
Use: Nasal decongestant.

DURATESTRIN. (Hauck) Testosterone cypionate 50
mg., estradiol cypionate 2 mg./ml. Vial 10 ml.
Use: Androgen and estrogen therapy.

DUREL-CORT. (Durel) Hydrocortisone ¼%, ½%,
1%/Gm. **Oint., Creme, Lotion:** Jar (¼%) 4 oz.,
(½%, 1%, 2.5%) 1 oz., 4 oz., pt.
Use: Treatment of various forms of allergic
dermatitis and other inflammatory skin diseases.

DUREL-CORT 'V'. (Durel) Hydrocortisone ¼%, ½%,
1%/Gm. and clioquinol 3%. **Oint. & Creme:** Jar
(¼%) 4 oz., pt.; (½%, 1%) 1 oz., 4 oz., 16 oz.
Use: Therapy for control of various acute and
chronic dermatologic disorders.

DURELERGIC EMOLLIENT LOTION. (Durel)
Acetylated lanolin, mineral oil, sorbitan
monostearates. Bot. 4 oz., pt., gal.
Use: Skin conditioner.

DURELERGIC EMOLLIENT LOTION PLUS. (Durel)

Menthol 0.25%, phenol 0.5% added to Durelergic emollient lotion. Bot. 4 oz., pt., gal.
Use: Antipruritic.

DUREZE OTIC DROPS. (O'Neal, Jones & Feldman) Hydrocortisone 1%, pramoxine HCl 2%, acetic acid 2%, benzalkonium cl. 0.02% parachlorometaxylenol 0.1%. Bot. 10 cc.
Use: Ear therapy.

DURICEF. (Mead Johnson) Cefadroxil. **Tab.:** 1 Gm./Tab. Bot. 24s, 100s. **Cap.:** 500 mg./Cap. Bot. 24s, 100s, 500s. **Susp.:** 125 mg./5 ml., 250 mg./5 ml., 500 mg./ 5 ml. Bot. 50 ml., 100 ml.

DUROLENE OINTMENT. (Durel) Glyceryl monostearate, petrolatum, cholesterol, polyoxyethyl sorb. monolaurate. Jars lb., 6 lb.
Use: Ointment base.

DUROMANTEL CREAM. (Durel) Spermaceti, cetyl alcohol, stearyl alcohol, glycerine, alcohol sulfates, aluminum acetate solution, purified water, methyl and propyl parasepts. Jar lb., 6 lb.

DUROSHAM. (Durel) Soapless shampoo concentrate. Bot. 6 oz., gal.

DURRAX. (Dermik) Hydroxyzine HCl 10 mg. or 25 mg./Tab. Bot. 100s.
Use: Treatment of tension, anti-anxiety and allergic dermatoses.

DUSOTAL. (Harvey) Sod. amobarbital ¾ gr., sod. secobarbital ¾ gr./Cap. Bot. 1000s. (3 gr.) Bot. 1000s.
Use: Sedative.

• **DUSTING POWDER, ABSORBABLE,** U.S.P. XXI. Starch-derivative dusting pow.
Use: Surgical aid (glove lubricant).

DUSTING POWDER, SURGICAL.
See: B-F-I Powder (Calgon).

DUTCH DROPS. Oil of Turpentine Sulfurated.

DUTCH OIL. Oil of Turpentine Sulfurated.

DUVOID. (Norwich Eaton) Bethanechol chloride 10 mg., 25 mg., 50 mg./Tab. Bot. 100s, Unit dose cartons 100s.
Use: Nonobstructive urinary retention.

D V CREAM. (Merrell Dow) Dienestrol 0.01% w/lactose, propylene glycol, stearic acid, diglycol stearate, TEA, benzoic acid, butylated hydroxytoluene, disodium edetate, buffered w/lactic acid to an acid pH. Tube 3 oz. w/applicator.
Use: Treatment of atrophic vaginitis and kraurosis vulvae associated with menopause.

D-VASO. (Dunhall) Pentylenetetrazole 50 mg., niacin 50 mg., dimenhydrinate 25 mg./Cap. Bot. 100s, 1000s.

D-VASO-S. (Dunhall) Pentylenetetrazole 50 mg., niacin 50 mg., dimenhydrinate 25 mg., alcohol 18%, sherry wine vehicle. Bot. pt.

D V SUPPOSITORIES. (Merrell Dow) Dienestrol 0.7 mg./Suppos. w/lactose, polyethylene glycol 400, polysorbate 80, polyethylene glycol 3350, glycerin, butylated hydroxytoluene, buffered w/lactic acid to an acid pH., inert glycerin-gelatin covering. Pkg. 16s. w/inserter.
Use: Treatment of atrophic vaginitis and kraurosis vulvae associated with menopause.

DWIATOL. (Kenyon) Hyoscyamine HBr 0.256 mg., hyoscine HBr 0.0144 mg., atropine sulfate 0.048 mg., phenobarbital ½ gr./Tab. Bot. 100s, 1000s.
Use: Antispasmodic.

DYAZIDE. (SmithKline) Triamterene 50 mg., hydrochlorothiazide 25 mg./Cap. Bot. 100s, 1000s. Unit Pak 100s.
Use: Diuretic, edema, hypertension.

DYCILL. (Beecham Labs) Dicloxacillin disodium 250 mg. & 500 mg./Cap. Bot. 100s.
Use: Antibiotic.

DYCLONE. (Astra) Dyclonine HCl 0.5% or 1.0% Solution. Bot. 1 oz.
Use: Topical anesthetic.

• **DYCLONINE HCl,** U.S.P. XXI. Gel, Topical Sol., U.S.P. XXI. 4'-Butoxy-3-piperidinopropiophenone HCl.
Use: Topical anesthetic.
See: Dyclone, Sol. (Astra)
W/Neomycin sulfate, polymyxin B sulfate, hydrocortisone acetate.
See: Neo-polycin HC, Oint. (Merrell Dow)

DYCOLATE. (Amfre-Grant) Dyphylline 200 mg., guaifenesin 50 mg./Tab. Bot. 100s, 1000s.
Use: Bronchial dilator.

DYCOMENE. (Hance) Hydrocodone bitartrate ⅙ gr., pyrilamine maleate 1½ gr./Fl. Oz. Bot. 3 oz., 1 gal.
Use: Sedative for coughs due to colds.

• **DYDROGESTERONE,** U.S.P. XXI. Tabs., U.S.P. XXI. 9β, 10-α-Pregna-4,6-diene-3,20-dione. Isopregnenone.
Use: Progesterone agent.

DYES.
See: Antiseptic, Dyes. Diagnostic Agents

DYFLEX-200 TABLETS. (Econo Med) Dyphylline 200 mg./Tab. Bot. 100s.
Use: Bronchial asthma.

DYFLEX-400 TABLETS. (Econo Med) Dyphylline 400 mg./Tab. Bot. 100s, 500s.
Use: Bronchodilator for relief of acute bronchial asthma.

DYFLEX-G TABLETS. (Econo Med) Dyphylline 200 mg., guaifenesin 200 mg./Tab. Bot. 100s, 1000s.
Use: Treatment of acute and chronic bronchitis.

DYFLEX-G ELIXIR. (Econo Med) Dyphylline 100 mg., guaifenesin 100 mg./15 ml Bot. pt.
Use: Chronic or acute bronchitis.

DYFLOS. B.A.N. Di-isopropyl phosphorofluoridate. Di-isopropyl fluorophosphonate.
Use: Treatment of glaucoma.
See: DFP

DYLATE. Clonitrate.
Use: Coronary vasodilator.

DYLINE. (Seatrace) Dyphylline 250 mg./ml. Vial 10 cc.

DYLINE-GG LIQUID. (Seatrace) Diphylline 100 mg., guaifenesin 100 mg./5 ml. Bot. Pt., gal.
Use: Anti-asthmatic.

DYLINE-GG TABLETS. (Seatrace) Diphylline 200 mg., guaifenesin 200 mg./Tab. Bot. 100s, 1000s.

• **DYMANTHINE HYDROCHLORIDE.** USAN. N,N-dimethyloctadecylamine hydrochloride.
Use: Anthelmintic.

DYMELOR. (Lilly) Acetohexamide 250 mg. or 500 mg./Tab. Bot. 50s, 200s, 500s. Blister Pkg. 10 × 10s.
Use: Maturity-onset diabetes.

DYMENATE. (Keene) Dimenhydrinate, 50 mg./ml. Vial 10 ml.
Use: Motion sickness.

DYNACORYL.
See: Nikethamide, Prep. (Various Mfr.)

DYNAPEN. (Bristol) Sod. dicloxacillin. **Cap.:** 125 mg., 250 mg. Bot. 24s, 100s. **Susp.:** 62.5 mg./5 ml. Bot. 80 ml., 100 ml., 200 ml.
Use: Infections due to penicillinase-producing staphylococci.

DYNAPLEX. (Alton) Vitamin B complex. Bot. 100s, 1000s.
Use: Dietary supplement.

DYNARSAN.
See: Acetarsone, Tab.

DYNOSAL. (Mallard) Acetaminophen 130 mg., aspirin 260 mg., caffeine anhydrous 16 mg./Tab. Bot. 100s.
Use: Analgesic.

DY-O-DERM. (Owen) Purified water, isopropyl alcohol, acetone, dihydroxyacetone, FD&C yellow No. 6, FD&C blue No. 1, D&C Red No. 33. Bot. 4 oz.
Use: Water-soluble vitiligo stain.

• **DYPHYLLINE,** U.S.P. XXI. Inj., Tab., U.S.P. XXI. 7-(2,3-Dihydroxypropyl) Theophylline, Hyphylline.
Use: Vasodilator, bronchodilator.
See: Brophylline, Inj., Granucaps (Reid-Provident)
  Dilor, Prep. (Savage)
  Dilorex, Inj. (Tunex)
  Droxine, Tab. (Shear-Kershman)
  Emfabid TD, Tab. (Saron)
  Lardet, Inj. (Standex)
  Lufyllin, Tab. (Mallinckrodt)
  Neothylline, Tab. (Lemmon)
  Prophyllin, Oint., Pow. (Rystan)
W/Chlorpheniramine maleate, guaifenesin, dextromethorphan HBr, phenylephrine HCl.
See: Hycoff-A, Syr. (Saron)
W/Ephedrine HCl, phenobarbital, guaifenesin.
See: Lufyllin-EPG, Tab., Elix. (Mallinckrodt)
W/Guaifenesin.
See: Bronkolate-G, Tab. (Parmed)
  Dilor-G, Liq., Tab. (Savage)
  Embron, Syr., Cap. (Amid)
  Emfaseem, Cap., Elix., Inj. (Saron)
  Neothylline GG, Liq. (Lemmon)
W/Guaifenesin, ephedrine HCl, phenobarbital.
See: Dilacap, Cap. (Coastal)

DYRENIUM. (SmithKline) Triamterene 50 mg./Cap. Bot. 100s, Unit packs 100s; 100 mg./Cap. Bot. 100s, 1000s. Unit packs 100s.
Use: Diuretic.

DYSENAID JR. (Jenkins) Paregoric 5 min., bismuth subgallate 1 gr., kaolin 1 gr., pectin ⅛ gr./Tab. Bot. 1000s.
Use: Diarrhea.

DYSPEL. (Dover) Acetaminophen, ephedrine sulfate, atropine sulfate 0.06 mg./Tab. Sugar and salt free. Unit dose 500s.

Use: Analgesic for minor muscle pains, cramps and dysmenorrhea.

DYVON. Metriphonate, B.A.N.

E

E-1 OPHTHALMIC SOL. (Alcon) Epinephrine bitartrate 1%, equiv. to 0.5% of base. Drop. Bot. 15 cc.
Use: Wide angle glaucoma.

EACA (Lederle) Epsilon aminocaproic acid.
Use: Antifibrinolytic agent.
See; Amicar (Lederle)

EARDRO. (Jenkins) Benzocaine 15 gm., antipyrine 0.70 gm., glycerol q.s./½ oz. Liq. Dropper Bot. ½ oz.
Use: Temporary relief of earache.

EAR DROPS. (Weeks & Leo) Carbamide peroxide 6.5% in an anhydrous glycerin base. Bot. 1 oz.
Use: Hygenic ear care.

EAR DROPS (OTC). (Columbia) Carbamide, glycerine, propylene, chlobutanol 0.5%. Bot. ½ oz.
Use: Softening wax in ear canal.

EAR DROPS (Rx). (Columbia) Antipyrine 3.2%, benzocaine 0.85%, glycerol. Bot. ½ oz.

EAR-DRY. (Scherer) Isopropyl alcohol & boric acid 2.75% Bot. 1 oz.
Use: Prevention of swimmer's ear.

EAREX EAR DROPS. (Approved) Benzocaine 0.15 Gm., antipyrine 0.7 Gm./½ oz. Bot. ½ oz.

EAR-EZE. (Hyrex) Hydrocortisone alcohol 1%, pramoxine HCl 1%, parachlorometaxylenol 0.1%. Bot. 15 ml.
Use: Antibacterial, antifungal, analgesic for ears.

EAR-OL. (Metro Med) Bot. ½ oz., 12s.
Use: Ear solution.

EARTHNUT OIL. Peanut Oil

EASPRIN. (Parke-Davis) Aspirin 15 gr./Enteric Coated Tab. Bot. 100s.
Use: Long-termed palliative treatment of mild to moderate pain, and inflammation of arthritic conditions.

EAST-A. (Eastwood) Lotion-therapeutic. Bot. 16 oz.

EAST-GESIC. (Eastwood) Tab. Bot. 100s.

EASTINIC. (Eastwood) Tab. Bot. 100s.

EAST-IRON. (Eastwood) Tab. Bot. 100s.

EAST-NATA. (Eastwood) Tab. Bot. 100s.

EAST-SERPINE. (Eastwood) Tab. Bot. 100s.

EASTWOOD HEMATINIC. (Eastwood) Tab. Bot. 100s.

EASY-LAX. (Walgreen) Docusate sodium 100 mg./Cap. Bot. 60s.
Use: Fecal softener.

EASY-LAX PLUS. (Walgreen) Docusate sodium 100 mg., casanthranol 30 mg./Cap. Bot. 60s.
Use: Fecal softener & laxative.

EAZOL. (Mallard) Fructose, dextrose, orthophosphoric acid. Bot. pts.
Use: Relief of upset stomach and nausea.

EBV-VCA. (Wampole-Zeus) Epstein-Barr virus, viral capsid antigen antibody test. Tests 100s.
Use: Qualitative and semi-quantitative detection of EBV antibody in human serum.

EBV-VCA IgM. (Wampole-Zeus) Epstein-Barr virus, viral

capsid antigen IgM antibody Test 50s.
Use: Qualitative and semiqualitative detection of
EBV-VCA IgM antibody in human serum.
ECBOLINE. Ergotoxine.
ECEE PLUS. (Edwards) Vitamin E 200 I.U., ascorbic
acid 100 mg., magnesium sulfate 70 mg., zinc
sulfate 80 mg./Tab. Bot. 100s.
Use: Vitamin deficiency; fibrocystic breast disease.
• **ECHOTHIOPHATE IODIDE.** U.S.P. XXI. Ophth. Sol.
U.S.P. XXI. Ethanaminium, 2-[(diethoxyphosphinyl)-
thio]-N,N,N-trimethyl-, iodide. (2-Mercaptoethyl)-
trimethylammonium iodide S-ester with O,O-diethyl
phosphorothioate. Bot. 100s.
Use: Glaucoma; cholinergic.
See: Echodide, Opth. Sol. (Alcon)
    Phospholine Iodide, Pow. (Ayerst)
ECLABRON. (U.S. Ethicals) Guaithylline. 240 mg./15
ml. Bot. 120 ml.
Use: Symptomatic treatment of bronchospasms.
ECLASUFED SR. (U.S. Ethicals) Pseudoephedrine
HCl.
Use: Temporary relief of nasal congestion.
ECLIPSE AFTER SUN. (Dorsey) Purified water, oleth-
3 phosphate, petrolatum, cetyl esters wax, glycerin,
carbomer 934, imidazolidinyl urea, benzyl alcohol,
sodium hydroxide. Bot. 6 oz.
Use: Moisturizer.
ECLIPSE LIP AND FACE PROTECTANT. (Dorsey)
Padimate 0, oxybenzone. SPF 15. Stick 12×0.15
oz. 24×0.15 oz.
Use: Sunscreen.
ECOLID. Chlorisondamine Chloride, B.A.N.
ECOMYTRIN. Amphomycin, B.A.N.
• **ECONAZOLE.** USAN.
Use: Antifungal.
• **ECONAZOLE NITRATE.** USAN.
Use: Antifungal.
ECONOCHLOR. (Alcon) Chloramphenicol 0.5% boric
acid, sodium borate 0.017%, thimerosal,
hydroxymethylcellulose 0.5%. Droptainer 15 ml.
Use: Bacterial infections of the eye.
ECONOCHLOR OINTMENT. (Alcon) Chloramphenicol
1% in sterile ophthalmic ointment. Tube 3.5 Gm.
Use: Bacterial infections of the eye.
ECONOPRED. (Alcon) Prednisolone acetate 0.125%,
0.25% or 0.5%, benzalkonium chloride 0.01%
w/hydroxymethyl cellulose. Droptainer 5 ml., 10 ml.
Use: Ophthalmic anti-inflammatory.
ECONOPRED PLUS. (Alcon) Prednisolone acetate
1%, benzalkonium chloride 0.01%,
w/hydroxymethyl cellulose. Droptainer 5 ml., 10 ml.
Use: Ophthalmic anti-inflammatory.
ECOSONE CREAM. (Star) Hydrocortisone 0.5% in a
water-soluble cream base. Tube 1 oz.
Use: Management of allergic dermatoses.
ECOTHIOPATE IODIDE. B.A.N. S-2-Dimethylamino-
ethyl diethyl phosphorothioate methiodide.
Use: Treatment of glaucoma.
See: Phospholine Iodide
ECOTRIN. (Menley & James) Aspirin 5 gr./Coated
Tab. Bot. 36s, 100s, 250s, 1000s.
Use: Antipyretic, anti-inflammatory.

ECOTRIN MAXIMUM STRENGTH. (Menley & James)
Aspirin 7.5 gr./Coated Tab. Bot. 24s, 60s, 150s.
Use: Analgesic, antipyretic, anti-inflammatory.
E CREAM. (Image) Vitamin E cream 3000 I.U. Tube 2
oz.
ECTASULE III. (Fleming) Ephedrine sulfate 15 mg.,
amobarbital 8 mg./T.D. Cap. Bot. 100s, 1000s.
ECTASULE JUNIOR. (Fleming) Ephedrine sulfate 30
mg., amobarbital 15 mg./T.D. Cap. Bot. 100s,
1000s.
ECTASULE SENIOR. (Fleming) Ephedrine sulfate 60
mg., amobarbital 30 mg./T.D. Cap. Bot 100s,
1000s.
ECTASULE MINUS III. (Fleming) Ephedrine sulfate
15 mg./Cap. Bot. 100s, 1000s.
ECTASULE MINUS JR. (Fleming) Ephedrine sulfate
30 mg./T.D. Cap. Bot. 100s, 1000s.
ECTASULE MINUS SR. (Fleming) Ephedrine sulfate
60 mg./T.D. Cap. Bot. 100s, 1000s.
ECTIMAR. Etisazole, B.A.N.
ECTOL. (Approved) Chlorpheniramine maleate,
pyrilamine maleate, diperodon, hexachlorphene,
benzalkonium, menthol, camphor. Tube 1 oz.
Use: Allergy-itching.
ECTYLUREA. B.A.N. (2-Ethylcrotonoyl)urea.
Use: Sedative.
See: Nostyn
• **ECTYLUREA.** 2-Ethyl-ciscrotonylurea.
EDATHAMIL. Edetate ethylenediaminetetraacetic
acid.
See: Nullapons (General Aniline)
EDATHAMIL CALCIUM-DISODIUM. Calcium Disod.
Ethylenediamine tetraacetate.
See: Calcium Disodium Versenate, Amp. & Tab.
(Riker)
EDATHAMIL DISODIUM. Disod. salt of ethylene
diamine tetraacetic acid.
See: Endrate, Amp. (Abbott)
EDECRIN. (Merck Sharp & Dohme) Ethacrynic acid
25 mg. or 50 mg./Tab. Bot. 100s. I.V. Inj. 50
mg./Vial.
Use: Diuretic.
EDECRIN, SODIUM.
See: Sodium Edecrin
• **EDETATE CALCIUM DISODIUM,** U.S.P. XXI. Inj.,
U.S.P. XXI. Calciate (2-), [[N,N'-1,2-ethanediylbis[N-
(carboxymethyl)-glycinato]](4-)-N,N',O,O',-O″,O‴]-,
disodium, hydrate, (OC-6-21)-. Disodium
(ethylenedinitrilo)tetraceto calciate (2-) hydrate.
Use: Chelating agent.
See: Calcium Disod. Versenate, Amp., Tab. (Riker)
• **EDETATE DISODIUM,** U.S.P. XXI. Inj., U.S.P. XXI.
Glycine, N,N'-1,2-ethanediylbis[N-(carboxymethyl)-,
disodium salt, dihydrate. Disodium
(ethylenedinitrilo)tetraacetate dihydrate.
Use: Pharm. aid (chelating agent).
See: Disotate, Inj. (Fellows-Testagar)
    Endrate, Amp. (Abbott)
    Sodium Versenate (Riker)
W/Benzalkonium chloride, boric acid, potassium
chloride, sodium carbonate anhydrous.
See: Swim-Eye Drops (Savage)

W/Phenylephrine HCl, methapyrilene HCl, benzalkonium chloride, sod. bisulfite.
See: Allerest Nasal Spray (Pharmacraft)

W/Phenylephrine HCl, benzalkonium chloride, sod. bisulfate.
See: Sinarest, Aerosol (Pharmacraft)

W/Potassium chloride, benzalkonium chloride, isotonic boric acid.
See: Dacriose (Smith, Miller & Patch)

W/Prednisolone sodium phosphate, niacinamide, sodium bisulfite, phenol.
See: P.S.P. IV. Inj. (Reid-Provident)
Solu-Pred, Vial (Kenyon)

W/Sodium thiosulfate, salicylic acid, isopropyl alcohol, propylene glycol, menthol, colloidal alumina.
See: Tinver Lotion (Barnes-Hind)

• **EDETATE DIPOTASSIUM.** USAN.
Use: Pharmaceutic aid (chelating agent).

• **EDETATE SODIUM.** USAN. Tetrasodium (ethylenedinitrilo)-tetraacetate, or tetrasodium ethylenediaminetetraacetate.
Use: Chelating agent.
See: Disodium Versenate (Riker)
Vagisec, Liq. (Julius Schmid)

• **EDETATE TRISODIUM.** USAN. Trisodium hydrogen (ethylenedinitrilo) tetraacetate, or trisodium hydrogen ethylenediaminetetraacetate.
Use: Chelating agent.

EDETIC ACID. B.A.N. Ethylenediamine-NNN'N'-tetra-acetic acid.
Use: Chelating agent.
See: Versene Acid

• **EDETIC ACID,** N.F. XVI. (Ethylenedinitrilo) tetraacetic acid.
Use: Pharmaceutic aid (metal-complexing agent).

• **EDETOL.** USAN.
Use: Alkalizing agent.

EDITHAMIL.
See: Edathamil

EDOGESTRONE. B.A.N. 17-Acetoxy-3,3-ethylene-dioxy-6-methylpregn-5-en-20-one.
Use: Progestational steroid.

EDROFURADENE. Name used for Nifurdazil.

EDROPHONIUM CHLORIDE. B.A.N. Ethyl-(3-hydroxy-phenyl)dimethylammonium chloride.
Use: Diagnosis of myasthenia gravis.

• **EDROPHONIUM CHLORIDE,** U.S.P. XXI. Inj. U.S.P. XXI. Dimethylethyl (3-hydroxyphenyl) ammonium chloride. Ethyl (m-hydroxyphenyl)di-methyl-ammonium chloride. Benzenaminium, N-ethyl-3-hy-droxy-N,N-dimethyl-, chloride.
Use: Antidote to curare principles; diagnostic aid (myasthenia gravis).
See: Tensilon Chloride, Vial (Roche)

EDTA.
See: Edathamil (Var. Mfr.)

E-DUST. (Hollister-Stier) Allergenic extract dust concentrate 1:40 w/v in 50% glycerin. Vial 10 ml.
Use: Dust allergy immunotherapy.

E.E.S. (Abbott) Erythromycin ethylsuccinate representing mg. of erythromycin activity. **Tab.:** E.E.S. Chewable Tablets 200 mg. Bot. 50s; E.E.S.

400 Filmtab 400 mg. Bot. 100s; **Drops:** 100 mg./2.5 ml. when reconstituted. Bot. 50 ml.; **Granules:** 200 mg./5 ml. when reconstituted. Bot. 60 ml., 100 ml., 200 ml. Abbo-Pac.; **Liquid-200 & 400:** 200 mg./5 ml. Bot. 100 ml., pt.; 400 mg./5 ml. Bot. 100 ml., pt.
Use: Antibiotic.
See: EES Prods. (Abbott)

E.E.S. 400 FILMTAB. (Abbott) Erythromycin ethylsuccinate representing 400 mg. erythromycin activity/Tab. Bot. 100s, 500s. Unit dose 100s.
Use: Antibiotic.

E.E.S. CHEWABLE TABLETS. (Abbott) Erythromycin ethylsuccinate representing erythromycin activity of 200 mg./Chewable Tab. Bot. 50s.
Use: Antibiotic.

E.E.S. DROPS. (Abbott) Erythromycin ethyl succinate representing 100 mg. erythromycin activity/2.5 ml. when reconstituted w/water. Bot. 50 ml.
Use: Antibiotic.

E.E.S. GRANULES. (Abbott) When mixed according to directions, contains erythromycin ethyl succinate representing 200 mg. erythromycin activity/5 ml. of oral suspension. **Granules** Bot. 60 ml., 100 ml., 200 ml, Abbo-Pac.
Use: Infections susceptible to erythromycin.

E.E.S. LIQUID-200 & 400. (Abbott) Erythromycin ethyl-succinate representing 200 mg. erythromycin activity/5 ml. Bot. 100 ml., pt. 400 mg./5 ml. Bot. 100 ml., pt.

EFED. (Alto) Ephedrine sulfate 8.1 mg., secobarbital 16.2 mg./Tab. Bot. 100s, 500s.
Use: Anti-asthmatic.

EFED-II. (Alto) Caffeine 200 mg./Cap. Box 24s. Bot. 100s.
Use: Stimulant.

EFEDRON HYDROCHLORIDE. (Hyrex) Ephedrine HCl 0.6% & chlorobutanol 0.5% w/Sod. chloride, menthol & cinnamon oil in a water-soluble jelly base. Nasal-tipped collapsible tubes 20 Gm.
Use: Shrinkage of nasal mucous membranes.

EFEROL. (O'Neal, Jones & Feldman) dl-Tocopherol ac-etate. Cap. (30 and 100 I.U.) Bot. 100s, 500s, 1000s. 200 & 400 I.U. Bot. 50s, 100s, 500s, 1000s. 800 I.U. Bot. 100s, 500s. Parenteral: 200 mg./cc. Vial 10 cc.
Use: Vitamin E therapy.

EFEROL AQUEOUS. (O'Neal, Jones & Feldman) Vitamin E 25 U./ml. Vial 2 ml.
Use: Vitamin E deficiency.

EFEROL OINTMENT. (O'Neal, Jones & Feldman) d-alpha Tocopherol acetate 30 I.U./Gm. Tube 1.5 oz. Jar 2 oz., and 1 lb.

E-FEROL SPRAY. (Fellows) Alpha tocopherol equiva-lent to 30 I.U. Vit. E/cc. Can 6 oz.

E-FEROL SUCCINATE. (Fellows) d-alpha Tocopherol acid succinate, equiv. to Vit. E. 100 or 400 I.U./Cap. Bot. 100s, 500s, 1000s. 200 I.U./Cap. Bot. 50s, 100s, 500s, 1000s. 50 I.U./Tab. Bot. 100s, 500s, 1000s.
Use: Orally, vitamin E therapy.

E-FEROL VANISHING CREAM. (Fellows) Alpha tocopherol. Jar 2 oz.

EFFECTIN TABLETS. (Winthrop Products) Bitoltoril mesylate.
Use: Bronchodilator.

EFFERSYLLIUM INSTANT. (Stuart) Psyllium hydrocolloid 3 Gm. in rounded tsp. (7 Gm.), Pow. Bot. 9 oz., 16 oz. Convenient packets 12s, 24s.
Use: Effervescent natural fiber bulking agent in treatment of constipation, diverticulitis, spastic colon and colitis.

EFFICIN. (Adria) Magnesium salicylate 500 mg./Tab. Bot. 36s.
Use: Analgesic.

EFO DINE OINTMENT. (Fougera) Povidone-iodine ointment. Foilpac 1/32 oz., Tube 1 oz. Jar 1 lb.

EFRICEL. (Softcon) Phenylephrine HCl 1/8%, w/benzalkonium chloride 1:25,000 as preservative; 2½% w/benzalkonium chloride 1:10,000 as preservative; 10% w/benzalkonium chloride 1:10,000 as preservative. Bot. 15 cc.
Use: Produce pupil dilation.

EFRICON EXPECTORANT. (Lannett) Codeine phosphate 1 gr., phenylephrine HCl 30 mg., chlorpheniramine maleate 12 mg., ammonium chloride 8 gr., Pot. guaiacol sulf. 8 gr., Sod. citrate 5 gr./fl. oz. Bot. 1 pt., gal.
Use: Antihistaminic nasal decongestant.

EFUDEX. (Roche) Fluorouracil. **Soln:** Fluorouracil 2% or 5%, w/propylene glycol, hydroxypropyl cellulose, parabens and disodium edetate, in Drop Dispensers 10 ml. **Cream:** fluorouracil 5%, in vanishing cream base consisting of white petrolatum, stearyl alcohol, propylene glycol, polysorbate 60 and parabens, Tubes 25 Gm.
Use: Treatment of solar keratoses or multiple actinic; 5% in treatment of superfical basal cell carcinoma, when conventional methods are impractical.

EGO. (Coastal) Vitamin E 200 I.U./Tab. Bot. 100s, 500s.

EGRAINE. A protein binder from oats.

• **EGTAZIC ACID.** USAN.
Use: Pharmaceutic aid.

EHRLICH 594.
See: Acetarsone, Tab.

EHRLICH 606.
See: Arspheramine (Various Mfr.)

E-IONATE P A. (Reid-Provident) Estradiol cypionate 5 mg., chlorobutanol 0.5% in cottonseed oil/cc. Vial 10 cc. 1s, 6s, 12s.
Use: Estrogen therapy.

EKG. (Alcon) Cream.
Use: Electrode contact agent.

• **ELANTRINE.** USAN.
Use: Anticholinergic.

ELAQUA XX. (Elder) Urea 20% Tube 1.5oz.
Use: Moisturizing cream.

ELASE-CHLOROMYCETIN OINTMENT. (Parke-Davis) Fibrinolysin 10 u., desoxyribonuclease 6666 u., chloramphenicol 100 mg., thimerosal 0.04 mg. as preservative, sucrose and sod. chloride/10 Gm.
Tube 10 Gm. Fibrinolysin 30 u., desoxyribonuclease 20,000 u., chloramphenicol 300 mg., thimerosal 0.12 mg./30 Gm. w/liq. petrolatum polyethylene, sucrose, sod. chloride. Tube 10 Gm., 30 Gm.

ELASE OINT. & PWD. FOR SOL. (Parke-Davis)
Pow.: Fibrinolysin 25 u., desoxyribonuclease 15,000 u., thimerosal 0.1 mg./Vial as lyophilized powder. May be reconstituted with 10 cc. of isotonic NaCl Sol. **Oint.:** Fibrinolysin 30 u., desoxyribonuclease 20,000 u., thimerosal 0.12 mg./30 Gm. Tube. Fibrinolysin 10 u., desoxyribonuclease 6,666 u./10 Gm., thimerosal 0.04 mg. as preservative. Tube avail w/V-Applicator pkg. 6s. Ointment base of liq. petrolatum, polyethylene w/sucrose and sod. chloride. Tube 10 Gm., 30 Gm.
Use: Proteolytic enzyme combination in gynecologic complications.

• **ELASTOFILCON A.** USAN.
Use: Contact lens material.

ELAVIL. (Merck Sharp & Dohme) Amitriptyline HCl 10 mg., 25 mg./Tab. Bot. 100s, 1000s, 5000s; 50 mg./Tab. Bot. 100s, 1000s; 75 mg. 100 mg./Tab. Bot. 100s; 150 mg./Tab. Bot. 30s, 100s; Inj. Vial 10 mg./ml. w/dextrose 44 mg., methylparaben 1.5 mg., propylparaben 0.2 mg./ml w/water for injection. All strengths in Unit dose Pkg. 100s.
Use: Antidepressant therapy.

ELDEC. (Parke-Davis) Vit. A 1667 I.U., C 66.7 mg., B-1 10 mg., B-2 0.87 mg., B-6 0.67 mg., Nicotinamide 16.7 mg., dl-Panthenol 10 mg., Fe 16.7 mg., Ca 66.7 mg., E 10 mg., B-12 2 mcg., Folic Acid 0.33 mg./Kapseal. Bot. 100s.
Use: Vitamin and mineral supplement.

ELDECORT 1%. (Elder) Hydrocortisone 1% in a water washable cream base. Tube ½ oz, 1 oz.
Use: Relief of inflammatory and pruritic manifestations of corticosteroid responsive dermatoses.

ELDECORT 2.5%. (Elder) Hydrocortisone 2.5% in a water washable cream base. Tube 1 oz.
Use: Relief of inflammatory and pruritic manifestations of corticosteroid responsive dermatoses.

ELDERCAPS. (Mayrand) Vit. A 4000 I.U., D-2 400 I.U., E 200 mg., ascorbic acid 200 mg., thiamine mononitrate 10 mg., riboflavin 5 mg., pyridoxine HCl 2 mg., niacinamide 25 mg., d-calcium pantothenate 10 mg., zinc sulfate 110 mg. magnesium sulfate 70 mg., manganese sulfate 5 mg., folic acid 1 mg./Cap. Bot. 100s.
Use: Nutritional supplement.

ELDER'S RVP. Red Vet. Petrolatum.
Use: Dermatoses.

ELDERTONIC ELIXIR. (Mayrand) Vit. B-1 2 mg., B-2 2 mg., B-6 0.5 mg., Vit. B-12 (as cobalamin conc.) 2 mcg., d-panthenol 5 mg., niacinamide 10 mg./fl. oz. w/pentylenetetrazol, alcohol 13.5%. Bot. pt., gal.
Use: Stimulant tonic.

ELDO-B & C. (Canright) Vit. C 250 mg., B-1 25 mg., B-2 10 mg., niacinamide 150 mg., B-6 5 mg., d-calcium pantothenate 20 mg./Tab. Bot. 100s, 1000s.
Use: B vitamins and Vit. C deficiencies.

ELDOFE. (Canright) Ferrous fumarate 225 mg./Chewable Tab. Bot. 100s, 1000s.
Use: Iron supplement.

ELDOFE-C. (Canright) Ferrous fumarate 225 mg., ascorbic acid 50 mg./Tab. Bot. 100s.
Use: Iron and Vit. C supplement.

ELDONAL. (Canright) Pentobarbital sod. ¼ gr., hyoscyamine sulfate 0.1075 mg., atropine sulfate 0.0195 mg., hyoscine HBr. 0.0070 mg./Tab. or 5 cc. Tab. Bot. 100s, 1000s. Elix. Bot. 1 pt.
Use: Sedative spasmolytic.

ELDONAL-L.A. (Canright) Hyoscyamine sulfate 0.3225 mg., atropine sulfate 0.0585 mg., hyoscine HBr 0.0210 mg., pentobarbital sod. ¾ gr./Cap. Bot. 50s.
Use: Antispasmodic, sedative spasmolytic.

ELDONAL-S. (Canright) Hyoscyamine sulfate 0.1075 mg., atropine sulfate 0.0195 mg., hyoscine HBr 0.0070 mg., pentobarbital sod. 32.5 mg./Tab. Bot. 100s, 1000s.
Use: Antispasmodic, sedative spasmolytic.

ELDOPAQUE. (Elder) Hydroquinone 2% in a tinted sunblocking cream base. Tube 0.5 oz., 1 oz.
Use: Gradual bleaching of hyperpigmented skin conditions and other unwanted areas of melanin hyperpigmentation

ELOPAQUE FORTE. (Elder) Hydroquinone 4% in a tinted sunblocking cream base. Tube 0.5 oz., 1 oz.
Use: Gradual bleaching of hyperpigmented skin conditions and other unwanted areas of melanin hyperpigmentation.

ELDOQUIN. (Elder) Hydroquinone 2% in a vanishing cream base. Tube 0.5 oz., 1 oz.
Use: Gradual bleaching of hyperpigmented skin conditions.

ELDOQUIN FORTE. (Elder) Hydroquinone 4% in vanishing cream base. Tube 0.5 oz., 1 oz.
Use: Gradual bleaching of hyperpigmented skin conditions.

ELDOQUIN LOTION. (Elder) Hydroquinone 2% in lotion base. Bot. 0.5 oz.
Use: Gradual bleaching of hyperpigmented skin conditions.

ELDOVITE. (Canright) Vitamin-mineral formula. Bot. 100s.

ELECAL. (Western Research) Calcium 250 mg., magnesium 15 mg./Tab. Bot. 1000s.

ELECTROCORTIN. Aldosterone. B.A.N.

ELECTROLYTE #48 INJECTION. Pediatric maintenance electrolyte solution. Dextrose 5% in elecatrolyte #48 w/Na 25 mEq., K 20 mEq., Mg 3 mEq., Cl 22 mEq., lactate 23 mEq., H PO₄ 3 mEq./L.
Use: Water, caloric, electrolyte source for maintenance in pediatrics.

ELECTROLYTE #75 INJECTION. (Cutter) Maintenance electrolyte solution. Dextrose 5% in electrolyte #75 w/Na 40 mEq., K 35 mEq., Cl 40 mEq., lactate 20 mEq., H PO₄ 17 mEq., Fructose 5% in Electrolyte #75 Injection. Bot. 250 ml., 500 ml., 1000 ml.
Use: Water, caloric, electrolyte source for maintenance in adults, replacement in pediatrics.

■**ELECTROLYTE THERAPY.**
See: K.M.C., Amp. (Ingram)
Lytren, Ready-to-Use, Liq. (Mead Johnson)

ELECTROLYTIC REPLENISHER. (Invenex) Pot. chloride 186 mg., magnesium chloride 47.6 mg., calcium chloride 55.5 mg., phenol red 0.1 mg./cc. Vial 10 cc.

ELEGEN-G. (Grafton) Amitryptiline 10 mg., 25 mg., 50 mg./Tab. Bot. 100s, 1000s.
Use: Antidepressant.

ELEKAP CAPSULES. (Western Research) Oyster shell calcium 250 mg., magnesium oxide 15 mg., Vit. D 133 I.U./Cap. Bot. 1000s, 10 × 10s.
Use: Dietary supplement.

ELEVITES. (Barth's) Vit. A 6000 I.U., D 400 I.U., B-1 1.5 mg., B-2 3 mg., C 60 mg., B-12 10 mcg., niacin 1 mg., E 10 I.U., malt diastase 15 mg., Fe 15 mg., Ca 381 mg., P .172 mg., citrus bioflavonoid complex 15 mg., rutin 15 mg., nucleic acid 3 mg., red bone marrow 30 mg., peppermint leaves 10 mg., wheat germ 30 mg./Tab. or Cap. Bot. 100s, 500s, 1000s.

• **ELFAZEPAM.** USAN.
Use: Appetite stimulant.

ELITE. (Badger) Fluoride (as sodium free) in 2% soln. Bot. 1 oz., pt.
Use: Oral fluoride.

ELIXICON SUSPENSION. (Berlex) Anhydrous theophylline 100 mg./5 ml. Bot 237 ml.
Use: Bronchial asthma treatment.

ELIXIRAL. (Vita Elixir) Phenobarbital 16.20 mg., hyoscyamine sulfate 0.1037 mg., atropine sulfate 0.194 mg., hyoscine HB 0.0065 mg./5 cc. Liq. pt., gal.
Use: Sedative, antispasmodic.

ELIXOMIN. (Cenci) Theophylline 80 mg., alcohol 20%/15 ml. Bot. Pts., Gal.
Use: Bronchial asthma treatment.

ELIXOPHYLLIN CAPSULES, DYE-FREE. (Berlex) Anhydrous theophylline 100 mg., 200 mg./Cap. 100 mg. Bot. 100s. 200 mg. Bot. 100s, 500s. Unit dose 100s.
Use: Bronchial asthma, chronic bronchitis & chronic obstructive pulmonary emphysema.

ELIXOPHYLLIN ELIXIR. (Berlex) Anhydrous theophylline 80 mg., alcohol 20%/15 ml. Bot. 473 ml., 946 ml., 3785 ml.
Use: Bronchial asthma, chronic bronchitis & chronic obstructive pulmonary emphysema.

ELIXOPHYLLIN-GG. (Berlex) Theophylline 100 mg., guaifenesin 100 mg./15 ml. Bot. 237 ml., 473 ml.
Use: Asthma & bronchospasm associated with chronic bronchitis, emphysema.

ELIXOPHYLLIN-KI ELIXIR. (Berlex) Anhydrous theophylline 80 mg., potassium iodide 130 mg., alcohol 10%/15 ml. Bot. 237 ml., gal.
Use: Excessive tenacious mucus in chronic asthma, severe chronic and allergic bronchitis, chronic obstructive pulmonary emphysema.

ELIXOPHYLLIN SR CAPSULES. (Berlex) Anhydrous theophylline 125 mg. or 250 mg./Sustained Released Cap. Bot. 100s, 500s, 1000s. Unit dose 100s.
Use: Bronchial asthma treatment.

ELLESDINE. (Janssen) Pipenperone.
Use: Tranquilizer.

ELLIMAN'S EMBROCATION LINIMENT. (CMC) Bot. 4 oz.
Use: Muscle pain, chest colds, rheumatism, lumbago.

ELON. p-Methylaminophenol.

ELOXYL. (Elder) Benzoyl peroxide 5% and 10% in gel base. Tubes 2 oz.
Use: Acne vulgaris treatment.

ELPHEMET. (Canright) Phendimetrazine tartrate 35 mg./Tab. Bot. 100s, 1000s.
Use: Anorexiant.

ELPRECAL. (Canright) Vit. A 5000 I.U., D 400 I.U., B-1 3 mg., B-2 2 mg., B-6 0.1 mg., B-12 1 mcg., C 50 mg., E 2 I.U., Ca pantothenate 2.5 mg., niacinamide 15 mg., inositol 5 mg., choline 5 mg., Ca lactate 500 mg., ferrous sulfate 50 mg., Cu 1 mg., Mn 1 mg., Mg 2 mg., K 2 mg., Zn 0.5 mg., S 1 mg./Cap. Bot. 100s.

ELSERPINE. (Canright) Reserpine 0.25 mg./Tab. Bots. 100s, 1000s.
Use: Hypotensive-tranquilizing agent.

ELSPAR. (Merck Sharp & Dohme) Asparaginase 10,000 I.U., mannitol 80 mg./vial.
Use: Acute lymphocytic leukemia therapy.

• **ELUCAINE.** USAN.
Use: Anticholinergic.

ELVANOL. (Du Pont) Polyvinyl Alcohol.

EMAGRIN. (Otis Clapp) Salicylamide, caffeine, aspirin/Tab. Sugar and salt free. Bot. 60s, 100s. Unit Box 20s.
Use: Analgesic, anti-inflammatory.

EMAGRIN FORTE. (Otis Clapp) Phenylephrine HCl, atropine sulfate, acetaminophen, caffeine/Tab. Sugar and salt free. Safety Pkg. 1000s. Bot. 100s, 1000s. AidPaks 100s. Unit boxes 8s, 16s.
Use: Analgesic, decongestant for colds, hay fever, sinusitis relief.

EMAGRIN PROFESSIONAL STRENGTH. (Otis Clapp) Aspirin, salicylamide, caffeine. Sugar and salt free. Safety packs 1000s, Medipaks 200s, Aidpaks 100s, Unit boxes 10s, 20s. Bot. 1000s.
Use: Analgesic, anti-inflammatory.

EMBECHINE. Aliphatic chloroethylamine.
Use: Treatment of cancer.

EMBEQUIN. Di-iodohydroxyquinoline, B.A.N.

EMBRAMINE. B.A.N. N-2-(4-Bromo-α-methylbenzhy-dryloxy)ethyldimethylamine.
Use: Antihistamine.
See: Mebryl (hydrochloride)

EMBRON CAPSULES. (T. E. Williams) Dyphylline 200 mg., guaifenesin 100 mg./Cap. Bot. 100s, 1000s.
Use: Bronchodilator-expectorant.

EMBUTRAMIDE. B.A.N. N-[2-Ethyl-2-(3-methoxy-phenyl)butyl]-4-hydroxybutyramide.
Use: Narcotic analgesic.

EMCYT. (Roche) Estramustine phosphate sodium 140 mg. Cap. Bot. 100s.
Use: Palliative treatment of patients with metatstatic and/or progressive carcinoma of the prostate.

EMDOL. (Approved) Salicylamide, para-aminobenzoic acid, sod. cal. succinate, Vit. D-1250. Bot. 100s, 1000s.
Use: Arthritis, rheumatism.

EMEPRONIUM BROMIDE. B.A.N. Ethyldimethyl-1-methyl-3,3-diphenylpropylammonium bromide.
Use: Anticholinergic.
See: Cetiprin.

EMERGENCY ANA-KIT. (Hollister-Stier). 1 sterile syringe containing 1 cc. epinephrine 1:1000. Each cc. contains 1 mg. epinephrine as hydrochloride, 5 mg. chlorobutanol (chloral derivative), 8.5 mg. sodium chloride and 1.5 mg. sodium bisulfite as preservative.
Use: Insect sting kit.

EMEROID. (Delta) Zinc oxide 5%, diperodon HCl 0.25%, bismuth subcarbonate 0.2%, pyrilamine maleate 0.1%, phenylephrine HCl 0.25%, in a petrolatum base containing codliver oil/1¼ oz. Tube 1¼ oz.
Use: Hemorrhoid relief.

EMERSAL. (Medco Lab) Ammoniated mercury 5%, salicylic acid 2.5%, castor oil 23%, liquid petrolatum, polyoxyl 40 stearate, polysorbate 80, and water. Plastic bot. 4 oz.
Use: Psoriasis of the scalp, isolated psoriatic lesions, and seborrheic dermatitis.

EMESIS. (Kenyon) Levulose and dextrose 57.6 Gm., orthophosphoric acid 0.5 Gm./100 cc. Bot. 4 oz., pt., gal.

EMETAN, 6′,7′,10,11-TETRAMETHOXY-,DIHYDRO-CHLORIDE. Emetine Hydrochloride, U.S.P. XXI.

EMETE-CON. (Roerig) Benzquinamide HCl 25 mg., 25 mg./ml. Citric acid 1%. Vial 50 mg. 10s.
Use: Antiemetic.

EMETICON. (Roerig) Benzquinamide.

EMETICS.
See: Apomorphine HCl
Cupric Sulf.
Ipecac Syr.

EMETINE BISMUTH IODIDE.
Use: Same as Emetine HCl.

• **EMETINE HYDROCHLORIDE,** U.S.P. XXI. Inj., U.S.P. XXI. Emetan, 6′, 7′, 10,11-tetramethoxy-,diHCl.
Use: Antiamebic.

EMETROL. (Rorer) Oral Soln. containing balanced amounts of levulose (fructose) and dextrose (glucose) with orthophosphoric acid, stabilized at an optimal pH. Bot. 3 oz., 1 pt.
Use: Antinauseant.

EMFASEEM. (Saron) **Liquid:** Dyphylline 100 mg., guaifenesin 50 mg./15 ml. w/alcohol 5%. Bot. pt. **Cap.:** Dyphylline 200 mg., guaifenesin 100 mg./Cap. Bot. 100s, 1000s. Unident 100s. **Inj.** Vial 10 cc.
Use: Asthma therapy.

EM-GG. (Econo Med) Guaifenesin 100 mg./5 cc. Bot. Pts.
Use: Expectorant.

• **EMILIUM TOSYLATE.** USAN.
Use: Cardiac depressant.

EM-K-10%. (Econo Med) Potassium 40 meq./30 ml. Bot. Pts.
Use: Potassium chloride supplement.

EMKO BECAUSE CONTRACEPTOR.
(Emko-Schering) Nonoxynol-9 (8% concentration).
Contraceptor container w/applicator. Tube 10 Gm.
Use: Vaginal contraceptive.
EMKO PRE-FIL. (Emko-Schering) Nonoxynol-9(8%
concentration). Aerosol Can 30 Gm. Refill 60 Gm.
Use: Vaginal contraceptive.
EMKO VAGINAL FOAM. (Emko-Schering) Nonoxynol-9
(8% concentration). Kit. Aerosol w/applicator. 45
Gm. Refill 45 Gm., 90 Gm.
Use: Vaginal contraceptive.
EMOLLIA-CREME. (Gordon) Cetylalcohol, lubricating
oils in water-soluble base. Jar 4 oz., 5 lbs.
Use: Non-soap cleansing agent, treatment dry skin.
EMOLLIA-LOTION. (Gordon) Water-dispersable
waxes, lubricating bland oils in a water-soluble lotion
base. Bot. 1 oz., 4 oz., gal.
Use: Dry, scaly skin, especially over extensive areas.
EMPIRIN ASPIRIN TABLETS. (Burroughs Wellcome)
Aspirin 325 ml./Tab. Bot. 25s, 50s, 100s, 250s.
Use: Oral analgesic.
EMPIRIN COMPOUND. (Burroughs Wellcome)
Product discontinued from market.
EMPIRIN WITH CODEINE. (Burroughs Wellcome)
Aspirin 325 mg. with codeine phosphate 15 mg., 30
mg., 60 mg./Tab. **No. 2** codeine phosphate 15 mg.
(¼ gr.). Bot. 100s, 1000s **No. 3** codeine
phosphate 30 mg. (½ gr.) Bot. 100s, 500s, 1000s.
Dispenserpak 25s. **No. 4** codeine phosphate 60
mg. (1 gr.). Bot. 100s, 500s, 1000s. Dispenserpak
25s.
Use: Orally; analgesic & antipyretic.
EMPRACET WITH CODEINE NO. 3. (Burroughs
Wellcome) Acetaminophen 300 mg., codeine
phosphate 30 mg./Tab. Bot. 100s, 500s.
Dispenserpak 25s.
Use: Narcotic analgesic for moderate to severe
pain.
EMPRACET WITH CODEINE NO. 4. (Burroughs
Wellcome) Acetaminophen 300 mg., codeine
phosphate 60 mg./Tab. Bot. 100s, 500s.
Use: Narcotic analgesic for moderate to severe
pain.
EMTRYL. Dimetridazole, B.A.N.
EMTRYL SOLUBLE POWDER. (Salsbury)
Dimetridazole 36.4 Gm./18.2 Gm. pouch.
Use: Blackhead treatment for turkeys.
EMULAVE. (CooperCare)
See: Aveenobar Oilated (CooperCare)
EMUL-O-BALM. (Pennwalt) Menthol, camphor, methyl
salicylate. Bot. 2 oz., 8 oz., gal.
Use: Topical analgesic.
EMULSOIL. (Paddock) Castor oil. Bot. 2 oz.
Use: Laxative.
E-MYCIN. (Upjohn) Erythromycin **250 mg.**/Tab. Bot.
100s, 500s. Unit-dose 100s. Unit-of-Use 40s. **333 mg.**
/Tab. Bot. 100s, 500s. Unit dose 100s.
Use: Antibacterial.
E-MYCIN E. (Upjohn) Erythromycin ethylsuccinate
equivalent to erythromycin 200 mg./5 ml. or 400
mg./5 ml. Bot. 500 ml.
Use: Antibiotic.

EMYLCAMATE. B.A.N. 1-Ethyl-1-methylpropyl carba-
mate.
Use: Tranquilizer; muscle relaxant.
See: Striatran
• **ENALAPRIL MALEATE.** USAN.
Use: Antihypertensive.
• **ENALAPRILAT.** USAN.
ENARAX (Beecham Labs) Oxyphencyclimine HCl 5
mg. or 10 mg., hydroxyzine HCl 25 mg./Tab. Bot.
60s.
Use: Anticholinergic; anti-anxiety.
E-NATURAL. (Columbia) Natural Vit. E Cream. Jar 2 oz.
Use: Hand, face and body care.
ENBUCRILATE. B.A.N. Butyl 2-cyanoacrylate.
Use: Surgical tissue adhesive.
See: Histoacryl
ENCAINIDE HYDROCHLORIDE. (Mead Johnson)
(USAN)
Use: Investigative: Antiarrhythmic.
• **ENCAINIDE HYDROCHLORIDE.** USAN.
Use: Cardiac depressant.
ENCARE. (Thompson Medical) Vaginal contraceptive
suppository w/noroxynol-9 (2.3%).
Use: Contraceptive.
EN-CEBRIN. (Lilly) Vit. A 4000 I.U., B-1 3 mg., B-2 2 mg.,
niacinamide 10 mg., B-6 1.7 mg., B-12 5 mcg., panto-
thenic acid 5 mg., C 50 mg., D 400 I.U., Ca
carbonate 250 mg., ferrous fumarate 30 mg., iodine
0.15 mg., Cu 1 mg., Mg 5 mg., Mn 1 mg., Zn 1.5
mg./Pulvule. Bot. 100s.
Use: Prenatal vitamin and mineral supplement.
EN-CEBRIN F. (Lilly) Vit. A 4000 I.U., B-1 3 mg., B-2 2
mg., niacinamide 10 mg., B-6 2 mg., folic acid 1 mg.,
B-12 5 mcg., Ca pantothenate 5 mg., C 50 mg., D 400
I.U., Ca carbonate 250 mg., ferrous fumarate 30
mg., iodine 0.15 mg., Cu 1 mg., Mg 5 mg., Mn 1
mg., Zn 1.5 mg./Pulvule. Rx Pak 100s.
Use: Vitamin-mineral deficiencies associated with
pregnancy and lactation.
• **ENCLOMIPHENE.** USAN.
• **ENCYPRATE.** USAN. Ethyl N-benzylcyclopropane-
carbamate.
Use: Antidepressant.
END-AKE ANALGESIC CREAM. (Columbia) Methyl
nicotinate, salicylamide, histamine dihydrochloride,
dipropylene glycol salicylate, capsicum oleoresin.
Tube 1¼ oz.
Use: Muscular aches, simple neuralgia.
END-A-KOFF 6-WAY COUGH SYRUP. (Columbia) Dextromethorphan 15 mg., guaifenesin 50 mg.,
chlorpheniramine maleate 2 mg., phenylephrine HCl
5 mg., acetaminophen 120 mg., alcohol 10%/2
teaspoonfuls. Bot. 4 oz.
Use: Cough-suppressant, antihistamine.
ENDAL. (UAD Labs) Phenylephrine HCl 20 mg.,
chlorpheniramine maleate 4 mg., guaifenesin 300
mg./Timed Release Tab., dye free. Bot. 100s.
Use: Nasal decongestant.
ENDAL EXPECTORANT. (UAD Labs) Codeine
phosphate 10 mg., phenylpropanolamine HCl 5
mg., phenylephrine HCl 5 mg., chlorpheniramine

maleate 2 mg., guaifenesin 100 mg., alcohol 5%/5 ml. Bot. Pts.
Use: Common cold therapy.

ENDECON. (Du Pont) Acetaminophen 325 mg., phenylpropanolamine HCl 25 mg./Tab. Bot. 60s.
Use: Decongestant analgesic and antipyretic.

ENDEP. (Roche) Amitriptyline HCl 10 mg., 25 mg., 50 mg., 75 mg., 100 mg. or 150 mg./Tab. Bot. 100s, 500s; Tel-E-Dose 100s; Pak 60s (10 mg., 25 mg., 50 mg.) or 30s (75 mg., 100 mg., 150 mg.); Tray 10s.
Use: Antidepressant.

ENDOBENZILINE BROMIDE. N,N-(dimethyl)-amino-ethyl-α-(bicyclo[2.2.1]-5-neptenyl) mandelate methyl bromide.
Use: Anticholinergic.

ENDOCAINE. Pyrrocaine.
Use: Local anesthetic.

ENDOLOR. (Keene) Butalbital 50 mg., caffeine 40 mg., acetaminophen 325 mg./Cap. Bot. 100s.
Use: Analgesic, sedative.

ENDOJODIN.
See: Entodon

ENDOMYCIN. A new antibiotic obtained from cultures of *Streptomyces endus*. Under study.

ENDOPHENOLPHTHALEIN. (Roche) Diacetyldioxyphenylisatin-Isacen-Bisatin.
Use: Laxative.
See: Diacetylhydroxphenylisatin, Prep. (Various Mfr.)

ENDOTUSSIN-NN. (Du Pont) Dextromethorphan HBr 10 mg., pyrilamine maleate 7.5 mg., ammonium chloride 40 mg./5 ml. w/alcohol 4%. Syrup Bot. 4 oz.
Use: Antitussive, antihistaminic.

ENDOTUSSIN-NN PEDIATRIC SYRUP. (Du Pont) Dextromethorphan HBr 5 mg., ammonium chloride 60 mg., alcohol 4%/5 ml. Syrup, Bot. 4 fl. oz.
Use: Antitussive, antihistaminic.

ENDOXANA. Cyclophosphamide, B.A.N.
• **ENDRALAZINE MESYLATE.** USAN.
Use: Antihypertensive.
• **ENDRYSONE.** USAN.
Use: Anti-inflammatory.

ENDURON. (Abbott) Methyclothiazide 2.5 mg./Tab. Bot. 100s, 1000s. 5 mg. Bot. 100s, 1000s, 5000s. Abbo-Pac 100s.
Use: Antihypertensive.

ENDURONYL. (Abbott) Methyclothiazide 5 mg., deserpidine 0.25 mg./Tab. Bot. 100s, 1000s. Abbo-Pac 100s.
Use: Antihypertensive.

ENDURONYL FORTE. (Abbott) Methyclothiazide 5 mg., deserpidine 0.5 mg./Tab. Bot. 100s, 1000s.
Use: Antihypertensive.

ENERJETS. (Chilton) Caffeine 65 mg./Loz. Pkg. 10s.
Use: CNS stimulant.

ENFAMIL. (Mead Johnson) Vit. A 2000 I.U., D 400 I.U., E 20 I.U., C 52 mg., B-1 0.5 mg., B-2 1.0 mg., B-6 0.4 mg., B-12 1.5 mcg., niacin 8 mg., Ca 440 mg., P 300 mg., folic acid 100 mcg., pantothenic acid 3 mg., inositol 30 mg., biotin 15 mcg., K-1 55 mcg., choline 100 mg., Fe 1.4 mg., K 650 mg., Cl 400

mg., Cu 0.6 mg., iodine 65 mcg., Na 200 mg., Mg 50 mg., Zn 5 mg., Mn 100 mg./Qt. Con. Liq. 13 fl. oz., Inst. Pow. 1 lb.
Use: Infant feeding formula containing vitamins and minerals.

ENFAMIL READY TO USE. (Mead Johnson) Ready-to-use Enfamil infant formula 20 kcal./fl. oz. Cans 8 fl. oz., 6-can pack; 32 fl. oz., 6 cans per case.

ENFAMIL WITH IRON. (Mead Johnson) Iron 12 mg./Qt. Pkg. Con. Liq. 13 fl. oz. 24s. Pow. 1 lb. 12s.
Use: Infant feeding.

ENFAMIL W/IRON READY TO USE. (Mead Johnson) Ready-to-use Enfamil with Iron infant formula 20 kcal./fl. oz. Cans 8 fl. oz., 6-can pack; 32 fl. oz. 6 cans per case.

ENFAMIL NURSETTE. (Mead Johnson) Glass formula bottle filled with ready-to-feed Enfamil, 20 kcal./fl. oz. 4 fl. oz., 6 fl. oz., and 8 fl. oz., four bottles/sealed carton. W/Iron. Ready to use. Bot. 6 fl. oz. 4s, 24s.

• **ENFLURANE,** U.S.P. XXI. 2-Chloro-1,1,2-trifluoroethyl difluoromethyl ether. Ethrane (Ohio Medical)
Use: Anesthetic (inhalation).

ENGRAN-HP. (Squibb) Vit. A 8000 I.U., D 400 I.U., B-1 1.7 mg., B-2 2 mg., B-6 2.5 mg., B-12 8 mcg., niacinamide 20 mg., C 60 mg., E 30 I.U., folic acid 0.8 mg., Ca 650 mg., iodine 0.15 mg., Fe 18 mg., Cu 2 mg., Mg 100 mg./2 Tabs. Bot. 100s.
Use: Vitamin and mineral supplement for pregnant or lactating women.

• **ENILCONAZOLE.** USAN.
Use: Antifungal.
• **ENISOPROST.** USAN.

ENISYL. (Person & Covey) L-Lysine monohydrochloride 334 mg. or 500mg./Tab. Bot. 100s, 250s.
Use: Dietary supplement.

ENNEX OINTMENT. (Ennex) Aloe vera ext. 37.5%. **Skin Oint.:** Zinc oxide 12.5%, coal tar 1.5%, alcohol 4.5%. Tube 1 oz. **Hemorrhoidal Oint.:** Tube 1 oz.
Use: Anti-inflammatory, astringent, antipruritic.

ENO. (Beecham Products) Sodium tartrate, sodium citrate. Bot. 3 ⅞ oz., 7 ¾ oz.
Use: Acid indigestion.

• **ENOLICAM SODIUM.** USAN.
Use: Anti-inflammatory, antirheumatic.

ENOVID. (Searle) Norethynodrel and mestranol. **Tab. 5 mg.:** Norethynodrel 5 mg., mestranol 0.075 mg./Tab. Bot. 100s. **Tab. 10 mg.:** Norethynodrel 9.85 mg., mestranol 0.15 mg./Tab. Bot. 50s.
Use: Oral contraceptive (5 mg.); endometriosis, hypermenorrhea, production of cyclic withdrawal bleeding (5 mg., 10 mg.).

ENOVID-E 21. (Searle) Norethynodrel 2.5 mg., mestranol 0.1 mg./Tab. Compack disp. 21s, 6×21. Refills 21s, 12×21.
Use: Oral contraceptive.

ENOVIL. (Hauck) Amtriptyline HCl 10 mg./ml. Vial 10 ml.
Use: Antidepressant.

• **ENOXACIN.** USAN.

ENOXOLONE. B.A.N. 3β-Hydroxy-11-oxo-olean-12-en-30-oic acid.
Use: Treatment of skin diseases.
See: Biosone

ENPIPRAZOLE. B.A.N. 1-(2-Chlorophenyl)-4-[2-(1-methylpyrazol-4-yl)ethyl]piperazine.
Use: Psychotropic drug.

• **ENPROMATE.** USAN.
Use: Antineoplastic.

• **ENPROSTIL.** USAN.

ENSIDON. (Geigy) Opipramol HCl.

ENSURE. (Ross) Each 32 fl. oz. contains: Protein 35.2 Gm., fat 35.2 Gm., carbohydrate 137.2 Gm., Vit. A 2500 I.U., D 200 I.U. E 30 I.U., K 140 mcg., C 0.15 Gm., folic acid 0.20 mg., B-1 1.5 mg., B-2 1.7 mg., B-6 2.0 mg., B-12 6.0 mcg., niacin 20 mg., choline 0.50 Gm., biotin 0.15 mg., pantothenic acid 5.0 mg., Na 0.80 Gm., potassium 1.5 Gm., Cl 1.36 Gm., P 0.50 Gm., Mg. 0.20 Gm., iodine 0.075 mg., Mn 2.0 Gm., Cu 1.0 mg., Zn 15 mg., Ca. 0.50 Gm., Fe. 9.0 mg./32 oz. W/corn syrup solids, sucrose, corn oil, soy protein isolate, soy lecithin, carrageenan, artificial flavoring. **Bot.:** 8 oz. Gavage set. Case 24s; **Cans:** 8 oz., 32 oz. Case 24s. **Powder:** 14 oz. cans. **Gavage Feeding Set:** 8 oz. Bot.
Use: Dietary supplement providing complete balanced nutrition for full liquid diet, liquid supplement or tube feeding.

ENSURE OSMOLITE. (Ross)
See: Osmolite, (Ross)

ENSURE PLUS. (Ross) Each 32 fl. oz. contains: Protein 52.0 Gm., fat 50.4 Gm., carbohyrate 189.2 Gm., Vit. A 3560 I.U., D 280 I.U., E 42.8 I.U., K 200 mcg., C 152 mg., folic acid 300 mg., B-1 2.5 mg., B-2 2.6 mg., B-6 3.0 mg., B-12 9.0 mcg., niacin 30 mg., biotin 224 mcg., choline 500 mg., pantothenic acid 8.0 mg., Na 1.08 Gm., potassium 2.2 Gm., Cl 1.9 Gm., Ca 0.60 Gm., P 0.60 Gm., Mg 300 mg., Mn 2.0 mg., iodine 100 mcg., Cu 1.5 mg., Fe 13.5 mg., Zn 22.5 mg./32 oz. W/corn syrup solids, sodium and calcium caseinates, corn oil, sucrose, soy protein isolate, soy lecithin, carrageenan, artificial flavoring. Cans 8 oz.
Use: Complete dietary supplement.

ENTAB-650. (Mayrand) Aspirin 650 mg./Enteric coated tab. Bot. 100s.
Use: Pain of arthritis and rheumatism.

ENTAMIDE. Diloxanide, B.A.N.

ENTEROTUBE. (Roche) Culture-identification method for enteriobacteriacea ACA. Test Kit 25s.

ENTEX. (Norwich Eaton) Phenylephrine HCl 5 mg., phenylpropanolamine HCl 45 mg., guaifenesin 200 mg./Cap. Bot. 100s, 500s.
Use: Decongestant.

ENTEX LA. (Norwich Eaton) Phenylpropanolamine HCl 75 mg., guaifenesin 400 mg., /T.R. Tab. Bot. 100s.
Use: Long acting decongestant.

ENTEX LIQUID. (Norwich Eaton) Phenylphrine HCl 5 mg., phenylpropanolamine HCl 20 mg., guaifenesin 100 mg./5 cc. Alcohol 5%. Elix. Bot. pt.
Use: Decongestant.

ENTIRE B W/C. (Pharmex) Vitamin B complex with Vitamin C. Cap. Bot. 100s, 1000s.

ENTODON. Propiodal, Entoidoin, Endojodin, 2-Hydroxy-trimethylene-bis-(trimethylammonium iodide)

ENTOIDOIN.
See: Entodon

ENTOZYME. (Robins) Pepsin 250 mg., pancreatin 300 mg., bile salts 150 mg./Tab. Bot. 100s, 500s.
Use: Digestant.

• **ENTSUFFEN SODIUM.** USAN.
Use: Detergent.

E.N.T. SYRUP. (Springbok) Brompheniramine maleate 4 mg., phenylephrine HCl 5 mg., phenylpropanolamine HCl 5 mg./5 ml. Bot. 16 oz., Gal.
Use: Nasal decongestant, antihistaminic.

E.N.T. TABLETS. (Springbok) Phenylephrine HCl 25 mg., phenylpropanolamine HCl 50 mg., chlorpheniramine maleate 8 mg./S.A. Tab. Bot. 100s, 500s.
Use: Nasal decongestant, antihistaminic.

ENTUSS. (Hauck) **Tab.:** Hydrocodone bitartrate 5 mg., guaifenesin 300 mg./Tab. Bot. 100s. **Liquid:** Hydrocodone bitartrate 5 mg., guaifenesin 300 mg./5 ml. Bot. 4 oz., 16 oz. Sugar Free.
Use: Expectorant.

ENUCLENE. (Alcon) Tyloxapol 0.25%, benzalkonium chloride 0.02%, hydroxypropyl methyl cellulose 0.85%. Soln. Drop-tainers of 15 cc.
Use: Lubricant; ocular prosthesis aid.

• **ENVIRADENE.** USAN.
Use: Antiviral.

• **ENVIROXIME.** USAN.
Use: Antiviral.

ENZACTIN CREAM. (Ayerst) Triacetin 250 mg./Gm. Tube 1 oz.
Use: Athlete's foot & other superficial fungus infections.

ENZEST. (Barth's) Seven natural enzymes and 250 mg., Ca. carbonate/Tab. Bot. 100s, 250s, 500s.

▪ **ENZYMES.**
See: Alpha Chymar, Vial (Armour)
Ananase, Tab. (Rorer)
Cholinesterase (Various Mfr.)
Chymotrypsin
Cotazym, Cap. (Organon)
Diastase (Various Mfr.)
Dornavac, Vial (Merck Sharp & Dohme)
Fibrinolysin
Hyaluronidase (Various Mfr.)
Neutrapen, Vial (Riker)
Pancreatin (Various Mfr.)
Papain (Var. Mfr.)
Papase, Tab. (Warner-Chilcott)
Penicillinase (Var. Mfr.)
Pepsin (Various Mfr.)
Plasmin
Rennin (Various Mfr.)
Taka-Diastase, Prep. (Parke-Davis)

Travase, Oint. (Flint)
Tri-Cone, Cap. (Glaxo)
Thrombolysin, I.V. Inj. (Merck Sharp & Dohme)
Varidase, Prep. (Lederle)
ENZYME FORMULA #E-2. (Barth's) Amylase 30 mg.,
lipase 25 mg., bile salts 1 gr., wilzyme 10 mg.,
pepsin 2 gr., pancreatin 0.5 gr., Ca carbonate 4
gr./Tab. Bot. 100s, 250s.
Use: Digestive aid.
ENZYMET. (O'Neal, Jones & Feldman) Pancreatin
300 mg., pepsin 200 mg., taurocholic acid 40
mg./Tab. Bot. 72.
Use: Indigestion.
ENZYPAN. (Norgine) Peptic potency equiv. to pepsin
0.009 Gm., amylolytic potency equiv. to pancreatin
0.276 Gm. proteolytic potency equiv. to pancreatin
0.372 Gm., lipolytic potency equiv. to pancreatin
0.370 Gm., ox bile desic. 0.056 Gm./Tab. Vial
120s, 500s.
Use: Digestive enzyme deficiencies.
• **EPHEDRINE,** U.S.P. XXI. l-α-[1-(Methylamino)-ethyl]-
benzyl alcohol. (Various Mfr.) (−)-erythro-α-[1-(Me-
thylamino)ethyl]benzyl Alcohol.
Use: Adrenergic (bronchodilator).
See: Bofedrol Inhalant (Bowman)
Racephedrine HCl (Various Mfr.)
W/Procaine.
See: Ephedrine and Procaine, Rx "A", Amp. (Lilly)
W/Pyrilamine maleate, guaifenesin, theophylline.
W/Theophylline, guaifenesin, phenobarbital.
See: Duovent, Tab. (Riker)
EPHEDRINE & AMYTAL. (Lilly) Ephedrine sulfate 25
mg. & Amytal 50 mg./Pulvule. Bot. 100s.
EPHEDRINE HYDROCHLORIDE, U.S.P. XXI. l-a-[1-
(Methylamino) ethyl]benzyl alcohol hydrochloride.
(−)-erythro-α-[1-(Methylamino)ethyl]-benzyl Alcohol
hydrochloride. (Various Mfr.); Cryst. Box ⅛ oz., ¼
oz., 4 oz.
Use: Adrenergic (bronchodilator)
EPHEDRINE HCl W/COMBINATIONS.
See: Airet R, Tab. (Baylor)
Airet Y, Tab., Elix. (Baylor)
Amphed, Cap. (Wolins)
Anoids Rectal, Supp. (Scrip)
Asmadil-S Susp. (Reid-Provident)
Asma-lief, Tab., Susp. (Columbia)
Asthmacon, Cap. (CMC)
Bofedral, Liq. (Bowman)
Bronchobid, Cap. (Glaxo)
Brondilate, Tab. (Walker)
Bron-Sed, Elix. (Southern Pharm.)
Calcidrine, Syr. (Abbott)
Ceepa, Tab. (Geneva)
Codel, Syr. (Elder)
Coryza Brengle, Cap. (Mallard)
Co-Xan, Elix. (Central)
Dainite-Day, Tab. (Mallinckrodt)
Dainite-KI, Tab. (Mallinckrodt)
Derma Medicone (Medicone)
Derma Medicone HC, Oint. (Medicone)
Dilacap, Cap. (Coastal)
Duovent, Tab. (Riker)

Ectasule, Ectasule Minus, Cap. (Fleming)
Emphysal, Cap. (Douglas)
Epragen, Pulv. (Lilly)
Fedacaps, Cap. (Freeport)
Golacal, Syr. (Arcum)
Hemocaine, Oint. (Mallard)
Histamead E.C., Liq. (Spencer-Mead)
Kie, Tab., Syr. (Laser)
Lardet Expectorant, Tab. (Standex)
Lardet, Tab. (Standex)
Luftodil, Tab. (Mallinckrodt)
Lufyllin-EP, Tab. (Mallinckrodt)
Lufyllin-EPG, Tab., Elix. (Mallinckrodt)
Mudrane GG, Tab. (Poythress)
Mudrane, Tab. (Poythress)
Myringacaine, Liq. (Upjohn)
Panaphyllin, Susp. (Panamerican)
Phedral, Tab. (Vortech)
Pyrralan DM, Expect. (Lannett)
Quadrinal, Tab., Susp. (Knoll)
Quelidrine, Syr. (Abbott)
Quibron Plus (Mead Johnson)
Tedfern, Tab. (Ferndale)
Tedral-25, Tab. (Warner-Chilcott)
T.E.P., Tab. (Kirkman)
T-E-P Compound, Tab. (Stanlabs)
Thalfed, Tab. (Beecham Labs)
Theofed, Tab. (Sutliff-Case)
Theofedral, Tab. (Redford)
Theofenal, Susp., Tab. (Spencer-Mead)
Theo-Kaps, Caps. (Scrip)
Theo-Span, Cap. (Scrip)
EPHEDRINE HYDROCHLORIDE NASAL JELLY.
See: Efedron Hydrochloride, Oint. (Hart)
EPHEDRINE and PHENOBARBITAL. (Jenkins)
Phenobarbital ¼ gr., ephedrine HCl ⅜ gr./Tab.
Bot. 1000s.
EPHEDRINE-RELATED COMPOUNDS.
See: Sympathomimetic Agents
• **EPHEDRINE SULFATE,** U.S.P. XXI. Caps., Inj.,
Nasal Soln., Syrup, Tabs., U.S.P. XXI.
(−)-erythro-α-[1-(Methylamino)ethyl]-benzyl Alcohol.
Benzenemethanol, α-[1-(methylamino)ethyl]-, sulfate
(2:1) (salt). (Various Manufacturers). **Inj.:** (Abbott)
50 mg./1 ml. ampul.
Use: Adrenergic (bronchodilator, nasal
decongestant).
Use: Adrenergic, bronchodilator.
See: Ectasule Minus, Jr. & Sr., Caps. (Fleming)
Isofedrol, Isotonic Solution (Blue Line)
Slo-Fedrin, Cap. (Dooner)
EPHEDRINE SULFATE W/COMBINATIONS
See: Asminorel (Reid-Provident)
Asminyl, Tab. (Cole)
Bifed, Cap. (Alto)
B.M.E., Elix. (Brothers)
Bronkaid, Tab. (Winthrop Products)
Bronkolixir, Elix. (Winthrop-Breon)
Bronkotabs (Winthrop-Breon)
C.P.C. Cough Syr. (Coastal)
Ectasule, Cap. (Fleming)
Ectasule Minus, Cap. (Fleming)

Ephed-Organidin, Elix. (Wallace)
Eponal, Prep. (Cenci)
Fednal, Cream (Blue Line)
Flavihist, Cap. (American Labs)
Hycoff-X, Expect. (Saron)
Iso-Asminyl, Tab. (Cole)
Isuprel Compound, Elix. (Winthrop-Breon)
Luasmin, Cap. (Cooper)
Marax DF, Syr. (Roerig)
Marax, Tab., Syr. (Roerig)
Maso-Thylline, Tab. (Mason)
Neogen, Supp. (Premo)
Nyquil, Liq. (Vicks)
Pazo, Oint., Supp. (Bristol-Myers)
Pheno-Fed, Tab. (Wendt-Bristol)
PBZ w/Ephedrine, Expect, Tab. (Geigy)
PBZ Expect. w/Ephedrine and Codeine (Geigy)
Rectacort, Supp. (Century)
Thymodyne, Tab. (Noyes)
Tri-Hist-Cap (Burgin-Arden)
Va-Tro-Nol, Nose Drops (Vicks)
Wyanoids, Preps. (Wyeth)

• **EPHEDRINE SULFATE AND PHENOBARBITAL
CAPSULES,** U.S.P. XXI.
Use: Adrenergic (bronchodilator).

EPHEDRINE TANNATE
W/Carbetapentane tannate, chlorpheniramine
tannate, phenylephrine tannate.
See: Rynatuss, Tab., Susp. (Mallinckrodt)

1-EPHENAMINE PENICILLIN G. Compenamine.

EPHENYLLIN. (CMC) Theophylline 130 mg.,
ephedrine HCl 24 mg., phenobarbital 8 mg./Tab.
Bot. 100s, 500s, 1000s.
Use: Antiasthmatic, decongestant, sedative.

EPHRINE NASAL SPRAY. (Walgreen) Phenylephrine
HCl ¼%, ½%. Bot. 20 ml.
Use: Decongestant.

EPHRINITE NO. 1. (Kenyon) Phenylephrine HCl 5
mg., prophenpyridamine 12.5 mg./Tab. Bot. 100s.

• **EPICILLIN.** USAN. 6-(D-α-Aminocyclohexa-1,4-dien-
1-ylacetamido)penicillanic acid.
Use: Antibiotic.
See: Dexacillin

EPICORT LOTION. (Blue Line) Hydrocortisone 0.5%
or 1%, benzalkonium chloride 0.1% in a washable
base w/petrolatum, methylcellulose, glycerin,
polyethylene glycol ethers & perfume. Squeeze bot.
15 cc.
Use: Anti-inflammatory.

EPIFOAM. (Reed & Carnrick) Hydrocortisone acetate
1% g. pramoxine HCl, 1% in base of propylene
glycol, cetyl alcohol, PEG-100 stearate, glyceryl stearate, laureth-23, polyoxyl-40 stearate, methylparaben,
propylparaben, trolamine, or hydrochloric acid to
adjust pH, purified water, butane and propane inert
propellant. Aerosol container 10 Gm.
Use: Corticosteroid responsive dermatoses.

EPIFORM-HC. (Delta) Hydrocortisone 1%, iodohydroxyquin 3% in cream base. Tubes 20 Gm.
Use: Dermatological disorders.

EPIFRIN. (Allergan) Levo-epinephrine (as HCl) ½%,
1%, 2%. W/benzalkonium chloride, sod. metabisulfite,

edetate disodium, purified water. Bot. 5 ml., 15 ml. ¼%
also contains sodium chloride. Bot. 15 ml.
Use: Treatment of open angle glaucoma.

EPIFRIN OPHTHALMIC SOLUTION. (Allergan) Levo-
epinephrine HCl 0.25%, 0.5%, 1% or 2%. Bot.
w/dropper 5 ml. or 15 ml.
Use: Treatment of simple or chronic glaucoma.

■ **EPILEPSY.**
See: Anticonvulsants.

E-PILO. (CooperVision) Pilocarpine HCl 1%, 2%, 3%,
4%, & 6%, epinephrine bitartrate 1%,
benzalkonium chloride 0.01%, edetate disodium
0.01%. Bot. 10 cc. w/dropper-tip plastic vial.
Use: Chronic primary open-angle glaucoma.

• **EPIMESTROL.** USAN. 3-Methoxy-estra-1,3,5(10)-
triene-16α, 17α-diol. Stimovul (Organon).
Use: Anterior pituitary activator.

EPIMYCIN A. (Delta) Polymyxin B sulfate 5000 u.,
bacitracin 400 u., neomycin sulfate 3.5 mg.,
diperodon HCl 10 mg./Gm. Oint. Tube ½ oz.
Use: Antibacterial ointment.

EPINAL. (Alcon) Epinephrine as borate complex,
benzalkonium chloride 0.01%, ascorbic acid,
acetylcysteine, boric acid, sod. carborate. Dropper
Bot. 7.5 cc. ¼%, ½% or 1% strengths.
Use: Treatment of open-angle glaucoma.

EPINEPHRAN.
See: Epinephrine, Prep. (Various Mfr.)

• **EPINEPHRINE,** U.S.P. XXI. Inh., Soln., Aerosol, Inj.,
Nasal Soln., Ophth. Soln., Aerosol Soln., Inj.,
XXI. (−)-3,4-Dihydroxy-alpha-[(methylamino)methyl]-
benzyl Alcohol. 1,2-Benzenediol,4-[1-hydroxy-2-(methylamino)ethyl]-Inhalation. Adnephrine, adrenal,
adrenamine, adrenine, epinephran, eptreman,
hemisine, hemostatin, nephridine, levorenine,
paranephrin, renaglandin, renalina, supra-capsulin,
suprarenaline, suprarenin, renoform, renostypticin,
renostyptin, styptirenal, supradin, supranephrane,
surrenine, takamina, vasoconstrictine, vasotonin,
hypernephrin, renaleptine, scurenaline, nieraline.
Pediatric Inj.: (Abbott) Solution 0.01 mg./ml.; 5 ml.
single-dose Abboject Syr.
Use: Asthma, hay fever, acute allergic states,
cardiac arrest, acute hypersensitivity reactions.
See: Asthma Meter, Aerosol (Rexall)
  Asmolin, Vial (Lincoln)
  Emergency Ana-Kit (Hollister-Stier).
  Sus-Phrine, Inj. (Berlex)
W/Lidocaine HCl.
See: Ardecaine 1%, 2%, Inj. (Burgin-Arden)

• **EPINEPHRINE BITARTRATE,** U.S.P. XXI. Inhalation
Aerosol, Ophth. Soln., for Ophth. Soln., U.S.P. XXI.
Use: Adrenergic (ophthalmic).
See: Epitrate, Liq. (Averst)
W/Banzalkonium chloride.
See: Mytrate, Liq. (Softcon)
W/Pilocarpine HCl.
See: E-Pilo, Liq. (Smith, Miller & Patch)

EPINEPHRINE HYDROCHLORIDE.
Use: Adrenergic (ophthalmic).
See: Adrenalin Chloride, Sol. (Parke-Davis)
  Epifrin, Ophth. Sol. (Allergan)

Epinal, Opth. Sol. (Alcon)
Sus-Phrine, Amp., Vial (Berlex)
Vaponefrin Solution & Nebulizer, Vial (Fisons)
W/Benzalkonium Cl, sodium chloride, sodium
metabisulfite.
See: Glaucon, Sol. (Alcon)
W/Pilocarpine HCl.
See: Epicar, Sol. (Barnes-Hind)

EPINEPHRINE, RACEMIC.
See: Asthmanefrin Solution (Norcliff-Thayer)

EPINEPHRINE-RELATED COMPOUNDS.
See: Sympathomimetic Agents

• **EPINEPHRYL BORATE.** F.D.A. Cyclic (-)-4-[l-hydroxy-
2-(methylamino)ethyl]-o-phenylene borate.

• **EPINEPHRYL BORATE OPHTHALMIC SOLUTION,**
U.S.P. XXI. (−)-3,4-Dihydroxy-α-[(methyl-amino)me-
thyl]benzyl alcohol, cyclic 3,4-ester w/boric acid.
Use: Adrenergic (ophthalmic).
See: Epinal (Alcon)
Eppy (Barnes-Hind)

EPIOSTRIOL. B.A.N. Estra-1,3,5(10)-triene-3,16β,17β-
triol. 16-epiEstriol
Use: Estrogen.
See: Actriol

EPIPEN AUTO-INJECTOR. (Center) Epinephrine
injection 1:1000. Delivers dose of 0.3 mg. Pkg.
1s, 2s.
Use: Insect sting emergency.

EPIPHENETHICILLIN.   L-(a-phenoxy-propionamido)
penicillanic acid.

• **EPIPROPIDINE.** USAN. 1,1'-Bis(2,3-epoxypropyl)-4,4'
-bipiperidine. Eponate.
Use: Antineoplastic.

EPIRENAN.
See: Epinephrine (Various Mfr.)

• **EPIRIZOLE.** USAN.
Use: Analgesic, anti-inflammatory.

EPISONE. (Delta) Hydrocortisone 10 mg. in a base
containing steryl alcohol, white petrolatum, mineral
oil, propylene glycol, polyoxyl 40 stearate, purified
water and perserved with methyl & propyl
parabens. Tube 1 oz.
Use: Steroid.

• **EPITETRACYCLINE HYDROCHLORIDE,** U.S.P.
XXI.
Use: Antibiotic.

• **EPITHIAZIDE.** USAN. 3-[(2,2,2-Trifluoroethylthio)me-
thyl]-6-chloro-3,4-dihydro-2H-1,2,4-benzothiadiazine-
7-sulfonamide 1,1-dioxide.
Use: Hypotensive and diuretic.

EPITRATE. (Ayerst) Epinephrine bitartrate ophthalmic
solution 2%, equiv. to 1.1% base w/chlorobutanol
(chloral derivative 0.55%), sod. bisulfite, sod.
chloride, polyoxypropylene-polyoxyethylene-diol,
disodium edetate. Drop. Bot. 7.5 ml.
Use: Treatment of chronic simple (open-angle)
glaucoma.

E-PLUS. (Drug Industries) Vit. E 100 I.U., niacin 20 mg.,
lemon bioflavonoid complex 25 mg., C 50 mg.,
B-6 2 mg., B-1 5 mg./Tab. Bot. 100s, 500s.
Use: Vitamin E therapy.

E.P. MYCIN. (Edwards) Oxytetracycline HCl 250
mg./Cap. Bot. 100s.
Use: Antibiotic.

EPONAL. (Cenci) Theophylline 2 gr., ephedrine
sulfate ⅜ gr., phenobarbital ⅛ gr./Tab. Bot. 100s,
1000s.
Use: Asthma.

EPONAL-G. (Cenci) Theophylline 2 gr., ephedrine sulfate ⅜ gr., phenobarbital ⅛ gr., guaifenesin 1½
gr./Tab. Bot. 100s, 1000s.
Use: Anti-asthmatic.

• **EPOPROSTENOL.** USAN.
Use: Inhibitor.

• **EPOPROSTENOL SODIUM.** USAN.
Use: Inhibitor.

**EPOXYAMINOXYTROPINE TROPATE
HYDROBROMIDE.** Genoscopolamine HBr, Pellets.
(C.M.C.)

**4,5α-EPOXY-3-METHOXY-17-METHYLMORPHINAN-
6-ONE TARTRATE (1:1) HYDRATE (2:5).** Hydrocodone Bitartrate, U.S.P. XXI.

**6β,7β-EPOXY-1αH,5αH-TROPAN-3α-OL(−)-TRO-
PATE (ESTER)HYDROBROMIDE TRIHYDRATE.**
Scopolamine Hydrobromide, U.S.P. XXI.

EPOXYTROPINE TROPATE METHYLBROMIDE.
See: Methscopolamine Bromide. (Various Mfr.)

EPSAL. (Press) 80% Saturated sol. epsom salts in
oint. form. Jar 0.5 oz., 2 oz.
Use: Drawing ointment.

EPSIKAPRON. Aminocaproic Acid, B.A.N.

EPSILAN-M. (Adria) d-Alpha-Tocopherol acetate. Vit. E
Cap. (100 I.U.) Bot. 100s.

EPSIVITE 100. (Standex) Vit. E 100 I.U./Cap. Bot.
100s.

EPSIVITE 200. (Standex) Vit. E 200 I.U./Cap. Bot.
100s.

EPSIVITE 400. (Standex) Vit. E 400 I.U./Cap. Bot.
100s.

EPSIVITE FORTE. (Standex) Vit. E 1000 I.U./Cap.
Bot. 100s.
Use: Orally; hyaluronidase for collagen diseases.

EPSOM SALT.
See: Magnesium Sulfate.

EPTOIN.
See: Phenytoin Sodium (Var. Mfr.)

EQUAGESIC. (Wyeth) Meprobamate 200 mg., Aspirin
325 mg./Tab. Bot. 100s. Redi-pak 25s, 100s.
Use: Relief of pain accompanied by anxiety and
tension.

EQUAL. (Searle) Aspartame. **Packets** 0.035 oz. (1
Gm.). Box 50s, 100s, 200s. **Tab.** Bot. 100s.
Use: Low calorie sweetener.

EQUANIL. (Wyeth) Meprobamate 200 mg. or 400
mg./Tab. **200 mg.:** Bot. 50s, 100s, 500s. Redipax
25s, 100s. **400 mg.:** Bot. 50s, 100s, 500s, 1000s.
Redi Pak 25s, 100s. Wyseal 400 mg./Tab. Bot.
50s.
Use: Sedative and tranquilizing agent.

EQUIBOLIN-50. (Vortech) Nandrolone phenpropionate
50 mg./ml. Vial 2 ml. Box 1s.
Use: I.M.: androgen, anabolic agent.

EQUIGARD. Dichlorvos, B.A.N.

EQUILET. (Mission) Calcium carbonate 500 mg./Tab. Strip packed in 50s, 100s.
Use: Antacid.
• **EQUILIN,** U.S.P. XXI. Estra-1, 3-5 (10), 7-tetraen-17 one, 3 hydroxy-3-Hydroxestra-1,3,5 (10), 7-tetraen-17-one.
EQUIMATE SODIUM SALT. Fluprostenol, B.A.N.
EQUINE-ATOM ELIXIR. (Vortech) Vit. B-1 50 mg., B-2 16 mg., B-6 3 mg., B-12 25 mcg., niacinamide 200 mg., panthenol 10 mg., folic acid 1 mg., inositol 60 mg., choline chloride 150 mg., iron ammonium citrate 720 mg., alcohol 5%, palatable elix. q.s./cc. Bot., Gal.
EQUIPERTINE CAPSULES. (Winthrop Products) Oxypertine.
Use: Anxiolytic.
EQUIZOLE. (MSD AGVET) Thiabendazole: **Pellets:** 13.2%; **Powder:** 10 Gm./oz. **Suspension:** 4 Gm./oz.
Use: Anthelmintic, veterinary medicine.
EQUIZOLE A. (MSD AGVET) **Liquid:** thiabendazole 2 Gm., piperazine 2.5 Gm./oz.; **Powder:** thiabendazole 6.67 Gm., piperazine 8.33 Gm./oz.
Use: Anthelmintic, veterinary medicine.
EQUIZOLE B. (MSD AGVET) Thiabendazole 20 Gm., trichlorfon 18 Gm./package. Powder 0.42 oz. pkg.
Use: Anthelmintic & for bots, veterinary medicine.
EQVALAN. (MSD AGVET) Ivermectin injectable solution, paste: 200 mcg./Kg.
Use: Antiparasitic, veterinary medicine.
ERADACIL CAPSULES. (Winthrop Products) Rosoxacin.
Use: Antigonoccal agent.
ERASEN. (Winston) Phenobarbital 16 mg., Vit. B-1 5 mg./Tab. Bot. 100s, 1000s.
Use: Sedative w/Vit. B-1 therapy.
ERCAL. (Blue Line) Ergotamine tartrate 2 mg./Sublingual tab. 12s.
ERGAMISOL. (Janssen) Levamisole HCl.
Use: Anthelmentic (veterinary).
ERGOBEL. (Wolins) Ergotamine tartrate 0.3 mg., hyoscyamine 0.1 mg., phenobarbital 20 mg./Tab. Bot. 250s, 1000s.
ERGOCAF. (Robinson) Ergotamine tartrate, caffeine. Bot. 100s, 500s, 1000s.
ERGO CAFFEIN. (CMC) Ergotamine tartrate 1 mg., caffeine alkaloid USP 100 mg./Tab. Bot. 100s, 1000s.
Use: Terminating attacks of migraine headaches.
• **ERGOCALCIFEROL,** U.S.P. XXI. Cap., Tab., Oral Soln. U.S.P. XXI. 9, 10-Secoergosta-5,7,10(19),22-tetraen-3-ol, (3β-. Irradiated Ergosta-5,7,22-trien-3-beta-ol. Use: Vitamin D (Antirachitic).
See: Calciferol.
Drisdol, Liq., Cap. (Winthrop-Breon)
Geltabs, Cap. (Upjohn)
ERGOCORNINE. (Various Mfr.) Ergot alkaloids.
Use: Peripheral vascular disorders.
ERGOCRISTINE. (Various Mfr.) Ergot alkaloid.
Use: Vascular disorders.
ERGOCRYPTINE. (Various Mfr.) Ergot alkaloid.
Use: Peripheral vascular disorders.

ERGOLINE-8-CARBOXAMIDE,9,10-DIDE-HYDRO-N-[1-(HYDROXY-METHYL)PROPYL]-1,6-DI-METHYL-,(8β-, (Z)-2-BUTANEDIOATE (1:1) (salt). Methysergide Maleate.
ERGOMAR. (Fisons) Ergotamine Tartrate 2 mg./Sublingual Tab. Pkg. 20s.
Use: Migraine and vascular headaches.
• **ERGOLOID MESYLATES.** U.S.P. XXI. Oral Soln., Tab., U.S.P.XXI. (Lederle) **0.5 mg.:** Dihydroergocornine 0.167 mg., dihydroergocristine 0.167 mg., dihydroergocryptine 0.167 mg./0.5 mg. Sublingual Tab.; **1 mg.;** dihydroergocornine 0.333 mg., dihydroergocristine 0.333 mg., dihydro-ergocryptine 0.333 mg./1 mg. Tab. Bot. 100s, 1000s.
Use: Treatment of elderly.
See: Deapril-ST, Tab. (Mead Johnson)
Hydergine Prods. (Sandoz)
ERGOMETRINE MALEATE.
See: Ergonovine (Various Mfr.)
ERGONAL. (Vita Elixir) Ergot powder 259.2 mg., aloin 8.1 mg., apiol fluid green 290 mg., oil pennyroyal 28 mg./Cap. Bot. 24s.
Use: Oxytocic.
ERGONOVINE. (Various Mfr.) Ergobasine, erolklinine, ergometrine, ergostetrine, ergotocine.
See: Ergonovine Maleate
• **ERGONOVINE MALEATE,** U.S.P. XXI. Inj., Tab., U.S.P. XXI. 9,10-Didehydro-N-[(S)-2-hydroxy-1-methylethyl]-6-methylergoline-8β-carboxamide maleate.
Use: I.V., I.M., orally; oxytocic.
See: Ergotrate Maleate, Preps. (Lilly)
ERGOSTAT. (Parke-Davis) Ergotamine tartrate 2 mg./Sublingual Tab. Vial 24s.
Use: Migraine and cluster headache treatment.
ERGOSTEROL, ACTIVATED OR IRRADIATED.
See: Ergocalciferol, U.S.P. XXI.
ERGOSTETRINE.
See: Ergonovine. (Various Mfr.)
ERGOTAMAN-3′,6′,18-TRIONE,12′-HYDROXY-2′-METHYL-5′-(PHENYLMETHYL)-2,3-DIHYDROXYBU-TANEIOATE (2:1) (SALT). Ergotamine Tartrate, U.S.P. XXI.
• **ERGOTAMINE TARTRATE,** U.S.P. XXI. Inj., Inhalation Aerosol, Tab., U.S.P. XXI. Ergotaman-3′,6′, 18-trione, 12′-hydroxy-2′-methyl-5′-(phenylmethyl)-2,3-dihydroxybutanedioate (2:1) (salt). Femergin.
Use: Analgesic (specific in migraine).
See: Ergomar, Tab. (Fisons)
Ergostat, Tab. (Parke-Davis)
Gynergen, Amp., Tab. (Sandoz)
Medihaler-Ergotamine, Vial (Riker)
W/Belladonna alkaloids, acetophenetidin & caffeine.
See: Wigraine, Tab., Supp. (Organon)
W/Belladonna alk. & pentobarbital.
See: Cafergot P-B, Supp., Tab. (Sandoz)
W/Belladonna alk. & phenobarbital.
See: Bellergal, Tab. (Dorsey)
W/Caffeine.
See: Cafergot, Tab., Supp. (Sandoz)
Ergothein, Tab. (Wolins)

W/Caffeine, homatropine methylbromide.
See: Ergotatropin, Tab. (Cole)
W/Cyclizine HCl, caffeine.
See: Migral Tab. (Burroughs Wellcome)
W/1-Hyoscyamine sulfate, phenobarbital.
See: Ergkatal, Tab. (Gilbert)
Ergobel, Tab. (Wolins)
• **ERGOTAMINE TARTRATE AND CAFFEINE
SUPPOSITORIES,** U.S.P. XXI.
Use: Vascular headache.
See: Cafergot, Supp. (Sandoz)
• **ERGOTAMINE TARTRATE AND CAFFEINE
TABLETS,** U.S.P. XXI.
Use: Vascular headache.
See: Cafergot, Tab. (Sandoz)
Ergocaf, Tab. (Robinson)
Ergo Caffein, Tab. (CMC)
Lanatrate, Tab. (Lannett)
ERGOTHEIN. (Wolins) Ergotamine tartrate 1 mg.,
caffeine 100 mg./Tab. Bot. 100s, 500s,
1000s.
ERGOT, FLUID EXTRACT. (Various Mfr.) Ergot 1
Gm./cc. Bot. 4 oz., pt.
ERGOTIDINE.
See: Histamine (Various Mfr.)
ERGOTOCINE.
See: Ergonovine (Various Mfr.)
ERGOTRATE.
See: Ergonovine (Various Mfr.)
ERGOTRATE-H.
See: Ergonovine (Various Mfr.)
ERGOTRATE MALEATE. (Lilly) Ergonovine maleate.
Amp.: (0.2 mg.) 1 ml., Pkg. 6s, 100s; **Tab.:** 0.2 mg.
Bot. 100s, 1000s. Blister pkg. 10 × 10s.
Use: I.V., I.M., orally; oxytocic.
■ **ERGOT-RELATED PRODUCTS.**
See: Cafergot, Supp., Tab. (Sandoz)
Deapril-ST, Tab. (Mead Johnson)
Cafergot P-B, Tab. & Supp. (Sandoz).
DHE-45, Amp. (Sandoz)
Ergonovine (Various Mfr.)
Ergotamine (Various Mfr.)
Ergotrate (Various Mfr.)
Gynergen, Amp., Tab. (Sandoz)
Hydergine, Sub. Tab. (Sandoz)
Hydro-Ergot, Tab. (Interstate)
Methergine, Amp., Tab. (Sandoz)
Trigot, Sublingual Tab. (Squibb)
Wigraine, Supp. & Tab. (Organon)
ERGOZIDE. (Jenkins) Carbolic acid 2.25%, ergot ext.
2.5%, zinc oxide 10%, balsam Peru 1.25%, oil
cade 0.3%. Supplied 1 lb.
ERIDIONE. (Eric, Kirk & Gary) Phenindione. 50
mg./Tab. Bot. 100s, 1000s.
Use: Anticoagulant.
ERIODICTIN.
See: Vitamin P & Rutin
• **ERIODICTYON,** N.F. XVI. Flext., Aromatic Syrup,
N.F. XVI.
Use: Pharmaceutic aid (flavor)
See: Vitamin P & Rutin

E-R-O. (Scherer) Propylene glycol and glycerol. Bot.
w/dropper tip 15 cc.
Use: For softening and facilitating the removal of
ear wax.
ERTINE. (Approved) Hexachlorophene, benzocaine,
cod liver oil, allantoin, boric acid, lanolin.
Tube 1½ oz.
Use: Burn and first aid remedy.
ERYC. (Parke-Davis) Erythromycin 250 mg./Cap.
containing enteric-coated pellets. Bot. 100s, 500s.
Unit dose 100s.
Use: Antibiotic.
ERYDERM. (Abbott) Erythromycin topical solution
2%. Bot. 60 ml.
Use: Treatment of acne.
ERYMAX. (Herbert) Erythromycin 2%. Bot. 4 oz.
Use: Topical control of acne vulgaris.
ERYPAR. (Parke-Davis) Erythromycin stearate 250
mg./Filmseal, Bot. 100s, 500s, Unit dose 100s. 500
mg./Filmseal. Bot. 100s.
Use: Antibiotic.
ERYPED. (Abbott) Erythromycin ethylsuccinate for
oral suspension representing erythromycin activity
of 400 mg./5 ml. Bot. 60, 100, 200 and 5 ml. unit
dose.
Use: Antibiotic.
ERY-TAB. (Abbott) Erythromycin enteric coated 250
333 mg. or 500 mg./Tab. **250 mg.:** Bot. 100s,
500s, Unit Dose 100s. **333 mg.:** Bot. 100s. Units
Dose 100s. **500 mg.:** Bot. 100s. Unit Dose 100s.
Use: Antibiotic.
• **ERYTHRITYL TETRANITRATE, DILUTED,** U.S.P.
XXI.
Use: Coronary vasodilator.
• **ERYTHRITYL TETRANITRATE TABLETS,** U.S.P.
XXI. (Various Mfr.) Erythritol, erythrol tetranitrate,
nitroerythrite, tetranitrin, tetranitrol.
Use: Coronary vasodilator.
See: Anginar, Tabs. (Pasadena Research Labs.)
Cardilate, Tab. (Burroughs Wellcome)
W/Phenobarbital.
See: Cardilate-P, Tab. (Burroughs Wellcome)
ERYTHROCIN. (Abbott) Erythromycin. **Erythrocin
Ethylsuccinate:** EES products are supplied as
chewable tablets, drops, granules, Filmtab tablets,
liquids. **Erythrocin Lactobionate:** Injectables.
Erythrocin stearate: Filmtab tablets, 250 mg., 500
mg. Bot. 100s.
Use: Antibiotic.
ERYTHROCIN LACTOBIONATE, I.V. (Abbott)
Erythromycin lactobionate, 500 mg./vial w/benzyl
alcohol 90 mg.; 1 Gm./vial w/benzyl alcohol 180
mg. Pkg. 5 & 25 vials.
Use: Antibiotic.
ERYTHROCIN LACTOBIONATE PIGGYBACK.
(Abbott) Erythromycin lactobionate for injection, 500
mg./dispensing vial. 5 mg./ml. of erythromycin after
reconstitution w/90 mg. benzyl alcohol. Sterile
lyophilized powder in 100 ml. dispensing vial.
Use: I.V. antibiotic.
ERYTHROCIN STEARATE. (Abbott) Erythromycin

stearate 250 mg./Tab. Bot. 20s, 100s, 500s. Abbo-
Pac 100s; 500 mg. Bot. 100s.
Use: Antibiotic.
• **ERYTHROMYCIN,** U.S.P. XXI. Caps., Oint., Ophth.
Oint., Tab., Topical Sol., U.S.P. XXI. An antibiotic
from *Streptomyces erythreus.* (Upjohn) Tab.: 100
mg., Bot. 100s; 250 mg., peach color. Bot. 25s,
100s.
Use: Antibiotic.
See: Dowmycin E, Tab. (Merrell Dow)
    E-Mycin, Tab. (Upjohn)
    Erymax, Sol. (Herbert)
    EryDerm, Sol. (Abbott)
    Erythrocin, Prep. (Abbott)
    Erythromycin Base Filmtab. (Abbott)
    Ethril 500, Tab. (Squibb)
    Ilotycin, Prep. (Dista)
    Robimycin, Tab. (Robins)
    RP-Mycin, Tab. (Reid-Provident)
ERYTHROMYCIN BASE FILMTAB. (Abbott)
Erythromycin base 250 mg. Bot. 100s. Abbo-Pac
100s. 500 mg./Tab. Bot. 100s.
Use: Antibiotic.
• **ERYTHROMYCIN ESTOLATE,** U.S.P. XXI. Cap.,
Oral Susp., for Oral Susp., Tab., U.S.P. XXI. Supp.,
Erythromycin 2'-propionate dodecyl sulfate. Lauryl
sulfate salt of the propionic acid ester of
erythromycin.
Use: Antibiotic
See: Ilosone, Prep. (Dista)
ERYTHROMYCIN ESTOLATE. B.A.N. Erythromycin
propionyl ester lauryl sulfate.
Use: Antibiotic.
See: Ilosone
• **ERYTHROMYCIN ETHYLSUCCINATE,** U.S.P. XXI.
Inj., Tabs., for Oral Susp., Oral Susp., Sterile, U.S.P.
XXI. Erythromycin 2'-(Ethylsuccinate).
Use: Antibiotic.
See: E.E.S. Prods. (Abbott)
    E-mycin E, Liq. (Upjohn)
    Pediamycin Prods. (Ross)
    Pediazole, Liq. (Ross)
    Wyamycin-E, Liq. (Wyeth)
• **ERYTHROMYCIN ETHYLSUCCINATE AND
SULFISOXAZOLE ACETYL FOR ORAL
SUSPENSION,** U.S.P. XXI.
Use: Antibiotic, anti-infective
See: Pediazole, Susp. (Ross)
• **ERYTHROMYCIN GLUCEPTATE, STERILE,** U.S.P.
XXI.
Use: Antibacterial.
See: Ilotycin Gluceptate, Amp. (Lilly)
ERYTHROMYCIN GLUCOHEPTONATE.
See: Erythromycin Gluceptate, U.S.P. XXI.
    Ilotycin Glucoheptonate, Amp. (Dista)
• **ERYTHROMYCIN LACTOBIONATE FOR
INJECTION,** U.S.P. XXI.
Use: Antibacterial.
See: Erythrocin Lactobionate, Vial (Abbott)
**ERYTHROMYCIN 2'-PROPIONATE DODECYL
SULFATE.** Erythromycin Estolate, U.S.P. XXI.

ERYTHROMYCIN PROPIONATE LAURYL SULFATE.
See: Erthromycin Estolate
    Ilosone, Prep. (Dista)
• **ERYTHROMYCIN STEARATE,** U.S.P. XXI. Tabs.,
for Oral Susp., U.S.P. XXI.
Use: Antibacterial.
See: Bristamycin, Tab. (Bristol)
    Dowmycin-E, Tab. (Merrell Dow)
    Erythrocin Stearate Prods. (Abbott)
    Erypar Filmseal, Tab. (Parke-Davis)
    Ethril, Tab. (Squibb)
    SK-Erthromycin, Tab. (SmithKline)
    Wyamycin-S, Tab. (Wyeth)
ERYTHROMYCIN SULFATE.
Use: Antibacterial.
• **ERYTHROSINE SODIUM,** U.S.P. XXI. Topical Sol.,
Soluble Tab., U.S.P. XXI.
Use: Diagnostic aid (dental disclosing agent).
ESANGEN. (Blue Line) Testosterone cypionate 50
mg., estradiol cypionate 2 mg., chlorobutanol 0.5%
in cottonseed oil/cc. Vial 10 cc.
ESBATAL SULPHATE. Bethanidine, B.A.N.
ESCLABRON. Guaithylline.
Use: Antiasthmatic.
ESCOT. (Reid-Provident) Bismuth aluminate 100 mg.,
magnesium trisilicate 160 mg., aluminum hydroxide
and magnesium carbonate coprecipitate 130
mg./Cap. Bot. 100s.
Use: Antacid for heartburn, sour stomach, acid
indigestion.
ESERINE. (physostigmine as alkaloid, salicylate or
sulfate salt).
ESERINE SALICYLATE (PHYSOSTIGMINE). (Alcon)
½%. Steri-Unit 2 cc. 24s (Mesco) 0.5%. Bot. 3.5 Gm.
**ESERINE SULFATE STERILE OPHTHALMIC
OINTMENT.** (CooperVision) Eserine sulfate 0.25%.
Tube 3.5 Gm.
Use: Treatment of primary glaucoma.
ESERINE SULFATE. Physostigmine sulfate.
(Robinson) ¼%. Tube ⅛ oz.
Use: Ophthalmic ointment for treatment of primary
glaucoma.
ESGIC CAPSULES. (Gilbert) Butalbital 50 mg.,
caffeine 40 mg., acetaminophen 325 mg./Tab. Bot.
100s.
Use: Analgesic, sedative.
ESGIC TABLETS. (Gilbert) Butalbital 50 mg., caffeine
40 mg., acetaminophen 325 mg./Tab. Bot. 100s.
Use: Analgesic, sedative.
ESIDRIX. (Ciba) Hydrochlorothiazide 25 mg., or 50
mg./Tab. Bot. 100s, 1000s, 5000s; Accu-Pak 25 mg.,
50 mg. Blister units 100s; Consumer Packs 25 mg.
in 100s, in 30s, 60s; 100 mg. Tab. Bot.
100s.
Use: Diuretic and antihypertensive.
W/Apresoline.
See: Apresoline-Esidrix, Tab. (Ciba)
ESIMIL. (Ciba) Hydrochlorothiazide 25 mg.,
guanethidine monosulfate 10 mg./Tab. Bot. 100s;
Consumer Packs of 100s; Accu-Pak 100s.
Use: Diuretic, hypertensive.
ESKACEF. Cephradine, B.A.N.

ESKALITH. (SmithKline) Lithium carbonate **Cap:** 300
mg./Cap. Bot. 100s, 500s; **Tab:** 300 mg./Tab.
(scored). Bot. 100s. Controlled Release Tab. 450
mg./Tab. Bot. 100s.
Use: Control of manic episodes in manic-depressive
psychosis.

ESKALITH CR. (SmithKline) Lithium carbonate 450
mg./Controlled Release Tab. Bot. 100s.
Use: Treatment of manic episodes of
manic-depressive illness.

• **ESMOLOL HYDROCHLORIDE.** USAN.

E-SON. (Eastwood) Bot. 100s.

ESOPHOTRAST. (Armour) Barium sulfate 560
mg./Gm. in cream base containing suspending
agents and flavoring. Tube 1 lb. Ctn. 12s.
Use: Diagnostic agent for use in radiologic
examination of esophagus.

ESOTERICA DRY SKIN TREATMENT LOTION.
(Norcliff Thayer) Bot. 13 fl. oz.
Use: Skin moisturizer.

ESOTERICA MEDICATED FADE CREAM FACIAL.
(Norcliff Thayer) Hydroquinone 2% padimate O
3.3%, oxybenzone 2.5% in cream base. Jar 3 oz.
Use: Skin lightener.

**ESOTERICA MEDICATED FADE CREAM,
FORTIFIED.** (Norcliff Thayer) Hydroquinone 2%,
padimate O 3.3%, oxybenzone 2.5% cream.
Unscented jar 3 oz., scented jar 3 oz.
Use: Skin lightener.

ESOTERICA MEDICATED FADE CREAM, REGULAR.
(Norcliff Thayer) Hydroquinone 2% cream.
Jar 3 oz.
Use: Skin lightener.

ESPERSON. Desoxymethasone, B.A.N.

ESPOTABS. (Combe) Yellow phenolphthalein/Tab.
Bot. 6s, 20s, 50s, 85s.
Use: Laxative.

E.S.P.R. (Wolins) N-acetyl-aminophenol 1½ gr., salicylamide, aspirin, caffeine/Tab. Bot. 100s, 1000s.

• **ESPROQUIN HYDROCHLORIDE.** USAN.
Use: Adrenergic.

ESSENTIAL-8. Liquid amino acid protein supplement.
Use: Protein supplement.
See: Essential-8, Liquid (Medics)
Vivonex Diets, Liquid (Norwich Eaton)

ESTAQUA "S." (Kay) Estrogenic substances 2
mg./cc. Vial 30 cc.

ESTAR. (Westwood) Tar equivalent to 5% Coal Tar
U.S.P. in a hydro-alcoholic gel w/alcohol 13.8%. Tube
3 oz.
Use: All tar responsive dermatoses including
psoriasis & eczema.

ESTATE. (Savage) Estradiol valerate 10 mg., benzyl
alcohol 2% sesame oil q.s./ml. Vial 10 ml.
Use: Estrogen therapy.

• **ESTERIFILCON A.** USAN.
Use: Contact lens material.

ESTERIGYN. (Pasadena Research) Esterified
estrogen 0.625 mg., 1.25 mg./Tab. Bot. 100s,
500s.

ESTILBEN.
See: Diethylstilbestrol Dipropionate. (Various Mfr.)

ESTINYL. (Schering) Ethinyl estradiol. Tab., coated
(0.02 mg. & 0.05 mg.) Bot. 100s, 250s; Tab. (0.5
mg.) Bot. 100s.
Use: Orally; estrogen therapy.

ESTIVIN. (Alcon) A specially processed aq. infusion
of *Rosa gallica* (rose petals). Bot. w/dropper 0.25
fl. oz.
Use: To relieve ocular symptoms of hay fever.

ESTOLATE. Erythromycin.
See: Erythromycin Propionate Lauryl Sulfate

ESTOMUL-M LIQUID. (Riker) Aluminum hydroxide-
magnesium carbonate 918 mg./15 ml. Bot. 12 oz.

ESTOMUL-M TABLETS. (Riker) Aluminum hydroxide-
magnesium carbonate 500 mg., magnesium oxide
45 mg./Tab. Bot. 100s.

ESTOPEN.
See: Benzylpenicillin 2-diethylaminoethyl ester HI

ESTRA-C INJECTION. (Amfre-Grant) Estradiol cypionate 5 mg./ml. Vial 10 ml.
Use: Hormone.

ESTRA-V. (Amfre-Grant) Estradiol vaerate 20 mg./ml.
Vial 10 ml.
Use: Hormone.

ESTRACE. (Mead Johnson) 17β-Estradiol Micronized.
1 or 2 mg./Tab. Bot. 100s.
Use: Estrogen replacement therapy.

ESTRACE VAGINAL CREAM. (Mead Johnson) 17β
Estradiol 0.1 mg./Gm. Tube 42.5 Gm.
Use: Estrogen replacement therapy.

ESTRACON. (Freeport) Conjugated estrogens 1.25
mg./Tab. Bot. 1000s.
Use: Menopausal syndrome.

ESTRA-D. (Seatrace) Estradiol cypionate 5 mg./ml.
Vial 10 cc.

• **ESTRADIOL,** U.S.P. XXI. Pellets, Sterile Susp., Tab.,
U.S.P. XXI. Estra-1,3,5(10)-triene-3,17-β-diol. Beta-
estradiol, agofollin, dihydroxyestrin, dihydrotheelin,
gynergon, gynoestryl. The form now known to be
physiologically active is the "beta" form rather than
the "alpha" form.
Use: Estrogen-replacement therapy.
See: Aquagen, Vial, Aq. (Remsen)
Estrace, Tab. (Mead Johnson)
Femogen, Susp., Tab. (Fellows-Testagar)
Progynon, Pellets (Schering)
W/Estriol and estrone.
See: Estro Plus, Tab., Vial (Rocky Mtn.)
Hormonin No. 1 & 2, Tab. (Carnrick)
W/Estrone, estriol.
See: Sanestro Tab. (Sandia)
W/Estrone, pot. estrone sulfate.
See: Tri-Estrin, Inj. (Keene)
W/Progesterone, testosterone, procaine HCl, procaine
base.
See: Horm-Triad, Vial. (Bell)
W/Testerone.
See: Testrolix, Inj. (Vortech)
W/Testosterone & chlorobutanol in cottonseed oil.
See: Depo-Testadiol, Vial (Upjohn)

ESTRADIOL BENZOATE. 1,3,5(10)-Estratriene-3,17-
β-diol 3-Benzoate. Estra-1,3,5,(10)-triene-3,17-di-
ol,(17β)-,3-benzoate. Beta-estradiol benzoate, ben-

zogynoestryl, benzoestrofol difolliculin, follicormon, follidrin. Estradiol 3-Benzoate. (Various Mfr.)
Use: Estrogen therapy.

ESTRADIOL CYCLOPENTYLPROPIONATE, Estradiol 17-beta(3-cyclopentyl)propionate. Estradiol Cypionate, U.S.P. XXI.
W/Testosterone cypionate.
See: Depo-Testadiol, Vial (Upjohn)

• **ESTRADIOL CYPIONATE,** U.S.P. XXI. Inj. U.S.P. XXI. Estradiol 17-β-(3-Cyclopentyl)propionate Estradiol 17-cyclopentanepropionate. Estra-1,3,5-(10)-triene-3,17-diol,(17 beta)-, 17-cyclopentane-propanoate.
Use: Estrogen.
See: Estradiol cyclopentylpropionate
Dep-Estradiol, Inj. (Rocky Mtn.)
Depo-Estradiol Cypionate, Inj. (Upjohn)
Depogen, Inj. (Hyrex)
D-Est, Inj. (Burgin-Arden)
Estra-C, Inj. (Amfre-Grant)
Estra-Ionate, Inj. (Tunex)
Estro-Cyp, Vial (Keene)
Estrogen-810, Inj. (Blue Line)
Estroject-L.A., Vial (Mayrand)
Hormogen Depot, Inj. (Mallard)
Span-F, Inj. (Scrip)
W/Testosterone cypionate.
See: D-Diol, Inj. (Burgin-Arden)
Dep-Tesestro, Inj. (ICN)
Dep-Testradiol, Inj. (Rocky Mtn.)
Duo-Cyp, Vial (Keene)
Duo-Ionate, Inj. (Tunex)
Duracrine, Inj. (Ascher)
Estran-C, Inj. (Amfre-Grant)
Menoject, L.A., Vial (Mayrand)
T.E. Ionate P.A., Inj. (Reid-Provident)
W/Testosterone cypionate, chlorobutanol.
See: Depo-Testadiol (Upjohn)
Esagen, Sol. (Blue Line)
Span F.M., Inj. (Scrip)
T.E. Ionate P.A., Inj. (Reid-Provident)
Testadiale-Depo, Vial (Kay)

ESTRADIOL DIPROPIONATE. Estra-1,3,5(10)-triene-3,17 β-diol dipropionate. Ovocyclin Dipropionate.

• **ESTRADIOL ENANTHATE.** USAN. Estradiol 17-enanthate.

ESTRADIOL, ETHINYL.
See: Ethinyl Estradiol

ESTRADIOL MONOBENZONATE.
See: Estradiol Benzoate

ESTRADIOL PHOSPHATE.
See: Estradurin, Secule (Ayerst)

• **ESTRADIOL UNDECYLATE.** USAN. Estradiol 17-undecanoate.
Use: Estrogen.
See: Delestrec

• **ESTRADIOL VALERATE,**U.S.P. XXI. Inj., U.S.P. XXI. Estra-1,3,5(10)-triene-3,17-diol (17β)-,17-pentano-ate. Estradiol 17-valerate.
Use: Estrogen.
See: Ardefem 10,20, Inj. (Burgin-Arden)
Delestrogen, Vial (Squibb)

Depogen, Inj. (Sig)
Dioval, Preps. (Keene)
Duratrad, Inj. (Ascher)
Estate, Inj. (Savage)
Estra-L, Inj. (Pasadena Research)
Estra-V, Inj. (Amfre-Grant)
Estraval, vial (Kay)
Estra-Vate, Inj. (Tunex)
Estravel-P.A., Estraval-2X, IM (Reid-Provident)
Femogen,L.A., Inj. (Fellows-Testagar)
Repo-Estro Med., Vial (Medics)
Retestrin, Inj. (Rocky Mtn.)
Span-Est, Inj. (Scrip)
Valergen, Inj. (Hyrex)
W/Benzyl alcohol.
See: Estate, Vial (Savage)
Reposo E-40., Vial (Paddock)
W/Chlorobutanol.
See: Estraval, Vial (Kay)
W/Hydroxyprogesterone caproate.
See: Hy-Gestradol, Inj. (Pasadena-Research)
Hylutin-Est, Inj. (Hyrex)
W/Testosterone cypionate.
See: Depo-Testadiol, Inj. (Upjohn)
W/Testosterone enanthate.
See: Ardiol 90/4, 180/8, Inj. (Burgin-Arden)
Bi-Nate, Inj. (Tunex)
Deladumone, Vial (Squibb)
Delatestadiol, Vial (Dunhall)
Duoval-P.A., I.M. (Reid-Provident)
Estran-E.V., Inj. (Amfre-Grant)
Estra-Testrin, Inj. (Pasadena Research)
Repo-Duo Med., Vial (Medics)
Retadiamone, Inj. (Rocky Mtn.)
Span-Est-Test 4, Inj. (Scrip)
Teev, Inj. (Keene)
Tesogen L.A., Inj. (Sig)
Testanate, Vial (Kenyon)
Valertest, Inj. (Hyrex)
W/Testosterone enanthate, benzyl alcohol, sesame oil.
See: Duogen L.A., Inj. (Vortech)
Repose-TE. (Paddock)
Testadiate, Vial (Kay)

ESTRADOL. (Kenyon) Ethinyl estradiol. **No. 1:** 0.02 mg./Tab. **No. 2:** 0.05 mg./Tab. Bot.
Use: Estrogen therapy.

ESTRADURIN. (Ayerst) Polyestradiol phosphate. Amp. (40 mg.) w/2 ml. sterile diluent.
W/polyestradiol phosphate 40 mg., phenylmercuric nitrate 0.02 mg., sod. phosphate 5.2 mg., niacinamide 25 mg., propylene glycol 4 mg.
Use: I.M., treatment of prostatic carcinoma.

ESTRAGUARD. (Reid-Provident) Dienestrol cream 0.01%. Tube 3 oz.
Use: Estrogen vaginal therapy.

ESTRA-IONATE. (Tunex) Estradiol cypionate 5 mg./ml. w/chlorobutanol 0.5%, cottonseed oil. Vial 5 cc
Use: Long acting progestational agent.

ESTRA-L. (Pasadena Research) Estradiol valerate in sesame oil 20 mg. Vial 10 cc. 40 mg./ml. Vial 5 cc.

ESTRALUTIN.
  See: Relutin (Reid-Provident)
• **ESTRAMUSTINE.** USAN. Estradiol 3-bis
  (2-chloroethyl) carbamate 17-(dihydrogen
  phosphate), disodium salt.
  Use: Antineoplastic agent.
  See: Emcyt, Cap. (Roche)
• **ESTRAMUSITINE PHOSPHATE SODIUM.** USAN.
  Use: Antineoplastic.
ESTRAN-C. (Amfre-Grant) Testosterone cypionate 50
  mg., estradiol cypionate 2 mg./ml. Vial 10 ml.
  Use: Hormone.
ESTRAN-E.V. (Amfre-Grant) Testosterone enanthate
  90 mg., estradiol valerate 4 mg./ml. Vial 10 ml.
  Use: Hormone.
ESTRATAB. (Reid-Provident) **Tab.:** Esterified estrogens
  principally sodium estrone sulfate 0.625 mg., 1.25
  mg. or 2.5 mg./Tab. Bot. 100s, 1000s. 0.3
  mg./Tab. Bot. 100s.
  Use: Estrogen replacement therapy.
ESTRATEST. (Reid-Provident) Esterified estrogens
  1.25 mg., methyltestosterone 2.5 mg./Tab. Bot.
  100s, 1000s.
  Use: Androgen-estrogen therapy.
ESTRATEST H.S. (Reid-Provident) Esterified estrogens
  0.625 mg., methyltestosterone 1.25 mg./Tab. Bot.
  100s.
  Use: Androgen-estrogen therapy.
ESTRA-TESTRIN. (Pasadena Research) Testosterone
  enanthate 90 mg., estradiol valerate 4 mg., benzyl
  alcohol 2%/ml. Vial 10 cc.
ESTRA-1,3,5(10)-TRIENE-3,17-DIOL,(17β)-,17-
CYCLOPENTANEPROPANOATE. Estradiol
  Cypionate, U.S.P. XXI.
ESTRA-1,3,5(10)-TRIENE-3,17-DIOL   (17β)-,17-PEN-
TANOATE. Estradiol Valerate, U.S.P. XXI.
ESTRAVAL. (Kay) Estradiol valerate 10.0 mg., benzyl
  alcohol 2%, sesame oil/ml. Vial, 10 cc.
  Use: Conditions requiring estrogen therapy.
ESTRAVAL-P.A. (Reid-Provident) Estradiol valerate 10
  mg./cc. in oil. Vial 10 cc. 1s, 6s, 12s.
ESTRAVAL-2X. (Reid-Provident) Estradiol valerate 20
  mg. ethyl oleate/cc. in sesame oil. Vial 10 cc. 1s,
  6s, 12s.
ESTRA-VATE. (Tunex) Estradiol valerate 20 mg./ml.
  w/benzyl benzoate 20%, benzyl alcohol 2%. Vial
  10 cc. Estradiol valerate 40 mg./ml. w/benzyl
  benzoate 40%, benzyl alcohol 2%. Vial 10 cc.
  Use: Amenorrhea, menopausal syndrome.
• **ESTRAZINOL HYDROBROMIDE.** USAN. dl-trans-
  3-Methoxy-8-aza-19-nor-17a-pregna-1,3,5-trien-20-
  yn-17-ol hydrobromide.
  Use: Estrogen.
ESTRIN.
  See: Estrone
• **ESTRIOL,** U.S.P. XXI.
W/Estrone, estradiol.
  See: Estro Plus, Tab. (Rocky Mtn.)
ESTRIOL-SQUIBB. (Squibb) Radioimmune assay kit for
  estradiol. 200 tests/kit.
  Use: Radioimmune assay.
ESTRITONE NO. 1. (Kenyon) Conjugated estrogens

equine 0.625 mg., methyltestosterone 5 mg./Tab.
  Bot. 100s, 1000s.
ESTRITONE NO. 2. (Kenyon) Conjugated estrogens
  equine 1.25 mg., methyltestosterone 10 mg./Tab.
  Bot. 100s, 1000s.
ESTROATE. (Kay) Conjugated estrogens 0.625 or
  1.25 mg./Tab. Bot. 100s, 500s, 1000s.
  Use: Female hormone therapy.
ESTROBENE DP.
  See: Diethylstilbestrol Dipropionate (Various Mfr.)
ESTROCON. (Savage) Conjugated estrogens 0.625
  mg. or 1.25 mg./Tab.
  Bot. 100s.
  Use: Estrogen replenishment therapy.
ESTRO-CYP. (Keene) Estradiol cypionate 5 mg./ml. Vial
  10 ml.
ESTROFEM. (Pasadena Research) Estradiol
  cypionate 5 mg./cc. Vial 10 cc.
ESTROFOL. (Reid-Provident) 20,000 I.U./cc. Aq. Susp.
  Vial. 10 cc., 30 cc. In oil vials 30 cc.
• **ESTROFURATE.** USAN. (1)21, 23-Epoxy-19-24-dinor-
  17α-chola-1,3,5(10),7,20,22-hexaene-3,17-diol-3-ace-
  tate; (2) 17-(3-furyl) estra-1,3,5-(10),7-tetraene-3,17β
  -diol-3-acetate.
  Use: Estrogen.
■ **ESTROGENIC SUBSTANCES, CONJUGATED,**
  (Water-soluble.) A mixture containing the sodium salts
  of the sulfate esters of the estrogenic substances,
  principally estrone & equilin that are of the type
  excreted by pregnant mares.
  Cream.
  See: Premarin Vaginal Cream (Ayerst)
  Intravenous.
  See: Estroject, Vial (Mayrand)
    Premarin (Ayerst)
  Tablets.
  See: Aquagen, Inj. (Remsen)
    Ces (ICN)
    Co-Estro, Tab. (Robinson)
    Estroquin, Tab. (Sheryl)
    Estrosan, Tab. (Recsei)
    Evestrone, Tab. (Delta)
    Femogen, Oil, Tab., Sus. (Fellows-Testegar)
    Genisis, Tab. (Organon)
    Menotabs, Tab. (Fleming)
    Orapin (Standex)
    Prelestrin, Tab. (Pasadena Research)
    Premarin, Tab. (Ayerst)
    Tag-39 H, Tab. (Reid-Provident)
  W/α-Estradiol.
  See: Makrogen Aqueous Susp. (O'Neal)
  W/Ethinylestradiol.
  See: Demulen, Tab. (Searle)
  W/Meprobamate.
  See: Milprem, Tab. (Wallace)
    PMB 200, Tab. (Ayerst)
    PMB 400, Tab. (Ayerst)
  W/Methyltestosterone.
  See: Menotab-M #1 & 2, Tab. (Fleming)
    Premarin with Methyltestosterone, Tab. (Ayerst)
ESTROGENIC SUBSTANCES IN AQUEOUS
  SUSPENSION. (Ayerst) Sterile estrone suspension
  2 mg./ml. Vials 10 ml.

Use: Menopausal symptoms, atrophic vaginitis, Kraurosis vulvae, prostatic carcinoma.
■ **ESTROGENIC SUBSTANCES MIXED.** May be a crystalline or an amorphous mixture of the naturally occurring estrogens obtained from the urine of pregnant mares.
Aq. Susp.
See: Gravigen Injection (Bluco)
　Lanestrin, Vial (Lannett)
Capsules.
See: Urestrin, Cap. (Upjohn)
W/Androgen therapy, vitamins & iron, & d-desoxyephedrine HCl.
See: Mediatric, Prep. (Ayerst)
W/Methyltestosterone.
See: Premarin w/methyltestosterone, Tab. (Ayerst)
W/Testosterone
See: Andrestraq, Vial (Central)
ESTROGEN-ANDROGEN THERAPY.
See: Androgen-Estrogen Therapy
ESTROGEN-810 INJECTION. (Blue Line) Estradiol cypionate 5 mg., chlorobutanol 0.5% in cottonseed oil/cc. Vial 10 cc.
• **ESTROGENS, CONJUGATED,** U.S.P. XXI. Inj. U.S.P. XXI.
Use: Estrogen.
See: Conest, Tab. (Century)
　Congens, Tab. (Blaine)
　Congesterone, Tab. (Kenyon)
　Estrocon, Tab. (Savage)
　Ganeake, Tab. (Geneva)
　Menotab, Tab. (Fleming)
　PMB, Tab. (Ayerst)
　Premarin, Tab., I.V. (Ayerst)
　Premarin Vaginal Cream (Ayerst)
　Premarin with Methyltestosterone, Tab. (Ayerst)
　Sodestrin and Sodestrin-H, Tab. (Reid-Provident)
　Tag-39, Tab. (Reid-Provident)
　Zeste, Tab. (Ascher)
■ **ESTROGENS EQUINE.**
See: PMB, Tab. (Ayerst)
　Premarin, Tab., I.V. (Ayerst)
　Premarin Vaginal Cream (Ayerst)
　Premarin with Methyltestosterone, Tab. (Ayerst)
• **ESTROGENS, ESTERIFIED,** U.S.P. XXI. Tabs., U.S.P. XXI.
Use: Estrogen.
See: Amnestrogen, Tab. (Squibb)
　Evex, Tab. (Syntex)
　Menest, Tab. (Beecham Labs)
　Ms-Med, Tab. (Dunhall)
■ **ESTROGENS, NATURAL.**
Use: Estrogen.
See: Depogen, Vial (Hyrex)
　Estradiol, Prep. (Various Mfr.)
　Estrone, Prep. (Various Mfr.)
　Estrogenic Substance (Various Mfr.)
　PMB, Tab. (Ayerst)
　Premarin, Tab., I.V. (Ayerst)
　Premarin Vaginal Cream (Ayerst)
　Premarin with Methyltestosterone, Tab. (Ayerst)

ESTROGENS, SYNTHETIC.
See: Dienestrol, Prep. (Various Mfg.)
　Diethylstilbestrol, Prep. (Various Mfr.)
　Hexestrol, Prep. (Various Mfr.)
　Meprane, Tab. (Reed & Carnrick)
　TACE, Cap. (Merrell Dow)
　Vallestril, Tab. (Searle)
ESTROGESTIN A. (Harvey) Estrogenic substance 1 mg., progesterone 10 mg./cc. in peanut oil. Vial 10 ml.
ESTROGESTIN C. (Harvey) Estrogenic substance 1 mg., progesterone 12.5 mg./cc. in peanut oil. Vial 10 ml.
ESTROJECT. (Mayrand) Estrogenic substances 2 mg., 5 mg./ml. Vial 10 ml. 2 mg./ml. Vial 30 ml.
ESTROJECT-LA. (Mayrand) Estradiol cypionate 5 mg./ml. Vial 10 ml.
ESTROL. (Kay) Estrogen. Vial 10 ml. or 30 ml.
Use: Hormone supplement.
ESTROLAN. (Lannett) Estrogenic sub. natural in oil 10,000 iu./cc. Vial 30 cc.
• **ESTRONE,** U.S.P. XXI. Inj., Sterile Susp., U.S.P. XXI. 3-Hydroxy-estra-1,3,5(10)-trien-17-one. Oil Inj., Femidyn, follicular hormone, folliculin, follicunodis, cristallovar, glandubolin, hiestrone, ketohydroxy-estratriene, ketohydroxyestrin. 1 mg. equals 10,000 I.U.
Use: Estrogen
See: Bestrone Suspension, Inj. (Bluco)
　Estrogenic Substances in Aqueous Suspension (Ayerst)
　Follestrol, Vial, Aq. (Blue Line)
　Foygen, Vial (Foy)
　Gynlin, Inj. (Tunex)
　Menagen, Cap. (Parke-Davis)
　Menformon (A), Vial (Organon)
　Nestronaq, Inj. (Noyes)
　Par-Supp, Vag. Supp. (Parmed)
　Propagon-S, Inj. (Spanner)
　Theelin, Vial, Aq. & Oil (Parke-Davis)
W/Hydrocortisone acetate.
See: Estro-V HC, Supp. (Webcon)
W/Estradiol, pot. estrone sulfate.
　Tri-Orapin (Standex)
W/Estradiol, Vit. B-12.
See: Ovest, Tab. (Trimen)
　Ovulin, Inj. (Sig)
W/Estriol and estradiol.
See: Estro Plus, Tab., Vial (Rocky Mtn.)
　Hormonin, Tab. (Carnrick)
W/Estrogens.
　Estrogenic Mixtures, Prep. (Various Mfr.)
　Estrogenic Substances, Prep. (Various Mfr.)
W/Lactose.
See: Estrovag. Supps. (Fellows-Testagar)
W/Potassium estrone sulfate.
See: Dura-Keelin, Vial (Pharmex)
　Estro Plus, Inj. (Rocky Mtn.)
　Gynlin R. P. Inj. (Tunex)
　Mer-Estrone, Inj. (Keene)
　Sodestrin, Inj. (Reid-Provident)
　Spanestrin-P, Vial (Savage)

W/Progesterone.
See: Duovin-S, Inj. (Spanner)
W/Testosterone.
See: Andesterone, Vial (Lincoln)
Anestro, Inj. (Mallard)
Di-Hormone, Susp. (Paddock)
Di-Met Susp. (Organon)
Diorapin (Standex)
Dl-Steroid, Vial (Kremers-Urban)
Estratest, Tab. (Reid-Provident)
Estrone-Testosterone, Vial (Maurry)
W/Testosterone, progesterone.
See: Tripole-F, Inj. (Spanner)
W/Testosterone, sod. carboxymethylcellulose, sod. chloride.
See: Tostestro, Inj. (Bowman)
W/Testosterone, vitamins.
See: Android-G, Vial (Brown)
Geratic Forte, Inj. (Keene Pharm.)
Geriamic, Tab. (Vortech)
Geritag, Inj., Cap. (Reid-Provident)
W/Testosterone, vitamin & mineral formula, amino acids.
See: Geramine, Tab. & Inj. (Brown)
W/Testosterone propionate.
ESTRONE-A. (Kay) Estrone 2 mg./ml. Vial 10 ml.
Use: Estrogen.
ESTRONE SULFATE, PIPERAZINE.
See: Ogen, Tab., Vaginal Cream (Abbott).
ESTRONE SULFATE, POTASSIUM.
See: Estrogens, Vial (Med. Chem.)
Kaytron, Inj. (Pasadena Research)
ESTRONE SULFATE POT. W/ESTRONE.
See: Dura-Keelin, Vial (Pharmex)
ESTRONOL AQUEOUS. (Central) Estrone 2 mg./ml. w/preservatives and stabilizers. Vial 10 ml., 30 ml. For I.M. use.
Use: Estrogen therapy.
• **ESTROPIPITATE,** U.S.P. XXI. Vaginal Cream, Tab., U.S.P. XXI. Estrone hydrogen sulfate compound with piperazine (1:1).
Use: Estrogen agent.
See: Ogen, Tab., Vag. Cream. (Abbott)
ESTRO PLUS. (Rocky Mtn.) **Inj.:** Estrone 2 mg., potassium estrone sulfate 1 mg./cc. Vial 10 cc.
Tab.: Estrone 0.7 mg., estriol 0.135 mg., estradiol 0.3 mg./Tab. Estrone 1.4 mg., estriol 0.27 mg., estradiol 0.6 mg./ #2 Tab. Bot. 100s.
Use: Menopausal syndrome.
ESTROQUIN TABLET. (Sheryl) 1.25 mg. of purified conjugated estrogens/Tab. Bot. 100s.
ESTROVIS. (Parke-Davis) Quinestrol 100 mcg./Tab. Bot. 100s.
Use: Moderate to severe vasomotor symptoms of menopause; atrophic vaginitis; kraurosis vulvae; female hypogonadism; female castration; primary ovarian failure.
• **ETAFEDRINE HCL.** USAN.
Use: Bronchodilator.
See: Mercodol w/Decapryn, Liq. (Merrell Dow)
Nethamine (Merrell Dow)
• **ETAFILCON A.** USAN.

Use: Contact lens material.
ETALENT. (Roger) Ethaverine HCl 100 mg./Cap. Bot. 50s, 500s.
Use: Smooth muscle relaxant.
ETAMIPHYLLINE. B.A.N. 7-(2-Diethylaminoethyl)-theophylline.
Use: Smooth muscle relaxant.
See: Millophylline (camsylate)
E-TAPP ELIXIR. (Edwards) Brompheniramine maleate 4 mg., phenylephrine HCl 5 mg., phenylpropanolamine HCl 5 mg., alcohol 2.3%. Bot. pt., gal.
Use: Decongestant, antihistaminic.
• **ETAZOLATE HYDROCHLORIDE.** USAN.
Use: Antipsychotic.
ETENZAMIDE. B.A.N. 2-Ethoxybenzamide.
Use: Analgesic.
See: Lucamid
ETERNA 27 CREAM. (Revlon) Pregnenolone acetate 0.5% in cream base.
Use: Skin moisurization in aged skin.
• **ETEROBARB.** USAN.
Use: Anticonvulsant.
ETHABID DURACAP. (Meyer) Ethaverine HCl 150 mg./T.R. Cap. Bot. 100s.
• **ETHACRYNATE SODIUM FOR INJECTION,** U.S.P. XXI. Sodium [2,3-dichloro-4-(2-methylenebutyryl)-phenoxy]acetate.
Use: Diuretic.
See: Edecrin Sodium I.V. Inj. (Merck Sharp & Dohme)
ETHACRYNIC ACID. B.A.N. 2,3-Dichloro-4-(2-ethyla-cryloyl)phenoxyacetic acid.
Use: Oral diuretic.
• **ETHACRYNIC ACID,** U.S.P. XXI. Tab., U.S.P. XXI. Acetic acid, [2,3-dichloro-4-(2-methylene-1-oxobutyl)-phenoxy].
Use: Diuretic
See: Edecrin, Tab. (Merck Sharp & Dohme)
ETHAMBUTOL. B.A.N. (+)-NN'-Di-(1-hydroxymethyl-propyl)ethylenediamine. NN'-Ethylenedi-(2-aminobu-tan-1-ol).
Use: Treatment of tuberculosis.
• **ETHAMBUTOL HCl,** U.S.P. XXI. Tab., U.S.P. XXI. (+)-2,2'-(Ethylenediimino)-di-1-butanol Di HCl.
Use: Antitubercular.
See: Myambutol Hydrochloride (Lederle)
ETHAMICORT.
See: Hydrocortamate
ETHAMIVAN. B.A.N. NN-Diethylvanillamide.
Use: Central nervous system stimulant.
See: Vandid
• **ETHAMSYLATE.** USAN. Diethylammonium 2,5-dihy-droxybenzenesulfonate. Dicynene.
Use: Hemostatic.
ETHANAMINE,2-[4-(2-CHLORO-1,2-DIPHENYL-ETHENYL)-PHENOXY]-N,N-DIETHYL-,2-HY-DROXY-1,2,3-PROPANE-TRICARBOXYLATE(1:1). Clomiphene Citrate, U.S.P. XXI.
ETHANAMINE,2-(DIPHENYLMETHOXY)-N,N-DIMETHYL-,HYDROCHLORIDE. Diphenhydramine Hydrochloride, U.S.P. XXI.

ETHANAMINIUM,2,2',2''-[1,2,3-BENZENETRIYLTRIS-(OXY)]-TRIS-[N,N,N-TRIETHYL]-,TRIIODIDE. Gallamine Triethiodide, U.S.P. XXI.

ETHANAMINIUM,2-[(DIETHOXYPHOSPHINYL)THIO]-N,N,N-TRIMETHYL-,IODIDE. Echothiophate Iodide, U.S.P. XXI.

ETHANAMINIUM,2,2'-(1,4-DIOXO-1,4-BUTANEDIYL)-BIS (OXY)BIS-N,N,N-TRIMETHYL-,DICHLORIDE. Succinylcholine Chloride, U.S.P. XXI.

ETHANE,2-BROMO-2-CHLORO-1,1,1-TRI-FLUORO-. Halothane, U.S.P. XXI.

1,2-ETHANEDIAMINE,N,N-DIMETHYL-N'-(PHENYL-METHYL)-N'-2-PYRIDINYL-, Tripelennamine, Citrate or Hydrochloride, U.S.P. XXI.

1,1-ETHANEDIOL,2,2,2-TRICHLORO-. Chloral Hydrate, U.S.P. XXI.

ETHANOL. (Various Mfr.) Alcohol, anhydrous. Alcohol, U.S.P. XXI.

ETHANOL,2-[[4-[(7-CHLORO-4-QUINOLINYL)-AMINO]PENTYL]ETHYLAMINO]-, SULFATE(1:1) SALT. Hydroxychloroquine Sulfate, U.S.P. XXI.

ETHANOLAMINE. Olamine.

ETHAQUIN. (Ascher) Ethaverine HCl 100 mg./Tab. Bot. 100s, 500s, 1000s, 2500s, 5000s.
Use: Peripheral vascular insufficiency.

ETHASULFATE SODIUM. Sod. 2-Ethyl-1-hexanol sulfate.

ETHATAB. (Glaxo) Ethaverine HCl 100 mg./Tab. Bot. 100s, 500s, 5000s. Unit dose 100s.
Use: Smooth muscle relaxant.

ETHAV. (Amfre-Grant) Ethaverine HCl 100 mg./Tab. Bot. 100s, 1000s.
Use: Cardiovascular.

ETHAVERINE HYDROCHLORIDE. The ethyl analog of papaverine HCl, 6,7-diethoxy-1-(3',4'-diethoxybenzyl) isoquinoline HCl. Diquinol HCl, Preparin HCl, Perperine HCl. The tetraethyl homolog of papaverine is 2 to 4 times more active and less than half as toxic as the parent drug. This compound is not a narcotic.
(Lincoln) Tab. (½ gr.) Bot. 100s, 300s.
Vial (15 mg./cc.) 10 cc.
Use: I.V., Antispasmodic.
See: Cebral, Cap. (Kenwood)
Circubid, Cap. (W. F. Merchant)
Etalent, Cap. (Roger)
Ethaquin, Tab. (Ascher)
Ethatab, Tab. (Glaxo)
Isovex, Cap. (Medics)
Neopavrin, Tab., Elix. (Savage)
Pavaspan, Cap. (Jamieson-McKames)
Roldiol, Tab. (Robinson)
Spasodil, Tab. (Rand)
(Pharmex) Vial 15 mg., 20 mg., 45 mg., 75 mg./ml.
W/Pentaerythritol tetranitrate.
Use: Intramuscular, antispasmodic.
See: Papavatral, Tab. (Kenwood)

ETHAVEROL "75". (Pharmex) Ethaverine HCl 75 mg./cc. Vial 10 cc.

ETHAVEX-100 TABLETS. (Econo Med) Ethaverine HCl 100 mg./Tab. Bot. 100s.

Use: Arterial spasmolytic for peripheral and cerebral vascular insufficiency.

• **ETHCHLORVYNOL,** U.S.P. XXI. Cap., U.S.P. XXI. 1-Chloro-3-ethyl-1-penten-4 yn-3-ol.
Use: Hypnotic, sedative.
See: Arvynol
Placidyl, Cap. (Abbott)
Serensil, Prod. (Ciba).

ETHCHLORVYNOL. B.A.N. 1-Chloro-3-ethyl-pent-1-en-4-yn-3-ol.
Use: Hypnotic; sedative.

ETHEBENECID. B.A.N. 4-Diethylsulamoylbenzoic acid.
Use: Uricosuric.
See: Urelim

ETHENOL, HOMOPOLYMER. Polyvinyl Alcohol, U.S.P. XXI.

ETHENZAMIDE. o-Ethoxybenzamide.

• **ETHER,** U.S.P. XXI. Ethyl ether
Use: General anesthetic.

ETHEREA ENVIRONMENTAL PROTECTION LOTION. (Revlon) Padimate O, Oxybenzone in lotion base. SPF #6
Use: Daytime moisturizer & sunburn preventitive.

ETHIAZIDE. B.A.N. 6-Chloro-3-ethyl-3,4-dihydro-1,2,4-benzothiadiazine-7-sulfonamide 1,1-dioxide.
Use: Diuretic.

• **ETHINAMATE,** U.S.P. XXI. Cap., U.S.P. XXI. 1-Ethynylcyclohexanoyl carbamate.
Use: Hypnotic.
See: Valmid, Tab. (Dista)
Valmidate

• **ETHINYL ESTRADIOL,** U.S.P. XXI. Tab., U.S.P. XXI. 17-Ethinyl-3,17-estradiol. 19-Norpregna-1,3,5(10)-trien-20-yne-3,17-diol,(17α)-. 19-Nor-17α-pregna-1, 3,5-(10)-trien-20-yne-3,17-diol.
Use: Estrogen.
See: Estinyl, Tab. (Schering)
Feminone, Tab. (Upjohn)
Lynoral, Tab. (Organon)
Menolyn, Tab. (Arcum)
Ovogyn, Tab. (Pasadena Research)

ETHINYL ESTRADIOL W/COMBINATIONS
See: Ardiatric, Tab. (Burgin-Arden)
Brevicon, Tab. (Syntex)
Demulen, Tab. (Searle)
Diatric, Tab. (Pasadena Research)
Geramine, Tab., Inj. (Brown)
Geritag, Cap. (Reid-Provident)
Gynetone, Tab. (Schering)
Halodrin, Tab. (Upjohn)
Hormox Plus, Tab. (Parmed)
Loestrin ¹/₂₀, Tab. (Parke-Davis)
Loestrin 1.5/30, Tab. (Parke-Davis)
Min-Gera, Tab. (Scrip)
Modicon 21 and 28, Tab. (Ortho)
Neosterol, Tab. (Winston)
Nordette, Tab. (Wyeth)
Norinyl, Prods. (Syntex)
Norlestrin, Tab. (Parke-Davis)
Norlestrin FE., Tab. (Parke-Davis)
Ortho-Novum 1/35, 21 and 28 (Ortho)
Os-Cal-Mone, Tab. (Marion)

Ovcon-35 Tablets (Mead Johnson)
Ovcon-50 Tablets (Mead Johnson)
Ovlin, Vial (ICN)
Ovral, Tab. (Wyeth)
Vee-Gera Basic, Cap. (Mericon)
Vimah, Vial, Tab. (Hyrex)
Viromone, Tabs. (Western Research Labs.)
Zorane, Tab. (Lederle)
Zorane 1/20, 1/50, 1.5/30 (Lederle)

ETHINYL ESTRENOL.
See: Lynestrenol (Organon)
ETHINYL ESTRADIOL AND DIMETHISTERONE TABLETS.
Use: Estrogen-progestin.
17α-ETHINYL-19-NORTESTERONE. Norethindrone Acetate, U.S.P. XXI.
ETHINYL (17)-19-NORTESTOSTERONE.
See: Norlutin, Tab. (Parke-Davis)
ETHIODOL. (Savage) Ethiodized oil. Fatty acid ethyl ester of poppy-seed oil w/37% iodine. Amp. 10 cc., Box 2s.
Use: Diagnostic agent, roentgenography.
• **ETHIODIZED OIL INJECTION,** U.S.P. XXI.
Use: Diagnostic aid (Radiopaque medium)
See: Ethiodol, Inj. (Savage)
• **ETHIODIZED OIL I-131.** USAN. Radioactive iodine addition to ethyl ester of poppyseed oil. Ethiodal-131.
Use: Anti-oncotic agent.
• **ETHIOFOS.** USAN.
Formerly gammaphos.
Use: Radioprotector
ETHIONAMIDE. B.A.N. 2-Ethylisonicotinthioamide.
Use: Treatment of tuberculosis.
See: Trescatyl
• **ETHIONAMIDE,** U.S.P. XXI. Tab., U.S.P. XXI. 2-Ethyl-thioisonicotinamide.   4-Pyridinecarbothioamide,   2-ethyl.
Use: Tuberculostatic.
See: Trecator S.C., Tab. (Ives)
ETHISTERONE. 17-Hydroxy-17a-pregn-4-en-20-yn-3-one.
See: Anhydrohydroxyprogesterone. (Various Mfr.)
ETHOCAINE.
See: Procaine Hydrochloride (Various Mfr.)
ETHOCYLORVYNOL. β-Chlorovinyl ethyl ethynyl carbinol. Ethchlorvynol, U.S.P. XXI.
ETHODRYL.
See: Diethylcarbamazine Citrate
ETHOGLUCID. B.A.N. 1,2:15,16-Diepoxy-4,7,10,-13-tetraoxahexadecane.
Use: Antineoplastic agent.
See: Epodyl
ETHOHEPTAZINE. B.A.N. Ethyl hexahydro-1-methyl-4-phenylazepine-4-carboxylate.
Use: Analgesic.
ETHOHEPTAZINE CITRATE. Ethyl Hexahydro-1-methyl-4-phenylazepine-4-carboxylate Dihydrogen citrate. Ethyl Hexahydro-1-methyl-4-phenyl-1H-azepine-4-carboxylate Citrate (1:1)
ETHOHEXADIOL. Ethyl hexanediol, 2-ethylhexane-1,3-diol, Rutgers 612. Used in Comp. Dimethyl Phthalate.

Use: Insect repellent.
ETHOMOXANE. B.A.N. 2-Butylaminomethyl-8-ethoxy-1,4-benzodioxan.
Use: Adrenaline antagonist.
• **ETHONAM NITRATE.** USAN. Ethyl 1-(1,2,3-4-tetrahydro-1-naphthyl)imidazole-5-carboxylate nitrate.
Use: Fungicide.
ETHOPROPAZINE. B.A.N. 10-(2-Diethylaminopropyl)-phenothiazine. Profenamine (I.N.N.)
Use: Treatment of the Parkinsonian syndrome.
See: Lysivane (hydrochloride)
• **ETHOPROPAZINE HYDROCHLORIDE,** U.S.P. XXI.
Tab. U.S.P. XXI. 10H-Phenothiazine-10-ethanamine, N,N-diethyl-α-methyl-,monohydrochloride. 10-[2-(Diethylamino)propyl]-phenothiazine monohydrochloride. Lysivane.
Use: Antiparkinsonian.
See: Parsidol HCl, Tab. (Warner-Chilcott)
ETHOSALAMIDE. B.A.N. 2-(2-Ethoxyethoxy) benzamide.
Use: Analgesic; antipyretic.
• **ETHOSUXIMIDE,** U.S.P. XXI. Cap., U.S.P. XXI. 2-Ethyl-2-methyl-succinimide.
Use: Anticonvulsant.
See: Zarontin, Cap., Syr. (Parke-Davis)
ETHOSUXIMIDE. B.A.N. 2-Ethyl-2-methylsuccinimide.
Use: Anticonvulsant.
See: Capitus
  Emeside
  Simatin
  Zarontin
ETHOTOIN. 3-Ethyl-5-phenylhydantoin.
See: Peganone, Tab. (Abbott)
ETHOTOIN. B.A.N. 3-Ethyl-5-phenylimidazoline-2,4-dione.
Use: Anticonvulsant.
See: Peganone, Tab. (Abbott)
ETHOVAN. Ethyl Vanillin.
• **ETHOXAZENE HYDROCHLORIDE.** USAN. 4-[(p-Ethoxy-phenyl)azo]-m-phenyl-enediamine HCl 2,4-Diamino-4'-ethoxyazobenzene hydrochloride.
Use: Urinary analgesic.
See: Serenium, Tab. (Squibb)
6-ETHOXY-2-BENZOTHIAZOLESULFONAMIDE.
Ethoxzolamide, U.S.P. XXI.
ETHOXZOLAMIDE. 6-Ethoxy-2-benzothiazolesulfonamide.
Use: Carbonic anhydrase inhibitor.
ETHRANE. (Ohio Medical) Enflurane.
ETHRIL. (Squibb) Erythromycin stearate 250 mg./Tab. Bot. 100s, 500s; 500 mg./Tab. Bot. 50s.
Use: Antibiotic.
ETHYBENZTROPINE. B.A.N. 3-Benzhydryloxy-8-ethyl-nortropane.
Use: Anticholinergic.
• **ETHYBENZTROPINE.** USAN. 3-(diphenylmethoxy)-8-ethylnortropane. Panolid. Methylbenztropine.
Use: Anticholinergic.
• **ETHYL ACETATE,** N.F. XVI.
Use: Flavor.
ETHYL AMINOBENZOATE. Anesthesin, anesthrone, benzocaine, parathesin.

Use: Surface anesthetic.
See: Benzocaine (Var. Mfr.)
ETHYL BISCOUMACETATE. B.A.N. Ethyl di(4-hydroxy-ycoumarin-3-yl)acetate.
Use: Anticoagulant.
See: Pelentan
ETHYL BISCOUMACETATE. 3,3'-(Carboxymethylene) bis (4-hydroxycoumarin) ethyl ester. Ethyl Bis (4-hydroxy-2-oxo-2H-1-benzopyran-3-yl) acetate.
ETHYL BROMIDE. (Various Mfr.) Bromoethane.
Use: Inhalation anesthetic.
5-ETHYL-5-n-BUTYLBARBITURIC ACID.
See: Butethal (Var. Mfr.)
ETHYL CARBAMATE.
See: Urethan (Var. Mfr.)
• **ETHYLCELLULOSE,** N.F. XVI.
Use: Tablet binder.
ETHYL CHAULMOOGRATE.
Use: Hansen's disease, sarcoidosis.
• **ETHYL CHLORIDE,** U.S.P. XXI.
Chloroethane
Use: Local anesthetic.
See: Gebauer-Spra-Pak
Stratford-Cook-Spray, 100 Gm.
2-ETHYLCROTONYLUREA.
See: Ectylurea
ETHYL 1-(3-CYANO-3,3-DIPHENYLPROPYL)-4-PHENYLISO-NIPECOTATE MONOHYDROCHLO-RIDE. Diphenoxylate Hydrochloride, U.S.P. XXI.
• **ETHYL DIBUNATE.** USAN. Ethyl 2,7-di-t-butyl-naphthalene-1-sulfonate.
Use: Cough suppressant.
ETHYL DIIODOBRASSIDATE. Iodobrassid. Lipoiodine.
ETHYLDIMETHYLAMMONIUM BROMIDE.
See: Ambutonium Bromide
5-ETHYL-3,5-DIMETHYL-2,4-OXAZOLIDINEDIONE. Paramethadione, U.S.P. XXI.
ETHYLENE. (Various Mfr.) Ethene.
Use: Inhalation anesthetic.
• **ETHYLENEDIAMINE,** U.S.P. XXI. Component of Aminophylline.
ETHYLENEDIAMINE SOLUTION. (67% w/v).
Use: Solvent (Aminophylline Inj.).
ETHYLENEDIAMINETETRAACETIC ACID.
See. Edathamil, EDTA (Var. Mfr.)
ETHYLENEDIAMINE TETRAACETIC ACID-DISODIUM SALT.
See: Endrate Disodium, Amp. (Abbott)
1-N-ETHYLEPHEDRINE HYDROCHLORIDE.
Use: Bronchodilator & vasoconstrictor.
See: Nethamine Hydrochloride, Prep. (Var. Mfr.)
• **ETHYLESTRENOL.** F.D.A. 19-Nor-17 alphapregn-4-en-17 beta-ol.
• **ETHYLESTRENOL.** USAN. 17α-Ethyl- 17β-hydroxy-estr-4-ene.
Use: Anabolic steroid.
See: Maxibolin, Tab., Elix. (Organon)
(+)-**13-ETHYL-17α-ETHYNYL-17-HYDROXYGON-4-EN-3-ONE.** Norgestrel, U.S.P. XXI.
2-ETHYLHEXANE-1,3-DIOL.
See: Ethohexadiol.

ETHYLHYDROCUPREINE HCI. O⁶′
Ethylhydrocupreine monohydrochloride.
Use: Antiseptic.
13-ETHYL-17-HYDROXY-18,19-DINOR,17 alpha-PREGN-4-EN-3-ONE. Genabol.
ETHYL 10-(IODOPHENYL)UNDECANOATE.
See: Iophendylate, U.S.P. XXI.
ETHYL(m-HYDROXYPHENYL)DIMETHYL-AMMONIUM CHLORIDE. Edrophonium Chloride, U.S.P. XXI.
5-ETHYL-5-ISOAMYL BARBITURIC ACID.
See: Amobarbital (Var. Mfr.)
ETHYLMETHYLTHIAMBUTENE. B.A.N. 3-Ethyl-methylamino-1,1-di-(2-thienyl)but-1-ene.
Use: Narcotic analgesic.
2-ETHYL-2-METHYLSUCCINIMIDE. Ethosuximide, U.S.P. XXI.
ETHYLMORPHINE HYDROCHLORIDE. 7,8-Didehydro-4,5α-epoxy-3-ethoxy-17-methyl-morphinan-6α-ol Hydrochloride. Dionin.
Use: Narcotic.
ETHYL NITRITE SPIRIT. Ethyl nitrite. Sweet Spirit of Niter. Spirit of Nitrous Ether.
• **ETHYLNOREPINEPHRINE HCI,** U.S.P. XXI. Inj., U.S.P. XXI.
See: Bronkephrine, Amp. (Winthrop-Breon)
ETHYLESTRENOL. B.A.N. 17α-Ethylestr-4-en-17β-ol.
Use: Anabolic steroid.
See: Orabolin
• **ETHYL OLEATE,** N.F. XVI.
Use: Pharmaceutic aid (vehicle).
ETHYL OXIDE; ETHYL ETHER,
Use: Solvent.
ETHYLPAPAVERINE HCI.
See: Ethaverine HCI. (Var. Mfr.)
• **ETHYLPARABEN,** N.F. XVI. Ethyl p-Hydroxybenzoate.
Use: Pharm. aid (antifungal preservative).
ETHYL PYROPHOSPHATE. B.A.N. Tetraethyl pyrophosphate.
Use: Treatment of myasthenia gravis.
5-ETHYL-SEC-BUTYLBARBITURIC ACID.
See: Butabarbital (Var. Mfr.)
ETHYLSTIBAMINE. Astaril, neostibosan.
Use: Antimony therapy.
2-ETHYLTHIOISONICOTINAMIDE. Ethionamide, U.S.P. XXI.
ETHYL VANILLATE. Ethyl-hydroxy-methoxy-benzoate.
• **ETHYL VANILLIN,** N.F. XVI. 3-Ethoxy-4-hydroxybenzaldehyde.
Use: Flavor.
• **ETHYNERONE.** USAN.
Use: Progestin.
ETHYNODIOL. B.A.N. 19-Nor-17α-pregn-4-en-20-yne-3β,17-diol.
Use: Progestational steroid.
• **ETHYNODIOL DIACETATE,** U.S.P. XXI. 19-Nor-17α-pregn-4-en-20-yne-3B,17-diol diacetate; 17α-ethynyl-4-estrene-3β,17β-diol diacetate.
Use: As Progesterone.
See: Ovulen, Tab. (Searle)
W/Ethinyl estradiol.
See: Demulen, Preps. (Searle)

W/Mestranol.
See: Ovulen, Tab. (Searle)
• **ETHYNODIOL DIACETATE AND ETHINYL ESTRADIOL TABLETS,** U.S.P. XXI.
Use: Oral contraceptive.
• **ETHYNODIOL DIACETATE AND MESTRANOL TABLETS,** U.S.P. XXI.
Use: Oral contraceptive.
ETHYNLESTRADIOL.
See: Ethinyl Estradiol, U.S.P. (Various Mfr.)
Mestranol (Var. Mfr.)
17α-ETHYNYLESTRADIOL 3-METHYL ETHER. Mestranol, U.S.P. XXI.
ETHYNYLESTRADIOL 3-METHYL ETHER.
See: Enovid, Tab. (Searle)
N-ETHYL-2-PHENYL-N-(4-PYRIDYLMETHYL)HYDRA-CRYLAMIDE. Tropicamide, U.S.P. XXI.
• **ETIBENDAZOLE.** USAN.
Use: Anthelmintic.
ETICYLOL. (Ciba) Ethinyl estradiol.
• **ETIDOCAINE.** USAN. (+)-2-(N-Ethylpropylamino)-butyro-2',6'-xylidide.
Use: Local anesthetic.
See: Duranest (base and hydrochloride)
• **ETIDRONATE DISODIUM,** U.S.P. XXI. The disodium salt of (1-Hydroxyethylidene) diphosphonic acid.
Use: Treatment of symptomatic Pagent's disease of bone (osteitis deformans).
See: Didronel, Tab. (Procter & Gamble)
• **ETIDRONIC ACID.** USAN. (1-Hydroxy-ethylidene) diphosphonic acid.
Use: Bone calcium regulator.
• **ETIFENIN.** USAN.
Use: Diagnostic aid.
ETIFOXINE. B.A.N. 6-Chloro-2-ethylamino-4-methyl-4-phenyl-4H-3,1-benzoxazine.
Use: Tranquilizer.
• **ETINTIDINE HYDROCHLORIDE.** USAN.
Use: Antagonist.
ETISAZOLE. B.A.N. 3-Ethylamino-1,2-benzisothiazole.
Use: Fungicide, veterinary medicine.
See: Ectimar
ETISUL. Ditophal, B.A.N.
ETNAPA ELIXIR. (U.S. Ethicals) Acetaminophen 120 mg./5 ml. Bot. 120 ml.
Use: Anti-pyretic, analgesic for children.
• **ETOCRYLENE.** USAN.
Use: Ultraviolet screen.
• **ETODOLAC.** USAN.
Use: Anti-inflammatory.
• **ETOFORMIN HYDROCHLORIDE.** USAN.
Use: Antidiabetic.
• **ETOMIDATE.** USAN.
Use: Hypnotic.
ETOMIDE HYDROCHLORIDE. Bandol. Carbiphene HCl.
ETONITAZENE. B.A.N. 1-(2-Diethylaminoethyl)-2-(4-ethoxybenzyl)-5-nitrobenzimidazole.
Use: Narcotic analgesic.
ETOPHYLATE. Acepifylline, B.A.N.
• **ETOPOSIDE.** USAN.
Use: Antineoplastic.

See: Vepesid, Inj. (Bristol)
• **ETOPRINE.** USAN.
Use: Antineoplatic.
ETOQUINOL SODIUM. Name used for Actinoquinol sodium.
ETORPHINE. B.A.N. 7,8-Dihydro-7α-[1(R)-hydroxy-1-methylbutyl]-0⁶-methyl-6,14-endoethenomorphine.
Use: Narcotic analgesic.
ETOVAL.   •
See: Butethal, N.F. (Various Mfr.)
• **ETOXADROL HYDROCHLORIDE.** USAN.
Use: Anesthetic.
ETOXERIDINE. B.A.N. Ethyl 1-[2-(2-hydroxyethoxy)e-thyl]-4-phenylpiperidine-4-carboxylate.
Use: Narcotic analgesic.
• **ETOZOLIN.** USAN.
Use: Diuretic.
ETRAFON (2-25). (Schering) Perphenazine 2 mg. amitriptyline HCl 25 mg./Tab. Bot. 100s, 500s. Unit dose 100s.
Use: Antidepressant, tranquilizer.
ETRAFON (2-10). (Schering) Perphenazine 2 mg., amitriptyline HCl 10 mg./Tab. Bot. 100s, 500s. Unit dose 100s.
Use: Tranquilizer, antidepressant.
ETRAFON-A (4-10). (Schering) Perphenazine 4 mg., amitriptyline HCl 10 mg./Tab. Bot. 100s, 500s. Unit dose 100s.
Use: Tranquilizer, antidepressant.
ETRAFON FORTE TABLETS (4-25). (Schering) Perphenazine 4 mg., amitriptyline HCl 25 mg./Tab. Bot. 100s, 500s. Unit dose 100s.
Use: Tranquilizer, antidepressant.
ETRENOL INJECTION. (Winthrop Products) Hycanthone (as mesylate).
Use: Antibilharziasis.
• **ETRETINATE.** USAN.
Use: Antipsoriatic.
ETRYNIT. Propatyl nitrate.
Use: Coronary
ETRYPTAMINE. B.A.N. 3-(2-Aminobutyl)-indole. a-Ethyltryptamine. Monase [acetate]
Use: Antidepressant.
• **ETRYPTAMINE ACETATE.** USAN. 3-(2-Aminobutyl)-indole Acetate.
Use: Central stimulant.
See: Monase (Upjohn)
ETTRIOL TRINITRATE.
See: Propatyl nitrate.
E.T. VITAMINS. (Squibb) Vit. A 5,000 I.U., D 400 I.U., E 30 I.U., C 60 mg., folic acid 0.4 mg.; thiamine 1.5 mg., riboflavin 1.7 mg., niacin 20 mg., B-6 2 mg., B-12 6 mcg/Chewable Tab. Bot. 60s.
Use: Childrens chewable vitamin.
E.T. VITAMINS WITH IRON. (Squibb) Vitamin A 5,000 I.U., D 400 I.U., E 30 I.U., C 60 mg., folic acid 0.4 mg., Thiamine 1.5 mg., riboflavin 1.7 mg., niacin 20 mg., B-6 2 mg., B-12 6 mcg.; iron 18 mg./Chewable Tab. Bot. 60s.
Use: Childrens chewable vitamin with iron.
ETYBENZATROPINE. Ethybenztropine.
ETYNODIOL ACETATE. Ethynodiol Diacetate.

EUBASIN.
See: Sulfapyridine (Various Mfr.)
EUCAINE HCl. 2,2,6-Trimethyl-4-piperidinol benzoate HCl.
EUCALYPTOL. 1,8-Epoxy-p-menthane.
Use: Pharmaceutic aid (flavor), antitussive, nasal decongestant.
See: Vicks Sinex, Nasal Spray (Vicks)
Vicks Va-Tro-Nol, Nose Drops (Vicks)
Vicks Prods. (Vicks)
• **EUCALYPTUS OIL,** N.F. XVI.
Use: Flavor, antitussive, nasal decongestant, expectorant, topical analgesic.
See: Vicks Prods. (Vicks)
Victors Regular & Cherry Loz. (Vicks)
EUCAPINE SYRUP. (Lannett) Ammonium chloride 10 gr., pot. guaiacol sulf. 8 gr., in white pine & wild cherry syrup. Bot. 1 pt., 1 gal.
Use: Cough expectorant.
EUCATROPINE. B.A.N. 1,2,2,6-Tetramethyl-4-piperidyl mandelate. Euphthalmine
Use: Mydriatic.
• **EUCATROPINE HYDROCHLORIDE,** U.S.P. XXI.
Ophth. Soln., U.S.P. XXI. 1,2,2,6-Tetramethyl-4-piperidyl mandelate HCl. Benzeneacetic acid, alpha-hydroxy-, 1,2,2,6-tetramethyl-4-piperidinyl ester hydrochloride. (Glogau) Cryst., Bot. 1 Gm.
Use: Pharm. necessity for ophthalmic dosage form.
EUCERIN. (Beiersdorf) Emulsion of equal parts Aquaphor and water. 1 lb. jar. 5 oz. tin.
EUCODAL.
See: Oxycodone (No Mfr. currently lists)
EUCORAN.
See: Nikethamide (Various Mfr.)
EUCUPIN DIHYDROCHLORIDE.
Isoamylhydrocupreine dihydrochloride.
EUDEMINE. Diazoxide, B.A.N.
EUFLAVINE.
See: Acriflavine (Various Mfr.)
• **EUGENOL,** U.S.P. XXI. (Various Mfr.) 4-Allyl-2-methoxy-phenol. Phenol, 2-methoxy-4-(2-propenyl)-.
Use: Dental analgesic, oral anesthetic.
See: Benzodent, Oint. (Vicks)
EUKADOL.
See: Dihydrohydroxycodeinone, Preps. (No Mfr. currently lists)
EULCIN. (Leeds) Methscopolamine bromide 2.5 mg., butabarbital sod. 10 mg., aluminum hydroxide gel dried 250 mg., Mag. trisilicate 250 mg./Tab. Bot. 100s.
Use: Gastric & duodenal ulcer therapy.
EULISSIN. Decamethonium Iodide, B.A.N.
EUMYDRIN DROPS. (Winthrop Products) Atropine methonitrate.
Use: Antispasmodic.
EUNERYL.
See: Phenobarbital (Various Mfr.)
EUPHORBIA COMPOUND. (Sherwood) Euphorbia pilulifera fl. ext. 1.5 cc., lobelia tr. 2.2 cc., nitroglycerin spirit 0.29 cc., Sod. iodide 1.04 Gm., Sod. bromide 1.04 Gm., alcohol 24%/30 cc. Bot. 1 pt., 1 gal.

Use: Sedative & expectorant.
EUPHORBIA PILULIFERA.
W/Cocillana, squill, antimony potassium tartrate, senega.
See: Cylana, Syr. (Bowman)
W/Phenyl salicylate & various oils.
See: Rayderm, Oint. (Velvet Pharmacal)
EUPRACTONE. (Travenol) Dimethadione.
EUPRAX. Albution.
• **EUPROCIN HCl.** USAN. O⁶′-Isopentylhydrocupreine dihydrochloride.
Use: Topical anesthetic.
See: Eucupin HCl
EUQUININE. Quinine ethyl carbonate.
Use: Orally; antimalarial & antipyretic.
EURAX CREAM. (Westwood) Crotamiton 10% in vanishing-cream base of glyceryl monostearate, lanolin, PEG 6-32, glycerin, polysorbate 80, water, benzyl alcohol, mineral oil, white wax, quaternium-15 and fragrance. Tube 60 Gm.
Use: Antipruritic & scabicide.
EURAX LOTION. (Westwood) Crotamiton 10% in emollient-lotion base of glyceryl monostearate, lanolin, PEG 6-32, glycerin, Polysorbate 80, water, benzyl alcohol, light mineral oil, Na carboxymethylcellulose, simethicone, quaternium-15 and fragrance. Bot. 60 Gm., 454 Gm.
Use: Antipruritic & scabicide.
EUTHROID. (Parke-Davis) Liotrix (sod. levothyroxine & sod. liothyronine) Tabs. ½ gr., 1 gr., 2 gr., & 3 gr. Bot. 100s. Tab. 1 gr. Bot. 1000s.
Use: Thyroid therapy.
EUTONYL. (Abbott) Pargyline Hydrochloride. 10 mg., 25 mg./Tab. Bot. 100s.
Use: Antihypertensive agent.
EUTRON FILMTAB. (Abbott) Pargyline HCl 25 mg., methylclothiazide 5 mg./Tab. Bot. 100s.
Use: Antihypertensive agent.
EVAC-Q-KIT. (Adria) Each kit contains: (1)**Evac-Q-Mag:** Magnesium citrate, citric acid, potassium citrate. (2) **Evac-Q-Tabs:** 2 tabs containing 2 gr. phenolphthalein/Tab. (3) **Evac-Q-Sert:** 2 Supps. containing potassium bitartrate, sodium bicarbonate/Supp. in polyethylene glycol base. (4) Patient instruction sheet.
Use: Bowel evacuant.
EVAC-Q-KWIK. (Adria) Each kit contains: **Evac-Q-Mag.:** Magnesium citrate, citric acid, potassium citrate in cherry-flavored base, **Evac-Q-Tabs.:** 2 Tab. phenolphthalein 2 gr. **Evac-Q-Kwik Supp.:** 10 mg. bisacodyl
Use: Bowel evacuant.
EVAC SUPPOSITORIES. (Burgin-Arden) Sodium bicarbonate, sodium biphosphate, dioctyl sodium sulfosuccinate 50 mg./Supp.
Use: Laxative.
EVAC TABLETS. (Burgin-Arden) Guar gum 300 mg., danthron 50 mg., sodium 100 mg./Tab.
Use: Laxative.
EVACTOL. (Delta) Dihydroxyanthraquinone 75 mg., docusate sodium 100 mg., sodium carboxymethyl

cellulose 200 mg./Cap. Pkg. 10s, Bot. 10s, 30s, 100s.
Use: Laxative.

EVAC-U-GEN. (Walker) Yellow phenolphthalein 97.2 mg./Tab. Pkg. 35s, Bot. 100s, 1000s, 6000s.
Use: Laxative.

EVAC-U-LAX. (Mallard) Phenolphthalein, yellow 80 mg./Wafer. Bot. 100s.
Use: Laxative.

• EVANS BLUE, U.S.P. XXI. Inj., U.S.P. XXI. 1,3-Naph-thalenedisulfonic acid, 6,6'-[(3,3'-dimethyl[1,1'-bi-phenyl]-4,4'-diyl)bis(azo)]bis[4-amino-5-hydroxy]-, tetrasodium salt. Azovan Blue, B.A.N. (Harvey) Pure diazo dye. Amp. (0.5%) 5 ml. 12s, 25s, 100s.
Use: Diagnostic aid, (blood-volume determination).

EVERONE. (Hyrex) Testosterone enanthate 100 mg. or 200 mg., benzyl alcohol 2%/ml. Vial 10 ml.
Use: Long acting male hormone.

EVEX. (Syntex) Purified esterified orally active water soluble estrogens expressed as sodium estrone sulfate. Tab. 0.625 mg., 1.25 mg. Bot. 100s.
Use: Estrogen replacement therapy.

EVICYL TABLETS. (Winthrop Products) Inositol hexanicotinate.
Use: Hypolipedimic, peripheral vasodilator.

EVIRON. (Delta) Ferrous fumarate 160 mg., copper 1 mg., ascorbic acid 75 mg./Tab.
Use: Hematinic.

EVIRON FA. (Delta) Ferrous fumarate 160 mg., copper 1 mg., Vit. C 75 mg., folic acid 1.5 mg./Tab.
Use: Hematinic.

EVIRON FT. (Delta) Ferrous fumarate 160 mg., copper 1 mg., Vit C 50 mg., cyanocobalamin 7.5 mcg.
Use: Hematinic.

E-VISTA. (Seatrace) Hydroxyzine HCl 50 mg./ml. Vial 10 cc.

E-VITABON. (Pasadena Research) Vit. E 200 I.U., C 100 mg., B-1 2 mg., B-2 2 mg., B-6 5 mg., B-12 10 mcg., d-panthenol 5 mg., niacinamide 10 mg./Tab. Bot. 60s, 100s, 500s.

E-VITAL. (Pasadena Research) d-Alpha tocopheryl succinate 100 I.U., 200 I.U./Cap. Bot. 100s, 1000s. 400 I.U. Bot. 100s, 500s.

E-VITAL CREME. (Pasadena Research) Vit. E 100 I.U., A 250 I.U., D 100 I.U., d-panthenol 0.2%, allantoin 0.1%/Gm. Jar 2 oz., 1 lb.

E-VITES. (Columbia) Vit. E (from dl-alpha tocopheryl acetate) 100 I.U., 200 I.U., 400 I.U., 1000 I.U./Cap. Bot. 100s.

EWIN NINOS TABLETS. (Winthrop Products) Aspirin.
Use: Analgesic, antipyretic.

• EXAPROLOL HYDROCHLORIDE. USAN.
Use: Antiadrenergic.

EX-AQUA. (Edward J. Moore) Ext. buchu, ext. uva ursi, ext. corn silk, ext. juniper, caffeine/Tab. Bot. 80s.
Use: Diuretic.

EX-CALORIC WAFERS. (Eastern Research) Carboxymethylcellulose 181 mg., methylcellulose 272 mg./Wafer. Bot. 100s, 500s, 5000s.
Use: Diet control.

EXCEDRIN CAPSULES. (Bristol-Myers) Aspirin 250 mg., acetaminophen 250 mg., caffeine 65 mg./Cap. Bot. 24s, 40s, 60s.
Use: Analgesic.

EXCEDRIN TABLETS. (Bristol-Myers) Acetaminophen 250 mg., caffeine 65 mg., aspirin 250 mg./Tab. Bot. 12s, 36s, 60s, 100s, 165s, 225s, 375s. Tins 12s.
Use: Analgesic.

EXCEDRIN P.M.. (Bristol-Myers) Acetaminophen 500 mg., diphenhydramine citrate 38 mg./Tab. Bot. 10s, 30s, 50s, 80s.
Use: Analgesic, sleep aid.

EX-LAX. (Ex-Lax) Yellow phenolphthalein 90 mg./ chocolated Tab. or unflavored pill. Chocolated Tab. 6s, 18s, 48s, 72s. Unflavored pills 8s, 30s, 60s.
Use: Laxative.

EX-LAX EXTRA GENTLE. (Ex-Lax) Phenolphthalein 65 mg., docusate sodium 75 mg./Tab. Pkg. 24s, 48s.
Use: Laxative, stool softener.

EXNA. (Robins) Benzthiazide 50 mg./Tab. Bot. 100s, 500s.
Use: Diuretic, antihypertensive.

EX-OBESE. (Kay) Phendimetrazine tartrate 35 mg./Tab. Bot. 100s, 1000s, 5000s.
Use: Anorexigenic agent.

EXOCAINE. (Commerce) Methyl salicylate 25%. Tube 1.3 oz.
Use: Minor pains of arthritis and rheumatism.

EXOCAINE ODOR FREE. (Commerce) Triethanolamine salicylate 10%. Tube 3 oz.
Use: Relief from minor pain of arthritis, rheumatism, backache, muscular aches.

EXOCAINE PLUS. (Commerce) Methyl salicylate. Jar 4 oz. Tube 1.3 oz.
Use: Temporary relief of minor pain of arthritis, rheumatism, muscular aches, bursitis, neuritis.

EXO-KOL. (Inwood) Phenylephrine HCl 5 mg., chlorpheniramine maleate 1 mg., salicylamide 3½ gr., phenacetin 1½ gr., caffeine 10 mg., Vit. C 20 mg./Tab. Bot. 50s, 1000s.
Use: Antihistaminic w/analgesic.

EXO-KOL COUGH SYRUP. (Inwood) Dextromethorphan HBr 10 mg., cetylpyridinium chloride 0.25%, phenyltoloxamine dihydrogen citrate 25 mg., sodium citrate/5 cc. Bot. 4 oz. Also Exo-Kol Pediatric Cough Syrup available. Bot. 4 oz.
Use: Coughs.

EXO-KOL NASAL SPRAY. (Inwood) Phenylephrine HCl 0.5%, pyrilamine maleate 0.15%, cetyl-dimethyl benzyl ammonium chloride 0.04%. Bot. 1 oz.
Use: Nasal-spray. Decongestant, antihistaminic.

EXOL. Di-isobutyl ethoxy ethyl dimethyl benzyl ammonium chloride.
W/Benzocaine, menthol, calamine, pyrilamine maleate.

EXONIC OT. Dioctyl Sodium Sulphosuccinate.
Use: Laxative.

EXORBIN. (Various Mfr.) Polyamine-methylene resin.

EXPECTICO COUGH SYRUP. (Coastal) Dihydrocodeinone bitartrate 30 mg., guaifenesin

600 mg., sod. citrate 900 mg., chlorpheniramine maleate 12 mg./Fl. oz. Bot. 16 oz., gal.
Use: Antitussive, antihistaminic, expectorant.

EXPECTICO PED. COUGH SYRUP. (Coastal) Dihydrocodeinone bitartrate 15 mg., guaifenesin 300 mg., sod. citrate 450 mg., chlorpheniramine maleate 6 mg., phenylephrine HCl 12 mg./Fl. oz. Bot. 16 oz., gal.
Use: Antitussive, antihistaminic, expectorant, decongestant.

EXPECTO HIST. (Wolins) Guaifenesin 100 mg., phenylephrine HCl, chlorpheniramine maleate 1 mg./Tab. Bot. 1000s.
Use: Antihistaminic, expectorant, decongestant.

EXPECTORANT COUGH SYRUP. (Weeks & Leo) Dextromethorphan HBr 15 mg., guaifenesin 100 mg./5 ml. w/alcohol 7.125%. Bot. 6 oz.
Use: Relief of cough and chest congestion.

EXPENDABLE BLOOD COLLECTION UNIT—ACD. (Travenol) Citric acid 540 mg., sodium citrate 1.49 Gm., dextrose 1.65 Gm./67.5 ml.
Use: Anti-coagulant.

EXSEL. (Herbert) Selenium sulfide 2.5% in shampoo base. Lotion. Bot. 4 fl. oz.
Use: Seborrheic dermatitis.

EXTEN STRONE 10. (Schlicksup) Estradiol valerate 10 mg./cc. Vial 10 cc.

EXTEND. (Edward J. Moore) Benzocaine, dibucaine. Tube 1 oz.
Use: Desensitizer.

EXTEND 12. (Robins) Dextromethorphan resin complex equivalent to 30 mg. Dextromethorphan H Br. Bot. 2 oz., 4 oz.
Use: Antitussive.

EXTENDAC. (Vitarine) Belladonna alk. 0.2 mg., phenylpropanolamine HCl 50 mg., chlorpheniramine maleate 1 mg., pheniramine maleate 12.5 mg./T.R. Cap. Pkg. 12s.
Use: Extended action cold capsules.

EXTENDRYL CHEWABLE TABLETS. (Fleming) Chlorpheniramine maleate 2 mg., phenylephrine HCl 10 mg., methscopolamine nitrate 1.25 mg./Chewable Tab. Bot. 100s, 1000s.
Use: Cold treatment.

EXTENDRYL JUNIOR. (Fleming) Chlorpheniramine maleate 4 mg., phenylephrine HCl 10 mg., methscopolamine nitrate 1.25 mg./T.D. Cap.
Use: Cold treatment.

EXTENDRYL SENIOR. (Fleming) Chlorpheniramine maleate 8 mg., phenylephrine HCl 20 mg., methscopolamine nitrate 2.5 mg./T.D. Cap. Bot. 100s, 1000s.
Use: Decongestant, cold treatment.

EXTENDRYL SYRUP. (Fleming) Chlorpheniramine maleate 2 mg., phenylephrine HCl 10 mg., methscopolamine nitrate 1.25 mg./5 cc. Bot. pt., gal.
Use: Decongestant, cold treatment.

EXTIL HYDROGEN MALEATE. Carbinoxamine, B.A.N.

EXTRALIN. (Lilly) Liver-stomach concentrate 50 mg./Pulvule. Bot. 84s.

Use: Pernicious anemias.

EXTRA STRENGTH ASPIRIN CAPSULES. (Walgreen) Aspirin 500 mg./Cap. Bot. 80s.
Use: Analgesic.

EXTRA STRENGTH SINUS FORMULA (Eckerd) Acetaminophen 500 mg., chlorpheniramine maleate 2 mg., pseuodoephedrine HCl 30 mg./Tab. Bot. 24s.
Use: Analgesic, decongestant, antihistaminic.

EXUL. (Yorktown Products Co.) Nupra (non-hormonic, nonsteridic extract of beef organs, liver, brain, adrenals) 2000 Standard Chick units, dehydrated milk (55% fat) 14 Gm., thiamine HCl 0.6 mg., niacinamide 1.2 mg., ferrous gluconate 8.7 mg., cocoa, coconut oil, casein, sucrose, ethyl vanillin malt ext./Wafer. Bot. 25s.
Use: Gastric or duodenal ulcer.

EXZIT MEDICATED CLEANSER. (Miles Pharm) Colloidal sulfur & salicylic acid cleanser. Dome Dispensajar 4 oz.
Use: Treatment of acne.

EXZIT MEDICATED CREME & LOTION. (Miles Pharm) Colloidal sulfur & resorcinol monoacetate. Creme 1 oz., tube, lotion. Bot. 2 oz.
Use: Treatment of acne.

EYE FACE AND BODY WASH STATION. (Lavoptik) Sodium Cl. 0.49 Gm., sodaium biphosphate 0.40 Gm., sodium phosphate 0.45 Gm./100 ml. w/benzalkonium Cl 0.005%. Bot. 32 oz.
Use: Emergency wash for face and body.

EYE MO. (Winthrop Products) Boric acid, benzalconium Cl, phenelephrine HCl, zinc sulfate.
Use: Opthalmic solution.

EYE-SED OPHTHALMIC SOLUTION. (Scherer) Boric Acid 2.17%, zinc sulfate 0.217%, chlorobutanol 0.25% in purified water. Bot. ½ fl. oz.
Use: Astringent eye wash for use in some common types of blepharitis, especially conjunctivitis, commonly known as pink eye.

EYE-STREAM. (Alcon) Sod. chloride, potassium chloride, calcium chloride, magnesium chloride, benzalkonium chloride 0.013% sod. citrate, sod. acetate. Bot. 1 oz., 4 oz.
Use: Foreign body irrigation, emergency flushing of eyes.

EZE PAIN. (Halsey) Acetaminophen 2½ gr., salicylamide, caffeine/Cap. Bot. 21.
Use: Analgesic.

EZOL. (Stewart-Jackson) Butalbital 50 mg., caffeine 40 mg., acetaminophen 325 mg./Cap. Bot. 100s.
Use: Treatment of stress-headache, mild to moderate pain.

EZOL #3. (Stewart-Jackson) Butalbital 50 mg., caffeine 40 mg., acetaminophen 325 mg., codeine 30 mg./Tab. Bot. 100s.
Use: Treatment of mild to moderate pain.

F

FACT HOME PREGNANCY TEST KIT. (Ortho) 1 test per kit.

Use: Accurate test for pregnancy in 45 minutes, for use as early as 3 days after a missed period.

FACTORATE. (Armour) Antihemophilic factor (human) dried for intravenous administration only. Average potency ranges of 225 I.U., 275 I.U., 325 I.U., 375 I.U., 500 I.U., 700 I.U. and 1000 I.U. w/diluent and needles. Administration Kit 1s.
Use: Classical hemophilia treatment.

FACTORATE GENERATION II. (Armour) Antihemophilic factor (human) dried for I.V. administration only. 250 I.U., 500 I.U., 1000 I.U. or 1500 I.U. w/diluent and needles. Kit 1s.
Use: Classical hemophilia treatment.

• **FACTOR IX COMPLEX,** U.S.P. XXI.
Use: Hemostatic.

FACTREL. (Ayerst) Gonadorelin HCl 100 mcg. or 500 mcg./Vial w/Ampul of 2 ml. sterile diluent.
Use: Evaluation of hypothalamic-pituitary gonadotropic function.

FALGOS TABLETS. (Winthrop Products) Acetylsalicylic acid.
Use: Analgesic, antipyretic, antiinflammatory.

FALMONOX. (Winthrop Products) Teclozan available as suspension and tablets.
Use: Intestinal amebicide.

• **FAMOTIN HCL.** USAN. 1-[(p-Chlorophenoxy)-methyl] - 3, 4-dihydroisoquinoline HCl.
Use: Antiviral.

FAMPROFAZONE. B.A.N. 4-Isopropyl-2-methyl-3-[N-methyl-N-(α-methyl-phenethyl)aminomethyl]-1-phenyl-5-pyrazolone.
Use: Analgesic; antipyretic.

• **FANETIZOLE MESYLATE.** USAN.
Use: Immunoregulator.

FANSIDAR. (Roche) Sulfadoxine 500 mg., pyrimethamine 25 mg./Tab. Box 25s.
Use: Treatment of malaria due to susceptible strains of plasmodia.

FANTHRIDONE. B.A.N. 5-(3-Dimethylaminopropyl)-phenanthridone. AGN 616 is the hydrochloride.
Use: Antidepressant.

• **FANTRIDONE HCL.** USAN. 5-[3-(Dimethylamino)-propyl]-6(5H)-phenanthridinone monohydrochloride monohydrate.
Use: Antidepressant.

FARA-GEL ANTACID TABLETS. (Faraday) Tab. Bot. 100s.

FARAMALS. (Faraday) Vit. A 10,000 I.U., D 2,000 I.U., B-1 6 mg., B-2 4 mg., B-6 0.5 mg., folic acid 0.1 mg., C 100 mg., Ca pantothenate 5 mg., niacinamide 30 mg., E 5 I.U., B-12 3 mcg./Tab. Bot. 100s, 250s, 500s, 1000s.
Use: Vitamin supplement.

FARAMALS-M. (Faraday) Faramals plus Ca 103 mg., Co 0.1 mg., Cu 1 mg., iodine 0.15 mg., Fe 10 mg., Mg 6 mg., molybdenum 0.2 mg., P 80 mg., K 5 mg., Zn 1.2 mg./Tab Bot. 100s, 250s, 500s, 1000s.
Use: Vitamin and mineral supplement.

FARAMINS. (Faraday) Vit. B-1 20 mg., B-2 6 mg., C 40 mg., niacinamide 20 mg., Ca pantothenate 3 mg., B-6 0.5 mg., pow. whole dried liver 125 mg., dried debittered yeast 125 mg., choline dihydrogen citrate

20 mg., inositol 20 mg., dl-methionine 20 mg., folic acid 0.1 mg., B-12 10 mcg., ferrous gluconate 30 mg., dicalcium phos. 250 mg., Cu sulf. 5 mg., Mg sulf. 10 mg., Mn sulf. 5 mg., Co sulf. 0.2 mg., pot. chloride 2 mg., pot. iodide 0.15 mg. Tab. Bot. 100s, 250s, 500s, 1000s.
Use: Multiple vitamin, mineral supplement.

FARA-SIN. (Faraday) Tab. Bot. 50s.
Use: Pain relief of sinus & common colds.

FARATAC. (Faraday) Flat 10 (contac). Cap. Flat 10.

FARATOL. (Faraday) Vit. A 12,500 I.U., D 1000 I.U., B-1 20 mg., B-2 6 mg., B-6 0.5 mg., B-12 15 mcg., folic acid, 0.1 mg., niacinamide 10 mg., Ca pantothenate 3 mg., C 60 mg., E 5 I.U., choline dihydrogen citrate 20 mg., inositol 20 mg., dl-methionine 20 mg., whole dried liver 100 mg., dried debittered yeast 100 mg., dicalcium phos. 200 mg., ferrous gluconate 30 mg., pot. iodide 0.2 mg., Mg. sulf. 7.2 mg., Cu sulf. 5 mg., Mn sulf. 3.4 mg., Co sulf. 0.2 mg., pot. chloride 1.3 mg., Zn sulf. 2 mg., molybdenum 0.2 mg., in a base of alfalfa. Tab. Bot. 100s, 250s, 500s, 1000s.
Use: Vitamin, mineral supplement.

FARATUSS. (Faraday) Cough syrup. Coca-Cola base. Bot. 4 oz., 8 oz.

FARATUSS JR. (Faraday) Cough syrup. Coca-Cola base. Bot. 4 oz.
Use: Cough preparation.

FARNOQUINONE. 2-Difarnesyl-3-methyl-1, 4-naphthoquinone.

FASTIN. (Beecham Labs) Phentermine HCl 30 mg./Cap. Bot. 100s, 450s. Pack 150s. (5 × 30s).
Use: Anorexiant.

FATHER JOHN'S MEDICINE. (Medtech) Cod liver oil 19%. Bot. 4 oz., 8 oz.
Use: Coughs due to colds, Vit A & D source.

FATHER JOHN'S PLUS. (Medtech) Dextromethorphan 45 mg. Bot. 4 oz.
Use: Colds & allergies.

FATTIBASE. (Paddock) Preblended fatty acid suppository base composed of triglycerides of cocoanut oil and palm kernel oil. Jar 1 lb., 5 lb.
Use: Fatty acid suppository base.

FAT, UNSATURATED.
See: Arcofac, Emul. (Armour)
Lufa, Cap. (USV Pharm.)

FATTY ACIDS, UNSATURATED.
See: Fats, Unsaturated
Linolestrol, Oint. (Vortech)
Undecylenic Acid (Various Mfr.)

FAZADINIUM BROMIDE. 1,1'-Azobis(3-methyl-2-phenylimidazo[1,2-α]pyridinium bromide).
Use: Neuromuscular blocking agent.

F.C.A.H. CAPSULES. (Scherer) Chlorpheniramine maleate 4 mg., acetaminophen 162 mg., salicylamide 162 mg., atropine sulfate 0.130 mg./Cap. Bot. 100s, 500s.
Use: Antihistaminic, analgesic.

• **FEBANTEL.** USAN.
Use: Anthelmentic.

FEBERIN. (Arcum) Ferrous gluconate 3 gr., C 25 mg.,

B-1 2 mg., B-6 1 mg., B-2 1 mg., niacinamide 5 mg./Tab. Bot. 100s, 1000s.
Use: Iron deficiency.
FEBRAMINE HYDROCHLORIDE. Cetoxime, B.A.N.
FEBREX ELIXIR. (Pan American) Acetaminophen 125 mg./5 ml. Bot. 16 oz.
Use: Analgesic.
FEBRILE ANTIGENS. (Laboratory Diagnostics) Group O antigens (somatic) are dyed blue and group H antigens (flagellars) are dyed red for clear identification. Vials 5 ml.
Use: Detection of presence of bacterial agglutinins, bacterial infection.
FEBRIN. (Jenkins) Acetophenetidin 0.1 Gm., acid acetylsalicylic 0.12 gm., caffeine 15 mg., camphor monobromated 60 mg./Tab. Bot. 1000s.
Use: Colds and muscular soreness.
FEBRINETTS. (Jenkins) Acetophenetidin ½ gr., acid acetylsalicylic 1 gr., camphor monobromated ¼₀ gr., caffeine ¹⁄₂₀ gr./Tab. Bot. 1000s.
Use: Analgesic.
FEBRINOL. (Vitarine) Acetaminophen 325 mg./Tab. Bot. 100s.
Use: Analgesic.
FE-BRONE. (Fellows) Vit. B-12 1 I.U., folic acid 1 mg., ferrous sulfate exsic. (powd.) 200 mg., ferrous sulfate exsic. (timed) 200 mg., Vit. C acid 100 mg., B-6 0.5 mg., B-1 2 mg., B-2 1 mg., Cu 0.9 mg., Zn 0.5 mg., Mn 0.3 mg./Cap. Bot. 30s, 100s, 1000s.
Use: Vitamin, mineral supplement.
FECO-T. (Blaine) Ferrous fumarate 300 mg./T.R. Cap. Bot. 100s.
FEDAHIST EXPECTORANT. (Rorer) Guaiafenesin 100 mg., pseudoephedrine HCl 30 mg., chlorpheniramine maleate 2 mg./5 ml. Nonalcoholic. Bot. 4 oz.
Use: Antihistaminic, decongestant, expectorant.
FEDAHIST GYROCAPS. (Rorer) Pseudoephedrine HCl 65 mg., chlorpheniramine maleate 10 mg./T.R. Cap. Bot. 100s.
Use: Antihistaminic, decongestant.
FEDAHIST SYRUP. (Rorer) Pseudoephedrine HCl 30 mg., chlorpheniramine maleate 2mg./5 ml. Nonalcoholic. Bot. 4 oz.
Use: Antihistaminic, decongestant.
FEDAHIST TABLETS. (Rorer) Pseudoephedrine HCl 60 mg., chlorpheniramine maleate 4 mg./Tab. Bot. 100s.
Use: Antihistaminic, decongestant.
FEDNAL. (Blue Line) Ephedrine sulfate 1%, camphor 2½%, menthol 0.5% in petrolatum ointment base. Tube ⅔ oz., 12S.
Use: Nasal cream.
FEDRAZIL. (Burroughs Wellcome) Pseudoephedrine HCl 30 mg., chlorcyclizine HCl 25 mg./Tab. Bot. 24s, 100s.
Use: Respiratory tract congestion.
FEDREX. (Blue Line) Ephedrine HCl, potassium guaiacolsulfonate, sodium bromide in a glycerinated and aromatized cane sugar syrup. Alcohol 3%. Bot. gal.
Use: Cough preparation.

FEDRINAL. (H.L. Moore) Ephedrine HCl 12 mg., phenobarbital 12 mg., potassium iodide 160 mg., theophylline anhydrous 31.2 mg./5 ml. Bot. Pts., Gal.
Use: Respiratory conditions.
FEEN-A-MINT GUM. (Plough)Yellow phenolphthalein 97.2mg. Chewing gum Tab. Box 5s, 16s, 40s.
Use: Laxative.
FEEN-A-MINT MINT. (Plough) Yellow phenolphthalein 97.2 mg./Mint Tab. Box 20s.
Use: Laxative.
FEEN-A-MINT PILLS. (Plough) Yellow phenolphthalein 65 mg., docusate sodium 100 mg./Pill. Box 15s, 30s, 60s.
Use: Stool softener & laxative.
FEET TREAT. (DeWitt) Water, stearic acid, isopropyl myristate, propylene glycol, lanolin, triethanolamine, p-Chloro-m-xylenol, menthol, mag. alum. silicate, allantoin. Bot. 8 oz.
Use: Soften hard skin & callouses.
FEET TREET CREAM. (DeWitt) Stearic acid, isoprop myristate, propylene glycol, lanolin, triethanolamine, p-Chloro-m-Xylenol, menthol, Mg. aluminum silicate, allantoin. Bot. 8 oz.
Use: Soften hard skin and callouses.
FEG-L. (Western Research) Ferrous gluconate 300 mg./Tab. Handicount 28s (36 bags of 28 tab.)
FELDENE. (Pfizer Laboratories) Piroxicam. 10 mg./Cap. Bot 100s. **20mg.**/Cap. Bot. 100s, 500s. Unit dose 100s.
Use: Osteoarthritis and rheumatoid arthritis.
FELLOBOLIC INJECTION. (Fellows) Methandriol dipropionate 50 mg./cc. Vial 10 cc.
FELLO-SED. (Fellows) Chloral hydrate 0.625 Gm., cal. bromide 0.625 Gm., atropine sulfate 0.156 mg./5 cc. Bot. 8 oz., gal.
Use: Sedative & hypnotic.
FELLOWS COMPOUND SYRUP. (Fellows) Strychnine hypophosphite 1.25 mg., quinine sulfate 3.75 mg., potassium hypophosphite 10 mg., sod. hypophosphite 10 mg., cal. hypophosphite 25 mg., manganese hypophosphite 10 mg., iron pyrophosphate 10 mg./5 cc. Bot. 7 oz., gal.
FELLOZINE. (Fellows) Promethazine HCl 25 mg., 50 mg./cc. Vial 10 cc. Amp. 1 cc., 25s.
Use: Antihistaminic.
FELSULES. (Fellows) Chloral hydrate 0.25 Gm./Cap. Bot. 100s, 500s, 0.5 Gm./Cap. Bot. 50s, 100s, 250s, 500s. Unit dose 100s.
Use: Sedative.
• **FELYPRESSIN.** USAN. 2-(Phenylalanine)-8-lysine vasopressin.
Use: Vasoconstrictor.
FELYPRESSIN.   B.A.N.   2-Phenylalanine-8-lysinevasopressin.
Use: Vasoconstrictor.
See: Octapressin.
FEMAGENE. (Tennessee) Boric acid, sod. borate, lactic acid, menthol, methylbenzethonium chloride, parachlorometaxylenol, lactose, surface-active agents. Pow. 6 oz.
Use: Feminine hygiene.

FEMCAPS. (Buffington) Acetaminophen, caffeine, ephedrine sulfate, atropine sulfate /Tab. Dispens-a-kit 500s. Aidpaks 100s.
Use: Temporary relief of minor menstrual pains and cramps.

FEMERGIN.
See: Ergotamine Tartrate (Various Mfr.)

FEMEZE. (Stanlabs) Acetaminophen, salicylamide, caffeine alk., ammonium chloride, Vit. B-1, homatropine HBr/Tab. Carton 14s.
Use: Analgesic: periodic pain reliever.

FEMGUARD VAGINAL CREAM. (Reid-Provident) Sulfanilamide 15%, aminacrine hydrochloride 0.2%, allantoin 2.0%. w/lactose, stearic acid, cetyl alcohol, triethanolamine, sod. lauryl sulfate, glycerine, methylparaben, propylparaben, and buffered w/lactic acid. Tubes 4 oz. w/App.
Use: Treatment of vaginal infections.

FEMID GREEN LABEL. (Cenci) Sod. bicarbonate, sod. borate, sod. chloride, sod. perborate, menthol. Pow. Bot. 7 oz., 15 oz.
Use: Vaginal cleansing & deodorant.

FEMID PINK LABEL. (Cenci) Sodium lauryl sulfate, aluminum ammonium sulf., boracic acid, citric acid, menthol. Pow. Bot. 7 oz.
Use: Vaginal cleansing and deodorant.

FEMIDINE. (A.V.P.) Povidone-iodine. Bot. 8 oz.
Use: Cleansing douche (dilute with water).

FEMIDYN.
See: Estrone (Various Mfr.)

FEMINONE. (Upjohn) Ethinyl estradiol. 0.05 mg./Tab. Bot. 100s.
Use: Estrogen supplement.

FEMIRON. (Beecham Products) Iron 20 mg./Tab. Bot 40s, 120s.
Use: Iron supplement.

FEMIRON MULTI-VITAMINS AND IRON. (Beecham Products) Iron 20 mg., Vit. A 5,000 I.U., D 400 I.U., B-1 1.5 mg., riboflavin 1.7 mg., niacinamide 20 mg., C 60 mg., B-6 2 mg., B-12 6 mcg., calcium pantothenate 10 mg., folic acid 0.4 mg., E 15 I.U./Tab. Bot. 35s, 60s, 90s.
Use: Iron and vitamin supplement.

FEMOGEN-L.A. (Fellows) Estradiol valerate 10 mg., 20 mg./cc. Inj. 10 cc. 40 mg./cc. Inj. 5 cc.

FEMOTRONE. (Bluco) Progesterone in oil 50 mg./ml. Vial 10 ml.
Use: Progestin supplement.

FEMSPAN. (Fellows) Pot. estrone sulfate 1 mg., estrone 2 mg./cc. Vial 10 ml.
Use: Menopausal symptoms.

• **FENALAMIDE.** USAN. (1) Ethyl N-[2-(diethylamino)-ethyl]-2-ethyl-2-phenylmalonamate; (2) Phenylethyl-malonic acid monoethyl ester diethylaminoethylamide.
Use: Smooth muscle relaxant.

FENAMISAL. Phenyl aminosalicylate.

• **FENAMOLE.** USAN. 5-Amino-1-phenyl-1H-tetrazol.
Use: Anti-inflammatory agent.

FENAPRIN TABLETS. (Winthrop Products) Aspirin, chlormezanone.
Use: Analgesic, muscle relaxanat.

FENAROL. (Winthrop Products) Chlormezanone 100 mg., 200 mg./Tab. Bot. 100s.
Use: Central relaxant and tranquilizer.

FENARSONE.
See: Carbarsone (Various Mfr.)

• **FENBENDAZOLE.** USAN.
Use: Anthelmintic.

• **FENBUFEN.** USAN.
Use: Anti-inflammatory.

FENCAMFAMIN. B.A.N. N-Ethyl-3-phenylbicyclo-[2.2.1]hept-2-ylamine.
Use: Central nervous system stimulant; appetite suppressant.
See: Euvitaol [hydrochloride].

FENCHLORPHOS. B.A.N. OO-Dimethyl O-(2,4,5-tri-chlorophenyl) phosphorothioate.
Use: Insecticide, veterinary medicine.
See: Nankor
 Ronnel
 Trolene.

• **FENCILBUTIROL.** USAN.
Use: Choleretic.

• **FENCLOFENAC.** USAN. 2-(2,4-Dichlorophenoxy)-phenylacetic acid.
Use: Anti-inflammatory.

• **FENCLONINE.** USAN. dl-3-(p-Chlorophenyl)-alanine. Under study by Pfizer.
Use: Serotonin biosynthesis inhibitor.

• **FENCLORAC.** USAN.
Use: Anti-inflammatory.

FENCLOZIC ACID. B.A.N. 2-(4-Chlorophenyl)-thiazol-4-ylacetic acid.
Use: Anti-inflammatory.

FEND. (Mine Safety Appliances)
A-2—Water soluble cream which forms a physical barrier to water insoluble irritants. Tube 3 oz., Jar 1 lb.
E-2—This cream combines the functions of the water soluble Fend A-2 and water insoluble Fend I-2 creams. Tube 3 oz., Jar 1 lb.
I-2—Water insoluble cream which forms a physical barrier to water soluble irritants. Tube 3 oz., Jar 1 lb.
S-2—A silicone cream which forms a barrier against a combination of water soluble and water insoluble irritants. Tube 3 oz., Jar 1 lb.
X—Industrial cold cream which rubs well into the skin and serves as a skin conditioner. Tube 3 oz., Jar 1 lb.
Use: Protective creams against irritants of industrial and household origin.

FENDOL. (Buffington) Salicylamide, caffeine, acetaminophen, phenylephrine HCl, atropine sulfate/Tab. Sugar and salt free. Dispens-A-Kit 500s. Bot. 100s.
Use: Analgesic and decongestant for relief of the common cold symptoms.

• **FENDOSAL.** USAN.
Use: Anti-inflammatory.

• **FENESTREL.** USAN. 5-Ethyl-6-methyl-4-phenyl-3-cy-clohexene-1-carboxylic acid. Under study.
Use: Nonsteroid estrogen.

FENETHYLLINE. B.A.N. 7-[2-(α-Methylphenethyl-amino)ethyl]theophylline.
Use: Cerebral stimulant.
• **FENETHYLLINE HYDROCHLORIDE.** USAN. 7-[2-[(α-Methylphenethyl)-amino]-ethyl]theophylline hydrochloride.
Use: Stimulant.
FENFLURAMINE. B.A.N. 2-Ethylamino-1-(3-trifluoromethylphenyl)propane. N-Ethyl-α-methyl-3-trifluoromethylphenethylamine.
Use: Appetite suppressant.
See: Ponderax [hydrochloride].
• **FENFLURAMINE HYDROCHLORIDE.** USAN. N-ethyl-α-methyl-m-(trifluoro-methyl)-phenethylamine hydro-chloride.
Use: Sympathomimetic (anorexic).
See: Pondimin, Tab. (Robins)
Pendimin, Tab.
• **FENIMIDE.** USAN. 3-Ethyl-2-methyl-2-phenylsuccinimide.
Use: Tranquilizer.
• **FENISOREX.** USAN. (±)-cis-7-Fluoro-1-phenylisochroman-3-ylmethylamine.
Use: Anorexigenic.
• **FENMETOZOLE HYDROCHLORIDE.** USAN.
Use: Antidepressant, antagonist.
• **FENMETRAMIDE.** USAN.
Use: Antidepressant.
• **FENNEL OIL.** N.F. XVI.
Use: Pharmaceutic aid (flavor).
• **FENOBAM.** USAN.
Use: Sedative.
• **FENOCTIMINE SULFATE.** USAN.
Use: Gastric antisecretory.
• **FENOLDOPAM MESYLATE.** USAN
• **FENOPROFEN.** USAN. 2-(3-Phenoxyphenyl)-propionic acid. (±)-m-Phenoxyhydratropic acid; (2) dl-2-(3-phenoxyphenyl)-propionic acid.
Use: Anti-inflammatory; analgesic.
• **FENOPROFEN CALCIUM,** U.S.P. XXI. Cap., Tab., U.S.P. XXI.
Use: Anti-inflammatory, analgesic.
FENOSTIL. B.A.N. Dimethindene.
• **FENOTEROL.** USAN. (1)3,5-Dihydroxy-α-[[(p-hydroxy-α-methylphenethyl) amino] methyl]-benzyl alcohol; (2) 1-(3,5-Dihydroxyphenyl)-2-[[1-(4-hydroxy-benzyl)ethyl]amino] ethanol.
Use: Bronchodilator.
• **FENPIPALONE.** USAN.
Use: Anti-inflammatory.
FENPIPRAMIDE. B.A.N. 2,2-Diphenyl-4-piperidonobutyramide.
Use: Spasmolytic.
FENPIPRANE. B.A.N. 1-(3,3-Diphenylpropyl)-piperidine.
Use: Spasmolytic.
• **FENPRINAST HYDROCHLORIDE.** USAN.
Use: Anti-allergic bronchodilator.
• **FENPROSTALENE.** USAN.
Use: Luteolysin.
• **FENQUIZONE.** USAN.
Use: Diuretic.
• **FENSPIRIDE HYDROCHLORIDE.** USAN.
Use: Bronchodilator, anti-adrenergic.

FENTANYL. B.A.N. 1-Phenethyl-4-(N-propionylanilino)-piperidine.
Use: Narcotic analgesic.
See: Sublimaze.
• **FENTANYL CITRATE,** U.S.P. XXI. Inj. U.S.P. XXI. N-(1-phenethyl-4-piperidyl) propionanilide citrate. Propanamide, N-phenyl-N-[1-(2-phenyl-ethyl)-4-piperidinyl]-, 2-hydroxy-1,2,3-propanetricarboxylate (1:1).
Use: Narcotic analgesic.
See: Innovar, Inj. (Janssen)
Sublimaze, Inj. (Janssen)
• **FENTICLOR.** USAN. Di-(5-chloro-2-hydroxyphenyl)-sulfide.
Use: Antiseptic, fungicide.
• **FENTICONAZOLE NITRATE.** USAN.
Use: Antifungal.
FENTON ELIXIR. (Winthrop Products) Ferrous Gluconate.
Use: Hematinic, dietary supplement.
FENYLHIST. (Mallard) Diphenhydramine HCl 50 mg./Cap. 25 mg./Capsule. **Cap.:** Bot. 1000s.
Use: Antihistamine with anticholinergic and sedative effects.
FENYRAMIDOL HCl. Phenyramidol HCl.
• **FENYRIPOL HYDROCHLORIDE.** USAN. α-(2-Pyrimidinylaminomethyl) benzyl alcohol hydrochloride.
Use: Skeletal muscle relaxant.
FENZOL. Dichloralphenazone, B.A.N.
FEOCYTE. (Dunhall) Ferrous fumarate 260 mg., ferrous gluconate 65 mg., Vit. C 100 mg., B-6 2 mg., cyanocobalamin 50 mcg., copper sulf. 2 mg., desiccated liver 15 mg., ferrous sulf. 65 mg./Time Cap. Bot. 100s, 1000s. T.D. Tab. Bot. 100s, 1000s.
Use: Hematinic.
FEOCYTE INJECTABLE. (Dunhall) Peptonized iron 15 mg., B-12 200 mcg., liver inj. N.F. beef, 10 u., sod. citrate 10 mg., benzyl alcohol 2%/ml. Vial 10 ml.
Use: Hematinic.
FEOSOL ELIXIR. (Menley & James) Ferrous sulfate 220 mg./5 cc. w/alcohol 5%. Bot. 12 oz.
Use: Iron-deficiency anemias and simple iron deficiency.
FEOSOL PLUS. (Menley & James) Vit. B-1 2 mg., B-12 5 mcg., B-2 2 mg., niacin 20 mg., B-6 2 mg., C 50 mg., folic acid 0.2 mg., dried-ferrous sulfate 200 mg./Cap. Bot. 100s.
Use: Iron deficiency anemias and simple iron deficiency.
FEOSOL SPANSULE CAPSULES. (Menley & James) Dried ferrous sulfate 159 mg. Bot. 30s, 100s, 500s. Unit dose 100s.
Use: Sustained release action of ferrous sulfate in the treatment of iron deficiency anemias.
FEOSOL TABLETS. (Menley & James) Dried ferrous sulfate 200 mg./Tab. Bot. 100s, 1000s, Unit Dose 100s.
Use: Iron deficiency anemias and simple iron deficiency.
FEOSTAT. (O'Neal, Jones & Feldman) Iron 50 mg./ml. Vial 10 ml.
FEOSTAT. (O'Neal, Jones & Feldman) **Tab.:** Ferrous

fumarate 100 mg., or 200 mg./Chewable Tab. Bot. 100s. **Drops:** Ferrous fumarate 45 mg./0.6 ml. Bot. 2 oz.
Use: Iron deficiency anemia.

FEOSTAT SUSPENSION. (O'Neal, Jones & Feldman) Ferrous fumarate 100 mg./5 cc. Bot. 8 oz.
Use: Anemia.

F-E-P CREME. (Boots) Hydrocortisone 1.0%, pramoxine HCl 0.5%. Tube 15 Gm.
Use: Relief of inflammatory & pruritic dermatoses.

FE-PLUS. (Miller) Iron (as an iron-protein complex) 50 mg./Tab. Bot. 100s.
Use: Anemia.

FEPRAZONE. B.A.N. 4-(3-Methylbut-2-enyl)-1,2-diphenylpyrazolidine-3,5-dione.
Use: Analgesic; anti-inflammatory.

FERANCEE. (Stuart) Elemental iron 67 mg. (from 200 mg. ferrous fumarate), Vit. C 150 mg./Tab. Bot. 100s.
Use: Chewable tablet for treatment of iron deficiency anemia.

FERANCEE-HP. (Stuart) Elemental iron 110 mg. (from 330 mg. ferrous fumarate), Vit. C 600 mg./Tab. Bot. 60s.
Use: Treatment of iron deficiency anemia.

FERATE-C. (Vale) Ferrous fumarate 150 mg., ascorbic acid 200 mg., docusate sodium 25 mg./Tab. Bot. 100s, 500s, 1000s.
Use: Hematinic.

FERATIN. (Pasadena Research) Iron 70 mg., Vit. B-12 10 mcg., C 60 mg., B-1 5 mg., B-2 3.5 mg., B-6 1 mg., niacinamide 50 mg., Ca pantothenate 5 mg., copper 0.1 mg., liver desic. 390 mg./Tab. Bot. 100s, 1000s.

FERGON. (Winthrop-Breon) Pure ferrous gluconate. **Tab.** 320 mg. equal to approximately 36 mg. ferrous iron/Tab. Bot. 100s, 500s, 1000s, 5000s, 50,000s. **Elixir** (6%), 300 mg./5 ml. Bot. 16 fl. oz. **Cap.** 435 mg. Bot. 30s.
Use: Hematinic.

FERGON COMPOUND ELIXIR. (Winthrop-Breon) Ferrous gluconate, thiamine, riboflavin, pyridoxine, cyanocobalamin, niacinamide, d-panthenol, alcohol.
Use: Hematinic.

FERGON PLUS. (Winthrop-Breon) Ferrous gluconate 500 mg., vit. B-12 w/intrinsic factor conc. 0.5 u., ascorbic acid 75 mg./Caplet. Bot. 100s.
Use: Hematinic.

FER-IN-SOL. (Mead Johnson) **Drops:** Elemental Iron 15 mg./0.6 ml. Bot. w/dropper 50 ml. **Syr:** 18 mg./5 ml. Bot. 16 fl. oz. **Cap:** 60 mg./Cap. Bot. 100s. **Caps.** Bot. 100s.
Use: Dietary supplement of iron.

FER-IRON DROPS. (Bay) Ferrous sulfate 125 mg.,/1 cc. Bot. 50 cc.
Use: Iron supplement.

FERMALOX. (Rorer) Ferrous sulfate 200 mg., magnesium and aluminum hydroxides (Maalox) 200 mg./Tab. Bot. 100s.
Use: Hematinic.

FERMETONE COMPOUND CAPSULES. (Winthrop Products) Pancreatin.
Use: Pancreatic deficiency, dyspepsia.

FERNCORT LOTION. (Ferndale) Hydrocortisone acetate 0.5% in lotion base. Bot. 120 ml.
Use: Anti-inflammatory, anti-pruritic.

FERNISOLONE. (Ferndale) Prednisolone 5 mg./Tab. Bot. 100s, 1000s. Susp. (25 mg./cc.) Vial 10 cc.
Use: Steroid hormone.

FERO-FOLIC 500. (Abbott) Ferrous sulfate 525 mg. controlled release (Equiv. to 105 mg. Iron), Vit. C 500 mg., folic acid 800 mcg./Filmtab. Bot. 100s, 500s.
Use: Iron and folic acid supplement.

FERO-GRAD 500 FILMTAB. (Abbott) Vit. C 500 mg., ferrous sulfate controlled release 525 mg./Filmtab Bot. 30s, 100s, 500s. Abbo-Pac. 100s.
Use: Iron-deficiency anemias.

FERO-GRADUMET FILMTAB. (Abbott) Ferrous Sulfate controlled release 525 mg./Filmtab. Bot. 100s.
Use: Treatment of iron-deficiency anemia.

FEROLATE. (Pasadena Research) Ferric Cl 2.5 gr., sod. cacodylate 5 gr. in Ringer's soln./10 cc. Amp. 25s.

FEROLIX. (Century) Ferrous sulfate 5 gr., alcohol 5%/10 cc. Elix. Bot. 8 oz., pint, gal.

FERONATE. (Pasadena Research) Ferrous gluconate 1 gr./ml. Amp. 1 cc., 25s.

FEROSAN FORTE. (Sandia) Ferrous fumarate 300 mg., liver-stomach concentrate 150 mg., Vita. B-12 w/intrinsic factor concentrate 7.5 mcg., intrinsic factor concentrate 150 mg., B-12 7.5 mcg., ascorbic acid 75 mg., folic acid 1 mg., sorbitol 50 mg./Tab. Bot. 100s.
Use: Multiple vitamin, mineral supplement.

FEROSAN SYRUP. (Sandia) Ferrous fumarate 91.2 mg., B-1 10 mg., B-6 3 mg., B-12 25 mcg./5 cc. 16 oz., gal.

FEROWEET. (Barth's) Vit. B-1 6 mg., B-2 12 mg. niacin 4 mg., Fe 30 mg., B-12 10 mcg., B-6 95 mcg., pantothenic acid 50 mcg./3 Cap. Bot. 100s, 500s, 1000s.
Use: Iron and vitamin supplement.

FERRACOMP. (Hauck) Liver 2 mcg., B-12 15 mcg., B-1 10 mg., B-2 5 mg., B-6 1 mg., Ca pantothenate 1 mg., niacinamide 10 mg., iron 31.3 mg./ml. Vial 30 ml.
Use: Hematinic & tonic.

FERRALET PLUS. (Mission) Ferrous gluconate 400 mg., ascorbic acid 400 mg., folic acid 1 mg., Vit. B-2 25 mcg./Tab. Bot. 100s.
Use: Hematinic.

FERRALYN. (Lannett) Ferrous sulf. 150 mg./Tab. E.C. Bot. 500s, 1000s.

FERRANOL. (Robinson) Ferrous fumarate 3 gr. or 5 gr./Tab. Bot. 100s, 1000s.

FERRATIHIC. (Wolins) Ferrous sulfate 200 mg., magnesium hydroxide 100 mg., aluminum hydroxide 100 mg. Bot. 100s, 1000s.
Use: Hematinic.

FER-REGULES. (Columbia) Ferrous fumarate 150 mg., docusate sodium 100 mg./timed rel. Cap. Bot. 100s, 1000s.
Use: Hematinic, iron deficiency anemia.

FERRIC AMMONIUM CITRATE. Ammonium iron $(3+)$ citrate.
Use: Hematinic.

FERRIC AMMONIUM SULFATE. (Various Mfr.).
Use: Astringent & styptic.
FERRIC AMMONIUM TARTRATE. (Various Mfr.).
Use: Iron deficiency
FERRIC-B Jr. (Jenkins) Vit. B-12 5 mcg., B-1 2 mg., C
30 mg., iron peptonate. 60 mg./Tab. Bot. 1000s.
Use: Nutritional deficiencies
FERRIC CACODYLATE. (Various Mfr.).
Use: Leukemias & iron deficiency
FERRIC CHLORIDE. (Various Mfr.)
Use: Astringent for skin disorders.
• **FERRIC CHLORIDE Fe 59.** USAN.
Use: Radioactive agent.
FERRIC CITROCHLORIDE TINCTURE. Iron $(3+)$
chloride citrate.
Use: Hematinic.
• **FERRIC FRUCTOSE.** USAN. Fructose iron complex
with potassium (2:1).
Use: Hematinic
FERRIC GLYCEROPHOSPHATE. Glycerol phosphate
iron $(3+)$ salt.
Use: Pharmaceutic necessity.
FERRIC HYPOPHOSPHITE. Iron $(3+)$ phosphinate.
Use: Pharmaceutic necessity.
• **FERRICLATE CALCIUM SODIUM.** USAN.
Use: Hematinic.
• **FERRIC OXIDE, RED,** N.F. XVI.
• **FERRIC OXIDE, YELLOW,** N.F. XVI.
FERRIC "PEPTONATE." (Various Mfr.)
See: Iron Peptonized.
FERRIC PYROPHOSPHATE, SOLUBLE. Iron $(3+)$
citrate pyrophosphate.
FERRIC QUININE CITRATE, "GREEN." (Various
Mfr.)
Use: For iron deficiency.
FERRIC QUININE & STRYCHNINE CITRATE.
(Various Mfr.)
Use: As a tonic.
FERRIC SUBSULFATE SOLUTION. (Various Mfr.)
Use: Local use on the skin.
FERRINAL-C. (Cenci) Ferrous fumarate 3 gr., Vit. C 150
mg./Tab. Bot. 100s, 1000s.
Use: Iron deficiency anemia.
FERRINAL CHRONCAP. (Cenci) Ferrous fumarate
330 mg., thiamine chloride 5 mg./S.R. Cap. Bot.
30s, 100s.
Use: Iron deficiency anemia and dietary
supplement.
FERRINAL TABLETS. (Cenci) Ferrous fumarate 3
gr./Tab. Bot. 100s, 1000s.
Use: Iron deficiency anemia.
FERRIZYME. (Abbott) Test kit 100s.
Use: Enzyme immunoassay for qualitative
determination of ferritin in human serum or plasma.
FERROCHOLATE.
See: Ferrocholinate
FERROCHOLINATE. Ferrocholate. Ferrocholine. A
chelate prepared by reacting equimolar quantities
of freshly precipitated ferric hydroxide with choline
dihydrogen citrate.
Use: Iron deficiency anemia.
See: Chel-Iron, Prep. (Kinney)

FERROCHOLINE.
See: Ferrocholinate
Kelex, Tabseal. (Nutrition)
FERRO-CYTE. (Spanner) Iron peptonate 20 mg., liver
injection (20 mg./cc.) 0.25 cc., Vit. B-1 22 mg., B-2 0.5
mg., B-6 2.5 mg., B-12 30 mcg., niacinamide 25 mg.,
panthenol 1 mg./cc. Multiple dose vial 10 cc. For
I.M. inj.
Use: Iron deficiency.
FERRODYL CHEWABLE TABLETS. (Arcum) Ferrous
fumarate 320 mg., Vit. C 200 mg./Tab. Bot. 100s,
1000s.
Use: Iron deficiency.
FERROGEN. (Tunex) Ferrous gluconate 30 mg., citric
acid 8.2 mg., sodium citrate 11.8 mg., folic acid 0.5
mg., liver inj. equiv. to cyanocobalamin 2.5
mcg./ml. Vial 30cc.
Use: Iron deficiency and nutritional anemias.
FERRO LEXAMIN. (Eckerd) Bot. 100s.
FERROMAX (INTRAMUSCULAR IRON). (Kenyon)
Iron peptonized 100 mg., copper gluconate 0.2 mg.,
cobalt Cl 4 mg., pectin 10 mg./cc. Vial 10 cc.
FERRON-100 IRON DEXTRAN COMPLEX. (Vortech)
Low hydroxide in complex w/ a low molecular
weight dextran fraction equiv. to 100 mg. elemental
iron, phenol 0.5%/ml. Vial 10 ml.
FERRONEED. (Hanlon) Ferrous gluconate 300 mg.,
ascorbic acid 60 mg./Cap. Bot. 100s.
FERRONEED T-CAPS. (Hanlon) Ferrous fumarate 250
mg., thiamine HCl 5 mg., ascorbic acid 50 mg./T.D.
Cap. Bot. 100s.
Use: Iron deficiency anemia.
FERRONEX. (Pasadena Research) Liver inj. (10
mcg./ml.) 0.2 ml., B-12 15 mcg., ferrous gluconate 50
mg., B-1 10 mg., B-2 0.5 mg., B-6 1 mg., d-panthenol
1 mg., niacinamide 50 mg., procaine 0.5%, sod.
citrate 1%, phenol 0.1%, benzyl alcohol 2%/cc.
Vial 30 cc.
Use: Iron deficiency and vitamin therapy.
FERRO-SEQUELS. (Lederle) Ferrous fumarate 150 mg.
(Equiv. to 50 mg. Elemental Iron), dioctyl sod.
sulfosuccinate 100 mg./Cap. T.D. Bot. 30s, 100s,
1000s. Unit dose 10×10s.
Use: Treatment of iron deficiency anemia.
FERROSPAN CAPSULES. (Imperial Lab.) Ferrous
fumarate 200 mg., ascorbic acid 100 mg./Tab. Bot.
100s, 1000s.
Use: Treatment of iron deficiency anemias.
FERROSYN INJECTION. (Standex) Cyanocabalamine
30 mcg., liver 2 mcg., ferrous gluconate 100 mg.,
riboflavin 1.5 mg., panthenol 2.5 mg., niacinamide
100 mg., procaine 2%. Vials 30 cc.
Use: Vitamin supplement.
FERROSYN S.C. (Standex) Iron 60 mg., Vit. B-12 5
mcg., Mg 0.6 mg., Cu 0.3 mg., Mn 0.1 mg., K 0.5
mg., Zn 0.15 mg./Tab. Bot. 100s, 1000s.
FERROSYN SEE TABS. (Standex) Iron 34 mg.,
ascorbic acid 80 mg./Tab. Bot. 100s, 1000s.
Use: Hematinic with ascorbic acid.
FERROSYN TAB. (Standex) Iron 60 mg., Vit. B-12 5
mcg., Mg 0.6 mg., Cu 0.3 mg., Mn 0.1 mg., K 0.5
mg., Zn 0.15 mg./Tab. Bot. 100s.

FERROUS BROMIDE. (Various Mfr.)
Use: In chorea & tuberculous cervical adenitis.
FERROUS CARBONATE MASS. Vallet's mass.
(Various Mfr.).
Use: For iron deficiency.
FERROUS CARBONATE, SACCHARATED. (Various Mfr.)
Use: For iron deficiency.
• **FERROUS CITRATE Fe-59 INJECTION,** U.S.P. XXI.
Use: Radioactive agent.
• **FERROUS FUMARATE,** U.S.P. XXI. Tabs., U.S.P. XXI.
Use: Hematinic.
See: Arne-C, Chew. Tab. (Haag)
Cefera, Tab. (Haag)
Childron, Susp. (Fleming)
Eldofe, Tab. (Canright)
El-Ped-Ron, Liq. (Elder)
Farbegen, Cap. (Hickam)
Feco-T., Cap. (Blaine)
Fumasorb, Tab. (Marion)
Fumerin, Tab. (Laser)
Hemocyte, Tab., Liq. (Medics)
Ircon, Tab. (Key)
Laud-Iron, Tab., Susp. (Amfre-Grant)
Maniron, Meltab. (Bowman)
Toleron, Tab., Susp. (Mallinckrodt)
W/Ascorbic Acid.
See: C-Ron, Prep. (Rowell)
Cytoferin, Tabs. (Ayerst)
Eldofe-C, Tab. (Canright)
Ferancee, Tab. (Stuart)
Ferancee-HP, Tab. (Stuart)
Ferrodyl Chewable Tab. (Arcum)
Hema-C Meta-Kaps, Cap. (Sutliff & Case)
Min-Hema Chewable, Tab. (Scrip)
W/Ascorbic acid, copper sulfate.
See: Ferrobid, Cap. (Glaxo)
W/Ascorbic acid, & folic acid.
See: C-Ron F.A., Tab. (Rowell)
W/Docusate sodium.
See: Fer-Regules, Cap. (Columbia)
Ferro-Sequels, Cap. (Lederle)
W/Norethindrone, mestranol.
See: Ortho Novum 1/80 Fe 28, 1/50 Fe-28, 1 mg. Fe-28, Tabs. (Ortho)
W/Thiamine.
See: Arner Timesules, Caps. (Haag)
W/Vitamins and minerals.
See: Cohema, Tabs. (Sutliff & Case)
Stuart Formula, Tab. (Stuart)
Stuart Prenatal, Tab. (Stuart)
Stuartnatal 1 + 1, Tab. (Stuart)
Theron, Tab. (Stuart)
Vitanate, Tab. (Century)
• **FERROUS GLUCONATE.** U.S.P. XXI. Cap., Elixir, Tab., U.S.P. XXI. Iron (2+) Gluconate.
Use: Iron deficiency.
See: Entron, Cap., Tab. (LaCrosse)
Fergon Prods. (Winthrop-Breon)
Ferrous-G, Elix. (Kenwood)

W/Ascorbic acid, desiccated liver, vitamin B complex.
See: I.L.X. w/B-12, Tab. (Kenwood)
Stuart Hematinic, Liq. (Stuart)
W/Polyoxyethylene glucitan monolaurate.
See: Simron, Cap. (Merrell Dow)
FERROUS IODIDE. (Various Mfr.)
Use: In chronic tuberculosis.
FERROUS IODIDE SYRUP. (Various Mfr.)
Use: In chronic tuberculosis.
FERROUS LACTATE. (Various Mfr.)
Use: For iron deficiency.
• **FERROUS SULFATE,** U.S.P. XXI. Tab., Dried, Syr., Oral Soln., U.S.P. XXI.
Use: Iron deficiency
See: Feosol, Spansule, Tab., Elix. (Menley & James)
Ferralyn, Cap. (Lannett)
Fero-Gradumet, Tab. (Abbott)
Ferolix, Elix. (Century)
Ferrous Sulfate Filmseals, Tab. (Parke-Davis)
Fesotyme SR, Cap. (Elder)
Irospan Cap., Tab. (Fielding)
Mol-Iron, Prods. (Schering)
Telefon, Cap. (Kenyon)
W/Ascorbic acid.
See: Fero-Grad-500, Tab. (Abbott)
Mol-Iron W/Vit. C, Tab., Chronosules (Schering)
W/Ascorbic acid, folic acid.
See: Fero-Folic-500, Tab. (Abbott)
W/Cyanocobalamin, ascorbic acid, folic acid.
See: Intrin, Cap. (Merit)
W/Folic acid.
See: Folvron, Cap. (Lederle)
W/Maalox
See: Fermalox, Tab. (Rorer)
FERROUS SULFATE FILMSEALS. (Parke-Davis)
Ferrous Sulfate 5 gr./d release Tab. Bot. 1000s.
Unit dose 100s.
Use: Iron deficiency.
• **FERROUS SULFATE Fe 59.** USAN.
Use: Radioisotope.
FERTILITY TAPE. (Weston Labs.) Regular, extrasensitive, less-sensitive. Pkg. 60 tests.
Use: W/Fertility Testor, cervical glucose test.
FERUSAL. (Vitarine) Ferrous sulfate 325 mg./Tab.
Use: Dietary supplement.
FESTAL II. (Hoechst) Lipase 6000 U., amylase 30,000 U., protease 20,000 U./Tab. Bot. 100s, 500s.
Use: Enzymes for digestion.
FESTALAN. (Hoechst) Lipase 6,000 U., amylase 30,000 U., protease 20,000 U., in inner core/Tab.w/outer layer containing atropine methylnitrate 1 mg. Bot. 100s, 1000s.
Use: Treatment of intestinal disorders.
FESTEX. (Blue Cross) Benzalkonium Cl., diperodon HCl 0.5%, carbolic acid, ichthammol, thymol, camphor, juniper tar. Tube 1.5 oz.
Use: Drawing salve.
FETOXYLATE. B.A.N. 2-Phenoxyethyl 1-(3-cyano-3,3-diphenylpropyl)-4-phenylpiperidine-4-carboxylate.
Use: Antidiarrheal.

- **FETOXYLATE HYDROCHLORIDE.** USAN.
  Use: Relaxant.
- **FEZOLAMINE FUMARATE.** USAN.

FIBERMED HIGH-FIBER SUPPLEMENT. (Purdue Frederick) Each supplement contains 5 Gm. dietary fiber. Box 14s.
Use: High-fiber dietary supplement.

FIBRIN HYDROLYSATE.
See: Aminosol, Sol. (Abbott)

FIBROGEN (HUMAN). Partially purified fibrinogen prepared by fractionation from normal human plasma.
Use: Coagulant (clotting factor).
See: Parenogen, (I.V.) Vial (Cutter)

- **FIBRINOGEN I-125.** USAN.
  Use: Diagnostic aid.

FIBRINOLYSIN (HUMAN). Plasmin. An enzyme prepared by activating a human blood plasma fraction with streptokinase.
See: Thrombolysin (Merck Sharp & Dohme)
W/Desoxyribonuclease.
See: Elase, Oint., Pow. (Parke-Davis)

FIBRINOLYSIS INHIBITOR.
See: Amicar Syr., Tab., Vial (Lederle)

FILAXIS. (Amlab) Vit. A 25000 I.U., D 1250 I.U., C 150 mg., E 5 I.U., B-1 12 mg., B-2 5 mg., B-6 0.5 mg., B-12 5 mcg., Ca pantothenate 5 mg., niacinamide 100 mg., Fe 15 mg., iodine 0.15 mg., Mg. 10 mg., K 5 mg., Ca 75 mg., P 60 mg./Tab. Bot. 30s, 100s. Available w/B-12. Bot. 30s, 60s, 100s.
Use: Therapeutic vitamin formula.

FILIBON. (Lederle) Vit. A 5000 I.U., D 400 I.U., B-1 1.5 mg., B-6 2 mg., niacinamide 20 mg., B-2 1.7 mg., B-12 6 mcg., ferrous fumarate 18 mg., iodine 150 mcg., Mg 100 mg., calcium carbonate 125 mg./Tab. Bot 100s.
Use: Prenatal care.

FILIBON F.A.. (Lederle) The basic Filibon prenatal formulation plus folic acid 1 mg/Tab. Bot. 100s.
Use: Prenatal care.

FILIBON FORTE. (Lederle) A 8,000 I.U., D 400 I.U., E 45 I.U., C 90 mg., niacinamide 30 mg., B-6 3 mg., B-1 2 mg., B-2 2.5 mg., folic acid 1 mg., B-12 12 mcg., calcium 300 mg., iron 45 mg., Mg 100 mg., iodine 200 mcg./Tab. Jar 100s.
Use: Prophylaxis of anemias of pregnancy.

FILIBON OT. (Lederle) The basic Filibon prenatal formulation plus docusate sodium 100 mg./Tab. Jar 100s.
Use: Dietary supplement during pregnancy and lactation.

- **FILIPIN.** USAN.
  Use: Antifungal.

FINAC. (C & M Pharmacal) Sulfur 2%, methylbenzethonium chloride, isopropyl alcohol 8%, in a powderfilm forming, flesh-tone base. Bot. 2 oz. lotion.
Use: Anti-acne cover-up lotion.

FINAJET ACETATE. Trenbolone, B.A.N.

FIOGESIC. (Sandoz) Calurin 382 mg. equiv. to aspirin 300 mg., phenylpropanolamine HCl 25 mg., pheniramine maleate 12.5 mg., pyrilamine maleate 12.5 mg./Tab. Bot. 100s.

Use: Analgesic, sinus and nasal congestion.

FIORINAL. (Sandoz) Butalbital (Sandoptal) 50 mg., caffeine 40 mg., aspirin 325 mg./Tab. or Cap. **Tab.:** Bot. 100s, 1000s. Sandopak 100s. **Cap.:** Bot. 100s, 500s. Control Pak 25s.
Use: Analgesic sedative.

FIORINAL WITH CODEINE CAPSULES. (Sandoz) Butalbital (Sandoptal) 50 mg., caffeine 40 mg., aspirin 325 mg./Cap. **No. 1:** ⅛ gr. codeine phosphate. Bot. 100s **No. 2:** ¼ gr. codeine phosphate. Bot. 100s **No. 3:** ½ gr. codeine phosphate. Bot. 100s. Control Pak 25s.
Use: Analgesic sedative.

FIRMDENT. (Moyco) Formerly Moy. Karaya gum 94.6%, sodium borate 5.36% Pkg. ¼ oz., ¾ oz., 2 oz., 4¼ oz.
Use: Denture adhesive.

FIRST AID CREAM. (Johnson & Johnson) Cetyl alcohol, glyceryl stearate, isopropyl palmitate, stearyl alcohol, synthetic beeswax. Tube 0.8 oz., 1.5 oz., 2.5 oz.
Use: Skin wound protectant.

FIRST AID CREAM. (Walgreen) Benzocaine, allantoin, benzyl alcohol, phenol. Tube 1.5 oz.
Use: Ointment for minor cuts and burns.

FITACOL. (Standex) Atropine sulfate 0.2 mg., phenylpropanolamine 12.5 mg., chlorpheniramine maleate 0.5 mg., chlorbutanol 0.5 mg., water q.s./cc. Bot. pt.

FITACOL STANKAPS. (Standex) Belladonna alkaloidal salts 0.16 mg. (atropine sulfate 0.024 mg., scopolamine HBr 0.014 mg., hyoscyamine sulfate 0.122 mg.), phenylpropanolamine HCl 50 mg., chlorpheniramine maleate 1 mg., pheniramine maleate 12.5 mg./Cap. Bot. 100s.

523 TABLETS. (Enzyme Process) Pancreatin 200 mg. 4x/Tab. Tryspin, chymoprypsin, amylase, lipase enzymes from pancreatin, raw beef pancreas. Bot. 100s, 250s.
Use: Digestive aid.

FIXODENT. (Vicks Prods) Calcium sodium poly (vinyl methyl ether-maleate) and carboxymethylcellulose sodium in a petrolatum base. Pkg. ¾ oz., 1½ oz., 2½ oz.
Use: Denture adhesive cream.

FLACID. (Amfre-Grant) Simethicone 25 mg., aluminum hydroxide, magnesium carbonate 282 mg., Magnesium hydroxide 85 mg./Tab. Bot. 100s, 1000s.
Use: Antacid/antiflatulents.

FLAGYL. (Searle) Metronidazole 250 mg./Tab. Bot. 100s, 250s, 500s. 1000s. Unit dose 100s; 500 mg./Tab. Bot. 100s, 500s. Unit dose 100s.
Use: Trichomonacidal agent, amebicide, anaerobic infections.

FLAGYL I.V. (Searle) Metronidazole HCl sterile lyophilized powder in single-dose vials equivalent to 500 mg. metronidazole. Cartons 10s.
Use: Anaerobic infections.

FLAGYL I.V. RTU. (Searle) Metronidazole ready-to-use, premixed, 500 mg. /100 ml. Sol. Vials: glass, Box 6s; plastic, Box 24s.
Use: Anaerobic infections.

FLATUS. (Foy) Nux vomica extract ¼ gr., cascara extract 1 gr., ginger ¾ gr., capsicum ⅛ gr./Tab. w/asfetida qs. Bot. 1000s.
Use: Stomachic, carminative, mild laxative.

FLAV-A-D. (Kirkman) Vit. A 5000 I.U., D 1000 I.U., C 100 mg./Tab. Bot. 100s, 1000s. Also w/fluoride Bot. 100s, 1000s.
Use: Dietary supplement for children and adults.

FLAVIHIST CAPSULE. (American Labs.) Ephedrine sulfate 10 mg., pheniramine maleate 6.25 mg., pyrilamine maleate 8.33 mg., salicylamide 227 mg., acetaminophen 130 mg., caffeine 32.4 mg., atropine sulfate, ascorbic acid 50 mg./Cap. Pkg. 16s, 40s.
Use: Antihistamine.

FLAVIHIST LOZENGE. (Amlab) Neomycin, tyrothricin, cetyl dimethyl benzyl ammonium chloride, benzocaine/Lozenge Vial 12s.
Use: Minor throat irritations.

FLAVINE.
See: Acriflavine Hydrochloride (Var. Mfr.)

FLAVINOID-C. (Barth's) Tab. Vit. C 150 mg., hesperidin complex 10 mg., citrus bioflavonoid 50 mg., rutin 20 mg./Tab. Bot. 100s, 500s, 1000s. Liq: Vit. C 100 mg., bioflavonoid complex 100 mg./5 ml. Bot. 4 oz.

FLAVITAB TABLETS. (Ferndale) Hesperidin methyl chalcone 50 mg., hesperidin complex 150 mg., ascorbic acid 200 mg./Tab. Bot. 100s, 1000s.
Use: Supplementary source of Vit. C and bioflavanoids.

• **FLAVODILOL MALEATE.** USAN.
Use: Antihypertensive.

FLAVOLUTAN.
See: Progesterone (Various Mfr.)

FLAVONOID COMPOUNDS.
See: Bio-Flavonoid Cpds. Vit. P.

FLAVOR CHEWS. (Towne) Vit. A acetate 5,000 I.U., D 400 I.U., B-1 1 mg., B-2 1.5 mg., B-6 1 mg., B-12 2 mcg., C 50 mg., niacinamide 10 mg., Ca pantothenate 2 mg./Tab. Bot. 100s, 300s.

FLAVOR CHEWS W/IRON. (Towne) Vit. A 5,000 I.U., D 400 I.U., B-1 2 mg., B-2 2.5 mg., B-6 1 mg., B-12 1 mcg., C 50 mg., niacinamide 20 mcg., iron 10 mg./Tab. Bot. 100s.

FLAVOXATE. B.A.N. 2-Piperidinoethyl 3-methylflavone-8-carboxylate.
Use: Antispasmodic.
See: Urispas [hydrochloride]

• **FLAVOXATE HCl.** USAN. 2-Piperidinoethyl-3-methyl-4-oxo-2-phenyl-4H-1-benzopyran-8-carboxylate HCl.
Use: Urinary antispasmodic.
See: Urispas, Tab. (SmithKline)

FLAVUROL. Merbromin.

FLAXEDIL TRIETHIODIDE. Gallamine triethiodide soln.
Use: Similar to curare. Relax skeletal muscle.

• **FLAZALONE.** USAN. p-Fluoro-phenyl 4-(p-fluoro-phenyl)-4-hydroxy-1-methyl-3-piperidyl ketone.
Use: Anti-inflammatory.

• **FLAZALONE.** USAN. 3-(4-Fluorobenzoyl)-4-(4-fluoro-phenyl)-1-methylpiperidin-4-ol.
Use: Anti-inflammatory.

• **FLECAINIDE ACETATE.** USAN.
Use: Cardiac depressant.

FLEET RELIEF ANESTHETIC HEMORRHOIDAL OINTMENT. (Fleet) Pramoxine HCl 1%. Six Disposable pre-filled applicators. Tube 1 oz.
Use: Direct temporary relief of rectal pain or itching.

FLEET BABYLAX. (Fleet) Glycerin 4 ml. in disposable pre-lubricated rectal applicator. 6/pkg.
Use: Pediatric laxative.

FLEET BAGENEMA. (Fleet) Castile soap or Fleets bisacodyl prep.
Use: Disposable large volume enema set.

FLEET BISACODYL. (Fleet) Bisacodyl. Tab.: 5 mg./Tab. Bot. 24s, 100s, 1000s. Suppos.: 10 mg./Supos. Box 4s, 50s, 100s. Enema: 10 mg./30 ml. Disposable enema 37 ml.
Use: Laxative.

FLEET BISACODYL PREP PACKETS. (Fleet) Bisacodyl 10 mg./10 ml. packet. 36 packets/box.
Use: Laxative.

FLEET DETECATEST. (Fleet) Three guaiac impregnated slides. Test kit.
Use: Home occult blood test for feces.

FLEET ENEMA. (Fleet) Sod. biphosphate 16 Gm., sod. phosphate 6 Gm./100 cc. Bot. w/rectal tube 4.5 oz. Pediatric size 2.25 oz.
Use: Laxative.

FLEET FLAVORED CASTOR OIL EMULSION. (Fleet) 1 oz. delivers 30 ml. castor oil. Bot. 1.5 oz., 3 oz.
Use: Laxative.

FLEET MINERAL OIL ENEMA. (Fleet) Mineral oil 4.5 fl. oz. in an unbreakable vinyl squeeze bottle.
Use: To soften stools.

FLEET PREP KIT. (Fleet) A series of different laxative kits for use prior to barium enema, bowel surgery, proctoscopy, colonoscopy, etc. w/complete patient instruction form:
Prep Kit #1: 1.5 oz. Fleet® Phospho-Soda, 4×5 mg. Fleet® Bisacodyl Tablets, 1×10 mg. Fleet® Bisacodyl Suppository.
Prep Kit #2: 1.5 oz. Fleet® Phospho-Soda, 4×5 mg. Fleet® Bisacodyl Tablets, 1 Fleet® Bagenema set for large volume enema, including optional Castile Soap Packet.
Prep Kit #3: 1.5 oz. Fleet® Phospho-Soda, 4×5 mg. Fleet® Bisacodyl Tablets, 1×37 ml. Fleet® Bisacodyl Enema.
Prep Kit #4: 1.5 oz. Fleet® Flavored Castor Oil Emulsion, 4×5 mg. Fleet® Bisacodyl Tablets, 1× 10 mg. Fleet® Bisacodyl Suppository.
Prep Kit #5: 1.5 oz. Fleet® Flavored Castor Oil Emulsion, 4×5 mg. Fleet® Bisacodyl Tablets, 1 Fleet® Bagenema set for large volume enema, including optional Castile Soap Packet.
Prep Kit #6: 1.5 oz. Fleet® Flavored Castor Oil Emulsion, 4×5 mg. Fleet® Bisacodyl Tablets, 1× 37 ml. Fleet® Bisacodyl Enema.

• **FLETAZEPAM.** USAN.
Use: Relaxant.

FLETCHER'S CASTORIA. (Glenbrook) Senna equiv. 6.5%. Liq. Bot. 2½ oz., 5 oz.
Use: Laxative for children ages 1 month to 15 yrs.

FLEX ANTI-DANDRUFF SHAMPOO. (Revlon) Zinc pyrithione 1% in liquid shampoo.
Use: Anti-Dandruff shampoo.

FLEX-CARE. (Alcon) Sterile solution of sodium Cl., sodium borate, boric acid. Bot. 12 oz., 8 oz.
Use: Soft contact lens rinsing, storage, disinfection.

FLEXERIL. (Merck Sharp & Dohme) Cyclobenzaprine HCl 10 mg./Tab. Bot. 100s. Unit dose pkg. 100s. Unit of Use 30s.
Use: Short-term relief of painful muscle spasms.

FLEXOJECT. (Mayrand) Orphenadrine citrate 30 mg./ml. Vial 10 ml.
Use: Muscle relaxant.

FLEXON. (Keene) Orphenadrine citrate inj. 30 mg./ml. Vial 2 ml.
Use: Muscle relaxant.

FLEXOR. (Amfre-Grant) Orphenadrine citrate 30 mg./ml. Vial 10 ml.
Use: Muscle relaxant.

FLEXSOL. (Alcon) Sterile, buffered, isotonic aqueous sol. of sodium chloride, sodium borate, boric acid, adsorbobase. Bot. 6 oz.
Use: Soft contact lens solution for disinfecting & storage.

FLINTSTONES. (Miles) Vit. A 2500 I.U., E 15 I.U., C 60 mg., folic acid 0.3 mg., B-1 1.05 mg., B-2 1.2 mg., niacin 13.5 mg., B-6 1.05 mg., B-12 4.5 mcg., D 400 I.U./Tab. Bot. 60s, 100s.
Use: Multivitamin supplement.

FLINTSTONES COMPLETE. (Miles) Vit. A 5000 I.U., D 400 I.U., E 30 I.U., C 60 mg., folic acid 0.4 mg., B-1 1.5 mg., B-2 1.7 mg., niacin 20 mg., B-6 2 mg., B-12 6 mg., biotin 40 mcg., pantothenic acid 10 mg., iron 18 mg., calcium 100 mg., phosphorus 100 mg., iodine 150 mcg., magnesium 20 mg., manganese 2.5 mg., zinc 15 mg./Chewable Tab. Bot. 60s.
Use: Multivitamin and mineral supplement.

FLINTSTONES WITH EXTRA C. (Miles) Vit. A 2500 I.U., D 400 I.U., E 15 I.U., C 250 mg., folic acid 0.3 mg., B-1 1.20 mg., niacin 13.50 mg., B-6 1.05 mg., B-12 4.5 mcg./Tab. Bot. 60s.
Use: Chewable multivitamin supplement with extra vitamin C.

FLINTSTONES WITH IRON. (Miles) Vit. A 2500 I.U., E 15 I.U., C 60 mg., folic acid 0.3 mg., B-1 1.05 mg., B-2 1.2 mg., niacin 13.5 mg., B-6 1.05 mg., B-12 4.5 mcg., D 400 I.U., iron 15 mg./Tab. Bot. 60s, 100s.
Use: Multivitamin supplement with iron.

• **FLOCTAFENINE.** USAN.
Use: Analgesic.

FLORAJEN. (Jenkins) Fluoride 0.5 mg., Vit. A 4000 I.U., Vit. D 400 I.U., ascorbic acid 75 mg., Vit. B-1 2 mg., Vit. B-2 2 mg., niacinamide 18 mg., B-6 1 mg., calcium pantothenate. dextro 5 mg., cyanocobalamin 2 mcg./Tab. Bot. 100s, 500s, 1000s.

FLORANTYRONE. Gamma-Fluoranthen-8-yl-gamma-oxybutyric acid.

FLORANTYRONE. B.A.N. 4-(Fluoranthen-8-yl)-4-oxobutyric acid.
Use: Stimulation of bile acid secretion.
See: Zanchol

FLORAPLEX. (Barry-Martin) Vit. B-1 100 mg., B-2 1 mg.,

B-6 2 mg., niacinamide 50 mg., Ca pantothenate 2 mg./cc. Vial 30 cc.

FLORAQUIN. Di-iodohydroxyquinoline, B.A.N.

FLOR-D CHEWABLE TAB. (Derm Pharm.) Fluoride 1 mg., Vit. A 4000 I.U., D 400 I.U., C 75 mg., B-1 1.5 mg., B-2 1.8 mg., niacinamide 15 mg., B-6 1 mg., B-12 3 mcg., calcium pantothenate 10 mg./Tab. Bot. 100s.
Use: Dietary supplement.

FLOR-D DROPS. (Derm Pharm.) Fluoride 0.5 mg., Vit. A 3000 I.U., D 400 I.U., C 60 mg., B-1 1 mg., B-2 1.2 mg., niacinamide 8 mg./0.6 cc. Bot. 60 cc.
Use: Dietary supplement.

• **FLORDIPINE.** USAN.
Use: Antihypertensive.

FLORICAL. (Mericon) Sodium fluoride 8.3 mg., calcium carbonate 364 mg./Cap. Bot. 100s, 500s.
Use: Dietary supplement.

FLORIDA FOAM. (Hill) Benzalkonium chloride, aluminum subacetate, boric acid 2%. Bot. 8 oz.
Use: Soap substitute, seborrhea, fungi, acne.

FLORINEF ACETATE TABLETS. (Squibb) Fludrocortisone acetate. Tab. 0.1 mg. Bot. 100s.
Use: Treatment of Addison's disease and adrenal hyperplasia.

FLORITAL. (Cenci) Butabital 50 mg., aspirin 200 mg., phenacetin 130 mg., caffeine 40 mg./Tab. Bot. 100s.
Use: Sedative and analgesic.

FLORONE CREAM. (Dermik) Diflorasone diacetate 0.5 mg./Gm. (0.05%) w/stearic acid, sorbitan monooleate, polysorbate 60, sorbic acid, citric acid, propylene glycol, and purified water. Tube 15 Gm., 30 Gm., 60 Gm.
Use: Anti-inflammatory, antipruritic, antimiotic.

FLORONE OINTMENT. (Dermik) Diflorasone diacetate 0.5 mg./Gm. (0.05%) W/polyoxypropylene 15-stearyl ether, stearic acid, lanolin alcohol and white petrolatum. Tube 15 Gm., 30 Gm., 60 Gm.
Use: Anti-inflammatory, antipruritic, antimiotic.

FLOROPRYL. (Merck Sharp & Dohme) Isoflurophate. Ophthalmic use only. Opth. Oint. 0.025%, sterile ointment in polyethylene & mineral oil gel. Tube 3.5 Gm.
Use: Miotic, cholinesterase inhibitor for glaucoma.

FLORVITE CHEWABLE TABLETS. (Everett) Vitamins, fluoride 0.5 mg./Chewable Tab. Bot 50s, 100s.
Use: Vitamin supplement & fluoride to reduce dental caries.

FLORVITE DROPS. (Everett) Vitamins and fluoride. Bot. 50 ml.
Use: Vitamin supplement and fluoride to help reduce dental caries.

FLORVITE & IRON DROPS. (Everett) Vitamins, iron, fluoride. Bot. 50 cc.
Use: Vitamin supplement with iron & fluoride to help reduce dental caries.

FLORVITE & IRON CHEWABLE. (Everett) Vitamins, fluoride 1 mg., iron 12 mg./Chewable Tab. Bot. 100s.

Use: Reduce dental caries and iron deficiency.
FLORVITE TABLETS. (Everett) Vitamins, fluoride 1 mg./Chewable Tab. Bot. 100s, 1000s.
Use: Vitamin supplement and fluoride to help reduce dental caries.
FLOWAWAY WATER TABLETS. (DeWitt) Potassium nitrate, uva ursi, buchu leaves, caffeine. Blister paks 24s, 48s.
Use: Mild diuretic.
• **FLOXACILLIN.** USAN.
Use: Antibacterial.
• **FLOXURIDINE,** U.S.P. XXI. Sterile, U.S.P. XXI. 2'-Deoxy-5-fluorouridine.
Use: Antiviral agent.
See: FUDR, Vials (Roche)
FLUANISONE. B.A.N. 4-Fluoro-γ-[4-(2-methoxyphenyl)piperazin-1-yl]butyrophenone.
Use: Neuroleptic.
FLUAX. (Merck Sharp & Dohme) Influenza virus vaccine. 1982–1983 formulation: A/Brazil 11/78 (H₁N₁), 15 mcg.; A/Bangkok/1/79 (H₃N₂), 15 mcg.; B/Singapore 22/79, 15 mcg. Vial 5 ml, (10 doses).
Product deleted for 1983–84.
Use: Influenza immunization.
• **FLUAZACORT.** USAN.
Use: Anti-inflammatory.
• **FLUBANILATE HYDROCHLORIDE.** USAN. Ethyl N-[2(dimethylamino)ethyl]-m-(trifluoromethyl)carbanilate HCl.
Use: Antidepressant.
• **FLUBENDAZOLE.** USAN.
Use: Antiprotozpal.
FLUCARBRIL. 1-Methyl-6-(trifluromethyl)carbostyril.
Use: Muscle relaxant and analgesic.
• **FLUCINDOLE.** USAN.
Use: Antipsychotic.
FLUCLOROLONE ACETONIDE. B.A.N. 9α,-11β-Dichloro-6α-fluoro-21-hydroxy-16α, 17α-isopropylidenedioxypregna-1,4-diene-3,20-dione.
Use: Corticosteroid.
See: Topilar Flucloronide.
• **FLUCLORONIDE.** USAN. 9, 11β-Dichloro-6α-fluoro-16α, 17, 21-trihydroxypregna-1, 4-diene-3, 20-dione cyclic 16, 17-acetal with acetone.
Use: Glucocorticoid.
FLUCLOXACILLIN. B.A.N. 6-[3-(2-Chloro-6-fluorophenyl)-5-methylisoxazole-4-carboxamido]-penicillanic acid.
Use: Antibiotic.
See: Floxapen
• **FLUCRYLATE.** USAN. 2,2,2-Trifluoro-1-methylethyl-2-cyanoacrylate.
Use: Surgical aid (tissue adhesive).
• **FLUCYTOSINE,** U.S.P. XXI. Cap. U.S.P. XXI. 5-Fluorocytosine.
Use: Antifungal.
See: Ancobon, Cap. (Roche)
• **FLUCYTOSINE.** USAN. 4-Amino-5-fluoro-1,2-dihydropyrimidin-2-one. 5-Fluorocytosine.
Use: Antifungal.
See: Alcobon

• **FLUDARABINE PHOSPHATE.** USAN.
Use: Antineoplastic.
• **FLUDAZONIUM CHLORIDE.** USAN.
Use: Anti-infective, topical.
• **FLUDALANINE.** USAN.
Use: Antibacterial.
• **FLUDOREX.** USAN.
Use: Anorexic, anti-emetic.
FLUDROCORTISONE. B.A.N. 9α-Fluoro-11β,-17α,21-trihydroxypregn-4-ene-3,20-dione. 9α-Fluorohydrocortisone. Alflorone, Florinef, and Fludrocortone are the 21-acetate
Use: Corticosteroid.
• **FLUDROCORTISONE ACETATE.** U.S.P. XXI. Tab. U.S.P. XXI. 9-alpha-Fluorohydrocortisone. Pregn-4-ene-3,20-dione,21-(acetyloxy)-9-fluoro-11,-17-dihydroxy-, (11 beta)-. 9-Fluoro-11 beta, 17,21-trihydroxypregn-4-ene-3,20-dione 21-acetate.
Use: Adrenocortical steroid (salt-regulation).
See: Florinef Acetate, Tab. (Squibb)
• **FLUFENAMIC ACID.** USAN. N-(α, α, α-Trifluoro-m-tolyl) anthranilic acid.
Use: Anti-inflammatory agent.
• **FLUFENSIAL.** USAN.
Use: Analgesic.
FLUGESTONE. B.A.N. 9α-Fluoro-11β,17-dihydroxypregn-4-ene-3,20-dione.
Use: Progestational steroid.
See: Flurogestone
FLUIDEX. (O'Connor) Natural botanical ingredients. Tabs. Bot. 36s, 72s.
Use: Diuretic
FLUIDEX PLUS. (O'Connor) Phenylpropanolamine HCl 25 mg./Tab. natural botanical ingredients Bot. 36s, 72s.
Use: Diuretic/appetite suppressant.
FLUIDEX WITH PAMABROM. (O'Connor) Pamabrom 50 mg./Cap. Pkg 3s, 12s, 24s.
Use: Premenstrual diuretic.
FLUIDIL. (Adria) Cyclothiazide 2 mg./Tab. Bot. 100s.
Use: Diuretic.
FLUITRAN. Trichlormethiazide.
FLUMEDROXONE. B.A.N. 17α-Hydroxy-6α-trifluoromethylpregn-4-ene-3,20-dione.
Use: Treatment of migraine.
See: Demigran [acetate]
• **FLUMEQUINE.** USAN.
Use: Antibacterial.
• **FLUMERIDONE.** USAN.
Use: Anti-emetic.
• **FLUMETHASONE.** USAN. 6α,9α-Difluoro-11β, 17α,21-trihydroxy-16α-methylpregna-1,4-diene-3,20-dione. 6α,9α-Difluoro-16α-methylprednisolone.
Use: Corticosteroid.
See: Locorten [21-pivalate] (Ciba)
• **FLUMETHASONE PIVALATE,** U.S.P. XXI. Cream, U.S.P. XXI. 6α-9α-difluoro-16α-methylprednisolone 21 pivalate. 6α,9-Difluoro-11β,17,21-trihydroxy-16-me-thylpregna-1,4-diene-3,20-dione-21 pivalate.
Use: Steroid.
See: Locorten, Cream (Ciba)

FLUMETHIAZIDE. 6-Trifluoromethyl-7-sulfamyl-1,2, 4-benzothiadiazine-1, 1-dioxide.
Use: Diuretic.
See: Rautrax, Tab. (Squibb)

FLUMETHIAZIDE. B.A.N. 6-Trifluoromethyl-1,2,4-benzothiadiazine-7-sulphonamide 1,1-dioxide.
Use: Diuretic.

• **FLUMETRAMIDE.** USAN.
Use: Relaxant.

• **FLUMEZAPINE.** USAN.
Use: Antipsychotic, neuroleptic.

• **FLUMINOREX.** USAN.
Use: Anorexic.

• **FLUMIZOLE.** USAN.
Use: Anti-inflammatory.

• **FLUNARIZINE HCl.** USAN. (E)-1-[Bis-(p-fluorophenyl)methyl]-4-cinnamyl-piperazine dihydrochloride.
Use: Vasodilator.

• **FLUNIDAZOLE.** USAN.
Use: Antiprotozoal.

• **FLUNISOLIDE,** U.S.P. XXI. Nasal Soln., U.S.P. XXI.
Use: Symptoms of seasonal and perennial rhinitis.
See: Nasalide, Liq. (Syntex)

• **FLUNISOLIDE ACETATE.** USAN. Fluoxolonate.

• **FLUNITRAZEPAM.** USAN. 5-Fluorophenyl-1,3-dihydro-1-methyl-7-nitro-2H-1,4-benzodiazepin-2-one.
Use: Hynoptic.

• **FLUNIXIN.** USAN.
Use: Anti-inflammatory, analgesic.

FLUOCINOLIDE. Fluocinonide, U.S.P. XXI.

FLUOCINOLONE. B.A.N. 6α,9α-Difluoro-11β,16α, 17α,21-tetrahydroxypregna-1,4-diene-3,20-dione. 6α,9α-Difluoro-16α-hydroxy-prednisolone. Synandone [acetonidel].
Use: Corticosteroid.
See: Synalar
     Synemol, Cream (Syntex)

• **FLUOCINOLONE ACETONIDE,** U.S.P. XXI. Cream, Oint., Topical Soln. U.S.P. XXI. Pregna-1,4-diene-3,20-dione,6,9-difluoro-11,21-dihydroxy-16,17-[(1-methylethylidene)bis(oxy)], (6α,11β,-16α)-. 9a-Difluoro-16a-hydroxyprednisolone-16, 17-acetonide. 6α,9α-Difluoro-11β,16α,17,21-tetrahydroxypregna-1,4-diene-3,20-dione. Cyclic 16,17-Acetal with Acetone.
Use: Adrenocortical steroid (topical anti-inflammatory).
Use: Glucocorticoid.
See: Fluonid, Cream, Oint., Sol. (Herbert)
     Synalar, Cream, Oint., Sol. (Syntex)
W/Neomycin sulfate.
See: Neo-Synalar. (Syntex)

• **FLUOCINONIDE,** U.S.P. XXI. Cream, Gel, Oint., U.S.P. XXI. F.D.A. 6α, 9α-Difluoro-11β-16α, 17α-21-tetrahydroxypregna-1,4-diene-3,20-dione, cyclic 16, 17-acetal with acetone, 21-acetate. B.A.N. 21-Acetoxy-6α,9α-difluoro-11β-hydroxy-16α, 17α-isopropylidene-dioxypregna-1,4-diene-3,20-dione. Fluocinolone 16α, 17α-acetonide 21 acetate
Use: Corticosteroid.
See: Lidex, Cream, Oint. (Syntex)
     Lidex-E, Cream (Syntex)

Metosyn
Topsyn, Gel (Syntex)

• **FLUOCORTIN BUTYL.** USAN. Butyl-6α-fluoro-11β-hydroxy-16α-methyl-3,20-dioxopregna-1,4-dien-21oate.
Use: Anti-inflammatory.

• **FLUOCORTOLONE.** USAN. 6α-Fluoro-11β,21-dihydroxy-16α-methylpregna-1,4-diene-20-dione. (Berlin) 6α-Fluoro-11β, 21-dihydroxy-16α-methylpregna-1, 4-diene-3, 20-dione.
Use: Corticosteroid.
See: Ultralanum [21-hexanoate]

• **FLUOCORTOLONE CAPROATE.** USAN.
Use: Glucocorticoid.

FLUOGEN. (Parke-Davis) Influenza virus vaccine, trivalent—Immunizing antigen, ether extracted. Vials 5 ml. The 5 ml. vial contains sufficient product to deliver ten 0.5 ml. doses.
Use: Influenza immunizing agent.

FLUONID. (Herbert) Fluocinolone Acetonide. **Cream:** 0.01%. Tube 15 Gm., 60 Gm. Jar 425 Gm.; 0.025%. Tube 15, 60 Gm. **Ointment:** 0.025% Tube 15 Gm., 60 Gm. **Solution:** 0.01% Bot. 20 ml., 60 ml.
Use: Anti-inflammatory for dermatoses.

FLUOPROMAZINE. B.A.N. 10-(3-Dimethylaminopropyl)-2-trifluoromethylpiamothiazine. Triflupromazine (I.N.N.)
Use: Tranquilizer.
See: Vespral
     Vesprin [hydrochloride]

FLUORAL. (CooperCare) Paste containing 2.3% fluoride from sodium fluoride. Tube 15 Gm.
Use: Topical application to aid in treatment of dentin hypersensitivity.

• **FLUORESCEIN,** U.S.P. XXI.
Use: Diagnostic aid (corneal trauma indicator).

• **FLUORESCEIN SODIUM,** U.S.P. XXI. Ophth. Strip, Inj. U.S.P. XXI. Spiro[isoberzofuran-1(3H), 9-[9H]xanthene]-3-one, 3'6'-dihydroxy, disodium salt. (Various Mfr.) Soluble fluorescein. Bot. 1 oz.
Use: 2% sol. in diagnosis of eye conditions. (circulation time).
See: Fluor-I-Strip. (Ayerst)
     Fluoreseptic, Sol. (Softcon)
     Funduscein, Amp. (CooperVision)
     Plak-Lite Sol. (Internat. Pharm.)

FLUORESCEIN SODIUM I.V.
See: Fluorescite, Amp. (Alcon)

FLUORESCEIN SODIUM 2% SOLUTION. (Alcon) Drop-Tainer 15 cc. Steri-Unit 2 cc. 24s; (CooperVision) Dropperette 1 cc. 10s.
Use: Diagnostic agent in ophthalmology.

FLUORESCEIN SODIUM 2%. (CooperVision) A sterile aqueous solution containing fluorescein sodium 2%. Dropperette 1 ml. Box 12s.
Use: Diagnostic for topical application.

FLUORESCITE. (Alcon) Fluorescein as Sod. salt **5%** Sol. Amp. 10 ml. Box 12s; **10%** Sol. Amp. 5 ml. Box 12s, Disp. Syringe 5 ml., 12s; **25%** Sol. Amp. Box 12s.

Use: Diagnostic aid, injectable ophthalmic.

FLUORESEPTIC. (Softcon) A sterile, buffered solution containing fluorescein sodium 2% w/phenylmercuric borate 1:25,000 as preservative, sod. bicarbonate. Plastic container in 7½ cc., 15 cc.
Use: Diagnostic agent.

FLUORIDE SODIUM.
See: Dentafluor Chewable, Tab. (Western Pharm.)
Karidium, Top. Soln., Tab. (Lorvic)
Karigel, Gel (Lorvic)

■ **FLUORIDE THERAPY.**
See: Adeflor preps. (Upjohn)
Cari-Tab, Softab Tab. (Stuart)
Coral Prod. (Lorvic)
Fluorineed, Chew. Tab. (Hanlon)
Fluorinse, Liq. (Pacemaker)
Fluora, Loz. (Kirkman)
Gal-Kam, Preps. (Scherer)
Luride Preps. (Hoyt)
Mulvidren-F, Softab Tab. (Stuart)
Point Two, Rinse (Hoyt)
Poly-Vi-Flor, Drops, Tab. (Mead Johnson)
Soluvite-F, Drops (Pharmics)
Tri-Vi-Flor, Drops, Tab. (Mead Johnson)

FLUORI-METHANE SPRAY. (Gebauer)
Dichlorodifluoromethane 15%, trichloromonofluoromethane 85%. Bot. 4 oz.
Use: "Painful motion" syndromes.

FLUORINEED. (Hanlon) Fluoride 1 mg./Chew. Tab. Bot. 100s, 1000s.
Use: Reduce caries in children.

FLUORINSE. (CooperCare) Sodium fluoride 0.2%. Bot. 16 oz.
Use: Fluoride mouthrinse.

FLUORINSE. (Pacemaker) Fluoride mouthwash. Pack. Fluoride ion level 0.05% & 0.2%. Unit dose Bot. 32 oz. Conc. 1 oz., 4 oz., gal.

FLUOR-I-STRIP. (Ayerst) Fluorescein sodium ophthalmic strips. Pkg. 300s.
Use: Ophthalmic diagnostic agent.

FLUOR-I-STRIP-A.T. (Ayerst) Fluorescein sodium ophthalmic strips. 100 envelopes, each with two sterile applicators. Box 300 (150 × 2).
Use: Applicator tonometry.

FLUORITAB. (Fluoritab) Sodium fluoride 2.2 mg. equivalent to 1 mg. of fluorine (as fluoride ion) w/inert organic filler 75.8 mg./Tab. Bot. 100s; Liq. dropper bot. (fluorine 0.25 mg./Drop) 19 cc.
Use: Fluoride supplement.

5-FLUOROCYTOSINE.
See: Ancobon, Cap. (Roche)

FLUOROGESTONE ACETATE. 9-Fluoro-11β, 17-dihydroxypregn-4-ene-3, 20-dione, 17-acetate.
Use: Progestin.

FLUOROHYDROCORTISONE ACETATE. 9-α-Fluorohydrocortisone.
See: Fludrocortisone Acetate (Var. Mfr.)

• **FLUOROMETHOLONE,** U.S.P. XXI. Cream, Ophth. Susp., U.S.P. XXI. Pregna-1,4-diene-3,20-diene, 9-fluoro-11,17-dihydroxy-6-methyl-,(6α,11β)-. 6α-Methyl-9α-fluoro-21-desoxyprednisolone. 9-Fluo-

ro-11β, 17-dihydroxy-6α-methylpregna-1, 4-diene-3, 20-dione. B.A.N. 9α-Fluoro-11β-17α-dihydroxy-6α-methylpregna-1,4-diene-3,20-dione.
Use: Glucocorticoid.
See: FML Liquifilm, Ophth. Susp. (Allergan)
Oxylone, Cream Ophth. Susp. (Upjohn)
W/Neomycin sulfate.
See: Neo-Oxylone, Oint. (Upjohn)

FLUOROPHENE.
Use: Antiseptic agent.

FLUOROPLEX CREAM. (Herbert) 5-Fluorouracil 1% in a propylene glycol base. Plastic bot. W/dropper 30 ml. Fluorouracil 1% in emulsion base w/benzyl alcohol 0.5%, ethoxylated stearyl alcohol, mineral oil, isopropyl myristate, sodium hydroxide and purified water. Tube 30 Gm.
Use: Treatment of multiple actinic keratoses.

• **FLUOROSALAN.** USAN. 3, 5-dibromo-3'-trifluoromethyl salicylanilide. Fluorophene.
Use: Antiseptic.

FLUOROSEPTIC. (Softcon) Fluoroscein sodium 2% 7.5 ml., 15 ml.
Use: To demonstrate surface irregularities and changes in epithelial thickness and for detecting points of pressure in fitting contact lens.

FLUOR-O-SOL. (Hoyt) Fluoride 1.2% with silicon dioxide abrasive. Jars 50 Gm. Carton 6s.
Use: Clean & polish teeth.

FLUOTHANE. (Ayerst) Halothane. Bot. 125 ml., 250 ml.
Use: Inhalation anesthetic.

FLUOROTHYL. Bis (2, 2, 2-trifluoroethyl) ether.
See: Flurothyl.

• **FLUOROURACIL,** U.S.P. XXI. Cream, Inj., Topical Soln., U.S.P. XXI. 5-Fluorouracil. (Roche) Amp. 10 ml., 500 mg. Box 10s.
Use: Malignancies, antineoplastic.
See: Adrucil, Inj. (Adria)
Efudex, Sol. & Cream (Roche)
Fluoroplex, Sol., Cream (Herbert Labs.)

• **FLUOTRACEN HYDROCHLORIDE.** USAN.
Use: Antipsychotic, antidepressant.

• **FLUOXETINE.** USAN.
Use: Antidepressant.

• **FLUOXYMESTERONE,** U.S.P. XXI. Tab., U.S.P. XXI. 9-α-Fluoro-11-β-hydroxy-17-α-methyltestosterone. 9-Fluoro-11β, 17β-dihydroxy-17-methylandrost-4-en-3-one.
Use: Androgen.
See: Android-F, Tab. (Brown)
Halotestin, Tab. (Upjohn)
Ora-Testryl, Tab. (Squibb)
W/Ethinyl estradiol.
See: Halodrin, Tab. (Upjohn)

FLUOXYMESTERONE. B.A.N. 9α-Fluoro-11β, 17 β-dihy 17α-methylandrost-4-en-3-one. 9α-Fluoro-11 β-hydroxymethyltestosterone.
Use: Androgen; anabolic steroid.
See: Ultandren

FLUPENTHIXOL. B.A.N. 9- 3-[4-(2-Hydroxyethel)-piperazin-1-yl]propylidene -2-trifluoromethylthioxanthene.
Use: Tranquilizer.

See: Depixol decanoate
- **FLUPERAMIDE.** USAN.
  Use: Antiperistaltic.

FLUPEROLONE. B.A.N. 9α-Fluoro-11β, 17α, 21-trihydroxy-21-methylpregna-1,4-diene-3,20-dione. 9α-Fluoro-21-methylprednisolone.
  Use: Corticosteroid.
  See: Methral acetate

- **FLUPEROLONE ACETATE.** USAN. 9α-Fluoro-21-methylprednisolone, 9α-Fluoro-11β,17α,21-trihydroxy-21-methylpregna-1:4-diene-3:20-dione acetate. Methral.
  Use: Corticosteroid.

FLUPHENAZINE. B.A.N. 10- 3-[4-(2-Hydroxyethyl)piperazin-1-yl]propyl -2-trifluoromethylphenothiazine.
  Use: Tranquilizer.
  See: Modecate (decanocate)
       Moditen
       Prolixin (dihydrochloride)

FLUPHENAZINE DECANOATE.
  See: Prolixin Decanoate, Sol. (Squibb)

- **FLUPHENAZINE ENANTHATE,** U.S.P. XXI. Inj., U.S.P. XXI. 4-(3-(2-(Trifluoromethyl)phenothiazine-10-yl)-propyl)-1-piperazine-ethanol.
  Use: Tranquilizer.
  See: Prolixin Enanthate Prods. (Squibb)

- **FLUPHENAZINE HYDROCHLORIDE,** U.S.P. XXI. Elixir, Inj., Oral Soln., Tab., U.S.P. XXI. 1-(2-Hydroxyethyl)-4-[3-(2-trifluoromethyl)-10H-Phenothiazinyl-propyl]-piperazine diHCl. 4-(3-(2-(Trifluoromethyl) phenothiazine-10-yl) propyl)-1-piperazine-ethanol Dihydrochloride.
  Use: Tranquilizer.
  See: Permitil, Prep. (Schering)
       Prolixin, Tab., Elix., Vials (Squibb)

FLUPREDNIDENE. B.A.N. 9α-Fluoro-11β-17 α,21-trihydroxy-16-methylenepregna-1,4-diene-3, 20-dione.
  Use: Glucocorticosteroid.

- **FLUPREDNISOLONE.** USAN. 6αFluoro-11β, 17α, 21-trihydroxypregna-1, 4-diene-3,20-dione;b) 6α-fluoroprednisolone.
  Use: Corticosteroid
  See: Alphadrol, Tab. (Upjohn)

- **FLUPREDNISOLONE VALERATE.** USAN. 6-Fluoro-11β, 17, 21-trihydroxypregna-1, 4-diene-3,20-dione 17-valerate.
  Use: Glucocorticoid.

FLUPROFEN. B.A.N. 2-(2'-Fluorobiphenyl-4-yl)-propionic acid.
  Use: Anti-inflammatory; analgesic.

- **FLUPROQUAZONE.** USAN.
  Use: Analgesic.

FLUPROSTENOL. B.A.N. (±)-7-(1R,2R,3R,5S)-3,5-Dihydroxy-2-[(3R)-3-hydroxy-4-(3-trifluoromethylphenoxy)but-1-(E)-enyl]cyclopent-1-yl hept-5-(Z)-enoic acid.
  Use: Infertility, veterinary medicine.
  See: Equimate (sodium salt)

- **FLUPROSTENOL SODIUM.** USAN.
  Use: Prostaglandin.

- **FLUQUAZONE.** USAN.
  Use: Anti-inflammatory.

- **FLURADOLINE HYDROCHLORIDE.** USAN.
  Use: Analgesic.

FLURA DROPS. (Kirkman) Sodium fluoride 2.21 mg./4 drops. (4 drops q.s. one quart provides 1 part per million of fluorine ion.) Bot. 24 ml.
  Use: Prevention of dental caries.

FLURA-LOZ. (Kirkman) Sod. fluoride 2.21 mg./Lozenge. Bot. 100s, 1000s.

- **FLURANDRENOLIDE,** U.S.P. XXI. Cream, Oint., Lotion, Tape, U.S.P. XXI.
  Use: Adrenocortical steroid (topical anti-inflammatory).
  See: Cordran, Preps. (Dista)

FLURANDRENOLONE. 6α-Fluoro-16α-hydroxyhydrocortisone 16, 17-acetonide.
  Use: Topical corticoid compound.

FLURANDRENOLONE. B.A.N. 6α-Fluoro-11β,-21-dihydroxy-16α, 17α-isopropylidenedioxypregn-4-ene-3,-20-dione. 6α-Fluoro-16α, 17α-isopropylidenedioxyhydrocortisone. Fludroxycortide (I.N.N.)
  Use: Corticosteroid.
       Drenison
       Haelan

FLURA-PREN. (Kirkman) Vit. A 4000 I.U., D 400 I.U., B-1 3 mg., B-2 2 mg., B-6 10 mg., niacinamide 10 mg., Vit. C 100 mg., K 0.5 mg., calcium carbonate 625 mg., ferrous fumarate 125 mg., Vit. B-12 w/intrinsic factor ⅛ oral u., sodium fluoride 2.21 mg./Tab. Bot. 100s.
  Use: Nutritional supplement.

FLURA-TABLETS. (Kirkman) Sod. fluoride 2.21 mg., equiv. to 1 mg. fluoride ion/Tab. Bot. 100s, 1000s.

FLURA-VITE. (Kirkman) Flavored Multiple-vitamin tablet, chewable, for children. Bot. 100s.

- **FLURAZEPAM HYDROCHLORIDE,** U.S.P. XXI. Cap., U.S.P. XXI. 7-Chloro-1-[2-(diethylamino)ethyl]-5-(o-fluorophenyl)-3,-dihydro-2H-1,4-benzodiazepin-2-one dihydrochloride. B.A.N. 7-Chloro-1-(2-diethylamino-ethyl)-5-(2-fluorophenyl)-1,3-dihydro-2H-1,4-benzodiazepin-2-one.
  Use: Hypnotic.
  See: Dalmane, Cap. (Roche)

- **FLURBIPROFEN.** USAN. 2-(2-Fluorobiphenyl-4-yl)-propionic acid.
  Use: Anti-inflammatory; analgesic.

FLURESS. (Barnes-Hind) Fluorescein sodium 0.25%, benoxinate HCl 0.4% in isotonic boric acid soln., chlorobutanol 1.0%. Bot. 5 cc.
  Use: Applanation tonometry; disclosing agent.

- **FLURETOFEN.** USAN.
  Use: Anti-inflammatory, antithrombotic.

- **FLURFAMIDE.** USAN.
  Use: Enzyme inhibitor.

- **FLUROCITABINE.** USAN.
  Use: Antineoplastic.

FLURO-ETHYL. (Gebauer) Ethyl chloride 25%, dichlorotetrafluoroethane 75%. Aerosol can 255 Gm.
  Use: Topical anesthetic.

- **FLUROGESTONE ACETATE.** USAN.
  Use: Progestin.

- **FLUROTHYL,** U.S.P. XXI. Bis (2,2,2-trifluoroethyl)

ether. Hexafluorodiethyl ether. B.A.N. Di-(2,2,2-tri-
fluoroethyl) ether. Bis(2,2,2-trifluoroethyl)ether.
Use: Central nervous system stimulant, shock
inducing agent (convulsant).
See: Indoklon
• **FLUROXENE.** USAN. 2,2,2-Trifluoroethyl vinyl ether.
Fluoromar.
Use: General inhalation anesthetic.
• **FLUSPIPERONE.** USAN.
Use: Antipsychotic.
FLUSPIRILENE. USAN. 8-[4, 4-bis(p-Fluorophenyl)-
butyl]-1-phenyl-1,3,8-triazaspiro-[4.5] decan-4-one.
Imap (McNeil).
Use: Tranquilizer.
• **FLUTAMIDE.** USAN.
• **FLUTIAZIN.** USAN.
Use: Anti-inflammatory.
FLUTRA. Trichlormethiazide.
Use: Diuretic.
• **FLUTROLINE.** USAN.
Use: Antipsychotic.
• **FLUZINAMIDE.** USAN.
FLUZONE. (Squibb-Connaught) Influenza virus vaccine.
Vial 5 ml. (10 doses).
Use: Prevention of influenza.
FML LIQUIFILM. (Allergan) Fluorometholone 0.1%,
polyvinyl alcohol 1.4% w/benzalkonium chloride,
edetate disodium, sod. chloride, sod. phosphate
monobasic, monohydrate, sod. phosphate dibasic,
anhydrous, polysorbate 80, purified water, sod.
hydroxide to adjust pH. Dropper bot. 5 ml., 10 ml.,
15 ml. Unit dose, 1 ml.
Use: Ocular anti-inflammatory.
FOAM-RICH TRAVEL PACK. (Matthew) Caps. 20s.
FOLABEE. (Vortech) Liver inj. equiv. to B-12 50 mcg.,
folic acid 10 mg., niacinamide 75 mg., phenol
0.5%/cc. Vial 10 cc.
FOLACINE.
See: Folic acid. (Var. Mfr.)
FOLATE, SODIUM.
See: Folvite, Sol. (Lederle)
FOLEX. (Adria) Methotrexate sodium 25 mg., 50 mg.,
100 mg./Vial. For injection.
Use: Antineoplastic.
• **FOLIC ACID,** U.S.P. XXI. Inj., Tab. U.S.P. XXI.
Pteroylglutamic acid. N-[p-[[(2-Amino-4-hydroxy-6-
pteridinyl)-methyl]-amino] benzoyl]-L-glutamic acid. L-
Glutamic acid, N-[4-[[(2-amino-1,4-dihydro-4-oxo-6-
pteridinyl)methyl]-amino]benzoyl]-. Vitamin Bc.
Use: Vitamin therapy.
See: Folvite, Tab., Sol. (Lederle)
FOLIC ACID ANTAGONISTS.
See: Methotrexate Inj., Tab. (Lederle)
FOLIC ACID SALTS.
See: Folvite, Tab., Sol. (Lederle)
FOLINIC ACID. Leucovorin Calcium, U.S.P. XXI.
Various Mfg.
FOLIPLEX-C. (Galen) Vit. B-1 3 mg., B-2 3 mg., B-6 0.5
mg., B-12 w. intrinsic factor conc. representing 3 mcg.
cyanocobalamin, Ca pantothenate 1 mg.,
niacinamide 5 mg., ferrous fumarate 40 mg., Cu 1

mg., yeast autolysate 1 gr., liver, whole desic. 2.67
gr., folic acid 0.05 mg./Cap. Bot. 100s.
Use: Oral hematinic and vit. supp.
FOLIVER "12." (Pharmex) Vit. B-12 activity from liver inj.
equiv. to cyanocobalamin 10 mcg., folic acid 1 mg.,
Vit. B-12 100 mcg./cc. Vial 10 cc. Univial 10 cc.
FOLIV-B-12 FORTE. (Rocky Mtn.) Liver inj. 10 mcg.,
folic acid 1 mg., B-12 100 mcg./cc. Univial 10 cc.
Use: Liver & vitamin therapy.
FOLLESTROL. (Blue Line) **Aq. susp.** Estrone 20,000
I.U./cc. (2 mg./cc.) & 50,000 I.U./cc. (5 mg./cc) 10
cc. **Tab.** Conjugated 1.25 mg. Bot. 100s, 1000s.
Use: Estrogen therapy.
FOL-LI-BEE. (Foy) Liver inj. equiv. to cyanocobalamin
10 mcg., folic acid 1 mg., cyanocobalamin 100
mcg./cc., phenol 0.5% pH adjusted w/sod.
hydroxide and/or HCl. Vial 10 cc. multi-dose, Monovi-
als.
FOLLICLE STIMULATING HORMONE, HUMAN.
Menotropins, Pergonal.
FOLLICORMON.
See: Estradiol Benzoate. (Various Mfr.)
FOLLICULAR HORMONES.
See: Estrone (Various Mfr.)
FOLLICULIN.
See: Estrone (Various Mfr.)
FOLLUTEIN. (Squibb) Chorionic gonadotropin. 10,000
units Pow. 10 ml. diluent. (W/NaCl 83 mg., sodium
hydroxide, phenol 0.5%).
Use: Cryptorchidism.
FOLTRIN. (Vitarine) Hematinic concentrate with
intrinsic factor.
Use: Hematinic.
FOLVITE. (Lederle) Folic Acid (as sodium folate).
Sol.: (Sequestrene sod. 0.2%, water for injection,
sod. hydroxide, benzyl alcohol 1.5%). 5 mg./ml.
Vial 10 ml. **Tab.:** 1 mg. Bot. 100s, 1000s. Unit dose
10 × 10s.
Use: Megaloblastic anemias of folate deficiency.
FOMAC FOAM. (Dermik) Salicylic acid 2% in a soap-
free protein/polyvinylpyrrolidone complex system.
Bot. 3 oz.
Use: Treatment for acne & oily skin.
FOMOCAINE. B.A.N. 4-(3-Morpholinopropyl)-benzyl
phenyl ether.
Use: Local anesthetic.
FONATOL.
See: Diethylstilbestrol (Various Mfr.)
• **FONAZINE.** USAN. Dimethothiazine.
Use: Serotonin inhibitor
FONAZINE MESYLATE. 10-[2-Dimethylamino)propyl]-
N, N-dimethylphenothiazine-2-sulfonamide methane-
sulfonate.
Use: Antihistamine, antiserotonin, antibradykinin.
FONTARSOL.
See: Dichlorophenarsine Hydrochloride.
FORALICON PLUS ELIXIR. (Forbes) Vit. B-12 16.7
mcg., B-6 4 mg., iron 200 mg. (equiv. to elemental iron
24 mg.), niacinamide 40 mg., folic acid 0.8 mg.,
sorbitol sol. q.s./15 ml. Bot. 8 oz., 16 oz.
Use: Vit. B-12, B-6, or iron deficiencies.
FORBUTOL. (Vangard) A.P.C. w/butalbital 50 mg.,

aspirin 200 mg., phenacetin 130 mg., caffeine 40 mg./Tab. Bot. 100s, 1000s.
Use: Headache.

FORDUSTIN. (Sween) Methylbenzethonium chloride, sodium bicarbonate, corn starch. Body pow. Plastic Bot. 9 Oz.
Use: Topical bacteriostatic.

FOR FACES ONLY. (Plough) Padimate O in lotion base with SPF values of 2, 4, 6, 15. Tubes. 2 oz.
Use: Ultraviolet sunblock, sunscreen.

FOR FACES ONLY FACE AND LIP SUN PROTECTION COMPACT. (Plough) Sun protectant. **Cream:** Compact 0.13 oz. **Lip Gloss:** Compact 0.14 oz.
Use: Ultraviolet sunscreen.

FORMADON SOLUTION. (Gordon) Formalin solution (10% of U.S.P. strength) in an aqueous perfumed base. Bot. 1 oz., 4 oz., 0.5 gal., gal.
Use: Bromidrosis, hyperhidrosis.

FORMADRIN. (Kenyon) Chlorpheniramine maleate 12 mg., pot. guaiacol sulfonate 8 gr., ammonium chloride 8 gr., tartar emetic 1/12 gr., dl-desoxyephedrine HCl 2 mg./oz. Bot. 4 oz.
Use: Treatment of cold symptoms.

• **FORMALDEHYDE SOLUTION,** U.S.P. XXI. A 37% aqueous solution.
Use: For poison ivy, fungus infections of the skin, hyperhidrosis & as an astringent disinfectant.

FORMALIN.
See: Formaldehyde Solution (Various Mfr.)

FORMEBOLONE. B.A.N. 2-Formyl-11α, 17β-dihydroxy-17α-methylandrosta-1,4-dien-3-one.
Use: Anabolic steroid.

FORMIC ACID.
W/Silicic acid.
See: Nyloxin, Inj. (Hyson, Westcott & Dunning)

FORMINITRAZOLE. B.A.N. 2-Formamido-5-nitrothiazole.
Use: Treatment of trichomoniasis.
See: Aroxine

• **FORMOCORTAL.** USAN. 3-(2-Chloroethoxy)-9-fluoro-11β, 16α, 17, 21-tetrahydroxy-20-oxopregna-3, 5-diene-6-carboxaldehyde, cyclic 16, 17-acetal with acetone, 21-acetate.
Use: Glucocorticoid.

FORMOCORTAL. B.A.N. 21-Acetoxy-3-(2-chloroethoxy)-9α-fluoro-6-formyl-11β-hydroxy-16α,-17α-isopropylidenedioxypregna-3,5-dien-20-one.
Use: Topical corticosteroid.
See: Deflamene

FORMULA "K." (Pharmex) Calcium gluconate 1.5 Gm., potassium chloride 4.47 Gm., Mg sulf. 60 mg./cc. Vial 30 cc.

FORMULA II COUGH SYRUP WITH d-METHORPHAN. (Walgreen) Dextromethorphan HBr, doxylamine succinate, sodium citrate, alcohol 10% by vol. Bot. 4 oz., 6 oz.
Use: Temporary relief of cough due to cold.

FORMULA 44 COUGH CONTROL DISCS. (Vicks)
See: Vicks Formula 44 Cough Discs (Vicks)

FORMULA 44 COUGH MIXTURE. (Vicks)
See: Vicks Formula 44 Cough Mixture (Vicks)

FORMULA 44D DECONGESTANT COUGH MIXTURE. (Vicks)
See: Vicks Formula 44D Decongestant Cough Mixture (Vicks)

FORMULA NO. 81. (Fellows) Liver (beef) for inj. 1 mcg., ferrous gluconate 100 mg., niacinamide 100 mg., B-2 1.5 mg., panthenol 2.5 mg., B-12 3.0 mcg., procaine HCl 25/2 cc. Vial 30 cc.

FORMULA 1207. (Thurston) Iodine, liver fraction No. 2, caseinates/Tab. Bot. 100s, 250s.
Use: Dietary supplement.

FORMULA NO. 3656. (Blue Line) Phenacetin 2½ gr., aspirin 3½ gr., phenolphthalein ¼ gr., caffeine ½ gr./Tab. Bot. 1000s.

FORMULA NO. 3948. (Blue Line) Phenobarbital 16 mg., phenacetin 162 mg., aspirin 227 mg./Tab. Bot. 1000s.

2-FORMYL-1-METHYLPYRIDINIUM CHLORIDE OXIME. Pralidoxime Chloride, U.S.P. XXI.

FORMYL TETRAHYDROPTEROYLGLUTAMIC ACID. Leucovorin Calcium, U.S.P. XXI.

FORTA-FLORA. (Barth's) Whey-lactose 90%, pectin. **Pow.** Jar 1 lb. **Wafers** Bot. 100s.

FORTAGESIC TABLETS. (Winthrop Products) Paracetamol, pentazocine.
Use: Analgesic.

FORTERRA—OBLONG RED TAB. (Panray) Vit. A 5000 I.U., D 1000 I.U., B-1 3 mg., B-2 2.5 mg., B-6 1.5 mg., B-12 2.5 mcg., C 50 mg., niacinamide 20 mg., cal. pantothenate 5 mg., Vit. E 3 I.U., dical. phos 747 mg., ferrous sulf. 45.56 mg., manganese sulf. 4.72 mg., zinc sulf. 3.9 mg., magnesium sulf. 54 mg., potassium sulf. 11.2 mg./Tab. Bot. 100s.
Use: Vitamin, mineral supplement.

FORTE L.I.V. (Foy) Cyanocobalamine 15 mcg. Liver injection equivalent to Vit. B-12 activity 1 mcg., ferrous gluconate 50 mg., B-2 0.75 mg., panthenol 1.25 mg., niacinamide 50 mg., citric acid 8.2 mg., sodium citrate 118 mg./ml. w/procaine HCl 2%. Bot. 30 ml.
Use: Multivitamin supplement.

FORTRAL. (Winthrop Products) Pentazocine as solution and tablets.
Use: Analgesic.

FORTRAMIN. (Thurston) Vit. E 200 I.U., A 6000 I.U., D 600 I.U., B-1 4.5 mg., B-2 4.5 mg., B-6 4.5 mg., B-12 5 mcg., C 2.75 mg., rutin 8 mg., hesperidin complex 10 mg., lemon bioflavonoids 15 mg., d-calcium pantothenate 50 mg., para-aminobenzoic acid 7.5 mg., biotin 10 mg., folic acid 24 mcg., niacinamide 20 mg., desicc. liver 25 mg., Fe 3 mg., Ca 75 mg., P 34 mg., Mn 10 mg., Cu 0.5 mg., Zn 0.5 mg., iodine 0.375 mg., K 500 mg., Mg 5.0 mg./Tab. Bot. 100s, 250s.
Use: Vit. supplement.

• **FOSAZEPAM.** USAN. 7-Chloro-1-dimethylphosphinylmethyl-1,3-dihydro-5-phenyl-2H-1,4-benzodiazepin-2-one.
Use: Hypnotic.

FOSFESTROL. B.A.N. trans-$\alpha\alpha'$-Diethylstilbene-4,4'-diol bis(dihydrogen phosphate).
Use: Treatment of carcinoma of the prostate.

See: Honvan (tetrasodium salt)

• **FOSFOMYCIN.** USAN.
Use: Antibacterial.

• **FOSFONET SODIUM.** USAN.
Use: Antiviral.

• **FOSPIRATE.** USAN.
Use: Anthelmintic.

FOSFREE. (Mission) Calcium lactate 250 mg., calcium gluconate 250 mg., calcium carbonate 300 mg., calcium 175.7 mg., Vit. D-2 150 I.U., Vitamin A acetate 1500 I.U., ferrous gluconate 125 mg. (iron 14.5 mg.), Vitamin B-12 2.0 mcg., C 50 mg., B-6 3.0 mg., B-1 5.0 mg., B-2 2.0 mg., niacinamide (B-3) 10 mg., d-calcium pantothenate (B-5) 1.0 mg./Tab. Bot. 100s.
Use: Prenatal, postpartum or geriatric supplement.

• **FOSTEDIL.** USAN.

FOSTEX CM. (Westwood) Sulfur 2% in a flesh-tinted greasless base. Tube 1 oz.
Use: Acne medication & cover up.

FOSTEX CREAM AND MEDICATED CLEANSER. (Westwood) Sulfur 2%, salicylic acid 2% w/soapless cleansers and wetting agents. **Cream:** tube 4 oz. **Medicated Cleanser:** plastic bot. 5 oz.
Use: Acne skin cleanser.

FOSTEX BPO GEL. (Westwood) Benzyl peroxide 5%. Tube 1.5 oz.
Use: Topical aid for control of acne.

FOSTEX MEDICATED CLEANSING BAR. (Westwood) Sulfur 2%, salicylic acid 2% in base of soapless cleansers and wetting agents. Bar 3.75 oz.
Use: Acne skin cleanser.

FOSTEX 10% BPO CLEANSING BAR. (Westwood) Benzoyl peroxide 10%. Bar 3.75 oz.
Use: Acne skin cleanser.

FOSTRIL. (Westwood) Sulfur 2% in greaseless base. Lot. Tubes 1 oz.
Use: Topical aid for control of acne.

FOTOTAR CREAM. (Elder) Coal tar 1.6% in emollient moisturizing cream base. Tube 3 oz.
Use: Chronic skin disorders.

FOTOTAR STIK. (Elder) Coal tar 5.0% in a hydrophilic wax base. Stick 0.5 oz.
Use: Chronic skin disorders.

FOUR ANTIHISTAMINES. (Wolins) Pyrilamine maleate 6¼ mg., phenyltoloxamine dihydrogen citrate 6¼ mg., prophenpyridamine maleate 6¼ gr./Tab. Bot. 1000s.
Use: Antihistaminic.

FOUR-B. (Pasadena Research) Vit. B-1 100 mg., B-2 10 mg., B-6 50 mg., nicotinamide 100 mg./cc. Vial 30 cc.
Use: Vitamin supplement.

4-WAY COLD TABS. (Bristol-Myers) Aspirin 324 mg., phenylpropanolamine HCl 12.5 mg., Chlorpheniramine maleate 2.0 mg./Tab. Bot. 15s, 36s, 60s.
Use: Analgesic, decongestant, antihistaminic.

4-WAY LONG ACTING NASAL SPRAY. (Bristol-Myers) Oxymetazoline HCl 0.05% in isotonic buffered soln. w/0.005% thimerosal preservative. Spray Bot. 0.5 oz.
Use: Long acting nasal decongestant.

4-WAY NASAL SPRAY. (Bristol-Myers) Phenylephrine HCl 0.5%, naphazoline HCl 0.05%, pyrilamine maleate 0.2% w/buffered isotonic aqueous sol., thimerosal 0.005%.
w/Atomizer 0.5 oz., 1 oz. Mentholated 0.5 oz., 1 oz.
Use: Decongestant/antihistamine.

FOURSALCO. (Jenkins) Salicylic acid ½ gr., sod. bicarbonate 3 gr., mag. salicylate 2 gr., strontium salicylate 2 gr., acetophenetidin ¼ gr. w/methyl salicylate, pancreatin ¹⁄₄₀ gr., diastase ¹⁄₄₀ gr./Tab. Bot. 1000s.
Use: Treatment of rheumatic conditions.

FOVANE. Benzthiazide, B.A.N.

FOWLER'S SOLUTION. Potassium Arsenite Solution (Various Mfr.)

FOXALIN. (Standex) Digitoxin 0.1 mg. w/Sod. carboxymethylcellulose/Cap. Bot. 100s.
Use: Orally; digitalis glycoside for rapid digitalization.

FOXGLOVE.
See: Digitalis (Var. Mfr.)

FRAMYCETIN. B.A.N. An antibiotic produced by Streptomyces decaris.
See: Framygen
Soframycin (sulfate)

FRANODIL. (Winthrop Products) Ephedrine sulfate, theophylline, anhydrous, chlormezanone.
Use: Antiasthmatic.

FRANOL. (Winthrop Products) Theophylline anhydrous, ephedrine sulfate, phenobarbital, thenyldiamine HCl.
Use: Antiasthmatic.

FREAMINE III. (American McGaw) Amino acid 3%, 8.5% or 10%.
Use: Amino acid solution.

FREAMINE HBC. (American McGaw) High branched 6.9% amino acid formulation for hypercatabolic patients.

FREEZONE. (Whitehall) Salicylic acid 13.6%, alcohol 20.5%, ether 64.8% in flexible collodion base. Bot. .13 oz.
Use: Corn Remover.

• **FRENTIZOLE.** USAN.
Use: Immunoregulator.

FRESH. (Pharmacraft) Aluminum chloride and aluminum chlorhydrate complex. **Cream:** Jar ¾ oz., 1.2 oz., **Roll-on:** 1 oz., 1.5 oz.
Use: Deodorant, antiperspirant.

• **FRUCTOSE,** U.S.P. XXI. Inj., U.S.P. XXI. (Abbott) (Cutter) 10% soln. Bot. 1000 ml.
See: Frutabs, Tab. (Pfanstiehl)

• **FRUCTOSE AND SODIUM CHLORIDE INJECTION,** U.S.P. XXI.
Use: Fluid, nutrient and electrolyte replenisher.

FRUIT-SAVER. (Stanlabs) Pow. Bot. 3 oz.

FRUSEMIDE. 4-Chloro-N-furfuryl-5-sulfamoylanthranilic acid. Lasix.

FRUSEMIDE. B.A.N. 4-Chloro-N-furfuryl-5-sulphamoylanthranilic acid. Furosemide (I.N.N.)
Use: Diuretic.
See: Lasix

FRUTABS. (Pfanstiehl) Fructose tablets. 2 Gm. Bot. 100s.
Use: Quick energy source for athletes, workers, etc.

FRUT-PAK. (Eckerd) Vitamin C 250 mg., 500 mg./Tab. Bot. 100s, 200s.
Use: Vitamin C supplement.

FTA-ABS. (Wampole-Zeus) Fluorescent treponemal antibody-absorbed test. Tests 100s.
Use: An *in vitro* diagnostic aid for confirming a positive reagin test for syphillis.

FTA-ABS/DS. (Wampole-Zeus) Fluorescent treponemal antibody absorbed test. Tests 100s.
Use: An *in vitro* diagnostic aid for confirming a positive reagin test for syphilis.

• **FUCHSIN, BASIC,** U.S.P. XXI. Basic Fuchsin is a mixture of rosaniline and pararosaniline HCl. Basic Magenta.
Use: Ingredient in Carbo-Fuchsin Sol.

FUDR. (Roche) Floxuridine. 2-Deoxy-5-fluorouridine. Vial 500 mg. 5 ml.
Use: Management of carcinoma.

FULFIL. (Mead Johnson) Nutritionally complete high calorie formula containing 355 calories/8 fl. oz. representing 40% from fat, 38% from carbohydrates and 22% from protein. Cans 8 oz.
Use: Nutritional supplement.

FUL-GLO. (Barnes-Hind) Fluorescein sod. 0.6%. Box 300 strips.
Use: Opthalmic strips; diagnostic agent.

FULVICIN P/G. (Schering) Griseofulvin ultramicrosize 125 mg., 165 mg., 250 mg., 330 mg./Tab. Bot. 100s.
Use: Antifungal.

FULVICIN-U/F. (Schering) Griseofulvin microsize 250 mg., 500 mg./Tab. Bot. 60s, 250s.
Use: Antifungal.

FUMAGILLIN. B.A.N. A cryst. antibiotic produced during the growth of a strain of Aspergillus fumigatus.

FUMARAL ELIXIR. (Vortech) Alcohol 5%, ferrous sulfate 5 gr./10 ml. Vial 4 oz., gal.
Use: Iron deficiency anemia.

FUMARAL SPANCAP. (Vortech) Iron 330 mg., Vitamin C 200 mg./Cap. Bot. 100s, 1000s.
Use: Iron supplement w/vitamin C.

• **FUMARIC ACID.** N.F. XVI. 2-Butenedioic acid.
Use: Acidifier.

FUMATINIC CAPSULES. (Laser) Ferrous fumarate 275 mg., Vit. C 100 mg., B-12 15 mcg., folic acid 1 mg. /Cap. Bot. 100s, 1000s.
Use: Hypochromic microcytic anemia, nutritional macrocytic anemia, nutritional macrocytic or microcytic anemia of pregnancy, tropical and nontropical sprue.

FUMATRIN-FORTE. (Reid-Provident) Elemental iron 100 mg., Vit. B-12 12 mcg., C 100 mg., B-1 3 mg., desiccated liver 100 mg., folic acid 0.5 mg./Tab. Bot. 60s, 500s.
Use: Hematinic.

FUMERIN. (Laser) Ferrous fumarate 195 mg./Tab. Bot. 100s, 1000s.

Use: Iron deficiency anemia.

FUMERON. (Vitarine) Ferrous fumarate 330 mg., Vit. B-1 5 mg./TR. Cap.
Use: Hematinic.

FUMEX. (CMC) Silver acetate 6 mg., cocarboxylase 0.025 mg., NH₄Cl 25 mg./oz. Bot. 24s.
Use: To break the smoking habit.

FUNDUSCEIN. (CooperVision) Sodium fluorescein 10%. Amp. 5 ml. 12s, 25% Amp. 3 ml. 12s.
Use: Aid in ophthalmic angiography.

FUNGACETIN OINTMENT. (Blair) Triacetin (glyceryl triacetate) 25% in a water-miscible ointment base. Tube 1 oz.
Use: Topically, fungus infections.

■ **FUNGICIDES.**
See: Aftate, Prods. (Plough)
Arcum, Preps. (Arcum)
Asterol
Basic Fuchsin (Var. Mfr.)
Coparaffinate
Desenex, Prods. (Pharmacraft)
Dichlorophene
Nifuroxime (Var. Mfr.)
Nitrofurfuryl Methyl Ether (Var. Mfr.)
Phenylmercuric Preps. (Various Mfr.)
Propionate, Sodium (Various Mfr.)
Propionic Acid (Various Mfr.)
Salicylanilide (Doak)
Undecylenic Acid (Various Mfr.)

• **FUNGIMYCIN.** USAN.
Use: Antifungal

FUNGIZONE CREAM, LOTION, OINT. (Squibb) Amphotericin B 3%, Thimerosal, titanium dioxide. **Lot.** Plastic Sq. Bot. 30 cc. **Cream & Oint.** Tube 20 Gm.
Use: Monilial infections.

FUNGIZONE INTRAVENOUS. (Squibb) Amphotericin B 50 mg., sodium desoxycholate 41 mg., sodium phosphate 25.2 mg./Vial. Lypholized.
Use: Mycotic infections.

FUNGIZONE FOR LABORATORY USE IN TISSUE CULTURE. (Squibb) Amphotericin B 50 mg., sodium desoxycholate 41 mg./vial of 20 cc.
Use: Laboratory.

FUNGOID CREME. (Pedinol) Cetyl pyridinium, triacetin, Cl, chloroxylenol in vanishing cream base. Tube 1 oz.
Use: Topical treatment for fungus, yeast and bacterial infections of the skin.

FUNGOID TINCTURE. (Pedinol) Cetyl pyridinium Cl, triacetin, chloroxylenol, glacial acetic acid, sodium propionate, propionic acid, isopropyl alcohol, benzyl alcohol, acetone, propylene glycol, eucalyptol. Bot. 1 oz., pt.
Use: Treatment of nail fungus, onychomycosis.

FUNGOID SOLUTION. (Pedinol) Cetyl pyradinium Cl, triacetin, chloroxylenol. Bot. 15 cc.
Use: Topical treatment for fungus, yeast, bacterial infections of the skin.

FUN MATES. (Vitarine) Fruit flavored multiple vitamin tablets.
Use: Multivitamin supplement.

FURACIN SOLUBLE DRESSING. (Norwich Eaton) Nitrofurazone 0.2% in a water-soluble, nondrying, ointmentlike base of polyethylene glycols. Jar 135 Gm., 454 Gm., 5 lb. Tube 28 Gm., 56 Gm.
Use: Topical application in surface infections.

FURACIN TOPICAL CREAM. (Norwich Eaton) Furacin 0.2% in a water miscible, self-emulsifying cream w/glycerin, cetyl alcohol, mineral oil, an ethoxylated fatty alcohol, methylparaben, propylparaben and water. Tube 14 Gm. & 28 Gm. Jar 368 Gm.
Use: Topical antibacterial agent in surface infections.

FURADANTIN. (Norwich Eaton) Nitrofurantoin 50 mg., 100 mg./Tab. Bot. 100s, 500s. Unit dose 100s.
Use: Antibacterial for urinary tract infections.

FURADANTIN ORAL SUSPENSION. (Norwich Eaton) Nitrofurantoin. Bot. (5 mg./ml.) 60 ml., 470 ml.
Use: Antibacterial for urinary tract infections.

FURALAN. (Lannett) Nitrofurantoin 50 mg., 100 mg./Tab. Bot. 100s, 500s, 1000s.
Use: Urinary tract antibacterial.

FURALAZINE HYDROCHLORIDE. 3-Amino-6-[2-(5-nitro-2-furyl)vinyl]-as-triazine hydrochloride.
Use: Anti-microbial compound.

FURALTADONE. (±)-5-Morpholinomethyl-3-[(5-nitrofurfurylidene)amino]-2-oxazolidinone.

FURAMIDE 2-FUROATE. Diloxanide, B.A.N.

2(3H)-FURANONE, 3-ETHYLDIHYDRO-4-[(1-METH-YL-1H-IMIDAZOL-5-YL)METHYL]-,MONOHYDROC-HLORIDE, (3S-cis)-. OR MONONITRATE. Pilocarpine Hydrochloride, or Nitrate. U.S.P. XXI.

FURANTOIN. (Vortech) Nitrofurantoin 50 mg./Tab. Bot. 100s, 1000s.
Use: Urinary tract infections.

• **FURAPROFEN.** USAN.
Use: Anti-inflammatory.

• **FURAZOLIDONE,** U.S.P. XXI. 2-Oxazolidone, 3-(((5-nitro-2 furanyl) methyl-ene)amino). 3[(5-Nitrofurfurylidene)-amino]-2-oxazolidinone.
Use: Antimicrobial agent.
See: Furoxone Tab., Susp. (Norwich Eaton)

• **FURAZOLIUM CHLORIDE.** USAN.
Use: Antibacterial.

• **FURAZOLIUM TARTRATE.** USAN.
Use: Antibacterial.

FURAZOSIN HCl. 1-(4-Amino-6, 7-dimethoxy-2-quin-azolinyl)-4-(2-furoyl)piperazine   monohydrochloride. Under study.
Use: Antihypertensive.

FURAZYME. (Jenkins) Nitrofurazone 0.2%. Tube. 1 oz., 1 lb.
Use: Soluble dressing.

FURETHIDINE. 1-(2-Tetrahydrofurfuryloxyethyl)-4-phe-nylpiperidine-4-carboxylic acid ethyl ester.

FURETHIDINE. B.A.N. Ethyl 4-phenyl-1-[2-(tetrahy-drofurfuryloxy)ethyl]piperidine-4-carboxylate.
Use: Narcotic analgesic.

• **FURODAZOLE.** USAN.
Use: Anthelmintic.

FU-RON. (Metro Med) Ferrous fumarate Tabs. Bot. 100s, 1000s.
Use: Hemoglobin regeneration.

FURONATALFA. (Metro Med) Bot. 60s, 1000s.
Use: Prenatal vitamins and minerals.

• **FUROSEMIDE.** U.S.P. XXI. Inj., Tab., U.S.P. XXI. 4-Chloro-N-(furfuryl-)-5-sulfamoylanthranilic acid. Ben-zoic acid, 5-(aminosulfonyl)-4-chloro-2[(2-furanylme-thyl)amino]-. (Abbot) 10 mg./ml. Injection. Single dose syr. 2 ml., 5 ml., 10 ml. Single dose vial 2 ml., 10 ml. 4 ml. partial fill single dose vial.
Use: Diuretic.
See: Lasix, Tab., Inj. (Hoechst-Roussel)

FUROXONE. (Norwich Eaton) Furazolidone. **Tab.** 100 mg./Tab. Bot. 20s, 100s. **Liq.** 50 mg./15 cc. Bot. 60 cc., 473 cc.
Use: Antimicrobial agent.

• **FURSALAN.** USAN. 3, 5-Dibromo-N-(tetrahydrofur-furyl)- salicylamide. Under study.
Use: Germicide.

FUSAFUNGINE. B.A.N. An antibiotic produced by Fusarium lateritium.

• **FUSIDATE SODIUM.** USAN. (I) Sodium 3α, 11α, 16β-trihydroxy-29-nor-8α,9β,13α,14β-dammara-17(-20),24-dien-21-oate 16-acetate. Fucidine (Squibb).
Use: Antibacterial
See: Fucidine (Squibb)

• **FUSIDIC ACID.** USAN. An antibiotic produced by a strain of Fusidium. cis-16β-Acetoxy-3α,-11 α-dihy-droxy-4α,8, 14-trimethyl-18-nor-5α,-8α,9β,13α,14β-cholesta-17(20),24-dien-21-oic acid.
Use: Antibacterial.

FYBRANTA. (Norgine) Miller's bran, calcium phosphate, sugar, corn starch, magnesium stearate. Bot. 100s.
Use: Balance roughage-poor diet.

G

G-1. (Hauck) Acetaminophen 500 mg., butalbital 50 mg., caffeine 40 mg./Cap. Bot. 100s. Unit dose 100s.
Use: Analgesic associated with nervous tension & anxiety.

G-2. (Hauck) Acetaminophen 500 mg., butalbital 50 mg., codeine phosphate 15 mg./Cap. Bot. 100s. Unit dose 100s.
Use: Analgesic.

G-3. (Hauck) Acetaminophen 500 mg., butalbital 50 mg., codeine phosphate 30 mg./Cap. Bot. 100s. Unit dose 100s.
Use: Analgesic.

G-4.
See: Dichlorophene.

G-11. (Givaudan) Hexachlorophene Pow. for mfg.
See: Hexachlorophene, U.S.P. XXI.

G-200. (Bock) Guaifenesin 200 mg./Cap. Bot. 100s, 1000s.
Use: Antitussive and expectorant.

2/G. (Merrell Dow) Guaifenesin 100 mg./5 ml. w/alcohol 3.5%. Bot. 4 oz.
Use: Expectorant

2G/DM. (Merrell Dow) Guaifenesin 100 mg., dextromethorphan HBr 15 mg./5 ml. w/alcohol 5%. Bot. 4 oz.
Use: Expectorant, antitussive.

GACID TAB. (Arcum) Mg trisilicate 500 mg., aluminum hydroxide 250 mg./Tab. Bot. 100s, 1000s.
Use: Antacid.

GALACTOSE INJECTION. (Horton & Converse) Galactose 50% in sterile distilled water. Vial 50 cc., 1s, 12s, 25s.
Use: Diagnostic agent.

GALLAMINE. B.A.N. 1,2,3-Tri-(2-diethylamino-ethoxy)-benzene.
Use: Neuromuscular blocking agent.
See: Flaxedil (Davis & Geck)

• **GALLAMINE TRIETHIODIDE,** U.S.P. XXI. Inj. U.S.P. XXI. [v-Phenenyltris(oxyethylene)] tris[triethylam-monium] Triiodide. Ethanaminium, 2,2′,2″-[1,2,3-benzenetriyltris(oxy)]tris-[N,N,N-triethyl]-,triiodide.
Use: Skeletal muscle relaxant.
See: Flaxedil (Davis & Geck)

• **GALLIUM CITRATE Ga-67 INJECTION,** U.S.P. XXI.
Use: Diagnostic aid (radiopaque medium).

GALLOCHROME.
See: Merbromin (Various Mfr.)

GALLOTANNIC ACID.
See: Tannic Acid, Preps. (Var. Mfr.)

GAMASTAN. (Cutter) Immune serum globulin (human) U.S.P. Vial 2 ml., 10 ml.
Use: Prophylaxis and attenuation of measles, poliomyelitis and viral hepatitis.

• **GAMFEXINE.** USAN. N,N-Dimethyl-γ-phenyl-cyclo-hexanepropylamine.
Use: Antidepressant.

GAMIMUNE. (Cutter) Immune globulin intravenous 5% in 10% maltose sterile 5 plus or minus 1% sol. of human protein stabilized w/0.1 M glycine. Single dose vial 50 or 100 ml.
Use: Immune globulin.

GAMMA BENZENE HEXACHLORIDE. B.A.N.γ-1,2,3,-4,5,6-Hexachlorocyclohexane. Lindane, U.S.P. XXI.
Use: Antiparasitic.
See: Lorexane
Quellada

GAMMAR. (Armour) Immune Serum Globulin, Human U.S.P. Vial 2 ml., 10 ml.

GAMOLENIC ACID. B.A.N. cis, cis, cis-Octadeca-6,9,-12-trienoic acid.
Use: Treatment of hypercholesterolemia.

GAMOPHEN ANTIBACTERIAL SOAP. (Arbrook) Hexachlorophene 2% in soap base. Bars 2 oz., 4 oz.
Use: Bacteriostatic skin cleanser.

GAMOPHEN HAND CLEANSING LEAVES. (Arbrook) 2% hexachlorophene in detergent base. One time use in rectangular leaves. Leaf refills 1000s.
Use: Bacteriostatic skin cleanser.

G.A.M.P.A.K. (Fellows) Gastric mucin 10 gr., aminoacetic acid 4.5 gr., magnesium trisilicate 30 gr., aluminum hydroxide gel 31.21 gr., kaolin colloidal 194.50 gr./oz. Bot. 4 oz., 8 oz.

GAMULIN Rh. (Armour) Rho (D) Immune globulin (Human). Vials, 1 dose, Vial crossmatched material.
Use: Rh negative mothers after delivery of an Rh-positive infant.

G AND W PRODUCTS. (G&W) G and W markets. The following products under their G & W brand name:
Aminophylline Rectal Suppos., 250 mg., 500 mg.
Aspirin Rectal Suppos., 125 mg., 300 mg., 600 mg.
Bisacodyl Suppos., 10 mg.
Glycerin Suppos., Adult and Infant Sizes
Hemorrhoidal Rectal Ointment.
Hemorrhoidal Rectal Suppos., Formula C-116 and Formula C-119.
Hemorrhoidal Rectal Suppos. w/Hydrocortisone Acetate 10 mg. or 25 mg./Suppos.
Vaginal Sulfa Cream.

GANEAKE. (Geneva) Estrogens, Conjugated 0.625 mg., 1.25 mg., 2.5 mg./Tab. Bot. 100s, 1000s.

■ **GANGLIONIC BLOCKING AGENTS.**
See: Arfonad, Amp. (Roche)
Dibenzyline HCl, Cap. (SmithKline)
Hexamethonium Chloride & Bromide (Various Mfr.)
Hydergine, Amp., Tab. (Sandoz)
Inversine, Tab. (Merck Sharp & Dohme)
Priscoline HCl, Tab., Vial (Ciba)
Regitine, Amp., Tab. (Ciba)

GANPHEN EXPECTORANT W/CODEINE. (Reid-Provi-dent) Promethazine HCl 5 mg., codeine phos. 10 mg., fl. ext. ipecac 0.17 min., potassium guaiacolsulfonate 44 mg., citric acid (anhydrous) 60 mg., sodium citrate 197 mg., alcohol 7%/5 cc. Bot. pt.

GANTANOL. (Roche) Sulfamethoxazole **Tab.:** 0.5 Gm./Tab. Bot. 100s, 500s. Tel-E-Dose 100s. **Susp.** (10%) 0.5 Gm./Tsp. Cherry flavored Bot. 1 pt.
Use: Antibacterial
W/Phenazopyridine.
See: Azo Gantanol, Tabs. (Roche) 100s, 500s.

GANTANOL DS. (Roche) Sulfamethoxazole 1 Gm./Tab. Bot. 100s. Tel-E-Dose 100s.
Use: Antibacterial.

GANTREX. (Coastal) Sulfisoxazole 500 mg./Tab. Bot. 100s, 1000s.

GANTRISIN. (Roche) Sulfisoxazole. **Ophth. Oint.** w/white petrolatum, mineral oil and phenylmercuric nitrate 1:50,000. (4%) Tube ⅛ oz. **Ophth. Sol.** phenylmercuric nitrate 1:100,000 added as preservative. (40 mg./ml.) Bot. w/dropper ½ oz. **Tab.:** (0.5 Gm.) Bot. 100s, 500s, 1000s. Drum 5000s. Prescription Pak 100s. Tel-E-Dose 100s (10 × 10). **Amp.:** (5 ml.) containing 2 Gm. Gantrisin, in ready-to-use solution in the form of Gantrisin diola-mine 10s.
Use: Antibacterial, sulfonamide therapy.
W/Phenylazo-diamino-pyridine HCl.
See: Azo Gantrisin, Tab. (Roche)

GANTRISIN, AZO.
See: Azo Gantrisin, Tab. (Roche)

GANTRISIN, LIPO. (Roche) Acetyl Sulfisoxazole.
Use: Sulfonamide therapy.

See: Lipo Gantrisin, Susp. (Roche)
GANTRISIN DIETHANOLAMINE OPHTHALMIC SOLUTION & OINTMENT. (Roche) Both Gantrisin ophthalmic oint. & sol. are stable antibacterial prep. containing 4% Gantrisin in the form of Gantrisin diethanolamine. Ophth. Oint. Tube ⅛ oz.; Sol. Bot. ½ oz.
Use: Antibacterial, sulfonamide therapy.
GANTRISIN DIOLAMINE. (Roche) Sulfisoxazole diolamine.
Use: Sulfonamide therapy.
GANTRISIN PEDIATRIC SUSPENSION. (Roche). Acetyl Sulfisoxazole 0.5 Gm./5 ml. Bot. 4 oz., pt.
Use: Sulfonamide therapy.
GANTRISIN SYRUP. (Roche) Acetyl Sulfisoxazole 0.5 Gm./5 ml. Bot. pt.
Use: Sulfonamide therapy.
GANTRISIN TEL-E-DOSE. (Roche) Sulfisoxazole 0.5 Gm./Tab. Pkg. 100s (10 strips of 10).
GARAMYCIN. (Schering) **Cream:** Gentamicin sulfate 1.7 mg. (equiv. to gentamicin base 1 mg.). Methylparaben 1 mg. and butylparaben 4 mg. as preservatives, stearic acid, propylene glycol monostearate, isopropyl myristate, propylene glycol, polysorbate 40, sorbitol sol., and water/Gm. Tube 15 Gm. **Oint.** Gentamicin sulfate 1.7 mg. (equiv. to gentamicin base 1 mg.), methylparaben 0.5 mg., propylparaben 0.1 mg. in petrolatum base/Gm. Tube, 15 Gm.
Use: Topical dermatologic antibiotic.
GARAMYCIN INJECTABLE. (Schering) Gentamicin sulfate equiv. to 40 mg. gentamicin base, methylparaben 1.8 mg., propylparaben 0.2 mg., as preservatives, sod. bisulfite 3.2 mg., disodium edetate 0.1 mg./ml. Vials 2 ml. (80 mg.), 20 ml. (800 mg.); Syringes 1.5 ml. (60 mg.), 2.0 ml. (80 mg.); **Pediatric Inj.;** 10 mg./ml. w/methylparaben 1.3 mg., propylparaben 0.2 mg., sod. bisulfite 3.2 mg., edetate disodium 0.1 mg./ml. Vials 2 ml. (20 mg.)
Use: Parenteral antibiotic.
GARAMYCIN INTRATHECAL INJECTION. (Schering) Gentamicin sulfate equiv. to 2 mg./ml. gentamicin base, 8.5 mg. Na Cl/ml: Amp. 2 ml. Box 25s.
Use: Antibiotic.
GARAMYCIN I.V. PIGGYBACK. (Schering) Gentamicin sulfate equivalent to 1 mg. gentamicin base, 8.9 mg. sodium Cl, no preservatives. 60 mg., 80 mg. Bot. 100 ml.
Use: Parenteral antibiotic.
GARAMYCIN OPHTHALMIC OINTMENT-STERILE. (Schering) Gentamicin sulfate equiv. to 3 mg., gentamicin, methylparaben & propylparaben as preservatives/cc. in petrolatum base. Tube ⅛ oz.
Use: Antibiotic.
GARAMYCIN OPHTHALMIC SOLUTION, STERILE. (Schering) Gentamicin sulfate equiv. to 3 mg., gentamicin, disodium phosphate, monosodium phosphate, sodium chloride & benzalkonium as preservative/ml. Plastic dropper bot. 5 ml. Sterile.
Use: Antibiotic.
GARDAC. (Vitarine) Belladonna alkaloids 0.13 mg.,

phenylpropanolamine HCl 50 mg., chlorpheniramine maleate 1 mg., pheniramine maleate 12.5 mg./S.R. Cap.
Use: Relief of nasal congestion due to common cold.
GARDAN. (Winthrop Products) Dipyrone.
Use: Analgesic, antipyretic, anti-inflammatory.
GARDENAL.
See: Phenobarbital. (Various Mfr.)
■ **GARDINOL TYPE DETERGENTS.** Aurinol, Cyclopon, Dreft, Drene, Duponol, Lissapol, Maprofix, Modinal, Orvus, Sandopan, Sadipan.
Use: Detergents.
GARDOL. Sod. Lauroyl Sarcosinate.
GARFIELD HEADACHE POWDERS. (Medtech) Acetaminophen 5 gr. w/caffeine. Bot. 72s.
Use: Relief of simple headache.
GARFIELDS TEA. (Last) Senna leaf powder 68.3%. Bot. 2 oz.
Use: Stimulant laxative.
GARITABS. (Blue Cross) Iron 50 mg., B-1 5 mg., B-2 5 mg., C 75 mg., niacinamide 30 mg., B-5 2 mg., B-6 0.5 mg., B-12 3 mcg. Bot. 1000s.
GARI-TONIC HEMATINIC. (Blue Cross) B-1 5 mg., niacinamide 100 mg., B-2 5 mg., pantothenic acid 4 mg., B-6 1 mg., B-12 6 mcg., choline bitartrate 100 mg., iron 100 mg./30 ml. Bot. 16 oz.
Use: Hematinic.
GARLIC. Allium.
Use: Intestinal antispasmodic.
See: Allimin, Tab. (Mosso)
GARLIC CONCENTRATE.
W/Parsley Concentrate.
See: Allimin, Tab. (Mosso)
GARLIC OIL.
See: Natural Garlic Oil, Cap. (Spirt)
GARLIC OIL CAPSULES. (Kirkman) Bot. 100s.
GARRATHION. Carbophenothion, B.A.N.
GARTRONE. (Eric, Kirk & Gary) Veratrum Viride Alk. 250 mg./30 cc. Vials.
Use: I.M.
GAS-EZE. (Edward J. Moore) Aluminum hydroxide, magnesium hydroxide, calcium carbonate, glycine, mannitol, oil peppermint/Tab. Bot. 50s, Pak 36s.
Use: Indigestion; gas pain.
GASTRIC MUCIN.
(Wilson)—Gran. 8 oz. & 1 lb.
Use: Orally, ulcers.
W/Mg glycinate, Al hydroxide gel.
See: Mucogel, Tab. (Inwood)
W/Magnesium trisilicate, magnesium hydroxide, aluminum hydroxide.
See: Mucotin, Tab. (Warner-Chilcott)
GASTROGRAFIN. (Squibb) Diatrizoate methyl-glucamine 66%. Sodium Diatrizoate 10%. Radiopaque medium. Bot. 4 fl. oz.
Use: Roentgenographic study of the gastrointestinal tract.
GASTRON. (Winthrop Products) Pancreatin.
Use: Pancreatic deficiency, dyspepsia.
GASTROVIST. (Berlex) Diatrizoate meglumine 660

mg., diatrizoate sodium 100 mg./ml. Bot. 100 ml.
Use: Oral radiopaque medium for radiographic
examination of the GI tract.

GAS-X. (Creighton) Simethicone 80 mg./Tab. Pkg.
12s, 30s.
Use: Antiflatulent.

• **GAUZE, ABSORBENT,** U.S.P. XXI.
Use: Surgical aid.

• **GAUZE, PETROLATUM,** U.S.P. XXI.
Use: Surgical aid.

GAVISCON. (Marion) Aluminum hydroxide dried gel
80 mg., magnesium trisilicate 20 mg./Tab. Bot.
100s.Box of 30s.
Use: Antacid.

GAVISCON-2. (Marion) Aluminum hydroxide gel 160
mg., magnesium trisilicate 40 mg./Tab. Box of 48.
Use: Antacid.

GAVISCON LIQUID. (Marion) Aluminum hydroxide 95
mg., magnesium carbonate 412 mg./15 ml. Bot. 2
oz, 6 oz., 12 oz.
Use: Antacid.

GAYSAL-S. (Geriatric) Sodium salicylate 300 mg.,
acetaminophen 180 mg., aluminum hydroxide gel
60 mg./Tab. Bot. 100s, 1000s.
Use: Antiarthritic.

G.B.H. LOTION. (Century) Gamma benzene
hexachloride 1%. Bot. 2 oz., pt., gal.
Use: Antaparasitic.

G.B.-PREP EMULSION. (Gray) Corn oil in 50% aqueous
dispersion. Bot. 2 oz.
Use: Oral cholecystokinetic.

G.B.S. (O'Neal, Jones & Feldman) Dehydrocholic acid
125 mg., phenobarbital 8 mg., homatropine methylbromide 2-5 mg./Tab.
Use: Biliary stasis & insufficiency.

GEBAUER'S 114. (Gebauer)
Dichlorotetraflouroethane 100%. Can 227 Gm.
Use: Topical anesthesia for minor surgical
procedures.

GEBAUER ETHYL CHLORIDE. (Gebauer) Ethyl
chloride. Bot. 106 Gm. Metal tube 100 Gm.
Use: Topical anesthetic.

GEE-GEE. (Bowman) Guaifenesin 200 mg./Tab. Bot.
100s, 1000s
Use: Expectorant.

GEFARNATE. B.A.N. A mixture of steroisomers of
3,7-dimethylocta-2,6-dienyl 5,9,13-trimethyl-tet-
radeca-4,8,12-trienoate. Geranyl farnesylacetate.
Gefarnil.
Use: Treatment of peptic ulcer.

GEL II 1.23% APF TOPICAL GEL. (CooperCare)
Acidulated phosphate fluoride 1.23%. Bot. 16 oz.
Use: Topical application to aid in prevention of
dental caries.

GEL II HOME TREATMENT. (CooperCare) Acidulated
phosphate fluoride 0.5%. Tube 2 oz.
Use: Topical application to aid in prevention of
dental caries.

GEL-A-CAP. (Kenyon) Gelatin 10 gr./Cap. Bot. 100s,
1000s.

GELADINE. (Barth's) Gelatin, protein, Vit. D/Cap. Bot.
100s, 500s.

GELAMAL. (Halsey) Magnesium-aluminum hydroxide
gel. Bot. 12 oz.
Use: Antacid.

• **GELATIN,** N.F. XVI.
Use: Pharmaceutic aid.

• **GELATIN FILM, ABSORBABLE,** U.S.P. XXI.
Use: Local hemostatic.
See: Gelfilm (Upjohn)

• **GELATIN SPONGE, ABSORBABLE,** U.S.P. XXI.
Use: Local hemostatic.
See: Gelfoam, Paks (Upjohn)

GELATIN, ZINC.
See: Zinc gelatin. (Var. Mfr.)

GEL-CLEAN. (Barnes-Hind) Gel formulated with nonionic surfactant. Tube 30 Gm.
Use: Hard contact lens cleaner.

GELFILM. (Upjohn) Sterile, nonantigenic, absorbable
gelatin film. Env. 1s. 100 mm. × 125 mm. Also
available as Ophth. Sterile 25 × 50 mm. Box 6s.
Use: Aid in surgical closure.

GELFOAM. (Upjohn)
Sterile Sponges:
Size 12-3mm. 20 × 60 mm. (12 sq. cm) × 3 mm.
Boxes of 4 sponges in ind. envelopes.
Size 12–7 mm. 20 × 60 mm. (12 sq. cm.) × 7
mm.
Boxes of 12 sponges in ind. envelopes, and jars
of 4 sponges.
Size 50. 62.5 × 80 mm. (50 sq. cm.) × 10 mm.
Boxes of 4 sponges in ind. envelopes.
Size 100. 80 × 125 mm. (100 sq. cm.) × 10 mm.
Boxes of 6 sponges in ind. envelopes.
Size 200. 80 × 250 mm. (200 sq. cm.) × 10 mm.
Boxes of 6 sponges in ind. envelopes.
Compressed size 100 (intended primarily for
application in the dry state). 80 × 125 mm.
Boxes of 6 sponges in ind. envelopes.
Packs:
Packs size 2 cm. (designed particularly for nasal
packing). 2 × 40 cm. Single jar. (packing
cavities).
Size 6 cm. 6 × 40 cm. Boxes of 6 sponges in ind.
envelopes.
Use: Hemostasis in neurosurgery, otolaryngology,
bone surgery, malignancy, dental surgery, and
abdominal surgery.

GELFOAM COMPRESSED. (Upjohn) Size 100 (12.5
cm. × 8 cm.) Box 6s.
Use: Topically, hemostatic.

GELFOAM DENTAL PACK. (Upjohn) Size 4, 20 mm.
× 20 mm. × 7 mm. Jar 15 sponges. Size 2, 10
mm. × 20 mm. (2 sq. cm.) × 7 mm. Jars 15
sponges.
Use: Control bleeding.

GELFOAM POWDER. (Upjohn) Sterile Jar 1 Gm.
Use: Hemostatic.

GELFOAM PROSTATECTOMY CONES. (Upjohn)
Prostatectomy cones (for use with Foley
catheter). 13 cm. in diameter & 18 cm. in diameter.
Box 6s.
Use: Hemostatic for use in surgical procedures.

GEL JET GELATIN CAPSULES. (Kirkman) Bot. 100s, 250s.

GEL-KAM. (Scherer) Water-free gel 0.4% stannous fluoride. Cinnamon, grape, red berry, mint, non-flavored and mixed fruit flavors. Bot. w/applicator tip 2.3 oz., 4.3 oz., 7 oz.
Use: Prevention of decalcification and dental caries.

GELOCAST. (Beiersdorf) Zinc oxide, calamine and gelatin bandage. 10 yd. × 4 in. & 10 yd. × 3 in. 12s.
Use: Unna's cast dressing.

GELOX LIQUID. (Xttrium) Mg. hydroxide 90 mg., aluminum hydroxide-magnesium carbonate co-dried gel 1.5 Gm./5 cc. Bot. 12 oz.

GELOX TABLETS. (Xttrium) Aluminum hydroxide-magnesium carbonate co-dried gel 400 mg./Tab. Bot. 100s, 1000s.

GELPIRIN TABLETS. (Schuemann) Aspirin 240 mg., acetaminophen 125 mg., caffeine 32 mg., gelsinate 50 mg./Tab. Bot. 100s, 1000s. Packet 2s. Use: Analgesic.

GELSAF SUPER. (Robinson) Safflower oil 750 mg./Cap. Bot. 100s, 1000s. Pkg. 30s. Bulk pkg. 5000s.

GELSAF SUPER W/B-6. (Robinson) Safflower oil 912 mg., B-6 0.5 mg./Cap. or Safflower oil 1150 mg., B-6 3 mg./Cap. Bot. 100s, 250s, 1000s.

GELSEMIUM. (Various Mfr.) Pkg. 1 oz.
Use: For neuralgia.
W/APC.
See: APC Combinations.

GELSEMIUM W/COMBINATIONS.
See: Briacel, Tab. (Briar)
    Bricor, Tab. (Briar)
    Cystitol, Tab. (Briar)
    Lanased, Tab. (Lannett)
    Ricor, Tab. (Vortech)
    Sodadide, Tab. (Scrip)
    UB, Tab. (Scrip)
    Urisan-P, Tab. (Sandia)
    Uriseptic w/Gelsemium, Tab. (Spencer-Mead)
    Uritol, Tab. (Kenyon)
    Urothyn Improved, Tab. (Reid-Provident)
    Urseptic, Tab. (Century)
    U-Tract, Tab. (Bowman)

GELSODYNE. (Blue Line) Aspirin 3½ gr., acetophenetidin 2½ gr., caffeine ½ gr./Tab. Bot. 100s, 1000s.
Use: Analgesic & antipyretic.

GELUMAC CHEWABLE. (Vitarine) Magnesium trisilicate 7.5 gr., dried aluminum hydroxide gel. 4 gr./Tab.
Use: Antiacid.

GELUSIL. (Parke-Davis) Magnesium hydroxide 200 mg., aluminum hydroxide 200 mg., simethicone 25 mg./5 ml. or Tab. **Susp.** Bot. 6 oz., 12 oz. **Tab.** Bot. 165s. Strips in boxes 50s, 100s, 1000s.
Use: Gastric hyperacidity, peptic ulcer, flatulence, hiatal hernia.

GELUSIL II. (Parke-Davis) Magnesium hydroxide 400 mg., aluminum hydroxide 400 mg., simethicone 30

mg./5 ml. or Tab. **Liq.:** Bot. 12 oz. **Tab.:** Strips of 80s.
Use: Double strength antacid for heartburn, acid indigestion, peptic ulcers, hiatal hernia, peptic esophagitis.

GELUSIL M. (Parke-Davis) Magnesium hydroxide 200 mg., aluminum hydroxide 300 mg., simethicone 25 mg./5 ml. or Tab. **Liq.:** Bot. 12 oz. **Tabs.:** Strips in boxes of 100.
Use: Peptic ulcer, heartburn, flatulence, gastric hyperacidity, hiatal hernia.

• **GEMCADIOL.** USAN.
Use: Antihyperlipoproteinemic.

• **GEMEPROST.** USAN.
Use: Prostaglandin.

• **GEMFIBROZIL,** U.S.P. XXI. Cap. U.S.P. XXI. 2,2-Di-methyl-5-(2,5-xyly-loxy) valeric acid.
Use: Treatment of hypercholesterolemia.
See: Lopid, Cap. (Parke-Davis)

GEMNISYN. (Rorer) Aspirin 325 mg., acetaminophen 325 mg./Tab. Bot. 100s.
Use: Analgesic, antipyretic, anti-inflammatory.

GEMONIL. (Abbott) Metharbital 100 mg./Tab. Bot. 100s.
Use: Grand mal, petit mal and myoclonic epilepsy & in mixed types of seizures.

GENAPAX. (Key) Gentian violet 5 mg./sanitary-type tampon. Box 12s.
Use: Treatment of monilial and non-specific vaginitis.

GENATROPINE HCl. Atropine-N-oxide HCl. Aminoxy-tropine Tropate HCl.
See: X-tro, Cap. (Xttrium)

GENERICACE. (Fellows) Docusate sodium 100 mg., casanthranol 30 mg./Cap. Bot. 100s, 1000s.

GENESIS B-hCG. (Wampole) Monoclonal antibody radi-oimmunoassay for the qualitative detection and quantitative determination of B-hCG/hCG in serum and qualitative detection of B-hCG/hCG in urine. Kits 125s.
Use: Aid in the diagnosis of pregnancy.

GENOPHYLLIN.
See: Aminophylline (Various Mfr.)

GENOPTIC OPHTHALMIC SOLUTION. (Allergan) Gentamicin sulfate equivalent to 3.0 mg. gentamicin/ml. w/disodium phosphate, monosodium phosphate, sodium Cl., benzalkonium Cl. Bot. 5 ml.
Use: Ocular antibiotic.

GENOPTIC S.O.P. STERILE OPHTHALMIC OINTMENT. (Allergan) Gentamicin sulfate equivalent to 3.0 mg. gentamicin/Gm. w/white petrolatum, methyl-paraben, propylparaben. Tube 3.5 Gm.
Use: Ocular antibiotic.

GENOSCOPOLAMINE. (CMC) Scopolamine aminoxide HBr, scopolamine-N-oxide HBr, epox-yaminoxytropine tropate HBr. Pellets 0.5 mg. Box 60s.
Use: Orally, hypnotic & sedative.
See: Scopodex, Pellet. (CMC)

GENSALATE SODIUM. Sod. gentisate. (Sod. salt of 2,5-dihydroxybenzoic acid)

Use: Analgesic & antipyretic.
GENTAMICIN, B.A.N. An antibiotic produced by *Micromonospora purpurea.*
See: Cidomycin
Garamycin
Genticin (sulfate).
• **GENTAMICIN SULFATE,** U.S.P. XXI. Cream, Oint., Inj., Ophth. Oint., Ophth. Soln., Sterile, U.S.P. XXI. (Schering) Produced by *Micromonospora purpurea.*
Use: Antibacterial.
See: Apogen, Inj. (Beecham Labs)
Garamycin, Prep. (Schering)
Genoptic, Prep. (Allergan)
• **GENTIAN VIOLET,** U.S.P. XXI. Topical Soln., Cream, U.S.P. XXI. Methylrosaniline chloride.
Bismuth Violet.
Use: Topical anti-infective.
See: Genapax, tampon. (Key)
GVS, Vag. cream & inserts. (Savage)
W/Surfactants.
See: Hyva, Vag. Tab. (Holland-Rantos)
GENTISATE SODIUM. 5-Hydroxysalicylate sod., 2,5-Dihydroxy benzoate sodium
GENTLAX-B GRANULES. (Blair) Standardized senna concentrate w/guar gum. 1 Can 6 oz.
Use: Laxative.
GENTLAX S TABLETS. (Blair) Standardized senna concentrate, docusate sodium. Bot. 30s, 60s.
Use: Treatment of constipation.
GENTLE SHAMPOO. (Ulmer) Bot. 8 oz., gal.
Use: Mild, neutral shampoo.
GENTRAN. (Travenol) Dextran-75 6%, Sod. chloride 0.9%, Bot. 500 ml; in 10% Travert (Invert sugar) 500 ml. Dextran-40 10% in saline Bot. 500 ml. Dextran-40 10% w/Dextrose 10% Bot. 500 ml.
Use: Plasma volume expander.
GENTZ RECTAL WIPES. (Roxane) Pramoxine HCl 1%, alcloxa 0.2%, cetylpyridinium chloride 0.05%, hamamelis water (nonalcoholic) 50%. Box 7s, 20s, 100s individually wrapped disposable wipes. Dispenser 50s. Jelly, Tubes—single dose, 12s.
Use: Anal/perianal itching and discomfort.
GENUINE BAYER ASPIRIN. (Glenbrook) Aspirin 325 mg./Tab. film coated. Bot. 24s, 50s, 200s, 300s, 12s.
Use: Analgesic, antipyretic, anti-inflammatory, antiplatelet.
GEOCILLIN. (Roerig) Carbenicillin indanyl sodium 382 mg./Tab. Bot. 100s. Unit Dose 100s.
Use: Antibiotic.
GEOPEN. (Roerig) Carbenicillin Disodium 1 Gm., 2 Gm., 5 Gm./Vial; 2 Gm., 5 Gm. and 10 Gm. Piggyback Vial; 30 Gm. Bulk Pharmacy Pack for I.V. use.
Use: Antibiotic for susceptible anaerobes & gram negative aerobes.
GERA-B. (Towne) Vit. A palmitate 7,500 I.U., D 400 I.U., B-1 18 mg., B-2 9 mg., B-6 1 mg., B-12 5 mcg., C 75 mg., niacinamide 50 mg., Ca pantothenate 5 mg., E 5 I.U., choline bitartrate 100 mg., inositol 100 mg., biotin 25 mcg., desic. liver 100 mg., iron 10 mg., pancreatin 500 mg./Captab. Bot. 100s.

GERALIX LIQUID. (Vortech) Vit. B-1 10 mg., B-2 5 mg., B-6 2 mg., choline bitartrate 100 mg., inositol 100 mg., Ca glycerophosphate 100 mg., Mn 1 mg., Mg 1 mg., Zn 1 mg., alcohol 15%/45 cc. Bot. 6 oz., gal.
Use: Dietary supplement.
GERAVITE. (Hauck) Lysine monohydrochloride 150 mg., B-1 1 mg., B-2 1.2 mg., niacinamide 100 mg., B-12 10 mcg./15 ml. w/alcohol 15%. Bot. 16 oz., gal.
Use: Stimulant, antidepressant, tonic.
GERI-ALL-D. (Barth's) Vit. A 10,000 I.U., D 400 I.U., B-1 7 mg., B-2 14 mg., C 200 mg., niacin 4.17 mg., B-12 25 mcg., E 50 I.U., B-6 0.35 mg., pantothenic acid 0.63 mg., plus trace minerals and other factors. 2 Cap. Bot. 1 mo., 3 mo., and 6 mo. supply of Geri-All regular and Geri-All-D.
Use: Vitamin, mineral therapy.
GERIAMIC. (Vortech) Ferrous sulfate 50 mg., B-12 3 mcg., B-1 5 mg., B-2 5 mg., B-6 0.5 mg., niacinamide 30 mg., Ca pantothenate 2 mg., C 75 mg./Tab. 100s.
Use: Vitamin.
GERIATRAZOLE. (Kenyon) Vit. B-12 50 mg., B-2 2 mg., liver-painless 2 mcg., dl-methionine 10 mg., inositol 20 mg., d-panthenol 20 mg., B-1 20 mg., B-6 5 mg., niacinamide 75 mg., pentylenetetrazole 10 mg./cc. Vial 30 cc.
Use: Vitamin (geriatric).
GERIATRIC ELIXIR. (CMC) Methamphetamine HCl 1 mg. Vit. B-1, B-2, B-6, B-12, niacinamide, Ca pantothenate choline, inositol, Fe, Cu, Ca, P/15 cc., alcohol 12% in sherry wine flavored base. Bot. Pt., Gal.
Use: CNS stimulant, vitamin therapy (geriatric).
GERIATRIC MULTIVITAMIN. (Zenith) Iron 50 mg., Vit. B-1 5 mg., B-2 5 mg., C 75 mg., niacinamide 30 mg., Ca pantothenate 2 mg., B-6 0.5 mg., B-12 3 mcg., inositol 20 mg., methionine 25 mg., choline bitartrate 25 mg., debittered brewers dried yeast 50 mg./Tab. Bot. 100s.
Use: Vitamin, mineral therapy (geriatric).
GERIATROPLEX. (Morton) Cyanocobalamin 30 mcg., liver inj. 0.1 cc. B-12 activity 2 mcg., ferrous gluconate 50 mg., B-2 1.5 mg., Ca pantothenate 2.5 mg., niacinamide 100 mg., citric acid 16.4 mg., sod. citrate 23.6 mg./2 cc. Vial 30 cc.
Use: Geriatric.
GERIBOM. (Bowman) Vit. A 10,000 I.U., D 400 I.U., B-1 5 mg. B-2 2.5 mg., B-6 1 mg., B-12 2 mcg., C 75 mg., niacinamide 40 mg., Ca pantothenate 4 mg., E 2 I.U., dicalcium phosphate anhydrous 260 mg., choline bitartrate 31.4 mg., inositol 15 mg., ferrous sulfate 102 mg., manganese sulfate dried 1.573 mg., potassium sulfate 4.458 mg., zinc sulfate dried 1.388 mg., magnesium sulfate dried 21.583 mg./Cap. Bot. 100s, 500s, 1000s.
GERI-BON. (Inwood) Vit. B-1 2 mg., B-2 2 mg., C 75 mg., niacinamide 30 mg., Ca pantothenate 2 mg., B-6 0.5 mg., B-12 3 mcg., inositol 20 mg., methionine 25 mg., choline bitartrate 25 mg., iron 50 mg., debittered brewer's yeast 50 mg./Tab. Bot. 100s.
GERIDEN. (Kenyon) Methyltestosterone 2 mg., ethinyl

estradiol 0.01 mg., rutin 10 mg., Vit. C 30 mg., B-12 2 mcg., A 5000 I.U., D 500 I.U., E 2 I.U., Ca. pantothenate 3 mg., B-1 2.5 mg., B-6 0.5 mg., niacinamide 15 mg., Fe 15 mg., Cu 0.2 mg., Mn 1 mg., Mg 5 mg., K 2 mg., choline bitartrate 40 mg., PABA 10 mg., inositol 20 mg./Cap. Bot. 100s, 1000s.

GERI-DERM. (Barth's) Vit. A 400,000 I.U., D 40,000 I.U., E 200 I.U., panthenol 800 mg./4 oz. Jar 4 oz.
Use: Skin supplement.

GERIFORT PLUS. (A.P.C.) Vit. A 10,000 I.U., B-1 5 mg., B-2 6 mg., B-6 2 mg., C 75 mg., Vit. D-2 1,000 I.U., niacinamide 60 mg., Fe 10 mg., Ca 115 mg., P 83 mg., iodine 0.1 mg., Ca pantothenate 10 mg., d-alpha tocopheryl acid succinate 3 I.U., cobalamin conc. 3 mcg., choline bitartrate 70 mg., inositol 35 mg., biotin 15 mcg., Cn 0.2 mg., Mg 2 mg., Mn 0.5 mg., potassium 0.15 mg./Amcap. Bot. 100s.

GERIGARD. (Eckerd) Vit. B-1, B-2, B-6, B-12, niacinamide, Ca pantothenate, biotin, Vit. A, D, C & E, calcium, phosphorus, iron, iodine, Cu, Mg, Mn, Zn./Cap. Bot. 60s, 150s.

GERIJEN IMPROVED. (Jenkins) Testosterone 10 mg., estrone 1 mg., cyanocobalamin 50 mcg., niacinamide 50 mg., inositol 5 mg., methionine 5 mg., choline chloride 5 mg./cc., pectin 0.25%. Vial 10 cc.

GERILETS. (Abbott) Vit. A 5000 I.U., D 400 I.U., E 45 I.U., C 90 mg., folic acid 0.4 mg., B-1 2.25 mg., B-2 2.6 mg., niacin 30 mg., B-6 3 mg., B-12 9 mcg., biotin 0.45 mg., pantothenic acid 15 mg., Fe 27 mg./Tab. Bot. 100s.
Use: Vitamin, iron supplement (geriatric).

GERILIQUID. (Key) Niacin 75 mg., glycine 750 mg., tsp. (5 ml.) in sherry wine base w/alcohol 5%. Bot. 16 oz.
Use: Poor peripheral circulation.

GERILITE ELIXIR. (Vitarine) Vit. B-1 5 mg., B-2 5 mg., B-6 1 mg., B-12 3 mcg., panthenol 4 mg., niacinamide 100 mg., iron 100 mg., choline bitartrate 100 mg., dl-methionine 100 mg./Fl. Oz. Bot. 12 oz.
Use: Nutritional fortifier.

GERILITE TAB. (Vitarine) Vit. B-1 5 mg., B-2 5 mg., B-6 0.5 mg., B-12 3 mcg., C 75 mg., niacinamide 30 mg., Ca pantothenate 2 mg., iron 50 mg./Tab. Bot. 100s, 250s.
Use: Dietary supplement.

GERIMED. (Fielding) Vitamin & minerals. Bot. 60s.
Use: Dietary supplement.

GERINEED. (Hanlon) Vit. A 5000 I.U., B-1 20 mg., B-2 5 mg., niacinamide 20 mg., B-6 0.5 mg., Ca pantothenate 5 mg., B-12 5 mcg., rutin 25 mg., Vit. C 50 mg., Vit. E 10 I.U., choline 50 mg., inositol 50 mg., Ca lactate 1.64 mg., Fe sulfate 10 mg., Cu 1 mg., iodine 0.5 mg., Mn & Mg sulfate 1 mg., pot. sulfate 5 mg., Zn sulfate 0.5 mg./Cap. Bot. 100s.

GERIPAN. (Image) Bot. 100s.
Use: Vitamin supplement.

GERI-PEN ELIXIR. (Fellows) Pentylenetetrazol 100 mg., nicotinic acid 50 mg., alcohol 5%/5 cc. Bot. pt., gal.

GERI-PEN TABLETS. (Fellows) Pentylenetetrazol 100 mg., nicotinic acid 50 mg./Tab. Bot. 100s, 1000s.

GERIPLEX. (Parke-Davis) Vit. A 5000 I.U., B-1 5 mg., B-2 5 mg., B-12 2 mcg., nicotinamide 15 mg., Vit. C 50 mg., choline dihydrogen citrate 20 mg., Vit. E 5 I.U., taka-distase 2½ gr., ferrous sulfate 30 mg., copper sulfate 4 mg., Mang. sulfate 4 mg., zinc sulfate 2 mg., dicalcium phosphate (anhydrous) 200 mg./Kapseal Bot. 100s, 500s.
Use: Vitamin-mineral combination.

GERIPLEX-FS. (Parke-Davis) Same as Geriplex, plus docusate sodium 100 mg./Kapseal Bot. 100s.

GERIPLEX-FS LIQUID. (Parke-Davis) Vit. B-1 1.2 mg., B-2 1.7 mg., B-6 1 mg., B-12 5 mcg., niacinamide 15 mg., iron 15 mg., pluronic F-68 200 mg./30 ml., alcohol 18%. Bot. 1 pt.

GERI-PLUS. (Approved) Vit. A 12,500 I.U., D 1200 I.U., B-1 15 mg., B-2 10 mg., C 75 mg., niacinamide 30 mg., Ca pantothenate 2 mg., B-6 0.5 mg., E 5 I.U., Brewer's yeast 10 mg., B-12 15 mcg., iron 11.58 mg., desiccated liver 15 mg., choline bitartrate 30 mg., inositol 30 mg., Ca 59 mg., Phos. 45 mg., Zn 0.68 mg., Fr. dicalcium phos. 200 mg., Mn 1.11, Mg. 1 mg., enzymatic factors and amino acids/Cap. Bot. 50s, 100s, 1000s.
Use: Geriatric formula.

GERI-PLUS ELIXIR. (Approved) Vit. B-1 25 mg., B-2 10 mg., B-6 1 mg., niacinamide 100 mg., Ca pantothenate 5 mg., B-12 20 mcg., iron ammonium citrate 100 mg., choline 200 mg., inositol 100 mg., Mg chloride 2 mg., Mn citrate 2 mg., Zn acetate 2 mg., amino acids/Fl. Oz. Bot. pt.
Use: Supplement.

GERISOL. (Amfre-Grant) Testosterone 10 mg., estrone 0.5 mg., Vit. B-12 100 mcg., liver injection 2 mcg., thiamine HCl 50 mg., niacinamide 50 mg., riboflavin sodium phosphate 1 mg., pyridoxine HCl 5 mg., panthenol 10 mg./ml. w/lidocaine HCl 2%. Vial 10 ml.
Use: Hormone, vitamin supplement.

GERISPAN. (Robinson) Vit. A 12,500 I.U., D 1000 I.U., B-1 5 mg., B-2 2.5 mg., niacinamide 40 mg., B-6 1 mg., Ca pantothenate 4 mg., B-12 2 mcg., C 75 mg., E 2 I.U., choline bitartrate 31.4 mg., inositol 15 mg., Ca 75 mg., phosphorus 58 mg., Fe 30 mg., Mg 3 mg., Mn 0.5 mg., Pot. 2 mg., Zn 0.5 mg./Cap. Bot. 100s, 1000s. Bulk Pack 5000s.
Use: Dietary supplement for older persons and convalescents.

GERITINIC. (Geriatric) Vit. A 5000 I.U., D 400 I.U., B-12 5 mcg., niacinamide 10 mg., inositol 20 mg., choline bitartrate 30 mg., amino acetic acid 30 mg., Cal. pantothenate 1 mg., desic. liver 22.4 mg., conc. yeast 22.4 mg., Pot. acetate 30 mg., ferrous sulfate 195 mg., phyllins/Tab. Bot. 42s, 500s.
Use: Nutritional anemias.

GERITOL. (Beecham Products) Liq. Bot. 4 oz., 12 oz., 1 pt. 8 oz. Tab. Bot. 14s, 24s, 40s, 80s, 100s, 180s, 300s.

GERITOL LIQUID HIGH POTENCY IRON AND VITAMIN TONIC. (Beecham Products) Iron 100 mg., Vit. B-1 5 mg., B-2 5 mg., niacinamide 100 mg., panthenol 4 mg., pyridoxine 1 mg., B-12 1.5 mcg., methionine 50 mg., choline bitartrate 100

mg./0.5 oz. (Tablespoonful). Bot. 4 oz., 12 oz., 24 oz.
Use: Prevent deficiency in iron & specific vitamins.

GERITOL TABLETS HIGH POTENCY IRON & VITAMIN TABLETS. (Beecham Products) Iron 50 mg., Vit. B-1 5 mg., B-2 5 mg., C 75 mg., niacinamide 30 mg., calcium pantothenate 2 mg., pyridoxine 0.5 mg. cyanocobalamin 3 mcg./Tab. Bot. 14s, 24s, 40s, 80s, 100s, 180s, 300s.
Use: Iron and vitamin deficiency or supplement.

GERITONIC INJ. (Kenyon) Vit. B-12 50 mcg., d-panthenol 5 mg., niacinamide 50 mg., choline chloride 5 mg., inositol 5 mg., methionine 5 mg., estrone 1 mg., testosterone 10 mg. Liver-painless (B-12 equiv.) 1 mcg./cc. Vial 30 cc.
Use: B complex with hormones.

GERITONIC LIQUID. (Geriatric) Thiamine chloride 1 mg., riboflavin 1 mg., Vit. B-12 3 mcg., niacinamide 10 mg., pyridoxine HCl 0.1 mg., Mag. as sulfate 1 mg., iron as ammonium citrate 35 mg., Mang. as sulfate 0.5 mg., Cal. as glycerophosphate 10 mg., Phos. as Cal. glycerophosphate 8 mg., Pot. as sulfate 1 mg., aminoacetic acid 60 mg., yeast conc. 125 mg., liver fraction-1 125 mg./5 cc. Bot. 8 oz., 1 gal.
Use: Nutritional deficiencies.

GERIX ELIXIR. (Abbott). Vit. B-1 6 mg., B-2 6 mg., niacin 100 mg., iron 15 mg., B-6 1.64 mg., cyanocobalamin 6 mcg./30 ml. Bot. pt.
Use: Hematinic.

GERLIPO. (Kenyon) Choline bitartrate 250 mg., methionine 150 mg., inositol 100 mg., whole liver desic. 100 mg., B-cotrate 100 mg., B-1 1.5 mg., B-2 1 mg., B-6 0.1 mg., d-calcium pantothenate 2 mg., niacinamide 15 mg./3 Tabs. Bot. 100s, 1000s.

GERMANIN.
See: Suramin Sodium (Naphuride Sod.)

GERMICIN. (CMC) Alkylbenzyldimethyl chloride 17% Bot. pt., 1 gal. 50% Bot. gal.
Use: (diluted) Antiseptic.

GER-O-FOAM. (Geriatric) Methylsalicylate 30%, benzocaine 3%, and volatile oils. Aerosol can 4 oz.
Use: Anesthetic-analgesic.

GERREN. (Wren) Pentylenetetrazol 100 mg., niacin 50 mg./Tab. Bot. 100s, 1000s.
Use: Geriatric therapy.

GERTEROL DEPO. (Fellows) Medroxyprogesterone acetate 50 mg., 100 mg./cc. Vial 5 cc.

GESIC. (Lexalabs) Aspirin 226.8 mg., caffeine 32.4 mg., codeine 32.4 mg./Tab. Bot. 100s.
Use: Analgesic.

• **GESTACLONE.** USAN. (1) 17β-Acetyl-6-chloro-1β, 1a,2β,8β,9α,10,11,12,13,14α-,15,16β,16a,17-tetradecahydro-10β,13β-dimethyl-3H-dicyclopropa[1,2:16,-17]cyclopenta-[a]-phenanthren-3-one.
Use: Progestin.

GESTANIN. Allylestrenol, B.A.N. (Organon)

GESTEROL 50. (O'Neal, Jones & Feldman) Progesterone 50 mg. in aq. susp. or oil/cc. Vial 10 cc.

GESTEROL L.A. (O'Neal, Jones & Feldman) Hydroyprogesterone caproate 125 mg./cc. Vial 10 cc. 250 mg./cc. Vial 5 cc.

GESTIN. (Dalin) Formerly G.I. 8. Bot. 4 oz., 8 oz.

• **GESTODENE.** USAN.
Use: Progestin.

GESTONEED. (Hanlon) Ca. lactate 1069 mg., Vit. C 100 mg., nicotinic acid 18 mg., Vit. B-2 2.4 mg., Vit. B-1 1.8 mg., Vit. B-6 9 mg., Vit. D 500 I.U., Vit. A 6000 I.U./Cap. Bot. 100s.
Use: Prenatal dietary supplement.

• **GESTONORONE CAPROATE.** USAN. 17-Hydroxy-19-norpregn-4-ene-3,20-dione hexanoate.
Use: Progestin.

• **GESTRINONE.** USAN.
Use: Progestin.

GESTRONOL, B.A.N. 17-Hydroxy-19-norpregn-4-ene-3,20-dione.
Use: Progestational steroid.
See: Gestonorone (I.N.N.)
  Depostat hexanoate

GEVRABON. (Lederle) Vit. B-1 5 mg., B-2 2.5 mg., Vit. B-12 1 mcg., niacinamide 50 mg., Vit. B-6 1 mg., pantothenic acid 10 mg., choline 100 mg., inositol 100 mg., Zn 2 mg., iodine 100 mcg., Mg 2 mg., Mn 2 mg., Fe mg./30 ml. w/alcohol 18%. Bot. 16 fl. oz., 1 gal.
Use: Vitamin & mineral deficiencies.

GEVRAL. (Lederle) Vit. A acetate 5000 I.U., D 162 I.U., B-1 1.5 mg., B-2 1.7 mg., B-6 2 mg., B-12 6 mcg., C 60 mg., E 30 I.U., niacinamide 20 mg., Ca 162 mg., P 125 mg., elemental iron 18 mg., Mg 100 mg., iodine 150 mcg./Tab. Bot. 100s.
Use: Vitamin and mineral supplement.

GEVRAL PROTEIN. (Lederle) Protein 60%, carbohydrate 24%, fat 2%, sodium 0.02%, Vit. A 2167 I.U., D 217 I.U., B-1 2.2 mg., B-2 2.2 mg., B-6 0.22 mg., B-12 0.87 mcg., Ca pantothenate 2.2 mg., niacinamide 6.5 mg., C 22 mg., E 4.3 I.U., choline 21 mg., inositol, 22 mg., lysine 1.1 mg., Ca 359 mg., Cu 0.4 mg., iodine 0.04 mg., Fe (as ferrous fumarate) elemental 4.3 mg., Mg 0.4 mg., Mn 0.4 mg., P 52.8 mg., Na less than 20 mg., Zn 0.22 mg., 26 Gm. alcohol 1% w/Ca caseinate, lactose, artificial flavors, malt ext., sucrose, yeast, sod. saccharin, polysorbate 80. Can. 0.5 lb., 5 lb.
Use: Therapeutic-nutritional supplement.

GEVRAL T. (Lederle) Vit. A acetate 5,000 I.U., D 400 I.U., B-1 2.25 mg., B-2 2.6 mg., B-6 3 mg., B-12 9 mcg., C 90 mg., E 45 I.U., niacinamide 30 mg., Ca 162 mg., P 125 mg., elemental iron 27 mg., Mg 100 mg., iodine 225 mcg., Cu 1.5 mg., Zn 22.5 mg./Cap. Bot. 100s.
Use: Severe vitamin deficiencies.

GG-CEN CAPSULES. (Central) Guaifenesin 200 mg./Cap. Bot. 100s.
Use: Temporary relief of dry nonproductive cough.

GG-CEN SYRUP. (Central) Guaifenesin 100 mg., alcohol 10%/5 ml. Bot. 4 oz., pt., gal.
Use: Expectorant.

G.G.I. EXPECTORANT. (Amfre-Grant) Guaifenesin 100 mg., Cal. iodide 150 mg./5 cc. Bot. 16 oz., gal.
Use: Bronchial asthma, bronchitis, pulmonary emphysema.

GG-TUSSIN. (Vitarine) Guaifenesin syrup.

Use: Expectorant.

GISPASMIN. (Winston) Phenobarbital 16 mg., magnesium hydroxyaminoacetate 250 mg., hyoscyamine sulf. 0.052 mg., hyoscine HBr 0.003 mg. atropine sulf. 0.01 mg./Tab. Bot. 100s, 1000s.
Use: Antispasmodic with sedative.

GITALIN. A cardioactive glycoside derived from digitalis purpurea.
Use: Cardiotonic.

GITALIN (AMORPHOUS).
Use: Cardiotonic.

GL-2 SKIN ADHERENT. (Gordon) Bot. pt., qt., gal. Ready to use.

G-L 7 SKIN ADHERENT. (Gordon) A plastic material which may be used full strength or diluted with 3 to 10 parts 99% isopropyl alcohol, acetone or naphtha. Pkg. pt., qt., gal.

GLANDUBOLIN.
See: Estrone (Various Mfr.)

GLAUBER'S SALT.
See: Sodium Sulfate (Var. Mfr.)

GLAUCON, Soln. (Alcon) 1-epinephrine HCl, ½%, 1%, 2%; benzalkonium chloride, 0.02%; sodium chloride, 0.2% sodium metabisulfite, 0.3% (as preservative). Drop. Bot. 10 ml.
Use: Glaucoma, miotic therapy.

GLAUCOSTAT. (Kinghill) Acelidine.
Use: Parasympathomimetic.

• **GLAZE, PHARMACEUTICAL,** N.F. XVI.
Use: Pharmaceutic aid (tablet coating).

• **GLEPTOFERRON.** USAN.
Use: Hematinic.

• **GLIAMILIDE.** USAN.
Use: Antidiabetic.

GLIBENCLAMIDE. B.A.N. 1- 4-[2-(5-Chloro-2-methoxybenzamido)ethyl]benzenesulphonyl-3-cyclohexylurea.
Use: Oral hypoglycemic agent.
See: Daonil
     Euglucon

• **GLIBORNURIDE.** USAN. endo-1-[(IR)-(2-Hydroxy-3-bornyl)]-3-(p-tolysulfonyl) urea. Glutril.
Use: Oral hypoglycemic.

• **GLICETANILE SODIUM.** USAN.
Use: Antidiabetic.

• **GLIFLUMIDE.** USAN.
Use: Antidiabetic.

GLIM.
See: Gardinol Type Detergents (Various Mfr.)

• **GLIPIZIDE.** USAN.
Use: Antidiabetic.

GLIQUIDONE. B.A.N. 1-Cyclohexyl-3-p-[2-(3,4-dihydro-7-methoxy-4,4-dimethyl-1,3-dioxo-2(1H)-isoquinolyl)ethyl]phenylsulfonylurea.
Use: Oral hypoglycemic.

GLISOXEPIDE. B.A.N. 3-[4-(Perhydroazepin-1-ylureidosulfonyl)phenethylcarbamoyl]-5-methylis-oxazole.
Use: Oral hypoglycemic agent.

GLOBIN ZINC INSULIN INJECTION. Globin zinc insulin, insulin w/globin & zinc chloride added.
Use: S.C., insulin therapy.

• **GLOBULIN, ANTI-HUMAN SERUM,** U.S.P. XXI.

GLOBULIN, GAMMA.
See: Gamma Globulin (Various Mfr.)
     Poliomyelitis Immune Globulin, Human, Vial. (Var. Mfr.)

GLOBULIN, HEPATITIS B IMMUNE.
See: H-BIG, Vial (Abbott)

• **GLOBULIN, IMMUNE,** U.S.P. XXI.
Use: I.M., measles prophylactic & polio; passive immunizing agent.
See: Gammagee, Vial (Merck Sharp & Dohme)
     Generic, Vials 2 & 10 ml. (Cutter)
     Generic, Vial 2 ml. (Lederle)

• **GLOBULIN, Rho(D) IMMUNE,** U.S.P. XXI.
Use: Immunosuppressive.

GLOBULIN, POLIOMYELITIS IMMUNE. Human.
See: Poliomyelitis Immune Globulin (Var. Mfr.)

• **GLOXAZONE.** USAN. 3-Ethoxybutane-1,2-dione bis(-thiosemicarbazone).
Use: Antiprotozoan, veterinary medicine.
See: Contrapar

GLUBIONATE CALCIUM.
See: Neo-Calglucon, Syrup (Dorsey)

• **GLUCAGON,** U.S.P. XXI. Inj., U.S.P. XXI. (Lilly) 1 unit w/1 ml. diluent. 10 units w/10 ml. diluent. Glucagon HCl 1 mg. or 10 mg. w/diluent; soln. contains lactose, glycerin 1.6% w/phenol 0.2% as a preservative. Vials.
Use: Hypoglycemic shock.

• **GLUCEPTATE SODIUM.** USAN.
Use: Pharmaceutic aid.

D-GLUCITOL, 1-DEOXY-1-(METHYLAMINO). Meglumine, U.S.P. XXI.

d-GLUCITOL (d-Sorbitol)/Homatropine methylbromide.
See: ProBilagol, Liq. (Purdue Frederick)

■ **GLUCO-CORTICOIDS.**
See: Cortical Hormone Products.

GLUCOMETER. (Ames) Electronic meter for blood glucose testing. Use at home by lay diabetics to read dextrostix reagent strips.
Use: For blood glucose monitoring.

D-GLUCONIC ACID, CALCIUM SALT. Calcium Gluconate, U.S.P. XXI.

GLUCONIC ACID SALTS.
See: Calcium Gluconate
     Ferrous Gluconate
     Magnesium Gluconate
     Potassium Gluconate

α-**D-GLUCOPYRANOSIDE,β-D-FRUCTO-FURANOSY-L-.** Sucrose, N.F. XVI.

• **GLUCOSAMINE.** USAN. 2-Amino-2-deoxy-β-D-glucopyranose.
W/Nystatin, oxytetracycline.
See: Terrastatin, Cap., Sol. (Pfizer)
W/Tetracycline HCl, nystatin.
See: Tetrastatin Cap., Susp. (Pfizer)
W/Tetracycline.
See: Tetracyn, Cap., Syr. (Roerig)
W/Oxytetracycline.
See: Terramycin, Prep (Pfizer)

GLUCOSE.
See: Pal-A-Dex, Pow. (Baker)

• **GLUCOSE ENZYMATIC TEST STRIP,** U.S.P. XXI.
Use: Diagnostic aid (in vitro, reducing sugars in urine).

• **GLUCOSE, LIQUID,** N.F. XVI. (Various Mfr.)
Cerelose, Dextrose.
Use: 5-50% sol. as nutrient; for acute hepatitis and dehydration; to increase blood volume; pharm. aid (tablet binder, coating agent).

D-GLUCOSE, MONOHYDRATE. Dextrose, U.S.P. XXI.

GLUCOSE-40 OPHTHALMIC OINTMENT.
(CooperVision) Liquid glucose 40%. Tube 3.5 Gm.
Use: Treatment of corneal edema.

GLUCOSE OXIDASE. W/peroxidase, pot. iodide.
See: Diastix, Vial, Tab. (Ames)

GLUCOSE POLYMERS.
See: Polycose, Pow., Liq. (Ross)

GLUCOSE TEST.
See: Combistix (Ames)

GLUCOSE TOLERANCE TEST PREPARATION.
See: Glucola (Ames)

GLUCOSOL LIQUID. (Lannett) Liq. pt., gal.

GLUCOSULFONE SODIUM, INJ.
See: Sodium Glucosulfone Injection

GLUCOVITE. (Vale) Ferrous gluconate 260 mg., B-1 1 mg., B-2 0.5 mg., C 10 mg./Tab. Bot. 100s, 1000s, 5000s.

GLUCUROLACTONE. Gamma lactone of glucofuranuronic acid.
See: Preltron-Oral, Tab. (Pasadena Research)

GLUCURONATE SODIUM.
See: Preltron, Inj. (Pasadena Research)

GLU-K. (Western Research) Potassium gluconate 486 mg./Tab. Bot. 1000s.
Use: Supplement.

GLUKOR. (Hyrex) Chorionic gonadotropin 200 I.U., Vit. B-1 25 mg., glutamic acid 52.5 ppm, procaine HCl 1%/cc. Vial 10 cc., 25 cc.
Use: I.M., androgen deficiency, uterine disorders.

GLUSIDE.
See: Saccharin (Var. Mfr.)

GLUTAMATE SODIUM.
W/Niacin, Vit., Minerals.
See: L-Glutavite, Cap. (Cooper)

L-GLUTAMIC ACID, N-[4-[[(2-AMINO-1,4-DIHYDRO-4-OXO-6-PTERIDINYL)-METHYL]AMINO]BENZOY-L]-. Folic Acid, U.S.P. XXI.

L-GLUTAMIC ACID, N-[4-][2,4-DIAMINO-6-PYERIDI-NYL)METHYL]-METHYLAMINO]BENZOYL]-. Methotrexate, U.S.P. XXI.

GLUTAMIC ACID HYDROCHLORIDE. Acidogen, aciglumin, glutasin.
Use: The hydrochloride for achlorhydria & hypochlorhydria.
See: Acidulin, Pulvules (Lilly)
W/Cellulase, Pepsin, Pancreatin, Ox Bile Extract.
See: Kanulase, Tab. (Dorsey)

GLUTAMIC ACID SALTS.
See: Calcium Glutamate (Various Mfr.)

• **GLUTARAL CONCENTRATE,** U.S.P. XXI.
Use: Disinfectant.
See: Cidex (Surgikos)

GLUTARALDEHYDE. (City Chem.) Glutaraldehyde 25% in water. Pkg. 3 kg.; (Ayerst) Sonacide Sol., Gal., 5 Gal.

GLUTEST. (Leland) Testosterone 10 mg., thiamine HCl 25 mg., glutamic acid 52.5 ppm, procaine HCl 1%, benzyl alc. 2%/cc. Vial 10 cc., 25 cc.
Use: I.M.; female climacteric.

GLUTEST. (Leland) Methyltestosterone 2 mg., thiamine mononitrate 5 mg., mono sodium glutamate 300 mg./Tab. Bot. 100s, 500s.
Use: Testosterone therapy.

GLUTETHIMIDE. B.A.N. 2-Ethyl-2-phenylglutatimide.
Use: Non-barbiturate hypnotic.
See: Doriden, Tab. (USV)

• **GLUTETHIMIDE,** U.S.P. XXI. Cap., Tab., U.S.P. XXI.
Alpha-ethyl-alpha-phenyl-glutarimide. 2-Ethyl-2-phenylglutarimide.
Use: Non-barbiturate hypnotic.
See: Dorimide, Tab. (Cenci)
Doriden, Cap. (USV)
Rolathimide, Tab. (Robinson)

GLUTOFAC. (Kenwood) *Saccharomyces siccum* 390 mg., Vit C 250 mg., B-1 15 mg., B-2 10 mg., niacinamide 50 mg., B-6 50 mg., Ca-pantothenate 20 mg., Mg sulfate 70 mg., Zn 80 mg./Tab. Bot. 90s, 500s.
Use: Nutritional supplement.

GLUTOL. (Paddock) Dextrose 100 Gm./180 ml. Bot. 180 ml.
Use: Glucose tolerance test.

GLUTOSE. (Paddock) Concentrated glucose for insulin reactions. Bot. 2 oz.
Use: Hypoglycemic states.

GLUTRIL. Glibornuride, B.A.N.

• **GLYBURIDE.** USAN.
Use: Antidiabetic
See: Diabeta (Hoechst)
Micronase, Tab. (Upjoin)

GLYCALOX. B.A.N. A polymerized complex of glycerol and aluminum hydroxide. Glucalox (I.N.N.)
Use: Treatment of gastric hyperacidity.
See: Manalox AG.

GLYCARNINE IRON.
See: Ferronord, Tab. (Cooper)

GLYCATE CHEWABLES. (O'Neal, Jones & Feldman) Glycine 150 mg., calcium carbonate 300 mg./Tab. Bot. 100s.

• **GLYCERIN,** U.S.P. XXI. Ophth. Soln., Oral Soln., U.S.P. XXI. 1,2,3-Propanetriol.
Use: Pharm. aid.
See: Corn Huskers Lotion (Warner-Lambert)
Glyrol, Liq. (CooperVision)
Osmoglyn (Alcon)
W/Urea.
See: Kerid Ear Drops (Blair)

• **GLYCERIN SUPPOSITORIES,** U.S.P. XXI. (Various Mfr.) Glycerin, sodium stearate.
Use: Rectal evacuant; cathartic.

• **GLYCEROL, IODINATED.** USAN.
Use: Expectorant.

GLYCERYL GUAIACOLATE.
Use: Expectorant.

See: Guaifenesin, U.S.P. XXI.
GLYCERYL GUAIACOLATE CARBAMATE.
Methocarbamol.
See: Robaxin, Tab., Inj. (Robins)
Robaxin 750, Tab. (Robins)
GLYCERYL GUAIACOL ETHER.
See: Guaifenesin.
• **GLYCERYL MONOSTEARATE,** N.F. XVI. (Various
Mfr.) Monostearin.
Use: Pharm. aid (emulsifying agent).
GLYCERYL-T. (Rugby) Theophylline 150 mg.,
guaifenesin 90 mg./Cap. Bot. 100s, 1000s.
Use: Bronchial dilator.
GLYCERYL TRIACETIN. (Various Mfr.) Triacetin.
See: Enzactin, Aer., Pow., Cream (Ayerst)
Fungacetin, Oint., Liq. (Blair Labs.)
GLYCERYL TRINITRATE OINTMENT.
See: Nitrol, Oint. (Kremers-Urban)
GLYCERYL TRINITRATE TABLETS.
See: Nitroglycerin (Var. Mfr.)
Nitroglyn, Tab. (Key Corp.)
GLYCETS-ANTACID TABLETS. (Weeks & Leo)
Calcium carbonate 350 mg., simethicone 25
mg./Chewable Tab. Bot. 100s.
Use: Antacid.
GLYCINATO DIHYDROXYALUMINUM HYDRATE.
See: Dihydroxyaluminum Aminoacetate, U.S.P. XXI.
• **GLYCINE,** U.S.P. XXI. Irrigation, U.S.P. XXI.
Aminoacetic Acid.
Use: Myasthenia gravis treatment, irrigating
solution.
W/Aluminum hydroxide-magnesium carbonate co-
precipitated gel.
See: Glycogel, Tab., Susp. (Central)
W/Alum. & mag. hydroxide, mag. trisilicate,
belladonna ext.mannitol, oil peppermint.
See: Gas-Eze, Tab. (Edward J. Moore)
W/Calcium Carbonate.
See: Antacid No. 6, Tab. (Bowman)
Antacid Tab. (Sutliff & Case)
Glycate Chewables, Tab. (O'Neal)
P.H. Tabs. (Scrip)
Titralac, Liq., Tab. (Riker)
Wol-Lac, Tab. (Wolins)
W/Calcium carbonate, amylolytic, proteolytic
cellulolytic enzymes.
See: Co-gel, Tab. (Arco)
W/Chlortrimeton & sod. salicylate.
See: Corilin, Liq. (Schering)
W/Glutamic acid, alanine.
See: Prostall, Cap. (Metabolic Prods.)
W/Magnesium trisilicate, calcium carbonate.
See: P.H. Tabs., Chewable, Mix (Scrip)
W/Vit. B Complex, C, & iron.
See: Bironate-B, Cap. (Coastal)
GLYCINE, ALUMINUM SALT.
See: Dihydroxyaluminum Aminoacetate, U.S.P. XXI.
GLYCINE, N-(4-AMINOBENZOYL)-. Aminohippuric
Acid, U.S.P. XXI.
**GLYCINE, N,N'-1,2-ETHANEDIYLBIS[N-(CAR-
BOXYMETHYL)-], DISODIUM SALT, DIHYDRATE.**
Edetate Disodium, U.S.P. XXI.

GLYCINE HYDROCHLORIDE. (Various Mfr.)
Use: Recommended for achlorhydria.
• **GLYCOBIARSOL.** U.S.P. XXI. Tab., U.S.P. XXI.
Bismuthyl-N-Glycolylarsanilate, Chemo Puro, Pow. for
Mfr. (Hydrogen N-glycoloylarsanilato) oxobismuth.
Use: Amebiasis, Trichomonas vaginalis, Monilia
albicans.
GLYCOBIARSOL. (I.N.N.) Bismuth Glycollylarsanilate,
B.A.N.
GLYCOCOLL. Glycine.
See: Aminoacetic Acid (Various Mfr.)
GLYCOCYAMINE. Guanidoacetic acid.
GLYCO IOPHEN SOLUTION. (Wade) Tr. iodine,
phenol 2%, glycerine q.s., oil peppermint. Bot. 2
oz., 4 oz., pt., gal.
Use: Antiseptic.
• **GLYCOL DISTERATE.** USAN.
Use: Pharmaceutic aid.
GLYCOL MONOSALICYLATE.
W/Oil of mustard, camphor, menthol, methyl
salicylate.
See: Musterole, Oint., Cream (Plough)
GLYCOPHENYLATE BROMIDE.
See: Mepenzolate Methylbromide.
• **GLYCOPYRROLATE,** U.S.P. XXI. Inj., Tab., U.S.P.
XXI. 1-Methyl-3-pyrrolidyl a-phenylcyclopentaneg-
lycolate methobromide. 3-Hydroxy-1,1-dimethylpyr-
rolidinium bromide α-cyclopentylmandelate.
See: Robinul, Tab., Inj. (Robins)
Robinul Forte, Tab. (Robins)
GLYCOPYRRONIUM BROMIDE. B.A.N. 3-α-Cyclopen-
tylmandeloyloxy-1,1-dimethylpyrrolidinium bromide.
Use: Anticholinergic.
See: Glycopyrrolate
Robinul
GLYCOTUSS. (Vale) Guaifenesin 100 mg./Tab. or 5
ml. **Syr.** pt., gal. **Tabs.** 100s, 500s, 1000s.
Use: Expectorant.
GLYCOTUSS-dM. (Vale) Guaifenesin 100 mg., dex-
tromethorphan HBr 10 mg./Tab. or 5 cc. **Tab.**
100s, 500s, 1000s. **Syr.** pt., gal.
Use: Expectorant/antitussive.
• **GLYCYRRHIZA,** U.S.P. XXI. Pure Extract,
Fluidextract, U.S.P. XXI. Licorice root.
Use: Flavoring agent.
• **GLYCYRRHIZA EXTRACT, PURE,** U.S.P. XXI.
Use: Flavoring agent.
• **GLYCYRRHIZA FLUIDEXTRACT,** N.F. XVI.
W/Camphorated opium tincture, tartar emetic,
glycerin.
See: Brown Mixture. (Bowman)
W/Pepsin-papain complex, pancreas, malt diastase,
charcoal, ox bile.
See: Pepsocoll, Tabs. (Western Research Labs.)
GLYDANILE SODIUM. (1)5'-Chloro-2-[p-[(5-isobutyl-
2-pyrimidinyl)sulfamoyl]-phenyl]-o-acetanilidide
monosodium salt; (2) 4-[N-(5-isobutyl-2-pyrimidinyl)-
sulfamoyl] phenylacetic acid-5-chloro-2-methoxyani-
lide sodium salt.
Use: Oral hypoglycemic.
• **GLYHEXAMIDE.** USAN.
Use: Antidiabetic.

GLYMIDINE. B.A.N. Sodium salt of 2-benzenesulfonamido-5-(2-methoxy-ethoxy)pyrimidine.
Use: Oral hypoglycemic agent.
See: Gondafon
Lycanol
• **GLYMIDINE SODIUM.** USAN.[N-[5-(2-Methoxyethoxy)-2-idinyl] benzene-sulfonamido]-sodium.
Use: Oral hypoglycemic.
GLYMOL.
See: Petrolatum Liquid (Various Mfr.)
GLYNAZAN EXPECTORANT. (Scherer) Theophylline sod. glycinate, 60 mg. (equiv. to 30 mg., theophylline), guaifenesin 50 mg., sod. citrate 100 mg./5 cc. Bot. pt.
Use: Management of non-productive cough due to the common cold.
• **GLYOCTAMIDE.** USAN. 1-Cyclooctyl-3(p-tolylsulfonyl) urea.
Use: Hypoglycemic agent.
GLY-O-TUSSIN. (Research Pharmacal Lab.) Guaifenesin 100 mg./tsp. Bot., gal.
Use: Cough syrup.
GLY-OXIDE. (Marion) Carbamide peroxide 10% in flavored anhydrous glycerol. Plas. bot. 0.5 fl. oz., 2 fl. oz.
Use: Oral inflammation.
GLYOXYLDIUREIDE.
See: Allantoin (Various Mfr.)
• **GLYPARAMIDE.** USAN. 1-(p-Chlorophenylsulfonyl)-3-(p-dimethylaminophenyl) urea.
Use: Oral hypoglycemic.
GLYPHODYL B INJ. (Torigian) Iron cacodylate 0.020 Gm., sod. glycerophosphate 0.2 Gm., strychnine glycerophosphate 0.001 Gm./cc. Amp. 1 cc. 12s, 25s, 100s.
GLYROL. (CooperVision) Glycerin 75% v/v in a solution of citric acid and purified water. Glass Bot. 4 oz.
Use: Oral osmotic agent to reduce intraocular pressure.
GLYTABS. (Pharmics) Amino acetic acid 100 mg., calcium carbonate 300 mg., aluminum hydroxide, magnesium carbonate 200 mg./Chew. Tab. Bot. 100s, 1000s.
Use: Antacid.
GLYTINIC. (Boyle) Ferrous gluconate 13.5 gr., glycine 1.3 gm., B-12 10 mcg., B-1 7.5 mg., B-6 2.25 mg., niacinamide 45 mg., panthenol 6.5 mg., liver fraction 5 gr./fl. oz. Bot. pt., gal.
Use: Hematinic.
GLYTINIC TABLET. (Boyle) Ferrous gluconate 3.4 gr., glycine 325 mg., B-12 2.5 mcg., B-1 1.9 mg., B-2 1.9 mg., B-6 0.56 mg., niacinamide 11.25 mg., panthenol 1.63 mg., liver desic. 1.25 gr./Tab. Bot. 100s.
Use: Potent hematinic.
GLY-TRATE. (Sutliff & Case) Nitroglycerin 2.5 mg./Meta-Kap. Bot. 100s.
Use: Management of angina pectoris.
GLYTUSS. (Mayrand) Guaifenesin 200 mg./Tab. Bot. 100s, 500s.
Use: Antitussive-expectorant.

GLYVENOL. (Ciba) Tribenoside. Not available in U.S.
Use: Venoprotective agent.
G-MYCIN CAPS & G-MYCIN-S SYRUP. (Coast) Tetracycline HCl 250 mg., 500 mg./Cap. Bot. 100s. 500 mg. 1000s. 125 mg./5 cc. Syr. 16 oz.
Use: Anti-infective.
GOLACOL. (Arcum) Codeine sulfate 30 mg., papaverine HCl 30 mg., emetine HCl 2 mg., ephedrine HCl 15 mg. syrup orange q.s./30 cc alcohol 6.25%. Bot. 4, 16 oz., gal.
Use: Cough syrup.
GOLD (Au198) Colloid Radio.
Use: Antineoplastic Agent.
See: Radio Gold (Au198)
GOLD Au 198 INJECTION.
Use: Antineoplastic; diagnostic for liver scanning.
■ **GOLD COMPOUNDS.**
See: Aurocein-10, Vial (Christina)
Gold Sodium Thiosulfate (Various Mfr.)
Myochrysine, Amp. (Merck Sharp & Dohme)
Solganal, Vial. (Schering)
GOLD, MERCAPTOBUTANEDIOATO(1-)-, DISODIUM SALT, MONOHYDRATE. Gold Sodium Thiomalate, U.S.P. XXI.
• **GOLD SODIUM THIOMALATE,** U.S.P. XXI. Inj., U.S.P. XXI. Gold, mercaptobutanedioato(1-)-, disodium salt, monohydrate. (Disodium mercaptosuccinato) gold monohydrate.
Use: Rheumatoid arthritis.
See: Myochrysine, Amp. (Merck Sharp & Dohme)
GOLD SODIUM THIOSULFATE. Sterile, Auricidine, Aurocidin, Aurolin, Auropin, Aurosan, Novacrysin, Solfocrisol & Thiochrysine.
Use: Rheumatoid arthritis.
GOLD THIOGLUCOSE.
See: Aurothioglucose, U.S.P. XXI.
GOLD, (1-THIO-d-GLUCOPYRANOSATO)-. Aurothioglucose, U.S.P. XXI.
GOLDEN BALM. (Jenkins) Methyl salicylate, menthol, camphor/Fl. oz. Bot. 3 oz., pt., gal.
GOLDEN BOUNTY VITAMIN PRODUCTS. (Squibb)
See: Squibb Golden Bounty Products.
GOLDEN-WEST COMPOUND. (Golden-West) Gentian root, licorice root, cascara sagrada, damiana leaves, senna leaves, psyllium seed, buchu leaves, crude pepsin. Box 1½ oz.
Use: Laxative.
GOLDICIDE CONCENTRATE. (Pedinol) N-Alkyl-dimethylbenzylammonium chloride. Bot. (Conc.) 1 oz. Ctn. 10s.
Use: Chemical disinfection of surgical and podiatry instruments.
■ **GOMENOL PREPARATIONS.**
Note: Products withdrawn from market.
GONACRINE.
See: Acriflavine (Various Mfr.)
GONADEX. (Continental) Chroionic gonadotropin 10,000 u w/mannitol 100 mg., benzyl alcohol 0.9%, sod. phosphate dibasic and monobasic. Vial. 10 cc.
Use: Precocious puberty.
GONADORELIN. B.A.N. L-Pyroglutamyl-L-histidyl-L-tryp-

tophyl-L-seryl-L-tyrosyl-glycyl-L-leucyl-L arginyl-L-pro-
lyl-L-glycinamide.
Use: Luteinizing hormone- and follicle stimulating hor-
mone-releasing hormone.
• **GONADORELIN ACETATE.** USAN.
Use: Gonad-stimulating principle.
See: Cryptolin Prods. (Hoechst)
• **GONADORELIN HYDROCHLORIDE.** USAN.
Use: Gonad-stimulating principle.
GONADOTROPIC SUBSTANCE.
See: Gonadotropin Chorionic
• **GONADOTROPIN, CHORIONIC,** U.S.P. XXI. For
Inj., U.S.P. XXI. Human Pregnancy Urine.
Use: In the female: Chronic cystic mastitis,
functional sterility, dysmenorrhea, premenstrual
tension, & threatened abortion. In the male:
Cryptorchidism, hypogenitalism, dwarfism,
impotency, enuresis.
See: Android HCG, Inj. (Brown)
    Antuitrin "S", Vial (Parke-Davis)
    A.P.L., Secules (Ayerst)
    Chopion-Plus, Vial (Pharmex)
    Corgonject, Vial (Mayrand)
    Dura-Chroion Plus, Vial (Pharmex)
    Follutein Powd. (Squibb)
    Gonadamine 5000, Vial (Torigian)
    Harvatropin, Vial (Harvey)
    Libigen, Vial (Savage)
    Pregnyl, Amp. (Organon)
W/Vit. B-1, glutamic acid, procaine HCl.
See: Glukor, Vial. (Brown)
GONADOTROPIN, PITUITARY ANT. LOBE.
Extracted from anterior lobe of equine pituitaries
(not pregnant mare urine) (rat unit = 1 Fevold-Hisaw
unit).
GONADOTROPIN SERUM. Pregnant Mare's Serum.
GONADOTROPIN SPECIAL DILUENT. (Kenyon) Sod.
succinate 0.5%, sod. nicotinate 1.0%, glutamic acid
52.5 ppm, propylparaben 0.02%, chlorobutanol
0.5%. Vial 10 cc.
GONIC. (Hauck) Chorionic gonadotropin 10,000 units.
Vial 10 ml. /w diluent.
GONIO GEL. (Muro) Methylcellulose 2½% in gel
base. Tube 3.5 Gm.
Use: Gonioscopic examination.
GONIOSCOPIC HYDROXYPROPYL
METHYLCELLULOSE.
See: Goniosol Lacrivial, Sol. (Smith, Miller & Patch)
GONIOSOL. (CooperVision) Gonioscopic
hydroxypropyl methylcellulose 2.5%. Bot. 0.5 oz.
GONOZYME. (Abbott) Test kit 100s.
Use: Enzyme immunoassay for detection of
Neisseria gonorrhoeae in urogenital swab
specimens.
GOOD SAMARITAN OINTMENT. (Good Samaritan)
Tin 1.7 oz.
Use: Promotes healing of irritated or burned skin.
GO PAIN. (DePree) **Cream:** Methyl salicylate,
chlorobutanol, menthol, camphor, thymol. Tube 1½
oz., 4 oz. **Oral Gel:** Benzocaine, eugenol. Tube ⅜
oz. **Throat spray** 4 oz.

GO PAIN EXTRA STRENGTH BALM. (DePree)
Methyl salicylate Jar 3¾ oz.
Use: External analgesic.
GO-PAIN LOTION. (Eckerd) Methyl nicotinate, methyl
salicylate, menthol, camphor. Bot. 5 oz.
GO PAIN THROAT LOZENGES. (Eckerd)
Benzocaine, menthol, eucalyptus.
Use: Sore throat pain.
GORDOBALM. (Gordon) Chloroxylenol, methyl
salicylate, menthol, camphor, thymol, eucalyptus oil,
isopropyl alcohol 16%, fast-drying gum base. Bot. 4
oz., gal.
GORDOCHOM. (Gordon) Undecylenic acid 25%,
dichlorophene 1%, penetrating oil base. Bot. 0.5
oz., 1 oz.
Use: Superficial fungus condition, calloused nail
grooves.
GORDOFILM. (Gordon) Salicylic acid 16.7%, lactic
acid 16.7% in flexible collodian.
Use: Keratolytic for removal of verrucae.
GORDOGESIC CREAM. (Gordon) Methyl salicylate
10% in absorbtion base. Jar 2.5 oz., 1 lb.
Use: Muscular aches, pains, and strains, simple
neuralgia.
GORDOMATIC CRYSTALS. (Gordon) Sod. borate,
sod. bicarbonate, sod. chloride, thymol, menthol, oil
of eucalyptus. Jar 8 oz., 7 lb.
Use: Aromatic, soothing foot soak.
GORDOMATIC LOTION. (Gordon) Menthol, camphor,
propylene glycol, isopropyl alcohol. Bot. 1 oz., 4
oz., gal.
Use: Burning aching, tired feet.
GORDOMATIC POWDER. (Gordon) Menthol, thymol
camphor, oil of eucalyptus, salicylic acid, alum
bentonite, talc. Shaker can 3.5 oz. Can 1 lb., 5 lbs.
Use: Cooling, soothing powder.
GORDOPHENE. (Gordon) Neutral coconut oil soap
15% and glycerin. Bot. 4 oz., gal.
Use: Surgical soap for office and at home use.
GORDO-POOL WHIRLPOOL CONCENTRATE.
(Gordon) Septi-Chlor (trichlorohydroxy diphenyl ether)
broad spectrum antimicrobial and bacteriostatic
agent. Bot. 4 oz., pt., gal.
Use: Water softener and de-scumming agent.
GORDO-VITE A CREME. (Gordon) Vit. A 100,000
I.U./oz. in water soluble base. Jar 0.5 oz., 2.5 oz.,
4 oz., lb., 5 lb.
Use: Dry skin and fissures, treatment for diabetic
and geriatric skin.
GORDO-VITE A LOTION. (Gordon) Vit. A 100,000
I.U./oz. Plastic Bot. 4 oz., gal.
Use: Treatment of diabetic and geriatric skin.
GORDO-VITE E CREME. (Gordon) Vit. E 1500
I.U./oz., water soluble base. Jar 2.5 oz., lb.
Use: Skin care; helpful for dryness after surgery.
GORD-UREA. (Gordon) Urea 22% or 40% in
petrolatum base. Jars 1 oz.
Use: Devitalized nail tissue cleansing, loosening
and debriding; non-surgical avulsion of nails.
GORMEL CREAM. (Gordon) Urea 20% in emollient
base. Jar 2.5 oz., 4 oz., 1 lb.

Use: Hyperkeratotic for dry skin conditions and fissures.

GOTAMINE. (Vita Elixir) Ergotamine tartrate 1 mg., caffeine 100 mg./Tab.
Use: Migraine therapy.

• **GRAMICIDIN,** U.S.P. XXI.
Use: Antibacterial.
W/Neomycin.
See: Spectrocin Ointment (Squibb)
W/Neomycin sulfate, polymyxin B sulfate, thimerosal.
See: Neo-Polycin Ophthalmic Solution (Merrell Dow)
W/Neomycin sulf., polymyxin B sulf., benzocaine.
See: Tricidin, Oint. (Amlab)
W/Neomycin, triamcinolone, nystatin.
See: Mycolog Cream, Oint. (Squibb)
W/Polymyxin B sulfate, neomycin sulfate.
See: Neosporin, Ophth. Sol. (Burroughs Wellcome)
Neosporin-G. Cream (Burroughs Wellcome)
W/Polymyxin B sulfate, neomycin sulfate & hydrocortisone acetate.
See: Cortisporin, Cream (Burroughs Wellcome)

GRAMIMUNE. (Cutter) Immune globulin intravenous 5% in 10% maltose. Single dose vials 50 ml., 100 ml.
Use: IgG antibody deficient patients.

GRAMINEAE POLLENS.
See: Allergenic Extracts, Timothy and Related Pollens (Parke-Davis)

GRANULEX. (Hickam) Trypsin 0.1 mg., balsam peru 72.5 mg., castor oil 650.0 mg. w/emulsifier/0.82 cc. Spray can, 2 oz., 4 oz.
Use: Wound healing.

GRAPEFRUIT DIET PLAN with DIADAX CAPSULES. (O'Connor) Natural grapefruit ext. 50 mg., Vit. C 30 mg., E 15 I.U., phenylpropanolamine HCl 30 mg./Cap. Bot. 20s, 50s.
Use: Vitamin fortified appetite suppressant.

GRAPEFRUIT DIET PLAN with DIADAX EXTRA STRENGTH CAPSULES. (O'Connor) Natural grapefruit Ext. 100 mg., Vit. C 60 mg., E 30 I.U., phenylpropanolamine HCl 75 mg./Cap. Bot. 10s, 24s.
Use: Vitamin fortified appetite suppressant.

GRAPEFRUIT DIET PLAN with DIADAX TABLETS. (O'Connor) Natural grapefruit ext. Vit. C 10 mg., E 5 I.U., phenylpropanolamine HCl 10 mg./Tab. Bot. 42s, 90s.
Use: Vitamin fortified appetite suppressant.

GRAPEFRUIT DIET PLAN with DIADAX EXTRA STRENGTH TABLETS. (O'Connor) Natural grapefruit ext., Vit. C 20 mg., E 10 I.U., phenylpropanolamine HCl 25 mg./Tab. Bot. 30s, 72s.
Use: Vitamin fortified appetite suppressant.

GRATUS STROPHANTHIN.
See: Ouabain (Various Mfr.)

GRAVIGEN INJECTION. (Bluco) Estrogenic sub. in aq. susp. or oil. 20,000 u./cc. Vial 30 cc.

GRAVINEED. (Hanlon) Vit. C 100 mg., Vit. E 10 I.U., Vit. B-1 3 mg., Vit. B-2 2 mg., Vit. B-6 10 mg., Vit. B-12 5 mcg., Vit. A 4000 I.U., Vit. D 400 I.U., niacin 10 mg., folic acid 0.1 mg., iron fumarate 40 mg., Ca. 67 mg./Cap. Bot. 100s.

Use: Prenatal dietary supplement.

GRAVOL. Dimenhydrinate, B.A.N.

GREEN MINT. (Block) Urea, glycine, polysorbate 60, sorbitol, alcohol 12.2%, peppermint oil, menthol, chlorophyllin-copper complex. Bot. 7 oz., 12 oz.
Use: Mouthwash and gargle.

GREEN SOAP, U.S.P. XXI.
Use: Detergent.

GRIFULVIN V. (Ortho) Griseofulvin microsize. **Tab.** 250 mg./Tab. Bot. 100s; 500 mg./Tab. Bot. 50s, 100s, 500s. **Susp.:** 125 mg./5 cc. Bot. 4 oz.
Use: Fungus infections of skin, hair & nails (oral).

GRILLODYNE TABLETS. (Fellows) Aspirin 3½ gr., phenacetin 2½ gr., caffeine alkaloid ½ gr., phenobarbital ¼ gr./Tab. Bot. 1000s.

GRISACTIN. (Ayerst) Griseofulvin microsize. 125 mg./Cap. Bot. 100s; 250 mg./Cap. Bot. 100s, 500s. 500 mg./Tab. Bot. 60s.
Use: Ringworm infections.

GRISACTIN ULTRA. (Ayerst) Grisofulvin ultramicrosize 125 mg., 250 mg. or 330 mg./Tab. Bot. 100s.
Use: Ringworm infections.

• **GRISEOFULVIN,** U.S.P. XXI. Cap., Oral Susp., Tab., Ultramicrosized Tab., U.S.P. XXI. An antibiotic. 7-Chloro-4,6-dimethoxy-coumaran-3-one-2-spiro-1'-(2'-methoxy-6'-methylcyclohex-2'-en-4'-one). 7-Chloro-2',4,6-trimethoxy-6'-methylspiro[benzofuran-2(3H), 1'-[2]-cyclohexene]-3,4'-dione. Spiro[benzofuran-2(3H)-1'-[2]cyclohexene]-3,4'-dione,7-chloro-2',4,6-trimethoxy-6'-methyl-, (1's-trans)-. Fulcin, Grisovin
Use: Antifungal (antibiotic).
See: Fulvicin P/G. Tab. (Schering)
Fulvicin-U/F, Tab. (Schering)
Grifulvin V, Tab., Susp. (Ortho)
Grisactin, Cap., Tab. (Ayerst)
Grisactin Ultra, Tab. (Ayerest)

GRISEOFULVIN MICROCRYSTALLINE.
See: Fulvicin U/F, Tab. (Schering)
Grifulvin V, Tab., Susp. (Ortho)
Grisactin, Cap., Tab. (Ayerst)

GRISEOFULVIN ULTRAMICROSIZE.
See: Fulvicin P/G. Tab. (Schering)
Gris-Peg Tablets (Dorsey)

GRIS-PEG TABLETS. (Herbert) Griseofulvin ultramicrosize 125 mg. or 250 mg./Tab. Bot. 100s, 500s.
Use: Antifungal.

GROFAS. Quindoxin, B.A.N.

GRO. (Coastal) Sterilized bone meal 16 gr., Vit. A 400 u., D 400 u., red bone marrow 20 mg./Tab. Bot. 100s.

GROUP A STREP. (Wampole-Zeus) Direct fluorescent test for group A Streptocci. 72 × 10 wells.
Use: Identification of Group A streptococci from cultures.

GROWTH HORMONE. B.A.N. Extract of human pituitaries containing predominantly growth hormone.
See: Crescormon.

G-STROPHANTHIN.
See: Ouabain (Various Mfr.)

G-TUSSIN SYRUP. (Columbia) Guaifenesin 100 mg./ cc. Bot. pt., gal.

Use: Coughs.

G-TUSSIN DM SYRUP. (Columbia) Guaifenesin 100 mg., dextro-methorphan HBr 15 mg., alcohol 1.4%/5 ml. Bot. pt., gal.
Use: Expectorant.

GUAIACOHIST. (Pharmex) Potassium guaiacol-sulfonate 40 mg., sod. iodide 50 mg., chlorpheniramine maleate 5 mg./cc. Vial 30 cc.

GUAIACOL. (Various Mfr.) Methylcatechol.
Use: Chronic infections of the respiratory tract.
W/Cacodylic acid.
See:
W/Methyl Salicylate.
See: Guiatex, Oint. (Scrip)
W/Naiouli oil, eucalyptol, iodoform, camphor.
See: Guaidol Compound, Vial (Medical Chem.; Kenyon)
Kleer, Inj. (Scrip)

GUAIACOL. (Jenkins) Guaiacol 0.1 Gm., eucalyptol 0.08 Gm., iodoform 0.02 Gm., camphor 0.05 Gm., sesame oil q.s./2 cc. Vial 10 cc.
W/Methyl salicylate, menthol.
See: Guaiamen, Cream (Lannett)

GUAIACOL CARBONATE. (Various Mfr.) (Duotal).
Use: Expectorant.

GUAIACOL GLYCERYL ETHER.
See: Guaifenesin

GUAIACOL POTASSIUM SULFONATE.
See: Bronchial, Syr. (DePree)
W/Ammonium Cl, sod. citrate, benzyl alcohol, carbinoxamine maleate.
See: Clistin Expectorant, Syr. (McNeil)
W/Dextromethorphan HBr.
Bronchial DM, Syr. (DePree)
W/Dextromethorphan HBr, chlorpheniramine maleate, ammonium Cl, tartar emetic.
See: Duomine, Syr. (Kenyon)
W/Pheniramine maleate, pyrilamine maleate, codeine phosphate.
See: Tritussin Syrup (Towne)

GUAIADOL. (Medwick) Aqueous. Vial 30 cc.

GUAIADOL COMPOUND. (Medical Chem.) Naiouli oil 100 mg., eucalyptol 80 mg., guaiacol 100 mg., iodoform 20 mg., camphor 50 mg./2 cc. Aqueous or in oil. Vial 30 cc.

GUAIADOL COMPOUND. (Medwick) Oil. Vial 30 cc.

GUAIAJEN. (Jenkins) Phenylephrine HCl 5 mg., pyrilamine maleate 12.5 mg., guaifenesin 100 mg./Tab. Bot. 1000s.
Use: Cold symptoms.

GUAIAMEN. (Lannett) Methyl salicylate, guaiacol, menthol in greaseless base. 4 oz., 1 lb.

GUAIAMINE SOLU-CAPS. (Sutliff & Case) Caffeine 32.5 mg., chlorpheniramine maleate 2 mg., phenylephrine HCl 5 mg., guaifenesin 50 mg., salicylamide 3 gr., acetaminophen 2 gr./Cap. Bot. 100s, 1000s.
Use: Colds.

GUAIANESIN.
See: Guaifenesin (Various Mfr.)
Use: Cough suppressant.

• **GUAIAPATE.** USAN.
Use: Antitussive.

GUAIFED. (Muro) Guaifenesin 250 mg., pseudoephedrine HCl 120 mg./TR Cap. Bot. 100s.
Use: Allergy therapy.

• **GUAIFENESIN,** U.S.P. XXI. Cap., Syrup, Tab., U.S.P. XXI. Methphenoxydiol. 3-(o-methoxyphenoxy)-1,2-propanediol.
Synonyms:
Guaifenesin
Glyceryl Guaiacol Ether
Guaianesin
Guaifylline
Guaiphenesin, B.A.N.
Guayanesin
Use: Expectorant.
See: Anti-tuss, Liq. (Century)
Consin-GG, Syr. (Wisconsin)
Dilyn, Liq., Tab. (Elder)
2/G, Liq. (Merrell Dow)
G-100, Syr. (Bock)
G-200, Cap. (Bock)
GG-Cen, Syr. (Central)
Glycotuss, Tab., Syr. (Vale)
Gly-O-Tussin, Liq. (Research Pharmacal Lab.)
Glytuss, Tab. (Mayrand)
G-Tussin, Syr. (Columbia)
Hytuss, Tab., Cap. (Hyrex)
Robitussin, Syr. (Robins)
Tursen, Tab. (Wren)
Wal-Tussin, Syr. (Walgreen)
W/Combinations.
See: Actified C Expectorant, Liq. (Burroughs Wellcome)
Actol Exp., Syr., Tab. (Beecham Labs)
Adatuss, Syr. (W.F. Merchant)
Airet G.G., Cap., Elix. (Baylor Labs.)
Ambenyl-D, Liq. (Marion)
Anti-tuss D.M., Liq. (Century)
Antitussive Guaiacolate, Syr. (Med. Chem.)
Asbron G, Tab., Elix. (Dorsey)
Asma. Syr. (Coastal)
Bur-Tuss Expectorant (Burlington)
Brexin, Cap., Liq. (Savage)
Bri-stan, Liq. (Briar)
Bronchohist, Syr. (Sutliff & Case)
Broncholate, Cap., Elix. (Bock)
Bronchovent, Tab. (Mills)
Bronkolate-G, Tab. (Parmed)
Bronkolixir, Elix. (Winthrop-Breon)
Bronkotabs, Tab. (Winthrop-Breon)
Bro-Tane, Exp. (Scrip)
C.D.M., Expect. (Lannett)
Cerylin, Liq. (Spencer-Mead)
Cheracol-D, Syr. (Upjohn)
Chlor-Trimeton, Expect. (Schering)
Colrex, Expectorant (Rowell)
Conar-A, Susp., Tab. (Beecham Labs)
Conar Expectorant, Liq. (Beecham Labs)
Consin-DM, Syr. (Wisconsin)
Coricidin Children's Cough Syrup (Schering)
Cortane D.C., Exp. (Standex)
Dextro-Tuss GG, Liq. (Ulmer)
Diabetussin, Expect. (Research Pharm.)
Dilacap, Cap. (Coastal)

Dilaudid, Syr. (Knoll)
Dilor-G, Tab., Liq. (Savage)
Dilyn, Liq. (Elder)
Dimacol, Cap. (Robins)
Dimetane Expectorant, Liq. (Robins)
Dimetane Expectorant-DC, Liq. (Robins)
DM Plus, Liq. (West-Ward)
Donatussin, Syr. (Laser)
Duovent, Tab. (Riker)
Emfaseem, Liq., Tab. (Saron)
Entex, Caps., Liq. (Norwich Eaton)
Expectico Cough Syrup (Coastal)
Expecto Hist, Tab. (Wolins)
Fedahist, Expect. (Dooner)
Formula 44D Decongestant Cough Mixture, Syr.
   (Vicks)
G-100/DM, Syr. (Bock)
G-Bron Elixir (Laser)
2G/DM, Liq. (Merrell Dow)
Glycotuss-DM, Tab. (Vale)
G-Tussin-DM, Syr. (Columbia)
Guaiamine, Cap. (Sutliff & Case)
Guiatussin w/Codeine. Liq. (Spencer-Mead)
Guistrey Fortis, Tab. (Bowman)
Gylanphen, Tab. (Lannett)
Histussinol, Syr. (Bock)
Hycoff-A, Syr. (Saron)
Hycotuss Expect., Liq. (Du Pont)
Hylate, Tab., Syr. (Hyrex)
Isoclor. Expect. (American Critical Care)
Lanatuss, Expect. (Lannett)
Lardet Expectorant, Tab. (Standex)
Lufyllin-EPG, Tab., Elix., (Mallinckrodt)
Mudrane GG, Tab., Elix. (Poythress)
Neospect, Tab. (Lemmon)
Novahistine Cough Formula, Liq. (Merrell Dow)
Novahistine DMX, Liq. (Merrell Dow)
Novahistine, Expect. (Merrell Dow)
Panaphyllin, Susp. (Panamerican)
Partuss-A, Tab. (Parmed)
Partuss AC (Parmed)
Pedituss Syrup (Sutliff & Case)
Phenatuss, Liq. (Dalin)
PMP, Expect. (Schlicksup)
PMP, Syrup (Schlicksup)
Polaramine Expect. (Schering)
Poly-Histine Expect. (Bock)
Polytuss-DM, Liq. (Rhode)
P.R. Syrup, Liq. (Fleming)
Queltuss, Syr., Tab. (Westerfield)
Quibron, Cap., Liq. (Mead Johnson)
Quibron-300, Cap. (Mead Johnson)
Quibron Plus, Cap., Elix. (Mead Johnson)
Quilate, Cap. (Wolins)
Rentuss, Cap., Syr. (Wren)
Rhinex DM (Lemmon)
Robitussin AC, CF, DAC, DM, PE (Robins)
Robitussin-DM Cough Calmers, Loz. (Robins)
Rondec-DM, Syr. (Ross)
Rymed, Prods. (Edwards)
Ryna-Cx, Liq. (Mallinckrodt)
Ryna-tussadine, Tab., Liq. (Mallinckrodt)

Santussin, Caps. (Sandia)
Scotcof, Liq. (Scott/Cord)
Silexin, Cough Syr. (Clapp)
Slo-Phyllin GG, Cap., Syr. (Dooner)
Sorbase Cough Syr. (Fort David)
Sorbase II Cough Syr. (Fort David)
Spen-Histine Expect. (Spencer-Mead)
Sudafed Cough Syrup (Burroughs Wellcome)
Theofed, Tab. (Sutliff & Case)
Theo-Guaia, Cap., Liq. (Sutliff & Case)
Tolu-Sed, Liq. (Scherer)
Tolu-Sed DM, Liq. (Scherer)
Trihista-Phen, Liq. (Recsei)
Tri-Histin Expect. (Recsei)
Tri-Mine, Expect. (Spencer-Mead)
Trind-DM, Liq. (Mead Johnson)
Trind, Liq. (Mead Johnson)
Tussafed, Exp. (Calvital)
Tussar-2, Syr. (Armour)
Tussend, Liq. (Merrell Dow)
Verequad, Tab., Susp. (Knoll)
Vicks Cough Syrup (Vicks)
Vicks Formula 44D Decongestant Cough Mixture,
   Syr. (Vicks)
Wal-Tussin DM, Syr. (Walgreen)

GUAIODOL AQUEOUS. (Kenyon) Potassium guaiacol
   sulf. 40 mg., sod. iodide 50 mg. in saturated
   aqueous naiouli, guaiacol, eucalyptol, menthol/cc.
   Vial 30 cc.
GUAIODOL COMPOUND. (Kenyon) Naiouli oil 0.10
   Gm., eucalyptol 0.08 Gm., guaiacol 0.1 Gm.,
   iodoform 0.02 Gm., camphor 0.05 Gm./2 cc. Vial
   30 cc.
GUAIODOL-PLUS AQUEOUS. (Kenyon) Potassium
   guaiacolsulfonate 40 mg., sod. iodide 50 mg.,
   chlorpheniramine maleate 5 mg., sod. bisulfite 1
   mg. in saturated aqueous naiouli, guaiacol,
   eucalyptol, menthol/cc. Vial 30 cc.
GUAIPHENESIN. B.A.N. 3- -Methoxyphenoxy-propane-
   1:2-diol. Guaiacol glycerol ether.
   Use: Cough suppressant.
   See: Guaifenesin U.S.P. XXI.
GUAIPHENYL. (Bowman) Guaifenesin 100 mg.,
   phenylephrine HCl 10 mg., chlorpheniramine
   maleate 1 mg./Tab.
   Use: Decongestant, expectorant, antihistaminic.
GUAIPHOTOL. (Foy) Iodine 1/30 gr., calcium cresoate
   4 gr./Tab. Bot. 1000s.
   Use: Expectorant for use in bronchitis.
• **GUAITHYLLINE.** USAN. 3-(o-Methoxy-phenoxy)-1,2-
   propanediol w/theophylline.
   Use: Antiasthmatic.
GUAMECYCLINE. B.A.N. N-(4-Guanidinoformi-midoyl-
   piperazin-1-ylmethyl)tetracycline.
   Use: Antibiotic.
GUAMIDE.
   See: Sulfaguanidine. (Various Mfr.)
• **GUANABENZ.** USAN.[(2,6-Dichlorobenzylidene)-
   amino] guanidine.
   Use: Antihypertensive.
   See: Wytensin, Tab. (Wyeth)

GUANACLINE. B.A.N. 1-(2-Guanidinoethyl)-1,-2,3,6-tetrahydro-4-picoline.
Use: Hypotensive.

GUANADREL SULFATE. USAN. (1,4-Dioxaspiro[4.5]dec-2-ylmethyl)guanidine sulfate (2:1).
Use: Antihypertensive.
See: Hylorel, Tab. (Pennwalt)

GUANABENZ ACETATE. USAN.
Use: Antihypertensive.

GUANCYDINE. USAN.
Use: Antihypertensive.

GUANETHIDINE. B.A.N. 1-(2-Guanidinoethyl)-azacyclo-octane.
Use: Hypotensive.
See: Ismelin sulfate, Tab. (Ciba)

GUANETHIDINE MONOSULFATE, U.S.P. XXI. Tab., U.S.P. XXI. [2-(Hex-ahydro-1(2H)-azocinyl)-ethyl]-guanidine sulfate (2:1), or [2-(hexahydro-1(2H)-azocinyl)-ethyl] guanidine hydrogen sulfate.
Use: Hypotensive.
W/Hydrochlorothiazide.
See: Esimil, Tab. (Ciba)

GUANETHIDINE SULFATE, U.S.P. XXI. Tab. U.S.P. XXI. Guanidine, 2-(hexahydro-1(2H)-azocinyl)ethyl-, sulfate (2:1). [2-(Hexahydro-1-(2H)-azocinyl)ethyl] guanidine sulfate.
Use: Hypotensive agent.
See: Ismelin, Tab. (Ciba)
W/Hydrochlorothiazide.
See: Esimil, Tab. (Ciba)

GUANFACINE HYDROCHLORIDE. USAN.
Use: Antihypertensive.

GUANIDINE HCl. (Key) Guanidine HCl 125 mg./Tab. Bot. 100s.
Use: Parasympathetic stimulant.

GUANIDINE, [2-(HEXAHYDRO-1(2H)-AXOCINYL)-ETHYL]-, SULFATE (2:1). Guanethidine Sulfate, U.S.P. XXI.

GUANISOQUIN. 7-Bromo- 3,4-dihydro-2-(1H)-iso-quinoline carboxamidine Sulfate (2:1).
Use: Antihypertensive agent.

GUANISOQUIN SULFATE. USAN.
Use: Antihypertensive.

GUANOCLOR. B.A.N. [2-(2,6-Dichlorophenoxy)-ethyl]aminoguanidine.
Use: Hypotensive.
See: Vatensol sulfate

• GUANOCLOR SULFATE. USAN.[[2-(2,6-Di-chlorophenoxy)-ethyl]amino] guanidine sulfate.
Use: Antihypertensive.
See: Vatensol

• GUANOCTINE HYDROCHLORIDE. USAN.
Use: Antihypertensive.

• GUANOXABENZ. USAN.
Use: Antihypertensive.

GUANOXAN. B.A.N. 2-Guanidinomethyl-1,4-benzodioxan.
Use: Hypotensive.
See: Envacar sulfate

• GUANOXAN SULFATE. USAN. (1,4-Benzodioxane-2-ylmethyl)-guanidine sulfate. Envacar.
Use: Antihypertensive.

• GUANOXYFEN SULFATE. USAN. (3-Phenoxypropyl) guanidine sulfate.
Use: Hypotensive and antidepressant.

GUARDAL. (Morton) Vit. A 10,000 I.U., B-1 20 mg., B-2 8 mg., C 50 mg., niacinamide 10 mg., Ca d-pantothenate 5 mg., Fe 10 mg., dried whole liver 100 mg., yeast 100 mg., choline bitartrate 30 mg., B-6 0.5 mg., B-12 8 mcg., mixed tocopherols 5 mg., dicalcium phosphate anhydrous 150 mg., Mg sulfate dried 7.2 mg., Na 1 mg., pot. chloride 1.3 mg./Tab. Bot. 100s.

GUARDEX. (Archer-Taylor) Tube 4 oz., 1 lb., 4½ lb.
Use: Protective cream.

• GUAR GUM, N.F. XVI.
Use: Pharm. aid (tablet binder; tablet disintegrant).
W/Danthron, docusate sodium.
See: Guarsol, Tab. (Western Research)
W/Docusate sodium, prune conc.
See: D-S-S Compound, Cap. (Wolins)
W/Standardized senna concentrate.
See: Gentlax B, Granules, Tab. (Blair)

GUARSOL TABLETS. (Western Research) Guar gum 300 mg., danthron 50 mg., docusate sodium 100 mg./Tab. 2 Handicount 28 (36 bags of 28).
Use: Bulk laxative, stool softener.

GUAYANESIN.
Use: Cough suppressant.
See: Guaifenesin (Various Mfr.)

GUIAMID AC EXPECTORANT. (Vangard) Guaifenesin 100 mg., codeine phosphate 10 mg./5 ml. Bot. pt., gal.
Use: Cough expectorant, depressant.

GUIAMID DM EXPECTORANT. (Vangard) Guaifenesin 100 mg., dextromethorphan HBr. 15 mg./5 ml. w/alcohol 1.4%. Bot. pt.
Use: Cough expectorant, depressant.

GUIAMID EXPECTORANT. (Vangard) Guaifenesin 100 mg./5 ml. w/alcohol 3.5%: Bot. pt., gal.
Use: Cough expectorant.

GUIATUSCON. (CMC) Guaifenesin 100 mg./5 cc. Vial.

GUIATUSCON. (CMC) Liq. Bot. 4 oz., pt., gal.

GUIATUSCON A.C. (CMC) Liq. Bot. 4 oz., pt., gal.

GUIATUSCON D.M. (CMC) Syr. Bot. 4 oz., pt., gal.

GUIATUSS BERTUSS COUGH SYRUP. (Alton) Bot. 4 oz., 8 oz., 16 oz., gal.
Use: Cough relief.

GUIATUSS DM BERTUSS COUGH SYRUP. (Alton) Bot. 4 oz., 8 oz., 16 oz., gal.
Use: cough relief.

GUIDO. (Rocky Mtn.) Camphor 0.025 Gm., guaiacol 0.05 Gm., iodoform 0.01 Gm., eucalyptol 0.04 Gm. Vial 30 cc.
Use: Expectorant.

GUISTREY FORTIS. (Bowman) Guaifenesin 100 mg., phenylephrine HCl 10 mg., chlorpheniramine maleate 1 mg./Tab. Bot. 100s, 1000s.
Use: Cold symptoms.

GUM-ZOR. (DeWitt) Lot. Bot. ½ oz.

GUNCOTTON, SOLUBLE. Pyroxylin.

GUSTALAC. (Geriatric) Cal. carbonate 300 mg.,

GUSTASE

282

defatted skim milk pow. 200 mg./Tab. Bot. 100s, 250s, 1000s.
Use: Antacid in the treatment of peptic ulcers.

GUSTASE. (Geriatric) Gerilase (standard amylolytic enzyme) 30 gm., geriprotase (standard proteolytic enzyme) 6 mg., gericellulase (standard cellulolytic enzyme) 2 mg./Tab. Bot. 42s, 100s, 500s.
Use: Digestion.

GUSTASE PLUS. (Geriatric) Phenobarbital 8 mg., homatropine methylbromide 2.5 mg., gerilase 30 mg., geriprotase 6 mg., gericellulase 2 mg./Tab. Bot. 42s, 100s, 500s.
Use: Antispasmodic and a sedative.

• **GUTTA PERCHA,** U.S.P. XXI.
Use: Dental restoration agent.

G-VITAMIN.
See: Riboflavin (Various Mfr.)

GLYNAPHEN TABLETS. (Lannett) Phenobarbital ⅛ gr., ext. hyoscyamus ¹/₁₀ gr., terpin hydrate 2 gr., guaifenesin 1 gr., calcium lactate 1 gr./Tab. Bot. 1000s.

GYN. (Amfre-Grant) Mag. gluconate 0.5 Gm./Tab. Bot. 100s, 1000s.
Use: Antispasmodic in treatment of primary dysmenorrhea.

GYNECORT. (Combe) Hydrocortisone acetate 0.5%. Tube 0.5 oz., 1.0 oz.
Use: Pruritus vulvae.

GYNE-LOTRIMIN VAGINAL CREAM 1%. (Schering) Clotrimazole 50 mg./applicatorful. Tube 45 Gm.
Use: Vulvovaginal candidiasis.

GYNE-LOTRIMIN VAGINAL TABLETS. (Schering) Clotrimazole 100 mg./Tab. Box 7 Tab. w/applicator.
Use: Vulvovaginal candidiasis.

GYNERGEN. (Sandoz) Ergotamine tartrate 1.0 mg./Tab. Bot. 100s.
Use: Orally, treatment of migraine.

GYNERGON.
See: Estradiol (Various Mfr.)

GYNE-SEC. (Marlyn) Diiodohydroxyquinoline 100 mg., sulfadiazine 500 mg., sorbic acid 5 mg., stilbestrol 0.1 mg., methylbenzethonium chloride 7.5 mg., boric acid 100 mg., sod. lauryl sulfate 5 mg., lactose 300 mg., tartaric acid 5 mg./insert. Box 20s, 50s w/applicator.
Use: Vaginal infections.

GYNLIN. (Tunex) Estrone 2 mg./ml. in aq. susp. Vial 30 cc.
Use: Estrogen deficiency.

GYNLIN R.P. (Tunex) Estrone 2 mg., potassium estrone sulfate 1 mg./ml. in aq. susp. Vial 10cc.
Use: Rapid & prolonged estrogen therapy.

GYNOGEN. (O'Neal, Jones & Feldman) Estrogenic substance 2 mg./ml. Vial 30 ml.

GYNOGEN L.A. 10. (O'Neal, Jones & Feldman) Estradiol valerate in sesame oil 10 mg./ml. Vial 10 ml.

GYNOGEN L.A. 20. (O'Neal, Jones & Feldman) Estradiol valerate in sesame oil 20 mg./ml. Vial 10 ml.

GYNOGEN R. P. (O'Neal, Jones & Feldman) Estrone 2 mg., estradiol 0.1 mg./ml. Vial 10 ml.

GYNOL II CONTRACEPTIVE JELLY. (Ortho) Nonxynol-9 in 2% concentration. Starter (2.85 oz. tube w/applicator) Refill (4.44 oz. tube).
Use: Contraceptive jelly for use with diaphragm.

GYNO-PETRARYL. (Janssen) Econazole nitrate.
Use: Antifungal.

H

HACHIMYCIN. B.A.N. An antibiotic produced by *Streptomyces hachijoensis.*
Use: Antibiotic used in the treatment of trichomoniasis.
See: Trichomycin

HAEMATE P. (Hoechst) Factor VIII (Human). Packs of 250 I.U., 500 I.U. or 1000 I.U. for Inj.
Use: Hemophilia therapy.

• **HALAZEPAM,** USAN.
Use: Sedative.
See: Paxipam, Tab. (Schering)

• **HALAZONE,** U.S.P. XXI Tab. for Soln., U.S.P. XXI. p-(Dichlorosulfamoyl)benzoic acid. (Abbott) Tab. 4 mg. Bot. 100s.
Use: Disinfectant.

• **HALCINONIDE.** USAN. Corticosteroid halcinonide. 21-Chloro-9-fluoro-11,16,17-trihydroxy-pregna-4-ene -3,20-dione, cyclic 16,17 acetal.
Use: Anti-inflammatory.
See: Halciderm Cream (Squibb)
      Halog Cream Oint., Sol. (Squibb)

HALCINONIDE. B.A.N. 21-Chloro-9α-fluoro-11β-hydroxy-16α, 17 α-isopropylidenedioxypregn-4-ene-3, 20-dione.
Use: Corticosteroid.

HALCION. (Upjohn) Triazolam 0.25 mg. or 0.5 mg./Tab. Bot. 100s. Unit dose 100s.
Use: Hypnotic for insomnia.

HALDOL. (McNeil Pharm) Haloperidol. **Tab.:** 0.5 mg., 1 mg., 2 mg./Tab. Bot. 100s, 1000s. 5 mg., 10 mg. Bot. 100s, 1000s. 20 mg. Bot. 100s. Blister Pack 10×10s in all sizes.**Conc. Soln.:** 2 mg./cc. Bot. 15 cc. 120 cc. **Inject.:** (w/methylparaben 1.8 mg. propylparaben 0.2 mg., lactic acid) ampul 5 mg./cc. Box 10×1 ml. & multidose vial of 10 ml. Prefilled Syringe 10×1 ml.
Use: Antipsychotic.

HALDRONE. (Lilly) Paramethasone acetate 1 mg./Tab. Bot. 100s. 2 mg./Tab. Bot. 100s.
Use: Steroid therapy, anti-inflammatory agent.

HALENOL. (Blue Cross) Acetaminophen 325 mg./Tab. Bot. 100s.
Use: Analgesic.

HALENOL ELIXIR. (Blue Cross) Acetaminophen 120 mg./5 ml. w/alcohol 7%. Bot. 4 oz.
Use: Analgesic for children.

HALENOL EXTRA STRENGTH CAPSULES. (Blue Cross) Acetaminophen 500 mg./Cap. Bot. 100s.
Use: Analgesic, antipyretic

HALENOL EXTRA STRENGTH TABLETS. (Blue Cross) Acetaminophen 500 mg./Tab. Bot. 100s.
Use: Analgesic, antipyretic

HALETHAZOLE. B.A.N. 5-Chloro-2-[4-(2-diethyl-amino-ethoxy)phenyl]benzothiazole.
Use: Antifungal agent.
See: Episol

HALEY'S M-O. (Winthrop Products) Mineral oil (25%) & milk of magnesia in emulsion base. Bot. 8 oz., 1 pt., 1 qt. Flavored and regular.
Use: Laxative.

HALFORT-T. (Blue Cross) Vit. C 300 mg., B-1 15 mg., B-2 10 mg., Niacin 100 mg., B-6 5 mg., B-12 4 mcg., pantothenic acid 20 mg./Tab. Bot. 100s.
Use: Vitamin supplement.

HALI-BEST. (Barth's) Vit. A 10,000 I.U., D 400 I.U./Cap. Bot. 100s, 500s.

HALIBUT LIVER OIL.
Use: Vitamin A & D deficiencies.

HALIVER OIL.
See: Halibut Liver Oil (Various Mfr.)

HALIVER OIL WITH VIOSTEROL.
See: Halibut Liver Oil with Viosterol

HALLS MENTHO-LYPTUS DECONGESTANT COUGH FORMULA. (Warner-Lambert) Dextromethorphan HBr 15 mg., phenylpropanolamine HCl 37.5 mg., menthol 14 mg., eucalyptus oil 12.7 mg./10 ml. w/alcohol 22%. Bot. 3 oz. 6 oz.
Use: Antitussive, decongestant.

HALL'S MENTHO-LYPTUS COUGH TABLETS.
(Warner-Lambert) Menthol and eucalyptus oil in varying amounts. Regular, honey-lemon, cherry flavor and ice blue. Stick-Pack 9s. Bags 30s.
Use: Antitussive.

HALODRIN. (Upjohn) Fluoxymesterone 1 mg., ethinyl estradiol 0.02 mg./Tab. Bot. 100s.
Use: Hormone preparation.

• **HALOFANTRINE HYDROCHLORIDE.** USAN.
Use: Antimalarial.

• **HALOFENATE.** USAN. 2-Acetamidoethyl (4-chlorophenyl) (3-trifluoromethylphenoxy)-acetate.
Use: Hypolipemic agent.
See: Livipas (Merck Sharp & Dohme).

HALOFUGINONE. B.A.N.DL-trans-7-Bromo-6-chloro-3-[3-(3-hydroxy-2-piperidyl)-2-acetonyl]-quinazolin-4-one.
Use: Antiprotozoan, veterinary medicine.

• **HALOFUGINONE HYDROBROMIDE.** USAN.
Use: Anti-protozoal.

HALOGAN. (Blue Cross) Chloroxylenol, acetic acid, glycerin, benzalkonium Cl. Ear drops Bot. 0.5 oz.
Use: Remove ear wax.

HALOG CREAM. (Squibb) Halcinonide 0.025% and 0.1%, in specially formulated cream base consisting of glyceryl monostearate, cetyl alcohol, myristyl stearate, isopropyl palmitate, polysorbate 60, propylene glycol and purified water. Tube 15 Gm., 30 Gm., 60 Gm., Jar 240 Gm.
Use: Topical corticosteroid therapy.

HALOG E CREAM. (Squibb) Halcinonide 0.1 mg. in hydrophylic vanishing cream base consisting of propylene glycol dimethicone 350, castor oil, cetearyl alcohol, ceteareth-20, propylene glycol stearate, white petrolatum, water. Tubes 15, 30, 60 Gm.
Use: Topical corticosteroid therapy.

HALOG OINTMENT. (Squibb) Halcinonide 0.1%, in Plastibase (plasicized hydrocarbon gel), PEG 400, PEG 6000 distearate, PEG 300, PEG 1540, and butylated hydroxy toluene. Tube 15 Gm., 30 Gm., 60 Gm., Jar 240 Gm.
Use: Anti-infammatory, antipruritic, vasoconstrictor.

HALOG SOLUTION. (Squibb) Halcinonide 0.1 mg./ml. w/edetate disodium, PEG 300, purified water and butylated hydroxy toluene as preservative. Bot. 20 ml., 60 ml.
Use: Topical corticosteroid therapy.

• **HALOPEMIDE.** USAN.
Use: Antipsychotic.

HALOPENIUM CHLORIDE. B.A.N. 4-Bromo-benzyl-3-(4-chloro-2-isopropyl-5-methyl-phenoxy)-propyldim-ethylammonium chloride.
Use: Antiseptic.

• **HALOPERIDOL,** U.S.P. XXI. Tab., Inj., Oral Soln. U.S.P. XXI. 4[-4-p-Chlorophenyl-4-hydroxy-piperidi-no]-4'-fluorobutyrophenone. Serenace Sol.
Use: Antipsychotic, tranquilizer.
See: Haldol, Tab., Conc., Inj. (McNeil)

• **HALOPERIDOL DECANOATE.** USAN.
Use: Antipsychotic.

• **HALOPREDONE ACETATE.** USAN.
Use: Anti-inflammatory.

• **HALOPROGESTERONE.** USAN. 6α-Fluoro-17α-bromo-progesterone.
Use: Progestin.

• **HALOPROGIN,** U.S.P. XXI. Cream, Top. Soln., U.S.P. XXI. 3-Iodo-2-propynyl-2, 4, 5-trichlorophenyl ether. Under study.
Use: Antimicrobic.
See: Halotex, Cream & Sol. (Westwood)

HALOPYRAMINE. B.A.N. 2-(4-Chloro-N-2-pyridylben-zylamino)ethyldimethylamine. Chloropyramine (I.N.N.)
Use: Antihistamine.
See: Synopen hydrochloride

HALORTON. (Vita Elixir) #1 chlorprophenpridamine 4 mg./Time Rel. Cap; #2 chlorprophenpridamine 8 mg./Timed Rel. Cap.; #3 chlorprophenpridamine 12 mg./Timed Rel. Cap.
Use: Antihistaminic.

HALOTESTIN. (Upjohn) Fluoxymesterone, 2 mg./Tab. Bot. 100s; 5 mg./Tab. Bot. 100s; 10 mg./Tab. Bot. 100s. Unit-of-Use Bot. 30s.
Use: Androgenic and anabolic agent.
W/Ethinyl estradiol.
See: Halodrin, Tab. (Upjohn)

HALOTEX CREAM. (Westwood) Haloprogin 1% in water dispersible, base composed of PEG-400, PEG-4000, diethyl sebacate, polyvinylpyrrolidone. Tube 15 Gm., 30 Gm.
Use: Treatment of superficial fungal infections of the skin.

HALOTEX SOLUTION. (Westwood) Haloprogin 1% in a vehicle of diethyl sebacate w/alcohol 75%. Bot. 10 ml., 30 ml.
Use: Treatment of superficial fungal infections of the skin.

• **HALOTHANE,** U.S.P. XXI. 2-Bromo-2-chloro-1-1,1-
trifluoroethane. Fluothane.
Use: General anesthetic (inhalation).
See: Fluothane, Liq. (Ayerst)
Halothane, 250 ml. Liquid (Abbott)
HALOTUSSIN. (Blue Cross) Guaifenesin 100 mg./5
ml. Bot. 4 oz.
Use: Expectorant.
HALOTUSSIN-DM. (Blue Cross) Guaifenesin 100 mg.,
dextromethorphan HBr 15 mg./5 ml.
Use: Expectorant, cough suppressant.
HALOXON. B.A.N. Bis(2-chloroethyl)3-chloro-4-methyl-
coumarin-7-yl-phosphate.
Use: Anthelmintic, veterinary medicine.
See: Loxon
HALQUINOL. B.A.N. A mixture of the chlorinated
products of 8-hydroxyquinoline containing about 65
per cent of 5,7-dichloro-8-hydroxyquinoline.
Use: Anti-infective.
See: Quixalin
• **HALQUINOLS.** USAN. 5, 7-Dichloro-8-quinolinol; 5-
chloro-8-quinolinol and 7-chloro-8-quinolinol in pro-
portions resulting naturally from chlorination of 8-
quinolinol. Trade mark, Quinolor (active ingredient
of) & Tarquinor.
Use: Topical antimicrobial.
HAMA. Hydroxy-aluminum magnesium aminoacetate.
• **HAMYCIN.** USAN.
Use: Antifungal.
HANDORA CREAM. (Torch) Greaseless, water-wash-
able cream, fatty alcohol glycerine, natural fatty
acid in hydrophillic base.
Use: Restore & maintain normal skin tone when
exposed to irritants.
HANG-OVER-CURE. (Silvers) Calcium carbonate,
glycine, thiamine HCl, pyridoxine HCl, aspirin. Cont.
6 Tab.
Use: Hangover treatment.
HANIFORM. (Hanlon) Vit. A 25,000 I.U., D 1,000 I.U.,
B-1 10 mg., B-2 5 mg., C 150 mg., niacinamide 150
mg./Cap. Bot. 100s.
Use: Dietary supplement.
HANIPLEX. (Hanlon) Vit. B-1 20 mg., B-2 10 mg., B-6
1 mg., Ca pantothenate 10 mg., B-12 5 mcg., niacin
20 mg., liver conc. 50 mg., Vit. C 150 mg./Cap.
Bot. 100s.
Use: Dietary supplement.
■ **HANSEN'S DISEASE.** Leprosy.
See: Diasone, Sod., Tab. (Abbott)
Ethyl Chaulmoograte (Various Mfr.)
Isoniazid (Various Mfr.)
HAPONAL. (Jenkins) Atropine sulfate 0.96 mg.,
hyoscine HBr 0.02 mg., hyoscyamine sulfate 0.30
mg., phenobarbital 50 mg./Cap. Bot. 1000s.
Use: Antispasmodic.
HAPONAL. (Kenyon) Atropine sulfate 0.0195 mg.,
hyoscine HBr 0.0065 mg., hyoscyamine sulfate
0.1040 mg., phenobarbital ¼ gr./Tab. Bot. 100s,
1000s.
Use: Antispasmodic.
HARBOLIN. (Arcum) Hydralazine HCl 25 mg.,

hydrochlorothiazide 15 mg., reserpine 0.1 mg./Tab.
Bot. 100s, 1000s.
HARCYTE. (Harvey) Estradiol benzoate 2.5 mg.,
progesterone 25 mg./cc. sesame oil. Vial 10 cc.
HARMAR. (Zemmer) Propoxyphene HCl 65 mg./Cap.
Bot. 500s.
HARMONYL. (Abbott) Deserpidine 0.1 mg./Tab. Bot.
100s; 0.25 mg./Tab. Bot. 100s, 1000s.
Use: Treatment of hypertension.
HARTSHORN. Ammonium Carbonate
HARVADEN. (Harvey) Adenosine-5-monophosphoric
acid 25 mg., Vit. B-12 60 mcg./cc. Vial 10 cc.
Use: I.M., neuritis and pruritus.
W/Phenobarbital. (Durst) Atropine methyl nitrate 1/60
gr., phenobarbital ¼ gr./Tab. Bot. 100s, 1000s,
5000s.
Use: Antispasmodic with sedative.
HARVATROPIN. (Harvey) Chorionic gonadotropin
1000 I.U./cc. when diluted. Vial 10 cc., w/diluent.
Use: Treatment of cryptorchidism.
HAUGASE. (Madland) Trypsin, chymotrypsin. Bot.
50s, 250s.
Use: Enzyme therapy.
HAUTOSONE. (Fellows) Hydrocortisone 0.5% in
Triusol (three polyols) 15 Gm. Box 6s.
HAVAB. (Abbott) Test kits 100s.
Use: Radioimmunoassay or enzyme immunoassay
for detection of antibody to hepatitis A virus.
HAVAB-M. (Abbott) Test kits 100s. Uses radioim-
munoassay or enzyme immunoassay for the
detection of specific IgM antibody to hepatitis A
virus in human serum or plasma.
HAYNON. Chlorpheniramine, B.A.N.
HAZOGEL BODY AND FOOT RUB. (Nortech) Witch
hazel 70%, isopropanol 20% in a neutralized resin
vehicle. Bot. 4 oz.
Use: Relief of topical itching; soothing body and
foot rub.
H-BIG HEPATITIS B IMMUNE GLOBULIN (HUMAN).
(Abbott) Hepatitis B immune globulin (human) Vials
4, 5 ml.
Use: Immune globulin.
HC DERMA-PAX. (Recsei) Hydrocortisone 0.5% in liq-
uid base. Dropper Bot. 2 oz.
Use: Treatment of poison oak, poison ivy, insect
bites, cold sores.
HC-FORM. (Recsei) Hydrocortisone 1%, clioquinol 3%,
chlorobutanol 1%. Jelly ½ oz., 1 oz., 1 lb.
Use: Contact and atopic dermatitis.
HC-JEL. (Recsei) Hydrocortisone 1%, chlorobutanol
1%. Jelly ½ oz., 1 oz., 1 lb.
Use: Dermatitis, pruritus.
HCV CREME. (Saron) Hydrocortisone alcohol 1%,
clioquinol 3%. Tube 15 Gm., 45 Gm.
Use: Antibacterial, anti-inflammatory.
HEAD & CHEST CAPSULES. (Procter & Gamble)
Phenylpropanolamine HCl 25 mg., guaifenesin 200
mg./Cap. Bot. 12s, 24s.
Use: Decongestant/expectorant cold medicine.
HEAD & CHEST LIQUID. (Procter & Gamble)
Phenylpropanolamine HCl 12.5 mg., guaifenesin
100 mg./5 ml. w/alcohol 5%. Bot. 4 oz., 8 oz.

Use: Decongestant, expectorant cold medicine.

HEAD & CHEST TABLETS. (Procter & Gamble) Phenylpropanolamine HCl 25 mg., guaifenesin 200 mg./Tab. Bot. 18s, 36s.
Use: Decongestant, expectorant cold medicine.

HEAD & SHOULDERS. (Procter & Gamble) Zinc 2-pyridinethiol-1-oxide 2% in cream or lotion detergent shampoo. **Cream** Tube 2.5 oz., 4 oz., 7 oz. **Lotion** 4 oz., 7 oz., 11 oz., 15 oz.
Use: Dandruff treatment and seborrheic dermatitis of the scalp.

HEALON. (Pharmacia) Sodium hyaluronate 10 mg./ml. Syringes 0.4, 0.75, or 2.0 ml.
Use: Surgical aid in cataract extraction, IOL implantation, corneal transplant, glaucoma filtration, retinal attachment surgery.

HEART MUSCLE DEPRESSANT.
See: Pronestyl HCl, Cap., Vial (Squibb)

HEART MUSCLE EXTRACTS, Adenosine-5-Monophosphate sodium.

HEATROL. (Cross) Sodium Cl., potassium Cl, calcium phosphate, mg. carbonate. Safety pks. 1000s. Medipaks 200s. Aidpaks 100s. Dispensers 350s.
Use: Replacement of electrolytes lost from perspiration.

HEAVY METAL POISONING, ANTIDOTE.
See: BAL., Amp. (Hynson, Westcott & Dunning)
Calcium Disodium Versenate, Amp., Tab. (Riker)

HEB CREAM BASE. (Barnes-Hind) Washable, hypoallergenic, odorless base. Jar 1 lb.
Use: For the incorporation of many of the medicinals used in dermatology.

HEDAQUINIUM CHLORIDE. B.A.N.
Hexadecamethylenedi-(2-isoquinolinium chloride).
Use: Antifungal agent.
See: Teoquil

HEDEX CAPLETS. (Winthrop Products) Paracetamol.
Use: Analgesic.

HEDULIN. (Merrell Dow) Phenindione 50 mg./Tab. Bot. 100s.
Use: Anticoagulant. **Note: Manufacture voluntarily stopped in 1983.**

HEET LINAMENT. (Whitehall) Methyl salicylate 15%, camphor 3.6%, oloeoresin capsicum 0.025%, alcohol 70%. Bot. 2⅓ oz., 5 oz.
Use: External analgesic.

• **HEFILCON A.** USAN.
Use: Contact lens material.

• **HELFILCON B.** USAN.
Use: Contact lens material.

HEISKELL'S OINTMENT. (Guild) Pkg. 1 oz.

HEISKELL'S SKIN SOAP. (Guild) Cake 3½ oz., 5 oz.

• **HELIUM,** U.S.P. XXI.
Use: Diluent for gases.

HELMATAC. Parbendazole, B.A.N.

HEMABEX. (Barry-Martin) Vit. B-1 40 mg., B-2 16 mg., B-6 1 mg., niacinamide 20 mg., B-12 18 mcg., Ca pantothenate 10 mg., inositol 50 mg., ferric ammonium citrate 720 mg., choline dihydrogen citrate 150 mg./Fl. oz. Bot. pt., gal.
Use: Vit. B complex.

HEMA-CHEK. (Ames) Fecal occult blood test containing slide tests, developer and applicators. Pkg. 100s, 300s, 1000s.
Use: Fecal occult blood test.

HEMA-C META-KAPS. (Sutliff & Case) Ferrous fumarate 300 mg. (100 mg. iron), ascorbic acid 200 mg./long acting Granucap. Bot. 100s, 1000s.

HEMA-COMBISTIX. (Ames) Four-way strip test of urinary pH, glucose, protein and occult blood. Strips. Bot. 100s.

HEMAFATE T.D. CAPSULES. (Knight) Bot. 60s.
Use: Sustained-action hematinic.

HEMAFERRIN TABLETS. (Western Research) Ferrous fumarate 150 mg., desiccated liver 50 mg., docusate sodium 25 mg., betaine HCl 100 mg., folic acid 0.4 mg., Vit. C 50 mg., B-6 2 mg., manganese 2 mg., B-12 5 mcg., copper 1 mg., zinc 2 mg., molybdenum 0.4 mg./Tab. 28 Pack 1000s.
Use: Non-constipating hematinic.

HEMAFOLATE. (Canright) Ferrous gluconate 293 mg., liver fraction II 250 mg., gastric sub. 100 mg., Vit. C 50 mg., B-12 10 mcg./Tab. Bot. 100s, 1000s.
Use: Hematinic agent.

HEMA-FORTE. (Stayner) Vit. B-1 5 mg., B-2 5 mg., B-6 1 mg., Ca pantothenate 2 mg., niacinamide 25 mg., liver desiccated 300 mg., iron 25 mg., inositol 25 mg., choline bitartrate 25 mg., B-12 5 mcg., C 50 mg./Tab. Bot. 100s, 1000s.
Use: B vitamin-iron supplement.

HEMAGLO. (Seatrace) Cyanocobalamin 15 mcg./ml. Vial 30 cc.

HEMALIVE LIQUID. (Barth's) Vit. B-1 3.15 mg., B-2 3.33 mg., niacin 22.5 mg., B-6 0.81 mg., B-12 6 mcg., biotin 3.6 mcg., iron 60 mg., choline, inositol, liver fraction No. 1, pantothenic acid./15 cc. Bot. 8 oz., 24 oz.
Use: Iron and vitamin supplement.

HEMALIVE TABLETS. (Barth's) Vit. B-12 25 mcg., iron 75 mg., B-1 2.5 mg., B-2 5 mg., niacin 1.4 mg., C 30 mg., liver 240 mg., B-6, pantothenic acid, aminobenzoic acid, choline, inositol, biotin, Mg, Mn, Cu/3 Tab. Bot. 100s, 500s, 1000s.
Use: Iron and vitamin supplement.

HEMANEED. (Hanlon) Hematinic B-12, intrinsic factor, iron/Cap. Bot. 100s.

■ **HEMAPOIETIC AGENTS.**
See: Iron products
Lipotropic Preparations
Liver Products
Vitamins

HEMASPAN. (Bock) Ferrous fumarate 275 mg., Vit. C 100 mg., docusate sodium 20 mg./Cap. Bot. 100s, 1000s.
Use: Anemia.

HEMASPAN-FA. (Bock) Ferrous fumarate 275 mg., ascorbic acid 100 mg., docusate sodium 20 mg., folic acid 1 mg./Cap. Bot. 100s, 1000s.
Use: Anemia treatment.

HEMASTIX. (Ames) A cellulose strip, impregnated with a peroxide and orthotolidine. Bot. 50s.
Use: Detection hematuria and hemoglobinuria.

HEMAT. (Kenyon) Iron 57.4 mg., Vit. B-1 3 mg., B-2 2 mg., B-12 1 mcg., niacinamide 5 mg., liver desic. 2 gr., stomach substance 50 mg./Tab. Bot. 100s, 1000s.
Use: Hematinic.

HEMATEST. (Ames) Strontium peroxide, o-Tolidin, tartaric acid & Cal. acetate. Tab. Bot. 100s.
Use: Diagnostic aid for the test of blood in the feces.

HEMATINIC. (Canright) Ferrous gluconate 180 mg., liver desic. 200 mg., Vit. B-12 1 mcg., copper gluconate 0.3 mg., Vit. C 25 mg., B-1 3.3 mg./Tab. Bot. 100s, 1000s.
Use: Anemias.

HEMATINIC CAPSULES. (Robinson) Vit. B-1 1 mg., B-2 2 mg., iron 40 mg., Vit. B-12 1 mcg., liver desic. 200 mg./Cap. Bot. 100s, 1000s.

■ **HEMATINICS.**
See: Iron Products
    Ferric Compounds
    Ferrous Compounds
    Liver Products
    Vitamin B-12
    Vitamin Products

HEMATOVALS. (Ulmer) Vit. C 75 mg., B-1 3 mg., B-2 3 mg., Niacin 10 mg., B-6 1 mg., B-12 3 mcg., pantothenic acid 5 mg., iron 75 mg./Cap. Bot. 100s.
Use: Dietary supplement.

HEMATRAN. (Hauck) Iron dextran 50 mg./ml. Bot 10 ml.
Use: Hematinic.

HEMATRIN. (Towne) Iron 50 mg., Vit. B-12 10 mcg., copper 0.25 mg., B-1 10 mg., B-2 10 mg., B-6 2 mg., C 150 mg., niacinamide 50 mg., calcium pantothenate 5 mg., liver desic. 200 mg./Captab. Bot. 60s, 100s.

HEMATRIN NO. 1. (Kenyon) Ferrous sulfate ex. 200 mg., desic. liver N.F. 200 mg., stomach substance 100 mg., C 50 mg., folic acid 1 mg., B-12 w/intrinsic factor conc. 0.25 I.U., B-12 N.F. (from cobalamin conc.) 6.26 mcg./Tab. Bot. 100s.

HEMATRIN NO. 2. (Kenyon) Intrinsic factor w/Vit. B-12 ½ I.U., liver stomach conc. 175 mg., Vit. B-12 conc. 10 mcg., folic acid 0.2 mg., ferrous sulfate exsic. 400 mg., Vit. C 75 mg./Cap. Bot. 100s, 1000s.
Use: Hematinic.

HEMET OINTMENT. (Blue Cross) Zinc oxide 5%, diperodon HCl 0.25%, bismuth subcarbonate 0.2%, pyrilamine maleate 0.1%, phenylephrine HCl 0.25% in petroleum base. Tube 1.5 oz.
Use: Rectal anesthetic.

HEMET SUPPOSITORIES. (Blue Cross) Bismuth subgallate, zinc oxide, boric acid, bismuth resorcin comp., balsam, benzocaine/Supp. Box. 12s.
Use: Hemorrhoid treatment.

HEMEX. (Vogarell) Ointment Tube 1¼ oz., Suppositories Box 12s.
Use: Relief of piles and minor rectal irritations.

HEMISINE.
See: Epinephrine (Various Mfr.)

HEMISUCCINOXYPREGNENOLONE, DELTA-5-Panzalone.

HEMOCAINE. (Mallard) Benzocaine 1%, phenol 1%, tannic acid 3%, thymol iodide 1%, ephedrine HCl 0.15%, zinc oxide 10%, peru balsam 2%. Jar 1 oz., 1 lb.
Use: Relief of itching and irritation from hemorrhoids.

HEMOCYTE. (U.S. Chemical) Ferrous fumarate 324 mg./Tab. Bot. 100s. Vial 10 cc.
Use: Anemia.

HEMOCYTE-F. (U.S. Chemical) Ferrous fumarate 325 mg., folic acid 1 mg./Tab.
Use: Hematinic, anti-anemic.

HEMOCYTE PLUS. (U.S. Chemical) Ferrous fumarate 324 mg., sodium ascorbate 200 mg., Vit. B-1 10 mg., B-2 6 mg., B-6 5 mg., B-12 15 mcg., Folic acid 1 mg., niacinamide 30 mg. Ca pantothenate 10 mg., Zn sulfate 80 mg., Mg sulfate 70 mg., Mn sulfate 4 mg., Cu sulfate 2 mg./Tabule. Bot. 100s.
Use: Anemia treatment.

HEMOFIL. (Hyland) Antihemophilic factor (human), method four, dried, concentrated. Vial W/Diluent. 10 ml., 30 ml.
Use: Antihemophilia therapy.

HEMOFIL T. (Hyland) Antihemophilia Factor (Human), method four, dried, heat-treated 225–375 IU/10 ml.; 450–650 IU/20 ml.; 675–999 IU/30 ml.; 1000–1600 IU/30 ml.
Use: Treatment of Hemophilia A, for prevention & control of hemorrhagic episodes.

HEMOFORM. (Spanner) Iron, arsenic, Cu. Ampul 10 cc. 100s.

HEMOGEST. (Mills) Betaine HCl 50 mg., ferrous fumarate 100 mg., folic acid 0.05 mg., zinc gluconate 5 mg., copper gluconate 10 mg., manganese gluconate 5 mg., Vit. B-1 1 mg., B-2 1 mg., B-6 0.5 mg., Vit. B-12 1 mcg., niacinamide 10 mg./Tab. Bot. 100s.
Use: Hematinic.

HEMORRHOIDAL OINTMENT. (Towne) Benzocaine 2%, Peruvian balsam 1.25%, zinc oxide 10%, 8-hydroxyquinoline benzoate 0.5%, menthol 0.4%, methylparaben 0.1%, propylparaben 0.1%, petrolatum base. Tube 1½ oz.

HEMORRHOIDAL UNISERTS. (Upsher-Smith) Bismuth subgallate 2.25%, bismuth resorcin compound 1.75%, benzyl benzoate 1.2%, peruvian balsam 1.8%, zinc oxide 11%/Suppos. Cartons 12s, 50s.
Use: Treatment of hemorrhoids.

HEMORRHOIDAL-HC UNISERTS. (Upsher-Smith) Hydrocortisone acetate 10 mg., bismuth subgallate 2.25%, bismuth resorcin compound 1.75%, benzyl benzoate 1.2%, peruvian balsam 1.8%, zinc oxide 11%/Suppos. Cartons 12s, 50s.
Use: Treatment of hemorrhoids.

HEMOSTATICS, LOCAL.
See: Absorbable Gelatin Sponge (Upjohn)
    Gelfilm (Upjohn)
    Gelfoam, Preps. (Upjohn)

Oxidized Cellulose
Thrombin (Various Mfr.)

■ **HEMOSTATICS, SYSTEMIC.**
See: Adrenosem Salicylate, Prep. (Beecham-Massengill)
Carbazochrome Salicylate

HEMOSTATIN.
See: Epinephrine (Various Mfr.)

HEMO-VITE. (Drug Industries) Ferrous fumarate 240 mg., Cu sulfate 1 mg., C 150 mg., B-1 5 mg., B-2 5 mg., B-6 1 mg., Ca pantothenate 10 mg., niacinamide 50 mg., folic acid 0.2 mg., intrinsic factor, B-12 0.5 I.U./-Tab. Bot. 100s, 500s. Liq. Bot. pt.
Use: Vitamin supplement to treat anemias.

HEMOVITE LIQUID. (Drug Industries) Vit. B-12 crystallin 8.34 mcg., B-6 2.0 mg., ferric pyrophosphate soluble 100 mg., folic acid 0.25 mg., niacinamide 13.3 mg./5cc. Bot. 473cc
Use: Vitamin supplement to treat anemias.

HEMOZYME ELIXIR. (Barrows) Vit. B-1 5 mg., B-2 5 mg., B-6 1 mg., panthenol 4 mg., niacinamide 100 mg., B-12 3 mcg., iron 100 mg., choline bitartrate 100 mg., dl-methionine 100 mg., yeast extract and alcohol 12%/fl. oz. Bot. 12 oz.
Use: Iron tonic.

HENBANE.
See: Hyoscyamus (Various Mfr.)

HENYDIN-M. (Arcum) Thyroid desic. powd. ½ gr., B-1 1 mg., B-2 0.5 mg., B-6 0.5 mg., niacinamide 2.5 mg./Tab. Bot. 100s, 1000s.

HENYDIN-R. (Arcum) Thyroid desic. powd. 1 gr., B-1 2 mg., B-2 1 mg., B-6 1 mg., niacinamide 5 mg./Tab. Bot. 100s, 1000s.

HEPAHYDRIN, Tab. (Comatic) Dehydrocholic acid 3.75 Gm./Tab. Bot. 100s.

HEPANE-LS EXTRA. (Kenyon) Vit. B-12 activity 40 mcg./cc. Vial 10 cc.

■ **HEPARIN ANTAGONIST.**
See: Protamine Sulfate (Various Mfr.)

HEPARIN CALCIUM.
Use: Anticoagulant
See: Calciparine, Inj. (American Critical Care)

HEPARIN LOCK FLUSH SOLUTION. (Winthrop-Breon) 10 USP Units/1 ml. in 2 ml. cartridge or 100 USP Units/1 ml. in 2 ml. cartridge. Carpuject.
Use: Maintain patency of indwelling venipuncture device.

HEPARIN LOCK FLUSH SOLUTION. (Wyeth) Heparin sodium 10 u. or 100 u./1 ml. vial. Pkg. 50 Tubex 1 ml., 2 ml.
Use: Clearing intermittent infusion sets.

• **HEPARIN SODIUM,** U.S.P. XXI. Inj., Lock Flush Sol., U.S.P. XXI. (Upjohn) 1,000 Units/ml. Vial 10 ml., 30 ml. 5,000 Units/ml. Vial 1 ml., 10 ml. 10,000 Units/ml. Vial 1 ml., 4 ml. (Winthrop) 5,000 USP Units/1 ml. Carpuject 1 ml. fill in 2 ml. cartridge.
Use: I.M., I.V. or S.C., anticoagulant in prevention & treatment of thrombosis or embolism. Note: Protamine sulfate is antidote.
See: Hepathrom, Amp., Vial (Fellows-Testagar)
Heprinar, Inj. (Armour)
Lipo-Hepin, Amp., Vial (Riker)

Lipo-Hepin/BL, Amp., Vial (Riker)
Liquaemin, Vial (Organon)
W/Choline chloride, Vit. B-12, folic acid & niacinamide.
Hep-Plex, Vial (Kenyon)
W/Vit. B-12, folic acid, niacinamide, choline chloride.
See: Heparin-B, Vial (Medical Chem.)

• **HEPARIN CALCIUM,** U.S.P. XXI. Inj., U.S.P. XXI.
Use: Anticoagulant.

HEPATHROM. (Fellows) Heparin sodium. 1000 u. equals 10 mg. supplied: (1000 u./cc.) Vials Amp.1 cc., 10 cc., 30 cc. (5000 u./cc.) Amp. 1 cc., Vials 10 cc. (10,000 u./cc.) Amps. 1 cc., Vial 4 cc., 10 cc. (20,000 u./cc.) Vial 1 cc., 4, 5 & 10 cc. (40,000 u./cc.) Vials 1, 4 & 10 cc.

• **HEPATITIS B IMMUNE GLOBULIN,** U.S.P. XXI.
Use: Passive immunizing agent.

• **HEPATITIS B VIRUS VACCINE INACTIVATED,** U.S.P. XXI.
Use: Active immunizing agent.

HEP-B-GAMMAGEE. (Merck Sharp & Dohme) Hepatitis B Immune Globulin. Vial 5 ml.
Use: Post exposure prophylaxis for those exposed to HBsAg positive materials.

HEPFOMIN INJECTION. (Keene) Liver inj. equiv. to Cyanocobalamin 10 mcg., folic acid 1 mg., cyanocobalamine 100 mcg., niacinamide 75 mg. Vial 10 ml.

HEP-FORTE. (Marlyn) Bot. 100s, 500s.
Use: Vitamin-liver dietary supplement.

HEPICEBRIN. (Lilly) Vit. B-1 2 mg., Vit. B-2 3 mg., ascorbic acid 75 mg., niacinamide 20 mg., Vit. A 5000 I.U., D 400 I.U./Tab. Pkg. 100s. Blister pkg. 10 × 10s.
Use: Vitamin deficiencies.

HEP-PLEX. (Kenyon) Heparin sod. 2500 u., Vit. B-12 50 mcg., choline Cl 100 mg., folic acid 2 mg., niacinamide 50 mg. in isotonic saline/cc. Vial 10 cc.

HEPROFAX.
See: Mucoplex (Stuart)

HEPRON WITH MULTI-VITAMINS. (Norgine) Liver fraction #2 600 mg., vit. B-12 10 mcg., ferrous sulf. exsic. 180 mg., vit. A 10,000 I.U., D 1000 I.U., B-1 3 mg., B-2 5 mg., C 90 mg., niacinamide 30 mg./6 Tabs. Bot. 100s, 500s.
Use: Hematinic.

HEPTABARBITONE. B.A.N. 5-(Cyclohept-1-enyl)-5-ethylbarbituric acid.
Use: Hypnotic; sedative.
See: Medomin

HEPATAMINE. (American McGaw) Amino acid injection 8%. Bot. 500 ml.
Use: Nutritional support for liver diseased patients.

HEPTAMINOL. B.A.N. 6-Amino-2-methylheptan-2-ol.
Use: Coronary vasodilator.

3-HEPTANONE,6-DIMETHYLAMINO-4,4-DIPHENYL-HYDROCHLORIDE. Methadone Hydrochloride, U.S.P. XXI.

HEPATIC-AID. (American McGaw) Instant drinks & puddings.
Use: For hepatic disease patients.

HEP-LOCK. (Elkins-Sinn) Sterile heparin sodium solu-

tion in saline 10 U. or 100 U. Dosette 1 ml., 2 ml. Multiple dose vial 10 ml., 30 ml.
Use: Maintenance of patency of heparin lock catheters.

HEP-LOCK PF. (Elkins-Sinn) Preservative-free heparin flush sol. 10 U./ml. or 100 U./ml. Vial 1 ml.
Use: Maintenance of patency of heparin lock catherters.

HEPTAVAX-B. (Merck Sharp & Dohme) Hepatitis B vaccine. Vial 3 ml.
Use: Hepatitis immunization.

HEPTO. (Zenith) Meprobamate 150 mg., ethoheptazine citrate 75 mg., aspirin 250 mg./Tab.
Use: Relief of pain accompanied by anxiety and tension.

HEPTO-M. (Zenith) Meprobamate 200 mg., aspirin 325 mg./Tab. Bot. 50s
Use: Short term treatment of pain with anxiety.

HEPTUNA PLUS. (Roerig) B-1 3.1 mg., B-2 2 mg., B-6 1.6 mg., niacinamide 15 mg., calcium pantothenate 0.9 mg., B-12 5 mcg., with intrinsic factor conc. 25 mg., C 150 mg., liver des. 50 mg., ferrous sulfate, dried 311 mg., copper 1 mg., molybdenum 0.2 mg., calcium 37.4 mg., iodine 0.05 mg., manganese 0.033 mg., magnesium 2 mg., phosphorus 29 mg., potassium 1.7 mg./Cap. Bot. 100s.
Use: Nutritional deficiency.

HEROIN. Forbidden in U.S.A. by Federal statute because of its addiction-causing nature.
See: Diacetylmorphine.

HERPECIN-L. (Campbell) Pyridoxine HCl, allantoin, octyl p-(dimethylamino)-benzoate (Padimate O), titanium dioxide in a balanced, acidic lipid system. Tube 2.5 Gm.
Use: Cold sore lip balm.

HERPLEX LIQUIFILM. (Allergan) Idoxuridine 0.1%, polyvinyl alcohol 1.4%. Plast. Bot. w/dropper 15 ml.
Use: Ocular lesions produced by herpes simplex virus.

HESACORB. (Jenkins) Citrus bioflavonoids comp. 100 mg., C 100 mg./Cap. Bot. 1000s.

HES-BIC. (Kenyon) Hesperidin purified 100 mg., ascorbic acid 100 mg./Cap. Hesperidin purified 200 mg., ascorbic acid 200 mg./Tab. Bot. 100s, 1000s.
Use: Hemorrhage and capillary fragility.

HESPAN INJECTION. (American Critical Care) Hetastarch 6.0 Gm., sodium chloride 0.90 Gm./100 ml. w/water for injection. Bot. 500 ml.
Use: Plasma volume expander.

HESPER BITABS. (Merrell Dow) Hesperidin complex 200 mg./Tab. Bot. 100s.

HESPER CAPSULES. (Merrell Dow) Hesperidin complex 100 mg./Cap. w/lactose, calcium stearate, gelatin Bot. 100s.

HESPERIDIN.
Use: Capillary fragility and permeability, and hemorrhage.
See: Vitamin P; also Rutin
W/Combinations.
See: A.C.N., Tab. (Person & Covey)

Acna-Vite, Cap. (Cenci)
Ceebec, Tab. (Person & Covey)
Citrobic, Tab. (Blue Line)
HesBic, Cap., Tab. (Kenyon)
Hesper Bitabs, Tab. (Merrell Dow)
Nialex, Tab. (Mallard)
Norimex-Plus, Cap. (Vortech)
Ominal, Tab. (Kenwood)
Pregent, Tab. (Beutlich)
Vita Cebus, Tab. (Cenci)

HESPERIDIN W/C. (Various Mfr.)
Use: Vitamin P and C therapy.
See: Min-Hest, Cap. (Scrip)

HESPERIDIN METHYL CHALCONE.
Use: Deficiency of Vitamin P.

HETACILLIN. B.A.N. 6-(2,2-Dimethyl-5-oxo-4-phenylimidazolidin-1-yl)penicillanic acid.
Use: Antibiotic.

• **HETACILLIN,** U.S.P. XXI. For Oral Susp., Tab., U.S.P. XXI. 6-(2,2-Dimethyl-5-oxo-4-phenyl-1-imidazolidinyl)-3, 3-dimethyl-7-oxo-4-thia-1-azabicyclo[3.2.0] heptane-2-carboxylic acid.
Use: Antibiotic.
See: Versapen, Tab., Susp., Drops (Bristol)

• **HETACILLIN POTASSIUM,** U.S.P. XXI. Cap., Sterile, U.S.P. XXI.
See: Versapen-K, Vial, Cap. (Bristol)

• **HETAFLUR.** USAN.
Use: Dental caries prophylactic.

• **HETASTARCH.** USAN.
Use: Plasma volume extender. Hespan, Inj. (American Critical Care)

• **HETERONIUM BROMIDE.** USAN. $(\pm)$-3-Hydroxy-1, 1-dimethypyrrolidinium bromide, α-phenyl-2-thiopheneglycolate. Hetrum Chloride.
Use: Anticholinergic.

HEXABAX. (Kirkman) Antibacterial skin cleanser. Bot. pt.

HEXACHLORCYCLOHEXANE.
See: Benzene Hexachloride, Gamma.

γ**-1,2,3,4,5,6-HEXACHLOROCYCLOHEXANE.** Benzene Hexachloride, Gamma.

• **HEXACHLOROPHENE.** U.S.P. XXI. Phenol, 2,2′-methylenebis[3,4,6-trichloro-. 2.2′-Methylenebis (3,4,6-trichlorophenol). Di-(3,5,6-trichloro-2-hydroxyphenyl)methane. Hexachlorophene (I.N.N.)
Use: Antiseptic.
See: Derl
Gamophen, Leaves, Bar (Arbrook)
pHisohex Prods. (Winthrop-Breon)
W/Soya protein complex.
See: Soy-Dome Cleanser, Liq. (Miles Pharm)

• **HEXACHLOROPHENE CLEANSING EMULSION,** U.S.P. XXI.
Use: Anti-infective, topical detergent

• **HEXACHLOROPHENE LIQUID SOAP, DETERGENT LIQUID,** U.S.P. XXI.
See: pHisoHex Liq. Prods. (Winthrop-Breon)
Use: Anti-infective, topical detergent.

HEXACOSE. Mixture of C-6 alcohols derived from oxidation of tetracosane—$C_{24}H_{50}$.
See: Hexathricin, Aerospra (Lincoln)

HEXACREST. (Nutrition) Vit. B-6 100 mg./cc., benzyl alcohol 1.5% Vial 10 cc.
Use: Source of B-6.

HEXACYCLONATE SODIUM. (Warner-Lambert) Sodium 3,3-pentamethylene-4-hydroxybutyrate. Treatment of alcoholism. Under Study.

HEXADECADROL.
See: Dexamethasone.

HEXADECANOIC ACID, 2- (2,2-DICHLOROACETYL-)AMINO-3-HYDROXY-3-(4-NITROPHENYL)PROPYL ESTER. Chloramphenicol Palmitate, U.S.P. XXI.

HEXADERM. (Amfre-Grant) Hydrocortisone free alcohol 0.5%, hexachlorophene 0.5%, menthol 0.125%. Tube 1 oz.
Use: Acute dermatosis.

HEXADERM-I.Q. (Amfre-Grant) Hydrocortisone 0.5%, hexachlorophene 0.5%, clioquinol 3%. Tube 1 oz.
Use: Antifungal, antieczematous, antibacterial.

HEXADIENOL. Hexacose.

HEXADIMETHRINE BROMIDE. B.A.N. Poly-(NNN′N′-tetra-methyl-N-trimethylenehexamethylenediammonium dibromide). Polybrene.
Use: Heparin antagonist.

HEXADROL. (Organon) Dexamethasone **Tab.:** 0.5 mg./Tab. Bot. 100s, 500s. Strips 10 x 10; 0.75 mg./Tab. Bot. 100s, 500s. Strips 10 x 10; 1.5 mg./Tab. Bot. 100s. Strips 10 x 10; 4.0 mg./Tab. Bot. 100s. Strips 10 x 10. **Elixir:** 0.5 mg./5 ml. w/alcohol 5%. Bot. 4 oz. **Cream:** 0.04% Tube 30 Gm.
Use: Corticosteroid.

HEXADROL PHOSPHATE. (Organon) Dexamethasone sodium phosphate 4 mg./ml.,10 mg./ml., 20mg./ml. w/benzyl alcohol as preservative. **4 mg./ml.:** Vial 1 ml., 5 ml. Disposable syringe 1 ml. **10 mg./ml.:** Vial 10 ml. Disposable syringe 1 ml. **20 mg./ml.:** Vial 5 ml. Disposable syringe 5 ml.
Use: Corticosteroid.

• **HEXAFLUORENIUM.** F.D.A. Hexamethylene bis-[9-fluorenyldimethylammonium ion]
Use: Muscle relaxant.

• **HEXAFLUORENIUM BROMIDE,** U.S.P. XXI. Inj., U.S.P. XXI. Hexamethyl-enebis-[fluoren-9-yldi-methylammonium] dibromide.
Use: Muscle relaxant; potentiator (succinylcholine).
See: Mylaxen, Vial (Mallinckrodt)

HEXAFLUORODIETHYL ETHER. Name used for Flurothyl.

HEXAFLUORONIUM BROMIDE. Hexafluorenium bromide.

1-(HEXAHYDRO-1H-AZEPIN-1-YL)-3-(p-TOLYLSULFONYL)-UREA. Tolazamide, U.S.P. XXI.

[2-(HEXAHYDRO-1(2H)-AZOCINYL)ETHYL] GUANIDINE SULFATE. Guanethidine Sulfate, U.S.P. XXI.

1,2,2,3a,β,8,8a,β-HEXAHYDRO-1,3a,8-TRI-METHYLPYRROLO[2,3,-b]-INDOL-5YL   METHYLCARBAMATE. Physostigmine, U.S.P. XXI.

HEXAHYDROXYCYCLOHEXANE.
See: Inositol, Prep. (Various Mfr.)

5,6,9,17,19,21-HEXAHYDROXY-23-METHOXY-2,4,12,-15,18,20,22-HEPTAMETHYL-8-[N-(4-METHYL-1-PIPERAZINYL)-FORMIMIDOYL-2,7-(EPOXYPENT-ADECA]1,11,13]TRIENIMINO)NAPHTHO[2,1-b]FU-RAN-1,11-(2H)-DIONE 21 ACETATE. Rifampin, U.S.P. XXI.

HEXAKOSE. Mixture of tetracosanes & oxidation products.
See: Hexathricin, Aerospra (Lincoln)
W/Benzethonium chloride, p-chloro-m-xylenol, ethyl p-aminobenzoate & tyrothricin.
See: Hexathricin, Aeropak (Lincoln)

HEXALOL. (Central) Atropine sulf. 0.03 mg., hyoscyamine 0.03 mg., methenamine 40.8 mg., phenyl salicylate 18.1 mg., benzoic acid 4.5 mg., methylene blue 5.4 mg./Tab. Bot. 100s, 1000s.
Use: Urinary antiseptic, antispasmodic.

HEXAMARIUM BROMIDE. (Hexamethylene bis(3-pyridyl N-methylcarbamate) dimethyl bromide.

HEXAMETHONIUM.
W/Rauwiloid.
See: Rauwiloid w/hexamethonium, Tab. (Riker)

HEXAMETHONIUM BROMIDE. B.A.N. Vegolysen. Hexamethylene (bistrimethyl ammonium) bromide.
Use: Hypotensive.

HEXAMETHONIUM CHLORIDE. (Various Mfr.) Hexamethylene (bistrimethylammonium) chloride.

HEXAMETHONIUM IODIDE. B.A.N. Hexamethylenedi(trimethylammonium iodide).
Use: Hypotensive.
See: Hexathide

HEXAMETHONIUM TARTRATE. B.A.N. Hexamethylenedi(trimethylammonium hydrogen tartrate).
Use: Hypotensive.
See: Vegolysen T

HEXAMETHYLENAMINE.
See: Methenamine (Various Mfr.)

HEXAMETHYLENAMINE MANDELATE. (CMC) 0.25, 0.5, 1.0 Gm./Tab. Bot. 100s, 1000s.
See: Mandelamine, Tab., Susp. (Parke-Davis)

HEXAMETHYLENETETRAMINE.
See: Methenamine, U.S.P. XXI.
Hexamethylenetetramine Mandelate.

HEXAMETHYLPARAROSANILINE CHLORIDE.
See: Bismuth Violet, Sol. (Table Rock)

HEXAMETHYLROSANILINE CHLORIDE.
See: Gentian Violet

HEXAMIC ACID. Cyclamic Acid, B.A.N.

HEXAMINE HIPPURATE. B.A.N. A 1:1 complex of hexamine and hippuric acid.
Use: Antiseptic.
See: Hiprex

HEXAMIN. (Galen) Vit. A 5000 I.U., D 400 I.U., B-1 1.5 mg., B-2 2 mg., B-6 0.1 mg., Ca pantothenate 1 mg., niacinamide 20 mg., C 37.5 mg./Cap. Bot. 100s.
Use: Vitamin deficiencies.

HEXAMINE.
See: Methenamine (Various Mfr.)

HEXAPROFEN. B.A.N. 2-(4-Cyclohexylphenyl)-propionic acid.

Use: Anti-inflammatory; antipyretic; analgesic.

HEXAPROPYMATE. B.A.N. 1-(2-Propynyl)cyclohexanol carbamate. Merinax.
Use: Sedative hypnotic.

HEXAPRADOL HCl. a-(1-Aminohexyl)benzhydrol HCl.
Use: Central nervous system stimulant.

HEXASEPT. (Med. Chem.; Kenyon) Hexachlorophene 3% in high-sudsing soap-free lotion base. Bot. 5 oz., pt., gal.
Use: Skin cleanser.

HEXATE. (Davis & Sly) Atropine sulfate 1/2000 gr., Ext. hyoscyamus ¼ gr., methylene blue 1/10 gr., methanamine ½ gr., benzoic acid ½ gr., salol ½ gr./Tab. Bot. 1000s.
Use: Renal discomfort.

HEXATHRICIN AEROSPRA. (Lincoln) Hexadienol 8 Gm., benzethonium chloride 80 mg., p-chloro m-xylenol 800 mg., tyrothricin 40 mg., ethyl-p-aminobenzoate 1.6 Gm./6 oz. Aeropak 3 oz.
Use: Topically, burns, pyodermas & fungal infections.

HEXATHRICIN EPISIOTOMY AEROSPRA. (Lincoln) Hexakose (hexadienol) 4.2 Gm., p-chloro-m-xylenol 420 mg., benzethonium chloride 55 mg., ethyl-p-aminobenzoate 2.77 Gm./3 oz. can. Aerospra can 3 oz.

HEXATHRICIN OTIC. (Lincoln) Benzocaine 50 mg., p-chloro-m-xylenol 40 mg., benzethonium chloride 1 mg./cc. Bot. 15 cc.
Use: Fungus infections of ear.

• **HEXAVITAMIN CAPSULES and TABLETS,** U.S.P. XXI. Vit-A 5000 I.U., B-1 2 mg., B-2 3 mg., C 75 mg., D 400 I.U., nicotinamide 20 mg./Tab. or Cap. Bot. 100s, 1000s, 5000s. (Various Mfr.)
See: Hepicebrin, Tab. (Lilly)

HEXAVITAMIN. (Panray) Vit. A 5000 I.U., D 400 I.U., C 75 mg., B-1 2 mg., B-2 3 mg., nicotinamide 20 mg./Tab. Bot. 1000s.

HEXAVITAMIN. (Upsher-Smith) Tab. Bot. 100s, 1000s. Unit Dose 100s.

HEXAVITAMIN TABLETS, N.F. (Fellows) Vit. A 1.5 mg., D 10.0 mcg., C 75 mg., B-1 2 mg., B-2 3 mg., nicotinamide 20 mg./S.C. Tab. Bot. 1000s.

HEXAVITAMIN TABLETS. (Stanlabs) Vit. A 5000 u., D 400 u., C 75 mg., B-1 2 mg., B-2 3 mg., niacinamide 20 mg./Tab. Bot. 100s, 1000s. (Vitarine) Tab. Bot. 100s, 200s.

HEXAZOLE. B.A.N. 4-Cyclohexyl-3-ethyl-1,2,4-triazole.
Use: Central nervous system stimulant.
See: Azoman

HEXCARBACHOLINE BROMIDE (I.N.N.). Carbolinium Bromide, B.A.N.

HEXCARBACHOLINE   BROMIDE.   1,6-Hexamethylenebiscarbaminoylcholine bromide.

• **HEXEDINE.** USAN. 2,6-bis(2-Ethylhexyl)hexahydro-7a-methyl-1H imidasol[1,5c]imidazole.
Use: Antibacterial.

HEXENE-OL. Hexacose.

HEXENOL. Hexacose.

HEXESTROL. Dihydro-diethylstilbestrol. Hexoestrol. Meso-3,4-bis(p-hydroxyphenyl)-n-hexane. (CMC) 3 mg./Tab. Bot. 100s, 1000s.

Use: Estrogen therapy. (200 mcg. to 3 mg. I.M.)

HEXESTROL AND PHENOBARBITAL. (Jenkins) Hexestrol 1 mg., phenobarbital ¼ gr./Tab. Bot. 1000s.

HEXETHAL SODIUM. (Hebaral) Sod. ethylhexylbarbiturate.
Use: Sedative & hypnotic.

HEXETIDINE. B.A.N. 5-Amino-1,3-bis(beta-ethylhexyl)-5-methylhexahydropyrimide. Triocil.
Use: Bactericide; fungicide.
See: Oraldene; Sterisil

HEXOBARBITAL.
See: Sombulex, Tab. (Riker)
W/Acetaminophen, salicylamide, d-amphetamine sulfate, secobarbital sod., butabarbital sod., phenobarbital.
See: Sedragesic, Tab. (Lannett)
W/Dihydrohydroxycodeinone HCl, dihydrohydroxycodeinone terephthalate, homatropine terephthalate, aspirin, phenacetin, caffeine.
See: Percobarb, Cap. (Du Pont)
W/Dihydrohydroxycodeinone terephthalate, dihydrohydroxycodeinone HCl, homatropine terephthalate, aspirin, phenacetin, caffeine.
See: Percobarb-Demi, Cap. (Du Pont)

• **HEXOBARBITAL,** U.S.P. XXI. Tab., U.S.P. XXI. (Cyclonal Sod., Dorico Soluble, Evipan Sod., Hexanastab, Hexobarbitone Sod., Methenexyl Sod.). N-methyl-5-cyclohexenyl-5-methylbarbiturate.
Use: Sedative.
See: Sombucaps, Caps (Riker)
Percobarb, Prods (Du Pont)

• **HEXOBENDINE.** USAN. Hexobendine HCl. 1,2-Di-[N-methyl-3-(3,4,5-trimethoxybenzoyloxy)propylamino]ethane.
Use: Coronary vasodilator.

HEXOCYCLIUM METHYLSULFATE. B.A.N. N-β-Cyclohexyl-β-hydroxy-β-phenylethyl)-N'-methylpiperazine dimethylsulfate.
Use: Anticholinergic.

HEXOESTROL.
See: Hexestrol (Various Mfr.)

HEX-ON. (Sween) 30 cc., vials w/Drop top cap.
Use: Odor-antagonist.

HEXOPAL. (Winthrop Products) Inositol hexanicotinate.
Use: Hypolipedimic, peripheral vasodilator.

HEXOPRENALINE. B.A.N. NN'-Di-[2-(3,4-dihydroxyphenyl)-2-hydroxyethyl]hexamethylenediamine.
Use: Bronchodilator.

• **HEXYLCAINE HYDROCHLORIDE,** U.S.P. XXI. Topical Soln., U.S.P. XXI. 1-(Cyclohexylamino)-2-propanol benzoate (ester) HCl.
Use: Injectable (Veterinary) and local (Human) anesthetic.
See: Cyclaine Topical Solution (Merck Sharp & Dohme)

• **HEXYLRESORCINOL,** U.S.P. XXI. Pill, U.S.P. XXI. 4-Hexylresorcinol. (Various Mfr.)
Use: Anthelmintic (intestinal roundworms and trematodes) and minor throat irritations.

See: Jayne's P.W., Tab. (Glenbrook)
Listerine Antiseptic Throat Lozenges (Warner-Lambert)
Sucrets Sore Throat Lozenge (Calgon)
W/Benzocaine, camphor, menthol.
See: Auristil, Dropule (Blue Line)

HEXYPHEN-2. (Robinson) Trihexyphenidyl HCl 2 mg./Tab. Bot. 100s.
Use: Anticholingergic, antiparkinsonian.

HEXYPHEN-5. (Robinson) Trihexyphenidyl HCl 5 mg./Tab. Bot. 100s, 1000s.
Use: Anticholinergic, antiparkinsonian.

H.H.R. (Towne) Hydralazine HCl 25 mg., hydrochlorothiazide 15 mg., reserpine 0.1 mg./Tab. Bot. 100s, 1000s.
Use: Hypertension treatment.

HI and DRY. (Revlon) Aluminum chlorohydrate in lotion base. Roll on bottle.
Use: Anti-perspirant.

HI-BEE W/C. (Vortech) Vit. B-1 15 mg., B-2 10 mg., B-6 5 mg., C 300 mg., niacinamide 50 mg., D-calcium pantothenate 10 mg./Cap. Bot. 50s, 100s, 1000s.
Use: Vit. B & C replacement therapy.

HIBICLENS. (Stuart) Chlorhexidine gluconate 4%, isopropyl alcohol 4%, in a non alkaline base. Bot. 4 oz., 8 oz., 16 oz., 32 oz., 1 gal. Packette 15 ml.
Use: Surgical hand scrub, health-care personnel handwash, skin wound cleanser, preoperative cleansing.

HIBICLENS SPONGE BRUSH. (Stuart) Chlorhexidine gluconate impregnated sponge-brush. Unit-of-use 22 ml. sponge-brushes.
Use: Antimicrobial skin cleanser.

HIBISCRUB. Chlorhexidine gluconate, B.A.N.
Use: Surgical handscrub.

HIBISTAT. (Stuart) Chlorhexidine gluconate 0.5%, isopropyl alcohol 70% with emollients. Bot. 4 oz., 8 oz.
Use: Germicidal hand rinse.

HIBITANE. Chlorhexidine, B.A.N.

HIBOL. (Amfre-Grant) Methandriol dipropionate 50 mg./ml. Vial 10 ml.
Use: Anabolic.

HI B & C. (Vitarine) High potency Vit. B complex with Vit. C.
Use: Dietary supplement.

HI B PLEX. (Standex) Vit. B-1 100 mg., B-2 2 mg., B-3 100 mg., panthenol 2 mg./ml. Vial 30 ml.
Use: Vitamin.

HI-COR 1.0. (C & M Pharmacal) Hydrocortisone 1.0% in a nonionic, ester-free, fat-free, paraben-free washable base. Tube 20 Gm. Jar 2 oz., 16 oz., 96 oz.
Use: Derma-steroid.

HI-COR-2.5. (C & M Pharmacal) Hydrocortisone 2.5% in a nonionic, ester-free, fat-free, paraben-free washable base. Tube 20 Gm. Jar 2 oz., 16 oz., 96 oz.
Use: Derma-steroid.

HIESTRONE.
See: Estrone (Various Mfr.)

HIGH B-12. (Barth's) Vit. B-12, desic. liver. Cap. Bot. 100s, 500s.

HIGH POTENCY COLD CAP. (Weeks & Leo) Salicylamide 325 mg., chlorpheniramine maleate 4 mg., dextromethorphan HBr. 15 mg., caffeine 16.2 mg./Tab. Bot. 18s.
Use: Colds, coughs, hayfever.

HIGH POTENCY PAIN RELIEVERS. (Weeks & Leo) Acetaminophen 300 mg., salicylamide 300 mg./Cap. Bot. 20s, 40s.
Use: Analgesic.

HIGH POTENCY VITAMINS AND MINERALS. (Burgin-Arden) Vit. A 25,000 I.U., D 400 I.U., B-1 10 mg., B-2 5 mg., C 150 mg., niacinamide 100 mg., Ca 103 mg., P 80 mg., Fe 10 mg., Vit. B-6 1 mg., B-12 5 mcg., Mg 5.5 mg., Mn 1 mg., K 5 mg., Zn 1.4 mg./Tab. Bot. 100s, fever.
Use: Multivitamin with minerals.

HIGH POTENCY VIT. CAP. (Scrip) Vit. A 25,000 I.U., D 400 I.U., B-1 10 mg., B-2 10 mg., C 200 mg., sod. ascorbate 100 mg., B-6 5 mg., Ca pantothenate 20 mg., B-12 5 mcg., E 15 I.U./Cap. Bot. 100s.

HILL-CORTAC LOTION. (Hill) Hydrocortisone 0.5%, sulfur 5%, isopropyl alcohol 5%, oat powd. 20%, zinc oxide 20% Lot. Bot. 2 oz.
Use: Acne vulgaris and acne rosacea.

HILL-SHADE LOTION. (Hill) Para-aminobenzoic acid, alcohol 65%. Sun protective factor 22.
Use: Sunscreen.

HILOMID. Tribromsalan, B.A.N.

HINKLE'S PILLS. (Stanlabs) Aloin, belladonna, cascara and podophyllum. Bot. 100s, 1000s.

HI-POTENCY B-COMPLEX. (Kenyon) Vit. B-1 20 mg., B-2 12 mg., B-6 2 mg., B-12 3 mcg., C 50 mg., Ca pantothenate 5 mg., folic acid 0.1 mg., niacinamide 25 mg., liver fraction II 30 mg., yeast 175 mg., iron gluconate 30 mg., iron reduced 10 mg., choline bitartrate 20 mg., inositol 20 mg., d1-methionine 20 mg./Tab. Bot. 100s, 1000s.

HI-POTENCY B-COMPLEX W/C. (Zenith) Vit. C 500 mg., niacinamide 100 mg., Ca pantothenate 20 mg., B-1 15 mg., B-2 10 mg., B-6 5 mg., B-12 4 mcg./Tab. Bot. 100s.

HI-POTENCY VITAMINS/MINERALS. (Zenith) Vit. B-1 15 mg., B-2 10 mg., B-6 2 mg., pantothenic acid 10 mg., niacinamide 100 mg., B-12 7.5 mcg., C 150 mg., E 5 mg., A 3 mg., D 10 mcg., Fe 15 mg., Cu 1 mg., iodine 0.15 mg., Mn 1 mg. Mg 5 mg., Zn 1.5 mg./Tab. Bot. 100s.
Use: Multivitamin with minerals.

HIPPRAMINE.
See: Methenamine hippurate.

HIPPUTOPE. (Squibb) Radio-iodinated sodium iodohippurate (131I) Injection Bot. 1 m Ci, 2 m Ci.
Use: Diagnostic.

HIPREX. (Merrell Dow) Methenamine hippurate 1 Gm./Tab. Bot. 100s.
Use: Prophylactic or long-term suppressive treatment of urinary tract infections.

HI-PRO WAFERS. (Mills) Casein-lactalbumin fusion 13.3 gr., dl-methionine 5 mg., l-lysine monohydrochloride 16.7 mg., l-cystine 5 mg./Tab. Bot. 336s.

HI-RIBO. (Kenyon) Vit. B-2 riboflavin-5-phos, 50 mg./cc. Vial 10 cc.

HISPRIL. (SmithKline) Diphenylpyraline HCl 5 mg./Spansule. Bot. 50s.
Use: Relief from hay fever, allergic rhinitis, urticaria.

HIST-A-BALM MEDICATED LOTION. (Columbia) Pyrilamine maleate 0.75%, diperodon HCl 0.25%, benzalkonium chloride 0.1%, menthol, camphor. Bot. 4 oz.
Use: Anesthetic-antiseptic, antihistamine.

HISTA-C. (Eckerd) D-methorphan HBr 10 mg., phenylephrine HCl 5 mg., pyrilamine maleate 12.5 mg., Vit. C 75 mg., pot. salicylate 3.75 gr., caffeine 0.25 gr./Cap.

HISTA-C SYRUP. (Eckerd) D-methorphan 10 mg., phenylephrine HCl 2.5 mg., pyrilamine maleate 8 mg., Vit. C 30 mg., NAPAP 81 mg., glyceryl guaiacol ether 50 mg./5 cc. Bot. 3 oz.

HISTACHLOR. (Kenyon) Chlorpheniramine maleate 4 mg./Tab. Bot. 100s, 1000s.

HISTACHLOR D-8, D-12. (Kenyon) Chlorpheniramine maleate 8 mg., 12 mg./Delayed Action Tab. Bot. 1000s.

HISTACHLOR T-8, T-12. (Kenyon) Chlorpheniramine maleate 8 mg., 12 mg./Time release Cap. Bot. 100s, 1000s.

HISTACHLOR W/A.P.C. (Kenyon) Chlorpheniramine maleate 2 mg., salicylamide 3.5 gr., phenacetin 2.5 gr., caffeine ½ gr./Tab. Bot. 100s, 1000s.

HISTA-COMPOUND #5. (Vortech) Acetaminophen 150 mg., salicylamide 175 mg., chlorpheniramine maleate 2 mg./Tab. Bot. 100s, 1000s.
Use: Antihistaminic, analgesic.

HISTACOMP SYRUP. (Approved) Thenylpyramine HCl 80 mg., ammonium chloride 10 gr., Sod. citrate 5 gr., antimony Pot. tartrate ¼₄ gr., menthol & aromatics q.s./fl. oz. Bot., Syr. 4 oz., 8 oz. Also available w/dextromethorphan. Bot. 4 oz.
Use: Allergic & asthmatic coughs.

HISTACOMP TABLETS. (Approved) Pyrilamine maleate 25 mg., aspirin 3½ gr., phenacetin 2½ gr., caffeine ½ gr./Tab. Bot. 30s, 100s, 1000s.
Use: Allergic symptoms & the common cold.

HISTACON. (Marsh-Emory) Chlorpheniramine maleate 12 mg., ephedrine hydrochloride 15 mg., atropine sulfate 0.24 mg./S.R. Tab. Bot. 100s, 1000s.
Use: Antihistaminic, decongestant.

HISTACON SYRUP. (Marsh-Emory) Chlorpheniramine maleate 3 mg., ephedrine HCl 4 mg., atropine sulfate 0.06 mg., alcohol 5%/5 cc. Bot. pt.
Use: Allergic, respiratory conditions.

HISTA-DERFULE. (O'Neal, Jones & Feldman) Chlorpheniramine maleate 4 mg., acetaminophen 325 mg., phenylpropanolamine HCl 25 mg., powdered opium 2 mg./Cap. Bot. 100s, 1000s.
Use: Analgesic.

HISTADYL E.C. (Lilly) Codeine phosphate 60 mg., ephedrine HCl 30 mg., chlorpheniramine maleate 12 mg., ammonium chloride 660 mg., menthol 3.9 mg./30 ml. w/alcohol 5%. Bot. 4 oz., pt., gal.

Use: Antitussive, antihistaminic, decongestant, expectorant.

HISTAGESIC D.M. (Bowman) Phenylpropanolamine HCl 25 mg., chlorpheniramine maleate 4 mg., dextromethorphan HBr 10 mg, acetaminophen 324 mg./Tab. Bot. 100s, 1000s.
Use: Analgesic, decongestant, antihistaminic, antitussive.

HISTAGESIC MODIFIED. (Bowman) Acetaminophen 324 mg., phenylephrine HCl 10 mg., chlorpheniramine maleate 4 mg./Tab.
Use: Analgesic, decongestant, antihistaminic.

HISTAJECT. (Mayrand) Atropine, chlorphemiramine maleate. Vial 10 ml.

HISTAJEN. (Jenkins) Codeine phosphate 10 mg., pyrilamine maleate 12 mg., ammonium chloride 175 mg., potassium citrate 131 mg., alcohol 2%/5 cc. Syr. Bot. 3, 4 oz., gal.
Use: Common cold, hay fever.

HISTAJEN JR. (Jenkins) Chlorpheniramine maleate 1 mg., acetophenetidin 75 mg., caffeine 15 mg., salicylamide 105 mg./Tab. Bot. 1000s.
Use: Colds and allergies.

HISTALET. (Reid-Provident) **Syrup:** Pseudoephedrine HCl 45 mg., chlorpheniramine maleate 3 mg./5 ml. Bot. pt. **Forte:** Phenylephrine HCl 10 mg., pyrilamine maleate 25 mg., chlorpheniramine maleate 4 mg., phenylpropanolamine HCl 50 mg./Sustained Release Tab. Bot. 100s, 250s. **Histalet DM:** Pseudoephedrine HCl 45 mg., chlorpheniramine maleate 3 mg., dextromethorphan HBr 15 mg./5 ml. Syr. Bot. 1 pt.
Use: Treatment, common cold.

HISTALET X. (Reid-Provident) **Syrup:** Pseudoephedrine HCl 45 mg., chlorpheniramine maleate 3 mg., guaifenesin 200 mg./5 ml. Bot. 16 oz. **Tab.:** Pseudoephedrine HCl 120 mg., chlorpheniramine maleate 8 mg., guaifenesin 200 mg./Tab. Bot. 100s.
Use: Treatment of common cold, bronchitis, croup, emphysema.

HISTALOG. (Lilly) Betazole HCl. 50 mg./ml. Amp. 1 ml., pkg. 6s.
Use: Clinical testing of gastric secretion.

HISTALOG HYDROCHLORIDE. Ametazole, B.A.N.

HISTAM #2, IMPROVED ELIXIR. (Vortech) Dextromethorphan HBr 10 mg., chlorpheniramine maleate 4 mg., phenylephrine HCl 5 mg., guaifenesin 100 mg., ephedrine sulfate 3 mg./5 cc. Vial 5 cc.

HISTAMIC TABS. (Metro Med) Chlorpheniramine maleate 4 mg., pseudoephedrine HCl 15 mg./Tab. Bot. 100s, 1000s.

HISTAMINE. 2-(4-Imidazolyl) ethylamine.
Use: Diagnostic agent.

HISTAMINE ACID PHOSPHATE.
See: Histamine Phosphate, U.S.P. XXI.

HISTAMINE DIHYDROCHLORIDE.
W/Methyl nicotinate, oleoresin capicum, glycomonosalicylate.
See: Akes-N-Pain Rub, Oint. (Edward J. Moore)

W/Menthol, thymol, methyl salicylate.
  See: Imahist Unction (Gordon)
• **HISTAMINE PHOSPHATE,** U.S.P. XXI. Inj. U.S.P.
  XXI. 1H-Imidazole-4-ethanamine, phosphate (1:2). 4-
  (2-Aminoethyl) imidazole Bis (Dihydrogen Phos-
  phate).
  Use: S.C., I.V., allergy therapy & diagnostic aid.
HISTANTIN HYDROCHLORIDE. Chlorcyclizine,
  B.A.N.
HISTAPCO. (Apco) Chlorpheniramine maleate 4 mg.,
  ipecac and opium powd. ¼ gr., (contains opium
  0.025 gr.), camphor monobromated ⅛ gr.,
  salicylamide 2 gr., phenacetin 1½ grs., caffeine
  alkaloid ⅛ gr., atropine sulfate ¹/₅₀₀ gr./Tab.
  Use: Analgesic, antipyretic, antihistaminic, and
  nasal antisecretory.
HISTAQUAD. Cap. (Richlyn) Phenylpropanolamine
  HCl 25 mg., pyrilamine maleate 12.5 mg.,
  pheniramine maleate 12.5 mg., phenylephrine HCl
  2.5 mg./Cap. Bot. 1000s.
HISTAQUAD. Tab. (Richlyn) Pyrilamine maleate 6¼
  mg., phenyltoloxamine dihydrogen citrate 6¼ mg.,
  prophenpyridamine maleate 6¼ mg./Tab. Bot.
  1000s.
HISTARON-4. (Approved) Chloroprophenpyridamine
  maleate 4 mg./Tab. Bot. 100s, 500s, 1000s.
HISTARON-12. (Approved) Chloroprophenpyridamine
  maleate 12 mg./Cap. Bot. 100s, 500s, 1000s.
HISTASPAN-D. (USV Labs.) Chlorpheniramine maleate
  8 mg., phenylephrine HCl 20 mg., methscopolamine
  nitrate 2.5 mg.,/Cap. in sustained-release micro-dialysis cells. Bot. 100s, 1000s.
  Use: Antihistaminic with decongestant.
HISTASPAN-PLUS. (USV Labs.) Chlorpheniramine
  maleate 8 mg., phenylephrine HCl 20 mg./Cap. in
  sustained-release micro-dialysis cells. Bot. 100s.
  Use: Antihistaminic and decongestant for relief of
  nasal congestion.
HISTATAB PLUS. (Century) Chlorpheniramine
  maleate 2 mg., phenylephrine HCl 5 mg./Tab. Bot.
  100s, 1000s.
  Use: Antihistaminic, decongestant.
HISTATAPP ELIXIR. (Upsher-Smith) Brompheniramine
  maleate 4 mg., phenylephrine HCl 5 mg.,
  phenylpropanolamine HCl 5 mg./5 cc. Bot. 4 oz.,
  pt., gal.
  Use: Antihistamine, nasal decongestant.
HISTATAPP T.D. (Upsher-Smith) Brompheniramine
  maleate 12 mg., phenylephrine HCl 15 mg.,
  phenylpropanolamine HCl 15 mg./Tab. Bot. 100s,
  500s, unit dose 100s.
  Use: Antihistamine, nasal decongestant.
HISTATROL. (Center) Histamine phosphate control
  1:1000 and 1:10,000. 2 ml. dropper vial 1:1000 or
  vial 1:100,000 intradermal.
  Use: Skin test control.
HISTA-VADRIN SYRUP. (Scherer) Phenylpropanolamine HCl 20 mg., chlorpheniramine maleate 2 mg.,
  phenylephrine HCl 2.5 mg., alcohol 2%/5 cc. Bot.
  pt.
  Use: Upper respiratory decongestant.
HISTA-VADRIN TABLETS. (Scherer) Phenylpropanola-

mine HCl 40 mg., chlorpheniramine maleate 6 mg.,
  phenylephrine HCl 5 mg./Tab. Bot. 100s.
  Use: Antihistaminic-Decongestant.
HISTA-VADRIN T.D. CAPSULES. (Scherer) Phenyl-
  propanolamine HCl 50 mg., chlorpheniramine
  maleate 4 mg., belladonna alkaloids 0.2 mg./Cap.
  Bot. 50s, 250s.
  Use: Nasal congestion relief.
HISTEX. (Mallard) Chlorpheniramine maleate, 12
  mg./T.D. Cap. Pkg. 100s, 1000s.
  Use: Antihistaminic.
HISTEX HYDROCHLORIDE. Diphenhydramine,
  B.A.N.
• **HISTIDINE,** U.S.P. XXI. $C_6H_9N_3O_2$. L-histidine.
  Use: Amino acid.
HISTINE-1. (Freeport) Diphenhydramine HCl 10 mg., al-
  cohol 12-14%/4 cc. Bot. 4 oz.
  Use: Antihistaminic with anticholinergic,
  antitussive, antiemetic & sedative affects.
HISTINE-2. (Freeport) Diphenhydramine HCl 12.5
  mg./5 ml. w/alcohol 5%. Bot. 4 oz.
  Use: Antitussive, expectorant for control of cough
  due to colds or allergy.
HISTINE-4. (Freeport) Chlorpheniramine maleate 4
  mg./Tab. Bot. 1000s.
  Use: Antihistaminic.
HISTINE-8. (Freeport) Chlorpheniramine maleate 8
  mg./T.R. Tab. Bot. 1000s.
  Use: Antihistaminic.
HISTINE-12. (Freeport) Chlorpheniramine maleate 12
  mg./T.R. Tab. Bot. 1000s.
  Use: Antihistminic.
HISTINE-25. (Freeport) Diphenhydramine HCl 25
  mg./Cap. Bot. 1000s.
  Use: Antihistaminic with antitussive, antiemetic, &
  sedative effects.
HISTINE-50. (Freeport) Diphenhydramine HCl 50
  mg./Cap. Bot. 1000s.
  Use: Antihistaminic with anticholinergic, antitussive,
  antiemetic, sedative effect.
HISTJEN CAPSULE. (Jenkins) Phenylpropanolamine
  HCl 25 mg., pyrilamine maleate 12.5 mg.,
  prophenpyridamine maleate 12.5 mg.,
  phenylephrine HCl 2.5 mg./Cap. Bot. 1000s.
HISTIDINE MONOHYDROCHLORIDE. Beta-4-Imidazo-
  lyl-1-amino propionic acid HCl.
  Use: I.M., peptic & jejunal ulcers.
HISTIVITE-D. (Vitarine) Dextromethorphan HBr 30 mg.,
  ammonium Cl 8 gr., ephedrine sulfate ⅜ gr.,
  menthol, methapyrilene fumarate 75 mg./oz.
  w/alcohol (by volume) 4.8%. Bot. 4 oz.
  Use: Coughs due to colds.
HISTOACRYL. Enbucrilate, B.A.N.
HISTOGESIC. (Century) Phenylpropanolamine HCl 25
  mg., pyrilamine maleate 10 mg., chlorpheniramine
  maleate 2 mg., terpin hydrate 2½ gr.,
  acetaminophen 5 gr./Tab. Bot. 100s, 1000s.
  Use: Cold symptoms.
HISTOLYN-CYL. (Berkeley Biologicals) Histoplasmin
  sterile filtrate from yeast cells of *Histoplasma
  capsulatum.* Vial 1.3 ml.
  Use: Skin test.

• **HISTOPLASMIN,** U.S.P. XXI. (Parke-Davis) An aqueous solution containing standardized sterile culture filtrate of *Histoplasma capsulatum* grown on liquid synthetic medium. Vial 1 ml. to give 10 tests.
Use: Diagnostic aid in testing for histoplasmosis.

HISTOR-D. (Hauck) **Timecelles:** Chlorpheniramine maleate 8 mg., phenylephrine HCl 20 mg., methscopalamine 2.5 mg./Cap. Bot. 100s, 500s.
Syrup: chlorpheniramine maleate 2 mg., phenylephrine HCl 5 mg./5 ml. w/alcohol 2%. Bot. 16 oz.
Use: Symptoms of cold, allergy and sinusitis.

HISTORAL. (Merchant) Chlorpheniramine maleate 12 mg., pseudoephedrine HCl 60 mg., methscopolamine nitrate 2.5 mg./Cap. Bot. 100s.
Use: Antihistaminic, decongestant, vasoconstrictor.

HISTORAL LIQUID. (Merchant) Chlorpheniramine maleate 2 mg., pseudoephedrine HCl 30 mg., methscopolamine nitrate 0.5 mg., alcohol 5%/5 cc. Bot. 16 oz.
Use: Antihistamine.

HISTOSAL. (Ferndale) Pyrilamine maleate 12.5 mg., phenylpropanolamine HCl 20 mg., acetaminophen 324 mg., caffeine 30 mg./Tab. Bot. 100s.
Use: Antihistaminic, analgesic, antipyretic.

HISTOSTAB HYDROCHLORIDE OR MESYLATE. Antazoline, B.A.N.

HISTOSTAT. (Salsbury) Nitarsone.

HISTREY. (Bowman) Chlorpheniramine maleate 4 mg./Tab. Bot. 100s, 1000s.
Use: Antihistaminic.

HISTRYL. Diphenylpyraline, B.A.N.

HIST-SPAN. (Kenyon) Pyrilamine maleate 25 mg., phenylpropanolamine HCl 25 mg., prophenpyridamine maleate 10 mg./T.R. Cap. Bot. 100s, 1000s.

HIST-SPAN NO. 2. (Kenyon) Pyrilamine maleate 25 mg., phenylpropanolamine HCl 25 mg., prophenpyridamine maleate 10 mg., phenylephrine HCl 10 mg./T.R. Cap. Bot. 100s, 1000s.

HISTUNEX. (Tunex) Atropine sulfate 0.2 mg., chlorpheniramine 5 mg./ml. Vial 10 cc.
Use: Decongestant.

HI-TOR. (Barth's) Vit. B-12 15 mcg., niacin 1.5 mg., B-1 6 mg., B-2 12 mg., B-6 54 mcg., pantothenic acid 150 mcg., choline 3.75 mg., inositol 5.25 mg./Tab. Bot. 100s, 500s, 1000s.

HI-TOR 900. (Barth's) Vit. B-1 13.5 mg., B-2 5.2 mg., niacin 15 mg., B-6 0.6 mg., pantothenic acid 1.2 mg., biotin, B-12 2.5 mcg., iron 0.9 mg., protein 7.5 Gm., inositol 50 mg., choline 40 mg., aminobenzoic acid 0.15-2.4 mg./15 Gm. Bot. 1 lb., 3 lb.

HIWOLFIA. (Bowman) Rauwolfia 25 mg., 50 mg., or 100 mg./Tab. Bot. 100s, 1000s.
Use: Antihypertensive.

HMS LIQUIFILM. (Allergan) Medrysone 1.0%, Liquifilm (polyvinyl alcohol) 1.4%. W/benzalkonium chloride, edetate disodium, sod. chloride, pot. chloride, sod. phosphate monobasic monohydrate, sod. phosphate dibasic anhydrous, hydroxypropyl methylcellulose, purified water, sod. hydroxide or hydrochloric acid. Ophth. Susp. Dropper Bot. 5 ml., 10 ml.

Use: Ocular anti-inflammatory.

H₂OEX. (Fellows) Benzthiazide 50 mg./Tab. Bot. 100s, 1000s.
Use: Diuretic.

HOLD. (Beecham Products) Dextromethorphan HBr 7.5 mg./Loz. Plastic tube 10 loz.
Use: Cough suppressant.

HOLOCAINE HYDROCHLORIDE. (Various Mfr.) Phenacaine HCl.
Use: Topically, local anesthetic.

HOMAPIN-5. (Mission) Homatropine methylbromide 5 mg./Tab. Bot. 100s.
Use: Antispasmodic-antichloinergic.

HOMAPIN-10. (Mission) Homatropine methylbromide 10 mg./Tab. Bot. 100s.
Use: Antispasmodic-anticholinergic.

HOMARYLAMINE HYDROCHLORIDE. N-Methyl-3,4-methylenedioxyphenethylamine HCl.

HOMATROCEL. (Softcon) Sterile buffered Methulose solution containing homatropine hydrobromide 2% & 5% w/benzalkonium chloride 1:15,000, monobasic & dibasic sod. phosphate, sod. chloride. Bot. 15 cc. sterile bufopto plastic containers.
Use: Mydriatic and cycloplegic.

• **HOMATROPINE HYDROBROMIDE,** U.S.P. XXI. Ophth. Sol., U.S.P. XXI. Benzeneacetic acid, α-hydroxy-, 8-methyl-β-azabicyclo-[3.2.1]-oct-3-yl ester, HBr, endo-($\pm$)-. 1αH, 3αH-Tropan-3α-ol mandelate (ester) HBr.
Use: Mydriatic & cycloplegia.
See: Homatrocel, Sol. (Softcon)
    Murocoll, Liq. (Muro)

HOMATROPINE HYDROCHLORIDE.
Use: Topically, mydriatic & cyclopegic; anticholinergic.

• **HOMATROPINE METHYLBROMIDE,** U.S.P. XXI. Tab., U.S.P. XXI. 3α-Hydroxy-8-methyl-1αH, 5αH-tropanium bromide mandelate.
Use: Anticholinergic.
See: Mesopin, Elix., Tab. (Du Pont)
    Novatrin, Liq., Tab. (Ayerst)
    Sed-Tens SE, Tab. (Lemmon)

HOMATROPINE METHYLBROMIDE W/COMBINATIONS
See: Aloxed, Liq. (N. Amer.)
    Aridol, Tabs. (MPL)
    Atrocholin, Tab. (Blue Line)
    Biloric, Caps. (Arcum)
    Butabel HMB, Tab. (Saron)
    DIA-Quel Liq. (Inter. Pharm.)
    Digesplen, Tab., Elixir (Med. Prod.; Panamericana)
    Dranochol, Tab. (Marin)
    Femicin, Tab. (Norcliff Thayer)
    Hepahydrin, Tab. (Comatic)
    Homachol, Tab. (Lemmon)
    Homapin, Tab. (Mission)
    Hycodan, Tab., Pow., Syr. (Du Pont)
    Hycomine Syr., Tab. (Du Pont)
    Maracid, Tab. (Marin)
    Matropinal, Elix., Inserts (Comatic)
    Matropinal Forte, Tab. (Comatic)

Matropinal Forte, Inserts (Comatic)
Mephenesal, Tab. (Richlyn)
Mesopin-PB, Tab., Elixir (Du Pont)
Nau-Aid 15, Supp. (Scrip)
Neocholan, Tab. (Merrell Dow)
Obesa-Mead #15, Tab. (Spencer-Mead)
Obesa-Mead, Tab., Cap. (Spencer-Mead)
Obe-Slim, Tab. (Jenkins)
Pancobile, Tab. (Reid-Provident)
Panitol H.M.B., Tab. (Wesley)
Periodic, Cap. (Towne)
Probilagol, Liq. (Purdue-Frederick)
Sinulin Tablets (Carnrick)
Spasticol S.A., PB, Tab. (Key Pharm.)
Spasmatol, Tab. (Pharmed)
Stim-10/50, Tab. (Scrip)
Stopp-15, 90, Supp. (Keene)
Tapuline, Tab. (Wesley)

HOMATROPINE METHYLBROMIDE AND PHENOBARBITAL COMBINATIONS
See: Bilamide, Tab. (Norgine)
Gustase-Plus, Tab. (Geriatric)
Lanokalin, Tab. (Lannett)
Matropinal, Tab., Elix. (Comatic)
Mesopin-PB, Tab., Elix. (Du Pont)
Novatrin w/Phenob., Tab. (Ayerst)
Oxi-Barb, Tab. (Scrip)
S.B.P. Plus, Tab. (Lemmon)
Spasmed Jr., Tab. (Jenkins)

HOMICEBRIN. (Lilly) Vit. A 2500 U.S.P. units, Vit. B-1 1 mg., B-2 1.2 mg., B-6 0.8 mg., niacinamide 10 mg., B-12 3 mcg., C 60 mg., D 400 U.S.P. units/5ml. w/alcohol 5%. Bot. 16 fl. oz.
Use: Vitamin deficiencies.

HOMOCHLORCYCLIZINE. B.A.N. 1-(p-Chlorobenzhydryl)-4-methylhomopiperazine. 1-(4-Chlorobenzhydrylhexahydro-4-methyl-1,4-diazepine.
Use: Antihistamine.

HOMOGENE-S. (Spanner) Testosterone 25 mg., 50 mg. or 100 mg./cc. Vial 10 cc.
Use: Androgen therapy.

• **HOMOSALATE.** USAN.
Use: Ultraviolet sunscreen.
W/Combinations.
See: Coppertone, Prods. (Plough)

HOMOSULFANILAMIDE HCl.
See: Sulfbenzamine HCl, Pow. (Flint; Eaton)

HOMO-TET. (Savage) Tetanus Immune Globulin-Human 250 u./cc. Vial 1 cc. Syringe, Disposable, 250 u.
Use: Biologic.

HOMPRENORPHINE. B.A.N. N-Cyclopropylmethyl-7,8-dihydro-7α-[1(R)-hydroxy-1-methylpropyl]-0³0⁶-dimethyl-endoethenonormorphine.
Use: Analgesic.

• **HOQUIZIL HCl.** USAN. 2-Hydroxy-2-methylpropyl 4-(6,7-dimethoxy-4-quinazolinyl)-1-piperazinecarboxylate monohydrochloride.
Use: Bronchodilator.

HORMOFOLLIN.
See: Estrone (Various Mfr.)

HORMOGEN-A. (Mallard) Natural estrogens 20,000 I.U./cc. Vial 30 cc.
HORMOGEN DEPOT. (Mallard) Estradiol cypionate 5 mg./cc. Vial 10 cc.
HORMOPLETE. (Key) Conjugated estrogenic substance 0.25 mg., methyltestosterone 2.5 mg., A 12,500 I.U., D 1000 I.U., B-1 10 mg., B-2 3 mg., B-6 2 mg., niacinamide 25 mg., nicotinic acid 5 mg., Ca pantothenate 5 mg., C 75 mg., E 2 I.U., B-12 2 mcg., ferrous sulfate 50 mg., pancreatin 100 mg., dl-methionine 15 mg., inositol 20 mg., choline bitartrate 40 mg., Ca 60 mg., phosphorus 30 mg., Cu 0.45 mg., Mn 0.5 mg., Pot. 2 mg., Zn 0.5 mg., Mg 3 mg./Tab. Bot. 50s, 500s.
Use: Vitamin, mineral, hormone supplement.
Homosalate w/combinations
See: Coppertone, Liq. (Plough)

HOSPITAL FOAM CLEANER. (Aeroceuticals) 0-phenylphenol 0.10%, 4-chloro-2-cyclopentylphenol 0.08%, lauric diethanolamide 0.20%, triethanolamine dodecylbenzenesulfonate 0.30%.
Use: Germicidal, disinfectant foam cleaner.

HOSPITAL LOTION. (Paddock) Diisobutylcresoxyethoxy-ethyl dimethyl benzyl amm. chloride, menthol, lanolin, mineral and vegetable oils. Bot. 4 oz., 8 oz., gal.

"HOT WEATHER" TABLETS. (Pharmex) Salt, dextrose. Tab. Bot. 100s, 1000s.

HOURNAZE. (Delta) Chlorpheniramine maleate 8 mg., phenylephrine HCl 20 mg./Cap. Bot. 100s.
Use: Oral antihistaminic, decongestant.

H.P. ACTHAR GEL. (Armour) Respiratory corticotropin injection highly purified 40 U.S.P. Units/1 ml. Vial 1 ml., 5 ml.; 80 U.S.P. Units/1 ml. Vial 1 ml., 5 ml.
Use: I.M. or S.C. stimulation of adrenal cortex & diseases related to it.

H-R LUBRICATING JELLY. (Holland-Rantos) Tube 5 oz.
Use: Lubricating jelly.

HRC-PRENATAL TABLETS. (Cenci) Comprehensive, well-balanced, vitamin-mineral formula. Tab. Bot. 90s, 500s.
Use: Prenatal supplement.

HRC-TYLAPRIN ELIXIR. (Cenci) Acetaminophen 120 mg., alcohol 7%/5 cc. Bot. 2 oz., 4 oz.
Use: Analgesic.

H.S. NEED. (Hanlon) Chloral hydrate 3¾ gr., 7½ gr./Cap. Bot. 100s.
Use: Sedative.

HSV-1. (Wampole-Zeus) Herpes Simplex virus type I test system. Tests 100s.
Use: For the qualitative and semi-quantitative detection of HSV-1 antibody in human serum.

HSV-2. (Wampole-Zeus) Herpes simplex virus type II antibody test. Tests 100s.
Use: For the qualitative and semi-quantitative detection of HSV-2 antibody in human serum.

H.T. FACTORATE. (Armour) Antihemophilic factor (human) dried, heat-treated for I.V. administration only. Single-dose vial w/diluent and needles. Kit 1s.
Use: Classical hemophilia treatment.

H.T. FACTORATE GENERATION II. (Armour)
Antihemophilic factor (human) dried heat treated for
I.V. administration only. Single dose vial w/diluent
and needles. Kit 1s.
Use: Classical hemophilia treatment.
HTO STAINLESS OINTMENT. (DeWitt) Ointment.
Tube 1 oz.
Use: Treatment hemorrhoids.
HTSH RIABEAD. (Abbott) Human thyroid stimulating
hormone radioimmunoassay. Test units 100s.
Use: Determination of concentration of human
thyroid stimulating hormone in serum.
HUMAN ANTOHEMOPHILIC FACTOR.
See: Antihemophilic factor
HUMAN COAGULATION. Fraction II, IX and X.
B.A.N. A preparation of human blood containing
coagulating factors II, IX and X.
Use: Treatment of hemophilia B deficiency.
HUMAN INSULIN. Insulin Human, U.S.P. XXI.
Use: Hypoglycemic.
See: Humulin Prods. (Lilly)
HUMAN MEASLES IMMUNE SERUM.
See: Immune Globulin, U.S.P. XXI.
HUMAN SERUM ALBUMIN.
See: Albumotope (Squibb)
HUMATIN CAPSULES. (Parke-Davis) Paromycin sul-
fate 250 mg./Cap. Bot. 16s.
Use: Treatment of intestinal amebiasis.
HUMIST. (Scherer) Sodium chloride 0.65%,
chlorobutanol 0.35%. Bot. 15 cc, 45 cc.
Use: Nasal spray.
HUMORSOL. (Merck Sharp & Dohme) Demecarium
bromide 0.125% and 0.25% ophthalmic soln.
w/sod. chloride, water, benzalkonium chloride
1:5,000. Sol. 5 ml. Ocumeter.
Use: Treatment of glaucoma, miotic, cholinesterase
inhibitor.
HUMULIN N. (Lilly) NPH human insulin (recombinant
DNA origin) 100 u./ml. Vial 10 ml.
Use: Diabetes treatment.
HUMULIN R. (Lilly) Regular human insulin
(recombinant DNA origin) 100 u./ml. Vial 10 ml.
Use: Diabetes treatment.
HURRICAINE. (Beutlich) Benzocaine 20%. Liquid or
Gel. Bot. 1 oz.
Use: Topical anesthetic.
HURRICAINE LIQUID PACK. (Beutlich) Benzocaine
20%. Unit dose 0.25 cc. packets. Box 50s.
Use: Topical anesthetic.
HURRICAINE TOPICAL ANESTHETIC SPRAY.
(Beutlich) Benzocaine 20%. Aerosol can 2 oz.
Use: Topical anesthetic for oral or mucosal
application.
HURRICAINE TOPICAL ANESTHETIC SPRAY KIT.
(Beutlich) Benzocaine 20%. Aerosol can 2 oz. plus
200 disposable extension tubes.
Use: Topical anesthetic.
HU-TET. (Hyland) Tetanus immune globulin (human)
sterile 16.5% soln., gamma globulin fraction of the
plasma of persons who have been immunized
w/tetanus toxoid. Vials and syringes 250 u.
Use: Injured persons who run the risk of tetanus

infection and need the immediate protection offered
by tetanus antitoxin.
H.V.B. CREAM. (Bowman) Clioquinol 3%,
hydrocortisone acetate 1%, coal tar sol. 5%
Use: Anti-inflammatory, anti-infective.
HYACIDE. (Niltig) Benzethonium chloride 0.1% with
sod. nitrite 0.55%. Bot. 1 oz.
Use: Germicidal solution.
HYALEX. (Miller) Magnesium salicylate 4 gr.,
magnesium p-aminobenzoate 2½ gr., Vit. A 1500 I.U.,
Vit. D 500 I.U., Vit. E 3 I.U., Vit. B-12 2 mcg., magne-
sium ascorbate 30 mg., calcium pantothenate 5
mg., zinc 0.7 mg., magnesium oxide 5 mg./Tab.
Bot. 100s.
Use: Arthritis, bursitis, neuritis & rheumatism.
HYALIDASE.
See: Hyaluronidase (Various Mfr.)
• HYALURONIDASE INJECTION, U.S.P. XXI.
Hyalidase, Hydase Enzymes which depolymerize
hyaluronic acid. Hyalase, Rondase.
Use: Hypodermoclyses & promote diffusion.
See: Alidase, Vial (Searle)
Wydase, Vial (Wyeth)
• HYALURONIDASE FOR INJECTION, U.S.P. XXI.
HYAMAGNATE. Hydroxy-Aluminum-Magnesium-Amin-
oacetate, Sodium-free.
HYAMATE. (Xttrium) Buramate.
Use: Tranquilizer.
HYAMINE 10-X. (Rohm & Haas) Di-isobutyl cresoxy
ethoxy ethyl dimethyl benzyl ammonium chloride.
W/Sulfur, salicylic acid.
See: Derma-Cover, Liq. (Scrip)
HYAMINE 1622. (Rohm & Haas)
See: Benzethonium Chloride U.S.P. XXI.
HYAMINE 2389. (Rohm & Haas) Mainly methyl
dodecyl benzyl trimethyl ammonium chloride.
Use: Disinfection and deodorization.
HYAMINE 3500. (Rohm & Haas)
See: Benzalkonium Chloride U.S.P. XXI.
HYATAL ELIXIR. (Winsale; Kenyon) Phenobarbital 16
mg., hyoscyamine sulfate 0.1037 mg., atropine
sulfate 0.0194 mg., scopolamine hyoscine HBr
0.0065 mg./5 cc. Bot. pt., gal.
HYBALAMIN. (Mallard) Crystalline hydroxocobalamin
1000 mcg./cc. Vial 10 cc.
HYBEC FORTE. (Amlab) Vit. B-1 100 mg., B-2 20 mg.,
B-6 2.5 mg., niacinamide 25 mg., C 200 mg., B-12 10
mcg., Ca pantothenate 5 mg., iron 10 mg., choline
bitartrate 24 mg., inositol 10 mg., biotin 5 mcg.,
liver 50 mg., yeast 100 mg./Tab. Bot. 30s, 100s.
Use: Water-soluble-vitamin deficiencies.
HYBEPHEN ELIXIR. (Beecham Labs) Phenobarbital
15 mg., hyoscyamine sulf. 0.1277 mg., atropine
sulf. 0.233 mg., scopolamine HBr 0.0094 mg./5 ml.
w/alcohol 16.5%, Orange color & citris flavor. Bot.
pt., gal.
Use: Antispasmodic and sedative.
HYBEPHEN TABLETS. (Beecham Labs)
Phenobarbital 15 mg., hyosyamine sulf. 0.1277 mg.,
atropine sulf. 0.0233 mg., scopolamine HBr 0.0094
mg./Tab. Bot. 100s, 1000s.

Use: Antispasmotic and sedative.

HYBOLIN. (Hyrex) Methylandrostenediol 50 mg., in sod. phosphate buffer, sod. carboxymethylcellulose 0.29, thimerosal 1:20,000/cc. Vial 10 cc. in oil. Aqueous, Vial 10 cc.
Use: Anabolic effects.

HYBOLIN DECANOATE. (Hyrex) Nandrolone decanoate 50 mg., 100 mg./ml. Vial 2 ml.
Use: Anabolic maintenance.

HYBOLIN IMPROVED. (Hyrex) Nandrolene phenpropionate 25 mg./ml. Vial 5 ml. 50 mg./ml. Vial 2 ml.
Use: Anabolic maintenance.

HYCAL. (Beecham Labs) Calories 280, carbohydrates 49.5%, fat-not more than 0.02%, protein-not more than 0.03%, water 69 ml./3.8 fl. oz. Bot. 3.8 oz. Case 24 bot.
Use: Low-electrolyte, limited-liquid volume, high carbohydrate source of calories.

• **HYCANTHONE.** USAN. 1-[(2-(Diethylamino)-ethyl)-amino]-4-(hydroxymethyl)thioxanthen-9-one.
Use: Schistosomacide.

HYCLORITE. Sod. Hypochlorite Sol., U.S.P. XXI.

HYCODAN. (Du Pont) Hydrocodone bitartrate 5 mg., homatropine methylbromide 1.5 mg./5 ml. or Tab. Syr. Bot. 1 pt., 1 gal., Tab. Bot. 100s, 500s, 1000s.
Use: Antitussive.

HYCODAPHEN. (Ascher) Hydrocodone bitartrate 5 mg., acetaminophen 500 mg./Tab. Bot. 100s.
Use: Pain relief.

HYCOFF-A-NN LIQUID. (Saron) Dextromethorphan HBr 15 mg., pseudoephedrine HCl 45 mg., dyphlline 100 mg./15 ml. Alcohol free. Bot. pt.
Use: Antitussive, decongestant, bronchodilator.

HYCOFF X-NN. (Saron) Dextromethorphan HBr 10 mg., pseudoephedrine HCl 30 mg./5 ml. Alcohol and sugar free. Bot. pt.
Use: Antitussive, decongestant.

HYCOMINE. (Du Pont) Hydrocodone bitartrate 5 mg., phenylpropanolamine HCl 25 mg./5 ml. Syr. Bot. 1 pt., 1 gal.
Use: Orally, antitussive and antihistaminic.

HYCOMINE COMPOUND. (Du Pont) Hydrocodone bitartrate 5 mg., chlorpheniramine maleate 2 mg., phenylephrine HCl 10 mg., acetaminophen 250 mg., caffeine 30 mg./Tab. Bot. 100s, 500s.
Use: Antihistaminic for treatment of respiratory tract infections.

HYCOMINE PEDIATRIC. (Du Pont) Hydrocodone bitartrate 2.5 mg., phenylpropanolamine HCl 12.5 mg./5 ml. Bot. 1 pt., 1 gal.
Use: Orally, antitussive.

HYCORTOLE. (Premo) Hydrocortisone. **Cream:** ½%, 5 Gm., 20 Gm.; 1%, 5 Gm, 20 Gm., & 4 oz. 2.5% Tube 5 Gm., 20 Gm.; **Oint.:** 1%, 2.5% Tube 5 Gm., 20 Gm.

HYCOTUSS EXPECTORANT. (Du Pont) Hydrocodone bitartrate 5 mg., guaifenesin 100 mg., alcohol 10% v/v/5 ml. Bot. pt.
Use: Antitussive.

HYDANTOIN DERIVATIVES.
Use: Anticonvulsant.

See: Dilantin, Prep. (Parke-Davis)
Diphenylhydantoin Sod., U.S.P.
Ethotoin
Mesantoin, Tab. (Sandoz)
Phenantoin

HYDASE.
Use: Hypodermoclyses & promote diffusion.
See: Hyaluronidase (Various Mfr.)

HYDELTRA-T.B.A. (Merck Sharp & Dohme) Prednisolone tebutate 20 mg. w/sod. citrate 1 mg., polysorbate 80-1 mg., sorbitol soln. 0.5 ml. (equiv. to 450 mg. d-sorbitol), water q.s., benzyl alcohol 9 mg./ml. Aqeous Susp. Vial 1 ml., 5 ml.
Use: Corticosteroid (glucocorticoid).

HYDELTRASOL. (Merck Sharp & Dohme) Prednisolone sodium phosphate. **Ophth. Sol.:** 5 mg./ml. w/creatinine, sod. citrate, polysorbate 80, disodium edetate, pot. phosphate, HCl, benzalkonium chloride 0.02%, phenylethanol 0.25%, sterile water for injection. Dropper Bot. 5 ml. **Inj.:** 20 mg./ml. w/niacinamide 25 mg., sod. hydroxide, disodium edetate 0.5 mg., water for injection, sod. bisulfite 1mg., phenol 5 mg. Vial 2 ml., 5 ml.
Use: Corticosteroid (glucocorticoid).

HYDELTRONE. (MSD AGVET) Prednisolone sodium phosphate and neomycin sulfate equivalent to 2.5 mg. prednisolone 21-phosphate and 3.5 mg. neomycin base/Gm.
Use: Ophthalmic ointment, veterinary medicine.

HYDELTRONE-T.B.A. (MSD AGVET) Prednisolone tebutate susp. 20 mg./cc.
Use: Anti-inflammatory agent, veterinary medicine.

HYDERGINE LC LIQUID CAPSULES. (Sandoz) Ergoloid mesylates 1 mg./Cap. Bot. 100s, 500s.
Use: Selected symptoms in elderly patients.

HYDERGINE LIQUID. (Sandoz) Equal parts of dihydroergocornine, dihydroergocristine, dihydroergocryptine as the mesylates. (Ergoloid Mesylates) 1 mg./ml. Bot. 100 ml. w/dropper.
Use: Selected symptoms in the elderly patients.

HYDERGINE, ORAL. (Sandoz) Equal parts of dihydroergocornine, dihydroergocristine, dihydroergocryptine (Ergoloid Mesylates). 1 mg./Tab. Bot. 100s, 500s. SandoPak (unit dose) 100s, 500s.
Use: Selected symptoms in elderly patients.

HYDERGINE, SUBLINGUAL. (Sandoz) Equal parts of dihydroergocornine, dihydroergocristine, dihydroergocryptine as the mesylates (Ergoloid Mesylates). 0.5 mg. and 1.0 mg./Tab. Tab. Bot. 100s, 1000s. SandoPak (unit dose) 100s.
Use: Selected symptoms in elderly patients.

HYDEX. (Moore Kirk) Methamphetamine HCl 5 or 10 mg./Tab. Bot. 1000s.
Use: For mild depression and anxiety states; appetite control in obesity.

HYDEXTRAN. (Hyrex) Iron dextran complex 50 mg./ml. Vial 10 ml.
Use: Anemia.

HYDORIL. (Cenci) Hydrochlorthiazide 25 or 50 mg./Tab. Bot. 100s, 1000s.

Use: Diuretic.

HYDOXIN. (Mallinckrodt) Pyridoxine HCl 25 & 50 Mg./Tab. Bot. 1000s.
Use: Treatment of pyridoxine deficiencies.

HYDRABAMINE PHENOXYMETHYL PENICILLIN.
See: Penicillin V Hydrabamine.

HYDRABASE. (Summers) Hydrophilic oint. Jar. 1 lb.

HYDRACRYLIC ACID BETA LACTONE.
See: Propiolactone

HYDRAL. (Reid-Provident) **25/25:** Hydralazine HCl 25 mg., hydrochlorothiazide 25 mg./Cap. **50/50:** Hydralazine HCl 50 mg., hydrochlorothiazide 50 mg/Cap. **100/50:** Hydralazine HCl 100 mg., hydrochlorothiazide 50 mg./Cap. Bot. 100s.
Use: Anti-hypertensive.

HYDRALAZIDE. (Zenith) Hydralazine 25 mg., hydrochlorothiazide 15 mg./Tab. Bot. 100s.
Use: Antihypertensive.

• **HYDRALAZINE HCl,** U.S.P. XXI. Inj., Tab., U.S.P. XXI. 1-Hydrazinophthalazine HCl. Phthalazine, 1-hydrazino-, HCl.
Use: Antihypertensive.
See: Apresoline, Amp. & Tab. (Ciba)
    Dralzine, Tab. (Lemmon)
    Hydralyn, Tab. (Kenyon)
W/Hydrochlorothiazide.
See: Apresazide, Cap. (Ciba)
    Apresoline-Esidrix, Tab. (Ciba)
    Hydralazide, Tab. (Zenith)
    Hydroserpine Plus, Tab. (Zenith)
W/Reserpine.
See: Dralserp, Tab. (Lemmon)
    Serpasil-Apresoline, Tab. (Ciba)
W/Reserpine, hydrochlorothiazide (Esidrix).
See: Harbolin, Tab. (Arcum)
    Ser-Ap-Es, Tab. (Ciba)
    Serapine, Tab. (Cenci)
    Serpahyde TM, Tab. (Wolins)
    Thia-Serpa-Zine, Tab. (Robinson)
    Unipres, Tab. (Reid-Provident)

HYDRALLAZINE. B.A.N. 1-Hydrazinophthalazine. Hydralazine (I.N.N.) Apresoline hydrochloride.
Use: Hypotensive.

HYDRALYN. (Kenyon) Hydralazine HCl 25 mg., 50 mg./Tab. Bot. 100s, 1000s.
Use: Hypertension.

HYDRARGAPHEN. B.A.N. 2,2'-(Binaphthalene-3-sulfonyloxyphenylmercury). Phenylmercury 2:2'-dinaphthylmethane-3:3'-disulfonate.
Use: Antiparasitic; anti-infective.
See: Penofome
    Penotrane (Ward Blenkinsop in England)

HYDRASERP. (Geneva) Hydrochlorothiazide 25 mg., 50 mg., reserpine 0.1 mg./Tab. Bot. 100s, 1000s.

HYDRA-SPRAY L.A. (Vortech) Xylometazoline HC1. Bot. 20 ml.
Use: Nasal decongestant.

HYDRASTINE. (Penick) Alkaloid. Bot. 1 oz.

HYDRASTINE HYDROCHLORIDE. (Penick) Pow., Bot. 1 oz.
Use: Uterine hemostatic.

HYDRATE. (Hyrex) Dimenhydrinate 50 mg./ml.

w/propylene glycol 50%, benzyl alcohol 5%. Amp. 1 ml. Boxes 25s, 100s; Vials 10 cc.
Use: Antinauseant, antihistamine.

I-HYDRAZINOPHTHALAZINE MONOHYDROCHLORIDE. Hydralazine Hydrochloride, U.S.P. XXI.

HYDRAZOL. (Softcon) Acetazolamide 250 mg./Tab. Bot. 100s.
Use: Carbonic anhydrase inhibitor.

HYDRAZONE. 3-(4-Methyl-piperazinyliminomethyl)rifamycin SV.
Use: Pulmonary tuberculosis.
See: Rimactane, Cap. (Ciba)

HYDREA. (Squibb) Hydroxyurea. 500 mg./Cap. Bot. 100s.
Use: Antineoplastic agent.

HYDRIL. (Blaine) Diphenhydramine HCl 80 mg., ammonium chloride 12 gr., sodium citrate 5 gr., menthol 1/10 gr., alcohol 5%/oz. Bot. Pts., 4 oz.
Use: Expectorant.

HY-DRINE. (Zemmer) Benzthiazide 50 mg./Tab. Bot. 1000s.

HYDRIODIC ACID. (Various Mfr.)
Use: Iodide therapy.

HYDRIODIC ACID SYRUP. (Lilly) Hydriodic acid 1.4 Gm./100 ml. Bot. 16 fl. oz.

HYDRIODIC ACID THERAPY.
See: Aminoacetic Acid HI

HYDRISALIC GEL. (Pedinol) Salicylic acid 6%, isopropanol, propylene glycol, hydroxypropyl cellulose. Tube 1 oz.
Use: Keratolytic.

HYDRISEA LOTION. (Pedinol) Dead sea salts concentrate 8%, sodium, potassium, calcium magnesium Chloride, propylene glycol stearate, polysorbate 40, silicone oil, coloring agent. Bot. 4 oz.
Use: Hyperkeratotic and dry skin conditioner.

HYDRISINOL CREME AND LOTION. (Pedinol) Sulfonated hydrogenated castor oil. **Cream:** Jar 4 oz., 1 lb. **Lotion:** Bot. 8 oz.
Use: Skin moisturizer, particularly for diabetics.

HYDRO-12. (Table Rock) Crystalline hydroxocobalamin 1000 mcg./cc. Pkg. 10 cc.

HYDROBEXAN. (Keene) Hydroxocobalamin 1000 mcg./ml. Vial 10 ml.

HYDRO-CHLOR. (Vortech) Hydrochlorthiazide 50 mg./Tab. Bot. 100s, 1000s.
Use: Diuretic.

HYDROCHLORATE. Same as Hydrochloride.

• **HYDROCHLORIC ACID,** N.F XVI. Diluted, N.F. XVI. (Various Mfr.) Muriatic Acid), Absolute 38%. Diluted 10%.
Use: Well diluted, achlorhydria; pharm. aid (acidifying agent).

■ **HYDROCHLORIC ACID THERAPY.**
Use: Gastric acidifier.
See: Betaine HCl (Various Mfr.)
    Glutamic Acid HCl (Various Mfr.)
    Glycine HCl (Various Mfr.)

HYDROCHLOROSERPINE. (Freeport) Hydralazine HCl. 25 mg., Hydrochlorthiazide 15 mg., reserpine 0.1 mg./Tab. Bot. 1000s.

Use: Antihypertensive.

• **HYDROCHLOROTHIAZIDE,** U.S.P. XXI. Tab. U.S.P. XXI. 2H-1,2,4-Benzothiadiazine-7-sulfonamide, 6-chloro-3,4-dihydro-,1,1-dioxide. 6-Chloro-3,4-dihydro-2H-1,2,4-Benzothiadiazene-7-sulfonamide 1, 1-dioxide.
Use: Diuretic.
See: Chlorzide, Tab. (Foy)
Delco-Retic, Tab. (Delco)
Diu-Scrip, Cap. (Scrip)
Esidrix, Tab. (Ciba)
Hydromal, Tab. (Mallard)
HydroDiuril, Tab. (Merck Sharp & Dohme)
Hydrozide Inj. (MSD AGVET)
Hydrozide-50, Tab. (Mayrand)
Kenazide-E,-H, Tab. (Kenyon)
Oretic, Tab. (Abbott)
Ro-Hydrazide, Tab. (Robinson)
SK-Hydrochlorothiazide, Tab. (SmithKline)
Thiuretic, Tab. (Parke-Davis)
Zide, Tab. (Reid-Provident)
W/Deserpidine.
See: Oreticyl, Tab. (Abbott)
W/Guanethidine monosulfate.
See: Esimil, Tab. (Ciba)
W/Hydralazine HCl.
See: Apresazide, Cap. (Ciba)
Apresoline-Esidrix, Tab. (Ciba)
Hydralazide, Tab. (Zenith)
W/Methyldopa.
See: Aldoril, Tab. (Merck Sharp & Dohme)
W/Propranolol.
See: Inderide, Tab (Ayerst)
W/Reserpine.
See: Aquapres-R, Tab. (Castal)
Hydropine, Tab. (Wolins)
Hydropres, Tab. (Merck Sharp & Dohme)
Hydroserp, Tab. (Zenith)
Hydroserpine, Tab. (Geneva)
Hydrotensin-50, Tab. (Mayrand)
Hyperserp, Tab. (Elder)
Mallopress, Tab. (Mallard)
Serpasil-Esidrix, Tab. (Ciba)
Thia-Serp-25, Tab. (Robinson)
Thia-Serp-50, Tab. (Robinson)
W/Reserpine, Hydralazine HCl.
See: Harbolin, Tab. (Arcum)
Hydroserpine Plus, Tab. (Zenith)
SER-AP-ES, Tab. (Ciba)
Serapine, Tab. (Cenci)
Serpahyde TM, Tab. (Wolins)
Thia-Serpa-Zine, Tab. (Robinson)
Unipres, Tab. (Reid-Provident)
W/Spironolactone.
See: Aldactazide, Tab. (Searle)
W/Timolol maleate.
See: Timolide, Tab. (Merck Sharp & Dohme)
W/Triamterene.
See: Dyazide, Cap. (SmithKline)
■ **HYDROCHOLERETICS.**
See: Bile Salts (Various Mfr.)
Dehydrocholic Acid (Various Mfr.)

Desoxycholic Acid (Various Mfr.)
Ox Bile Ext. (Various Mfr.)
HYDROCIL INSTANT. (Rowell) Blond psyllium coating containing psyllium 3.5 Gm/3.7 Gm. dose. Tan granular, instant mix, sugar-free, low sodium, low potassium powder. Unit dose packets. Jar 250 Gm.
Use: Bulk forming laxative.
HYDRO COBEX. (Pasadena Research) Hydroxocobalamin 1000 mcg. Vial 10 cc.
HYDROCODONE. B.A.N. Dihydrocodeinone (Various Mfr.) 7,8-Dihydro-0³-methylnormorphine.
Use: Cough suppressant.
HYDROCODONE RESIN COMPLEX.
Use: Cough suppressant.
W/Phenyltoloxamine resin complex.
See: Tussionex, Prods. (Pennwalt)
• **HYDROCODONE BITARTRATE,** U.S.P. XXI. Tab., U.S.P. XXI. Dihydrocodeinone bitartrate. 4,5α-Epoxy-3-methoxy-17-methylmorphinan-6-one tartrate (1:1) hydrate (2:5).
Use: Antitussive.
See: Anodynos-DHC, Tab. (Berlex)
Dicodethal, Elix. (Lannett)
W/Combinations.
See: Vicodin, Tab. (Knoll)
HYDROCORT. (Kenyon) Hydrocortisone 1%, clioquinol 3%, pramoxine HCl 0.5% in a cream base. Jar 20 Gm.
Use: Anti-inflammatory (topical).
HYDROCORTAMATE HCl. 17-Hydroxycorticosterone-21-diethylaminoacetate HCl.
Use: Anti-inflammatory (topical).
See: Ulcortar, Oint. (Ulmer)
HYDROCORTEX. (Kenyon) Hydrocortisone 1% in a cream base. Jar. 20 Gm.
• **HYDROCORTISONE,** U.S.P. XXI. Cream, Sterile, Susp., Oint., Gel., Tab. Lot., Enema, U.S.P. XXI. Pregn-4-ene-3,20-dione, 11,17,21-trihydroxy-, (11β)-Hydrocortisone. 11β, 17, 21-Trihydroxypregn-4-ene-3, 20-Dione. Compound F. Cortisol. (Upjohn) Micronized non-sterile powder for prescription compounding.
Use: Anti-inflammatory (topical).
See: Acticort Lotion 100. (Cummins)
Aeroseb-HC, Aersol (Herbert)
Alphaderm, Cream (Norwich Eaton)
Cetacort, Lot. (Owen)
Cort-Dome, Cream, Lot., Supp. (Miles Pharm)
Cortef, Tab., Cream, Oint. (Upjohn)
Cortenema, Enema (Rowell)
Cortinal, Tube (Kenyon)
Cortril, Oint. (Pfipharmecs)
Cremesone, Cream (Dalin)
Delacort, Lot. (Mericon)
Dermacort, Cream, Lot. (Rowell)
Dermolate, Prods. (Schering)
Durel-Cort, Creme, Oint., Lot. (Durel)
Ecosone, Cream (Star)
HC Derma-Pax, Liq. (Recsei)
HI-COR-1.0, Cream, (C&M Pharmacal)
HI-COR-2.5, Cream (C&M Pharmacal)

Hycortole, Cream, Oint. (Premo)
Hydrocortex, Tube (Kenyon)
Hydrocortone, Tab. (Merck Sharp & Dohme)
Hytone, Cream, Oint., Lot. (Dermik)
Lexocort, Pow., Lot. (Lexington)
Lipo-Adrenal Cortex, Vial (Upjohn)
Maso-Cort, Lot. (Mason)
Microcort, Lotion (Alto Pharm.)
My Cort, Cream (Scrip)
Optef, Sol. (Upjohn)
Proctocort, Oint. (Rowell)
Rocort, Lot. (Rocky Mtn.)
Signef, Supp. (Fellows-Testagar)
Synacort, Cream (Syntex)
Tarcortin, Cream (Reed & Carnrick)
Texacort 25, & 50, Lot. (Cooper)
Ulcort, Cream, Lot. (Ulmer)

HYDROCORTISONE W/COMBINATIONS

See: Achromycin W/Hydrocortisone, Oint., Ophth.
Oint. (Lederle)
Acrisan w/Hydrocortisone, Liq. (Recsei)
Aural Acute, Ear Drops (Saron)
Bafil, Cream. (Scruggs)
Barseb HC, Scalp Lot. (Barnes-Hind)
Barseb Thera-spray, Aerosol (Barnes-Hind)
Biscolan HC, Supp. (Lannett)
Bro-Parin, Otic Susp. (Riker)
Calmurid HC, Cream (Pharmacia)
Caquin, Cream (O'Neal, Jones, Feldman)
Carmol HC, Cream (Ingram)
Coidocort, Cream (Coast)
Cor-Tar-Quin, Cream, Lot. (Miles Pharm)
Cortef, Preps. (Upjohn)
Corticaine Cream (Glaxo)
Corticoid, Cream (Jenkins)
Cortin, Cream (C&M Pharm.)
Cortisporin, Prep. (Burroughs Wellcome)
Derma-Cover-HC, Liq., Oint. (Scrip)
Dermarex, Cream (Hyrex-Key)
Dicort, Cream, Supp. (Hickam)
Doak Oil Forte, Liq. (Doak)
Drotic No. 2, Drops (Ascher)
Durel-Cort 'V,' Cream, Oint., Lot. (Durel)
Eldecort, Cream (Elder)
Fostril HC, Lot. (Westwood)
HC-Form, Jelly (Recsei)
HC-Jel, Jelly (Recsei)
Heb-Cort., Cream, Lot. (Barnes-Hind)
Heb-Cort MC, Cream (Barnes-Hind)
Heb-Cort V, Cream, Lot. (Barnes-Hind)
Hexaderm, Hexaderm-I.Q., Cream (Amfre-Grant)
Hi-Cort N Cream (Blaine)
Hill-Cortac, Cream, Lot. (Hill)
Hydrocort, Tube (Kenyon)
Hydroquin, Cream, Oint. (Robinson)
Hysone, Oint. (Mallard)
Kencort, Cream (Kenyon)
Kleer, Spray (Scrip)
Lanvisone, Cream (Lannett)
Loroxide-HC, Lot. (Dermik)
Maso-Form, Cream (Mason)
Mity-quin, Cream (Reid-Provident)

Myci-Cort, Liq., Spray (Misemer)
My-Cort, Drops, Lot., Oint., Spray (Scrip)
Neocort, Oint. (H.V.P.)
Neo-Cort Dome, Cream, Lot., Drops (Miles Pharm)
Neo Cort Top, Oint. (Standex)
Neo-Domeform-HC, Cream, Lot., Susp. (Miles Pharm)
Nutracort, Cream, Gel., Lot. (Owen)
1 + 1 Creme, 1 + 1-F Creme (Dunhall)
Ophthel, Liq. (Elder).
Ophthocort, Oint. (Parke Davis)
Orlex HC Otic (Baylor)
Oto, Drops (Reid-Provident)
Otobiotic, Soln. (Schering)
Otocalm-H Ear Drops (Parmed)
Otostan H.C. (Standex)
Panhydrosone, Tab., Pow. (Panray)
Pyocidin-Otic, Sol. (Berlex)
Quinsone, Cream (Sutliff & Case)
Racet Forte, Cream (Lemmon)
Racet LCD, Cream (Lemmon)
Rectal Medicone-HC (Medicone)
Sherform-HC, Creme (Sheryl)
Stera-Form, Creme (Mayrand)
Steramine Otic, Drops (Mayrand)
Syntar HC Cream, Oint. (Elder)
Tarcortin, Cream (Reed & Carnrick)
Tar-Quin-HC, Oint. (Jenkins)
Tenda HC, Cream (Dermik)
Terra-Cortril, Prep. (Pfipharmecs)
Theracort, Lot. (C&M Pharm.)
T-Spray, Spray (Saron)
Vanoxide-HC, Lot. (Dermik)
V-Cort, Cream (Scrip)
Vioform-Hydrocortisone, Prep. (Ciba)
Vio-Hydrocort, Oint., Cream (Columbia)
Vytone, Cream, (Dermik)

• **HYDROCORTISONE ACETATE,** U.S.P. XXI. Sterile Susp., Lotion, Ophth. Oint., Ophth. Susp., Oint., Cream, U.S.P. XXI. Pregn-4-ene-3,20-dione, 21-(acetyloxy)-11,17-dihydroxy-, (11β)-. Hydrocortisone 21-acetate. 17-Hydroxycorticosterone-21-acetate, comp.F. (Upjohn) Micronized non-sterile powder for prescription compounding.
Use: Adrenocortical steroid (topical anti-inflammatory).
See: Anusol-HC, Supp. (Warner-Chilcott)
Biosone, Vial (Kay)
Caldecort, Cream (Pharmacraft)
Cortef Acetate, Ophth. Oint., Inj. (Upjohn)
Cortifoam, Aerosol (Reed & Carnrick)
Cortiprel, Cream (Pasadena Research)
Cortril Acetate, Aq. Susp., Oint. (Pfipharmecs)
Ferncort, Lotion (Ferndale)
Fernisone Inj., Vial (Ferndale)
Gynecort, Oint. (Combe)
Hydro-Can (Paddock)
Hydrocort, Vial (Dunhall)
Hydrocortone Acetate, Prep. (Merck Sharp & Dohme)
Hydrosone, Inj. (Sig)
My-Cort, Lot. (Scrip)

Pramosone Cream, Lot. (Ferndale)
Span-Ster, Inj. (Scrip)
Tucks-HC (Parke-Davis)
HYDROCORTISONE ACETATE W/COMBINATIONS
See: Anusol-HC, Cream, Supp. (Warner-Chilcott)
Biotic-Opth W/HC, Oint. (Scrip)
Biotres HC, Cream (Central)
Biscolan HC, Supp. (Lannett)
Carmol HC, Cream (Ingram)
Chloromycetin-Hydrocortisone Ophth. Susp.
(Parke-Davis)
Coly-Mycin-S Otic, Sol. (Warner-Chilcott)
Cor-Oticin, Liq. (Maurry)
Cortaid, Cream, Lot., Oint. (Upjohn)
Cortef Acetate, Inj., Oint., Susp. (Upjohn)
Derma Medicone-HC, Oint. (Medicone)
Dicort, Supp. (Hickam)
Doctient HC, Supp. (Suppositoria)
Epifoam, Aerosol (Reed & Carnrick)
Estro-V HC, Supp. (Webcon)
Eye-Cort, Sol. (Mallard)
Furacin-HC Otic (Eaton)
Furacin HC Urethral Inserts (Eaton)
Furacort Cream (Eaton)
Komed HC, Lotion (Barnes-Hind)
Lida-Mantle HC, Cream (Miles Pharm)
Mantadil, Cream (Burroughs Wellcome)
Neo-Cortef, Preps. (Upjohn)
Neo-Hytone Cream (Dermik)
Neopolycin-HC, Oint., Ophth. Oint. (Merrell Dow)
Ophthocort, Ointment (Parke-Davis)
Ortho, Eye-Ear Drops (Vortech)
Proctofoam-HC, Aer. (Reid and Carnrick)
Pyracort, Liq. (Lemmon)
Quinsone, Oint. (Sutliff & Case)
Racet Forte, Cream (Lemmon)
Rectacort, Supp. (Century)
Rectal Medicone-HC, Supp. (Medicone)
Wyanoids HC, Suppos. (Wyeth)
• **HYDROCORTISONE BUTYRATE.** USAN.
Use: Glucocorticoid.
• **HYDROCORTISONE CYPIONATE,** U.S.P. XXI. Oral
Susp. U.S.P. XXI. Hydrocortisone 21-cyclopentane-
propionate. Hydrocortisone Cypionate.
Use: Glucocorticoid.
• **HYDROCORTISONE HEMISUCCINATE,** U.S.P. XXI.
• **HYDROCORTISONE SODIUM PHOSPHATE,** U.S.P.
XXI. Inj., U.S.P. XXI. Pregn-4-ene-3,20-dione, 11,17-
dihydroxy-21-(phosphonoxy)-, disodium salt,
(11β)-. Hydrocortisone 21-(disodium phosphate). Hy-
drocortisone Sodium Phosphate
Use: Adrenocortical steroid (anti-inflammatory).
• **HYDROCORTISONE SODIUM SUCCINATE,** U.S.P.
XXI. Inj., U.S.P. XXI. Pregn-4-ene-3,20-dione, 31-(3-
carboxy-l-oxopropoxy)-11,17-dihydroxy-, (11β)-. Hy-
drocortisone 21-(sodium succinate). Hydrocortisone
Sodium Succinate.
Use: Adrenocortical steroid (anti-inflammatory).
See: A-hydroCort, Vial (Abbott)
Solu-Cortef, Vial (Upjohn)
HYDROCORTISONE DIETHYLAMINOACETATE HCl.
See: Hydrocortamate

HYDROCORTISONE DYPROPIONATE.
See: Cortef, Fluid (Upjohn)
HYDROCORTISONE I.V.
See: A-Hydro Cort, Vial (Abbott)
Solu-Cortef, Vial (Upjohn)
HYDROCORTISONE PHOSPHATE.
See: Hydrocortone Phosphate, Inj. (Merck Sharp &
Dohme)
• **HYDROCORTISONE VALERATE,** U.S.P. XXI.
Cream, U.S.P. XXI.
Use: Glucocorticoid.
See: Westcort Cream (Westwood)
HYDROCORTONE ACETATE. (Merck Sharp &
Dohme) Hydrocortisone Acetate, U.S.P. **Ophth.
Oint.** 15 mg./Gm. in a white petrolatum and
mineral oil base. Tube 3.5 Gm.; **Saline Susp.** 25
mg./ml. 50 mg./ml., w/sod. chloride 9 mg.,
polysorbate 80 4 mg., sod. carboxymethylcellulose
5 mg./ml. w/water for injection, benzyl alcohol 9
mg. Vial 5 ml. Use: Rheumatoid and osteo-arthritis.
Topical Oint. 1%, w/zinc stearate, propylene
glycol, polyethylene glycol, purified water,
benzalkonium chloride 0.025%. Tube 15 Gm., 30
Gm.
Use: Relief of the inflammatory manifestations of
corticosteroid-responsive dermatoses.
HYDROCORTONE PHOSPHATE INJECTION. (Merck
Sharp & Dohme) Hydrocortisone sodium phosphate
equivalent to 50 mg./ml. w/creatinine 8 mg., sod.
citrate 10 mg./ml. w/sod. hydroxide, sod. bisulfite
3.2mg., methylparaben 1.5mg., propylparaben
0.2mg., water for injection q.s./ml. Vial 2ml. multiple
dose, 10 ml. multiple dose. Disp. syringe 2 ml.
single dose.
Use: Adrenocortical steroid.
HYDROCORTONE TABLETS. (Merck Sharp &
Dohme) Hydrocortisone 10 mg., 20 mg./Tab. Bot.
100s.
HYDRO-D TABLETS. (Blue Cross)
Hydrochlorothiazide 25 mg. or 50 mg./Tab. Bot.
1000s.
Use: Diuretic.
HYDRODIURIL. (Merck Sharp & Dohme)
Hydrochlorothiazide 25 mg./Tab. Bot. 100s, 1000s;
Unit dose pkg. 100s; 50 mg./Tab. Bot. 100s,
1000s, 5000s. Unit dose pkg. 100s; 100 mg./Tab.
Bot. 100s.
Use: Diuretic, antihypertensive.
HYDRO-ERGOT. (Interstate) Hydrogenated ergot
alkaloids 0.5 mg. or 1.0 mg./Tab. Bot. 100s.
• **HYDROFILCON A.** USAN.
Use: Contact lens material.
• **HYDROFLUMETHIAZIDE,** U.S.P. XXI. Tab., U.S.P.
XXI. 3,4-Dihydro-6-tri-fluoromethyl-7-sulfamoylbenzo-
1,2,4-thiadiazine1,1 dioxide,3,4-Dihydro-6-(tri-
fluoromethyl)-2H-1,2,4-benzo-thiadiazine-7-sulfonami-
de-1,1-Dioxide. Di-Ademil; Hydrenox; Naclex; Rontyl
Use: Antihypertensive; diuretic.
See: Diucardin, Tab. (Ayerst)
Saluron, Tab. (Bristol)
W/Reserpine.

See: Salutensin, Tab. (Bristol)
    Salutensin-Demi, Tab. (Bristol)
HYDROGEN DIOXIDE.
    See: Hydrogen Peroxide.
• **HYDROGEN PEROXIDE CONCENTRATE,** U.S.P. XXI.
• **HYDROGEN PEROXIDE TOPICAL SOLUTION,**
    U.S.P. XXI. (Various Mfr.) (3%). 4 oz., 8 oz., pt.
    Use: Antiseptic.
HYDROGEN PEROXIDE SOLUTION 30%, Perhydrol.
    Hydrogen pioxide. Bot. ¼ lb., ½ lb., 1 lb.
    Use: Dentistry & preparing the 3% solution.
HYDROGESIC. (Edwards) Hydrocodone birtartrate 7.5
    mg., acetaminophen 650 mg./Tab. Bot. 100s.
    Use: Mild to moderate pain.
HYDROMAL. (Mallard) Hydrochlorothiazine 50
    mg./Tab. Bot. 1000s
HYDROMAX SYRUP. (Blue Cross) Ephedrine sulfate
    6.25 mg., theophylline 32.5 mg., hydroxyzine HCl
    2.5 mg./5 ml. Bot. 16 oz.
    Use: Bronchodilator for use in asthma.
HYDROMORPHINOL. B.A.N. 7,8-Dihydro-14-hydroxy-
    morphine. Numorphan Oral
    Use: Narcotic analgesic.
HYDROMORPHONE. B.A.N. 7,8-Dihydromorphinone.
    Dilaudid hydrochloride
    Use: Narcotic analgesic.
HYDROMORPHONE. 4,5-Epoxy-3-hydroxy-17-methyl-
    morphinan-6-one.
    Use: Analgesic (narcotic).
• **HYDROMORPHONE HYDROCHLORIDE,** U.S.P.
    XXI. Inj., Tab., U.S.P. XXI. Dihydromorphinone HCl.
    4,5α-Epoxy-3-hydroxy-17-methylmorphinan-6-one
    HCl.
    Use: Analgesic; Narcotic.
    See: Dilaudid Prods. (Knoll)
W/Sod. citrate, antimony pot. tartrate and chloroform.
    Inj.
    See: Dilocol, Liq. (Table Rock)
HYDROMORPHONE SULFATE. 4,5-Epoxy 3-hydroxy-
    17-methylmorphinan-6-one sulfate (2:1).
    Use: Analgesic (narcotic).
HYDROMOX. (Lederle) Quinethazone. 7-Chloro-2-eth-
    yl-1,2,3,4-tetrahydro-4-oxo-6-sulfamylquinazoline 50
    mg./Tab. Bot. 100s, 500s.
    Use: Treatment of edema & hypertension.
HYDROMOX-R. (Lederle) Quinethazone 50 mg., reser-
    pine 0.125 mg./Tab. Bot. 100s, 500s.
HYDROPANE. (Blue Cross) Hydrocodone bitartrate 5
    mg., homatropine methylbromide 1.5 mg./5 ml. Bot.
    16 oz.
    Use: Cough syrup.
HYDROPEL. (C & M Pharmacal) Silicone 30%,
    hydrophobic starch derivative 10%, petrolatum. Jar.
    2 oz., 1 lb.
    Use: Protective silicone ointment.
HYDROPHILIC OINTMENT, U.S.P. XXI. Stearyl
    alcohol, white petrolatum, propylene glycol, sod.
    lauryl sulfate & water. 1 lb. jar (Fougea)
HYDROPHILIC OINTMENT BASE. Oil in water
    emulsion bases. (Emerson) 1 lb.
    See: Aquaphilic Ointment (Medco)

Cetaphil, Cream, Lot. (Texas Pharmacal)
Dermovan, Cream (Texas Pharmacal)
Lanaphilic Ointment (Medco)
Monobase, Oint. (Torch)
Polysorb, Oint. (Savage)
Unibase, Oint. (Parke-Davis)
HYDROPINE #1. (Wolins) Hydrochlorothiazide 25
    mg., reserpine 0.125 mg./Tab. Bot. 100s, 1000s.
HYDROPINE #2. (Wolins) Hydrochlorothiazide 50
    mg., reserpine 0.125 mg./Tab. Bot. 100s, 1000s.
HYDROPLUS. (Reid-Provident) Hydrocholorothiazide
    50 mg., reserpine 0.125 mg./Tab. Bot. 1000s.
    Use: Hypertension treatment.
HYDROPRES-25 & 50. (Merck Sharp & Dohme) Hydro-
    chlorothiazide 25 mg., reserpine 0.125 mg./Tab.
    Also hydrochlorothiazide 50 mg., reserpine 0.125
    mg./Tab. Bot. 100s & 1000s.
    Use: Antihypertensive.
HYDROPRIN. (Cenci) Hydrochlorothiazide 25 mg.,
    reserpine 0.125 mg./Tab. or 50 mg./Tab. Bot.
    100s, 1000s.
    Use: Hypertension treatment.
HYDROQUIN. (Robinson) Hydrocortisone 1%,
    clioquinol 3%. Cream: Tube 5 Gm., 20 Gm. Jar 4
    oz., 8 oz., 1 lb. Ointment: Jar 4 oz., 1 lb.
    Use: Adrenocortical steroid therapy.
HYDROQUIN W/COAL TAR SOLUTION. (Robinson)
    Hydrocortisone ½%, clioquinol 1%, coal tar sol.
    3%. Tube ½ oz.
• **HYDROQUINONE,** U.S.P. XXI. Cream, Topical Soln.,
    U.S.P. XXI. 1,4-Benzenediol.
    Use: Depigmenting agent.
    See: Artra Skin Tone Cream (Plough)
        Black and White Bleaching Cream (Plough)
        Derma-Blanch, Cream (Chattem)
        Eldopaque Cream, Oint. (Elder)
        Eldopaque Forte Cream, Oint. (Elder)
        Eldoquin, Cream, Lot. (Elder)
        Esoterica Medicated Cream Prods. (Norcliff
        Thayer)
HYDROQUINONE MONOBENZYL ETHER.
    See: Benoquin, Oint., Lot. (Elder)
HYDROSAL. (Hydrosal Co.) A colloidal susp. of
    aluminum acetate 5%. **Susp.:** Bot. 16 oz., 1 gal.
    Oint.: 54 Gm., 113.4 Gm. Jars 54 Gm., 454 Gm.
HYDROSERP. (Zenith) Hydrochlorothiazide 25 mg., or
    50 mg., reserpine 0.125 mg. or 0.1 mg./Tab. Bot.
    100s, 1000s.
    Use: Antihypertensive.
HYDROSERP-50. (Freeport) Hydrochlorothiazide 50
    mg., reserpine 0.125 mg./Tab. Bot. 1000s.
    Use: Antihypertensive.
HYDROSERPINE. (Geneva) Hydrochlorothiazide 25
    mg., 50 mg., reserpine 0.125 mg./Tab. Bot. 100s.
    Use: Antihypertensive.
HYDROSERPINE No. 1. (Zenith) Hydrochlorothiazide
    25 mg., reserpine 0.125 mg./Tab. Bot. 100s,
    1000s.
    Use: Antihypertensive, diuretic.
HYDROSERPINE No. 2. (Zenith) Hydrochlorothiazide
    50 mg., reserpine 0.125 mg./Tab. Bot. 100s,
    1000s.

Use: Antihypertensive, diuretic.
HYDROSERPINE No. 3. (Zenith) Hydrochlorothiazide
25 mg., reserpine 0.1 mg./Tab. Bot. 100s, 1000s.
Use: Antihypertensive, diuretic.
HYDROSERPINE No. 4. (Zenith) Hydrochlorothiazide
50 mg., reserpine 0.1 mg./Tab. Bot. 100s, 1000s.
Use: Antihypertensive diuretic.
HYDROSERPINE PLUS. (Zenith) Hydralazine HCl 25
mg., hydrochlorothiazide 15 mg., reserpine 0.1
mg./Tab. Bot. 100s, 1000s.
Use: Hypertension.
HYDROSOL. (Rocky Mtn.) Prednisolone 21
phosphate 20 mg./cc. Vial 10 cc.
Use: Steroid.
HYDROSONE. (Sig) Hydrocortisone acetate 25 mg.,
50 mg./ml. Vial 5 mg.
Use: Anti-inflammatory.
HYDROTALCITE. B.A.N. Aluminum magnesium
hydroxide carbonate hydrate. Altacite.
Use: Antacid.
HYDROTENSIN-50. (Mayrand) Hydrochlorothiazide 50
mg., reserpine 0.125 mg./Tab. Bot. 100s, 1000s.
Use: Treatment of hypertension.
HYDROTOIN CREAM. (Knight) Hydrocortisone 0.5%.
Tube ½ oz.
Use: Antifungal, antibacterial, antipruritic.
HYDROXACEN. (Central) Hydroxyzine HCl 50
mg./ml. w/benzyl alcohol 0.9%, sodium hydroxide.
Vial 10 ml.
Use: I.M. tranquilizer, antihistaminic.
HYDROX B-12. (Rocky Mtn.) Hydroxocobalamin 1000
mcg./cc. Vial 10 cc.
HYDROXAL. (Blue Line) Aluminum hydroxide susp.
Bot. 1 gal.
Use: Orally, antacid.
HYDROXAMETHOCAINE. B.A.N. 2-Dimethyl-amino-
ethyl 4-butylaminosalicylate. Hydroxytetracaine
(I.N.N.)
Use: Local anesthetic.
HYDROXINDASOL HCl. 5-Hydroxy-1-(p-methoxy-ben-
zyl)-2-methyltryptamine HCl.
• **HYDROXOCOBALAMIN,** U.S.P. XXI. Inj., U.S.P.
XXI. α-(5,6-Dimethylbenzimidazolyl) hydroxocoba-
mide. Vit. B 12a and B 12b. Hydrovit; Neo-Cytamen.
Use: Treatment of megaloblastic anemia.
See: Alphamin, Inj. (Vortech)
　 AlphaRedisol, Vial (Merck Sharp & Dohme)
　 Alpha-Ruvite, Vial (Savage)
　 Cobavite L.A., Vial (Lemmon)
　 Droxomin, Inj. (Reid-Provident)
　 Droxovite, Vial (Kay)
　 Hydrobexan, Vial (Keene)
　 Rubesol-L.A. 1000, Inj. (Central)
　 Span-12, Inj. (Scrip)
　 Sytobex-H, Vial (Parke-Davis)
　 Twelve-Span, Vial (Foy)
4'-HYDROXYACETANILIDE. Acetaminophen, U.S.P.
XXI.
HYDROXY BIS(ACETATO)ALUMINUM. Aluminum
Subacetate Topical Solution, U.S.P. XXI.
HYDROXYAMPHETAMINE. B.A.N. 4-(2-Amino-propyl)-
phenol. Paredrine.

Use: Sympathomimetic; mydriatic.
• **HYDROXYAMPHETAMINE HYDROBROMIDE,**
U.S.P. XXI. Ophth. Soln., U.S.P. XXI. dl-p-(2-Amino-
propyl) phenol HBr.
Use: Adrenergic (ophthalmic).
See: Paredrine Hydrobromide, Sol. (SmithKline)
**17β-HYDROXYANDROST-4-EN-3-ONE HEPTANO-
ATE, OR PROPIONATE.** Testosterone Enanthate, or
Propionate. U.S.P. XXI.
2-HYDROXYBENZAMIDE.
See: Salicylamide.
**HYDROXYBIS(SALICYLATO)ALUMINUM
DIACETATE.**
See: Aluminum aspirin
HYDROXYCHLOROQUINE. B.A.N. 7-Chloro-4-[4-(N-
ethyl-N-2-hydroxyethylamino)-1-methyl-butylamino]q-
uinoline.
Use: Antimalarial.
See: Plaquenil sulfate (Winthrop-Breon)
• **HYDROXYCHLOROQUINE SULFATE,** U.S.P. XXI.
Tab., U.S.P. XXI. Ethanol, 2-4-(7-chloro-4-quinolinyl)-
amino pentyl ethylamino-, sulfate (1:1) salt. 7-Chloro-
4- 4-[ethyl(2-hydroxyethyl)-amino]-1-methyl-
butylamino quinoline sulfate. 2-[[4-[(7chloro-4-quino-
lyl)amino]-pentyl]ethylamino]ethanol Sulfate (1:1).
Use: Antimalarial; lupus erythematosus
suppressant.
See: Plaquenil, Tab. (Winthrop-Breon)
17-HYDROXYCORTICOSTERONE-21-ACETATE. Hydrocortisone Acetate, U.S.P. XXI.
HYDROXYDIONE SODIUM. 21-Hydroxy-pregnane-
dione sod. succinate.
HYDROXYDIONE SODIUM SUCCINATE. B.A.N. Sod.
21-hydroxypregnane-3,20-dione succinate.
Presuren; Viadril.
Use: Anesthetic.
17β-HYDROXYESTER-4-EN-3-ONE DECANOATE.
See: Deca-Durabolin, Amp., Vial (Organon)
**2-HYDROXYETHANESULFONIC ACID, 2-HYDROXY-
4,4'-STILBENEDICARBOXAMIDINE COMPOUND
(2:1).** Hydroxystilbamidine Isethionate, U.S.P.
XXI.
2-HYDROXYETHYL BENZYLCARBAMATE. Bura-
mate.
• **HYDROXYETHYL CELLULOSE,** N.F.XVI.
Use: Topical protectant, thickening agent.
**(2-HYDROXYETHYL)DIISOPROPYLMETHYL-AMMO-
NIUM BROMIDE XANTHENE-9-CARBOXYLATE.**
Propantheline Bromide, U.S.P. XXI.
**I-(2-HYDROXYETHYL)-2-METHYL-5-NITRO-MIDAZO-
LE.** Metronidazole, U.S.P. XXI.
**8-HYDROXY-4', 5',6,7-FUROCOUMARIN, AMMOIDIN,
XANTHOTOXIN.** Methoxsalen, U.S.P. XXI.
**I-(2-HYDROXYETHYL)-4-[3-(2-TRIFLUOROMETHYL)-
10-PHENOTHIAZINYL-PROPYL]-PIPERAZINE
DIHYDROCHLORIDE.** Fluphenazine Hydrochloride,
U.S.P. XXI.
HYDROXYISOINDOLIN. Under study.
Use: Hypertension treatment.
**17-HYDROXY-7α-MERCAPTO-3-OXO-17α-PREGN-
4-ENE-21-CARBOXYLIC ACIDα-LACTONE ACE-
TATE.** Spironolactone, U.S.P. XXI.

2-HYDROXY-4-METHOXYBENZOPHENONE. Oxybenzone, U.S.P. XXI.

l-m-HYDROXY-α-[(METHYLAMINO)METHYL]-BENZYL ALCOHOL HYDROCHLORIDE. Phenylephrine Hydrochloride, U.S.P. XXI.

11,β-HYDROXY-6α-METHYLPREGN-4-ONE-3,20DIONE. (Allergan; Upjohn)

1-(HYDROXYMERCURI-¹⁹⁷Hg)-2-PROPANOL.
See: Merprane

17β-HYDROXY-17-METHYLANDROST-4-EN-3-ONE
Methyltesterone, U.S.P. XXI.

17-HYDROXY-6α-METHYLPREGN-4-ENE-3,20DIONE 17 ACETATE. Medroxyprogesterone Acetate, U.S.P. XXI.

17-β-HYDROXY-6α-METHYL-17-(1-PRO-PYNYL)-ANDROST-4-EN-3-ONE.
See: Oracon, Tab. (Mead Johnson)

N-[I-(HYDROXYMETHYL)PROPYL]-I-METHYL-D-LYSERGAMIDE BIMALEATE. Methysergide Maleate, U.S.P. XXI.

3-HYDROXY-I-METHYLPYRIDINIUM BROMIDE DIMETHYLCARBAMATE. Pyridostigmine Bromide, U.S.P. XXI.

HYDROXYMYCIN. An antibiotic substance obtained from cultures of *Streptomyces paucisporogenes.*

HYDROXYPETHIDINE. B.A.N. Ethyl 4-(3-hydroxy-phenyl)-1-methylpiperidine-4-carboxylate.
Use: Narcotic analgesic.

• **HYDROXYPHENAMATE.** USAN. 2-Hydroxy-2-phenyl-butyl carbamate.
Use: Tranquilizer.

(M-HYDROXYPHENYL) TRIMETHYLAMMONIUM BROMIDE DIMETHYL CARBAMATE. Neostigmine Bromide, U.S.P. XXI.

(m-HYDROXYPHENYL) TRIMETHYL AMMONIUM METHYL SULFATE DIMETHYL CARBAMATE. Neostigmine Methylsulfate, U.S.P. XXI.

17-HYDROXY-19-NOR-17α-PREGN-4-EN-20-YN-3-, ONE ACETATE. Norethindrone Acetate, U.S.P. XXI.

17-HYDROXY-19-NOR-17α-PREGN-4-EN-20-YN-3-ONE. Norethindrone, U.S.P. XXI.

17-HYDROXYPREGN-4-ENE-3,20-DIONE HEXANOATE. Hydroxyprogesterone Caproate, U.S.P. XXI.

HYDROXYPROCAINE. B.A.N. 2-Diethylamino-ethyl 4-aminosalicylate.
Use: Local anesthetic.

HYDROXYPROGESTERONE. B.A.N. 17α-Hydroxy-pregn-4-ene-3,20-dione. Primolut Depot [hexanoate].
Use: Progestogen.

• **HYDROXYPROGESTERONE CAPROATE,** U.S.P. XXI. Inj., U.S.P. XXI. 17α-Hydrogypregn-4-ene-3,20-dione. Pregn-4-ene-3,20-dione,17-[(l)oxohexyl)-oxy]-.
Use: Progestin.
See: Delalutin, Vial (Squibb)
    Hy-Gestrone, Vial (Pasadena Research)
    Hylutin, Inj. (Hyrex)
    Hyprogest 250, Inj. (Keene)
    Hyproval-P.A., Inj. (Reid-Provident)
    Pro-Depo, Inj. (Vortech)
W/Estradiol valerate.
See: Hy-Gestradol, Inj. (Pasadena Research)
    Hylutin-Est., Inj. (Hyrex)

• **HYDROXYPROPYL CELLULOSE,** N.F. XVI.
Use: Topical protectant, tablet coating agent.

• **HYDROXYPROPYL METHYLCELLULOSE,** U.S.P. XXI. Ophth. Sol. U.S.P. XXI. Cellulose, 2-hydroxypro-pyl methyl ether. Cellulose hydroxypropyl methyl ether. The propylene glycol ether of methylcellulose available in the 2208, 2906 and 2910 forms.
Use: Suspending agent; ophth, topical protectant.
See: Anestacon (Alcon)
    Econopred, Susp. (Alcon)
W/Benzalkonium chloride.
See: Goniosol (Smith, Miller & Patch)
    Isopto Tears (Alcon)
    Ultra Tears, Sol. (Alcon)

• **HYDROXYPROPYL METHYLCELLULOSE PHTHALATE 200731,** N.F. XVI.

• **HYDROXYPROPYL METHYLCELLULOSE PHTHALATE 200824,** N.F. XVI.

8-HYDROXYQUINOLINE COMB.
See: Ammens Medicated Powder, Spray (Bristol-Myers)
    Foille, Spray, Liq., Oint. (Carbisulphoil)

8-HYDROXYQUINOLINE SULFATE. (Mallinckrodt; City Chem.)
Use: As an antiseptic.
See: Oxyquinoline Sulfate (Various Mfr.)

5-HYDROXYSALICYLIC ACID. Gentisic Acid. (Various Mfg.)

HYDROXYSTEARIN SULFATE. Sulfonate hydrogenated castor oil.

HYDROXYSTILBAMIDINE. B.A.N. 4,4'-Diamidino-2-hydroxystilbene.
Use: Treatment of leishmaniasis and trypanosomiasis.

• **HYDROXYSTILBAMIDINE ISETHIONATE,** U.S.P. XXI. Sterile, U.S.P. XXI. Benzenecarboximidamide, 4-[2-[4-(aminoiminomethyl)phenyl]ethnyl]-3-hydroxy-bis(2-hydroxyethanesulfonate). 2-Hydroxy-4,4'-stil-benedicarboxamidine bis(2-hydroxyethanesul-fonate)(Salt). 2-Hydroxyethanesulfonic acid, 2-hy-droxy-4,4'-stilbenedicarboxamidine compound (2:1) (Merrell Dow) Amp. (225 mg.) 20 cc. Box 1s.
Use: Antileishmanial; I.V. 225 mg., may be repeated at 24-hour intervals; blastomycosis Indian kalaa-zar.

2-HYDROXY-4,4'-STILBENEDICARBOXAMIDINE BIS (2-HYDROXY-ETHANESULFONATE)(SALT). Hy-droxystilbamidine Isethionate, U.S.P. XXI.

HYDROXYTOLUIC ACID. B.A.N. 2-Hydroxy-m-toluic acid. 3-Methylsalicylic acid.
Use: Analgesic.

6-HYDROXY-β,2,7-TRIMETHYL-5-BENZOFURANAC-RYLIC ACID, β-**LACTONE W/4,**-5,8-trimethylpsor-alen. Trisoralen.

• **HYDROXYUREA,** U.S.P. XXI. Cap., U.S.P. XXI.
Hydroxycarbamide (I.N.N.)
Use: Antineoplastic agent.
See: Hydrea, Cap. (Squibb)

HYDROXYZINE. B.A.N. 1-4-(Chlorobenzhydryl)-4-[2-(2-hydroxyethoxy)ethyl]piperazine-.
Use: Tranquilizer.

See: Atarax hydrochloride.
 Equipose embonate.
HYDROXYZINE HCI, U.S.P. XXI. Inj., Syrup, Tab.,
 U.S.P. XXI. 2-[2-[-4-(p-Chloro-α-phenylbenzyl-)-1-
 piperazinyl]ethoxy]ethanol dihydrochloride. **Inj.:** (Ab-
 bott) 100 mg./2 ml. amp. or Abboject syringe, 500
 mg./10 ml. vial.
 Use: Tranquilizer, antihistaminic.
 See: Atarax, Syr., Tab. (Roerig)
  Hyzine-50, Inj. (Hyrex)
  Vistarex 50, Inj. (Tunex)
  Vistazine 25, Inj. (Keene)
  Vistazine 50, Inj. (Keene)
  Isoject Vistaril. (Pfizer Laboratories)
W/Ephedrine sulf., theophylline.
 See: Marax DF, Syr. (Roerig)
  Marax Tab. (Roerig)
  Theo-Drox, Tab. (Columbia)
W/Oxyphencyclimine HCl.
 See: Vistrax 5 & 10, Tab. (Pfizer Laboratories)
W/Pentaerythritol tetranitrate.
 See: Cartrax 10, 20, Tab. (Roerig)
HYDROXYZINE PAMOATE, U.S.P XXI. Cap., Oral
 Susp., U.S.P. XXI. 1,1'-Methylene bis(2-hydroxy-3-
 naphthalene-carboxylic acid salt of 1-p-chlorobenzhy-
 dryl)-4-[2-2-hydroxy-ethoxyethyl]piperazine. 2-(2-(4-
 (piperazine.   2-(2-(4-(p-Chloro-α-phenyl-benzyl)-1-
 piperazinyl)ethoxy)ethanol   4,4'-Methylenebis-(3-hy-
 droxy-2-napthoate) (1:1).
 Use: Tranquilizer; antihistaminic.
 See: Vistaril, Cap., Susp. (Pfizer Laboratories)
HYDROZIDE. (MSD AGVET) Hydrochlorothiazide Inj.
 25 mg./cc.
 Use: Diuretic, veterinary medicine.
HYDROZIDE-Z-50. (Mayrand) Hydrochlorothlazide 50
 mg./Tab. Bot. 100s, 1000s.
 Use: Treatment of hypertension.
HY-E-PLEX. (Nutrition) Nat. Vit. E 400 I.U./Cap. Vial.
 Bot. 100s.
HY-FLOW. (CooperVision) Polyvinyl alcohol, hydroxye-
 thycellulose, potassium chloride, sodium chloride,
 benzalkonium chloride 0.01%, edetate disodium
 0.025%. Bot. 2 oz.
 Use: Wetting solution for hard contact lenses.
HYGEFEM DOUCHE. (Blue Line) **Pow.** Benzalkonium
 chloride, citric acid, sod. phosphate, K alum,
 aromatics, excipient, colors. Bot. 4 oz., .38 oz. Box
 6s, 12s.
 Use: Astringent and acidic vaginal douche.
HY-GESTRONE. (Pasadena Research) Hydroxyprogesterone caproate 125 mg./ml. Vial 10 cc. 250
 mg./ml. Vial 5 cc.
HYGIENIC POWDER.
 See: Bo-Car-Al, Pow. (Calgon)
HYGROTON. (USV Labs.) Chlorthalidone 25 mg., 50
 mg., 100 mg./Tab. Bot. 100s, 1000s. Strip
 dispenser 100s. Bot. 5000s for 50 mg. and 100 mg.
 strengths.
 Use: Diuretic, antihypertensive.
HYLOREL. (Pennwalt) Guanadrel sulfate 10 mg. or
 25 mg./Tab. Bot. 100s.
 Use: Hypertension, step II therapy.

HYLUTIN INJECTABLE. (Hyrex) Hydroxyproges-
 terone caproate in oil 250 mg./ml. Vial 5 ml.
 Use: Long acting progesterone for endometriosis,
 infertility, amenorrhea, menstrual cycle.
HYMECROMONE. USAN.
 Use: Choleretic.
HYMETIC. (Hyrex) Trimethobenzamide HCl 100
 mg./ml. Vial 20 ml. I.M. administration.
 Use: Treatment of nausea & vomiting.
HY-N.B.P. OINTMENT. (Bowman) Bacitracin zinc 400
 u., neomycin sulfate 5 mg., polymixin B sulfate
 10,000 u./Gm. Tube ⅛ oz.
 Use: Topical antibiotic.
HYOSCINE AMINOXIDE HBr.
HYOSCINE HYDROBROMIDE. Scopolamine HBr,
 U.S.P. XXI.
 Use: Intestinal antispasmodic.
HYOSCINE-HYOSCYAMINE-ATROPINE.
 Use: Anticholinergic.
 See: Atropine w/hyoscyamine w/hyoscine
HYOSCINE METHOBROMIDE. B.A.N.
 Use: Treatment of peptic ulcer.
 See: Methscopolamine Bromide
HYOSCYAMINE, U.S.P. XXI. Tab., U.S.P. XXI. 1α
 H,5αH-Tropan-3α-ol(−)-tropate (ester). Levo form of
 atropine.
 Use: Anticholinergic.
 See: Bellafoline, Amp., Tab. (Sandoz)
  Cysto-Spaz, Tab. (Webcon)
HYOSCYAMINE-ATROPINE-HYOSCINE.
 Use: Anticholinergic.
 See: Atropine w/hyoscyamine w/hyoscine
HYOSCYAMINE HYDROBROMIDE, U.S.P. XXI. 1α
 H,5αH-Tropan-3α-ol(−)-tropate HBr. Daturine HBr.
 (Various Mfr.)
 Use: Anticholinergic.
W/Physostigmine salicylate.
 See: Pyatromine-H Inj. (Kremers-Urban)
HYOSCYAMINE HYDROCHLORIDE. (Various Mfr.)
HYOSCYAMINE MALEATE.
 See: Bellafoline, Amp., Tab. (Sandoz)
HYOSCYAMINE SALTS.
 Use: Anticholinergic.
W/Atropine salts.
 See: Atropine W/Hyoscyamine.
HYOSCYAMINE SULFATE, U.S.P. XXI. Elixir, Inj.,
 Oral Soln., Tab., U.S.P. XXI. 1αH,5αH-Tropan-3α-
 ol-(−)-tropate (ester) sulfate (2:1) dihydrate.
 Use: Anticholinergic.
 See: Anaspaz, Tab. (Ascher)
  Cystospaz-M, Cap. (Webcon)
W/Atropine sulfate, hyoscine HBr, phenobarbital.
 See: Bar-Cy-Amine, Elix. (Sutliff & Case)
  Bar-Cy-A, Tabs. (Sutliff & Case)
  DeTal, Elix., Tab. (DeLeon)
  Donnatal, Prods. (Robins)
  Hyatal, Elix., Liq. (Kenyon)
  Hyonal C.T., Tab. (Paddock)
  Maso-Donna, Elix., Tab. (Mason)
  Peece, Tab. (Scrip)
  Sedamine, Tab. (Dunhall)

Spasaid, Cap. (Century)
Spasmolin, Tab. (Kenyon)
Spasquid, Elix. (Geneva)
W/Atropine sulf, hyoscine HBr, phenobarbital, pepsin, pancreatin, bile salts.
See: Donnazyme, Tab. (Robins)
W/Atropine sulfate. Scopolamine HCl, phenobarbital.
See: Ultabs, Tab. (Burlington)
W/Belladonna Alkaloids.
See: Belladonna Products
W/Butabarbital.
See: Cystospaz-SR, Cap. (Webcon)
W/Methenamine, atropine sulfate, methylene blue, salol, benzoic acid, gelsemium.
See: Uriprel, Tab. (Pasadena Research)
W/Phenobarbital.
See: Levsin/PB, Tab., Elix., Drops, Inj. (Kremers-Urban)
W/Phenobarbital, simethicone, atropine sulfate, scopolamine HBr.
See: Kinesed, Tab. (Stuart)

HYOSCYAMUS EXTRACT.
W/A. P. C.
See: Valacet Junior, Tab. (Vale)
W/A. P. C., gelsemium ext.
See: Valacet, Tab. (Vale)

HYOSCYAMUS PRODUCTS AND PHENOBARBITAL COMBINATIONS.
Use: Anticholinergic, sedative.
See: Anaspaz PB, Tab. (Pasadena Research)
Donnacin, Elixir, Tab. (Pharmex)
Donnatal, Preps. (Robins)
Elixiral, Elixir (Vita Elixir)
Floramine, Tab. (Lemmon)
Gylanphen, Tab. (Lannett)
Kinesed, Tab. (Stuart)
Neoquess, Tab. (O'Neal)
Nevrotose, Cap. (Vale)
Restophen, Tab. (Noyes)
Sedajen, Tabs. (Jenkins)
Sedatromine, Tab. (Sutliff & Case)

HYOSED T.D. (Galen) Hyoscyamine HBr 0.256 mg., hyoscine HBr 0.0144 mg., atropine sulfate 0.0480 mg., phenobarbital 32.0 mg./Timed disintegration tab. Bot. 100s, 1000s.
Use: Sedative, intestinal antispasmodic.

HY-PAM 25. (Lemmon) Hydroxyzine pamoate 25 mg./Cap. Bot. 100s, 500s, 1000s.
Use: Relief of anxiety & tension, allergic dermatoses.

HY-PAM 50. (Lemmon) Hydroxyzine pamoate 50 mg./Cap. Bot. 100s, 500s, 1000s.
Use: Relief of anxiety & tension, allergic dermatoses.

HY-PANTHRON. (High) Danthron (1,8 Dihydroxyanthraquinone) 7 mg., d-calcium pantothenate 25 mg./Tab. Bot. 100s, 1000s.
Use: Constipation; rehabilitation of the lower bowel.

HYPAQUE-76. (Winthrop-Breon) Diatrizoate meglumine 66%, diatrizoate sodium 10%, iodine 370 mg./ml. Vials 30 ml. Box. 25s; Vials 50 ml. Box 25s, Vials 100 ml. Box. 10s; Bot. 200 ml. Box 10s; Dilution Bot. 200 ml. containing 100 ml. drug. Box 10s.

Use: Urography, aortography, angiography, venography, angiocardiography, arteriography, contrast enhancement of computed tomographic head imaging and intravenous digital arteriography.

HYPAQUE-CYSTO. (Winthrop-Breon) Diatrizoate meglumine 30% solution. 250 ml. in 500 ml. dilution bottle. **Pediatric:** 100 ml. in 300 ml. dilution bottle.
Use: Retrograde cystourethrography.

HYPAQUE-M 75%. (Winthrop-Breon) Diatrizoate meglumine 50%, diatrizoate sodium 25%, 385 mg. iodine/ml. Vials 20 ml., 50 ml. Box 25s.
Use: Angiocardiography, angiography, aortography & urography.

HYPAQUE-M 90%. (Winthrop-Breon) Diatrizoate meglumine 60% & diatrizoate sodium 30%. Vial 50 ml. Box 25s.
Use: Angiocardiography, angiography, aortography, urography, hysterosalpingography.

HYPAQUE MEGLUMINE 30%. (Winthrop-Breon) Diatrizoate meglumine 30%. Bot. 300 ml. w/ & w/o I.V. infusion set.
Use: Infusion urography, CT scan enhancement.

HYPAQUE MEGLUMINE 60%. (Winthrop-Breon) Diatrizoate meglumine 60%. which contains 47.06% iodine. **Vial:** 20 ml. Box 25s. 30 ml. Box 25s. 50 ml. Box 25s. 100 ml. Box 10s. **Dilution Bottle:** 200 ml. w/hanger containing 150 ml. Hypaque meglumine 60%. w/10 intravenous infusion sets. Box 10s.; 200 ml. w/hanger containing 200 ml. Hypaque meglumine 60%, rubber stoppered. Box 10s; 200 ml. w/hanger containing 100 ml. Hypaque meglumine 60% w/10 intravenous infusion sets. Box 10s.
Use: Excretory urography, cerebral angiography, peripheral arteriography, venography, direct cholangiography, splenoportography, anthrography & discography.

HYPAQUE (R)-131 SODIUM.
See: Sodium Diatrizoate

HYPAQUE ORAL. (Winthrop-Breon) **Powder:** Diatrizoate sodium oral powder containing 600 mg. iodine/Gm. Cans 250 Gm. Bot. 10 Gm. **Liquid:** A 41.66% solution. Bot. 120 ml.
Use: Contrast radiology of G.I. tract (orally & enema).

HYPAQUE SODIUM. (Winthrop-Breon) Diatrizoate sodium and contains 59.87% iodine. Sodium 3,5-diacetamido 2,4,6-triiodobenzoate.
Use: Radiopaque medium.
See: Hypaque, Prod. (Winthrop-Breon)

HYPAQUE SODIUM 20%. (Winthrop-Breon) Diatrizoate sodium 20% containing 120 mg. iodine/ml. Multidose vials 100 ml. Box 1s.
Use: Retrograde pyelography.

HYPAQUE SODIUM 25%. (Winthrop-Breon) Diatrizoate sodium 25% containing 150 mg. iodine/ml. Bot. 300 ml., w/ and w/out intravenous infusion set.
Use: Urography and CT scan enhancement.

HYPAQUE SODIUM 50%. (Winthrop-Breon) Diatrizoate sodium. **Vial:** 50% 30 ml., 20 ml. Box 25s, Vial 50 ml. Box 25s. **Dilution Bottle:** 200 ml. w/hanger

containing 100 ml. Hypaque sodium 50% w/10
intravenous infusion sets.; 200 ml. w/hanger
containing 150 ml. Hypaque sodium 50% w/10
intravenous infusion sets; 200 ml. w/hanger
containing 200 ml. Hypaque sodium 50%, rubber
stoppered. Box 10s.
Use: Cerebral and peripheral angiography,
aortography, excretory urography, direct
cholangiography, hysterosalpingography,
intraosseous venography, splenoportography.

HYPERAB. (Cutter) Rabies immune globulin (Human).
Vial 2 ml., 10 ml.
Use: I.M., passive immunization.

HYPERACID. (Wolins) Dihydroxyaluminum
aminoacetate 0.5 Gm./Tab. Bot. 100s, 1000s.

HYPERHEP. (Cutter) Hepatitis B immune globulin
(Human) Vial 250 unit, prefilled syringe 250 unit.
Use: Passive immunity, I.M.

HYPERINE. (Sutliff & Case) Reserpine 0.25 mg./Tab.
Bot. 100s, 1000s.
Use: Antihypertensive.

HYPEROPTO 5%. (Professional Pharmacal) Sterile
5% sodium chloride ointment. Tube 3.5 gm.
Use: Eye therapy.

HYPEROPTO OINTMENT. (Professional Pharmacal)
Sodium HCl 50 mg., D.I. water 150 mg., anhydrous
lanolin 150 mg., liquid petrolatum 50 mg., white
petrolatum 599 mg., methyl paraben 7 mg., propyl
paraben 3 mg./Gm. Tube 3.5 gm.
Use: Reducing edema.

HYPER-RAUW. (Sutliff & Case) Rauwolfia serpentine
100 mg./Tab. Bot. 100s, 1000s.
Use: Antihypertensive.

HYPERSAL. (Softcon) Sodium chloride 5%,
0.002% thimerosal, 0.05% disodium edetate.
Bot. 15 ml.
Use: Reduction of corneal edema.

HYPERSTAT I.V. INJECTION. (Schering) Diazoxide
300 mg. pH adjusted to approx. 11.6 with sod.
hydroxide./20 ml. Amp.
Use: Antihypertensive for hospital use only.

HYPERTEN. (Kenyon) Phenobarbital ¼ gr.,
nitroglycerin 1/300 gr., sod. nitrate 1 gr., veratrum
viride ¾ gr./Tab. Bot. 100s, 1000s.
Use: Hypertension treatment.

HYPERTENSIN-CIBA. Angiotensin Amide, B.A.N.

HYPERTENSION DIAGNOSIS.
See: Regitine, Amp., Tab. (Ciba)

■ **HYPERTENSION THERAPY.**
See: Aldoclor, Tab. (Merck Sharp & Dohme)
Aldomet, Tab. (Merck Sharp & Dohme)
Aldomet Ester HCl, Amp. (Merck Sharp &
Dohme)
Aldoril, Tab. (Merck Sharp & Dohme)
Alkavervir
Alseroxylon
Apresoline, Amp., Tab. (Ciba)
Apresoline, Apresoline Esidrix, Amp., Tab.
(Ciba)
Arfonad, Amp. (Roche)
Corgard, Tab. (Squibb)
Cryptenamine

Deserpidine
Dibenzyline HCl, Cap. (SmithKline)
Diupres, Tab. (Merck Sharp & Dohme)
Diutensen & Diutensen-R, Tab. (Wallace)
Dyazide, Cap. (SmithKline)
Enduron, Tab. (Abbott)
Enduronyl, Tab. (Abbott)
Enduronyl Forte, Tab. (Abbott)
Esidrix, Tab. (Ciba)
Eutonyl, Tab. (Abbott)
Eutron, Tab. (Abbott)
Exna & Exna-R, Tab. (Robins)
Hesperidin Methyl Chalcone (Various Mfr.)
Hexamethonium Chloride & Bromide (Various
Mfr.)
Hydropres, Tab. (Merck Sharp & Dohme)
Hygroton, Tab. (USV)
Hyperstat, I.V. Inj. (Schering)
Inversine, Tab. (Merck Sharp & Dohme)
Lopressor, Tab. (Geigy)
Metatensin, Tab. (Merrell Dow)
Moderil, Tab. (Pfizer)
Naturetin, Tab. (Squibb)
Naquival, Tab. (Schering)
Oretic, Tab. (Abbott)
Oreticyl, Tab. (Abbott)
Priscoline HCl, Preps. (Ciba)
Protoveratrines A & B
Raudixin, Tab. (Squibb)
Rautrax, Tab. (Squibb)
Rautrax-N, Tab. (Squibb)
Rauwolfia Serpentina (Various Mfr.)
Rauzide, Tab. (Squibb)
Regroton, Tab. (USV)
Renese-R, Tab. (Pfizer)
Rescinnamine, Tab. (Var. Mfr.)
Reserpine (Various Mfr.)
Rutin, Tab. (Various Mfr.)
Tetraethylammonium Chloride (Various Mfr.)
Vasodilators
Veratrum Alba
Veratrum Viride
Wytensin, Tab. (Wyeth)
Zaroxolyn, Tab. (Pennwalt)

HYPER-TET. (Cutter) Tetanus immune globulin
(Human) U.S.P. Vial 250 u., Disp. Syringe 250 u.
Use: For immediate injection after injury.

HYPERTHYROIDISM.
See: Antithyroid agents

HYPER-ZEM. (Zemmer) Sod. nitrite 60 mg., pot. nitrate
60 mg., ox bile desic. 8 mg., sod. bicarbonate 110
mg./Tab. Bot. 100s, 1000s.
Use: Orally, vasodilator.

HYPHYLLINE. Dyphylline. (7-Dihydroxy-propyl-theop-
hylline).
See: Neothylline, Elix., Amp., Tab. (Lemmon)

HYPLEX VARI DOSE. (Hyrex) Sterile injectable
solution of Vitamins. **Sol. #1:** B-1 3 mg., B-2 3.6 mg.,
B-6 4 mg., niacin 40 mg., pantothenic acid 15 mg., C
100 mg., biotin 60 mcg./ml. **Sol. #2:** Vit. B-12 5 mcg.,
folic acid 400 mcg./ml.
Use: Multivitamin.

HYPNALDYNE. (Vortech) Phenobarbital 16.2 mg., hyoscyamine sulfate 0.104 mg., atropine sulfate 0.019 mg., scopolamine HBr 0.0065 gr./Tab. Bot. 100s, 1000s.
Use: Sedative w/antispasmodic.

HYPNOGENE.
See: Barbital (Various Mfr.)

HYPNOMIDATE. (Janssen) Etomidate.
Use: Hypnotic.

HYPNO-SED. (Jenkins) Bromisovalum 1 gr., carbromal 3 gr., thiamine mononitrate 9 mg./Tab. Bot. 1000s.

■ **HYPNOTICS.**
See: Sedatives

"HYPO."
See: Sodium Thiosulfate (Various Mfr.)

HYPO-BEE. (Towne) Vit. B-1 50 mg., B-2 20 mg., B-6 5 mg., B-12 15 mcg., niacinamide 25 mg., Ca pantothenate 5 mg., Vit. C 300 mg., E 200 I.U., iron 10 mg./Tab. Bot. 30s, 100s, 250s.

HYPOCHLORITE PREPS.
See: Antiformin
Dakin's Soln.
Hyclorite

■ **HYPOGLYCEMIC AGENTS.**
See: Chlorpropamide
Diabinese, Tab. (Pfizer)
Dymelor, Tab. (Lilly)
Orinase, Tab., Vial (Upjohn)
Phenformin HCl
Tolbutamide
Tolinase, Tab. (Upjohn)

HYPOMINS. (Pasadena Research) Vit. A 5000 I.U., D 400 I.U., C 50 mg., B-1 5 mg., B-2 5 mg., B-6 1 mg., Ca pantothenate 5 mg., niacinamide 20 mg., E 2 I.U., B-12 2 mcg., Fe 10 mg., iodine 0.1 mg., Ca 100 mg., Cu 0.2 mg./Tab. Bot. 100s, 1000s.

α-**HYPOPHAMINE.** Oxytocin.

• **HYPOPHYOSPHOROUS ACID,** N.F. XVI.
Use: Antioxidant.

HYPOTEARS. (CooperVision) Polyvinyl alcohol 1%. Bot. 15 ml. or 30 ml.
Use: Ocular lubricant.

■ **HYPOTENSIVE AGENTS.**
See: Hypertension Therapy

HypRho-D. (Cutter) Rho (D) Immune globulin (Human). Kit of pre-filled single dose syr., prep swab, crossmatch dropper vial and lab forms.

HYPROGEST 250. (Keene) Hydroxyprogesterone caproate inj. 250 mg./ml. Vial 5 ml.
Use: I.M. Long acting progestational agent.

HYPROMELLOSE. B.A.N. A partial mixed methyl and hydroxypropyl ether of cellulose.
Use: Surface active agent.
See: Isopto

HYPROVAL P.A. (Reid-Provident). Hydroxyprogesterone caproate 250 mg., benzyl benzoate 46%, benzyl alcohol 2%, in castor oil base. Vial 5 ml.
Use: I.M. progestin therapy.

HYREX-105. (Hyrex) Phendimetrazine tartrate 150 mg./Cap. Bot. 100s.
Use: Anorexiant.

HYREXIN. (Hyrex) Diphenhydramine HCl 50 mg./cc. Vial 10 cc.
Use: Antihistamic.

HYROXON. (Kay) Hydroxyprogesterone caproate 250 mg./ml. Vial 5 ml.
Use: Progestin.

HYRUNAL. (Kenyon) Rutin 20 mg., mannitol hexanitrate ½ gr., phenobarbital ¼ gr./Tab. Bot. 100s, 1000s.
Use: Hypertension.

HYRUNAL W/VERATRUM VIRIDE. (Kenyon) Phenobarbital ¼ gr., mannitol hexanitrate ½ gr., rutin 10 mg., veratrum viride 100 mg./Tab. Bot. 100s, 1000s.

HYSCORBIC PLUS. (Bock) Vit. E 45 I.U., C 600 mg., folic acid 400 mcg., B-1 20 mg., B-2 10 mg., niacinamide 100 mg., B-6 10 mg., B-12 25 mcg., pantothenic acid 25 mg., copper 3 mg., zinc 23.9 mg./Tab. Bot.
Use: High potency vitamin formula.

HYSERP. (Freeport) Reserpine alkaloid 0.25 mg./Tab. Bot. 1000s.
Use: Antihypertensive.

HYSKON. (Pharmacia) Clear, viscid, sterile, solution of 32% dextran 70 in dextrose. Bot. 100 ml., 250 ml.
Use: Distending the uterine cavity and in irrigating and visualizing its surfaces.

HYSONE. (Mallard) Iodoquinol 3%, hydrocortisone 1% in a water soluble base w/sodium lauryl sulfate, propylene glycol, cetyl alcohol, white petrolatum, water. Oint. Tube 15 Gm.
Use: Treatment of contact or atopic dermatitis.

HYTAKEROL. (Winthrop-Breon) Dihydrotachysterol (Hydrocalciferol) 0.125 mg./Cap. Bot. 50s. Sol. in oil, 0.25 mg./cc. Bot. 15 cc.
Use: Tetany therapy, hypoparathyroidism.

HYTINIC. (Hyrex) Polysaccharide-iron complex 150 mg./Cap. Bot. 50s, 500s. Unit dose 100s.
Use: Iron deficiency anemia.

HYTINIC ELIXIR. (Hyrex) Polysaccharide-iron 100 mg./Tsp. Bot. 8 oz.
Use: Iron deficiency anemia.

HYTINIC INJECTION. (Hyrex) Ferrous gluconate 30 mg., citric acid 8.2 mg., sodium citrate 11.8 mg., folic acid 0.5 mg., liver equivalent to Vit. B-12 2.5 mcg.
Use: Iron-vitamin therapy.

HYTONE CREAM. (Dermik) Hydrocortisone in cream base. 0.5%, Tube 1 oz.; 1%, Tube 1 oz., Jar 4 oz.; 2.5% Tube 1 oz., 2 oz.
Use: Anti-inflammatory for dermatoses.

HYTONE LOTION 1%. (Dermik) Hydrocortisone 1% (10 mg./ml.). Bot. 4 oz.
Use: Anti-inflammatory for dermatoses.

HYTONE LOTION 2.5%. (Dermik) Hydrocortisone 2 1/2% (25 mg./ml.) in lotion base. Bot. 2 oz.
Use: Anti-inflammatory for dermatoses.

HYTONE OINTMENT. (Dermik) Hydrocortisone in ointment base. 0.5%. Tube 1 oz.; 1%, Tube 1 oz., 2.5%, Tube 1 oz.

Use: Anti-inflammatory for dermatoses.

◀YTUSS TABLETS. (Hyrex) Guaifenesin 100 mg./Tab. Bot. 100s, 1000s.
Use: Expectorant.

◀YTUSS-2X. (Hyrex) Guaifenesin 200 mg./Cap. Bot. 100s, 1000s.
Use: Expectorant.

◀YWOLFIA-S.C. Orange. (Jenkins) Pow. whole root rauwolfia serpentina 50 mg./Tab. Bot. 1000s. Also red, yellow, 100 mg./Tab. Bot. 1000s.

◀YZINE-50. (Hyrex) Hydroxyzine HCl 50 mg./cc. Vial 10cc.
Use: Tranquilizer, antihistaminic.

I

◀BENZMETHYZIN. Name used for Procarbazine Hydrochloride.

◀BERET. (Abbott) Controlled release, ferrous sulfate 525 mg., ascorbic acid 150 mg., Vit. B-12 25 mcg., B-1 6 mg., B-2 6 mg., niacinamide 30 mg., B-6 5 mg., Ca pantothenate 10 mg./Filmtab. Bot. 60s, 500s.
Use: Iron-deficiency anemias.

◀BERET-500. (Abbott) Ascorbic acid 500 mg., controlled release ferrous sulfate 525 mg., vit. B-12 25 mcg., B-1 6 mg., B-2 6 mg., niacinamide 30 mg. B-6 5 mg., Ca pantothenate 10 mg./Filmtab. Bot. 60s, 500s. Abbo-Pac.
Use: Iron deficiency anemias.

BERET-FOLIC-500 FILMTAB. (Abbott) Controlled release, ferrous sulfate 105 mg., Vit. C 500 mg., niacinamide 30 mg. Ca pantothenate 10 mg., thiamine mononitrate 6 mg., B-2 6 mg., B-6 5 mg., folic acid 800 mcg., B-12 25 mcg./Filmtab. Bot. 30s, 60s.
Use: Iron deficiency anemia.

BERET LIQUID. (Abbott) Elem. iron 26.25 mg., Vit. C 37.5 mg., B-12 6.25 mcg., B-1 1.5 mg., B-2 1.5 mg., niacinamide 7.5 mg., B-6 1.25 mg., dexpanthenol 2.5 mg./5 ml. Liquid Bot. 8 fl. oz.
Use: Iron deficiency anemia.

BERET-500 LIQUID, ORAL SOLUTION. (Abbott) Elem. iron 26.25 mg., Vit. B-12 6.25 mcg., B-1 1.5 mg., B-2 1.5 mg., niacinamide 7.5 mg., dexpanthenol 2.5 mg., B-6 1.25 mg., C 125 mg./5 ml. Bot. 8 oz.
Use: Iron deficiency anemia.

◀BEROL. (Abbott) B-12 12.5 mcg., Iron (as 525 mg. ferrous sulf.) 105 mg., Vit. C 75 mg., B-1 3 mg., B-2 3 mg., niacinamide 15 mg., B-6 1.5 mg., Ca pantothenate 3 mg./Filmtab. Bot. 100s.
Use: Treatment of anemias.

◀BEROL-F. (Abbott) Vit. B-12 12.5 mcg., Iron (as Ferrous sulf.) 105 mg., folic acid 0.2 mg., Vit. C 75 mg., B-1 3 mg., B-2 3 mg., niacinamide 15 mg., Vit. B-6 1.5 mg., Ca pantothenate 3 mg./Filmtab. Bot. 100s.
Use: Anemias.

• IBOPAMINE. USAN.
Use: Dopaminergic agent (peripheral).

• IBUFENAC. USAN. (p-Isobutylphenyl-acetic acid).
Use: Antirheumatic (anti-inflammatory, analgesic & antipyretic).
See: Dytransin.

• IBUPROFEN, U.S.P. XXI. Tab., U.S.P. XXI. (3) 2-(p-Isobutyl phenyl) propionic acid; p-Isobutylhydratropic acid. 2-(4-Isobutylphenyl)propionic acid. Brufen.
Use: Anti-inflammatory.
See: Motrin, Tab. (Upjohn)

• IBUPROFEN ALUMINUM. USAN.
Use: Anti-inflammatory.

ICE MINT. (Westwood) Stearic acid, syn. cocoa butter, lanolin oil, camphor, menthol, beeswax, mineral oil, sodium borate, aromatic oils, emulsifiers, water. Jar 4 oz.
Use: Cream for burning feet, chapped skin, detergent hands, sunburn.

• ICHTHAMMOL, U.S.P. XXI. Oint., U.S.P. XXI. Ichthynate. Isarol Oint.
Use: Mild antiseptic in skin disorders.
W/Aluminum acetate, phenol, zinc oxide, boric acid, eucalyptol.
See: Lanaburn, Oint. (Lannett)
W/Aluminum hydroxide, phenol, zinc oxide, camphor, eucalyptol.
See: Almophen, Oint. (Bowman)
W/Benzocaine, resin cerate, carbolic acid, thymol, camphor, juniper tar, hexachlorophene.
See: Boil-Ease Anesthetic Drawing Salve (Commerce)
W/Benzocaine, tetracaine, resin cerate, thymol iodide.
See: Boilaid, Oint. (Edward J. Moore)
W/Hydrocortisone acetate, benzocaine, oxyquinoline sulfate, ephedrine HCl.
See: Derma Medicone-HC (Medicone)
W/Naftalan, calamine, amber pet.
See: Naftalan, Oint. (Paddock)
W/Phenol, benzocaine, balsam peru, alum. exsic., cade oil, eucalyptus oil, carbolic acid.
See: Alucaine, Oint. (Jenkins)

ICHTHYNATE.
See: Ichthammol

ICHTHYOL OINTMENT. (Stiefel) Ichthyol 10% in an ointment base. Tube 1 oz.
Use: Eczemas, dermatoses, psoriasis seborrhea.

• ICTASOL. USAN.
Use: Disinfectant.

ICTOTEST. (Ames) p-Nitrobenzene diazonium p-toluene sulfonate. Reagent Tab., Bot. 100s.
Use: Test for urinary bilirubin.

ICY HOT RUB. (Searle) Methyl salicylate 12%, menthol 9%. Tubes 1.25 oz, 3 oz.
Use: Counterirritant, analgesic rub.

ICY HOT BALM. (Searle) Methyl salicylate 29%, menthol 8%. Jars 3.5 oz., 7 oz.
Use: Counterirritant, analgesic balm.

IDO-CORTISTAN OINTMENT. (Standex) Hydrocortisone alcohol 10 mg., clioquinol 30 mg., methylparaben 0.5 mg., propylparaben 0.5 mg./½ oz. Tube ½ oz.

IDOTEIN. (Sig) Sod. iodide 40 mg., peptone 20 mg./ml. Vial 30 ml.

• IDOXURIDINE, U.S.P. XXI. Ophth. Oint., Soln., U.S.P. XXI. 5-Iodo-2′-deoxyuridine. Uridine; Dendroid; Kerecid; Ophthalmidine.
Use: Herpes simplex; antiviral.

See: Dendrid, Ophth. Sol. (Alcon)
  Herplex Ophth. Soln. (Allergan)
  Stoxil, Ophth. Sol., Oint. (SmithKline
• **IFOSFAMIDE.** USAN. (Mead Johnson)
  Use: Investigative: Antineoplastic.
IGEPAL Co-430. (General Aniline & Film) Non-oxynol 4.
IGEPAL Co-730. (General Aniline & Film) Non-oxynol 15.
IGEPAL Co-880. (General Aniline & Film) Non-oxynol 30.
IHSA I-125. (Mallinckrodt) Albumin, Iodinated I 125 Serum.
IHSA I-131. (Mallinckrodt) Albumin, Iodinated I 131 Serum.
ILETIN I. (Lilly) Regular and modified insulin products.
  Protamine Zinc: 40, 100 u./cc. Vial 10 cc.
  Regular: 40, 100 u./cc. Vial 10 cc.
  Lente: 40, 100 u./cc. Vial 10 cc.
  Semilente: 40, 100 u./cc. Vial 10 cc.
  Ultralente: 40, 100 u./cc. Vial 10 cc.
  NPH: 40, 100 u./cc. Vial 10 cc.
  Use: Diabetes.
ILETIN II. (Lilly) Special insulin products prepared from purified beef and purified pork.
  Regular: 100 u./cc. Vial 10 cc.
  Lente: 100 u./cc. Vial 10 cc.
  NPH: 100 u./cc. Vial 10 cc.
  Protamine Zinc: 100 u./cc. Vial 10 cc.
  Use: Diabetes.
ILETIN II CONCENTRATED. (Lilly) Purified pork regular insulin 500 u./cc. Vial 20 cc.
  Use: Diabetes.
ILIDAR PHOSPHATE. Azapetine, B.A.N.
ILOPAN. (Adria) Dexpanthenol 250 mg./cc. w/Chlorobutanol 0.5%. Amp. 2 cc. Box 12s, 25s, 100s. Stat-Pak Disp. Syringe 2 cc. and Vial 10 cc.
  Use: Intestinal atony and distention.
ILOPAN- CHOLINE. (Adria) Ilopan 50 mg., choline bitartrate 25 mg./Tab. Bot. 100s, 500s.
  Use: Antiflatulent.
ILOSONE. (Dista) Erythromycin estolate. **Cap.:** (Erythromycin base) 125 mg., 250 mg./Pulvule. 125 mg. Bot. 24s, 100s. 250 mg. Bot. 24s, 100s. Blister pkg. 10 × 10s. **Liq.:** (250 mg. or 125 mg./5 ml.) Bot. 100 ml., 16 fl. oz. **Tab:** 500 mg./Tab. Bot. 50s. **Ready-Mixed Drops. Susp.:** 100 mg./ml. Bot. 10 ml. **For Oral Susp.** 125 mg./5 ml. Bot. 60 ml., 150 ml.
  Use: Most common bacterial infections.
ILOSONE CHEWABLE. (Dista) Erythromycin estolate 125 mg., 250 mg./Tab. Bot. 50s.
  Use: Bacterial infections.
ILOTYCIN. (Dista) Erythromycin Oint. 10 mg./Gm. Tube 0.5 oz., 1 oz., Jar 1 lb. **Ophth. Oint.** 5 mg./Gm. Tube 0.12 oz., 1 Gm.
  Use: Antibiotic therapy against gram-positive & gram-negative organisms.
ILOTYCIN TABS. (Dista) Erythromycin 250 mg./Tab. Bot. 24s, 100s, 500s.
  Use: Antibiotic.
ILOTYCIN GLUCEPTATE I.V. (Dista) Erythromycin gluceptate. Vial. I.V. (250 mg.) 30 ml. 1s, (500 mg.) 30 ml. 1s; (1 Gm.) 30 ml. Box 1s.

Use: I.V.; antibiotic therapy.
ILOZYME. (Adria) Pancrelipase equiv. to lipase 11000 u., protease 40,000 u., amylase 40,000 u./Tab. Bot. 250s.
  Use: Exocrine pancreatic insufficiency.
I.L.X. ELIXIR. (Kenwood) Liver fraction 1 98 mg., iron 102 mg., B-1 5 mg., B-2 2 mg., nicotinamide 10 mg. B-12 10 mcg./15 cc. w/alcohol 8% Bot. 12 oz.
  Use: Hematinic, multivitamin. Iron & ammonium citrate 18 gr., liver fraction No. 1, 3 gr., Vit. B-1 10 mg. B-2 4 mg., nicotinamide 20 mg., Vit. B-12 20 mcg./3 cc., alcohol 8%. Bot. 12 oz.
  Use: Anemias.
I.L.X. B-12 TABLETS. (Kenwood) Iron (as ferrous gluconate) 5 gr., Vit. C 60 mg., B-12 10 mcg., liver 2 gr. thiamine HCl 2 mg., riboflavin 2 mg., niacinamide 20 mg./Tab. Bot. 100s.
  Use: Hematinic, multivitamin.
• **IMAFEN HYDROCHLORIDE.** USAN.
  Use: Antidepressant.
IMBRETIL. Carbolonium Bromide, B.A.N.
• **IMCARBOFOS.** USAN.
  Use: Anthelmintic.
IMENOL. (Sig) Guaiacol 0.10 Gm., eucalyptol 0.08 Gm., iodoform 0.02 Gm., camphor 0.05 Gm./ml. Vial 30 ml.
  Use: Mucous liquefaction and respiratory antibacterial.
IMFERON. (Merrell Dow) An iron-dextran complex containing 50 mg. iron/ml. Amp. 2 ml. Box 10s. Vial (w/phenol 0.5%), 10 ml. Box 2s.
  Use: IM/IV Iron deficiency state not amenable to oral iron therapy.
1H-IMIDAZOLE,4,5-DIHYDRO-2-(1-NAPHTHALENYL METHYL)-MONOHYDROCHLORIDE. Naphazoline Hydrochloride, U.S.P. XXI.
IH-IMIDAZOLE-4-ETHANAMINE, PHOSPHATE (1:2) Histamine Phosphate, U.S.P. XXI.
IH-IMIDAZOLE-1-ETHANOL,2-METHYL-5-NITRO-. Metronidazole, U.S.P. XXI.
2H-IMIDAZOLE-2-THIONE,1,3-DIHYDRO-1-METHYL-. Methimazole, U.S.P. XXI.
2,4-IMIDAZOLIDINEDIONE,5,5-DIPHENYL-. Phenytoin, U.S.P. XXI.
m-[N-(2-IMIDAZOLIN-2-YLMETHYL)-p-TOLUIDINO]P HENOL MONOMETHANESULFONATE (SALT). Phentolamine Mesylate, U.S.P. XXI.
2,4-IMIDAZOLIDINEDIONE,1-[[(5-NITRO-2-FURANY L)METHYLENE]AMINO]-. Nitrofurantoin, U.S.P. XXI
• **IMIDECYL IODINE.** USAN. 1-Carboxymethylene-1-(2-ethanol)-2-alkyl(C_7 to C_{17})-2-imidazolinium chloride-tridecyl polyoxyethylene-ethanol-iodine complex
  Use: Antiseptic agent.
IMIDOCARB. B.A.N. 3,3'-Di-(2-imidazolin-2-yl)carbanilide.
  Use: Antiprotozoan, veterinary medicine.
• **IMIDOCARB HCl.** USAN. 3,3'-Di-2-imidazolin-2-ylcar banilide dihydrochloride.
  Use: Antiprotozoal.
IMIDODICARBONIMIDIC   DIAMIDE,N-(2-PHENYLE THYL)-MONOHYDROCHLORIDE. Phenformin Hy drochloride.

- **IMIDOLINE HYDROCHLORIDE.** USAN. 1-(m-Chloro-phenyl)-3-(2-(dimethylamino)ethyl)-2-imidazolidinone hydrochloride.
  Use: Tranquilizer.
- **IMIDUREA,** N.F. XVI.
- **IMIPEMIDE.**
  Use: Antibacterial.
  See: Imipenem, USAN.
- **IMIPENEM.** USAN.
  Use: Antibacterial.
- **IMIPRAMINE HCl.** U.S.P. XXI. Inj., Tab., U.S.P. XXI. 5H-Dibenz [b,f] azepine-5-propanamine, 10,11-dihy-dro-N,N-dimethyl-, HCl. 5-(3-Dimethyl-aminopropyl)-10,11,dihydro-5H-dibenz-(b,f) azepine HCl. Praminil. Berkomine, IA-Pram, Impamin, Iprogen, Norpramine, & Tofranil HCl salts.
  Use: Antidepressant.
  See: Janimine, Tab. (Abbott)
      Presamine, Tab. (USV)
      SK-Pramine, Tab. (SmithKline)
      Tofranil, Tab., Amp. (Geigy)
      W.D.C., Tab. (Reid-Provident)
- **IMIRON INJECTION.** (Amfre-Grant) Iron dextran 50 mg./ml. Vial 10 ml.
  Use: Hematinic.
- **IMIPRAMINE PAMOATE.** bis 5-[3-(Di-methylamino) propyl]-10,11-dihydro-5H-dibenz [b,f] azapine com-pound (2:1) with 4,4-methylenebis-[3-hydroxy-2-naph-thoic acid].
  Use: Antidepressant.
  See: Tofranil-PM, Cap. (Geigy)
- **IMMOLIN.** (Schmid) Methoxypolyoxyethyleneglycol 550 laurate 5%, nonylphenoxpolyethoxyethanol 1% in creamjel emulsion base. Tube 75 Gm.
  Use: Contraceptive.
- **IMMUGLOBIN.** (Savage) Soln. of gamma globulin standardized for measles & polio antibody con-tent. 16.5% ± 1.5% Gamma Globulin/cc. Vial 10 cc.
  Use: Gamma globulin deficiency.
- **IMMUNE GLOBULIN,** U.S.P. XXI. Immune Serum Globulin Human. Gamma-globulin fraction of normal human plasma. Vial 10 cc. Tubex 1 cc., 2 cc. w/thimerosal 1:10,000.
  Use: Modification of active measles, prophylaxis of hepatitis, treatment of immune deficiencies.
  See: Gamastan, Vial (Cutter)
      Gamimune, Vial (Cutter)
      Gammagee, Vial (Merck Sharp & Dohme)
      Gammar, Vial (Armour)
      Generic, Vial 2 ml., 10 ml. (Merck Sharp & Dohme)
      Immuglobin, Vial (Savage)
- **IMMUNE GLOBULIN, Rh₀ (D).**
  See: Gamulin Rh (Parke-Davis)
      HypRho-D (Cutter)
      RhoGAM (Ortho Diagnostics)
- **IMMUNE SERUMS.**
  See: Human Measles Immune Serum (Var. Mfr.)
      Immune Serum Globulin (Human)
- **IMMUNE SERUM (ANIMAL).**
  See: Botulism Antitoxin, Vial (Lederle)

      Diphtheria Antitoxin
      Gas Gangrene Antitoxin
      Tetanus Antitoxin
      Tetanus Antitoxin—Gas Gangrene Combined
- **IMMUNE SERUM (HUMAN).**
  See: Hypertussis, Vial (Cutter)
      Poliomyelitis Immune Globulin (Various Mfr.)
- **IMMUNEX CRP.** (Wampole) Two-minute latex agglutination slide test for the qualitative detection of C-Reactive protein in serum. Kit 100s.
  Use: An aid in the diagnosis of inflammatory conditions.
- **IMMUNOREX.** (Barry) Treatment set of 4 serially diluted vials w/concentration of 1:60 w/v pollen units.
  Use: Restore allergic balance.
- **IMODIUM CAPSULES.** (Janssen) Loperamide 2 mg./Cap. Bot. 100s, 500s.
  Use: Acute, non-specific, chronic diarrhea and reduc-ing volume of discharge from ileostomies.
- **IMOGAM RABIES IMMUNE GLOBULIN.** (Merieux Institute) Rabies immune globulin (human) 150 I.U./ml. Vial 2 ml. or 10 ml. in tamper proof box.
  Use: For post-exposure rabies treatment.
- **IMOLAMINE.** B.A.N. 4-(2-Diethylaminoethyl)-5-imino-3-phenyl-1,2,4-oxadiazoline.
  Use: Treatment of angina pectoris.
  See: Angolon hydrochloride
- **IMOVAX RABIES VACCINE.** (Merieux Institute) Merieux rabies vaccine, Wistar rabies virus strain PM-1503-3M grown in human diploid cell cultures.
  Use: Pre & post exposure to rabies.
- **IMPACT.** (Approved) Belladonna alkaloids 0.16 mg., phenylpropanolamine HCl 50 mg., chlorpheniramine maleate 1 mg., pheniramine maleate 12.5 mg./Cap. Pack 12s, 24s. Vial 15s, 30s, Bot. 1000s.
  Use: Decongestant.
- **IMPROMEN.** (Janssen) Bromperidol decanoate.
  Use: Anti-psychotic.
- **IMPROMEN DECANOAS.** (Janssen) Bromperidol decanoate.
  Use: Antipsychotic.
- **IMURAN.** (Burroughs Wellcome) **Tab.:** Azathioprine. 50 mg./Tab. Bot. 100s. **Inj.:** Azathioprine 100 mg./20 ml. Vial.
  Use: Immunosuppression agent for renal transplantation, rheumatoid arthritis.
- **IMPROMIDINE HYDROCHLORIDE.** USAN.
  Use: Diagnostic aid.
- **IMPROVED SINUSTAT.** (Vitarine) Acetaminophen 325 mg., phenylpropanolamine HCl 25 mg., phenyltoloxamine citrate 22 mg./Tab.
  Use: Temporary relief of sinus headache & nasal congestion.
- **IMUNIVY.** (Kay) Poison ivy extract. Vial 1 ml.
  Use: Prophylactic sensitization for poison ivy.
- **IMUNOAK.** (Kay) Poison oak extract. Vial 1 ml.
  Use: Prophylactic sensitization for poison oak.
- **INACTIVATED DIAGNOSTIC DIPHTHERIA TOXIN.**
  See: Diphtheria Toxin for Schick Test, U.S.P. XXI.
- **INAPSINE.** (Janssen) Droperidol 2.5 mg./cc. Amp. 2 cc., 5 cc Box 10s. Multi-dose Vial w/methylparben 1.8

mg., propylparaben 0.2 mg., lactic acid/10 cc. Box 10s.
Use: Tranquilizer.
W/Fentanyl citrate.
Use: Tranquilizer.
See: Innovar, Inj. (Janssen)
INCORPOHIST. (Blue Line) Pyrilamine maleate 10 mg., prophenpyridamine maleate 5 mg./Tab. Bot. 1000s.
Use: Triple antihistaminic.
INCREMIN W/IRON. (Lederle) l-Lysine HCl 300 mg., Vit. B-12 25 mcg., B-1 10 mg., B-6 5 mg., ferric pyrophosphate soluble 30 mg., sorbitol 3.5 Gm., alcohol 0.75%/5 cc. Syr. Bot. 4 fl. oz. & 16 fl. oz.
Use: An appetite stimulant.
• INDACRINONE. USAN.
Use: Antihypertensive, diuretic.
INDALITAN. Clorindione, B.A.N.
INDALONE.
See: Butopyronoxyl (Various Mfr.)
• INDAPAMIDE. USAN.
Use: Antihypertensive, diuretic.
• INDECAINIDE HYDROCHLORIDE. USAN.
• INDELOXAZINE HYDROCHLORIDE. USAN.
Use: Antidepressant.
INDERAL. (Ayerst) Propranolol HCl. **Tab.:** 10 mg., 20 mg., 40 mg., 60 mg., or 80 mg./Tab. Bot. 100s, 1000s. Unit dose 100s. Bot. 5000s for 10 mg., 20 mg., and 40 mg. **Inj.:** 1 mg./ml. Amp. Box 10s.
Use: Arrhythmia, angina pectoris, hypertension, migraine treatment.
INDERAL-LA. (Ayerst) Propranolol HCl 80 mg., 120 mg. or 150 mg./SR Cap. Bot. 100s, 1000s, unit dose.
Use: Angina pectoris, hypertension, migraine treatment.
INDERIDE.(Ayerst) Propranolol HCl 40 mg., hydrochlorothiazide 25 mg./Tab. Bot 100s, 1000s. Unit Dose 100s. Propranolol HCl 80 mg., hydrochlorothiazide 25 mg./Tab. Bot. 100s, 1000s. Unit Dose 100s.
Use: Hypertension management.
INDIAN GUM.
See: Karaya Gum
INDIGO CARMINE. (CMC) Sod. indigotindisulfate 0.8% Amp. 5 cc. 100s.
INDIGO CARMINE. (Hynson, Westcott & Dunning) Sod. indigotindisulfonate 8 mg./ml. Amp. 5 ml. Box 10s, 100s.
Use: Localizing ureteral orifices during cystoscopy.
See: Sod. indigotindisulfonate
• INDIGOTINDISULFONATE SODIUM, U.S.P. XXI. Inj., U.S.P. XXI. 1H-Indole-5-sulfonic acid, 2-(1,3-dihydro-4-oxo-5-sulfo-2H-indol-2-ylidene)-2,3-dihydro-3-oxo-, sod. salt. Indigo Carmine, Amp. (Various Mfr.)
Use: Diagnostic aid (cystoscopy).
See: Sodium Indigotindisulfonate
• INDIUM In 111 PENTETRATE INJECTION, U.S.P. XXI.
INDOCIN. (Merck Sharp & Dohme) Indomethacin. 25 mg./Cap. Bot. 100s, 1000s. Unit dose pkg. 100s. Unit of use 100s; 50 mg./Cap. Bot. 100s. Unit dose pkg. 100s. Unit of use 60s, 100s.

Use: Anti-inflammatory agent.
INDOCIN SR. (Merck Sharp & Dohme) Indomethacin 75 mg./S.R. Cap. Unit of Use 30s, 60s.
Use: Anti-inflammatory agent.
• INDOCYANINE GREEN, U.S.P. XXI. Sterile, U.S.P. XXI. A tricarbocyanine dye. 1H-Benz [e] indolium, 2-[7-[1,3-dihydro-1,1-dimethyl-3-(4-sulfobutyl)-2H-benz [e] indol-2-ylidene]-1,3,5-heptatrienyl]-1,1-dimethyl-3-(4-sulfobutyl)-, hydroxide, inner salt, sodium salt.
Use: Diagnostic aid.
See: Cardio-Green, Inj. (Hynson, Westcott & Dunning)
INDOGESIC. (Century) Acetaminophen 32.5 mg., butalbital 50 mg./Tab. Bot. 100s, 1000s.
Use: Analgesic, sedative.
INDOKLON. Hexafluorodiethyl ether. Flurothyl. Bis-(2,2,2-trifluorethyl)ether.
Use: Shock inducing agent (convulsant).
• INDOLAPRIL HYDROCHLORIDE. USAN.
• INDOMETHACIN, U.S.P. XXI. Cap., U.S.P. XXI. 1-(p-Chlorobenzoyl)-5-methoxy-2-methyl-indole-3-acetic acid.
Use: Anti-inflammatory agent (nonsteroid).
See: Indocin, Cap., S.R. Cap. (Merck Sharp & Dohme)
• INDOPROFEN. USAN.
Use: Analgesic, anti-inflammatory.
• INDORAMIN. USAN. N-[1-(2-Indol-3-ylethyl)-4-piperidyl]benzamide. 3-[2-(4-Benzamidopiperidino)ethyl]indole.
Use: Antihypertensive.
• INDORENATE HYDROCHLORIDE. USAN.
Use: Antihypertensive.
• INDOXOLE. USAN.
Use: Antipyretic, anti-inflammatory.
• INDRILINE HYDROCHLORIDE. USAN.
Use: Stimulant.
INFACAPS A & D. (Lannett) Vitamin A 3000 I.U., D 800 I.U./Cap. Bot. 1000s, 5000s.
INFALYTE. (Pennwalt) Provides (per liter) sodium 50 mEq., chloride 40 mEq., Bicarbonate 30 mEq., potassium 20 mEq., D-glucose 111 m.moles/24 Gm. packet to be dissolved in 32 fl. oz. of water.
Use: Oral electrolyte replenisher.
INFANTOL PINK. (Scherer) Paregoric (equivalent) contains 15 mg. opium/fl. oz w/bismuth subsalicylate, Ca carageenan, pectin, Zn phenolsulfonate, alcohol 2%. Suspension. Bot. 4 oz., 8 oz., pt.
Use: Antidiarrheal.
INFANTOVIT PLUS. (CMC) Vit. A 5000 I.U., D 1000 I.U., C 60 mg., B-1 1.5 mg., B-2 1 mg., B-6 0.5 mg., Ca pantothenate 3 mg., nicotinamide 10 mg., B-12 1 mcg., folic acid 0.05 mg./Chewable sphere. Bot. 30s, 100s, 250s, 1000s.
Use: Dietary supplement.
INFARUB CREAM. (Whitehall) Methylsalicylate 35%, menthol 10% in vanishing cream base. Tube 1.25 oz., 3.5 oz.
Use: External analgesic.
INFATUSS. (Scott/Cord) Dextromethorphan HBr 7.20 mg., chlorpheniramine maleate 1.10 mg.,

phenylpropanolamine HCl 4.80 mg., ammonium chloride 50.00 mg./5 cc. Bot. 4 oz., pt., gal.
Use: Cough due to colds.

NFATUSSIS. (Blue Line) Pot. citrate, squill fl. ext. ipecac syr., tolu syr., honey & alcohol. Bot. 1 pt., 1 gal.
Use: Cough, expectorant.

NFLAMASE MILD 1/8% OPHTHALMIC SOLUTION. (CooperVision) Prednisolone sod. phosphate 0.125% (equiv. to prednisolone phosphate 0.11%). Bot. 5 ml. and 10 ml. w/dropper tip.
Use: Anti-inflammatory.

NFLAMASE FORTE 1% OPHTHALMIC SOLUTION. (CooperVision) Prednisolone sod. phosphate 1.0% (equiv. to prednisolone phosphate 0.91%), benzalkonium chloride. Bot. 5 ml., 10 ml.
Use: Anti-inflammatory.

• **INFLUENZA VIRUS VACCINE,** U.S.P. XXI.
Use: Active immunizing agent.
See: Fluzone, Inj. (Squibb-Connaught)

INFLUENZAE TYPE B SERUM (RABBIT) ANTIHEMOPHILUS. (Various Mfr.) The sterile suspension of formaldehyde-killed influenza virus, type A, Asian strain grown in the extra-embryonic fluid of chick eggs.
Use: Immunization.

INFLUENZA VIRUS VACCINE.
Lederle—Bivalent types A and B. A/Port Chalmers/1/73 (h3n2)-700 CCA Units, B/Hong-Kong/5/72-500 CCA Units. Vial 5 ml.
Wyeth—Types A & B Tubex Cartridge-Needle Unit 0.5cc., 10s. Vial 5 cc.
Merck Sharp & Dohme—Types A & B 200 CCA/dose, Vial 5 cc. 10s Syringe 0.5 cc.
Use: Prevention of influenza.
See: Fluax, (Merck Sharp & Dohme)
Fluzone, Inj. (Squibb-Connaught)

INH. (Ciba) Isoniazid 300 mg./Tab. Bot.
Use: Tuberculosis treatment.
See: Rimactane/INH, Dual Pack (Ciba)

INHAL-AID. (Key)
Use: Drug delivery system for metered dose inhalers.

INNERCLEAN HERBAL LAXATIVE. (Last) Senna leaf powder, psyllium seed, buckthorne, anise seed, fennel seed. Bot. 1 oz., 2 oz.
Use: Stimulant laxative.

INNERTABS. (Last) Senna leaf powder 88.5 mg., psyllium seed 10.5 mg./Tab. Bot. 80s, 200s.
Use: Stimulant laxative.

INNER RINSE. (Block) Sodium lauryl sulfate, sodium borate, edetate disodium, triethanolamine, ethyl alcohol, aromatics, citric acid buffer. Bot. 2 oz., 4 oz.
Use: Vaginal douche concentrate.

INNOVAR INJECTION. (Janssen) Fentanyl citrate 0.05 mg., droperidol 2.5 mg./cc. Amp. 2 cc., 5 cc. Box of 10s.
Use: Tranquilizer, analgesic

INOPHYLLINE.
See: Aminophylline (Various Mfr.)

INOSIT.
See: Inositol, (Var. Mfr.)

INOSITOL. 1,2,3,5/4,6-Cyclohexanehexol. Commercial solvents (Bios 1,Hexahydroxycyclohexane, Inosit, Dambose).
Use: Alterations in lipid metabolism.
W/Choline bitartrate, vitamins, minerals.
W/Choline chloride, dl-methionine, B-12.
Cho-Meth, Vial (Kenyon)
See: Lypo-B, Vial (Rocky Mtn.)
W/Methionine, choline bitartrate, liver desic., Vit. B-12.
See: Limvic, Tab. (Briar)
W/Panthenol, choline chloride, vitamins, minerals, estrone, testosterone.
See: Geramine, Inj. (Brown)
W/Panthenol, choline chloride, vitamins, minerals, estrone, testosterone, polydigestase.
See: Geramine, Tab. (Brown)

• **INOSITOL NIACINATE.** USAN. Myo-Inositol hexanicotinate. Meso-inositol hexanicotinate, hexanicotinate. Meso-inositol hexanicotinate. Hexopal; Meso-nex
Use: Peripheral Vasodilator.

INOSITOL NICOTINATE. Inositol Niacinate.

INPERSOL W/DEXTROSE. (Abbott) Dextrose 1.5%, 2.5% & 4.25% w/sodium chloride 140.5 mEq., Ca chloride 3.5 mEq., Mg chloride 1.5 mEq., sod. lactate 445 mEq./100 ml. **1.5% Dextrose:** 250 ml./500 ml.; 500 ml., 1000 ml.; 1000 ml./2000 ml.; or 1500 ml./2000 ml. partial fill single-dose container and 3000 ml. container. **2.5% Dextrose:** 250 ml./500 ml.; 500 ml./1000 ml.; 1000 ml./2000 ml.; or 1500 ml./2000 ml. partial fill single-dose container and 3000 ml. single-dose container. **4.25% Dextrose:** 250 ml./500 ml.; 500 ml./1000 ml.; 1000 ml./2000 ml.; or 1500 ml./2000 ml. partial fill single-dose container and 3000 ml. single-dose container.
Use: Peritoneal dialysis solution.

INPERSOL-LM. W/DEXTROSE. (Abbott) Inpersol-LM w/1.5% or 2.5% Dextrose. **1.5% Dextrose:** Single-dose flexible container 2000 ml. **2.5% Dextrose:** Partial fill single-dose container 2000 ml./3000 ml.
Use: Peritoneal dialysis solution.

INPROQUONE. B.A.N. 2,5-Di(aziridin-1-yl)-3,6-di-propoxy-1,4-benzoquinone.
Use: Antineoplastic agent.

INSECT ANTIGEN. (Hollister-Stier) Potent extracts from whole insect body of honey bee, bumblebee, hornet, yellowjacket, wasp, mosquito, ant, flea, moth, fly, locust, and household insects. Scratch (1:10) and Intradermal (100 PNU/cc.) tests.
Use: Diagnosis and desensitizing of stinging insect venom.

INSECT ANTIGEN, STINGING 108. (Barry) Combined antigens of bumble bee, honey bee, wasp, hornet, and yellow jacket/5 cc.; three 5 cc. serial dilution vials. Vial 5 cc., 10 cc. 1:100.
Use: Hyposensitization against common insect venom reactions.

INSERFEM. (Blue Line) Iodoquinol 100 mg., benzalkonium Cl 1 mg., tartaric acid 5 mg., lactose

& liquid glucose 1.1 Gm./Vag. Tab. Bot. 60s w/ or
w/o plastic inserters.
Use: Vaginitis, particularly with trichomonas
infection.

INSPIREASE. (Key)
Use: Drug delivery system for metered-dose
inhalers.

INSTAFREEZE SPRAY. (Century) Fluorinated and
chlorinated hydrocarbons. Bot. 7 oz.

INSTA-GLUCOSE. (ICN) Undiluted USP glucose. Unit
dose tube containing 31 Gms. of liquid glucose.
Use: Insulin reactions.

INST-E-VITE. (Barth's) Vit. E 100 I.U./Cap. Bot 100s,
500s, 1000s. 200 I.U./Cap. Bot. 100s, 250s, 500s.

INSULATARD NPH. (Nordisk) Isophane purified pork
insulin suspension 100 I.U./ml.
Use: Diabetes care (IDDM).

• **INSULIN.** U.S.P. XXI. Inj., U.S.P. XXI.
See: Iletin Prod. (Lilly)
Insulin Prod. (Squibb)

INSULIN. (Nordisk) Insulatard NPH Mixtard Velosulin

INSULIN. (Lilly)
Human-100 u./ml.
Isophane—40 u., 100 u./ml.
Protamine Zinc—40u., 100 u./ml.
Regular—40u., 100 u./ml.
Semilente—Zinc insulin 40 u., 100 u./ml.
Ultralente—Zinc insulin 40 u., 100 u./ml.
Lente—Zinc insulin 40 u., 100 u./ml. Vial 10 ml.
Use: Hypoglycemia.

• **INSULIN, DALANATED.** USAN.
Use: Antidiabetic.

INSULIN, GLOBIN ZINC INJECTION.
Use: Antidiabetic.

• **INSULIN HUMAN,** U.S.P. XXI. Inj., U.S.P. XXI.
Use: Antidiabetic.

• **INSULIN I-125.** USAN.
Use: Radioactive agent.

• **INSULIN I-131.** USAN.
Use: Radioactive agent.

• **INSULIN INJECTION,** U.S.P. XXI. Insulin, insulin HCl.
Use: Antidiabetic.

• **INSULIN, NEUTRAL.** USAN.
Use: Antidiabetic.

INSULIN NOVO RAPITARD. Biphasic Insulin
Injection, B.A.N.

• **INSULIN, PROTAMINE ZINC SUSPENSION,** U.S.P.
XXI. 40, 100 u./cc. Vials 10 cc.
Use: Antidiabetic.

• **INSULIN ZINC SUSPENSION,** U.S.P. XXI.
Use: Antidiabetic.
See: Lente Insulin, Vial (Lilly)

• **INSULIN ZINC SUSPENSION, EXTENDED,** U.S.P.
XXI.
Use: Antidiabetic.

• **INSULIN ZINC SUSPENSION, PROMPT,** U.S.P.
XXI.
Use: Antidiabetic, Hypoglycemic.

INTAL CAPSULES. (Fisons) Cromolyn sodium 20
mg., lactose powder 20 mg./Cap. Box 60s, 120s.
Use: Bronchial asthma inhibitor.

INTAL NEBULIZER SOLUTION. (Fisons) Cromolyn
sodium 20 mg. in 2 ml. distilled water for use with a
power operated nebulizer unit. Box 48s, 2 ml.
ampules.
Use: Anti-asthmatic.

INTERCEPT CONTRACEPTIVE INSERTS. (Ortho)
Nonoxynol-9 5.56% at pH 4.5. Starter 12 inserts
w/applicator. Refill 12 inserts.
Use: Contraceptive insert.

INTEGRIN CAPS. (Winthrop Products) Oxypertine.
Use: Anxiolytic, tranquilizer.

• **INTERFERON.** USAN. A protein formed by the
interaction of animal cells with viruses capable of
conferring on animal cells resistance to virus
infection. A drug derived from human white blood
cells and originally used in Finland.
Note: An investigational drug in the U.S.A.
Use: Antineoplastic, antiviral. Treatment of breast
cancer lymphoma, multiple melanoma & malignant
melanoma

INTRADEX. Dextran, B.A.N.

INTRALIPID 10% I.V. FAT EMULSION. (Cutter) I.V.
fat emulsion containing soybean oil 10%, egg yolk
phospholipids 1.2%, glycerin 2.25% & water for
injection. I.V. Flask 100ml., 500 ml.
Use: Calories & fatty acids for prolonged nutrition.

INTRALIPID 20% I.V. FAT EMULSION. (Cutter) I.V.
fat emulsion containing soybean oil 20%, egg yolk
phospholipids 1.2%, glycerin 2.25% and water for
injection. I.V. Flask 100 ml., 500 ml.
Use: Calories and fatty acids for prolonged
nutrition.

INTRA-SUL. (Torigian) Sod. thiosulfate, sod. sulfide, sulfur. Amp. 2 cc. 6s, 25s, 100s.

INTRAVAL SODIUM.
See: Pentothal Sodium, Prep. (Abbott)

• **INTRAZOLE.** USAN. 1-(p-Chlorobenzoyl)-3-(1H-tetrazol-5-ylmethyl) indole.
Use: Anti-inflammatory.

• **INTRIPTYLINE HYDROCHLORIDE.** USAN.
Use: Antidepressant.

INTRON-C. (Pharmics) Ferrous fumarate 300 mg., Vit. C
500 mg./Cap. Bot. 1000s.
Use: Iron deficiency anemia.

INTROPIN 200 mg. (American Critical Care)
Dopamine HCl 40 mg./ml. w/sodium bisulfite 1%
as an antioxidant. Vial 5 ml. Box 20s; Amp. 5 ml.
Box 20s; Prefilled additive Syr. 5 ml. Box 5s.
Use: Treatment of shock.

INTROPIN 400 mg. (American Critical Care)
Dopamine HCl 80 mg./ml. w/sodium bisulfite 1%
as an antioxidant. Vial 5 ml. Box 20s.; Prefilled
additive Syringe 5 ml. Box 5s.
Use: Treatment of shock.

INTROPIN 800 mg. (American Critical Care)
Dopamine HCl 160 mg./ml. w/sodium bisulfite 1%
as an antioxidant. Vial 5 ml. Box 20s.; Prefilled
additive syringe 5 ml. Box 5s.
Use: Treatment of shock.

INULIN. (American Critical Care) Purified inulin 5
Gm./50 ml. Sod. chloride 0.9%, sod. hydroxide to
adjust pH. Amps. 50 ml.

Use: Diagnostic aid, kidney function, glomerular filtration rate.

INVENEX INJECTABLES. (Invenex) A wide variety of generic injectable products.

INVENOL. Carbutamide, B.A.N.

INVERSINE. (Merck Sharp & Dohme) Mecamylamine HCl. 2.5 mg./Tab. Bot. 100s. 10 mg./Tab. Bot. 100s.
Use: Antihypertensive.

INVERT SUGAR. (Abbott) 10% solution. Bot 1000 ml.
Use: Nutritional.
See: Emetrol, Liq. (Rorer)
Travert, Sol. (Travenol)

• **IOBENZAMIC ACID.** USAN. N-3-(3-Amino-2,4,6-triiodobenzoyl)-N-phenyl-β-alanine. Osbil. (Mallinkcrodt)
Use: Contrast medium for cholecystography.

• **IOCARMATE MEGLUMINE.** USAN.
Use: Diagnostic aid.

• **IOCARMIC ACID.** USAN. 5,5'-(Adipoyldiamino)-bis-(2,4,6-tri-iodo-N-methylisophthalamic acid). Dimer X is a sterile solution of the meglumine salt.
Use: Radio-opaque substance.

• **IOCETAMIC ACID,** U.S.P. XXI. Tab., U.S.P. XXI. N-Acetyl-N-(3-amino-2,4,6-triiodophenyl)-2-methylalanine. 3-(N-3-Amino-2,4,6-tri-iodophenyl)acetamido-2-methylpropionic acid.
Use: Diagnostic aid (radiopaque medium).
See: Cholebrine, Tab. (Mallinckrodt)

IOCON GEL. (Owen) Polyoxyethylene ethers, coal tar solution, Iopol (a cationic polymer), alcohol 1%, benzalkonium chloride in a non-ionic/amphoteric base. Tube 3.5 oz.
Use: Scalp dermatoses.

IOCORTAR. (Doak) Microfine hydrocortisone w/clioquinol 3%, solution of coal tar 3%. **Cream:** ½% Tube 1 oz; 1% Tube 1 oz. **Lotion:** ¼% 4 oz.; ½% 1 oz.; 1% 1 oz. **Oint.:** 1% 1 oz.
Use: Dermatologic.

• **IODAMIDE.** USAN. 3-Acetamido-5-(acetamidomethyl)-2,4,6-triiodobenzoic acid. α,5-Di(acetamido)-2,4,6-tri-iodo-m-toluic acid.
Use: Radiopaque.

• **IODAMIDE MEGLUMIDE.** USAN.
Use: Radiopaque, diagnostic aid.
W/Combinations:
See: Renovue-65, Vial (Squibb)
Renovue-Dip, Vial (Squibb)

IODEX. (Medtech) Iodine 4.7% in petrolatum ointment base. Jar 1 oz., 1 lb.
Use: Topical anti-infective.

IODEX W/METHYL SALICYLATE. (Medtech) Iodine 4.7%, methyl salicylate 4.8% in petrolatum ointment base.
Use: Local analgesic, topical anti-infective.

• **IODIDIDE, SODIUM, I-123 CAPSULES,** U.S.P. XXI.
• **IODIDE, SODIUM, I-123 TABLETS,** U.S.P. XXI.
• **IODIDE, SODIUM, I-125 CAPSULES,** U.S.P. XXI.
• **IODIDE, SODIUM, I-125 SOLUTION,** U.S.P. XXI.
• **IODIDE, SODIUM, I-131 CAPSULES,** U.S.P. XXI.
• **IODIDE, SODIUM, I-131 SOLUTION,** U.S.P. XXI.
• **IODINATED GLYCEROL.** B.A.N. A mixture of iodinated dimers of glycerol.

Use: Mucolytic expectorant.
See: Organidin, Elix., Sol., Tab. (Wampole)

• **IODINATED I-125 ALBUMIN INJECTION,** U.S.P. XXI.
• **IODINATED I-131 ALBUMIN AGGREGATED INJECTION,** U.S.P. XXI.
• **IODINATED I-131 ALBUMIN INJECTION,** U.S.P. XXI.

IODINATED HUMAN SERUM ALBUMIN.
See: Albumotope (Squibb)

• **IODINE,** U.S.P. XXI. Topical Sol., Strong Soln., Tincture, U.S.P. XXI.
Use: Topical anti-infective; source of iodine.
See: Kelp Tablets (Columbia)

IODINE 131: CAPSULES DIAGNOSTIC-CAPSULES THERAPEUTIC-SOLUTION THERAPEUTIC ORAL.
See: Iodotope (Squibb)

IODINE CACODYLATE, COLLOIDAL. Cacodyne Iodine.

IODINE COMBINATION.
See: Calcidrine Syr. (Abbott)

IODINE-IODOPHOR.
See: Betadine, Prep. (Purdue Frederick)
Isodine, Preps. (Blair)

IODINE POVIDONE.
See: Efodine, Oint. (Fougera)
Iodophor
Mallsol, Liq. (Mallard)

▪ **IODINE PRODUCTS, ANTI-INFECTIVE.**
See: Anayodin
Betadine, Prep. (Purdue Frederick)
Chiniofon
Diodoquin, Tab. (Searle)
Diiodo-Hydroxyquinoline (Various Mfr.)
Isodine, Preps. (Blair)
Prepodyne, Sol., Scrub (West)
Quinoxyl
Surgidine, Liq. (Continental)
Vioform, Prep. (Ciba)

▪ **IODINE PRODUCTS, DIAGNOSTIC.**
See: Chloriodized Oil (Var. Mfr.)
Ethyl Iodophenylundecylate (Var. Mfr.)
Iodized Oil
Iodoalphionic Acid (Various Mfr.)
Iodobrassid
Iodohippurate Sodium (Var. Mfr.)
Iodopanoic Acid (Var. Mfr.)
Iodophthalein Sodium (Various Mfr.)
Iodopyracet, Prep. (Var. Mfr.)
Lipiodol Lafay, Amp., Vial (Savage)
Methiodal Sodium (Var. Mfr.)
Pantopaque, Amp. (Lafayette)
Sodium Acetrizoate (Var. Mfr.)
Sodium Iodomethamate (Var. Mfr.)
Telepaque, Tab. (Winthrop-Breon)

▪ **IODINE PRODUCTS, NUTRITIONAL.**
See: Calcium Iodobehenate (Various Mfr.)
Entodon
Hydriodic Acid (Var. Mfr.)
Iodobrassid (Various Mfr.)
Organidin, Elix., Sol., Tab. (Wampole)
Orgaphen, Elix., Tab. (Wampole)
Potassium Iodide (Various Mfr.)
Syniodin, Tab. (Blue Line)

IODINE RATION, (Barth's) Iodine (from kelp) 0.15 mg., trace minerals/Tab. Bot. 90s, 180s, 360s.
IODINE RATION. (Nion) Iodine (from kelp) 0.15 mg./3 Tab. Bot. 175s, 500s.
Use: Dietary supplement.
IODINE SOLUBLE.
See: Burnham Soluble Iodine, Sol. (Burnham)
IODINE SURFACE ACTIVE COMPLEX.
See: Ioprep, Sol. (Arbrook)
• **IODINE TINCTURE, STRONG,** U.S.P. XXI.
• **IODIPAMIDE,** U.S.P. XXI. Benzoic acid, 3,3'-[(1,6-dioxo-1,6-hexanediyl)diimino]bis[2,4,6-triiodo-. NN'-Di-(3-carboxy-2,4,6-tri-iodophenyl)-adipamide. Adipiodone (I.N.N.)
Use: Pharm. necessity for Iodipamide Meglumine Injection.
• **IODIPAMIDE MEGLUMINE INJECTION,** U.S.P. XXI. Benzoic acid, 3,3'-[(1,6-dioxo-1,6-hexanediyl)diimino] bis [2,4,6-triiodo-, compound with 1-deoxy-1-(methylamino)-d-glucitol (1:2).
Use: Diagnostic aid (radiopaque medium).
IODIPAMIDE METHYLGLUCAMINE. N,N'-Adipyl-bis(3-amino-2,4,6-triiodobenzoic acid). Also sodium salt inj. W/Diatrizoate methylglucamine.
See: Sinografin, Vial (Squibb)
• **IODIPAMIDE SODIUM I-131.** USAN.
Use: Radioactive agent.
IODIPAMIDE SODIUM INJECTION.
See: Cholografin Sod., Sol. (Var. Mfr.)
IODIZED OIL. A vegetable oil containing not less than 38% and not more than 42% of organically combined iodine.
Use: Diagnostic aid (radiopaque, hysterosalpingography.
See: Lipiodol Lafay, Amp., Vial (Savage)
IODIZED POPPY-SEED OIL.
See: Lipiodol Lafay, Amp., Vial (Savage)
IODOALPHIONIC ACID. 3-(4-Hydroxy-3,5-Diiodophenyl)-2-phenylpropionic acid. Biliselectan dikol, pheniodol.
• **IODOANTIPYRINE I-131.** USAN.
Use: Radioactive agent.
IODOBEHENATE CALCIUM. Calcium iododocosanoate.
Use: Antigoitrogenic.
IODOBRASSID. Ethyl Diiodobrassidate. Lipoiodine.
• **IODOCETYLIC ACID I-123.** USAN.
Use: Diagnostic aid.
• **IODOCHOLESTEROL I-131.** USAN.
Use: Radioactive agent.
• **IODOCHLORHYDROXYQUIN.** Clioquinol, U.S.P. XXI.
IODOCORT CREAM. (Ulmer) Hydrocortisone 1%, clioquinol 3%. Tube 20 Gm.
IODO CREAM. (Day-Baldwin) Clioquinol 3%. Tube 1 oz., Jar 1 lb.
IODOFORM. (Various Mfr.) Triiodomethane. Pow., Bot. ⅛ oz., 1 oz., ¼ lb., 1 lb.
Use: For dressing wounds.
W/Guaiacol, eucalyptol, camphor.
See: Camusol, Vial (Central)
Guaiphoto, Vial (Foy)

Guiaform, Inj. (Vortech)
Guido, Vial (Rocky Mtn.)
Imenol, Inj. (Sig)
Kleer, Vial (Scrip)
Respirex, Vial (Savage)
IODOGENOL PEPIN. (C.M.C.) Organic iodide preparation, 1¾ oz.
IODO H-C. (Day-Baldwin) Clioquinol 3%, hydrocortisone 1%. **Oint:** Tube. 20 Gm. Jar. 1 lb. **Cream:** Tube. 20 Gm. Jar 1 lb.
• **IODOHIPPURATE SODIUM I-125.** USAN.
See: Hipputope I 125 (Squibb)
• **IODOHIPPURATE, SODIUM I-131 INJECTION,** USAN. U.S.P. XXI. Glycine, N-(2-iodo-^{131}1-benzoyl)-, sod. salt.
Use: Diagnostic aid (renal function determination).
See: Hippuran, Pow. (Mallinckrodt)
Hipputope (Squibb)
IODO-HIPPURIC ACID.
See: Hipputope (Squibb)
7-IODO-8-HYDROXYQUINOLINE-5-SULFONATE, SODIUM.
See: Chiniofon, Tab. (CMC)
IODOL. 2,3,4,5-Tetraiodopyrrole.
IODO-NIACIN TABLETS. (O'Neal, Jones & Feldman) Pot. iodide 135 mg., niacinamide HCl 25 mg./Tab. Bot. 100s, 500s, 1000s.
Use: Iodine therapy.
IODO OINTMENT. (Day-Baldwin) Clioquinol 3%. Tube 1 oz., Jar 1 lb.
IODOPANOIC ACID.
Use: Diagnostic aid (radiopaque medium).
IODOPHENE. Iodophthalein.
IODOPHENE SODIUM.
See: Iodophthalein Sodium. (Various Mfr.)
IODOPHOR.
See: Betadine, Prep. (Purdue Frederick)
Isodine, Preps. (Blair)
IODOPHTHALEIN SODIUM. Tetraiodophenolphthalein Sod., Tetraiodophthalein Sod., Tetiothalein Sod. (Antinosin, Cholepulvis, Cholumbrin, Foriod, Iodophene, Iodorayoral, Nosophene Sod., Opacin, Photobiline, Piliophen, Radiotetrane.)
Use: Radiopaque medium for cholecystography.
IODO-PRO. (Fellows) Sod. iodide 40 mg., peptone 20 mg./cc. Vial 30 cc.
IODOPROPYLIDENE GLYCEROL.
See: Organidin, Elix., Tab., Sol. (Wampole)
• **IODOPYRACET I-125.** USAN.
Use: Radioactive agent.
• **IODOPYRACET I-131.** USAN.
Use: Radioactive agent.
See: Diodrast (R)-131
IODOPYRACET INJ. (Diatrast, Diodone, Iopyracil, Neo-Methiodal, NeoSkiodan) 3,5-Diiodo-4-oxo-1(4H)-pyridineacetic Acid 2,2-Iminodiethanol (1:1) Compound.
Use: Radiopaque medium.
IODOPYRACET COMPOUND. Diodrast.
IODOPYRACET CONCENTRATED. Diodrast
IODOPYRINE. Antipyrine "iodide."
Use: Iodides & analgesic.

• **IODOQUINOL,** U.S.P. XXI. Tab., U.S.P. XXI. 8-Quinoli-
nol-5,7-diiodo. Diiodohydroxyquinoline, (Embequin,
Enterosept)5,7-Diiodo-8-quinolinol.
Use: Anti-amebic.
See: Diodoquin (Searle)
   Floraquin (Searle)
   Inserfem, Vag. Tabs. (Blue Line)
   Sebaquin, Shampoo (Summers Labs.)
W/9-Aminoacridine HCl.
See: Vagitric, Cream (Elder)
   Yodoxin, Tab., Pow. (Glenwood)
W/Diiodohydroxyquin
See: Panaquin, Tab. (Panray)
W/Hydrocortisone alcohol.
See: Vytone, Cream (Dermik)
W/Hydrocortisone, coal tar solution.
See: Cor-Tar-Quin, Cream, Lot. (Miles Pharm)
W/Stilbestrol, sulfadiazine, tartaric acid, boric acid,
etc.
See: Gynben, Vag. Insert, Cream (ICN)
   Gynben Insufflate, Pow. (ICN)
W/Sulfadiazine, diethylstilbestrol.
See: Benegyn, Vag. Insert, Cream (Vortech)
W/Surfactants.
See: Lycinate, Supp. (Hoechst)
W/Sulfanilamide, diethylstilbestrol.
See: Amide V/S, Vag Ins. (Scrip)
   D.I.T.I. Creme (Dunhall)
IODOSONE CREAM. (Century) Hydrocortisone 1%,
clioquinol 3%, promoxine HCl 0.5%. Tube ½ oz.
IODOTHIOURACIL. B.A.N. 1,2-Dihydro-5-iodo-2-thiox-
opyrimidin-4-one. 5-Iodo-2-thiouracil
Use: Antithyroid substance.
See: Itrumil [sodium derivative]
IODOTOPE I-131. (Squibb) Sodium Radio-Iodide-I-131
for oral use. 8,15, 30, 50, 100 u Ci/Vial of 5, 10,
15, 20 Caps.
IODOTOPE. (Squibb) Sodium Iodide I-131. 6 m Ci
Caps./5, 10, 15, 20, 50, 75 m Ci solution.
Use: Therapeutic agent.
• **IODOXAMATE MEGLUMINE.** USAN.
Use: Diagnostic aid.
• **IODOXAMIC ACID.** USAN. NN'-(1,16-Dioxo-4,-7,10,-
13-tetraoxahexadecane-1,16-diyl)di-(3-amino-2,4,6-
tri-iodobenzoic acid).
Use: Contrast medium.
IODOXYL.
See: Sodium Iodomethamate (Var. Mfr.)
• **IOGLICIC ACID.** USAN.
Use: Diagnostic aid.
• **IOGLUCOL.** USAN.
Use: Diagnostic aid.
• **IOGLUCOMIDE.** USAN.
Use: Diagnostic aid.
• **IOGLYCAMIC ACID.** USAN. 3,3-(Diglycoloyl-
diimino)-bis-[2,4,6-triiodobenzoic acid]. Biligram,
Bilivistan.
Use: Radiopaque (cholecystographic and
cholangiographic).
• **IOGULAMIDE.** USAN.
Use: Diagnostic aid (radiopaque medium).

• **IOHEXOL.** USAN.
Use: Diagnostic aid.
IOHYDRO CREAM. (Freeport) Hydrocortisone 1%,
clioquinol 3%, pramoxine HCl 0.5%/½ oz. Tubes
½ oz.
Use: Broad control of various dermatologic disorders.
• **IOMETHIN I-125.** USAN. 4-[[3-(Dimethylamino)propyl-
]amino]-7-iodo-^{125}I-quinoline.
Use: Diagnostic aid (neoplasm).
• **IOMETHIN I-131.** USAN. 4-[[3-Dimethylamino)propyl-
]amino]-7-iodo-^{131}I-quinoline.
Use: Diagnostic aid (neoplasm).
IONAMIN. (Pennwalt) Phentermine. Phenyl-tert-butyla-
mine as resin complex 15 mg. and 30 mg./Cap.
Bot. 100s, 400s.
Use: Appetite suppressant.
IONAX ASTRINGENT CLEANSER. (Owen) Isopropyl
alcohol 48%, Owenethers, (polyoxyethylene
ethers), acetone, salicylic acid, allantoin. Bot. 8 oz.
Use: Astringent skin cleanser.
IONAX FOAM. (Owen) Polyoxyethylene ethers,
benzalkonium Cl, purified water, isobutane,
propylene glycol, myristamide. DEA, PEG 1000,
D&C No. 5. Aerosol cans 2½ oz, 5 oz.
Use: Aerosol oily skin cleanser.
IONAX SCRUB. (Owen) Polyethylene granules,
polyoxyethylene ethers, alcohol 10%, benzalkonium
Cl. Tubes 2 oz., 4 oz.
Use: Abradant cleanser for oily skin.
IONAZE.
See: Propazolamide
ION-EXCHANGE RESINS.
See: Polyamine Methylene Resin
   Resins, Sodium Removing
IONIL RINSE. (Owen) Conditioners with benzalkonium
Cl in water base. Bot. 16 oz.
Use: Rinse.
IONIL SHAMPOO. (Owen) Salicylic acid,
benzalkonium Cl, alcohol 12%, polyoxyethylene
ethers. Plas. Bot. w/disp. cap 4 oz., 8 oz., 16 oz.,
32 oz.
Use: Anti-seborrheic.
IONIL T. (Owen) A nonionic/cationic foaming
shampoo w/coal tar. salicylic acid, benzalkonium
chloride, alcohol 12%, polyoxyethylene ethers.
Plas. bot. 4 oz., 8 oz., 16 oz., 32 oz.
Use: Anti-seborrheic.
IONOSOL B W/DEXTROSE 5%. (Abbott) Sod.
chloride 180 mg., pot. chloride 100 mg., Mg
chloride, anhy. 25 mg., dipotassium phosphate,
anhy. 100 mg., monosodium phosphate anhy. 14
mg., sod. lactate 280 mg., dextrose 5 Gm., sod.
bisulfite 30 mg./100 ml. Bot. 250 ml., 500 ml., 1000
ml.
IONOSOL B W/INVERT SUGAR 10%. (Abbott) Sod.
chloride 180 mg., pot. chloride 100 mg., Mg
chloride, anhy. 25 mg., dipotassium phosphate
anhy. 100 mg., monosodium phosphate, anhy. 14
mg., sod. lactate 246 mg., invert sugar 10 Gm.,
sod. bisulfite 30 mg./100 ml. Bot. 1000 ml.
IONOSOL D-CM. (Abbott) Sod. chloride 516 mg., pot.
chloride 89.4 mg., cal. chloride, anhy. 27.8 mg., Mg

chloride, anhy. 14.2 mg., sod. lactate 560 mg./100 ml. Bot. 1000 ml.

IONOSOL D-CM W/DEXTROSE 5%. (Abbott) Sod. chloride 516 mg., pot. chloride 89.4 mg., cal. chloride, anhy. 27.8 mg., Mg chloride, anhy. 14.2 mg., sod. lactate 560 mg., dextrose 5 Gm., sod. bisulfite 50 mg./100 ml. Bot. 1000 ml.
Use: Duodenal use.

IONOSOL D (MODIFIED) W/INVERT SUGAR 10%. (Abbott) Sod. chloride 117 mg., pot. chloride 268 mg., cal. chloride, anhy. 25.5 mg., Mg chloride, anhy.13.3mg.,sod.lactate672mg.,invertsugar10Gm., sod. bisulfite 41.6 mg./100 ml. Bot. 1000 ml.

IONOSOL G W/DEXTROSE 10%. (Abbott) Sod. chloride 370 mg., pot. chloride 126 mg., ammonium chloride 377 mg., dextrose 10 Gm. sodium bicarbonate (buffer) 4.5 mg., sodium bisulfite 30 mg./100 ml. Bot. 1000 ml.
Use: Gastric use.

IONOSOL G W/INVERT SUGAR 10%. (Abbott) Sod. chloride 350 mg., pot. chloride 127 mg., ammonium chloride 375 mg., invert sugar 10 Gm., sod. bisulfite 60 mg., sod. bicarbonate 4.5 mg./100 ml. Bot. 1000 ml.

IONOSOL MB W/DEXTROSE 5%. (Abbott) Pot. chloride 141 mg., Mg chloride, anhy. 14.2 mg., monopotassium phosphate, anhy. 15 mg., monosodium phosphate, anhy. 21.4 mg., sod. lactate 260 mg., dextrose 5 Gm., sod. bisulfite 22 mg./100 ml. Bot. 250 ml., 500 ml., 1000 ml.

IONOSOL T W/DEXTROSE 5%. (Abbott) Sod. chloride 146 mg., pot. chloride 111 mg., monosodium phosphate, anhy. 181 mg., pot. lactate 256 mg., dextrose 5 Gm., sod. bisulfite 23 mg./100 ml. Bot. 250 ml., 500 ml., 1000 ml.

• **IOPAMIDOL.** USAN.
Use: Diagnostic aid.

• **IOPANOIC ACID,** U.S.P. XXI. Tabs. U.S.P. XXI. Benzenepropanoic acid, 3-amino-α-ethyl-2,4,6-triiodo-. 2-(3-Amino-2,4,6-tri-iodobenzyl)-butyric acid. 3-Amino-a-ethyl-2,4,6 Triiodohydrocinnamic acid.
See: Telepaque, Tab. (Winthrop-Breon)

IOPHED SYRUP. (Marsh-Emory) Ephedrine HCl 12 mg., calcium iodide hexahydrate 167 mg., chloral hydrate 300 mg./5 cc. Bot. pt.
Use: Bronchial & cardiac asthma & status asthmaticus.

• **IOPHENDYLATE,** U.S.P. XXI. Benzenedecanoic acid, iodo-t-methyl-, ethyl ester.
Use: Diagnostic aid (radiopaque medium).

• **IOPHENDYLATE INJECTION,** U.S.P. XXI. Ethiodan, Myodil. Ethyl Iodophenylundecylate.
Use: Diagnostic aid (radiopaque medium).
See: Pantopaque, Amp. (LaFayette)

IOPHENOXIC ACID. Tabs. a-(2-4,6-Triiodo-3-hydroxybenzyl) butyric acid.

IOPODATE SODIUM.
See Ipodate Sodium.

IOPREP. (Arbrook) Nonylphenoxypolyethylenoxy (4) ethanol and nonylphenoxypolyethyleneoxy (15) ethanol iodine complex 5.5%, nonylphenoxypolyethyleneoxy (30) ethanol 10%.

Solution provides 1% available iodine. Bot. plastic, gal.
Use: Antiseptic.

• **IOPROCEMIC ACID.** USAN.
Use: Diagnostic aid.

• **IOPRONIC ACID.** USAN.
Use: Diagnostic aid.

• **IOPYDOL.** USAN. 1-(2,3-Dihydroxypropyl)-3,5-diiodo-4(1H)-pyridone.
Use: X-ray contrast medium for bronchography.

• **IOPYDONE.** USAN. 3,5-Diiodo-4-(1H)-pyridone.
Use: X-ray contrast medium for bronchography.

• **IOSEFAMIC ACID.** USAN. 5,5'-(Sebacoyldiimino) bis[2,4,6-triiodo-N-methylisophthalamic acid]
Use: Contrast medium.

• **IOSERIC ACID.** USAN.
Use: Diagnostic aid.

• **IOSULAMIDE MEGLUMINE.** USAN.
Use: Diagnostic aid.

• **IOSUMETIC ACID.** USAN.
Use: Diagnostic aid.

• **IOTASUL.** USAN.
Use: Diagnostic aid.

• **IOTETRIC ACID.** USAN.
Use: Diagnostic aid.

• **IOTHALAMATE MEGLUMIDE AND IOTHALMATE SODIUM INJECTION,** U.S.P. XXI.

• **IOTHALAMATE MEGLUMINE INJECTION,** U.S.P. XXI. Benzoic acid, 3-(acetylamino)-2,4,6-triiodo-5-[(methylamino)carbonyl]-, compound with 1-deoxy-1-(methylamino)-d-glucitol (1:1).
Use: Diagnostic aid (radiopaque medium).

• **IOTHALAMATE SODIUM I-125.** USAN.

• **IOTHALAMATE SODIUM I-131.** USAN.

• **IOTHALAMATE SODIUM INJECTION,** U.S.P. XXI. Benzoic acid, 3-(acetylamino)-2,4,6-triiodo-5-[(me-thylamino)carbonyl]-, sod. salt. 5-Acetamido-2,4,6-triiodo-N-methylisophthalamic acid, sod. salt. Sod. Iothalamate.
Use: Diagnostic aid (radiopaque medium).

• **IOTHALAMIC ACID,** U.S.P. XXI. (Mallinckrodt) Benzoic acid, 3-(acetylamino)-2,4,6-triiodo-5-[(me-thylamino)carbonyl]-. 5-Acetamino-2,4,6-triiodo-N-methylisophthalamic acid.
Use: Radiopaque; pharm. necessity for Iothalamate Meglumine Injection, Iothalamate Meglumine and Iothalamate Sodium Injection, and Iothalamate Sodium Injection.
See: Conray, Amp., Vial (Mallinckrodt)
Conray 400, Amp., Vial (Mallinckrodt)

IOTHIOURACIL SODIUM. Sod. salt of 5-iodo-2-thiouracil.

IOTIS. (Research Pharmacal Lab.) Iodine crystals 0.03, carbamide 1%, benzyl alcohol 3%, glycerine (dehydrated) Bot. 15 cc.
Use: Chronic otitis externa.

• **IOTROL.** USAN.

• **IOTROXIC ACID.** USAN.
Use: Diagnostic aid.

• **IOTYROSINE 1-131.** USAN.
Use: Radioactive agent.

• **IOXAGLATE MEGLUMINE.** USAN.

Use: Diagnostic agent (radiopaque medium).
- **IOXAGLATE SODIUM.** USAN.
  Use: Diagnostic agent (radiopaque medium).
- **IOXAGLIC ACID.** USAN.
  Use: Diagnostic agent (radiopaque medium).
- **IOXOTRIZOIC ACID.** USAN.
  Use: Diagnostic aid.
IPATERP. (Fellows) Terpin hydrate 2 gr., ammonium chloride 1 gr., licorice extract ½ gr., ipecac ¹/₁₀ gr./Tab. Bot. 1000s.
  Use: Antitussive, expectorant.
- **IPECAC,** U.S.P. XXI. Powd., Syr. U.S.P. XXI.
  Use: Emetic.
W/Comb.
  See: Balmial Cough Syrup, Syr. (Clapp)
    Creozets, Loz. (Creomulsion Co.)
    Derfort, Cap. (Cole)
    Diatrol, Tab. (Otis Clapp)
    Dophenco, Cap. (Blue Line)
    Ipedote, Syrup (Panray)
    Ipsatol/DM, Cough Syr. (Key)
    Ipsatol, Syr. (Key)
    Mallergan, Liq. (Mallard)
    Neo-Bronchoid, Tab. (Moore-Kirk)
    Phenatrocaps, Cap. (O'Neal)
    Phenatrohist, Cap. (O'Neal)
    Polyectin, Liq. (Amid)
    Proclan, Preps. (Cenci)
    Romilar, CF, Syr. (Block)
    Rhubarb, Ipecac & Soda, Tab. (Noyes)
    Rubacac, Tab. (Scrip)
    Spenlaxo, Tab. (Spencer-Mead)
    Terpium, Tab. (Scrip)
IPEDOTE SYRUP. (Panray) Syrup of ipecac. Bot. 30 ml.
  Use: Emetic.
- **IPEXIDINE MESYLATE.** USAN.
  Use: Dental caries prophylactic.
- **IPODATE CALCIUM,** U.S.P. XXI. Oral Susp., U.S.P. XXI. Benzenepropanoic acid, 3-[[(dimethylamino)methylene]amino]-2,4,6-triiodo-, calcium salt.
  Use: Diagnostic aid (radiopaque medium).
  See: Oragrafin cal., Granules (Squibb)
- **IPODATE SODIUM,** U.S.P. XXI. Cap., U.S.P. XXI. Benzenepropanoic acid, 3-[[(dimethylamino)-methylene] amino]-2,4,6-triiodo-, sod. salt.
  Use: Diagnostic aid (radiopaque medium).
  See: Bilivist, Cap. (Berlex)
    Oragrafin sod., Cap., Vial (Squibb)
- **IPRATROPIUM BROMIDE.** USAN. 8-Isopropyl-3-(±)-tropoyloxy-1αH,5αH-tropanium bromide. N-Isopropylatropinium bromide.
  Use: Bronchodilator.
  See: Atrovent
- **IPRINDOLE.** USAN. 5-[3-(Dimethylamino)-propyl]-6,-7,8,9,10,11-hexahydro-5H-cyclo-oct[β]-indole. 5-(3-Dimethylaminopropyl)-6,7,8,9,10-11-hexahydrocyclo-oct[β]indole. Prondol hydrochloride.
  Use: Antidepressant.
- **IPROCINODINE HYDROCHLORIDE.** USAN.
  Use: Antibacterial.

IPROCLOZIDE. B.A.N. 4-Chlorophenoxy-2'-isopropylacetohydrazide.
  Use: Monoamine oxidase inhibitor.
- **IPROFENIN.** USAN.
  Use: Diagnostic aid.
IPRONIAZID. B.A.N. I-isonicotinyl-2-isopropylhydrazine phosphate. 2'-Isopropylisonicotinohydrazide.
  Use: Monoamine oxidase inhibitor.
  See: Marsilid phosphate.
- **IPRONIDAZOLE.** USAN. 2-Isopropyl-1-methyl-5-nitroimidazole. Ipropran (Hoffman-LaRoche).
  Use: Antiprotozoal (Histomanas).
- **IPROPLATIN.** USAN.
IPROVERATRIL. Name used for Verapamil.
- **IPROXAMINE HYDROCHLORIDE.** USAN.
  Use: Vasodilator.
IPSATOL. (Key) Ipecac alkaloids 0.24 mg., ammonium chloride 22 mg./5 ml. in tolu balsam syrup base. Bot. 4 oz.
  Use: Pediatric expectorant.
IPSATOL/DM. (Key) Dextromethorphan HBr 10 mg./5 ml. in addition to the Ipsatol formulation. Bot. 4 fl. oz.
  Use: Antitussive, expectorant.
IRCON. (Key) Ferrous fumarate 200 mg./Tab. Bot. 100s.
  Use: Hematinic.
IRCON-FA. (Key) Ferrous fumarate 250 mg., folic acid 1 mg./Tab. Bot. 100s.
IRGASAN CF3. Cloflucarban. Under study.
  Use: Antiseptic.
- **IRIDIUM IR-192.** USAN.
  See: Iriditope (Squibb)
IRIGATE. (Ketchum) Bot. 4 oz.
  Use: Eyewash.
IRISIN. A polysaccharide found in several species of iris.
IROCAINE.
  See: Procaine Hydrochloride (Various Mfr.)
IRODEX. (Keene) Iron dextran complex 50 mg./ml. Vial 10 ml.
  Use: Iron deficiency anemia.
IRODEX. (Tunex) An iron-dextran complex 50 mg./ml. Vial 10cc.
  Use: Iron deficiency anemia.
IROMIN-G. (Mission) Ferrous gluconate 333.3 mg. (Iron 38.6 mg.), Vit. B-12 (crystalline on resin) 2.0 mcg., C 100 mg., A acetate 4000 I.U., D-2 400 I.U., B-1 5.0 mg., B-2 2.0 mg., B-6 25 mg., niacinamide 10 mg., cal. pantothenate 1.0 mg., folic acid 0.8 mg., calcium gluconate 100 mg., calcium lactate 100 mg., calcium carbonate 70 mg. (calcium 50 mg.)/Tab. Bot. 100s.
  Use: Hematic supplement.
IRON, ARSENIC AND COPPER INJ. (Torigian) Iron cacodylate 0.065 Gm., sod. cacodylate 0.15 Gm., copper sulfate 0.5 mg./5 cc. Amp. 5 cc.
IRON BILE SALTS.
  See: Bilron, Pulvules (Lilly)
IRON CACODYLATE. (CMC) 0.03 Gm./cc., 1 gr./2 cc., 1 gr./5 cc. Amp. 100s.
IRON CACODYLATE. (Torigian) Metallic iron 12%, organically combined arsenic as ferric salt of

dimethylarsonate. Amp. ½ gr. 1 cc., 25s, 100s. 1 gr. 2 cc. 5 cc., 25s, 100s.

IRON CARBONATE COMPLEX.
See: Polyferose

IRON CHOLINE CITRATE COMPLEX.
See: Chel-Iron, Tab. (Kinney)
  Kelex, Tabseals. (Nutrition Control)

IRONCO-B. (Vale) Ferrous sulfate 194.4 mg., manganese sulfate 21.6 mg., dicalcium phosphate 129.6 mg., B-1 1 mg., B-2 1 mg., niacin 6.0 mg.,Vit. D 100 I.U./Tab. Bot. 100s, 500s, 1000s.

• **IRON-DEXTRAN INJECTION.,** U.S.P. XXI.
Use: Hematinic.
See: Ferrodex, Inj. (Keene Pharm.)
  Hydextran, Inj. (Hyrex)
  Imferon, Amp., Vial (Merrell Dow)

IRON-FOLIC ACID-LIVER. (Medwick) Vial 30 cc.

"IRON FOR WOMEN". (Pharmex) Ferrous fumarate 5 gr./Tab. Bot. 90s.

IRON (2+) FUMARATE. Ferrous Fumarate, U.S.P. XXI.

IRON (2+) GLUCONATE.
See: Ferrous Gluconate, U.S.P. XXI.

IRON OXIDE MIXTURE WITH ZINC OXIDE.
Calamine, U.S.P. XXI.

IRON PEPTONIZED.
See: Saferon, Tab. (Elder)

IRON PROTEIN COMPLEX.

• **IRON SORBITEX.** USAN. A sterile, colloidal solution of a complex of trivalent iron, sorbitol, and citric acid, stabilized with dextrin and sorbitol.
Use: Hematinic.

• **IRON SORBITEX INJECTION,** U.S.P. XXI. (Formerly iron sorbitol)
Use: Iron supplement.
See: Jectofer Amp. (Astra)

IRON SULFATE. W/Maalox.
See: Fermalox, Tab. (Rorer)

IRON w/PRO SOF SG. (Vangard) Ferrous fumarate 150 mg., docusate sodium 100 mg./Cap. Bot. 100s.
Use: Vitamin w/stool softener.

IRON WITH VITAMIN C. (Squibb) Iron 50 mg., Vit. C 25 mg./Tab. Bot. 100s. (Formerly called Feramel)
Use: Hematinic.

IROPHOS D. (Lannett) Dicalcium phosphate anh. 330 mg., ferrous sulf. 30 mg., Vit. D 333 I.U./Cap. Bot. 500s, 1000s.
Use: Hematinic.

IROSPAN. (Fielding) Ferrous sulfate 200 mg., Vit. C 150 mg./Cap. Bot. 60s. Tab. Bot. 100s.
Use: Iron deficiency anemia.

IRRADIATED 7-DEHYDROCHOLESTEROL.
See: Activated 7-Dehydrocholesterol.

IRRADIATED ERGOSTEROL.
See: Calciferol.

IRRIGATE. (Professional Pharmacal) Boric acid 1.2%, potassium Cl. 0.38%, sodium carbonate 0.014%, benzalkonium Cl. 0.01%, disodium edetate 0.05%. Bot. 0.5 oz., 4 oz.
Use: Ocular cleanser.

ISACEN.
See: Oxyphenisatin, Prep. (Various Mfr.)

• **ISAMOXOLE.** USAN.
Use: Anti-asthmatic.

ISAVERINE HCl. Methindizate, B.A.N.

ISMELIN. (Ciba) Guanethidine sulfate, 10 mg. and 25 mg./Tab. Bot. 100s, 1000s; Consumer Packs of 100s.
Use: Hypertension treatment.

ISMOTIC. (Alcon) Isosorbide solution.
Use: Reduce intraocular pressure.

ISO-ALCOHOLIC ELIXIR.
Use: Vehicle.

ISOAMINILE. B.A.N. (Robins) 4-Dimethylamino-2-isopropyl-2-phenylvaleronitrile. Dimyril citrate.
Use: Antitussive.

ISOAMYLHYDROCUPREINE DIHYDROCHLORIDE.
See: Eucupin Dihydrochloride

ISOAMYL NITRATE.
See: Amyl Nitrite, U.S.P. XXI.

ISOAMYNE.
See: Amphetamine (Various Mfr.)

ISO-BID. (Geriatric) Isosorbide dinitrate 40 mg./Cap. Bot. 30s, 100s, 500s.
Use: Prophylaxis in angina pectoris.

ISOBORNYL THIOCYANOACETATE, TECHNICAL.
Use: Pediculicide.
See: Barc, Liq. (Commerce)
W/Anhydrous soap.
W/Docusate sodium and related terpenes.
See: Barc, Cream (Commerce)

• **ISOBUCAINE HYDROCHLORIDE,** U.S.P. XXI. 2-Isobutylamino-2-methylpropyl benzoate HCl. 2-(Isobutylamino)-2-methyl-1-propanol benzoate (ester) HCl.
Use: Local anesthetic (dental).

• **ISOBUCAINE HCl & EPINEPHRINE INJECTION,** U.S.P. XXI.
Use: Local anesthetic (dental).

• **ISOBUTAMBEN,** USAN. Isobutyl p-aminobenzoate. Isocaine. Cycloform.
Use: As a surface anesthetic.

• **ISOBUTANE,** N.F. XVI.

ISOBUTYLALLYLBARBITURIC ACID.
W/Aspirin, phenacetin, caffeine.
See: Buff-A-Comp, Tab., Cap. (Mayrand)
  Fiorinal, Cap., Tab. (Sandoz)
  Lanorinal, Cap. (Lannett)
  Palgesic, Tab., Cap. (Pan Amer.)
  Sedagesic, Tab. (Kay)
  Tenstan, Tab. (Standex)
  Wolgraine, Tab. (Wolins)
W/Aspirin, phenacetin, caffeine, codeine phosphate.
See: Fiorinal w/codeine, Cap. (Sandoz)

ISOBUTYL p-AMINOBENZOATE. Isobutamben, U.S.A.N.

4-ISOBUTYLPHENYLACE-ACID. Ibufenac

ISOBUZOLE. B.A.N. 5-Isobutyl-2-(4-methoxybenzenesulphonamido)-1,3,4-thiadiazole. Glysobuzole (I.N.N.)
Use: Oral hypoglycemic agent.
See: Stabinol

ISOCAINE. Isobutamben, U.S.A.N.

ISOCAL. (Mead Johnson) Lactose-free isotonic liquid

containing as a % of the calories 13% protein as casein and soy protein; 37% fat as soy oil and medium chain triglycerides; 50% carbohydrate as corn syrup solids w/vitamins and minerals for the tube fed patient. Vitamins, and minerals. Cans 8 fl. oz., 12 fl. oz., 32 fl. oz., Bot. 8 fl. oz.
Use: Complete enteral liquid diet, nutritionally balanced and lactose free to meet nutritional needs of tube fed patients.

ISOCAL HCN. (Mead Johnson) High calorie, nitrogen nurtitionally complete food. Protein 15%, fat 40%, carbohydrate 45%. Cans 8 fl. oz.
Use: Complete, concentrated nutrition.

• **ISOCARBOXAZID,** U.S.P. XXI. Tab., U.S.P. XXI. 1-Benzyl[-2-(5-methyl-3-isoxazolyl-carbonyl)hydra-zine. 5-Methyl-3-isoxazolecarboxylic acid 2-benzyl-hydrazide. 3-(2-Benzylhydrazinocarbonyl)-5-meth-ylisoxazole. 2'-Benzyl-5-methylisoxazole-3-carbohy-drazide.
Use: Antidepressant.
See: Marplan, Tab. (Roche)

ISOCOCAINE. Pseudococaine.

• **ISOCONAZOLE.** USAN.
Use: Antibacterial, antifungal.

ISO D. (Dunhall) Isosorbide dinitrate. **Cap.** 40 mg. Bot. 100s, 1000s. **Tab.** (sublingual) 5 mg. Bot. 100s.

ISODINE ANTISEPTIC. (Blair) Povidone-iodine. **Soln:** Bot. 1 oz. **Mouth Wash:** Bot. 6 oz.
Use: Topical antiseptic.

ISOEPHEDRINE HCl. d-Isoephedrine HCl.
See: Pseudoephedrine HCl.
W/Chlorpheniramine maleate.
See: Isoclor, Tab., Expect., Timesule, Liq. (Arnar-Stone)
W/Chlorprophenpyridamine maleate.
See: Isoclor, Tab. (Arnar-Stone)
W/Theophylline sodium glycinate & guaifenesin.
See: Iso-Tabs 60 Tab. (Rowell)

D-ISOEPHEDRINE SULFATE.
See: Pseudoephedrine Sulfate.

• **ISOETHARINE,** USAN. 3,4-Dihydroxy α-(l-iso-propylamino-propyl)benzyl alcohol. 1-(3,4-Dihydroxy-phenyl)-2-isopropylaminobutan-1-ol. Numotac hydro-chloride.
Use: Bronchodilator.

• **ISOETHARINE HYDROCHLORIDE,** U.S.P. XXI.
Use: Bronchodilator.
See: Bronkosol, Sol. (Winthrop-Breon)

• **ISOETHARINE INHALATION SOLUTION,** U.S.P. XXI.
Use: Bronchodilator.

• **ISOETHARINE MESYLATE,** U.S.P. XXI. Inhalation Aerosol, U.S.P. XXI.
Use: Bronchodilator
See: Bronkometer, Aerosol (Winthrop-Breon)

ISOFEDROL. (Blue Line) Ephedrine sulfate 1% in an isotonic sol. Bot. ¾ oz.
Use: Nasal vasoconstrictor.

ISOFIL. (Seatrace) Theophylline 200 mg., noscapine 30 mg./Tab. Bot. 100s, 1000s.
Use: Long-acting bronchodilator.

• **ISOFLUPREDONE ACETATE.** USAN.
Use: Anti-inflammatory.

• **ISOFLURANE.** U.S.P. XXI.
Use: Anesthetic.

• **ISOFLUROPHATE,** U.S.P. XXI. Ophth. Oint., U.S.P. XXI. Phosphorofluoridic acid, bis(1-methylethyl)ester. Diisopropyl phosphorofluoridate.
Use: Cholinergic (ophthalmic).
See: Floropryl, Oint. (Merck Sharp & Dohme)

ISOGREGNENONE. Dydrogesterone.
See: Duphaston, Tab. (Philips Roxane)

ISO-IODEIKON.
See: Phentetiothalein Sodium (No Mfr. currently lists.)

ISOJECT. (Pfipharmecs) A purified, sterile, disposable injection system.
Permapen (benzathine pencillin G.) aqueous solution, 1,200,000 u./2 cc. 10s.
Terramycin (oxytetracycline) Intramuscular solution 250 mg./2 cc. 10s.

• **ISOLEUCINE,** U.S.P. XXI. $C_6H_{13}NO_2$, L-isoleucine. DL-Isoleucine. (Pfaltz & Bauer)—Pow. 10 Gm.
Use: Nutrient.

ISOMEPROBAMATE.
See: Carisoprodol (Var. Mfr.)

• **ISOMEROL.** USAN.
Use: Antiseptic.

ISOMETHADONE. B.A.N. 6-Dimethylamino-5-methyl-4,4-diphenylhexan-3-one.
Use: Narcotic analgesic.
See: Isoamidone

ISOMETAMIDIUM. B.A.N. 8-m-Amidinophenyl-diazoamino-3-amino-5-ethyl-6-phenylphenanthridiniu-m chloride.
Use: Antiprotozoan, veterinary medicine.
See: Samorin HCl.

ISOMETHEPTENE BITARTRATE.
See: Tega-Nyl, Vial (Ortega)

ISOMETHEPTENE HCl. Methyl-isooctenylamine mu-cate or tartrate. Also available as Hydrochloride.
W/N-acetyl-p-aminophenol, dichloralphenazone.
See: Midrin, Cap. (Carnrick)

ISOMETHEPTENE MUCATE.
See: Midrin, Cap. (Carnick)
Octinum, Tab. (Knoll)

ISOMETHEPTENE TARTRATE.
See: Tri-Grain, Vial (Pharmex)

ISOMIL. (Ross) Soy protein isolate formula. Each liter contains: protein 20.0 g, fat 36.0 g, carbohydrate 68.0 g, Ca 0.70 g, P 0.50 g, Na 0.30 g, K 0.71 g, Cl 0.53 g, Mg 50 mg., Zn 5.0 mg., Cu 0.50 mg., Fe 12 mg., iodine 0.10 mg., Mn 0.20 mg., Vit. A 2500 IU, D 400 IU, E 20 IU, C 55 mg., B-1 0.40 mg., B-2 0.60 mg., B-6 0.40 mg., niacin 9.0 (mg. Eq.), folic acid 0.10 mg., B-12 3.0 mcg., pantothenic acid 5.0 mg., biotin 30 mcg., K-1 0.15 mg./Liter. Concentrated liquid 13 fl. oz. cans; ready-to-feed (20 Cal/fl. oz.) 4 oz. and 8 oz. bottles, 32 oz. cans; "as fed" 20 cal/fl. oz. Use: For milk sensitive and lactose intolerant infants and children.

ISOMIL SF. (Ross) Low osmolar sucrose free soy protein isolate formula; concentrated liquid 13 fl oz

cans, ready-to-feed (20 cal/fl oz) 4 oz and 8 oz bottles, 32 oz cans; "as fed" 20 cal/fl oz; per liter: protein 20.0 Gm., fat 36.0 Gm., carbohydrate 68.0 Gm., Ca 0.70 Gm., P 0.50 Gm., Na 0.30 Gm., K 0.71 Gm., Cl 0.53 Gm., Mg 50 mg, Zn 5.0 mg, Cu 0.50 mg, Fe 12 mg, Iodine 0.10 mg, Mn 0.20 mg, Vit. A 2500 IU, Vit. D 400 IU, Vit. E 20 IU, Vit. C 55 mg, thiamine 0.40 mg, riboflavin 0.60 mg, Vit. B-6 0.40 mg, niacin 9.0 (mg eq), folic acid 0.10 mg, Vit. B-12 3.0 mcg, pantothenic acid 5.0 mg, biotin 30 mcg, Vit. K-1 0.15 mg per liter.
Use: For milk sensitive and lactose intolerant infants and children.

ISOMUNE-LD. (Roche) Rapid immunochemical separation method of the heart specific LD-1 isoenzyme for quantitation when used with an appropriate LD substrate reagent. 40 and 100 test kits.

ISOMUNE-CK. (Roche) Rapid immunochemical separation method of the heart specific CK-MB isoenzyme for quantitation when used with an appropriate CK substrate reagent. 100 and 250 test kits.

• **ISOMYLAMINE HCl.** USAN. 2-(Diethylamino)ethyl 1-isopentylcyclohexanecarboxylate HCl.
Use: Smooth muscle relaxant.

ISOMYN.
See: Amphetamine (Various Mfr.)

• **ISONIAZID,** U.S.P. XXI. Inj., Syr., Tab. U.S.P. XXI. Isonicotinic acid hydrazide, isonicotinyl hydrazide. Cotinazin; I.N.H.; Mybasan; Neumandin; Nicetal; Nydrazid; Pycazide; Rimifon; Tubomel; Vazadrine.
Use: Antibacterial (tuberculostatic).
See: Dow-Isoniazid, Tab. (Merrell Dow)
   INH, Tab. (Ciba)
   Laniazid, Tab. (Lannett)
   Niconyl, Tab. (Parke-Davis)
   Nydrazid, Tab., Inj. (Squibb)
   Panzid, Tab., Pow. (Panray)
   Rolazid, Tab. (Robinson)
   Teebaconin, Tab., Pwd. (Consol. Mid.)
   Triniad, Tab. (Kasar)
   Uniad, Tab. (Kasar)
W/p-Aminosalicylic acid.
   See: Di-Isopacin, Tab. (CMC)
   Isopacin, Tab. (CMC)
W/Calcium paraminosalicylate.
   See: Calpas-INH, Tab. (Amer. Chem. & Drug)
W/Calcium p-aminosalicylate, Vit. B-6.
   See: Calpas Isoxine, Tab. (American Chem. & Drug)
   Calpas-INAH-6, Tabs. (Amer. Chem. & Drug)
W/Pyridoxine HCl. (Vit. B6)
   See: Hyzyd + B-6, Tab. (Mallinckrodt)
   Niadox, Tab. (Barnes-Hind)
   P-I-N Forte, Syr., Tab. (Lannett)
   Teebaconin w/B6 (Consol. Mid.)
   Triniad Plus 30, Tab. (Kasar)
   Uniad-Plus, Tab. (Kasar)
W/Pyridoxine HCl, sodium aminosalicylate.

See: Pasna, Tri-Pack 300, Granules (Barnes-Hind)
W/Rifampin.
   See: Rimactane/INH DuoPack (Ciba)
W/Sodium aminosalicylate, pyridoxine.
   See: Pasna Tri-Pack, Granules (Barnes-Hind)
W/Sodium para-aminosalicylate.
   See: Isopacin, Double-Isopacin, Tab. (CMC)

ISONICOTINIC ACID HYDRAZIDE.
See: Isoniazid, U.S.P. XXI. (Var. Mfr.)

ISONICOTINYL HYDRAZIDE.
See: Isoniazid, U.S.P. XXI. (Var. Mfr.)

ISONIPECAINE HYDROCHLORIDE.
See: Meperidine Hydrochloride, U.S.P. XXI. (Var. Mfr.)

ISOPAQUE. (Winthrop Products) Metrozoic acid.
Use: Diagnostic radiopaque medium.

ISOPENTAQUINE.
Use: Curative & prophylactic in malaria.

• **ISOPHANE INSULIN SUSPENSION,** U.S.P. XXI.
Use: Hypoglycemic agent.
See: NPH Iletin, Vial (Lilly)

ISOPHYLLINE. Diprophylline, B.A.N.

ISOPREDNIDENE. B.A.N. $11\beta,17\alpha,21$-Trihydroxy-16-methylenepregna-4,6-diene-3,20-dione.
Use: ACTH inhibitor.

ISOPREGNENONE.
See: Duphaston, Tab. (Philips Roxane) Dydrogesterone

ISOPRENALINE. B.A.N. $(\pm)$-1-(3,4-Dihydroxy-phenyl)-2-isopropylaminoethanol. Isopropylnoradrenaline.
Use: Sympathomimetic.
See: Isoproterenol HCl

• **ISOPROPAMIDE IODIDE,** U.S.P. XXI. Tab., U.S.P. XXI. (3-Carbamoyl-3,3-diphenylpropyl) diisopropyl-methylammonium iodide. Tyrimide.
Use: Anticholinergic.
See: Darbid, Tab. (SmithKline)
W/Prochlorperazine maleate.
   See: Iso-Perazine, Cap. (Lemmon)

ISOPROPHENAMINE HCl. Name used for Clorprenaline HCl.

ISOPROPICILLIN POTASSIUM. Potassium 3,3-dimethyl-6-(2-methyl-2-phenoxypropionamido)-7-oxo-4-thia-1-azabicyclo [3.2.0]heptane-2-carboxylate.
Use: Antibiotic.

N-ISOPROPOYL-α-(2-METHYLHYDRAZI-NO)-p-TOL-UAMIDE HCl. Procarbazine HCl. U.S.P. XXI.

• **ISOPROPYL ALCOHOL,** U.S.P. XXI.
Use: Local anti-infective; pharm. aid (solvent).

• **ISOPROPYL ALCOHOL, AZEOTROPIC,** U.S.P. XXI.

ISOPROPYLARTERENOL HYDROCHLORIDE.
Use: Asthma, vasoconstrictor & allergic states.

ISOPROPYLARTERENOL SULFATE.
See: Isoproterenol Sulf.

1-(ISOPROPYLAMINO)-3-(1-NAPHTHYLOXY)-2-PRO-PANOL HCl. Propanolol HCl, U.S.P. XXI.

• **ISOPROPYL MYRISTATE,** N.F. XVI.
Use: Pharm. aid (emollient)

ISOPROPYL-NORADRENALINE HCl.

See: Isoproterenol HCl, U.S.P. XXI.
• **ISOPROPYL PALMITATE,** N.F. XVI.
  Use: Pharmaceutic aid (oleaginous vehicle).
ISOPROPYL PHENAZONE. 4-Isopropyl antipyrine.
  Larodon
• **ISOPROPYL RUBBING ALCOHOL,** U.S.P. XXI.
  Use: Rubefacient, solvent.
ISOPROTERENOL.
  See: Norisidrine (Abbott)
W/Butabarbital, theophylline, ephedrine HCl.
  See: Medihaler-Iso, Vial (Riker)
• **ISOPROTERENOL HYDROCHLORIDE,** U.S.P. XXI.
  Inhalation, Tab. Inj.; U.S.P. XXI. 1,2-Benzenediol,4-
  [1-hydroxy-2-[(1-methylethyl)-amino]ethyl]-, HCl. 3,4-
  Dihydroxy-α-[(isopropylamino)methyl]benzyl alcohol
  hydrochloride. Oleudrin-Proternol. 1:5,000 5 ml and
  10 ml in Univ. Add. Syr.; 1:5,000 1 mg and 2 mg
  pintop vials; 1:50,000 10 ml with Abboject Syr.
  (21G × 1 ½").
  Use: Adrenergic (bronchodilator).
  See: Isuprel HCl, Prods. (Winthrop-Breon)
    Norisodrine, Aerotrol, Syrup (Abbott)
    Proternol, Tab. (Key Pharm.)
    Vapo-Iso, Sol. (Fisons)
W/Acetylcysteine.
  See: Mucomyst with Isoproterenol, Sol. (Mead
  Johnson)
W/Aminophylline, ephedrine sulfate, phenobarbital.
  See: Asminorel, Tab. (Reid-Provident)
W/Clopane (clopentamine) HCl, propylene glycol,
  ascorbic acid.
  See: Aerolone Compound, Sol. (Lilly)
W/Phenobarbital, ephedrine sulfate, theophylline, pot.
  iodide.
  See: Isophed, Tab. (Jamieson-McKames)
    Isuprel Compound, Elix. (Winthrop-Breon)
W/Phenobarbital sod., ephedrine sulfate, theophylline
  hydrous.
  See: Iso-asminyl, Tab. (Cole)
W/Phenylephrine bitartrate.
  See: Duo-Medihaler, Vial (Riker)
• **ISOPROTERENOL INHALATION SOLUTION,**
  U.S.P. XXI.
  Use: Bronchodilator.
• **ISOPROTERENOL HYDROCHLORIDE AND
  PHENYLEPHRINE BITARTRATE INHALATION
  AEROSOL,** U.S.P. XXI.
  Use: Adrenergic (bronchodilator)
  See: Duo-Medihaler, Vial (Riker)
• **ISOPROTERENOL SULFATE,** U.S.P. XXI. Inhal.
  Aerosol, Inhal. Sol., U.S.P. XXI.
  See: Luf-Iso Inhalation (Mallinckrodt)
    Medihaler-Iso, Vial (Riker)
W/Calcium iodide (anhydrous), alcohol.
  See: Norisodrine, Syr. (Abbott)
ISOPTIN IV. (Knoll) Verapamil HCl 5 mg., sodium Cl.
  17 mg./2 ml. Amp. 2 ml.
  Use: Calcium ion influx inhibitor.
ISOPTIN TABLETS. (Knoll) Verapamil HCl 80 mg. or
  120 mg./Tab. Bot. 100s. Unit Dose 10 × 10s.
  Use: Calcium ion influx inhibitor for treatment of
  angina.

ISOPTO ALKALINE. (Alcon) 1% Methylcellulose
  sterile ophth. sol. Dropper Bot. 15 cc.
  Use: Ophthalmic emollient & lubricant, artificial
  tears.
ISOPTO ATROPINE. (Alcon) Atropine sulfate in
  methylcellulose solution. Drop-tainer 0.5% and 3.0%
  5 cc. 1.0% 5 cc., 15 cc.
  Use: Mydriatic and cycloplegic.
ISOPTO CARBACHOL. (Alcon) Carbachol U.S.P.
  0.75%, 1.5%, 2.25%, 3%, in a sterile buffered
  solution of 1% methylcellulose. Drop-Tainer 15 cc.,
  0.75%, 1.5%, 3%, 30 cc.
  Use: Glaucoma, contraindications, corneal injuries.
ISOPTO CARPINE. (Alcon) Pilocarpine HCl in stable
  sterile 0.5% methylcellulose sol. w/isotonicity of
  lacrimal fluid. Bot. Drop-Tainer (0.25%, 0.5%, 1%,
  1.5%, 2%, 3%, 4%, 5%, 6%, 8% & 10%
  pilocarpine HCl) 15 cc.; 0.5%, 1%, 1.5%, 2%, 3%,
  4%, 6% 30 cc.
  Use: Glaucoma.
ISOPTO CETAMIDE. (Alcon) Sod. Sulfacetamide
  15% in buffered pH 7.4, 0.5% methylcellulose sol.
  Drop-Tainer 5 cc.
  Use: Conjunctival infections.
ISOPTO CETAPRED. (Alcon) Sulfacetamide sod.
  U.S.P. 10%, prednisolone U.S.P. 0.25%,
  methylcellulose 0.5% in a sterile, buffered and
  stable suspension. Drop-Tainer 5 cc.,
  15 cc.
  Use: Chronic and allergic blepharitis and
  conjunctivitis.
ISOPTO ESERINE. (Alcon) Eserine salicylate 0.25%
  & 0.5% in stable sterile 0.5% methyl cellulose
  solution. Drop-Tainer 15 cc.
  Use: Treatment & control of glaucoma.
ISOPTO FRIN. (Alcon) 0.12% Phenylephrine HCl in a
  methylcellulose sol. Drop-Tainer 15 cc.
  Use: Ocular decongestant.
ISOPTO HOMATROPINE. (Alcon) Homatropine HBr
  2.0% and 5.0% in methylcellulose solution. Drop-
  Tainer 5 cc., 15 cc.
ISOPTO HYOSCINE. (Alcon) Hyoscine HBr 0.25%
  in a methylcellulose solution. Drop-Tainer 5 cc.,
  15 cc.
ISOPTO P-ES. (Alcon) Pilocarpine 2%, eserine salicy-
  late 0.25%, sterile buffered, isotonic vehicle
  containing 0.5% methylcellulose. Plastic Drop-Tainer
  15 cc.
  Use: Glaucoma treatment.
ISOPTO PLAIN. (Alcon) Methylcellulose 0.5% Drop-
  Tainer 15 cc.
  Use: Ophthalmic lubricant and emollient, artificial
  tears.
ISOPTO TEARS. (Alcon) Hydroxypropyl
  methylcellulose 0.5%, benzalkonium chloride
  1:10,000. Bot. Drop-Tainer 15 cc., 30 cc.
  Use: Artificial tears.
ISORDIL CHEWABLE TABLETS. (Ives) Isosorbide
  dinitrate 10 mg./chewable Tab. Bot. 100s.
  Clinipak.
  Use: For angina pectoris.
ISORDIL SUBLINGUAL. (Ives) Isosorbide dinitrate

2.5 mg./Tab. Bot. 100s, 500s. Clinipak; 5 mg./Tab. Bot. 100s, 250s, 500s Clinipak; 10 mg./Tab. Bot. 100s. Clinipak.
Use: Angina pectoris and coronary insufficiency.

ISORDIL TEMBIDS. (Ives) Isosorbide dinitrate 40 mg./Tab. or Cap.
Tab. Bot. 100s, 500s, 1000s. **Cap.** Bot. 100s., 500s.
Use: For Angina pectoris.

ISORDIL TITRADOSE TABLETS. (Ives) Isosorbide dinitrate. 5 mg./Tab. Bot. 100s, 500s, 1000s. Clinipak; 10 mg./Tab. Bot. 100s, 500s, 1000s. Clinipak; 20 mg./Tab. Bot. 100s, 500s. Clinipak; 30 mg./Tab. Bot. 100s.
Use: Control of angina pectoris and coronary insufficiency.

ISORGEN-G. (Grafton) Isosorbide 5 mg., 10 mg./Tab. Bot. 1000s.

ISOSORB-5. (Robinson) Isosorbide dinitrate oral 10 mg./Tab. Bot. 100s, 1000s.
Use: Coronary vasodilator; antianginal.

ISOSORB-10. (Robinson) Isosorbide dinitrate 10 mg./Tab. Bot. 100s, 1000s.
Use: Coronary vasodilator; anti-anginal.

• **ISOSORBIDE.** USAN.
Use: Diuretic.

• **ISOSORBIDE CONCENTRATE,** U.S.P. XXI.
Use: Diuretic.

• **ISOSORBIDE ORAL SOLUTION,** U.S.P. XXI.
Use: Diuretic.

• **ISOSORBIDE DINITRATE, DILUTE,** U.S.P. XXI.
Tab., U.S.P. XXI. D-Glucitol, 1,4:3,6-dianhydro-, dinitrate.
Use: Coronary vasodilator; anti-anginal.
See: Dilatrate-SR, Cap. (Reed & Carnrick)
Iso-Bid, Cap. (Geriatric)
Iso-D, Cap., Tab. (Dunhall)
Isordil, Tab. (Ives)
Isordil Tembids Cap., Tabs. (Ives)
Isosorb Prods. (Robinson)
Onset, Tab. (Bock)
Sorbitrate, Tab. (Stuart)
Sorquad., Tab. (Reid-Provident)
W/Phenobarbital.
See: Isordil w/Phenobarbital, Tab. (Ives)
Sorbitrate w/Phenobarbital, Tab. (Stuart)

• **ISOSTERYL ALCOHOL.** USAN.
Use: Pharmaceutic aid.

• **ISOSULFAN BLUE.** USAN.
Use: Diagnostic aid.

ISOTEIN HN. (Doyle) Vanilla Flavor. Maltodextrin, delactosed lactalbumin, partially hydrogenated soy oil with BHA, fructose, medium chain triglycerides, artificial flavor, sodium caseinate, mono and diglycerides, sodium chloride, vitamins and minerals. Powder 2.9 oz. packets.
Use: Total feeding, oral or tube.

ISOTHIPENDYL. B.A.N. 10-(2-Dimethylamino-propyl)-10H-pyrido[3,2-b]-[1,4]benzothiazine.
Use: Antihistamine.
See: Nilergex
Theruhistin (HCl)

ISOTRATE. (Hauck) Isosorbide dinitrate 40 mg./Timecelle. Bot. 100s, 500s. Unit dose 100s.
Use: Coronary vasodilator.

• **ISOTRETINOIN.** USAN.
Use: Keratolytic.

• **ISOTRETINOIN.** USAN. 13-cis-retinoic acid.
Use: Treatment of severe recalcitrant cystic acne.
See: Accutane, Cap. (Roche)

ISOVEX. (U.S. Chemical) Ethaverine HCl. 100 mg./Cap. Bot. 100s, 1000s.
Use: Smooth muscle relaxant, vasorelaxant.

3-ISOXAZOLIDINONE, 4-AMINO-. Cycloserine, U.S.P. XXI.

• **ISOXEPAC.** USAN.
Use: Anti-inflammatory.

• **ISOXICAM.** USAN.
Use: Anti-inflammatory.

ISOXSUPRINE. B.A.N. 1-(4-Hydroxyphenyl)-2-(1-methyl-2-phenoxyethylamino)propan-1-ol.
Use: Peripheral vasodilator.
See: Dilavase
Duphaspasmin (lactate)
Duvadilan
Vasodilan
Vasotran (HCl)

• **ISOXSUPRINE HCl,** U.S.P. XXI. Inj., Tab., U.S.P. XXI. 1-(p-Hydroxy-phenyl)-2-(1'-methyl-2'-phenoxy ethylamino) propanol-1 HCl. p-Hydroxy-α-[1-[(1-methyl-2-phenoxyethyl)amino ethyl benzyl alcohol HCl.
Use: Vasodilator.
See: Rolisox-10, Tab. (Robinson)
Rolisox-20, Tab. (Robinson)
Vasodilan, Tab., Amp. (Mead Johnson)

ISUPREL. (Winthrop-Breon) Isoproterenol HCl. Available in various dosage forms.

ISUPREL COMPOUND ELIXIR. (Winthrop-Breon) Isoproterenol HCl, 2.5 mg., ephedrine sulfate 12 mg., theophylline 45 mg., phenobarbital 6 mg., potassium iodide 150 mg./15 ml. Bot. pt., gal.
Use: Bronchodilator

ISUPREL GLOSSETS. (Winthrop-Breon) Isoproterenol HCl 10 mg., 15 mg./Tab. Bot. 50s.
Use: Bronchodilator.

ISUPREL INHALATION SOLUTION. (Winthrop-Breon) Isoproterenol HCl inhalation Sol. 1:200 and 1:100. Bot. 10 ml., 60 ml.
Use: Bronchodilator

ISUPREL MISTOMETER. (Winthrop-Breon) Isoproterenol HCl. Complete nebulizing unit of aerosol soln. containing 15 ml. or 22.5 ml. of isoproterenol HCl w/inert propellants, alcohol 33% and ascorbic acid. Measured dose of approximately 131 mcg. Aerosol Unit. Bot. 15 ml., 22.5 ml. Refill 15 ml., 22.5 ml.
Use: Bronchodilator.

ISUPREL STERILE INJECTION. (Winthrop-Breon) Isoproterenol HCl 0.2 mg., lactic acid 0.12 mg., sodium lactate 1.8 mg., sodium chloride 7 mg. and not more than 1 mg. sodium bisulfite as preservative/ml. of 1:5000 sol. **Amp.** 1 ml. Boxes 25s; 5 ml. Boxes 10s.

Use: Adjunct treatment of shock, cardiac standstill, etc.

ISUPRENE.
See: Isoproterenol (Var. Mfr.)

ITCHI-KOOL. (Eckerd) Zirconium oxide 5%, benzocaine, chlorobutanol, pyrilamine maleate, benzethonium Cl, calamine, zinc oxide. Tube 1.5 oz.
Use: Antipruritic, local anesthetic, antihistiminic, antispeptic.

ITCHAWAY. (Moyco) Zinc undecylenate 20%, undecylenic acid 2%. Powder, Cans 1.5 oz.
Use: Antifunal foot powder for athelete's foot.

ITOBARBITAL.
W/Acetaminophen.
See: Panitol, Tab. (Wesley)

ITRAMIN TOSYLATE. B.A.N. 2-Nitratoethylamine toluene-p-sulfonate.
Use: Angina pectoris; Vasodilator.
See: Nilatil

IVADANTIN. (Norwich Eaton) Nitrofurantoin sodium 180 mg./Vial.
Use: Urinary anti-infective for I.V. use only.

• **IVERMECTIN.** USAN. (MSD AGVET) 22,23-Dihydroaver-mectin B-1, (80% or more "a" component, 20% or less "b" component). Ivomec and Eqvalan.
Use: Antiparasitic, veterinary medicine.

IVERSAL HYDRATE. Ambazone, B.A.N.

I.V. ESTRO. (Rocky Mtn.) Potassium estrone sulfate 4 mg./cc. Vial 10 cc. Amp. 5 cc. Box 6s.
Use: I.M. or I.V. functional uterine bleeding.

IVOCORT. (Winston) Micronized hydrocortisone alcohol 5 mg./Gm. Bot. 4 oz.
Use: Dermatoses.

IVOMEC. (MSD AGVET) Ivermectin injectable solution, suspension 200 mg./Kg.
Use: Antiparasitic, veterinary medicine.

IVY-CHEX. (Bowman) Polyvinylpyrrolidone-vinyl acetate & benzylkonium chloride 1:1000 in alcohol acetone base. Aerosol can 4 oz.
Use: Treatment or prevention of Poison Ivy, Poison Oak, Poison Sumac dermatitis.

IVY DRY. (Ivy) Tannic acid 10%, isopropyl alcohol 12.5% Liq. 4 oz., Cream 1 oz. Super 6 oz.
Use: Relief of itching.

IVY-RID. (Mallard) Polyvinylpyrrolidone-vinylacetate, benzalkonium chloride. Spray can 3 oz.
Use: Relief of itching and discomfort of poison ivy, poison oak and poison sumac.

J

JACOBSON'S SOLUTION WITH VIT. A. (CMC) Benzyl alcohol 2%, benzyl cinnamate 1.6%, ethyl cinnamate 0.5% in olive oil w/Vit. A. 10,000 I.U. Amp. 1 cc. Box 12s, 50s.
Use: Resolution of localized inflammation.

JALOVIS.
See: Hyaluronidase (Various Mfr.)

JANIMINE. (Abbott) Imipramine HCl 10 mg., 25 mg., 50 mg./Tab. Bot. 100s, 1000s.
Use: Antidepressant.

JAPAN AGAR.
See: Agar (Various Mfr.)

JAPAN GELATIN.
See: Agar (Various Mfr.)

JAPAN ISINGLASS.
See: Agar (Various Mfr.)

JECTO SAL. (Mallard) Sodium thiosulfate 50 mg./ml. Vial 30 ml.
Use: Analgesic, antipyretic.

JEL DROX LIQUID. (Coastal) Aluminum hydroxide 4%, magnesium hydroxide 1%/5 cc. Bot. 12 oz., 16 oz.
Use: Antacid.

JENAMICIN. (Hauck) Gentamicin sulfate 40 mg./ml. Vial 2 ml.
Use: Antibiotic.

JEN-BALM. (Jenkins) Methyl salicylate 15%, oil of eucalyptus 3%, menthol 2%. Jar, 1 oz., 1 lb.
Use: Analgesic balm for muscular aches, bursitis.

JEN-DIRIL. (Jenkins) Hydrochlorothiazide 50 mg./Tab. Bot. 1000s.
Use: Diuretic.

JENKAPS. (Jenkins) Vit. B-1 1.5 mg., B-2 2 mg., nicotinamide 10 mg., B-6 0.1 mg., cal. pantothenate 1 mg., B-12 1 mcg., liver desiccated 50 mg. dried yeast 100 mg./Cap. Bot. 100s, 1000s.

JEN-LAX. (Jenkins) Bile salts ½ gr., ext. cascara sagrada ½ gr., phenolphthalein yellow ½ gr., aloin ⅛ gr., podophyllin ¹⁄₂₀ gr./Tab. Bot. 1000s.

JENSENEX. (Jenkins) Nicotinic acid 50 mg., salicylamide 0.3 Gm., B-12 activity 3 mcg., C 15 mg./Tab. Bot. 1000s.
Use: Geriatric energizer.

JEN-VITE. (Jenkins) Vit. A 5000 I.U., D 1000 I.U., B-1 2.5 mg., B-2 2.5 mg., nicotinamide 20 mg., B-6 1 mg., cal. pantothenate 5 mg., B-12 2 mcg., C 40 mg., E 2 I.U./Cap. Bot. 100s, 1000s.
Use: Vitamin supplement.

JERI-BATH. (Dermik) Concentrated moisturizing bath oil. Plastic Bot. 8 oz.

JERI-LOTION. (Dermik) Concentrated moisturizing lotion. Plastic Bot. 6 oz.

JETRIUM. Dextromoramide, B.A.N.

JIFFY. (Block) Benzocaine, menthol, eugenol in glycerin-water base with alcohol. Bot. 0.125 oz.
Use: Toothache drops.

J-LIBERTY. (J Pharmacal) Chlordiazepoxide HCl 5, 10, or 25 mg./Cap.
Use: Relief of anxiety & tension.

JOHNSON's MEDICATED POWDER. (Johnson & Johnson) Bentonite, kaolin, talc, zinc oxide. Pow. Sm., Med., Lg.
Use: Diaper rash & prickly heat remedy.

• **JOSAMYCIN.** USAN.
Use: Antibacterial.

JUBALON HYDROCHLORIDE. Carbiphene, B.A.N.

JUNICOID. (Jenkins) Dextromethorphan HBr 5 mg., cocillana comp., 88 mg., pot. guaiacolsulfonate 66 mg., citric acid 22 mg./5 cc. Syr. Bot. 3 oz., 4 oz., gal.

• **JUNIPER TAR,** U.S.P. XXI. Oil of cade.
Use: Local anti-eczematic.

JUNYER-ALL. (Barth's) Vit. A 6000 I.U., D 400 I.U., B-1 3 mg., B-2 6 mg., C 120 mg., niacin 1 mg., E 12 I.U., B-12 10 mcg., Ca 217 mg., P 97.5 mg., red bone marrow 10 mg., organic iron 15 mg., iodine 0.1 mg., beef peptone 20 mg./2 Vit. and mineral caps. Bot. 10 mo., 3 mo., 6 mo. supply.
Use: Vitamin supplement.

JUVOCAINE.
See: Procaine Hydrochloride (Various Mfr.)

K

K-10 SOLUTION. (Cenci) Pot. chloride 10% in a sugar-less nonalcoholic solution (20 mEq/15 cc.) Bot. pt., gal.

K 34. Hexachlorophene.

KABIKINASE. (Kabi) Streptokinase 250,000 or 600,000 I.U./Vial.
Use: Thrombolytic agent.

KABIKINASE. (Pharmacia) Streptokinase 250,000 I.U., 600,000 I.U., 750,000 I.U./Vial. Box 10 × 5 ml.
Use: Lysis of vascular thrombi and emboli.

KAERGONA.
See: Menadione (Various Mfr.)

• **KALAFUNGIN.** USAN.
Use: Antifungal.

KALCINATE. (Kay) Calcium gluconate 1 Gm., calcium D-saccharate 0.004 Gm./10 cc. Amp. 10 cc, 25s, 100s.

KALLIDINOGENASE. B.A.N. An enzyme that splits the kinin, kallidin, from kininogen.
Use: Vasodilator.
See: Glumorin; Depot-Glumorin

KALOL. (Jenkins) Boric acid, sodium biborate, sodium chloride, menthol, thymol, oil of eucalyptus, methyl salicylate (synthetic), carbolic acid/Tab. Bot. 1000s.

KALORY-PLUS. (Tyler) Thyroid 3 gr., amphetamine sulfate 15 mg., atropine sulfate 1/180 gr., aloin ¼ gr., phenobarbital ¼ gr./Timed release cap. Bot. 100s, 1000s.
Use: Anorexient.

KAMABEL. (Towne) Colloidal kaolin 6 Gm., pectin 142.8 mg., hyoscyamine sulfate 0.1037 mg., atropine sulfate 0.0194 mg., hyoscine HBr 0.0065 mg./fl. oz. Bot. 4 oz.
Use: Antidiarrheal.

KAMAGEL. (Towne) Opium 15 mg., colloidal kaolin 6 Gm., pectin 300 mg., milk of bismuth 5 ml./fl. oz. Bot. 4 oz.
Use: Antidiarrheal.

KAMFOLENE. (Wade) Camphor, menthol, methyl salicylate, oils turpentine and eucalyptus, carbolic acid 2%, calamine, zinc oxide in lanolin base. Jar 2 oz., lb.
Use: Antiseptic.

KANALKA TABLETS. (Lannett) Phenobarbital sod. ¼ gr., benzocaine ¼ gr., mag. carbonate 2 gr., calcium carbonate 3 gr./Tab. Bot. 100s, 1000s.
Use: Antacid w/sedative.

KANAMYCIN. B.A.N. An antibiotic produced by *Streptomyces kanamyceticus.*
Use: Antibiotic.
See: Kannasyn; Kantrex (sulfate)

• **KANAMYCIN SULFATE,** U.S.P. XXI. Caps., Inj., Sterile, U.S.P. XXI. D-Streptamine, 0-3-amino-3-deoxy-α-d-glucopyranosyl-(1→6)-0-6-amino-6-deoxy-α-d-gluco-pyranosyl-(1→4)-2-deoxy-, sulfate (1:1). An antibiotic obtained from *Streptomycin kanamyceticus.*
Use: Antibacterial.
See: Kantrex, Cap., Vial (Bristol)
Klebcil, Inj. (Beecham)

KANKEX. (Edward J. Moore) Benzocaine, tannic acid, benzyl alcohol, diisobutyl crosoxy ethoxy ethyl dimethyl benzyl ammonium chloride, in propylene base. Bot. ½ oz. w/applicator.
Use: Toothaches, teething pains, cold sores, fever blisters.

KANTREX. (Bristol) Kanamycin sulf. **Cap.** (0.5 Gm.) Bot. 20s, 100s. **Vial** (0.5 Gm./2 cc.) or (1.0 Gm./3 cc.) **Pediatric Inj.,** 75 mg./2 ml. **Disposable Syr.** 500 mg./2 ml.
Use: Infections from gram-positive and gram-negative bacteria.

KANULASE. (Dorsey) Cellulase (Dorase) standardized to 9 mg., pepsin 150 mg., glutamic acid HCl 200 mg., lipase 1,000 U., amylase 1,000 U., protease 12,000 U. ox bile extract 100 mg./Tab. Bot. 50s.
Use: Digestant.

KAOCASIL. (Jenkins) Kaolin colloidal 60 mg., calcium carbonate 0.1 Gm., magnesium trisilicate 60 mg., bismuth subgallate 15 mg., papain 8 mg., atropine sulphate 1/2000 gr./Tab. Bot. 1000s.
Use: Antacid and adsorbent.

KAOCHLOR 10% LIQUID. (Adria) Potassium and chloride 20 mEq each, 15 cc. alcohol 5%, sugar, saccharin, flavoring, FD&C Yellow No. 5. Bot. 4 oz., pt., gals. Stat-Pak: 15 ml. 100s.
Use: Treatment and prevention of hypokalemia.

KAOCHLOR-EFF. (Adria) Elemental potassium 20 mEq and chloride 20 mEq/Tab. supplied by: potassium chloride 0.6 Gm., potassium citrate 0.22 Gm., potassium bicarbonate 1 Gm., betaine HCl 1.84 Gm., saccharin 20 mg., artificial fruit flavor and color/Tab. Sugar free. Carton 60s, 1000s.
Use: Treatment and prevention of hypokalemia.

KAOCHLOR S-F 10% LIQUID. (Adria) Potassium 20 mEq and chloride 20 mEq/15 ml. w/saccharin, flavoring, alcohol 5%. Sugar free. Unit dose 15 ml. 100s. Bot. 4 oz., pt., gal.
Use: Treatment and prevention of hypokalemia.

• **KAOLIN,** U.S.P. XXI. (Various Mfr.)
Use: Adsorbent for diarrhea.
W/Alumina gel, pectin.
See: Kalpec, Susp. (Wyeth)
W/Aluminum hydroxide, pectin.

See: Kao-pectin, Tab. (Wolins)
  Kenpectin, Susp. & Kenpectin-P, Susp. (Kenwood)
W/Atropine sulfate, phenobarbital.
  See: Alkasans, Tab. (Noyes)
W/Belladonna, phenobarbital.
  See: Bellkata, Tab. (Ferndale)
W/Bismuth compound.
  See: Kaomine, Pow. (Lilly)
W/Bismuth subgallate.
  See: Diastop, Liq. (Elder)
W/Bismuth subgallate, pectin, zinc phenolsulfonate
  opium pow.
  See: Amogel, Tab. (Vortech)
    Diastay, Tab. (Elder)
W/Bismuth subgallate, Zinc phenolsulfonate,
  powdered opium.
  See: B-K-Z Tablets, Chewable, Tab. (Sutliff and Case)
W/Bismuth subsalicylate, salol, methyl salicylate,
  benzocaine, pectin.
W/Calcium carbonate, magnesium trisilicate, bismuth
  subgallate, papain, atropine sulphate.
  See: Kaocasil, Tab. (Jenkins)
W/Cornstarch, camphor, zinc oxide, eucalyptus oil.
  See: Mexsana, Pow. (Plough)
W/Furazolidone, pectin.
  See: Furoxone, Liq. (Eaton)
W/Hyoscyamine sulfate, sod. benzoate, atropine
  sulfate, hyoscine HBR, pectin.
  See: Donnagel, Susp. (Robins)
W/Neomycin sulfate, pectin.
  See: Pecto-Kalin, Liq. (Harvey)
W/Opium pow., bismuth subgallate, pectin, and zinc
  phenolsulfonate.
  See: Bismuth, Pectin & Paregoric (Lemmon)
W/Opium pow., pectin, hyoscyamine sulfate, atropine
  sulfate, hyoscine HBr, alcohol.
  See: Donnagel P.G., Susp. (Robins)
W/Paregoric, aluminum hydroxide, bismuth
  subcarbonate, pectin.
  See: Kapinal, Tab. (Jenkins)
W/Pectin.
  See: Baropectin, Susp. (Barry-Martin)
    Kaopectate, Liq. (Upjohn)
    Kapectin, Liq. (Approved)
    Keotin, Liq. (Blue Line)
    Pecto-Kalin, Susp. (Lemmon)
    Pectokay Mixture (Bowman)
W/Pectin, belladonna alkaloids.
  See: Kapectolin, Liq. (GMC)
W/Pectin, bismuth subcarbonate.
  See: B-K-P Mixture, Liq. (Sutliff & Case)
W/Pectin, bismuth subcarbonate, belladonna.
  See: Kay-Pec, Liq. (Case)
W/Pectin, bismuth subcarbonate, opium pow.
  See: KBP/O, Cap. (Cole)
W/Pectin, bismuth subsalicylate.
W/Pectin, bismuth subsalicylate, paregoric, zinc
  sulfocarbolate.
W/Pectin, hyoscyamine sulfate, atropine sulfate,
  hyoscine HBr.
  See: Kapigam, Liq. (Reid-Provident)
    Palsorb Improved, Liq. (Hauck)

W/Pectin, pow. opium ext.
  See: Keoparic, Susp. (Blue Line)
    Pecto-Kalin, Susp. (Lemmon)
W/Pectin, opium powd., bismuth subgallate, zinc
  phenolsulfonate.
  See: Cholactabs, Tab. (Philips Roxane)
    B.P.P., Tab. (Lemmon)
W/Pectin, paregoric (equivalent)
  See: Duosorb, Liq. (Reid-Provident)
    Kaoparin, Liq. (McKesson)
    Kapectin, Liq. (Approved)
    Ka-Pek w/Paregoric, Liq. (APC)
    Parepectolin, Susp. (Rorer)
W/Pectin, zinc phenolsulfonate.
  See: Pectocel, Susp. (Lilly)
    Pectocomp, Liq. (Lannett)
W/Phenobarbital, atropine sulfate, aluminum
  hydroxide gel.
  See: Kao-Lumin, Tab. (Philips Roxane)
W/Salol, zinc sulfocarbolate, aluminum hydroxide,
  bismuth subsalicylate, pectin.
  See: Wescola Antidiarrheal-Stomach Upset (Western
  Research)
KAODONNA PG SUSPENSION. (Vangard) Kaolin 6
  Gm., pectin 142.8 mg., hyoscyamine sulfate 0.0137
  mg., atropine sulfate 0.0194 mg., hyoscine HBr
  0.0065 mg., sodium benzoate 60 mg., powdered
  opium 24 mg./30 ml. w/alcohol 5%. Bot. pt., gal.
  Use: Antidiarrheal.
KAODONNA SUSPENSION. (Vangard) Kaolin 6 Gm.,
  pectin 142.8 mg., hyoscyamine sulfate 0.0137 mg.,
  atropine sulfate 0.0194 mg., hyoscine HBr 0.0065
  mg., sodium benzoate 60 mg./30 ml. w/alcohol
  3.8%. Bot. pt., gal.
  Use: Antidiarrheal.
KAOLIN COLLOIDAL.
W/Bismuth subcarbonate.
  See: Bisilad, Susp. (Central)
W/Magnesium trisilicate, aluminum hydroxide dried
  gel.
  See: Kamadrox, Tab. (Elder)
    Kathmagel, Tab. (Mason)
W/Opium, pectin, milk of bismuth.
  See: Kamagel Liq. (Towne)
W/Paregoric, pectin, milk of bismuth, methyl para-
  hydroxybenzoate, alcohol.
  See: Mul-Sed, Susp. (Webcon)
W/Pectin, aromatics.
  See: Paocin, Susp. (Beecham-Massengill)
W/Pectin, belladonna alkaloids.
  See: Kamabel Liq. (Towne)
W/Phenobarbital, homatropine methylbromide.
  See: Lanokalin, Tab. (Lannett)
KAON CL CONTROLLED RELEASE TABLETS.
  (Adria) Potassium chloride 500 mg./Tab. w/FDD&C
  Yellow No. 5. Bot. 100s, 250s, 1000s. Stat-Pak
  100s.
  Use: Potassium supplement.
KAON CL-10 CONTROLLED RELEASE TABLETS.
  (Adria) Potassium Cl 750 mg./Tab. Bot. 100s, 500s,
  Stat-Pak 100s.
  Use: Potassium supplement.

KAON CL 20%. (Adria) Potassium and chloride 40 mEq. to potassium chloride 3 Gm., saccharin and flavoring. 15 ml. alcohol 5%. Bot. 4 oz., pt., gal.
Use: Treatment and prevention of hypokalemia.

KAON ELIXIR. (Adria) 20 mEq. elemental pot. (as 4.68 Gm. pot. gluconate)/15 cc. w/aromatics, saccharin, grape and lemon-lime flavors, alcohol 5%. Unit pkg. 4 oz., pt., gal. Stat-Pak 15 ml. 100s.
Use: Treatment and prevention of hypokalemia.

KAON TABLETS. (Adria) 5mEq. elemental potassium obtained from 1.17 Gm. potassium gluconate/S.C. Tab. Bot. 100s & 500s. Stat-Pak 100s. (10 × 10).
Use: Treatment and prevention of hypokalemia.

KAO-NOR ELIXIR. (Vortech) Elemental potassium 20 mEq. as pot. gluconate 4.68 Gm./15 ml. w/saccharin, alcohol 5%. Bot. 4 oz., gal.
Use: Potassium deficiency.

KAOPECTATE. (Upjohn) Kaolin 90 gr., pectin 2 gr./oz. Bot. 8 oz., 12 oz., 1 gal. Unit dose pkg. 3 oz. Bilingual. Bot. 8 oz., 12 oz.
Use: Orally for symptomatic relief of diarrhea.

KAOPECTATE CONCENTRATE. (Upjohn) Kaolin 135 gr., pectin 3 gr./oz. Unit-dose 3 oz., Bot. 8 oz., 12 oz.
Use: Orally for symptomatic relief of diarrhea.

KAO-PECTIN. (Wolins) Aluminum hydroxide 1 gr., kaolin 2 gr., pectin ½ gr., aromatics/Tab. Bot. 1000s.

KAOPEN SUSPENSION. (Wayne) Bot. pt.

KAPECTIN. (Approved) Kaolin 90 gr., pectin 2 gr./Oz. Bot. gal.
W/Paregoric Liq. 4 oz.
Use: Diarrhea.

KAPECTOLIN P.G. (Century) Powdered opium 24 mg., kaolin 6 mg., pectin 142.8 mg., hyoscyamine sulfate 0.1037 mg., atropine sulfate 0.0194 mg., hyoscine hydrobromide 0.0065 mg., sodium benzoate preservative 65 mg. Bot. gal.
Use: Antidiarrheal.

KAPECTOLIN. (CMC) Kaolin 90 gr., pectin 2 gr./fl. oz. Bot. 4 oz., 8 oz., pt., gal.
Use: Antidiarrheal.
W/Belladonna. Kaolin 6000 mg., pectin 142.8 mg., hyoscyamine sulfate 0.1037 mg., atropine sulfate 0.194 mg., hyoscine HBr 0.0065 mg./fl. oz. Bot. 4 oz., pt., gal.
W/Paregoric 6%. Bot. 4 oz., pt., gal.

KA-PEK. (A.P.C.) Kaolin 90 gr., pectin 4½ gr./Fl. Oz. Bot. 6 oz., gal.
Use: Control of diarrhea.

KA-PEK WITH PAREGORIC. (APC) Paregoric 60 min., kaolin 90 gr., pectin 4½ gr./Fl. Oz. Bot. 4 oz.
Use: Control of diarrhea.

KAPILIN.
See: Menadione (Various Mfr.)

KAPINAL. (Jenkins) Paregoric 0.6 ml., (Pow. opium 0.0375 gr.), kaolin colloidal 0.3 Gm., aluminum hydroxide 0.12 Gm., bismuth subcarbonate 60 mg., pectin 60 mg., aromatics/Tab. Bot. 1000s.
Use: Antacid and adsorbent.

KARAYA GUM. (Penick) Indian Gum. Sterculia gum,
See: Tri-Costivin (Prof. Lab.)
W/Frangula
See: Saraka, Gran. (Plough)

W/Psyllium seed, plantago ovata, brewers yeast.
See: Plantamucin Granules (Elder)
W/Cortex rhamni frangulae.
See: Movicol (Norgine)
W/Refined psyllium mucilloid.
See: Hydrocil regular (Rowell)

KAREON.
See: Menadione (Various Mfr.)

KARIDIUM. (Lorvic) **Tab.:** Sodium fluoride 2.21 mg., sod. chloride 94.49 mg., disintegrant 0.5 mg./Tab. Bot. 180s, 1000s. **Liq.** Sodium fluoride 2.21 mg., sod. chloride 10 mg., purified water q.s./8 drops. Bot. 30 ml., 60 ml.
Use: Reduction of dental caries.

KARIGEL. (Lorvic) Fluoride ion 0.5%, 0.1 molar phosphate. Gel. Bot. 30 ml., 130 ml., 250 ml.
Use: Reduction of dental caries.

• **KASAL.** USAN. Approximately $Na_8AP_2(OH_2(PO_4)_4$ with about 30% of dibasic sodium phosphate; sodium aluminum phosphate, basic.
Use: Food additive.

KASDENOL. (Edward J. Moore) Clorpactin WCS-60. Jar 10 Gm.
Use: Germicidal mouthwash for relief of bleeding gums.

KASOF. (Stuart) Docusate potassium 240 mg./Cap. Bot. 30s, 60s.
Use: General constipation, anorectal disorders, stool softener.

KASUGAMYCIN. Under study.
Use: Antibiotic.

KA-THAL-PEC. (O'Neal, Jones & Feldman) Opium 7 mg., pectin 80 mg., kaolin 2,500 mg./15 ml. Bot. 8 oz.
Use: Antidiarrheal.

KAVACAPS. (Blue Line) Hyoscyamus ext. ⅛ gr., copaiba mass, methylene blue, and ext. kava kava/Tab. Bot. 100s, 1000s.

KAVITON.
See: Menadione, U.S.P. XXI. (Var. Mfr.)

KAYBOVITE "1000." (Kay) Cyanocobalamine 1000 mcg./cc. Vial 30 cc.
Use: Vitamin B-12 supplement.

KAY CIEL ELIXIR. (Berlex) Potassium chloride 1.5 Gm/15 ml. (20 mEq./15 ml.) w/alcohol 4%. Bot. 118 ml., 473 ml,, 3785 ml.
Use: Potassium replacement.

KAY CIEL POWDER. (Berlex) Potassium chloride. 1.5 Gm./Packette. (20 mEq./Packet). Box 30s, 100s, 500s.
Use: Potassium replacement.

KAYEXALATE. (Winthrop-Breon) Sod. polystyrene sulfonate. Jar 1 lb.
Use: Hyperkalemia.

KAYPECTOL. (Kay) Kaolin 90 gr., pectin 2 gr./1 oz. Bot. Pts., Gal.
Use: Antidiarrheal.

KAY POTE 10% Solution. (Vitarine) Potassium Cl. 40 mEq./30 ml. Cherry flavor.
Use: Treatment of potassium deficiency or potassium depletion.

KAY-POTE SOLUTION. (Vitarine) Pot. chloride 0.5 Gm.,

supplying 5 mEq. elemental potassium/5 cc. Bot. 5
oz., pt., gal.

Use: Treatment of potassium deficiency.

KAY POTE SUGAR FREE. (Vitarine) Potassium Cl 30
mEq./30 ml. Citrus flavor.

Use: Treatment of potassium deficiency or
depletion.

KAYTRATE. (Kay) Pentaerythritol tetranitrate. Tab.
(20 mg.) green. Bot. 100s, 1000s. Kaykaps (30
mg.) purple & yellow. Bot. 100s, 1000s.

KAYTRON. (Pasadena Research) Pot. estrone
sulfate, aqueous 20 mg./2 cc. Vial 20 cc., Amp. 2
cc. 25s, 100s.

KAY-VI-C. (Kay) Vit. C 300 mg., niacinamide 100 mg., B-
1 20 mg., B-2 10 mg., pyridoxine HCl 5 mg., D-calcium
pantothenate 20 mg., magnesium sulfate 70 mg.,
zinc sulfate 80 mg./Cap. Bot. 100s, 1000s.

Use: Vitamin supplement.

K-B-PLEX. (Kay) Water-soluble or oil soluble fractions
of B-complex. Vial 10 ml., 30 ml.

Use: Vitamin supplement.

KBP/O. (O'Neal, Jones & Feldman) Kaolin 350 mg.,
pectin 60 mg., pow. opium 3 mg., bismuth
subcarbonate 60 mg./Cap. Bot. 100s, 1000s.

Use: Diarrhea remedy.

K-C LIQUID. (Century) Kaolin 5.2 Gm., pectin 260 mg.,
bismuth subcarbonate 260 mg./oz. Bot. 4 oz., pt.,
gal.

KC-20 ELIXIR. (Scruggs) Bot. pt., gal.

KCL-20. (Western Research) Potassium chloride 1.5
Gm. (20 mEq. potassium, 20 mEq. chloride)/
Packet. Box 30s.

Use: Supplement.

K-CLORE-Y. (Kay) Potassium 20 mEq provided by potassium chloride 1.5 Gm./15 ml. w/sugar &
flavoring. Bot. Pts., Gal.

Use: Potassium supplement.

K.D.C. VAGINAL CREAM. (Kenyon) Sulfanilamide
15%, 9-aminoacridine HCl 0.2%, allantoin 2% in a
dispersible base containing stearic acid, diglycol,
stearate, triethanolamine, propylene glycol, lactic
acid, water.

KE.

See: Cortisone Acetate (Various Mfr.)

KEDRIN TABLET. (Dolcin) Analgesic compound. Bot.
100s.

Use: Analgesic without aspirin.

KEELAMIN. (Mericon) Zinc 20 mg., manganese 5
mg., copper 3 mg./Tab. Bot. 100s.

Use: Dietary supplement.

KEEP-A-WAKE. (Stayner) Vit. B-1 5 mg., B-2 2 mg.,
B-12 activity (cobalamin conc., 1.5 mcg.),
niacinamide 10 mg., caffeine citrate 2½ gr./Tab.
Bot. 24s.

Use: Ward off drowsiness & fatigue.

KEFERON. (Kay) Ferric hydroxide, dextran 0.9%
sodium Cl. Vial 2 ml., 5 ml. Amp.

Use: Iron supplement.

KEFGLYCIN. Cephaloglycin, B.A.N.

KEFLEX. (Dista) Cephalexin. **Pulvule** 250 mg., 500
mg. Bot. 20s, 100s. Blister pkg. 10 × 10s; **Tab.:** 1
Gm. Bot. 24s. Blister pkg. 100s. **For Susp.** 125

mg./5 ml. Bot. 60 ml., 100 ml., 200 ml. Unit dose 5
ml. × 100s; 250 mg./5 ml. Bot. 100 ml., 200 ml.
Unit dose 5 ml. × 100s.

Use: Antibiotic.

KEFLEX FOR PEDIATRIC DROPS. (Dista)
Cephalexin. 100 mg./ml. Dropper Bot. 10 ml.

KEFLIN, NEUTRAL. (Lilly) Cephalothin/sodium 1
Gm./10 ml., Vial 1s, 25s; 1 Gm./100 ml. Vial 10s; 2
Gm./20 ml. Vial 10s; 2 Gm./100 ml., Vial 10s; 4
Gm./50 ml., Vial 10s; 20 Gm./200 ml. Vial 6s.
Faspak 1 Gm. or 2 Gm. Vial 96s.

Use: Broad-spectrum bactericidal antibiotic.

KEFZOL. (Lilly) Cefazolin sodium. 250 mg./10 ml.,
Vial 1s; 500 mg./10 ml., Vial 1s, 25s; 500 mg./100
ml. Vial 10s; 1 Gm./10 ml., Vial 1s, 25s; 1 Gm./100
ml., Vial 10s; 10 Gm./100 ml., Vial 6s; Redi Vial
500 mg. 1s, 10s; Redi Vial 1 Gm. 1s, 10s; Faspak
500 mg. or 1 Gm./Vial. Box 96s.

Use: Antibiotic.

KELEX. (Nutrition) Iron choline citrate 360 mg.
providing approx. 40 mg. of elemental iron/Tabseal.
Bot. 90s.

Use: Anemia.

KELGIN. Algin.

KELL E. (Canright) di-α Tocopheryl 100 I.U. Bot. 100s,
200 I.U. Bot. 100s, 400 I.U. Bot. 100s.

KELLOGG'S TASTELESS CASTOR OIL. (Beecham
Products) Castor oil 100%. Bot. 2 oz.

Use: Laxative.

KELOCAINE. (Key) Lidocaine 1% or 2%. Vial 50 cc.

KELP. (Arcum) Tab. Bot. 100s, 1000s.

KELP. (Stanlabs) Tab. Bot. 100s.

KELP TABLETS. (Kirkman) Bot. 125s.

KELP TABLETS. (Columbia) Iodine 0.15 mg. Bot.
250s, 500s.

KELP TABLETS. (Faraday) Iodine from kelp 0.15
mg./Tab. Bot. 100s.

KELP-B-THIN. (Columbia) Vit. B-6 21 mg., soya lecithin
600 mg., iodine 225 mcg., dry cider vinegar 240
mg./6 Tabs or 6 Caps. Bot. 100s, 250s.

Use: Dietary supplement.

KELP PLUS. (Barth's) Iodine from kelp plus 16 trace
minerals/Tab. Bot. 100s, 500s, 1000s.

KELP (WITH IRON) TABLETS. (Eckerd) Bot. 250s.

KEMADRIN. (Burroughs Wellcome) Procyclidine HCl
5 mg./Tab. Bot. 100s.

Use: Parkinsonism.

KEMICETINE. Chloramphenicol, B.A.N.

KEMITHAL. Thialbarbital. 5-Allyl-5-cyclohex-2-enyl-2-
thiobarbituric acid.

KENACORT (Squibb) Triamcinolone 4 mg./Tab. Bot.
100s. 8 mg. Tab. Bot. 50s. Unimatic 100s.

Use: Oral corticosteroid.

KENACORT DIACETATE. (Squibb) Triamcinolone
diacetate equiv. to 4 mg., triamcinolone; buffered
with sodium citrate and sodium phosphate/5 cc.
Bot. 120 cc.

Use: Oral corticosteroid.

KENAHIST-S.A. (Kenyon) Phenylpropanolamine HCl 50
mg., pheniramine maleate 25 mg., pyrilamine
maleate 25 mg./Tab. Bot. 100s, 1000s.

Use: Cough and colds.

KENAKION. (Harriett Lane Home of Johns Hopkins Hospital) Vit. K-1 oxide.
Use: Vit. K-induced kernicterus.

KENALOG. (Squibb) Triamcinolone acetonide **0.1% Cream** Tubes 5 Gm., 15 Gm., 60 Gm., 80 Gm. Jar 240 Gm., 5.25 lb. in aqueous lotion base w/propylene glycol, cetyl and stearyl alcohols, glyceryl monostearate, sorbitan monopalmitate, polyoxyethylene sorbitan monolaurate, methylparaben, propylparaben, polyethylene glycol monostearate, simethicone and sorbic acid. **0.5% Cream** Tube 20 Gm, Lot. sq. bot. 15 cc., 60 cc. Oint. (w/base of polyethylene, mineral oil) Tube, 5 Gm., 15 Gm., 60 Gm., 80 Gm. Jar 240 Gm. 0.5% Tube 20 Gm., **Spray** (6.6 mg./100 Gm.) (50 Gm. or 150 Gm.)

KENALOG 0.025%. (Squibb) **Cream:** Tube, 15 Gm., 80 Gm. Jar, 240 Gm., 5.25 lb. **Lotion:** in aqueous lotion base w/propylene glycol, cetyl and stearyl alcohols, glyceryl monostearate, sorbitan monopalmitate, polyoxyethylene sorbitan monolaurate, methylparaben, propylparaben, polyethylene glycol monostearate, simethicone and sorbic acid, tinted in an isopropyl palmitate vehicle with alcohol (4.7%) Bot. 60 ml. **Spray:** w/ propellants (trichloromonofluoromethane and dichlorofluoromethane). Cans 23 GM., 63 Gm. **Ointment:** plastibase (w/base of polyethylene and mineral oil gel) 15, 80 & 240 Gm.
Use: Topical corticosteroid.

KENALOG H. (Squibb) Triamcinolone acetonide cream USP 0.1%. Each Gm. of cream provides 1.0 mg. of triamcinolone acetonide in a specially formulated hydrophilic vanishing cream base containing propylene glycol, dimethicone 350, castor oil, cetearyl alcohol and ceteareth-20, propylene glycol stearate, white petrolatum, purified water. Tube 15 Gm., 60 Gm.
Use: Topical corticorsteroid.

KENALOG-10 INJECTION. (Squibb) Sterile triamcinolone acetonide suspension 10 mg./cc., w/sod. chloride for isotonicity, 0.9% (w/v) benzyl alcohol as a preservative, 0.75% sod. carboxymethylcellulose, and 0.04% polysorbate 80. Sod. hydroxide or HCl acid may be present to adjust pH to 5.0 to 7.5. At the time of manufacture the air in the container is replaced by nitrogen. Vial 5 cc. Unimatic syringe 1 cc. Cartridge-needle units 1 ml.
Use: Anti-inflammatory, corticosteroid.

KENALOG-40 INJECTION. (Squibb). Sterile triamcinolone acetonide suspension 40 mg./cc., w/sod. chloride for isotonicity, 0.9% (w/v) benzyl alcohol as a preservative, 0.75% sod. carboxymethylcellulose, and 0.04% polysorbate 80. Sod. hydroxide or HCl acid may be present to adjust pH to 5.0 to 7.5. At the time of manufacture the air in the container is replaced by nitrogen. Vial 1 cc., 5 cc., 10 cc.
Use: Anti-inflammatory, corticosteroid.

KENALOG IN ORABASE. (Squibb) Triamcinolone acetonide 0.1% in Orabase. 1 mg. triamcinolone acetonide per gram. Tube 5 Gm.
Use: Dental paste.

KENAZIDE-E. (Kenyon) Hydrochlorothiazide 50 mg./Tab. Bot. 100s, 1000s.
Use: Anti-hypertensive.

KENAZIDE-H. (Kenyon) Hydrochlorothiazide 50 mg./Tab. Bot. 100s, 1000s.
Use: Anti hypertensive.

KENCORT. (Kenyon) Hydrocortisone 1%, clioquinol 3% in bland, water washable base. Jar. 1 lb.

KENDALL'S "COMPOUND B."
See: Corticosterone (Various Mfr.)

KENDALL'S "COMPOUND E."
See: Cortisone Acetate (Var. Mfr.)

KENDALL'S "COMPOUND F."
See: 17-Hydroxycorticosterone (Various Mfr.)

KENDALL'S "DESOXY COMPOUND B."
See: Desoxycorticosterone Acetate (Var. Mfr.)

KENISONE DROPS. (Kenyon) Neomycin sulfate 6 mg., hydrocortisone 5 mg., parachlorometaxylenol 0.05%, pramoxine HCl 1%, alcohol 4.8%/cc. Bot. 15 cc.
Use: Ear infections.

KENPECTIN-P SUSPENSION. (Kenwood) Paregoric 1 dram, purified kaolin 90 gr., aluminum hydroxide 10 gr., pectin 3 gr./fl. oz. w/alcohol 6%. Bot. 4 oz.
Use: Treatment of diarrhea.

KENTONIC. (Kenyon) Vit. A 25,000 I.U., D 1000 I.U., B-1 10 mg., B-2 10 mg., B-6 5 mg., B-12 5 mg., C 200 mg., niacinamide 100 mg., Ca pantothenate 20 mg./Cap. Bot. 1000s.
Use: Multivitamin.

KEN-TUSS. (Kenyon) Dextromethorphan HBr 10 mg., phenylephrine HCl 5 mg., chlorpheniramine maleate 2 mg., salicylamide 227 mg., phenacetin 100 mg., caffeine alkaloid 10 mg., ascorbic acid 20 mg./Tab. Bot. 100s, 1000s.
Use: Cough and colds.

KEOPARIC SUSPENSION. (Blue Line) Pow. opium ext. 0.514 gr., kaolin 80 gr., pectin 6 gr., alcohol 1%/fl. oz. Bot. 4 fl. oz., 14 fl. oz.
Use: Diarrhea.

KEOTIN. (Blue Line) Kaolin 80 gr., pectin 8 gr./oz. Bot. 4 oz., 14 oz., 1 gal.
Use: Orally, intestinal disturbances.

KERALYT GEL. (Westwood) Salicylic acid 6% in a gel base of propylene glycol w/alcohol 19.4%, hydroxypropyl cellulose, water. Tube 1 oz.
Use: Dermatologic: Removal of excessive keratin and adjunctive therapy for fungal infections; Podiatric: Removal of excessive keratin on dorsal and planter hyperkeratotic lesions.

KERASOL. (Upsher-Smith) Therapeutic bath oil. Bot. 8 oz.

KERI CREME. (Westwood) Cream containing water, mineral oil, talc, sorbitol, ceresin, lanolin alcohol, magnesium stearate, glyceryl oleate/propylene glycol, isopropyl myristate, methylparaben, propylparaben, fragrance, quaternium-15. Tube 2.25 oz.
Use: Moisturizer, emollient.

KERID EAR DROPS. (Blair) Urea and glycerin in propylene glycol. Bot. w/dropper 8 ml.
Use: Ear wax remover.

KERI FACIAL CLEANSER. (Westwood) Water, glycerin, squalane, propylene glycol, glyceryl stearate, PEG-100 stearate, stearic acid, steareth-20, lanolin alcohol, magnesium aluminium silicate, cetyl alcohol, beeswax, PEG-20 sorbitan, beeswax, methylparaben, propylparaben, quaternium-15, fragrance. Bot. 4 oz.
Use: Soapless facial cleanser.

KERI FACIAL SOAP. (Westwood) Bar consisting of Na tallowate, Na cocoate, water, mineral oil, octyl hydroxystearate, fragrance, glycerin, titanium dioxide, PEG-75, lanolin oil, docusate Na, PEG-4 dilaurate, propylparaben, PEG-40 stearate, glyceryl monostearate, PEG-100 stearate, NaCl, BHT. EDTA. Bar 3.25 oz.
Use: Gentle facial skin cleanser.

KERI LIGHT LOTION. (Westwood) Water, stearyl alcohol, ceteareath-20, cetearyl octaneoate, glycerin, stearyl heptanoate, stearyl alcohol, Carbomer 934, sodium hydroxide, squalane, methylparaben, propylparaben, and fragrance. Bot. 6½ oz. 13 oz.
Use: Moisturizer.

KERI LOTION. (Westwood) Mineral oil, lanolin oil, water, propylene glycol, glyceryl stearate PEG-100 stearate, PEG 40 stearate, PEG-4 dilaurate, laureth-4, parabens, docusate sodium, triethanolamine, quaternium 15. Carbomer 934 and fragrance. Bot. 6½ oz., 13 oz., 20oz.
Use: Skin lubricant, moisturizer.

KEROCAINE.
See: Procaine Hydrochloride (Various Mfr.)

KERODEX. (Ayerst)
No. 51: Water-miscible, Tube 4 oz., Jar 1 lb.
No. 71: Water-repellent, Tube 4 oz., Jar 1 lb.
Use: Skin protective.

KEROHYDRIC. A de-waxed, oil-soluble fraction of lanolin.
Use: Emollient, cleanser.
See: Alpha-Keri, Soap, Spray (Westwood)
Keri, Cream, Lot., (Westwood)
W/Docusate sodium, sod. alkyl polyether sulfonate, sod. sulfoacetate, sulfur, salicylic acid, hexachlorophene.
See: Sebulex, Cream, Liq. (Westwood)

KERR INSTA-CHAR. (Kerr) **Adult:** Aqueous suspension activated charcoal 50 gm./250 ml. **Pediatric:** Aqueous suspension activated charcoal 15 Gm./120 ml. pediatric.
Use: Toxic substance antidote.

KERR TRIPLE DYE. (Kerr) Gentian violet, proflavine hemisulfate, brilliant green in water. Dispensing Bot. 15 ml.
Use: Umbilical area antiseptic.

KESSADROX. (McKesson) Magnesium-aluminum hydroxide gel. bot. 12 oz.
Use: Antacid.

KESSOTAPP ELIXIR. (McKesson) Brompheniramine maleate, phenylephrine HCl, phenylpropanolamine HCl/5 ml. Bot. pt., gal.

Use: Decongestant.

KESSO-TETRA. (McKesson) Tetracycline HCl 250 mg. or 500 mg./Cap. Bot. 100s, 1000s, 5000s.
Use: Antibiotic.

KESTOLATE. (Key) Sod. thiosalicylate. Vial 50 cc.

KESTRIN. (Hyrex) Estrogens 20,000 u. (2 mg.) in oil or aqueous/cc. Vial 10 cc., 30 cc. I.V. 4 mg./5 cc. Vial 5 cc.
Use: Estrogen therapy.

KESTRONE AQUEOUS. (Hyrex) 5 mg./cc. Vial 10 cc.
Use: Estrogen therapy.

KETAJECT. (Bristol) Ketamine HCl w/Benzethonium chloride 0.1 mg./ml., **10 mg./ml.** Vial 50 ml.; **50 mg./ml.** Vial 10 ml; **100 mg./ml.** Vial 5 ml.
Use: Anesthetic.

KETALAR. (Parke-Davis) Ketamine HCl with sod. chloride, benzethonium chloride 0.1 mg./ml. as preservative. 10 mg./ml. Vial. 20 ml. Pkg. 10s. 50 mg./ml. Vial 50 ml. Pkg. 10s; 100 mg./ml. Vial 5 ml. Pkg. 10s.
Use: Rapid acting general anesthetic.

• **KETAMINE HCl,** U.S.P. XXI. Inj., U.S.P. XXI. (+)-2-(o-Chlorophenyl)-2-(methylamino) cyclohexanone HCl.
Use: Anesthetic.
See: Ketaject, Vial (Bristol)
Ketalar, Inj. (Parke-Davis)

• **KETANSERIN.** USAN.
Use: Serotonin antagonist.

• **KETAZOCINE.** USAN.
Use: Analgesic.

• **KETAZOLAM.** USAN.
Use: Tranquilizer.

• **KETHOXAL.** USAN.
Use: Antiviral.

• **KETIPRAMINE FUMARATE.** USAN. 5-[3-Diethylamino)propyl]-5,11-dihydro-10H-dibenz[b, f]-azepin-10-one fumarate (1:1).
Use: Antidepressant.

KETOBEMIDONE. B.A.N. 4-(3-Hydroxyphenyl)-1-methyl-4-propionylpiperidine. Cliradon.
Use: Narcotic analgesic.

KETOCHOLANIC ACID. 90% oxidized cholic acid of natural bile acids.
See: Dehydrocholic acid (Various Mfr.)

• **KETOCONAZOLE.** USAN.
Use: Antifungal.

• **KETOCONAZOLE,** U.S.P. XXI. 1-acetyl-4 (4-((2-2(2,4 dichlorophenyl)-2-(1-H-imidazol-1-yimethyl)-1,3-dioxolan-4-yl)methoxy) phenyl) piperazine.
Use: Broad spectrum antifungal.
See: Nizoral, Tab. (Janssen)

KETODESTRIN.
See: Estrone (Various Mfr.)

KETO-DIASTIX. (Ames) Dip and read reagent strip test for glucose and ketones in urine. Two test areas: glucose levels from 30 mg. to 5000 mg/dL; Ketone test (acetoacetic acid) negative 5, 40, 80, 160 mg./dL. Bot 100s. Bot. 50, 100 strips.
Use: Diagnostic and monitoring diabetic patients.

• **KETORFANOL.** USAN.
Use: Analgesic.

KETOHEXAZINE. 4, 6-Diethyl-3(2H)-pyridazinono (Lederle).
Use: Hypnotic.

KETOHYDROXYESTRATRIENE.
See: Estrone

KETOHYDROXYESTRIN.
See: Estrone (Var. Mfr.)

KETOLAN. (Galen) Mixed oxidized bile acids 180 mg., desoxycholic acid 60 mg., homatropine methylbromide 2 mg./Tab. Bot. 100s, 1000s.
Use: Hydrocholeretic, choleretic, fat emulsifier.

• **KETOPROFEN.** USAN.
Use: Anti-inflammatory.

KETOSTIX. (Ames) Sod. nitroprusside, sod. phosphate, glycine. Stick test for ketones in urine (measures acetoacetic acid) Bot. 50s, 100s.
Use: Urine-ketone estimation.

• **KETOTIFEN FUMARATE.** USAN.
Use: Anti-asthmatic.

KEY-PLEX INJECTABLE. (Hyrex) Thiamine 100 mg., Riboflavin 2 mg., pyridoxine 2 mg., panthenol 2 mg., niacinamide 100 mg./ml. Vial 30 ml.
Use: Vitamin deficiency.

KEY-PRED. (Hyrex) Prednisolone. Parenteral, 25 mg./cc., Vial 10 cc., 30 cc.; 50 mg./cc., Vial 10 cc.; 100 mg./cc., Vial 10 cc.
Use: Steroid therapy.

KEY-PRED-SP. (Hyrex) Prednisolone sodium phosphate 20 mg./ml.
Use: Steroid therapy.

K-FLEX. (Kay) Orphenadrine citrate 30 mg./ml. Vial 10 ml.
Use: Treatment of Parkinson's syndrome.

K-FORTE. (O'Connor) Potassium 39 mg. (from potassium gluconate, potassium citrate and potassium chloride), Vit. C 10 mg./Tab. Bot. 90s.
Use: Potassium supplement.

K-FORTE MAXIMUM STRENGTH. (O'Connor) Potassium 99 mg., Vit. C 25 mg./Tab. Bot. 60s.
Use: Potassium supplement.

KHAROPHEN.
See: Acetarsone (Var. Mfr.)

KHELLIN. 5,8-dimethoxy-2-methyl-4′,5′-furano-6,7-chromone.
Use: Coronary vasodilator.

KIDDIE POWDER. (Gordon) Pure fine Italian talc. Can 3.5 oz.
Use: Foot powder.

KIDDIES SIALCO. (Foy) Chlorpheniramine maleate 2 mg., phenylephrine HCl 2.5 mg., acetaminophen 62.5 mg., salicylamide 75 mg./Tab. Bot. 1000s.
Use: Analgesic, antihistaminic.

KIDDI-VITES, Improved. (Geneva) Vit. A 5000 I.U., D 500 I.U., B-1 1 mg., B-2 1.5 mg., B-12 2 mcg., C 50 mg., B-6 1 mg., pantothenate 2 mg., niacinamide 10 mg./Tab. Bot. 100s, 1000s.
Use: Multivitamin.

KIDETT. (Kay) Vit. A 5000 I.U. D 400 I.U., B-1 1.5 mg., B-2 1.5 mg., C 37.5 mg., Niacinamide 20 mg., B-6 0.1 mg., Ca pantothenate 1 mg., B-12 1.0 mcg., E 1 I.U., /Cap. Bot. 100s, 1000s.
Use: Vitamin supplement.

■ **KIDNEY FUNCTION AGENTS.**
See: Hippuran, Pow. (Mallinckrodt)
Indigo Carmine Sol. (Var. Mfr.)
Inulin, Amp. (Arnar-Stone)
Iodohippurate, Sod.
Mannitol Sol., Amp. (Merck Sharp & Dohme)
Methylene Blue (Various Mfr.)
Phenolsulfonphthalein (Various Mfr.)

KIE SYRUP. (Laser) Pot. iodide 150 mg., ephedrine HCl 8 mg./5 ml. Syr. Bot. pt., gal.
Use: Bronchodilator, expectorant.

KINATE. Hexahydrotetra hydroxybenzoate salt, quinic acid salt.

KINDER-DARE. (Sween) Bot. 16 oz., gal.
Use: Skin care cream.

KINESED. (Stuart) Phenobarbital 16 mg., hyoscyamine sulf. 0.1 mg., atropine sulf. 0.02 mg., scopolamine hydrobromide 0.007 mg./Tab. Bot. 100s.
Use: Antispasmodic, sedative.

KINEVAC. (Squibb) Sincalide 5 mcg./vial.
Use: Diagnostic for gall bladder, pancreatic secretion and cholecystography.

KINSMAN'S ASTHMA CIGARETTES & POWDER. (Guild) Cigarettes 50/Pkg. Pow. 3 oz.

KIN WHITE. (Whiteworth) Triamcinolone acetonide.
Cream: 0.025%, 1%. Tube 15 Gm., 80 Gm.
Ointment: 1%. Tube 15 Gm., 80 Gm.
Use: Anti-inflammatory steroid.

KIRKMASSAGE. (Kirkman) 8 oz., gal.

• **KITASAMYCIN.** USAN. An antibiotic substance obtained from cultures of *Streptomyces kitasatoensis*. Under study.
Use: Antibiotic.

KLARON LOTION 2.0%. (Dermik) Salicylic acid 2%, sulfur colloid 5%, in a hydro-alcoholic suspension w/colloidal magnesium aluminum silicate, alkyl-aryl sulfonic acid salts, propylene glycol, silicone emulsion, cellulose gum, tetrasodium EDTA, 2-bromo-2-nitropropane-1,3-diol, lauric myristic diethanolamine, butyl paraben, fragrance, alcohol 13.1%. Bot. 2 oz. plas. sq.
Use: Seborrhea, acne and related conditions.

KLAVIKORDAL. (U.S. Ethicals) Nitroglycerin 2.6 mg./S.R. Tab. Bot. 100s, 1000s.
Use: Vasodilator for anginal attacks.

KLEBCIL. (Beecham Labs) Kanamycin sulfate 500 mg./2 ml. vial or 1 Gm./3 ml. Vial. **Ped. Inj.** 75 mg./2 ml. Vial in 10s; 500 mg./2ml. disposable syringe in 25s.
Use: Antibiotic.

KLEBSIELLA PNEUMONIAE.
W/*Haemophilus influenzae, Neisseria catarrhalis, streptococci, staphylococci, pneumococci,* killed.
See: Mixed Vaccine No. 4 W/H. Influenzae (Lilly)

KLEER CHEWABLE. (Scrip) Phenylphrine HCl 5 mg., chlorpheniramine maleate 2 mg., d-methorphan HBr 2.5 mg., Vit. C 15 mg./Chewable Tab. Bot. 100s.

KLEER COMPOUND. (Scrip) Acetaminophen. 300 mg., phenylpropanolamine HCl 35 mg., caffeine 10 mg./Tab. Bot. 100s.

KLEER IMPROVED. (Scrip) Atropine sulfate 0.2 mg., chlorpheniramine maleate 5 mg./cc.

KLEER MILD. (Scrip) Phenylpropanolamine HCl 75 mg./Cap. Bot. 100s.

KLENSEB. (Durel) Mild astringent and facial cleanser. Bot. 4 oz., gal.

KLER-RO LIQUID. (Ulmer) Surgical cleanser and laboratory detergent. Bot. gal.

KLER-RO POWDER. (Ulmer) Surgical cleanser and laboratory detergent. Can 2 lb., Bot. 6 lb., Drum 45 lb.

K-LOR. (Abbott) Potassium chloride equiv. to potassium 20 mEq. and chloride 20 mEq./2.6 Gm. for oral solution. Pkg. 30s, 100s. 15 mEq/2 Gm. Pkg. 100s.
Use: Potassium chloride supplement.

KLOR-10% SOLUTION. (Upsher-Smith) Potassium chloride 10%. Bot. 4 oz., pt., gal.

KLOR-CON POWDER. (Upsher-Smith) Potassium chloride for oral solution 20 mEq/Packet. Packets 1.5 Gm. Box 30s, 100s.
Use: Potassium supplement.

KLOR-CON/25 POWDER. (Upsher-Smith) Potassium Cl. for oral sol. 25 mEq./Pkt. Cartons 30s, 100s, 250s.
Use: Potassium supplement.

KLOR-CON SOLUTION. (Upsher-Smith) Potassium chloride 20% oral solution. Bot. 4 oz., pt., gal.

KLORIDE. (Amfre-Grant) K chloride 1.5 Gm./15 cc. Elix. Bot., pt., gal.
Use: Treatment of potassium deficiency.

KLORLYPTUS. (High) Chemical cpd. of eucalyptus oil & chlorine in a petroleum ointment and light oil base. **Oint.:** Jars 1 oz., 1 lb. **Oil:** Bot. 30 ml., 1 pt.
Use: Topical dressing.

KLOROMIN. (Blue Cross) Chlorpheneramine maleate 4 mg./Tab. Bot. 1000s.
Use: Decongestant.

KLORVESS EFFERVESCENT GRANULES. (Sandoz) Potassium 20 mEq. & chloride 20 mEq. supplied by KCl 1.125 Gm., potassium bicarbonate 0.5 Gm., L-lysine monohydrochloride 0.913 Gm./Packet. Box 30s.
Use: Potassium & chloride supplement.

KLORVESS EFFERVESCENT TABLETS. (Sandoz) Pot. chloride 1.125 Gm., pot. bicarb. 0.5 Gm., 1-lysine HCl 0.913 Gm./Eff. Tab. Sodium & sugar free. Pkg. 60s, 1000s.
Use: Potassium & chloride supplement.

KLORVESS LIQUID. (Sandoz) Potassium chloride 1.5 Gm., (20 mEq.)/15 ml., alcohol 0.7%. Bot. pt. Unit dose 15 ml. Box 100s.
Use: Potassium & chloride supplement.

KLOTRIX. (Mead Johnson) Potassium chloride 10 mEq. KCl/Tab. Slow-release Tab. Bot. 100s, 1000s. Unit dose 100s.
Use: Potassium supplement.

K-LYTE. (Mead Johnson) Pot. bicarbonate and citrate 25 mEq. potassium/Tab., individually wrapped effervescent tabs.; Flavors: Lime, Orange. Pkg. 30s, 100s, 250s.
Use: Treatment of potassium loss accompanying body fluid disorders.

K-LYTE/CL. (Mead Johnson) Pot. chloride 25 mEq.-/Dose. Pkg. 30s, 100s, 250s; Individually wrapped effervescent tabs.; Bulk powder 225 Gm./Can. Available in citrus and fruit punch flavors.
Use: Potassium and chloride replacement therapy.

K-LYTE/CL 50. (Mead Johnson) Potassium Cl. 50 mEq/Dose. Pkg. 30s, 100s. Available in citrus and fruit punch flavors.
Use: Potassium & chloride replacement therapy.

K-LYTE DS. (Mead Johnson) Potassium bicarbonate & citrate 50 mEq. Potassium/Effervescent Tab. Pkg. 30s, 100s, individually foil wrapped. Available in lime and orange flavors.
Use: Potassium replacement therapy, treatment of potassium loss.

KNIBEL TABLETS. (Knight) Bot. 100s, 500s.
Use: Antispasmodic.

KNIBEL T.D. CAPSULES. (Knight) Bot. 100s.
Use: Sustained action antispasmodic.

KNIHALANT SPRAY. (Knight) Bot. 20 cc.
Use: Nasal congestion.

KNIMINE T.D. CAPSULES. (Knight) Bot. 100s.
Use: Antihistamine decongestant.

KNIMINE TABLETS. (Knight) Bot. 100s.
Use: Antihistamine decongestant.

KNISED TABLETS. (Knight) Bot. 100s.
Use: Sedative.

KNISERP TABLETS. (Knight) Bot. 100s.
Use: Antihypertensive and calmative.

KNITRON TABLETS. (Knight) Bot. 100s.
Use: Hematinic.

KNITUSSIN SYRUP. (Knight) Bot. pt.
Use: Antitussive, antihistamine expectorant.

KOATE. (Cutter) Antihemophilic Factor (Human) comprises factors VIII, AHF and AHG; each 10 ml. contains approx. 250 AHF units. Vial 10 ml., 20 ml., 40 ml., w/sterile diluent and filter needle.
Use: Antihemophilic.

KODONYL EXPECTORANT. (Blue Cross) Bromodiphenhydramine HCl 3.75 mg., diphenhydramine HCl 8.75 mg., ammonium Cl. 80 mg. potassium guaiacolsulfonate 80 mg., menthol 0.5 mg./5 ml. Bot. 16 oz.
Use: Expectorant, antihistaminic.

KOHLER HEADACHE POWDERS. (Guild) Pkg. 8s.

KOHLER ONE NIGHT CORN SALVE. (Guild)

KOLANTYL GEL. (Merrell Dow) Aluminum hydroxide 150 mg., magnesium hydroxide 150 mg./5 ml. Bot. 12 oz.
Use: Antacid.

KOLANTYL WAFERS. (Merrell Dow) Magnesium hydroxide 170 mg., aluminum hydroxide 180 mg./wafer. Box 32s.
Use: Antacid.

KOLYUM LIQUID AND POWDER. (Pennwalt) Potassium ion 20 mEq., chloride ion 3.4 mEq. from pot. gluconate 3.9 Gm., pot. chloride 0.25 Gm./15 ml. or 5 Gm. **Liquid:** Bot. pt., gal. **Powder:** Packets 5 Gm. 30s.
Use: Potassium deficiency.

KOMED LOTION. (Barnes-Hind) Sodium thiosulfate 8%, salicylic acid 2%, w/Isopropyl alcohol 25%

menthol, camphor, colloidal alumina. Squeeze Bot.
1.75 oz.
Use: Treatment of acne associated with oily skin.
KOMED HC. (Barnes-Hind) Hydrocortisone acetate 0.-
5%, sodium thiosulfate 8%, salicylic acid 2%,
isopropyl alcohol 25%, menthol, camphor, colloidal
alumina, disodium edetate. Lotion, Plastic Bot. 2 oz.
Use: Acne therapy.
KOMEX. (Barnes-Hind) Sodium tetraborate decahy-
drate. Jar 75 Gm.
Use: Aid in reducing oily skin conditions associated
with acne.
KONAKION. (Roche) Phytonadione-synthetic vitamin
K-$_1$ w/polysorbate 80, phenol, propylene glycol, sod.
acetate, glacial acetic acid. Amp.: 1 mg./0.5 ml.
Box 10s.
Use: Prevention and treatment of
hypoprothrombinemia.
KONDON'S NASAL JELLY. (Kondon) Tube 20 Gm.
W/Ephedrine alkaloid. Tube 20 Gm.
KONDREMUL. (Fisons) Plain: Mineral oil 55% w/Irish
moss, emulsion. Bot. 1 pt., 8 oz. Unit dose 2 oz.
Use: Laxative.
W/Phenolphthalein 2.2 gr./Tbsp. Bot. 1 pt.
W/Cascara 0.66 Gm./15 cc. Bot. 14 oz.
KONSTO. (Freeport) Docusate sodium 100 mg./Cap.
Bot. 1000s.
Use: Fecal softener.
KONSYL POWDER. (Lafayette) Psyllium hydrophyllic
mucilloid.
Use: Bulk producing laxative.
KONSYL-D POWDER. (Lafayette) Psyllium hydrophilic
mucilloid with dextrose.
Use: Bulk producing laxative.
KONYNE. (Cutter) Stable, dried, purified plasma
fraction comprising coagulation factors II, VII, IX
and X with a minimal amount of total protein; 500
clinical units of Factor IX/20 ml. Vial w/sterile
diluent and filter needle.
Use: To correct or prevent bleeding.
KOOL FOOT CREAM LOTION. (Wade) Menthol,
camphor, acid boracic, glycerine, methyl salicylate,
isopropyl alcohol. Bot. 2 oz., 4 oz., pt.
KOREAN GINSENG. (Kirkman) Bot. 60s.
KORIZOL. (Sutliff & Case) Methapyrilene HCl 0.2%,
Naphazoline HCl 0.05%, Cetylpyridinium chloride
0.02%, thimerosal 0.005%. Bot. w/dropper 20 cc.
Use: Acute & chronic sinusitis.
KORO-FLEX. (Holland-Rantos) (Diaphragm, Arcing) Improved contouring spring natural latex diaphragm.
60-95 mm.
KOROMEX. (Holland-Rantos) **Cream:** Octoxynol
3.0%, base of purified water, propylene glycol, stearic
acid, sorbitan stearate, polysorbate 60, boric acid,
and fragrance, pH buffered and adjusted to 4.5.
Tube 45 Gm. w/ or w/out measured dose
applicator; refill 128 Gm. **Jelly:** Nonoxynol-9 3% in
base of purified water, propylene glycol, cellulose
gum, boric acid, sorbitol, starch, simethicone,
fragrance, pH buffered and adjusted to 4.5. Tube
81 Gm., 126 Gm. **Foam:** Nonoxynol-9 12.5%. Aerosol
can 40 Gm.

Use: Spermicide, contraceptive & vaginal lubricant
with diaphragm.
**KOROMEX CONTRACEPTIVE CRYSTAL CLEAR
GEL.** (Holland-Rantos) Nonoxynol-9 2% in base of
purified water, propylene glycol, cellulose gum,
boric acid, sorbitol, simethicone w/pH 4.5. Tube
126 Gm. w/applicator
Use: Contraceptive for use with diaphragm.
KOROMEX COIL SPRING DIAPHRAGM. (Holland-
Rantos) Diaphragm made of pure latex rubber,
cadmium plated coil spring is tension adjusted. As
kit w/Koromex Contraceptive Jelly and Koromex
Contraceptive Cream. Sizes 50 mm.-95 mm. at
graduations of 5 mm.
KOROMEX COMBINATION. (Holland-Rantos)
Diaphragm 50-95 mm., Koromex Jelly and Cream/
Kit.
KOROSTATIN. (Holland-Rantos) Nystatin 100,000
u./Vaginal Tab. Boxes 15s, 30s.
Use: Vulvovaginal candidiasis.
KORO-SULF VAGINAL CREAM. (Holland-Rantos) Sulfisoxazole 10% in a cream base of stearic acid,
polysorbate 60, sorbitan monostearate boric acid,
glycerin, methylparaben, propylparaben and water.
Vag. cream. Tube 3 oz. w/applicator.
Use: Treatment of hemophilus vaginalis vaginitis.
KORUM. (Geneva) Acetominophen 5 gr./Tab. Bot.
1000s.
KORYZA TAB. (Fellows) Phenylephrine HCl 15 mg.,
phenylpropanolomine HCl 25 mg., chlorpheniramine
maleate 4 mg., acetaminophen 300 mg.,
hyoscyamine HBr 0.134 mg., hyoscine HBr 0.008
mg., atropine sulfate 0.020 mg./Tab. Bot.
1000s.
KOTABARB. (Wesley) Phenobarbital 1/4 gr./Tab.
Bot. 1000s.
Use: Sedative.
K-PAVA. (Kay) Papaverine HCl 150 mg./Cap. (Kaykap)
Bot. 100s, 500s, 1000s.
K-PHEN. (Kay) Promethazine HCl 50 mg./cc. Vial 10 cc.
Expect.: w/codeine, pt., gal.
K-PHOS M.F. (Beach) Potassium acid phosphate
155 mg., sodium acid phosphate 350 mg./Tab.
Bot. 100s, 500s.
Use: Acidify the urine.
K-PHOS NEUTRAL. (Beach) Dibasic sodium
phosphate 852 mg., potassium acid phosphate 155
mg., sodium acid phosphate 130 mg./Tab. Bot.
100s, 500s.
Use: Lowers urinary calcium levels, phosphorus
supplement.
K-PHOS NO. 2 (Beach) Potassium acid phosphate
305 mg., sodium acid phosphate, anhydrous 700
mg./Tab. Bot. 100s, 500s.
Use: Urinary acidifier.
K-PHOS ORIGINAL. (Beach) Potassium acid
phosphate 500 mg./Tab. Bot. 100s, 500s.
Use: Acidify the urine, useful in idiopathic
hypercalciuria.
K-P SUSPENSION. (Century) Kaolin 5.2 Gm., pectin 260
mg./oz. Bot. 4 oz., pt, gal.

Use: Antidiarrheal.

KRONOFED-A-JR. (Ferndale) Pseudoephedrine HCl 60 mg., chlorpheniramine maleate 4 mg./Cap. Bot. 100s, 500s.
Use: Antihistaminic, decongestant.

KRONOFED-A KRONOCAPS. (Ferndale) Pseudoephedrine HCl 120 mg., chlorpheniramine maleate 8 mg./Cap. Bot. 100s, 500s.
Use: Antihistaminic, decongestant.

KRONOHIST KRONOCAPS. (Ferndale) Chlorpheniramine maleate 4 mg., pyrilamine maleate 25 mg., phenylpropanolamine HCl 50 mg./Cap. Bot. 100s, 1000s.
Use: Antihistaminic-decongestant.

KRUSCHEN SALTS. (CMC) Mineral spa-type supplement. Bot. 4 oz.

• **KRYPTON CLATHRATE Kr 85.** USAN.
Use: Radioactive agent.

• **KRYPTON Kr 81m,** U.S.P. XXI.
Use: Radioactive agent.

K-TAB. (Abbott) Potassium chloride (10 mEq) 750 mg./Slow Release Tab. Bot. 100s, 1000s. Abbo-Pac 100s.
Use: Potassium supplement.

K.T.V. TABLETS. (Knight) Vitamin B-12 and minerals. Bot. 50s.

KUDROX (Double Strength) SUSP. (Rorer) Susp. of aluminum hydroxide & magnesium hydroxide, d-sorbitol. Bot. 12 oz.
Use: Antacid.

KUTAPRESSIN. (Rorer) Liver derivative complex. Vial 20 cc.
Use: Subcutaneous, I.M. reduces inflammation in a variety of skin conditions.

KUTRASE. (Rorer) Amylolytic enzyme 30 mg., proteolytic enzyme 6 mg., lipolytic enzyme 75 mg., cellulolytic enzyme 2 mg., phenyltoloxamine citrate 15 mg., hyoscyamine sulfate 0.0625 mg./Cap. Bot. 100s, 500s.
Use: Enzymatic digestant with antispasmodic/calmative.

KU-ZYME. (Rorer) Amylolytic enzyme 30 mg., proteolytic enzyme 6 mg., lipolytic enzyme 75 mg., cellulolytic enzyme 2 mg./Cap. Bot. 100s, 500s.
Use: Enzymatic digestant.

KU-ZYME-HP. (Rorer) Lipase 8,000 u., protease 30,000 u., amylase 30,000 u./Cap. Bot. 100s.
Use: Enzymatic digestant.

KWELL. (Reed & Carnrick) Lindane 1%. **Lot.** W/Glyceryl monostearate, cetyl alcohol, stearic acid, trolamine, 2-amino-2-methyl-1-propanol, methyl p-hydroxybenzoate, butyl p-hydroxybenzoate, irish moss extract. Bot. 2 oz., 16 oz. **Shampoo.** W/Polyethylene sorbitan monostearate, TEA-Lauryl sulfate, acetone and purified water. Bot. 2 oz., pt., gal. **Cream.** W/Stearic acid, lanolin, glycerin, 2-amino-2-methyl-1-propanol, perfume and purified water. Tube 2 oz., Jar 1 lb.
Use: Topically, scabies & pediculosis.
Shampoo: Pediculosis.

L

LA-12. (Hyrex) Hydroxocobalamin 1000 mcg./cc. Vial 10 cc., 30 cc.
Use: Anemia.

• **LABETALOL HYDROCHLORIDE.** USAN.
Use: Anti-adrenergic.

LABID. (Norwich Eaton) Theophylline anhydrous 250 mg./Tab. Bot. 100s.
Use: Relief of symptoms of asthma.

LABSTIX. (Ames) Urine screening in 30 sec. pH values, protein, glucose, ketones, occult blood. Bot. 100s.
Use: Diagnostic.

LACLEDE CLEANER. (Laclede) 2 lb. Container.
Use: Detergent for instruments and trays.

LACLEDE DISCLOSING SWAB. (Laclede) 6″ Swabs. 100s, 500s, 1000s.
Use: Dental swab.

LACLEDE PROFIE. (Laclede) Enzyme-action prophylaxis. **Paste:** Jar. 13.5 oz. **Liq.:** Bot. pt. **Tab.:** Bot. 500s.
Use: Removal of calculus.

LACLEDE ROOM DEODORIZER. (Laclede) Can 16 oz.
Use: Neutralize odors.

LACLEDE SKIN LUBRICANT. (Laclede) Tube 1.5 oz.
Use: Skin lubricant for lips, face and intra-oral use.

LACLEDE TOPI-FLUOR A.P.F. TOPICAL CREAM. (Laclede) Fluoride ion 1.23% (from sod. fluoride) in orthophosphoric acid 0.98%. Jar 50 ml., 500 ml., 1000 ml., 2000 ml.
Use: Dental cream.

LACOTEIN. (Christina) Protein digest 5% w/preservatives. Vial 30 cc. w/iodochin Vial 30 cc.
Use: I.M., nonspecific protein therapy.

LACRIL ARTIFICAL TEARS. (Allergan) Hydroxypropyl methylcellulose & gelatin A in a sterile buffered isotonic solution w/chlorbutanol 0.5%. Drop bot. 15 ml.

LACRI—LUBE S.O.P. (Allergan) White petrolatum, mineral oil, nonionic lanolin derivatives, chlorobutanol. Tube 3.5 Gm., 7.5 Gm.
Use: Ocular lubricant.

LACRISERT. (Merck Sharp & Dohme) Hydroxypropyl cellulose 5 mg./Lacrisert insert. Pkg. contains 60 unit doses, 2 reusable applicators and storage container.
Use: Dry eye syndromes.

LACTALBUMIN HYDROLYSATE.
See: Aminonat

LACTATED PEPSIN ELIXIR. (Lilly) Alcohol 15%. Elixir. Bot. 16 fl. oz. (Parke-Davis) 1.75 Gm./100 ml. Alcohol 15%. Elix. Bot. 16 fl. oz.

• **LACTATED RINGER'S INJECTION,** U.S.P. XXI.

• **LACTIC ACID,** U.S.P. XXI. Propanoic acid, 2-hydroxy.
Use: Pharm. necessity for Sodium Lactate Injection, U.S.P. XXI.
W/Sodium pyrrolidone carboxylate.
See: LactiCare (Stiefel)

LACTICARE LOTION. (Stiefel) Lactic acid 5%, sodium pyrrolidone carboxylate 2.5% in an emollient lotion base. Bot. 8 oz.
Use: Dry skin treatment.

LACTINEX. (Hynson, Westcott & Dunning) *Lactobacillus acidophilus & Lactobacillus bulgaricus* mixed culture. Tab. 250 mg., Bot. 50s. Granules 1 Gm. pk. Box 12s.
Use: Orally, to restore intestinal flora.

LACTOBACILLUS ACIDOPHILUS. Preparation made from acid-producing bacterium.
Use: Antidiarrheal.
See: Bacid (Fisons)
DoFUS (Miller)

LACTOBACILLUS ACIDOPHILUS & BULGARICUS MIXED CULTURE.
See: Lactinex, Tab., Granules (Hynson, Westcott & Dunning)

LACTOBACILLUS ACIDOPHILUS, VIABLE CULTURE.
See: DoFus, Tab. (Miller)
Lactinex Granules, Tab. (Hynson, Westcott & Dunning)
Neo-Cultol, Jelly (Fisons)

LACTOCAL-F. (Laser) Vit. A 8000 I.U., D 400 I.U., E 30 I.U., C 100 mg., Folic acid 1 mg., B-1 3 mg., B-2 3.4 mg., nicotinamide 20 mg., B-6 5 mg., B-12 12 mcg., Ca 200 mg., iodine 0.15 mg., iron 65 mg., Mg. 25 mg., Cu 2 mg., Zn 15 mg./Tab. Bot. 100s, 1000s.
Use: Vitamin and mineral supplement for pregnancy and lactation.

LACTOFLAVIN.
See: Riboflavin, U.S.P. XXI. (Var. Mfr.)

• **LACTOSE,** N.F. XVI. Milk sugar.
Use: Pharm. aid (tablet and capsule diluent).
See: Natur-Aid powder (Scott/Cord)

LACTRASE. (Rorer) Lactase 125 mg./Cap. Bot. 100s.
Use: Lactose intolerance.

• **LACTULOSE,** U.S.P. XXI. Concentrate, Syr, U.S.P. XXI. 4-0-β-D-Galactopyranosyl-D-fructose. Duphalac.
Use: Treatment of hepatic coma and chronic constipation.
See: Cephulac, Syr. (Merrell Dow)
Chronulac, Liq. (Merrell Dow)

LADOGAL. (Winthrop Products) Danazol.
Use: Gonadotropin inhibitor.

LADY ESTHER 4 PURPOSE FACE CREAM. (Norcliff Thayer) Jar 4 oz., 8 oz.

LADY ESTHER FACE POWDER. (Norcliff Thayer) Box 1 oz.

L.A.E. 20. (Seatrace) Estradiol valerate 20 mg./ml. Vial 10 cc.

L.A.E. 40. (Seatrace) Estradiol valerate 40 mg./ml. Vial 10 cc.

■ **LAETRILE.** Substance obtained from apricot pits and thought by some to arrest certain forms of cancer. Contains amygdalin (a cyanogenic glycoside) as the major component. Currently legal in many states.

LAGOL OIL. (Last) 8 Hydrooxyquinoline 0.038% in oil base. Bot. 1 oz., 2 oz., 4 oz., 16 oz.
Use: Soothing, cleansing oil.

LAGOL OINTMENT. (Last) Allantoin 1%, benzocaine 5%. Jar 1 oz., 8 oz., 16 oz., 5 lb.
Use: Soothing, dressing ointment.

LAKTOMOL. (Durel) Whole milk, dewaxed lanolin esters. Bot. pt., gal.
Use: Pediatric and gereatric skin conditioner, prophylatic for normal skin.

LAMOTANE-X. (Myers) Trichlorethylamino-glycol-benzoate (ethylaminobenzoate-chloralhydrate derivative). Bot. 4 oz., 6 oz., 8 oz., pt., qt., gal.
Use: Antiseptic, anesthetic, antipruritic.

LAMPRENE. Clofazimine, B.A.N.

LANABAC. (Lannett) Aspirin 0.3 gr., caffeine 15 mg., potassium bromide 15 mg., sodium bromide 15 mg./Tab. Bot. 1000s.

LANABARB. (Lannett) **No. 1:** Sod. amobarbital ¾ gr., sod. secobarbital ¾ gr./Cap. Bot. 500s, 1000s. **No. 2:** Sod. amobarbital 1½ gr., sod. secobarbital 1½ gr./Cap. Bot. 500s, 1000s.
Use: Sedative.

LANABEE-C. (Lannett) Vit. B-1 15 mg., B-1 10 mg., B-6 5 mg., niacinamide 50 mg., calcium pantothenate 10 mg., C 300 mg./Cap. Bot. 100s, 1000s.

LANABROM ELIXIR. (Lannett) 60 gr. of combined bromides of sod., pot., strontium, ammonium/fl. oz. Bot. 1 pt., 1 gal.

LANABURN OINT. (Lannett) Aluminum basic acetate, phenol, zinc oxide, boric acid, ichthammol, eucalyptol, Jar 1 lb.

LANACANE CREME. (Combe) Benzocaine, chlorothymol, resorcin. Tube 1¼ oz., 2½ oz. Spray Can 3 oz.
Use: Topical anesthetic.

LANACILLIN. (Lannett) Penicillin G potassium 200,000 u./5 cc. Bot. 100 cc. 400,000 u./5 cc. Bot. 100 cc., 150 cc.
Use: Antibiotic.

LANACILLIN VK TABLETS. (Lannett) Potassium phenoxymethyl penicillin 400,000 u. (250 mg.), 800,000 u. (500 mg.)/Tab. Bot. 100s.
Use: Antibiotic.

LANACILLIN VK POWDER. (Lannett) Potassium phenoxymethyl penicillin 125 mg./5 cc. (200,000 u.), 250 mg./5 cc. (400,000 u.), Bot. 100 cc.

LANACORT CREAM. (Combe) Hydrocortisone acetate 0.5%. Tube 0.5 oz., 1.0 oz.
Use: Topical anti-inflammatory.

LANAMINS. (Lannett) Combination of vitamins (11)/Cap. Bot. 100s, 1000s.

LANAPHILIC OINTMENT. (Medco Lab) Sorbitol, isopropyl palmitate, stearyl alcohol, white petrolatum, oil soluble lanolin, sodium lauryl sulfate, propylene glycol, methylparaben, propylparaben. Jar 16 oz. Also available w/Urea 10% or 20%.
Use: Prescription compounding and dry skin.

LANASED. (Lannett) Atropine sulfate 0.03 mg., hyoscyamine 0.03 mg., methenamine 408 mg., methylene blue 5.4 mg., phenyl salicylate 18.1 mg., gelsemium 6.1 mg., benzoic acid 4.5 mg./Tab. Bot. 1000s.

LANATOSIDE C. B.A.N. 3-(3″-Acetyl-4″-β -glucosyl-tridigitoxosido)-digoxogenin.

Use: Myocardial stimulant.
See: Cedilanid, Tab. (Sandoz)

LANATRATE. (Lannett) Ergotamine tartrate 1 mg., caffeine alkaloid, 100 mg./Tab. Bot. 100s, 500s, 1000s.
Use: Relief of different throbbing and recurrent headaches.

LANATUSS. (Lannett) Guaifenesin 100 mg., phenylpropanolamine HCl 5 mg., chlorpheniramine maleate 2 mg., sodium citrate 197 mg., citric acid 60 mg./5 cc. Bot. pts., gal.
Use: Cough, decongestant.

LANAURINE. (Lannett) Antipyrine & Benzocaine in glycerin. Bot. ½ oz., 4 oz.
Use: Otitis media.

LANAVITE. (Lannett) Vitamins A 5000 I.U., D 1000 I.U., B-1 1.5 mg., B-2 2 mg., B-6 0.1 mg., C 37.5 mg., B-12 1 mcg., niacinamide 20 mg., Ca pantothenate 1 mg. E 1 I.U./Cap. Bot. 500s, 1000s.

LANAVITE DROPS. (Lannett) Vit. A 3000 I.U., D 400 I.U., B-1 1 mg., B-2 1.2 mg., niacinamide 8 mg., C 60 mg./0.6 cc. Drop. bot. 15 cc., 60 cc.

LANAZETS. (Lannett) Cetylpyridinium 1 mg., benzocaine 5 mg./Loz. Bot. 500s, 1000s.

LANES PILLS. (Last) Casanthranol 45 mg./Tab. Bot. 20s.
Use: Laxative.

LANESTRIN. (Lannett) Estrogenic sub. natural in aq. susp. 20,000 u./cc. Vial 30 cc.

LANIAZID C.T. (Lannett) Isoniazid 50 mg. Tab. Bot. 500s, 1000s. 100 mg./Tab. Bot. 100s, 500s, 1000s.
Use: Tuberculosis.

LANNATES ELIXIR. (Lannett) Sodium glycerophosphate 2 gr., calcium glycerophosphate 2 gr., phosphoric acid 1½ min., wine base/fl. oz. Bot. pt., gal.

LANOKALIN. (Lannett) Phenobarbital 15 mg., homatropine methyl bromide 5 mg., colloidal kaolin 300 mg./Tab. Bot. 1000s.
Use: Antacid, absorbant.

• **LANOLIN,** U.S.P. XXI. Anhydrous U.S.P. XXI.
Use: Water-in-oil emulsion ointment base; absorbent ointment base.
See: Kerohydric (Westwood)
W/Coconut oil, pine oil, castor oil, cholesterols, lecithin and parachlorometaxylenol.
See: Sebacide, Liq. (Paddock)
W/Diiosbutylcresoxyethoxyethyl, dimethyl benzyl ammonium chloride, menthol.
See: Hospital Lotion (Paddock)

• **LANOLIN ALCOHOLS,** N.F. XVI.
Use: Pharmaceutic aid (ointment base ingredient).

LANOLINE. (Burroughs Wellcome) Perfumed emollient ointment. Tube 1.75 oz.
Use: Derma emollient.

LANO-LO BATH OIL. (Whorton) 8 oz.

LANOLOR. (Squibb) Cream. Jar 8 oz. Tube 2 oz.

LANOPHYLLIN ELIXIR. (Lannett) Anhydrous theophylline 80 mg., alcohol 20%/15 cc. Bot. pt., gal.

LANOPHYLLIN INJ. (Lannett) Theophylline 250 mg./cc. Inj. 10 cc. vial.

LANOPLEX ELIXIR. (Lannett) Vit. B-1 4 mg., B-6 mg., nicotinamide 40 mg., B-6 2 mg./fl. oz. Bot. pt., gal.

LANOPLEX FORTE CAPSULES. (Lannett) Vit. B-1 25 mg., B-2 12.5 mg., nicotinamide 50 mg., C 250 mg., B-6 3 mg., B-12 5 mcg., Ca pantothenate 10 mg./Cap. Bot. 100s, 500s, 1000s.

LANOPLEX INJECTION. (Lannett) Vitamins B-1 100 mg., B-2 1 mg., B-6 2 mg., niacinamide 50 mg., cal. pantothenate 10 mg., benzyl alcohol 1%, urea 10%, chlorobutanol 0.5%/cc. Vial 30 cc.

LANORINAL. (Lannett) Isobutylallylbarbituric acid 50 mg., caffeine 40 mg., aspirin 200 mg., phenacetin 130 mg./Cap. or Tab. **Cap.** Bot. 100s, 1000s. **Tab.** Bot. 1000s.
Use: Tension headache.

LANOTHAL PILLS. (Lannett) Phenolphthalein ½ gr., aloin ¼ gr., ipecac 1/15 gr., belladonna ext. 1/12 gr./Pill. Bot. 1000s.

LANOXICAPS. (Burroughs Wellcome) Digoxin solution in capsules. Digoxin 0.05 mg., 0.1 mg. or 0.2 mg./Cap. Bot. 100s.
Use: Digitalization, cardiotonic.

LANOXIN. (Burroughs Wellcome) Digoxin. **Tab.** 0.125 mg., Bot. 100s, 1000s; 0.25 mg., Bot. 100s, 500s, 1000s, 5000s. Unit dose 1000s. Unit of Use Bot. 100s, 0.5 mg., Bot. 100s. **Pediatric Elixir** (0.05 mg./ml.) Bot. 60 ml. **Inj.** (w/propylene glycol 40%, alcohol 10%, sod. phosphate 0.3%, anhydrous citric acid 0.08%) Amp. 0.5 mg./2 ml. Amp. 12s, 100s. **Pediatric Inj.** 0.1 mg./ml. Amp. 1 ml. 50s.
Use: Digitalization, cardiotonic.

LANTEEN JELLY. (Medtech) Ricinoleic acid 0.5%, hexylresorcinol 0.1%, chlorothymol 0.0077% w/sod. benzoate & glycerin in tragacanth base. Tube 3 oz., with or without applicator. Refill only, 3 oz., 5 oz.
Use: Vaginal jelly and lubricant.

LANTRISUL. (Lannett) Sulfamerazine, sulfadiazine, sulfamethazine 2½ gr. each/Tab. Bot. 100s, 500s, 1000s. **Susp.** Bot. pt., gal.
Use: Triple sulfa therapy.

LANTURIL. (Winthrop Products) Oxypertine.
Use: Anxiolytic, tranquilizer.

LANUM. (Various Mfg.) Lanolin.

LANVISONE CREAM. (Lannett) Hydrocortisone 1%, clioquinol 3%. Tube 20 Gm. Jar 16 oz.

LAPAV. (Amfre-Grant) **Cap.:** Papaverine HCl 150 mg./Cap. Bot. 100s, 1000s. **Elixir:** Papaverine HCl 100 mg./15 cc. Bot. 4 oz., 16 oz., 1 Gal.
Use: Relief of cerebral and peripheral ischemia.

LAPUDRINE HYDROCHLORIDE. Chlorproguanil, B.A.N.

• **LAPYRIUM CHLORIDE.** USAN.
Use: Pharmaceutic aid.

LARDET. (Standex) Phenobarbital 8 mg., theophylline 130 mg., ephedrine HCl 24 mg./Tab. Bot. 100s.

LARDET EXPECTORANT. (Standex) Phenobarbital 8 mg., theophylline 130 mg., ephedrine HCl 24 mg., guaifenesin 100 mg./Tab. Bot. 100s.

LARGACTIL HYDROCHLORIDE. Chlorpromazine B.A.N.

LARGON. (Wyeth) Propiomazine HCl 20 mg./ml. w/ sodium formaldehyde sulfoxylate, sodium acetate buffer. Amp. 1 cc., 2 cc. Pkg. 25s. 20 mg./Tubex 1 cc., 10s.
Use: Tranquilizing agent.

LAROBEC. (Roche) Vit. B-1 15 mg., B-2 15 mg., niacinamide 100 mg., Ca pantothenate 20 mg., B-12 5 mcg., folic acid 0.5 mg., C 500 mg./Tab. Bot. 100s.
Use: Nutritional supplementation for patients under treatment w/levodopa.

LARODOPA CAPSULES. (Roche) Levodopa 250 mg./Cap. Bot. 100s, 500s; 500 mg./Cap. Bot. 100s, 500s.
Use: Treatment of Parkinson's disease and syndrome.

LARODOPA TABLETS. (Roche) Levodopa 100 mg./Tab. Bot. 100s; 250 mg./Tab. Bot. 100s, 500s; 500 mg./Tab. Bot. 100s, 500s.
Use: Treatment of Parkinson's disease and syndrome.

LAROTID. (Roche) Amoxicillin. **Cap.:** 250 mg. Bot. 18s, 100s, 500s. Tel-E-Dose 100s. 500 mg. Bot. 18s, 50s, 500s. Tel-E-Dose 100s. **Oral Suspension:** 125 mg. or 250 mg. (as trihydrate)/5 ml. Bot. 80 ml., 100 ml., 150 ml. **Pediatric drops:** 50 mg. (as trihydrate)/1 ml. Bot. 15 ml.

LAROXYL HYDROCHLORIDE. Amitriptyline, B.A.N.

LARYLGAN THROAT SPRAY. (Ayerst) Antipyrine 0.3%, pyrilamine maleate 0.05%, sodium caprylate 0.50%, w/alcohol 1%, methyl salicylate, benzyl alcohol 0.05%, methylparaben, propylparaben, gentian violet, menthol, isobornyl acetate, aromatics, glycerin, sod. saccharin. Bot. 28 ml. (0.94 fl. oz.)
Use: Throat spray.

LARYNEX. (Dover) Benzocaine lozenges. Sugar and salt free. Unit dose 500s.
Use: Sore throat relief.

• **LASALOCID.** USAN.
Use: Coccidiostat.

LASAN CREAM. (Stiefel) Anthraline 0.1%, 0.2%, or 0.4%. Tube 65 Gm.
Use: Psoriasis treatment.

LASAN HP-1 CREAM. (Stiefel) Anthralin 1%. Tube 65 Gm.
Use: Psoriasis treatment.

LASAN NASAL SPRAY. (Eastwood) Bot. 2/3 oz.

LASAN UNGUENT. (Stiefel) Anthralin 0.4% in a base of cetyl alcohol, mineral oil, sodium lauryl sulfate and petrolatum with salicylic acid preservative. Jar 4 oz.
Use: Psoriasis treatment.

LASIX. (Hoechst) Furosemide **Tab.:** 20 mg., 40 mg./Tab. Bot. 100s, 500s, 1000s. Unit Dose 100s; 40 mg./Tab. Unit of Use 100s; 80 mg./Tab. Bot. 50s. Unit Dose 100s. **Inj.:** 2 ml./Amp. Box 5s, 25s; 4 ml./Amp. Box 5s, 25s; 10 ml./Amp. Box 5s, 25s; Syringes 2 ml., 4 ml., 10 ml. Box 5s. **Oral Soln.:** Drop. Bot 60 ml.; Bot. 120 ml. w/spoon. mg./cc.
Use: Diuretic, antihypertensive.

LASSAR'S PASTE.
See: Zinc Oxide Paste, U.S.P. XXI. (Various Mfr.)

LAUDACIN. (Sutliff and Case) Opium 10 mg./15 cc. Syr. Bot. 3 oz., pt., gal.
Use: Diarrhea.

LAUDEXIUM METHYLSULFATE. B.A.N.
Decamethylene-α, ω-bis-(1-(3', 4'-dimethoxybenzyl)-1,-2,3,4-tetrahydro-6,7-dimethoxy-2-methylisoquinolinium methosulfate. Laudolissin.
Use: Neuromuscular blocking agent.

LAUD-IRON. (Amfre-Grant) Ferrous fumarate 5 gr./Tab. Bot. 100s, 1000s. Liq. Bot. 4 oz.
Use: Iron deficiency anemia.

LAUD-IRON-C. (Amfre-Grant) Ferrous fumarate 200 mg., ascorbic acid 150 mg./Gradual. Bot. 100s.

LAUD IRON FOLIC TABLETS. (Amfre-Grant) Ferrous fumarate 320 mg., folic acid 800 mcg., ascorbic acid 500 mg./Tab. Bot. 100s, 1000s.
Use: Iron supplement.

LAUD-IRON FORTE. (Federal) Ferrous fumarate 5 gr., Vit. B-12 50 mcg., B-12 w/Intrinsic Factor concentrate 0.5 I.U., C 100 mg., folic acid 1 mg., B-1 7.5 mg., B-2 5 mg., B-6 5 mg., niacinamide 25 mg., pantothenic acid 5 mg./Tab. Bot. 100s, 500s. Sol. Vial 30 cc.
Use: Hematinic.

LAUD-IRON PLUS. (Amfre-Grant) Ferrous fumarate 100 mg., B-12 5 mcg., D-sorbitol 500 mg./Chewable Tab. Bot. 100s, 1000s.
Use: Iron deficiency anemia.

LAUD-IRON SUSPENSION. (Amfre-Grant) Ferrous fumarate 100 mg./5 cc. Bot. pt.
Use: Hematinic.

• **LAURETH 4.** USAN.
Use: Pharmaceutic aid.

• **LAURETH 9.** USAN. Mixture of polyoxyethylene lauryl ethers having a statistical average of 9 ethylene oxide groups per molecule.
Use: Surfactant, emulsifier, spermaticide.

• **LAURETH 10S.** USAN.
Use: Spermaticide.

• **LAUROCAPRAM.** USAN.

LAURO EYE WASH. (Otis Clapp) Boric acid, sodium chloride. Bot. ½ oz., 4 oz., irrigator bot.
Use: Eye wash and tear substitute.

LAUROLINIUM ACETATE. B.A.N. 4-Amino-1-dodecylquinaldinium acetate. Laurodin.
Use: Surface active agent.

LAUROMACROGOL 400. Laureth 9.

• **LAURYL ISOQUINOLINIUM BROMIDE.** USAN.
Use: Anti-infective.

LAURYL SOLUTION. (Knight) Bot. pt.
Use: Acid vaginal douche.

LAURYL SULFOACETATE.
See: Lowila, Cake, Liq., Oint. (Westwood)

LAVACOL. (Parke-Davis) Ethyl alcohol 70%. Plastic Bot. 1 pt.

LAVATAR. (Doak) Coal tar distillate 25.5% in a bath oil base. Liq. Bot. 4 oz., 1 pt.
Use: Treatment of dermatoses, and psoriasis of the scalp.

• **LAVENDER OIL,** N.F. XVI.
Use: Perfume.

LAVOPTIK EMERGENCY WASH. (Lavoptik) Eye, face, body wash. 32 oz./Emergency station.

Use: Emergency wash for eyes, face, body.

LAVOPTIK EYE WASH. (Lavoptik) Sodium chloride 0-49 Gm., sodium biphosphate 0.40 Gm., sodium phosphate 0.45 Gm./100 ml. w/benzalkonium chloride 0.005%. Bot. 6 oz.
Use: Eye wash, eye drop, irrigation liquid.

LAVORIS. (Vicks Prods) Zinc chloride, glycerin, poloxamer 407, saccharin, polysorbate 80, flavors, clove oil, alcohol, citric acid, water. Bot. 6, 12, 18, 24 fl. oz.
Use: Mouthwash and gargle.

LAXATAB. (Freeport) Danthron 75 mg., docusate sodium 100 mg., D-calcium pantothenate 25 mg./Tab. Bot. 1000s.
Use: Laxative.

LAXATIVE CAPS. (Weeks & Leo) Docusate sodium 100 mg., casathranol 30 mg./Cap. Bot. 30s, 60s.
Use: Management of chronic or temporary constipation.

■ **LAXATIVES.**
See: Agar-Gel (Various Mfr.)
Aloe (Various Mfr.)
Aloin (Various Mfr.)
Bile Salts (Various Mfr.)
Bisacodyl, Tab., Supp. (Various Mfr.)
Bisacodyl Tannex (Barnes-Hind)
Carboxymethylcellulose Sodium (Various Mfr.)
Casanthranol, Cap., Tab. (Various Mfr.)
Cascara Sagrada (Various Mfr.)
Cascara Sagrada Fluidextract, Liq. (Parke-Davis)
Cascara Tablets (Various Mfr.)
Castor Oil (Various Mfr.)
Correctol, Tab. (Plough)
Danthron, Tab. (Various Mfr.)
Docusate Sodium (Various Mfr.)
Ex-Lax, Tab., Powder (Ex-Lax. Inc.)
Feen-a-Mint, Gum, Mints (Plough)
Karaya Gum (Penick)
Liquid Petrolatum, Liq. (Var. Mfr.)
Magnesia Magma (Various Mfr.)
Maltsupex (Wallace)
Methylcellulose (Various Mfr.)
Mucilloid of Psyllium Seed W/Dextrose (Searle)
Natures Remedy (Norcliff Thayer)
Nujol, Liquid (Plough)
Oxyphenisatin Acetate (Various Mfr.)
Petrolatum, Liquid (Various Mfr.)
Petrolatum, Liquid, Emulsion (Various Mfr.)
Phenolphthalein (Various Mfr.)
Plantago ovata, Coating (Various Mfr.)
Poloxalkol, Cap., Sol. (Various Mfr.)
Prune Concentrate, Tab., Cap. (Various Mfr.)
Prune Preps. (Various Mfr.)
Psyllium Granules W/Dextrose (Med. Chem.)
Psyllium Husk Powder (Upjohn)
Psyllium Hydrocolloid, Pow. (Stuart)
Psyllium Hydrophilic Mucilloid (Various Mfr.)
Psyllium Seed, Gel, Granules (Various Mfr.)
Regutol, Tab. (Plough)
Sakara, Gran. (Plough)
Senna, Alexandrian, Liq., Tab. (Various Mfr.)
Senna, Cassia angustifolia, Tab. (Brayten)

Senna Conc., Standardized, Gran., Tab., Pow., Supp. (Various Mfr.)
Senna Fruit Extract, Liq. (Various Mfr.)
Sennosides A&B, Tab. (Dorsey)
Sodium Biphosphate (Various Mfr.)
Sodium Phosphate (Various Mfr.)

LAXOBERAL. Sodium Picosulphate, B.A.N.

LAXONALIN DIACETATE. Bisoxatin, B.A.N.

LAYOR CARANG.
See: Agar (Various Mfr.)

LC-65 DAILY CONTACT LENS CLEANER. (Allergan) Daily cleaning solution for all hard, soft (hydrophilic), Polycon and Paraperm oxygen gas permeable contact lenses. Plastic dropper bottle 0.5 oz., 2 oz.

L-CAINE. (Century) Lidocaine HCl 1% Inj.: 20, 50 ml. or 2%, 50 ml. Topical Liq. 4%, 50 cc.
Use: Local anesthetic.

L-CAINE E. (Century) Lidocaine HCl 1% or 2%, epinephrine 1:100,000/cc. Inj. 20 cc., 50 cc.
Use: Local anesthetic.

L.C.D. (Almay) Cream Modified and Soln. Alcohol extractions of crude coal tar for eczemas, psoriasis, pruritus, etc. Bot. 4 oz., 1 pt.
See: Coal Tar Topical Soln., U.S.P. XXI.

LEBER TABULAE. (Paddock) Aloe 0.09 Gm., extr. rhei 0.03 Gm., myrrh 0.01 Gm., frangula 5 mg., galbanum 2 mg., olibanum 3 mg./Tab. Bot. 100s, 500s, 1000s.

LEBER TAURINE. (Paddock) Sod. salicylate 8 gr., ox bile 2¼ gr., ext cascara 1:4 4½ gr., pancreatin 1¼ gre., pepsin 1:10,000 ³⁄₁₀ gr./fl. oz. Bot. pt., gal.

LEC-E-PLEX. (Barth's) Vit. E 100 I.U., 200 I.U. or 400 I.U./Cap. w/lecithin. Bot. 100s, 500s, 1000s.

• **LECITHIN,** N.F. XVI.
(Arcum) 1200 mg./Cap. Bot. 100s, 1000s.
Gran.Bot. 8 oz. Pow. Bot. 4 oz.
(Barth's) 8 gr./Cap. Bot. 100s, 500s, 1000s. Gran.
Can 8 oz., 16 oz. Pow. Can 10 oz.
(Cavendish) Tab. (½ gr.) Bot. 500s.
(CMC) 1200 mg./Cap. Bot. 100s, 1000s.
(Columbia) 1200 mg., Caps. 100s.
(De Pree) Cap. Bot. 100s.
(Pfanstiehl) 25 Gm., 100 Gm., 500 Gm./Pkg.
W/Choline base, cephalin, lipositol.
See: Alcolec Cap., Granules (American Lecithin)
W/Coconut oil, pine oil, castor oil, lanolin, cholesterols, parachlorometaxylenol.
See: Sebacide, Liq. (Paddock)
W/Vitamins.
See: Acletin, Cap. (Associated Concentrates)
Lec-E-Plex, Cap. (Barth's)

LEC-KELP. (Western Research) Lecithin 100 mg., kelp 25 mg., Vit. B-6 3.5 mg., cider vinegar 40 mg./Cap. Bot. 1000s.

LECTRO. (Guild) Bot. 4 oz.

LEDERCILLIN VK. (Lederle) Penicillin V potassium.
Sol.: 125 mg. & 250 mg./5 ml. 100 ml., 150 ml., 200 ml. **Tab.:** 250 mg./Tab. Bot. 100s, 1000s.
Dose 100s.; 500 mg./Tab. Bot. 100s. Unit dose 100s.

Use: Antibiotic.

LEDERMYCIN. Demeclocycline, B.A.N.

LEDERPLEX CAPSULES. (Lederle) Vit. B-1 2 mg., B-2 2 mg., niacinamide 10 mg., B-6 0.2 mg., Ca pantothenate 3 mg., choline 20 mg., inositol 10 mg., insoluble liver fraction 340 mg., B-12 1 mcg./Cap. Bot. 100s.
Use: Anemias.

LEDERPLEX LIQUID. (Lederle) Vit. B-1 2 mg., B-2 2 mg., niacinamide 10 mg., pantothenic acid 2 mg., Vit. B-6 0.2 mg., B-12 5 mcg., liver 470 mg., inositol 10 mg., choline 20 mg./4 ml. Bot. 12 oz.
Use: Hematinic w/vitamin B complex.

LEDERPLEX TABLETS. (Lederle) Vit. B-1 2 mg., B-2 2 mg., niacinamide 10 mg., B-6 0.1 mg., Ca pantothenate 3 mg., insoluble liver fraction 250 mg., B-12 1 mcg./Tab. Bot. 100s.
Use: Anemias.

LEGIONELLA. (Wampole-Zeus) Direct fluorescent test for legionella organisms.
Use: An *in vitro* diagnostic aid for the identification of various legionella bacteria in tissue specimens, sputum, cultures.

LEGIONELLA, INDIRECT. (Wampole-Zeus) Indirect fluorescent antibody test for legionella pneumophila.
Use: An immunofluorescent procedure for the detection of *L. penumophila* antibodies in human serum.

• **LEMON OIL,** N.F. XVI.
Use: Pharmaceutic aid (flavor).

LENATE. (Maurry) Phenol 2.75%, iodine & potassium iodide 3.1%, menthol 0.55%, guaifenesin, glycerol, alcohol 2.5%. Bot. 1 oz., 4 oz., 8 oz., pt.
Use: Analgesic and antiseptic.

LENETRAN. Mephenoxalone.
Use: Tranquilizer.

LENICET.
See: Aluminum Acetate, Basic (Various Mfr.)

• **LENIQUINSIN.** USAN. 6,7-Dimethoxy-4-(veratrylideneamino) quinoline. Under study.
Use: Antihypertensive.

LENIUM MEDICATED SHAMPOO. (Winthrop Products) Selenium sulphide
Use: Medicated shampoo.

• **LENPERONE.** USAN.
Use: Antipsychotic.

LENSEN. (Geneva) Diphenhydramine HCl 25 mg., 50 mg./Cap. Bot. 1000s.

LENSINE 5. (CooperVision) Poloxamer 407, sodium chloride, potassium chloride, hydroxyethylcellulose, polyvinyl alcohol, polyethylene glycol, benzalkonium Cl 0.01%, edetate disodium 0.05%. Bot. 2 oz., 4 oz.
Use: Hard contact lens soaking, wetting & cleaning solution.

LENSINE EXTRA STRENGTH CLEANER. (CooperVision) Cleaning agent, benzalkonium Cl, edetate disodium. Bot. 1.5 fl. oz.
Use: Hard contact lens cleaner.

LENS MATE. (Alcon) Plastic Bot. 2 oz., 6 oz.
Use: All-purpose contact lens solution.

LENSRINS. (Allergan) Sterile preserved saline solution for heat disinfection, rinsing and storage of soft hydrophilic contact lenses; rinsing solution for chemical disinfection. Bot. 8 oz.

LENS-WET. (Allergan) Bot. 0.5 fl. oz.
Use: Lubricate & rewet hard & soft (hydrophilic) contact lenses.

LENTE INSULIN. Susp. of zinc insulin crystals.
See: Iletin Lente, Vial (Lilly)

LENTE INSULIN. (Squibb/Novo) Insulin zinc suspension U-40 (40 u./cc), U-80 (80 u./cc.), and U-100 (100 u./cc) in 10 cc. vials.
Use: An intermediate acting form of insulin.

LENTIZOL HYDROCHLORIDE. Amitriptyline, B.A.N.

LEPROSY THERAPY.
See: Hansen's Disease

LEPTAZOL.
See: Pentylenetetrazol.

LERGOBAN HYDROCHLORIDE. Diphenylpyraline, B.A.N.

• **LERGOTRILE MESYLATE.** USAN.
Use: Enzyme inhibitor.

LERTON OVULES. (Vita Elixir) Caffeine 250 mg./Cap.
Use: Stimulant.

LESTEROL. (Dram) Nicotinic acid 500 mg./Tab. Bot. 250s.
Use: Hypercholesteremia and hyperlipemia.

LETHOPHEROL. (Nutrition) Vitamin E 100 I.U./Kapule. Bot. 100s.
Use: Dietary supplement.

• **LETIMIDE HCl.** USAN. 3-[2-(Diethylamino)-ethyl]-2H-1,3-benzoxazine-2,4-(3H)-dione monohydrochloride.
Use: Analgesic.

LETUSIN. Naphthalene-2-sulfonate ester of levopropoxyphene. Levopropoxyphene (Lilly)

• **LEUCOVORIN CALCIUM,** U.S.P. XXI. Inj., U.S.P. XXI. L-Glutamic acid, N-[[(2-amino-5-formyl-1,4,5,6,-7,8-hexahydro-4-oxo-6-pteridinyl)-methyl]amino]benzoyl]-, calcium salt (1:1), pentahydrate. Folinic acid-S.F. Formyl tetrahydropteroylglutamic acid, a derivative of folic acid as calcium salt. (Lederle) Injection: **Amp.** 3 mg./1ml. Box 6s. **Vial** 10 mg./ml. after reconstitution w/5 ml. sterile
Use: Antagonist of aminopterin & other folic-acid antagonists. Anti-anemic (folate-deficiency); antidote to folic acid antagonists.
See: Leucorvin Calcium, Prods. (Lederle).

■ **LEUKEMIA AGENTS.**
See: Antineoplastics.

LEUKERAN. (Burroughs Wellcome) Chlorambucil 2 mg./Tab. Bot. 50s.
Use: Orally, for the treatment of chronic lymphocyctic leukemia and malignant lymphomas.

• **LEUPROLIDE ACETATE.** USAN.
Use: Antineoplastic.

LEUROCRISTINE.
See: Vincristine Sulfate (Lilly)

LEUROCRISTINE SULFATE (1:1) (SALT). Vincristine Sulfate, U.S.P. XXI.

• **LEUCINE,** U.S.P. XXI. $C_6H_{13}NO_2$. L-leucine.
Use: Amino acid.

LEVALLORPHAN, B.A.N. 1-3-Hydroxy-N-allylmorphinan.(—)-N-Allyl-3-hydroxymorphinan.
Use: Narcotic antagonist.
See: Lorfan, Vial, Amp. (Roche)
• **LEVALLORPHAN TARTRATE,** U.S.P. XXI. Inj., U.S.P. XXI. 1-3-Hydroxy-n-allylmorphinan tartrate. 17-Allylmorphinan-3-ol tartrate (1:1).
See: Lorfan, Amp., Vial (Roche)
LEVAMFETAMINE. F.D.A. (—)-α-Methylphenethylamine.
LEVAMFETAMINE.
See: Levamphetamine (Various Mfr.)
LEVAMISOLE. B.A.N. (—)-2,3,5,6-Tetrahydro-6-phenylimidazo[2,1-b]thiazole. Ketrax.
Use: Anthelmintic.
• **LEVAMISOLE HYDROCHLORIDE.** USAN.
Use: Anthelmintic.
LEVAMPHETAMINE. B.A.N. levo-Amphetamine. Levamfetamine. Cydril succinate.
Use: Sympathomimetic.
• **LEVAMPHETAMINE SUCCINATE.** USAN. (l-isomer), 1-phenyl-2-amino propane succinate. Amphetamine, levo. 1-a-methylphenethylamine succinate.
Use: Anorexiant.
See: Amodril, Cap. (North Amer. Pharmacal)
LEVARTERENOL BITARTRATE.
See: Norepinephrine Bitartate, U.S.P. XXI.
LEVIRON. (Approved) Liver desiccated 7 gr., iron and ammonium citrate 3 gr., B-1 1 mg., B-2 0.5 mg., B-6 0.5 mg., Ca pantothenate 0.3 mg., niacinamide 2.5 mg., B-12 1 mcg./Cap. Bot. 100s, 1000s.
Use: Supplement.
LEVO-AMPHETAMINE. Alginate (l-isomer) alpha-2-phenylaminopropane succinate.
See: Levamphetamine
LEVO-AMPHETAMINE SUCCINATE.
See: Pedestal, Cap. & Tab. (Len-Tag)
• **LEVODOPA.** U.S.P. XXI. Cap., Tab., U.S.P. XXI. L-Tyrosine, 3-hydroxy-. (—)-3-(3,4-Dihydroxyphenyl)-L-alanine. Berkdopa; Brocadopa; Veldopa
Use: Treatment of the Parkinsonian syndrome.
See: Bio Dopa, Cap. (Bio-Deriv.)
Dopar, Cap. (Norwich Eaton)
Larodopa, Tab. or Cap. (Roche)
Levopa, Cap. (ICN)
Parda, Cap. (Parke-Davis)
Rio-Dopa Caps., (D.D.R. Pharm.)
W/Carbidopa
See: Sinemet, Tab. (Merck Sharp & Dohme)
LEVO-DROMORAN. (Roche) Levorphanol tartrate, levo-3-Hydroxy-n-methylmorphinan tartrate. Amp. (2 mg./ml.; methyl and propyl parabens 0.2%, sod. hydroxide) 1 ml., Box 10s. Vial (2 mg./ml.; phenol 0.45%, sod. hydroxide) 10 ml. Tab. (2 mg.) Bot. 100s.
Use: Narcotic, analgesic.
LEVO-EPINEPHRINE BITARTRATE.
See: Lyophrin, Sol. (Alcon)
• **LEVOFURALTADONE.** USAN. 1-5-Morpholinomethyl-3-[(5-nitrofurfurylidene)amino]-2-oxazolidinone.
Use: Antibacterial; antiprotozoal.

LEVOID. (Nutrition) Levothyroxine sodium 0.1 mg., or 0.2 mg./Tab. Bot. 90s, 500s. I.M. or I.V. 0.1 mg./ml. (w/sod. formaldehyde sulfoxylate 0.1%, phenol 0.5%, sod. hydroxide, glycine buffer) Vial 10 ml.
Use: Thyroid deficiencies.
• **LEVOBUNOLOL HYDROCHLORIDE.** USAN.
Use: Anti-adrenergic.
• **LEVOMETHADYL ACETATE.** USAN.
Use: Analgesic, narcotic.
LEVOMETHORPHAN. B.A.N. (—)-3-Methoxy-N-methyl-morphinan.
Use: Cough suppressant.
LEVOMORAMIDE. B.A.N. (—)-1-(3-Methyl-4-morpholino-2,2-diphenylbutyryl)pyrrolidine.
Use: Narcotic analgesic.
• **LEVONANTRADOL HYDROCHLORIDE.** USAN.
Use: Analgesic.
• **LEVONORGESTREL.** USAN.
Use: Progestin.
W/Ethinyl estradiol. See: Nordette, Tab. (Wyeth)
• **LEVONORDEFRIN,** U.S.P. XXI. l-1-(1-Aminoethyl)3,4-Dihydroxy benzyl alcohol. Levonordefrin. (-)-α-(1-Aminoethyl)-3,4-dihydroxybenzyl Alcohol.
Use: Adrenergic (vasoconstrictor).
LEVOPHED BITARTRATE. (Winthrop-Breon) Norepinephrine bitartrate 1 mg./ml. w/sod. chloride, sod. bisulfite. 2 mg./ml. Amp. 4 ml. Box 10s.
Use: To maintain blood pressure in acute hypotensive states, adjunct in treatment of cardiac arrest & profound hypotension.
LEVOPHENACYLMORPHAN. B.A.N. (—)-3-Hydroxy-N-phenacylmorphinan.
Use: Narcotic analgesic.
LEVOPROME. (Lederle) Methotrimeprazine, 20 mg./ml. w/benzyl alcohol 0.9% w/v, disodium edetate 0.065% w/v, sod. metabisulfite 0.3% w/v. Vial, 10 ml., Amps. 1 ml., 25s.
Use: Analgesic, sedative.
• **LEVOPROPOXYPHENE.** USAN. Letusin α-(—)-4-Dimethylamino-3-methyl-1:2-diphenyl-2-propionyloxy-butane. α-(—)-1-Benzyl-3-dimethylamino-2-methyl-1-phenylpropyl propionate. Letusin napsylate.
Use: Cough suppressant.
• **LEVOPROPOXYPHENE NAPSYLATE,** U.S.P. XXI. Cap., Oral Susp., U.S.P. XXI. 2-Naphthalenesulfonic acid compound with (—)-α-[2-(dimethylamino)-1-methylethyl]-α-phenylphenethyl propionate (1:1) monohydrate. α-1-4-Dimethylamino-1,2-diphenyl-3-methyl-2-butanol propionate 2-naphthalene-sulfonate hydrate. (—)-α-4-(Dimethylamino)-3-methyl-1,2-diphenyl-2-butanol Propionate (ester) 2-Naphthalen-sulfonate (salt).
Use: Antitussive.
• **LEVOPROPYLCILLIN POTASSIUM.** USAN. (1) Potassium 3,3-Dimethyl-7-oxo-6-(—)-(2-phenoxy-ybutyramido)-4-thia-1-azabicyclo[3.2.0]-heptane-2-carboxylate; (2) Potassium 6-(—)-(2-phenoxy-ybutyramido) penicillinate.
Use: Antibacterial.
LEVORENINE.
See: Epinephrine, U.S.P. XXI. (Various Mfr.)

LEVOROXINE. (Bariatric) Sodium levothyroxine 0.05 mg./Tab., red; 0.1 mg., pink; 0.2 mg., yellow; 0.3 mg., dark blue. Bot. 100s, 500s.
Use: Thyroid therapy.

LEVORPHAN TARTRATE.

LEVORPHANOL. B.A.N. (—)-3-Hydroxy-N-methylmorphinan. Levorphan. Dromoran hydrogen tartrate.
Use: Narcotic analgesic.

• **LEVORPHANOL TARTRATE,** U.S.P. XXI. Inj., Tab., U.S.P. XXI. 1-3-Hydroxy-N-methyl-morphinan bitartrate. 17-Methylmorphinan-3-ol Tartrate (1:1)
Use: Analgesic (narcotic).
See: Levo-Dromoran, Amp., Tab., Vial (Roche)

LEVOTHROID. (USV Labs.) Levothyroxine sodium.
Tab.: 0.025 mg., 0.05 mg, 0.1 mg., 0.125 mg., 0.15 mg., 0.175 mg., 0.2 mg., 0.3 mg./Tab. Bot. 100s, 1000s. Unit dose 100s. **Inj.:** 200 mcg. or 500 mcg./6 ml. Vial. Formerly marketed as Letter.
Use: Thyroid deficiency.

• **LEVOTHYROXINE SODIUM,** U.S.P. XXI. Tabs. U.S.P. XXI. L-Tyrosine, 0-(4-hydroxy-3,5-diiodo-phenyl)-3,5-diiodo-, monosodium salt, hydrate. Sodium L-3-[4-(4-Hydroxy-3,5-diiodophenoxy)-3,5-diiodopheny]-alanine.
Use: Thyroid hormone.
See: Cytolen, Tab. (Len-Tag)
  Levoid, Tab., Vial (Nutrition Control Products)
  Noroxine, Tab. (Vortech)
  Synthroid, Tab., Inj. (Flint)
W/Mannitol.
See: Synthroid, Inj. (Flint)
W/Sod. liothyronine.
Use: Thyroid hormone.
See: Thyrolar, Tab. (Armour)

• **LEVOXADROL HYDROCHLORIDE.** USAN. l-2(2,2-Diphenyl-1,3-dioxolan-4-yl) piperidine hydrochloride. levo form of dioxadrol HCl.
Use: Local anesthetic.

LEVSIN. (Rorer) **Tab.** Hyoscyamine sulfate 0.125 mg./Tab. Bot. 100s, 500s. w/Phenobarbital 15 mg./Tab. Bot. 100s, 500s. **Elixir:** Hyoscyamine sulfate 0.125 mg./5 cc., w/phenobarb. 15 mg./5 cc. Bot. 1 pt.; **Injectable:** Hyoscyamine sulfate 0.5 mg./ml. Amp. 1 ml. Box 5s. Vial 10 ml. **Drops:** Bot. (0.125 mg./cc.) 15 ml. w/phenobarb. Bot. (Levsin 0.125 mg., phenobarbital 15 mg./cc.) 15 ml.
Use: Anticholinergic and sedative.

LEVSINEX TIMECAPS. (Rorer) Hyoscyamine sulf. 0.375 mg./long action Cap. Bot. 100s, 500s. Also with phenobarbital 45 mg./Cap. Bot. 100s, 500s.
Use: Anti-cholinergic.

LEVUCAL. (Kay) Calcium levulinate 1 Gm./10 cc. Ampules 10 cc. 25s.
Use: Calcium supplement.

LEVULOSE. Fructose.

LEVULOSE-DEXTROSE.
See: Invert Sugar.

LEVULOSE W/DEXTROSE.

LEXOCORT POWDER. (Lexington) Hydrocortisone 0.1% in a talc base. Pkg. 20 Gm.
Use: Anti-inflammatory.

LEXTRON. (Lilly) Liver-stomach conc. 50 mg., iron 30 mg., Vit. B-12 (activity equiv.) 2 mcg., B-1 1 mg., B-2 0.25 mg. w/other factors of Vit. B complex present in the liver-stomach conc./Pulvule. Bot. 84s.
Use: B complex therapy.

LEXTRON FERROUS. (Lilly) Liver-stomach conc. 50 mg., ferrous sulfate, anhy., 35 mg., Vit. B-12 (activity equiv.) 2 mcg., B-1 1 mg., B-2 0.25 mg., w/other factors of Vit. B complex present in the liver-stomach conc./Pulvule. Bot. 84s.
Use: B complex therapy with iron.

L.F.B. 12-100 INJECTION. (Ulmer) Liver injection equivalent to Cyanocobalamin 10 mcg., Folic Acid 1 mg., cyanocobalamine 100 mcg./ml. 10 ml. Vial.
Use: Anemia.

L-GLUTAVITE CAPSULES. (Berlex) Vit. B-1 0.96 mg., B-2 1.92 mg., niacin 45 mg., B-6 1.0 mg., B-12 6 mcg., iron 10.2 mg./6 Caps. Bot. 100s.
Use: Vitamin & mineral supplement.

L'HOMME. (Geneva) Vit. A 4000 I.U., D 400 I.U., B-1 1 mg., B-2 1.2 mg., B-12 2 mcg., Ca Pan. 5 mg., B-3 10 mg., C 30 mg., Ca 100 mg., P 76 mg., Fe 10 mg. Mn 1 mg., Mg 1 mg., Zn 1 mg. Bot. 100s.
Use: Multiple vitamin.

LI BAN SPRAY. (Pfipharmecs) Synthetic pyrethroid 0.500%, related compounds 0.065%, aromatic petroleum hydrocarbons 0.664%. Bot. 5 oz. Box 6s.
Use: Control of lice, louse, fleas on bedding, furniture, etc. (Not to be used on humans or animals).

LIBCO-12 INJECTION. (Blue Line) Liver injection 2.0 mcg., Vit. B-12, crystalline 15.0 mcg., iron peptonate 23.0 mg., Vit. B-1 10.0 mg., B-2 0.5 mg., B-6 1.0 mg., Ca pantothenate 1.0 mg., niacinamide 10.0 mg., phenol 0.5%, benzyl alcohol 2.0%, sodium citrate 1.0%/cc. 10 cc.

LIBIDINAL. (Everett) Vit. E 400 I.U., zinc gluconate 150 mg./Cap. Bot. 60s.
Use: Dietary supplement.

LIBIGEN 10,000 AND DILUENT. (Savage) Chorionic gonadotropin 1,000 I.U./cc. Vials 10 cc. with 10 cc. diluent.

LIBRAX. (Roche) Clidinium bromide (Quarzan) 2.5 mg., chlordiazepoxide HCl (Librium) 5 mg./Cap. Bot. 100s, 500s. Prescription Pak. 50s. Teledose 100s (10 strips of 10).
Use: Gastrointestinal disorders.

LIBRITABS. (Roche) Chlordiazepoxide 5 mg., 10 mg., 25 mg./Tab. Bot. 100s, 500s.
Use: Relief of anxiety, tension, withdrawal symptoms of acute alcoholism.

LIBRIUM. (Roche) Chlordiazepoxide, HCl 5 mg., 10 mg. or 25 mg./Cap. Bot. 100s, 500s; Prescription Pak. 50s; Teledose (10 strips of 10; 4 rolls of 25) in RNP (Reverse Numbered Package); Amp. 100 mg., 10s.
Use: Relief of anxiety, apprehensions and nervous tension, withdrawal symptoms of acute alcoholism.

LIBRIUM INJECTABLE. (Roche) Chlordiazepoxide HCl 100 mg./Dry filled Amp. Special I.M. Diluent, 2 ml. for I.M. benzyl alcohol 1.5%, polysorbate 80 4%, propylene glycol 20%, w/maleic acid and

sodium hydroxide to adjust pH to 3. Amp. 5 ml.,
Box 10s.
Use: Relief of anxiety and tension, withdrawal
symptoms of acute alcoholism.

LICOPLEX. (Mills) Desiccated whole bile 2 gr., dried
whole pancreatic substance ¾ gr., dl-methionine 2
gr., choline bitartrate 3 gr./Tab. Bot. 100s.
Use: Bile laxative and cholagogue.

LICOPLEX DS. (Keene) Cyanocobalamin 15 mcg.,
liver inj. equiv. to cyanocobalamin activity 1 mcg.,
ferrous gluconate 25 mg., riboflavin 0.75 mg.,
calcium pantothenate 1.25 mg., niacinamide 50 mg.
Vial 30 ml.
Use: Multivitamin.

• **LICRYFILCON A.** USAN.
Use: Contact lens material.

• **LICRYFILCON B.** USAN.
Use: Contact lens material.

LIDA-MANTLE CREME. (Miles Pharm) Lidocaine 3% in
vehicle buffered to the pH range of normal skin.
Tube 1 oz.
Use: Topical anesthetic.

• **LIDAMIDINE HYDROCHLORIDE.** USAN.
Use: Antiperistaltic.

LIDEX. (Syntex) Fluocinonide 0.05%. **Cream base:**
stearyl alcohol, polyethylene glycol 8000, propylene
glycol, 1,2,6-hexanetriol, citric acid. **Ointment base:**
Amerchol CAB, white petrolatum, propylene
carbonate, propylene glycol. Cream, Ointment.
Tube 15 Gm., 30 Gm., 60 Gm., 120 Gm.
Use: Topical steriod.

LIDEX-E. (Syntex) Fluocinonide 0.05% in aqueous
emollient base of stearyl alcohol, cetyl alcohol,
mineral oil, propylene glycol, sorbitan
monostearate, polysorbate 60, citric acid, purified
water. Tube 15 Gm., 30 Gm., 60 Gm., 120 Gm.
Use: Topical steroid.

• **LIDOCAINE,** U.S.P. XXI. Oint., Oral Topical Sol.,
Sterile, Topical Aerosol, U.S.P. XXI. 2-Diethylamino-
2',6'-acetoxylidide. Acetamide, 2-(diethylamino)-N-
(2,6-dimethylphenyl)-
Use: Local anesthetic.

• **LIDOCAINE HYDROCHLORIDE,** U.S.P. XXI. Inj.,
Jelly, Topical Sol., U.S.P. XXI. Acetamide, 2-
(diethylamino)-N-(2,6-dimethylphenyl)-, HCl. 2-Die-
thylamino-2',6'-acetoxylidide HCl.
Use: Cardiac depressant (anti-arrhythmic); local anesthetic.
(Abbott) **0.2%, 0.4% or 0.8%:** w/5% Dextrose. 250
ml. single-dose containers; **1% or 2%.** Abboject syringes 5 ml.; 1 Gm, 2 Gm. Vial. Premixed: 0.2%,
0.4% in 5% dextrose inj./500 ml. Flex. or glass
containers. **1%:** 2 ml. or 5 ml. single-dose amp. **1.5%:**
20 ml. single-dose amp. **2%:** 10 ml./20 ml. vial (for
dilution to prepare I.V. drip soln.) **5%:** w/ 7.5%
Dextrose amp. 2 ml.
(CMC) 1%, 2%. Vial 50 cc.
(Maurry) 2%. Vial.
(Pharmex) 1%, 2%. Vial 50 cc.
Use; Injection for infiltration block anesthesia and
I.V. drip for cardiac arrhythmias.

See: Anestacon, Liq. (Webcon)
   Ardecaine 1%, 2%, Inj. (Burgin-Arden)
   Dolicaine, I.M. (Reid-Provident)
   L-Caine, Inj., Liq. (Century)
   Nervocaine, Inj. (Keene)
   Norocaine, Inj. (Vortech)
   Rocaine, Inj. (Rocky Mtn.)
   Stanacaine (Standex)
   T-CAIN, Inj. (Tunex)
   Xylocaine Hydrochloride, Prep. (Astra)
W/Benzalkonium chloride.
   See: Medi-Quik, Aerosol (Lehn & Fink)
      Medi-Quick Pump Spray (Lehn & Fink)
W/Benzalkonium chloride, phenol, menthol, eugenol,
   oil thyme, oil eucalyptus.
   See: Unguentine Spray (Norwich)
W/Cetyltrimethylammonium bromide,
   hexachlorophene.
   See: Aerosept, Aerosol (Dalin)
W/Hydrocortisone, clioquinol.
   See: Bafil, Lot. (Scruggs)
      Hil-20 Lotion (Reid-Provident)
W/Dextrose.
   See: Xylocaine HCl for Spinal Anesthesia, Amp.
      (Astra)
W/Epinephrine.
   See: L-Caine E, Vial (Century)
      Norocaine 1%, 2% w/Epinephrine. (Vortech)
      Xylocaine W/Epinephrine, Sol. (Astra)
W/Methylparaben, sodium chloride.
   See: Nulicaine, Vial (Kay)
W/Methyl parasept.
   See: L-Caine, Inj. (Century)
W/Methyl parasept, epinephrine.
   See: L-Caine-E, Inj. (Century)
W/Orthohydroxyphenyl mercuric chloride, menthol,
   camphor, allantoin.
   See: Kip First Aid preps. (Youngs Drug)
W/Parachlorometaxylenol, phenol, zinc oxide.
   See: Unguentine Plus, Cream (Norwich)
W/Polymyxin B sulfate.
   See: Lidosporin, Otic Soln. (Burroughs-Wellcome)
W/Testosterone, estrone, liver inj., niacinamide,
   panthenol, Vit. B complex.

• **LIDOCAINE HYDROCHLORIDE AND DEXTROSE
INJECTION,** U.S.P. XXI.

• **LIDOCAINE HYDROCHLORIDE AND
EPINEPHRINE BITARTRATE. INJECTION,** U.S.P.
XXI.

• **LIDOCAINE HYDROCHLORIDE AND
EPINEPHRINE INJECTION,** U.S.P. XXI.

• **LIDOFENIN.** USAN.
Use: Diagnostic aid.

• **LIDOFILCON A.** USAN.
Use: Contact lens material.

• **LIDOFILCON B.** USAN.
Use: Contact lens material.

• **LIDOFLAZINE.** USAN. 4-[4,4-bis(p-Fluro-phenyl)-
butyl]-1-piperazineaceto-2',6'-xylidide. 4-[3-(4,4'-Di-
fluorobenzhydryl)propyl]piperazin-1-ylacet-2',6'-
xylidide.
Use: Cardiovascular agent.

LIDOJECT-1. (Mayrand) Lidocaine HCl 1%. Vial 50 ml.
Use: Local anesthetic.

LIDOJECT-2. (Mayrand) Lidocaine HCl 2%. Vial 50 ml.
Use: Local anesthetic.

LIDOXIDE. (Interstate) Chlordiazepoxide HCl 5 mg., clidinium bromide 2.5 mg./Tab. Bot. 100s, 500s.
Use: Gastrointestinal disorders.

LIFE PLEX. (Burgin-Arden) Vit. B-12 5 mcg., liver fraction 1 300 mg., B-1 20 mg., B-2 5 mg., B-6 1 mg., panthenol 5 mg., niacinamide 100 mg., inositol 100 mg., choline 100 mg., l-lysine 100 mg., betaine 100 mg., iron 10 mg./30 cc. alcohol 12%. Bot. pt.
Use: Multivitamin with iron.

LIFER-B. (Burgin-Arden) Cyanocobalamin 30 mcg., liver inj. 0.1 cc., ferrous gluconate 100 mg., riboflavin 1.5 mg., panthenol 2.5 mg., niacinamide 100 mg., citric acid 16.4 mg., sodium citrate 23.6 mg./cc. Vial 30 cc.

LIFE SPANNER. (Spanner) Vit. A 12,500 I.U., D 400 I.U., E 5 I.U., B-1 10 mg., B-2 5 mg., B-6 2 mg., B-12 5 mcg., niacinamide 50 mg., Ca pantothenate 10 mg., biotin 10 mcg., C 100 mg., hesperidin complex 10 mg., rutin 20 mg., choline bitartrate 40 mg., inositol 30 mg., betaine anhydrous 15 mg., l-lysine monohydrochloride 25 mg., Fe 30 mg., Cu 1 mg., Mn 1 mg., K 5 mg., Ca 105 mg., P 82 mg., Mg 5.56 mg., Zn 1 mg./Cap. Bot. 100s.
Use: Nutritional supplement.

• **LIFIBRATE.** USAN.
Use: Antihyperlipoproteinemic.

LIFOCORT-100. (Hauck) Hydrocortisone sodium succinate 100 mg./Mono-mix vial. Vial 2 ml.
Use: Glucocorticoid.

LIF-O-GEN. (Lif-O-Gen) Oxygen 24 L., 58 L., 100 L., 220 L. at 400 p.s.i.g. & 2265 p.s.i. (70° F.) Unit complete with disposable mask. Refill for Model 400.
Use: First-aid treatment; emergency oxygen treatment.

LIFOJECT. (Mayrand) Liver, folic acid, Vit. B-12. Vial 10 ml.

LIFOL-B. (Burgin-Arden) Liver Inj. 10 mcg., folic acid 1 mg., cyanocobalamin 100 mcg., phenol 0.5%/cc. Vial 10 cc.

LIFOLBEX. (Central) Cyanocobalamin 100 mcg., folic acid 1.0 mg., liver inj. 0.5 ml./ml. w/phenol 0.5%. Vial 10 cc. Box 12s.
Use: Triple antimacrocytic-anemia preparation.

LIFOLEX. (Pasadena Research) Liver inj. 10 mcg., cyanocobalamin 100 mcg., folic acid 5 mg./cc. Vial 10 cc.

LIFOMIN. (Kay) Liver, beef (equiv. to cyanocobalamin 10 mcg.), folic acid 10 mg., B-12 crystalline 100 mcg., phenol 0.5%/ cc. Multiple dose sterile vial 10 cc.

LIGNOCAINE. B.A.N. N-(Diethylaminoacetyl)-2,6-xylidine. Duncaine; Lidothesin; Lignostab; Xylocaine; Xylotox.
Use: Local anesthetic.
See: Lidocaine, Oint. U.S.P. XXI. (Various Mfr.)

LILLY BULK PRODUCTS. (Lilly) The following products are supplied by Eli Lilly under the U.S.P., N.F. or chemical name as a service to the health professions:
Ammoniated Mercury Ointment
Amyl Nitrite
Analgesic Balm
Apomorphine Hydrochloride
Aromatic Elixir
Aromatic Ammonia
Aromatic Cascara
Atropine Sulfate
Bacitracin Ointment
Belladonna Extract, Tablets
Belladonna Tincture
Benzoin
Boric Acid
Calcium Gluceptate
Calcium Gluconate
Calcium Gluconate with Vitamin D
Calcium Hydroxide
Calcium Lactate
Carbarsone
Cascara, Aromatic, Fluidextract
Cascara Sagrada Fluidextract
Citrated Caffeine
Cocaine Hydrochloride
Codeine Phosphate
Codeine Sulfate
Colchicine
Compound Benzoin
Dibasic Calcium Phosphate
Diethylstilbestrol
Ephedrine Sulfate
Ferrous Gluconate
Ferrous Sulfate
Folic Acid
Glucagon for Injection
Green Soap Tincture
Heparin Sodium
Histamine Phosphate
Ipecac
Isoniazid
Isopropyl Alcohol, 91%
Liver, Vials for Injection
Magnesium Sulfate
Mercuric Oxide, Yellow
Methadone Hydrochloride
Methenamine and Sodium Biphosphate
Methenamine for Timed Burning
Methytestosterone
Milk of Bismuth
Morphine Sulfate
Mumps Skin Test Antigen
Myrrh
Neomycin Sulfate
Niacin
Niacinamide
Nitroglycerin
Opium (Deodorized)
Ox Bile Extract
Pancreatin
Papaverine Hydrochloride
Paregoric

Penicillin G Potassium
Phenobarbital
Phenobarbital Sodium
Potassium Chloride
Potassium Iodide
Powder Papers (Glassine)
Progesterone
Propylthiouracil
Protamine Sulfate
Pyridoxine Hydrochloride
Quinidine Gluconate
Quinidine Sulfate
Quinine Sulfate
Reserpine
Riboflavin
Silver Nitrate
Sodium Bicarbonate
Sodium Chloride
Sodium Iodide
Sodium Salicylate
Streptomycin Sulfate
Sulfadiazine
Sulfapyridine
Sulfur
Terpin Hydrate
Terpin Hydrate and Codeine
Testosterone Propionate
Thiamine Hydrochloride
Thyroid
Tubocurarine Chloride
Tylosterone
Whitfield's Ointment
Wild Cherry Syrup
Zinc Oxide
Zinc Oxide Paste
LIMARSOL.
See: Acetarsone (City Chemical)
LIMBITROL 5-12.5. (Roche) Chlordiazepoxide 5 mg.,
amitriptyline HCl 12.5 mg./Tab. Bot. 100s, 500s.
Tel-E-Dose 100s. Prescription paks 50s. Rolls (4
rolls of 25).
Use: Treatment of moderate to severe depression
associated with anxiety.
LIMBITROL 10-25. (Roche) Chlordiazepoxide 10 mg.,
amitriptyline HCl 25 mg./Tab. Bot. 100s, 500s.
Tel-E-Dose 100s. Prescription paks 50s. Rolls (4
rolls of 25).
Use: Treatment of moderate to severe depression
associated with anxiety.
LIMBO. (Eckerd) All-purpose liniment for sore muscles.
Bot. 4 oz.
• **LIME,** U.S.P. XXI.
Use: Pharmaceutical necessity.
• **LIME SOLUTION, SULFURATED,** U.S.P. XXI.
Use: Scabicide.
LIME SULFUR SOLUTION. Calcium polysulfide and
calcium thiosulfate.
Use: Scabicide.
See: Vlem-Dome, Liq. Conc. (Miles Pharm)
LIMIT. (Bock) Phendimetrazine tartrate 35 mg./Tab.
Bot. 100s, 500s.
Use: Obesity.

LINCOCIN. (Upjohn) Lincomycin HCl 500 mg./Cap.
Bot. 24s, 100s. **Pediatric.** 250 mg./Cap. Bot. 24s.
Use: Antibiotic against *staphylococci, streptococci,
pneumococci.*
LINCOCIN STERILE SOLUTION. (Upjohn)
Lincomycin HCl equiv. to 300 mg. lincomycin base,
benzyl alcohol 9.45 mg./ml. Lincomycin HCl 600
mg., benzyl alcohol 9.45 mg./ml. Vials 2 ml., 10 ml.
U-Ject. 2 ml. in 5s, 25s, 100s.
Use: Treatment of serious infections.
LINODIL CAPSULES. (Winthrop Products) Inositol
hexanicotinate.
Use: Hypolipedemic, peripheral vasodilator.
• **LINOGLIRIDE FUMARATE.** USAN.
Use: Antidiabetic.
• **LINCOMYCIN.** USAN. Antibiotic produced by
Streptomyces lincolnensis. Methyl 6,8-Di-deoxy-6-
(1-methyl-4-propyl-L-2-pyrrolidine-carboxamido)-1-
thio-D-Erythro-α-D-galacto-octopyranoside.
Use: Antiobiotic-infections due to gram positive or-
ganisms.
• **LINCOMYCIN HYDROCHLORIDE,** U.S.P. XXI. Inj.,
Cap., Sterile, Syrup, U.S.P. XXI. D-erythro-α-D-galac-
to-Octopyranoside, methyl-6,8-dideoxy-6-[[1-methyl-
4-propyl-2-pyrrolidinyl)carbonyl]amino]-1-thio, HCl.
Use: Antibacterial.
See: Lincocin, Cap., Sol., Syr. (Upjohn)
• **LINDANE,** U.S.P. XXI. Cream, Lot., Shampoo,
U.S.P. XXI. Gamma-benzene-hexachloride, hexa-
chlorocyclohexane.
Fidelity Lab.—Pow. 50%, Pkg. 1 lb., 5 lb.
Imperial—Pow. 50%, Pkg. 1 lb., 4 lb.; 12%, Pkg. 1
lb., 4 lb.
Use: Pediculicide, scabicide.
See: Kwell, Cream, Lot. & Shampoo (Reed &
Carnrick)
LINDORA. (Westwood) Sodium laureth sulfate, water,
cocamide DEA, NaCl, lactic acid, tetra sodium
EDTA, benzophenone-4, FD&C Blue #1 and fra-
grance. Bot. 8 oz.
Use: Soap free lathering cleanser for sensitive skin.
LINIMENTO NO. 1. (D'Franssia)
Use: Arthritis, rheumatism cold aid.
LINOLENIC ACID W/VIT. E.
See: Petropin, Cap. (Lannett)
LINOLESTROL. (Vortech) Jar. 1 oz., 16 oz.
Use: Allergic skin conditions.
LINUCEE TABLETS. (Fellows) Vit. B-1 15 mg., B-2 10
mg., B-6 10 mg., nicotinic acid 100 mg., pantholate 25
mg., B-12 10 mcg., biotin 50 mcg./Tab. Bot. 100s.
LIORESAL. (Geigy) Baclofen 10 mg. or 20 mg./Tab.
Bot. 100s. Unit Dose 100s.
Use: Muscle relaxant, antispasmodic.
LIOTHYRONINE. B.A.N. 3-[4-(4-Hydroxy-3-iodo-
phenoxy)-3,5-di-iodophenyl]- -alanine. (—)-Tri-iodo-
thyronine. Cynomel and Tertroxin sodium derivative.
Use: Thyroid hormone.
• **LIOTHYRONINE I-125.** USAN.
Use: Radioactive agent.
• **LIOTHYRONINE I-131.** USAN.
Use: Radioactive agent.

LIOTHYRONINE RESIN.
- **LIOTHYRONINE SODIUM,** U.S.P. XXI., Tabs. U.S.P. XXI. L-Tyrosine, 0-(4-hydroxy-3-iodophenyl)-3,5-dii-odo-, sod. salt. Sod. L-triiodo-thyronine. Sod. L-4-(3-iodo-4-hydroxphenoxy)-3,5-diiodo-phenylalanine.
  Use: Thyroid hormone.
  See: Cytomel, Tab. (SmithKline)
- **LIOTRIX,** U.S.P. XXI. A combination of sod. levothyroxine & sod. 1-triiodothyronine in a ratio of 4 to 1 by weight.
  Use: Thyroid hormone.
  See: Euthroid, Tab. (Parke-Davis)
  Thyrolar, Tab. (Armour)

LIPASE. W/Amylase, Protease.
  Use: Digestive enzyme.
  W/Amylase, bile salts, wilzyme, pepsin, pancreatin, calcium.
  See: Enzyme, Tab. (Barth's)
  W/Amylase, protease, cellase, hyoscine HBr,
  See: Am-Zyme, Tab. (Vortech)
  W/Amylase, protease, simethicone.
  See: Tri-Cone, Cap. (Meyer)
  W/Alpha-amylase W-100, proteinase W-300, cellase W-100, estrone, testosterone, vitamins, minerals.
  See: Geramine, Tab. (Brown)
  W/Alpha-Amylase, proteinasa, cellase
  See: Kutrase (Kremers-Urban)
  Ku-Zyme (Kremers-Urban)
  W/Amylolytic, proteolytic, cellulolytic enzymes.
  See: Arco-Lase, Tab. (Arco)
  W/Amylolytic, proteolytic, cellulolytic enzymes, phenobarbital, hyoscyamine sulf., atropine sulf.
  See: Arco-Lase Plus, Tab. (Arco)
  W/Pancreatin, protease, amylase.
  See: Dizymes, Caps. (Recsei)
  W/Pepsin, homatropine methyl Br, amylase, protease, bile salts.
  See: Digesplen, Tab., Elix., Drops (Med. Prod. Panamericana)

LIPKOTE. (Plough) Homosalate, petrolatum in ointment base. Unflavored, mint, grape, cherry. Tube 0.14 oz.
  Use: Ultraviolet sunscreen lip balm.

LIPKOTE SPF 15 ULTRA SUNSCREEN LIPBALM. (Plough) Tube 0.15 oz.
  Use: Ultraviolet sunscreen.

LIPOCHOLINE. See: Choline dihydrogen citrate. (Various Mfr.)

LIPODERM. (Spirt) Pancreas, whole hog 500 mg., Vit. B-6 3 mg., Cap. Bot. 180s, 500s.
  Use: Orally, treatment of psoriasis.

LIPOFLAVANOID CAPSULES. (CooperVision) Choline, inositol, B-1, B-2, niacinamide, pantothenic acid, B-6, B-12, C, lemon bioflavonoid complex./Cap. Bot. 100s, 500s.
  Use: Vitamin supplement.

LIPO GANTRISIN. (Roche) Acetyl Sulfisoxazole 1 Gm./5 ml. in a palatable, readily digestible vegetable oil emulsion. Bot. 16 oz.
  Use: Systemic and urinary tract infections.

LIPO-HEPIN. (Riker) Heparin sodium injection, U.S.P.

aqueous derived from porcine intestial mucosa. Amp, Vial
  Use: Anticoagulant.

LIPO-HEPIN/BL. (Riker) Heparin sodium injection, U.S.P. aqueous. Derived from beef lung. Amp. Vial.
  Use: Anticoagulant.

LIPO-K CAPSULES. (Marcen) Epinephrine-neutralizing factor 25 u., pancreatic lipotropic factor 1.2 mg., Cy-mucopolysaccharides 2.5 mg., choline bitartrate 100 mg., dl-methionine 50 mg., inositol 25 mg., bile extract 5 mg./Cap. Bot. 100s, 500s, 1000s.
  Use: Treatment of circulatory disturbances.

LIPO-K INJECTABLE. (Marcen) Pancreatic lipotropic factor 1.2 mg., epinephrine-neutralizing factor 25 u., Cy-mucopolysaccharides 0.5 mg., sod. citrate 10 mg., inositol 5 mg., phenol 0.5%/cc. multidose vials 10 cc., 30 cc.
  Use: Treatment of circulatory disturbances.

LIPOLYTIC ENZYME.
  W/Proteolytic enzyme, amylolytic enzyme, cellulolytic enzyme, methyl polysiloxane, ox bile, betaine HCl.
  See: Zymme, Cap. (Scrip)

LIPOMUL. (Upjohn) Corn oil 10 Gm./15 ml. w/d-Alpha tocopheryl acetate, butylated hydroxy-anisole, poly-sorbate 80, glyceride phosphates, sod. saccharin, sod. benzoate 0.05%, benzoic acid 0.05%, sorbic acid 0.07%. Bot. pt.
  Use: Underweight in the malnourished.

LIPO-NICIN/100 mg. (Brown) Nicotinic acid 100 mg., niacinamide 75 mg., Vit. C 150 mg., B-1 25 mg., B-2 2 mg., B-6 10 mg./Tab. Bot. 100s, 500s.
  Use: Vasodilator, peripheral.

LIPO-NICIN/250 mg. (Brown) Nicotinic acid 250 mg., niacinamide 75 mg., Vit. C 150 mg., B-1 25 mg., B-2 2 mg., B-6 10 mg./Tab. Bot. 100s, 500s.

LIPO-NICIN/300 mg. Timed Caps. (Brown) Nicotinic acid 300 mg., Vit. C 150 mg., B-1 25 mg., B-2 2 mg., B-6 10 mg./T.R. Cap. Bot. 100s, 500s.

LIPOSYN. (Abbott) Intravenous fat emulsion containing safflower oil 10%, egg phosphatides 1.2%, glycerin 2.5% in water for injection. **10%:** Single-dose containers 50 ml., 100 ml., 200 ml., or 500 ml. Syringe Pump Unit 50 ml. single-dose. **20%:** Single-dose containers 200 ml. or 500 ml. Syringe Pump Unit 25 ml. or 50 ml. single-dose.
  Use: Parenteral source of essential fatty acids; parenteral nutrition.

LIPOTIN. (Galen) Ferric ammonium citrate 500 mg., Vit. B-1 12 mg., B-2 6 mg., B-6 0.6 mg., folic acid 0.5 mg., Ca pantothenate 6 mg., niacinamide 15 mg., Mg 2 mg., Mn 1 mg., Co 0.1 mg., Zn 2 mg., choline 100 mg., inositol 100 mg., alcohol 12%/fl. oz. Bot. pt.

LIPOTIN TABLETS. (Galen) Choline bitartrate 83.3 mg., dl-methionine 50 mg., inositol 33.3 mg., whole desic. liver 33.3 mg., B-cotrate 33.3 mg., Vit. B-1 0.5 mg., B-2 0.3 mg., B-6 0.03 mg., d-calcium pantothenate 1.6 mg., niacinamide 5 mg./Tab. Bot. 100s, 1000s.

LIPOTRIAD CAPSULES. (CooperVision) Vit. B-1, B-2, B-6, B-12, niacin, choline, pantothenic acid, inositol. See label strength. Bot. 100s, 1000s.

Use: Vitamin supplement.

LIPOTRIAD LIQUID. (CooperVision) Vit. B-1, B-6, B-12, niacin, choline, pantothenic acid, inositol, niacinamide. See label strength. Bot. 16 oz.
Use: Vitamin supplement.

■ **LIPOTROPIC AGENTS.**
See: Betaine Products (Var. Mfr.)
Choline Products (Various Mfr.)
Cho-Meth, Vial (Med. Chem.)
Cytellin, Susp. (Lilly)
Inositol Products (Various Mfr.)
Lecithin Products (Various Mfr.)
Methionine Products (Various Mfr.)

LIPOZYME TABLETS. (Inwood) Choline, methionine, and inositol 1 Gm. total/Tab. Bot. 100s.
Use: Reduction of blood cholesterol level.

LIPPES LOOP. (Ortho) Intrauterine double-S. Sizes A, B, C, D.
Use: Contraceptive.

LIQUAEMIN SODIUM. (Organon) Heparin sod. aq. sol. **Vial** (20,000 u./ml.) 1 ml., 2 ml., 5 ml. 1 ml.; (5,000 u./ml.) 1 ml., 10 ml.; (10,000 u./ml.) 1 ml., 4 ml.; (1000 u./ml.) 10 ml., 30 ml., Box 25s. (40,000 u./ml.) .
Use: I.V., Sub. Q.: Anticoagulant.

LIQUAMAR. (Organon) Phenprocoumon 3 mg./Tab. Bot. 100s.
Use: Anticoagulant.

LIQUID ANTIDOSE. (U.S. Products) Liquid activated charcoal 40 Gm./200 ml. of suspension.
Dispensing jar.
Use: Poison antidote.

LIQUID LUBRICATING JELLY. (Paddock) Boric acid, glycerine, propylene glycol, methylparaben, propylparaben, irish moss ext., methylcellulose. Bot. 4 oz., 16 oz.

LIQUI-DOSS. (Ferndale) Docusate sodium 60 mg., mineral oil. Bot. pt.
Use: Stool softener.

LIQUID LATHER. (Ulmer) Gentle wash for hands, body face, hair. Bot. 8 oz., Gal.
Use: Cleanser.

LIQUID PETROLATUM EMULSION.
See: Mineral Oil Emulsion, U.S.P. XXI.

LIQUID PRED. (Muro) Prednisone 5 mg./5 ml. Bot. 120 ml., 240 ml.
Use: Anti-inflammatory effects in allergic states.

LIQUIFILM FORTE. (Allergan) Enhanced artificial tears w/polyvinyl alcohol 3%, thimerosal 0.002%, edetate disodium in a buffered sterile, isotonic solution. Bot. 0.5 fl. oz., 1 fl. oz.
Use: Artificial tears.

LIQUIFILM TEARS. (Allergan) Polyvinyl alcohol 1.4%, chlorobutanol 0.5% w/sod. chloride and purified water. Bot. 15 ml., 30 ml.

LIQUIFILM WETTING SOLUTION. (Allergan) Polyvinyl alcohol, hydroxypropyl methylcellulose, edetate disodium, NaCl, KCl and benzalkonium chloride. Bot. 20 ml., 60 ml.
Use: Hard contact lens wetting solution.

LIQUIMAT. (Owen) Sulfur 5%, alcohol 22%, in drying make-up base. Plastic Bot. 1.5 oz. 5 Shades.

Use: Medicated cover-up for pimples, oily skin & acne.

LIQUI-NOX. (Alconox) 1 qt., 1 gal.
Use: Optimum combination of anionic and nonionic detergents and wetting agents.

LIQUIPRIN. (Norcliff Thayer) Acetaminophen 80 mg./1.66 ml. Solution. Bot. 35 ml. w/dropper.
Use: Analgesic; antipyretic.

LIQUOID BLOOD CULTURE BOTTLE. (Roche) Sodium polyanethol sulfonate, tryptic soy broth. Bot. 12 × 45 ml.
Use: Diagnostic agent.

LIQUOPHYLLINE. (Paddock) Theophylline 80 mg., alcohol 20%/15 ml. Bot. pt., ½ gal., gal.
Use: Asthma.

LIQUOR CARBONIS DETERGENS.
See: Coal Tar Topical Soln., U.S.P. XXI. (Various Mfr.)

LIRON B-12 1000. (Kenyon) Vit. B-12 1000 mcg., liver 2 mcg., iron peptonate 20 mg., cobalt Cl 0.2 mg., Vit. B-1 10 mg., B-6 1 mg., B-2 1 mg./cc. Vial 10 cc.

LIRON B-12 50. (Kenyon) Same formula as Liron B-12 1000, except B-12 50 mg./cc. Vial 10 cc.

LISACORT. (Fellows) Prednisone 5 mg./Tab. Bot. 100s, 1000s, 5000s.
Use: Rheumatoid arthritis and other rheumatic disorders.

• **LISINOPRIL.** USAN.

LISIUM HYDROCHLORIDE. Chlorhexidine, B.A.N.

LISTEREX SCRUB MEDICATED LOTION. (Warner-Lambert) Salicylic acid 2% lotion. Golden & Herbal. Bot. 4 oz., 8 oz.
Use: Acne cleansing scrub.

LISTERINE ANTISEPTIC. (Warner-Lambert) Thymol, eucalyptol, methyl salicylate, menthol. Bot. 3 oz., 6 oz., 12 oz., 18 oz., 24 oz., 32 oz.
Use: Oral antiseptic.

LISTERINE ANTISEPTIC THROAT LOZENGES. (Warner-Lambert) Hexylresorcinol 2.4 mg./Loz. Regular and lemon-mint flavors. Boxes 24s.
Use: Relieve minor sore throat pain.

LISTERMINT WITH FLUORIDE. (Warner-Lambert) Sodium fluoride 0.02% w/water, alcohol, glycerin, poloxamer 407, sodium lauryl sulfate, sodium citrate, sodium saccharine, ZN chloride, citric acid, flavors and colors. Bot. 6 oz., 12 oz., 18 oz., 24 oz., 32 oz.
Use: Anticavity dental rinse & mouthwash.

LITHANE. (Miles Pharm) Lithium carbonate 300 mg./Tab. Bot. 100s, 1000s.
Use: Manic-depressive illness.

• **LITHIUM CARBONATE,** U.S.P. XXI. Cap., Tab.
U.S.P. XXI. Carbonic acid, dilithium salt.
Use: Antidepressant.
See: Eskalith, Cap., Tab. (SmithKline)
Lithane, Tab. (Miles Pharm)
Lithobid, Tab. (Ciba)
Lithotabs, Tab. (Rowell)

LITHIUM CARBONATE CAPSULES. (Roxane) Lithium carbonate 300 mg./Cap. Bot. 100s, 1000s.
Use: Control of manic episodes in manic-depressive psychosis.

• **LITHIUM CITRATE,** U.S.P. XXI. Syrup U.S.P. XXI. CH$_2$ (COO Li) C (OH)(COOLi) CH$_2$ COO Li.x. H$_2$O.C$_6$H$_5$Li$_3$O$_7$
Use: Manic-depressive states.
See: Cibalith-SiLiq. (Ciba)
   Lithonate-S, Liq. (Rowell)

• **LITHIUM HYDROXIDE,** U.S.P. XXI. LiOH.x.H$_2$O. Lithium hydroxide monohydrate.
Use: Manic-depressive states.

LITHOBID. (Ciba) Lithium carbonate 300 mg./Tab. (slow release). Bot. 100s, 1000s. Unit Dose 100s.
Use: Manic depressive states.

LITHONATE. (Rowell) Lithium carbonate 300 mg./Cap. Bot. 100s, 1000s. Unit dose 100s.
Use: Control of manic episodes in manic-depressive psychosis.

LITHOSTAT. (Mission) Acetohydroxamic acid 250 mg./Tab. Bot. 120s.
Use: Urease inhibitor.

LITHOTABS. (Rowell) Lithium carbonate 300 mg./Tab. Bot. 100s, 1000s.
Use: Control of manic episodes in manic-depressive psychosis.

LIVA. (Vortech) Ferrous gluconate 50 mg., citric acid 8.2 mg., sod. citrate 11.8 mg., Vit. B-2 0.75 mg., niacinamide 50 mg., Ca pantothenate 1.25 mg., liver inj. 0.05 cc. (Vit. B-12 activity 1 mcg.), dl-methionine 5 mg., l-cysteine HCl 0.5 mg., procaine HCl 2%, benzyl alcohol 2%, cyanocobalamin 15 mcg./cc. Vial 30 ml.
Use: Dietary supplement.

LIVEC. (Enzyme Process) Vit. A 5000 I.U., B-1 1.5 mg., B-2 1.7 mg., niacin 20 mg., C 60 mg., B-6 2 mg., pantothenic acid 10 mg., E 30 I.U., B-12 6 mcg., calcium 250 mg., iron 5 mg., D 400 I.U. folacin 0.075 mg./3 Tabs. Bot. 100s, 300s.
Use: Dietary supplement.

LIVER. (Lilly; CMC) Amp. inj. 2 mcg./ml. Bot. 10 ml., 2 mcg./ml. Bot. 30 ml., 10 mcg./ml. Bot. 10 ml., 20 mcg./ml. Bot. 10 ml.
See: Tonic 10 & 20. (Scrip)

LIVERBEX. (Spanner) Liver 2 mcg., B-1, B-2, B-6, B-12, niacinamide, pantothenate/cc. Vial 30 cc.

LIVER, B-12 AND FOLIC ACID. (Lincoln) Vit. B-12 activity 5 mcg., cyanocobalamin 35 mcg., cyanocobalamin 5 mg., folic acid, w/phenol 5%, sodium citrate 0.25%, disodium sequestrene 0.01%, sodium bisulfite 0.025%/cc. Vial 15 cc.

LIVER, B12 AND FOLIC ACID FORTE. (Lincoln) Vit. B-12 activity 10 mcg., cyanocobalamin 150 mcg., cyanocobalamin 10 mg., folic acid, w/phenol 0.5%, sodium citrate 0.5%, disodium sequestrene 0.01%, sodium bisulfite 0.05%/cc. Vial 15 cc.

LIVER, CRUDE. (Lilly) 2 mcg./ml. Vials 10 ml., 30 ml.; (Medwick) 2 mcg./cc. Vial 30 cc.; (Vortech) 2 mcg./cc. Vial 30 ml.
Use: General hematinic.

LIVER DESICCATED. Desic. liver substance.

LIVER EXTRACT. Dry liver ext. W/Vit. B-12 & folic acid.

LIVER-FOLIC ACID B-12. (Sandia; CMC) Vit. B-12 10 mcg., folic acid 10 mg., cyanocobalamin 100 mcg./cc. Vial 10 cc. (Medwick) Vit. B-12 10 mcg., folic

acid 1 mg., cyanocobalamin 100 mcg./cc. Vial 30 cc.

■ **LIVER FUNCTION AGENTS.**
See: Bromsulphalein, Amp. (Hynson, Westcott and Dunning)
   Iodophthalein (Various Mfr.)
   Sulfobromophthalein Sodium, Amp. U.S.P. XXI. (Gotham)

LIVERGRAN. (Rawl) Desiccated whole liver 9 Gm., Vit. B-1 18 mg., B-2 36 mg., niacinamide 90 mg., choline bitartrate 216 mg., B-6 3.6 mg., calcium pantothenate 3.6 mg., inositol 90 mg., biotin 6 mcg., Vit. B-12 5.4 mcg., methionine 198 mg., arginine 242 mg., cystine 72 mg., glutamic acid 675 mg., histidine 99 mg., isoleucine 333 mg., leucine 495 mg., lysine 297 mg., phenylalanine 189 mg., threonine 333 mg., tryptophan 45 mg., tyrosine 180 mg., valine 306 mg./3 Tsp. Bot. 15 oz.
Use: Nutritional supplement.

LIVER INJECTION. Liver ext. for parental use. (Various Mfr.)

LIVER INJECTION. (Arcum; Lederle) B-12 20 mcg./cc. Vial 10 cc.

LIVER-IRON-B COMPLEX WITH VITAMIN B-12. (Maurry) Liver inj. 2.0 mcg., B-12 15.0 mcg., ferrous gluconate 31.1 mg., B-1 10.0 mg., B-2 0.5 mg., B-6 1.0 mg., cal. pantothenate 1.0 mg., niacinamide 10.0 mg., d-Glucose 1.0%, chlorobutanol 0.5%, benzyl alcohol 2.0%/inj.
Use: Treat Vitamin B deficiencies and anemias.

LIVER, IRON, FOLIC & COBALT. (Kenyon) Liver refined (B-12 eqv.) 10 mcg., iron peptonate 59 mg., cobalt gluconate 9 mg., folic acid 5 mg., procaine HCl 1%/2 cc. Vial 30 cc.

LIVER IRON VITAMINS INJ. (Arcum) Liver inj. (10 mcg. B-12 Activity/cc.) 0.1 cc., crude liver inj. (2 mcg. B-12 Activity/cc.) 0.125 cc., green ferric ammonium citrate 20 mg., niacinamide 50 mg., Vit. B-6 0.3 mg., B-2 0.3 mg., procaine HCl 0.5%, phenol 0.5%/2 cc. Vial 30 cc.

LIVER, IRON, VITAMINS. (CMC) Liver (B-12 eqv.) 1.0 mcg., iron gluconate 59 mg., B-2 0.3 mg., B-6 0.3 mg., niacinamide 50 mg./2 cc. Vial 30 cc.

LIVER, IRON, VITAMINS. (Kenyon) Liver (B-12 eqv.) 1 mcg., iron gluconate 59 mg., niacinamide 50 mg., Vit. B-2 (as 5-phos.) 0.3 mg., B-6 0.3 mg., sod. dicitrate 10 mg./2 cc. procaine HCl 1% Vial 30 cc.

LIVER, IRON & VITAMINS. (Pharmex) Liver inj. (equiv. to 1 mcg. B-12) 100 mg., B-12 5 mcg., B-2 0.3 mg., B-6 0.3 mg., niacinamide 50 mg., iron peptonate 19.5 mg., sod. citrate 1%, phenol 0.5%/3 cc. Vial 30 cc.

LIVER, IRON, VITAMINS AND AMINO ACIDS. (Kenyon) Liver B-12 Eqv., 1 mcg., ferrous gluconate 50 mg., B-2 (as 5-phos.) 0.5 mg., d-panthenol 2.5 mg., niacinamide 100 mg., dl-methionine 10 mg., choline chloride 5 mg./2 cc. Vial 30 cc.

LIVER, IRON, VITAMINS WITH B-12. (CMC) Liver (B-12 eqv.) 2 mcg., B-12 15 mcg., ferrous gluconate 20 mg., B-1 10 mg., B-2 0.5 mg., B-6 1 mg., d-panthenol 1 mg., niacinamide 10 mg., choline chloride 20 mg./cc., procaine HCl 0.5% Vial 30 cc.

LIVER, IRON, VITAMINS WITH B-12. (Kenyon) Liver (B-12 eqv.) 2 mcg., Vit. B-12 15 mcg., ferrous lactate 20 mg., B-1 10 mg., B-2 (as 5-phos.) 9.5 mg., B-6 1 mg., d-panthenol 1 mg., niacinamide 10 mg., choline chloride 0.5 mg./cc. Vial 30 cc.

LIVER-P (PAINLESS). (Vortech) Vit. B-12 activity 2; mcg./cc. Vial 10 cc.

LIVER, RAW.
W/Duodenum.
See: Jayron, Pow., Cap. (VioBin)

LIVER, REFINED. (Medwick) 20 mcg./cc. Vial 10 cc., 30 cc.

LIVER VASOCONSTRICTOR.
See: Kutapressin, Vial, Amp. (Kremers-Urban)

LIV-FER-B. (Sutliff & Case) Liver fraction No. 1 0.6 Gm., ferrous gluconate 0.06 Gm., mang. gluconate 10 mg., copper gluconate 0.001 Gm., zinc sulfate 0.003 Gm., Vit. B-1 2 mg., B-2 2 mg., B-12 2 mcg., alcohol 12%
niacinamide 10 mg., sod. citrate 0.6 Gm./Fl. oz., alcohol 12%. Elix. 6 oz., 1 pt., 1 gal.
Use: Hematinic.

LIV-FER-BLEX. (Sutliff & Case) Ferrous gluconate 0.022 Gm., liver conc. 0.227 Gm., thiamine HCl 1 mg., riboflavin 1 mg., niacin 10 mg., brewer's yeast 0.194 Gm./Tab. Bot. 100s, 1000s.
Use: Iron-deficiency anemias.

LIVIFOL. (Dunhall) Vit. B-12 activity from liver inj. equivalent to cyanocobalamin 10 mcg., folic acid 1 mg., cyanocobalamin 100 mcg./ml. Vial 10 ml.
Use: Vitamin, iron supplement.

LIVIPAS. Halofenate, B.A.N.

LIVI-PLEX FORTIFIED. (Rocky Mtn.) Vit. B-12 30 mcg., liver inj. 1.0 cc., ferrous gluconate 50 mg., riboflavin 1.5 mg., calcium pantothenate 2.5 mg., niacinamide 100 mg., citric acid 16.4 mg., sodium citrate 23.6 mg., benzyl alcohol 2%, procaine HCl 2%/2 cc. Vial 30 cc.

LIVITAMIN. (Beecham Labs) Ferrous fumarate 100 mg., Vit. B-1 3 mg., B-2 3 mg., B-6 3 mg., C 100 mg., niacinamide 10 mg., Ca pantothenate 2 mg., B-12 5 mcg., Cu 0.66 mg., desic. liver 150 mg./Cap. Bot. 100s.
Use: Iron and vitamin deficiency anemias.

LIVITAMIN CHEWABLE TABLETS. (Beecham Labs) Ferrous fumarate 50 mg., Vit. C 100 mg., B-1 3 mg., B-2 3 mg., niacinamide 10 mg., B-6 3 mg., Ca pantothenate 2 mg., cyanocobalamin 5 mcg., copper 0.33 mg./Tab. Bot. 100s.
Use: Iron and vitamin supplement.

LIVITAMIN W/INTRINSIC FACTOR. (Beecham Labs) Desic. liver 150 mg., ferrous fumarate 100 mg., B-1 3 mg., C 100 mg., B-2 3 mg., niacinamide 10 mg., B-12 5 mcg., B-6 3 mg., Ca pantothenate 2 mg., Cu 0.66 mg., B-12 w/intrinsic factor ⅓ u./Cap. Bot. 100s.
Use: Pernicious anemia & geriatrics.

LIVITAMIN LIQUID. (Beecham Labs) Iron peptonized N.F. 210 mg., liver fraction No. 1 0.5 Gm., B-1 3 mg., B-2 3 mg., niacinamide 10 mg., B-6 HCl 3 mg., pantothenic acid 2 mg., Vit. B-12 5 mcg., Cu 0.66 mg./15 cc. Bot. 8 oz., 1 pt., 1 gal.
Use: General hematinic.

LIVITAMIN PRENATAL. (Beecham Labs) Vit. D 400 USP units, A 6000 USP units, B-1 3 mg., B-2 3 mg., niacinamide 20 mg., pantothenic acid 5 mg., B-6 10 mg., C 100 mg., B-12 5 mcg., folic acid 0.5 mg., calcium 350 mg., Iron as Fe fumarate 50 mg./Tab. Bot. 100s.

LIVITOL. (CMC) Vit. A 2500 I.U., D 250 I.U., B-12 3 mcg., C 37.5 mg., folic acid 0.5 mg., iron 15 mg., cobalt 0.1 mg., copper 0.25 mg., liver fr. 250 mg., liver pow. 25 mg., gastric mucosa 75 mg./Vial. Mixovial 10 cc.
Use: Anemias.

LIVITOL INJ. W/VIT. C, B-12, IRON. (CMC) Vit. B-1 20 mg., B-2 3 mg., B-6 5 mg., B-12 20 mcg., C 100 mg., d-panthenol 5 mg., cyanocobalamin 5 mcg., ferrous gluconate 25 mg./cc. Mixovial 10 cc.

LIV-O-VITE. (Jenkins) Ferrous fumarate 3 gr. (elemental iron 1 gr.), desiccated liver 2 gr., thiamine HCl 3 mg., riboflavin 3 mg., cyanocobalamin 3 mcg./Tab. Bot. 1000s.

LIV-O-REX. (Nutrition) Liver, desiccated 1.4 gr., green iron & ammonium citrate 3 gr., B-1 1.5 mg., B-2 0.5 mg., calcium pantothenate 0.25 mg., B-6 0.15 mg., niacinamide 10 mg./Cap. Bot. 100s, 1000s.

LIVOREX W/B-12. (Reid-Provident) Liver inj. N.F. 20 mcg., iron and ammonium citrate 60 mg., niacinamide 50 mg., B-2 0.3 mg., B-6 0.3 mg., B-12 5 mcg., procaine HCl 1%/2 cc. Vials 30 cc.

LIVREX. (CMC) Liver extracts. Vit. B-12 2 mcg., 10 mcg. 20 mcg./cc.

LIVREX-BB. (CMC) Vit. B-12 activity eqv. to 10 mcg. cyanocobalamin, B-12 5 mcg., B-1 5 mcg./cc.

LIVREX-BF. (CMC) Vit. B-12 activity eqv. to 2 mcg. cyanocobalamin, Vit. B-12 15 mcg., folic acid 5 mg./cc.

LIVREX-BF (5-5-25). (CMC) Cyanocobalamin 5 mcg., Vit. B-12 cryst. 25 mcg., folic acid 5 mg./cc.

LIVREX-BF (10-10-50). (CMC) Cyanocobalamin 10 mcg., Vit. B-12 50 mcg., folic acid 10 mg./cc.

LIVREX-BF (10-10-100). (CMC) Cyanocobalamin 10 mcg., B-12 100 mcg., folic acid 10 mg./cc.

LIVROBEN. (O'Neal, Jones & Feldman) Liver 10 mcg., folic acid 1 mg., cyanocobalamin 100 mcg./ml. Vial 10 ml.

LIVTRINSIC. (Vitarine) Liver-stomach concentrate 240 mg., Vit. B-12 15 mcg., iron 110 mg., Vit. C 75 mg./Cap.
Use: Hematinic.

LIXAMINOL ELIXIR. (Ferndale) Aminophylline 250 mg. with alcohol, 30% by volume/15 cc. Bot. pt.
Use: Coronary vasodilator, diuretic.

LIXOIL. (Lixoil Labs.) Sulfonated fatty oils and one or more esters of higher fatty acids. Bot. 16 oz.
Use: Dermatologic.

LKGB. (Image) Vitamins. Bot. 100s.
Use: Supplement.

LLD FACTOR.
See: Vitamin B-12, Prep. (Various Mfr.)

LMD. (Abbott) Low Molecular Weight Dextran. LMD 10% w/v in D5-W and LMD 10% w/v in Saline 0.9%, 500 ml. each.

Use: Enhancement of blood flow, plasma volume expander.

LMWD-DEXTRAN 40. (Pharmachem) Normal saline 0.9%, dextrose 10%.
Use: Plasma expander.

LOBAC. (Seatrace) Chlorzoxazone 250 mg., acetaminophen 300 mg./Cap. Bot. 40s, 100s, 1000s.
Use: Muscle relaxant, analgesic.

LOBANA BODY LOTION. (Ulmer) Bot. 4 oz., 8 oz., 1 gal.
Use: Skin lotion.

LOBANA BODY POWDER. (Ulmer) All purpose body powder. Pkg. 8 oz.

LOBANA BODY SHAMPOO. (Ulmer) Bot. 8 oz., Gal.
Use: Hair & body cleanser.

LOBANA CONDITIONING SHAMPOO. (Ulmer) Bot. 8 oz., Gal.
Use: Shampoo for hair and scalp.

LOBANA DERM-ADE CREAM. (Ulmer) Vitamin A, D, E cream. Jar 2 oz., 8 oz.
Use: Red, irritated skin problems.

LOBANA LIQUID HAND SOAP. (Ulmer) 14 oz. dispenser, 16 oz. refill. Bot. 1 gal.
Use: cleanser.

LOBANA PERI-GARD. (Ulmer) Water-resistant ointment containing vitamin A & D. Jar 2 oz., 8 oz.
Use: Protect the skin from urine, feces or drainage.

LOBANA PERINEAL CLEANSE. (Ulmer) 4 oz. sprayer. Bot. 1 gal.
Use: Urine, feces, vomit cleanse.

LOBELIA FLUIDEXTRACT.
W/Hyoscyamus fl. ext., grindelia fl. ext., pot. iodide.
See: L.S. Mixture, Liq. (Paddock)

LOBELINE SULFATE.
See: Lobidram, Tab. (Dram)
Nikoban, Loz., Gum. (Thompson)
No-Kotin, Tab. (Walker)

• **LOBENDAZOLE.** USAN.
Use: Anthelmintic.

LOBIDRAM. (Dram) Lobeline sulfate 2 mg./Tab. Pkg. 15s, 30s.
Use: Withdrawal symptoms of smoking.

LOCOID. (Owen) Hydrocortisone butyrate 0.1%. Tubes 15 Gm., 45 Gm.
Use: Topical anti-inflammatory.

LOCORTEN. (Ciba) Flumethasone pivalate 0.03% in water-washable cream base containing cetyl alcohol, sod. lauryl sulfate, propylene glycol, methyl- and propylparabens. Tube 15 Gm., 60 Gm.
Use: Anti-inflammatory, antipruritic.

• **LODOXAMIDE ETHYL.** USAN.
Use: Anti-asthmatic, anti-allergic.

• **LODOXAMIDE TROMETHAMINE.** USAN.
Use: Anti-asthmatic, anti-allergic.

LODRANE. (Poythress) Theophyllin anhydrous 130 mg. or 260 mg./S.R. Cap. Bot. 100s.
Use: Treatment of asthma.

LOESTRIN 21 1/20. (Parke-Davis) Norethindrone acetate 1 mg., ethinyl estradiol 20 mcg./white Tab. Petipac compacts 21 Tab.
Use: Oral contraceptive.

LOESTRIN 21 1.5/30. (Parke-Davis) Norethindrone acetate 1.5 mg., ethinyl estradiol 30 mcg./green Tab. Petipac compacts.
Use: Oral Contraceptive.

LOESTRIN Fe 1/20. (Parke-Davis) White Tab.: Norethindrone acetate 1 mg., ethinyl estradiol 20 mcg. White Tab.; Brown Tab: ferrous fumarate 75 mg./Brown Tab. (7 tabs.) Carton 5 petipac compacts of 28 Tab., carton of 5 refills 28 Tab.
Use: Oral contraceptive.

LOESTRIN Fe 1.5/30. (Parke-Davis) Green Tab.: Norethindrone acetate 1.5 mg., ethinyl estradiol 30 mcg./Green Tab. Brown Tab.: ferrous fumarate 75 mg./Brown Tab. (7 tabs.). Carton 5 petipac compacts 28 Tab., carton of 5 refills 28 tab.
Use: Oral contraceptive.

• **LOFEMIZOLE HYDROCHLORIDE. USAN.**

LOFENALAC. (Mead Johnson) Low phenylalanine food: Corn syrup solids 49.2%, casein hydrolysate 18.7% (enzymic digest of casein containing amino acids and small peptides & processed to remove most of the phenylalanine) corn oil 18%, modified tapioca starch 9.57%, Protein equiv. 15%, fat 18%, carbohydrate 60%, minerals (ash) 3.6%, phenylalanine 80 mg./100 Gm. pow. Vit. A 1600 I.U., D 400 I.U., E 10 I.U., C 52 mg., folic acid 100 mcg., B-1 0.5 mg., B-2 0.6 mg., niacin 8 mg., B-6 0.4 mg., B-12 2.0 mg., Biotin 0.05 mg., pantothenic acid 3 mg., Vit. K-1 100 mcg., choline 85 mg., inositol 30 mg., Ca 600 mg., P 450 mg., iodine 45 mcg., Fe 12 mg., Mg 70 mg., Cu 0.6 mg., Zn 4 mg., Mn 1 mg., Cl 450 mg., K 650 mg., Na 300 mg./qt. at normal dilution of 20 k cal/fl. oz. Can 2 ½ lb.
Use: Dietary management of phenylketonuria.

LOFENE. (Lannett) Diphenoxylate HCl 2.5 mg., atropine sulfate 0.025 mg. Bot. 100s, 500s, 1000s.
Use: Antiperistaltic.

• **LOFENTANIL OXALATE.** USAN.
Use: Analgesic, narcotic.

LOFEPRAMINE. B.A.N. 5- 3-[N-(4-Chlorophenacyl)methylamino]propyl -10, 11-dihydrobenz[b,f]azepine. Lopramine (I.N.N.)
Use: Antidepressant.

L.O.L. LOTION. (O'Leary) Bot. 4 oz., 8 oz., 16 oz.
Use: Prevention and treatment of blackheads, enlarged pores, pimples and acne.

• **LOMETRALINE HYDROCHLORIDE.** USAN.
Use: Antipsychotic, antiparkinson

• **LOMOFUNGIN.** USAN.
Use: Antifungal.

LOMOTIL. (Searle) Diphenoxylate HCl 2.5 mg., atropine sulfate 0.025 mg./Tab. or 5 cc. **Tabs.** Bot. 100s, 500s, 1000s, 2500s. Unit Dose 100s. **Liq.** Bot. w/dropper 2 oz.
Use: In diarrhea management as adjunctive therapy.

• **LOMUSTINE.** USAN. CCNU; NSC-79037. 1-(2-Chloroethyl)-3-cyclohexyl-1-nitrosourea.
Use: Antineoplastic.
See: CeeNu, Cap. (Bristol)

LONALAC. (Mead Johnson) High protein, low sodium powder containing as a % of the calories 21%

protein as casein, 49% fat as coconut oil, 30%
carbohydrate as lactose, Vit. A 1440 I.U., B-1 0.6 mg.,
B-2 2.6 mg., niacin 1.2 mg., Ca 1.69 Gm., P 1.5 Gm.,
Cl 750 mg., K 1.88 Gm., Na 38 mg., Mg 135
mg./qt., Pow. Can 16 oz.
Use: Low sodium, high protein supplement for use
when dietary restriction is prescribed.

LONG ACTING NEO-SYNEPHRINE II NOSE DROPS.
(Winthrop Products) Xylometazoline HCl 0.1% Adult
strength and 0.05% Child strength. Bot. 1 oz.
Use: Nasal decongestant.

LONG ACTING NEO-SYNEPHRINE II VAPOR SPRAY.
(Winthrop Products) Xylometazoline HCl 0.1%.
Mentholated. Spray Bot. ½ fl. oz.
Use: Nasal decongestant.

LONG ACTING NASAL SPRAY. (Weeks & Leo)
Oxymetazoline 0.1% nasal solution. Bot. 0.75 oz.
Use: Nasal decongestant.

LONGIFENE DIHYDROCHLORIDE. Buclizine, B.A.N.

LONITEN. (Upjohn) Minoxidil 2.5 mg./Tab. Unit-of-Use
Bot. 100s; 10 mg./Tab. Unit-of-Use Bot. 100s.
Use: Peripheral vasodilator used as
antihypertensive.

LO/OVRAL. (Wyeth) Norgestrel 0.3 mg., ethinyl
estradiol 30 mg./Tab. 6 Pilpak dispensers, 21
Tabs.
Use: Oral contraceptive.

LO/OVRAL-28. (Wyeth) 21 white tab. each containing
0.3 mg. norgestrel with 0.03 mg. ethinyl estradiol &
7 inert Tab. 6 Pilpak dispensers. 28 Tabs.
Use: Oral contraceptive.

LOPERAMIDE. B.A.N. 4-(4-p-Chlorophenyl-4- hydrox-
ypiperidino)-NN-dimethyl-2,2-diphenyl-butyramide.
See: Imodium, Tab. (Janssen)

• **LOPERAMIDE HCL,** U.S.P. XXI. Cap., U.S.P. XXI.
Use: Antiperistaltic.
See: Imodium, Cap. (Ortho)

LOPID. (Parke-Davis) Gemfibrozil 300 mg./Cap. Bot.
100s. Lipid regulating agent.
Use: Routine treatment of elevated blood lipids for
the prevention of coronary heart disease.

LOPRESSOR. (Geigy) Metoprolol tartrate. **Tab.:** 50
mg., 100 mg./Tab. Bot. 100s, 1000s. Unit dose
100s. Gy-Pak 60s, 100s. **Ampul:** 5 mg./5 ml.
Use: Antihypertensive beta blocker, myocardial
infarction.

LOPROX. (Hoechst) Ciclopirox olamine 1% in cream
base. Tube 15 Gm., 30 Gm.
Use: Topical, broad-spectrum antifungal.

LOPURIN. (Boots) Allopurinol 100 mg. or 300
mg./Tab. Bot. 100s, 500s, 1000s.
Use: Treatment of gout, uric acid nephropathy, uric
acid stone formation.

LOQUA. (Columbia) Hydrochlorothiazide 50 mg./Tab.
Bot. 100s, 1000s.
Use: Diuretic and antihypertensive.

• **LORAJMINE HYDROCHLORIDE.** USAN.
Use: Cardiac depressant.

• **LORAZEPAM.** USAN. 7-Chloro-5-(o-chlorophenyl)-
1,3-dihydro-3-hydroxy-2H-1,4-benzodiazepin-2-one.
Use: Minor tranquilizer.
See: Ativan, Tab., Inj. (Wyeth)

• **LORBAMATE.** USAN.
Use: Muscle relaxant.

• **LORCAINIDE HYDROCHLORIDE.** USAN.
Use: Cardiac depressant.

LORELCO. (Merrell Dow) Probucol 250 mg./Tab. Bot.
120s.
Use: Cholestorol reducing agent.

LORFAN. (Roche) Levallorphan tartrate. 1 mg./ml.
w/methyl and propyl parabens 0.2%, phenol
0.45%. Amp. 1 ml. Box 10s. Vial 10 ml.
Use: I.V. or I.M., overdosage of narcotics.

• **LORMETAZEPAM.** USAN.
Use: Sedative, hypnotic.

LOROXIDE. (Dermik) Benzoyl peroxide 5.5%
w/propylene glycol, cetyl alcohol,
hydroxyethylcellulose, kaolin, caramel, talc,
cholesterol and related sterols, propylene
glycolstearate, polysorbate 20, lanolin alcohol,
propylparaben, methylparaben, tetrasodium EDTA,
pH buffers, antioxidants, silicone emulsion, silica,
decyl oleate, vegetable oil, purcelline oil syn.,
titanium dioxide, cyclohexanediamine tetraacetic
acid, calcium phosphate. Lot. Bot. 25 Gm.
Use: Severe recalcitrant acne.

LORPHEN. (Geneva) **Cap.:** Chlorpheniramine maleate
8 mg., 12 mg./Cap. Bot. 100s. **Tab.** 4 mg./Tab.
Bot. 100s.

LORVIC'S 2-TONE DISCLOSING SOLUTION. (Lorvic)
Dropper Bot. 2 oz.

• **LORZAFONE.** USAN.
Use: Minor tranquilizer.

LO-SAL. (Glenbrook) Calcium carbonate 585 mg., magnesium hydroxide 120 mg./Tab. Boxes 2s, 12s,
36s, 48s, 96s.
Use: Antacid, low sodium.

LOTALBA CREAM. (Durel) Lotalba oint. 30%, zinc
oxide 10%, sulfur pot. 5%, greaseless ointment
base 55%. Jars 3 oz., lb.
Use: Acne vulgaris, acne rosacea.

LOTALBA OINTMENT. (Durel) Stabilized lotio alba,
glycerine, mineral gums. Jars 3 oz., lb.
Use: Acne vulgaris, acne rosacea.

LOTAWIN CAPSULES. (Winthrop Products)
Oxypertine.
Use: Anxiolytic, tranquilizer.

LOTIO ALBA. White Lotion.
Use: Acne vulgaris, seborrhea.
W/Sulfur, calamine, alcohol.
See: Sulfa-Lo, Lot. (Whorton)

LOTIO ALSULFA. (Doak) Colloidal sulfur 5%. Bot. 4
oz.
Use: Acne vulgaris, seborrhea.

LOTOCREME. (C.S. Dent) Bot. 8 oz.
Use: Body rub.

LOTRIMIN. (Schering) Clotrimazole 1%, **Cream:** Tube
15 Gm., 30 Gm., 45 Gm., 90 Gm. **Sol.** 1% Bot. 10
ml., 30 ml.
Use: Antifungal.

LO-TROL. (Vangard) Diphenoxylate HCl 2.5 mg., atropine sulfate 0.015 mg./5 ml. Bot. 60 ml.
Use: Antidiarrheal.

LO-TROP. (Vangard) Diphenoxylate HCl 2.5 mg., atropine sulfate 0.025 mg./Tab. Bot. 100s, 1000s.
Use: Antidiarrheal.

LOTUSATE. (Winthrop-Breon) Talbutal 120 mg./Cap. Bot. 100s.
Use: Hypnotic.

LOUCEVERIN CALCIUM. Calcium 5-formyl-5, 6, 7, 8-tetrahydroteroylglutamate.

LOVE LONGER. (Youngs Drug) Benzocaine 7.5% in water soluble lubricant base. Tube ½ oz.
Use: Desensitizing lubricant for premature ejaculation.

LOWILA CAKE. (Westwood) Sodium lauryl sulfoacetate, dextrin, boric acid, urea, sorbitol, mineral oil, PEG 14 M, lactic acid, cellulose gum, docusate sodium, fragrance. Cake 3¾ oz.
Use: Soap-free skin cleanser.

LOW-QUEL. (Blue Cross) Diphenoxylate HCl 2.5 mg., atropine sulfate 0.025 mg./Tab. Bot. 100s.
Use: Intestinal antispasmotic.

• **LOXAPINE.** USAN. 2-Chloro-11-(4-methyl-1-piperazinyl) dibenz [b,f] [1,4] oxazepine.
Use: Tranquilizer.

LOXAPINE HYDROCHLORIDE.
Use: Tranquilizer.
See: Daxolin Concentrate, Liq. (Miles Pharm)
Loxitane-C Oral Concentrate (Lederle)
Loxitane, Inj. (Lederle)

• **LOXAPINE SUCCINATE.** USAN. (1)2-Chloro-11-(4-methyl-1-piperazinyl) dibenz-[b,f] [1,4]-oxazepine succinate; (2) Succinic acid compound with 2-chloro-11-(4-methyl-1-piperazinyl) dibenz-[b,f] [1,4] oxazepine.
Use: Tranquilizer.
See: Loxitane, Cap. (Lederle)

LOXITANE CAPSULES. (Lederle) Loxapine succinate 5 mg./Cap. Bot. 100s. Unit.Dose 10 × 10s. 10 mg., 25 mg., 50 mg./Cap. Bot. 100s, 1000s. Unit Dose 10 × 10s.
Use: Tranquilizer.

LOXITANE-C. (Lederle) Loxapine HCl oral concentrate 25 mg./ml. 120 ml. Bot. w/dropper.
Use: Tranquilizer.

LOXITANE IM. (Lederle) Loxitane HCl 50 mg./ml. Vial 10 ml.
Use: Anti-psychotic.

LOXON. Haloxon, B.A.N.

LOZOL. (USV Labs.) Indapamide 2.5 mg./Tab. Bot. 100s, 1000s.
Use: Diuretic, antihypertensive.

L-PAM. p-Di(2-chloroethyl) amino-L-phenylalamine. An alkylating antineoplastic agent. Under study.

L-SARCOLYSIN.
See: Alkeran, Tab. (Burroughs Wellcome)

LUBAFAX. (Burroughs Wellcome) Surgical lubricant, sterile; water-soluble, non-staining. Foil wrapper 2.7 Gm., 5 Gm. Box 144s.
Use: Surgical lubricant.

LUBATH. (Warner-Lambert) Mineral oil, PPG-15, stearyl ether, oleth-2, nonoxynol-5; fragrance, D&C Green No. 6. Bot. 4 oz., 8 oz., 16 oz.
Use: Bath oil for dry skin.

LUBINOL. (Purepac) Light, heavy, and ext. heavy mineral oil. Bot. pt., qt., gal. Ext. heavy. Bot. 8 oz., pt., qt., gal.
Use: Emollient.

LUBRASEPTIC JELLY. (Guardian) Water-soluble amyl phenyl phenol complex 0.12%, phenylmercuric nitrate, 0.007%. Bellows type tubes, 10 Gm., 24s.
Use: Urethral instillation, urologic and proctologic exams.

LUBRIDERM CREAM. (Warner-Lambert) Water, mineral oil, petrolatum, glycerin, glyceryl stearate, PEG-100 stearate, squalane, lanolin, lanolin alcohol, lanolin oil, cetyl alcohol, sorbitan laurate, fragrance (if scented), methylparaben, butylparaben, propylparaben, quaternium-15. Tube: scented 1.5 oz., 4 oz.; unscented 4 oz.
Use: For extremely dry skin.

LUBRIDERM LOTION. (Warner-Lambert) Water, mineral oil, petrolatum, sorbitol, lanolin, lanolin alcohol, stearic acid, TEA, cetyl alcohol, fragrance (if scented), butylparaben, methylparaben, propyl paraben, sodium chloride. Bot. scented, 4 oz., 8 oz., 16 oz.; unscented 8 oz., 16 oz.
Use: For dry skin.

LUCANTHONE. B.A.N. F.D.A. 1-[[2-(Diethylamino)ethyl]amino]-4-methylthioxanthen-9-one. Miracil D; Nilodin hydrochloride
Use: Treatment of filariasis and schistosomiasis.

• **LUCANTHONE HYDROCHLORIDE.** USAN. 1-[[2-(Diethylamino)ethyl] amino]-4-methylthioxanthen-9-one Monohydrochloride.
Use: Antischistosomal.

LUCOFEN HYDROCHLORIDE. Chlorphentermine, B.A.N.

LUDENS COUGH DROPS. (Luden's) Honey lemon, honey licorice, menthol, strong flavor menthol, strong flavor eucalyptus or wild cherry flavored lozenges. Square-Pack. Box. Bag.

LUDIOMIL. (Ciba) Maprotiline 25 mg., 50 mg. or 75 mg./Tab. Bot. 100s, 1000s.
Use: Antidepressive.

LUFA CAPSULES. (Armour) Nutrients. Bot. 100s.

LUFYLLIN. (Wallace) Dyphylline Injection. **Amp.:** (500 mg./2 ml.) Box 25s. **Elix.:** (100 mg./15 ml.; alcohol 20%) Bot. pt., gal. **Tab.:** (200 mg./Tab.) Bot. 100s, 1000s. Unit dose 100s.
Use: Bronchodilator.

LUFYLLIN-400. (Wallace) Dyphylline 400 mg./Tab. Bot. 100s, 1000s.
Use: Bronchodilator and expectorant.

LUFYLLIN-EPG. (Wallace) Ephedrine HCl 16 mg., dyphylline 100 mg., phenobarbital 16 mg., guaifenesin 200 mg./Tab. or 10 ml. **Tab.** Bot. 100s. **Elix.,** (alcohol 5.5%) Bot. pt.
Use: Bronchodilator.

LUFYLLIN-GG. (Wallace) **Tab.:** Dyphylline 200 mg., guaifenesin 200 mg./Tab. Bot. 100s, 1000s. **Elixir:** Dyphylline 100 mg., guaifenesin 100 mg., alcohol 17%/15 ml. Elix. Bot. pt., gal.
Use: Bronchodilator and expectorant.

LUGOL'S SOLUTION. Strong Iodine Solution, U.S.P. XXI. (Lyne) Iodine 5.0 Gm., pot. iodide 10 Gm., in enough purified water to make 100 ml. Bot. 15 ml. (Wisconsin) Bot. pt.

LUMINAL. (Winthrop-Breon) Phenobarbital. **Ovoids:** 16 mg. (¼ gr.) or 32 mg. (½ gr.). **Inj.:** 1 ml. (130 mg.)/Amp. Box 100s.
Use: Sedative, hypnotic, anticonvulsant.

LUMOPAQUE CAPSULES. (Winthrop Products) Tyropanoate sodium.
Use: Oral chloecystographic medium.

LUPO-TEC. (Wampole) Radioimmunoassay for the quantitative determination of antibodies to double-stranded DNA in serum. Kits 60s.
Use: Aid in diagnosis of systemic lupus erythematosus (SLE).

LURIDE DROPS. (Hoyt) Sodium fluoride equiv. to 0.125 mg. of fluoride/Drop. Plastic dropper bottle 30 ml.
Use: Aid in the protection against dental caries.

LURIDE-F LOZI TABLETS. (Hoyt) Sodium fluoride in Lozi base tablet available as fluoride. **0.25 mg.:** Bot. 120s; **0.5 mg.:** Bot. 120s, 1200s; **1.0 mg.:** Bot. 120s, 1000s, 5000s.
Use: Dental caries preventive.

LURIDE PROPHYLAXIS PASTE. (Hoyt) Acidulated phosphate sodium fluoride containing 0.4% fluoride ion w/silicon dioxide abrasive. Unit dose 3 Gm. Jars 50 Gm.
Use: Clean and polish teeth.

LURIDE-SF LOZI TABLETS. (Hoyt) Sodium fluoride containing 1.0 mg fluoride/Tab. Special formula with no color or flavor. Bot. 120s.
Use: Dental caries preventive.

LURIDE TOPICAL GEL. (Hoyt) Acidulated phosphate sodium fluoride containing 1.2% fluoride ion at pH 3.0 to 4.0 in gel base. Bot. 32 oz., 250 ml.
Use: Dental caries preventive.

LURIDE TOPICAL SOLUTION. (Hoyt) Acidulated phosphate sodium fluoride w/pH 3.2. Bot. 250 ml.
Use: Dental caries preventive.

LUSTOZYME. (Kenyon) Lucelzyme (cellulolytic enzyme) 1 mg., lumylzyme (amylolytic enzyme) 25 mg., luprozyme (proteolytic enzyme) 10 mg., dehydrocholic acid 100 mg., hyoscyamine HBr 0.1 mg., hyoscine HBr 0.0065 mg., atropine sulfate 0.02 mg./Tab. Bot. 100s, 1000s.
Use: Flatulence.

LUTEOGAN.
See: Progesterone (Various Mfr.)

LUTEOSAN.
See: Progesterone (Various Mfr.)

LUTOCYLOL. (Ciba) Ethisterone.

LUTOLIN-F. (Spanner) Progesterone 25 mg. or 50 mg./cc. Vial 10 cc.

LUTOLIN-S. (Spanner) Progesterone 25 mg./cc. Vial 10 cc.

• **LUTRELIN ACETATE.** USAN.

LUTREN.
See: Progesterone (Various Mfr.)

LUTUTRIN.
See: Lutrexin, Tab. (Hynson, Westcott & Dunning)

• **LYAPOLATE SODIUM.** USAN. Sodium ethenesulfonate polymer. Peson (Hoechst).

Use: Anticoagulant.

• **LYCETAMINE.** USAN.
Use: Antimicrobial.

LYCINE HYDROCHLORIDE.
See: Betaine Hydrochloride (Various Mfr.)

LYCOLAN ELIXIR. (Lannett) Glycocoll 28 gr., lysine 100 mg. in Tokay wine base/Tbsp. Bot. pt.
Use: Geriatric vitamin.

LYDIA E. PINKHAM TABLETS. (CooperVision) 72s, 250s.

LYDIA E. PINKHAM VEGETABLE COMPOUND. (CooperVision) Bot. 8 fl. oz., 16 fl. oz.

• **LYDIMYCIN.** USAN.
Use: Antifungal.

LYMECYCLINE. B.A.N. A water-soluble combination of tetracycline, lysine and formaldehyde. Armyl; Mucomycin; Tetralysal.
Use: Antibiotic.

LYMPHAZURIN. (Hirsch) Isosulfan blue 10 mg., sodium monohydrogen phosphate 6.6 mg., potassium dihydrogen phosphate 2.7 mg./ml. Vials 5 ml.
Use: Contrast agent.

• **LYMPHOGRANULOMA VENEREUM ANTIGEN,** U.S.P. XXI. Lymphogranuloma venereum skin test antigen.
Use: Diagnostic aid (dermal reactivity indicator).

• **LYNESTRENOL.** USAN. (1) 19-Nor-17α-pregn-4-en-20-yn-17-ol; (2) 17α-Ethinyl-17β-hydroxyestr-4-ene. Orgametril.
Use: Progestin.

LYNOESTRENOL. Lynestrenol.

LYOPINE. (Hyrex) Atropine sulfate lyophilized 10 mg./10 ml. vial w/diluent 10 ml.
Use: Anticholinergic, antidote to cholinesterase inhibitors.

LYPO-B. (Rocky Mtn.) Choline chloride 200 mg., dl-methionine 50 mg., inositol 100 mg., B-12 cryst. 20 mcg./2 cc. Vial 30 cc.

• **LYPRESSIN NASAL SOLUTION,** U.S.P. XXI. 8-Lysine vasopressin. Syntopressin.
Use: Antidiuretic.
See: Diapid Nasal Spray (Sandoz)

LYSERGIDE. B.A.N. NN-Diethyl-lysergamide. Lysergic acid diethylamide LSD, Delysid.
Use: Psychotomimetic.

LYSIDIN. Methyl glyoxalidin.

LYSINE. USAN.
Use: Nutrient & rapid weight gain.

• **LYSINE ACETATE,** U.S.P. XXI. $C_6H_{14}N_2O_2 \cdot C_2H_4O_2$
Use: Amino acid.

• **LYSINE MONOHYDROCHLORIDE,** U.S.P. XXI. $C_6H_{14}N_2O_2 \cdot HCl$
Use: Amino acid.
See: Enisyl, Tab. (Person & Covey).

LYSITONE. (Jenkins) l-Lysine HCl 300 mg., iron peptonate 200 mg., cobalamine conc. 10 mcg., B-1 10 mg., niacinamide 20 mg., B-2 2.5 mg., B-6 2 mg., panthenol 2 mg., d-sorbitol 1.83 Gm., alcohol 11%/Fl. Oz. Bot. 3 oz., 8 oz., gal.
Use: Reconstructive nutritional tonic.

LYSIVANE.
See: Parsidol, Tab. (Warner-Chilcott)
LYSMINS. (Miller) l-Lysine 20 mg., dl-methionine 150 mg., Cu 1.0 mg., iodine 0.015 mg., Mn 2.0 mg., Fe 10.0 mg., K 20.0 mg., Zn 2.0 mg., Mg 20.0 mg./Tab. Bot. 100s.
Use: Adults, orally as a dietary supplement.
LYSODREN. (Bristol) Mitotane. 500 mg./Tab. Bot. 100s.
Use: Inoperable adrenal cortical carcinoma.
• **LYSOSTAPHIN.** USAN. Antibiotic derived from *Staphylococcus staphylolyticus.*
Use: Antibiotic.
LYSURIDE. B.A.N. 9-(3,3-Diethylureido)-4,6,-6a,7,8,9-hexahydro-7-methylindolo[4,3-f,g]-quinoline.
Use: Prophylaxis of migraine.
See: Lysenyl.
LYTEERS. (Barnes-Hind) Isotonic, viscous liquid adjusted to pH of tears. Balanced amounts of sodium and potassium ions, cellulose derivative, benzalkonium chloride 0.01% and disodium edetate 0.05%. Plas. Bot. 15 cc.
Use: Optic; artificial tear fluid.
LYTREN. (Mead Johnson) Water, corn syrup solids, dextrose, Na citrate, KCl, citric acid, Na biphosphate, K citrate, Ca chloride and Mg sulfate. Ready-To-Use Bot. 8 fl. oz.
Use: Orally, electrolyte and fluid balance.

M

MAAGEL. (Approved) Aluminum and Mg hydroxide. Bot. 12 oz., gal.
Use: Gastric hyperacidity.
MAALOX. (Rorer) Suspension of magnesium hydroxide 200 mg., and aluminum hydroxide 225 mg./5 ml. Sodium content (0.06 mEq) 1.35 mg./5 ml. Bot. 5 oz., 12 oz., 26 oz. Unit dose 15 ml., 30 ml.
Use: Antacid.
MAALOX NO. 1 TABLETS. (Rorer) Magnesium hydroxide 200 mg., dried aluminum hydroxide gel 200 mg./Tab. Sodium content (0.03 mEq) 0.84 mg./Tab. Bot. 100s.
Use: Antacid.
MAALOX NO. 2 TABLETS. (Rorer) Magnesium hydroxide 400 mg., dried aluminum hydroxide gel 400 mg./Tab.
Sodium content (0.07 mEq) 1.84 mg./Tab. Bot. 50s, 250s.
Strip 24s, 100s.
Use: Antacid.
MAALOX PLUS. (Rorer) Suspension of magnesium hydroxide 200 mg., aluminum hydroxide 225 mg., simethicone 25 mg./5 ml. Sodium content (0.06 mEq) 1.3 mg./5 ml. Bot. 12 oz. Unit dose 15 ml., 30 ml.
Use: Antacid, antiflatulent.
MAALOX PLUS TABLETS. (Rorer) Magnesium hydroxide 200 mg., dried aluminum hydroxide gel 200 mg., simethicone 25 mg./Tab. Sodium content

(0.03 mEq.) 1.0 mg./Tab. Bot. 50s. Strip 100s. Pocket Packs 12s. Roll Packs 12s.
Use: Antacid, antiflatulent.
MAALOX TC (THERAPEUTIC CONCENTRATE). (Rorer) Suspension of magnesium hydroxide 300 mg., aluminum hydroxide 600 mg./5 ml. Sodium content (0.03 mEq.) 0.8 mg./5 ml. Bot. 12 oz.
Use: Concentrated antacid.
MACRISALB (^{131}I) INJECTION. B.A.N.
Macroaggregated iodinated (^{131}I) human albumin injection.
Use: Examination of pulmonary perfusion.
MACROAGGREGATED ALBUMIN.
See: Albumotope-LS. (Squibb)
MACRODANTIN. (Norwich Eaton) Nitrofurantoin macrocrystals 50 or 100 mg./Cap. Bot. 30s, 100s, 500s, 1000s. Hospital Unit Dose 100s. 25 mg./Cap. Bot. 100s.
Use: Antibacterial for urinary tract infections.
MACRODEX. (Pharmacia) Dextran 6% w/v in normal saline and 6% w/v in 5% dextrose in water. Bot. 500 ml.
Use: Treatment of shock due to trauma, hemorrhage, burns and surgery.
MACROGOL 400. B.A.N. Polyoxyl stearate.
Use: Surface active agent.
See: Polyethylene glycol 400
MACROGOL 4000. B.A.N.
Use: Surface active agent.
See: Polyethylene glycol 4000
MACROGOL STEARATE 2000. Polyoxyl 40 Stearate.
MACROTIN W/Phenobarbital, hyoscyamus ext., caulophyllin, helonin, pulsatilla ext.
See: Tranquilans, Tab. (Noyes)
• **MAFENIDE,** USAN. α-Aminotoluene-p-sulfonamide. Marfanil [HCl], Sulfomyl [propionate], Sulfamylon [acetate].
Use: Antibacterial agent.
• **MAFENIDE ACETATE,** U.S.P. XXI. Cream, U.S.P. XXI. α-Aminotoluene-p-sulfonamide monoacetate.
See: Sulfamylon Cream (Winthrop-Breon)
• **MAFILCON A.** USAN.
Use: Contact lens material.
MAFYLON CREAM. (Winthrop Products) Mafenide acetate.
Use: Topical antibacterial agent for burns.
• **MAGALDRATE,** U.S.P. XXI. Oral Susp., Tab., U.S.P. XXI. (Ayerst) Monalium Hydrate. Aluminum Magnesium Hydroxide.
Use: Antacid.
See: Monalium Hydrate
Riopan, Tab. & Susp. (Ayerst)
MAGAN. (Adria) Magnesium salicylate (anhydrous) 545 mg./Tab. Bot. 100s, 500s.
Use: Salicylate therapy.
MAGDROX. (Vita Elixir) Magnesium hydroxide, aluminum hydroxide.
Use: Gastric antacid.
MAGLAGEL. (Kenyon) Mg-Al hydroxide gel. Bot. 12 oz., pt., gal.
MAG-LUM. (Kenyon) Magnesium trisilicate 7.5 gr., dried Al hydroxide gel 4 gr. Tab. Bot. 100s, 1000s.

MAGMA ALBA. (Durel) Sulfurated lime solution (Vleminckx's) 60.0%, saturated zinc sulfate solution 40.0%. Jars 3 oz., lb.
Use: Acne vulgaris, acne cystica, acne rosacea, rosacealike tuberculid (Lewandowsky).

MAGMALIN SUSPENSION. (Vale) A colloidal suspension of aluminum hydroxide gel and magnesium hydroxide. Bot. pt., gal.

MAGMALIN LOZENGE. (Vale) Magnesium hydroxide 0.2 Gm., aluminum hydroxide gel, dried 0.2 Gm./Loz. Bot. 100s, 500s, 1000s.

MAGNAGEL. (Mallard) Aluminum hydroxide-magnesium carbonate 325 mg./Tab. **Tab.** Bot. 100s.
Use: Antacid.

MAGNA-GEL LIQUID. (Vortech) Magnesium-aluminum hydroxide gel. Bot. 12 oz., gal.
Use: Antacid.

MAGNALETS. (Towne) Vit. A acetate 10,000 I.U., D 400 I.U., B-1 15 mg., B-2 10 mg., B-6 5 mg., B-12 12 mcg., C 250 mg., niacinamide 100 mg., Ca pantothenate 20 mg., E 15 I.U., Fe 10 mg., iodine 0.1 mg., Mn 1 mg., K 5 mg., Cu 1 mg., Zn 1.5 mg., Mg 6 mg./Captab. Bot. 100s, 50s.

MAGNALUM. (Richlyn) Magnesium hydroxide 3.75 gr., aluminum hydroxide 2 gr./Tab. Bot. 1000.
Use: Antacid.

MAGNATRIL. (Lannett) Aluminum hydroxide gel dried 4 gr., magnesium trisilicate 7 gr., magnesium hydroxide 2 gr./Tab. Bot. 50s, 100s.
Use: Antacid, adsorbant.

MAGNATRIL SUSPENSION. (Lannett) Magnesium trisilicate 4 gr., colloidal susp. of magnesium and aluminum hydroxides/5 cc. Bot. 12 fl. oz.
Use: Relief and control of pain in gastric hyperacidity and for treatment of peptic ulcer.

• **MAGNESIA TABLETS,** U.S.P. XXI.
Use: Antacid.

• **MAGNESIA & ALUMINA ORAL SUSPENSION.** U.S.P. XXI. (Philips Roxane) Oral Susp. 6 fl. oz. 25s.
Use: Antacid.
See: Maalox, Liq. (Rorer)

• **MAGNESIA & ALUMINA TABLETS,** U.S.P. XXI.
Use: Antacid.
See: Maalox, Tab. (Rorer)

MAGNESIA MAGMA. Milk of Magnesia, U.S.P. XXI.
Use: Antacid, cathartic.
See: Magnesium Hydroxide, Prep.

MAGNESIUM ACETYLSALICYLATE. Apyron, Magnespirin, Magisal, Novacetyl.
Use: Like acetylsalicylic acid.

MAGNESIUM ALUMINATE HYDRATED.
Use: Antacid.
See: Riopan, Susp., Tab. (Ayerst)

MAGNESIUM ALUMINUM HYDROXIDE.
Use: Antacid.
See: Maalox, Susp. (Rorer)
    Maglagel (Kenyon)
    Malogel, Gel (Columbia)
    Medalox, Gel (Med. Chem.)
W/APC.
See: Buffadyne, Tab. (Lemmon)

W/Calcium carbonate.
See: Camalox, Susp. (Rorer)
W/Magnesium trisilicate.
See: Magnatril Susp. (Lannett)
W/Simethicone.
See: Maalox Plus, Susp. (Rorer)

• **MAGNESIUM ALUMINUM SILICATE,** U.S.P. XXI.
Use: Suspending agent.

• **MAGNESIUM CARBONATE,** U.S.P. XXI. (Baker, J. T.) Pow. 4 oz., 1 lb., 5 lb.
Use: Antacid.

• **MAGNESIUM CARBONATE AND SODIUM BICARBONATE FOR ORAL SUSPENSION,** U.S.P. XXI.
Use: Antacid.

MAGNESIUM CARBONATE W/COMBINATIONS.
Use: Antacid.
See: Alised, Tab. (Elder)
    Alkets, Tab. (Upjohn)
    Antacid, Tab. (Mallard)
    Antacid No. 2, Tab. (Bowman)
    Bismatesia, Can (Noyes)
    Bufferin, Tab. (Bristol-Myers)
    Buffertabs, Tab. (O'Neal)
    Buffinol, Tab. (Otis Clapp)
    Di-Gel, Tab., Liq. (Plough)
    Dimacid, Tab. (Otis Clapp)
    Dristan, Tab. (Whitehall)
    Glycogel, Tab. (Central)
    Glytabs, Chew. Tab. (Pharmics)
    Hycidol, Pow. (Mallard)
    Kanalka, Tab. (Lannett)
    Magnagel, Liq., Tab. (Mallard)
    Marblen, Susp., Tab. (Fleming)
    Maygel, Tab. (Century)
    Panacarb, Tab. (Lannett)
    Ratio, Tab. (Adria)
    Romach, Tab. (Ror Chem.)
    Spasased, Tab. (Wolins)
    Spastosed, Tab. (Vortech)

• **MAGNESIUM CHLORIDE,** U.S.P. XXI. Magnesium chloride hexahydrate.
Use: Electrolyte replenisher, pharmaceutical necessity for hemodialysis & peritoneal dialysis.
W/Pot. chloride, calcium chloride, phenol red.
See: Electrolytic Replenisher, Vial (Invenex)

• **MAGNESIUM CITRATE ORAL SOLUTION,** U.S.P. XXI. 1,2,3-Propanetricarboxylic acid, hydroxymagnesium salt (2:3).
Use: Cathartic.

• **MAGNESIUM GLUCONATE.** U.S.P. XXI. Tab., U.S.P. XXI.
Use: Magnesium deficiencies
See: Almora, Tab. (O'Neal)
    Gyn, Tab. (Amfre-Grant)

MAGNESIUM GLUCONATE. (Western Research) Magnesium gluconate 500 mg./Tab. Bot. 1000s.
Use: Magnesium deficiencies.

MAGNESIUM GLYCINATE.
W/Aspirin, magnesium carbonate.
See: Buffinol, Tab. (Otis Clapp)

W/Gastric mucin; Al hydroxide gel.
  See: Mucogel, Tab. (Inwood)
• **MAGNESIUM HYDROXIDE,** U.S.P. XXI.
  Use: Antacid; cathartic.
  See: Magnesia Magma
    Milk of Magnesia
MAGNESIUM HYDROXIDE W/COMBINATIONS.
  See: Aludrox, Susp., Tab., Vial (Wyeth)
    Aluscop, Cap., Susp. (Westerfield)
    Anachloric A, Tab. (Upjohn)
    Ascriptin, Tab. (Rorer)
    Ascriptin A/D, Tab. (Rorer)
    Ascriptin w/Codeine, Tab. (Rorer)
    Aspadine, Tab. (Vortech)
    Banacid, Tab. (Buffington)
    Camalox, Susp., Tab. (Rorer)
    Congespirin, Tab. (Bristol-Myers)
    Creamalin, Tab. (Winthrop Products)
    Delcid, Susp. (Merrell Dow)
    Fermalox, Tab. (Rorer)
    Ferratinic, Tab. (Wolins)
    4-Way Cold Tabs., Tab. (Bristol-Myers)
    Gas-Eze, Tab. (Edward J. Moore)
    Haley's M.O., Liq. (Winthrop Products)
    Jel Drox, Liq. (Coastal)
    Kamadrox Jel Liquid, Liq. (Elder)
    Kolantyl, Gel, Wafer (Merrell Dow)
    Kudrox, Susp., Tab. (Kremers-Urban)
    Laxsil Liquid, Liq. (Reed & Carnrick)
    Maalox, Susp., Tab. (Rorer)
    Maalox Plus, Susp., Tab. (Rorer)
    Magnatril, Susp., Tab. (Lannett)
    Magoleum, Liq. (Blue Line)
    Magwol #1, Tabs. (Wolins)
    Mint Acid Tablets, Tab. (Kenyon)
    Mylanta, Mylanta II, Liq., Tab. (Stuart)
    Neutralox, Susp. (Lemmon)
    Oxaine-M, Susp. (Wyeth)
    Simeco, Liq. (Wyeth)
    Trialka, Liq., Tab. (Commerce)
    Trigelma H.M., Tab., Liq. (O'Neal)
    WinGel, Liq., Tab. (Winthrop Products)
MAGNESIUM NICOTINATE.
W/Theobromine Mg oleate.
  See: Athemol-N, Tab. (Glaxo)
MAGNESIUM OROTATE.
  (Nutrition) 500 mg./Tab. Bot. 100s.
  See: Magora, Tab. (Miller)
• **MAGNESIUM OXIDE,** U.S.P. XXI.
  (Manne) 420 mg./Tab. Bot. 250s, 1000s.
  (Stanlabs) 10 gr./Tab. Bot. 100s, 1000s.
  Use: Pharm. aid (sorbant).
  See: Mag-Ox, Tab. (Blaine)
    Mag-Ox 400, Tab. (Blaine)
    Niko-Mag, Cap. (Scruggs)
    Oxabid, Cap. (Jamieson-McKames)
    Par-Mag, Cap. (Parmed)
    Uro-Mag, Cap. (Blaine)
W/Calcium, Vit. D.
  See: Elekap, Caps. (Western Research)
W/Glutamic acid magnesium complex, N-acetyl-P-
    aminophenol, ascorbic acid, dl-methionine,

lemon bioflavonoid complex, dl-α-tocopheryl ac-
    etate, glycine, soybean flour.
  See: Ulcimins, Tab. (Miller)
W/Magnesium carbonate, Ca carbonate.
  See: Alkets, Tab. (Upjohn)
W/Ox bile (desic.), hog bile (desic.).
  See: Hyper-Cholate, Tab. (Mallard)
W/Phenobarbital, atropine sulfate.
  See: Magnox, Tab. (Bowman)
• **MAGNESIUM PHOSPHATE,** U.S.P. XXI.
  Use: Antacid.
• **MAGNESIUM SALICYLATE.** U.S.P. XXI. Tab. U.S.P.
  XXI.
  Use: Analgesic, antipyretic, antirheumatic.
  See: Analate, Tab. (Winston)
    Efficin, Tab. (Adria)
    Causalin, Tab. (Amfre-Grant)
    Magan, Tab. (Adria)
W/Phenyltoloxamine citrate.
  See: Mobigesic, Tab. (Ascher)
• **MAGNESIUM SILICATE,** N.F. XVI.
  Use: Pharmaceutic aid (tablet excipient).
• **MAGNESIUM STEARATE,** N.F. XVI.
  Use: Pharmaceutic aid (lubricant).
• **MAGNESIUM SULFATE,** U.S.P. XXI. Inj. U.S.P. XXI.
  Epsom salt.
  Use: Pow. or crystals cathartic: Inj. anticonvulsant,
  electrolyte replenisher.
  (Abbott)—50% Amp. 2 ml. Box 25s, 100s.
  Abboject Syringe (20 G $\times$ 2½″) 5 ml., 10 ml.;
  12.5% in Pintop Vial, 8 ml., 20 ml.
  (Atlas)—10% Amp. 10 cc. Box 100s; 1 Gm., 2 cc.
  Box 100s.
  (Baxter)—10% Vial 10 cc., 20 cc.
  (CMC)—1 Gm./2 cc., 10% Amp. 10 cc., 20 cc.
  25% Amp. 10 cc. 50% Vial 30 cc.
  (Columbia)—50% Amp. 2 cc., 100s.
  (Lilly)—10% Amp. 20 cc. Box 6s, 25s; 50% 1 Gm.
  Amp. 2 cc., Box 12s, 100s.
  (Parke-Davis)—50% Amp. 2 ml., 10s.
  (Torigian)—50% Amp. 2 cc. 12s, 25s, 100s.
  (Trent)—50% Amp. 2 cc., 10 cc.
• **MAGNESIUM TRISILICATE,** U.S.P. XXI. Magnesium
  silicate hydrate.
  Use: Antacid.
  See: Trisomin, Tab. (Lilly)
MAGNESIUM TRISILICATE W/COMBINATIONS.
  See: Alsorb Gel C.T., Gel (Standex)
    Antacid, Tab. (Panray)
    Antacid, Tab. (Reid-Provident)
    Antacid, Tab. (Zenith)
    Antacid G, Tab. (Walgreen)
    Arcodex Tablets, Tab. (Arcum)
    Azolid-A, Cap. (USV)
    Banacid, Tab. (Buffington)
    Barosil, Susp. (Barry-Martin)
    Butazolidin Alka, Cap. (Geigy)
    Equilet, Tab. (Mission)
    Escot, Cap. (Reid-Provident)
    Gacid, Tab. (Arcum)
    Gaviscon, Tab. (Marion)
    Kaocasil, Tab. (Jenkins)

Kathmagel, Tab. (Mason)
Kolantyl, Wafer (Merrell Dow)
Magnased, Tab. (Century)
Magnatril, Susp., Tab. (Lannett)
Magnesil w/Calcium Carbonate, Tab. (Bowman)
Malcogel, Liq. (Upjohn)
Maracid-2, Tab. (Marin)
Marblen, Tab., Susp. (Fleming)
Mint Acid Tablets, Tab. (Kenyon)
Mucotin, Tab. (Warner-Chilcott)
Neutracomp, Tab., Liq. (CMC)
Neutralox, Liq., Tab. (Lemmon)
Noralac, Tab. (Vortech)
Pama, Tab. (Vortech)
P.H. Plus, Tab. (Scrip)
Silmagel, Tab. (Lannett)
Triactin, Tab. (Norwich)
Trigelma H.M., Tab. (O'Neal)
Trilox, Susp., Tab. (Blue Line)
Trisogel, Liq. Pulv. (Lilly)

MAGNESIUM ZINC SHAKE LOTION. (Durel)
Magnesium carbonate, zinc oxide, lime water,
menthol, phenol 0.5%. Bot. 8 oz., gal.
Use: Generalized and widely disseminated
erythematous, vesicular and papular eruptions.

MAGNIPIN. (Kenyon) Atropine sulfate $1/500$ gr.,
nitroglycerin $1/500$ gr., magnesium sulfate 5 gr., ext.
ox bile 1 gr. Tab. Bot. 100s, 1000s.

MAGOLEUM. (Blue Line) Mineral oil 25%, milk of
Mag. 75%. Bot. gal.
Use: Orally, laxative & antacid.

MAGONATE. (Fleming) Magnesium gluconate 500
mg./Tab. Bot. 100s, 1000s.
Use: Magnesium deficiencies.

MAGORA. (Miller) Mg (as magnesium orotate) 65
mg./Tab. Bot. 100s.

MAG-OX. (Blaine) Magnesium oxide 400 mg./Tab. Bot.
100s, 1000s.
Use: Antacid, calcium oxalate urinary stone
prevention.

MAGSAL. (U.S. Chemical) Magnesium salicylate 600
mg., phenyltoloxamine citrate 25 mg./Tab. Bot.
100s.
Use: Analgesic, anti-arthritic, dysmenorrhea.

MAGWOL #1 TABS. (Wolins) Aluminum hydroxide
gel 200 mg., magnesium hydroxide 200 mg./Tab.
Bot. 100s, 1000s.

MAINTENANCE VITAMIN FORMULA W/MINERALS.
(Towne) Vit. A palmitate 10,000 I.U., D 400 I.U.,
B-1 5 mg., B-2 2.5 mg., C 75 mg., niacinamide 40 mg.,
B-6 1 mg., Ca pantothenate 4 mg., B-12 2 mcg., E 2
I.U., choline bitartrate 31.4 mg., inositol 15 mg., Ca
75 mg., P 58 mg., Fe 30 mg., Mg 3 mg., Mn 0.5
mg., K 2 mg., Zn 0.5 mg./Cap. Bot. 100s.

MAIZE PRO-GEN. Arsanilic acid, B.A.N.

MAJEPTIL. Thioproperazine. Psychopharmacologic
agent; pending release.

MALAGRIDE.
See: Acetarsone.

MALARAQUIN. (Winthrop Products) Chloroquine
phosphate.
Use: Antimalarial agent.

MALATONIC ELIXIR. (Blue Line) Peptonized iron 8
gr., fl. ext. cascara sagrada 12 mins., fl. ext.
gentian 6 mins./fl. oz. alcohol 8% Bot. gal.
Use: Iron tonic.

• **MALETHAMER.** USAN. Maleic anhydride ethylene
polymer.
Use: Antidiarrheal, antiperistaltic.

• **MALIC ACID,** N.F. XVI.

MALIC ACID WITH PECTIN.
See: Mallo-Pectin, Liq. (Mallard)

MALIDONE. Aloxidone, B.A.N.

MALLAMINT. (Mallard) Calcium carbonate 420
mg./Tab. Bot. 100s.

MALLISOL. (Mallard) Povidone-iodine.
Use: Germicidal, antiseptic surgical scrub soap.

MALLOPRESS. (Mallard) Hydrochlorothiazide 25 mg.,
reserpine 0.125 mg./Tab. Bot. 1000s.

MAL-O-FEM 90/4 L.A. IN OIL INJ. (Fellows) Testosterone enanthate 90 mg., estradiol valerate 4 mg./cc.
Vial 10 cc.

MAL-O-FEM 180/8 L.A. IN OIL INJ. (Fellows) Testosterone enanthate 180 mg., estradiol valerate 8
mg./cc. Vial 10 cc.

MAL-O-FEM. (Fellows) Aq.—Testosterone 25 mg., estrone 2 mg./cc. Vial 10 cc.
Use: I.M., estrogen and androgen therapy.

MAL-O-FEM CYP. (Fellows) Testosterone cypionate 50
mg., estradiol cypionate 2 mg./cc. Vial 10 cc.

MALOGEL. (Columbia) Magnesium-Aluminum hydroxide gel. Bot. 12 oz., gal.
Use: Adsorbent-antacid.

MALOGEN INJECTION AQUEOUS. (Fellows)
Testosterone. (25 mg./cc.) 10 cc., 30 cc.; (50
mg./cc.) 10 cc.; (100 mg./cc.) 10 cc.
Use: I.M., male hormone therapy.

MALOGEN 100 L.A. IN OIL INJ. (Fellows)
Testosterone enanthate 100 mg./cc. 10 cc.

MALOGEN 200 L.A. IN OIL INJ. (Fellows)
Testosterone enanthate 200 mg./cc. 10 cc.

MALOGEN CYP. (Fellows) Testosterone cypionate in
oil 100 mg., 200 mg./cc. Vial 10 cc.

MALONAL.
See: Barbital (Various Mfr.)

MALOTRONE AQUEOUS INJECTION. (Bluco)
Testosterone, USP 25 mg., 50 mg./cc. in aq. susp.
Vial 10 cc.

MALOTUSS. (Mallard) Guaifenesin 100 mg./5 cc.
Bot. 3 oz.
Use: Non-narcotic expectorant cough syrup.

MALTSUPEX. (Wallace) Laxative derived from natural
barley malt extract for relief of constipation in
children and adults. **Liq.**. Bot. 8 oz., 1 pt. **Pow.**,
dry, Jar. 8 oz., lb. **Tab.** Malt Soup ext. 750
mg./Tab. Bot. 100s.
W/Psyllium seed husks.
Use: Orally, laxative.
See: Syllamalt, Pow. (Wallace)

MAMMOL OINTMENT. (Abbott) Bismuth subnitrate
40%, castor oil 30%, lanolin 20%, ceresin wax 7%,
balsam peru 3%. Tube $7/8$ oz., 12s.
Use: Dressing for nipples of nursing mothers.

MANALAX. (Jenkins) Phenolphthalein 0.12 Gm.,

atropine sulfate 0.12 mg., w. mannitol, sodium
glycocholate, sodium taurocholate, ext.
cascara/Tab. Bot. 100s, 1000s.
Use: Constipation.

MANCHANIL. (D'Franssia)
Use: Bleaching creme.

MANDELAMINE. (Parke-Davis) **Tab.** contains 0.25
Gm. (3¾ gr.) methenamine mandelate. Bot. 100s,
1000s. **Susp.** (250 mg./5 ml.) Bot. 4 oz., 1 pt. (500
mg./5 ml.) Bot. 8 oz., 16 oz. **Granules.** 0.5
Gm./Packet 56s. 1.0 Gm./Packet 56s.
Use: Urinary antiseptic.

MANDELAMINE "HAFGRAMS." (Parke-Davis)
Methenamine mandelate 0.5 Gm./Tab. Bot. 100s,
1000s. Unit dose 100s.
Use: Urinary antiseptic.

MANDELAMINE 1 GM. (Parke-Davis) Methenamine
mandelate 1 Gm./Tab. Bot. 100s, 1000s. Unit dose
100s.

MANDELAMINE SUSPENSION FORTE. (Parke-Davis)
Methenamine mandelate susp. 500 mg./5 cc. Bot.
8 oz., pt.
Use: Urinary antiseptic.

MANDELETS. (Columbia) Methenamine mandelate
0.5 Gm. or 1.0 Gm./Tab. Bot. 100s, 1000s.

MANDELIC ACID.
Use: Orally, urinary antiseptic.

MANDELIC ACID SALTS.
See: Calcium mandelate (Var. Mfr.)

MANDELYLTROPEINE.
See: Homatropine Salts (Var. Mfr.)

MANDEX. (Vale) Methenamine mandelate 250 mg.,
salicylamide 120 mg., ext. belladonna 5 mg./Tab.
Bot. 100s, 500s, 1000s.
Use: Urinary antiseptic.

MANDOL. (Lilly) Cefamandole nafate. Vials: 500
mg./10 ml. Traypak: 25s; 1 Gm./10 ml. Traypak:
25s; 1 Gm./100 ml. Traypak: 10s; 2 Gm./20 ml.
Traypak: 10s; 2 Gm./100 ml. Traypak: 10s; 10
Gm./100 ml. Ctn. 6s; Traypak: 1 Gm. or 2 Gm.,
Pkg 96s.
Use: Antibiotic.

• **MANGANESE CHLORIDE,** U.S.P.XXI. Inj., U.S.P.
XXI.
Use: Manganese deficiency treatment.
See: Mangatrace, Inj. (Armour)

MANGANESE GLUCONATE. (Western Research)
45.45 mg./Tab. Bot. 1000s.

MANGANESE GLYCEROPHOSPHATE. Glycerol
phosphate manganese salt.
Use: Pharmaceutical necessity.

MANGANESE HYPOPHOSPHITE. Manganese (2+)
phosphinate.
Use: Pharmaceutic necessity.

• **MANGANESE SULFATE.** U.S.P. XXI. Inj, U.S.P. XXI.
W/Thyroid, ferrous sulfate, ferrous gluconate, sod.
ferric pyrophosphate, ext. of nux vomica.
See: Hemocrine, Tab. (Mallard)

MANGATRACE. (Armour) Manganese chloride
injection containing manganese 0.1 mg./ml. Vial 10
ml. Box 25s.
Use: Dietary supplement to I.V. Solutions for
manganese deficiency.

MANIRON. (Bowman) Ferrous fumarate 3 mg./Tab.
Bot. 100s, 1000s, 5000s.
Use: Anemias.

MANITERA. (Vitarine) High potency multiple vitamins.
Use: Dietary supplement.

MANIVIM. (Vitarine) Vit. A 10,000 I.U., D 1000 I.U., E
5 I.U., B-1 20 mg., B-2 6 mg., B-12 10 mcg., B-6 0.5
mg., C 30 mg., biotin 1 mcg., niacinamide 10 mg.,
Ca pantothenate 3 mg., choline bitartrate 20 mg.,
inositol 20 mg., dl-methionine 20 mg., pd. wh. dried
liver 100 mg., dried debit. yeast 100 mg., dicalcium
phosphate 200 mg., ferrous gluconate 50 mg., pot.
iodide 0.15 mg., Mg sulfate 7.2 mg., Cu sulfate 5
mg., Mn sulfate 3.4 mg., Zn sulfate 5 mg., pot.
chloride 25 mg./Cap. Bot. 100s.
Use: Vitamin-mineral supplement.

MANNA SUGAR.
See: Mannitol (Various Mfr.)

MANN A.R.P. SOLUTION. (Mann) Bot. pt., qt., ½
gal., gal.
Use: Prevention of rust in sterilizers.

**MANN ASTRINGENT MOUTH WASH
CONCENTRATE.** (Mann) Bot. 4 oz., qt., ½ gal.,
gal. Also mint flavored. Bot. qt., ½ gal., gal.

MANN BODY DEODORANT. (Mann) Bot. 4 oz., 8 oz.,
pt., qt., gal.

MANN BREATH DEODORANT. (Mann) Bot. 1 oz., 4
oz., 8 oz., pt., qt., gal.

MANN EMOLLIENT. (Mann) Jar. 100 Gm.
Use: Preoperative protective application.

MANN EUGENOL U.S.P. EXTRA. (Mann) ¼ lb., ½
lb., 1 lb.
Use: With zinc oxide as protective pack.

MANN GERMICIDAL SOLUTION. (Mann) Bot. gal., 6
gal. **Conc.** 12.8%. Bot. pt., qt., ½ gal., gal.

MANN HAND LOTION. (Mann) Twin Pack, gal.

MANNHEMOSTATIC. (Mann) Bot. 4 oz., 8 oz., pt., qt.
Use: Stop capillary bleeding.

MANN LIQUID SOAP. (Mann) Concentrated
cococastile. Bot. qt., ½ gal., gal.

MANN LUBRICANT AND CLEANSER. (Mann) Bot.
pt., qt.

MANN SUPERFATTED BAR SOAP. (Mann) Rich in
lanolin. Cake. 12s.

MANN TALBOT'S IODINE. (Mann) Glycerin base.
Bot. 4 oz., 8 oz., pt., qt., gal.

MANN TOPICAL ANESTHETIC. (Mann) Bot. 4 oz., 8
oz., pt., qt., gal. W/stain to indicate area treated.
Bot. 4 oz., 8 oz., pt., qt.
Use: Local surface anesthetic.

MANNITE.
See: Mannitol, U.S.P. XXI.

• **MANNITOL,** U.S.P. XXI. Inj. U.S.P. XXI. Manna
Sugar, D-Mannitol, Mannite.
See: Osmitrol (Travenol)
W/Aluminum hydroxide, magnesium hydroxide,
glycine, calcium carbonate, oil of peppermint.
See: Gas-Eze, Tab. (Edward J. Moore)
W/Sorbitol.
See: Cystosol, Liq. (Travenol)
Cytal, Liq. (Cutter)

• **MANNITOL INJECTION,** U.S.P. XXI. (Abbott) 20%,

15%. Abbo-Vac Single dose container 500 ml.; 10%, 5%. Abbo-Vac Single dose container 1000 ml. diuretic.
Use: Diagnostic aid (renal function determination); diuretic.
See: Mannitol Solution, Amp. (Merck Sharp & Dohme)

MANNITOL HEXANITRATE.
Use: Orally, coronary vasodilator.
See: Vascunitol, Tabs. (Apco)
W/Reserpine, rutin, ascorbic acid.
See: Ruhexatal W/Reserpine, Tab. (Lemmon)

MANNITOL HEXANITRATE & PHENOBARBITAL TAB. (Bowman; Columbia; Jenkins; Kenyon) Mannitol hexanitrate ½ gr., phenobarbital ¼ gr./Tab. Bot. 1000s. (Kenyon): Bot. 100s, 1000s.

MANNITOL HEXANITRATE WITH PHENOBARBITAL COMBINATIONS.
See: Hyrunal, Tab. (Kenyon)
Manotensin, Tab. (Dunhall)
Ruhexatal, Tab. (Lemmon)
Vascused, Tabs. (Apco)
Vermantin, Tab. (Trout)

• **MANNITOL & SODIUM CHLORIDE INJECTION,** U.S.P. XXI.
Use: Diuretic.

MANNOMUSTINE. B.A.N. 1,6-Di-(2-chloroethyl-amino)-1,6-dideoxy-D-mannitol. Degranol dihydrochloride.
Use: Antineoplastic agent.

MANOLA. (Manola Co.) Thiamine HCl 10 mg., riboflavin 3 mg., niacinamide 2.5 mg., iron citrate 3 gr., conc. sols. of glycerophosphates of Sod., Pot. & Cal. 12 min. in palatable aromatic menstruum & 15% alcohol/fl. oz. Bot. pt., 1 gal.
Use: Deficient nutrition.

MANOTENSIN. (Dunhall) Mannitol hexanitrate 32 mg., phenobarbital 16 mg./Tab. Bot. 100s, 1000s.
Use: Vasodilator.

MANOXOL OT. B.A.N. Docusate Sodium.

MANTADIL. (Burroughs Wellcome) Chlorocyclizine HCl 2%, hydrocortisone acetate 0.5%, liq. and white petrolatum, wax, methylparaben 0.25%. Cream Tubes 15 Gm.
Use: Antipruritic, anti-inflammatory, anesthetic.

MANTOMIDE. Chlorbetamide, B.A.N.

MANTOUX TEST.
See: Tuberculin, U.S.P. XXI. Test (Parke-Davis)

MANVENE. 3-Methoxy-16a-methyl-1,3,5: 10-estra-triene-16B, 17B-diol.
Use: Treatment of prostatic cancer.

MANVITOL. (Vitarine) High potency Vitamin B complex w/iron and Vit. B-12, C and E. Cap. Bot. 100s.
Use: Supplement.

MANZAN. (DeWitt) Ointment Tube 1 oz., 2 oz. Supp. 12s.
Use: Antihemorrhoidal.

MAOLATE TABLETS. (Upjohn) Chlorphenesin carbamate 400 mg./Tab. Bot. 50s, 500s. Unit-Dose 100s.
Use: Muscle relaxant, mild tranquilizer.

MAPHENIDE. p-Sulphamoylbenzylamine HCl.
See: Sulfbenzamine HCl

MAPROFIX.
See: Gardinol Type Detergents (Various Mfr.)

• **MAPROTILINE.** USAN. N-Methyl-9, 10-ethanoanthra-cene-9(10H)-propylamine. 3-(9, 10-Dihydro-9, 10-ethanoanthracen-9-yl)propylmethylamine.
Use: Antidepressant.
See: Ludiomil, Tab. (Ciba).

• **MAPROTILINE HYDROCHLORIDE,** U.S.P. XXI. Tab., U.S.P. XXI. 9,10-Ethanoathracene-9(10H)-propanamine, N-methyl-, hydrochloride.
Use: Antidepressant.

MARACID-2. (Marin) Magnesium trisilicate 150 mg., aluminum hydroxide dried gel 90 mg., aminoacetic acid 75 mg./Tab. Bot.
Use: Antacid, adsorbant.

MARANOX. (C.S. Dent) Phenacetin 100 mg., acetaminophen 60 mg., salicylamide, caffeine/Tab. Bot.: 9 Tab. (6 white for prompt action and 3 orange for delayed action), 18 Tab. (12 white and 6 orange).
Use: Analgesic.

MARAX DF SYRUP. (Roerig) A colorless dye free syrup containing hydroxyzine HCl 2.5 mg., ephedrine sulfate 6.25 mg., theophylline 32.5 mg., alcohol 5%/5 cc. Bot. Pt.
Use: Bronchodilator.

MARAX TAB. (Roerig) Hydroxyzine HCl 10 mg., ephedrine sulf. 25 mg., theophylline 130 mg./Tab. Bot. 100s, 500s.
Use: Bronchodilator.

MARAZIDE. (Vortech) Benzthiazide 50 mg./Tab. Bot. 100s, 1000s.
Use: Diuretic.

MARAZIDE II. (Vortech) Trichloromethazide 4 mg./Tab. Bot. 100s, 1000s.
Use: Diuretic.

MARBAXIN-750. (Vortech) Methocarbamol 750 mg./Cap. Bot. 500s.
Use: Skeletal muscle relaxant.

MARBEC. (Marlyn) High potency B and C vitamins. Tabs. Bot. 100s, 1000s.

MARBLEN LIQUID. (Fleming) Magnesium carbonate 400 mg., calcium carbonate 520 mg./5 cc. Bot. pt., gal.
Use: Antacid.

MARBLEN TABLETS. (Fleming) Magnesium and calcium carbonate 21 gr./Tab. Bot. 100s, 1000s.
Use: Antacid.

MARCAINE. (Winthrop-Breon) Bupivacaine in sterile isotonic solution containing sod. chloride, pH adjusted 4.0 to 6.5 w/sod. hydroxide or hydrochloric acid.Multiple-dose vials also contain methylparaben. 1 mg./ml. as preservative . **0.25%:** Amp. 50 ml. Box 5s. Vial: single dose 10 ml., 30 ml. Box 10s; multiple dose 50 ml. Box 1s.**0.5%:** Amp. 30 ml. Box 1s, 5s. Vial: single dose 10 ml., 30 ml. Box 10s. multiple dose 50 ml. Box 1s.
0.75%: Amp. 30 ml. Box 5s. Vial (single dose) 10 ml., 30 ml. Box 10s.
Use: Local anesthetic (injectable) for peripheral nerve block, infiltration, sympathetic block, caudal or epidural block, retrobulbar block (see package insert for complete use recommendations).

MARCAINE WITH EPINEPHRINE (1:200,000).
(Winthrop-Breon) **Bupivacaine 0.25%:** with epinephrine 1:200,000: in sterile isotonic solution containing
sodium chloride. Each 1 ml contains 2.5 mg
bupivacaine hydrochloride and 0.0091 mg
epinephrine bitartrate, with 0.5 mg sodium bisulfite,
0.001 ml monothioglycerol, and 2 mg ascorbic acid
as antioxidants, 0.0017 ml 60% sodium lactate
buffer and 0.1 mg edetate calcium disodium as
stabilizer. In Multiple Dose Vials, each 1 ml also
contains 1 mg methylparaben as antiseptic
preservative. pH adjusted to between 3.4 and 4.5
with sodium hydroxide or hydrochloric acid. Amp.
50 ml. 5s, Single Dose Vials, 10 ml, 30 ml. 10s,
Multiple Dose Vials, 50 ml. 1s. **Bupivacaine 0.5%:**
with epinephrine 1:200,000: in sterile isotonic
solution containing sodium chloride. Each 1 ml
contains 5 mg bupivacaine hydrochloride and
0.0091 mg epinephrine bitartrate, with 0.5 mg
sodium bisulfite, 0.001 ml monothioglycerol and 2
mg ascorbic acid as antioxidants, 0.0017 ml 60%
sodium lactate buffer, and 0.1 mg edetate calcium
disodium as stabilizer. In Multiple Dose Vials, each
1 ml also contains 1 mg methylparaben as
antiseptic preservative. pH adjusted to between 3.4
and 4.5 with sodium hydroxide or hydrochloric acid.
Amp. 3 ml. 10s, 30 ml. 5s, Single Dose Vials 10 ml,
30 ml 10s, Multiple Dose Vials 50 ml. 1s.
Bupivacaine 0.75%: with epinephrine 1:200,000: in
sterile isotonic solution containing sodium chloride.
Each 1 ml. contains 7.5 mg bupivacaine
hydrochloride and 0.0091 mg epinephrine bitartrate
with 0.5 mg sodium bisulfite, 0.001 ml
monothioglycerol and 2 mg ascorbic acid as
antioxidants, 0.0017 ml 60% sodium lactate buffer
and 0.1 mg edetate calcium disodium as stabilizer.
pH adjusted to between 3.4 and 4.5 with sodium
hydroxide or hydrochloric acid. Amp 30 ml. 5s.
Use: Local anesthetic (injectable) for peripheral
nerve block (see package insert for complete use
recommendations).
MARDON. (Geneva) Propoxyphene HCl 32 mg./Cap.
Bot. 100s, 1000s. 65 mg./Cap. Bot. 100s, 500s,
1000s.
MARDON COMPOUND. (Geneva) Propoxyphene
comp. 65 mg., aspirin 3½ gr., phenacetin 2½ gr.,
caffeine ½ gr./Cap. Bot. 100s, 500s, 1000s.
MAREZINE INJECTION. (Burroughs Wellcome)
Cyclizine lactate. Amp. (50 mg./ml.) 1 ml., Box
100s.
Use: Antinauseant for motion sickness.
MAREZINE TABLETS. (Burroughs Wellcome)
Cyclizine HCl 50 mg./Tab. Bot. 100s, 1000s. Box
12s.
Use: Antinauseant for motion sickness.
W/Ergotamine tartrate, caffeine.
See: Migral, Tabs. (Burroughs Wellcome)
MARFANIL.
See: Sulfbenzamine HCl (Var. Mfr.)
MARFLEX INJECTION. (Vortech) Vial 10 ml.
Use: Skeletal muscle relaxant.

MARFLEX TABLETS. (Vortech) Orphenadrine citrate
100 mg./Tab. Bot. 100s,
500s.
Use: Skeletal muscle relaxant.
MARGESIC COMPOUND 65. (Vortech) Propoxyphene
HCl 65 mg., aspirin 227 mg., phenacetin 162 mg.,
caffeine 32 mg./Cap. Bot. 500s.
Use: Analgesic.
MARGESIC IMPROVED. (Vortech) Propoxyphene HCl
65 mg. Bot. 100s, 1000s.
Use: Analgesic.
MARHIST. (Marlop) Chlorpeniramine maleate 20 mg.,
phenylephrine HCl 2.5 mg., methscopolamine
nitrate in special base/Cap. Bot. 30s, 100s. Expect.
Bot. 4 oz., pt., gal.
Use: Relief of cold symptoms and hay fever
symptoms.
MARMINE. (Vortech) Dimenhydrinate 50 mg./Tab.
Bot. 1000s.
Use: Antinauseant, motion sickness.
MARMINE INJECTION. (Vortech) Dimenhydrinate 50
mg./cc. Vial 10 ml.
Use: Antinauseant, motion sickness.
MARNAL. (Vortech) Allylisobutyl-barbituric acid 50 mg.,
aspirin 200 mg., phenacetin 130 mg., caffeine 40
mg./Tab. or Cap. Bot. 1000s.
Use: Analgesic, sedative.
MARPLAN. (Roche) Isocarboxazid 10 mg./Tab. Bot.
100s.
Use: Amine oxidase regulator, mental depression.
MARSHALL'S CUBEB CIGARETTES. (Guild) Pkg. 8s.
MARUATE-25. (Vortech) Diethylpropion HCl 25
mg./Tab. Bot. 100s, 1000s.
Use: Appetite suppressant.
MARUATE SPANTAB. (Vortech) Diethylpropion HCl
75 mg./Cap. Bot. 100s, 1000s.
Use: Anorectic.
MARZINE HYDROCHLORIDE. Cyclizine, B.A.N.
MASSE BREAST CREAM. (Ortho) Water, glyceryl
monostearate, glycerin, cetyl alcohol, lanolin,
peanut oil, Span-60, stearic acid, Tween-60, sodium
benzoate, propylparaben, methylparaben,
potassium hydroxide.
Use: Nipple care.
MASSENGILL FEMININE DEODORANT SPRAY.
(Beecham Products) Aerosol Bot. 3 oz.
Use: Vaginal deodorant.
MASSENGILL DISPOSABLE DOUCHE. (Beecham
Products) Water, alcohol, lactic acid, sodium
lactate, octoxymol-9, cetylpyridium chloride,
imidazolidinyl urea, disodium EDTA, fragrance, color.
Bot. 6 oz.
Use: Liquid douche.
MASSENGILL LIQUID. (Beecham Products) Lactic
acid, water, sodium lacate, methyl salicylate,
eucalyptol, menthol, thymol, octoxynol-9, color, alco-
hol. Bot. 4 oz., 8 oz.
Use: Vaginal douche.
MASSENGILL MEDICATED. (Beecham Products)
Povidone iodine 0.23% when added to sanitized
fluid. Bot. 6 oz.
Use: Medicated douche for vaginal therapy.

MASSENGILL POWDER. (Beecham Products)
Sodium Cl., ammonium alum, PEG-8, methyl salicylate, eucalyptus oil, menthyl, thymol, phenol. Jar 4 oz., 8 oz., 16 oz., 22 oz. Packette 10s, 12s.
Use: Vaginal cleanser.

MASSENGILL VINEGAR-WATER DISPOSABLE DOUCHE. (Beecham Products) Water and vinegar solution. Bot. 6 oz.
Use: Disposable liquid douche.

MASTER FORMULA. (Barth's) Vit. A 10,000 I.U., D 400 I.U., C 180 mg., B-1 7 mg., B-2 14 mg., niacin 4.6 mg., B-6 292 mcg., pantothenic acid 210 mcg., B-12 25 mcg., biotin 2.9 mcg., E 50 I.U., calcium 800 mg., P 387 mg., iron 10 mg., iodine 0.1 mg., choline 7.78 mg., inositol 11.6 mg., aminobenzoic acid 35 mcg., rutin 30 mg., citrus bioflavonoid complex 30 mg./4 Tab. Bot. 120s, 600s, 1200s.

MASTISOL. (Ferndale) Nonirritating medical adhesive. Bot. 4 oz.
Use: Skin dressing adhesive.

MATERNA 1.60. (Lederle) Vit. A 8000 I.U., D 400 I.U., E 30 I.U., C 120 mg., folic acid 1.0 mg., B-1 3 mg., B-2 3.4 mg., B-6 4 mg., niacinamide 20 mg., B-12 12 mcg., Ca 350 mg., iodine 0.3 mg., Mg 100 mg., Fe 60 mg., Cu 2 mg., Zn 15 mg./Tab. Bot. 100s.
Use: Prenatal supplement.

MATERNAVITE CAPSULES. (Knight) Bot. 100s.
Use: Prenatal vitamin.

MATULANE. (Roche) Procarbazine HCl 50 mg./Cap. Bot. 100s.
Use: Palliative treatment of Hodgkin's disease.

MAURRY'S FUNGICIDE. (Maurry) Nitromersol 37 mg., alcohol 70-74%/oz. Bot. 1 oz., pt.
Use: External fungus infection.

MAXAFIL CREAM. (CooperCare) Cinoxate 4%, methyl anthranilate 5% in cream base. Tube 1 oz.
Use: Sunscreen.

MAXAMAG SUSPENSION. (Vitarine) Magnesium hydroxide, aluminum hydroxide gel.
Use: Antacid.

MAXIBOLIN. (Organon) Ethylestrenol 2 mg./Tab. Bot. 100s. Elixir 2 mg./5 ml. Bot. 4 oz.
Use: Anabolic agent.

MAXIDEX. (Alcon) Dexamethasone 0.1% in a 0.5% solution, methylcellulose vehicle/5 cc. Bot. 5 cc. & 15 cc.
Use: Opthalmic anti-inflammatory.

MAXIFLOR CREAM & OINTMENT. (Herbert) Diflorasone diacetate 0.05%. Tubes 15 Gm., 30 Gm., 60 Gm.
Use: Steroid responsive dermatoses.

MAXIGESIC. (Merchant) Codeine phosphate 30 mg., acetaminophen 325 mg., promethazine HCl 6.25 mg./Cap. Bot. 100s.
Use: Analgesic.

MAXIMUM STRENGTH NO-ASPIRIN SINUS MEDICATION. (Walgreen) Acetaminophen 500 mg., pseudoephedrine HCl 30 mg./Tab. Bot. 50s.
Use: Analgesic, decongestant.

MAXITON.
See: Amphetamine (Various Mfr.)

MAXITROL OINTMENT. (Alcon) Dexamethasone

0.1%, neomycin 3.5 mg., polymyxin B sulfate 10,000 u./Gm. Tubes 3.5 Gm.
Use: Ocular infections.

MAXITROL OPHTHALMIC SUSPENSION. (Alcon) Dexamethasone 0.1%, neomycin (as sulfate) 3.5 mg., polymyxin B sulfate 10,000 u./cc. Bot. 5 cc. droptainer.
Use: Infectious ocular inflammations.

MAYASEN. (Janssen) Astemizole
Use: Anti-allergenic, antihistaminic.

• **MAYTANSINE.** USAN.
Use: Antineoplastic.

MAZANOR. (Wyeth) Mazindol 1 mg./Tab. Bot. 30s.
Use: Anorectic agent.

• **MAZINDOL,** U.S.P. XXI. Tab., U.S.P. XXI. 5-(p-Chlorophenyl)-2,3-dihydro-5,H-imidazo [2,1-a]isoindol-5-ol.
Use: Anorexic; appetite suppressant.
See: Mazanor, Tab. (Wyeth)
Sanorex, Tab. (Sandoz)

MAZON MEDICATED CREAM. (Norcliff Thayer) Coal tar 0.18%, salicylic acid 1%, resorcinol 1%, benzoic acid 0.5%. Jar 1.75 oz., 3 oz.
Use: Dermatologic.

MBF. (Gerber) Meat Base Formula Liquid hypoallergenic infant feeding formula. Made from beef hearts, water, cane sugar, sesame oil, modified tapioca starch, w/tricalcium phosphate, calcium citrate, potassium chloride, iodized salt, Mg chloride, Na ascorbate, ferrous sulfate, zinc sulfate, Mn sulfate, biotin, cupric sulfate, potassium iodide and Vit. A, B-2, B-6, B-12, niacinamide, calcium pantothenate, folic acid, D, E, and K. Cans 15 oz.
Use: Hypoallergenic infant formula, specifically for milk intolerance or lactose intolerance, and other non-specific food intolerances.

M-CAPS. (Mill-Mark) Methionine 200 mg./Cap. Bot. 50s, 1000s.
Use: Diaper rash and odor control.

M-CILLIN B-400 POWDER. (Misemer) Bot. 80 cc, 150 cc.

MCT OIL. (Mead Johnson) Triglycerides of medium chain fatty acids. Lipid fraction of coconut oil; fatty acid shorter than C-8 <6%, C_8(octanoic) 67%, C_{10}(decanoic) 23%, longer than C_{10} <4%. Bot. qt.
Use: Easily absorbed dietary fat.

MDP-SQUIBB. (Squibb) Technetium Tc 99 medronate. Pkg. 10 reaction vials.
Use: Bone imaging agent to delineate areas of altered osteogenesis..

MEADININ. Mixture of Amoidin & Amidin alk. of Ammi Majus Linn.

MEASLES CONVALESCENT SERUM.
See: Measles Immune Human Serum

MEASLES IMMUNE GLOBULIN (HUMAN). Sterile soln. of gamma globulin derived from pooled normal human plasma.
Use: In conjunction with live attenuated measles virus vaccine, to attenuate symptoms.

MEASLES PROPHYLACTIC SERUM.
See: Immune Serum Globulin (Human)

• **MEASLES & MUMPS VIRUS VACCINE LIVE,** U.S.P. XXI.

MEASLES, MUMPS AND RUBELLA VIRUS VACCINE LIVE, U.S.P. XXI.

MEASLES AND RUBELLA VIRUS VACCINE LIVE, U.S.P. XXI.
See: M-R-Vax, Inj. (Merck Sharp & Dohme)

• **MEASLES VIRUS VACCINE, LIVE,** U.S.P. XXI.
Modified live-virus measles vaccine (Schwarz strain).
Use: One-shot vaccine for common measles (rubeola).
Use: Active immunizing agent.
See: Attenuvax, Inj. (Merck Sharp & Dohme)
Lirugen, Inj. (Merrell Dow)
M-Vac, Inj. (Lederle)
W/Mumps virus vaccine, rubella virus vaccine.
See: Lirutrin, Vial (Merrell Dow)
W/Rubella virus vaccine.
See: Lirubel, Vial (Merrell Dow)

MEASLES VIRUS VACCINE, LIVE ATTENUATED.
Moraten line derived from Enders' attenuated Edmonston strain grown in cell cultures of chick embryos.
See: Attenuvax, Inj. (Merck Sharp & Dohme)
W/Mumps virus vaccine, rubella virus vaccine.
See: M-M-R., Vial (Merck Sharp & Dohme)
W/Rubella virus vaccine.
See: M-R-Vax, Inj. (Merck Sharp & Dohme)

MEASURIN. (Winthrop-Breon) Aspirin 10 gr. in sustained-release form/Tab. Bot. 60s.
Use: Analgesic.

MEBADIN. Dehydroemetine, B.A.N.

MEBANAZINE. B.A.N. α-Methylbenzylhydrazine. Actomol
Use: Monoamine oxidase inhibitor.

MEBARAL. (Winthrop-Breon) Mephobarbital. Tab. 0.5 gr. Bot. 250s, 1000s. 0.75 gr., 1.5 gr., 3 gr. Bot. 250s.
Use: Sedative, anticonvulsant for treatment petit mal and grand mal epilepsy.

• **MEBENDAZOLE,** U.S.P. XXI. Tab., U.S.P. XXI.
Methyl 5-benzoyl-2-benzimidazolecarbanate.
Use: Anthelmintic.
See: Vermox, Tab. (Janssen)

MEBEVERINE. B.A.N. 4-[N-Ethyl-2-(4-methoxy-phenyl)-1-methylethylamino]butyl-3,4-dimethoxy-benzoate.
Colofac; Duspatal; Duspatalin hydrochloride.

• **MEBEVERINE HYDROCHLORIDE.** USAN. 4-[Ethyl (p-methoxy-α-methyl-phenethyl) amino] butyl veratrate hydrochloride.
Use: Spasmolytic agent.

MEBEZONIUM IODIDE. B.A.N. 4,4'-Methylenedi-(cyclohexyltrimethylammonium iodide).
Use: Neuromuscular blocking agent.

MEBHYDROLIN. B.A.N. 5-Benzyl-1,2,3,4-tetrahydro-2-methyl-γ-carboline. Fabahistin napadisylate
Use: Antihistamine.

MEBINOL. Clefamide, B.A.N.

• **MEBROFENIN.** USAN.
Use: Diagnostic aid (hepatobiliary function determination).

• **MEBUTAMATE.** USAN. 2-Carbamoyloxymethyl-2,3-dimethyl carbamate. Capla.

Use: Hypotensive.

MECADOX. Carbadox, B.A.N.

MECAMYLAMINE. B.A.N. 2,2,3-Trimethyl-3-methylaminobicyclo[2.2.1]heptane. Inversine; Mevasine hydrochloride.
Use: Hypotensive.

• **MECAMYLAMINE HYDROCHLORIDE,** U.S.P. XXI.
Tab., U.S.P. XXI. N, 2, 3, 3-Tetramethyl-2-norbornanamine HCl. 3-Methylaminoiso-camphane HCl. N-Methyl-di-isobornylamine HCl.
Use: Antihypertensive.
See: Inversine, Tab. (Merck Sharp & Dohme)

• **MECHLORETHAMINE HYDROCHLORIDE,** U.S.P. XXI. Inj. U.S.P. XXI. 2,2'-Dichloro-n-methyl-diethylamine HCl. Trituration. Dichloren.
Use: Antineoplastic.
See: Mustargen, Vial (Merck Sharp & Dohme)

MECHOL INJ. (Manne) Vial 30 cc.

MECHOL TABS. (Manne) dl B-6 5 mg., soy protein 100 mg.; Vit. B-1 5 mg.; B-2 2mg.; C 75 mg.; niacinamide 20 mg.; pantothenic acid 2 mg.; brewer's yeast 2.5 gr./Tabs. Bot. 100s, 120s, 1000s.
Use: Metabolic tonic.

MECHOLIN HCl.
See: Methacholine Chloride, U.S.P. XXI.

MECHOLYL OINTMENT. (Gordon) Methacholine Cl 0.25%, methyl salicylate 10% in ointment base. Jar 4 oz., lb., 5 lb.
Use: Minor muscular aches and pains, simple neuralgia.

MECILLINAM. B.A.N. (2S,5R,6R)-6-(Perhydro-azepin-1-ylmethyleneamino)penicillanic acid.
Use: Antibiotic.

MECLAN. (Ortho) Meclocycline sulfosalicylate cream 1%. Tube 20 Gm., 45 Gm.
Use: Acne vulgaris treatment.

MECLASTINE. Clemastine.

• **MECLIZINE HYDROCHLORIDE,** U.S.P. XXI. Tab. U.S.P. XXI. 1(p-Chloro-α-phenylbenzyl)-4-m-(methylbenzyl)piperazine 2 HCl.
Use: Antinauseant.
See: Antivert, Tab., Chewable (Roerig)
Bonine, Tab. (Pfizer)

• **MECLOCYCLINE.** USAN. 7-Chloro-4-(di-methylamino)-1, 4, 4a, 5, 5a, 6, 11, 12a-octahydro-3, 5, 10, 12, 12a-pentahydroxy-6-methylene-1, 11-dioxo-2-naphthacenecarboxamide.
Use: Antibiotic.

• **MECLOCYCLINE SULFOSALICYLATE,** U.S.P. XXI. Cream, U.S.P. XXI.
Use: Antibiotic
See: Meclan, Cream (Ortho)

• **MECLOFENAMATE SODIUM,** U.S.P. XXI. Cap., U.S.P. XXI. Benjoic acid, 2-(2, 6-dichloro-3-methylphenyl) amino)-, monosodium salt, monohydrate.
Use: Anti-inflammatory.

• **MECLOFENAMIC ACID.** USAN. N-(2,6-Dichloro-m-tolyl)-anthranilic acid.
Use: Anti-inflammatory.

MECLOFENOXATE. B.A.N. 2-Dimethylamino-ethyl 4-chlorophenoxyacetate. Lucidril hydrochloride
Use: Cerebral stimulant.

MECLOMEN. (Parke-Davis) Meclofenamate sodium

monohydrate equiv. to 50 or 100 mg. meclofenamic acid/Cap. Bot. 100s, 500s (100 mg.). Unit dose 100s.
Use: Non-steroidal anti-inflammatory.

• **MECLOQUALONE.** USAN. 3-(o-Chlorophenyl)-2-methyl-4 (3 H)-quinazolinone.
Use: Sedative, hypnotic.

• **MECLORISONE DIBUTYRATE.** USAN.
Use: Anti-inflammatory.

• **MECOBALAMIN.** USAN.
Use: Vitamin.

MECLOZINE. B.A.N. 1-(4-Chlorobenzhydryl)-4-(3-methylbenzyl)piperazine. Ancolan dihydrochloride.
Use: Antihistamine.

MECOBALAMIN. B.A.N. α-(5,6-Dimethylbenzimidazol-1-yl)cobamide methyl.
Use: Treatment of vitamin B-12 deficiency.

MECODRIN.
See: Amphetamine (Various Mfr.)

• **MECRYLATE.** USAN. Methyl 2-cyanoacrylate.
Use: Surgical aid (tissue adhesive).

MECYSTEINE. Methyl Cysteine.

MEDA CAP. (Circle) Acetaminophen 500 mg./Cap. Bot. 100s.
Use: Analgesic, antipyretic.

MEDA-HIST ELIXIR. (Medwick) Bot. 4 oz., pt., gal.
Use: Decongestant.

MEDA-HIST EXPECTORANT. (Medwick) Bot. 4 oz., pt., gal.
Use: Decongestant, antitussive.

MEDA-HIST DH. (Medwick) Bot. 4 oz., pt., gal.
Use: Decongestant, antitussive.

MEDALOX. (Med. Chem; Medwick) Magnesium alum. hydroxide gel. Bot. 12 oz., pt., gal.
Use: Antacid.

MED-APAP ELIXIR. (Medwick) Bot. 4 oz., pt., gal.

MEDA-TEX. (Sutliff & Case) Ethinyl estradiol 0.01 mg., methyltestosterone 2.0 mg., Vit. A 5000 I.U., D 400 I.U., E 2 I.U., C 30 mg., B-1 3 mg., B-2 2 mg., B-6 0.5 mg., B-12 1 mcg., niacinamide 20 mg., calcium pantothenate 3 mg., Fe 60 mg., Cu 1 mg., Mn 3 mg., iodine 0.15 mg., Zn 1 mg., Mg 5 mg., Ca 48 mg., P 37 mg./3 Tabs. Bot. 100s, 1000s.

MEDA-TUSS. (Medwick) Bot. 4 oz., pt., gal.

MEDA-TUSS A-C. (Medwick) Bot. 4 oz., pt., gal.

MEDA-TUSS DM. (Medwick) Bot. 4 oz., pt., gal.

MEDA-TUSS PE. (Medwick) Bot. 4 oz., pt., gal.

MEDAZEPAM. B.A.N. 7-Chloro-2,3-dihydro-1-methyl-5-phenyl-1H-1,4-benzodiazepine. Nobrium.
Use: Tranquilizer.

• **MEDAZEPAM HCl.** USAN. 7-Chloro-2, 3-dihydro-1-methyl-5-phenyl-lH-1, 4-benzodiazepine mono-HCl. Under study.
Use: Tranquilizer.

MEDENT. (Stewart-Jackson) Pseudoephedrine HCl 120 mg., guaifenesin 500 mg./Tab. Bot. 100s.
Use: Temporary relief of nasal congestion and nonproductive cough.

MEDI-AID FIRST AID SPRAY. (Wisconsin) Bot. 4 oz.
Use: Minor cut and burn treatment.

MEDIATRIC CAPS & TABS. (Ayerst) Conjugated Estrogens 0.25 mg., methyltestosterone 2.5 mg., Vit. C 100 mg., thiamine mononitrate 10 mg., Vit. B-12 2.5 mcg., ferrous sulfate exsic. 30 mg., B-2 5

mg., B-6 3 mg., niacinamide 50 mg., Ca pantothenate 20 mg., methamphetamine HCl 1 mg./Cap. & Tab. **Cap.** Bot. 100s. **Tabs.** Bot. 100s.
Use: For use in aging patients of both sexes.

MEDIATRIC LIQUID. (Ayerst) Conjugated estrogens 0.25 mg., methyltestosterone 2.5 mg., Vit. B-1 5 mg., B-12 1.5 mcg., methamphetamine HCl 1 mg./15 ml. Bot. 1 pt.
Use: For use in aging patients of both sexes.

MEDIBRIN-T FORMULA. (Image) Multiple vitamin. Bot. 100s.
Use: Supplement.

MEDICAINE CREAM. (Walgreen) Benzocaine & resorcinol. Tube 1.25 oz.
Use: Antipruritic.

MEDICATED POWDER. (Johnson & Johnson) Zinc oxide, talc, fragrance, menthol. Plastic containers 3 oz., 6 oz., 11 oz.
Use: Minor skin irritations.

MEDI CEPTIX FIRST AID SPRAY. (Eckerd) Alcohol 3.17%, octoxynol-9 1%, benzethonium chloride 0.-5%. Bot. 4 oz.
Use: Topical antiseptic.

MEDI-CON CAPS. (Image) Bot. 100s.
Use: Supplement.

MEDICONE DRESSING. (Medicone) Cod liver oil 125 mg., zinc oxide 125 mg., 8-hydroxyquinoline-sulfate 0.5 mg., benzocaine 5 mg., menthol 1.8 mg./Gm. w/petrolatum, lanolin, talcum, paraffin, perfume. Tube 1 oz., 3 oz.; Jar 1 lb.
Use: Antiseptic skin preparation.

MEDICONE-HC RECTAL. (Medicone) Hydrocortisone acetate 10 mg., benzocaine 2 gr., oxyquinoline sulfate ¼ gr., zinc oxide 3 gr., menthol ½ gr., balsam peru 1 gr., in a cocoa butter base/Supp. Box 12s. W/out H.C. Box 12s, 24s.
Use: Anorectal inflammation, pruritus and hemorrhoids.

MEDICONET. (Medicone) Benzalkonium chloride 0.02%, ethoxylated lanolin 0.5%, methylparaben 0.15%, hamamelis water 50%, glycerin 10%. Cloth wipe. Boxes 20s.
Use: Treatment of anal discomfort as a cleanser of the affected area.

MEDIGESIC PLUS. (U.S. Chemical) Butalbital 50 mg., acetaminophen 325 mg., caffeine 40 mg./Cap.
Use: Analgesic-sedative.

MEDIHALER-DUO. Now Duo-Medihaler.(Riker)

MEDIHALER-EPI. (Riker) Epinephrine bitartrate 7.0 mg./ml. solution. Pkg. Medihaler in inert propellant. Oral adapter w/15 ml. vial. Refill Vial 15 ml.
Use: Inhalation, bronchial asthma therapy.

MEDIHALER-ERGOTAMINE. (Riker) Ergotamine tartrate 9.0 mg./ml. 0.36 mg. is delivered with each inhalation. Oral adapter w/2.5 ml. Vial.
Use: Recurrent-type headache including migrainous headache.

MEDIHALER-ISO. (Riker) Isoproterenol sulfate 2.0 mg./ml. solution. Oral adapter w/15 ml. vial; Oral adapter w/22.5 ml vial. Refill vials 15 ml. and 22.5 ml.
Use: Inhalation, bronchial asthma therapy.

MEDI-JECT UNIT DOSE VIALS. (Century) Tamperproof

rubber stoppered vial containing 1 ml. sterile
solution. Single dose use.
See: Ulti-ject disposable syringe products.
  Atropine sulfate. 0.4 mg./ml.
  Atropine sulfate. 1.2 mg./ml.
  Scopolamine HBr. 400 mcg./ml.
MEDIPAK. (Geneva) First aid kit.
MEDI-PHITE. (Med. Chem.) Vitamin B-1 & B-12 syrup.
Bot. 4 oz., pt., gal.
MEDIPLEX TABULES. (U.S. Chemical) B-complex, Vit.
C, Vit. E, trace minerals, zinc/Tab. Bot. 100s.
Use: Stress, alcoholism, geriatrics.
MEDIQUE EAR DROPS. (Edward J. Moore)
Carbamide peroxide in anhydrous glycerol.
Use: Antiseptic ear drops.
MEDIQUELL. (Warner-Lambert) Dextromethorphan
HBr 15 mg./Chewy square. Pkg. 12s, 24s.
Use: Cough suppressant.
MEDI-QUIK AEROSOL. (Lehn & Fink) Lidocaine 2.5%,
benzalkonium chloride 0.1%, ethanol 38%. Aerosol
3 oz.
Use: Antiseptic, anesthetic first-aid spray.
MEDI-QUICK PUMP SPRAY. (Lehn & Fink) Lidocaine
2.5%, benzalkonium chloride, 0.1%, ethanol 38%,
isopropyl alcohol. Bot. 4 oz.
Use: Antiseptic, anesthetic first-aid spray.
MEDI-SPAS ELIXIR. (Medical Chemicals; Medwick)
Phenobarbital 16.2 mg., hyoscyamine sulfate
0.1037 mg., atropine sulfate 0.0194 mg., hyoscine
hydrobromide 0.0065 mg., alcohol 23%/5 cc. Bot.
4 oz., pt., gal.
Use: Antispasmodic and sedative.
MEDI-TAL. (Medi-Rx) Phenobarbital 16 mg., hyoscyamine sulfate 0.1037 mg., atropine sulfate 0.0194
mg., scopolamine HBr 0.0065 mg., alcohol 23%/5
cc. Bot. pt., gal. Tabs., Bot. 100s, 1000s.
Use: Antispasmodic and sedative.
MEDITUSSIN-X LIQUID. (Hauck) Codeine phosphate
50 mg., ammonium chloride 520 mg., potassium
guaiacolsulfonate 520 mg., pyrilamine maleate 50
mg., phenylpropanolamine HCl 50 mg., dl-desox-
yephedrine HCl 2 mg., tartar emetic 5 mg.,
phenyltoloxamine dihydrogen citrate 30 mg./30 cc.
Bot. gal., pt.
Use: Antitussive antihistaminic expectorant.
MEDI-ZINC. (Image) Zinc supplement. Bot. 100s.
Use: Supplement.
MEDIZINC. (U.S. Chemical) Zinc sulfate 220 mg./Tab.
Use: Zinc deficiencies.
MEDODORM. Chlorhexadol, B.A.N.
MEDOTAR. (Medco Lab) Coal tar 1%, polysorbate 80
0.5%, octoxynol 5, zinc oxide, starch, white
petrolatum. Jar 1 lb.
Use: Psoriasis and eczema, neurodermatitis,
occupational and contact dermatitis.
■ **MEDOTOPES.** (Squibb) Radiopharmaceuticals.
See: A-C-D Solution Modified (Squibb)
  Acid Citrate Dextrose Anticoagulant Solution
    Modified (Squibb)
  Aggregated Albumin (Squibb)
  Albumotope (Squibb)
  Angiotensin Immutope Kit (Squibb)
  Cobalt-Labeled Vitamin B-12 (Squibb)
  Cobalt Standards for Vitamin B-12 (Squibb)
  Cobatope (Squibb)
  Digoxin (^{125}I) Immutope Kit (Squibb)
  Gastrin (^{125}I) Immutope Kit (Squibb)
  Gold-198 (Squibb)
  Hipputope (Squibb)
  Human Serum Albumin (Squibb)
  Iodine 131: Capsules Diagnostic-Capsules Thera-
    peutic-Solution Therapeutic Oral (Squibb)
  Iodinated Human Serum Albumin (Squibb)
  Iodo-hippuric Acid (Squibb)
  Macroaggregated Albumin (Squibb)
  Macrotec (Squibb)
  Minitec (Squibb)
  Phosphorus-32: Solution Oral, Therapeutic-Sodium
    Phosphate Solution U.S.P. for oral or IV use
    therapeutic or diagnostic (Squibb)
  Red Cell Tagging Solution (Squibb)
  Renotec (Squibb)
  Rose Bengal (Squibb)
  Rubratope-57: Diagnostic Capsules-Diagnostic Kit
    (Squibb)
  Rubratope-60: Diagnostic Capsules-Diagnostic Kit
    (Squibb)
  Selenomethionine (Squibb)
  Sethotope (Squibb)
  Technetium 99m (Squibb)
  Technetium 99m-Iron-Ascorbate (DTPA) (Squibb)
  Technetium 99m Sulfur Colloid Kit (Squibb)
  Tesuloid (Squibb)
  Thyrostat-FTI (Squibb)
  Thyrostat-3 (Squibb)
  Thyrostat 4 FTI (Squibb)
MEDRALONE 40. (Keene) Methylprednisolone
acetate 40 mg./ml. Vial 5 ml.
Use: Anti-inflammatory.
MEDRALONE 80. (Keene) Methylprednisolone
acetate 80 mg/ml. Vial 5 ml.
Use: Anti-inflammatory.
• **MEDROGESTONE.** USAN. Formerly Metrogestone.
Dimethyl pregna-4, 6 diene-3, 20-dione.
Use: Oral progestin.
See: Colprone (Ayerst)
MEDROL. (Upjohn) Methylprednisolone. **Tabs.:** 2 mg.
Bot. 100s; 4 mg. Bot. 30s, 100s, 500s. Unit-Dose
100s; 8 mg. Bot. 25s; 16 mg. Bot. 50s; 24 mg. Bot.
25s; 32 mg. Bot. 25s. **Dosepak:** 4 mg. Pkg. 21s.
Alternate Daypak: 16 mg. Pkg. 14s.
Use: An anti-inflammatory corticosteroid.
MEDROL ACETATE TOPICAL. (Upjohn)
Methylprednisolone acetate 2.5 mg. or 10 mg.,
methylparaben 4 mg., butylparaben 3 mg./Gm.
0.25% Tube 7.5 Gm., 30 Gm. ; 1% Tube 7.5 Gm.,
30 Gm.
Use: Allergic dermatoses and inflammatory skin
diseases.
MEDROL ENPAK. (Upjohn) Methylprednisolone
acetate 40 mg. w/sod. chloride, polysorbate 80
Bot. when reconstituted as directed. Pak 6 Bot. & 1
administration unit. Refill Pk. 12s.
Use: Retention enema for adjunctive treatment of
ulcerative colitis.
• **MEDRONATE DISODIUM.** USAN.

Use: Pharmaceutic aid.
• **MEDRONIC ACID.** USAN.
Use: Pharmaceutic aid.
MEDRONE. (Kay) Methylprednisolone acetate 20 mg./ml. Vial 5 ml.; 40 mg./ml. Vial 5 ml., 10 ml.; 80 mg./ml. Vial 5 ml.
Use: I.M. Glucocorticosteroid.
MEDROSPHOL Hg-197. 1-(Hydroxymercuri-197 Hg)-2-propanol.
See: Merprane
• **MEDROXALOL.** USAN.
Use: Antihypertensive.
• **MEDROXALOL HYDROCHLORIDE.** USAN.
Use: Antihypertensive.
MEDROXYPROGESTERONE. B.A.N. 17 α-Hydroxy-6α-methylpregn-4-ene-3,20-dione. Provera acetate.
Use: Progestational steroid.
• **MEDROXYPROGESTERONE ACETATE,** U.S.P.XXI. Sterile Susp., Tab., U.S.P.XXI. 17-Hydroxy-6α-methylpregn-4-ene-3, 20-dione 17-Acetate. (CMC) 50 mg., 100 mg./ml. Vial 5 ml.
See: Amen, Tab. (Carnrick)
   Curretab, Tab. (Reid-Provident)
   depCorlutin (O'Neal, Jones & Feldman)
   Depo-Provera, Vials (Upjohn)
   P-Medrate-P.A., Inj. (Reid-Provident)
   Provera, Tab. (Upjohn)
• **MEDRYSONE,** U.S.P.XXI. Ophthalmic Suspension U.S.P.XXI. 11 β-Hydroxy-6α-methylpregn-4-ene-3,20-dione.
Use: Topical anti-inflammatory agent.
See: HMS Liquifilm, Ophth. Sol. (Allergan)
MED-TANE ELIXIR. (Medwick) Brompheniramine maleate. Bot. 4 oz., pt., gal.
MED-TANE EXPECTORANT DC. (Medwick) Brompheniramine maleate. Bot. 4 oz., pt., gal.
MED-TAPP ELIXIR. (Medwick) Bot. 4 oz., pt., gal.
• **MEFENIDIL.** USAN.
Use: Cerebral vasodilator
• **MEFENIDIL FUMARATE.** USAN.
Use: Cerebral vasodilator
• **MEFENAMIC ACID.** USAN. N-(2,3-Xylyl) anthranilic acid. Ponstan.
Use: Anti-inflammatory agent.
See: Ponstel, Kapseals (Parke-Davis)
MEFENOREX HCl. USAN. N-(3-chloropropyl)-α-methylphenethylamine HCl. Under study.
Use: Anorexiant.
• **MEFEXAMIDE.** USAN.
Use: Stimulant.
• **MEFLOQUINE.** USAN.
Use: Antimalarial.
MEFOXIN. (Merck Sharp & Dohme) Sterile cefoxitin sodium 1 Gm. and 2 Gm./Vial. **1 Gm.:** Vials, Tray of 25. Infusion bottles, Tray of 10 bottles. **2 Gm.:** Vials, Tray of 25. Infusion bottles, Tray of 10 bottles.
Use: Broad spectrum antibiotic by I.V. or I.M. administration.
MEFRUSIDE. USAN. (FBA) 4-Chloro-N'-methyl-N'-(tetrahydro-2-methylfurfuryl)-m-benzenedisulfonamide. Baycaron.
Use: Diuretic.

MEGA-B. (Arco) Vit. B-1 100 mg., B-2 60 mg., B-6 100 mg., B-12 100 mcg., niacinamide 100 mg., folic acid 100 mcg., pantothenic acid 100 mg., d-biotin 100 mcg., PABA 100 mg./Tab. Bot. 30s, 100s, 500s.
MEGACE. (Mead Johnson) Megestrol acetate. 20 mg., 40 mg./Tab. Bot. 100s.
Use: Palliative treatment of advanced carcinoma of the breast or endometrium.
MEGACLOR. Clomocycline, B.A.N.
MEGADOSE. (Arco) Vit. A 25,000 USP U., D 1000 USP U, C 250 mg., E 100 I.U., folic acid 400 mcg., B-1 80 mg., B-2 80 mg., niacinamide 80 mg., B-6 80 mg., B-12 80 mcg., biotin 80 mcg., pantothenic acid 80 mg., choline bitartrate 80 mg., inositol 80 mg., para-aminobenzoic acid 80 mg., rutin 30 mg., citrus bioflavonoids 30 mg., betaine HCl 30 mg., glutamic acid 30 mg., hesperidin complex 5 mg., iodine 0.15 mg., Ca gluconate 10 mg., ferrous gluconate 10 mg., Mg gluconate 7 mg., Mn gluconate 6 mg., Cu gluconate 0.5 mg./Cap. Bot. 100s, 250s.
Use: Dietary supplement.
• **MEGALOMICIN POTASSIUM PHOSPHATE.** USAN.
Use: Antibacterial.
MEGATON. (Hyrex) Thiamine HCl 2.5 mg., riboflavin 2.5 mg., pyridoxine HCl 1.0 mg., Vit. B-12 5.0 mcg., dexpanthenol 5 mg., niacin 10.0 mg., ferric pyrophosphate 20 mg./30 ml. W/alcohol 15%. Bot. 16 oz.
Use: Geriatric supplement.
MEGA-VITA. (Saron) Vit. C 500 mg., niacinamide 500 mg., B-6 50 mg., B-1 25 mg., B-2 10 mg., B-12 50 mcg., folic acid 150 mcg., E 200 I.U., pantothenic acid 10 mg., A 2500 I.U., D 333 I.U., magnesium oxide 10 mg., zinc sulfate 50 mg./3 Tabs. Bot. 100s.
Use: Multivitamins with minerals.
MEGA-VITA HEMATINIC. (Saron) Mega-Vita formula with iron 50 mg., Vit A 1000 I.U., Cu 2 mg., Mn 1.8 mg., iodine 0.1 mg., K 10 mg./3 Tabs.
Use: Multivitamin and mineral supplement.
MEGA-VITA TONIC. (Saron) Vit. B-12 25 mcg., B-6 6 mg., niacin 25 mg., aminoacetic acid 750 mg./15 ml. w/alcohol 17%.
Use: Vitamin supplement.
MEGESTROL. B.A.N. 17 α-Hydroxy-6-methylpregna-4,6-diene-3,20-dione.
Use: Progestogen.
• **MEGESTROL ACETATE.** U.S.P. XXI. Tab., U.S.P. XXI. 17 α-acetoxy-6-methylpregna-4,6-diene-3, 20-dione.
Use: Palliative treatment of advanced carcinoma of the breast or endometrium.
See: Megace (Mead Johnson)
   Pallace, Tab. (Bristol)
MEGIMIDE. Bemegride, B.A.N.
MEGLUMINE, U.S.P. XXI. 1-Deoxy-1-methyl-amino glucitol. 1-Methylamino-1-deoxy-D-glucitol.
Use: Pharmaceutical aid.
• **MEGLUMINE, DIATRIZOATE INJ.,** U.S.P. XXI. N-Meglumine salt of 3, 5 diacetamido-2, 4, 6-triiodo-benzoic acid. Methylglucamine Diatrizoate. D-Glucitol, 1-deoxy-1-(methylamino).
Use: Radiopaque medium.

See: Cardiografin, Vial (Squibb)
Cystografin, Vials (Squibb)
Gastrografin, Soln. (Squibb)
Hypaque-76, Inj. (Winthrop-Breon)
Hypaque-M 75%, Inj. (Winthrop-Breon)
Hypaque-M 90%, Inj. (Winthrop-Breon)
Hypaque Meglumine, Vials (Winthrop-Breon)
Reno-M-30, -60, Vial (Squibb)
Reno-M-Dip, Vial (Squibb)
W/Meglumine iodipamide.
See: Sinografin, Sol. (Squibb)
W/Sodium diatrizoate.
See: Gastrografin, Sol. (Squibb)
Renografin-60, Inj. (Squibb)
Renografin-76, Inj. (Squibb)
Renovist II, Inj. (Squibb)
• **MEGLUMINE, IODIPAMIDE INJ.,** U.S.P. XXI. 1-Deoxy-1-(Methyl amino) glucitol, D glucitol, 1-deoxy-1-(methylamino)
Use: Radiopaque medium.
See: Cholografin, Vial (Squibb)
W/Meglumine diatrizoate.
See: Sinografin, Sol. (Squibb)
• **MEGLUMINE, IOTHALAMATE INJ.,** U.S.P. XXI. 5-Acetamido-2,4,6-triiodo-N-methylisophthalamic acid, N-methylglucamine.
See: Conray, Vial, Amp. (Mallinckrodt)
W/Sod. iothalamate.
Use: Radiopaque medium.
See: Vascoray, Sol. (Mallinckrodt)
• **MEGLUTOL.** USAN.
Use: Antihyperlipoproteinemic.
MEJEPTIL.
See: Thioperazine (SmithKline)
MEJORAL-ACETAMINOPHEN. (Glendbrook) Acetaminophen 500 mg./Tab. Bot. 30s, 60s.
Use: Analgesic.
MEJORAL-ASPIRIN. (Glenbrook) Aspirin 500 mg., caffeine 30 mg./Tab. Bot. 30s, 60s.
Use: Analgesic.
MEJORALITO. (Glenbrook) Acetaminophen. **Tab.:**80 mg./Tab. Bot. 30s. **Liquid:** 80 mg./0.8 ml. Bot. 1 oz.
Use: Analgesic, antipyretic.
MEKTEC 99 AUTOMATIC LIQUID EXTRACTOR. (Imaj International) Soln. 99m Tc Sodium Pertechnetate.
Use: Radiodiagnostic.
MELADRAZINE. B.A.N. 2,4-Di(diethylamino)-6-hydrazino-1,3,5-triazine. Lisidonil (+)-tartrate
Use: Polysynaptic inhibitor.
MELANEX. (Neutrogena) hydroquinone 30 ml./ml. in solution containing 47.3% alcohol. Bot. 1 oz. w/Appliderm applicator.
Use: Hyperpigmentation.
MELARSONYL POTASSIUM. B.A.N. Dipotassium 2-[4-(4,6-diamino-1,3,5-triazin-2-ylamino)phenyl]-1,3,2-dithiarsolan-4,5-dicarboxylate. Trimelarsan
Use: Treatment of trypanosomiasis.
MELARSOPROL. B.A.N. 2-[4-(4,6-Diamino-1,3,5-triazin-2-ylamino)phenyl]-4-hydroxymethyl-1,3,2-dithiarsolan. Mel B

Use: Treatment of trypanosomiasis.
• **MELENGESTROL ACETATE.** USAN.
Use: Antineoplastic, progestin.
MELFIAT. (Reid-Provident) Phendimetrazine tartrate 35 mg./Tab. Bot. 100s, 1000s.
Use: Management of obesity.
MELFIAT 105 UNICELLES. (Reid-Provident) Phendimetrazine tartrate 105 mg./S.R. Cap. Bot. 100s.
Use: Management of obesity.
MELHORAL CHILD TABLET. (Winthrop Products) Acetylsalicylic acid.
Use: Analgesic, antipyretic.
MELITOXIN.
See: Dicumarol (Various Mfr.)
• **MELITRACEN HYDROCHLORIDE.** USAN.
Use: Antidepressant.
• **MELIZAME.** USAN.
Use: Sweetener.
MELLARIL CONCENTRATE. (Sandoz) Thioridazine HCl Solution 30 mg./ml. w/alcohol 3.0% Bot. 4 oz. Concentrate 100 mg./ml. Pk. 4 oz.
Use: Tranquilizer.
MELLARIL S. (Sandoz) Thioridazine oral suspension 25 mg./5 ml. or 100 mg./5 ml. Bot. pt.
Use: Tranquilizer.
MELLARIL TABLETS. (Sandoz) Thioridazine HCl 10 mg., 15 mg., 25 mg., 50 mg., 100 mg., 150 mg., 200 mg./Tab. Bot. 100s, 1000s. 10 mg., 15 mg., 25 mg., 50 mg., 100 mg., 200 mg./Tab. SandoPak pkgs. 100s.
Use: Tranquilizer.
MELLOBATH. (Beiersdorf) Water dispersible oil containing a lanolin fraction, polyethylene glycol oleate, light mineral oil, and perfume. Bot. 1 pt.
Use: Bath oil.
MELLOSE. Methylcellulose.
MELOIDS. (Boots) Throat pastille. Tube ½ oz.
Use: Hoarseness and throat irritation.
MELONEX. Metahexamide.
Use: Oral antidiabetic.
• **MELPHALAN,** U.S.P. XXI. Tabs., U.S.P. XXI. L-3-{p[bis(2-Chloroethyl)amino]phenyl} alanine.
Previously Sarcolysin.
Use: Antineoplastic.
See: Alkeran, Tab. (Burroughs Wellcome)
• **MEMOTINE HCl.** USAN. 3, 4-Dihydro-1-[(p-methoxyphen-oxy)methyl] isoquinoline HCl.
Use: Antiviral.
• **MEMOTINE HYDROCHLORIDE.** USAN.
Use: Antiviral.
• **MENABITAN HYDROCHLORIDE.** USAN.
Use: Analgesic.
• **MENADIOL SODIUM DIPHOSPHATE,** U.S.P. XXI. Inj., Tab., U.S.P. XXI. 1,4-Naphtha-lenediol,2-methyl-,bis(dihydrogen phosphate), tetrasodium salt, hexahydrate.
Use: Vitamin K therapy (Orally or I.M. 4 to 75 mg.)
See: Kappadione, Amp. (Lilly)
Synkayvite, Amp. & Tab. (Roche)
• **MENADIONE,** U.S.P. XXI. Inj., U.S.P. XXI. 2-Methyl-1,4-naphthoquinone (Menaphthone, Danitamon K, Aquinone, Aquaday, Menaquinone).

Use: Orally & I.M., Vit. K therapy.
W/Ascorbic acid.
  See: Rependo, Cap. (Scruggs)
W/Ascorbic acid, hesperidin.
  See: Hescor-K, Tab. (Madland)
W/Bioflavonoid citrus compound, ascorbic acid.
  See: C.V.P. W/Vitamin K, Syr., Tab. (USV Pharm.)
MENADIONE DIPHOSPHATE SODIUM.
  See: Menadiol Sodium Diphosphate.
MENADIONE SODIUM BISULFITE. 2-Methyl-1,4-naph-thoquinone sod. bisulfite. Sodium 1,2,3,4-tetrahydro-2-methyl-1,4-dioxo-2-naphthalenesulfonate.
  Use: Vit. K therapy.
MENADOXIME. B.A.N. Ammonium salt of 2-methyl-naphthaquinone-4-oxime O-carboxymethyl ether. Kapilon Soluble.
  Use: Treatment of hypoprothrombinemia.
MENAPHTHENE OR MENAPHTHONE.
  See: Menadione (Various Mfr.)
MENAQUINONE.
  See: Menadione (Various Mfr.)
MENEST. (Beecham Labs) Esterified estrogens, conjugated estrogens (equine) 0.3 mg./Tab. Bot. 100s. 0.625 mg.; 1.25 mg./Tab. Bot. 100s, 1000s. 2.5 mg./Tab. Bot. 50s.
  Use: Menopausal symptoms.
MENI-D. (Seatrace) Dimenhydrinate 25 mg., niacin 50 mg./Cap. Bot. 100s.
  Use: Vertigo treatment.
• **MENINGOCOCCAL POLYSACCHARIDE VACCINE GROUP A,** U.S.P. XXI.
• **MENINGOCOCCAL POLYSACCHARIDE VACCINE GROUPS A AND C COMBINE D.** U.S.P. XXI.
  See: Meningovax-AC, Inj. (Merck Sharp and Dohme)
  W/Groups A, C, Y, W-135 Combined.
  See: Menomune, Inj. (Squibb-Connaught)
MENINGOCOCCAL POLYSACCHARIDE VACCINE, GROUP A, GROUP C, GROUPS A AND C COMBINED AND GROUPS A, C, Y, W-135 COM-BINED.
  See: Menomune Inj. (Squibb-Connaught)
• **MENINGOCOCCAL POLYSACCHARIDE VACCINE GROUP C,** U.S.P. XXI.
MENINGOVAX-AC. (Merck Sharp & Dohme) Meningococcal polysaccharide vaccine, groups A & C 0.5 ml. 50 dose vial or 10 dose vial.
  Use: Immunization against infection caused by *Neisseria meningitidis.*
• **MENOCTONE.** USAN. 2-(8-Cyclohexyl-octyl)-3-hy-droxy-1, 4-naphthoquinone. Under study.
  Use: Antimalarial.
MENOGEN. (General Pharm.) Conjugated estrogens 1.25 mg./Tab. Bot. 100s.
  Use: Estrogen therapy.
MENOJECT L.A. (Mayrand) Testosterone cypionate, estradiol cypionate. Vial 10 ml.
MENOLYN. (Arcum) Ethinyl estradiol 0.05 mg./Tab. Bot. 100s, 1000s.
  Use: Hormone therapy.
MENOMUNE. (Squibb-Connaught) Meningococcal poly-

saccharide vaccine, Groups A and C, Groups A, C, Y, W-135. Vials 10 or 50 dose w/diluent.
  Use: Immunization against infection caused by *Neisseria meningitis.*
MENOMUNE-C VACCINE. Group-specific polysaccharide antigen from Neisseria meningitis, Group C. Bot. 10 & 50 dose vials.
  Use: Immunization.
• **MENOTROPINS,** U.S.P. XXI. For Inj., U.S.P. XXI.
  Use: Gonadotropin.
  See: Pergonal
MENRIUM. (Roche) **Menrium 5-2:** Chlordiazepoxide 5 mg., conjugated estrogens 0.2 mg./Tab. **Menrium 5-4:** Chlordiazepoxide 5 mg., conjugated estrogens 0.4 mg./Tab. **Menrium 10-4:** Chlordiazepoxide 10 mg., conjugated estrogens 0.4 mg./Tab. Bot. 100s.
  Use: Menopause syndromes.
MENSTRESS CAPS. (Pharmex) Cap. Bot. 15s.
  Use: Cramps.
MENTHALGESIC LIQUID. (Blue Line) Menthol, camphor, methyl salicylate. Bot. 2 oz. 12s, pt., gal.
  Use: Rubefacient liniment (external use).
MENTHALGESIC OINTMENT. (Blue Line) Chloral hydrate 1½%, methyl salicylate 12%, menthol 1½%, camphor 1½% in suitable ointment base. Jar 1 lb.
p-MENTHAN-3-OL. Menthol, U.S.P. XXI.
MENTHOL, U.S.P. XXI. Cyclohexanol, 5-methyl-2-(1-methylethyl). p-Menthan-3-ol.
  Use: Topical antipruritic, local analgesic, nasal decongestant, antitussive.
  See: Benzedrex Inhaler (SmithKline)
    Vicks Cough Silencers, Loz. (Vicks)
    Vicks Formula 44 Cough Control Discs, Loz. (Vicks)
    Vicks Inhaler (Vicks)
    Vicks Blue Mint, Lemon, Regular & Wild Cherry Medicated Cough Drops (Vicks)
    Vicks Medi-Trating Throat Lozenges (Vicks)
    Vicks Oracin Regular & Cherry, Loz. (Vicks)
    Vicks Sinex, Nasal Spray (Vicks)
    Vicks Vaporub, Oint. (Vicks)
    Vicks Vaposteam, Liq. (Vicks)
    Vicks Va-Tro-Nol, Nose Drops (Vicks)
    Victors Regular & Cherry, Loz. (Vicks)
  W/Combinations
    See: Halls Mentho-Lyptus, Prods. (Warner-Lambert)
    Listerine Antiseptic, Liq. (Warner-Lambert)
MENTHOLATUM. (Mentholatum) Menthol 1.35%, camphor 9%. Tube 1 oz., 0.4 oz. Jar. 1 oz., 3 oz.
  Use: External analgesic.
MENTHOLATUM DEEP HEATING LOTION. (Mentholatum) Menthol 6%, methyl salicylate 20%, lanolin derivative. Bot. 2 oz., 4 oz.
  Use: External analgesic.
MENTHOLATUM DEEP HEATING RUB. (Mentholatum) Menthol 5.9%, methyl salicylate 12.7%, eucalyptus oil, turpentine oil, lanolin anhydrous. Tube 1¼ oz., 3 ⅓ oz., 5 oz.
  Use: External analgesic.
MENTHOLIN. (Apco) Methyl salicylate 30%, chloroform 20%, hard soap 3%, camphor gum

2.2%, menthol 0.8%, alcohol 35%. Bot. 2 oz.
Use: External application for relief of superficial
muscular aches and pains.

MENTHYL VALERATE. Validol.
Use: Sedative.

MENTROLZ. (Mayer) Mayercin (Homatropine
methylbromide 0.5 mg. & amm. chloride 300 mg.),
caffeine alk. 32 mg., acetophenetidin 150 mg.,
salicylamide 225 mg. Tab. Bot. 16s.
Use: Analgesic.

• **MEOBENTINE SULFATE.** USAN.
Use: Cardiac depressant.

MEPARACRINE HYDROCHLORIDE.
See: Quinacrine Hydrochloride, U.S.P. XXI.

MEPARFYNOL. 2-Ethinylbutanol-2. Methylparafynol,
methylpentynol.

• **MEPARTRICIN.** USAN.
Use: Antifungal, antiprotozoal.

MEPAVLON.
See: Meprobamate, U.S.P. XXI.

MEPAZINE ACETATE & HCl. 10-[1-Methyl-3-(piperi-
dyl)methyl] phenothiazine acetate or HCl.

• **MEPENZOLATE BROMIDE,** U.S.P. XXI. Syrup, Tab.
U.S.P. XXI. N-methyl-3-hydroxypiperidine benzilate
methobromide.
Use: Anticholinergic.
See: Cantil, Tab., Liq. (Merrell Dow)
W/Phenobarbital.
See: Cantil w/phenobarbital (Merrell Dow)

MEPENZOLATE METHYL BROMIDE. Mepenzolate
bromide.
Use: Anticholinergic.

MEPERGAN. (Wyeth) promethazine HCl 25 mg.,
meperidine HCl 25 mg./ 10 cc. Tubex 50 mg./2 cc.
Box 10s.
Use: Analgesic and sedative.

MEPERGAN FORTIS. (Wyeth) Meperidine HCl 50
mg., promethazine HCl 25 mg./Cap. Bot. 100s.
Use: Analgesic and sedative.

• **MEPERIDINE HYDROCHLORIDE,** U.S.P. XXI. Inj.,
Syrup, Tab., U.S.P. XXI. (Various Mfr.) Ethyl-1-methyl-
4-phenylisonipecotate hydrochloride. (Parke-Davis)
50 mg./ml., 75 mg./ml., 100 mg./ml. as 1 ml. fill in
2 ml. Steri-dose syringe. (Dolantal, Dolantin, Dolosal,
Dolvanol, Endolate, Isonipecaine & Pethidine)
Use: Analgesic (narcotic).
See: Demerol Hydrochloride, Preps. (Winthrop-
Breon)
W/Acetaminophen.
See: Demerol APAP, Tab. (Winthrop-Breon)
W/Promethazine HCl.
See: Mepergan, Prep. (Wyeth)

MEPHENESIN. 3-o-Tolyloxypropane-1,2-diol. Lisse-
phen; Myanesin; Tolseram carbamate.
Use: Skeletal muscle relaxant.
See: Mervaldin, Tab. (Lannett)
    Myanesin
W/Acetaminophen, Vit. C, butabarbital.
See: T-Caps, Cap. (Burlington)
W/Mephobarbital, hyoscine HBr.
See: Tranquil, Tab. (Kenyon)
W/Pentobarbital.

See: Nebralin, Tab. (Dorsey)
W/Salicylamide, butabarbital sodium.
See: Metrogesic, Tab. (Metro Med)

MEPHENESIN CARBAMATE.
See: Methoxydone

MEPHENOXALONE. 5-(o-Methoxyphenoxy-methyl-)-
2-oxazolidinone.

MEPHENTERMINE. B.A.N. Nαα-Trimethyl-phenethyl-
amine. Mephine sulfate.
Use: Hypertensive.

• **MEPHENTERMINE SULFATE,** U.S.P. XXI. Inj.,
U.S.P. XXI. N,α,α-Trimethyl-phenethylamine sulfate.
Mephine.
Use: Vasoconstrictor and nasal decongestant. Also
I.V. or I.M.
See: Wyamine Sulfate Inl. (Wyeth)
W/Phenacetin, aspirin, promethazine HCl.
See: Synalgos, Cap. (Ives)

• **MEPHENYTOIN,** U.S.P. XXI. Tab., U.S.P. XXI. 5-Ethyl-
3-methyl-5-phenylhydantoin.
Use: Anticonvulsant.
See: Mesantoin, Tab. (Sandoz)

• **MEPHOBARBITAL,** U.S.P. XXI. Tab., U.S.P. XXI. 5-
Ethyl-5-phenyl N-methyl-barbituric acid. 5-Ethyl-1-
methyl-5-phenylbarbituric Acid.
Use: Anticonvulsant; sedative.
See: Mebaral, Tab. (Winthrop-Breon)
W/Acetaminophen.
See: Koly-Tabs (Scrip)
W/Homatropine methylbromide, atropine methylnitrate
& hyoscine HBr.
W/Mephenesin, hyoscine HBr.
See: Tranquil, Tab. (Kenyon)

MEPHONE.
See: Mephentermine.

MEPHYTON. (Merck Sharp & Dohme) Phytonadione
(vitamin K-1) 5 mg./Tab. Bot. 100s.
Use: Hemostatic agent.

MEPIBEN. (Schen Labs.) Methylpiperidyl benzhydryl
ether.
Use: Antihistaminic.

MEPIPERPHENIDOL BROMIDE. 1-(3 Hydroxy-5-
methyl-4-phenylexyl)-1-methyl piperidium bromide.
Use: Anticholinergic.

MEPIPRAZOLE. B.A.N. 1-(3-Chlorophenyl)-4-[2-(5-me-
thylpyrazol-3-yl)ethyl]piperazine.
Use: Psychotropic agent.

MEPIVACAINE. B.A.N. 1-Methyl-2-(2,6-xylyl-carbam-
oyl) piperidine. Carbocaine.
Use: Local anesthetic.

• **MEPIVACAINE HCl,** U.S.P. XXI. Inj. U.S.P. XXI. dl-
1-Methyl-2′,6′-pipecoloxylidide monohydrochloride.
(+)-1-Methyl-2′,6′-pipecoloxylidide Hydrochloride.
Use: Local anesthetic.
See: Carbocaine, Cartridge, Vial (Cook-Waite)
    Carbocaine, Vials (Winthrop-Breon)
    Cavacaine, Vial (Graham)

• **MEPIVACAINE HYDROCHLORIDE AND
LEVONORDEFRIN INJ.,** U.S.P. XXI.
Use: Local anesthetic.
See: Carbocaine, Cartridge, Vial (Cook-Waite)

MEPRED-40. (Savage) Methylprednisolone acetate suspension 40 mg./ml. Vial 5 ml.
Use: Corticosteroid.

MEPRED-80. (Savage) Methylprednisolone acetate suspension 80 mg./ml. Vial 5 ml.
Use: Corticosteroid.

MEPREDNISONE. 17,21-Dihydroxy-16β-methylpregna-1,4-diene-3,11,20-trione. Betaspred.
Use: Glucocorticoid.

• **MEPROBAMATE,** U.S.P. XXI. Oral Susp., Tab., U.S.P. XXI. 2-Methyl-2-n-propyl-1,3-propanediol dicarbamate. 2,2-Di(carbamoyloxymethyl)pentane. 2-Carbamoyloxymethyl-2-methylpentyl carbamate. Mepavlon.
Use: Minor tranquilizer, sedative.
See: Arcoban Tablets (Arcum)
Bamate, Tab. (Century)
Equanil Tab., Cap., (Wyeth)
Meprocon, Tab. (CMC)
Meprospan, Cap. (Wallace)
Miltown, Tab. (Wallace)
Pax-400, Tab. (Kenyon)
SK-Bamate, Tab. (SmithKline)
Tranmep, Tab. (Reid-Provident)
W/Benactyzine HCl.
See: Deprol, Tab. (Wallace)
W/Estrogens conjugated.
See: Milprem, Tab. (Wallace)
W/Ethoheptazine citrate, acetylsalicylic acid.
See: Equagesic, Tab. (Wyeth)
W/Pentaerythritol tetranitrate.
See: Miltrate, Tab. (Wallace)
Robam-Petn, Tab. (Robinson)
W/Premarin.
See: PMB-200, Tab. (Ayerst)
W/Tridihexethyl chloride.
See: Milpath, Tab. (Wallace)
Pathibamate—200, 400, Tab. (Lederle)

MEPROBAMATE, N-ISOPROPYL.
See: Carisoprodol

MEPROCHOL. B.A.N. (2-Methoxyprop-2-enyl)-trimethylammonium bromide. Esmodil.
Use: Parasympathomimetic.

MEPROCON. (CMC) Meprobamate 200 mg. or 400 mg./Tab. Bot. 100s, 500s, 1000s.
Use: Tranquilizer.

MEPROGESIC. (Lemmon) Meprobamate 150 mg., ethoheptazine citrate 75 mg., aspirin 250 mg./Tab. Bot 100s, 500s, 1000s.
Use: Muscle relaxant.

MEPROSPAN. (Wallace) Meprobamate in form of coated pellets which release drug continuously for 10-12 hours. 200 mg. or 400 mg./Cap. Bot. 100s.
Use: Anxiety and tension states.

MEPROTHIXOL. B.A.N. 9-(3-Dimethylamino-propyl)-9-hydroxy-2-methoxythiaxanthen.
Use: Analgesic; anti-inflammatory.

• **MEPRYLCAINE HYDROCHLORIDE,** U.S.P. XXI. 2-Methyl-2-propylaminopropyl Benzoate HCl. 2-Methyl-2-(propylamino)-1-propanol benzoate (Ester) Hydrochloride.

Use: Local anesthetic (dental).

• **MEPRYLCAINE HYDROCHLORIDE AND EPINEPHRINE INJ.,** U.S.P. XXI.
Use: Local anesthetic.

MEPTAZINOL. B.A.N. 3-Ethyl-3-(hydroxyphenyl)-1-methylhexahydroazepine.
Use: Analgesic.

MEPYRAMINE. B.A.N. N-4-Methoxybenzyl-N'N'-dimethyl-N-2-pyridylethylenediamine. 2-(N-p-Anisyl-N-2-pyridylamino)ethyldimethylamine. Anthical; Anthisan; Flavelix; Neo-antergan hydrogen maleate.
Use: Antihistamine.
See: Pyrilamine Maleate U.S.P. XXI.

MEPYRAPONE. 2-Methyl-1,2-dl-3-pyridyl-1-propane.
See: Metopirone, Tab., Amp. (Ciba)

• **MEQUIDOX.** USAN. 3-Methyl-2-quinozaline-methanol 1,4-dioxide. Under study.
Use: Antibacterial.

MEQUINOLATE. Name used for Proquinolate.

MERAGIDONE SODIUM. The sodium salt of anhydro-N-(beta-methoxy-gamma-hydroxymercuripropyl)-2-pyridone-5-carboxylic acid-theophylline.

• **MERALEIN SODIUM.** USAN.
Use: Topical anti-infective.
See: Sodium Meralein

MERALLURIDE. B.A.N. Equal amts. of theophylline and methoxyhydroxymercuripropyl succinylurea. [3-[3-(3-Carboxypropionyl)ureido]-2-methoxypropyl]hydroxy-mercury mixture with theophylline.
Use: Diuretic.
See: Mercuhydrin, Sod., Inj. (Lakeside)

MERBAPHEN. 2-(Carboxymethoxy)-3-chlorophenyl (5,5-diethylbarbiturato)mercury.

MERBENTYL. Dicyclomine, B.A.N.

MERBROMIN. Disodium 2,7-dibrom-4-hydroxy-mercurifluorescein. (Asceptichrome, Chromargyre, Cynochrome, Flavurol, Gallochrome Mercurocol, Mercurophage, Mercurome, Planochrome)
Use: Topical antiseptic.
See: Mercurochrome, Pow., Sol. (Hynson, Westcott & Dunning)

(2-MERCAPTOETHYL)TRIMETHYLAMMONIUM IODIDE S-ESTER WITH O, O-DIETHYL PHOSPHOROTHIOATE. Echothiophate Iodide, U.S.P. XXI.

MERCAPTOMERIN SODIUM. Disodium salt of N-(3-carboxymethyl-thio-mercuri-2-methoxypropyl)camphoramic acid. 3-(3-Carboxy-2,2,3-trimethylayclopentanecarboxamide)-2-methoxy propyl (hydrogen mercaptoaceto) mercury disodium salt.
Use: Diuretic.
See: Thiomerin Sodium, Inj. (Wyeth)

• **MERCAPTOPURINE,** U.S.P. XXI. Tab., U.S.P. XXI. 6-Mercaptopurine. Purine-6-thiol. monohydrate; 6H-purine-6-thione, monohydrate.
Use: Antineoplastic.
See: Purinethol, Tab. (Burroughs Wellcome)

6-MERCAPTOPURINE. Mercaptopurine, U.S.P. XXI.

D-3-MERCAPTOVALINE. Penicillamine, U.S.P. XXI.

MERCARBOLID. o-Hydroxy-phenylmercuric chloride.

MERCAZOLE.
　See: Methimazole U.S.P. XXI.
MERCLORAN. Chlormerodrin, B.A.N.
MERCOCRESOLS.
　See: Mercresin, Tr. (Upjohn)
• **MERCUFENOL CHLORIDE.** USAN.
　Use: Anti-infective.
MERCUMATILIN. 8-(2′Methoxy-3′-hydroxy-mercuri-
　propyl)coumarin-3-carboxylic acid. Cumertilin.
MERCUMATILIN SODIUM. 3-(3-Carboxy-2-oxo-2H-1-
　benzopyran-8-yl-2-methoxypropyl)hydroxymercury
　sodium salt compound with theophylline.
　Use: Diuretic.
MERCUPROCYL. (Inwood) Mersalyl 100 mg.,
　theophylline 50 mg., procaine borate 0.5%/cc.
　Amp. 2 cc. Box 100s. Vial 10 cc.
　Use: Mercurial diuretic.
MERCUPURIN.
　See: Mercurophylline Injection (Various Mfr.)
MERCURANINE.
　See: Merbromin (City Chem.)
MERCURIAL, ANTISYPHILITICS. Mercuric Oleate
　Mercuric Salicylate.
■ **MERCURIAL DIURETICS.**
　See: Dicurin Procaine, Vial (Lilly)
　　Meralluride
　　Mercaptomerin Sodium (Various Mfr.)
　　Mercumatilin
　　Mercupurin
　　Mercurophylline (Various Mfr.)
　　Mersalyl
　　Mersalyl & Theophylline, Inj. (Various Mfr.)
　　Mersalyn, Vial (Var. Mfr.)
　　Salyrgan
MERCURIC OLEATE. Oleate of mercury.
　Use: Parasitic skin diseases.
W/Coal tar crude, salicylic acid, phenol & p-nitrophenol.
　See: Prosol, Emulsion (Torch)
　　Estercol, Emulsion (less p-Nitrophenol) (Torch).
**MERCURIC OXIDE OPHTHALMIC OINTMENT,
YELLOW.**
　Use: Local anti-infective.
MERCURIC SALICYLATE. Mercury subsalicylate.
　Use: Parasitic & fungous skin diseases.
MERCURIC SUCCINIMIDE. BisSuccinimidato-mercury.
MERCURIC SULFIDE, RED. W/Colloidal sulfur, urea.
　See: Teenac Cream, Oint. (Elder)
MERCURIN. Sod. salt of β-methoxy-hydroxy-mercuri
　propylamide of camphoramic acid.
　Trimethylcyclopentanedicarboxylic acid. Combined
　with theophyline is mercurophylline sodium.
MERCUROCAL.
　See: Merbromin Sol. (Premo)
MERCUROL. (Durel) Oleate of mercury 0.5%, phenol
　0.5%, salicylic acid 3%, coal tar solution 1.2% in
　Moisturizing Hand and Body Lotion. Bot. 4 oz., pt.,
　gal.
　Use: Seborrheic dermatitis and psoriasis.
MERCUROME.
　See: Merbromin Sol. (City Chem.)
MERCUROPHYLLINE SODIUM. B.A.N. Sod. salt of
　(beta-methoxygamma-hydroxy-mercuri-propylamide
　of camphoramic acid)

trimethylcyclopentanedicarboxylic acid and
theophylline.
Mercuzanthin Inj. Amp. 2 cc., Box 6s, 25s, 100s.
Tab. Bot. 50s, 100s, 1000s.
Use: Diuretic.
See: Mercupurin. (Various Mfr.)
**MERCURY-197 Hg,[3-[(AMINOCARBONYL)-AMINO]-
2-METHOXYPROPYL]-CHLORO-.** Chlormerodrin
Hg 197 Injection.
• **MERCURY, AMMONIATED,** U.S.P. XXI. Oint.,
Ophth. Oint., U.S.P. XXI.
Use: Topical anti-infective.
MERCURY BICHLORIDE.
See: Diamond, Tab. (Lilly)
■ **MERCURY COMPOUNDS.**
See: Antiseptics, Mercurials
　Mercurial, Diuretics
MERCURY-197-203.
See: Chlormerodrin (Squibb)
MERCURY OLEATE. Mercury (2+) oleate.
Pharmaceutic aid.
MERDEX. (Faraday) Docusate sodium 100 mg./Tab.
Vial 60.
Use: Relief of constipation.
MERETHOXYLLINE PROCAINE.
W/Theophylline.
See: Dicurin Procaine, Vial (Lilly)
• **MERISOPROL ACETATE Hg 197.** USAN.
Use: Radioactive agent.
• **MERISOPROL ACETATE Hg 203.** USAN.
Use: Radioactive agent.
• **MERISOPROL Hg 197.** USAN.
Use: Diagnostic aid.
MERITAL. (Hoechst) Nomifensine.
Use: Oral anti-depressant.
MERITENE LIQUID. (Doyle) Vanilla Flavor:
Concentrated sweet skim milk, corn syrup solids,
corn oil, sodium caseinate, sucrose, artificial flavor,
cellulose flour, mono & diglycerides, salt, cellulose
gum, carrageenan, vitamins & minerals. Ready-to-
serve 250 ml. cans.
Use: Total or supplemental feeding oral or tube.
MERITENE POWDER. (Doyle) Vanilla Flavor:
Specially processed nonfat dry milk, corn syrup
solids, sucrose, fructose, calcium caseinate, sodium
chloride, natural & artificial flavors, lecithin, vitamins
& minerals. Can 1 lb, 4½ lb. 25 lb. Packets 1.14
oz.
Use: Supplemental oral or tube feedings.
MERLENATE OINTMENT. (Vortech) Phenylmercuric
nitrate 1.15%, undecylenic acid 0.5% in water
miscible base. Jars. 1 oz., 1 lb.
Use: Antipruritic for relief athlete's foot.
MEROCET. Cetylpyridinium Chloride, B.A.N.
MERODICEIN. Sodium meralein.
W/Saligenin.
See: Thantis, Loz. (Hynson, Westcott & Dunning)
MERPHENE. (Barry) Disinfectant concentrate. Plastic
Bot. 8 oz.
MERPHYLLINE. (Seatrace) Sodium mersalyl 100 mg.,
theophylline 50 mg./ml. Vial 30 cc.
MERPRANE. 1-(Hydroxymercuri-197 Hg)-2-propanol.
Use: Diagnostic agent.

MERSALINE. (Standex) Mersalyl 100 mg.,
theophylline 50 mg./cc. Vial 30 cc.
MERSALYL. (Various Mfr.) Mersalyl Sod., Salygran,
Sod. (ortho-[gamma-hydroxy- mercuri-beta-methoxy-
propylcarbamyl]phenoxy) acetate.
W/Theophylline.
  See: Mersaline (Standex)
W/Theophylline, methylparaben, propylparaben.
  See: Meprophyl, Vial (Lemmon)
MERSALYL SODIUM & THEOPHYLLINE.
  See: Mersalyl & Theophylline Inj.
MERSALYL AND THEOPHYLLINE INJECTION.
(CMC) Amp. 2 cc. (Medwick) Vial 30 cc. (Metro)
Mersalyl 0.2 Gm., theophylline 0.1 Gm., water for
inj. q.s./2 cc. Amp. 2 cc. Box 10s, 100s. (Torigian)
Amp. 2 cc. 12s, 25s, 100s. Vial 30 cc. (Reid-Provident)
Mersalyl 200 mg., theophylline 100 mg./2 ml.
Use: Diuretic.
  See: Aquanil (Sig.)
    Mercurasol, Vial (Medics)
    Mer-Im, Vial (Scrip)
    Mersaline, Inj. (Standex)
    Mersalyn, Vial (Bowman; Keene; Rocky Mtn.)
    Mersaphyllin, Vial (Pharmex)
    Theo-Syl R, Inj. (Kay)
MERSALYN. Mersalyl & Theophylline Inj.
Use: I.V. & I.M., diuretic.
  See: (Bowman) Mersalyl 100 mg., theophyllin 50
  mg./ml. Vial 10 cc.
    (Keene) Mersalyl 100 mg., theophylline
    50 mg./ml. Vials 10cc, 30cc.
    (Rocky Mtn.) Mersalyl sodium 100mg.,
    theophylline anhydrous 45 mg./ml. Vial 10cc.,
    30cc.
MERSAPHYLLIN. (Pharmex) Mersalyl sod. (equiv. to
40 mg. Hg) 100 mg., theophylline 50 mg./cc.,
methylparaben 0.18%, propylparaben 0.02%. Vial
30 cc.
MERSOL. (Century) Thimerosol tincture, N.F. $^1/_{1000}$. 1
oz., 4 oz., 1 pt., 1 gal.
MERTHIOLATE. (Lilly) Thimerosal.
  Aeropump: Tincture thimerosal 0.1 Gm., alcohol
  50%. Bot. 6 fl. oz.
  Glycerite: (1:1000) Thimerosal 0.1 Gm.,
  monoethanolamine 0.1 Gm./100 ml. Bot. gal.
  Powder: Bot. 1 oz.
  Soln.: 1:1000 4 fl. oz., 16 fl. oz., gal.
  Tincture.: 1:1000 0.75 oz., 4 fl. oz., 16 fl. oz., gal.
  50% alcohol.
  Use: Antiseptic.
MERUVAX II. (Merck Sharp & Dohme) Lyophilized,
live attenuated rubella virus of the Wistar Institute
RA 27/3 strain. Each dose contains approx. 25
mcg. of neomycin. Single dose Vial 0.5 ml. 1s, 10s,
w/Disp. Syringe containing diluent & fitted with a
25 gauge, ⅝″ needle.
W/Attenuvax.
  See: M-R-Vax II, Vial (Merck Sharp & Dohme)
W/Attenuvax, Mumpsvax.
  See: M-M-R II, Vial (Merck Sharp & Dohme)
W/Mumpsvax.
  See: Biavax II, Vial (Merck Sharp & Dohme))
MERVALDIN. (Lannett) Formerly Proloxin.

Mephenesin. 0.5 Gm./Tab. Bot. 500s, 1000s.
Use: Muscle relaxant.
MESANTOIN. (Sandoz) (Mephenytoin) Phenantoin, 3-
Methyl 5,5-phenylethylhydantoin 100 mg./Tab. Bot.
100s.
Use: Antiepileptic & anticonvulsant.
MESCOMINE.
  See: Methscopolamine bromide (Var. Mfr.)
• **MESECLAZONE.** USAN.
  Use: Anti-inflammatory.
• **MESIFILCON A.** USAN.
  Use: Contact lens material.
• **MESORIDAZINE.** USAN. 10-[-2-(1-Methyl-2-piperidyl)
ethyl]-2-(methylsulfinyl)phenothiazine. Lidanil.
Use: Tranquilizer.
• **MESORIDAZINE BESYLATE,** U.S.P. XXI. Inj., Oral
Soln., Tab., U.S.P. XXI. 10-2-(1-methyl-2-piperidyl)-
ethyl-2-(methylsulfinyl)phenothiazine monobenzene-
sulfonate.
Use: Antipsychotic agent.
  See: Serentil, Amp., Liq., Tab. (Boehringer-Ingelheim)
MESSAGE LOTION. (Sween) Bot. 8 oz., gal.
Use: Massage cream.
MESTANOLONE. B.A.N. 17 β-Hydroxy-17αmethyl-5α
androstan-3-one. Androstalone.
Use: Anabolic steroid.
• **MESTEROLONE.** USAN.
  Use: Androgen.
MESTIBOL. Monomestrol.
MESTINON. (Roche) Dimethylcarbamate of 3-hydroxy-
1-methyl-pyridinium bromide. Pyridostigmine bromide
60 mg./Tab. Bot. 100s, 500s. Timespan 180
mg./Tab. Bot. 100s.
Use: Myasthenia gravis treatment.
MESTINON INJECTABLE. (Roche) Pyridostigmine Br.
5 mg./ml., methyl and propyl parabens 0.2%,
sodium citrate 0.02%, citric acid. Amp. 2 ml., 10s.
Use: Treatment of myasthenia gravis.
MESTINON SYRUP. (Roche) Pyridostigmine bromide
60 mg./5 ml. w/alcohol 5%. Bot. pts.
Use: Myasthenia gravis in children and infants.
• **MESTRANOL.** U.S.P. XXI. 17 αEthynylestradiol 3-
methyl ether. 3-Methoxy-19-nor-17-alpha-pregna-1,-
3,5(10)-trien-20-yn-17-ol. 19 Norpregna-1,3,5(10)tri-
en-20-yn-17-ol,3-methoxy-, (17α)-.
Use: Estrogenic compound.
W/Ethynodiol Diacetate.
  See: Ovulen, Tab. (Searle)
    Ovulen-21, Tab. (Searle)
    Ovulen-28, Tab. (Searle)
W/Norethindrone.
  See: Norinyl, Tab. (Syntex)
    Norinyl-1 Fe 28 (Syntex)
    Ortho-Novum, Tab. (Ortho)
W/Norethindrone, ferrous fumarate.
  See: Ortho Novum $^1/_{80}$ Fe-28, $^1/_{50}$ Fe-28, 1 mg. Fe-
  28, Tabs. (Ortho)
W/Norethynodrel.
  See: Enovid, Tab. (Searle)
    Enovid-E, Tab. (Searle)
    Enovid-E 21, Tab. (Searle)
MESULPHEN. B.A.N. 2,7-Dimethylthianthren. Mitigal;
Sudermo.

Use: Treatment of skin infections.

• **MESUPRINE HYDROCHLORIDE.** USAN.
Use: Vasodilator, smooth muscle relaxant.

METABALM. (Noyes) Menthol, camphor, thymol, methyl salicylate, oils clove and cassia in a nonstaining vanishing base. Tube 1 oz., Jar 1 lb.

METABOLIN. (Thurston) Vit. A 833 I.U., D 66 I.U., B-1 833 mcg., B-2 500 mcg., B-6 0.083 mcg., Ca pantothenate 833 mcg., niacinamide 5 mg., folic acid 0.066 mcg., niacinamide 5 mg., p-aminobenzoic acid 0.416 mcg., inositol 833 mcg., B-12 500 mcg., C 5 mg., Ca 33.1 mg., phosphorus 14.6 mg., iron 2.5 mg., iodine 0.15 mg./Tab. Bot. 100s, 500s, 1000s.
Use: Pregnancy and lactation, dietary supplement.

• **METABROMSALEN.** USAN. 3,5-Dibromosalicylanilide.
Use: Germicide.

METABUTETHAMINE HYDROCHLORIDE. 2-Isobutylaminoethyl m-aminobenzoid HCl. 2-(Isobutylamino)ethanol m-Aminobenzoate (Ester) Monohydrochloride.
Use: Local anesthetic.

METABUTOXYCAINE HYDROCHLORIDE. 2'-Diethylaminoethyl 3-Amino-2-butoxybenzoate Hydrochloride.
Use: Local anesthetic.

METACARAPHEN HYDROCHLORIDE. Netrin.

METACETAMOL. B.A.N. 3-Acetamidophenol.
Use: Analgesic.

METACORDRALONE.
See: Prednisolone. (Various Mfr.)

METACORTALONE.
See: Meticortelone, Susp. (Schering)

METACORTANDRACIN.
See: Prednisone, Tab. (Various Mfr.)

METACORTIN.
See: Meticorten, Tab. (Schering)

META-DELPHENE. Diethyltoluamide U.S.P. XXI.

METAGLYCODOL. 2-m-Chlorophenyl-3-methyl-2,3-butanediol.
Use: Central nervous system depressant.

METAHEXAMIDE. B.A.N. N-Cyclohexyl-N'-(3-amino-4-methylbenzene Sulfonyl) urea. Euglycin. Melanex.
Use: Hypoglycemic agent.

METAHYDRIN. (Merrell Dow) Trichlormethiazide 2 mg. and 4 mg./Tab. Bot. 100s.
Use: Diuretic.

• **METALOL HYDROCHLORIDE.** USAN. 4'-[Hydroxy-2-(methylamino)-propyl methanesulfonanilide hydrochloride. Under study.
Use: Andrenergic β receptor antagonist.

METALONE T.B.A. (Foy) Prednisolone tertiary butylacetate 20 mg., sod. citrate 1 mg., polysorbate 80 1 mg., d-sorbitol 450 mg./cc., benzyl alcohol 0.9% water for inj. Vial 10 ml.

METAMFEPRAMONE (I.N.N.). Dimepropion, B.A.N.

METAMUCIL. (Searle) Psyllium hydrophilic mucilloid, sodium 1 mg., potassium 31 mg./Dose. **Regular Flavor:** w/ dextrose. Pow. Pkg. 7 oz., 14 oz., 21 oz. **Orange and Strawberry Flavors:** w/flavoring, sucrose and coloring. Pow. Pkg. 7 oz., 14 oz., 21 oz.
Use: Oral laxative.

METAMUCIL INSTANT MIX. (Searle) Psyllium hydrophilic mucilloid with citric acid, sucrose, potassium bicarbonate, Na bicarbonate. Powder when combined with water forms an effervescent, flavored liquid. **Regular Flavor:** w/calcium carbonate. Cartons of 16 & 30 packets of 6.4 Gm. **Orange Flavor:** w/flavoring and coloring. Ctn. 16 and 30 packets of 6.4 Gm.
Use: Oral laxative

METANDREN. (Ciba) Methyltestosterone. **Linquet** 5 mg., 10 mg. Bot. 100s. **Tab.** 10 mg., 25 mg. Bot. 100s.
Use: Androgen therapy.

METAPHENYLBARBITURIC ACID.
See: Mebaral, Tab. (Winthrop-Breon)

METAPHYLLIN.
See: Aminophylline (Var. Mfr.)

METAPREL INHALENT SOLUTION 5%. (Dorsey) Metaproterenol sulfate 50 mg./1 ml. Bot. 10 ml. w/dropper.
Use: Bronchodilator.

METAPREL METERED DOSE INHALER. (Dorsey) Metaproterenol sulfate 225 mg., micronized powder in inert propellant/ 15 ml. Metered Dose Inhaler. (Approx. 0.65 mg./Inhalation).
Use: Bronchodilator

METAPREL SYRUP. (Dorsey) Metaproterenol sulfate 10 mg./5 ml. Bot. Pint.
Use: Bronchodilator.

METAPREL TABLETS. (Dorsey) Metaproterenol sulfate 10 mg., 20 mg./Tab. Bot. 100s.
Use: Oral Bronchodilator.

• **METAPROTERENOL SULFATE.** USAN. 1,-(3,5-Dihydroxyphenyl)-2-isopropyl-amino-ethanol sulfate, Alupent.
Use: Bronchodilator.
See: Alupent Inhal. (Geigy)
Metaprel, Tab., Inhalation, Syr. (Dorsey)

METARAMINOL. B.A.N. (Invenex) Metaraminol bitartrate. (−)-2-Amino-1-(3-hydroxyphenyl)-propan-1-ol. 10 mg./ml. Vial 1 ml., 10 ml.
Use: Hypertensive.

• **METARAMINOL BITARTRATE,** U.S.P. XXI. Inj., U.S.P. XXI. 1-α-(1-Aminoethyl)-m-hydroxybenzyl alcohol bitartrate. Benzenemethanol, a-(1 aminoethyl)-3-hydroxy-R-(R*,R*)-2,3-dihydroxybutandioate (1:1) (salt).
Use: Sympathomimetic amine (vasopressor)
See: Aramine, Amp., Vial (Merck Sharp & Dohme)

METATENSIN. (Merrell Dow) Trichlormethiazide 2 mg. and 4 mg., each containing reserpine 0.1 mg./Tab. Bot. 100s.
Use: Antihypertensive.

• **METAXALONE.** USAN. 5-(3,5-Dimethylphenoxymethyl)-2-oxazolidinone.
Use: Skeletal muscle relaxant, tranquilizer.
See: Skelaxin, Tab. (Robins)

METAZOCINE. B.A.N. 1,2,3,4,5,6-Hexahydro-8-hydroxy-3,6, 11-trimethyl-2,6-methano-3-benzazocine.
Use: Narcotic analgesic.

METCARAPHEN HYDROCHLORIDE. 2-Diethylaminoethyl-1-(3′,4′dimethylphenyl) cyclopentanecarboxylate HCl.

METECLOPRAMIDE. 4-Amino-5-chloro-N-(2-diethylaminoethyl)-2-methoxybenzamide. Primperan is the hydrochloride.

METED SHAMPOO. (CooperCare) Salicylic acid 2%, sulfur 3%, detergents 45% as liquid. Bot. 4 oz.
Use: Shampoo and cleanser.

METED 2 SHAMPOO. (CooperCare) Colloidal sulfur 2.3%, salicylic acid 1%, PEG 400 5%, detergents 20%. Bot. 4 oz.
Use: Shampoo for dry, scaly dandruff.

• **METENEPROST.** USAN.
Use: Oxytocic, prostaglandin.

METETHOHEPTAZINE. Ethyl hexahydro-1,3-dimethyl-4-phenyl-1H-azepine-4-carboxylate.
Use: Analgesic.

• **METFORMIN.** USAN. 1,1-Dimethylbiguanide. Diguanil; Glucophage; Metiguanide; Obin [HCl].
Use: Oral hypoglycemic.

METHACHOLINE BROMIDE. Mecholin bromide. (2-Hydroxypropyl)-trimethylammonium bromide acetate. Mecholyl Bromide.
Use: Cholinergic.

• **METHACHOLINE CHLORIDE,** U.S.P. XXI. (2-Hydroxypropyl)-trimethylammonium chloride acetate. Methylacetyl choline. Amechol.
Use: Cholinergic.
See: Mecholyl Chloride, Amp. (J.T. Baker)
W/Camphor, menthol & methyl salicylate.
See: Surin, Oint. (McKesson)

• **METHACRYLIC ACID COPOLYMER,** N.F. XVI.

• **METHACYCLINE.** USAN. 6-Deoxy-6-demethyl-6-methylene-5-oxytetracycline.
Use: Antibiotic.
See: Rondomycin, Cap., Syr. (Wallace)

• **METHACYCLINE HYDROCHLORIDE,** U.S.P. XXI. Cap., Oral Susp., U.S.P. XXI.
Use: Antibacterial.
See: Rondomycin, Cap., Syr. (Wallace)

METHADOL. Dimepheptanol, B.A.N.

• **METHADONE HYDROCHLORIDE,** U.S.P. XXI. Inj., Oral Concentrate, Tab., U.S.P. XXI. 6-Dimethylamino-4,4-diphenyl-3-heptanone hydrochloride. 3 Heptanone, 6-(dimethylamino)-4,4-diphenyl hydrochloride. Amidon HCl, Butalgin, Diaminon HCl, Hoechst 10820, Miadone, Physeptone HCl, Polamidon HCl.
Use: Narcotic analgesic, narcotic abstinence syndrome suppressant.
See: Dolophine Hydrochloride, Prep. (Lilly)
W/Aspirin, phenacetin, caffeine.
See: Nodalin, Tab. (Table Rock)

• **METHADYLACETATE.** USAN. 6-(Dimethylamino)-4,4-diphenyl-3-heptanol acetate (ester). 1-Ethyl-4-dimethylamino-2,2-diphenylpentyl acetate. Acetylmethadol (I.N.N.)
Use: Narcotic analgesic.

METHAGUAL. (Gordon) Guaiacol 2%, methyl salicylate 8% in petrolatum. Oint. 2 oz., lb.
Use: Minor muscular pains and strains.

METHALAMIC ACID. Name used for Iothalamic Acid, U.S.P. XXI.

METHALGEN. (Schuemann) Camphor, menthol, oil mustard, methyl salicylate in non-greasy cream base. Bot. 2 oz., Jar 4 oz., 1 lb.
Use: Analgesic cream.

METHALLATAL. 5-Ethyl-5-(2-methylallyl)-2-thiobarbituric acid.

METHALLENESTRIL. B.A.N. 3-(6-Methoxy-2-naphthyl)-2,2-dimethylpentanoic acid.
Use: Estrogen.

• **METHALLIBURE.** USAN. 1-Methyl-6-(1-methylallyl)-2,5-dithiobiurea.
Use: Suppression of pituitary, ovarian, and adrenal function.

• **METHALTHIAZIDE.** USAN. 3-[(Allylthio)-methyl]-6-chloro-3,4-dihydro-2-methyl-2H-1,2,4-benzothiadiazine-7-sulfonamide 1,1-dioxide.
Use: Hypotensive & diuretic.

METHAMINODIAZEPOXIDE. Chlordiazepoxide HCl, U.S.P. XXI.
See: Librium, Cap., Amp. (Roche)

METHAMOCTOL. 2-Methyl-6-(methylamino)-2-heptanol.
Use: Adrenergic.

METHAMPEX. (Lemmon) Methamphetamine HCl 10 mg./Tab. Bot. 1000s, 5000s.
Use: CNS Stimulant, anorexiant.

METHAMPHAZONE. B.A.N. 4-Amino-6-methyl-2-phenyl-3((2H)-pyridazone.
Use: Analgesic; antirheumatic.

METHAMPHETAMINE HYDROCHLORIDE.
Deoxyephedrine hydrochloride; N-α-Dimethyl-phenethylamine hydrochloride.
Use: Orally, central nervous system stimulant.
See: Desoxyn, Gradumets & Tab. (Abbott)
Methampex, Tab. (Lemmon)
Methamphetamine HCl, Tab. (Various Mfr.)
W/Amobarbital; homatropine methylbromide.
See: Obe-Slim, Tab. (Jenkins)
W/dl-Methamphetamine HCl, butabarbital.
See: Span-RD, Tab. (Metro Med)
W/Pamabrom, pyrilamine maleate, homatropine methylbromide, hyoscyamine sulfate, scopolamine HBr.
See: Aridol, Tabs. (MPL)
W/Pentobarbital sod., vitamins, minerals.
See: Fetamin, Tab. (Mission)

dl-METHAMPHETAMINE HCl. dl-Desoxyephedrine HCl.
See: Oxydess, Tab. (North American)
Roxyn, Tab. (Rocky Mtn.)
W/d-Methamphetamine HCl, butabarbital.
See: Span-RD, Span RD-12, Tab. (Metro Med)
W/Pyrilamine maleate, phenyltoloxamine dihydrogen citrate, didesoxyephedrine HCl, codeine phosphate, ammonium chloride, pot. guaiacolsulfonate, chloroform, phenylpropanolamine tartar emetic.
See: Meditussin-X Liquid (Hauck)

METHAMPYRONE.
See: Dipyrone

METHANAMINIUM,1-CARBOXY-N,N,N-TRI-METHYL-,HYDROXIDE, INNER SALT, COMPD. W/ 2,2,2-TRICHLORO-1,1-ETHANE-DIOL. Chloral Betaine.

**METHANAMINIUM,N-[4-[BIS[4-DIMETHYLAMINO)-
PHENYL]METHYLENE]-2,5-CYCLOHEXADIEN-1-
YLIDENE]-N-METHYL-, CHLORIDE.** Gentian Violet,
U.S.P. XXI.
METHANDIENONE. B.A.N. 17 β-Hydroxy-17
α-methylandrosta-1,4-dien-3-one. Dianabol.
Use: Anabolic steroid.
METHANDRIOL. Methylandrostenediol. (Various Mfr.)
17-alpha-methyl-Δ^5-androstene-3-beta, 17 beta-diol.
Diolostene, Mestenediol, Methanabol. Spenbolic.
See: Anabol, Inj. (Keene Pharm.)
METHANDRIOL DIPROPIONATE.
See: Andriol Injection (Reid-Provident)
  Andronex, Inj. (Tunex)
  Arbolic, Inj. (Burgin-Arden)
  Crestabolic, Vial (Nutrition)
  Durandrol, Vial (Pharmex)
  Fellobolic, Vial (Fellows-Testagar)
  Hibol, Inj. (Amfre-Grant)
  Probolik (Hickam)
  Robolic, Vial (Rocky Mtn.)
  Steribolic, Vial (Kay)
METHANDROSTENOLONE. Δ^1-17 α-methyltestoster-
one. 17 α-Methyl-17 β-hydroxyandrosta-1,4-dien-3-
one. 17 β-Hydroxy-17-methylandrosta-1,4-dien-3-
one.
See: Dianabol, Tab. (Ciba)
**METHANONE, (2-HYDROXY-4-METHOXY-
PHENYL)(2-HYDROXYPHENYL)-.** Dioxybenzone,
U.S.P. XXI.
**METHANONE, (2-HYDROXY-4-METHOXYPHENYL)-
PHENYL-.** Oxybenzone, U.S.P. XXI.
METHANTHELINIUM BROMIDE. B.A.N. 2-Diethyl-
aminoethyl xanthen-9-carboxylate methobromide.
Banthine Bromide.
Use: Anticholinergic.
• **METHANTHELINE BROMIDE,** U.S.P. XXI. Sterile,
Tab., U.S.P. XXI. Diethyl (2-hydroxyethyl) methyl-am-
monium bromide xanthene-9-carboxylate.
Use: Parasympatholytic; anticholinergic.
See: Banthine, Vial & Tab. (Searle)
W/Phenobarbital.
See: Banthine w/Phenobarb., Tab. (Searle)
METHAPHENILENE. B.A.N. 2-(N-Phenyl-N-2-
thenylamino)ethyldimethylamine. Diatrin [hydrochlo-
ride].
Use: Antihistamine.
METHAPHOR. (Borden) Protein hydrolysate (l-leucine,
l-isoleucine, l-methionine, l-phenylalanine, l-tyrosine);
methionine, camphor, benzethonium chloride, in
Dermabase vehicle/Oint. Tube 1½ oz.
Use: Dermatologic, amino acid preparation.
METHAPYRILENE. B.A.N. NN-Dimethyl-N'-(2-pyridyl)-
N'-(2-thenyl)ethylenediamine.
NOTE: Due to recent legislation many products
are being reformulated to exclude oral use of
this drug.
Use: Antihistamine.
METHAPYRILENE FUMARATE. 2-[[2-(Dimethylamino)-
ethyl]-2-thenylamino pyridine fumarate (2:3)
NOTE: Due to recent legislation many products
are being reformulated to exclude oral use of

this drug. This drug is no longer official in the
U.S.P.
Use: Antihistaminic.
METHAPYRILENE HYDROCHLORIDE, 2-[[2-Diem-
thylamino)-ethyl]-2-thenylamino] pyridine hydrochlo-
ride. (Thenylpyramine, Teralin). Blue Line—Elixir
200 mg./fl. oz. Bot. 1 pt., 1 gal. CMC-Vial 30 cc. Ken-
yon-Vial 20 mg./cc.
NOTE: Due to recent legislation many products
are being reformulated to exclude oral use of
this drug. This drug is no longer official in the
U.S.P.
Use: Antihistamine.
**METHAPYRILENE HYDROCHLORIDE
W/COMBINATIONS.**
NOTE: Due to recent legislation many products
are being reformulated to exclude oral use of
this drug.
• **METHAQUALONE,** U.S.P. XXI. Tab., U.S.P. XXI. 2-
Methyl-3-o-tolyl-4(3H)-quinazolinone. Melsedin, Pax-
idorm, Sedaquin (HCl), Melsed, Quaalude, Revonal.
Use: Tranquilizer.
See: Mequin, Tab. (Lemmon)
  Parest, Cap. (Lemmon)
  Quaalude, Tab. (Lemmon)
• **METHAQUALONE HYDROCHLORIDE,** U.S.P. XXI.
Cap., U.S.P. XXI.
Use: Tranquilizer.
See: Optimil (Wallace)
  Parest (Parke Davis)
  Somnafac (CooperVision)
• **METHARBITAL,** U.S.P. XXI. Tab., U.S.P. XXI. 5,5'-
Diethyl-1-methylbarbituric acid.
Use: Anticonvulsant.
See: Gemonil, Tab. (Abbott)
METHARBITONE. B.A.N. 5,5-Diethyl-1-methylbarbituric
acid.
Use: Anticonvulsant.
METHAZINE. (Pharmex) Promethazine HCl 50
mg./cc. Vial 10 cc.
• **METHAZOLAMIDE,** U.S.P. XXI. Tab. U.S.P. XXI. N-
(4-Methyl-2-sulfamoyl-Δ^2-1,3,4-thiadiazolin-5-ylidene)-
acetamide. Acetamide, N-5-(aminosulfonyl)-3-methyl-
1,3,4-thiadiazol-2(3H)-ylidene-. 5-Acetylimino-4-meth-
yl-1,3,4-thiadiazoline-2-sulfonamide.
Use: Carbonic anhydrase inhibitor.
See: Neptazane
  Neptazane, Tab. (Lederle)
METH-DIA-MER SULFA TABLETS, Trisulfapyrimidines
Tab., U.S.P. XXI.
Use: Triple sulfonamide therapy.
See: Buffonamide (Reid-Provident)
  Chemozine, Tab. (Tennessee Pharm.)
  Neotrizine, Tab. (Lilly)
  Terfonyl, Susp., (Squibb)
  Trionamide, Tab., (O'Neal)
  Triple Sulfa, Tab. (Various Mfr.)
  Triple Sulfas, Tab. (Lederle)
  Trisem, Tab. (Beecham Labs)
METH-DIA-MER SULFONAMIDES.
Use: Triple sulfonamide therapy.
W/Sulfacetamide.

See: Sulfa-Plex Vaginal Cream (Rowell)
W/Sulfacetamide, hexestrol.
See: Vagi-Plex, Cream (Rowell)
METH-DIA-MER SULFONAMIDES SUSPENSION,
Trisulfapyrimidines Oral Suspension, U.S.P. XXI.
Use: Triple sulfonamide therapy.
See: Chemozine, Susp. (Tennessee Pharm.)
  Neotrizine, Susp. (Lilly)
  Terfonyl, Susp. (Squibb)
  Tri-Diazole, Liq. (Coastal)
  Triple Sulfa, Susp. (CMC)
  Trisem, Susp. (Beecham Labs)
METHDILAZINE, U.S.P. XXI. Tab., U.S.P. XXI. 10-(1-
Methylpyrrolidin-3-ylmethyl)phenothiazine.   Dilosyn
(hydrochloride)
See: Tacaryl Chewable Tab. (Westwood)
• **METHDILAZINE HCI,** U.S.P. XXI. Syrup, Tab.,
U.S.P. XXI. 10-(1-Methyl-pyrrolidinyl)phenothiazine
HCl.
Use: Antipruritic.
See: Tacaryl, Tab. (Westwood)
• **METHENAMINE,** U.S.P. XXI. Elixir, Tab., U.S.P. XXI.
(Hexamethyleneamine, Cystamin, Cystogen,
Hexamine, Hexamethylenetetramine.)
Use: Antibacterial (urinary).
METHENAMINE W/COMBINATIONS.
Use: Urinary tract anti-infective.
See: Cystamine, Tab. (Tennessee Pharm.)
  Cysto, Tab. (Freeport)
  Cystised, Tab. (Jenkins)
  Cystitol, Tab. (Briar)
  Cystorrhoids W/Atropine, Tab. (Noyes)
  Cystrea, Tab. (Moore Kirk)
  Formathyn, Tab. (Scrip)
  G-U-Sist, Tab. (Freeport)
  Hexalol, Tab. (Central)
  Lanased, Tab. (Lannett)
  UB, Tab. (Scrip)
  Uralene, Tab. (Sutliff & Case)
  Uramine, Tab. (Kay)
  Urelief, Tab. (Rocky Mtn.)
  Uricide, Tab. (Elder)
  Urilief, Tab. (Mallinckrodt)
  Urineaze, Tab. (Foy)
  Uriprel, Tab. (Pasadena Research)
  Urisan-P, Tab. (Sandia)
  Urised, Tab. (Webcon)
  Uriseptin, Tab. (Blaine)
  Uristat, Tab. (Lemmon)
  Uritabs, Tab. (Vortech)
  Urithol, Tab. (O'Neal)
  Uritin Modified Formula, Tab. (Wolins)
  Uritrol, Tab. (Kenyon)
  Uro Phosphate, Tab. (Poythress)
  Urothyn Improved, Tab. (Reid-Provident)
  Uro-Ves, Tab. (Mallard)
  Urseptic, Tab. (Century)
  UTA, Tab. (Bentex)
  U-Tract, Tab. (Bowman)
  U-Tran, Tab. (Scruggs)
**METHENAMINE AND MONOBASIC SODIUM
PHOSPHATE TABLETS,** U.S.P. XXI.

Use: Antibacterial (urinary).
METHENAMINE ANHYDROMETHYLENE CITRATE.
Formanol, Uropurgol, Urotropin.
• **METHENAMINE HIPPURATE,** U.S.P. XXI. Tab.,
U.S.P. XXI. A 1:1 complex of methenamine and
hippuric acid.
Use: Urinary antiseptic.
See: Hiprex, Tab. (Merrell Dow)
  Urex, Tab.(Riker)
• **METHENAMINE MANDELATE,** U.S.P. XXI. Tab.,
For Oral Soln., Oral Susp.; U.S.P. XXI.
Use: Urinary antibacterial.
See: Mandacon, Tab. (Webcon)
  Mandalay, Tab. (Beutlich)
  Mandelamine, Tab., Susp. (Parke-Davis)
  Mandelamine "Hafgram" Tab. (Parke-Davis)
  Mandelets, Tab. (Columbia)
  Methalate, Tab. (Vortech)
  Methavin, Tab. (Star)
  Renelate, Tab. (Fellows)
  Thendelate, Tab. (Blue Line)
METHENAMINE MANDELATE W/COMBINATIONS.
Use: Antibacterial (urinary).
See: Azolate, Tab. (Amfre-Grant)
  Azo-Methalate, Tab. (Vortech)
  Donnasep, Tab. (Robins)
  Levo-Uroqid, Tab. (Beach)
  Manacid, Tab. (Hyrex)
  Mandalay A.P., Tab. (Beutlich)
  Mandex, Tab. (Vale)
  Prov-U-Sep Forte, Tab. (Reid-Provident)
  Pyrisul Plus, Tab. (Kenyon)
  Renalgin, Tab. (Meyer)
  Thiacide, Tab. (Beach)
  Urisedamine, Tab. (Webcon)
  Uritral, Cap. (Central)
  Uropeutic, Tab. (Circle)
  Uroqid-Acid, Tab. (Beach)
METHENOLONE. B.A.N. 17β-Hydroxy-1-methyl-5 α-
androst-1-en-3-one. Primobolan acetate; Primobolan-
Depot enanthate
Use: Anabolic steroid.
• **METHENOLONE ACETATE.** USAN. 17 β-Hydroxy-
1-methyl-5 α-androst-1-en-3-one acetate. Primobo-
lan.
Use: Anabolic agent.
• **METHENOLONE ENANTHATE.** USAN. 17β-Hydroxy-
1-methyl-5αandrost-1-en-3-one heptanoate. Nibal in-
jection. Primobolan.
Use: Anabolic.
METHEPONEX. (Rawl) Choline 0.54 Gm., dl-methionine
1.80 Gm., inositol 0.27 Gm., whole liver desic. 8.10
Gm., Vit. B-1 18 mg., B-2 36 mg., niacinamide 90 mg.,
B-6 3.6 mg., Ca pantothenate 3.6 mg., biotin 10.8
mcg., B-12 5.4 mcg. & amino acid/daily therapeutic
dose. Caps. Bot. 100s, 500s.
Use: Liver disorders, diabetes.
METHEPTAZINE. Methyl hexahydro-1, 2-dimethyl-4-
phenyl-1H-azepine-4-carboxylate.
Use: Analgesic.
METHERGINE. (Sandoz) Methylergonovine maleate.
Amp. 0.2 mg./ml. w/tartaric acid 0.25 mg., NaCl

3.0 mg./ml. SandoPak 20s, 100s. **Tab:** 0.2 mg./Tab. Bot. 100s, 1000s. SandoPak pkgs. 100s.
Use: Orally, I.V. & I.M., oxytocic.

METHESTROL.
See: Promethestrol (Various Mfr.)

METHETHARIMIDE BEMEGRIDE. 3-Methyl-3-ethyl glutarimide.

• **METHETOIN.** USAN. 5-Ethyl-1-methyl-5-phenylimidazoline-2,4-dione. Deltoin.
Use: Anticonvulsant.

METHIBON CAPSULES. (Barrows) Choline dihydrogen citrate 278 mg., dl-methionine 111 mg., inositol 83.3 mg., B-12 2 mcg., liver conc. and liver desic. 86.6 mg./Cap. Bot. 100s.

METHICILLIN. B.A.N. 6-(2,6-Dimethoxy-benzamido)-penicillanic acid. Celbenin; Staphcillin (sodium salt)
Use: Antibiotic.

• **METHICILLIN SODIUM, STERILE,** U.S.P. XXI., Inj., U.S.P. XXI. Sod. 2,6-Dimethoxyphenyl penicillin. Dimethoxyphenyl pencillin sod.
Use: Antibiotic.
See:
Celbenin, Vial (Beecham Labs)
Staphcillin, Vial (Bristol)

• **METHIMAZOLE,** U.S.P. XXI. Tab., U.S.P. XXI. 1-Methylimidazole-2-thiol. Mercazole. 2H-imidazole-2-thione, 1,3-dihydro-1-methyl.
Use: Thyroid inhibitor. (5 to 20 mg.)
See: Tapazole, Tab. (Lilly)
Thiamazole (I.N.N.)

METHINDIZATE. B.A.N. 2-(1-Methyloctahydroindol-3-yl)ethyl benzilate. Present in Isaverine hydrochloride.
Use: Spasmolytic, veterinary medicine.

• **METHIODAL SODIUM,** U.S.P. XXI. Inj., U.S.P. XXI. Sod. monoiodomethanesulfonate. Abrodil, Radiographol, Diagnorenol.
Use: Radiopaque medium for urinary tract.

METHIOMEPRAZINE HCl. dl-10-(3-Dimethyl-amino-2-methylpropyl)-2-methylthiophenothiazine HCl. (SmithKline)
Use: Anti-emetic.

• **METHIONINE,** U.S.P. XXI. **Note:** Also see Racemethionine, U.S.P. XXI.
Use: Amino acid.

METHIOPLEX. (Lincoln) Methionine 25 mg., B-1 50 mg., niacinamide 100 mg., B-2 2 mg., choline 50 mg., B-6 2 mg., panthenol 2 mg., benzyl alcohol 1%, distilled water q.s./cc. Vial 30 cc.
Use: Lipotropic & vitamin therapy.

• **METHISAZONE.** USAN. N-methylisatin-β-thiosemicarbazone. 1-Methylindoline-2,3-dione 3-thiosemicarbazone. Marboran.
Use: Antiviral drug.

METHISCHOL CAPSULES. (Armour) Nutrients. Bot. 100s, 500s.

METHITURAL SODIUM. 5-(1-Methylbutyl)-5-[2-(methylthio)ethyl]-2-thiobarbituric acid sodium salt.
Use: Hypnotic; sedative.

METHIXENE. B.A.N. 9-(1-Methyl-3-piperidyl-methyl)-thiaxanthen. Tremonil (hydrochloride).
Use: Treatment of the Parkinsonian syndrome.

• **METHIXENE HYDROCHLORIDE.** USAN. I-Methyl-3-(thioxanthen-9-ylmethyl)-piperidine HCl.
Use: Antispasmodic.

METHNITE. (Kenyon) Methscopolamine nitrate 2.5 mg./Tab. Bot. 100s, 1000s.
Use: Antispasmodic.

• **METHOCARBAMOL,** U.S.P. XXI. Cap., Tab., U.S.P. XXI. 1,2-Propanediol, 3-(2-methoxy phenoxy)-, 1-carbamate. (2-Hydroxy-3-o-methoxyphenoxypropyl) carbamate. 3-(o-Methoxyphenoxy)-1,2-propanediol 1-carbamate.
Use: Skeletal muscle relaxant.
See: Delaxin, Tab. (Ferndale)
Robaxin, Tabs., Inj. (Robins)
Romethocarb, Tab. (Robinson)
S.K. Methecarbamol, Tab. (SmithKline)
W/Aspirin.
See: Robaxisal, Tab. (Robins)

METHOCEL. Methyl cellulose.

• **METHOHEXITAL,** U.S.P. XXI.
Use: Pharmaceutical necessity for Methohexital Sodium for Injection.

• **METHOHEXITAL SODIUM FOR INJECTION,** U.S.P. XXI. Alpha-(dl)-5-allyl-1-methyl-5-(1-methyl-2-pentynyl) barbituric acid. 2,4,6(IH,-3H,5H)-pyrimidinetrione,. 1-methyl-5-(1-methyl-2-pentynyl)-5-(2-propenyl)-, ($\pm$) monosodium salt.
Use: General anesthetic (intravenous).
See: Brevital, Amp., Pow. (Lilly)

METHOHEXITONE. B.A.N. α-5-Allyl-1-methyl-5-(1-methylpent-2-ynyl)barbituric acid.
Use: Anesthetic.
See: Brevital
Brietal

METHOIN. B.A.N. 5-Ethyl-3-methyl-5-phenylhydantoin. 5-Ethyl-3-methyl-5-phenylimidazoline-2,4-dione. Mephenytoin (I.N.N.)
Use: Anticonvulsant.
See: Mesantoin, Tab. (Sandoz)

• **METHOPHOLINE HCl.** USAN. 1-(p-Chlorophenethyl)-2-methyl-6, 7-dimethoxy-1,2,3,4-tetrahydroisoquinoline HCl.
Use: Analgesic.
See: Versidyne

METHOPTO ¼%. (Professional Pharmacal) Methylcellulose powder 2.5 mg. (¼% soln.), boric acid 12 mg., potassium Cl. 7.3 mg., benzalkonium Cl. 0.04 mg., glycerin 12 mg./ml. w/sodium carbonate to adjust pH and purified water. Bot. 15 or 30 ml.
Use: Tear replacement.

METHOPTO FORTE ½%. (Professional Pharmacal) Methylcellulose powder 5 mg. (½% soln.), boric acid 12 mg., potassium Cl. 7.3 mg., benzalkonium Cl. 0.4 mg., glycerin 12 mg./ml. w/sodium carbonate to adjust pH and purified water. Bot. 15 ml.
Use: Tear replacement.

METHOPTO FORTE 1%. (Professional Pharmacal) Methylcellulose powder 10 mg. (1% soln.), boric acid 12 mg., potassium Cl. 7.3 mg., benzalkonium Cl. sol 0.04 mg., glycerin 12 mg./ml. w/sodium

carbonate to adjust pH and purified water. Bot. 15 ml.
Use: Tear replacement.

METHOPYRAPHONE.
See: Metopirone, Tab., Amp. (Ciba)

METHORATE. Not listed.
See: Dextromethorphan HBr

METHORBATE S.C. (Standex) Methenamine 40.8 mg., atropine sulfate 0.03 mg., hyoscyamine sulfate 0.03 mg., salol 18.1 mg., benzoic acid 4.5 mg., methylene blue 5.4 mg./Tab. Bot. 100s.

d-METHORPHAN HBr.
See: Dextromethorphan HBr (Various Mfr.)

METHORPHINAN. •Racemorphan HBr. Dromoran.

l-METHORPHINAN LEVORPHANOL.
See: Levo-Dromoran, Amp., Tab., Vial (Roche)

METHOSERPIDINE. B.A.N. 10-Methoxydeserpidine.
Use: Hypotensive.
See: Decaserpyl

• **METHOTREXATE,** U.S.P. XXI. Tab., U.S.P. XXI. Amethopterin. 4-Amino-10-methylfolic acid. N-[p-[[(2,4-Diamino-6-pteridinyl)-methyl]-methylamino]benzoyl] glutamic acid. L-glutamic acid, N-[4-[[(2,4-diamino-6-pteridinyl)methyl] -me-thylamino]benzoyl].
Use: Leukemia in children, antineoplastic, antisporiatic.
See: Methotrexate, Tab., Inj. (Lederle)

• **METHOTREXATE SODIUM INJECTION.** U.S.P. XXI. 4-Amino-N¹⁰-methyl-pteroylglutamic acid sodium. (Lederle) 2.5 mg./ml. Vial 2 ml.; 25 mg./ml. Vial 2 ml. w/preservatives; 20 mg., 50 mg., 100 mg. Vials cryodesiccated, preservative free; 50 mg., 100 mg., 200 mg. Vials; 25 mg./ml. solution preservative free.
Use: Leukemia therapy., psoriasis.
See: Methotrexate, Inj., Pow. (Lederle)
     Mexate, Inj. (Bristol)

• **METHOTRIMEPRAZINE,** U.S.P. XXI. Inj., U.S.P. XXI. 2-Methoxy-10-(3-dimethylamino-2-methyl-propyl)phenothiazine. (—)-10-(3-(Dimethyl-amino)-2-methyl-propyl)-2-methoxyphenothiazine. Levomepromazine (I.N.N.) Veractil.
Use: Tranquilizer, non-addicting analgesic.
See: Levoprome, Amp., Vial (Lederle)

METHOXAMINE. B.A.N. 2-Amino-1-(2,5-dimethoxy-phenyl)propan-1-ol. Vasoxine; Vasylox (hydrochloride).
Use: Vasoconstrictor.

• **METHOXAMINE HYDROCHLORIDE,** U.S.P. XXI. Inj., U.S.P. XXI. α-(1-Aminoethyl)-2,5-dimethoxybenzyl alcohol hydrochloride. Benzenemethanol, α-(1-aminoethyl)-2,5-dimethoxy-,hydrochloride.
Use: Sympathomimetic, adrenergic (vasopressor).
See: Vasoxyl, Inj. (Burroughs Wellcome)

• **METHOXYSALEN,** U.S.P. XXI.
Use: Topical pigmenting agent.
See: Meloxine, (Upjohn)
     Oxsoralen, Cap., Lot. (Elder)

• **METHOXSALEN TOPICAL SOLUTION,** U.S.P. XXI. 8-Methoxypsoralen. 8-Hydroxy-4′,5′,6,7-furocoumarin, ammoidin, xanthotoxin. 7H-Furo[3,2-g][1] benzo-pyran-7-one,2-methoxy-9-methoxy-7H-Furo[3,2-g][1]-benzopyran-7-one.
Use: Topical pigmenting agent.

O-METHOXY-N,α-DIMETHYLPHENETHYLAMINE HCl. Methoxyphenamine HCl.

METHOXYDONE.
See: Mephenoxalone (Various Mfr.)

• **METHOXYFLURANE,** U.S.P. XXI. 2,2-Dichloro-1,1-difluoroethyl methyl ether.
Use: General inhalation anesthetic.
See: Penthrane, Liq. (Abbott)

METHOXYPHENAMINEI B.A.N. 1-o-Anisylethylme-thylamine. Orthoxine.
Use: Bronchodilator.

9-METHOXY-7H-FURO[3,2-g][1]BENZOPYRAN-7-ONE. Methoxsalen, U.S.P. XXI.

3-METHOXY-19-NOR-17-α-PREGNA-1,3,5,(10)-TRIEN-20-YN-17-OL. Mestranol, U.S.P. XXI.

• **METHOXYPHENAMINE HYDROCHLORIDE,** U.S.P. XXI. o-Methoxy-N, α-dimethylphenethylamino HCl.
Use: Adrenergic (bronchodilator).
W/Chlorpheniramine maleate, acetophenetidin, acetylsalicylic acid, caffeine.
See: Pyrroxate, Cap., Tab. (Upjohn)
W/Dextromethorphan HCl, orthoxine, sod. citrate.
See: Orthoxicol, Syr. (Upjohn)
W/Dextromethorphan HBr, phenylephrine HCl, chlorpheniramine maleate.
See: Statuss, Syr., Cap. (Elder)
W/Medrol.
See: Medrol, Tab. (Upjohn)

3-(o-METHOXYPHENOXY)-PROPANEDIOL-1,2.
See: Guaifenesin

o-METHOXYPHENYL GLYCERYL ETHER.
See: Guaifenesin, Guaifenesin.

METHOXYPROMAZINE MALEATE. 10-[3-(Dimethylamino)propyl]-2-methoxyphenothiazine maleate. Tentone.
Use: CNS depressant.

8-METHOXYPSORALEN.
See: Methoxsalen

• **METHSCOPOLAMINE BROMIDE,** U.S.P. XXI. Inj., Tab., U.S.P. XXI. Epoxytropine tropate methylbromide, scopolamine methylbromide, hyoscine methylbromide. 6β, 7β-Epoxy-3α-hydroxy-8-methyl-1αH, 5αH-tropanium bromide(−)-Tropate.
Use: Anticholinergic
See: Pamine, Tab., Vial (Upjohn)
     Scoline, Tab. (Westerfield)
W/Amobarbital.
See: Scoline-Amobarbital, Tab. (Westerfield)
W/Butabarbital Sod., aluminum hydroxide gel dried & mag. trisilicate.
See: Eulcin, Tab. (Leeds Pharmacal)
W/Phenobarbital.
See: Pamine PB, Prep. (Upjohn)
     Synt-PB, Tab. (Scrip)
W/Phenylpropanolamine HCl chlorpheniramine maleate.

See: Bobid, Cap. (Boyd)
  Symptrol, Cap. (Saron)
METHSCOPOLAMINE NITRATE. Scopolamine
Methyl Nitrate, Prep. (Various Mfr.) Mescomine.
  See: Allerspan, Cap. (Merit)
    Aluscop, Cap., Susp. (Westerfield)
    Cenahist, Cap. (Century)
    Chlorpel, Cap. (Santa)
    Conalsyn Chroncap, Cap. (Cenci)
    Dallergy, Cap., Tab., Syr. (Laser)
    Drinus Graduals, Cap. (Federal)
    Drize M, Cap. (Ascher)
    Extendryl, Cap., Syr., Tab. (Fleming)
    Histaspan-D, Cap. (USV Labs.)
    Historal, Cap., Liq. (W.F. Merchant)
    Hydrochol-Plus, Tab. (Elder)
    Kleer, Cap. (Scrip)
    Kleer Compound, Tab. (Scrip)
    Kleer-Tuss, Cap. (Scrip)
    Methnite, Tab., (Kenyon)
    MSC Triaminic, Tab. (Dorsey)
    Narine, T.R. Cap. (Dooner)
    Narspan, Cap. (Coast Labs.)
    Paraspan, Cap. (Fleming)
    Sanhist T.D. 12, Tab. (Sandia)
    Scotnord, Tab. (Scott/Cord)
    Sinaprel, Cap. (Pasadena Res.)
    Sinodec, Cap. (Primedics)
    Sinovan, Timed Cap. (Drug Ind.)
    Sinunil, Pellsule (Misemer)
    Spasmid, Elix., Tab. (Dalin)
    Symptrol, Cap. (Saron)
    Trisohist, Cap. (Riker)
• **METHSUXIMIDE,** U.S.P. XXI. Cap., U.S.P. XXI.
N,2-Dimethyl-2-phenylsuccinamide Mesuximide
(I.N.N.)
  Use: Anticonvulsant.
  See: Celontin Kapseal. (Parke-Davis)
METHULOSE. (Softcon) Methylcellulose ¼% and
benzalkonium chloride 1:25,000 as a preservative.
Bot. 15 cc., 30 cc.
  Use: Tear replacement and ophthalmic vehicle.
• **METHYCLOTHIAZIDE,** U.S.P. XXI. Tab., U.S.P. XXI.
6-Chloro-3-chloro-methyl-2-methyl-7-sulfamyl-3,4-dih-
ydro-1,2,4-benzothiadiazine-1,1-dioxide. 6-Chloro-
3-(chloromethyl)-3,4-dihydro-2-methyl-2H-1,2,4-benz-
othiadiazine-7-sulfonamide 1,1-Dioxide.
  Use: Diuretic; antihypertensive.
  See: Enduron, Tab. (Abbott)
W/Cryptenamine.
  See: Diutensen, Tabs. (Mallinckrodt)
W/Cryptenamine, reserpine.
  See: Diutensen-R, Tabs. (Mallinckrodt)
W/Deserpidine.
  See: Enduronyl, Tab. (Abbott)
    Enduronyl Forte, Tab. (Abbott)
W/Pargyline hydrochloride.
  See: Eutron, Tab. (Abbott)
W/Reserpine.
  See: Diutensen-R (Mallinckrodt)
METHYLACETYLCHOLINE.
  See: Methacholine

METHYL ALCOHOL, N.F. XVI.
  Use: Pharmaceutic acid (solvent).
**(−)-ERYTHRO-α-[1-(METHYLAMINO)-ETHYL]-
BENZYL ALCOHOL.** Ephedrine Sulfate.
**METHYLAMPHETAMINE HYDROCHLORIDE &
SULFATE.**
  See: Desoxyephedrine HCl (Var. Mfr.)
METHYLANDROSTENEDIOL.
  See: Hybolin, Vial (Hyrex)
    Methandriol
    Methyldiol, Prep. (North American Pharm)
W/Adrenal cortex ext., Vit. B-12.
  See: Geri-Ace, Inj. (Brown)
W/Carboxymethylcellulose sod., thimerosal.
  See: Cenabolic, Vial (Century)
W/Pentylenetetrazol, nicotinic acid, l-lysine, dl-
methionine, ethinyl estradiol, thiamine,
pyridoxine, riboflavin, Vit. B-12, Vit. A, Vit. D,
ascorbic acid.
  See: Ardiatric, Tab. (Burgin-Arden)
• **METHYL ATROPINE NITRATE.** USAN. Atropine
Methylnitrate. (Various Mfr.) 8-Methylatropinium ni-
trate. dl-Hyoscyamine methylnitrate.
  Use: Antispasmodic.
W/Aluminum hydroxide, pectin, osmokadin,
betalactose.
  See: Metropectin, Tab. (Pennwalt)
W/Butabarbital, methscopolamine nitrate.
  See: Scolate, Tab. (Central)
W/Oxidized bile acids, ox and hog bile ext.,
phenobarbital.
  See: G.B.S., Tab. (O'Neal)
W/Phenobarbital & dihydroxy aluminum aminoacetate.
  See: Harvatrate A, Tab. (O'Neal)
• **METHYLBENZETHONIUM CHLORIDE,** U.S.P. XXI.
Lotion, Oint., Powder, U.S.P. XXI. Benzyl-dimethyl-
2[2-(p-1,1,3-tetramethyl-butyl-cresoxy)ethoxy]-ethyl
ammonium chloride. (p-Tertiary octyl cresoxy ethoxy
ethyl dimethyl-benzyl ammonium chloride). Benzyl-
dimethyl[2[2-[[4-(1,1,3,3-tetramethylbutyl)tolyl]oxy]et-
hoxy]-ethyl]ammonium chloride.
  Use: Bactericide; Local anti-infective.
  See: Ammorid, Oint. (Kinney)
    Benephen, Prods. (Halsted)
    Cuticura Acne Cream (Purex)
    Cuticura Medicated First Aid Cream (Purex)
    Diaparene Prods. (Glenbrook)
    Fordustin, Pow. (Sween)
    Surgi-Kleen, Liq. (Sween)
W/Cod liver oil.
  See: Benephen, Prods. (Halsted)
    Sween Skin Care, Cream (Sween)
W/Magnesium stearate.
  See: Mennen Baby Pow. (Mennen)
W/Phenol, acetanilid, zinc oxide, calamine &
eucalyptol.
  See: Taloin, Oint. (Warren-Teed)
W/Phenylmercuric acetate, methylparaben.
  See: Lorophyn, Supp. (Eaton)
    Norforms, Aer., Supp. (Norwich)
W/Zinc oxide, calamine, eucalyptol.
  See: Taloin, Tube (Warren-Teed)

METHYL BENZOQUATE. B.A.N. Methyl 7-benzyloxy-6-butyl-1,4-dihydro-4-oxoquinoline-3-carboxylate. Nequinate (I.N.N.) Statyl.
Use: Antiprotozoan, veterinary medicine.
METHYLBENZTROPINE.
See: Ethybenztropine (Sandoz)
METHYLBROMTROPIN MANDELATE.
See: Homatropine Methylbromide, U.S.P. XXI.
• **METHYLCELLULOSE,** U.S.P. XXI. Ophth. Soln., Oral Soln.,Tab.,U.S.P.XXI.Cellulosemethylether.Mellose.
Use: Suspending agent.
See: Cellothyl, Tab. (International Drug)
Cologel, Sol. (Lilly)
Isopto-Plain, Liq. (Alcon)
Melozets, Wafer (Calgon)
Methulose, Sol. (Softcon)
Syncelose, Tab. (Blue Line)
Tearisol, Sol. (Smith, Miller & Patch)
Visculose, Sol. (Softcon)
W/Benzocaine, vitamins, minerals, niacinamide.
See: Rite-Diet, Cap. (Edward J. Moore)
W/Boric acid, glycerine, propylene glycol, methylparaben, propylparaben, irish moss ext.
See: Canfield Lubricating Jelly (Paddock)
W/Carboxymethylcellulose.
See: Ex-Caloric, Wafer (Eastern Research)
W/Dicyclomine HCl, magnesium trisilicate, aluminum hydroxide-magnesium carbonate dried.
See: Triactin Tab. (Norwich)
W/Dicyclomine HCl, aluminum hydroxide & magnesium hydroxide.
See: Triactin Liq. (Norwich)
W/Phenylephrine HCl.
See: Vernacel (Professional Pharmacal)
W/Phenylephrine HCl, benzalkonium chloride.
See: Efricel ⅛% (Professional Pharmacal)
W/Polysorbate 80, boric acid.
See: Lacril Artificial Tears (Allergan)
METHYL 7(S)-CHLORO-6,7,8-TRIDEOXY-6-trans-(1-METHYL-4-PROPYL-L-2-PYRROLIDINECARBOXA-MIDE)-1-THIO-L-THREO-α-D-GALACTO-OCTOPY-RANOSIDE MONOHYDROCHLORIDE. Clindamycin Hydrochloride, U.S.P. XXI.
METHYLCHROMONE. B.A.N. 3-Methyl-(4H)-chromen-4-one.
Use: Coronary vasodilator.
See: Crodimyl
METHYL CYSTEINE. B.A.N. Methyl 2-amino-3-mercaptoproprionate. Mecysteine (I.N.N.) Acdrile; Visclair [hydrochloride]
Use: Vasoconstrictor.
METHYL CYSTEINE HYDROCHLORIDE. Cysteine methyl ester hydrochloride.
Use: Mucolytic agent.
METHYLDESORPHINE. B.A.N. 6-Methyl-Δ⁶-deoxymorphine.
Use: Narcotic analgesic.
METHYL 6,8-DIDEOXY-6-(I-METHYL-TRANS-4-PRO-PYL-L-2-PYRROLIDINECARBOXAMIDE)-I-THIO-D-ERYTHRO-ALPHA-D-GALACTO-OCTOPYRANO-SIDE MONOHYDROCHLORIDE MONOHYDRATE.

Lincomycin Hydrochloride, U.S.P. XXI.
METHYLDIOL IN OIL. (Vortech) Methandriol dipropionate 50 mg., benzyl alcohol 5% in sesame oil/cc. Vial 10 cc.
Use: Anabolic steroid.
METHYLDIOL TABLETS. (Vortech) Methylandrostendiol 2 mg./Tab. Bot. 100s, 1000s.
Use: Anabolic steroid.
• **METHYLDOPA,** U.S.P. XXI. Oral Susp., Tabs. U.S.P. XXI. Levo-3-(3,4-dihydroxyphenyl)-2-methylalanine.
Use: Antihypertensive.
See: Aldomet, Tab. (Merck Sharp & Dohme)
W/Chlorothiazide.
See: Aldoclor, Tab. (Merck Sharp & Dohme)
• **METHYLDOPA AND HYDROCHLORTHIAZIDE TABLETS,** U.S.P. XXI.
Use: Antihypertensive.
See: Aldoril, Tab. (Merck Sharp & Dohme)
• **METHYLDOPATE HCl,** U.S.P. XXI. Inj. U.S.P. XXI. (Merck Sharp & Dohme) Ethyl ester of levo-3-(3,4-dihydroxyphenyl)-2-methylalanine HCl. l-Tyrosine, 3-hydroxy-α-methyl-,ethyl ester hydrochloride-.
Use: Anti-hypertensive agent.
See: Aldomet Ester HCl, Inj. (Merck Sharp & Dohme)
3,3′-METHYLENEBIS (4-HYDROXYCOUMARIN).
See: Bishydroxycoumarin (Var. Mfr.)
Dicumarol, U.S.P. XXI. (Various Mfr.)
• **METHYLENE BLUE,** U.S.P. XXI. Inj. U.S.P. XXI. (Various Mfr.) Methylthionine chloride. 3,7-Bix-(Dimethyl-amino)phenzathionium chloride.
Use: Antimethemoglobinemic, antidote to cyanide poisoning.
See: Urolene Blue, Tab. (Star)
Wright's Stain, Liq. (Hynson, Westcott & Dunning)
METHYLENE BLUE W/COMBINATIONS.
See: Cysto, Tab. (Freeport)
Cystrea, Tab. (Moore Kirk)
G-U-Sist, Tab. (Freeport)
Hexalol, Tab. (Central)
Lanased, Tab. (Lannett)
Renalgin, Tab. (Meyer)
Uramine, Tab. (Kay)
Urilief, Tab. (Mallinckrodt)
Urineaze, Tab. (Foy)
Uriprel, Tab. (Pasadena Research)
Urised, Tab. (Webcon)
Uristat, Tab. (Lemmon)
Uritabs, Tab. (Vortech)
Uritin Modified Formula, Tab. (Wolins)
Urostat Forte, Tab. (Elder)
Urothyn Improved, Tab. (Reid-Provident)
Uro-Ves, Tab. (Mallard)
UTA, Tab. (ICN)
U-Tract, Tab. (Bowman)
2,2′-METHYLENEBIS[3,4,6-TRICHLOROPHENOL].
Hexachlorophene, U.S.P. XXI.
• **METHYLENE CHLORIDE,** N.F. XVI.
Use: Pharmaceutic aid (solvent).
METHYLERGOMETRINE. B.A.N. N-(+)-1-(Hydroxymethyl)propyl-(+)-lysergamide.

Use: Uterine stimulant.
See: Methergin hydrogen maleate
• **METHYLERGONOVINE MALEATE,** U.S.P. XXI. Inj., Tab., U.S.P. XXI. 9,10-Didehydro-N-[(S)-1-(hydroxymethyl) propyl]-6-methylergoline-8-carboxamide maleate (1:1).
Use: Oxytocic.
See: Methergine, Amp. & Tab. (Sandoz)
METHYLETHYLAMINO-PHENYLPROPANOL HCl.
See: Nethamine HCl. (Var. Mfr.)
METHYLGESIC. (Kay) Methyl nicotinate, methyl salicylate, menthol, camphor, dipropyleneglycol salicylate, oil of cassia, oleoresins capsicum and ginger. Lotion Bot. 4 oz., pt., gal.
Use: Analgesic, counterirritant, vasodilator.
METHYLGLUCAMINE DIATRIZOATE, INJ., A water-soluble radiopaque iodine cpd. N-methylglucamine salt of Diatrizoate.
See: Diatrizoate (Var. Mfr.)
Diatrizoate Meglumine Inj. U.S.P. XXI.
METHULGLUCAMINE IODIPAMIDE, INJ.
See: Meglumine Iodipamide, Inj. U.S.P. XXI. (Var. Mfr.)
W/Diatrizoate methylglucamine.
See: Sinografin, Vial (Squibb)
METHYLGLYOXAL-BIS-GUANYLHYDRAZONE. Methyl GAG.
METHYL 18β-HYDROXY-11,17α-DIMETHOXY-3β,20 α-YOHIMBAN-16β-CARBOXYLATE 3,4,5-TRIME-THOXYBENZOATE (ESTER)- Reserpine, U.S.P. XXI.
METHYL 3β-HYDROXY-1α-H,5αH-TROPAN-2β-CAR-BOXYLATE, BENZOATE (ESTER) HYDRO-CHLORIDE. Cocaine Hydrochloride, U.S.P. XXI.
1-METHYLIMIDAZOLE-2-THIOL. Methimazole, U.S.P. XXI.
N-METHYLISATIN BETA-THIOSEMICARBAZONE. Under study.
Use: Smallpox protection.
• **METHYL ISOBUTYL KETONE,** N.F. XVI. 4-Methyl-2-pentanone.
Use: Pharmaceutic aid (alcohol denaturant).
METHYLISO-OCTENYLAMINE.
See: Isomethepene HCl (Var. Mfr.)
1-METHYL-D-LYSERGIC ACID BUTANOLAMIDE.
See: Sansert, Tab. (Sandoz)
METHYLMERCADONE. Name used for Nifuratel.
2-METHYL-1,4-NAPHTHOQUINONE.
See: Menadione (Var. Mfr.)
METHYL NICOTINATE.
W/Histamine dihydrochloride, oleoresin capsicum, glycomonosalicylate.
See: Akes-N-Pain Rub., Oint. (Moore)
W/methyl salicilate, menthol
See: Musterole Deep Strenght Oint. (Plough)
W/Methyl salicylate, menthol, camphor, dipropylene glycol salicylate, cassia oil, oleoresins capsium, & ginger.
See: Arthaderm, Lot. (Paddock)
Scrip-Gesic, Oint. (Scrip)
2-METHYL-5-NITROMIDAZOLE-1-ETHANOL. Metronidazole, U.S.P. XXI.
6-[(1-METHYL-4-NITROIMIDAZOL-5-YL)-THIO]PU-RINE. Azathioprine, U.S.P. XXI.

METHYLONE. (Paddock) Methylprednisolone acetate 40 mg./cc. Vials 5 cc.
Use: Corticosteroid.
• **METHYL PALMOXIRATE.** USAN.
See: Antidiabetic.
• **METHYLPARABEN,** N.F. XVI. (Various Mfr.) Methyl p-hydroxybenzoate. Methyl Chemosept.
Use: Pharm. aid (anti-fungal preservative).
METHYLPARAFYNOL. 3-Methyl-pentyne-1-ol-3. Oblivon, Somnesin.
METHYLPENTYNOL. B.A.N. 3-Methylpent-1-yn-3-ol. Atempol, Insomnol, Meparfynol, Methylparafynol, Oblivon, Somnesin, & Oblivon-C Carbamate.
Use: Tranquilizer.
METHYLPHENETHYLAMINE. 1-alpha-Methylphenethylamine.
See: Amphetamine HCl (Var. Mfr.)
METHYLPHENIDATE. B.A.N. Methyl α-phenyl-2-piperidylacetate.
Use: Central nervous system stimulant.
• **METHYLPHENIDATE HCl,** U.S.P. XXI. Tabs., U.S.P. XXI. Methyl a-phenyl-2-piperidine-acetate hydrochloride.
Use: Central stimulant.
See: Ritalin HCl, Tab., Vial (Ciba)
METHYLPHENIDYLACETATE HCl. Methyl 1-phenyl-2-piperidylacetate.
See: Methylphenidate HCl (Var. Mfr.)
METHYLPHENOBARBITAL. N-Methyl-5-ethyl-5-phenylbarbituric Acid.
See: Mebaral, Tab. (Winthrop-Breon)
d-METHYLPHENYLAMINE SULFATE.
See: Dextroamphetamine Sulfate, U.S.P. XXI. (Var. Mfr.)
METHYL PHENYLETHYLHYDANTOIN.
See: Mesantoin, Tab. (Sandoz)
5-METHYL-3-PHENYL-4-ISOXAZOLYL PENICILLIN. Oxacillin Sodium, U.S.P. XXI.
METHYLPHENYLSUCCINIMIDE.
See: Milontin, Kapseal, Susp. (Parke-Davis)
METHYL POLYSILOXANE.
See: Mylicon, Tab., Drops (Stuart)
Phasil, Tab. (Reed & Carnrick)
Silain, Tab. (Robins)
Simethicone
METHYLPRED-40. (Seatrace) Methylprednisolone acetate 40 mg./ml. Vial 5 cc.
• **METHYLPREDNISOLONE,** U.S.P. XXI. Tab., U.S.P. XXI. 11 α,17,21-Trihydroxy-6-α-methyl-pregna-1,4-diene-3,20-dione. Medrone, Metastab.
Use: Glucocorticoid.
See: A-Methapred, Inj. (Abbott)
Dura-Meth, Inj. (Foy)
Medralone 40, Inj. (Keene)
Medralone 80, Inj. (Keene)
Medrol, Tab. (Upjohn)
W/Neomycin sulfate.
See: Neo-Medrol, Oint. (Upjohn)
W/Sod. succinate.
See: Solu-Medrol, Vial (Upjohn)
• **METHYLPREDNISOLONE ACETATE,** U.S.P. XXI. Cream, For Enema, Sterile Susp., U.S.P. XXI. 6-α-methylprednisolone-21-acetate.

Use: Glucocorticoid.
See: Dep-med 40 Inj. (Tunex)
  Depo-Medrol, Inj., Rectal (Upjohn)
  Depo-Pred., Vial (Hyrex)
  Medrol Preps., Cream (Upjohn)
  Mepred-40, Susp. (Savage)
  Mepred-80, Susp. (Savage)
  Neo-Medrol, Preps. (Upjohn)
  Rep-Pred, Vial (Central)
• **METHYLPREDNISOLONE ACETATE FOR ENEMA,**
U.S.P. XXI.
Use: Glucocorticoid.
• **METHTLPREDNISOLONE HEMISUCCINATE,**
U.S.P. XXI.
Use: Adrenocortical steroid.
• **METHYLPREDNISOLONE SODIUM PHOSPHATE.**
USAN.
Use: Glucocorticoid.
• **METHYLPREDNISOLONE SODIUM SUCCINATE,**
U.S.P. XXI. For Inj., U.S.P. XXI. Methylprednisolone
21-(Hydrogen Succinate) sodium salt.
Use: Adrenocorticoid steroid.
See: Solu-Medrol, Mix-O-Vial (Upjohn)
METHYLPROMAZINE. 10-(3-Dimethylaminopropyl)-
2-methylphenethiazine.
METHYLPYRIMAL.
See: Sulfamerazine (Various Mfr.)
METHYLROSANILINE CHLORIDE.
Use: Anthelmintic & anti-infective.
See: Gentian Violet, U.S.P. XXI. (Various Mfr.)
• **METHYL SALICYLATE,** N.F. XVI. (Various Mfr.) Oil
of wintergreen.
Use: Pharm. aid (flavor).
METHYL SALICYLATE W/COMBINATIONS.
Use: Rubefacient rub (external).
See: Analbalm, Liq. (Central)
  Analgesic Balm (Various Mfr.)
  Analgesic Ointment "Lannett," Oint. (Lannett)
  Analgesine, Liq. (Elder)
  Analgex, Oint. (Bowman)
  Banalg, Liniment (Cole)
  Chloral-Methylol, Oint. (Ulmer)
  Chloro-Salicylate, Oint. (Kremers-Urban)
  Cydonol, Lot. (Gordon)
  Emul-o-balm, Liq. (Pennwalt)
  Gordobalm, Oint. (Gordon)
  Guaiamen, Cream (Lannett)
  Listerine Antiseptic, Liq. (Warner-Lambert)
  Methagul, Oint. (Gordon)
  Musterole, Oint. (Plough)
  Pixacol, Liq. (Pixacol)
  Sloan's Linament, Liq. (Warner-Lambert)
  Stimurub, Cream (Otis Clapp)
  Thi-Cin, Cap. (Warren-Teed)
METHYL SULFANIL AMIDOISOXAZOLE.
Sulfamethoxazole.
See: Gantanol, Tab., Susp. (Roche Lab.)
• **METHYLTESTOSTERONE,** U.S.P. XXI. Tab., Cap.,
U.S.P. XXI. Buccal, Tab. 17-Methyltestosterone. 17β
-Hydroxy-17-methylandrost-4-en-3-one. (Anertan,
Glasso-Sterandryl, Testoviron)
Use: Androgen.
See: Android-5, 10, 25, Tab. (Brown)

Arcosterone, Tabs. (Arcum)
Metandren, Linguet, Tab. (Ciba)
Neo-Hombreol-M, Tab. (Organon)
Oreton-M, Tab., Buccal Tab. (Schering)
Ostone, Tab. (Rowell)
Testred, Cap. (ICN)
METHYLTESTOSTERONE W/COMBINATIONS.
Use: Androgen.
See: Android-5, 10, 25, Tab. (Brown)
  Diatric, Tab. (Pasadena Research)
  Esdone, Cap., Tab. (Westerfield)
  Estritone, Tab. (Kenyon)
  Femogen W/Methyltestosterone, Tab. (Fellows-
  Testagar)
  Formatrix, Tab. (Ayerst)
  Geramine, Tab., Inj. (Brown)
  Gera-Pet, Tab. (Vortech)
  Geritag, Cap. (Reid-Provident)
  Gynetone, Tab. (Schering)
  Mediatric, Cap., Liq., Tab. (Ayerst)
  Menotab-M #1 & 2, Tab. (Fleming)
  Neosterol, Tab. (Winston)
  Os-Cal-Mone, Tab. (Marion)
  Premarin W/Methyltestosterone, Tab. (Ayerst)
  Tylosterone, Tab., Amp. (Lilly)
  Vimah, Cap. (Hyrex)
  Virilon, Cap. (Star)
METHYLTHIONINE CHLORIDE. Name used for
Methylene Blue.
METHYLTHIONINE HCl. Name used for Methylene
Blue.
• **METHYLTHIOURACIL,** U.S.P. XXI. 6-Methyl-2-thi-
ouracil. 4-Methyl-2-thiouracil. Antibason, Methiocil.
Use: Thyroid inhibition.
METHYL VIOLET.
See: Gentian Violet, Crystal Violet,
Methylrosanaline chloride
METHYNDAMINE. Name used for Tetrydamine.
• **METHYNODIOL DIACETATE.** USAN.
Use: Oral progestin.
• **METHYPRYLON,** U.S.P. XXI. Cap., Tab., U.S.P. XXI.
3,3-Diethyl-5-methyl-2,4-piperidinedione.
Use: Hypnotic.
See: Noludar, Cap. & Tab. (Roche)
METHYRIDINE. B.A.N. 2-(2-Methoxyethyl)pyridine. Pro-
mintic.
Use: Anthelmintic, veterinary medicine.
• **METHYSERGIDE.** USAN.
Use: Vasoconstrictor.
• **METHYSERGIDE MALEATE,** U.S.P. XXI. Tab.,
U.S.P. XXI. N-[1-(Hydroxymethyl)propyl]-1-methyl-
D-lysergamide bimaleate. 1-Methyl-D-lysergic acid
butanolamide. (+)-9,10-Didehydro-N-[1-(hydroxyme-
thyl)-propyl]-1,6-dimethylergoline-8β-carboxamide
Maleate (1:1).
Use: Analgesic (specific in migraine).
See: Sansert, Tab. (Sandoz)
• **METIAMIDE.** USAN. Histamine H_2 antagonist. 1-Meth-
yl-3-[2-(5-methylimidazol-4-
ylmethylthio)ethyl]thiourea.
Use: Treatment for peptic ulcer.
• **METIAPINE.** USAN.
Use: Antipsychotic.

METICLOPINDOL. Name used for Clopidol.
METICORTEN. (Schering) Prednisone 1 mg., 5
mg./Tab. Bot. 1 mg. 100s. 5 mg. 100s.
Use: Anti-inflammatory steroid.
METI-DERM. (Schering) Prednisolone 5 mg./Gm.
of cream. Tube 10 Gm., 25 Gm.
Use: Topical anti-inflammatory steroid.
METIMYD OPHTHALMIC OINT. STERILE. (Schering)
Prednisolone acetate 0.5% (5 mg.), sod.
sulfacetamide 10% (100 mg.) in an emollient
petrolatum and mineral oil base w/methylparaben
0.5 mg., propylparaben 0.1 mg. Tube ⅛ oz.
Use: Topical ophthalmic anti-inflammatory.
METIMYD OPHTH. SUSP. STERILE. (Schering)
Prednisolone acetate 5 mg., sulfacetamide sod.
100 mg./ml. Bot. dropper 5 ml.
Use: Topical ophthalmic anti-inflammatory.
• **METIOPRIM.** USAN.
Use: Antibacterial.
• **METIZOLINE.** F.D.A. 2-[(2-Methylbenzo[b]-thien-3-
yl)methyl]-2-imidazoline.
Use: Nasal decongestant.
See: Benazoline.
• **METIZOLINE HYDROCHLORIDE.** USAN.
Use: Adrengeric.
• **METKEPHAMID ACETATE.** USAN.
Use: Analgesic.
• **METOCLOPRAMIDE HYDROCHLORIDE.** USAN. 4-
Amino-5-chloro-n-[2-(diethyl-amino)-ethyl]-o-anisami-
de dihydrochloride hydrate.
4-amino-5-chloro-N-[2-(diethylamino)
ethyl]-2-methoxybenzamide monohydrochloride
monohydrate.
Use: Antiemetic.
See: Reglan, Amp. (Robins)
• **METOCURINE IODIDE,** U.S.P. XXI. Inj., U.S.P. XXI.
(+)-O,O′-Dimethylchondro-curarine diiodide.
Use: Skeletal muscle relaxant.
See: Metubine Iodid, Vial (Lilly)
METOFOLINE. B.A.N. 1-(4-Chlorophenethyl)-1,2,3,4-
tetrahydro-6,7-dimethoxy-2-methylisoquinoline.
Use: Analgesic.
METOFURONE. Name used for Nifurmerone.
• **METOGEST.** USAN.
Use: Hormone.
• **METOLAZONE.** USAN. 7-Chloro-1,2,3,4-tetrahydro-
2-methyl-4-oxo-3-o-tolyl-6-quinazolinesulfonamide.
Use: Diuretic, antihypertensive.
See: Diulo, Tab. (Searle)
Zaroxolyn, Tab. (Pennwalt)
• **METOPIMAZINE.** USAN. 10-[3-(4-Carbamoyl-
piperidino)propyl]-2-methanesulfonylphenothiazine.
Use: Antiemetic.
METOPIRONE. (Ciba) Metyrapone 250 mg./Tab. Bot.
18s.
Use: Diagnostic aid for pituitary function
determination.
METOPON. B.A.N. Methyldihydromorphinone 7,8-Dihy-
dro-5-methylmorphinone.
Use: Analgesic.
• **METOPRINE.** USAN.
Use: Antineoplasti

• **METOPROLOL.** USAN. (+)-1-Isopropylamino-3-p-
(2-methoxyethyl)phenoxypropan-2-ol.
Use: Beta-adrenergic blocking agent.
• **METOPROLOL TARTARATE.** USAN.
Use: Anti-adrenergic.
See: Lopressor, Tab. (Geigy)
• **METOPROLOL TARTRATE,** U.S.P. XXI. Tab.,
U.S.P. XXI.
Use: Beta-adrenergic blocking agent.
See: Lopressor, Tab. (Geigy)
METOQUINE.
Use: Antimalarial.
See: Quinacrine Hydrochloride (Var. Mfr.)
Atabrine HCl, Tab. (Winthrop-Breon)
• **METOQUIZINE.** USAN. 4,7-Dimethyl-9-(3,5-dimethyl-
pyrazole-1-carboxamido)-4,6,6a,7,8,9,10,-10a-octahy-
droindolo-[4,3-fg]quinoline.
Use: Anti-ulcer agent.
METOSERPATE. B.A.N. Methyl O-methyl-18-epireser-
pate. Avicalm hydrochloride.
Use: Tranquilizer, veterinary medicine.
• **METOSERPATE HYDROCHLORIDE.** USAN.
Use: Sedative.
METRA. (O'Neal, Jones & Feldman) Phendimetrazine
35 mg./Tab. Bot. 1000s.
Use: Anorexic.
METRETON OPHTHALMIC SOLUTION. (Schering)
Prednisolone sodium phosphate 5.5 mg./ml. Bot. 5
ml.
Use: Topical ophthalmic anti-inflammatory.
METRIC 21. (Fielding) Metronidazole 250 mg./Tab.
Bot. 100s.
Use: Antitrichomonal.
METRIPHONATE. B.A.N. Dimethyl 2,2,2-trichloro-1-
hydroxyethylphosphonate. Trichlorphon. Dipterex;
Dyvon; Neguvon; Tugon.
Use: Insecticide; unthelmintic, veterinary medicine.
• **METRIZAMIDE.** USAN. 2-[3-Acetamido-2, 4, 6-triiodo-
5-(N-methylacetamido) benzamido]-2-deoxy-D-
glucopyranose.
Use: Myelography.
See: Amipaque, Inj. (Winthrop-Breon)
• **METRIZOATE SODIUM.** USAN.
Use: Diagnostic aid (radiopaque medium).
See: Sodium metrizoate.
METROGESIC. (Metro Med) Salicylamide 325 mg.,
acetaminophen 162 mg., phenacetin 65 mg., Tab.
Bot. 100s, 1000s. **No. 2** (w/codeine phosphate
16.2 mg.) Bot. 50s, 1000s. **No. 3** (w/codeine
phosphate 32.5 mg.) Bot. 50s, 1000s.
Use: Analgesic w/Sedative.
METROGESTONE. 6,17-Dimethylpregna-4,6-diene-3,
20-dione.
Use: Oral progestin.
METRO I.V. (American McGaw) Metronidazol 500
mg./100 ml. Bot. 100 ml.
Use: Antibacterial.
METROJEN. (Jenkins) Metrate 1 mg., triple barb 12
mg. (representing 33⅓% each, pentobarbital, sod.
butabarbital, sod. phenobarbital)/Tab. Bot. 1000s.
Use: Sedative, hypnotic.

METRONID. (Ascher) Metronidazole 250 mg./Tab.
Bot. 100s.
Use: Amebicide, antitrichomonal.
• **METRONIDAZOLE, U.S.P. XXI.** Inj., Tab.; U.S.P.
XXI. 1-(2-Hydroxethyl)-2-methyl-5-nitromidazole. 2-
Methyl-5-nitromidazole-1-ethanol.
Use: Antitrichomonal.
See: Flagyl, Tab. (Searle)
    Flagyl I.V., Vial (Searle)
    Flagyl I.V. RTU, Vial (Searle)
    Metronid, Tab. (Ascher)
    Metryl, Tab. (Lemmon)
• **METRONIDAZOLE HYDROCHLORIDE.** USAN.
Use: Antibacterial.
See: Flagyl I.V. (Searle)
• **METRONIDAZOLE PHOSPHATE.** USAN.
Use: Antibacterial, antiprotozoal.
METRYL. (Lemmon) Metronidazole 250 mg./Tab. Bot.
100s, 250s, 500s. Unit dose 100s.
Use: Trichomonacidal agent, amebicide.
METRYL 500. (Lemmon) Metronidazole 500 mg./Tab.
Bot. 50s. Unit dose 100s.
Use: Trichomonacidal agent.
METUBINE IODIDE. (Lilly) Metocurine iodide 2
mg./ml. Vial 20 ml.
Use: Skeletal-muscle relaxant.
• **METUREDEPA.** USAN. Formerly Dimethyl
urethimine. Ethyl [bis(2,2-dimethyl-aziridinyl)-phos-
phinyl]-carbamate. Turloc.
Use: Anti-neoplastic.
METUSSIN. (Faraday) d-Methorphan. Bot. 4 oz.
Use: Non-narcotic cough syrup.
METUSSIN JR. (Faraday) d-Methorphan. Bot. 4 oz.
Use: Children's non-narcotic cough syrup.
• **METYRAPONE, U.S.P. XXI.** Tabs. U.S.P. XXI. 2-Meth-
yl-1,2-di-3-pyridyl-1-propanone.
Use: Diagnostic aid (pituitary function determination).
See: Metopirone, Tab. (Ciba)
METYRAPONE DITARTRATE. 2-Methyl-1,2-di-3-pyri-
dyl-1-propanone ditartrate. Methopyrazone
Use: Diagnostic test of pituitary function.
Adrenocortical enzyme inhibitor.
See: Metopirone, Amp. (Ciba)
• **METYRAPONE TARTRATE.** USAN.
Use: Diagnostic aid.
METYRAPONE TARTRATE INJECTION. 2-methyl-
1,2-di-3-pyridyl-1-propanone tartrate
(1:2).
Use: Diagnostic test of pituitary function.
• **METYROSINE, U.S.P. XXI.** Cap., U.S.P. XXI. L-Tyro-
sine, a-methyl-,(-)-.
Use: Antihypertensive.
See: Demser (Merck, Sharp & Dohme)
METYZOLINE. B.A.N. 3-(2-Imidazolin-2-yl-methyl)-2-
methylbenzo[b]thiophene. Eunasin [hydrochloride.]
Use: Vasoconstrictor.
MEVANIN-C. (Beutlich) Vit. C 200 mg., hesperidin com-
plex 30 mg., calcium lactate 300 mg.,
cyanocobalamin 1 mcg., ferrous sulfate 65 mg.,
folic acid 0.1 mg., Vit. A 3000 I.U., D 300 I.U., B-1 2
mg., B-2 2 mg., B-6 0.5 mg., niacin 5 mg., Cu 0.33 mg.,

Zn 0.40 mg., Mn 0.33 mg., Mg 1 mg., potassium
1.5 mg., iodine 0.03 mg./Cap. Bot. 90s, 450s.
Use: Vitamin & mineral supplement.
MEXATE. (Bristol) Methotrexate for injection. Vial 20
mg., 50 mg., 100 mg., 250 mg.
Use: Antineoplastic agent.
MEXENONE. B.A.N. 2-Hydroxy-4-methoxy-4'-methyl-
benzophenone. Uvistat.
Use: Protection of skin from sunlight.
MEXILETINE. B.A.N. 1-Methyl-2-(2,6-xylyloxy)-ethyla-
mine.
Use: Anti-arrhythmic.
• **MEXRENOATE POTASSIUM.** USAN.
Use: Aidosterone antagonist.
MEXSANA MEDICATED POWDER. (Plough) Corn
starch, kaolin, triclosan, zinc oxide. Can 3 oz., 6.25
oz., 11 oz.
Use: Topical protectant.
MEXTRA. (Kenyon) Prednisolone ½ mg.,
acetylsalicylic acid 5 gr./Tab. Bot. 100s, 1000s.
Use: Arthritis.
MEXTRAFOR. (Kenyon) Acetylsalicylic acid 5 gr.,
prednisolone 1.5 mg./Cap. Bot. 100s, 1000s.
Use: Arthritis.
MEZLIN. (Miles Pharm) Mezlocillin sodium. Vials 1
Gm., 2 Gm. 3 Gm., 4 Gm. Infusion Bot. 2 Gm., 3
Gm., 4 Gm.
Use: Broad spectrum antibiotic.
• **MEZLOCILLIN.** USAN. 6-[D-2-(Methylsulfonyl-2-ox-
oimidazolin-1-ylcarboxamido)-2-phenylacetamido]pe-
nicillanic acid.
Use: Antibiotic.
• **MEZLOCILLIN SODIUM, STERILE, U.S.P. XXI.**
Use: Antibiotic
See: Mezlin, Inj. (Miles Pharm)
MG CAPSULES. (Blue Line) Vit. B-1 5 mg., Vit. A palmi-
tate 12,500 I.U., Fe 30 mg., D 400 I.U., C 75 mg.,
B-2 2.5 mg., P 58 mg., niacinamide 40 mg., B-6 1 mg.,
B-12 2 mcg., Mg 3 mg., Ca pantothenate 4 mg., E
2 I.U., choline bitartrate 31.4 mg., inositol 15 mg., Mn
0.5 mg., K 2 mg., Zn 0.5 mg./Cap. Bot. 100s.
Mg-PLUS. (Miller) (Magnesium-protein complex made
w/specially isolated soy protein and torula yeast)
60 mg./Tab. Bot. 100s.
Use: For patients deficient in magnesium.
Mg PLUS C. (Miller) Ascorbic acid 120 mg.,
magnesium 20 mg./Tab. Bot. 100s.
Use: Dietary supplement.
MGW. (Western Research) Magnesium gluconate 500
mg./tab. Bot. 1000s.
Use: Supplement.
M-GYN. (U.S. Products) Magnesium gluconate 500
mg./Tab. Bot. 100s, 1000s.
Use: Treatment of magnesium deficiency.
MIADONE.
See: Methadone HCl. (Var. Mfr.)
• **MIANSERIN HCl.** USAN. 1,2,3,4,10,14b-Hexahydro-
2-methyldibenzo[c,f]pyrazino-[1,2-a]-azepine
monohydrochloride. Under study.
Use: Antiserotonin, antihistamine.
MIAQUIN.
See: Camoquin, Tab. (Parke-Davis)

• **MIBOLERONE.** USAN.
  Use: Anabolic, androgen.
  See: Cheque (Upjohn)

MI-BON TABLETS. (Inwood) Vit. B-1 10 mg., B-2 5 mg., B-6 2 mg., pantothenic acid 10 mg., nicotinamide 30 mg., B-12 3 mcg., C 100 mg., E 5 mg., A 3 mg., D 25 mcg., Fe 1 mg., iodine 0.15 mg., Co 0.1 mg., boron 0.1 mg., Mn 1 mg., Mg 5 mg., Mo 0.2 mg., Zn (as chloride) 1.5 mg./Tab. Bot. 100s, 250s.

MI-BON-T TABLETS. (Inwood) Vit. B-1 15 mg., B-2 10 mg., B-6 2 mg., pantothenic acid 10 mg., nicotinamide 100 mg., B-12 7.5 mg., C 150 mg., E 5 mg., A 25,000 I.U., D 1000 I.U., Fe 15 mg., Cu 1 mg., Mn 1 mg., Mg 5 mg., Mo 0.2 mg., Zn 1.5 mg., iodine 0.15 mg., Co 0.1 mg./Tab. Bot. 100s, 250s, 1000s.

MICASORB. W/Red Veterinary Petrolatum.
  See: RV Plus, Oint. (Elder)

MICATIN. (Ortho) Miconazole nitrate 2%. **Cream.** Tube 0.5 oz., 1.0 oz. **Spray powder.** Aerosol 3 oz., **Powder.** Bot. 1.5 oz. **Spray Liquid Aerosol:** Bot. 3.5 oz.
  Use: Treatment athlete's foot, jock itch, ringworm.

MI-CEBRIN. (Dista) Vit. B-1 10 mg., B-2 5 mg., B-6 1.7 mg., pantothenic acid 10 mg., niacinamide 30 mg., Vit. B-12 (activity equiv.) 3 mcg., C 100 mg., E 5.5 I.U., Vit. A 10,000 I.U., D 400 I.U. Also containing iron 15 mg., copper 1 mg., iodine 0.15 mg., manganese 1 mg., magnesium 5 mg., zinc 1.5 mg./Tab. Pkg. 60s, 100s, 1000s. Blister pkg. 10 × 10s.
  Use: Vitamin & mineral deficiencies.

MI-CEBRIN T. (Dista) Vit. B-1 15 mg., B-2 10 mg., B-6 2 mg., pantothenic acid 10 mg., niacinamide 100 mg., B-12 7.5 mcg., C 150 mg., E 5.5 I.U., A 10,000 I.U., D 400 I.U., Fe 15 mg., Cu 1 mg., iodine 0.15 mg., Mn 1 mg., Mg 5 mg., Zn 1.5 mg./Tab. Bot. 30s, 100s, 1000s. Blister pkg. 10 × 10s.
  Use: Therapeutic vitamin-minerals.

MICOFUR. Anti 5-Nitro-2-Furaldoxime, Nifuroxime.
  Use: Antifungal, antibacterial (topical)
  See: Tricofuron, Vaginal Pow., Supp. (Eaton)

• **MICONAZOLE,** U.S.P. XXI. Inj., U.S.P. XXI. 1-[2,4-Dichloro-β-(2,4-dichlorobenzyloxy)phenethyl]imidazole.
  Use: Antifungal agent.
  See: Monistat IV, Inj. (Janssen)

• **MICONAZOLE NITRATE,** U.S.P. XXI. Cream, U.S.P. XXI. 1-[2,4-Dichloro-β-[(2,4-dichlorobenzyl)-oxy]-phenylmethyl]imidazole mononitrate.
  Use: Antifungal.
  See: Monistat, Cream, (Ortho)
    Monistat-Derm, Prods. (Ortho)
    Nibustat Prods. (Ortho)

MICOREN. (Geigy) n-Crotonyl α-Ethylaminobutyric acid diethylamine and n-crotonyl α-propylaminobutyric acid diethylamide in aqueous solution. A respiratory stimulant; pending release.

MICRhoGAM. (Ortho Diagnostic) RH_0 (D) immune globulin (Human) micro dose. Single-dose vials. Pkg. 50s single-dose vials.
  Use: Prevention of maternal Rh immunization (for up to twelve weeks gestation).

MICRAININ. (Wallace) Meprobamate 200 mg., aspirin 325 mg./Tab. Bot. 100s.
  Use: Analgesic and tranquilizer combination for treatment of muscle contraction (tension) headache.

MICRIDIUM. (Johnson & Johnson) Phenacridane (9-(p-hexyloxphenyl)-10-methyl-acridinium chloride).
  Use: Skin disorders in infants and children.

MICRIN PLUS. (Johnson & Johnson) Water, S.D. alcohol 38-B, glycerin, poloxamer 407, flavor, sodium saccharin, glutamic acid buffer, cetylpyridinium chloride F.D. & C. Yellow #5 and Blue #1. Bot. 12 oz., 24 oz.
  Use: Gargle & rinse.

MICROCORT. (Alto) Hydrocortisone alcohol ½% in water washable base. Lot. Pkg. 4 oz.
  Use: Dermatoses.

MICROCULT-GC TEST. (Ames) Miniaturized culture test for the detection of *Neisseria Gonorrhoeae.* Kits for 25 tests.
  Use: Diagnostic.

MICRO-K EXTENCAPS. (Robins) Potassium chloride (8 mEq) 600 mg./Cap. Bot. 100s, 500s, Dis-Co packs/100s.
  Use: Potassium supplement.

MICRONASE. (Upjohn) Glyburide 1.25 mg., 2.5 mg., or 5.0 mg./Tab. Bot.
  Use: Lower blood glucose in type II diabetes.

MICRONEFRIN. (Bird) Racemic methylaminoethanol catechol HCl 2.25 Gm., sodium chloride, sodium bisulfite, potassium metabisulfite 0.99 Gm., chlorobutanol 0.50 Gm., benzoic acid 0.50 Gm., propylene glycol 8.0 mg./100 ml. Bot. 7.5 ml., 15 ml., 30 ml.
  Use: Croup, peripheral airway diseases.

MICRONOR. (Ortho) Norethindrone 0.35 mg./Tab. Dialpak 28s.
  Use: Progestin only contraceptive.

MICROSOL. (Star) Sulfamethizole 0.5 Gm. or 1.0 Gm./Tab. Bot. 100s, 1000s.
  Use: Urinary antibacterial.

MICROSOL-A. (Star) Phenazopyridine 50 mg., sulfamethizole 0.5 Gm./Tab. Bot. 100s, 1000s.
  Use: Urinary antibacterial for pain and burning.

MICROSTIX CANDIDA. (Ames) Box 25s.
  Use: Test for Candida species in vaginal specimens.

MICROSTIX-NITRITE REAGENT STRIPS. (Ames) Box of 3 reagent strips.
  Use: Dip and read test for nitrite in urine.

MICROSTIX INCUBATOR. (Ames) For use with Microstix reagent strips.

MICROSTIX-3 REAGENT STRIPS. (Ames) For immediate recognition of nitrite in urine and for semi-quantitation of bacterial growth. Bot. 25s w/25 incubation pouches.

MICROSUL. (Star) Sulfamethizole 0.5 Gm. 1.0 Gm./Tab. Bot. 100s, 1000s.
  Use: Urinary tract infections.

MICROSUL-A. (Star) Sulfamethizole 0.5 Gm., phenazopyridine HCl 50 mg./Tab. Bot. 100s, 1000s.
  Use: Urinary tract infections.

MICROSULFON. (CMC) Sulfadiazine 0.5 Gm./Tab. Bot. 100s, 250s, 1000s.
Use: Gram-positive bacteria infections.

MICTINE. Aminometradine, B.A.N.

MICTONE 25. (Kenyon) Bethanecol Cl 25 mg./Tab. Bot. 100s, 1000s.

MICTRIN. (Econo Med) Hydrochlorothiazide 50 mg./Tab. Bot. 100s, 1000s.
Use: Diuretic.

• **MIDAFLUR.** USAN. 4-Amino-2,2,5,5-tetrakis-(trifluoromethyl)-3-imidazoline.
Use: Sedative.

MIDAHIST DH EXPECTORANT. (Vangard) Codeine phosphate 10 mg., phenylpropanolamine HCl 18.75 mg., chlorpheniramine maleate 2 mg./5 ml. w/alcohol 5%. Bot. pt., gal.
Use: Antitussive; decongestant; antihistamine.

MIDAHIST EXPECTORANT. (Vangard) Codeine phosphate 10 mg., phenylpropanolamine HCl 18.75 mg., guaifenesin 100 mg./5 ml. w/alcohol 7.5%. Bot. pt., gal.
Use: Antitussive, decongestant, expectorant.

MIDAMALINE HCl. N-(5-chloro-2-benzimidazolylmethyl)-N-phenyl-N′N′-dimethyl-ethylene-diamine HCl.
Use: Local anesthetic.

MIDAMOR. (Merck Sharp & Dohme) Amiloride 5 mg./Tab. Bot. 100s.
Use: Antikaliuretic diuretic, antihypertensive.

MIDANEED. (Hanlon) Vit. A 5000 I.U., D 500 I.U., B-1 5 mg., B-2 3 mg., B-6 0.5 mcg., B-12 5 mcg., C 100 mg., niacinamide 10 mg., Ca pantothenate 5 mg./Cap. Bot. 100s.
Use: Dietary supplement.

MIDATANE DC EXPECTORANT. (Vangard) Brompheniramine maleate 2 mg., guaifenesin 100 mg., phenylephrine HCl 5 mg., phenylpropanolamine HCl 5 mg., codeine phosphate 10 mg./5 ml. w/alcohol 3.5% Bot. pt., gal.
Use: Antihistamine, expectorant, antitussive, decongestant.

MIDATANE EXPECTORANT. (Vangard) Brompheniramine maleate 2 mg., guaifenesin 100 mg., phenylephrine HCl 5 mg., phenylpropanolamine HCl 5 mg./5 ml. w/alcohol 3.5%.
Use: Antihistamine, expectorant, decongestant.

MIDATAP TR TABLETS. (Vangard) Brompheniramine maleate 12 mg., phenylephrine HCL 15 mg., Phenylpropanolamine HCL 15 mg./Tab. Bot. 100s, 500s, 1000s.
Use: Antihistamine, Decongestant.

MIDATAP ELIXIR. (Vangard) Brompheniramine maleate 4 mg., phenylephrine HCL 5 mg., phenylpropanolamine HCL 5 mg./5 ml. w/alcohol 2.3%. Bot. pt., gal.
Use: Antihistamine, decongestant.

• **MIDAZOLAM HYDROCHLORIDE.** USAN.
Use: Injectable Anesthetic.

• **MIDAZOLAM MALEATE.** USAN.
Use: Anesthetic.

• **MIDODRINE HYDROCHLORIDE.** USAN.

Use: Antihypertensive, vasoconstrictor.

MIDOL. (Glenbrook) Cinnamedrine HCl 14.9 mg., aspirin 454 mg., and caffeine 32.4 mg./Tab. Bot. 30s, 60s. Strip pack 12s.
Use: Antispasmodic-analgesic for menstrual symptoms.

MIDRIN. (Carnrick) Isometheptene mucate 65 mg., acetaminophen 325 mg., dichloralphenazone 100 mg./Cap. Bot. 50s, 100s.
Use: Relief of migraine & tension headache.

MIFLEX. (Misemer) Chlorzoxazone 250 mg., acetaminophen 300 mg./Cap.
Use: Discomfort of musculoskeletal conditions.

• **MIFOBATE.** USAN.

MIGERGOT P-B. (G&W) Ergotamine tartrate, belladonna alkaloids, caffeine, pentobarbital/Suppository. Boxes 10s.
Use: Migraine headaches.

MIGRADE. (Crystal) Salicylamide 3 gr., methyl-iso-octenylamide mucate 1 gr., acetaminophen 3 gr./Tab. Bot. 100s.
Use: Anti-migraine.

MIKAMYCIN. B.A.N. An antibiotic produced by *Streptomyces mitakoensis*. Mikamycin B is Ostreogrycin B.

MILD SILVER PROTEIN.
See: Silver Protein, Mild

• **MILENPERONE.** USAN.
Use: Antipsychotic.

MILES NERVINE. (Miles) Diphenhydramine 25 mg./Tab. Pkg. 12s. Bot. 30s, 50s.
Use: Nighttime sleep aid.

MILIBIS. (Winthrop Products) Glycobiarsol.
Use: Amebicide.

• **MILIPERTINE.** USAN. 5,6-Dimethoxy-3-[2-[4(o-methoxy-phenyl)-1-piperazinyl]ethyl]-2-methyl-indole.
Use: Tranquilizer.

MILKINOL. (Rorer) Liquid petrolatum specially processed for instant aqueous mixing. Bot. 8 oz.
Use: Laxative.

• **MILK OF BISMUTH,** U.S.P. XXI. (Various Mfr.) Bismuth hydroxide & bismuth subcarb.
Use: Orally, intestinal disturbances.
W/Paregoric, kaolin & pectin, methyl parahydroxybenzoate.
See: Mul-Sed, Liq. (Webcon)

• **MILK OF MAGNESIA,** U.S.P. XXI.
Use: Cathartic, antiacid.
See: Magnesium hydroxide.

MILLICORTEN. Dexamethasone, B.A.N.

MILONTIN. (Parke-Davis) Phensuximide. 0.5 Gm./Kapseal. Bot. 100s.
Use: Anticonvulsant.

MILPAR. (Winthrop Products) Magnesium hydroxide, mineral oil.
Use: Laxative antacid, lubricant.

MILPATH. (Wallace) Meprobamate 200 mg., tridihexethyl chloride 25 mg./Tab. Bot. 100s. Meprobamate 400 mg., tridihexethyl chloride 25 mg./Tab. Bot. 100s, 500s.
Use: Tranquilizer and anticholinergic combination for treatment of gastrointestinal disorders.

MILPREM. (Wallace) Meprobamate 200 or 400 mg., conjugated estrogens (equine) 0.45 mg./Tab. Bot. 100s.
Use: Treatment of menopausal symptoms.

• **MILRINONE.** USAN.

MILROY ARTIFICIAL TEARS. (Milton Roy) Dr. Bot. 22 ml.
Use: Ocular lubricant and tear replacement.

MILTOWN. (Wallace) Meprobamate. Tab. 200 mg., Bot. 100s, 400 mg. Bot. 100s, 500s, 1000s. 600 mg./Tab. Bot. 100s.
Use: Tranquilizing agent.
See: Meprospan, (Wallace)

MILTRATE. (Wallace) Meprobamate 200 mg., pentaerythritol tetranitrate 10 mg. & 20 mg./Tab. Bot. 100s.
Use: Prophylactic treatment of angina pectoris.

• **MIMBANE HYDROCHLORIDE.** USAN. 1-Methyl-yohimbane hydrochloride.
Use: Analgesic.

MINABAR. (Minette) Tab. Bot. 100s, 500s.

• **MINAXOLONE.** USAN.
Use: Anesthetic.

MINCARD. Aminometradine. 1-Allyl-3-ethyl-6-aminotetrahydropyrimidinedione.
Use: Diuretic.

MINEPENTATE. B.A.N. 2-(2-Dimethylamino-ethoxy)ethyl 1-phenylcyclopentanecarboxylate.
Use: Treatment of the Parkinsonian syndrome.

MINERAL-CORTICOIDS.
See: Desoxycorticosterone Salts (Var. Mfr.)

• **MINERAL OIL,** U.S.P. XXI.
Use: Cathartic, pharmaceutic aid (solvent, oleaginous vehicle).
See: Petrolatum, Liquid.

• **MINERAL OIL EMULSION,** U.S.P. XXI.
Use: Cathartic.

• **MINERAL OIL, LIGHT,** N.F. XVI.
Use: Vehicle.

MINIBEX. (Faraday) Vit. B-1 6 mg., B-2 3 mg., B-6 0.5 mg., C 50 mg., niacinamide 10 mg., Ca pantothenate 3 mg., B-12 2 mcg., folic acid 0.1 mg./Cap. Bot. 100s, 250s, 1000s.

MINI-GAMULIN Rh. (Armour) Rho (D) Immune Globulin (Human) in one-sixth the quantity contained in a standard dose.

MINIPRESS. (Pfizer Laboratories) Prazosin HCl 1 mg., 2 mg., or 5 mg./Cap. 1 mg. and 2 mg.: Bot. 250s, 1000s. Unit dose 100s; 5 mg: Bot. 250s, 500s. Unit dose 100s.
Use: Antihypertensive agent.

MINITEC. (Squibb) Sodium pertechnetate Tc 99 m generator.
Use: Radiodiagnostic.

MINITEC GENERATOR (COMPLETE WITH COMPONENTS). (Squibb) Medotopes Kit.
Use: Diagnostic agent for cancer.

MINIT-RUB. (Bristol-Myers) Methyl salicylate 15%, methol 3.5%, camphor 2.3% in anhydrous/and in base. Tubes 1.5 oz., 3 oz.
Use: Analgesic ointment.

MINIZIDE. (Pfizer Laboratories) Prazosin HCl and polythiazide **Minizide 1:** prazosin 1 mg., polythiazide 0.5 mg./Cap. **Minizide 2:** prazosin 2 mg., polythiazide 0.5 mg./Cap. **Minizide 5:** prazosin 5 mg., polythiazide 0.5 mg./Cap. Bot. 100s.
Use: Antihypertensive.

MINOCIN. (Lederle) **Cap.:** Minocycline HCl 50 mg./Cap. Bot. 100s. Unit dose 100s. 100 mg./Cap. Bot. 50s, 100s. Unit dose 100s. **I.V.:** 100 mg./Vial.
Oral Susp.: 50 mg./5 ml. w/propylparaben 0.10%, butylparaben 0.06%, alcohol 5% v/v. Bot. 2 oz.
Tabs: 50 mg./Tab. Bot. 100s. 100 mg./Tab. Bot. 50s.
Use: Antibiotic.

• **MINOCYCLINE.** USAN.
Use: Antibacterial.
See: Minocyn (Lederle)

• **MINOCYCLINE HYDROCHLORIDE,** U.S.P. XXI.
Cap., Oral Susp., Sterile, Tab., U.S.P. XXI. 4,7-bis-(Dimethylamino)-1,4,4a,5,5a,6,11,12a-octahydro-3, 10, 12,12a,tetrahydroxy-1,11-dioxo-2-naphthacenecarboxamide.
Use: Antibiotic.
See: Minocin, Cap., Syr., Vial (Lederle)

• **MINOXIDIL.** USAN. 2,4-diamino-6-piperidinopyrimide-3-oxide.
Use: Antihypertensive peripheral vasodilator.
See: Loniten, Tab. (Upjohn)

MIN-PLEX. (Scrip) Vit. B-1 15 mg., B-2 10 mg., B-6 5 mg., nicotinamide 50 mg., calcium pantothenate 10 mg., ascorbic acid 300 mg./Cap. Bot. 100s.

MINRO-PLEX. (Mallard) Vit. A 5000 I.U., D 400 I.U., B-1 3 mg., B-2 2.5 mg., niacinamide 20 mg., B-6 1.5 mg., Ca pantothenate 5 mg., B-12 2.5 mcg., C 50 mg., E 3 I.U., Ca 215 mg., P 166 mg., Fe 13.4 mg., Mg 7.5 mg., Mn 1.5 mg., K 5 mg., Zn 1.4 mg./Cap. Bot. 50s, 1000s.

MINTEZOL. (Merck Sharp & Dohme) Thiabendazole. Susp. 500 mg./5 ml. Bot. 120 ml. Chewable Tabs. (500 mg.) Pkg. 36s.
Use: Anthelmintic.

MINT-O-FECTANT. (Lannett) Mint odor, phenol coefficient 5. Bot. pt., gal., 5 gal., 55 gal. drum.

MINURIC. Benzbromarone, B.A.N.

MIN-VITERAL. (Kay) Vit. A 5000 U.S.P. I.U., D 1000 I.U., B-1 3.0 mg., B-2 2.5 mg., nicotinamide 20 mg., B-6 0.75 mg., Ca pantothenate 5.0 mg., B-12 2.5 mcg., C 50 mg., E 3 I.U.; plus Ca, P, Fe, Mg, Mn, K, Zn. Bot. 100s, 500s, 1000s.
Use: Dietary supplement.

MIOCEL. (Softcon) Physostigmine salicylate ⅛%, pilocarpine HCl 2% and phenyl mercuric borate. 1:25,000, methylcellulose, sod. bisulfite, boric acid, sod. carbonate. Bot. dropper 5 cc., 15 cc., 30 cc.
Use: Control and treatment of glaucoma and miotic.

MIOCHOL. (CooperVision) Acetylcholine chloride 20 mg., mannitol 60 mg., sterile water for inj. (upper chamber) 2 ml./2 cc. univial. 1:100 intraocular.
Use: Miotic in cataract surgery.

• **MIOFLAZINE HYDROCHLORIDE.** USAN.

MIOSTAT INTRAOCULAR SOLUTION. (Alcon) Carbochol 0.01%. Vial 1.5 ml.
Use: Parasympathetic miotic.

MIRAL. (Geneva) Dexamethasone 0.75 mg./Tab. Bot. 100s, 1000s.
• **MIRINCAMYCIN HYDROCHLORIDE.** USAN.
Use: Antibacterial, antimalarial.
MIRAFLOW. (CooperVision) Extra-strength cleaning solution. Bot. 15 ml.
Use: Hard contact lens cleaner.
MIRASOL. (CooperVision) Sterile isotonic buffered aqueous sol. Bot. 8 oz., 12 oz.
Use: Cleaning, rinsing, heat disinfection, storage of soft contact lenses.
MISALOID. (Jenkins) N-acetyl-p-aminophenol 5.0 gr., salicylamide 3.0 gr., triple barb 8.0 mg., (representing 33⅓% each, pentobarbital sod., butabarbital sod., phenobarbital sod.)/Tab. Bot. 1000s.
• **MISONIDAZOLE.** USAN.
Use: Antiprotozoal (trichomonas).
• **MISOPROSTOL.** USAN.
Use: Anti-ulcerative.
MISSION PRENATAL. (Mission) Ferrous gluconate 333.3 mg. (iron 38.6 mg.), Vit. C 100 mg., B-1 5.0 mg., B-6 3.0 mg., B-2 2.0 mg., niacinamide 10 mg., d-calcium pantothenate 1.0 mg., B-12 2 mcg., A (acetate) 4,000 I.U., D-2 400 I.U., calcium carbonate 70 mg., calcium gluconate 100 mg., calcium lactate 100 mg. (Calcium 50 mg.) zinc 15 mg./Tab. Bot. 100s.
MISSION PRENATAL F.A. (Mission) Ferrous gluconate 333.3 mg. (iron 38.6 mg.), Vit. C 100 mg., B-1 5 mg., B-6 10 mg., B-2 2 mg., niacinamide 10 mg., B-12 2 mcg., folic acid 0.8 mg., Vit. A acetate 4000 I.U., D2 400 I.U., Ca carbonate 70 mg., Ca gluconate 100 mg., Ca lactate 100 mg., (Ca 50 mg.), d-calcium pantothenate 1 mg./Tab. Bot. 100s.
Use: Prenatal and postpartum supplement.
MISSION PRENATAL H.P. (Mission) Ferrous gluconate 333.3 mg. (iron 38.6 mg.) Vit. C 100 mg., B-1 5 mg., B-6 25 mg., B-2 2 mg., niacinamide 10 mg., Ca pantothenate 1 mg., B-12 2 mcg., folic acid 1 mg., Vit. A 4000 I.U., Vit. D 400 I.U., Ca carbonate 70 mg., Ca gluconate 100 mg., Ca lactate 100 mg./Tab. Bot. 100s.
Use: Prenatal and postpartum supplement.
MISSION PRESURGICAL. (Mission) Vit. C 500 mg., B-1 2.5 mg., B-2 2.6 mg., B-3 30 mg., B-5 16.3 mg., B-6 3.6 mg., B-12 9 mcg., A 5000 USP u., D-2 400 USP u., E 45 I.U., ferrous gluconate 233 mg., zinc 22.5 mg./Tab. Bot. 100s.
Use: Dietary supplement for pre-surgical and post-surgical patients.
MITCHUM ANTI-PERSPIRANT. (Revlon) Aluminum chlorohydrate and aluminum chloride or aluminum sesquichlorohydrate or aluminum zirconium tetrachlorohydrex. Roll-on, lotion, stick, cream, liquid dab-on, non-aerosol spray.
Use: Anti-perspirant.
MI-THERIC. (Columbia) Vit. A 10,000 I.U., D 400 I.U., C 150 mg., B-1 15 mg., B-2 10 mg., B-6 2 mg., B-12 7.5 mcg., niacinamide 100 mg., pantothenic acid 10 mg., E 5 mg., iron 15 mg., Cu 1 mg., Mn 1 mg., Mg 5 mg., Zn 1.5 mg./Tab. Bot. 100s, 1000s.
Use: Vitamin-mineral therapy.

MITHRACIN. (Miles Pharm) Mithramycin 2,500 mcg./Vial Units of 10 vials.
Use: Antineoplastic, antihypercalcemic.
• **MITHRAMYCIN.**
See: Plicamycin.
• **MITINDOMIDE.** USAN.
Use: Antineoplastic.
MITOBRONITOL. B.A.N. 1,6-Dibromo-1,6-dideoxy-D-mannitol. Myelobromol.
Use: Antineoplastic agent.
• **MITOCARCIN.** USAN. Antibiotic derived from *Streptomyces* species.
Use: Antineoplastic.
MITOCLOMINE. B.A.N. NN-Di-(2-chloroethyl)-4-methoxy-3-methyl-1-naphthylamine.
Use: Antineoplastic agent.
• **MITOCROMIN.** USAN. Produced by *Streptomyces virdochromogenes.*
Use: Antineoplastic.
• **MITOGILLIN.** USAN. An antibiotic obtained from an "unique strain" of *Aspergillus restrictus.*
Use: Antitumorigenic antibiotic.
• **MITOMALCIN.** USAN. Produced by *Streptomyces malayensis.* Under study.
Use: Antineoplastic.
• **MITOMYCIN,** U.S.P. XXI. For Inj., U.S.P. XXI. In literature as Mitomycin C. Antibiotic isolated from *Streptomyces caespitosis.*
Use: Antibiotic.
See: Mutamycin, Inj. (Bristol)
MITOPODOZIDE. B.A.N. 2'-Ethylpodophyllohydrazide.
Use: Antineoplastic.
• **MITOSPER.** USAN. Substance derived from *Aspergillus* of the *glaucus* group.
Use: Antineoplastic.
• **MITOTANE.** U.S.P. XXI. Tabs. U.S.P. XXI. 1,1-Dichloro-2-(o-chlorophenyl)-2-(p-chlorophenyl)-ethane. Lysodren. Benzene, 1-chloro-2-[2,2-dichloro-l-(4-chlorophenyl)ethyl]-.
Use: Antineoplastic.
Lysodren, Tab. (Bristol)
MITOTENAMINE. B.A.N. 5-Bromo-3-[N-(2-chloroethyl)ethylaminomethyl]benzo[b]thiophen.
Use: Antineoplastic agent.
• **MITOXANTRONE HYDROCHLORIDE.** USAN.
Use: Antineoplastic.
MITROLAN. (Robins) Calcium polycarbophil equivalent to polycarbophil 500 mg./Tab. Blister Pak 36s, 100s.
Use: Treatment of constipation and diarrhea.
MITY-MYCIN OINTMENT. (Reid-Provident) Bacitracin 400 u., neomycin sulfate 5 mg., polymyxin B sulfate 5000 u., diperodon 10 mg./Gm. Tubes 0.5 oz.
Use: Antibiotic, anesthetic.
MITY-QUIN CREAM. (Reid-Provident) Clioquinol (3%) 30 mg., hydrocortisone (0.5%) 5 mg./Gm. Tube 20 Gm.
Use: Antifungal, antibacterial, anti-inflammatory, antipruritic.
• **MIXIDINE.** USAN.
Use: Vasodilator (coronary).
MIXTARD. (Nordisk) Isophane purified pork insulin

suspension 70% and purified pork insulin injection 30%, 100 I.U./ml.
Use: Diabetes care (IDDM).

MIXTURE 612. Dimethyl Phthalate Solution, Compound.

MLT-ASPIRIN. (Kenyon) Acetylsalicylic acid 7.5 gr./multilayered Tab. Bot. 100s, 1000s.

M-M-R II. (Merck Sharp & Dohme) Lyophilized preparation of live attenuated measles virus vaccine (Attenuvax), live attenuated mumps virus vaccine (Mumpsvax), live attenuated rubella virus vaccine (Meruvax II). See details under Attenuvax, Mumpsvax and Meruvax II. Single dose vial 1s, 10s. w/diluent.
Use: Immunization against measles, mumps and rubella.

MOBAN. (Du Pont) Molindone HCl. **Liquid:** 20 mg./ml. concentrate. Bot. 4 oz./w dropper. **Tab.:** 5 mg., 10 mg., 25 mg., 50 mg. or 100 mg./Tab. Bot. 100s.
Use: Management of manifestations of schizophrenia.

MOBENOL.
See: Tolbutamide U.S.P. XXI.

MOBIDIN. (Ascher) Magnesium salicylate, anhydrous 600 mg./Tab., Bot. 100s, 500s.
Use: Anti-arthritic agent.

MOBIGESIC. (Ascher) Magnesium salicylate 300 mg., phenyltoloxamine citrate 30 mg./ Tab. Bot. 50s, 100s. Pkg. 18's.
Use: Analgesic.

MOBISYL CREME. (Ascher) Triethanolamine salicylate in vanishing creme base. Tubes 100 Gm.
Use: Topical analgesic.

MOCCASIN BITE.
See: Antivenin, Snake, Polyvalent (Wyeth)

• **MODALINE SULFATE.** USAN. 2-Methyl-3-piperidinopyrazine monosulfate.
Use: Antidepressant.

MODANE. (Adria) Danthron 75 mg./Tab. Pkg. 10s, 30s. Bot. 100s, 1000s. Stat-Pak 100s. (10 × 10).
Use: Orally, laxative.

MODANE BULK. (Adria) Powdered mixture of equal parts of psyllium and dextrose. Container 14 oz.
Use: Bulk laxative.

MODANE LIQUID. (Adria) Danthron 37.5 mg./5 ml. Bot. 16 oz.
Use: Orally, Laxative.

MODANE MILD. (Adria) Danthron 37.5 mg./Tab. or 5 cc. Bot. 100s, 1000s.
Use: Orally, laxative.

MODANE PLUS. (Adria) Danthron 50 mg., docusate sodium 100 mg./Tab. Bot. 100s, Box 30s.
Use: Laxative, stool softener.

MODANE SOFT. (Adria) Docusate sodium 120 mg./Cap. Unit. dose, Pkg. 30s.
Use: Stool Softener.

MODERIL. (Pfizer Laboratories) Rescinnamine Tab. (0.25 mg.) Bot. 100s. (0.5 mg.) Bot. 100s.
Use: Hypertension treatment.

MODICON 21. (Ortho) Norethindrone 0.5 mg., ethinyl estradiol 35 mcg./Tab. (white) Dialpak 21s.
Use: Oral contraceptive.

MODICON 28. (Ortho) Norethindrone 0.5 mg., ethinyl estradiol 35 mcg./Tab. (white) plus 7 inert Tab. Dialpak 28s.
Use: Oral contraceptive.

MODINAL.
See: Gardinol Type Detergents. (Various Mfr.)

MODORAL. (Winthrop Products) Penthienate.
Use: Anticholinergic.

MODUCAL. (Mead Johnson) Maltodextrin. Pow. Can 13 oz.
Use: Source of dietary carbohydrate.

MODUMATE. Arginine Glutamate, B.A.N.

MODURETIC. (Merck Sharp & Dohme) Hydrochlorthiazide 50 mg., amiloride 5 mg./Tab. Bot. 100s.
Use: Antikaliuretic diuretic, antihypertensive.

MOEBIQUIN. (CMC) Bot. 100s, 1000s.

MOEDIQUIN. (CMC) Iodoquinol 650 mg./Cap. Bot. 100s, 1000s.
Use: Amoebecide.

MOENOMYCIN. Phosphorus-containing glycolipide antibiotic. Active against Gram positive organisms. Under study.

M.O., HALEY'S. (Winthrop Products)
See: Haley's M.O., Liq. (Winthrop Products)

MOLAFIL TOOTHACHE PELLETS. (DeWitt) 24s.

MOLAR PHOSPHATE.
W/Fluoride ion.
See: Coral Prod. (Lorvic)
Karigel, Gel. (Lorvic)

MOLCER. Dioctyl Sodium Sulphosuccinate, B.A.N.

• **MOLINAZONE.** USAN. 3-Morpholino-1,2,3-benzotriazin-4(3H)-one.
Use: Analgesic.

MOLINDONE. B.A.N. 3-Ethyl-6,7-dihydro-2-methyl-5-(morpholinomethyl)indol-4(5H)-one HCl.
Use: Sedative, tranquilizer, antipsychotic.

• **MOLINDONE HYDROCHLORIDE.** USAN.
Use: Antipsychotic.
See: Lidone, Cap. (Abbott)
Lidone Concentrate, Liq. (Abbott)
Moban, Tab. (Du Pont)

MOL-IRON CHRONOSULES. (Schering) Ferrous sulfate 390 mg. (78 mg. elemental iron)/Cap. Bot. 30s, 250s.
Use: Iron deficiency anemias.

MOL-IRON TABLETS, LIQUID. (Schering) Ferrous sulfate 195 mg., (equivalent 39 mg. elemental iron)/Tab. Bot. 100s.
Use: Iron-deficiency anemias.
W/Vitamin C (Schering) Ferrous sulf. 195 mg., ascorbic acid 75 mg./Tab. Bot. 100s.

• **MOLSIDOMINE.** USAN.
Use: Anti-anginal, vasodilator.

MOLYCU. (Burns) Meprobamate 400 mg., copper 60 mg./ml.
Use: Molybdenum poisoning.

MOMENTUM. (Whitehall) Salsalate 5 gr., aspirin 2.5 gr., phenyltoloxamine citrate 12.5 mg./Tab. Bot. 24s, 48s.
Use: Analgesic.

MONACETYL PYROGALLOL. Eugallol. Pyrogallol
Monoacetate.
Use: Keratolytic in chronic dermatitis.
MONALIUM HYDRATE. Hydrated magnesium
aluminate. Magalorate.
See: Riopan, Tab. & Susp. (Ayerst)
• **MONENSIN.** USAN. (1) 2-[5-Ethyltetrahydro-5-[tet-
rahydro-3-methyl-5-[tetrahydro-6-hydroxy-6-(hydroxymethyl)-3,5-dimethyl-2H-pyran-2-yl]-2-furyl]-2-furyl]-
9-hydroxy-β-methoxy-α,γ,2,8,-tetramethyl-1,6-dioxas-
piro[4,5]decane-7-butyric acid. Coban (as sodium
salt)(Lilly).
Use: Antiprotozoal; antibacterial; antifungal.
MONISTAT IV. (Janssen) Miconazole 10 mg./ml.
w/PEG 40, castor oil, lactate, methylparaben,
propylparaben, water. Amp. 20 ml.
Use: Antifungal.
MONISTAT 7 VAGINAL CREAM. (Ortho) Miconazole
nitrate 2% in water-miscible cream. Tube 47 Gm.
w/dose applicator.
Use: Local treatment of vulvovaginal candidiasis.
MONISTAT 7 VAGINAL SUPPOSITORIES. (Ortho)
Miconazole nitrate 100 mg./Suppos. Pkg. 7 supp.
w/applicator.
Use: Local treatment of vulvovaginal candidiasis
(moniliasis).
MONISTAT-DERM CREAM. (Ortho) Miconazole
nitrate 2%. w/pegoxol 7 stearate, peglicol 5 oleate,
mineral oil, benzoic acid, butylated hydroxyanisole.
Tube 1 oz., 15 Gm., 85 Gm.
Use: Anti-fungal & anti-candidal.
MONISTAT-DERM LOTION. (Ortho) Miconazole
nitrate 2% w/pegoxol 7 stearate, peglicol 5 oleate,
mineral oil, benzoic acid, butylated hydroxyanisole.
Squeeze bot. 30 ml., 60 ml.
Use: Antifunal & anti-candidal.
■ **MONO-AMINE OXIDASE INHIBITORS.**
See: Marplan, Tab. (Roche)
Nardil, Tab. (Parke-Davis)
• **MONO AND DI-ACETYLATED MONOGLYCERIDES,**
N.F. XVI. A mixture of glycerin esterfied mono- and di-
esters of edible fatty acids followed by direct acetyla-
tion.
• **MONO AND DI-GLYCERIDES,** N.F. XVI. A mixture
of mono- and di-esters of fatty acids from edible
oils.
Use: Fatty acids.
MONOBASE. (Torch) Water-washable emulsion vehicle
of fatty alcohols, natural wax & PEG. Consistency
maintained over wide temperature range. Jar 1 lb.
Use: Ointment base for hydration of skin, vehicle
for dermatological medications. Incompatible with
Burow's solution.
• **MONOBENZONE,** U.S.P. XXI. Oint., U.S.P. XXI. p-
(Benzyloxy)phenol.
Use: Depigmenting agent.
See: Benoquin, Oint., Lot. (Elder)
MONOBENZYL ETHER OF HYDROQUINONE.
See: Benoquin, Oint., Lot. (Elder)
MONOBROMISOVALERYLUREA.
See: Bromisovalum. (Various Mfr.)
MONO-CALAFORMULA. (Eric, Kirk & Gary) Calcium

cabonate 500 mg., ferrous fumarate 90 mg., Vit. A
5000 I.U., Vit. D 400 I.U., Vit. B-1 1 mg., Vit. B-6 1 mg.,
Vit. B-12 3 mcg., Vit. C 50 mg., niacinamide 10 mg.,
Vit. B-2 1 mg., iodine 0.1 mg., Mn 1.5 mg., cobalt 0.1
mg., Cu 1 mg., Zn 1.4 mg., Mg 1 mg., K 5
mg./Tab. Bot. 30s, 100s, 180s, 1000s.
Use: Vitamin-mineral supplement.
MONOCETE SOLUTION. (Pedinol) Monochloracetic
acid 80% w/color. Bot. 15 ml.
Use: Removal of verrucae.
MONOCHLOR. (Gordon) Monochloracetic acid 80%.
Bot. 15 cc.
Use: Verruca cauterant.
MONOCID. (SmithKline) Cefonicid sodium 500 mg. or
1 Gm/10 ml. Vials 1 Gm./100 ml. piggyback. 10
Gm./100 ml. piggyback.
Use: Antiinfective.
MONOCYCLINE HYDROCHLORIDE.
See: Minocin I.V., Syr., Cap. (Lederle)
MONO-DIFF TEST. (Wampole) A two-minute hemag-
glutination slide test for the differential qualitative
and quantitative determination of infectious
mononucleosis and other heterophile antibioties in
serum or plasma. Test kit 20s.
Use: An aid in the differential diagnosis of
infectious mononucleosis.
• **MONOETHANOLAMINE,** N.F.XVI. 2-Aminoethanol.
Use: Pharmaceutic aid (surfactant).
MONO-GESIC TABLETS. (Central) Salicylsalicylic
acid 750 mg./Tab. Bot. 100s
Use: Treatment of rheumatoid arthritis.
MONOJEL. (Sherwood) Glucose 40% in a 25 gm.
unit dose.
Use: Insulin reactions.
MONOIODOMETHANESULFONATE SODIUM.
See: Methiodal Sodium, U.S.P. XXI.
MONOPAR. Stilbazium Iodide.
Use: Anthelmintic.
MONOPHEN. 2-(4-Hydroxy-3,5-diiodobenzyl)-cyclohex-
ane carboxylic acid.
Use: Orally; cholecystography.
• **MONOSODIUM GLUTAMATE,** N.F. XVI.
MONOSODIUM PHOSPHATE.
See: Sodium Biphosphate, U.S.P. XXI.
MONOSTEARIN. (Various Mfr.) Glyceryl
monostearate.
MONO-SURE. (Wampole) One-minute hemagglutina-
tion slide test for the differential qualitative
detection and quantitative determination of
infectious mononucleosis heterophile antibodies in
serum or plasma. Kit 20s.
Use: An aid in the diagnosis of infectious
mononucleosis.
MONOSYL. (Arcum) Secobarbital sod. 1 gr.,
butabarbital ½ gr./Tab. Bot. 100s, 1000s.
MONOTARD HUMAN INSULIN. (Squibb/Novo)
Human insulin zinc suspension 100 Units/ml. Vial
10 ml.
Use: Human insulin (intermediate action).
MONO-TEST. (Wampole) A 2-minute hemagglutination
slide test for the qualitative detection and
quantitative determination of infectious

mononucleosis heterophile antibodies in serum or plasma. Kits 40s, 100s.
Use: Diagnosis of infectious mononucleosis.

MONO-TEST FTB. (Wampole-Zeus) 2- minute hemagglutination slide test for the qualitative detection of infectious mononucleosis heterophile antibodies using fingertip blood. Kits 10s.
Use: Aid in the diagnosis of infectious mononucleosis.

• **MONOTHIOGLYCEROL,** N.F.XVI. 3-Mercapto-1,2-propanediol.
Use: Pharmaceutic aid (preservative).

MONO-VACC. (Lincoln) Device used for vaccination against smallpox. Box 12 without vaccine or 20 sterile units with vaccine.
Use: Scarifier.

MONO-VACC TEST O.T.. (Merieux) 5 tuberculin units administered by the mantoux method. Box 25s (tamper proof).
Use: Tuberculosis screening test.

MONOXYCHLOROSENE. A stabilized, buffered, organic hypochlorous acid derivative.
See: Oxychlorosene (Guardian Chem.)

MONSEL SOLUTION. (Wade) Bot. 2 oz., 4 oz.
Use: Styptic solution.

MORANTEL. B.A.N. (E)-1,4,5,6-Tetrahydro-1-methyl-2-[2-(3-methyl-2-thienyl)vinyl]-pyrimidine.
Use: Anthelmintic, veterinary medicine.

• **MORANTEL TARTRATE.** USAN. (E)-1,4,5,6-Tetrahydro-1-methyl-2-[2(3)methyl-2-thienyl-vinyl]pyrimidine tartrate.
Use: Anthelmintic.

MORANYL.
See: Suramin Sod.

MORAZONE. B.A.N. 2:3-Dimethyl-4-(3-methyl-2-phenylmorpholinomethyl)-1-phenylpyrazol-5-one.
Use: Analgesic.

MORCO. (Archer-Taylor) Cod-liver-oil ointment w/zinc oxide, benzethonium chloride, benzocaine 1%. Suppl. 1½ oz., 1 lb.
Use: First aid dressing.

• **MORICIZINE.** USAN.
Use: Cardiac depressant.

• **MORNIFLUMATE.** USAN.
Use: Anti-inflammatory.

MOROLINE. (Plough) Petrolatum. Jars 1.75 oz., 3.75 oz., 15 oz., 5 lbs.
Use: Topical protectant, lubricant.

MOROXYDINE. B.A.N. 4-Morpholine-carboxymidoyl guanidine. N-(Guanidinoformimidoyl)-morpholine.
Use: Antiviral agent.

MORPHERIDINE. B.A.N. Ethyl 1-(2-morpholino-ethyl)-4-phenylpiperidine-4-carboxylate. Morpholino-ethylnorpethidine.
Use: Narcotic analgesic.

MORPHINAN-6-ONE,4,5-EPOXY-3,14-DI-HYDROXY-17-(2-PROPENYL)-,HYDROCHLORIDE,(5α)-.
Naloxone Hydrochloride, U.S.P. XXI.

MORPHINE ACETATE.
W/Terpin hydrate, ammonium hypophosphite & Pot. guaiacol sulfonate.
See: Broncho-Tussin Sol. (First Texas)

MORPHINE AND ATROPINE SULFATES TABLETS.
Use: Analgesic, parasympatholytic.

MORPHINE HYDROCHLORIDE. (Various Mfr.) Pow., Bot. 1 oz., 5 oz.
Use: Analgesic.

• **MORPHINE SULFATE,** U.S.P. XXI. Inj., U.S.P. XXI. (Various Mfr.) Flake or Pow. Bot. ⅛ oz., 1 oz., 5 oz., H.T. ⅛ gr., ⅙ gr., ¼ gr., ½ gr., 1 gr.
Use: Narcotic, analgesic & sedative.
W/Tartar emetic, bloodroot, ipecac, squill, wild cherry.
See: Pectoral, Prep. (Noyes)

• **MORRHUATE SODIUM INJECTION.,** U.S.P. XXI.
Use: Sclerosing agent.

MOSCO. (Moss) Jar. 0.4 oz., 0.8 oz.
Use: Corn and callus removal.

MOTILIUM. (Janssen) Domperidone maleate
Use: Antifungal.

MOTION AID ELIXIR. (Vangard) Dimenhydrinate 12.5 mg./4 ml. Bot. 10 ml.
Use: Vertigo, motion sickness.

MOTION AID TABLETS. (Vangard) Dimenhydrinate 50 mg./Tab. Bot. 100s, 1000s. Unit dose 10×10s.
Use: Vertigo, motion sickness.

■ **MOTION SICKNESS AGENTS.**
See: Antinauseants
Bucladin, Softab Tab. (Stuart)
Dramamine, Prep. (Searle)
Emetrol, Liq. (Rorer)
Marezine, Tab., Amp. (Burroughs Wellcome)
Scopolamine HBr (Various Mfr.)

• **MOTRETINIDE.** USAN.
Use: Keratolytic.

MOTRIN. (Upjohn) Ibuprofen. **300 mg.**/Tab. Bot. 500s. Unit-0f-Use 60s; **400 mg.**/Tab. Bot. 500s. Unit-of-Use Bot. 100s. Unit dose 100s; **600 mg.**/Tab. Bot. 500s. Unit-of-Use 100s. Unit Dose 100s.
Use: Anti-inflammatory agent.

MOVICOL (Norgine) Gum karaya 3.4 Gm., cortex rhamni frangulae 0.3 Gm., Sugar 1.5 Gm./Heaping Tsp. Container 200 Gm., 500 Gm.
Use: Treatment of constipation.

• **MOXALACTAM DISODIUM.** USAN.
Use: Antibiotic
See: Moxam, Liq. (Lilly)

• **MOXALACTAM DISODIUM FOR INJECTION,** U.S.P. XXI.
Use: Anti-infective.

MOXAM. (Lilly) Moxalactam disodium 1 g/10 ml. Vial 10s; 2 Gm./20 ml. Vial 10s; 10 Gm./100 ml. Vial 6s.
Use: Antibiotic.

• **MOXAZOCINE.** USAN.
Use: Analgesic, antitussive.

MOXIPRAQUINE. B.A.N. 8- |6-[4-(3-Hydroxy-butyl)piperazin-1-yl]hexylamino| -6-methoxy-quinoline.
Use: Protozoacide.

• **MOXNIDAZOLE.** USAN.
Use: Antiprotozoal.

MOYCO FLUORIDE RINSE. (Moyco) Flavored rinse w/0.05% fluoride. Bot. 16 oz., 128 oz.
Use: As an aid in the prevention of dental caries.

M-R-VAX II. (Merck Sharp & Dohme) Live attenuated

measles virus vaccine (ATTENUVAX) and live attenuated rubella virus vaccine (MERUVAX II). See details under Attenuvax and Meruvax II. Single dose Vial w/diluent. Box 1s, 10s.
Use: Immunization against measles, rubella.

MS ANTIFOAM M. (Midsil) Simethicone.

M-TETRA. (Misemer) Tetracycline HCl 250 mg./Cap. Bot. 100s.
Use: Antibiotic.

MUCILLIUM. (Robinson) Refined psyllium mucilloid & dextrose. Bot. 8 oz.
Use: Laxative.

MUCILLIUM. (Whiteworth) Psyllium hydrophilic mucilloid. Bot. 14 oz., 21 oz.
Use: Bulk laxative.

MUCILLOID OF PSYLLIUM SEED.
W/Dextrose.
See: Metamucil, Liq. (Searle)

MUCILOSE. (Winthrop Products) Highly purified hemicellulose prepared from psyllium. **Powder** 14 oz. jar.
Use: Laxative.

MUCIN.
See: Gastric Mucin (Wilson)

MUCIN, VEGETABLE.
W/Yeast or alkalized.
See: Plantamucin, Granules (Elder)

MUCODYNE. Carboxymethylcysteine, B.A.N.

MUCOGEL TABLETS. (Inwood) Gastric mucin 160 mg., magnesium glycinate 250 mg., aluminum hydroxide gel 250 mg./Tab. Bot. 100s.
Use: Peptic ulcer and hyperacidity.

MUCOMYST. (Mead Johnson) A sterile 20% solution of acetylcysteine for nebulization or direct instillation into the lung as a mucolytic agent. Vials 4 ml. Ctn. 12s, 10 ml. Ctn. 3s with dropper, 30 ml. Ctn. 3s.
Use: Bronchopulmonary disorders.

MUCOMYST-10. (Mead Johnson) A sterile 10% solution of acetylcysteine for nebulization or direct instillation into the lung as a mucolytic agent. Vials 4 ml. Ctn. 12s, 10 ml. Ctn. 3s with dropper, 30 ml. Ctn. 3s.
Use: Bronchopulmonary disorders.

MUCOMYST WITH ISOPROTERENOL. (Mead Johnson) Acetyl-L-cysteine, isoproterenol HC sterile 10% sol. acetyl-L-cysteine, 0.05% isoproterenol HCl.Vial 4 ml.
Use: Adjuvant therapy for patients with viscid or inspissated mucus secretions who might react to inhaled acetyl-L-cysteine aerosol with increased airway obstruction.

MUCOPLEX. (ICN) Heprofax 750 mg., Vit. B2 1.5 mg., Vit. B12 5 mcg./Tab. Bot. 100s, 200s.
Use: Vit. B deficiencies.

MUDD. (Chattem Labs.) Natural hydrated magnesium aluminum silicate. Topical preparation.
Use: Cleansing agent.

MUDRANE. (Poythress) Aminophylline (anhydrous) 130 mg., phenobarbital 8 mg., ephedrine HCl 16 mg., Pot. iodide 195 mg./Tab. Bot. 100s, 1000s.
Use: Treatment of asthma.

MUDRANE-2. (Poythress) Potassium iodide 195 mg., aminophylline (anhydrous) 130 mg./Tab. Bot. 100s.
Use: Emphysema, asthma, bronchitis, bronchiectasis.

MUDRANE GG. (Poythress) Aminophylline (anhydrous) 130 mg., ephedrine HCl 16 mg., guaifenesin 100 mg., Phenobarb. 8 mg./Tab. Bot. 100s, 1000s.
Use: Bronchial asthma.

MUDRANE GG-2. (Poythress) Guaifenesin 100 mg., aminophylline (anhydrous) 130 mg./Tab. Bot. 100s.
Use: Emphysema.

MUDRANE GG ELIXIR. (Poythress) Theophylline 20 mg., ephedrine HCl 4 mg., guaifenesin 26 mg., phenobarbital 2.5 mg./5 cc., alcohol 20%, Bot. pt., 0.5 gal.
Use: Antiasthmatic.

MULTABOLIC. (Kenyon) Adrenal cortex ext. 50 mg., Vit. B-12 30 mcg., methylandrostenediol 10 mg., liver "pink" B-12 equiv. 10 mcg./cc. Vial 10 cc.

MULTA-GEN 12 + E. (Bowman) Vit. A 5000 I.U., D 400 I.U., B-1 2 mg., B-2 2 mg., B-6 0.5 mg., B-12 3 mcg., C 37.5 mg., E 15 I.U., folic acid 0.2 mg., nicotinamide 20 mg./Cap. Bot. 60 s, 500s, 1000s.
Use: Multiple vitamin.

MULTALAN. (Lannett) Vit. A 5,000 I.U., D 400 I.U., B-1 2.5 mg., B-2 2.5 mg., B-6 0.5 mg., B-12 2.0 mcg., C 50 mg., niacinamide 20 mg., calcium pantothenate 5 mg./Cap. Bot. 500s, 1000s.
Use: Multiple vitamin.

MULTI-B-PLEX. (Fellows) Vit. B-1 100 mg., B-2 1 mg., nicotinamide 100 mg., pantothenic acid 10 mg., B-6 10 mg./cc. Vial 10 cc., 30 cc.
Use: Multiple Vit. B deficiencies.

MULTI-B-PLEX CAPSULES. (Fellows) Vit. B-1 50 mg., B-2 5 mg., niacinamide 50 mg., Ca pantothenate 5.4 mg., B-6 0.2 mg., C 150 mg., B-12 1 mcg./Cap. Bot. 100s, 1000s.
Use: Multiple vitamin.

MULTICEBRIN. (Lilly) Vit. B-1 3 mg., B-2 3 mg., B-6 1.2 mg., pantothenic acid 5 mg., niacinamide 25 mg., Vit. B-12 (activity equiv.) 3 mcg., C 75 mg., E 6.6 I.U., Vit. A 10,000 I.U., D 400 I.U./Tab. Pkg. 100s. Blister pkg. 10 × 10s.
Use: Multiple vitamin deficiencies.

MULTIFLUOR. (Amfre-Grant) Vit. A acetate 4000 I.U., D-2 200 I.U., C 100 mg., B-1 1.2 mg., B-2 1.9 mg., niacinamide 20 mg., B-6 2 mg., folic acid 0.4 mg., cal. pantothenate 10 mg., cyanocobalamin 5 mcg., cal. carbonate 200 mg., ferrous fumarate 40 mg., sod. fluoride 2.2 mg./Tab. Bot. 100s.
Use: Dietary supplement.

MULTIFUGE CITRATE. (Blue Line) Piperazine citrate. Syr. 100 mg./cc. Bot. 4 fl. oz. 1 pt. & 1 gal. Tab. (500 mg.) Bot. 1000s.
Use: Vermifugal agent.

MULTI-GERM OIL. (Viobin) Corn, sunflower and wheat germ oils. Bot. 4 oz., 8 oz., pt., qt.

MULTI-JETS. (Kirkman) Vit. A 10,000 I.U., D-2 400 I.U., B-1 20 mg., B-2 8 mg., C 120 mg., niacinamide 10 mg., Ca pantothenate 5 mg., B-6 0.5 mg., E 50 I.U., desic. liver 100 mg., dried debittered yeast 100 mg.,

choline bitartrate 62 mg., inositol 30 mg., dlmethionine 30 mg., B-12 7 mcg., iron 2.6 mg., calcium (dical phos.) 58 mg., phosphorus (dical phos.) 45 mg., iodine (potassium iodide) 0.114 mg., magnesium sulf. 1 mg., copper sulf. 1.99 mg., manganese sulf. 1.11 mg., potassium chloride iodide 79 mg./Tab. Bot. 100s.
Use: Multivitamin with minerals.

MULTI-JETS-T. (Kirkman) Vit. A 25,000 I.U., D 1,000 I.U., B-1 10 mg., B-2 10 mg., B-6 2 mg., B-12 5 mcg., C 150 mg., E 5 I.U., niacinamide 100 mg., Ca pantothenate 5 mg., calcium 107 mg., phosphorus 82 Gm., Fe 15 mg., Mg 6 mg., K 5 mg., 10.15 mg., Cu 1 mg., Mn 1 mg., Zn 1.5 mg., choline bitartrate 25 mg., inositol 25 mg./Cap. Bot. 100s.
Use: Multivitamin with minerals.

MULTIPALS. (Faraday) Vit. A 5000 I.U., D 400 I.U., C 50 mg., B-1 3 mg., B-6 0.5 mg., B-2 3 mg., Ca pantothenate 5 mg., niacinamide 20 mg., B-12 2 mcg./Tab. Bot. 100s, 250s, 1000s.
Use: Multivitamin.

MULTIPALS-M. (Faraday) Vit. A 6000 I.U., D 400 I.U., B-1 3 mg., B-2 3 mg., B-6 0.5 mg., B-12 5 mcg., C 60 mg., E 2 I.U., niacinamide 20 mg., Ca pantothenate 5 mg., Fe 10 mg., Iodine 0.15 mg., Cu 1 mg., Mg 6 mg., Mn 1 mg., K 5 mg./Tab. Bot. 100s, 250s, 1000s.
Use: Multivitamin with minerals.

MULTIPLE VITAMIN MINERAL FORMULA. (Kirkman) Vit. A 5,000 I.U., D-2 400 I.U., C 50 mg., B-1 2.5 mg., B-2 2.5 mg., B-6 0.5 mg., B-12 1 mcg., niacinamide 15 mg., Ca pantothenate 5 mg., Vit. E 0.1 I.U., Ca 100 mg., Fe 7.5 mg., Mg 2.5 mg., K 2.5 mg., Zn 0.15 mg., Mn 0.5 mg., Iodine 0.07 mg./Tab. Bot. 100s.
Use: Multivitamin with minerals.

MULTIPLE VITAMINS CHEWABLE. (Kirkman) Vit. A 5,000 I.U., D 400 I.U., C 50 mg., B-1 3 mg., B-2 2.5 mg., B-6 1 mg., B-12 1 mcg., niacinamide 20 mg./Tab. Bot. 100s.
Use: Multiple vitamin.

MULTIPLE VITAMINS W/IRON. (Kirkman) Vit. A 5,000 I.U., D 400 I.U., C 50 mg., B-1 3 mg., B-2 2.5 mg., B-6 1 mg., B-12 1 mcg., niacinamide 20 mg., iron 10 mg./Tab. Bot. 100s.
Use: Multivitamin with iron.

MULTISTIX S. G. REAGENT STRIPS. (Ames) Reagent strip for urine test of pH, glucose, protein, ketones, bilirubin, blood and urobilinogen. Bot. 100s.
Use: Diagnostic aid.

MULTITEST CMI. (Merieux Institute) One applicator pre-loaded with seven glycerinated liquid antigens and glycerin negative control. 10 units/box.
Use: Skin test antigens for celluar hypersensitivity.

MULTITRACE CONCENTRATE. (Armour) Trace element mixture of zinc 5 mg., copper 1 mg., manganese 0.5 mg., chromium 10 mcg./ml. Vial 1 ml. Box 25s. Vial 5 ml. Box 10s.
Use: Supplement to I.V. solutions for mineral deficiency.

MULTITRACE SOLUTION. (Armour) Trace element

mixture of zinc 1 mg., copper 0.4 mg., manganese 0.1 mg., chromium 4 mcg./ml. Vial 10 ml. Box 25s. Vial 30 ml. Box 10s.
Use: Supplement to I.V. solutions for mineral deficiency.

MULTI-VITAMIN. (Western Research) Vit. A 5000 I.U., D 400 I.U., B-1 1 mg., B-2 1.5 mg., B-6 1 mg., B-12 2 mcg., C 50 mg., niacinamide 10 mg., Ca pantothenate 2 mg., iron 10 mg., calcium 70 mg./Tab.
Use: Multivitamin with minerals.

MULTI-VITAMINS CAPSULES. (Fellows) Vit. A 5,000 I.U., D 400 I.U., B-1 1.5 mg., B-2 2 mg., B-6 0.1 mg., C 37.5 mg., cal. pantothenate 1 mg., niacinamide 20 mg./Cap. Bot. 100s, 1000s, 5000s.

MULTIVITAMINS ROWELL. (Rowell) Vit. A 5000 I.U., D 400 I.U., B-1 2.5 mg., B-2 2.5 mg., C 50 mg., niacinamide 20 mg., B-6 0.5 mg., calcium pantothenate 5 mg., B-12 2 mcg., E 10 I.U./Cap. Bot. 100s, unit-dose 100s.
Use: Vitamin therapy.

MULTIZINE.
See: Trisulfapyrimidines Tab., U.S.P. XXI.

MULTOREX. (Approved) Vit. A 6000 I.U., D 1250 I.U., C 50 mg., E 5 I.U., B-1 3 mg., B-2 3 mg., B-6 0.5 mg., niacinamide 20 mg., cal. pantothenate 5 mg., B-12 5 mcg., cal. 59 mg., phos. 45 mg./Cap. Bot. 100s, 250s, 1000s.
Use: Supplement.

MULVIDREN-F. (Stuart) Fluoride 1 mg., Vit. A 4000 U., D 400 U., C 75 mg., B-1 2 mg., B-2 2 mg., B-6 1.2 mg., B-12 3 mcg., calcium pantothenate 3 mg., niacinamide 10 mg./Softab Tab. Bot. 100s.
Use: Vitamin supplement and aid in promoting development of caries-resistant teeth.

MULVITOL. (CMC) Vitamins A 5000 I.U., D 500 I.U., B-1 2.5 mg., B-2 2.5 mg., B-6 0.5 mg., B-12 1 mcg., C 37.5 mg., cal. pantothenate 5 mg., folic acid 0.1 mg., niacinamide 20 mg./Cap. Bot. 30s, 100s, 250s, 1000s.
Use: One daily. Avitaminosis.

MUMPS IMMUNE GLOBULIN, HUMAN.
See: Hyparotin, Inj. (Cutter)

• **MUMPS SKIN TEST ANTIGEN,** U.S.P. XXI. (Lilly) Antigen made from allantoic fluid of chick embryos. Vial 1 cc. (10 tests).
Use: Diagnostic aid.

MUMPSVAX. (Merck Sharp & Dohme) Live mumps virus vaccine, Jeryl Lynn strain. Single-dose vial w/disposable syringe containing diluent. 1s, 10s.
Use: Immunization against mumps.
W/Attenuvax, Meruvax II.
See: M-M-R II, Inj. (Merck Sharp & Dohme)
W/Meruvax II
See: Biavax II (Merck Sharp & Dohme).

• **MUMPS VIRUS VACCINE LIVE,** U.S.P. XXI.
Use: Active immunizing agent.
See: Mumpsvax, Inj. (Merck Sharp & Dohme)

MUMPS VIRUS VACCINE, LIVE ATTENUATED. Jeryl Lynn (B Level) strain.
W/Measles virus vaccine, rubella virus vaccine.
See: Lirutrin, Vial (Merrell Dow)
     M-M-R, Inj. (Merck Sharp & Dohme)

MURIATIC ACID.
See: Hydrochloric Acid, N.F. XVI.
MURI-LUBE. (Invenex) Mineral Oil "Light," Vial: 2 cc.,
10 cc., 30 cc. "Heavy," Vial: 10 cc.
Use: Lubricant in surgical procedures.
MURINE. (Abbott Products) Potassium chloride,
sodium chloride, sodium phosphate, (monobasic
and dibasic), water, glycerin, edetate disodium
0.05% and benzalkonium chloride 0.01%. Plastic
dropper Bot. 0.5 oz., 1.5 oz.
Use: Soothing isotonic collyrium.
MURINE EAR DROPS. (Abbott Products) Carbamide
peroxide 6.5% in anhydrous glycerin. Bot. 0.5 oz.
Use: Softening hardened ear wax.
MURINE EAR WAX REMOVAL SYSTEM. (Abbott
Products) Carbamide peroxide 6.5% in anhydrous
glycerin w/ear washing syringe. Bot. 0.5 oz. and
ear washer 1 oz.
Use: Softening excessive ear wax and removal by
washing with syringe.
MURINE PLUS. (Abbott Products) Tetrahydrozoline
HCl 0.05%, boric acid, sodium borate, edetate
disodium 0.1%, benzalkonium chloride 0.01%. Bot.
0.5 oz., 1.5 oz.
Use: Ophthalmic decongestant.
MURIPSIN. (Norgine) Glutamic acid HCl, 500 mg.,
pepsin 35 mg./Tab. Bot. 100s, 500s.
Use: Treatment of hydrochloric acid deficiencies.
MURO. (Muro) A line of sterile ophthalmics.
MURO #128 OINTMENT. (Muro) Sodium chloride
5% in sterile ointment base. Tube 3.5 Gm.
Use: Corneal edema treatment.
MURO #128 SOLUTION. (Muro) Methylcellulose
4000 CPS 0.9%, sodium chloride 5%. Bot. 15 ml.,
30 ml.
Use: Corneal edema treatment.
MUROCEL 1% SOLUTION. (Muro) Methylcellulose
1% 4000 cps. Bot. 15 ml., 30 ml.
Use: Tear replacement, lubricant, eye bath,
ophthalmic vehicle.
MUROCOLL-2. (Muro) Phenylephrine HCl 10%,
scopolamine HBR 0.3% Bot. 5 ml.
Use: Mydriatic.
MURO'S OPCON A SOLUTION. (Muro) Naphazoline
HCl 0.025% pheniramine maleate 0.3%. Bot. 15
ml.
Use: Ophthalmic.
MURO'S OPCON SOLUTION. (Muro) Naphazoline
HCl 0.1%. Bot. 15 ml.
Use: Ophthalmic.
MURO TEARS SOLUTION. (Muro) Hydroxypropyl
methylcellulose, dextran 40. Bot. 15 ml.
Use: Ophthalmic.
MUSCLE ADENYLIC ACID.. (Various Mfr.) Active
form of adenosine 5-monophosphate.
See: Adenosine 5-monophosphate, Prep. (Various
Mfr.)
■ **MUSCLE RELAXANTS.**
See: Curare (Various Mfr.)
Flaxedil Triethiodide, Vial (Davis & Geck)
Lioresal, Tab. (Geigy)
Mephenesin (Various Mfr.)

Meprobamate (Various mfr.)
Metubine Iodine, Vial (Lilly)
Neostig, Tab. (Freeport)
Norflex, Tab., Inj. (Riker)
Parafon Forte, Tab. (McNeil)
P-A-V, Cap. (Amid)
Rela, Tab. (Schering)
Robaxin, Tab., Inj. (Robins)
Soma, Tab., Cap. (Wallace)
Succinylcholine Chloride (Various Mfr.)
d-Tubocurarine Chloride (Various Mfr.)
MUSTARAL OIL.
See: Allyl Isothiocyanate.
MUSTARGEN. (Merck Sharp & Dohme)
Mechlorethamine HCl. Each vial containing 10 mg.
with sod. chloride q.s. 100 mg. Treatment sets of 4
Vials.
Use: Parenteral administration for certain forms of
neoplastic diseases.
MUSTEROLE. (Plough) Oil of mustard, camphor,
menthol, methyl salicylate, glycol monosalicylate.
Reg.: Jars 0.9 oz., 1 oz., 1¾ oz. **Extra strength:**
Jar 0.9 oz., 1 oz. Tubes 1 oz., 2¼ oz.
Use: Analgesic rub.
MUSTEROLE DEEP STRENGTH. (Plough) Methyl
salicylate 30%, menthol 3%, Methyl nicotinate
0.5%. Jar 1.25 oz., 3 oz.
Use: Analgesic rub.
MUSTIN.
See: Mechlorethamine HCl, Sterile, U.S.P.
MUSTINE. B.A.N. NN-Di-(2-chloroethyl) methylamine.
Chlormethine (I.N.N.)
Use: Antineoplastic agent.
MUSTONE. (Key) Adenosine, B-12. Vial 10 cc.
MUTALIN. (Spanner) Protein and iodine. Vial 30 cc.
MUTAMYCIN. (Bristol) Mitomycin 5 mg., 20 mg./Vial.
Use: Antineoplastic.
MUVICA. (Blue Line) Vit. A palmitate 5000 I.U., Vit. D
400 I.U., B-1 1.5 mg., B-2 2 mg., nicotinamide 15
mg., C 30 mg., B-6 0.1 mg., Ca pantothenate 1 mg.,
Vit. B-12 1 mcg., Vit. E 1 I.U./Cap. Bot. 100s, 1000s.
• **MUZOLIMINE.** USAN.
Use: Diuretic, antihypertensive.
M.V.I. (Armour) Vit. A 10,000 I.U., D 1000 I.U., E 5
I.U., C 500 mg., B-1 50 mg., B-2 10 mg., niacinamide
100 mg., B-6 15 mg., dexpanthenol 25 mg./10 ml.
Amp. 10 ml., 25s, 100s.
Use: I.V., infusion feeding.
M.V.I.-12. (Armour) **Vial 1:** Vit. A 3300 I.U., D 200 I.U.,
E 10 I.U., C 100 mg., B-1 3 mg., B-2 3.6 mg., B-6 4
mg., niacinamide 40 mg., dexpanthenol 15 mg./5
ml. **Vial 2:** Biotin 60 mcg., folic acid 400 mcg., Vit.
B-12 5 mgc./5 ml. Vials 1 and 2 used together. Box
25s. Ctn. 100s.Vial.
Use: I.V. infusion feeding.
M.V.I. CONCENTRATE. (Armour) Vit. A 10,000 I.U., D
1000 I.U., E 5 I.U., C 500 mg., B-1 50 mg.,
B-2 10 mg., B-6 15 mg., niacinamide 100 mg., dexpan-
thenol 25 mg./5 ml. Vial 100s.
Use: I.V. infusion feeding.
M.V.I.-12 LYOPHILIZED. (Armour) Vit. A 3,300 I.U., D
200 I.U., E 10 I.U., C 100 mg., B-1 3 mg., B-2 3.6 mg.,

B-6 4 mg., B-12 5 mcg., niacinamide 40 mg., dexpanthenol 15 mg., biotin 60 mcg., folic acid 400 mcg./Vial. Box 25s. Ctn. 100s.
Use: I.V. infusion feeding.

M.V.I. PEDIATRIC. (Armour) Vit. A 2,300 I.U., D 400 I.U., C 80 mg., E 7 I.U., B-1 1.2 mg., B-2 1.4 mg., B-6 1 mg., B-12 1 mcg., K 200 mcg., niacinamide 17 mg., dexpanthenol 5 mg. biotin 20 mcg., folic acid 140 mcg./Vial. Box 25s. Ctn. 100s.
Use: I.V. infusion feeding.

MYACHOL FORMULA. (Image) Multiple vitamin Bot. 100s.
Use: Supplemental.

MYADEC. (Parke-Davis) Vit. B-12 cryst. 6 mcg., B-2 10 mg., B-6 5 mg., B-1 mononitrate 10 mg., niacin 100 mg., Vit. C 250 mg., A 10,000 I.U., D 400 I.U., E 30 I.U., Fe 20 mg., iodine 0.15 mg., Mn 1.25 mg., Cu 2 mg., Zn 20 mg., Mg 100 mg., pantothenic acid 20 mg., folic acid 0.4 mg./Tab. Bot. 130s, 250s. Unit dose 100s.
Use: Nutritional agent.

MYAGEN. Bolasterone.
Use: Anabolic agent.

MYAMBUTOL. (Lederle) Ethambutol HCl Tabs. 100 mg., Bot. 100s, 1000s. 400 mg., Bot. 100s, 1000s. Unit dose 10 × 10s.
Use: Tuberculostatic.

MYANESIN.
See: Mephenesin (Various Mfr.)

MYCARTAI. (Winthrop Products) Pentaerythritol tetranitrate.
Use: Coronary vasodilator.

MYCELEX. (Miles Pharm) Clotrimazole. **Topical cream:** 1% Tube 15 Gm., 30 Gm. **Topical Soln.:** 1%. Bot. 10 ml., 30 ml.
Use: Antifungal.

MYCELEX-G. (Miles Pharm) Clotrimazole **Vag. Tab.:** 100 mg./Tab. Pkg. 7 tab. w/applicator. **Cream:** 1%. Tube 45 Gm.
Use: Vulvovaginal candidiasis treatment.

MYCHEL. (Pfizer Laboratories) Chloramphenicol 250 mg./Cap. Bot. 100s.
Use: Antibiotic.

MYCHEL-S. (Pfizer Laboratories) Sterile chloramphenicol sodium succinate. Vial 1 Gm. 15 cc. Box 10s.
Use: Antibiotic.

MYCIFRADIN. (Upjohn) Neomycin sulfate. **Tab.** 0.5 Gm./Tab. (equivalent to 0.35 Gm neomycin). Bot. 100s, 500s. **Oral Soln.:** 125 mg./5 ml. (equivalent to 87.5 mg neomycin). Bot. pt. **Sterile Powder:** 0.5 Gm./Vial (equivalent to 0.35 Gm. neomycin) for I.M. use.
Use: Antibiotic.

MYCIGUENT. (Upjohn) Neomycin sulfate. **Cream** 5 mg./Gm. Tube 0.5 oz. **Oint.** 5 mg./Gm. Tube 0.5 oz., 1 oz., 4 oz.
Use: Antibiotic.

MYCIL, CHLORPHENESIN, B.A.N.

MYCI-SPRAY. (Misemer) Phenylephrine HCl 0.25%, methapyrilene HCl 0.2%/cc. Bot. 20cc, 60cc.
Use: Nasal congestion.

MYCITRACIN. (Upjohn) Bacitracin 500 u., neomycin sulfate 5 mg., polymyxin B sulf. 5000 u./Gm. **Oint.** Tube 0.5 oz., 1 oz. Unit-Dose 1/32 oz., Box 144s. **Ophth. Oint.** Tube 3.5 Gm. w/applicator tip.
Use: Reinforced antibiotic therapy.

MYCOLOG CREAM AND OINTMENT. (Squibb) Triamcinolone acetonide 1.0 mg., neomycin 2.5 mg., gramicidin 0.25 mg., nystatin 100,000 u./Gm. Ointment base: w/Plastibase (polyethylene, mineral oil). Tube 15 Gm., 30 Gm., 60 Gm., Jar 120 Gm.
Use: Infected or inflamed skin.

MYCOMIST. (Gordon) Chlorophyll, formalin, benzalkonium chloride. Bot. 4 oz., Plastic Bot. 1 oz.
Use: Fungicide to sanitize and deodorize shoes and boots.

• **MYCOPHENOLIC ACID.** USAN. (E)-6-(4-Hydroxy-6-methoxy-7-methyl-3-oxo-5-phthalanyl)-4-methyl-4-hexenoic acid.
Use: Antineoplastic.

MY-CORT LOTION. (Scrip) Hydrocortisone acetate 0.5%. Bot. 1 oz.

MY-CORT OTIC. (Scrip) Hydrocortisone free alcohol 2.5 mg., polymyxin B sulfate 2000 u., neomycin (as sulfate) 3.5 mg., diperodon HCl 5 mg./ml. Bot. ½ oz.

MYCOSTATIN. (Squibb) Nystatin **Tab.:** (500,000 u.) Bot. 100s. **Cr.:** 100,000 u./Gm. Tube 15 Gm., 30 Gm. **Oint.:** (100,000 u./Gm.) In PLASTIBASE (polyethylene and mineral oil). Tube 15 & 30 Gm. **Susp.:** (100,000 u./ml.) In vehicle containing sucrose 50%) Bot. w/dropper 60 ml. **Vag. Tab.:** 100,000 u., lactose 0.95 Gm., ethyl cellulose, stearic acid, starch/Tab. Pkg. 15s, 30s, Unimatic Carton 50s. **Pwd.** (topical) 100,000 u./Gm. in talc. Shaker type bot. 50 Gm. 500,000 u./Gm. Vial 1 cc. for lab use.
Use: Oral, intestinal, vaginal or cutaneous moniliasis.

MYCO TRIACET CREAM & OINTMENT. (Lemmon) Nystatin 100,000 U., neomycin sulfate 2.5 mg., gramicidin 0.25 mg., triacinolone acetonide 1 mg./Gm. **Cream:** Tube 15 Gm., 30 Gm., 60 Gm. **Ointment:** Tube 15 Gm, 30 Gm, 60 Gm.
Use: Skin infections accompanied by inflammation.

MYDFRIN 2.5%. (Alcon) Phenylephrine HCl 2.5%. Bot. 5 ml.
Use: Mydriatic.

MYDRAPRED. (Alcon) Atropine sulf. 1%, prednisolone 0.25%, in a sterile, buffered, isotonic suspension. Plas. Bot. 5 cc.
Use: Mydriatic, cycloplegic, anti-inflammatory.

MYDRIACYL. (Alcon) N-Ethyl-2-phenyl-N-(4-pyridylmethyl) hydracrylamide. Tropicamide. Bistropamide 0.5% or 1.0% Sterile aqueous solution. 15 cc. Drop-Tainer.
Use: Mydriatic-cyloplegic action.

■ **MYDRIATICS.**
Parasympatholytic Types
Atropine Salts (Various Mfr.)
Homatropine Hydrobromide (Various Mfr.)
Scopolamine Salts (Various Mfr.)

Sympathomimetic Types
Amphetamine Sulfate 3% (Various Mfr.)
Clopane HCl, Liq. (Lilly)
Ephedrine Sulfate (Various Mfr.)
Epinephrine HCl (Various Mfr.)
Neo-Synephrine HCl, Prep. (Winthrop Products)
Phenylephrine HCl. (Various Mfr.)

MYDRILATE HYDROCHLORIDE. Cyclopentolate, B.A.N.

MYLANTA LIQUID. (Stuart) Magnesium hydroxide 200 mg., aluminum hydroxide 200 mg., simethicone 20 mg./5 ml. Bot. 5 oz., 12 oz. Unit dose 30 ml. 100s.
Use: Antacid/antiflatulent for management of routine hyperacidity and similar gastrointestinal disorders.

MYLANTA TABLETS. (Stuart) Magnesium hydroxide 200 mg., aluminum hydroxide, dried gel 200 mg., simethicone 20 mg./Chewable Tab. Boxes 40s, 100s. Bot. 180s. Convenience pack 48s.
Use: Antacid/antiflatulent for management of routine hyperacidity and similar gastrointestinal disorders.

MYLANTA-II LIQUID. (Stuart) Magnesium hydroxide 400 mg., aluminum hydroxide 400 mg., simethicone 30 mg./5 ml. Bot. 12 oz., Unit dose 30 ml., 100s.
Use: High potency antacid/antiflatulent for management of peptic ulcer and other gastrointestinal disorders related to acid hypersecretion.

MYLANTA-II TABLETS. (Stuart) Magnesium hydroxide 400 mg., aluminum hydroxide 400 mg., simethicone 30 mg./Chewable Tab. Box 60s.
Use: High-potency antacid/antiflatulent for management of peptic ulcer and other gastrointestinal disorders related to acid hypersecretion.

MYLASE 100. Alpha-amylase.
See: Diastase.
W/Prolase-300, dehydrocholic acid, hyoscyamine HBr, hyoscine HBr, atropine sulfate.
See: Almezyme, Cap. (Meyer)
W/Prolase, cellulase, calcium carbonate, magnesium glycinate.
See: Zylase Tab. (Vitarine)

MYLERAN. (Burroughs Wellcome) Busulfan 2 mg./Tab. Bot. 25s.
Use: Chronic myeloid leukemia.

MYLICON. (Stuart) Simethicone 40 mg./Chewable Tab. Bot. 100s, 500s. Unit dose 100s. **Drops.** (40 mg./0.6 ml.) Bot. 30 ml.
Use: Antiflatulent.

MYLICON-80. (Stuart) Simethicone 80 mg./Chewable Tab. Bot. 100s. Boxes 12s, 48s, Unit dose 100s.
Use: High-capacity antiflatulent.

MYO-B. (Sig) Adenosine-5-monophosphoric acid and Vit. B-12. Vial 10 ml.

MYOBID. (Laser) Papaverine HCl 150 mg./Cap. Bot. 100s, 1000s.
Use: Relief of ischemia.

MYOCALM. (Parmed) Acetaminophen 8 gr., salicylamide 2 gr., phenyltoloxamine citrate 40 mg./Tab. Bot. 100s, 1000s.

Use: Analgesic/calmative.

MYOCHRYSINE. (Merck Sharp & Dohme) Sterile aqueous soln. of gold sodium thiomalate 10 mg., 25 mg., 50 mg./ml. w/benzyl alcohol 0.5%. Amps. Box 6s. Vial 50 mg./ml. 10 ml.
Use: (I.M.) Rheumatoid arthritis.

MYODIL.
See: Iophendylate Inj., U.S.P. XXI.

MYOFLEX CREME. (Adria) Trolamine salicylate 10% in a vanishing cream base. Tube 2 oz., 4 oz. Jar 8 oz., 1 lb.
Use: Topically, analgesic.

MYOLIN. (Hauck) Orphenadrine citrate 30 mg./ml. Vial 10 ml.
Use: Muscle relaxant.

MYORGAL. Mysuran. Ambenonium chloride.
Use: Cholinergic.
See: Mytelase Chloride, Cap. (Winthrop-Breon)

MYOSAL. (Seatrace) Sodium thiosalicylate 50 mg./ml. Vial 30 cc.

MYOSPAZ. (Vortech) Propoxyphene HCl 65 mg., Aspirin 227 mg., phenacetin 162 mg., caffeine 32.4 mg./Cap. Bot. 100s.
Use: Muscle disorders.

MYOTALIS. (Vita Elixir) Digitalis 1½ gr./Tab.
Use: Digitalis therapy.

MYOTONACHOL. (Glenwood) Bethanechol chloride 5 mg., 10 mg., 25 mg./Tab. Bot. 100s.

MYOTOXIN. (Vita Elixir) # 1: Digitoxin 0.1 mg./Tab.; #2: digitoxin 0.2 mg./Tab.
Use: Cardiotonic.

MY OWN. (Emko-Schering) p-Chloro-m-xylenol 0.015% in can, 0.50% in deposited film, emollient vehicle/Spray. 3.5 oz. Hexachlorophene 0.10% in can, 1% in deposited film/Powder. Benzalkonium chloride 0.12% buffered aq. solution. Spray 2 oz.
Use: Antibacterial.

MYRALACT. B.A.N. N-(2-Hydroxyethyl)tetradecylammonium lactate.
Use: Antiseptic.

MYRIATIN DROPS. (Winthrop Products) Atropine methonitrate BP.
Use: Antispasmodic.

MYRISTICA OIL.
Use: Flavor.

MYRISTYL-γ-PICOLINIUM CHLORIDE.
See: Wet Tone, Soln. (Riker)

MYRJ 45. (ICI Americas) Mixture of free polyoxyethylene glycol and its mono- and di-stearates. *Polyoxyl 8 stearate.
Use: Surface-active agent.

MYRJ 52 and 52S. (ICI Americas) Polyoxyethylene 40 Stearate. Mixture of free polyoxyethylene glycol and its mono-and di-stearates.
Use: Surface-active agent.

MYROPHINE. B.A.N. O³-Benzyl-0⁶-tetradecanoylmorphine.
Use: Narcotic analgesic.

MYSOLINE. (Ayerst) Primidone. **Tab.** 250 mg./Tab. Bot. 100s, 1000s. Unit dose 100s. 50 mg./Tab. Bot. 100s, 500s. **Susp.** 250 mg./5 ml. Bot. 8 oz.

Use: Control of grand mal, psychomotor, and focal epileptic seizures.

MYSTECLIN-F. (Squibb) Tetracycline 250 mg., amphotercin B 50 mg./Cap. Bot. 16s, 100s. Unimatic 100s.

MYSTECLIN-F SYRUP. (Squibb) Tetracycline 125 mg., potassium metaphosphate, amphotericin B 25 mg./5 ml. Bot. 240 ml.
Use: Antibiotic.

MYSURAN. Ambenonium chloride.
Use: Treatment of myasthenia gravis.
See: Mytelase Chloride, Cap. (Winthrop-Breon)

MYTELASE. (Winthrop-Breon) Ambenonium chloride 10 mg./Cap. Bot. 100s.
Use: Myasthenia gravis treatment.

MYTRATE. (Softcon) Epinephrine bitartrate 1%, 2% w/Benzalkonium chloride 1:25,000, Methulose sol., sod. bisulfite, & disod. edetate. Plastic drop bot. 15 cc.
Use: Chronic simple glaucoma.

MYTREX CREAM & OINTMENT. (Savage) Nystatin 100,000 U., neomycin sulfate 2.5 mg. neomycin base, gramicidin 0.25 mg., triamcinolone acetonide 1 mg./1 Gm. in cream or ointment base. Tube 15 Gm., 30 Gm., 60 Gm., 120 Gm.
Use: Anti-inflammatory, anti-pruritic, anti-candidal, antibacterial.

MYVEROL. (Eastman) Glyceryl monostearate.

N

NAAL. (Haag) Chlorpheniramine maleate 9 mg., Phenylephrine HCl 21 mg./Cap. Bot. 50s, 250s.

NA-ANA-TAL. (Churchill) Phenobarbital 0.25 gr., phenacetin 2 gr., aspirin 3 gr., nicotinic acid 50 mg./Tab. Bot. 100s, Liquid Bot. 16 oz.
Use: Sedative-analgesic-tension.

• **NABAZENIL.** USAN.
Use: Anticonvulsant.

• **NABILONE.** USAN.
Use: Tranquilizer (minor).

• **NABITAN HYDROCHLORIDE.** USAN.
Use: Analgesic.

• **NABOCTATE HYDROCHLORIDE.** USAN.
Use: Antiglaucoma agent, antina.

NA-CO-AL. (High) Phenylephrine HCl 2 mg., phenylpropanolamine HCl 10 mg., pyrilamine maleate 7.5 mg./Tab. Bot. 100s, 1000s.
Use: Nasal decongestant and antihistaminic.

NACREM. (Jenkins) Ammonium chloride 1.5%, menthol, methyl salicylate, camphor, oil eucalyptus Tube ¼ oz.
Use: Sinus congestion, hay fever.

• **NADIDE.** USAN. 3-Carbamoyl-1-β-D-ribofuranosyl-pyridinium hydroxide. Nicotinamide adenine dinucleotide. 1-(3-Carbamoylpyridinio)-βD-ribofuranoside 5-(adenosine-5'-pyrophosphate). Ensopride. Codehydrogenase I.
Use: Treat alcoholism and drug addiction.

NADINOLA FOR DRY SKIN. (Strickland) Hydroquinone 2%. Bot. 1.25 oz., 2.25 oz.
Use: Depigmenting agent for skin.

NADINOLA (DELUXE) FOR OILY SKIN. (Strickland) Hydroquinone 2%. Bot. 1.25 oz., 2.25 oz.
Use: Depigmenting agent for skin.

NADINOLA (ULTRA) FOR NORMAL SKIN. (Strickland) Hydroquinone 2%. Bot. 1.25 oz., 3.75 oz. Tube 1.85 oz.
Use: Depigmenting agent for skin.

NADISAN. Carbutamide, B.A.N.

• **NADOLOL.** USAN.
Use: Antiadrenergic.

NAEPAINE HYDROCHLORIDE. 2-(Pentylamino)-ethanol-p-aminobenzoate HCl.
Use: Local anesthetic.

NADOLOL.
Use: Antihypertensive and antiangina beta-blocker.
See: Corgard, Tab. (Squibb)

• **NAFARELIN ACETATE.** USAN.

NAFCIL. (Bristol) Nafcillin sodium for inj. 500 mg., 1.0 Gm., 2.0 Gm./Vial; Bulk vial 10 Gm.; 500 mg., 1 Gm., 2 Gm. Piggyback vial.
Use: Anti-infective.

NAFCILLIN. B.A.N. 6-(2-Ethoxy-1-naphthamido)-penicillanic acid.
Use: Antibiotic.
See: Unipen, Vial, Cap., Pow., Tab. (Wyeth)

• **NAFCILLIN, SODIUM,** U.S.P. XXI. Caps., Inj., Oral Solution, Sterile, Tab., U.S.P. XXI. 4-Thia-1-azabicyclo[3.2.0]-heptane-2-carboxylic acid, 6-[[(2-ethoxy-1-naph-thalenyl)carbonyl]amino]-3,3-dimethyl-7-oxo-monosodium salt, monohydrate,[2S-($2\alpha,5\alpha,6\beta$)]. Monosodium 6-(2-ethoxy-1-naphthamido)-3,3-dimethyl-7-oxo-4-thia-1-azabicyclo [3.2.0.] heptane-2-carboxylate monohydrate. Sodium 6-(2-ethoxy-1-naphthamido)-penicillanate.
Use: Antibiotic.
See: Nafcil, Inj. (Bristol)
Unipen, Vial, Cap., Pow., Tab. (Wyeth)

NA-FEEN. (Pacemaker) Fluoride 1 mg./Dose. Bot. Tabs. 100s, 500s, 1000s; Liq. 2 oz.
Use: Control of dental caries.

• **NAFENOPIN.** USAN. 2-Methyl-2-[p-1,2,3,4-tetrahydro-1-naphthyl)phenoxy]propionic acid.
Use: Hypolipidemic.

• **NAFIMIDONE HYDROCHLORIDE.** USAN.

• **NAFLOCORT.** USAN.

• **NAFOMINE MALATE.** USAN.
Use: Muscle relaxant.

• **NAFOXIDINE HYDROCHLORIDE.** USAN.
Use: Anti-estrogen.

• **NAFRONYL OXALATE.** USAN. 2-(Diethylamino-ethyl tetrahydro-α-(1-naphthyl-methyl)2-furanpropionate oxalate. Dusodril.
Use: Vasodilator.

NAFTALAN
W/Ichthyol, calamine, amber petrolatum.
See: Nagtalan, Oint. (Paddock)

• **NAFTALOFOS.** USAN.
Use: Anthelmintic.

NAFTAZONE. B.A.N. 1,2-Naphthaquinone 2-semicarbazone. Haemostop
Use: Hemostatic.

NAFTIDROFURYL. B.A.N. 2-Diethylaminoethyl 2-(1-

naphthylmethyl)-3-(tetrahydro-2-furyl)propionate.
Praxilene [oxalate]
Use: Vasodilator.

• **NAFTIFINE HYDROCHLORIDE.** USAN.
Use: Antifungal.

NAGANOL.
See: Suramin Sodium. Naphuride Sodium.

NAGEST Times Tabs. (Leeds) Phenylpropanolamine
HCl 40 mg., phenylephrine HCl 10 mg.,
phenyltoloxamine dihydrogen citrate 15 mg.,
chlorpheniramine maleate 5 mg./sustained action
Tab. Bot. 50s, 100s.
Use: Decongestant-antihistamine.

NAIL-A-CAIN. (Medtech) Benzocaine 15% w/v, tannic
acid 4% w/v. Bot. 0.5 oz.
Use: Relief of pain of ingrown nails.

NAILICURE. (Purepac) Denatonium benzoate in a
clear nailpolish base. Bot. 0.33 oz.
Use: Nail biting deterrent.

NAIL PLUS. (Faraday) Gelatin Cap. Bot. 100s, 200s.

NAIL RITE. (Eckerd) Bot. ½ oz.

NAILIFE. (Columbia) Refined gelatin 10 gr./ 8 Cap.
Bot. 1000s. Jar 100s.
Use: Nail strengthener.

NALATE. (Kay) Sod. thiosalicylate 50 mg., sodium
bisulfite 0.1%, benzyl alcohol 2%/cc. Multiple dose
sterile solution 30 cc.
Use: Analgesic in arthritis or rheumatism.

• **NALBUPHINE HYDROCHLORIDE.** USAN. (−)-17-
(cyclobutylmethyl)-4, 5a-epoxymorphinan-3, 6a, 14-
triol, hydrochloride.
Use: Analgesic
See: Nubain, Vial (Du Pont)

NALDECON. (Bristol) Phenylephrine HCl 10 mg.,
phenylpropanolamine HCl 40 mg.; phenyltoloxamine
citrate, 15 mg.; chlorpheniramine, 5 mg./Tab., half
each ingredient in inner and half in outer layer. Bot.
100s, 500s.
Use: Hayfever, sinus, congestion.

NALDECON-CX SUSPENSION. (Bristol) Phenylpropanolamine 18 mg., guaifenesin 200 mg.,
codeine phosphate 10 mg./5 ml. Bot. 4 oz, 6 oz.
Use: Decongestant, expectorant, antitussive.

NALDECON-DX PEDIATRIC SYRUP. (Bristol) Phenylpropanolamine 9 mg., dextromethorphan 7.5 mg.,
guaifenesin 100 mg./5 ml. w/alcohol 5%. Bot. 4
oz., 16 oz.
Use: Decongestant, expectorant, antitussive.

NALDECON-EX PEDIATRIC DROPS. (Bristol) Phenylpropanolamine 9 mg., guaifenesin 30 mg./ml.
w/alcohol 0.6%. Bot. 30 ml.
Use: Decongestant, expectorant.

NALDECON PEDIATRIC DROPS. (Bristol)
Chlorpheniramine maleate 0.5 mg.,
phenyltoloxamine citrate, 2 mg.,
phenylpropanolamine HCl 5 mg., phenylphrine HCl
1.25 mg./1 ml. Bot. 20 ml.
Use: Decongestant.

NALDECON PEDIATRIC SYRUP. (Bristol)
Chlorpheniramine maleate 0.5 mg.,
phenyltoloxamine citrate 2 mg.,

phenylpropanolamine HCl 5 mg., phenylephrine HCl
1.25 mg./5 ml. syrup. Bot. 16 oz.
Use: Decongestant.

NALDECON SYRUP. (Bristol) Chlorpheniramine
maleate 2.5 mg., phenyltoloxamine citrate 7.5 mg.,
phenylpropanolamine 20 mg., phenylephrine HCl 5
mg./5 ml. Bot. pt.
Use: Antihistamine combinations & decongestant.

NALFON. (Dista) Fenoprofen calcium. **200** mg./Cap.
Rx Pak 100s. **300** mg./Cap. Bot. 100s, 500s. 600
mg./Tab. Bot. 100s, 500s.
Use: Antiarthritic, analgesic.

• **NALIDIXATE SODIUM.** USAN. Sodium 1-ethyl-1,4-
dihydro-7-methyl-4-oxo-1,8-naphthyridine-3-carboxyl-
ate monohydrate. Under study.
Use: Antibacterial.

• **NALIDIXIC ACID,** U.S.P. XXI. Oral Susp., Tab.,
U.S.P. XXI. 1-Ethyl-7-methyl-1,8-naphthyridin-4-one-
3-carboxylic acid, 1-Ethyl-1,4-dihydro-7-methyl-4-oxo-
1,8-naphthyridine-3-carboxylic Acid.
Use: Antibacterial.
See: NegGram, Caplet, Susp. (Winthrop-Breon)

NALLPEN. (Beecham Labs) Nafcillin sodium
monohydrate 500 mg., 1 Gm., 2 Gm./Vial.
Use: Antibacterial.

• **NALMETRENE.** USAN.
Use: Antagonist to narcotics.

NALLINE HYDROCHLORIDE. (MSD AGVET)
Nalorphine HCl 5 mg./cc. Injection.
Use: Narcotic antidote, veterinary medicine.

NALORPHINE. B.A.N. N-Allylnormorphine. Lethidrone
[hydrobromide]
Use: Narcotic analgesic.

NALORPHINE HYDROCHLORIDE. N-Allylnormorphine
HCl. 17-Allyl-7,8-didehydro-4,5-epoxymorphinan-3,6
diol hydrochlo-ride.
Use: Narcotic antagonist.

NALOXONE. B.A.N. F.D.A. (−)-17-Allyl-4,5α-epoxy-
3,14-dihydroxymorphinan-6-one.
Use: Narcotic antagonist.
See: Narcan, Amp. (Du Pont)

• **NALOXONE HYDROCHLORIDE,** U.S.P. XXI. Inj.
U.S.P. XXI. Morphinan-6-one, 4,5-epoxy-3,14-dihy-
droxy-17-(2-propenyl)-,hydrochloride.
Use: Narcotic antagonist.
See: Narcan, Amp. (Du Pont)

NALSA SPRAY. (Jenkins) Methapyrilene HCl 0.2%,
naphazoline HCl 0.05%, cetyl pyridinium chloride
0.02%, thimerosal as preservative 0.005%. Spray
Bot. 20 cc.

• **NALTREXONE.** USAN.
Use: Antagonist to narcotics.

NAMAZENE. Phenothiazine.

NAMOL XENYRATE. 2-(4-Biphenylyl) butyric acid, compound with 2-dimethyl-amino-
ethanol.
See: Namoxyrate.

• **NAMOXYRATE.** USAN. 2-[4-Biphenylyl]butyric acid
cpd. w/2-dimethylaminoethanol. Namol Xenyrate-
previous name.
Use: Analgesic.

See: Namol Xenyrate (Warner-Chilcott)
NAMURON.
See: Cyclobarbital Calcium (Var. Mfr.)
NANROBOLIC. (O'Neal, Jones & Feldman)
Nadrolone phenpropionate 25 mg./ml. Vial 5 ml.
Use: Control of metastatic breast cancer.
NANDROBOLIC L.A. (O'Neal, Jones & Feldman)
Nandrolone decanonate 100 mg./ml. 2 ml./Vial
Box 5s.
NANDROLIN. (Reid-Provident) Nandrolone phenpro-
pionate 25 mg./ml. Vial 5 ml.
Use: Control of metastatic breast cancer.
NANDROLONE. B.A.N. 17β-Hydroxyestr-4-en-3-one.
17β-Hydroxy-19-norandrost-4-en-3-one. Nortester-
one (I.N.N.)
Use: Anabolic steroid.
• **NANDROLONE CYCLOTATE.** USAN.
Use: Anabolic.
• **NANDROLONE DECANOATE,** U.S.P. XXI. Inj.,
U.S.P. XXI. 17β-Hydroxy-estr-4-en-3-one-decanoate.
Use: Androgen.
See: Anabolin LA-100, Vial (Alto)
Androlone-D, Inj. (Keene)
Androlone-D 50, Inj. (Keene)
Deca-Durabolin, Amp., Vial (Organon)
Hybolin Decanoate, Vial (Hyrex)
• **NANDROLONE PHENPROPIONATE,** U.S.P. XXI.
Inj. U.S.P. XXI. 19-nor-17-beta-Hydroxy-3-ketoan-
drost-4-ene-17-phenylpropionate. Norandrosteno-
lone phenylpropionate. 17β-Hydroxyestr-4-en-3-one
Hydrocinnamate.
Use: Androgen.
See: Anabolin IM, Vial (Alto)
Androlone, Inj. (Keene)
Androlone 50, Inj. (Keene)
Durabolin Inj. (Organon)
Hybolin Improved, Vial (Hyrex)
Nandrolin, Vial (Reid-Provident)
NANKOR. Fenchlorphos, B.A.N.
• **NANTRADOL HCL.** USAN.
Use: Analgesic.
NAOTIN. (Drug Products) Sod. nicotinate. Amp.
(equiv. to 10 mg., nicotinic acid/cc.) 10 cc., Box
25s, 100s.
Use: I.V. & I.M., nicotinic acid therapy.
• **NAPACTADINE HYDROCHLORIDE.** USAN.
Use: Antidepressant.
NAPAL. (T.E. Williams) N-Acetyl-p-aminophenol 5 gr.,
hyoscyamine sulfate 0.03 mg., phenyltoloxamine
dihydrogen citrate 6.25 mg./Cap. Bot. 24s, 100s.
Use: Analgesic, antispasmodic, antihistaminic.
NAPHAZOLINE. B.A.N. 2-(1-Naphthylmethyl)-2-
imidazoline.
Use: Vasoconstrictor.
• **NAPHAZOLINE HYDROCHLORIDE,** U.S.P. XXI.
Nasal Soln., Ophthalmic Soln., U.S.P. XXI. lH-Imida-
zole, 4,5-dihydro-2-(1-naphthalenylmethyl)-,monohy-
drochloride, 2-(1-Naphthylmethyl)-2-imidazoline
HCl.
Use: Adrenergic.
See: Allerest Eye Drops, Soln. (Pharmacraft)
Clear Eyes, Drops (Abbott)

Naphcon, Drops (Alcon)
Privine Hydrochloride, Sol., Spray (Ciba)
Vasocon Regular, Liq. (CooperVision)
W/Antazoline phosphate, boric acid, phenylmercuric
acetate, sod. chloride, sod. carbonate anhydrous.
See: Vasocon-A Ophthalmic, Sol. (CooperVision)
W/Antazoline phosphate, polyvinyl alcohol.
See: Albalon-A Liquifilm, Ophth. (Allergan)
W/Methapyrilene HCl, cetylpyridinum chloride,
thimerosal.
See: Korizol, Sol. (Sutliff & Case)
Vapocyn II Nasal Spray (Reid-Provident)
W/Pheniramine maleate.
See: Naphcon A, Liq. (Alcon)
W/Phenylephrine HCl, pyrilamine maleate,
phenylpropanolamine HCl.
See: 4-Way Nasal Spray (Bristol-Myers)
W/Polyvinyl alcohol.
See: Albalon, Ophth. Sol. (Allergan)
Albalon Liquifilm, Ophth. Soln. (Allergan)
NAPHCON. (Alcon) Naphazoline 0.012%. Drop-Tainer
Bot. 0.5 fl. oz.
Use: Ophthalmic decongestant.
NAPHCON A. (Alcon) Naphazoline HCl 0.025%,
pheniramine maleate 0.3%. Bot. 15 ml.
Use: Ocular decongestant, antihistamine.
NAPHCON FORTE. (Alcon) Naphazoline HCl 0.1%,
benzalkonium chloride 0.01%, boric acid, sod.
chloride, pot. chloride, disod. edetate, sod.
carbonate/ml. Drop-Tainer Bot. 15 ml.
Use: Ocular decongestant.
**2-NAPHTHACENECARBOXAMIDE, 4-(DIMETHYL-
AMINO)-1,-4,4a,5,5a,6,11,12a-OCTAHYDRO-3,5,6,-
10,12,12a-HEXAHYDROXY-6-METHYL-1,11-DI-
OXO-, MONOHYDROCHLORIDE, [4S-(4α,4aα,5α,-
5α,6β,12aα)]-.** Oxytetracycline Hydrochloride,
U.S.P. XXI.
**2-NAPHTHACENECARBOXAMIDE, 4-(DIMETHYL-
AMINO)-1,4,4a,5,5a,6,11,12a-OCTAHYDRO-3,6,10,-
12,12a-PENTAHYDROXY-6-METHYL-1,11,-DI-
OXO-.** Tetracycline, U.S.P. XXI.
**2-NAPHTHACENECARBOXAMIDE, 4-(DIMETHYL-
AMINO)-1,4,4a,5,5a,6,11,12a-OCTAHYDRO-3,5,10,-
12,12a-PENTAHYDROXY-6-METHYL-1,11-DI-
OXO-, MONOHYDRATE.** Doxycycline, U.S.P. XXI.
**2-NAPHTHACENECARBOXAMIDE,4,7-BIS-(DIMETH-
YLAMINO)-1,4,4a,5,5a,6,11,12a-OCTAHYDRO-
3,10,12,12a-TETRAHYDROXY-1,11-DIOXO-,
MONOHYDROCHLORIDE,[4S-(4α,4aα,5aα,12aα]-.**
Minocycline Hydrochloride, U.S.P. XXI.
**1,4-NAPHTHALENEDIONE,2-METHYL-3-(3,7,11,15-
TETRAMETHYL-2-HEXADECENYL)-,[R-[R*,R*-
(E)]]-.** Phytonadione, U.S.P. XXI.
**1,3-NAPHTHALENEDISULFONIC ACID,6,-6'-[(3,3'-
DIMETHYL[1,1'-BIPHENYL]-4,4'-DIYL)BIS(AZO)]B-
IS 4-AMINO-5-HYDROXY]-, TETRASODIUM SALT.**
Evans Blue, U.S.P. XXI.
NAPHTHALOPHOS. B.A.N. N-(Diethoxyphosphiny-
loxy)naphthalimide. Rametin.
Use: Anthelmintic, veterinary medicine.
NAPHTHONONE. (Robins) 2-(2-Hydroxynaphthy-l-yl)-
cyclohexanone.

Use: Antitussive.

O-2-NAPHTHYL m,N-DIMETHYLTHIO-CARBANI-LATE. Tolnaftate, U.S.P. XXI.

2-(1-NAPHTHYLMETHYL)-2-IMIDAZOLINE MONOHYDROCHLORIDE. Naphazoline Hydrochloride, U.S.P. XXI.

b-NAPHTHYL SALICYLATE. Betol, Naphthosalol, Salinaphthol.
Use: G.I. & G.U., antiseptic.

NAPHURIDE SODIUM. Suramin Sodium.

NAPLOPAN. (Vortech) D-pantothenyl alcohol 250 mg./ml. Vial 10 ml.
Use: Intestinal atony and distention.

NAPROSYN. (Syntex) Naproxen 250 mg./Tab. Bot. 100s, 500s. Blister pkg. 100s; 375 mg./Tab. Bot. 100s, 500s. Blister pkg. 100s; 500 mg./Tab. Bot. 100s, 500s.
Use: Non-steroid antiinflammatory

NAPROXEN, U.S.P. XXI. Tab., U.S.P. XXI. (+)-6-Methoxy-αmethyl-2-naphthaleneacetic acid. (+)-2-(6 Methoxy-2-naphthyl)propionic acid.
Use: Anti-inflammatory; analgesic; antipyretic.
See: Anaprox, Tab. (Syntex)
    Naprosyn, Tab. (Syntex)

• **NAPROXEN SODIUM,** U.S.P. XXI. Tab., U.S.P. XXI.
Use: Anti-inflammatory, analgesic, antipyretic.

• **NAPROXOL.** USAN. (−)-6-Methoxy-β-methyl-2-naphthaleneethanol.
Use: Anti-inflammatory; analgesic; antipyretic.

NAPTRATE TABLETS. (Vortech) Pentaerythritol tetranitrate 10 mg., 20 mg./Tab. Also 20 mg., w/phenobarbital 15 mg./Tab. Bot. 1000s.
Use: Angina pectoris.

NAQUA. (Schering) Trichlormethiazide 2 mg. or 4 mg./Tab. Bot. 100s, 1000s.
Use: Diuretic, hypotensive.
W/Reserpine.
See: Naquival, Tab. (Schering)

NAQUIVAL. (Schering) Trichlormethiazide (Naqua) 4 mg., reserpine 0.1 mg./Tab. Bot. 100s, 500s.
Use: Hypertension & diuretic.

• **NARANOL HCl.** USAN. 8,9,10,11,11α,-12-Hexahydro-8,10-dimethyl-7 αH-naphtho[1′,2′:5,-6]pyrano-[3,2-c]pyridin-7-α-ol HCl.
Use: Tranquilizer.

• **NARASIN.** USAN.
Use: Growth stimulant.

NARCAN. (Du Pont) Naloxone HCl. **Amp. 0.4 mg./ml.:** 1 ml. Box 10s. **Amp. 0.02 mg./ml.:** 2 ml. Box 10s.
Use: Narcotic antagonist.

NARCAN NEONATAL. (DuPont) Naloxone HCl 0.02 mg./ml. Box 10s.
Use: Narcotic antagonist for reversal narcotic respiratory depression in neonate.

NARDELZINE. (Warner-Lambert) Psychic energizer; pending release.

NARDIL. (Parke-Davis) Phenelzine sulfate 15 mg./Tab. Bot. 100s.
Use: Anti-depressant.

NARSPAN. (Coast) Chlorpheniramine maleate 8 mg.,

phenylephrine HCl 20 mg., methscopolamine nitrate 2.5 mg./T.R. Cap. Bot. 30s, 250s.

NASACON. (CMC) Bot. 0.5 oz.
Use: Long acting nasal spray.

NASADENT. (Scherer) Sodium metaphosphate, glycerin, distilled water, dicalcium phosphate dihydrate, sodium carboxymethylcellulose, oil of spearmint, sodium benzoate, saccharin.
Use: Ingestible dentifrice.

NASAHIST. (Keene) Dextromethorphan HBr 15 mg., chlorpheniramine maleate 1 mg., phenylephrine HCl 5 mg./5 ml. w/sorbitol base q.s. Bot. pt.
Use: Cough suppresant, decongestant.

NASAHIST CAPSULES. (Keene) Phenylpropanolamine HCl 40 mg., phenylephrine HCl 10 mg., chlorpheniramine maleate 12 mg./Cap. Bot. 100s.
Use: Decongestant, antihistaminic.

NASAHIST II INJECTABLE. (Keene) Atropine sulfate 0.2 mg., chlorpheniramine maleate 5 mg./ml. Vial 10 ml.
Use: Decongestant and antihistamine.

NASALCROM NASAL SOLUTION. (Fisons) Cromolyn sodium. Metered dose spray. Pkg. 13 ml.
Use: Anti-allergic rhinitis.

NASALIDE. (Syntex) Flunisolide 0.025% sol. Bot. 25 ml.
Use: Symptoms of seasonal and perennial rhinitis.

NASDRO. (Jenkins) Ephedrine sulfate 1%, chlorobutanol 5% with menthol, camphor, oil eucalyptus, thymol and oil red thyme. Bot. drop ½ oz., pt.
Use: Nose and throat drops or spray.

NASOPHEN. (Premo) Phenylephrine HCl 0.25%, 1%. Bot. 1 pt.
Use: Treatment of vasomotor rhinitis, sinusitis, allergic rhinitis, and as an adjuvant in the treatment of acute coryza.

NATABEC. (Parke-Davis) Vit. A 4000 I.U., D 400 I.U., B-1 3 mg., B-2 2 mg., B-6 3 mg., C 50 mg., B-12 5 mcg., niacinamide 10 mg., Ca carbonate 600 mg., ferrous sulfate 150 mg./Kapseal. Bot. 100s.
Use: Vitamin, iron & calcium deficiencies.

NATABEC-F.A.. (Parke-Davis) Same as Natabec, plus folic acid 0.1 mg./Kapseal. Bot. 100s.
Use: Dietary supplement during pregnancy and lactation.

NATABEC Rx. (Parke-Davis) Same as Natabec, plus folic acid 1 mg./Kapseal. Bot. 100s.

NATABEC WITH FLUORIDE. (Parke-Davis) Same formula as Natabec, plus fluoride 2.2 mg./Kapseal. Bot. 100s.
Use: Nutritional support.

NATACYN. (Alcon) Natamycin (5%) 50 mg./ml. Bot. 15 ml.
Use: Ophthalmic antifungal agent.

NATAFORT FILMSEAL. (Parke-Davis) Vit. A 6000 I.U., D 400 I.U., C 120 mg., B-1 3 mg., B-2 2 mg., B-6 15 mg., B-12 6 mcg., niacin 20 mg., Folic Acid 1 mg., E 30 I.U., Ca 350 mg., Mg. 100 mg., Zn 25 mg., Iodine 0.15 mg., Fe 65 mg./Tab. Bot. 100s.
Use: Prenatal vitamin and mineral supplement.

NATALINS. (Mead Johnson) Vit. A 8000 I.U., D 400 I.U., E 30 I.U., C 90 mg., B-1 1.7 mg., B-2 2.0 mg., B-6 4.0 mg., B-12 8 mcg., niacin 20 mg., folic acid 0.8 mg., iodine 150 mcg., Ca 200 mg., Fe 45 mg., Mg 100 mg./Tab. Bot. 100s, 1000s. Drum 36,000.
Use: Multivitamin and mineral supplement for pregnant or lactating women.

NATALINS RX. (Mead Johnson) Vit. A 8,000 I.U., D 400 I.U., E 30 I.U., C 90 mg., B-1 2.55 mg., B-2 3.0 mg., B-6 10 mg., B-12 8 mcg., niacin 20 mg., folic acid 1.0 mg., pantothenic acid 15 mg., biotin 0.05 mg., Ca 200 mg., Fe 60 mg., Mg 100 mg., Cu 2 mg., Zn 15.0 mg., iodine 150 mcg./Tab. Bot. 100s, 1000s.
Use: Multivitamin and mineral supplement for pregnant or lactating women.

• **NATAMYCIN,** U.S.P. XXI. Ophth. Susp., U.S.P. XXI. An antibiotic produced by *Streptomyces natalensis*. Pimafucin.
Use: Antibiotic.

NATA-PAR. (Pharmics) Ferrous fumarate 200 mg., C 75 mg., cal. carbonate 450 mg., A 4000 I.U., D 400 I.U., B-6 5 mg., B-1 5 mg., B-2 2 mg., niacinamide 15 mg., B-12 2.5 mcg., iodine 0.15 mg., K 0.05 mg., Mn 0.5 mg., Cu 0.25 mg., Zn 0.5 mg., Mg 1 mg./Cap. Bot. 100s, 1000s.
Use: Pregnancy and lactation.

NATAPLEX-C. (Galen) Vit. A 5000 u., D 400 u., B-1 3 mg., B-2 2 mg., B-6 e mg., C 100 mg., B-12 3 mcg., niacinamide 10 mg., folic acid 0.05 mg., Ca 575 mg., ferrous fumarate 100 mg., K.I. 0.1 mg., Mn 1 mg., Mg 1 mg., Zn 1 mg./Tab. Bot. 100s, 1000s.
Use: Vitamin-mineral supplementation during pregnancy and lactation.

NATA-SAN. (Sandia) Vit. A 4000 I.U., D 400 I.U., B-1 5 mg., B-2 4 mg., B-6 10 mg., nicotinic acid 10 mg., Vit. C 100 mg., B-12 activity 5 mcg., ferrous fumarate 200 mg. (elemental iron 65 mg.), cal. carbonate 500 mg. (calcium 196 mg.), copper (sulfate) 0.5 mg., magnesium (sulfate) 0.1 mg., manganese (sulfate) 0.1 mg., potassium (sulfate) 0.1 mg., zinc (sulfate) 0.5 mg./Tab. Bot. 100s, 1000s.

NATA-SAN F.A. (Sandia) Vit. A 4000 I.U., D 400 I.U., B-1 5 mg., B-2 4 mg., B-6 10 mg., nicotinic acid 10 mg., Vit. C 100 mg., B-12 activity 5 mcg., folic acid 1 mg., iron 65 mg., calcium 200 mg., copper (sulfate) 0.5 mg., magnesium (sulfate) 0.1 mg., manganese (sulfate) 0.1 mg., potassium (sulfate) 0.1 mg., zinc (sulfate) 0.5 mg./Tab. Bot. 100s, 1000s.

NATODINE. (Faraday) Iodine in organic form as found in kelp. 1 mg./Tab. Bot. 100s, 250s.

NATRICO. (Drug Products) Pot. nitrate 2 gr., Sod. nitrite 1 gr., nitroglycerin ¼ gr., crataegus oxycantha ¼ gr./Pulvoid. Bot. 100s, 1000s.
Use: Hypertension.

NATROGESTIVE. (Wolins) Sodium bicarbonate 10 gr., papain ½ gr., ginger, pancreatin/Tab. Bot. 1000s.

NATURACIL. (Mead Johnson) Psyllium seed husks 3.4 Gm./2 pieces Carton 24s, 40s.
Use: Bulk forming laxative.

NATUR-AID. (Scott/Cord) Lactose w/pectin-and Carob-lemon juice. Pow. 90%. Bot. 8 oz.

Use: Increase in normal intestinal flora.

NATURAL THERATAB. (Vortech) Bot. 30s, 100s.
Use: Natural & organic vitamins plus minerals.

NATURAL VITAMIN A IN OIL.
See: Oleovitamin A, U.S.P.

NATUR-"C" TABLETS. (Columbia) Vit. C 300 mg. Chewable Tab. Bot. 100s, 250s.
Use: Nutritional supplement.

NATURE CAL-D TABLETS. (Image) Bot. 100s.
Use: Supplement.

NATURE'S AID LAXATIVE TABS. (Walgreen) Docusate sodium 100 mg., yellow phenolphthalein 65 mg./Tab. Bot. 60s.
Use: Mild laxative & stool softener.

NATURE'S PANRAY BEE POLLEN TABLETS. (Panray) Bee pollen 500 mg./Tab. Bot. 100s.
Use: Dietary supplement.

NATURE'S PANTRY ROSE HIPS TABLETS. (Panray) Vitamin C from rose hips 500 mg., 100 mg./Tab. Bot. 100s.
Use: Dietary supplement.

NATURE'S REMEDY. (Norcliff Thayer) Aloe 100 mg., cascara sagrada 150 mg./Film coated Tab.; Foil backed blister pkg. Box 12s, 30s, 60s.
Use: Laxative.

NATURETIN. (Squibb) Bendroflumethiazide.2.5 mg./Tab. Bot. 100s. 5 mg./Tab. Bot. 100s, 1000s. **10 mg.**/Tab. Bot. 100s.
Use: Diuretic, hypotensive.

NATURETIN W/K. (Squibb) Bendroflumethiazide 5 mg., potassium chloride 500 mg./Tab. Bot. 100s.
Use: Diuretic and hypotensive.

NATURIL. (Kenyon) Pow. ext. uva ursi ½ gr., pow. ext. buchu leaves ½ gr., pow. ext. corn silk ½ gr., pow. ext. juniper ¼ gr., caffeine ¼ gr./Tab. Bot. 100s, 1000s.

NATUR-LAX TABLETS. (Faraday) Rhubarb root, cape aloes, ext. cascara sagrada, mandrake root, parsley, carrot/Tab. Protein coated tablets. Bot. 100s.
Use: Vegetable laxative.

NAUS-A-TORIES. (Table Rock) Pyrilamine maleate 25 mg., secobarbital 30 mg./Supp. Box 12s.
Use: Prevention or control of nausea.

NAUZINE. (Century) Dimenhydrinate 50 mg., propylene glycol 50%, benzyl alcohol 5%/cc. Inj. vial 10 cc.

NAVANE. (Roerig) Thiothixene. **Caps.** 1 mg., Bot. 100s. Unit dose. 100s. 2 mg., 5 mg., 10 mg., Bot. 100s, 1000s. Unit dose. 100s. 20 mg. Bot. 100s, 500s. Unit dose. 100s. **Liq.** 5 mg./cc. Bot. 1 oz., 4 oz. **Inj.** Parenteral I.M. Vial 2 mg./ml. Pkg. 10s.
Use: Antipsychotic agent, tranquilizer.

NAVANE LIOPHIL IM. (Roerig) Thiothixene HCl 5 mg./ml. Liophylized for reconstitution with 2.2 ml. sterile water. Vial 10 cc. Pkg. 10 vials.
Use: Antipsychotic agent.

NAVANE ORAL CONCENTRATE. (Roerig) Thiothixene HCl 5 mg./ml. Bot. 1 oz., 4 oz. x/calibrated dropper.
Use: Antipsychotic.

NAVIDREX. Cyclopenthiazide, B.A.N.

NAVIDRIX (NAVIDREX, CYCLOPENTHIAZIDE).
Cyclopenthiazide. 3-Cyclopentylmethyl derivative of hydrochlorothiazide.
Use: Oral diuretic.

NAVSEAST. (Eastwood) Tab. Bot. 100s.

N.B.P. OINTMENT. (Bowman) Bacitracin zinc 400 u., neomycin sulfate 5 mg., polymyxin B sulfate 10,000 u./Gm. Tube ⅛ oz., ½ oz.
Use: Topical antibiotic.

N.B.P. OINTMENT. (O'Neal, Jones & Feldman) Neomycin, bacitracin, polymixin ointment. Tube ⅛ oz., ½ oz.
Use: Antibiotic ointment.

N-CHLORO COMPOUND ANTISEPTICS.
See: Antiseptic, N-Chloro Compounds.

N D CLEAR. (Seatrace) Chlorpheniramine maleate 8 mg., pseudoephedrine HCl 120 mg./T.D. Cap. Bot. 100s, 1000s.
Use: Antihistaminic, nasal decongestant.

N-DIETHYL META-TOLUAMIDE.
W/Red Veterinary Petrolatum.
See: RV Pellent, Oint. (Elder)

ND-GESIC. (Hyrex) Acetaminophen 300 mg., pyrilamine maleate 12.5 mg., chlorpheniramine maleate 2 mg., phenindamine tartrate 5 mg./Tab. Bot. 100s, 1000s, 5000s.
Use: Analgesic, antihistaminic, vasoconstrictor.

ND-HIST. (Hyrex) Chlorpheniramine maleate 12 mg., phenylpropanolamine HCl 40 mg., phenylephrine HCl 10 mg./long acting Cap. Bot. 100s,
Use: Antihistaminic/decongestant.

nDNA. (Wampole-Zeus) Anti-native DNA test by IFA. Tests 48s.
Use: Confirmatory test for active SLE.

ND-STAT. (Hyrex) Atropine sulfate 0.2 mg., chlorpheniramine maleate 5 mg./cc. Vial 10 cc.
Use: Decongestant.

NEALBARBITONE. B.A.N. 5-Allyl-5-neopentylbarbituric acid. Censedal; Nevental
Use: Hypnotic; sedative.

NEBCIN. (Dista) Tobramycin sulfate 80 mg./2 ml. Vial 2 ml. Box 1s, 25s; 1.2 Gm./30 ml. Vial 30 ml. Box 6s; 1.2 Gm./40 ml. Vial 40 ml. Box 6s. **Pediatric.** 20 mg./2 ml. Vial 2 ml. **Hyporets.** 80 mg./2 ml., 60 mg./1.5 ml. Box 24s.
Use: Antibiotic.

• **NEBRAMYCIN.** USAN. A complex of antibiotic substances produced by *Streptomyces tenebrarius.*
Use: Antibacterial.

NEBU-PREL. (Mahon) Isoproterenol sulf. 0.4%, phenylephrine HCl 2%, propylene glycol 10%. Liq. Vial 10 cc.
Use: Bronchial asthma.

NECHLORIN. (Interstate) Chlorpheniramine 5 mg., phenylpropanolamine 40 mg., penylephrine 20 mg., phenyltoloxamine 15 mg./Tab. Bot. 100s.
Use: Antihistaminic, decongestant.

NECTA SWEET. (Procter & Gamble) Saccharin 12.3 mg./¼ gr. Tab.; 24.6 mg./½ gr. Tab.; 49.2 mg./1 gr. Tab. Bot. 500s, 1000s.
Use: Nonnutritive artificial sweetener.

• **NEFAZODONE HYDROCHLORIDE.** USAN.

NEFOPAM. B.A.N. 3,4,5,6-Tetrahydro-5-methyl-1-phenyl-1H-2,5-benzoxazocine.
Use: Muscle relaxant.

• **NEFOPAM HCl.** USAN. 3,4,5,6-Tetrahydro-5-methyl-1-phenyl-1H-2,5-benzoxazocine HCl.
Use: Muscle relaxant.

NEFROLAN. Clorexolone, B.A.N.

NEGACIDE. (Winthrop Products) Nalidixic acid.
Use: Urinary & intestinal infections.

NEGASOL SOLUTION. (Lydia O'Leary, Inc.) Glyceryl ester of para-aminobenzoic acid in aq. sol., 50% isopropyl alcohol. Bot. 2 fl. oz.
Use: Sun screen.

NEGATAN. (Savage) Negatol 45% in aq. sol. Bot. w/applicator 0.25 oz.

NEGGRAM. (Winthrop-Breon) Nalidixic acid 1 Gm./Caplet Bot. 100s, Unit Dose Pack 100s; 500 mg./Cap. Bot. 56s, 500s, 1000s, Unit Dose Pack 100s; 250 mg./Cap. Bot. 56s, Susp. 250 mg./5 ml. Bot. pt.
Use: Treatment of urinary infections.

NEGUVON. Metriphonate, B.A.N.

NEIMOTEC. (Mallinckrodt) Technetium Tc 99m.

NEISSERIA CATARRHALIS.

NEMAZINE. 3-(p-Chlorophenyl)-4-imino-2-oxo-1-imidazolidine acetonitrile. Under study.
Use: Anti-inflammatory.

NEMBUTAL ELIXIR. (Abbott) Pentobarbital 18.2 mg./5 ml. Alcohol 18% Bot. pt., gal.

NEMBUTAL SODIUM. (Abbott) Pentobarbital sodium. **Amp.:** (100 mg./2 ml. Box 25s.) **Vial:** 50 mg./ml. Vial 20 ml., 50 ml. **Cap.:** (30 mg.) Bot. 100s, (50 mg.) Bot. 100s, 500s, 1000s. (100 mg.) Bot. 100s, 500s, 1000s, Strip Pak 100s. Abbo-Pac 100 (10 × 10). **Supp.:** (½ gr., 1 gr., 2 gr., 3 gr.) Box 12s.
Use: Sedative and hypnotic.

NEOARSPHENAMINE. Sod. 3,3'-diamino-4,4'-dihydroxyarsenobenzene-N-methanal sulfoxylate. (Neosalvarsan, Neoarsenobenzol).

NEO-BENZ-ALL. (Xttrium) Benzalkonium Cl 20.1%. Packet 25 ml. 15s. to make gal. of 1:750 soln. Also Aqueous Neo-Benz-All 1:750 soln. Packet 20 ml., 50s.
Use: Antiseptic, germicidal.

NEOBIOTIC. (Pfipharmecs) Neomycin sulf. 500 mg./Tab. Bot. 100s.
Use: Antibiotic.

NEO-BRONCHOID TABLETS. (Moore Kirk) Histamor (brand of pyrilamine maleate) 10 mg., phenylephrine HCl 2 mg., potassium guaiacolsulfonate 2 gr., ammonium chloride 2 gr., ipecac ⅛ gr./Tab. Bot. 1000s.
Use: Colds, coughs, allergic rhinitis and expectorant.

NEOCALAMINE. (Various Mfr.) Red ferric oxide 30 Gm., yellow ferric oxide 40 Gm., zinc oxide 930 Gm.
Use: Astringent and mild antiseptic.

NEO-CALGLUCON. (Sandoz) Glubionate calcium 1.8 benzoic acid 5.0 mg./5 ml. Syr. Bot. pt.
Use: Calcium therapy.

NEOCASTADERM. (Lannett) Resorcin, boric acid, acetone. Bot. 1 oz., 4 oz., 16 oz.

Use: Treatment of fungal infections.

NEOCET. (Vale) Pyrilamine maleate 25 mg., acetaminophen 130 mg., salicylamide 130 mg./Tab. Ped. Tab. half-strength. Bot. 100s, 1000s, 5000s.
Use: Antihistaminic and analgesic.

NEO-CHOLEX. (Lafayette) Fat emulsion containing 40%/w/v pure vegetable oil. Bot. 60 cc.
Use: Produce maximum cholecystokinetic activity in roentgen study.

NEOCINCHOPHEN, B.A.N. Ethyl 6-methyl-2-phenyl-quinolin-4-carboxylate. Novatophan.
Use: Orally; analgesic, antipyretic & in gout.

NEO-COBEFRIN. levo-Nordefrin. 1-2, 4-dihydroxyphenyl-3-hydroxy-2-isopropylamine.
Use: Vasoconstrictor.

NEO-CORT-DOME. (Miles Pharm) Hydrocortisone alcohol ¼%, ½%, or 1% w/neomycin 5 mg./Gm. Cream base: glyceryl monostearate, cetyl alcohol, lanolin, isopropyl palmitate, propylene glycol, methyl and propyl parabens. Lotion base: isopropyl myristate, isopropyl palmitate, cetyl alcohol, polyethylene glycol ricinoleate, white petrolatum, thimerosal. ½% Tube ½ oz., Dispensajar 1 oz., 4 oz., 1% Tube ½ oz. Lot. ½% Bot. 1 oz.
Use: Anti-inflammatory.

NEO-CORT-DOME, OTIC. (Miles Pharm) Hydrocortisone alcohol 10 mg., neomycin sulfate 5 mg., acetic acid 2%, vehicle buffered to the pH range of normal skin w/glyceryl monostearate, stearic acid, propylene glycol, potassium sorbate, methyl and propyl parabens, sodium acetate. Bot. 10 cc. w/dropper.
Use: External otitis.

NEO-CORTEF CREAM. (Upjohn) Hydrocortisone acetate 10 mg. (1%), neomycin sulfate 5 mg./Gm. w/methylparaben 1 mg., butylparaben 4 mg., polysorbate 80, propylene glycol, cetyl palmitate, glyceryl monostearate, and emulsifier/Gm. When necessary, pH adjusted with sulfuric acid. Tube 20 Gm.
Use: Allergic & inflammatory skin conditions.

NEO-CORTEF OINTMENT. (Upjohn) **0.5%:** Hydrocortisone acetate 5 mg., neomycin sulfate 5 mg., methylparaben 0.2 mg., butylparaben 1.8 mg. in a bland base of white petrolatum, microcrystalline wax, mineral oil, and cholesterol/Gm. Tube 20 Gm. **1%:** Hydrocortisone acetate 10 mg., neomycin sulfate 5 mg./Gm. Oint., Tube 5 & 20 Gm. **2.5%:** Hydrocortisone acetate 25 mg., neomycin sulfate 5 mg./Gm., Oint., Tube 5 & 20 Gm.
Use: Broad range antibiotic w/anti-inflammatory effect.

NEO-CORTEF OPHTHALMIC OINTMENT. (Upjohn) Hydrocortisone acetate 5 mg./Gm. (0.5%) or 15 mg./Gm. (1.5%), neomycin sulfate 5 mg./Gm., anhydrous lanolin, mineral oil, white petrolatum, chlorobutanol 0.65%. Tube 3.5 Gm. w/applicator tip
Use: Ophthalmic anti-inflammatory and antibacterial.

NEO-CORTEF OPHTHALMIC SUSPENSION, 0.5%. (Upjohn) Hydrocortisone acetate 5 mg./ml. (0.5%), neomycin sulfate 5 mg./ml., myristyl-gamma-picolinium chloride, sodium citrate, polyethylene glycol 3350, povidone, sodium hydroxide and/or hydrochloric acid. In 5 ml. Drop Bot.
Use: Ophthalmic anti-inflammatory and antibacterial.

NEO-CORT TOP OINTMENT. (Standex) Neomycin sulfate 0.5%, hydrocortisone 1% Tube ½ oz.

NEO-CULTOL. (Fisons) Refined mineral oil jelly. Chocolate flavored. Bot. 6 oz.
Use: Laxative.

NEOCURB. (Pasadena Research) Phendimetrazine tartrate 35 mg./Tab. Bot. 100s, 1000s.
Use: Anorexient.

NEOCURTASAL. (Winthrop Products) Potassium chloride 92%, tribasic calcium phosphate, pot. glutamate, glutamic acid and calcium silicate. [Less than 10 mg. of Na per 100 Gm. or 0.5 mg. per teaspoonful.] Container 2 oz.; 8 oz.
Use: Table salt substitute.

NEO-CUTONE. (Sutliff & Case) Pyrilamine maleate 1%, calamine 8%, benzocaine 3%. Lot., Container 2 oz., 1 pt., 1 gal.
Use: Topically, antihistaminic w/local anesthetic.

NEOCYLATE. (Central) Pot. salicylate 280 mg., aminobenzoic acid 250 mg./Tab. Bot. 100s, 1000s.
Use: Analgesic in rheumatic conditions.

NEOCYTEN. (Central) Orphenadrine citrate 30 mg., sodium bisulfate 1 mg., sodium Cl 2.9 mg., benzethonium Cl 0.1 mg./ml. Vial 10 ml.
Use: Skeletal muscle relaxant, antihistaminic.

NeoDECADRON OCUMETER. (Merck Sharp & Dohme) Dexamethasone sod. phosphate equiv. to 1 mg. dexamethasone phosphate, neomycin sulfate equiv. to 3.5 mg. neomycin base/ml. w/creatinine, sod. citrate, sod. borate, polysorbate 80, disodium edetate, hydrochloric acid, sod. bisulfite 0.1%, benzalkonium chloride 0.02% and water for injection. Plastic Dispenser 5 ml.
Use: Anti-inflammatory.

NeoDECADRON OPHTHALMIC OINTMENT. (Merck Sharp & Dohme) Dexamethasone sod. phosphate equiv. to 0.5 mg. dexamethasone phosphate, neomycin sulfate equiv. to 3.5 mg. neomycin base/Gm. w/white petrolatum and mineral oil. Tube 3.5 Gm.
Use: Anti-inflammatory.

NeoDECADRON OPHTHALMIC SOLUTION. (Merck Sharp & Dohme) Dexamethasone sod. phosphate equiv. to 1 mg. dexamethasone phosphate, neomycin sulf, equiv. to 3.5 mg. neomycin base/ml. w/creatinine, sod. hydroxide, sod. bisulfite 0.32%, benzalkonium chloride 0.02%, sodium citrate, sodium borate, polysorbate 80 and water for injection. Dropper Bot. 2.5 ml., 5 ml.
Use: Anti-inflammatory.

NeoDECADRON TOPICAL CREAM. (Merck Sharp & Dohme) Dexamethasone sod. phosphate equiv. to 1 mg. dexamethasone phosphate, neomycin sulf. equiv. to 3.5 mg. neomycin base/Gm. w/stearyl alcohol, cetyl alcohol, mineral oil, polyoxyl 40 stearate, sorbitol soln, methyl polysilicone emul., creatinine, disodium edetate, sod. citrate, sod. hydroxide, purified water, methylparaben 0.15%,

sod. bisulfite 0.25%, sorbic acid 0.1%. Tube 15 Gm., 30 Gm.
Use: Anti-inflammatory.

NEODECYLLIN. (Penick) Neomycin undecylinate.
Use: Antibacterial & antifungal.

NEO-DELTA-CORTEF OINTMENT. (Upjohn) Prednisolone acetate 5 mg., neomycin sulfate 5 mg., methylparaben 0.2 mg., butylparaben 1.8 mg./Gm., base of white petrolatum, microcrystalline wax, mineral oil, cholesterol. Tube 20 Gm.
Use: Topically, allergic dermatitis & inflammatory skin diseases.

NEO-DELTA-CORTEF OPHTHALMIC OINTMENT. (Upjohn) **0.25%:** Prednisolone acetate 2.5 mg. neomycin sulfate 5 mg./Gm. w/anhydrous lanolin, mineral oil, white petrolatum, chlorobutanol 0.65%. Tube 3.5 Gm. w/applicator tip.
Use: Eye infections.

NEO-DELTA-CORTEF OPHTHALMIC SUSPENSION. (Upjohn) Prednisolone acetate 2.5 mg., neomycin sulfate 5 mg./ml. w/myristyl-gamma-picolinium chloride, sod. citrate, polyethylene glycol 3350, povidone, sod. hydroxide and/or hydrochloric acid/cc. Dropper Bot. 5 ml.
Use: Treatment of infections of the eye.

NEODEX SYRUP. (U.S. Ethicals) Dextromethorphan HBr, chlorpheniramine maleate, phenylephrine HCl, guaifenesin. Bot. 120 ml., 3840 ml.
Use: Antitussive, nasal decongestant, expectorant.

NEODRENAL.
See: Isoproterenol

NEO-DURABOLIC. (Hauck) Nandrolone decanoate 50 mg./ml. Vial 2 ml.
Use: Androgen; anabolic steroid.

NEO-FLO. (Softcon) Boric acid, sodium chloride, potassium chloride and sodium carbonate preserved with benzalkonium chloride 1:15,000. Plastic squeeze bot. 30 cc., 110 cc.
Use: Ophthalmic irrigating solution.

NEO FRANOL. (Winthrop Products) Theophylline monohydrate.
Use: Bronchodilator, sedative spasmolytic.

NEOGEN. (Premo) Theophylline 3 gr., aminophylline 4 gr., ephedrine sulfate ⅜ gr., pentobarbital 1 gr., benzocaine 3 gr./Supp. Also available ½ strength. Box 12s.
Use: Bronchodilator, mild sedative, local anesthesia.

NEO-GENIC. (Kay) Potassium estrone sulfate 1 mg., estrogenic substance 2 mg., thimerosal (preservative) 0.01%, polysorbate-80 (stabilizer) 0.15%/ml. Vial 10 cc.
Use: Menopausal syndrome, conditions involving deficiency in vaginal epithelium.

NEO-GERASTAN. (Standex) Pentylenetetrazol 100 mg., nicotinic acid (niacin) 50 mg., glutamic acid 100 mg./Tab. Bot. 100s.
Use: Geriatric stimulant.

NEO-HYDELTRASOL. (Merck Sharp & Dohme) **Ophth. Sol.:** Prednisolone sodium phosphate equiv. to 5 mg. prednisolone phosphate, neomycin sulf. equivalent to 3.5 mg. of neomycin base/ml.

w/creatinine, sod. citrate, polysorbate 80, disodium edetate, potassium phosphate, hydrochloric acid, water, benzalkonium chloride 0.02%. Bot. 5 ml., 2.5 ml.
Use: Ophthalmic use for inflammation & infection.

NEOLAX. (Central) Docusate sodium 50 mg., dehydrocholic acid 240 mg./Tab. Bot. 100s, 1000s. Unit dose 100s.
Use: Choleretic laxative and fecal softener.

NEOLOID. (Lederle) Castor oil 36.4% (emulsified) (w/w). Bot. 4 oz. Unit dose pack, 12×4 oz.
Use: Orally; laxative.

NEOMARK. (C & M Pharmacal) Salicylic acid 1.6%, LCD 2.0%, betanaphthol 1.0%, resorcin monoacetate 1.0%, castor oil, isopropyl alcohol 68%. Bot. 4.3 fl. oz. w/applicator tip.
Use: Anti-dandruff lotion.

NEO-MEDROL ACETATE TOPICAL. (Upjohn) Methylprednisolone acetate 2.5 mg. or 10 mg., neomycin sulfate 5 mg., methylparaben 4 mg., butylparaben 3 mg./Gm., Tube 7.5 Gm., 30 Gm., 1.5 oz.
Use: Treatment of skin lesions.

NEO-MERCAZOLE. Carbimazole, B.A.N.

NEO-MIST NASAL SPRAY. (A.P.C.) Phenylephrine HCl 0.50%, cetalkonium chloride 0.02%. Spray Bot. 20 cc.
Use: Decongestant, antiseptic.

NEO-MIST PEDIATRIC ¼% NASAL SPRAY. (A.P.C.) Phenylephrine HCl 0.25%, cetalkonium chloride 0.02%. Squeeze Bot. 20 cc.
Use: Decongestant, antiseptic.

NEOMIXIN. (Mallard) Zinc bacitracin 400 u., neomycin 3.5 mg., polymyxin B sulfate 5,000 u. in petrolatum base/Gm. Tube ½ oz.

NEOMYCIN. B.A.N. An antibiotic produced by a strain of *Streptomyces fradiae.* Expedil, Mycifradin, Myciguent, Neomin, Nivemycin [sulfate].

NEOMYCIN BASE.
Use: Antibiotic.
W/Combinations.
See: Biotic, Oint. (Scrip)
Biotic-Opth W/HC, Oint. (Scrip)
Biotic-Opth W/HC, Oint. (Scrip)
Bro-Parin, Susp. (Riker)
Maxitrol, Oint., Susp. (Alcon)
Mycolog, Cream, Oint. (Squibb)
My Cort Otic, Ear Drops (Scrip)
Necort A.V.P., Oint. (A.V.P. Pharm.)
Neo-Cort-Dome, Cream, Lot. (Miles Pharm)
Neotal, Oint. (Mallard)
Neothalidine, Granules (Merck Sharp & Dohme)

NEOMYCIN-HYDROCORTISONE CREAM. (Day-Baldwin) Neomycin 5 mg./Gm., hydrocortisone 0.5%. Tube ½ oz., 1 oz. W/hydrocortisone 1%. Tube ½ oz., 1 oz.
Use: Antibiotic, anti-inflammatory.

NEOMYCIN-HYDROCORTISONE OINTMENT. (Day-Baldwin) Neomycin 5 mg./Gm., hydrocortisone 0.5%. Tube 1 oz. w/hydrocortisone 1%, 20 Gm., 1 oz.
Use: Antibiotic, anti-inflammatory.

• **NEOMYCIN PALMITATE.** USAN.
Use: Antibiotic.

See: Biozyme, Oint. (Armour)
- **NEOMYCIN AND POLYMYXIN B SULFATES, BACITRACIN, AND HYDROCORTISONE ACETATE OINTMENT,** U.S.P. XXI.
  Use: Antibiotic, antifungal.
- **NEOMYCIN AND POLYMYXIN B SULFATES, BACITRACIN, AND HYDROCORTISONE ACETATE OPHTHALMIC OINTMENT,** U.S.P. XXI.
  Use: Antibiotic, antifungal.
- **NEOMYCIN AND POLYMYXIN B SULFATES AND BACITRACIN OINTMENT,** U.S.P. XXI.
  Use: Antibiotic.
- **NEOMYCIN AND POLYMYXIN B SULFATES AND BACITRACIN OPHTHALMIC OINTMENT,** U.S.P. XXI.
  Use: Antibiotic.
- **NEOMYCIN AND POLYMYXIN B SULFATES, BACITRACIN ZINC, AND HYDROCORTISONE ACETATE OPHTHALMIC OINTMENT,** U.S.P. XXI.
- **NEOMYCIN AND POLYMYXIN B SULFATES, BACITRACIN ZINC, AND HYDROCORTISONE OINTMENT,** U.S.P. XXI.
  Use: Antibiotic, anti-inflammatory.
- **NEOMYCIN AND POLYMIXIN B SULFATES, BACITRACIN ZINC, AND HYDROCORTISONE OPHTHALMIC OINTMENT,** U.S.P. XXI.
  Use: Antibiotic, anti-inflammatory.
- **NEOMYCIN AND POLYMYXIN B SULFATES AND BACITRACIN ZINC OINTMENT.** U.S.P. XXI.
  Use: Local anti-infective.
- **NEOMYCIN AND POLYMYXIN B SULFATES AND BACITRACIN ZINC OPHTHALMIC OINTMENT,** U.S.P. XXI.
  Use: Ophthalmic antibiotic.
- **NEOMYCIN AND POLYMYXIN B SULFATES AND BACITRACIN ZINC TOPICAL AEROSOL,** U.S.P. XXI.
  Use: Antibiotic.
- **NEOMYCIN AND POLYMYXIN B SULFATES AND BACITRACIN ZINC TOPICAL POWDER,** U.S.P. XXI.
  Use: Antibiotic.
- **NEOMYCIN AND POLYMYXIN B SULFATES AND DEXAMETHASONE OPHTHALMIC OINTMENT,** U.S.P. XXI.
  Use: Antibiotic, anti-inflammatory.
- **NEOMYCIN AND POLYMYXIN B SULFATES AND DEXAMETHASONE OPHTHALMIC SUSPENSION.** U.S.P. XXI.
  Use: Antibiotic, anti-inflammatory.
- **NEOMYCIN AND POLYMYXIN B SULFATES AND GRAMICIDIN CREAM,** U.S.P. XXI.
  Use: Antibiotic.
- **NEOMYCIN AND POLYMYXIN B SULFATES, GRAMICIDIN, AND HYDROCORTISONE ACETATE CREAM,** U.S.P. XXI.
  Use: Antibiotic, anti-inflammatory.
- **NEOMYCIN AND POLYMYXIN B SULFATES AND GRAMICIDIN OPHTHALMIC SOLUTION,** U.S.P. XXI.
  Use: Antibiotic.
- **NEOMYCIN AND POLYMYXIN B SULFATES AND HYDROCORTISONE ACETATE OPHTHALMIC SUSPENSION,** U.S.P. XXI.

Use: Antibiotic, anti-inflammatory.
- **NEOMYCIN AND POLYMIXIN B SULFATES AND HYDROCORTISONE OPHTHALMIC SUSPENSION,** U.S.P. XXI.
  Use: Antibiotic, anti-inflammatory.
- **NEOMYCIN AND POLYMYXIN B SULFATES AND HYDROCORTISONE OTIC SOLUTION,** U.S.P. XXI.
  Use: Antibiotic, anti-inflammatory.
- **NEOMYCIN AND POLYMYXIN B SULFATES AND HYDROCORTISONE OTIC SUSPENSION,** U.S.P. XXI.
  Use: Antibiotic, anti-inflammatory.
- **NEOMYCIN AND POLYMYXIN B SULFATES OPHTHALMIC OINTMENT,** U.S.P. XXI.
  Use: Antibiotic.
- **NEOMYCIN AND POLYMYXIN B SULFATES AND PREDNISOLONE ACETATE OPHTHALMIC SUSPENSION,** U.S.P. XXI.
  Use: Antibiotic, anti-inflammatory.
- **NEOMYCIN AND POLYMYXIN B SULFATES SOLUTION FOR IRRIGATION.** U.S.P. XXI.
  Use: Irrigating solution; topical antibacterial.
- **NEOMYCIN AND POLYMYXIN B SULFATES OPHTHALMIC SOLUTION.** U.S.P. XXI.
  Use: Ophthalmic antibiotic.
- **NEOMYCIN SULFATE,** U.S.P. XXI. Cream, Oint., Ophth. Oint., Oral Soln., Sterile, Tab., U.S.P. XXI.
  An antibiotic from *Streptomyces fradiae*: (Upjohn)
  Pow. micronized for compounding Bot. 100 Gm.
  Use: Antibacterial.
  See: Mycifradin Sulfate, Tab., Sol. (Upjohn)
  Myciguent, Oint., & Ophth. Oint., Cream (Upjohn)
  Neobiotic, Tab. (Pfizer)
  W/Combinations
  See: Aural Acute (Saron)
  Bacitracin Neomycin, Oint. (Various Mfr.)
  Baximin, Oint. (Columbia)
  Biotic, Oint. (Scrip)
  Biotres HC, Oint. (Central)
  B.N.P. Ophthalmic Oint. (Reid-Provident)
  B.P.N., Oint. (Norwich)
  Bro-Parin, Otic Susp. (Riker)
  Coracin, Oint. (Mallard)
  Cordran-N, Oint., Lot. (Dista)
  Cor-Oticin, Liq. (Maurry)
  Cortisporin, Prep. (Burroughs Wellcome)
  Duo-Aqua-Drin, Loz. (McKesson)
  Epimycin A, Oint. (Delta)
  Hi-Cort N, Cream (Blaine)
  Hysoquen Oint. (Reid-Provident)
  Maxitrol, Ophth., Oint., Susp. (Alcon)
  Mity-Mycin Ointment (Reid-Provident)
  Mycifradin Sulfate Sterile, Vial (Upjohn)
  Mycitracin, Oint., Ophth. Oint. (Upjohn)
  My-Cort, Oint., Cream, Sol. (Scrip)
  Necort, Oint. (A.V.P.)
  Neo-Cort Dome, Otic Sol. (Miles Pharm)
  Neo-Cortef, Preps. (Upjohn)
  Neo Cort Top, Oint. (Standex)
  Neo-Decadron, Preps. (Merck Sharp & Dohme)
  Neo-Delta-Cortef, Preps. (Upjohn)
  Neogel W/Sulfa, Tab. (Vortech)

Neo-Hydeltrasol, Oint., Sol. (Merck Sharp & Dohme)
Neo-Hytone, Cream (Dermik)
Neo-Medrol, Preps (Upjohn)
Neo-Nysta-Cort, Oint. (Miles Pharm)
Neo-Oxylone, Oint. (Upjohn)
Neo-Polycin, Ophthal., Sol., Oint. (Merrell Dow)
Neosone, Ophth. Oint. (Upjohn)
Neosporin, Prep. (Burroughs Wellcome)
Neo-Thrycex, Oint. (Commerce)
Otobione Sol. (Schering)
Otoreid-HC, Liq. (Reid-Provident)
P.B.N., Oint. (Jenkins)
Spectrocin, Oint. (Squibb)
Statrol Sterile Ophthalmic Ointment (Alcon)
Tigo, Oint. (Burlington)
Tri-Bow Oint. (Bowman)
Tricidin, Oint. (Amlab)
Trimixin, Oint. (Hance)
Triple Antibiotic Ointment, Tube (Kenyon)
• **NEOMYCIN SULFATE AND BACITRACIN OINTMENT,** U.S.P. XXI.
Use: Antibiotic.
• **NEOMYCIN SULFATE AND BACITRACIN ZINC OINTMENT,** U.S.P. XXI.
Use: Antibiotic.
• **NEOMYCIN SULFATE AND DEXAMETHASONE SODIUM PHOSPHATE CREAM,** U.S.P. XXI.
Use: Antibiotic, anti-inflammatory.
• **NEOMYCIN SULFATE AND DEXAMETHASONE SODIUM PHOSPHATE OPHTHALMIC OINTMENT,** U.S.P. XXI.
Use: Antibiotic, anti-inflammatory.
• **NEOMYCIN SULFATE AND DEXAMETHASONE SODIUM PHOSPHATE OPHTHALMIC SOLUTION,** U.S.P. XXI.
Use: Antibiotic, anti-inflammatory.
• **NEOMYCIN SULFATE AND FLUOCINOLONE ACETONIDE CREAM,** U.S.P. XXI.
Use: Antibiotic, anti-inflammatory.
• **NEOMYCIN SULFATE AND FLUOROMETHOLONE OINTMENT,** U.S.P. XXI.
Use: Antibiotic, anti-inflammatory.
NEOMYCIN SULFATE AND FLURANDRENOLIDE, U.S.P. XXI. Cream, Oint., U.S.P. XXI.
Use: Antibiotic, anti-inflammatory.
See: Cordran Prods. (Dista)
• **NEOMYCIN SULFATE AND GRAMICIDIN OINTMENT,** U.S.P. XXI.
Use: Antibiotic
NEOMYCIN SULFATE AND HYDROCORTISONE, U.S.P. XXI. Cream, Oint., U.S.P. XXI.
Use: Antibiotic, anti-inflammatory.
• **NEOMYCIN SULFATE AND HYDROCORTISONE ACETATE,** U.S.P. XXI. Cream, Oint., Ophth. Oint., Ophth. Susp., U.S.P. XXI.
Use: Antibiotic, anti-inflammatory.
• **NEOMYCIN SULFATE AND METHYLPREDNISOLONE ACETATE CREAM,** U.S.P. XXI.
Use: Antibiotic, anti-inflammatory.
• **NEOMYCIN SULFATE AND PREDNISOLONE ACETATE OINTMENT,** U.S.P. XXI.

Use: Antibiotic, anti-inflammatory.
• **NEOMYCIN SULFATE AND PREDNISOLONE ACETATE OPHTHALMIC OINTMENT,** U.S.P. XXI.
Use: Antibiotic, anti-inflammatory.
• **NEOMYCIN SULFATE AND PREDNISOLONE ACETATE OPHTHALMIC SUSPENSION,** U.S.P. XXI.
Use: Antibiotic, anti-inflammatory.
• **NEOMYCIN SULFATE AND PREDNISOLONE SODIUM PHOSPHATE OPHTHALMIC OINTMENT,** U.S.P. XXI.
Use: Antibiotic, anti-inflammatory.
• **NEOMYCIN SULFATE, SULFACETAMIDE SODIUM, AND PREDNISOLONE ACETATE OPHTHALMIC OINTMENT,** U.S.P. XXI.
Use: Antibiotic, anti-inflammatory.
• **NEOMYCIN SULFATE AND TRIAMCINOLONE ACETONIDE OPHTHALMIC OINTMENT,** U.S.P. XXI.
Use: Antibiotic, anti-inflammatory.
• **NEOMYCIN UNDECYLENATE.** USAN.
Use: Antibacterial.
See: Neodecyllin (Penick)
NEOMYCORSONE.
See: Neosone, Oint. (Upjohn)
NEO-NACLEX. Bendrofluazide, B.A.N.
NEO NOVALDIN. (Winthrop Products) Dipyrone.
Use: Analgesic, antipyretic, anti-inflammatory.
NEOPENYL. Clemizole Penicillin, B.A.N.
NEO PHYRIN DROPS. (Winthrop Products) Phenylephrine HCl.
Use: Nasal decongestant.
See: Phenylephrine HCl
NEO PICATYL. (Winthrop Products) Glycobiarsol.
Use: Intestinal amebicide.
■ **NEOPLASTIC AGENTS.**
See: Folic acid antagonists. Leukemia agents.
NEO-POLYCIN OINTMENT. (Merrell Dow) **Oint.:** Neomycin sulfate equiv. to 3.5 mg. neomycin base, zinc bacitracin 400 u., polymyxin B sulfate 5000 u./Gm. in special base. Tube 0.5 oz.
Use: Topical antibiotic.
NEO-PYRANISTAN. (Standex) Ascorbic acid 20 mg., phenylephrine HCl 2.5 mg., salicylamide 60 mg., acetaminophenol 60 mg., chlorpheniramine maleate 1.5 mg./Tab. Bot. 100s.
Use: Relief of sinus headache, cold symptoms.
NEOQUESS INJECTION. (O'Neal, Jones & Feldman) Dicyclomine HCl 10 mg./ml. Vial 10 ml.
NEOQUESS TABLETS. (O'Neal, Jones & Feldman) Phenobarbital 16.2 mg., hyoscyamine sulfate 0.1037 mg., scopolamine hydrobromide 0.0065 mg., atropine sulfate 0.0194 mg./Tab. Bot. 100s.
NEOQUINOPHAN.
See: Neocinchophen (Various Mfr.)
NEO QUIPENYL. (Winthrop Products) Primaquine phosphate.
Use: Antimalaria agent.
NEOSAR. (Adria) Cyclophosphamide. **100 mg.:** Cyclophosphamide 100 mg., sodium Cl 45 mg./Vial. Pkg. 12s. **200 mg.:** cyclophosphamide 200 mg., sodium Cl 90 mg./Vial. Pkg. 12s. **500 mg.:** cyclophosphamide 500 mg., sodium Cl. 225 mg./Vial. Pkg 12s. **1 Gm.:** Individual cartons.
Use: Antineoplastic.

NEO-SKIODAN.
Iodopyracet, Diodrast.

NEOSPORIN AEROSOL. (Burroughs Wellcome) Aerosporin brand polymyxin B sulfate 100,000 u., neomycin sulfate 100 mg., zinc bacitracin 8000 u., dispersed in inert propellant./Containers (aerosol spray) 90 Gm. Approx. spraying time: 100 seconds.
Use: Bacterial skin infections.

NEOSPORIN-G CREAM. (Burroughs Wellcome) Polymyxin B sulfate 10,000 units, neomycin sulfate 5 mg., gramicidin 0.25 mg./Gm., liq. and white petrolatum, propylene glycol, polyoxyethylene polyoxypropylene compound, wax, methyl paraben 0.25%. Cream. Tube 15 Gm.
Use: Treatment of dermatoses.

NEOSPORIN G. U. IRRIGANT. (Burroughs Wellcome) Neomycin sulfate 40 mg., polymyxin B sulfate 200,000 u./ml. Amps. 1 ml. Box 12s, 100s. MDV 20 ml.
Use: Antibiotic irrigant.

NEOSPORIN OINTMENT. (Burroughs Wellcome) Polymyxin B sulfate 5,000 u., bacitracin zinc 400 u., neomycin sulfate 5 mg./Gm. Tube 0.5 oz., 1 oz. Foil packet 1/32 oz. Box 144s.
Use: First aid antibiotic.

NEOSPORIN OPHTHALMIC OINTMENT, STERILE. (Burroughs Wellcome) Polymyxin B sulfate 10,000 u., bacitracin zinc 400 u., neomycin sulfate 5 mg./Gm., special white petrolatum base. Tube 1/8 oz.
Use: Ocular bacterial infections.

NEOSPORIN OPHTHALMIC SOLUTION, STERILE. (Burroughs Wellcome) Polymyxin B sulfate 10,000 u., neomycin sulfate 2.5 mg., gramicidin 0.025 mg./ml., alcohol 0.5%, thimerosal 0.001%, propylene glycol, polyoxyethylene polyoxypropylene cpd., sod chloride. Bot 10 ml.
Use: Topically, eye infections.

NEOSPORIN POWDER. (Burroughs Wellcome) Polymyxin B 5000 u., zinc bacitracin 400 u., neomycin sulfate 5 mg., lactose base./Gm. Shaker vial 10 Gm.
Use: External bacterial infections.

NEO-SPRAY. (Blue Cross) Xylometazoline Solution. Bot. 0.5 oz.
Use: Nasal spray.

NEOSTEROL TABLETS. (Winston) Ethinyl estradiol 0.01 mg., methyltestosterone 2.5 mg., Vits. A, D, B Complex, C, E, B-12, minerals and lipotropes. Bot. 100s, 1000s.
Use: Vitamin, mineral, hormone, geriatric supplement.

NEOSTIBOSAN. Ethylstibamine.

NEOSTIG. (Freeport) Salicylamide 200 mg., acetaminophen 300 mg., neostigmine Br. 1.5 mg., scopolamine HBr. 0.125 mg./Tab. Bot. 1000s.
Use: Relief of pain, skeletal muscle spasm.

• **NEOSTIGMINE BROMIDE,** U.S.P. XXI. Tab., U.S.P. XXI. Benzenaminium, 3-[[(dimethylamino)-carbonyl-]oxy]-N,N,N-trimethyl-, bromide. (m-Hydroxyphenyl)-trimethylammonium bromide dimethylcarbamate.
Use: Cholinergic.

See: Prostigmin Bromide, Tab. (Roche)

• **NEOSTIGMINE METHYLSULFATE,** U.S.P. XXI. Inj., U.S.P. XXI. Benzenaminium, 3-[[(dimethylamino)carbonyl]-oxy]-N,N,N-trimethyl-, methyl sulfate. (m-Hydroxyphenyl) trimethylammonium methylsulfate dimethylcarbamate.
Use: Parasympathomimetic agent, cholinergic.
See: Prostigmin methylsulfate, Vial (Roche Lab.)

NEO-STREPSAN.
See: Sulfathiazole (Various Mfr.)

NEO-SYNALAR. (Syntex) Fluocinolone acetonide 0.025%, neomycin sulfate 0.5%, in a water washable base w/stearic acid, propylene glycol, sorbitan monostearate and monooleate, polysorbate 60 w/methylparaben and propylparaben as preservatives. Cream Tube 15 Gm., 30 Gm., 60 Gm.
Use: Infected dermatoses.

NEO-SYNEPHRINE 12 HR. (Winthrop Products) Oxymetazoline HCl 0.05%. Bot. 1/2 oz. as spray or drops.
Use: Nasal decongestant.

NEO-SYNEPHRINE HYDROCHLORIDE. (Winthrop Products) **Spray:** 1/4% children and adult, 1/2% adult. Regular in squeeze bottles of 1/2 oz. 1/2% mentholated in squeeze bottles of 1/2 oz. **Drops:** 1/8% infant; 1/4% children and adult; 1/2% adult; 1% adult extra strength. Bot. 1 oz.; 1/4% and 1% also Bot. 16 oz. **Jelly:** 1/2%. Tube 5/8 oz.
Use: Nasal decongestant.

NEO-SYNEPHRINE HYDROCHLORIDE. (Winthrop-Breon) Phenylephrine HCl. **Amp.** 1%, 1 ml. 25s. **Ophthalmic** 2.5%, Mono-Drop Bot. 15 ml.; 10% Mono-Drop Bot. 5 ml.; 10% viscous solution, Mono-Drop Bot. 5 ml.
Use: **Amp:** vasoconstrictor; **Ophth:** vasoconstrictor & mydriatic.

NEO-SYNEPHRINE II, LONG ACTING. (Winthrop Products) Xylometazoline HCl **0.1%** Adult strength. Regular and mentholated. Spray: Bot. 0.5 oz. Drops: Bot. 1 oz. **0.05%** Child strength. Drops: Bot. 1 oz.
Use: Nasal decongestant.

NEO-SYNEPHRINOL DAY RELIEF CAPSULES. (Winthrop Products) Pseudoephedrine HCl 120 mg./T.R. Cap. Box 10s.
Use: Nasal decongestant.

NEOTAL. (Mallard) Zinc bacitracin 400 u., polymyxin B sulfate 5000 u., neomycin sulfate 5 mg., petrolatum and mineral oil base/Gm. Tube 1/8 oz.

NEO-TEARS. (Barnes-Hind) Sterile, isotonic sol. containing polyvinyl alcohol and hydroxyethylcellulose, sodium chloride, potassium chloride. Bot. 15 ml.
Use: Ophthalmic lubricating solution; artificial tear fluid.

NEOTEP GRANUCAPS. (Reid-Provident) Chlorpheniramine maleate 9 mg., phenylephrine HCl 21 mg./Granucap. Bot. 100s.
Use: Decongestant, antihistaminic.

NEO-THRYCEX OINT. (Commerce) Bacitracin, neomycin sulfate, polymyxin B sulfate. Tube 0.5 oz.
Use: Triple antibiotic ointment.

NEOTHYLLINE. (Lemmon) Dyphylline. **Tab.** (200 mg.) Bot. 100s, 1000s, (400 mg.) 100s, 500s. **Elix.** (160 mg./15 ml.) Bot. pt., gal. **Amp.** I.M. (500 mg.) Amp. 2 ml., Box 10s.
Use: Orally, diuretic vasodilator, bronchodilator and myocardial stimulant.
W/Guaifenesin & alcohol.
See: Neothylline-GG, Elix., Tab. (Lemmon)

NEOTRIZINE. (Lilly) Trisulfapyrimidines **Susp.:** Sulfadiazine 167 mg., sulfamerazine 167 mg., sulfamethazine 167 mg./5 ml. Bot. 16 fl. oz. **Tabs.:** Sulfadiazine 167 mg., sulfamerazine 167 mg., sulfamethazine 167 mg./Tab. Bot. 100s.
Use: Orally; triple sulfonamide therapy.

NEO-TROBEX INJECTION. (Fellows) Vit. B-1 150 mg., B-6 10 mg., riboflavin 5-phosphate sod. 2 mg., niacinamide 150 mg., panthenol 10 mg., choline chloride 20 mg., inositol 20 mg./cc. Vial 30 cc.

NEOTROL. (Hance) Phenylephrine HCl 0.25%, pyrilamine maleate 0.2%, cetalkonium chloride 0.05%, tyrothricin 0.03%, phenylmercuric acetate 1:50,000. Sol., Squeeze Bot. 20 cc.
Use: Nasal congestion.

NEO-VADRIN D-S-S. (Scherer) Docusate sodium 250 mg./Cap. Bot. 100s.
Use: Stool softener.

NEO-VADRIN PROTEIN CHEWABLE TAB. (Scherer) Protein 455 mg./Tab. Bot. 250s.
Use: Dietary supplement.

NEO-VADRIN STRESS FORMULA. (Scherer) Vit. B-1 15 mg., B-2 15 mg., C 600 mg., niacinamide 100 mg., B-6 5 mg., calcium panothenate 20 mg., B-12 12 mcg., E 30 I.U., biotin 45 mcg., folic acid 0.4 mg./Tab. Bot. 60s.
Use: Multivitamin

NEO VADRIN STRESS FORMULA WITH IRON AND FOLIC ACID. (Scherer) Vit. B-1 15 mg., B-2 15 mg., niacinamide 100 mg., C 600 mg., B-6 25 mg., panothenic acid 20 mg., B-12 12 mcg., E 30 I.U., biotin 45 mcg., folic acid 0.4 mg. iron 27 mg./Tab. Bot. 60s.
Use: Dietary multivitamin supplement.

NEO-VADRIN STRESS FORMULA VITAMINS PLUS ZINC. (Scherer) Vit. E 45 I.U., C 600 mg., folic acid 400 mcg., B-1 20 mg., B-2 10 mg., B-12 25 mcg., biotin 45 mcg., pantothenic acid 25 mg., copper 3 mg., zinc 23.9 mg./Tab. Bot. 60s.
Use: Dietary multivitamin supplement.

NEO-VADRIN TIME RELEASE VIT. C. (Scherer) Vit. C 500 mg./Cap. Bot. 50s, 100s; 250 mg./Cap. Bot. 50s.
Use: Dietary supplement.

NEO-VADRIN VITAMIN B-6 TR. (Scherer) Vit. B-6. 100 mg./Cap. Bot. 100s.
Use: Pyridoxine supplement.

NEOVAL. (Blue Cross) Vit. A 10,000 I.U., D 400 I.U., B-1 10 mg., B-2 5 mg., B-6 2 mg., B-12 3 mcg., C 100 mg., E 5 mg., pantothenic acid 10 mg., niacinamide 30 mg., iron 15 mg., copper 1 mg., Mg. 5 mg., Mn 1 mg., zinc 1.5 mg., iodine 0.15 mg./Tab. Bot. 100s.
Use: Multiple vitamin and mineral supplement.

NEOVAL T. (Blue Cross) Vit. A 10,000 I.U., D 400 I.U., B-1 15 mg., B-2 10 mg., B-6 2 mg., C 150 mg., B-12 7.5 mcg., E 5 mg., pantothenic acid 10 mg., E 5 mg., niacinamide 100 mg., iron 15 mg., Mg 5 mg., Mn 1 mg., zinc 1.5 mg., copper 1 mg./Tab. Bot. 1000s.
Use: High potency vitamin and mineral supplement.

NEOVICAPS. (Scherer) Vit. B-1 15 mg., B-2 10 mg., B-6 5 mg., niacinamide 50 mg., C 300 mg., zinc 15 mg./Cap. Bot. 50s, 100s.
Use: Dietary supplement.

NEO WHITE OINTMENT. (Whiteworth) Triple antibiotic ointment. Tube 0.5 oz., 1 oz.
Use: Antibiotic.

NEOZIN. (Softcon) Phenylephrine HCl ⅛%, zinc sulf. ¼% and benzalkonium chloride 1:25,000 as preservative. Bot. 5 fl. oz. Eye drops.
Use: Astringent, antiseptic & decongestant.

NEPHRAMINE. (American McGaw) Essential amino acid injection 5.4%.
Use: For renal disease patients.

NEPHRIDINE.
See: Epinephrine (Various Mfr.)

NEPHROCAPS. (Fleming) Multiple vitamin. Bot. 100s.
Use: Multiple vitamin especially for dialysis patients.

NEPHRON INHALANT AND VAPORIZER. (Nephron) Racemic epinephrine HCl 2.25%. Bot. ¼ oz., ½ oz, or 1 oz.
Use: Inhalant for bronchial asthma.

NEPHROX. (Fleming) Aluminum hydroxide 320 mg., mineral oil 10%/5 ml. Bot. pts., gal.
Use: Antacid.

NEPRESOL. Dihydrallazine, B.A.N.

NEPTAZANE. (Lederle) Methazolamide 50 mg./Tab. Bot. 100s.
Use: Carbonic anhydrase inhibitor, treatment of glaucoma.

• **NEQUINATE.** USAN.
Use: Coccidiostat.

NEQUINATE (I.N.N.). Methyl Benzoquate, B.A.N.

NERAVAL. Methitural Sod. 5-(1-Methylbutyl)-5-[2-(methylthio)ethyl]-2-thiobarbiturate.
Use: I.V., general anesthesia.

NERVINE. (Miles)
See: Miles Nervine

NERVOCAINE. (Keene) Lidocaine. 1%, 2%. Vial 50 ml.
Use: Local anesthetic.

NESACAINE. (Astra) **1% Conc.:** Chloroprocaine HCl 10 mg./ml. in sterile solution containing sodium bisulfite, sodium chloride w/preservatives and buffer. Vial 30 ml. **2% Conc.:** Vial 30 ml.
Use: Local anesthetic for infiltration and regional nerve block.

NESACAINE-CE. (Astra) **2% Conc.** Chloroprocaine HCl 20 mg./ml. in a sterile solution containing sodium bisulfite, sodium chloride, HCl. Vial 30 ml. **3% Conc.** Chloroprocaine HCl 30 mg./ml. in a sterile solution containing sodium bisulfite, sodium chloride, HCl. Vial 30 ml.
Use: Local anesthetic for infiltration and regional

nerve block including caudal and epidural anethesia.

NESA NINE CAP. (Standex) Vit. A 5000 I.U., D 400 I.U., C 37.5 mg., B-1 1.5 mg., B-2 2 mg., niacinamide 20 mg., B-6 0.1 mg., Ca pantothothenate 1 mg., E 2 I.U./Cap. Bot. 100s.

NESDONAL SODIUM.
See: Thiopental Sodium U.S.P. XXI.
Pentothal Sodium, Prods. (Abbott)

NESTABS. (Fielding) Prenatal vitamins and minerals. Bot. 100s.
Use: Dietary supplement.

NESTABS FA. (Fielding) Vit A 8000 U., D 400 U., E 30 U., C 120 mg., Folic acid 1 mg., thiamine 3 mg., riboflavin 3 mg., niacinamide 20 mg., pyridoxine 3 mg., B-12 8 mcg., Ca carbonate 500 mg., iodine 150 mcg., ferrous fumarate 110 mg., zinc 15 mg./Tab. Bot. 100s.
Use: Dietary supplement.

NESTREX. (Fielding) Pydridoxine 25 mg./Tab w/dextrose. Bot. 100s.
Use: Dietary supplement.

NETHAMINE. Etafedrine HCl. 1-N-ethylephedrine HCl, 2-methylethylamino-1-phenylpropanol-1 HCl.
W/Codeine phosphate, phenylephrine HCl, sodium citrate, doxylamine succinate.
See: Mercodol with Decapryn Syrup (Merrell Dow)

• **NETILMICIN SULATE,** U.S.P. XXI. Inj., U.S.P. XXI.
Use: Antibacterial
See: Netromycin (Schering)

NETRIN. Under Study.
Use: Anticholinergic.
See: Metcaraphen HCl

NETROMYCIN. (Schering) Netilmicin. **Inj.:** 100 mg/ml. Vial 1.5 ml. Box 10s, 25s. Multi-dose Vial 15 ml. Box 5s. Disposable Syringes 1.5 ml. Box 10s. **Pediatric Inj.:** 25 mg./ml. Vial 2 ml. Box 10s. **Neonatal Inj.** 10 mg./ml. Amp. 2 ml. Box 25s.
Use: Antibiotic.

NEULACTIL.
See: Pericyazine.

NEURAMATE. (Blue Cross) Meprobamate 400 mg./Tab. Bot. 100s.
Use: Tranquilizer.

NEUROGYN. (O'Neal, Jones & Feldman) Estrone 2 mg., estradiol 0.1 mg./ml. Vial 30 ml.

NEUROSIN.
See: Calcium glycerophosphate (Various Mfr.)

NEUROSINE. (Dios) Sod. bromide 30 gr., pot. bromide 30 gr., ammonium bromide 30 gr., zinc bromide 3/5 gr., hyoscyamus ext. 3/40 gr., belladonna fl. ext. 3/40 min., cascara 3/5 gr., humulus ext. 3/5 gr., in pleasantly flavored 4% alcoholic aq. vehicle/fl. oz. Bot. 4 & 8 oz. Tabs. Bot. 50s, 100s, 200s.
Use: Antispasmodic.

NEUT [SODIUM BICARBONATE 4% ADDITIVE SOLUTION]. (Abbott) Sodium bicarbonate 0.2 Gm./5 ml. Vial (2.4 mEq. each of sodium and bicarbonate), disodium edetate anhydrous 0.05% as stabilizer. Pintop Vials 5 ml. in 10 ml. vials. Box 25s, 100s.

NEUTRACOMP. (CMC) **Tabs.** Aluminum hydroxide 260 mg., magnesium trisilicate 488 mg./Tab. Bot. 30s, 100s, 250s, 500s, 1000s. **Liq.** 1 pt.
Use: Adsorbent, nonalkaline antacid.

NEUTRAL ACRIFLAVIN.
See: Acriflavin (Various Mfr.)

NEUTRALIN. (Dover) Calcium carbonate, magnesium oxide/Tab. Sugar and salt free. Unit dose 500s.
Use: Antacid.

NEUTRAL INSULIN INJECTION. B.A.N. A solution of insulin buffered at pH 7 Insulin Novo Actrapid; Nuso.
Use: Hypoglycemic agent.

NEUTRAL PROTAMINE HAGEDORN-INSULIN.
See: Insulin, N.P.H. Iletin (Lilly)

• **NEUTRAMYCIN.** USAN. A neutral macrolide antibiotic produced by a variant strain of *Streptomyces rimosus.*
Use: Antibacterial antibiotic.

NEUTRA-PHOS. (Willen) A combination of dibasic and monobasic sodium & potassium phosphates. **Powder:** Bot. 2.25 oz. reconstitutes to 1 Gal. of liquid. **Cap.:** 1.25 Gm./Cap. Bot. 48s. Each cap. reconstitutes to 2.5 oz. of solution which supplies 250 mg. phosphorus, 7.125 mEq., sodium and 7.125 mEq. potassium.
Use: Oral phosphorus supplement.

NEUTRA-PHOS-K. (Willen) A combination of monobasic & dibasic potassium phosphates. **Powder:** Bot. 2.5 oz. reconstitutes to 1 gal. of liquid. **Cap.:** 1.45 Gm./Cap. Bot. 48s. Each cap. reconstitutes to 2.5 oz. of solution which supplies 250 mg. phosphorus and 14.25 mEq. potassium.
Use: Oral phosphorus supplement sodium free.

NEUTRAPHYLLINE. Diprophylline, B.A.N.

NEUTROFLAVIN.
See: Acriflavine (Various Mfr.)

NEUTROGENA. (Neutrogena) A neutralized soap (pH 7.5) W/glycerine, triethanolamine, fatty acids. 100 Gm. Disposable Sponge Pads. Box 12s. Shampoo, Solid Bar 3.4 oz. Unscented soap, 3.5 oz.

NEUTROGENA BODY OIL. (Neutrogena) Isopropyl myristate, sesame oil, hexachlorophene 0.5%. In 8 oz. w/sponge applicator.

NEUTROGENA DISPOSABLES. (Neutrogena) Sulfur 1.5%, salicylic acid 2%, allantoin 1%/medicated pad. Pkg. 12s.
Use: Dried oily skin.

NEUTROGENA LOTION. (Neutrogena) Glycerine monostearate, triethanolamine, lactic acid, hexachlorophene 0.5%, delta and cetyl alcohol, oil in water base. In 8 oz.
Use: Emollient and protective lotion.

NEUTROGENA T/GEL. (Neutrogena) Coal tar extract equivalent to 2% crude coal tar. Bot. 4.4 oz.
Use: Treatment of scalp psoriasis, dandruff, seborrheic dermatitis and eczema.

NEVROTOSE #3. (Vale) Phenobarbital 32.4 mg., hyoscyamus 16.2 mg., passiflora ext. 16.2 mg., valerian ext. 16.2 mg., camphor monobromate 8.1 mg./Cap. Bot. 100s, 500s, 1000s.
Use: Sedative.

NEW BESEROL. (Winthrop Products) Aspirin, methocarbamol.
Use: Analgesic, tranquilizer.
NEWPHRINE. (Vitarine) Phenylephrine HCl 0.25%.
Bot. 1 oz., 1%, Bot. pt.
Use: Nasal decongestant.
NEW-SKIN. (Medtech) Alcohol 8.7%, Pyroxylin solution, oil of cloves, 8-hydroxy-quinoline. Bot. ½ oz., 1 oz. Spray Bot. 1 oz. Tube: 0.14 oz.
Use: Liquid bandage.
• **NEXERIDINE HYDROCHLORIDE.** USAN.
Use: Analgesic.
NIAC. (O'Neal, Jones & Feldman) Nicotinic acid 300 mg./S.R. Cap. Bot. 100s.
NIACAL. (Bowman) Calcium lactate 324 mg., niacin 25 mg./Tab. w/peppermint flavor. Bot. 100s, 1000s.
Use: Vasodilator, calcium supplement.
NIACAMIDE.
See: Nikethamide (Various Mfr.)
• **NIACIN,** U.S.P. XXI. Inj., Tab., U.S.P. XXI. 3-Pyridine-carboxylic acid.
Use: Vit. B-complex component.
See: Efacin, Tab. (Person & Covey)
Niac, Cap. (Cole)
Nicobid, Tab. (Armour)
Nico-400 (Marion)
Ni Cord XL, Caps. (Scott/Cord)
Nicotinex, Elix. (Fleming)
Nicotym, Cap. (Everett)
Ni-Span, Cap. (Vortech)
Span Niacin 300, Tab. (Scrip)
Vasotherm, Inj. (Nutrition Control Products)
Wampocap, Cap. (Wallace)
W/Pentylenetetrazol.
See: Aminobrain, Liq. (Med. Prod. Panamericana)
Atrazol, Tab., Liq. (Reid-Provident)
Gevizol (Saron)
Mentalert, Tab., Elix. (Keene Pharm.)
Nico-Metrazol, Bot. (Knoll)
Vasostim, Cap. (Dunhall)
NIACIN W/COMBINATIONS.
See: Adenocrest, Vial (Pharmex)
Antivert, Tab. (Roerig)
Ardiatric, Tab. (Burgin-Arden)
Arterine, Tab., Liq. (Paddock)
Athemol, Tab. (Meyer)
Athemol-N, Tab. (Meyer)
Benizol, Tab., Elix. (Bentex)
Benizol Plus, Elix., Tab. (ICN)
Cerebro-Nicin, Cap. (Brown)
Geroniazo, Tab., Liq. (Philips Roxane)
Geroniazol TT, Tab. (Philips Roxane)
Lipo-Nicin, Cap., Tab. (Brown)
Menic, Tab. (Geriatric)
Nascobarb Ovalet, Tab. (Mayrand)
Niapent, Tab., Elix. (Ferndale)
Norozol, Tab. (Vortech)
Pentinic, Liq. (Alto)
Phy-Vasco, Tab. (Scrip)
Senilex, Tab. (O'Neal)
Vasostim, Cap. (Dunhall)

• **NIACINAMIDE,** U.S.P. XXI. Inj., Tab., U.S.P. XXI. 3-Pyridinecarboxamide. Nicotinic acid amide. Nicotinamide.
Use: Enzyme co-factor vitamin.
See: Niacinamide (Various Mfr.)
W/Pentylenetetrazol, thiamine HCl, cyanocobalamin, alcohol.
See: Cenalene, Elix., Tab. (Central)
W/Pot. iodide.
See: Iodo-Niacin, Tab. (Cole)
W/Riboflavin.
See: Riboflavin & Niacinamide, Amp. (Lilly)
NIACINAMIDE HI.
W/Pot. iodide.
See: Iodo-Niacin, Tab. (Cole)
NIALAMIDE. B.A.N. N-Benzyl-α(isonicotinoyl hy-drazine)propionamide. Isonicotinic Acid 2-[2-(Benzyl-carbamoyl)ethyl]hydrazide.
Use: Monoamine oxidase inhibitor; antidepressant.
NIALEXO-C. (Mallard) Niacin 50 mg., Vit. C 30 mg./Tab. Bot. 100s.
NIAOULI COMPOUND. (Zemmer) Benzyl alcohol 2%, guaiacol 0.1 Gm., eucalyptol 0.08 Gm., iodoform 0.02 Gm., camphor 0.05 Gm./2 cc. Vial 30 cc.
NIARB. (Miller) Nicotinamide ascorbate 200 mg., magnesium ascorbate 200 mg./Tab. Bot. 100s.
Super: Bot. 100s.
NIAZO. Neotropin.
Use: Urinary antiseptic.
NIB BASE. (Cenci) Washable self-emulsifying base es-pecially developed for incorporation of many of the therapeutic agents used in dermatology. Pkg. 1 & 5 lbs.
NIBESOL-THERAPEUTIC CAPSULES. (Table Rock) Vit. A 25,000 I.U., D-2 1000 I.U., B-1 10 mg., B-2 10 mg., B-6 2 mg., Ca pantothenate 20 mg., niacinamide 100 mg., C 300 mg., B-12 4 mcg./Cap. Bot. 30s, 100s.
Use: Therapeutic multivitamin formula.
• **NIBROXANE.** USAN.
Use: Antimicrobial.
NIBUSTAT-DERM LOTION. (Ortho) Miconazole nitrate 2% w/pegoxol 7 stearate, peglicol 5 oleate, mineral oil, benzoic acid butylated hydroxyanisole. Bot. 30 ml., 60 ml.
Use: Anti-fungal, anti-candidal.
NICAMETATE. B.A.N. 2-Diethylaminoethyl nicotinate. Euclidan. [dihydrogen citrate].
Use: Peripheral vasodilator.
NICAMINDON.
See: Nicotinamide (Various Mfr.)
NICARB. (MSD AGVET) Nicarbazin, 25% medicated feed.
Use: Coccidiostat, veterinary medicine.
NICARBAZIN.
See: Nicarb Prods (MSD AGVET)
• **NICARDIPINE HYDROCHLORIDE.** USAN.
Use: Vasodilator.
N' ICE. (Beecham Products) Menthol in sugarless sorbitol base. Pkg. 8s, 16s.
Use: Cough lozenge.
• **NICERGOLINE.** USAN. 8β-(5-Bromonicotinoyl-oxy-methyl)-10-methoxy-1,6-dimethylergoline.

Use: Vasodilator.

NICERITROL. B.A.N. Pentaerythritol tetranicotinate.
Use: Treatment of hypercholesterolemia.

NICHOLS SYPHON POWDER. (Last) Sodium bicarbonate, sodium chloride, sodium borate. 12.2 Gm pouch (add to 32 oz. water to yield isotonic sol.)

NICLOCIDE. (Miles Pharm) Niclosamide 500 mg./ Chewable Tab. Box 4s.
Use: Anthelmintic.

NICLOFOLAN. 2,2'-Bis(4-chloro-6-nitrophenol). Bilevon
Use: Anthelmintic, veterinary medicine.

• **NICLOSAMIDE.** USAN. 2',5-Dichloro-4'-nitro-salicylanilide. Yomesan.
Use: Anthelmintic.
See: Niclocide, Tab. (Miles)

NICO-400. (Marion) Niacin 400 mg./Cap. Bot. 100s.
Use: Correction of nicotinic acid deficiencies.

NICOBID. (USV Labs.) Nicotinic acid 125, 250 mg., or 500 mg./Tempule time-released capsule. Bot. 100s, 500s, Unit dose 100s.
Use: Vitamin supplement.

NICOBION.
See: Nicotinamide (Various Mfr.)

NICOCODINE. B.A.N. O^3-Methyl-O^6-nicotinoylmorphine.
Use: Narcotic analgesic.

NICODICODINE. B.A.N. 7,8-Dihydro-O^3-methyl-O^6-nicotinoylmorphine.
Use: Antitussive.

NICODUOZIDE. A mixture of nicothazone and isoniazid.

NICOLAR. (USV Labs.) Niacin 500 mg./Tab. Bot. 100s.
Use: For patients with hyperlipidemia who do not respond adequately to diet and weight loss.

NICOMORPHINE. B.A.N. 3,6-Dinicotinoylmorphine.
Use: Narcotic analgesic.

• **NICORANDIL.** USAN.
Use: Coronary vasodilator.

NI CORD XL CAPS. (Scott/Cord) Nicotinic acid 400 mg./Cap. Bot. 100s, 500s.

NICORETTE. (Merrell Dow) Nicotine resin complex 2 mg./Chewing piece. Box 96s.
Use: Temporary aid in smoking cessation program.

NICO-SPAN. (Key) Nicotinic acid 400 mg./Sustained Action Cap. Bot. 100s, 1000s.
Use: Nicotinic acid deficiency.

NICOTAMIDE.
See: Nicotinamide (Various Mfr.)

NICOTHAZONE. Nicotinaldehyde thiosemicarbazone.

NICOTILAMIDE.
See: Nicotinamide (Various Mfr.)

NICOTINAMIDE. Niacinamide, U.S.P. XXI. Vit. B-3, Aminicotin, Dipegyl, Nicamindon, Nicotamide, Nicotilamide, Nicotinic Acid Amide.

NICOTINAMIDE ADENINE DINUCLEOTIDE. Name used for Nadide.

NICOTINATE, METHYL.

NICOTINEX ELIXIR. (Fleming) Niacin 50 mg./5 cc. w/alcohol 14%. Bot. plastic pt., gal.

NICOTINIC ACID. Niacin, U.S.P. XXI.

NICOTINIC ACID W/COMBINATIONS.
See: Niacin W/Combinations (Various Mfr.)

NICOTINIC ACID AMIDE. Niacinamide, U.S.P. XXI.
See: Niacinamide (Various Mfr.)

• **NICOTINYL ALCOHOL.** USAN. 3-Pyridine-methanol. beta-Pyridylcarbinol.
Use: Vasodilator.
See: Roniacol, Elix., Tab. (Roche)

NICOTINYL TARTRATE. 3-Pyridinemethanol tatrate.
See: Roniacol Timespan. Tabs. (Roche)

NICOTYM. (Everett) Niacin 400 mg./T.R. Cap. Bot. 60s.
Use: Dietary supplement.

NICOUMALONE. B.A.N. 3-[2-Acetyl-1-(4-nitro-phenyl) ethyl]-4-hydroxycoumarin. Acenocoumarol (I.N.N.) Sinthrome
Use: Anticoagulant.

NICO-VERT. (Edwards) Niacin 50 mg., dimenhydrinate 25 mg./Cap. Bot. 100s.
Use: Nausea, dizziness.

NICOZIDE. (Premo) Isonicotinic acid hydrazide. (Isoniazid) Tab. 100 mg. Bot. 100s, 1000s.
Use: Streptomycin-resistant tuberculosis.

NIDROXYZONE. 5-Nitro-2-furaldehyde-2-(2-hydroxy-ethyl)semicarbazone.

NIERALINE.
See: Epinepherine (Various Mfr.)

• **NIFEDIPINE,** U.S.P. XXI. Cap., U.S.P. XXI. Dimethyl 1,4-dihydro-2,6-dimethyl-4-(2-nitrophenyl)pyridine-3,5 -dicarboxylate.
Use: Coronary vasodilator.
See: Procardia, Cap. (Pfizer)

NIFENAZONE. B.A.N. 2,3-Dimethyl-4-nicotinamido-1-phenyl-5-pyrazolone. Thylin
Use: Anti-inflammatory; analgesic.

NIFEREX. (Central) **Elixir:** Iron 100 mg./5 cc. polysaccharide-iron complex. Alcohol 10%. Sugar Free. Bot. 8 oz. **Tab.:** 50 mg./Tab. Bot. 100s, 1000s.
Use: Hematinic.

NIFEREX-150. (Central) Polysaccharide iron complex equiv. to iron 150 mg./Cap. Bot. 100s, 1000s.
Use: Iron deficiency anemias.

NIFEREX FORTE ELIXIR. (Central) Iron 100 mg., folic acid 1 mg., Vit. B-12 25 mcg./5 ml. Bot. 4 oz.
Use: Hematinic.

NIFEREX-150 FORTE CAPSULES. (Central) Elemental iron as polysaccharide-iron complex 150 mg., Folic acid 1 mg., Vit B-12 25 mcg./Cap. Bot. 100s, 1000s.
Use: Iron deficiency anemias.

NIFEREX-PN. (Central) **Modified Formula:** Iron 60 mg., folic acid 1 mg., Vit. C 50 mg., B-12 3 mcg., A 4000 I.U., D-2 400 I.U., thiamine mononitrate 3 mg., B-2 3 mg., B-6 2 mg., niacinamide 10 mg., Zinc sulfate 80 mg., Ca carbonate 312 mg./Tab. Bot. 100s, 1000s.
Use: Prenatal vitamin-mineral supplement.

NIFEREX W/VITAMIN C. (Central) Iron 50 mg., Vit. C 100 mg., sod. ascorbate 168.75 mg./Tab. Bot. 50s.
Use: Iron deficiency anemia.

- **NIFLURIDIDE.** USAN.
  Use: Ectoparasiticide.
- **NIFUNGIN.** USAN. Substance derived from *Aspergillus giganteus.*
- **NIFURADENE.** USAN. 1-[(5-Nitrofurfurylidene)-amino]-2-imidazolidinone.
  Use: Antibacterial.
- **NIFURALDEZONE.** USAN. 5-Nitro-2-furaldehyde semioxamazone. Furamazone (Eaton).
- **NIFURATEL.** USAN. 5-[(Methylthio)methyl]-3-[(5-nitro furfurylidene)-amino]-2-oxazolidinone. Macmiror, Magmilor, Polmiror. Under study.
  Use: Antibacterial, antifungal, trichomonacidal.
- **NIFURATRONE.** USAN. N-(2-Hydroxy-ethyl)-α-(5-nitro-2-furyl)nitrone.
  Use: Antibacterial.
- **NIFURDAZIL.** USAN. 1-(2-Hydroxyethyl)-3-[(5-nitrofurfurylidene)-amino]-2-imidazolidinone.
  Use: Antibacterial.
- **NIFURETHAZONE.** 5-Nitro-2-furaldehyde-2-[2-(dimethylamino)ethyl] semicarbazone.
  Use: Antibacterial.
- **NIFURIMIDE.** USAN. ($\pm$-4-Methyl-1-[(5-nitro-furfurylidene)amino]-2-imidazolidinone.
  Use: Antibacterial.
- **NIFURMERONE.** USAN. Chloromethyl 5-nitro-2-fufryl ketone. Metofurone.
  Use: Antimycotic agent.
- **NIFUROXIME.** 5-Nitro-2-fural-doxime. (Z)-5-Nitro-2-furaldehyde Oxime.
  Use: Antifungal, antibacterial (topical), antiprotozoal.
  See: Micofur
  W/Furazolidone.
  See: Tricofuron, Pow., Supp. (Eaton)
- **NIFURPIRINOL.** USAN.
  Use: Antibacterial.
- **NIFURQUINAZOL.** USAN. 2,2'-[[2-(5-Nitro-2-furyl)-4-quinazolinyl]imino]diethanol. Under study.
  Use: Antibacterial.
- **NIFURSEMIZONE.** USAN. 5-Nitro-2-furaldehyde-2-ethyl-semicarbazone.
  Use: Poultry histomonostat.
- **NIFURSOL.** USAN. 3,5-Dinitrosalicylic acid (5-nitrofurfurylidene)hydrazide.
  Use: Histomonocide, vet. growth stimulant.
- **NIFURTHIAZOLE.** USAN. Formic acid 2-[4-(5-nitro-2-furyl)-2-thiazolyl]hydrazide.
  Use: Antibacterial (veterinary).
- **NIFURTIMOX.** B.A.N. Tetrahydro-3-methyl-4-(5-nitrofurfurylideneamino)-1,4-thiazine 1, 1-dioxide.
  Use: Treatment of trypanosomiasis.
- **NIGLYCON.** (CMC) Nitroglycerine ¹⁄₂₅ gr./Tab. Bot. 50s.
  Use: Treatment of angina.
- **NIGRIN.** Streptonigrin.
  Use: Antineoplastic.
- **NIGROIDS.** (CMC) Throat lozenges. Box 12s.
- **NIHYDRAZONE.** Acetic acid (5-nitrofurfurylidene) hydrazide. Veterinary.
- **NIKETHAMIDE.** (Anacardone, Cardiamid, Cormed,

Dynacoryl, Eucoran, Nicamide, Pyricardyl) N,N-Diethyl nicotinamide.
  Use: Central nervous system stimulant.
  See: Coramine, Amp., Liq. (Ciba)
- **NIKO-MAG.** (Scruggs) Magnexium oxide 500 mg./Cap. Bot. 100s, 1000s.
  Use: Temporary relief of constipation and gastric hyperacidity from overeating.
- **NILAIN.** (A.V.P.) Aspirin 227 mg., acetaminophen 227 mg., caffeine 32.4 mg./Cap. Bot. 100s.
  Use: Analgesic.
- **NILCOL ELIXIR.** (Health Care Industries) Phenylpropanolamine 25 mg., chlorpheniramine maleate 2 mg., guaifenesin 100 mg., dextromethorphan; H Br. 15 mg./15 ml.
  Use: Decongestant, antihistaminic, expectorant.
- **NILCOL TABLETS.** (Health Care Industries) Phenylpropanolamine 50 mg., chlorpheniramine maleate 4 mg., guaifenesin 200 mg., dextromethorphan H Br 30 mg./Tab. Bot. 100s.
  Use: Decongestant, antihistaminic, expectorant.
- **NILORIC.** (Ascher) Dihydroergocornine, dihydroergocristine, dihydroergocyptine osmelate equal parts to make 1 mg./Tab. Bot. 100s.
  Use: Selected symptoms in elderly patients.
- **NILPRIN.** (A.V.P. Pharmaceuticals) Acetaminophen 7½ gr./Tab. Bot. 100s.
  Use: Analgesic-antipyretic.
- **NILSPASM.** (Parmed) Phenobarbital 50 mg., hyoscyamine sulfate 0.31 mg., atropine sulfate 0.06 mg., scopolamine hydrobromide 0.0195 mg./Tab. Bot. 100s, 1000s.
  Use: Antispasmodic-sedative.
- **NILSTAT.** (Lederle) Nystatin 500,000 u./Tab., film coated. Bot. 100s, Unit dose 100s.
  Use: Treatment of candida albicans infections.
- **NILSTAT OINTMENT & CREAM.** (Lederle) Nystatin 100,000 u./Gm. **Cream base** w/Ethoxylated stearyl alcohol, isopropyl myristate, glycerin, lactic acid, sod. hydroxide, 0.2% sorbic acid as a preservative. Tube 15 Gm. Jar 240 Gm. **Ointment base:** Light mineral oil, plastibase 50 W. Tube 15 Gm.
  Use: Topical antibiotic.
- **NILSTAT ORAL SUSPENSION.** (Lederle) Nystatin 100,000 u./ml. w/methylparaben 0.12%, propylparaben 0.03%, cherry flavor. Bot. 60 ml. w/dropper, 16 fl. oz..
  Use: Antimycotic.
- **NILSTAT POWDER.** (Lederle) Nystatin powder 1 or 2 billion units/Bot.
  Use: Infections of the oral cavity caused by *Candida albicans.*
- **NILSTAT VAGINAL TABLETS.** (Lederle) Nystatin 100,000 u., starch, lactose, polyvinyl pyrrolidone, sorbitol, magnesium stearate./Tab. Pkg. 15s, 30s w/applicator.
  Use: Antimycotic.
- **NIL TUSS.** (Minnesota Pharm.) Dextromethorphan HBr 10 mg., chlorpheniramine maleate 1.25 mg., phenylephrine HCl 5 mg., ammonium chloride 83 mg./tsp. Syr.: Bot. 1 pt.

Use: Cough syrup, antitussive, vasoconstrictor, antihistaminic, expectorant.

NIL VAGINAL CREAM. (Century) Sulfanilamide 15%, 9-aminoacridine HCl 0.2%, allantoin 1.5%. Bot. 4 oz. w/applicator.

NILVERM HCI. Tetramisole, B.A.N.

• **NIMAZONE.** USAN. 3-(p-Chlorophenyl)-4-imino-2-oxo-1-imidazolidineacetonitrile.
Use: Anti-inflammatory.

• **NIMIDANE.** USAN.
Use: Acaricide.

• **NIMODIPINE.** USAN.
Use: Vasodilator.

NIMORAZOLE. B.A.N. 4-[2-(5-Nitroimidazol-1-yl)ethyl]-morpholine. Nitrimidazine. Naxogin; Nulogyl
Use: Treatment of trichomoniasis.

NIMO-TEX. (Sutliff & Case) Vit. A 5000 I.U., D 400 I.U., E 2 I.U., B-1 3 mg., B-2 2 mg., B-6 0.5 mg., B-12 1 mcg., cal. pantothenate 3 mg., niacinamide 20 mg., choline bitartrate 50 mg., inositol 10 mg., Vit. C 30 mg., ferrous sulf. 60 mg., Cu 1 mg., Mn 3 mg., iodine 0.15 mg., Mg 5 mg., Ca 48 mg., P 37 mg./Tab. Bot. 100s, 1000s.
Use: Vitamin & mineral supplement.

NINE-VITA. (Robinson) Vit. A 5000 I.U., D 1000 I.U., B-1 1.5 mg., B-2 2 mg., niacinamide 20 mg., B-6 0.1 mg., Ca pantothenate 1 mg., C 37.5 mg., E 2 I.U./Cap. Bot. 100s, 1000s. Bulk Pack 5000s.
Use: Dietary supplement.

NIODOL. (Horton & Converse) Camphor 50 mg., chlorobutanol 30 mg., eucalyptol 60 mg., guaiacol 100 mg., iodized oil 50 mg., menthol 60 mg., niaouli oil 100 mg./2 cc. Vial 30 cc. 1s, 12s, 25s.

NIPRIDE. (Roche) Nitroprusside, sodium, 50 mg./5 ml. Vial 5 ml.
Use: Antihypertensive.

NIRAM OINTMENT. (Guild) Pkg. 1 oz.

NIRATRON. (Progress) Chlorpheniramine maleate 4 mg./Tsp. Bot. Pts.
Use: Antihistaminic agent.

• **NIRIDAZOLE.** USAN. 1-(5-Nitrothiazol-2-yl)-imidazoli-din-2-one. Ambilhar
Use: Treatment of schistosomiasis.

NIRON. (Mills) Niacinamide 150 mg., Vit. B-1 10 mg., B-2 6 mg., Vit. B-12 25 mcg., iron 30 mg./prolonged action Tab. Bot. 100s.
Use: Vitamin therapy.

NISAVAL. (Vale) Pyrilamine maleate 25 mg./Tab. Bot. 100s, 1000s.

• **NISBUTEROL MESYLATE.** USAN.
Use: Bronchodilator.

NISENTIL. (Roche) Alphaprodine HCl 40 mg./ml. Vial box. 10s. 60 mg./ml. Vial 10 ml.
Use: Obstetric analgesia.

• **NISOBAMATE.** USAN. (1) 2-(Hydroxymethyl)-2,3-di-methylpentyl isopropylcarbamate carbamate (ester); (2)2-sec-Butyl-2-methyl-1,3-propanediol carbamate isopropylcarbamate.
Use: Minor tranquilizer; sedative; hypnotic.

• **NISOLDIPINE.** USAN.
Use: Vasodilator.

• **NISOXETINE.** USAN.
Use: Antidepressant.

NI-SPAN. (Vortech) Nicotinic acid 400 mg./Cap. Bot. 100s, 1000s.
Use: Nicotinic acid deficiency.

• **NISTERIME ACETATE.** USAN.
Use: Androgen.

• **NITARSONE.** USAN. p-Nitrobenzenearsonic acid.
Use: Veterinary histomonastat.

• **NITHIAMIDE.** USAN.
Use: Antibacterial.

• **NITRAFUDAM HYDROCHLORIDE.** USAN.
Use: Antidepressant.

• **NITRALAMINE HYDROCHLORIDE.** USAN. 2-[[o-Chloro-α-(nitromethyl)benzyl]-thio] ethyl-amine HCl.
Use: Fungicide.

• **NITRAMISOLE HYDROCHLORIDE.** USAN.
Use: Anthelmintic.

• **NITRAZEPAM.** USAN. 1,3-Dihydro-7-nitro-5-phenyl-2H-1,4-benzodiazepin-2-one. Mogadon.
Use: Hypnotic, sedative.

NITRAZINE PAPER. (Squibb) Phenaphthazine. Sod. dinitrophenyl-azo-naphthol disulfonate. 15 ft. roll with dispenser & color chart.
Use: Determine pH of a solution.

NITRAZONE. (Kenyon) Nitrofurazone **Cream** 2% in a water soluble base. Tube 1 oz. **Soluble Dressing** 0.2% in a water soluble base of polyethylene glycol.

NITRE. (Eckerd) Sweet spirits. Bot. 1 oz.

• **NITRENDIPINE.**
Use: Antihypertensive.

NITREX. (Star) Nitrofurantoin 50 mg., 100 mg./Tab. Bot. 100s, 1000s.
Use: Urinary tract infections.

• **NITRIC ACID.** N.F. XVI.
Use: Pharmaceutic aid (acidifying agent).

NITRIC ACID SILVER. Silver Nitrate, U.S.P. XXI.

NITRO-BID. (Marion) Nitroglycerin 2.5 mg., 6.5 mg./T.R. Cap. Bot. 60s, 100s.
Use: Angina pectoris.

NITRO-BID IV. (Marion) Nitroglycerin 5 mg./ml. 1 ml. box of 10s; 5 ml. box of 10s; 10 ml. box of 5s.
Use: Angina pectoris treatment.

NITRO-BID 9 mg. (Marion) Nitroglycerin 9 mg./T.R. Cap. Bot. 60s, 100s.
Use: Angina pectoris treatment.

NITRO-BID OINTMENT. (Marion) Nitroglycerin (glyceryl trinitrate) 2%, lactose in lanolinpetrolatum base. Tube 20 Gm., 60 Gm., 100 Gm.; Uni-Rx Paks 20 Gm., 60 Gm. Box 6s; Pouch 1 Gm. Box 100s.
Use: Angina pectoris.

NITROCAP. (Freeport) Nitroglycerin 2.5 mg./T.R. Cap. Bot. 100s.
Use: Treatment of anginal attacks.

NITROCAP T.D. (Vortech) Nitroglycerin 2.5 mg., 6.5 mg./Cap. Bot. 100s.
Use: Angina pectoris.

NITROCELS. (Winston) Nitroglycerin 2 mg., 0.4 mg./sublingual Tab. Duopak 60s. Bot. 100s.
Use: Angina therapy.

- **NITROCYCLINE.** USAN. 4-(Dimethylamino)-1-4,4α, 5,5α,6,11,12α-octahydro-3,10,12,12α-tetrahydroxy-7-nitro-1,11-dioxo-2-naphthacenecarboxamide.
  Use: Antibiotic.
- **NITRODAN.** USAN.
  Use: Anthelmintic.
- **NITRODAN.** (Century) Nitrofurantoin 100 mg./Tab. Bot. 100s, 1000s.
- **NITRO-DIAL.** (Rocky Mtn.) Nitroglycerin 2.5 mg./T.D. Cap. Bot. 50s, 250s.
- **NITRODISC.** (Searle) Nitroglycerin. Transcustaneous nitroglycerin discs releasing 5 mg./24 hrs. or 10 mg./24 hrs. Cartons 30s.
  Use: Prophylactic antianginal therapy.
- **NITRO-DUR TRNASDERMAL INFUSION SYSTEM.** (Key) Nitroglycerin Patches 5, 10, 15 and 20 square centimeters. Box 28 patches.
  Use: Cardiovascular diseases.
- **NITROFOR-50.** (Kenyon) Nitrofurantoin 50 mg./Tab. Bot. 100s, 1000s.
- **NITROFOR-100.** (Kenyon) Nitrofurantoin 100 mg./Tab. Bot. 100s, 1000s.
- **NITROFURANTOIN,** U.S.P. XXI. Tab., Inj., U.S.P. XXI. 2,4-Imidazolidinedione, 1-[[(5-nitro-2-furanyl)methylene]-amino]-. 1-[(5-Nitrofurfurylidene)amino]hydantoin. 1-(5-Nitro-furfurlyideneamino)imidazoline-2,4-dione. Berkfurin; Furadantin; Urantoin
  Use: Antibacterial for urinary tract infections.
  See: Furadantin, Preps. (Norwich Eaton)
    Furalan, Tab. (Lannett)
    Furantoin, Tab. (Vortech)
    Nitrex, Tab. (Star)
    Nitrofor-50, Tab. (Kenyon)
    Nitrofor-100, Tab. (Kenyon)
    Nitrofurantoin sodium, Vial (Norwich Eaton)
    Sarodant (Saron)
    Trantoin, Tab. (McKesson)
    Urotoin, Tab. (Scruggs)
- **NITROFURANTOIN MACROCRYSTALS.**
  Use: Antibacterial for urinary tract infections.
  See: Macrodantin, Cap. (Norwich Eaton)
- **NITROFURASTAN.** (Standex) Nitrofurazone 1 oz. Tube.
  Use: Topical antibacterial agent.
- **NITROFURAZONE,** U.S.P. XXI. Cream, Oint., Topical Sol., U.S.P. XXI. 5-Nitro-2-furaldehyde semicarbazone.
  Use: Bacteriostatic for surface wounds.
  See: Furacin, Preps. (Norwich Eaton)
    Nisept, Oint. (Blue Line)
    Nitrazone, Cr., Sol. dressing (Kenyon)
    Nitrofurastan, Oint. (Standex)
    Nitrozone, Oint. (Century)
  W/Allantoin, stearic acid.
  See: Eldezol, Oint. (Elder)
- **1-[(5-NITROFURFURYLIDENE)AMINO]-HYDANTOIN.** Nitrofurantoin, U.S.P. XXI.
- **NITROFURFURYL METHYL ETHER.** 2-(Methyloxymethyl)-5-nitrofuran.
  Use: Antifungal veterinary.

- **NITROGEN,** N.F. XVI.
  Use: Pharm. aid (air displacement).
- **NITROGEN MONOXIDE.** Laughing Gas, Nitrous Oxide.
  Use: Inhalation anesthetic & analgesic.
- **NITROGEN MUSTARD.**
  See: Mustargen, Vial (Merck Sharp & Dohme)
- **NITROGEN MUSTARD DERIVATIVES.**
  See: Leukemia Agents
    Leukeran, Tab. (Burroughs-Wellcome)
    Mustargen HCl, Vial (Merck Sharp & Dohme)
    Triethylene Melamine, Tab. (Lederle)
- **NITROGLYCERIN, DILUTED,** U.S.P. XXI.
  Use: Vasodilator.
- **NITROGLYCERIN INJECTION.** (Abbott) 25 mg./ 1 ml. Vials 5 ml., 10 ml.
  Use: Vasodilator, treatment of angina.
  See: Tridil, Inj. (American Critical Care)
- **NITROGLYCERIN OINTMENT,** U.S.P. XXI.
  Use: Vasodilator.
- **NITROGLYCERIN TABLETS,** U.S.P. XXI. 1,2,3-Propanetriol, trinitrate. (Various Mfr.) Glyceryl Trinitrate, Glonoin, Nitroglycerol, Trinitrin, Trinitroglycerol Tab. $\frac{1}{2000}$ gr., $\frac{1}{150}$ gr., $\frac{1}{100}$ gr., Sublingual tabs. (Key) $\frac{1}{100}$ gr., $\frac{1}{400}$ gr., $\frac{1}{200}$ gr., $\frac{1}{400}$ gr./Tab. Bot. 100s, 1000s.
  Use: Vasodilator.
  See: Ang-O-Span, Cap. (Scrip)
    Cardabid (Saron)
    Corobid, Cap. (Medics)
    Gly-Trate, Meta-Kap. (Sutliff & Case)
    Niglycon, Tab. (Consol. Midland)
    Nitrobid, Cap. (Marion)
    Nitrocap T.D., Cap. (Vortech)
    Nitrocels, Cap. (Winston)
    Nitro-Dial, T.D. Caps. (Rocky Mtn.)
    Nitrodyl, Cap. (Bock)
    Nitroglyn, Tab. (Key Pharm.)
    Nitrol Ointment, (Kremers-Urban)
    Nitro-Lyn, Cap. (Lynwood)
    Nitrong, Tab. (Wharton)
    Nitrospan, Cap. (USV Labs.)
    Nitrostat, Tab. (Parke-Davis)
    Nitrotym, Cap. (Kenyon)
    Nitro T.D., Cap. (Fleming)
    Trates, Caps. (Reid-Provident)
    Vasoglyn, Unicelles (Reid-Provident)
  W/Butabarbital.
    See: Nitrodyl-B, Cap. (Bock)
    Nitrotym-Plus, Cap. (Kenyon)
  W/Nicotinic acid.
    See: Nitrovas, Tab. (Amfre-Grant)
  W/Veratrum viride, Sod. nitrite, Pot. nitrate, aconite root.
    See: Nyomin, Tab. (Elder)
- **NITROGLYCEROL.**
  See: Nitroglycerin (Various Mfr.)
- **NITROGLYN.** (Key) Nitroglycerin $\frac{1}{25}$ gr. (2.6 mg.), $\frac{1}{10}$ gr. (6.5 mg.)/Tab. Bot. 100s, 1000s.
  Use: Angina pectoris.
- **NITROL IV.** (Rorer) Glyceryl trinitrate 0.8 mg.

nitroglycerin/ml. Amp. 1 ml. Box 25s; 10 ml. Box
10s; 30 ml. Box 5s.
Use: Control of blood pressure in perioperative
hypertension; angina pectoris.
NITROL OINTMENT. (Rorer) Glyceryl trinitrate 2% in
lanolin and petrolatum base. **Tubes:** 3 Gm., Pack
50s; 30 Gm. Pack 6s. 60 Gm. Pack 6s.
Use: Coronary & peripheral vasodilator.
NITRO-LYN. (Lynwood) Nitroglycerin 2.5 mg./Cap. Bot.
100s.
Use: Smooth muscle relaxant; arteriole-capillary dila-
tor.
NITROMANNITE.
See: Mannitol Hexanitrate (Various Mfr.)
NITROMANNITOL.
See: Mannitol Hexanitrate (Various Mfr.)
• **NITROMERSOL,** U.S.P. XXI. Topical Sol., Tincture,
U.S.P. XXI. 4-Nitro-3-hydroxy mercuri-o-cresol
anhydride. 5-Methyl-2-nitro-7-oxa-8-mercurabicyclo
(4.2.0) octa-1,3,5-triene. Metaphen.
Use: Local anti-infective.
• **NITROMIDE.** USAN. 3,5-Dinitrobenzamide.
Use: Coccidiostat & antibacterial.
• **NITROMIFENE CITRATE.** USAN.
Use: Anti-estrogen.
NITRONET. (U.S. Ethicals) Nitroglycerin 2.6 mg., or
6.5/Controlled Rel. Tab. Bot. 100s.
Use: Vasodilator for anginal attacks and coronary
artery disease.
NITRONG TABLETS. (Wharton) Nitroglycerin 2.6 mg.,
6.5 mg. or 9 mg./Controlled release Tab. Bot. 30s,
100s, 250s, 1000s.
Use: Vasodilator for anginal attacks due to
coronary artery disease.
NITRONG OINTMENT. (Wharton) Nitroglycerin 2%
ointment. Tube 30 Gm., 60 Gm. with dose
applicator.
Use: Vasodilator for anginal attacks due to
coronary artery disease.
p-NITROPHENOL.
See: Niphen, Liq. (Torch)
NITROPRESS. (Abbott) Sodium nitroprusside 50
mg./2 ml. Vial
Use: Hypotensive agent.
• **NITROSCANATE.** USAN.
Use: Anthelmintic.
NITROSPAN CAPSULES. (USV Labs)
Nitroglycerin 2.5 mg. or 6.5 mg./Sustained Release
Caps. 2.5 mg./Cap. Bot. 100s; 6.5 mg./Cap. Bot.
60s.
Use: Management and treatment of anginal
attacks.
NITROSTAT. (Parke-Davis) Nitroglycerin 0.15, 0.3,
0.4, and 0.6 mg./Tab. Bot. 25s, 100s.
Use: Treatment of anginal attacks.
NITROSTAT IV. (Parke-Davis) Nitroglycerin for infusion
0.8 mg./ml. Amp. 10 ml.
Use: Congestive heart failure, angina pectoris.
NITROSTAT OINTMENT. (Parke-Davis) Nitroglycerin
2%. Tubes 30 Gm., 60 Gm.
Use: Prevention and treatment of angina pectoris
due to coronary artery disease.

NITROSTAT SR. (Parke-Davis) Nitroglycerin 2.5 mg.,
6.5 mg., or 9 mg./SR Cap. Bot. 60s, 100s.
Use: Management, prophylaxis, or treatment of
anginal attacks.
p-NITROSULFATHIAZOLE. 2-(p-Nitrophenylsulfona-
mide) thiazole.
NITROTYM. (Kenyon) Nitroglycerin 2.5 mg./Cap. Bot.
100s, 1000s.
NITROTYM-PLUS. (Kenyon) Nitroglycerin 2.5 mg., buta-
barbital 48 mg./Cap. Bot. 100s, 1000s.
NITROUS ACID, SODIUM SALT. Sodium Nitrite,
U.S.P. XXI.
NITROUS ETHER.
• **NITROUS OXIDE,** U.S.P. XXI.
Use: General anesthetic (inhalation).
See: Nitrogen Monoxide.
NITROVIN. B.A.N. 1,5-Bis(5-nitro-2-furyl)penta-1,4-
dien-3-one amidinohydrazone. Payzone and Panazon
[hydrochloride]
Use: Growth promoter, veterinary medicine.
NITROXOLINE. B.A.N. 8-Hydroxy-5-nitroquinoline.
Nibiol
Use: Antibacterial.
NITROXYNIL. B.A.N. 4-Hydroxy-3-iodo-5-nitrobenzoni-
trile. Trodax [meglumine salt].
Use: Anthelmintic, veterinary medicine.
NITROZONE OINTMENT. (Century) Nitrofurazone
0.2%. 4 oz., 1 lb., 5 lb.
NIVAQUINE SULFATE. Chloroquine, B.A.N.
• **NIVAZOL.** USAN. 2′-(p-Fluorophenyl-2′H-17α-
pregna-2,4-dien-20-yno [3,2-c]pyrazol-17-ol.
Use: Glucocorticoid.
NIVEA OIL. (Beiersdorf) Emulsion of neutral aliphatic
hydrocarbons. **Liq.** Bot. 2 oz., 4 fl. oz., 1 pt., 1 qt.
Cream Tube 1 oz. & 2⅓ oz., Jar 4 oz., 6 oz. 1 lb. 5
lb. tin.**Soap:** bath or toilet size.
Use: Emollient.
See: Basic soap (Beiersdorf)
• **NIVIMEDONE SODIUM.** USAN.
Use: Anti-allergic.
• **NIZATIDINE.** USAN.
Use: Anti-ulcerative.
NIZORAL. (Janssen) Ketoconazole 200 mg./Tab. Bot.
60s. Box of 10 strips of 10 tablets.
Use: Broad spectrum antifungal agent.
N-MULTISTIX S. G. REAGENT STRIPS. (Ames) Dip-
and-read urine test for pH, protein, glucose, ketones,
bilirubin, blood, nitrite, urobilinogen and specific
gravity. Bot. 100s.
Use: Diagnostic.
N-N COUGH SYRUP. (Vitarine) Dextromethorphan HBr
60 mg., pot. guaiacolsulfonate 390 mg., ammonium
chloride 390 mg., chlorpheniramine maleate 3
mg./fl. oz. Bot. 4 oz.
Use: Antihistaminic, antitussive.
NO-ASPIRIN. (Walgreen) Acetaminophen 325
mg./Tab. Bot. 100s,
Use: Analgesic.
NO-ASPIRIN EXTRA STRENGTH. (Walgreen)
Acetaminophen 500 mg./Tab. or Cap. Bot. 60s,
100s. Cap. 50s.
Use: Analgesic.

• **NOCODAZOLE.** USAN.
Use: Antineoplastic.
NOCTEC. (Squibb) Chloral hydrate. **Syrup:** 500 mg./5
ml. Bot. 1 pt., 1 gal. Bot. 100s. **Cap.:** 250 mg. or
500 mg./Cap. Bot. 100s. Unimatic 25s, 100s.
Use: Nocturnal sedation.
NODALIN. (Table Rock) Methadon HCl 2½ mg.,
aspirin 3 gr., phenacetin 2 gr., caffeine ⅓ gr./Tab.
Bot. 100s, 500s.
Use: Analgesic.
NODEMA. (Towne) Ammonium chloride 486 mg./Tab.
Bot. 80s.
NODOZ, Keep Alert Tablets. (Bristol-Myers) Caffeine
100 mg./Tab. Bot. 60s. Box 15s, 36s.
Use: Stimulant.
• **NOGALAMYCIN.** USAN.
Use: Antineoplastic.
NO GEST. (Foy) Atropine sulfate 0.2 mg.,
phenylpropanolamine HCl 12.5 mg.,
chlorpheniramine maleate 5.0 mg./ml. w/benzyl
alcohol 2%. Vial 10 ml.
Use: Upper respiratory decongestant.
NO-HIST CAPSULES. (Dunhall) Phenylephrine HCl 5
mg., phenylpropanolamine HCl 40 mg.,
pseudoephedrine HCl 40 mg./Cap. Bot. 100s.
Use: Decongestant.
NO-HIST-S SYRUP. (Dunhall) Phenylephrine HCl 5 mg.,
phenylpropanolamine HCl 40 mg., pseudoephedrine
HCl 40 mg./5 ml. Bot. pt.
Use: Decongestant.
NOKANE. (Wren) Salicylamide 4 gr., N-acetyl-p-amino-
phenol 4 gr., caffeine ½ gr./Tab. Bot. 40s.
NOLAHIST. (Carnrick) Phenindamine tartrate 25
mg./Tab. Bot. 100s.
Use: Allergic rhinitis treatment.
NOLAMINE. (Carnrick) Chlorpheniramine maleate 4
mg., phenindamine tartrate 24 mg.,
phenylpropanolamine HCl 50 mg./Tab. Bot. 100s,
250s.
Use: Upper respiratory and nasal congestion.
• **NOLINIUM BROMIDE.** USAN.
Use: Anti-ulcerative, antisecretory.
NOLUDAR. (Roche) Methyprylon. **Tab.** 50 mg./Tab.
Bot. 100s; 200 mg. Bot. 100s. **Caps.** 300 mg./Cap.
Bot. 100s.
Use: Hypnotic.
NOLVADEX. (Stuart) Tamoxifen citrate equivalent to
10 mg. tamoxifen/Tab. Bot. 60s, 250s.
Use: Treatment of advanced breast cancer.
NOMETIC. Diphenidol.
Use: Antiemetic.
NOMIFENSINE. B.A.N. 8-Amino-1,2,3,4-tetrahydro-2-
methyl-4-phenylisoquinoline.
Use: Thymoleptic and central nervous system
stimulant.
See: Merital (Hoechst)
NONAMIN. (Western Research) Calcium 100 mg.,
chloride 90 mg., magnesium 50 mg., zinc 3.75 mg.,
iron 4.5 mg., copper 0.5 mg., iodine 37.5 mcg.,
potassium 100 mg., phosphorus 100 mg./Tab. Bot.
1000s.

NONE. (O'Neal, Jones & Feldman) Heparin sodium
1000 units/ml. Amps 5 ml. Box 25s.
Use: Anticoagulant.
NONOXYNOL. (Ortho)
Nonylphenoxypolyethoxyethanol.
Use: Spermatocide.
See: Emko, Preps. (Emko)
• **NONOXYNOL 4.** USAN. Nonylphenoxy-poly-
ethyleneoxyethanol. Igepal CO-430. Under study.
Use: Nonionic surfactant.
• **NONOXYNOL 9.** USAN. Poly (ethylene glycol) p-
nonylphenyl ether. Igepal CO-630.
Use: Spermatocide.
See: Conceptrol, Cream, Gel (Ortho)
Delfen, Foam (Ortho)
Emko Prods. (Emko-Schering)
Encare, Insert (Eaton-Merz)
Gynol II, Jelly (Ortho)
Intercept, Inserts (Ortho)
Ortho-Creme, Cream (Ortho)
Ortho-Gynol, Jelly (Ortho)
• **NONOXYNOL 10,** U.S.P. XXI.
Use: Spermatocide.
• **NONOXYNOL 15.** USAN. Nonylphenoxy-poly-
ethyleneoxyethanol. Igepal CO-880. Under
study.
Use: Nonionic surfactant.
• **NONOXYNOL 30.** USAN. Nonylphenoxy-poly-
ethyleneoxyethanol. Under study.
Use: Nonionic surfactant.
NONSPECIFIC PROTEIN THERAPY.
See: Protein, Nonspecific Therapy
NONSUL VAGINAL JELLY. (Misemer) Benzalconium
Cl. 1:2000, tragacanth, pectin, glycerin, methyl
paraben, propyl paraben.
Use: Treatment of Monilial, trichomonal,
non-sporulating bacterial infections.
NONYLPHENOXYPOLYETHOXY ETHANOL.
Nonoxynol.
Use: Contraceptive agent.
See: Delfen Vaginal Foam (Ortho)
W/Benzethonium chloride.
See: Because Birth Control Foam (Emko)
Dalkon Foam (Robins)
Emko Pre-Fil, Foam (Emko)
Emko Vaginal Foam (Emko)
NORACYMETHADOL. B.A.N. α-1-Ethyl-4-methyl-
amino-2,2-diphenylpentyl acetate.
Use: Narcotic analgesic.
• **NORACYMETHADOL HCl.** USAN. α-4, 4-Diphenyl-
6-methylamino-3-heptanol acetate HCl.
Use: Analgesic agent.
NORADRENALINE. B.A.N. (−)-2-Amino-1-(3,4-dihy-
droxyphenyl)ethanol. Levarterenol (I.N.N.)
Use: Hypertensive.
NORADRYL ELIXIR. (Vortech) Bot. 4 oz., gal.
Use: Antihistaminic.
NORADRYL EXPECTORANT. (Vortech) Bot. 4 oz.,
gal.
Use: Antihistaminic, expectorant.
NORALAC. (Vortech) Bismuth aluminate 100 mg., Al

hydroxide-Mg carbonate co-precipitate 300 mg., Mg trisilicate 100 mg., landalgine 50 mg./Tab.
Use: Antacid.
NORAMINIC EXPECTORANT. (Vortech) Bot. 4 oz., gal.
Use: Decongestant, expectorant.
NORAMINIC SYRUP. (Vortech) Phenylpropanolamine HCl 12.5 mg., pheniramine maleate 6.25 mg., pyrilamine maleate 6.25 mg., methylparaben 0.2%/5 cc. Bot. 4 oz., gal.
Use: Antihistaminic.
NORATUSS LIQUID. (Vortech) Potassium guaiacol sulfonate 32.4 mg., ammonium Cl 194.4 mg., terpin hydrate 32.4 mg., codeine phosphate 20 mg., ext. cocillana comp. 26.6 mg., sodium benzoate 0.1%/fl. oz. Bot. 4 oz., gal.
Use: Antitussive, expectorant.
NORAZINE HCl. (Vortech) Promazine HCl 50 mg./ml. Vial 10 ml.
Use: Tranquilizer.
• **NORBOLETHONE.** USAN. 13-Ethyl-17-hydroxy-18, 19-dinor-17α-pregn-4-en-3-one.
Use: Anabolic.
NORBUTRINE. B.A.N. 2-Cyclobutylamino-1-(3,4-dihydroxyphenyl) ethanol.
Use: Bronchodilator.
NORCODEINE. B.A.N. N-Demethyl-O^3-methylmorphine.
Use: Narcotic analgesic.
NORCYCLINE. 6-Demethyl-6-deoxytetracycline. Bonomycin. Sancycline.
Use: Antibiotic.
NORDETTE-21. (Wyeth) Levonorgestrel 0.15 mg., ethinyl estradiol 0.03 mg./Tab. 6 Pilpak dispensers, 21 Tabs.
Use: Oral contraceptive.
NORDETTE-28. (Wyeth) Levonorgestrel 0.15 mg., ethinyl estradiol 0.03 mg./White Tab. (21) with inert tablets (7). 6 Pilpak dispensers, 28 tab.
Use: Oral contraceptive.
NORDRYL. (Vortech) Diphenhydramine HCl **Cap.:** Diphenhydramine HCl 25 mg. or 50 mg./Cap. Bot. 1000s. **Elix.** 10 mg./4 cc. Bot. 4 oz., gal. **Expectorant:** 80 mg., menthol ¹⁄₁₀ gr., ammonium chloride 12 gr., sod. citrate 5 gr., alcohol 5%/cc. 4 oz., gal. **Parenteral:** 10 mg./cc. Vial 30 cc.
Use: Anti-allergic.
NOREL PLUS CAPSULES. (U.S. Chemical) Chlorpheniramine Maleate 4 mg., phenyltoloxamine dihydrogen citrate 25 mg., phenylpropanolamine HCl 25 mg., acetaminophen 325 mg./Cap.
Use: Antihistaminic, decongestant, analgesic.
dl-NOREPHEDRINE HYDROCHLORIDE. alpha-Hydroxy-beta-aminopropylbenzene HCl.
See: Phenylpropanolamine Hydrochloride. (Various mfr.)
Propadrine, Cap., Elix. (Merck Sharp & Dohme)
• **NOREPINEPHRINE BITARTRATE,** U.S.P. XXI. Inj., U.S.P. XXI. 1,2-Benzenediol, 4-(2-amino-1-hydroxyethyl)-, 2,3-dihydroxybutanedioate (1:1) (Salt), monohydrate l-a-(Aminomethyl)3,4-dihydroxybenzyl alcohol bitartrate.

Use: Adrenergic (vasopressor).
See: Levophed Bitartrate, Sol., Amp. (Winthrop-Breon)
NORETHANDROLONE, B.A.N. 17-Alphaethyl-17-hydroxynorandrostenone, 17-Hydroxy-19-nor-17α-pregn-4-en-3-one. Nileyar
Use: Anabolic steroid.
• **NORETHINDRONE,** U.S.P. XXI. Tab., U.S.P. XXI. 19-Norpregn-4-en-20-yn-3-one, 17-hydroxy-, (17α)-. 17-Hydroxy-19-nor-17-alpha-pregn-4-en-20-yn-3-one.
Use: Progestin.
See: Micronor, Tab. (Ortho)
Norlutin, Tab. (Parke-Davis)
Nor-Qd., Tab. (Syntex)
W/Ethinyl estradiol.
See: Brevicon 21 and 28, Tab. (Syntex)
Modicon 21 and 28, Tab. (Ortho)
Ortho-Novum 21 and 28 Prods (Ortho)
Ovcon-35 Tab. (Mead Johnson)
Ovcon-50 Tab. (Mead Johnson)
W/Mestranol.
See: Norinyl, Prods. (Syntex)
Ortho-Novum Prods. (Ortho)
W/Mestranol, ferrous fumarate.
See: Norinyl-I Fe 28 Prods. (Syntex)
• **NORETHINDRONE ACETATE,** U.S.P. XXI. Tab., U.S.P. XXI. 19-Norpregn-4-en-20-yn-3-one, 17-(acetyloxy)-, (17α)-, 17α-Ethinyl-19-nortestosterone. 17-Hydroxy-19-nor-17α-pregn-4-en-20-yn-3-one Acetate.
Use: Progestin.
See: Norlutate, Tab. (Parke-Davis)
• **NORETHINDRONE ACETATE AND ETHINYL ESTRADIOL TABLETS,** U.S.P. XXI.
Use: Oral contraceptive.
See: Brevicon, Tab. (Syntex)
Gestest, Tabs. (Squibb)
Loestrin, Prods. (Parke-Davis)
Norinyl, Prods. (Syntex)
Norlestrin, Prods. (Parke-Davis)
• **NORETHINDRONE AND ETHINYL ESTRADIOL TABLETS,** U.S.P. XXI.
Use: Oral contraceptive.
• **NORETHINDRONE AND MESTRANOL TABLETS,** U.S.P. XXI.
Use: Oral contraceptive.
NORETHISTERONE. B.A.N. 17β-Hydroxy-19-norpregn-4-en-20-yn-3-one. 17α-Ethynyl-17β-hydroxyoestr-4-en-3-one. 17α-Ethynyl-19-nor-testosterone. Micronor; Noriday; Primolut N; Norlutin-A [acetate]
Use: Progestational steroid.
See: Norethindrone (Var. Mfr.)
• **NORETHYNODREL,** U.S.P. XXI. 17-Hydroxy-19-nor-17α-pregn-5(10)-en-20-yn-3-one.
Use: Progesterone agent.
See: Enovid, Prods (Searle)
NORFERAN. (Vortech) Iron dextran 50 mg./ml. Vial 10 ml.
Use: Anemias.

NORFLEX. (Riker) Orphenadrine citrate 100 mg./Tab. Bot. 100s, 500s.
Use: Relief of discomfort of acute painful musculoskeletal conditions.

NORFLEX INJECTABLE. (Riker) Orphenadrine citrate 60 mg., sodium bisulfite 2 mg., sodium chloride 5.8 mg., water for injection qs 2 cc. Amp. 2 cc. 6s, 50s.
Use: Relief of discomfort of acute painful musculoskeletal conditions.

• **NORFLOXACIN.** USAN.

• **NORFLURANE.** USAN. 1,1,1,2-Tetrafluoroethane. Under study.
Use: Inhalation anesthetic.

NORFORMS. (Fleet) PEG 20, PEG 6, PEG 20 Palmitate, lactic acid, methylbenzethonium chloride/Supp. Regular and herbal scent. Box 6s, 12s, 24s.
Use: Vaginal deodorant suppository.

NORGESIC FORTE TABLETS. (Riker) Orphenadrine citrate 50 mg., Aspirin 770 mg., caffeine 60 mg./Tab. Bot. 100s, 500s.
Use: Relief of mild to moderate pain, acute musculo-skeletal disorders.

NORGESIC TABLETS. (Riker) Orphenadrine citrate 25 mg., aspirin 385 mg., caffeine 30 mg./Tab. Bot. 100s, 500s.
Use: Relief of mild to moderate pain of acute musculo-skeletal disorders.

• **NORGESTIMATE.** USAN.
Use: Progestin.

• **NORGESTOMET.** USAN.
Use: Progestin.

• **NORGESTREL.** U.S.P. XXI. Tab., U.S.P. XXI. 18,19-Dinorpregn-4-en-20-yn-3-one, 13-ethyl-17-hydroxy,-(17 α)-(+)-. (+)-13-Ethyl-17-hydroxy-18, 19-dinor-17α-pregn-4-en-20-yn-3-one. (+)-13-Ethyl-17α-ethynyl-17-hydroxygon-4-en-3-one.
Use: Oral contraceptive.
See: Ovrette, Tab. (Wyeth)

• **NORGESTREL AND ETHINYL ESTRADIOL TABLETS,** U.S.P. XXI.
Use: Oral contraceptive.
See: Lo/Ovral, Tab. (Wyeth)
Ovral-Prep. (Wyeth)

NORINYL 2 MG. (Syntex) Norethindrone 2 mg., mestranol 0.1 mg./Tab. Memorette Disp. of 20s. Refill folders of 20s.
Use: Oral contraceptive.

NORINYL 1 + 35. (Syntex) Norethindrone 1 mg., ethinyl estradiol 0.035 mg./Tab. 21 & 28 day (7 inert tabs) Wallette.
Use: Oral contraceptive.

NORINYL 1 + 50. (Syntex) Norethindrone 1 mg., mestranol 0.05 mg./Tab. 21 & 28 day (7 inert tabs) Wallette.
Use: Oral contraceptive.

NORINYL 1 + 80 (Syntex) Norethindrone 1 mg., Mestranol 0.08 mg./Tab. 21 & 28 day (7 inert tabs) Wallette.
Use: Oral contraceptive.

NORISODRINE AEROTROL. (Abbott) Norisodrine HCl (isoproterenol HCl) 0.25% (2.8 mg./ml.) in inert chlorofluorohydrocarbon propellants, alcohol 33%, ascorbic acid 0.1% as preservative. Aerotrol 15 ml. Box 12s.
Use: Management of severe attacks of bronchial asthma.

NORISODRINE WITH CALCIUM IODIDE SYRUP. (Abbott) Isoproterenol sulfate 3 mg., calcium iodide 150 mg./5 ml. w/alcohol 6% Bot. pt.
Use: Symptomatic control of bronchospasm and allied respiratory disorder.

NORLAC. (Rowell) Vit. A 8000 I.U., D-2 400 I.U., Ca 200 mg., Iron 60 mg., C 90 mg., B-1 2 mg., B-2 2 mg., B-6 4 mg., niacinamide 20 mg., E 30 I.U., B-12 8 mcg., Folic Acid 0.4 mg., Mg 100 mg., Zn 15 mg., Cu 2 mg., iodine 0.15 mg./RoSeal. Bot. 100s.
Use: Prenatal supplement.

NORLAC RX. (Rowell) Same formula as Norlac except folic acid 1 mg./Ro-Seal. Bot. 100s, 1000s.
Use: Prenatal supplement for high risk of folic acid deficiency.

NORLESTRIN-21 1/50 TABLETS. (Parke-Davis) Norethindrone acetate 1 mg., ethinyl estradiol 50 mcg./yellow tab. Compact 21s. Pkg. 5 compacts. Pkg. 5 refills; Ctn. 10×5 refills.
Use: Oral contraceptive.

NORLESTRIN-28 1/50 TABLET. (Parke-Davis) Norethindrone acetate 1 mg., ethinyl estradiol 50 mcg./yellow tab. Compact 21 yellow, 7 white (inert) tablets. Pkg. 5 compacts. Pkg. 5 refills; Ctn. 10×5 refills.
Use: Oral contraceptive.

NORLESTRIN-21 2.5/50 TABLETS. (Parke-Davis) Norethindrone acetate 2.5 mg., ethinyl estradiol 50 mcg./pink tablet. Compact 21s. Pkg. 5 compacts. Pkg. 5 refills; Ctn. 10×5 refills.
Use: Oral contraceptive.

NORLESTRIN Fe 1/50 TABLET. (Parke-Davis) Norethindrone acetate 1 mg., ethinyl estradiol 50 mcg./yellow tab. Compact 21 yellow tablets, 7 brown 75 mg. ferrous fumarate tab. Pkg. 5 compacts. Pkg. 5 refills; ctn. 10×5 refills.
Use: Oral contraceptive.

NORLESTRIN Fe 2.5/50 TABLETS. (Parke-Davis) Norethindrone acetate 2.5 mg., ethinyl estradiol 50 mcg./pink tab. Compact 21 pink Tab., 7 brown 75 mg. ferrous fumarate Tab. Pkg. 5 compacts. Pkg. 5 refills; Ctn. 10×5 refills.
Use: Oral contraceptive.

NORLEVORPHANOL. B.A.N. (−)-3-hydroxymorphinan.
Use: Narcotic analgesic.

NOR-LIEF. (Vortech) Phenylephrine HCl 5 mg., chlorpheniramine maleate 0.5 mg., ascorbic acid 15 mg./Tab. Bot. 1000s.
Use: Antihistamine decongestant.

NORLUTATE. (Parke-Davis) Norethindrone acetate 5 mg./Tab. Bot. 50s.
Use: Amenorrhea, menstrual irregularity.

NORLUTIN. (Parke-Davis) Norethindrone, 5 mg./Tab. Bot. 50s.
Use: Control of many menstrual disorders.

NORMADERM CREAM & LOTION. (Doak) Buffered lactic acid in vanishing bases. **Cream:** jar 3¾ oz.,

16 oz. **Lotion:** Bot. 4 oz., 16 oz., 128 oz.
Use: Lubricant & acid restorer for skin.
NORMAL HUMAN SERUM ALBUMIN. Albumin Human, U.S.P. XXI.
NORMATANE DC EXPECTORANT. (Vortech) Codeine phosphate 10 mg., brompheniramine maleate 2 mg., guaifenesin 100 mg., phenylephrine HCl 5 mg., phenylpropanolamine HCl 5 mg., menthol 1 mg., alcohol 3.5%/5 cc. Bot. 4 oz., gal.
Use: Antihistaminic, antitussive.
NORMATANE ELIXIR. (Vortech) Bot. 4 oz., gal.
Use: Antihistaminic, nasal decongestant.
NORMATANE EXPECTORANT. (Vortech) Brompheniramine maleate 2 mg., guaifenesin 100 mg., phenylephrine HCl 5 mg., phenylpropanolamine HCl 5 mg., menthol 1 mg., alcohol 3.5%/5 ml. Bot. 4 oz., gal.
Use: Antihistaminic, antitussive.
NORMATANE TD. (Vortech) Brompheniramine maleate 12 mg., phenylephrine HCl 15 mg., phenylpropanolamine HCl 15 mg./Tab. Bot. 100s, 1000s.
Use: Antihistaminic, decongestant.
NORMENON. Chlormadinone, B.A.N.
NORMETHADONE. B.A.N. 6-Dimethylamino-4,4-di-phenylhexan-3-one.
Use: Narcotic analgesic.
NORMETHANDRONE. 17-α-methyl-19-nortestoster-one. 17β-Hydroxy-17-methylestr-4-en-3-one. Methalutin. (Parke-Davis)
NOR-MIL LIQUID. (Vortech) Diphenoxylate HCl 2.5 mg., atropine sulfate 0.025 mg./5 ml. w/ethyl alcohol 15% Bot. 2 oz.
Use: Antidiarrheal.
NOR-MIL TABLETS. (Vortech) Diphenoxylate HCl 2.5 mg./Tab. Bot. 100s, 500s, 1000s.
Use: Antidiarrheal.
NORMODYNE. (Schering). Labetalol HCl. **Inj.:** 5 mg./ml. Amp. 20 ml. (100 mg.). **Tab.:** 100 mg./Tab. Bot. 100s. Unit dose 100s. Calendar paks 56s. 300 mg./Tab. Bot. 100s. Unit dose 100s. Calendar paks 56s.
NORMOL. (Alcon) Sterile, isotonic solution of sodium chloride, sodium borate, boric acid. Bot. 8 oz.
Use: Soft contact lenses rinsing solution.
NORMORPHINE. B.A.N. N-Demethylmorphine.
Use: Narcotic analgesic.
NORMOSOL-M in D5-W. (Abbott) Dextrose 5 Gm., sod. chloride 234 mg., pot. acetate 128 mg., magnesium acetate 21 mg., sodium bisulfite 30 mg./100 ml. Bot. 500 ml., 1000 ml. in Abbo-Voc (glass) or LifeCare (flexible) containers.
Use: Fluid and electrolyte maintenance, I.V.
NORMOSOL-M 900 CAL. (Abbott) Dextrose 5 Gm., fructose 15 Gm., alcohol 4 ml., sodium chloride 234 mg., pot. acetate 128 mg., magnesium acetate 21 mg., sodium bisulfate 30 mg./100 ml. Bot. 1000 ml.
Use: Fluid and electrolyte maintenance, caloric source.
NORMOSOL-R; NORMOSOL-R pH 7.4; 500 ml., 1000 ml. NORMOSOL-R D5-W. (Abbott) Sod. chloride 526 mg., sod. acetate 222 mg., sod. gluconate 502 mg.,

pot. chloride 37 mg., magnesium chloride 14 mg. pH of Normosol-R and Normosol R in D5-W adjusted with HCl/100 ml. Bot. 1000 ml., 500 ml. in LifeCare (flexible) containers.
Use: Fluid and electrolyte replacement, I.V.
NORMOTENSIN. (Marcen) I.M. sol. for inj.: Mucopolysaccharide 20 mg., sodium nucleate 25 mg., epinephrine-neutralizing factor 25 u., sodium citrate 10 mg., inositol 5 mg., phenol 0.5%/cc. multidose vials 10 cc., 30 cc.
Use: Lowers blood pressure.
NOROCAINE. (Vortech) Lidocaine HCl 1%, 2%, W/sod. Cl and methyl parasept/cc. Vial 50 ml.
Use: Local anesthetic.
NOROCAINE 1% W/EPINEPHRINE. (Vortech) Lidocaine HCl 1%, epinephrine 1:100,000/cc. Vial 50 ml.
Use: Local anesthetic.
NOROCAINE 2% W/EPINEPHRINE. (Vortech) Lidocaine 2%, epinephrine 0.01 mg./cc. Vial 50 ml.
Use: Local anesthetic.
NOROLON. (Winthrop Products) Chloroquine phosphate.
Use: Antimalaria agent.
NOROPHYLLINE LIQUID. (Vortech) Theophylline 80 mg., alcohol 20%/15 cc. Bot. pt.
Use: Bronchial asthma, bronchitis.
NOROZOL. (Vortech) Pentylenetetrazol 100 mg., niacin 50 mg./Tab. Bot. 100s, 1000s.
Use: Mental stimulant for elderly.
NORPACE. (Searle) Disopyramide phosphate 100 mg., 150 mg./Cap. Bot. 100s, 500s, 1000s. Unit Dose 100s.
Use: Treatment of specific ventricular arrhythmias.
NORPACE C.R. (Searle) Disopyramide phosphate 100 mg. or 150 mg./Controlled-Release Cap. Bot. 100s, 500s, 1000s.
Use: Treatment of ventricular arrhythmias.
NORPANTH. (Vortech) Propantheline bromide 15 mg./Tab. Bot. 1000s.
Use: Anticholinergic.
NORPHYL. (Vita Elixir) Aminophylline 1½ gr./Tab.
Use: Bronchial asthma, myocardial infarction.
NORPIPANONE. B.A.N. 4,4-Diphenyl-6-piperidinohexan-3-one.
Use: Analgesic.
NORPRAMIN. (Merrell Dow) Desipramine HCl. **10** mg./Tab. Bot. 100s; **25** mg./Tab. Bot. 100s, 1000s. Unit dose 100s; **50** mg./Tab. Bot. 100s, 1000s. Unit dose 100s; **75** mg./Tab. Bot. 100s; **100** mg./Tab. Bot. 100s. **150** mg./Tab. Bot. 50s.
Use: Antidepressant.
NOR-PRED S. (Vortech) Prednisolone sod. phosphate 20 mg./cc. Vial 10 cc.
Use: Adrenocortical steroid (anti-inflammatory).
NOR-PRED T.B.A. (Vortech) Prednisolone tertiary butyl acetate 20 mg., sod. citrate 1 mg., polysorbate 80 1 mg., d-sorbital 450 mg., benzyl alcohol 0.9%/cc. Vial 10 cc.
Use: Rheumatic arthritis.
19-NORPREGN-4-EN-20-YN-3-ONE, 17-HYDROXY-, (17α)-. Norethindrone, U.S.P. XXI.

19-NORPREGNA-1,3,5(10)TRIEN-20-YN-17-OL; 3-METHOXY-, (17α). Mestranol. U.S.P. XXI.
NOR-Q.D. (Syntex) Norethindrone 0.35 mg./Tab. Dispenser 42s.
Use: Progestin-only contraceptive, hypermenorrhea.
NORTESTERIONATE. 19-Nortestosterone cyclopentylpropionate.
NOR-TET. (Vortech) Tetracycline HCl 250 mg./Cap. orange/yellow; 500 mg./Cap. black/yellow Bot. 100s, 1000s.
Use: Antibiotic.
NORTRAN. Trifluomeprazine, B.A.N.
NORTRIPTYLINE. B.A.N. 3-(3-Methylaminopropylidene)dibenzo[a,d]cyclohepta-1,4-diene. Allegron, Altilev.
Use: Antidepressant.
• **NORTRIPTYLINE HCl,** U.S.P. XXI. Oral Sol., Cap. U.S.P. XXI. 5-(3-Methyl-aminopropylidene)-10,11-dihydro-5H-dibenzo [a,d] cycloheptene HCl. 10,11-Dihydro-N-methyl-5H-dibenzo(a,d)cycloheptene-Δ⁵, γ propylamine Hydrochloride.
Use: Antidepressant.
See: Aventyl HCl, Liq., Pulvule (Lilly)
  Pamelor, Cap., Liq. (Sandoz)
NORTUSSIN LIQUID. (Vortech) Guaifenesin 100 mg., alcohol 3.5%/5 cc. Bot. 4 oz., gal.
Use: Expectorant.
NORTUSSIN W/CODEINE LIQUID. (Vortech) Codeine phosphate 5 mg., guaifenesin 100 mg., alcohol 3.5%/5 cc. Bot. 4 oz., gal.
Use: Antitussive, expectorant.
NORVAL. Docusate sodium.
NORWICH ASPIRIN. (Procter & Gamble) Aspirin 325 mg./Tab. Bot. 100s, 250s, 500s.
Use: Pain relief of headache, minor aches and pains; antipyretic.
NORWICH EXTRA STRENGTH ASPIRIN. (Procter & Gamble) Aspirin 500 mg./Tab. Bot. 150s.
Use: Pain relief of headache, minor aches and pains; antipyretic.
NORWICH GLYCERIN SUPPOSITORIES. (Procter & Gamble) Jar adult: 12s, 24s, 50s. Infant: 12s.
Use: Laxative.
NOSALT SALT ALTERNATIVE. (Norcliff Thayer) Potassium Cl., potassium bitartrate, potassium glutamate, adipic acid, fumaric acid, polyethylene glycol 400, disodium inosinate. Container 11 oz.
Use: Salt substitute.
• **NOSCAPINE,** U.S.P. XXI. Narcotine.
Use: Antitussive.
See: Tusscapine, Susp. (Fisons)
NOSCAPINE HCl. l-Narcotine hydrochloride.
Use: Antitussive.
See: Conar Prods. (Beecham Labs)
W/Chlorpheniramine maleate, phenylephrine HCl, N-acetyl-p-aminophenol, salicylamide, Vit. C.
See: Noscaps, Cap. (Table Rock)
W/Phenylephrine HCl.
See: Conar Liq. (Beecham Labs)
W/Phenylephrine, acetylsalicylic acid, N-acetyl-p-aminophenol, caffeine, pyrilamine maleate.
See: Tussapap, Tab. (Sutliff & Case)

W/Phenylephrine HCl, guaifensin.
See: Conar, Expect. (Beecham Labs)
NOSCAPS. (Table Rock) Noscapine 7.5 mg., chlorpheniramine maleate 1 mg., phenylephrine HCl 5 mg., N-acetyl-p-aminophenol 150 mg., salicylamide 150 mg., Vit. C 20 mg./Cap. Bot. 100s, 500s.
Use: Relief of common cold.
• **NOSIHEPTIDE.** USAN.
Use: Growth stimulant.
NOSKOTE. (Plough) Homosalate, oxybenzone, SPF 8. Tube 7/16 oz., Jar 1 oz.
Use: Ultraviolet sunscreen.
NOSPAZ, IM. (Reid-Provident) Dicyclomine HCl 10 mg., sodium chloride 0.9%, chlorobutanol 0.5%, water q.s./cc. Vial 10 cc.
Use: Anticholinergic.
NOTENSIL MALEATE. Acepromazine, B.A.N.
NOVAFED. (Merrell Dow) Pseudoephedrine HCl 30 mg./5 ml., alcohol 7.5%, Bot. 4 oz.
Use: Decongestant.
NOVAFED A. (Merrell Dow) Pseudoephedrine HCl 30 mg., chlorpheniramine maleate 2 mg./5 ml., alcohol 5%. Bot. 4 oz.
Use: Decongestant, antihistamine.
NOVAFED A CAPSULES (Merrell Dow) Pseudoephedrine HCl 120 mg., chlorpheniramine maleate 8 mg./ controlled release capsule. Bot. 100s.
Use: Decongestant/antihistamine.
NOVAFED CAPSULES. (Merrell Dow) Pseudoephedrine HCl 120 mg./Controlled-Release Cap. Bot. 100s.
Use: Decongestant.
NOVAHISTINE COUGH & COLD FORMULA. (Merrell Dow) Dextromethorphan hydrobromide 10 mg., pseudoephedrine HCl 30 mg., chlorpheniramine maleate 2 mg./5 ml. w/alcohol 5%. Bot. 4 oz., 8 oz.
Use: Antitussive, decongestant, antihistamine for cough & cold symptoms.
NOVAHISTINE COUGH FORMULA. (Merrell Dow) Dextromethorphan HBr 10 mg., guaifenesin 100 mg./5 ml. w/alcohol 7.5%. Bot. 4 oz., 8 oz.
Use: Antitussive, expectorant.
NOVAHISTINE DMX. (Merrell Dow) Pseudoephedrine HCl 30 mg., dextromethorphan HBr 10 mg., guaifenesin 100 mg./5 ml. w/alcohol 10%. Bot. 4 oz., 8 oz.
Use: Antitussive, expectorant, decongestant.
NOVAHISTINE DH. (Merrell Dow) Pseudoephedrine HCl 30 mg., codeine phosphate 10 mg., chlorpheniramine maleate 2 mg./5 ml. w/alcohol 5%. Bot. 4 oz., pt.
Use: Antitussive, decongestant, antihistamine.
NOVAHISTINE ELIXIR. (Merrell Dow) Phenylephrine HCl 5 mg., chlorpheniramine maleate 2 mg./5 ml. w/alcohol 5%. Bot. 4 oz., 8 oz.
Use: Decongestant, antihistamine.
NOVAHISTINE EXPECTORANT. (Merrell Dow) Pseudoephedrine HCl 30 mg., codeine phosphate 10 mg., guaifenesin 100 mg./5 ml. w/alcohol 7.5%. Bot. 4 oz., Pt.

Use: Antitussive, decongestant, expectorant.
NOVAHISTINE FORTIS. (Merrell Dow) Phenylephrine HCl 10 mg., chlorpheniramine maleate 2.0 mg./Cap. Bot. 100s.
Use: Decongestant, antihistamine.
NOVAHISTINE L.P. (Merrell Dow) Phenylephrine HCl 20 mg., chlorpheniramine maleate 4 mg./Tab. Bot. 100s.
Use: Decongestant, antihistamine.
NOVAHISTINE TABLETS. (Merrell Dow) Phenylpropanolamine HCl 18.75 mg., chlorpheniramine maleate 2 mg./Tab. Pkg. 48s.
Use: Decongestant, antihistamine for treatment of cold and hay fever symptoms.
NOVALDIN. (Winthrop Products) Dipyrone. Available as Tabs., Amp., Drops.
Use: Analgesic, antipyretic, anti-inflammatory.
NOVALGIN.
See: Dipyrone (Various Mfr.)
NOVAMIDON.
See: Aminopyrine (Various Mfr.)
NOVAMINE. (Cutter) Amino acids injection. 8.5% in flasks of 500 ml., 1000 ml. 11.4% in flasks of 250 ml., 500 ml., 1000 ml.
Use: Source for amino acids in parenteral nutrition regimens.
NOVATOPHAN.
See: Neocinchophen (Various Mfr.)
NOVATROPINE.
See: Homatropine Methylbromide (Various Mfr.)
NOVERIL HYDROCHLORIDE. Dibenzepin, B.A.N.
NOVOBIOCIN, B.A.N. Streptonivicin. (Biotexin) An antibiotic from Streptomyces niveus and Streptomyces spheroides.
See: Albamycin, Cap. (Upjohn)
• **NOVOBIOCIN CALCIUM,** U.S.P. XXI. Oral Susp., U.S.P. XXI.
See: Cathomycin Calcium
NOVOBIOCIN MONOSODIUM SALT.
See: Sodium Novobiocin.
• **NOVOBIOCIN SODIUM,** U.S.P. XXI. Cap., U.S.P. XXI.
See: Albamycin, Cap. (Upjohn)
Cathomycin Sodium
NOVOCAIN. (Winthrop-Breon) Procaine HCl solution. **1%:** Amp. 2 ml. Box 25s, 6 ml. Box 50s; Vial 30 ml. Box 10s. **2%:** Vial 30 ml. Box 10s.
Use: Local anesthetic by infiltration injection, nerve block and other peripheral blocks.
NOVOCAIN FOR SPINAL ANESTHESIA. (Winthrop-Breon) Procaine HCl 10% solution. Amp. 2 ml. Box 25s.
Use: Spinal anesthesia.
NOVOHYDRIN. Ambuside, B.A.N.
NOXIPTYLINE, B.A.N. 3-(2-Dimethylaminoethyloxy-imino)dibenzo[a,d]cyclohepta-1,4-diene.
Use: Antidepressant.
NOXYTHIOLIN. B.A.N. N-Hydroxymethyl-N'-methylthiourea. Noxyflex
Use: Antifungal agent.
NOXZEMA 12-HOUR ACNE MEDICINE. (Noxell) Benzoyl peroxide 10%. Bot. 1 oz.

Use: Acne medicine.
NOXZEMA ANTISEPTIC SKIN CLEANSER. (Noxell) SD alcohol 63%. Bot. 4 oz., 8 oz.
Use: Oily skin cleanser.
NOXZEMA MEDICATED SKIN CREAM. (Noxell) Menthol, camphor, clove oil, eucalyptus oil, phenol. Jar 2.5 oz., 4 oz., 6 oz., 10 oz. Tube 4.5 oz. Bot. 6 oz.
Use: Soothing sunburn pain.
NP-27 AEROSOL. (Procter & Gamble) Zinc undecylenate, alcohol 20.5%. Spray Cans 4 oz.
Use: Dermatophytosis.
NP-27 CREAM. (Procter & Gamble) 8-hydroxyquinoline benzoate 2.5% in cream base. Tube 1.5 oz.
Use: Antifungal for relief of athlete's foot and ringworm.
NP-27 LIQUID. (Procter & Gamble) Undecylenic acid 10%, isopropyl alcohol 56%. Plastic bot. 2 oz.
Use: Dermatophytosis.
NTR NOSE DROPS. (Winthrop Products) Phenylephrine HCl.
Use: Nasal decongestant.
NTZ SOLUTION. (Winthrop-Breon) Oxymetazoline HCl 0.05% w/benzalkonium Cl and phenylmercuric acetate 0.002% as preservatives. Bot. 1 oz., 16 oz.; Spray Bot. 15 ml.
Use: Decongestant, antihistaminic.
NUBAIN. (Du Pont) Nalbuphine HCl **10 mg.**/ml. Ampul 1 ml., 2 ml. Vial 10 ml. **20 mg.**/ml. Ampul 1 ml. Syringes 1 ml. calibrated. Vial 10 ml.
Use: Analgesic.
NU-BOLIC. (Seatrace) Methandriol dipropionate 50 mg./cc. Vial 10 cc.
NUCITE.
See: Inositol (Various Mfr.)
■ **NUCLEIC ACID ANTAGONISTS.**
Use: Treatment certain forms of neoplastic diseases.
See: Leukeran, Tab. (Burroughs Wellcome) Mustargen, Vial (Merck Sharp & Dohme) Myleran, Tab. (Burroughs Wellcome) Purinethol, Tab. (Burroughs Wellcome) Triethylene Melamine, Tab. (Lederle)
NUCLEOSINE. (Pasadena Research) Adenosine-5'-monophosphate 25 mg., cyanocobalamin 60 mcg./cc. Vial 10 cc.
NUCLOMIN. (Miller) Vit. A 5,000 I.U., D 400 I.U., E 25 I.U., B-1 2.5 mg., B-2 5.0 mg., B-6 5 mg., niacinamide 25 mg., pantothenic acid 25 mg., Vit. C 50 mg., B-12 6 mcg., para-amino benzoic acid 10 mg., other factors natural to yeast ext., Cu 1 mg., Mn 2 mg., Fe 10 mg., Mg. 50 mg., Zn 2 mg./Tab. Tab. Bot. 100s.
Use: Dietary supplement.
NUCOFED. (Beecham Labs) Codeine phosphate 20 mg., pseudoephedrine HCl 60 mg/5 ml. or Cap. **Liq.:** Bot. pts.; **Cap.:** Bot. 60s.
Use: Antitussive, decongestant.
NU-DISPOZ. (Coastal) Diethylpropion HCl 25 mg./Tab. Bot. 100s, 1000s.
• **NUFENOXOLE.** USAN.
Use: Antiperist

nu-FLOW. (CooperCare) A blend of two synthetic detergents, an emollient complex, parachlorometaxylenol 2%, isopropanol 7.5% Bot. 120 ml.
Use: Concentrated, neutral, medicated shampoo.

NUGOFED EXPECTORANT. (Beecham Labs) Codeine phosphate 20 mg., pseudoephedrine HCl 60 mg., guaifenesin 200 mg./5 ml. w/alcohol 12.5%. Bot. pt.
Use: Antitussive, decongestant.

NU-IRON. (Mayrand) Polysaccharide-iron complex. **Cap.:** 150 mg. elemental iron. Bot. 100s, 500s. **Elixir:** 100 mg. elemental iron/5 cc., w/alcohol 10%. Bot. 8 oz.
Use: Iron deficiency anemia.

NU-IRON PLUS ELIXIR. (Mayrand) Polysaccharide iron complex 100 mg., folic acid 1 mg., Vit B-12 25 mcg./5 ml. w/alcohol 10%. Bot. 8 oz.
Use: Iron-vitamin supplement.

NU-IRON-V. (Mayrand) Polysaccharide iron 60 mg., folic acid 1 mg., ascorbic acid 50 mg., cyancobalamin 3 mcg., Vit. A 4000 I.U., D-2 400 I.U., B-1 3 mg., B-2 3 mg., niacinamide 10 mg., Cacarbonate 312 mg., B-6 HCl 2 mg./Tab. Bot. 100s.
Use: Vitamin iron supplement.

NUJOL. (Plough) Mineral oil. Bot. 8 oz., 1 pt.
Use: Laxative.

Nu'LEVEN. (Lemmon) Gastro-soluble layer: Pepsin 150 mg. Enteric coated inner core: pancreatic enzyme conc. 100 mg., ox bile ext. 100 mg., cellulase 10 mg./Tab. Bot. 1000s.
Use: Digestive aid.

NULICAINE. (Kay) Lidocaine HCl 10 mg. or 20 mg., methylparaben 1 mg., sodium chloride 6 mg./cc. Multiple dose sterile solution 50 cc.
Use: Minor nerve block anesthesia.

NULLAPONS. (General Aniline & Film) The whole group of chelating agents related to ethylenediaminetetraacetic acid. Pkg. according to demand.
Use: Sequestering agent.

NULLO. (Eckerd) Chlorophyllins 10 mg., ferrous sulfate 9.6 mg., Tab., Bot. 16s, 45s, 100s, 500s.
Use: Orally, to help prevent body odors, control of ileostomy and colostomy odors.

NUL-TACH. (Davis & Sly) Potassium 16 mg., magnesium 13 mg., ascorbic acid 250 mg./Tab. Bot. 100s.
Use: Paroxysmal tachycardia.

NUMORPHAN. (Du Pont) Oxymorphone HCl. **1 mg./ml.:** Amp. 1 ml. Box 10s, 100s. **1.5 mg./ml.:** Amp. 1 ml. Box 10s, 100s.; Vial 10 ml. Box 1s. **Rectal Suppos.:** Box 6s. 5 mg./Suppos.
Use: Relief of pain.

NUMOTIZINE. (Hobart) Guaiacol 0.52 Gm., beechwood creosote 2.60 Gm., methyl salicylate 0.52 Gm./100 Gm. **Liniment** Glass Bot. 1.16 oz. Pl. Bot. 2 oz., 8 oz. **Oint.** 24 oz., 3 lb.
Use: Analgesic and decongestant.

NUMOTIZINE CATAPLASM. (Hobart) Guaiacol 0.260 Gm., beechwood creosote 1.302 Gm., methyl salicylate 0.260 Gm./100 Gm. Jar. 4 oz.
Use: Relief of pain and soreness.

NUMOTIZINE COUGH SYR. (Hobart) Guaifenesin 5 gr., ammonium chloride 5 gr., sodium citrate 20 gr., menthol 0.04 gr./fl. oz. Bot. 3 oz., pt., gal.

NUMZIDENT. (Purepac) Benzocaine, clove oil, peppermint oil. ½ oz.
Use: Topical anesthetic.

NUMZIT. (Purepac) Glycerin, ethyl alcohol 10%. Gel. Bot. ¼ oz. **Lot** ¾ oz.
Use: Teething.

NU-NATAL FL. (Marlyn) Vit. A acetate 2000 I.U., D 200 I.U., B-1 1.5 mg., B-2 2.5 mg., C 50 mg., nicotinamide 10 mg., d-Ca pantothenate 5 mg., B-6 5 mg., B-12 1 mcg., folic acid 0.2 mg., hesperidin 25 mg., fluoride 0.5 mg., Ca 150 mg., Fe 30 mg./Tab. Bot. 100s.
Use: Prenatal Vitamin.

NUNOL.
See: Phenobarbital (Various Mfr.)

NUPERCAINAL. (Ciba) **Cream.** Dibucaine 0.5%, acetone, sod. bisulfite 37%. Tube 1½ oz. **Oint.** Dibucaine 1%, sod. bisulfite 0.5%. Tube 1 oz., 2 oz.
Use: Topically: local anesthetic, minor burns remedy. **Supp.** Zinc oxide 250 mg., bismuth subgallate 1 Gm., acetone, sod. bisulfite 0.5%. Box 12s, 24s.
Use: Hemorrhoids.

NUPERCAINE HYDROCHLORIDE. (Ciba) Dibucaine HCl Amp. 1:200, 10 mg. w/sod. chloride 10 mg., sod. phosphate monobasic 4 mg., sod. phosphate dibasic 0.9 mg./2 ml., 10s. Heavy Sol. (1:400) 5 mg., dextrose 100 mg./2 ml. Pkg. 10s. Amp. 1:1500 sod. chloride 100 mg., 20 ml. 12s.
Use: Spinal anesthetic.

N-URISTIX REAGENT STRIPS. (Ames) Bot 100s.
Use: Dip and read test for protein, glucose and nitrite in urine.

NURSOY. (Wyeth) Vit. A 2500 I.U., D-3 400 I.U., C 55 mg., B-1 0.67 mg., B-2 1 mg., E 9 I.U., niacin 9.5 mEq., B-6 0.4 mg., B-12 2 mcg., pantothenic acid 3 mg., K-1 0.1 mg., folic acid 50 mcg., choline 85 mg., inositol 26 mg., iodine, biotin, Ca, P, Na, K, Mg, Mn, Cl, Cu, Zn/qt. of formula. Conc. liq. Can 13 oz. Ready to feed Can 32 oz. Ready to feed Hospital Bot. 4 oz.

NU-THERA. (Kirkman) Vit. A 10,000 I.U., D 400 I.U., B-1 10 mg., B-2 5 mg., niacinamide 100 mg., B-6 1 mg., B-12 5 mcg., C 150 mg., Ca 103 mg., P 80 mg., Fe 10 mg., Mg 5.5 mg., Mn 1 mg., K 5 mg., Zn 1.4 mg./Cap. Bot. 100s.
Use: Dietary supplement for vitamin and mineral deficiency.

• **NUTMEG OIL,** N.F. XVI.
Use: Pharmaceutic aid (flavor).

NUTRACORT. (Owen) Hydrocortisone. **Cream:** 1%: Jars 2 oz., 4 oz., 1 lb., Tube 30 Gm. **Lotions:** 0.25%: 0.5%, 1%: Bot. 2 oz., 4 oz.
Use: Dermatologic anti-inflammatory.

NUTRACORT GEL. (Owen) Hydrocortisone 1.0% in vehicle of propylene glycol, alcohol 22%, hydroxypropyl cellulose and citric acid. Tube 15 gm., 60 gm.
Use: Inflammatory manifestations of corticosteroid-responsive dermatoses.

NUTRADERM

NUTRADERM. (Owen) Oil-in-water emulsion. **Lot.** Plastic Bot. 8 oz., 16 oz. **Cream:** Tube 1.5 oz., 3 oz., Jar 1 lb.
Use: Emollient.

NUTRADERM BATH OIL. (Owen) Mineral oil, PEG-4 dilaurate, lanolin oil, butylparaben, benzophenone-3, fragrance, D & C Green No. 6. Bot. 8 oz.
Use: Aid in the relief of dry, itchy skin.

NUTRAJEL. (Cenci) Aluminum hydroxide, 5 gr./5 cc. Bot. 12 oz.
Use: Antacid, duodenal ulcers.

NUTRAMAG. (Cenci) Colloidalized gel of aluminum and magnesium hydroxide. Bot. 12 oz.
Use: Antacid, nonconstipating demulcent.

NUTRAMENT LIQUID. (Drackett) Protein 16 Gm., fat 10 Gm., carbohydrates 52 Gm., and vitamins & minerals/360 calories/12½ oz. Can 12½ oz.
Use: Nutritional supplement.

NUTRAMIGEN. (Mead Johnson) Hypoallergenic formula that supplies 640 calories/qt. w/18 Gm. protein, 25 Gm. fat, 86 Gm. carbohydrate. Vit. A 2000 I.U., D 400 I.U., E 20 I.U., C 52 mg., folic acid 100 mcg., B-1 0.5 mg., B-2 0.6 mg., niacin 8 mg., B-6 0.4 mg., B-12 2 mcg., biotin 50 mcg., pantothenic acid 3 mg., Vit. K-1 100 mcg., choline 85 mg., inositol 30 mg., Ca 600 mg., P 400 mg., iodine 45 mcg., Fe 12 mg., Mg 70 mg., Cu 0.6 mg., Zn 5 mg., Mn 200 mcg., Cl 550 mg., K 700 mg., Na 300 mg./qt. of formula (4.9 oz. pow.), Cans 16 oz.
Use: Feeding of infants and children allergic to ordinary food proteins and/or lactose intolerant. Complete, nutritionally balanced diet.

NUTRAMIN. (Thurston) Vit. A 666 I.U., D 66 I.U., B-1 666 mcg., B-2 333 mcg., niacinamide 2 mg., folic acid 0.0444 mcg., Ca 16.6 mg., P 8.33 mg., Fe 1.33 mg., iodine 0.15 mg./Tab. Bot. 200s, 500s, 1000s.
Use: Dietary supplement.

NUTRAMIN GRANULAR. (Thurston) Vit. A 333 I.U., D 333 I.U., B-1 3.3 mg., B-2 1.6 mg., niacinamide 10 mg., folic acid 0.133 mg., Ca 250 mg., P 115 mg., Fe 6.6 mg., iodine 0.15 mg./5 Gm. Bot. 10 oz., 32 oz.
Use: Vitamin-mineral supplement.

NUTRAPLUS. (Owen) Urea 10% in emollient cream base or lotion base with preservatives. **Cream.** Tube 3 oz., Jar 1 lb.**Lot.** Bot. 8 oz., 16 oz.
Use: Moisturize dry, rough skin.

NUTRASPA BATH OIL. (Owen) Mineral oil, PEG-4 dilaurate, lanolin oil, butylparaben, benzophenone-3, fragrance, D&C green #6. Bot. 8 oz., 16 oz.
Use: Dry or pruritic skin conditions.

NUTRAVIMS. (Approved) Vit. A 6000 I.U., D 1250 I.U., C 50 mg., E 5 I.U., B-12 5 mcg., B-1 3 mg., B-2 3 mg., B-6 0.5 mg., niacinamide 20 mg., Ca pantothenate 5 mg., zinc 1.5 mg., Mn 1 mg., iodine 0.15 mg., pot. 5 mg., Mg 4 mg., iron 15 mg., Ca 59 mg., phos. 45 mg./Cap. Bot. 100s, 250s, 1000s.
Use: Daily supplement.

NUTRI-AID. (American McGaw) Complete isotonic liquid nutrition. Can 8 oz.
Use: Dietary supplement.

NUTRICOL. (Nutrition Control) Safflower oil 1530 mg.,

choline bitartrate 500 mg., soybean lecithin 600 mg., inositol 100 mg., natural tocopherols 20 mg., B-6 10 mg., B-12 5 mcg., panthenol 5 mg./Cap. Bot. 90s.
Use: Dietary supplement.

NUTRI-E. (Nutri Lab.) Vitamin E. Cream: 200 I.U./Gm. Jar 1 oz., 2 oz. Oil: 1 oz. Oint. 200 I.U./Gm. Tube 1 oz., 1½ oz. Cap. 200 I.U., Bot. 80s, 400 I.U., Bot. 60s, 100s. 800 I.U., Bot. 55s.

NUTRIGANIC. (Commerce) Multi-vitamin with minerals and amino acids. Tab. Bot. 50s.
Use: Vitamin supplement.

NUTRI-PLEX TABLETS. (Faraday) Vit. B-1 5 mg., B-2 5 mg., B-6 5 mg., pantothenic acid 25 mg., B-12 12.5 mcg., niacinamide 50 mg., Fe gluconate 30 mg., choline bitartrate 50 mg., inositol 50 mg., P.A.B.A. 15 mg., C 150 mg./2 Tabs. Bot. 100s, 250s.
Use: Protein therapy.

NUTRI-VAL. (Marcen) Vit. A 5000 I.U., D 500 I.U., B-1 10 mg., B-2 5 mg., B-12 activity 5 mcg., B-6 5 mcg., C 50 mg., hesperidin 5 mg., niacinamide 15 mg., folic acid 0.2 mg., Ca pantothenate 50 mg., choline bitartrate 50 mg., betaine HCl 25 mg., lipo-K 0.4 mg., duodenum substance 50 mg., pancreas substance 50 mg., inositol 25 mg., Cy-yeast hydrolysates 50 mg., rutin 5 mg., 1-lysine HCl 5 mg., E 5 I.U., Ossonate (glucuronic complex) 8 mg., glutamic acid 30 mg., lecithin 5 mg., iron 20 mg., iodine 0.15 mg., Ca 50 mg., P 40 mg., boron 0.1 mg., Cu 1 mg., Mn 1 mg., Mg 1 mg., Pot. 5 mg., Zn 0.5 mg., biotin 0.02 mg./Cap. Bot. 100s, 500s, 1000s.
Use: Dietary supplement and absorption aid.

NUTRI-VITE NATURAL MULTIPLE VITAMIN AND MINERALS. (Faraday) Vit. A 15,000 I.U., D 400 I.U., B-1 1.5 mg., B-2 3 mg., B-12 15 mcg., niacin 500 mcg., B-6 20 mcg., choline 1.75 mg., folic acid 13 mcg., pantothenic acid 50 mcg., p-aminobenzoic acid 12 mcg., inositol 1.72 mg., C 60 mg., citrus bioflavonoids 15 mg., E 50 I.U., Fe gluconate 15 mg., Ca 192 mg., P 85 mg., iodine 0.15 mg., red bone marrow 30 mg./3 Tabs. Protein coated Tab. Bot. 100s, 250s.

NUTRIZYME. (Enzyme Process) Vit. A 5000 I.U., D 400 I.U., C 60 mg., B-1 1.5 mg., B-2 1.7 mg., niacinamide 20 mg., B-6 2 mg., pantothenate 10 mg., B-12 6 mcg., E 30 I.U., iron 10 mg., Cu 1 mg., Zn 1 mg., Folacin 0.025 mg./Tab. Bot. 90s, 250s.
Use: Dietary supplement.

NUTROFEROL PLUS. (Winthrop Products) Ferrous gluconate.
Use: Hematinic.

NUX VOMICA EXTRACT. W/Bile salts, cascara sagrada, phenolphthalein, aloin, papain.
See: Taurocolate, Tab. (Vortech)
W/Iron oxide, cinchona, vitamin B-1, alcohol.
See: Briatonic, Liq. (Briar)
W/Methyl testosterone, yohimbine HCl.
See: Climactic, Tab. (Burgin-Arden)

NUZINE OINTMENT. (Hobart) Guaiacol 1.66 Gm., oxyquinoline sulf. 0.42 Gm., zinc oxide 2.5 Gm., glycerine 1.66 Gm., lanum (anhyd.) 43.76 Gm., petrolatum 50 Gm./100 Gm. Tube 1 oz.
Use: Hemorrhoidal pain, pruritus.
NYCOFF. (Dover) Dextromethorphan HBr./Tab. Unit dose 500s. Sugar and salt free.
Use: Cough suppressant.
NYCO-WHITE. (Whiteworth) Nystatin, neomycin, gramcidin, triamcinolone cream. Tube 15 Gm., 30 Gm., 60 Gm.
Use: Antibiotic cream.
NYCO-WORTH. (Whiteworth) Nystatin cream. Tube 15 Gm.
Use: Antibiotic cream.
NYCRALAN. (Lannett) Vit. B-1 10 mg., calcium lactate 10 gr./Tab. Bot. 100s.
NYDRANE. Beclamide. B.A.N.
NYDRAZID. (Squibb) Isoniazid. Tab. 100 mg., Bot. 100s, 1000s Inj. 100 mg./cc. w/chlorbutanol 0.25%, sodium hydroxide or hydrochloric acid to adjust pH. Vial 10 cc.
Use: Tuberculosis.
• **NYLESTRIOL.** USAN. 3-Cyclopentyloxy-19-nor-17 α -pregna-1,3,5(10)-trien-20-yne-16, 17β-diol.
Use: Estrogen.
NYLIDRIN HYDROCHLORIDE, U.S.P. XXI. Inj., Tab., U.S.P. XXI. p-Hydroxy-a-[1-[(1-methyl-3-phenyl-propyl)-amino]ethyl]benzyl alcohol HCl.
Use: Peripheral vasodilator.
See: Arlidin, Tab. (USV Labs.)
    Rolidrin-6, Tab. (Robinson)
    Rolidrin-12, Tab. (Robinson)
NYLMERATE II SOLUTION CONCENTRATE. (Holland-Rantos) SD alcohol 50%, purified water, acetic acid, boric acid, polysorbate 20, nonoxynol-9, sodium acetate, FD & C Blue # 1, D & C Yellow # 10 Bo. 16 oz.
Use: Acidic cleansing douche in dilution.
NYLONETS TRAVEL PACKET. (Matthew) Caps. 20s.
NYQUIL. (Vicks) Dextromethorphan HBr 30 mg., pseudoephedrine HCl 60 mg., doxylamine succinate 7.5 mg., acetaminophen 1000 mg./oz. w/alcohol 25%. FDC Yellow #5 tartrazine. Bot. 6 oz., 10 oz., 14 oz.
Use: Analgesic, decongestant, antitussive, antihistaminic cold medicine.
NYRAL. (Vale) Cetylpyridinium chloride 0.5 mg., benzocaine 5 mg./Lozenge w/parabens. Pkg. 100s, 1000s.
Use: Antiseptic.
NYSACETOL. (Kenyon) N-Acetyl-p-aminophenol 5 gr./Tab. Bot. 100s, 1000s.
NYSTAFORM. (Miles Pharm) Nystatin 100,000 U., clioquinol 1% in petrolatum base w/octylphenoxyethanol, wax. Oint. Tube ½ oz.
Use: Moniliasis treatment.
NYSTAFORM-HC. (Miles Pharm) Nystaform w/hydrocortisone alcohol 1%. Bot ½ oz.
Use: Treatment of moniliasis.
• **NYSTATIN,** U.S.P. XXI. Cream, For Oral Susp.,

Lotion, Oint., Topical Powder, Oral Susp., Tab., Vaginal Suppos., Vaginal Tab., U.S.P. XXI. An antifungal antibiotic derived from cultures of Streptomyces noursei.
Use: Antifungal.
See: Mycostatin Prep. (Squibb)
    Nilstat, Cream, Oint., Tabs. (Lederle)
    Nilstat Oral Drops (Lederle)
    Nilstat Vaginal Tab. (Lederle)
    Nystex, Cream, Oint. (savage)
    O-V Statin, Tab. (Squibb)
W/Clioquinol
    See: Nystaform, Oint. (Miles Pharm)
W/Demethylchlortetracycline.
    See: Declostatin, Caps., Tab. (Lederle)
W/Gramicidin, neomycin, triamcinolone.
    See: Mycolog Cream, Oint. (Squibb)
W/Neomycin base, gramicidin, triamcinolone acetonide.
    See: Mycolog Cream, Oint. (Squibb)
W/Oxytetracycline, glucosamine HCl.
    See: Terrastatin, Cap., Sol. (Pfizer)
W/Tetracycline phosphate buffered.
    See: Achrostatin-V, Cap. (Lederle)
W/Tetracycline phosphate complex.
    See: Tetrex-F, Cap. (Bristol)
• **NYSTATIN AND CLOROQUINOL OINTMENT,** U.S.P. XXI.
Use: Antifungal.
See: Nystaform, Oint. (Miles Pharm).
• **NYSTATIN, NEOMYCIN SULFATE, GRAMICIDIN AND TRIAMCINOLONE ACETONIDE,** U.S.P. XXI. Cream, Oint., U.S.P. XXI.
Use: Antifungal, antibacterial, anti-inflammatory.
See: Mycolog Prods (Squibb)
NYSTEX CREAM & OINTMENT. (Savage) Nystatin 100,000 units/Gm. Tubes 15 Gm., 30 Gm.
Use: Antifungal antibiotic therapy.
NYTILAX. (Mentholatum) Crystalline sennosides A & B calcium salts 12 mg./Tab. Bot. 12s, 24s.
Use: Laxative.
NYTIME COLD MEDICINE. (Rugby) Acetaminophen 1000 mg., doxylamine succinate 7.5 mg., pseudoephedrine HCl 60 mg., dextromethorphan HBr 30 mg./30 ml. w/alcohol 25%. Bot. 6 oz.
Use: Cold therapy.
NYTOL. (Block) Diphenhydramine HCl 25 mg./Tab. Bot. 16s, 32s, 72s.
Use: Sleep aid.

O

OASIS. (Zitar) Artificial saliva. Bot. 6 oz.
Use: To relieve xerostomia.
OATMEAL, GUM FRACTION.
See: Aveeno, Preps. (Cooper)
OBACIN. (Kenyon) Phendimetrazine tartrate 35 mg./Tab. Bot. 100s, 1000s.
Use: Control obesity.
OBALAN. (Lannett) Phendimetrazine tartrate 35 mg./Tab. Bot. 100s, 1000s.

Use: Treatment of obesity.

OBECALP-C. (Western Research) Placebo Capsule. Bot. 1000s.
Use: Placebo

OBECALP-T. (Western Research) Placebo Tablet. Bot. 1000s.
Use: Placebo.

OBEPAR. (Parmed) Phendimetrazine tartrate 35 mg./Tab. Bot. Bot. 100s.
Use: Appetite suppressant.

OBEPAR. (Tyler) Vit. A 3000 I.U., D 300 I.U., B-1 3 mg., B-2 2 mg., nicotinamide 10 mg., B-6 3 mg., Ca pantothenate 2 mg., B-12 3 mcg., C 37.5 mg., Ca 150 mg., Fe 5 mg., Mg 1 mg., Mn 0.1 mg., K 1 mg., Zn 0.15 mg./Cap. Bot. 100s.
Use: Phosphorus-free vitamin-mineral dietary supplement specially recommended for pregnancy.

OBERMINE. (O'Neal, Jones & Feldman) Phentermine HCl 30 mg./Cap. Bot. 1000s.
Use: Anorexiant.

OBESITY AGENTS.
See: Anti-Obesity Agents. (Various Mfr.)

OBE-SLIM. (Jenkins) Amobarbital 50 mg., homatropine methylbromide 7.5 mg., methamphetamine 10 mg./Tab. Bot. 1000s.

OBESTIN-30. (Ferndale) Phentermine HCl 30 mg. /Cap. Bot. 100s, 1000s.
Use: Anorectic.

OBE-TITE. (Scott/Cord) Phendimetrazine tartrate 35 mg./Tab. Bot. 100s, 500s.
Use: Control of obesity.

OBETRIM-T. (Sylvania) Methamphetamine HCl 15 mg., ascorbic acid 60 mg., phenobarbital 15 mg./Tab. or Cap. **Tab.** Bot. 30s, 100s. **Cap.** Bot. 30s, 100s.
Use: Appetite control in obesity.

OBETROL. (Obetrol) Dextroamphetamine saccharate, amphetamine aspartate, amphetamine sulfate, dextroamphetamine sulf. in equal parts. Tab. 10 or 20 mg. Bot. 100s, 500s, 1000s.
Use: Treatment of obesity.

OBETROL-10 TABS. (Obetrol) Dextroamphetamine saccharate 2.5 mg., amphetamine asparate 2.5 mg., amphetamine sulfate 2.5 mg., dextroamphetamine sulfate 2.5 mg./Tab. Bot. 100s, 500s, 1000s.
Use: Treatment of obesity.

OBETROL-20 TABS. (Obetrol) Methamphetamine saccharate 5 mg., amphetamine asparate 5 mg., amphetamine sulfate 5 mg., dextroamphetamine sulfate 5 mg./Tab. Bot. 100s, 500s, 1000s.
Use: Treatment of obesity.

OBEZINE. (Western Research) Phendimetrazine tartrate 35 mg./Tab. Handicount 28 (36 bags of 28s).
Use: Anorexic.

• **OBIDOXIME CHLORIDE.** USAN. 1,1'-(Oxydimethylene)-bis-[4-formylpyridinium]dichloride dioxime.
Use: Cholinesterase reactivator.

OBLATE PLUS. (Haag) Vit. A4000 I.U., D400 I.U., B-1 3 mg., B-2 2 mg., B-6 1 mg., C50 mg., niacinamide 10 mg., B-12 2 mcg., folic acid 1 mg., calcium 230 mg., iron 30 mg., magnesium 0.15 mg., potassium

0.835 mg., iodine 0.01 mg., copper 0.15 mg., manganese 0.05 mg., zinc 0.085 mg./Tab. Bot. 100s.

OB-NATAL. (Geneva) Prenatal multivitamins and minerals/T.R. Tab. Bot. 100s.
Use: Prenatal, lactating dietary supplement.

OB-NATAL PLUS. (Geneva) Prenatal multivitamins and mineral. Bot. 100s.
Use: Vitamin and mineral supplement for prenatal lactating women.

OBRICAL. (Canright) Ca lactate 500 mg., Vit. D 400 I.U., ferrous sulfate exsic. 35 mg., Vit. B-1 1 mg., B-2 1 mg., C 10 mg./Tab. Bot. 100s, 1000s.
Use: Nutritional needs during pregnancy, rapid growth in childhood, convalescence.

OBRICAL-F. (Canright) Ferrous sulf. 50 mg., cal. lactate 500 mg., Vit. D 400 I.U., B-1 1 mg., B-2 1 mg., C 10 mg., folic acid 0.67 mg./Tab. Bot. 100s, 1000s.
Use: Vitamin & mineral supplement.

OBRITE. (Milton Roy) Contact lens and eye glass cleaner. Plastic spray Bot. 30 ml., 55 ml.

OBTUNDIA CALAMINE CREAM. (Otis Clapp) Zinc oxide, calamine, camphorated meta-cresol, lime water. Tube 2 oz. Aidpak 0.11 oz. foilpaks, 36s. Unit box 0.11 oz. foilpaks, 6s.
Use: Topical antipruritic and skin protectant.

OBTUNDIA CREAM. (Otis Clapp) Camphorated meta-cresol, petrolatum, lanolin. Tubes 1¼ oz.; Jars 16 oz.; Aidpaks 0.11 oz. foil pkg. Box 36s.
Use: Bacterostatic, anesthetic, antifungal first aid cream.

OBTUNDIA FIRST AID SPRAY. (Otis Clapp) Camporated meta-cresol. Aerosol can 2.5 oz.
Use: Bactericidal, fungicidal, sporicidal, anesthetic spray.

OBTUNDIA SURGICAL DRESSING. (Otis Clapp) Camphorated meta-cresol. Bot. 0.5 oz., 4 oz. Swab Pads Box 10s; Aid Packs 100s.
Use: Bactericidal, fungicidal, sporicidal, anesthetic liquid.

OB-VIT. (Scrip) Vit. A 4000 I.U., D 400 I.U., B-1 2.0 mg., B-2 2.0 mg., C 100 mg., calcium 400 mg., iron 115 mg., oyster shell calcium carbonate 500 mg., folic acid 0.1 mg., B-12 2.0 mcg./Tab. Bot. 90s.

OBY-TRIM. (Rexar) Phentermine HCl 30 mg./Cap. Bot. 1000s
Use: Treatment of obesity.

OC-250. (Western Research) Vitamin C 250 mg./Chewable Tab. Handicount 28s (36 bags of 28s).
Use: Vitamin supplement.

O-CAL-FA. (Pharmics) Iron 66 mg., calcium 200 mg., A 8000 I.U., C 90 mg., D 400 I.U., B-6 4 mg., B-1 3 mg., B-2 2 mg., niacinamide 15 mg., B-12 2.5 mcg., folic acid 1 mg., sod. fluoride 1.1 mg., iodine 0.15 mg., manganese sulfate 0.5 mg., copper sulfate 0.25 mg., potassium iodide 0.05 mg., magnesium 1 mg., zinc sulfate 0.5 mg./Tab. Bot. 100s.
Use: Vitamin & mineral supplementation.

OCUSERT. (Ciba) Pilocarpine.
Pilo-20: Releases 20 mcg. pilocarpine/hour for one week. Pkg. 8s.

Pilo-40: Releases 40 mcg. pilocarpine/hour for one week. Pkg. 8s.
Use: Control of elevated intraocular pressure.
OCEAN. (Fleming) Sod. chloride 0.65% w/benzyl alcohol. Bot. 45 cc., pt., gal.
OCEAN PLUS. (Fleming) Caffeine 2.5% w/benzyl alcohol. Bot. 15 cc.
• **OCRYLATE.** USAN. Octyl 2-cyano-acrylate.
Use: Surgical aid (tissue adhesive).
• **OCTABENZONE.** USAN. 2-Hydroxy-4-(octyloxy) benzophenone. Spectra-Sorb UV 531. Under study.
Use: Sunscreen agent.
OCTACOSACTRIN. B.A.N. α- Corticotrophin
Use: Corticotrophic peptide.
9-OCTADECANOIC ACID. Oleic acid, N.F. XVI.
OCTADECANOIC ACID.
See: Stearic Acid, N.F. XVI.
OCTADECANOIC ACID, SODIUM SALT.
See: Sodium Stearate, N.F. XVI.
OCTADECANOIC ACID, ZINC SALT.
See: Zinc Stearate, N.F. XVI.
I-OCTADECANOL.
See: Stearyl Alcohol, N.F. XVI.
• **OCTANOIC ACID.** USAN.
OCTAPHONIUM CHLORIDE. B.A.N. Benzyldiethyl-2-[4-(1,1,3,3-tetramethylbutyl)phenoxy]-ethylammonium chloride. Octaphen; Phenoctide.
Use: Antiseptic.
OCTAREX. (Approved) Vit. A 5000 I.U., D 1000 I.U., B-1 1.5 mg., B-2 2 mg., B-6 0.1 mg., cal. pantothenate 1 mg., niacinamide 20 mg., C 37.5 mg., E 1 I.U., B-12 1 mcg./Cap. Bot. 100s, 1000s.
OCTATROPINE METHYLBROMIDE. B.A.N. Anisotropine methylbromide. 2-Propyl-pentanoylmethyltropinium bromide. 8-Methyl-O-(2-propylvaleryl)-tropinium bromide.
Use: Anticholinergic.
See: Valpin, Elix., Tab. (Du Pont)
OCTAVERINE. B.A.N. 6,7-Dimethoxy-1-(3,4,5-triethoxyphenyl)isoquinoline.
Use: Antispasmodic.
OCTAVIMS. (Approved) Vit. A 6000 I.U., D 1250 I.U., C 50 mg., E 5 I.U., B-1 3 mg., B-2 3 mg., B-6 0.5 mg., niacinamide 20 mg., Ca pantothenate 5 mg., B-12 5 mcg., calcium 59 mg., phosphorus 45 mg./Cap. Bot. 100s, 250s, 1000s.
• **OCTAZAMIDE.** USAN.
Use: Analgesic.
• **OCTENIDINE HYDROCHLORIDE.** USAN.
Use: Anti-infective, topical.
• **OCTICIZER.** USAN. 2-Ethylhexyl diphenyl phosphate. Santicizer 141 (Monsanto). SCAN Spray-On. (Johnson & Johnson)
Use: Pharmaceutic aid (plasticizer).
• **OCTOCRYLENE.** USAN.
Use: Ultraviolet screen.
• **OCTODRINE.** USAN. 1,5-Dimethylhexylamine. Under study.
Use: Vasoconstrictor, local anesthetic.
OCTOFOLLIN.
See: Benzestrol U.S.P. XXI.

L-threo-αD-galacto-OCTOPYRANOSIDE, METHYL 7-CHLORO-6,7,8-TRIDEOXY-6-[[(1-METHYL-4-PROPYL-2-PYRROLIDINYL)-CARBONYL]AMINO]-I-THIO, (2S-trans)-MONOHYDROCHLORIDE. Clindamycin Hydrochloride, U.S.P. XXI.
D-erythro-α-D-galacto-OCTOPYRANOSIDE, METHYL 6,8-DIDEOXY-6-[[(1-METHYL-4-PROPYL-2-PYRROLIDINYL)CARBONYL]-AMINO]-1-THIO, MONOHYDROCHLORIDE. MONOHYDRATE. Lincomycin Hydrochloride, U.S.P. XXI.
• **OCTOXYNOL 9,** N.F. XVI.
Use: Surfactant.
• **OCTRIPTYLINE PHOSPHATE.** USAN.
Use: Antidepressant.
• **OCTRIZOLE.** USAN.
Use: Ultraviolet screen.
N-OCTYL BICYALOHEPTENE DICARBOSIMIDE. W/N-N-diethyl-m-toluamide, 2,3,4,5-bis-(delta-2-butylene) tetrahydrofurfural, Di-n-propyl isocinchomeronate, other isomers, isopropanol.
See: Bansum, Bot. (Summers)
OCTYLPHENOXY POLYETHOXYETHANOL. A mono-ether of a polyethylene glycol. Igepal CA 630 (Antara).
W/Phenylmercuric acetate, methylparaben, sodium borate.
See: Lorophyn jelly, Supp. (Eaton)
W/Lactic acid, sodium lactate.
See: Jeneen premeasured liquid douche (Norwich)
OCU-BATH. (Commerce) Bot. 4 oz.
Use: Eye lotion.
OCU-DROP. (Commerce) Bot. 0.5 oz.
Use: Eye drops.
• **OCUFILCON A.** USAN.
Use: Contact lens material.
• **OCUFILCON B.** USAN.
Use: Contact lens material.
• **OCUFILCON C.** USAN.
Use: Contact lens material.
OCUMETER.
See: Decadron Phosphate, Prep. (Merck Sharp & Dohme)
Humorsol, Ophth. Sol. (Merck Sharp & Dohme)
Neo-Decadron, Prep. (Merck Sharp & Dohme)
OCURINS. (Softcon) Sod. chloride 0.85%, buffering agents, thimerosal 0.001%, disodium edetate 0.1%. Plastic squeeze Bot. 7½ fl. oz.
Use: Ophthalmic irrigating procedures.
OC-U-ZIN Ophth. Sol. (Blue Line) (w/v) Zinc sulfate 0.25%, boric acid 2%, phenylephrine HCl 0.12%, sodium borate with benzalkonium chloride 1:10,000. Plastic squeeze Bot. 15 cc.
Use: Superficial irritations of the eye.
ODALATE. (Kenyon) Chlorpheniramine maleate 8 mg., phenylpropanolamine HCl 50 mg., atropine sulfate 0.36 mg./Cap. Bot. 100s, 1000s.
ODARA. (Lorvic) Alcohol 48%, carbolic acid less than 2%, zinc chloride, potassium iodide, glycerin, methyl salicylate, oil eucalyptus, tinct. myrrh. **Conc. Liq.** Bot. 8 oz.
Use: Mouthwash, gargle and general antiseptic.

ODONIL. (Kenyon) dl-Methionine 200 mg./Cap. Bot. 100s, 1000s.

ODOR-SCRIP. (Scrip) Dl-methionine 0.3 Gm./Cap. Bot. 100s.
Use: Treatment of diaper rash in infants.

OESTERGON.
See: Estradiol (Various Mfr.)

OESTRADIOL.
See: Estradiol (Various Mfr.)

OESTRASID.
See: Dienestrol (Various Mfr.)

OESTRIN.
See: Estrone (Various Mfr.)

OESTRIOL SUCCINATE. B.A.N. Oestra-1,3,5-(10)-triene-3,16α,17β-triol 16,17-di(hydrogen succinate).
Use: Treatment of thrombocytopenic hemorrhage.

OESTRIOL SODIUM SUCCINATE. B.A.N. Oestra-1,3,-5(10)-triene-3,16α,17β-di(sodium succinate).
Use: Treatment of thrombocytopenic hemorrhage.

OESTROFORM.
See: Estrone (Various Mfr.)

OESTROMENIN.
See: Diethylstilbestrol (Various Mfr.)

OESTROMON.
See: Diethylstilbestrol (Various Mfr.)

OFF-EZY CORN REMOVER. (Commerce) Flexible collodion, salicylic acid, camphor. Bot. 0.45 oz.
Use: Corn remover.

OFF-EZY WART REMOVER. (Commerce) Flexible collodion, salicylic acid. Bot. 0.45 oz.

O-FLEX. (Seatrace) Orphenadrine citrate 30 mg./ml. Vial 10 cc.

OGEN. (Abbott) Estropipate. **Tab. 0.625:** 0.75 mg. Estropipate/Tab. Bot. 100s. **Tab. 1.25:** 1.5 mg. Estropipate/Tab. Bot. 100s. **Tab. 2.5:** 3 mg. Estropipate/Tab. Bot. 100s. **Tab. 5.:** 6 mg. Estropipate/Tab. Bot. 100s.
Use: Estrogen deficiency states.

OGEN VAGINAL CREAM. (Abbott) Estropipate 1.5 mg./Gm. Tube 1½ oz. w/applicator.
Use: Atrophic vaginitis and kraurosis vulvae.

OILATUM SOAP. (Stiefel) A neutral soap containing 7½% protein-free, low viscosity, readily absorbed polyunsaturated vegetable oil. Bars 4.0 oz. or 5.8 oz./Cake. Scented or unscented.
Use: Hypoallergenic cleansing of dry, tender or irritated skin.

OIL FOR USE. (DeWitt) Bot. ½ oz. w/dropper.
Use: Ear drops.

OIL OF CAMPHOR W/COMBINATIONS.
See: Sloan's Liniment, Liq. (Warner-Lambert)

OIL OF CLOVES W/ALCOHOL.
See: Buckley "Z.O.", Liq.(Crosby)

OIL OF PINE W/COMBINATIONS.
See: Sloan's Liniment, Liq. (Warner-Lambert)

OIL-O-SOL. (Health Care Industries) Corn oil 52%, Castor Oil 40.8%, camphor 6.8%, hexylresorcinol 0.1%. Bot. 1 oz., 2 oz., 4 oz.
Use: For minor cuts, scratches, surface abrasions, sunburn.

OINT-EAST OINTMENT. (Guild) Pkg. 2⅛ oz.

OINTMENT BASE, WASHABLE.
See: Absorbent Base (Upsher-Smith)
Cetaphil, Cream, Lot. (Owen)
Velvachol, Cream (Owen)

• **OINTMENT, HYDROPHILIC,** U.S.P. XXI.
Use: Pharm. aid (oil-in-water emulsion ointment base).

• **OINTMENT, WHITE,** U.S.P. XXI.
Use: Pharm. aid (oleaginous ointment base).

• **OINTMENT, YELLOW,** U.S.P. XXI.
Use: Ointment base.

• **OLAFLUR.** USAN.
Use: Dental caries prophylactic.

OLAMINE.
See: Ethanolamine

OLAQUINDOX. B.A.N. 2-(2-Hydroxyethylcarbamoyl)-3-methylquinoxaline 1,4-dioxide.
Use: Growth promoter; bactericide, veterinary medicine.

OLDEROL. (Doral) Vit. B-1 15 mg., B-2 10 mg., niacinamide 100 mg., B-6 5 mg., B-12 4 mcg., Capantothenate 20 mg., folic acid 150 mcg., C 750 mg., E 30 I.U.,/Cap. Bot. 60s.
Use: Therapeutic vitamin supplement.

OLEANDOMYCIN. B.A.N. An antibiotic from Streptomyces antibioticus.
See: Matromycin; Romicil

OLEANDOMYCIN PHOSPHATE. Phosphate of an antibacterial substance produced by *Streptomyces antibioticus*.
Use: Infections caused by susceptible gram-positive and gram-negative organisms.

OLEANDOMYCIN SALT OF PENICILLIN.
See: Pen-M (Pfizer) Under study.

OLEANDOMYCIN, TRIACETYL. Troleandomycin USP XX.

OLEIC ACID, N.F. XVI. 9-Octadecanoic acid.
Use: Pharm. aid (emulsion adjunct).

• **OLEIC ACID I-131.** USAN.
Raoleic Acid-131 (Abbott)
Use: Radioactive agent.

• **OLEIC ACID I-125.** USAN.
Use: Radioactive agent.

OLEIN OZONIDE.

OLEORESINS OF PLANTS. (Hollister-Stier) Oleoresins of plants in acetone or petrolatum, and in corn oil. Plant patch test materials in applicator vials, singly or in sets, regionalized or grouped for specific needs.
Use: Diagnosis of contact dermatitis from plants.

OLEOVITAMIN A, Vitamin A, U.S.P. XXI.

• **OLEOVITAMIN A & D,** U.S.P. XXI. Cap., U.S.P. XXI.
Use: Vit. A & D therapy.
See: Super-D, Perles, Liq. (Upjohn)

• **OLEOVITAMIN D, SYNTHETIC.**
Use: Vitamin D replacement therapy.
See: Viosterol in Oil.

• **OLEYL ALCOHOL,** N.F. XVI. (Z)-9-Octadecen-1-ol.
Use: Emulsifying agent; emollient.

OLIVE OIL, N.F. XVI.
Use: Emollient, pharm. aid (setting retardant for dental cements).

OMBRE EXTRA STRENGTH. (Edward J. Moore) Vit.

A palmitate, D, B-1, B-2, B-6, B-12, niacinamide, Ca pantothenate, ascorbic acid./Tab. Bot. 50s, 100s.

OMEGA OIL. (Block) Methyl nicotinate, methyl salicylate, capsicum oleoresin, histamine dihydrochloride, isopropyl alcohol 48%. Bot. 2½ oz., 4.85 oz.
Use: External analgesic.

OMNIBEL. (Delta) Butabarbital 15 mg., atropine sulfate 0.0194 mg., hyoscyamine sulfate 0.1037 mg., hyoscine hydrobromide 0.0065 mg., Tab. 100s.
Use: Antispasmodic, antisecretory sedative.

OMNICOL. (Delta) Dextromethorphan HBr 15 mg., chlorpheniramine maleate 4 mg., phenylephrine HCl 5 mg., phenindamine tartrate 4 mg., salicylamide 227 mg., acetaminophen 100 mg., caffeine alkaloid 10 mg., ascorbic acid 25 mg./Tab. Bot. 100s, Bot. Pt.
Use: Antitussive, decongestant, antihistaminic, analgesic.

OMNIHEMIN. (Delta) Iron 110 mg., C 150 mg., B-12 7.5 mcg., folic acid 1.0 mg., zinc 1.0 mg., Cu 1.0 mg., Mn 1.0 mg., Mg 1.0 mg./Tab. or 5 ml. **Tab.** Bot. 100s., **Soln.** Bot. pt.
Use: Hematinic.

OMNI-M TABLETS. (Blue Cross) Vitamins & Minerals for people 12 years old and older. Bot. 100s.
Use: Supplement.

OMNINATAL. (Delta) Iron 60 mg., copper 2 mg., zinc 15 mg., Vit. A 8000 I.U., D 400 I.U. C 90 mg., Ca 200 mg., folic acid 1.5 mg., B-1 2.5 mg., B-2 3 mg., niacinamide 20 mg., pyridoxine HCl 10 mg., pantothenic acid 15 mg., B-12 8 mcg./Tab. Bot. 100s.
Use: Vitamin-mineral supplement.

OMNIPEN. (Wyeth) Anhydrous ampicillin 250 mg./Cap. Bot. 100s, 500s; Redipak 100s, 500 mg./Cap. Bot. 100s, 500s; Redipak 100s. For oral suspension 125 mg. or 250 mg./5 cc. to make 80 cc., 100 cc., 150 cc., 200 cc. 500 mg./5 cc. to make 100 cc. Drops, 100 mg./cc. Bot. w/dropper to make 20 cc.
Use: Antibiotic.

OMNIPEN-N. (Wyeth) Sod. ampicillin 125 mg., 250 mg., 500 mg., 1 Gm. or 2 Gm./Vial. Pkg. 10s. 10 Gm./Vial. Pkg. 1s.
Use: Antibiotic.

OMNITABS. (Blue Cross) Vit A 5000 I.U., D 400 I.U., C 50 mg., B-1 3 mg., B-2 2.5 mg., niacin 20 mg., B-6 1 mg., B-12 1 mcg., pantothenic acid 0.9 mg./Tab. Bot. 100s.
Use: Vitamin supplement.

OMNITABS WITH IRON. (Blue Cross) Vit. A 5000 I.U., D 400 I.U., B-1 3 mg., B-2 2.5 mg., B-6 1 mg., B-12 1 mcg., C 50 mg., niacinamide 20 mg. calcium pantothenate 1 mg., iron 15 mg./Tab. Bot. 100s.
Use: Multivitamin with iron.

OMNITRATE. (Kenyon) Vit. A 6000 I.U., D 600 I.U., E 0.1 mg., B-1 1.0 mg., B-2 0.1 mg., B-6 0.1 mg., C 37.5 mg., B-12 1 mcg., niacinamide 15 mg., folic acid 0.067 mg., hesperidin 50 mg., Ca carbonate 400 mg., iron-ferrous iodide dried 20 mg., Mg 15 mg., iodine 0.15 mg., Mn 3 mg., Zn 3 mg./3 Cap. Bot. 1000s.
Use: Vitamin mineral supplement.

OMNIZOLE. (MSD AGVET) Thiabendazole. **Boluses:** 2 Gm., 15 Gm., **Crumbles:** 6.6%; **Paste:** 43%; **Suspension:** 4 Gm./oz.
Use: Anthelmintic, veterinary medicine.

OMNIZOLE-SIX. (MSD AGVET) Thiabendazole 6 Gm./oz. Suspension.
Use: Anthelmintic, veterinary medicine.

ONCOVIN. (Lilly) Vincristine sulfate injection. 1 mg./ml., 2 mg./2 ml. or 5 mg./5 ml.
Use: Treatment of acute leukemia in children.

ONDONID. Cyclofenil, B.A.N.

ONE-A-DAY ENRICHED B COMPLEX. (Miles) B-1 10 mg., B-2 9 mg., niacin 85 mg., B-6 9.5 mg., folic acid 400 mcg., B-12 30 mcg., biotin 30 mcg., pantothenic acid 18.5 mg., choline 5 mg., inositol 5 mg., phosphorus 100 mg./Tab. Bot. 100s.
Use: High potency B-complex supplement for adults.

ONE-A-DAY ENRICHED C 500. (Miles) Vit. C 500 mg., zinc 5 mg./Tab. Bot. 90s.
Use: Supplement for adults.

ONE-A-DAY ENRICHED E 400 WITH SELENIUM. (Miles) Vit. E 400 I.U., selenium 25 mcg./Tab. Bot. 60s.
Use: Supplement for adults.

ONE-A-DAY ESSENTIAL. (Miles) Vit. A 5000 I.U., E 30 I.U., C 60 mg., folic acid 0.4 mg., B-1 1.5 mg., B-2 1.7 mg., niacin 20 mg., B-6 2.0 mg., B-12 6.0 mcg., K 50 mcg.; pantothenic acid 10 mg., biotin 30 mcg., D 400 I.U./Tab. Bot., 60s, 100s, 250s, 365s.
Use: Multivitamin supplement.

ONE-A-DAY PLUS EXTRA C. (Miles) Vit. A 5000 I.U., E 30 I.U., C 500 mg., Folic acid 0.4 mg., B-1 1.5 mg., B-2 1.7 mg., niacin 20 mg., B-6 2 mg., B-12 6 mcg., K 50 mcg.; pantothenic acid 10 mg., biotin 30 mcg., D 400 I.U./Tab. Bot. 60s.
Use: High potency vitamin C with 9 essential vitamins.

ONE-A-DAY PLUS IRON. (Miles) Vit. A 5000 I.U., E 30 I.U., C 60 mg., folic acid 0.4 mg., B-1 1.5 mg., B-2 1.7 mg., niacin 20.0 mg., B-6 2.0 mg., B-12 6.0 mcg., K 50 mcg.; pantothenic acid 10 mg., biotin 30 mcg., D 400 I.U., iron 18 mg./Tab. Bot. 60s, 100s, 240s, 365s.
Use: Multivitamin supplement with iron.

ONE-A-DAY PLUS MINERALS. (Miles) Vit. A 5000 I.U., E 30 I.U., C 60 mg., folic acid 0.4 mg., B-1 1.5 mg., B-2 1.7 mg., niacin 20 mg., B-6 2 mg., B-12 6 mcg., K 50 mcg., D 400 I.U., pantothenic acid 10 mg., iron 18 mg., Ca 129.6 mg., P 100 mg., iodine 150 mcg., Mg 100 mg., Cu 2 mg., Cr 10 mcg., selenium 10 mcg., molybdenum 10 mcg., Mn 2.5 mg., potassium 37.5 mg., biotin 30 mcg., chloride 34 mg., Zn 15 mg./Tab. Bot. 30s, 60s, 100s.
Use: Vitamin and mineral supplement.

ONE-A-DAY STRESSGARD. (Miles) Vit. A 5000 I.U., C 600 mg., B-1 15 mg., B-2 10 mg., niacin 100 mg., D 400 I.U., E 30 I.U., B-6 5 mg., K 50 mc., folic acid 400 mcg., B-12 12 mcg., pantothenic acid 20 mg., iron 18 mg., zinc 15 mg., Cu 2 mg.
Use: Vitamin B complex plus C stress formula.

ONE ONLY VITAMIN TABLETS. (Robinson) Vit. A 5000 I.U., D 400 I.U., B-1 2 mg., B-2 2.5 mg., B-6 1

mg., B-12 1 mcg., niacinamide 20 mg., panthenol 1 mg./Tab. Bot. 100s, 250s, 1000s.
Use: Dietary supplement.

ONE ONLY VITAMIN TABLETS WITH IRON. (Robinson) Vit. A 5000 I.U., D 400 I.U., B-1 2 mg., B-2 2.5 mg., C 50 mg., B-6 1 mg., B-12 1 mcg., niacinamide 20 mg., calcium pantothenate 1 mg., iron 15 mg./Tab. Bot. 100s, 250s, 1000s.
Use: Dietary supplement.

1000-BC, IM OR IV. (Reid-Provident) Vit. B-1 25 mg., B-2 2.5 mg., B-6 5 mg., panthenol 5 mg., B-12 500 mcg., niacin-amide 75 mg., Vit. C 100 mg./cc. Vial 10 cc.
Use: Vitamin supplement.

1+1 CREME. (Dunhall) Pramoxine HCl 1%, hydrocortisone 1%. Tube 1 oz.
Use: Anesthetic, anti-inflammatory.

1+1-F CREME. (Dunhall) Hydrocortisone 1%, pramoxine HCl 1%, clioquinol 3%. Tube 1 oz.
Use: Anesthetic, anti-inflammatory, anti-fungal, anti-bacterial.

1-2-3 OINTMENT NO. 20. (Durel) Burow's solution, lanolin, zinc oxide (Lassar's paste). Jars 1 oz., lb., 6 lb.
Use: Nummular eczema, hand eczema, and other localized eczematous processes.

1-2-3 OINTMENT NO. 21. (Durel) Burow's solution 1 part, lanolin 2, zinc oxide (Lassar's paste) 1.5, cold cream 1.5. Jars 1 oz., lb., 6 lb.
Use: Nummular eczema, hand eczema, and other localized eczematous processes.

ONOTON TABLETS. (Winthrop Products) Pancreatin, hemicellulose, oxbile extracts.
Use: Pancreatic deficiency and dyspepsia.

ONSET-5 TABLETS. (Bock) Isosorbide dinitrate 5 mg./Chewable Tab. Bot. 100s, 1000s.
Use: Cardiovascular.

ONSET-10 TABLETS. (Bock) Isosorbide dinitrate 10 mg./Chewable Tab. Bot. 100s, 1000s.
Use: Cardiovascular.

ONTOSEIN.
See: Orgotein (Diagnostic Data)

OPHTHA LIPO CAPSULES. (Misemer) Bot. 100s.

OPHTHA P/S. (Misemer) Sodium sulfacetamide 100 mg., prednisolone acetate 5 mg./ml.
Use: Treatment eye infections.

OPHTHACET EYE DROPS. (Vortech) Sulfacetamide sod. 10%, methylcellulose 0.5%, boric acid with sod. bisulfite 0.1%, disodium EDTA 0.05%, thimerosal 0.01%. Bot. ½ oz. w/dropper.
Use: Antibacterial (ophthalmic).

OPHTHAINE HCl. (Squibb) Proparacaine 2-Diethylaminoethyl-3-amino-4-propoxybenzoate HCl 0.5%, glycerin 2.45%, chlorobutanol 0.2%, benzalkonium chloride, sod. hydroxide or hydrochloric acid to adjust pH. Sol Bot. w/dropper 15 cc.
Use: Topical anesthesia for the eye.

OPHTHALGAN. (Ayerst) Glycerin ophthalmic solution w/chlorobutanol (chloral derivative 0.55%) as preservative. Bot. 7.5 ml./Dropper screw cap.
Use: Corneal edema. Diagnostic.

OPHTHALMIC 0.5% AND 1.5%. (Columbia) Hydrocortisone acetate 5 mg. & 15 mg., neomycin sulfate 5 mg./Gm. Tube ⅛ oz.

OPHTHETIC OPHTHALMIC SOLUTION. (Allergan) Proparacaine HCl 0.5%, benzalkonium chloride. Dropper bot. 15 ml.
Use: Topical ophthalmic anesthesia.

OPHTHOCHLOR. (Parke-Davis) Chloramphenicol 5 mg./ml. in a boric acid-sod. borate buffer sol., with sod. hydroxide to adjust pH. Plastic Drop. Bot. 15 ml.
Use: Ophthalmic solution.

OPHTHOCORT. (Parke-Davis) Chloramphenicol 10 mg., hydrocortisone acetate 5 mg., polymyxin B sulfate 5,000 u./Gm. in liquid pet., polyethylene base. Tube 3.5 Gm.
Use: Ocular inflammation and infection.

OPIPRAMOL. B.A.N. 5- 3-[4-(2-Hydroxyethyl)-piperazin-1-yl]propyl -dibenz[b,f]azepine.
Use: Antidepressant.
See: Insidon dihydrochloride

• **OPIPRAMOL HYDROCHLORIDE.** USAN. 4-[3-(5H-Dibenz[b,f]azepin-5yl)-propyl]-1-piperazine-ethanol dihydrochloride.
Use: Antidepressant, tranquilizer.

• **OPIUM, U.S.P. XXI.**
Use: Pharm. necessity for powdered opium.

OPIUM ALKALOIDS, TOTAL, AS THE HYDROCHLORIDE SALT.
See: Pantopon, Amp. (Roche)

OPIUM AND BELLADONNA. (Wyeth) Powd. opium 60 mg., ext. belladonna 0.25 gr./Supp. Box 20s.

• **OPIUM POWDER.,** U.S.P. XXI.
Use: Pharmaceutical necessity for Paregoric.

W/Albumin tannate, colloidal kaolin, pectin.
See: Ekrised, Tab. (Mallard)

W/Atropine sulfate, alcohol.
See: Stopit Liq. (Scrip)

W/Belladonna extr.
See: B & O, Supp. (Webcon)

W/Bismuth subgallate, Zn phenolsulfonate, kaolin.
See: B-K-Z Tablets (Sutliff & Case)

W/Bismuth subgallate, kaolin, pectin, zinc phenolsulfonate.
See: Amogel, Tab. (Vortech)
Diastay, Tab. (Elder)
Laudacin, Liq. (Sutliff & Case)

W/Kaolin, pectin.
See: Keoparic, Susp. (Blue Line)

W/Kaolin, pectin, bismuth subcarbonate.
See: KBP/O, Cap. (Cole)

W/Kaolin, pectin, hyoscyamine sulfate, atropine sulfate, hyoscine HBr.
See: Donnagel-PG, Susp. (Robins)

W/Ipecac pow., acetophenetidin, atropine sulf., acetylsalicylic acid, camphor monobromated, caffeine.
See: Dophenco, Cap. (Blue Line)

W/Ipecac powder, phenacetin, aspirin, camphor monobromated, caffeine, anhydrous, atropine sulfate.
See: Phenatracops, Cap. (O'Neal)

W/Ipecac pow., phenacetin, atropine sulfate, monobromated camphor, methapyrilene HCl, salicylamide, caffeine.

See: Phenatrohist, Cap. (O'Neal)
• **OPIUM TINCTURE,** U.S.P. XXI.
W/Homatropine MBr, Pectin.
See: Dia-Quel, Liq. (I.P.C.)
W/Pectin.
See: Opecto, Elixir. (Bowman)
Parelixir, Liq. (Purdue Frederick)
OPIUM TINCTURE, CAMPHORATED.
Use: Antiperistaltic.
See: Paregoric, U.S.P. XXI.
W/Glycyrrhiza fl. ext., tartar emetic, glycerin.
See: Brown Mixture
OP-THAL-ZIN. (Alcon) Zinc sulfate 0.25%, in sterile buffered solution. Drop-Tainer Bot. 0.5 oz.
Use: Ophthalmic astringent.
OPTHOCORT OINT. (Parke-Davis) Chloramphenicol 1%, hydrocortisone acetate 0.5%, polymyxin B sulfate 5000 u./Gm., petrolatum and polyethylene base. Tube 3.5 Gm.
OPTI-BON EYE DROPS. (Barrows) Phenylephrine HCl, berberine sulfate, boric acid, sodium chloride, sodium bisulfite, glycerine, camphor water, peppermint water, thimerosal 0.004%. Bot. 1 oz.
Use: Ophthalmic sterile solution.
OPTICAPS. (Approved) Vit. A 32,500 I.U., D 3250 I.U., B-1 15 mg., B-2 5 mg., B-6 0.5 mg., C 150 mg., E 5 I.U., Ca. pantothenate 3 mg., niacinamide 150 mg., B-12 20 mcg., iron 11.26 mg., choline bitartrate 30 mg., inositol 30 mg., pepsin 32.5 mg., diastase 32.5 mg., Ca 30 mg., phos. 25 mg., Mg. 0.7 mg., Fr. dicalcium phos. 110 mg., Mn 1.3 mg., pot. 0.68 mg., Zn 0.45 mg., hesperidin comp. 25 mg., biotin 20 mcg., Brewer's yeast 50 mg., wheat germ oil 20 mg., hydrol. yeast 81.25 mg., protein digest. 47.04 mg., amino acids 34.21 mg./Cap. Bot. 30s, 60s, 90s, 1000s.
Use: Multiple vitamins with minerals.
OPTI-CLEAN. (Alcon) Thimerosal 0.004% w/surfactant and micropolymeric beads. Bot. 12 ml.
Use: Daily cleaning for soft & hard contact lenses.
OPTILETS-500. (Abbott) Vit. B-1 15 mg., B-2 10 mg., niacinamide 100 mg., pantothenate 20 mg., B-6 5 mg., C 500 mg., A 10,000 I.U., D 400 I.U., E 30 I.U., B-12 12 mcg./Filmtab. Bot. 30s, 100s.
OPTILETS-M-500. (Abbott) Vit. C 500 mg., niacinamide 100 mg., Ca pantothenate 20 mg., B-1 15 mg., Vit. A 10,000 I.U., B-2 10 mg., B-6 5 mg., D 400 I.U., B-12 12 mcg., E 30 I.U. Fe 20 mg., Mg 80 mg., Zn 1.5 mg., Cu 2 mg., Mn 1 mg., iodine 0.15 mg./Filmtab. Bot. 100s & 30s.
Use: Vitamin-mineral therapy.
OPTIMINE. (Schering) Azatadine maleate 1 mg./Tab. Bot. 100s.
Use: Antihistamine.
OPTIMYD. (Schering) Prednisolone phos. 0.5%, sod. sulfacetamide 10%, sod. thiosulfate, tyloxapol, disodium edetate, monobasic sod. phosphate, dibasic sod. phosphate, sod. hydroxide to adjust pH, purified water, benzalkonium chloride 0.025% and phenylethyl alcohol 0.5% as preservatives combined in a clear aqueous sol. Solution-Sterile. Plas. Drop Bot. 5 ml.
Use: Steroid ophthalmic solution.

OPTISED SOL. (Ketchum) Zinc sulfate 0.025%, phenylephrine HCl 0.12%. Bot. 15 cc.
Use: Decongestant emollient-astringent.
OPTO-MIST. (Ketchum) Sod. propionate, sod. chloride, camphor, peppermint oil. Bot. ½ oz.
OPTREX. (CMC) Eye bath Bot. 4 oz., 8 oz. Eye drops Bot. ½ oz.
OPTULLE. (CMC) Sterile dressings. 24s.
ORABASE. (Hoyt) Gelatin, pectin, sod. carboxy methylcellulose in hydrocarbon gel w/polyethylene and mineral oil. 0.75 gm Packet Boxs 100s. Tube 5 Gm., 15 Gm.
Use: Oral protective paste for minor irritations of mouth and gums.
ORABASE HCA. (Hoyt) Hydrocortisone acetate 0.5% in paste base. Packets 0.75 Gm. Box 100s. Tube 5 Gm., 15 Gm.
Use: Adjunctive treatment of oral lesions.
ORABASE WITH BENZOCAINE. (Hoyt) Benzocaine 20% in paste base. Packets 0.75 Gm. Box 100s. Tube 5 Gm., 15 Gm.
Use: Topical anesthetic and emollient for oral lesions
ORABILIX SODIUM. Buniodyl, B.A.N.
ORACIN. (Vicks) Benzocaine 6.25 mg., menthol 0.1%/Regular Loz. Menthol 0.08%/Cherry Loz. in sorbitol base. Contains FDC Yellow #5 tartrazine. Pkg. 18s.
Use: Cooling throat lozenges.
ORADERM LIP BALM. (Schattner) Sod. phenolate, sod. tetraborate, phenol, base containing an anionic emulsifier. ⅛ oz.
Use: Anesthetic & antiseptic.
ORADEX-C. (Commerce) Cetylpyridinium chloride 2.5 mg., benzocaine 10 mg./Troche. Bot. 10s.
Use: Antibacterial anesthetic throat troches.
ORADEXON. Dexamethasone, B.A.N.
ORADRATE. (Coast) Chloral hydrate 500 mg./Cap. Bot. 100s, 500s.
Use: Sedative-hypnotic.
ORAFIX MEDICATED. (Norcliff Thayer) Allantoin 0.2%, Benzocaine 2%. Tube 0.75 oz.
Use: Analgesic denture adhesive for denture sore gums.
ORAFIX ORIGINAL. (Norcliff Thayer) Denture adhesive. Tube 1.5 oz., 2.5 oz., 4 oz.
ORAFIX SPECIAL. (Norcliff Thayer) Denture adhesive. Tube 1.4 oz., 2.4 oz.
ORAFLEX. (Lilly) Benoxaprofen
Note: Withdrawn from market in 1982.
ORA-FRESH. (A.V.P.) Sugar-free non-alcoholic, non-toxic, flavored mouthwash. Bot. 1 oz. Unit dose cup.
Use: Mouthwash after oral surgery.
ORAGRAFIN CALCIUM GRANULES. (Squibb) Ipodate calcium 3 Gm./8 Gm. Pkg. 25 × 1 dose pkg.
Use: Radiopaque substance.
ORAGRAFIN SODIUM CAPSULES. (Squibb) Ipodate sodium 0.5 Gm./Cap. Bot. 100s. Unimatic pkg. 100s. Card 6s. Box 25s.
Use: Radiopaque substance.
ORAGULANT. Diphenadione, B.A.N.

ORAHEMA SOLU-CAPS. (Sutliff & Case) Ferrous fumarate 200 mg., Zn 1 mg., Mn 5 mg., Cu 0.25 mg., Vit. C 30 mg., B-12 1 mcg., B-1 1 mg., B-2 1.2 mg./Solu-cap. Bot. 100s, 1000s.
Use: Multivitamin with minerals.
W/Folic acid 0.5 mg. Bot. 100s, 1000s.
Use: Nutritional supplement.
ORAHESIVE POWDER. (Hoyt) Gelatin, pectin, sodium carboxymethylcellulose. Bot. 25 Gm.
Use: Denture adhesive.
ORAHIST TR. (Vangard) Chlorpheniramine maleate 8 mg., phenylpropanolamine HCl 50 mg., isopropanide iodide 2.5 mg./T.R. Cap. Bot. 100s, 1000s.
Use: Antihistamine, Decongestant.
ORA-JEL. (Commerce) Benzocaine in a special base. Tube 0.2 oz., 0.5 oz.
Use: Temporary relief of toothache pain.
ORA-JEL BABY. (Commerce) Benzocaine in a special base. Tube 0.5 oz.
Use: Teething pain.
ORAJEL BRACE-AID ORAL ANESTHETIC GEL. (Commerce) Benzocaine 20%, allantoin 0.5%. Tube 0.5 oz.
Use: Relieves pain, soreness and irritations due to braces.
ORAJEL BRACE-AID ORAL HYGIENIC RINSE. (Commerce) Carbamide peroxide 10% in anhydrous glycerin. Tube 1 oz.
Use: Cleanses and disinfects sore inflamed areas.
ORA-JEL CSM. (Commerce) Benzocaine, tannic acid, benzalkonium Cl in special base. Tube 0.5 oz.
Use: Relief of minor mouth & gum irritations.
ORA-JEL D. (Commerce) Benzocaine in a special "anti-irritant" adhesive base. Tube 0.5 oz.
Use: Relief from pain of denture irritation.
ORAJEL EXTRA STRENGTH. (Commerce) Benzocaine in special base. Tube 1/2 oz., 3/16 oz.
Use: Relief of toothache pain.
ORAL BARIUM. (Lafayette) Contains 96% barium sulfate. Drum 100 lb.
Use: Alimentary tract radiography.
ORALCID.
See: Acetarsone
■ **ORAL CONTRACEPTIVES.**
See: Demulen, Tab. (Searle)
Enovid-E, Tabs. (Searle)
Loestrin, Prods. (Parke-Davis)
Lo/Ovral, Prods. (Wyeth)
Miconor, Tab. (Ortho)
Modicon, Prods. (Ortho)
Nordette, Tab. (Wyeth)
Norinyl, Prods. (Syntex)
Norlestrin, Prods. (Parke-Davis)
Norquen, Tab. (Syntex)
Ortho-Novum, Prods. (Ortho)
Ovcon-35, Tab. (Mead Johnson)
Ovcon-50, Tab. (Mead Johnson)
Ovral, Tabs. (Wyeth)
Ovrette, Tab. (Wyeth)
Ovulen, Tab. (Searle)

ORAL DROPS/CANKER SORE RELIEF. (Weeks & Leo) Carbamide peroxide 10% in anhydrous glycerin base. Bot. 30cc.
Use: Relief of mouth and gum irritations, canker sores, denture sores.
ORALPHYLLIN LIQUID. (CMC) Theophylline 80 mg., alcohol 20%/15 cc. Bot. pt., gal.
Use: Antiasthmatic, bronchial and coronary dilator.
ORAMINIC. (Vortech) Atropine sulfate 0.2 mg., chlorpheniramine maleate 5 mg./ml. Inj. vial 10 ml.
Use: Decongestant, antispasmodic.
ORAMINIC SPANCAP. (Vortech)
Phenylpropanolamine HCl 50 mg., chlorpheniramine maleate 8 mg., atropine sulfate 1/180 gr./Spancap. Bot. 100s, 1000s.
Use: Decongestant, antispasmodic.
• **ORANGE FLOWER OIL,** N.F. XVI.
Use: Flavor; perfume, vehicle.
• **ORANGE FLOWER WATER,** N.F. XVI.
Use: Flavor; perfume.
ORANGE JU. C. (Image) Vitamin C 100 mg./Tab. Bot. 30s, 100s.
Use: Dietary supplement.
• **ORANGE OIL,** N.F. XVI.
Use: Flavor.
• **ORANGE PEEL TINCT., SWEET,** N.F. XVI.
Use: Flavor.
• **ORANGE SPIRIT, COMP.,** N.F. XVI.
Use: Flavor.
• **ORANGE SYRUP,** N.F. XVI.
Use: Flavored vehicle.
ORANYL. (Otis Clapp) Pseudoephedrine HCl 60 mg./Tab. Sugar and salt free. Safety packs 500s.
Use: Nasal and sinus decongestant.
ORAPHEN-PD. (Comatic) Acetaminophen 120 mg./5 ml. w/alcohol 5%. Bot. 4 oz.
Use: Analgesic, antipyretic.
ORAPIN. (Standex) Conjugated estrogen 0.625 mg., 1.25 mg./Tab. Bot. 100s.
ORAPIN INJ. (Standex) Estrogenic substance 20,000 u./30 cc. Susp. aq or oil.
ORARSAN.
See: Acetarsone.
ORASONE. (Rowell) Prednisone 1 mg., 5 mg., 10 mg., 20 mg./Tab. Bot. 100s, 1000s. Unit dose 100s. Prednisone 50 mg./Tab. Bot. 100s, Unit dose 100s.
Use: Steroid therapy.
ORASPAN. (Primedics) Iron fumarate 330 mg., B-1 5 mg., C 50 mg./Tab. Bot. 100s, 500s.
Use: Treatment of iron deficiency anemias.
ORA-TESTRYL. (Squibb) Fluoxymesterone. Tab. 5 mg., Bot. 50s.
Use: Anabolic agent.
ORATRAST. (Armour) Barium sulfate 92%, sucrose 3%, sodium saccharin and approved suspending agents. Containers 25 lb.
Use: Gastrointestinal X-ray diagnosis.
ORATUSS TR. (Vangard) Ceramiphen edisylate 20 mg., chlorpheniramine maleate 8 mg., phenylpropanolamine HCl 50 mg., isopropamide iodide 2.5 mg./T.R. Cap. Bot. 100s, 500s.

Use: Antihistamine, expectorant.

ORATUSSIN. (Panray) Guaifenesin 180 mg., ephedrine HCl 65 mg., ammonium chloride 600 mg., Vit. C 100 mg., sod. citrate 500 mg., citric acid 200 mg./30 cc. Bot. pt.

ORAZINC. (Mericon) Zinc sulfate 220 mg./Cap. Bot. 100s, 1000s.

ORBENIN. Sodium cloxacillin.
Use: Antibiotic.f

ORBENIN SODIUM SALT. Cloxacillin, B.A.N.

ORBETIC. (Cenci) Tolbutamide 0.5 g./Tab. Bot. 200s, 1000s.
Use: Oral anti-diabetic agent.

ORBIFERROUS. (Orbit) Ferrous fumarate 300 mg., Vit. B-12 12 mcg., Vit. C 50 mg., B-1 3 mg., defatted desiccated liver 50 mg./Tab. Bot. 60s, 500s.
Use: Anemias.

ORBIT. (Spanner) Vit. A 6,250 I.U., D 400 I.U., B-1 3 mg., B-2 3 mg., B-6 2 mg., B-12 5 mcg., C 75 mg., niacinamide 20 mg., Ca pantothenate 10 mg., Vit. E 15 I.U., biotin 15 mcg., iron 20 mg./Tab. Bot. 100s.

ORBIT WITH IRON. (Eckerd) Bot. 100s, 250s.

ORCIPRENALINE. B.A.N. 1-(3,5-Dihydroxyphenyl)-2-isopropylaminoethanol.
Use: Bronchodilator.
See: Alupent (sulfate)

• **ORCONAZOLE NITRATE.** USAN.
Use: Antifungal.

ORENZYME. (Merrell Dow) Trypsin 50,000 u., chymotrypsin 4000 u./Tab. Bot. 48s. Bitabs double strength Bot. 100s.
Use: Oral enzymes for adjunctive treatment of inflammation and edema.

ORETIC. (Abbott) Hydrochlorothiazide 25 mg. or 50 mg./Tab. Bot. 100s, 1000s. Strips 100s.
Use: Antihypertensive.

ORETICYL 25 and 50. (Abbott) **25:** Hydrochlorothiazide 25 mg., deserpidine 0.125 mg./Tab. Bot. 100s, 100s. **50:** Hydrochlorothiazide 50 mg., deserpidine 0.125 mg./Tab. Bot. 100s, 1000s.
Use: Hypotensive.

ORETICYL FORTE. (Abbott) Hydrochlorothiazide 25 mg., deserpidine 0.25 mg./Tab. Bot. 100s, 1000s.
Use: Hypotensive.

ORETON METHYL. (Schering) Methyltestosterone. **Buccal Tab.** 10 mg., Bot. 100s. **Tab.** 10 mg., 25 mg., Bot. 100s.
Use: Hormone therapy.

OREXIN. (Stuart) Vit. B-1 10 mg., B-6 5 mg., B-12 25 mcg./Softab Tab. Bot. 100s.
Use: Vitamin B-1, B-6 and B-12 deficiencies.

ORGANIDIN. (Wallace) Iodinated glycerol. Contains virtually no inorganic iodides and no free iodine and is stable in various media including gastric juice. **Elixir** 1.2%, 60 mg./5 cc., alcohol 21.75%. Bot. pt., gal. **Soln.** 50 mg., per cc., 30 cc. dropper bottles. **Tab.** 30 mg. Bot. 100s.
Use: Mucolytic expectorant.
W/Chlorpheniramine maleate & codeine phos.
See: Tussi-Organidin, Elix. (Wallace)
W/Dextromethorphan HBr, chlorpheniramine maleate.
See: Tussi-Organidin DM, Elix. (Wallace)

ORGATRAX. (Organon) Hydroxyzine HCl 25 mg./ml. Vial 10 ml. Disposable Syringe 1 ml. 50 mg./ml. Vial 1 ml.,
Use: Minor tranquilizer.

• **ORGOTEIN.** USAN. A group of soluble metalloproteins isolated from liver, red blood cells, and other mammalian tissues.
Use: Anti-inflammatory.

ORGOTEIN. (Diagnostic Data) Pure water soluble protein with a compact conformation maintained by 4 Gm. atoms of chelated divalent metals, produced from bovine liver as a Cu-Zn mixed chelate having superoxide dismutase activity. Ontosein, Palosein.

ORIGINAL ECLIPSE GEL. (Dorsey) Padimate O. SPF 10. Bot. 3 oz.
Use: Sunscreen.

ORIGINAL ECLIPSE LOTION. (Dorsey) Padimate 0, glyceryl PABA. SPF 10. Bot. 4 oz., 6 oz.
Use: Sunscreen.

ORIMUNE TRIVALENT. (Lederle) Poliovirus vaccine. Live, Oral, Trivalent. Sabin strains Types 1, 2, and 3. Dose of 0.5 ml. Dispette disposable pipette 1 dose. 10s. Pkg. 5s, 10s, 50s. Dose of 2 drops, Vial 10 doses. Pkg. 5s, 50s.

ORINASE. (Upjohn) Tolbutamide. 250 mg. & 500 mg./Tab. **250 mg.**/Tab. Bot. 100s; **500 mg.**/Tab. Bot. 200s, 500s, 1000s. Unit dose Box 100s. Unit-of-Use Bot. 50s, 100s.
Use: An oral hypoglycemic agent in the treatment of diabetes.

ORISUL. (Ciba) Sulfaphenazole. A sulfonamide under study.

ORMAZINE. (Hauck) Chlorpromazine HCl 25 mg./ml. Vial 10 ml.
Use: Tranquilizer.

• **ORMETROPRIM.** USAN. (1)2,4-Diamino-5-(6-methyl-veratryl)pyrimidine; (2)2,4-diamino-5-(4,5-dimethoxy-2-methylbenzyl)pyrimidine.
Use: Antibacterial.

ORNACOL. (Menley & James) Dextromethorphan HBr 30 mg., phenylpropanolamine HCl 25 mg./Cap. Pkg. 20s.
Use: Anti-tussive, nasal decongestant for relief of common cold and sinusitis.

ORNADE. (SmithKline) Phenylpropanolamine HCl 75 mg., chlorpheniramine maleate 12 mg./Spansule. Bot. 50s, 500s. Unit dose, 100s.
Use: Decongestant.

ORNEX. (Menley & James) Acetaminophen 325 mg., phenylpropanolamine HCl 18 mg./Cap. Blister Pak 24s, 48s. Bot. 100s.
Use: Temporary relief of nasal congestion, headache, aches, pains and fever due to colds, sinusitus, flu.

• **ORNIDAZOLE.** USAN.
Use: Anti-infective.

OROBEX. (Pasadena Research) Cobalamin concentrate 25 mcg./gelatin Cap. Bot. 100s, 1000s.

• **ORPANOXIN.** USAN.
Use: Anti-inflammatory.

ORPENEED VK. (Hanlon) Penicillin buffered 400,000 u./Tab. Bot. 100s.

Use: Antibiotic.

ORPHENADRINE. B.A.N. 2-(2-Methylbenzhydryloxy)-ethyldimethylamine.
Use: Treatment of the Parkinsonian syndrome.
See: Disipal, Ventromil (hydrochloride)
Norflex (citrate)

• **ORPHENADRINE CITRATE,** U.S.P. XXI. Inj., U.S.P. XXI. N,N-Dimethyl-2-(0-methyl-α-phenyl-benzyloxy)-ethylamine. N,N-Dimethyl-2-((o-methyl-α-phenylbenzyl)oxy)-ethylamine Citrate (1:1).
Use: Skeletal muscle relaxant; antihistaminic.
See: Flexon, Inj. (Keene)
Flexor, Inj. (Amfre-Grant)
Norflex, Tab., Amp. (Riker)
W/Aspirin, phenacetin, caffeine.
See: Norgesic, Tab. (Riker)
Norgesic Forte, Tab. (Riker)

ORPHENADRINE HYDROCHLORIDE. N,N-Dimethyl-2-(o-methyl-α-phenylbenzyloxy)ethylamine.
See: Disipal, Tab. (Riker)
W/Comb.
See: Estomul, Liq., Tab. (Riker)

ORTAC. (Ion) **Tab.:**Phenylephrine HCl 10 mg., guaifenesin 100 mg./Tab. Bot. 40s. **Liq.:**
phenylephrine HCl 5 mg., guaifenesin 100 mg./5 ml. Bot. 4 oz.
Use: Decongestant, expectorant.

ORTAC-DM. (Ion) Dextromethorphan HBr 15 mg., phenylephrine HCl 10 mg., guaifenesin 100 mg./Tab. Bot. 24s. **Liq.:**Dextromethorphan 10 mg., phenylephrine HCl 5 mg., guaifenesin 100 mg./5 ml. Bot. 4 oz.
Use: cough suppressant.

ORTAL SODIUM. Sod. 5-ethyl-5-hexylbarbiturate. Hexethal sodium.

ORTEDRINE.
See: Amphetamine (Various Mfr.)

ORTHESIN.
See: Benzocaine

ORTHO. (Ortho) Diaphragm kit, coil spring sizes 50, 55, 60, 65, 70, 75, 80, 85, 90, 95, 100, 105 mm.

ORTHO ALL-FLEX. (Ortho) Diaphragm kit (all flex arcing spring) in plastic compact, sizes 55, 60, 65, 70, 75, 80, 85, 90, 95 mm.

ORTHOCAINE. Orthoform. (No mfr. listed).

ORTHO-CREME CONTRACEPTIVE CREAM. (Ortho) Nonoxynol-9 2% in nonfatty acid cream base. Tube, 70 Gm. w/measured dose applicator. Tube only 70 Gm., 115 Gm.
Use: Contraceptive cream for use with diaphragm.

ORTHO DIAPHRAGM-WHITE. (Ortho) Diaphragm kit, flat spring sizes 55, 60, 65, 70, 75, 80, 85, 90, 95 mm.

ORTHO DIENESTROL CREAM. (Ortho) Dienestrol 0.01% Tube 78 Gm. with or without applicator.
Use: Intravaginal use.

ORTHO EAR DROPS. (Vortech) Hydrocortisone acetate 15 mg., neomycin sulfate 5 mg./cc. Bot. 5 ml. w/dropper.
Use: Anti-inflammatory (otic).

ORTHOFLAVIN. (Enzyme Process) Vit. C 150 mg., E 25 mg./Tab. Bot. 100s, 250s.

ORTHOFORM. No mfr. listed. Menthyl 3-amino-4-hydroxybenzoate.
Use: Local anesthetic.
W/Tyrothricin. (Columbus) Tyrothricin 0.5 mg., tetracaine HCl 0.5%, epinephrine 1/1000 sol. 2%/Gm. Oint., Tube ⅛ oz.
Use: Eye infections.

ORTHO-GYNOL CONTRACEPTIVE JELLY. (Ortho) p-diisobutyl-phenoxy-polyethoxy-ethanol 1.0%, in water-dispersible jelly at pH 4.5. Tube 81 Gm. w/measured-dose applicator. Tube only 81 Gm., 126 Gm.
Use: Contraceptive jelly for use with diaphragm.

ORTHO-HYDROXYBENZOIC ACID, Salicylic Acid, U.S.P. XXI.

ORTHOHYDROXYPHENYLMERCURIC CHLORIDE. (O-chloromercuriphenol)
Use: Antiseptic.
W/Benzocaine, ephedrine HCl.
See: Myrimgacaine, Liq. (Upjohn)
W/Benzocaine, parachlorometaxylenol, benzalkonium chloride and phenol.
See: Unguentine Aerosol (Norwich)
W/Benzoic acid, salicylic acid.
See: NP-27 Liq. (Norwich)

ORTHOHYDROXYPHENYLMERCURIC CHLORIDE.
W/Benzoic acid, salicylic acid, sec.-amyltricresols.
See: Salicresin, Liq. (Upjohn)
W/Zinc acetate, salicylic acid, phenol.
See: Zemacol, Medicated Skin Lotion (Norwich)

ORTHO-NOVUM 2 mg.-21. (Ortho) Norethindrone 2 mg., mestranol 100 mcg./Tab. Dialpak 21s.
Use: Oral contraceptive.

ORTHO-NOVUM 1/35-21. (Ortho) Norethindrone 1 mg., ethinyl estradiol 0.035 mg./Tab. Dialpak 21s.
Use: Oral contraceptive.

ORTHO-NOVUM 1/35-28. (Ortho) Norethindrone 1 mg., ethinyl estradiol 0.035 mg./Tab. plus 7 inert Tab. Dialpak 28s.
Use: Oral contraceptive.

ORTHO-NOVUM 1/50-21. (Ortho) Norethindrone 1 mg., mestranol 50 mcg./Tab. (yellow) Dialpak 21s.
Use: Oral contraceptive

ORTHO-NOVUM 1/50-28. (Ortho) Norethindrone 1 mg., mestranol 50 mcg./Tab. (yellow) plus 7 inert Tabs. Dialpak 28s.
Use: Oral contraceptive.

ORTHO-NOVUM 1/80-21. (Ortho) Norethindrone 1 mg., mestranol 80 mcg./Tab. (white) Dialpak 21s.
Use: Oral contraceptive.

ORTHO-NOVUM 1/80-28. (Ortho) Norethindrone 1 mg., mestranol 80 mcg./Tab. (white) plus 7 inert Tabs. Dialpak 28s.
Use: Oral contraceptive.

ORTHO-NOVUM 10/11 21 TABLETS. (Ortho) White Tab.: norethindrone 0.5 mg., ethinyl estradiol 0.035 mg./Tab. Peach Tab.: norethindrone 1 mg., ethinyl estradiol 0.035 mg./Tab. Dialpak 21s.

ORTHO-NOVUM 10/11 28 TABLETS. (Ortho) White Tab.: norethindrone 0.5 mg., ethinyl estradiol 0.035 mg., Peach Tab.: norethindrone 1 mg., ethinyl

estradiol 0.035 mg./Tab. Green Tab.: contains inert ingredients. Dialpak 28s.
Use: Oral Contraceptive.

ORTHO PERSONAL LUBRICANT. (Ortho) Greaseless, water soluble and non-staining aqueous hydrocolloid gel. Acid buffered to vaginal pH. Tube 2 oz., 4 oz.
Use: Lubricating gel.

ORTHOXICOL. (Upjohn) Dextromethorphan HBr 10 mg., methoxyphenamine HCl 17 mg./5 cc. Bot. 2 oz., 4 oz., pt.
Use: Coughs.

ORTHOXINE. Methoxyphenamine.

ORTICALM.
Use: Hypotensive and tranquilizing agent.
See: Serpasil, Prod. (Squibb)

OR TOPIC-M SUSPENSION. (Ortega) Sodium sulfacetamide 100 mg., prednisolone acetate 5 mg./ml. Bot. 5cc.
Use: Ophth. antibacterial, anti-inflammatory.

OR-TYL. (Ortega) Dicyclomine HCl 10 mg./ml. Vial 10 ml.
Use: Peptic ulcer therapy.

ORVUS.
See: Gardinol Type Detergents (Various Mfr.)

OSARSAL.
See: Acetarsone

OSBIL.
See: Iobenzamic acid (Mallinckrodt)

O.S.C. (Kenyon) Calcium (oyster shell) 250 mg., Vit. D-2 125 I.U./Tab. Bot. 100s, 1000s.

OS-CAL 250. (Marion) Oyster shell powder as calcium 250 mg., Vit. D 125 I.U. and trace minerals (Cu, Fe, Mg, Mn, Zn, silica)/Tab. Bot. 100s, 240s, 500s, 1000s.
Use: Calcium & Vit. D therapy.

OS-CAL 500. (Marion) Calcium 500 mg./Tab. Bot. 60s, 120s.
Use: Calcium supplement.

OS-CAL-FORTE. (Marion) Ca 250 mg., Fe 5 mg., Cu 0.3 mg., Mg 1.6 mg., Mn 0.3 mg., iodine 0.05 mg., Zn 0.5 mg., Vit. A 1668 I.U., D 125 I.U., B-1 1.7 mg., B-2 1.7 mg., B-6 2 mg., niacinamide 15 mg., Vit. C 50 mg., E 0.83 I.U./Tab. Bot. 100s.
Use: Calcium, vitamin & mineral supplement.

OS-CAL-GESIC. (Marion) Salicylamide 400 mg., Ca 100 mg., Vit. D 50 I.U.,/Tab. Bot. 100s.
Use: Arthritis.

OS-CAL PLUS. (Marion) Ca 250 mg., Vit. D 125 I.U., A 1666 I.U., C 33 mg., B-2 0.66 mg., B-1 0.5 mg., B-6 0.5 mg., niacinamide 3.33 mg., Zn 0.75 mg., Mn 0.75 mg., Cu 0.036 mg., Fe 16.6 mg., iodine 0.036 mg./Tab. Bot. 100s.
Use: Multivitamin & Multimineral therapy.

OSMITROL. (Travenol) Mannitol in water 5%—1000 ml., 10%—500 and 1000 ml., 15%—150 and 500 ml. 20%—250 and 500 ml. Mannit-l in 0.3% NaCl, 5% —1000 ml. Mannitol in 0.45% NaCl, 20%—500 ml.
Use: Osmotic diuretic.
See: Mannitol

OSMOGLYN. (Alcon) Glycerin 50% in flavored aqueous vehicle. Plastic Bot. 6 oz.

Use: Osmotic agent for reducing intraocular pressure.

OSMOLITE. (Ross) Medical/nutritional food for oral & tube feeding 1000 kcal/qt. Cans 8 oz., 32 oz.
Use: Oral & tube feedings especially designed for osmotic sensitive individuals.

OSPOLOT. Tetrahydro-2-(p-sulfa-molyphenyl)-1,2-thiazine-1,1-dioxide.
Use: Anticonvulsant drug; pending release.

OSSONATE CAPSULE. (Marcen) Cartilage mucopolysaccharide ext., chondroitin sulfate, 50 mg./Cap. Bot. 100s, 500s, 1000s.

OSSONATE-PLUS, CAPS. (Marcen) Ossonate-mucopolysaccharide ext. 50 mg., acetaminophen 300 mg., salicylamide 200 mg./Cap. Bot. 100s, 500s, 1000s.
Use: Prophylaxis or maintenance therapy of controlled arthritics.

OSSONATE-PLUS, INJ. (Marcen) Ossonate Cartilage mucopolysaccharide ext. 12.5 mg., casein hydrolysates 80 mg., sulfur 20 mg., sodium citrate 5 mg., benzyl alcohol 0.5%, phenol 0.5%/cc. Multidose 10 cc. vial.
Use: Skeletal muscle relaxant and pain reliever with specific antirheumatic action.

OSSONATE-75. (Marcen) Chondroitin sulfate 37.5 mg., benzylalcohol 0.5%, phenol 0.5%, sodium citrate 5 mg./cc. Vial 10 cc.
Use: Infantile and atopic eczemas, drug allergies, and dermatoses associated with intestinal toxemias.

OSTEOLATE INJECTION. (Fellows) Sodium thiosalicylate 50 mg., benzyl alcohol 2%/cc. Vial 30 cc.

OSTEON/D. (Pasadena Research) Calcium 600 mg., phosporous 400 mg., magnesium 240 mg., Vit. D 400 I.U./6 Tab. Bot. 180s.
Use: Dietary supplement.

OSTI-DERM LOTION. (Pedinol) Liquified phenol, glycerin, zinc oxide, magnesium carbonate, aluminum acetate solution, camphor water, in hydrated aluminum silicate gel. Tube 45 cc.
Use: Antipruitic, astringent.

OSTREOGRYCIN. B.A.N. Antimicrobial substances produced by *Streptomyces ostreogriseus.* (Specific substances are designated by a terminal letter; thus, Ostreogrycin B) Ostreocin is a mixture of Ostreogrycins B and G; Ostreogrycin B is Mikamycin B.

OSVARSAN.
See: Acetarsone

OTIC DOMEBORO. (Miles Pharm) Acetic acid 2%, aluminum acetate 1:10, buffered to pH 5. Soln. plastic drop. bot. 2 oz.
Use: Ear infections.

OTIC-HC. (Hauck) Chloroxylenol 1 mg., pramoxine HCl 10 mg., hydrocortisone alcohol 10 mg., benzalkonium Cl. 0.2 mg./ml. Bot. 12 ml.
Use: External ear infections.

OTIC-NEO-CORT DOME.
See: Neo-Cort Dome Otic Sol. (Miles Pharm)

OTIC-PLAIN. (Hauck) Chloroxylenol 1 mg., pramoxine

HCl 10 mg., benzalkonium Cl 0.2 mg./ml. Bot. 12 ml.
Use: External ear infections.
OTIC SOLUTION NO. 1. (Foy) Hydrocortisone alcohol
10 mg., pramoxine HCl 10 mg., benzalkonium
chloride 0.2 mg., acetic acid glacial 20 mg./ml.
w/propylene glycol q.s.
Use: Treatment of superficial infections of the
external auditory canal.
OTOBIONE. (Schering) Neomycin 3.5 mg., Polymixin
B sulfate 10,000 units, hydrocortisone 10 mg./ml.
in a vehicle of disodium edetate, povidone,
polysorbate 80, propylene glycol, glycerin and
water. Bot. 5 ml. w/dropper.
Use: Ear infections—anti-inflammatory, antibacterial.
OTOBIOTIC OTIC SOLUTION. (Schering) Polymixin
B and hydrocortisone in propylene glycol and
glycerin vehicle w/edetate disodium, sodium
bisulfite, anhydrous sodium sulfite, purified water.
Bot. w/dropper 15 ml.
Use: Otitis externa.
OTOCALM-H EAR DROPS. (Parmed) Pramoxine HCl
10 mg., hydrocortisone alcohol 10%, p-Chloro-m-
Xylenol 1 mg. benzalkonium chloride 0.2 mg.,
acetic acid glacial 20 mg., propylene glycol/ml. Bot.
10 ml.
Use: Superficial infections of the external auditory
canal.
OTOCORT STERILE. (Lemmon) Neomycin sulfate 5
mg., polymyxin B sulfate 10,000 U., hydrocortisone
10 mg./1 ml. w/propylene glycol, glycerin,
potassium metabisulfate and HCl. Bot. 10 ml.
Use: External ear infections.
OTO DROPS. (Vortech) Antipyrine 870 mg.,
benzocaine 230 mg., chlorbutanol 1%, glycerine
q.s./fl. oz. Bot. ½ oz. w/Dropper.
Use: Analgesic (ear drops).
OTO DROPS. (Standex) Benzocaine 0.85%,
antipyrine 3.2%, glycerol q.s./½ oz. Bot. ½ oz.
OTOLGESIC. (Blue Line) Phenol 4%, benzocaine
10%, clove 4%, menthol 4%, polyethylene glycol
400. 50 min./Dropule. Pkg. 12s.
Use: Inflammation of external ear canal
OTOMYCIN-HPN. (Misemer) Polymyxin B sulfate
10,000 u., neomycin sulfate 3.5 mg., hydrocortisone
10 mg./ml. Bot. 10 ml. w/dropper.
Use: Otic solution.
OTOREID-HC. (Reid-Provident) Hydrocortisone free alcohol 10 mg. (1%), polymyxin B sulfate 10,000 u.,
neomycin sulfate equiv. to neomycin base 3.5 mg.
Dropper Bot. 10 cc.
Use: Antibiotic ear drops.
OTOSTAN H.C. (Standex) Pramoxine HCl 1.0%,
hydrocortisone 1.0%, parachlorometaxylenol 0.1%,
benzalkonium chloride 0.02%, acetic acid 2.0%,
propylene glycol. Vial 10 cc.
OTRIVIN. (Geigy) Xylometazoline HCl **Nasal Drops:**
0.1% w/sod. chloride, phenylmercuric acetate
1:50,000. Dropper Bot. 20 ml. **Nasal Spray:** 0.1%
w/pot. phosphate monobasic, pot. chloride, sod.
phosphate dibasic, sod. chloride, benzalkonium
chloride 1:5,000. plastic squeeze spray 15 ml. **Ped.
Nasal Soln. Drops:** 0.05%. Bot. 20 ml.
Use: Nasal congestion.

OUABAIN. Card-20(22)-enolide, 3-[(6-deoxy-α-L-man-
nopyranosyl)-oxy]-1,5,11,14,19-pentahydroxy-, oc-
tahydrate, (1β,3β,5β,-
11α)-. Ouebain octahydrate G-Strophanthin.
(Lilly)—Amp. (0.5 mg.) 2 cc., Box 12s.
(Varick)—Amp. (0.25 mg.) 1 cc., Box 6s.
Use: Cardiac glycoside therapy.
OUABAIN OCTAHYDRATE. Ouabain, U.S.P. XXI.
OUTGRO. (Whitehall) Chlorobutanol 5%, tannic acid
25%, isopropyl alcohol 83%. Bot. .13 oz.
OVARIAN EXTRACT. Aq. ext. of whole ovaries of
cattle.
Use: I.M. & S.C.; estrogen therapy.
OVARIAN HORMONE, isolated from ovary.
See: Lutrexin, Tab. (Hynson, Westcott & Dunning)
OVARIAN SUBSTANCE. (Various Mfr.) Whole ovarian
substance from cattle, sheep or swine.
OVCON-35. (Mead Johnson) Norethindrone 0.4 mg.,
ethinyl estradiol 0.035 mg./Tab. Ctn. 6×21s.
Use: Oral contraceptive.
OVCON-35, 28 day. (Mead Johnson) 21 peach tablets
of norethindrone 0.4 mg. combined with ethinyl
estradiol 0.035 mg., followed by 7 green inert
tablets/Cart. 6×28s.
Use: Oral contraceptive.
OVCON-50. (Mead Johnson) Norethindrone 1 mg.,
ethinyl estradiol 0.05 mg./Tab. Ctn. 6×21s.
Use: Oral contraceptive.
OVCON-50, 28 day. (Mead Johnson) 21 yellow tablets
of norethindrone 1 mg. combined with ethinyl
estradiol 0.05 mg., followed by 7 green inert
tablets/Cart. 6×28s.
Use: Oral contraceptive.
OVIFOLLIN.
See: Estrone (Various Mfr.)
OVLIN. (Sig) **Tabs.** Ethinylestradiol 0.02 mg.,
conjugated estrogens 0.2 mg./Tab. Bot. 100s,
1000s.**Injectable.** estrone 2 mg., estradiol 0.05
mg., Vit. B-12 1000 mcg./cc. Vial 30 cc.
Use: Menopause, senile vaginitis, kraurosis
vulvae, pruritus vulvae, estrogen therapy.
OVOCYLIN DIPROPIONATE. (Ciba) Estradiol
Dipropionate.
OVOGYN. (Pasadena Research) Ethinyl estradiol 0.02
mg./Tab. Bot. 100s, 1000s. 0.05 mg./Tab. Bot.
100s, 1000s.
OVRAL. (Wyeth) Norgestrel 0.5 mg., ethinyl estradiol
0.05 mg./Tab. 6 Pilpak dispensers, 21 Tabs. Tripak
63s.
Use: Oral contraception.
OVRAL-28. (Wyeth) Norgestrel 0.5 mg., ethinyl estradiol
0.05 mg./White Tab. (21) plus inert Tabs. (7). 6
Pilpak dispenser, 21 Tabs +7 inert Tabs.
Use: Oral contraceptive.
OVRETTE. (Wyeth) Norgestrel 0.075 mg./Tab. 6
Pilpak dispensers, 28 Tabs.
Use: Oral contraception.
O-V STATIN. (Squibb) Nystatin. Oral/vaginal therapy
pack containing 42 Mycostatin Oral Tabs. (500,000
u./Tab.) and 14 Mycostatin Vaginal Tabs (100,000
u./Tab.)
Use: Vaginal candidiasis.

OVULEN-21. (Searle) Ethynodiol diacetate 1 mg., mestranol 0.1 mg./Tab. Compack Disp. 21s, 6×21. 24
×21. Refills 21s, 12×21
Use: Oral contraceptive.
OVULEN-28. (Searle) Ethynodiol diacetate 1 mg., mestranol 0.1 mg./Tab. Compack 28s: 21 active tabs, 7
placebo tabs. Compack disp. 28s, 6×28. Refills
28s, 12×28.
Use: Oral contraceptive.
OXABID. (Jamieson-McKames) Magnesium oxide 140
mg. or magnesium oxide heavy 400 mg./Cap. Bot.
100s.
OXACILLIN.   B.A.N.   6-(5-Methyl-3-phenyl-4-isox-
azolecarboxamido-penicillanic acid.
Use: Antibiotic.
• OXACILLIN, SODIUM, U.S.P. XXI. Cap., Inj., Sol.,
Sterile, U.S.P. XXI. 5-Methyl-3-phenyl-4-isoxazolyl
penicillin. Sodium 3,3-Dimethyl-6-(5-methyl-3-phenyl-
4-isoxazole-carboxamido)-7-oxocarboxylate.
Use: Antibiotic.
See: Bactocill, Cap., Vial (Beecham Labs)
Prostaphilin, Prep. (Bristol)
Sodium oxacillin
OXADIMEDINE HCl. N-(2-Benzoxazolyl)-N-benzyl-N',
N'-dimethylethylenediamine HCl.
Use: Antifibrillatory agent.
OXAFURADENE. Name used for Nifuradene.
Use: Platlet anti-aggretory agent.
• OXAGRELATE. USAN.
OXALID. (USV Labs.) Oxyphenbutazone 100
mg./Tab. Bot. 100s, 1000s.
Use: Anti-inflammatory.
• OXAMARIN HYDROCHLORIDE. USAN. 6,-7-bis[2-
(Diethylamino)-ethoxy]-4-methylcoumarin   dihydro-
chloride.
Use: Systemic hemostat.
• OXAMNIQUINE, U.S.P. XXI. Cap., U.S.P. XXI. 6-Hy-
droxymethyl-2-isopropylaminomethyl-7-nitro-1,2,3,4-
tetrahydroquino-line.
Use: Treatment of schistosomiasis.
See: Vansil, Cap. (Pfipharmecs)
OXANAMIDE. 2-Ethyl-3-propyl glycidamide.
Use: Tranquilizer.
• OXANDROLONE, U.S.P. XXI. Tab., U.S.P. XX (1)
Dodecahydro-3-hydroxy-6-(hydroxy-methyl)-3,3α,-6-
trimethyl-1H-benz[e]indene-7-acetic acid, α-lactone.
(2) 17 β-hydroxy-17-methyl-2-oxa-5α-androstan-3-
one.
Use: Anabolic.
See: Anavar, Tab. (Searle)
OXANTEL.   B.A.N.   1,4,5,6-Tetrahydro-1-methyl-2-
(trans-3-hydroxystyryl)pyrimidine.
Use: Anthelmintic.
• OXANTEL PAMOATE. USAN.
Use: Anthelmintic.
• OXAPROTILINE HYDROCHLORIDE. USAN.
Use: Antidepressant.
• OXAPROZIN. USAN. 3-(4,5-Diphenyloxazol-2-yl)-pro-
pionic acid.
Use: Anti-inflammatory.
2H-1,3,2-OXAZAPHOSPHORIN-2-AMINO, N,N-BIS-
(2-CHLOROETHYL)TETRAHYDRO-, 2-OXIDE,
MONOHYDRATE. Cyclophosphamide, U.S.P. XXI.

• OXARBAZOLE. USAN.
Use: Anti-asthmatic.
• OXATOMIDE. USAN.
Use: Anti-allergic, anti-asthmatic.
• OXAZEPAM, U.S.P. XXI. Cap., Tab., U.S.P. XXI. 7-
Chloro-1,3-dihydro-3-hydroxy-5-phenyl-2H-1,4-benzo-
dia-zepin-2-one. Serenid-D.
Use: Sedative.
See: Serax, Cap., Tab. (Wyeth)
2,4-OXAZOLIDINEDIONE,5-ETHYL-3,5-DIMETHYL-.
Paramethadione, U.S.P. XXI.
2,4-OXAZOLIDINEDIONE, 3,5,5-TRIMETHYL-. Trime-
thadione, U.S.P. XXI.
OX BILE EXTRACT. Purified oxgall.
See: Bile Extract, Ox
OXELADIN. B.A.N. 2-(2-Diethylaminoethoxy)-ethyl 2-
eethyl-2-phenylbutyrate. Pectamol citrate.
Use: Cough suppressant.
• OXETHAZAINE. USAN. 2-Di-(N-methyl-N-phenyl-tert.
butyl-carbamoyl-methyl)-aminoethanol; N,N-bis-(N-
methyl-N-phenyl-t-butyl-acetamido)-beta-hydroxethyl
-amino). 2,2'-[(2-Hydroxyethyl)imino]bis-[N-(α,α-
dimethylphenethyl)-N-methylacetamide]. 2-Di-[(Nαα-
trimethylphenethylcarbamoyl-methyl]-amino-
ethanol.
Use: Local anesthetic.
• OXETORONE FUMARATE. USAN.
Use: Analgesic specific for migraine.
• OXFENDAZOLE. USAN.
Use: Anthelmintic.
See: Synanthic (Syntex)
• OXFENICINE. USAN.
Use: Vasodilator.
• OXYFILCON A. USAN.
Use: Contact lens material.
OX GALL.
See: Bile Extract, Ox
• OXIBENDAZOLE. USAN.
Use: Anthelmintic.
OXIDIZED BILE ACIDS.
See: Bile Acids, Oxidized
• OXIDIZED CELLULOSE, U.S.P. XXI. Absorbable
cellulose. Cellulosic acid.
Use: Local hemostatic.
• OXIDOPAMINE. USAN.
Use: Adrenergic.
• OXIFUNGIN HYDROCHLORIDE. USAN.
Use: Antifungal.
• OXILORPHAN. USAN.
Use: Antagonist to narcotics.
OXINE.
See: Oxyquinoline sulfate (Various Mfr.)
• OXIPEROMIDE. USAN.
Use: Antipsychotic.
OXIPHEN. (Webcon) Sod. glycocholate ¼ gr., Sod.
taurocholate ¼ gr., phenolphthalein ½ gr., cascara
comp. ext. ½ gr., aloin ⅛ gr./Tab. Bot. 100s,
1000s.
Use: Laxative.
OXIPOR VHC PSORIASIS LOTION. (Whitehall) Coal
tar sol. 48.5%, salicylic acid 1.0%, benzocaine 2%,
alcohol 81%. Bot. 1.9 oz., 4 oz.
Use: Psoriasis treatment.

- **OXIRAMIDE.** USAN.
  Use: Cardiact depressant.
- **OXISURAN.** USAN. (Methyl-sulfinyl)-methyl-2-pyridyl ketone.
  Use: Antineoplastic.
- **OXMETIDINE HYDROCHLORIDE.** USAN.
  Use: Antagonist to histimine receptors.
- **OXMETIDINE MESYLATE.** USAN.
  Use: Antagonist to histimine receptors
- **OXOGESTONE PHENPROPIONATE.** USAN. #1: 20β-Hydroxy-19-norpregn-4-en-3-one hydrocinnamate. #2: 20β-hydroxy-19-nor-4-pregnen-3-one 20-phenylpropionate.
  Use: Progestogen.
- **OXOLAMINE.** (Arcum) Crystalline hydroxycobalamin 1000 mcg./cc. Vial 10 cc.
- **OXOLINIC ACID.** USAN. 5-Ethyl-5,8-dihydro-8-oxo-1,3-dioxolo-[4,5-g]quinoline-7-carboxylic acid.
  Use: Antibacterial.
- **OXOPHENARSINE HYDROCHLORIDE.** 2-Amino-4-arsenophenol hydrochloride.
- **OXPENTIFYLLINE.** B.A.N. 3,7-Dimethyl-1-(5-oxohexyl)xanthine. Pentoxifylline (I.N.N.).
  Use: Vasodilator.
  See: Trental (Hoechst)
- **OXPHENERIDINE.** 1-(β-phenyl-β-hydroxy-ethyl)-4-carbethoxy-4-phenylpiperidine.
- **OXPRENOLOL.** B.A.N. 1-(o-Allyloxyphenoxy)-3-isopropylaminopropan-2-ol. Trasicor hydrochloride.
  Use: Beta-adrenergic receptor blocking agent.
- **OXPRENOLOL HCI.** USAN. ($\pm$) 1-[o-(Allyloxy)-phenoxy]-3-(isopropylamino)-2-propanol HCl. Trasicor.
  Under study.
  Use: Coronary dilator.
- **OXSORALEN CAPSULES.** (Elder) Methoxsalen. 10 mg./Cap. Bot. 30s, 100s.
  Use: Symptomatic control of severe, recalcitrant, disabling psoriasis in conjunction with U.V. radiation.
- **OXSORALEN LOTION.** (Elder) Methoxsalen 1% in an inert lotion vehicle of alcohol 71%, propylene glycol, acetone, water. Bot. 1 oz.
  Use: Topical repigmenting agent in vitiligo in conjunction with U.V. light.
- **OXTRIPHYLLINE,** U.S.P. XXI. Elixir, Tab., U.S.P. XXI. Choline theophyllinate.
  Use: Bronchodilator.
  See: Choledyl, Tab., Elix. (Parke-Davis)
  W/Guaifenesin.
  See: Brondecon, Tab., Elix. (Parke-Davis)
- **OXY-5 ACNE-PIMPLE MEDICATION.** (Norcliff Thayer) Benzoyl peroxide 5% in lotion base. Bot. 1 fl. oz.
  Use: Acne treatment.
- **OXY-10 COVER MAXIMUM STRENGTH ACNE-PIMPLE MEDICATION.** (Norcliff Thayer) Benzoyl peroxide lotion 10%. Bot. 1 oz.
  Use: Acne treatment.
- **OXY-10 MAXIMUM STRENGTH ACNE-PIMPLE MEDICATION.** (Norcliff Thayer) Benzoyl peroxide 10% in lotion base. Bot. 1 fl. oz.
  Use: Acne treatment.
- **OXY-10 WASH ANTIBACTERIAL SKIN WASH.**

(Norcliff Thayer) Benzoyl peroxide 10%. Bot. 4 fl. oz.
  Use: Acne treatment.
- **OXYBENZONE,** U.S.P. XXI. 2-Hydroxy-4-methoxybenzophenone. Methanone, (2-hydroxy-4-methoxyphenyl)phenyl-. Cyasorb UV 9 (Lederle).
  Use: Ultraviolet screen.
  W/Dioxybenzone, benzophenone.
  See: Solbar, Lot. (Person & Covey)
- **OXYBENZONE WITH COMBINATIONS.**
  See: Coppertone, Prods. (Plough)
  Noskote, Cream (Plough
  Shade, Prods. (Plough)
  Sunger, Prods. (Plough)
  Super Shade, Lotion (Plough)
- **OXYBUPROCAINE.** B.A.N. 2-Diethylaminoethyl 4-amino-3-butoxybenzoate. Novesine hydrochloride.
  Use: Local anesthetic.
- **OXYBUTYNIN CHLORIDE.** USAN. 4-Diethylamino-2-butynyl-α-phenylcyclo-hexanegly-colate hydrochloride.
  Use: Anticholinergic.
  See: Ditropan Syrup, Tab. (Marion Lab.)
  Oxybutynin Chloride. (Mead Johnson)
- **OXYCAP.** (Hyrex) Dyphylline 200 mg., guaifenesin 200 mg./Cap. Bot. 100s, 1000s.
  Use: Vasodilator, bronchodilator, expectorant.
- **OXYCEL.** (Deseret) Cellulosic acid in absorbable hemostatic agent prepared from cellulose. Resembles ordinary surgical gauze or cotton. Pledgets 2 × 1 × 1 in. 10s. Pads 3 × 3 in. 8 ply. 10s. Strips 5 × ½ in. 4 ply. 18 × 2 in. 4 ply. 10s. 36 × ½ in. 4 ply.
  Use: Hemostatic.
- **OXYCINCHOPHEN.** B.A.N. 3-Hydroxy-2-phenyl-quinoline-4-carboxylic acid.
  Use: Uricosuric.
- **OXY-CHINOL.** (Ferndale) Pot. oxyquinoline sulfate 1 gr./Tab. Bot. 100s, 1000s.
  Use: Deodorizer, bacteriostatic.
- **OXYCHLOROSENE.** USAN. Monoxychlorosene. Hydrocarbon derivative containing fourteen carbons and hypochlorous acid. The hydrocarbon chain also has a phenyl substituent which in turn holds a sulfonic acid group.
  Use: Topical anti-infective.
  See: Clorpactin, Prod. (Scrip)
- **OXYCHLOROSEN SODIUM.** USAN. Sodium salt of the complex derived from hypochlorous acid and tetradecylbenzene sulfonic acid. Action of active chlorine.
  Use: Topical anti-infective.
- **OXYCLOZANIDE.** B.A.N. 3,3',5,5',6-Pentachloro-2'-hydroxysalicylanilide. Zanil
  Use: Anthelmintic, veterinary medicine.
- **OXYCODONE.** USAN. 7,8-Dihydro-14-hydroxy-O^3-methylmorphinone. Dihydrohydroxycodeineone Eucodal hydrochloride; Proladone pectinate.
  Use. Narcotic analgesic.
- **OXYCODONE HCI.** USAN. (1) ($-$)-4,5α-Epoxy-14-hydroxy-3-methoxy-17-methylmorphinan-6-one, (2) ($-$)-14-Hydroxydi-hydrocodeinone.

Use: Narcotic analgesic.
See: Dihydrohydroxycodeinone HCl
W/Acetaminophen & oxycodone terephthalate.
See: Percocet-5, Tab (Du Pont)
Tylox, Cap. (McNeil)
OXYETHYLATED TERTIARY OCTYLPHENOL-FOR-MALDEHYDE POLYMER.
See: Triton WR-1339. (Rohm & Haas)
OXYETHYLENE OXYPROPYLENE POLYMER.
See: Poloxalkol
W/Danthron, B-1, carboxymethyl cellulose.
See: Evactol, Cap. (Delta)
OXYFEDRINE. B.A.N. L-3-[(β-Hydroxy-α-methyl-phenethyl-amino]-3'-methoxypropiophenone. Ildamen hydrochloride.
Use: Coronary vasodilator.
• **OXYGEN,** U.S.P. XXI.
Use: Medicinal.
OXYGEN-CARBON DIOXIDE MIXTURES.
OXYMESTERONE. B.A.N. 4,17β-Dihydroxy-17α-methylandrost-4-en-3-one. 4-Hydroxy-17α-methyl-testosterone. Oranabol
Use: Anabolic steroid.
OXYMETAZOLINE. B.A.N. 2-(4-t-Butyl-3-hydroxy-2,6-dimethylbenzyl)-2-imidazoline. Afrin and Hazol hydrochloride.
Use: Vasoconstrictor.
• **OXYMETAZOLINE HYDROCHLORIDE,** U.S.P. XXI. Nasal Soln., U.S.P. XXI. Phenol, 3-[(4,5-dihydro-1H-imidazol-2-yl-)methyl]-6-(1,1-dimethyl-ethyl)-2,4-dimethyl-, monohydrochloride. 6-Tert-butyl-3-(2-imidazolin-2-ylmethyl)-2,4-dimethylphenol HCl.
Use: Decongestant, adrenergic.
See: Afrin, Nasal Spray, Soln. (Schering)
Duration Nasal Spray (Plough)
Duration Nose Drops (Plough)
Duration Nose Drops for Children (Plough)
St. Joseph Nasal Spray for Children (Plough)
St. Joseph Nose Drops for Children (Plough)
• **OXYMETHOLONE,** U.S.P. XXI. Tab., U.S.P. XXI. 17-beta-Hydroxy-2-(hydroxymethylene)-17-methyl-5α-androstan-3-one.
Use: Androgen.
See: Anadrol, Tab. (Syntex)
OXYMORPHONE. B.A.N. 7,8-Dihydro-14-hydroxy-morphinone. Numorphan hydrochloride.
Use: Narcotic analgesic.
• **OXYMORPHONE HCl,** U.S.P. XXI. Inj., Suppos., U.S.P. XXI. 14-Hydroxydihydromorphinone HCl. 4,5α-Epoxy-3,14-dihydroxy-17-methylmorphinan-6-one Hydrochloride.
Use: Analgesic, narcotic.
See: Numorphan Amp., Vial, Supp. (Du Pont)
OXYMYCIN. (O'Neal, Jones & Feldman) Oxytetracycline 50 mg., lidocaine 20 mg./ml. Vial 10 ml.
• **OXYPERTINE.** USAN. 5,6-Dimethoxy-2-methyl-3-[2-(4-phenyl-1-piperazinyl-ethyl]indole. 1-[2-(5,6-Dimethoxy-2-methylindol-3-yl)ethyl]-4-phenylpiperazine. Integrin hydrochloride.
Use: Psychotropic.

• **OXYPHENBUTAZONE,** U.S.P. XXI. Tab., U.S.P. XXI. 1-(p-Hy-droxyphenyl)-2-phenyl-4-butyl-3,5-pyrazolidin-e-dione. Oxazolidin. 4-Butyl-1-(p-hydroxyphenyl)-2-phenyl 3,5-pyrazolidinedione monohydrate.
Use: Antiarthritic, anti-inflammatory analgesic, antipyretic.
See: Oxalid, Tab. (USV Labs.)
Tandearil, Tab. (Geigy)
OXYPHENCYCLIMINE. B.A.N. 1,4,5,6-Tetrahydro-1-methylpyrimidin-2-ylmethyl α-cyclohexylmandelate. Daricon and Naridan hydrochloride.
Use: Antispasmodic.
• **OXYPHENCYCLIMINE HCl,** U.S.P. XXI. Tab., U.S.P. XXI. 1-Methyl-1,4,5,6-tetrahydro-2-pyrimidylmethyl-alpha-cyclohexyl-alpha-phenylglycolate HCl. (1,4,5,6-Tetrahydro-1-methyl-2-pyrimidinyl)methyl α-phenylcyclohexane-glycolate monohydrochloride.
Use: Antispasmotic.
See: Daricon, Tab. (Beecham Labs)
W/Hydroxyzine HCl.
See: Enarax, Tab. (Beecham Labs)
Vistrax 5 & 10 Tab. (Pfizer Laboratories)
W/Phenobarbital.
See: Daricon-PB, Tab. (Beecham Labs)
OXYPHENISATIN. B.A.N. 3,3-Di-(4-hydroxyphenyl)-indolin-2-one. Bydolax; Contax diacetate.
Use: Laxative.
• **OXYPHENISATIN ACETATE.** USAN. 3,3-bis(p-Hydroxyphenyl)2-indolinone diacetate. Diacetoxydiphenylisatin, Acetphenolisatin, Acetylphenylisatin, Diacetoxyphenyloxindol, Bisatin, Phenylisatin bis-(acetoxyphenyl) oxindol.
Use: Laxative.
See: Endophenolphthalein (Roche)
Isacen (No Mfr. currently lists.)
Prulet, Tab. (Mission)
Prulet Liquitab. (Mission)
OXYPHENONIUM BROMIDE. B.A.N. Diethyl (2-hydroxyethyl-methylammonium bromide-α-phenyl cyclohexyl glycolate. 2-α-(Cyclohexyl-mandeloyloxy) ethyldiethylmethylammonium bromide.
Use: Anticholinergic.
See: Antrenyl Bromide, Tab. (Ciba)
OXYPHENUDRINE. α-{[(p-Hydroxy-α-methylphenethyl)amino]methyl}proto-catechuyl alcohol.
• **OXYPURINOL.** USAN. 4,6-Dihydroxypyrazolo(3,4-d)pyrimidine. 1H-Pyrazolo[3,4-d]pyrimidine-4,6-diol.
Use: Xanthine oxidase inhibitor.
• **OXYQUINOLINE.** USAN.
Use: Disinfectant.
OXYQUINOLINE BENZOATE. (Mallinckrodt; Merck) Pkg. 1 lb. 8-Hydroxyquinoline benzoate.
W/Alkyl aryl sulfonate, disodium edetate, aminacrine HCl, copper sulfate, Na sulfate.
See: Triva, Vag. Jelly, Powd. (Boyle)
W/Benzoic acid, salicylic acid & sodium tetradecyl sulfate.
See: NP-27 Cream (Norwich)
• **OXYQUINOLINE SULFATE.** USAN. 8-Hydroxyquinoline sulfate.
Use: Disinfectant.
See: Chinosol, Tab., Pow., Vial (Vernon)

OXYQUINOLINE SULFATE W/COMBINATIONS.
See: Alochor Stypic, Liq. (Gordon)
Arnolds Rectal Supp. (Scrip)
Benzodent, Oint. (Vicks)
Dennt's Dental Poultice (C.S. Dent)
Derma Medicone Oint. (Medicone)
Derma Medicone-HC, Oint. (Medicone)
Foille, Prods. (Carbisulphoil)
Maseda Foot Powder, Pow. (Elder)
Medicone Dressing (Medicone)
Oxyzal Wet Dressing, Sol. (Gordon)
Rectal Medicone, Oint. (Medicone)
Rectal Medicone-HC, Oint. (Medicone)
Rectal Medicone Unguent, Oint. (Medicone)
Trapens, Tab. (Mills)
Triticoll, Tab. (Western Research)
Triva, Douche Pow. (Boyle)
V.A. Douche Powder (Norcliff-Thayer)
Zyanoid, Oint. (Elder)
OXY-SCRUB. (Norcliff Thayer) Abradant cleanser containing dissolving abradant particles of sodium tetraborate decahydrate. Tube 2.65 oz.
Use: Skin, cleanser to open plugged pores and removing excess oil.
OXYSORALEN. 8-Hydroxy-4',5',6,7-furocoumarin.
See: Methoxsalen
OXYSTAT. (Hyrex) Dyphylline 250 mg./ml. Vial 10 ml.
Use: Vasodilator, bronchodilator.
OXYTETRACLOR. (Kenyon) Oxytetracycline HCl 250 mg./Cap. Bot. 100s, 1000s.
Use: Antibiotic.
• **OXYTETRACYCLINE,** U.S.P. XXI. Inj., Sterile, Tab., U.S.P. XXI.
Use: Antibiotic.
See: Oxytetraclor, Cap. (Kenyon)
Terramycin, Prod. (Pfipharmecs)
Terramycin, Prod. (Pfizer Laboratories)
• **OXYTETRACYCLINE AND NYSTATIN CAPSULES,** U.S.P. XXI.
Use: Antibiotic, antifungal.
• **OXYTETRACYCLINE AND NYSTATIN FOR ORAL SUSPENSION,** U.S.P. XXI.
Use: Antibiotic, antifunal.
• **OXYTETRACYCLINE HYDROCHLORIDE AND HYDROCORTISONE OINTMENT,** U.S.P. XXI.
Use: Antibiotic, anti-inflammatory.
• **OXYTETRACYCLINE AND HYDROCORTISONE ACETATE OPTHALMIC SUSPENSION,** U.S.P. XXI.
Use: Antibiotic, anti-inflammatory.
• **OXYTETRACYCLINE CALCIUM,** U.S.P. XXI. Oral Susp., U.S.P. XXI.
Use: Antibiotic.
• **OXYTETRACYCLINE HYDROCHLORIDE,** U.S.P. XXI. Cap., For Inj., Sterile, U.S.P. XXI. 5-Hydroxytetracycline HCl. An antibiotic from *Streptomyces rimosus.*
Use: Antibiotic, antireckettsial.
See: Dalimycin, Cap. (Dalin)
Oxlopar, Cap. (Parke-Davis)
Oxy-Kesso-Tetra, Cap. (McKesson)
Terramycin Hydrochloride, Preps. (Pfizer Laboratories & Pfipharmecs)

Uri-tet, Cap. (American Urologicals)
Urobiotic (Roerig)
• **OXYTETRACYCLINE AND PHENAZOPYRIDINE HYDROCHLORIDES AND SULFAMETHIZOLE CAPSULES,** U.S.P. XXI.
Use: Antibiotic; urinary analgesic antispasmotic and anti-infective.
• **OXYTETRACYCLINE HYDROCHLORIDE AND POLYMYXIN B SULFATE,** U.S.P. XXI.
Use: Antibiotic.
• **OXYTETRACYCLINE HYDROCHLORIDE AND POLYMYXIN B SULFATE OPTHALMIC OINTMENT,** U.S.P. XXI.
Use: Antibiotic.
• **OXYTETRACYCLINE HYDROCHLORIDE AND POLYMYXIN B SULFATE TOPICAL POWDER,** U.S.P. XXI.
Use: Antibiotic.
• **OXYTETRACYCLINE HYDROCHLORIDE AND POLYMYXIN B SULFATE VAGINAL TABLETS,** U.S.P. XXI.
Use: Antibiotic.
OXYTETRACYCLINE-POLYMYXIN B. Mix of oxytetracycline HCl & polymyxin B sulfate.
Use: Antibiotic.
See: Terramycin Hydrochloride w/Polymyxin B Sulfate, Oint., Tab., Pow. (Pfizer Laboratories & Pfipharmecs)
OXYTOCICS.
See: Ergot Prep.
• **OXYTOCIN INJECTION,** U.S.P. XXI.
Use: Oxytocic.
See: Pitocin, Amp. (Parke-Davis)
Syntocinon, Amp. (Sandoz)
• **OXYTOCIN NASAL SOLUTION,** U.S.P. XXI.
Use: Oxytocic.
OXYTOCIN, SYNTHETIC.
See: Pitocin, Amp. (Parke-Davis)
Syntocinon, Amp. (Sandoz)
Syntocinon Nasal Spray (Sandoz)
OXYZAL WET DRESSING. (Gordon) Benzalkonium chloride 1:2000, oxyquinoline sulfate, distilled water. Dropper bot. 1 oz., 4 oz.
Use: Minor infections.
OYSTER SHELLS.
See: Os-Cal, Tab. (Marion)
W/Vit. D-2.
See: Ostrakal, Tab. (Elder)
• **OZOLINONE.** USAN.
Use: Diuretic.

P

P1E1;P2E1;P3E1;P4E1;P6E1. (Alcon) Pilocarpine HCl 1%,2%,3%,4%,6% respectively, epinephrine bitartrate 1%. Vial plastic drop. Vial 15 cc.
Use: Management of open angle glaucoma.
P.A. (Scrip) Phenobarbital ⅛ gr., atropine sulfate 1/250 gr./Tab. Bot. 100s.
P.A.A.M. (Kenyon) Acetylsalicylic acid 5 gr., para-aminobenzoic acid 5 gr., Vit. C 50 mg./Tab. Bot. 100s, 1000s.

Use: Arthritis.

PABA-"5". (Durel) P-amino benzoic acid in quick drying moisturizing base. Pl. Bot. 4 oz.
Use: Sunscreen lotion.

PABALAN. (Lannett) Potassium para-amino benzoate 5 gr., potassium salicylate 5 gr., ascorbic acid 50 mg./Tab. Bot. 100s, 1000s.

PABALATE. (Robins) Sod. salicylate 300 mg., sodium aminobenzoate 300 mg./E.C. Tab. Bot. 100s, 500s.
Use: Antirheumatic.

PABALATE-SF. (Robins) Potassium salicylate 300 mg., potassium aminobenzoate 300 mg./Tab. Bot. 100s, 500s.
Use: Antirheumatic.

PABANOL. (Elder) p-Aminobenzoic acid 5%, ethanol 70%. Bot. 4 oz.
Use: Sunburn preventative, sunscreen lotion.

PABAQUINONE CREAM. (Dermohr Pharmacal) Hydroquionone 4%, amyl dimethyl paba 3% in creamy base. Tube 1 oz.
Use: Gradual fading of "age spots".

PABASAL. (Wolins) Para-aminobenzoic acid, as sodium 5 gr., sodium salicylate 5 gr./Tab. Bot. 1000s.

PABA-SALICYLATE. (Various Mfr.) Sodium salicylate, p-aminobenzoate, Vit. C/Tab. Bot. 100s, 500s.
Use: Antirheumatic.

PABASAL N.S. (Wolins) Potassium salicylate 5 gr., potassium para-aminobenzoate 5 gr./Tab. Bot. 1000s.

PABA SODIUM. Sod. p-aminobenzoate. (Various Mfr.)
Use: Antirickettsial agent.

PABASONE. (Pinex) Sod. salicylate 5 gr., para-aminobenzoic acid 5 gr., ascorbic acid 20 mg./Tab. Bot. 100s.
Use: Arthritis, rheumatism.

P-A-C. Preparations of phenacetin, aspirin, and caffeine.
See: A.P.C. Preparations & Empirin Preparations

PACEMAKER PROPHYLAXIS PASTES WITH FLUORIDE. (Pacemaker) Silicone dioxide and diatomaceous earth, sodium fluoride 4.4%. Light abrasive, cinnamon/cherry. Medium abrasive, orange. Heavy abrasive, mint. Paste. Bot. 8 oz.

PACKER'S PINE TAR LIQUID SHAMPOO. (CooperCare) Bot. 6 fl oz.
Use: Treatment of dandruff and itchy scalp.

PACKER'S PINE TAR SOAP. (CooperCare) Bar 3.3 oz.
Use: Treatment of minor skin and scalp troubles.

PACLIN G. (Geneva) Penicillin G potassium 100M u., 200M u./Tab. Bot. 1000s. 250M u., 400M u./Tab. Bot. 100s, 1000s.

PACLIN VK. (Geneva) Penicillin phenoxymethyl 125 mg., 250 mg./Tab. Bot. 100s, 1000s.

P-A-C REVISED FORMULA ANALGESIC. (Upjohn) Aspirin 400 mg., caffeine 32 mg./Tab. Bot. 100s, 1000s.
Use: Analgesic.

• **PADIMATE A.** USAN.
Use: Ultraviolet screen.

• **PADIMATE O.** USAN.
Use: Ultraviolet screen.
See: Coppertone, Prods. (Plough)
  Eclipse Prods. (Dorsey)

Escalol 506 (Van Dyk)
Noskote, Prods. (Plough)
Pabafilm (Owen)
Shade, Prods. (Plough)
Sunger, Prods. (Plough)
Super Shade, Prods. (Plough)
Tropical Blend Sunscreen Lotion (Plough)

PAGITANE HYDROCHLORIDE. (Lilly) Cycrimine HCl 1.25 mg./Tab. Bot. 100s.
Use: Antispasmodic.

PAH.
See: Sodium Aminohippurate Inj. (Var. Mfr.)

PAIN-A-LAY. (Glessner) Antiseptic, anesthetic solution. Bot. 4 oz. w/sprayer, Bot. 4 oz., 8 oz., 1 pt.
Use: Relief of sore gums, minor sore throat.

PAIN & FEVER TABLET. (Lederle) Acetaminophen 325 mg./Tab. Bot. 100s, 1000s.
Use: Analgesic, antipyretic.

PAIN EXPELLER. (Guild) Tube 2½ oz.

PAIN EXPELLER BALM. (Guild) Tube ¼ oz.

PAIN-EZE. (Edward J. Moore) Benzocaine, menthol, oil of peppermint. Tube ⅛ oz., ¼ oz.
Use: Toothache and teething pain.

PAIN RELIEF OINTMENT. (Walgreen) Methylsalicylate 8.0%, menthol 7.2%. Tube 1.5 oz.
Use: Relief from pain of colds, muscle aches, neuralgia.

PAIN RELIEVERS-TENSION HEADACHE RELIEVERS. (Weeks & Leo) Acetaminophen 325 mg., phenyltoloxamine citrate 30 mg./Tab. Bot. 40s, 100s.
Use: Analgesic.

PALADAC LIQUID. (Parke-Davis) Vit. A 5000 I.U., D 400 I.U., B-1 3 mg., B-2 3 mg., B-6 1 mg., B-12 5 mcg., C 50 mg., niacinamide 20 mg., pantothenic acid 5 mg./5 ml. Bot. 4 oz., 1 pt.
Use: Multivitamin therapy.

PALADAC W/MINERALS. (Parke-Davis) Vit. A 4000 I.U., D 400 I.U., C 50 mg., E 10 I.U., B-1 3 mg., B-2 3 mg., B-6 1 mg., B-12 5 mcg., nicotinamide 20 mg., pantothenic acid 5 mg., Ca 23 mg., Fe 5 mg., P 17 mg., iodine 0.05 mg., K 2.5 mg., Mg 1 mg./Chewable Tab. Bot. 100s.
Use: Vitamin and mineral supplement.

PALAPRIN. Aloxiprin, B.A.N.

PALBAR. (Hauck) Phenobarbital 16.2 mg., atropine sulfate 0.012 mg., scopolamine HBr 0.005 mg., hyoscyamine HBr 0.18 mg./Tab. Bot. 100s, 1000s. Elixir 23% alcohol/5 cc. Bot. pt.
Use: Sedative-spasmolytic effect.

PALBAR NO. 2. (Hauck) Atropine sulfate 0.012 mg., scopolamine HBr 0.005 mg., hyoscyamine HBr 0.018 mg., phenobarbital 32.4 mg./Tab. Bot. 100s.
Use: Antispasmodic-anticholinergic.

PALESTROL.
See: Diethylstilbestrol (Various Mfr.)

PALFIUM HYDROGEN TARTRATE. Dextromoramide, B.A.N.

PALGESIC. (Pan American) Isobutylallylbarbituric acid ¾ gr., phenacetin 2 gr., aspirin 3 gr., caffeine ⅔ gr./Tab., Cap. Bot. 100s.
Use: Tension headache, as sedative-analgesic.

PALINUM.
Use: Hypnotic and sedative.

See: Cyclobarbital Calcium (Var. Mfr.)
PALLACE. (Bristol) Megestrol acetate 40 mg./Tab.
Bot. 100s.
Use: Antineoplastic.
PALMIDROL. N-(2-Hydroxyethyl)palmitamide.
PALMINATE-FA. (Hauck) Vit. A 4000 I.U., D 400 I.U.,
B-1 3 mg., B-2 3 mg., B-6 2 mg., B-12 3 mcg.,
niacinamide 10 mg., Vit. C 50 mg., calcium
carbonate 125 mg., ferrous fumarate 60 mg., folic
acid 1 mg./Tab. Bot. 100s.
Use: Dietary supplement.
PALMIRON. (Hauck) Ferrous fumarate 200 mg./Tab.
Bot. 100s.
Use: Anemias.
PALMIRON-C-TABS. (Hauck) Ferrous fumarate 200
mg., ascorbic acid 120 mg., Vit. B-6 5 mg./Chewable
Tab. Bot. 100s, 1000s.
Use: As hematinic.
• **PALMOXIRATE SODIUM.** USAN.
Use: Antidiabetic.
PAMABROM. 2-Amino-2-methyl-1-propanol salt of 8-
bromotheophyllinate.
W/Acetaminophen.
See: Pamprin, Tab. (Chattem Labs.)
W/Acetaminophen, pyrilamine maleate.
See: Cardui, Tab. (Chattem Labs.)
Sunril, Cap. (Emko)
W/Pyrilamine maleate, homatropine methylbromide,
hyoscyamine sulfate, scopolamine HBr,
methamphetamine HCl.
See: Aridol, Tab.s (MPL)
• **PAMATOLOL SULFATE.** USAN.
Use: Anti-adrenergic.
PAM-B-12 INJ. (Pan American) Cyanocobalamin 1000
mcg./cc. Amp. 10 cc., 30 cc.
Use: B-12 therapy, pernicious anemia.
PAMELOR. (Sandoz) Nortriptyline HCl. **Cap.:**
Nortriptyline HCl 10 mg., 25 mg. or 75 mg.
base/Cap. **10 mg.** Bot. 100s, SandoPak 100s; **25
mg.:** Bot. 100s, 500s, SandoPak 100s; **75 mg.:** Bot.
100s. **Liq.:** Nortriptyline HCl equiv. to 10 mg.
base/5 ml. Bot. Pts.
Use: Relief of symptoms of depression.
PAMINE. (Upjohn) Methscopolamine bromide. Tab.
2.5 mg. Bot. 100s, 500s.
Use: Antispasmodic.
PAMPRIN. (Chattem Labs.) Pamabrom 25 mg.,
acetaminophen 325 mg., pyrilamine maleate 12.5
mg./Tab. or Cap. Pkg. 12s, 24s, 48s.
Use: Premenstrual and menstrual symptoms.
PAMPRIN-MAXIMUM CRAMP RELIEF FORMULA.
(Chattem Labs.) Pamabrom 25 mg., acetaminophen
500 mg., pyrilamine maleate 15 mg./Cap. Pkg. 8s,
16s, 32s.
Use: Premenstrual and menstrual symptoms.
PAN A-C. (Eckerd) Vit. A palmitate 5000 I.U., C 150 mg.,
d-calcium pantothenate 25 mg./Cap. Bot. 100s, 200s.
PANACARB. (Lannett) Bismuth subnitrate, sod.
bicarb., mag. carb., papain, diastase/Tab. Bot.
1000s.
Use: Antacid.

PANACID. (Panray) Magnesium trisilicate 500 mg.,
aluminum hydroxide gel 250 mg./Tab. Bot. 100s,
500s.
Use: Antacid.
PANADEINE TABLETS. (Winthrop Products)
Paracetamol, codeine.
Use: Analgesic, antipyretic.
PANADEINE CO. TABLETS. (Winthrop Products)
Paracetamol, codeine.
Use: Analgesic, antipyretic.
PANADO. (Winthrop Products) Paracetamol, codeine.
Use: Analgesic, antipyretic.
PANADOL. (Glenbrook) Acetaminophen 500
mg./Tab. or Cap. Bot. Tab. 2s, 30s, 60s, 100s;
Cap. 10s, 24s, 48s.
Use: Analagesic, anti-pyretic.
PANADOL CHILDREN'S. (Glenbrook)
Acetaminophen. **Tab.**: 80 mg./Tab. Bot. 30s.
Liquid: 80 mg./0.8 ml. Bot. 2 oz., 4 oz. **Drops**: 80
mg./0.5 oz. Bot. 0.5 oz.
Use: Analgesic/antipyretic.
PANADOL WITH CODEINE. (Winthrop-Breon) **No 3**:
Codeine phosphate 30 mg. acetaminophen 300
mg./Tab.**No 4**: Codeine phosphate 60 mg.,
acetaminophen 300 mg./Tab. Bot. 100s, 500s,
1000s.
Use: Analgesic.
PANADYL. (Misemer) Pyrilamine maleate 25 mg.,
phenylpropanolamine HCl 25 mg.,
prophenpyridamine maleate 10 mg./Pelltab. Bot.
100s, 1000s.
Use: Decongestant, antihistaminic.
PANAFIL. (Rystan) Papain pow. 10%, urea 10%,
chlorophyll water sol. 0.5%, hydrophilic base. Oint.
Tube 1 oz., Jar 1 lb.
Use: For debridement and healing of skin lesions.
PANAFIL WHITE OINTMENT. (Rystan) Papain
10,000 u. enzyme activity, hydrophilic base/Gm.,
urea 10%. Tubes 1 oz.
Use: For debridement of skin lesions.
PANAFORT ELIXIR. (Pan American) Lysine mono
HCl 800 mg., Vit. B-12 30 mcg., B-1 2 mg., B-2 12 mg.,
B-6 12 mg., niacinamide 100 mg., panthenol 20 mg.,
alcohol 5%/15 cc. Bot. 8 oz.
Use: Dietary supplement, appetite stimulant.
PANAFORT TABLETS. (Pan American) Bot. 100s.
PANAHIST. (Panray) Chlorpheniramine Maleate 4 mg.
or 8 mg./Tab. Bot. 1000s.
Use: Antihistaminic
PANALGESIC. (Poythress) Methyl salicylate 55.78%,
aspirin 5.32%, menthol 0.95% & camphor 2.0%, in
alcohol 17% w/emollients and color. Bot. 4 oz., pt.,
0.5 gal.
Use: Analgesic & counterirritant.
PANAMIN. (Panray) Aminophylline 100 mg., or 200
mg./Tab. Bot. 100s, 1000s.
Use: Bronchial dilators.
PAN-APC. (Panray) Aspirin 3½ gr., phenacetin 2½ gr.,
caffeine ½ gr./Tab. Bot. 1000s.
Use: Analgesic.
PANAPHYLLIN. (Pan American) Theophylline 65 mg.,

ephedrine HCl 12 mg., guaifenesin 50 mg./5 cc.
Susp. Bot. 8 oz.
Use: Bronchodilator, vasoconstrictor, expectorant.
PANAQUIN. (Panray) Iodoquinol. 650 mg./Tab. Bot.
100s, 1000s.
Use: Amebicide.
PANASCORB. (Panray) Ascorbic acid 100 mg., 250
mg., 500 mg./Tab. Bot. 1000s.
Use: Vitamin therapy.
PANASOL. (Seatrace) Prednisone 5 mg./Tab. Bot.
100s.
Use: Adrenocortical steroid (anti-inflammatory).
PANASORB DROPS. (Winthrop Products)
Paracetamol, codeine.
Use: Analgesic, antipyretic.
PANASORB ELIXIR. (Winthrop Products)
Paracetamol, codeine.
Use: Analgesic, antipyretic.
PANASORB SUPPOSITORIES. (Winthrop Products)
Paracetamol, codeine.
Use: Analgesic, antipyretic.
PANASORB TABLETS. (Winthrop Products)
Paracetamol.
Use: Analgesic, antipyretic.
PANAZID. (Panray) Isoniazid powder 1 lb. container.
Tab. 50 mg., 100 mg., 300 mg./Tab. Bot. 100s,
1000s. Injection: 1 Gm./Vial. 50 cc./Vial.
Use: Anti-tuberculostatic.
PANAZID PLUS B-6. (Panray) Isoniazid 300 mg., Vit.
B-6 30 mg./Tab.; Isoniazid 100 mg., Vit. B-6 10
mg./Tab. Bot. 100s, 1000s.
Use: Anti-tuberculostatic with pyridoxine.
PANAZID TABLETS. (Panray) Isoniazid 50 mg., 100
mg., 300 mg./Tab. Bot. 100s, 1000s.
Use: Antibacterial (tuberculostatic).
PANAZON HCI. Nitrovin, B.A.N.
PAN-B-1. (Panray) Thiamin HCl 50 mg., 100 mg./Tab.
Bot. 1000s.
Use: Vitamin supplement.
PAN-B-6. (Panray) Pyridoxine HCl 25 mg., 50 mg., 100
mg./Tab. Bot. 1000s.
Use: Vitamin therapy.
PANCARD. (Pan American) Pentaerythritol tetranitrate
10 mg./Tab. Bot. 100s, 500s. Also available
w/phenobarbital. 20 mg./Tab. Bot. 100s.
PANCARD 30 TP. (Pan American) Pentaerythritol
tetranitrate 30 mg./long-acting Panseal. Bot. 60s.
Use: Coronary vasodilator.
PANCARD 30 TPA. (Pan American) Pentaerythritol
tetranitrate 30 mg., amobarbital 50 mg./long-acting
Panseal. Bot. 60s.
Use: Coronary vasodilator & sedative.
PANCET. (Pan American) Propoxyphene HCl 65 mg.,
acetaminophen 650 mg./Tab. Bot. 100s.
Use: Analgesic.
PANCOXIN HCI. Amprolium, B.A.N.
PANCREASE. (McNeil Pharm) Enteric coated
pancrelipase capsules. Bot. 100s, 250s.
Use: Pancreatic enzyme supplement.
PANCREASE EC. (McNeil Pharm) Lipase 4,000 NF
U., amylase 20,000 NF U., protease 25,000 NF
U./Cap. Bot. 100s, 250s.

Use: Digestive aid.
PANCREATIC DORNASE.
See: Dornavac for Inhalation, Vial (Merck Sharp &
Dohme)
PANCREATIC ENZYME.
W/Pepsin, ox bile.
See: Nu' Leven, Nu' Leven Plus, Tab. (Lemmon)
PANCREATIC SUBSTANCE. Substance from fresh
pancreas of hog or ox & contains enzymes
amylopsin, trypsin & steapsin.
W/Bile extract, dl-methionine, choline bitartrate.
See: Licoplex, Tab. (Mills)
W/Bile salts, lipase.
See: Cotazym-B, Tab. (Organon)
W/Bile, whole (desic.), oxidized bile acids,
homatropine methylbromide.
See: Pancobile, Tab. (Reid-Provident)
W/Cholic acid and ketocholanic acid.
See: Chobile, Tab. (Mallinckrodt)
W/dl-Methionine, choline bitartrate, ox bile.
See: Cholipan, Tab. (Western Research Labs.)
W/Lipase.
See: Cotazym, Cap., Packet (Organon)
• **PANCREATIN,** U.S.P. XXI. Cap., Tab., U.S.P. XXI.
Pancreatic enzymes obtained from hog or cattle
pancreatic tissue.
Use: Digestant.
See: Depancol, Tab. (Warner-Chilcott)
Elzyme, Tab. (Elder)
Panteric, Tab. (Parke-Davis)
PANCREATIN W/COMBINATIONS.
See: Aro-Pepsin, Tab. (Scrip)
Bile, Anthus Comp., Cap. (Scrip)
Bilogen, Tab. (Organon)
Bocresin, Liq. (Scrip)
Calsarbain, Tab. (Sutliff & Case)
Canz, Tab. (Cole)
Diethylstilbestrol Digestive Formula, Tab. (Wolins)
Digenzyme, Tab. (Burgin-Arden)
Digestozyme, Tab. (Wolins)
Digolase, Cap. (Boyle)
Dizymes, Cap. (Recsei)
Donnazyme, Tab. (Robins)
Entozyme, Tab. (Robins)
Enzobile, Tab. (Mallard)
Enzolax, Tab. (Kay)
Enzymet, Tab. (Westerfield)
Gastroenterase, Tabs. (Wampole)
Gourmase, Cap. (Rowell)
Ilozyme, Tab. (Adria)
Konzyme, Tab. (Brunswick)
Lever Taurine, Liq. (Paddock)
Maso-Gestive, Tab. (Mason)
Nu'Leven, Tab. (Lemmon)
Nu'Leven Plus, Tab. (Lemmon)
Pepsatal, Tab. (Kenyon)
Phazyme prod., Tab. (Reed & Carnrick)
Ro-Bile, Tab. (Rowell)
Sto-Zyme, Tab. (Jalco)
Zypan, Tab. (Standard Process)
• **PANCRELIPASE,** U.S.P. XXI. Cap., Tab., U.S.P. XXI.
Formerly Lipancreatin. Preparation of hog pancreas

with high content of steapsin and adequate amounts of pancreatic enzymes.
Use: Pancreatic enzymes preparation; digestive aid.
See: Accelerase, Cap. (Organon)
   Cotazym, Cap., Packet (Organon)
   Viokase, Pow., Tab. (Viobin)
W/Mixed conjugated bile salts, cellulase.
See: Accelerase, Cap. (Organon)
   Cotazym-B, Tab. (Organon)

PANCREOZYMIN. B.A.N. A hormone obtained from duodenal mucosa.
Use: Diagnostic aid.

PANCRETIDE. (Baxter) Pancreatic polypeptide in normal saline.
Use: Fibrinolytic conditions.

PANCURONIUM.
See: Poncuronium Bromide (Organon)

• **PANCURONIUM BROMIDE.** USAN. (1) 1,1'-(3α,17β-Dihydroxy-5α-androstan-2β,16β-ylene)bis-[1-methyl-piperidinium]dibromide diacetate: (2) 2β,16β-dipiperidino-5α-androstane-3α, 17 β-diol diacetate dimethobromide. Pavulon (Organon).
Use: Skeletal muscle relaxant.

P AND S PLUS. (Baker/Cummins) Coat tar sol. 8%, salicylic acid 2%. Bot. 3.5 oz.
Use: Tar gel for psoriasis and other scaling conditions.

PANEX. (Mallard) Acetaminophen 325 mg./Tab. Bot. 1000s.
Use: Analgesic.

PANFIL. (Pan American) Dyphyllin 200 mg./Tab. Bot. 100s.
Use: Treatment of bronchopulmonary insufficiency.

PANFIL-G. (Pan American) Dyphyllin 200 mg., guaifenesin 50 mg./Tab. Bot. 100s. Dyphyllin 100 mg., guaifenesin 50 mg./5 cc. Elix. Bot. pt.
Use: Treatment of bronchopulmonary insufficiency.

PANGYN. (Panray) Magnesium gluconate 0.5 mg./Tab. Bot. 100s, 1000s.
Use:

PANHEMATIN. (Abbott) Hemin 313 mg./43ml. Vial 100 ml.
Use: Amelioration of recurrent attacks of acute inermittent porphyria.

PANHIST. (Panray) Chlorpheniramine 8 mg./Tab. Bot. 1000s.
Use: Antihistaminic.

PANHYDROSONE. (Panray) Hydrocortisone 10 mg., 20 mg./Tab. Bot. 100s, 1000s. Powder 1 Gm., 5 Gm./Bot.
Use: Hormone.

PANIDAZOLE. B.A.N. 2-Methyl-5-nitro-1-[2-(4-pyridyl)ethyl]imidazole.
Use: Amebicide.

PANISOLONE. (Panray) Prednisolone powder 5 Gm., 1 Gm./Bot. Tab. 1 mg., 5 mg. Bot. 100s, 1000s.
Use: Adrenocortical steroid.

PANITOL. (Wesley) Allylisobutyl barbituric acid 15 mg., acetaminophen 300 mg./Tab. Bot. 100s, 1000s.
Use: Tension, pain.

PANITOL H.M.B.. (Wesley) Panitol formula plus homatropine methylbromide 2.5 mg./Tab. Bot. 100s, 1000s.

Use: Gastrointestinal spasms.

PAN-KLORIDE ELIXIR. (Panray) Potassium chloride 20 meq./15 cc. Bot. 16 oz, Gal.
Use: Potassium supplement.

PANMYCIN. (Upjohn) Tetracycline HCl. Cap. (250 mg.) Bot. 100s, 1000s. Tab. 500 mg. Bot. 100s.
Use: Antibiotic therapy.

PANOL. (O'Neal, Jones & Feldman) Dexpanthenol 250 mg./ml. Vial 10 ml.

PANOPHYLLINE FORTE. (Panray) Theophylline sodium glycinate 330 mg./15 cc. Bot. 16 oz., 1 Gal.
Use: Bronchial dilators.

PANOXYL ACNE GEL. (Stiefel) Benzoyl peroxide 5%, or 10%, alcohol 20%. w/polyoxyethylene lauryl ether in a hydroalcoholic gel base. Tube 2 oz., 4 oz.
Use: Antiseptic gel in treatment of acne.

PANOXYL AQ ACNE GEL. (Stiefel) Benzoyl peroxide 2½%, 5%, or 10% with polyoxyethylene lauryl ether in an aqueous gel base. Tube 2 oz., 4 oz.
Use: Antiseptic gel for treatment of acne.

PANOXYL BAR-5. (Stiefel) Benzoyl peroxide 5% in a mild surfactant cleansing base. Bar 4 oz.
Use: Acne wash.

PANOXYL BAR-10. (Stiefel) Benzoyl peroxide 10% in rich-lathering, mild surfactant. Bar 4 oz.
Use: Acne wash.

PANPARNIT HYDROCHLORIDE. Caramiphen HCl.
Use: Parkinson's syndrome.

PANPRES. (Pan American) Hydralazine HCl 25 mg., hydrochlorothiazide 15 mg., resperine 0.1 mg./Tab. Bot. 100s.
Use: Hypertension treatment.

PANRITIS. (Pan American) Salicylamide 250 mg., acetaminophen 250 mg./Tab. Bot. 100s.
Use: Analgesic and anti-rheumatic.

PANSCOL. (Baker/Cummins) Salicylic acid 3%, lactic acid 2%, phenol (less than 1%). Oint.: Jar 3 oz. Lot.: Bot. 4 oz.
Use: Treatment and management of dermatitis.

PANSHAPE M TP. (Pan American) Phentermine HCl 30 mg./Cap. Bot. 60s.
Use: Anorexiant.

PAN-SONE. (Panray) Prednisone powder 5 Gm., 1 Gm./Bot. Tab. 1 mg., 2.5 mg., 5 mg., Bot. 100s, 1000s.
Use: Adrenocortical steroid.

PAN-TALC. (Panray) Talc 25 mg., 50 mg., 75 mg., 100 mg./Tab. Bot. 1000s.
Use: Radioimmunoassay, laboratory use only.

PANTEMIC M. (Pan American) Tab.: Ferrous fumarate 300 mg./Tab. Bot. 100s. Susp. 100 mg./5 cc. Bot. 8 oz.
Use: Iron deficiency anemia.

• **PANTHENOL,** U.S.P. XXI. Alcohol corresponding to pantothenic acid. Pantothenol. Pantothenylol. (+)-2,4-Dihydroxy-N-(3-hydroxypropyl)-3,3-dimethylbutyramide.
Use: Treatment of paralytic ileus and postoperative distention.
See: Ilopan, Amp., Vial (Warren-Teed)
   Panadon, Cream (Gordon Labs.)

Pantenyl, Vial (Kay)
Panthoderm Cream (USV Pharm)
PANTHENOL W/COMBINATIONS.
See: Android-G, Vial (Brown)
B Complex w/C, Vial (Maurry)
Benizol Plus, Elix., Tab. (ICN Pharm.)
Geramine, Inj. (Brown)
Geramine Tablets (Brown)
Geriatrazole prod., Vial (Kenyon)
Geritag, Inj. (Reid-Provident)
Ilopan-Choline, Tab. (Warren-Teed)
Life Plex, Liq. (Burgin-Arden)
Lifer-B, Liq. (Burgin-Arden)
Liva, Inj. (Vortech)
LyoB-C prod., Pkg. (Merck Sharp & Dohme)
Minoplex, Vial (Savage)
Nutricol, Cap., Inj. (Nutrition Control)
Panfort, Elix. (Panamerican)
Pantho-F, Cream (USV Pharm.)
Savaplex, Vial (Savage)
Vi-Testrogen, Vial (Pharmex)
Zentinic, Pulvules (Lilly)
PANTHODERM CREAM. (USV Labs.) Dexpanthenol
2% in water-miscible cream. Tube 1 oz., Jar 2 oz., 1
lb.
Use: Antipruritic & healing aid.
PANTHOLIN. (Lilly) Calcium pantothenate. Tab. 10
mg., Bot. 100s.
Use: Orally; dietary supplement.
PANTIGEN. (Pasadena Research) Nonspecific
antigen. Vial 10 cc.
PANTISONE. (Panray) Cortisone acetate 5 mg., 25
mg./Tab. Bot. 100s, 1000s.
Use: Anti-inflammatory agent.
PANTOCAINE.
See: Tetracaine hydrochloride. (Various Mfr.)
PANTOCRIN-F. (Spanner) Plurigland, ovarian, ant, and
post. pituitary, adrenal, thyroid exts. Vial 30 cc.
PANTOPAQUE. (Lafayette) Iophendylate, ethyl
iodophenylundecanoate. Amp. 3 cc. 3s; 6 cc. 6s;
12 cc. 2s.
Use: Intrathecally for myelography.
PANTOPON. (Roche) Hydrochlorides of opium
alkaloids w/alcohol 6%, glycerin 136 mg., methyl
and propyl parabens 0.2%, acetic acid and/or sod.
hydroxide to adjust pH to 3.3. Amp.: 0.33 gr/ml.,
Box 10s.
Use: S.C. & I.M. as an analgesic.
PANTOTHENIC ACID. As Cal. or Sod. salt.
Use: Nonspecific protein therapy.
See: Vitamin preparations.
PANTOTHENIC ACID SALTS.
See: Calcium Pantothenate
Sodium Pantothenate
PANTOTHENOL.
See: Panthenol, Prep. (Various Mfr.)
PANTOTHENYL ALCOHOL.
See: Panthenol, Prep. (Various Mfr.)
PANTOTHENYLOL.
See: Panthenol, Prep. (Various Mfr.)
PAN ULTRA. (Cummins) Benzophenone in
moisturizing lotion or lipstick. Bot. 4 oz. Lipstick 4
Gm.

Use: Sun protective.
PANVITEX GERIATRIC CAPSULES. (Fellows)
Safflower oil 340 mg., Vit. A 10,000 I.U., D 400 I.U.,
Vit. B-1 5 mg., B-6 1 mg., B-2 2.5 mg., B-12 activity 2
mcg., C 75 mg., niacinamide 40 mg., Ca
pantothenate 4 mg., E 2 I.U., inositol 15 mg.,
choline bitartrate 31.4 mg., Ca 75 mg., P 58 mg.,
Fe 30 mg., Mn 0.5 mg., K 2 mg., Zn 0.5 mg., Mg 3
mg./Cap. Bot. 100s, 1000s.
Use: Vitamin and mineral supplement.
PANVITEX GERIATRIC INJ. (Fellows) Testosterone
10 mg., Vit. B-12 100 mcg., B-1 50 mg., nicotinamide
50 mg., B-6 5 mg., estrone 0.5 mg., liver inj. equiv. in
B-12 activity of cyanocobalamin 2 mcg., lidocaine 20
mg., panthenol 10 mg., B-2 5 mg./cc. Vial 30 cc.
PANVITEX G.H. (Fellows) Methyl testosterone 2 mg.,
ethinyl estradiol 0.01 mg., Vit. A 5000 I.U., D 400
I.U., E 10 I.U., B-1 2 mg., B-2 2 mg., B-6 0.3 mg.,
B-12 1 mcg., C 30 mg., niacinamide 20 mg., cal.
pantothenate 3 mg., choline bitartrate 40 mg.,
inositol 20 mg., methionine 20 mg., Fe sulfate 10
mg., Cu 0.2 mg., molybdenum 0.5 mg., Mn 1.0 mg.,
Zn 1.0 mg., Mg 5 mg., K 2 mg., iodine 0.15
mg./S.C. Tab. Bot. 100s, 1000s.
Use: Vitamin and mineral supplement.
PANVITEX PLUS MINERALS CAPSULES. (Fellows)
Vit. A 5000 I.U., D 400 I.U., B-1 3 mg., B-2 2.5 mg.,
niacinamide 20 mg., B-6 1.5 mg., Ca pantothenate 5
mg., B-12 2.5 mcg., C 50 mg., E 3 I.U., Ca 215 mg.,
P 166 mg., Fe 13.4 mg., Mg 7.5 mg., Mn 1.5 mg.,
K 5 mg., Zn 1.4 mg./Cap. Bot. 100s, 1000s.
Use: Vitamin and mineral supplement.
PANVITEX PRENATAL CAPSULES. (Fellows)
Ferrous fumarate 150 mg., cobalamin conc. 2 mcg.,
Vit. A 6,000 I.U., D 400 I.U., B-1 1.5 mg., B-2 2.5 mg.,
niacinamide 15 mg., B-6 3 mg., C 100 mg., calcium
250 mg., Ca pantothenate 5 mg., folic acid 0.2
mg./Cap. Bot. 100s, 1000s.
Use: Multivitamin with iron.
PANVITEX T-M. (Fellows) Vit. A 10,000 I.U., D 400 I.U.,
Vit. B-1 10 mg., B-6 1 mg., B-2 5 mg., B-12 5 mcg., C
150 mg., niacinamide 100 mg., Ca 103 mg., P 80
mg., Fe 10 mg., Mn 1 mg., K 5 mg., Zn 1.4 mg.,
Mg 5.56 mg./Cap. Bot. 100s, 1000s.
Use: Vitamin and mineral supplement.
PANWARFIN. (Abbott) Warfarin sodium 2 mg., 2½
mg., 5 mg., 7½ mg. and 10 mg./Tab. Bot. 100s.
Abbo-Pac.
Use: Anticoagulant.
PANZYME. (Hyrex) Hyoscyamine sulfate 0.0519 mg.,
homatropine methylbromide 0.2885 mg., hyoscine
HBr 0.0033 mg., phenobarbital 8.1 mg., pancreatin
300 mg., pepsin 150 mg./Tab. Bot. 100s, 1000s,
5000s.
Use: Functional G. I. disorders.
PAP. (Abbott) Test kit 100s.
Use: Enzyme immunoassay for measurement of
prostatic acid phosphatase.
PAP. (Zenith) Phenacetin 194 mg., aspirin 162 mg.,
phenobarbital 16.2 mg./Cap. Also w/codeine ¼,
½, 1 gr./Cap. Bot. 100s.
Use: Analgesic.

P.A.P. No. 1. (Jenkins) Phenobarbital 15 mg., acid acetylsalicylic 0.23 Gm., acetophenetidin 0.15 Gm./Tab. Bot. 1000s.
Use: Sedative and anodyne.

PAPA-CARIA. (Jenkins) Mg carbonate 100 gr., cal. carbonate 50 gr., sod. bicarbonate 120 gr., bismuth subnitrate 50 gr., cerium oxalate 25 gr., Mg trisilicate 70 gr., powd. ginger 4 gr., papain 11 gr., pancreatin 5½ gr./oz. Pkg. 2 oz.
Use: Antacid and digestive powder.

PAPACON. (CMC) Papaverine HCl 150 mg./Cap. Bot. 30s, 100s, 500s, 1000s.
Use: Cerebral and peripheral ischemia.

• **PAPAIN.** U.S.P. XXI. Tab. for Topical Soln., U.S.P. XXI. A proteolytic substance derived from *Carlica papaya.*
Use: Proteolytic enzyme.
See: Papase, Tab. (Parke-Davis)
    Softlens Enzymatic Contact Lens Cleaner (Allergan)

PAPAIN W/COMBINATIONS.
See: Baculin, Tab. (Amfre-Grant)
    Bilate, Tab. (Central)
    Calsarbain, Tab. (Sutliff & Case)
    Cerophen, Tab. (Wendt-Bristol)
    Diethylstilbestrol Digestive Formula, Tab. (Wolins)
    Digenzyme, Tab. (Burgin-Arden)
    Kaocasil, Tab. (Jenkins)
    Natrogestive, Tab. (Wolins)
    Panacarb, Tab. (Lannett)
    Panafil, Oint. (Rystan)
    Taurocolate, Tab. (Vortech)

PAP-A-LIX. (Freeport) n-Acetyl-aminophenol 120 mg., alcohol 10%/5 cc. Bot. 4 oz., Gal.
Use: Pediatric analgesic, antipyretic.

PAPASE. (Parke-Davis) Proteolytic enzyme from carica papaya 10,000 u./Tab. peppermint-flavored. Bot. 100s, 1000s.
Use: Symptomatology related to episiotomy.

PAPAVATRAL. (Kenwood) Ethaverine HCl 30 mg., pentaerythritol tetranitrate 10 mg., or 20 mg./Tab. Bot. 100s, 500s.
Use: Angina pectoris.

PAPAVATRAL L.A. (Kenwood) Ethylpapaverine HCl 30 mg., pentaerythritol tetranitrate 50 mg./Cap. Bot. 30s, 250s. Available w/Phenobarbital 45 mg./Cap. Bot. 30s, 250s.
Use: Agina pectoris.

• **PAPAVERINE HYDROCHLORIDE,** U.S.P. XXI. Inj., Tab., U.S.P. XXI. 6,7-Dimethoxy-l-veratrylisoquinoline Hydrochloride.
Use: Smooth muscle relaxant.
See: BP-Papaverine, Cap. (Burlington)
    Cerebid Capsules (Saron)
    Cerespan, Cap. (USV Labs.)
    Cirbed, Cap. (Boyd)
    Delapav, Time Cap. (Dunhall)
    Lapay, Graduals (Amfre-Grant)
    Myobid, Cap. (Laser)
    Papacon, Cap. (CMC)
    Papital T.R. (Zemmer)
    Pap-Kaps-150 Meta-Kaps, Cap. (Sutliff & Case)

Pavabid, Cap. (Marion)
Pavacap, Unicells (Reid-Provident)
Pavacaps, Cap. (Freeport)
Pavacen Cenules, Cap. (Central)
Pavaclor, Cap. (Pasadena Research)
Pavacron, Cap. (Cenci)
Pavadel, Cap. (Canright)
Pavadyl, Cap. (Bock)
Pavakey 300, Cap. (Key)
Pavakey S.A., Cap. (Key)
Pava-lyn, Cap. (Lynwood)
Pava Par, Cap. (Parmed)
Pava-Rx, Cap. (Blaine)
Pavasule, Cap. (Jalco)
Pavatest T.D., Cap. (Fellows-Testagar)
Pavatime, Cap. (Rocky Mtn.)
Pavatym, Cap. (Everett)
Pavatran T. D. Capsules (Mayrand)
Pava-Wol, Cap. (Wolins)
Paverolan, Lanacap. (Lannett)
Pavex, Cap. (Xxtrium)
Ro-Papav, Tab. (Robinson)
Vasocap, Cap. (Keene)
Vasospan, Cap. (Ulmer)
Vazosan, Tab. (Sandia)
W/Codeine sulfate.
See: Copavin, Pulvule, Tab. (Lilly)
W/Codeine sulfate, aloin & Sod. salicylate.
See: Copavin Compound, Elixir (Lilly)
W/Codeine sulfate, emetine HCl, ephedrine HCl.
See: Golacol, Syr. (Arcum)
W/Phenobarbital.
See: Pavadel-PB, Cap. (Canright)

PAPAVEROLINE. B.A.N. 1-(3,4-Dihydroxybenzyl)-6,7-dihydroxyisoquinoline.
Use: Vasodilator.

PAPITAL T.R. CAPSULES. (Zemmer) Papaverine HCl 150 mg./Cap. Bot. 100s, 1000s.

PAP-KAPS-150 META-KAPS. (Sutliff & Case) Papaverine HCl 150 mg./Cap. Bot. 100s, 1000s.

PAPZANS MODIFIED. (Bowman) Acetaminophen 160 mg., phenylephrine HCl 7.5 mg., chlopheniramine maleate 1 mg./Tab. Bot. 100s, 1000s.
Use: Analgesic, decongestant, antihistaminic.

PARA-AMINOBENZOIC ACID. Aminobenzoic Acid, U.S.P. XXI.
See: Pabafilm Gel (Owen)
    Paba-"5", Lot. (Durel)
    Pabagel, Gel. (Owen)
    Pabalate, Tab. (Robins)
    Pabanol, Lot. (Elder)
    Presun, Lotion, Gel (Westwood)
    Protan, Liq. (Westwood)
    Sunbrella, Liq. (Dorsey)
    Super Shade Lotion (Plough)
W/Acetylsalicylic acid, Vit. C.
See: P.A.A.M., Tab. (Kenyon)

PARA-AMINOSALICYLIC ACID. Aminosalicylic Acid, U.S.P. XXI.

PARABAXIN. (Parmed) Methocarbamol 500 or 750 mg./Tab. Bot. 100s.
Use: Muscle skeletal relaxant.

PARABROM.
See: Pyrabrom
PARABROMIDYLAMINE.
See: Brompheniramine, Dimetane, Preps. (Robins)
PARACAIN.
See: Procaine Hydrochloride (Various Mfr.)
PARACARBINOXAMINE MALEATE. Carbinoxamine.
PARACETALDEHYDE.
See: Paraldehyde, U.S.P. XXI.
PARACETAMOL. B.A.N. 4-Acetamidophenol.
Use: Analgesic; antipyretic.
See: Calpol
Eneril
Febrilix
Panadol
Panok
Tabalgin
PARACHLORAMINE HYDROCHLORIDE. Meclizine HCl, U.S.P. XXI.
See: Bonine, Tab. (Pfizer)
PARACHLOROMETAXYLENOL.
Use: Phenolic antiseptic.
See: D-Seb, Liq. (Cooper)
Nu-Flow, Liq. (Cooper)
W/9-aminoacridine HCl, methyl-dodecylbenzyl-trimethyl ammonium chloride, pramoxine HCl, hydrocortisone, acetic acid.
See: Drotic No. 2, Drops (Ascher)
W/Benzocaine.
See: TPO 20 (DePree)
W/Coconut oil, pine oil, castor oil, lanolin, cholesterols, lecithin.
See: Sebacide, Liq. (Paddock)
W/Hydrocortisone, pramoxine HCl, benzalkonium chloride, acetic acid.
See: Oto Drops (Reid-Provident)
W/Hydrocortisone, pramoxine HCl, benzalkonium chloride, acetic acid, propylene glycol.
See: Otostan H.C. (Standex)
W/Lidocaine, phenol, zinc oxide.
See: Unguentine Plus, Cream (Norwich)
W/Pramoxine HCl, hydrocortisone, benzalkonium chloride, acetic acid.
See: My Cort Otic #2, Drops (Scrip)
Steramine Otic, Drops (Mayrand)
W/Resorcinol, sulfur.
See: Rezamid, Lot. (Dermik)
W/Zinc undecylenate.
See: Cruex, Cream (Pharmacraft)
• **PARACHLOROPHENOL,** U.S.P. XXI. Camphorated, U.S.P. XX. Phenol, 4-chloro. p-Chlorophenol.
Use: Topical antibacterial.
W/Camphor.
See: Camphorated Parachlorophenol.
PARACODIN.
See: Dihydrocodeine
PARADIONE CAPSULES. (Abbott) Paramethadione 150 mg, or 300 mg./Cap. Bot. 100s.
Use: Anticonvulsant.
PARADIONE SOLUTION. (Abbott) Paramethadione oral solution 300 mg./ml. Bot. 50 ml. w/dropper.
Use: Anticonvulsant.

PARADYNE. (Spanner) Dipyrone injection 50%. Vial 10 cc.
PARAEUSAL LIQUID. (Paraeusal) Liquid Bot. 2 oz., 6 oz., 12 oz.
Use: Cuts, burns, sunburn, minor irritations of skin.
PARAEUSAL SOLID. (Paraeusal) Ointment Jar 1 oz., 2 oz., 16 oz.
Use: Burns, bedsores, keloids, skin infection, acne.
• **PARAFFIN,** N.F. XVI.
Use: Stiffening agent.
PARAFLEX. (McNeil Pharm) Chlorzoxazone 250 mg./Tab. Bot. 100s.
Use: Skeletal muscle relaxant.
PARAFON FORTE. (McNeil Pharm) Chlorzoxazone 250 mg., acetaminophen 300 mg./Tab. Bot. 100s, 500s. Blister pack 200s.
Use: Skeletal muscle relaxant.
PARAFORM. Paraformaldehyde. (No mfr. listed)
PARAFORMALDEHYDE.
Use: Essentially the same as formaldehyde.
See: Formaldehyde (Various Mfr.)
Trioxymethylene (an incorrect term for paraformaldehyde)
PARAGLYCYLARSANILIC ACID. N-Carbamylmethyl-p-aminobenzenearsonic acid, the free acid of tryparsamide.
PARA-HIST. (Pharmics) Chlorpheniramine maleate 8 mg., phenylephrine HCl 20 mg., phenylpropanolamine HCl 30 mg./Cap. T.R. Bot. 100s.
Use: Antihistamine decongestant.
PARA-HIST ANTITUSSIVE. (Pharmics) Diphenhydramine HCl 12 mg., phenylephrine HCl 2.5 mg., phenylpropanolamine HCl 10 mg., menthol 1 mg., potassium guaiacolsulfonate 60 mg., codeine phosphate 10 mg./5 cc. Syr. Bot. pt., gal.
Use: Antitussive.
PARA-JEL. (Approved) Benzocaine 5%, cetyl dimethyl benzyl ammonium chloride. Tube ¼ oz.
Use: Teething, toothache jel.
PARAL. (O'Neal, Jones & Feldman) Paraldehyde 15 gr./Cap. or cc. **Cap.:** Bot. 60s, 250s. **Amp.:** 2 cc., 5 cc., 10 cc. Boxes 12s, 25s. **Oral:** 30 cc./Bot. 12s, 25s.
Use: C.N.S. depressant.
• **PARALDEHYDE,** U.S.P. XXI. Sterile, U.S.P. XXI. 1,3,5-Trioxane, 2,4,6-trimethyl-.2,4,6-Trimethyl-s-trioxane. Paracetaldehyde. Bot. ¼ lb., 1 lb.-Amp.
Use: I.M., I.V. or Orally; Hypnotic & sedative.
See: Paral, Cap., Liq., Amp. (Fellows-Testagar)
PARAMEPHRIN.
See: Epinephrine (Various Mfr.)
• **PARAMETHADIONE,** U.S.P. XXI. Cap., Oral Soln., U.S.P. XXI. 2,4-Oxazolidinedione, 5-methyl-3,5-dimethyl-.5-Ethyl-3,5-dimethyl-2,4-oxazolidinedione.
Use: Anticonvulsant.
See: Paradione, Cap. & Sol. (Abbott)
PARAMETHASONE. B.A.N. 6α-Fluoro-11β,-17α, 21-trihydroxy-16α-methylpregna-1,4-diene-3,20-dione. 6 α-Fluoro-16α-methylprednisolone.
Use: Corticosteroid.

See: Haldrate Metilar [21-acetate]
- **PARAMETHASONE ACETATE,** U.S.P. XXI. Tab., U.S.P. XXI. 16α-Methyl-6α-fluoroprednisolone-21-acetate.6α-Fluoro-11β,17,21-trihydroxy-16α-methylpregna-1,4-diene-3,20-dione 21-Acetate.
Use: Glucorticoid.
See: Haldrone, Tab. (Lilly)
PARA-MONOCHLOROPHENOL.
See: Camphorated para-chlorophenol, Liq. (Novocol)
- **PARANYLINE HYDROCHLORIDE.** USAN.
Use: Anti-inflammatory.
- **PARAPENZOLATE BROMIDE.** USAN.
Use: Anticholingeric.
PARAROSANILINE EMBONATE. Pararosaniline Pamoate.
- **PARAROSANILINE PAMOATE.** USAN. Bis-[tris(p-Aminophenyl)methylium (4,4′-methylenebis[3-hydroxy-2-naphthoate])hydrate. Under study.
Use: Antischistosomal agent.
PARASAL SODIUM. (Panray) p-Aminosalicylate Sod. **Pow.:** Bot. 1 lb. **Tabs.:** Plain (0.5 Gm., 1 Gm.) Bot. 1000s. Lyophilized for laboratory use only 5 Gm./50 cc.
Use: Tuberculosis.
PARASITICIDE SHAMPOO. (Panray) Soap 30%, isobornyl thiocyanoacetate 5.125%, other related terpenes 1.125%. Bot. 16 oz.
Use: Antiparasitic.
- **PARASYMPATHOLYTIC AGENTS,** Cholinergic Blocking agents.
See: Anticholinergic Agents
Antispasmodics
Mydriatics
Parkinsonism
- **PARASYMPATHOMIMETIC AGENTS.**
See: Cholinergic Agents
PARA-THOR-MONE.
See: Parathyroid Inj. (Lilly)
PARATHYROID THERAPY. Dihydrotachysterol, U.S.P. XXI. Tachysterol.
See: Hytakerol, Sol., Cap. (Winthrop-Breon)
Parathyroid Injection (Various Mfr.)
PARA-TOX. (Eckerd) Pyrethrians 0.2%, peperonyl butoxide 2.0%, deodorized kerosene 5%.
Use: Treatment of body lice.
PARATROL LIQUID. (Walgreen) Pyrethrins 0.2%, piperonyl butoxide technical 2%, deodorized kerosene 0.8%. Bot. 2 oz.
Use: Kills head and body crab lice and eggs.
PARAXIN. Chloramphenicol, B.A.N.
PARAZONE. (Interstate) Chlorzoxazone 250 mg., acetaminophen 300 mg./Tab. Bot. 100s, 1000s.
Use: Skeletal muscle relaxant.
- **PARBENDAZOLE.** USAN. Methyl 5-butyl-2-benzimidazolecarbamate. Helmatac. Under study.
Use: Anthelmintic.
PARBUTOXATE. β-Dimethylaminoethyl-3-amino-4-butoxybenzoate.
PARCILLIN. (Parmed) Crystalline potassium penicillin G 240 mg., 400,000 u./Tab. Bot. 100s, 1000 s. Pow. for syr. 400,000/Tsp. 80 cc.
Use: Bacterial infections.

- **PARCONAZOLE HYDROCHLORIDE.** USAN.
Use: Antifungal.
PAR CREAM. (Parmed) Sulfanilamide 15%, 9-Aminoacridine HCl 0.2%, Allantoin 1.5% in a dispersible base. Tube 4 oz.
Use: Vulva, vaginal infections.
PAREDRINE. (SmithKline) Hydroxyamphetamine HBr. 1%, boric acid 2%, sod. ethyl mercurithiosalicylate 1:50,000. Bot. 0.5 oz.
Use: Ophthalmic solution; vasoconstrictor.
PAREDRINOL. p-(2-Methylaminopropyl) phenol (No Mfr. currently lists).
- **PAREGORIC.** U.S.P. XXI. (Various Mfr.)
Use: Antiperistaltic.
W/Bismuth subgallate, kaolin, pectin.
See: Dysenaid Jr., Tab. (Jenkins)
W/Glycyrrhiza fl. ext., antimony pot. tartrate.
See: Brown Mixture, Liq. (Lilly)
W/Kaolin (colloidal), aluminum hydroxide, bismuth subcarbonate, pectin.
See: Kapinal, Tab. (Jenkins)
W/Kaolin, pectin.
See: Kaoparin, Susp. (McKesson)
Kenpectin-P, Susp. (Kenwood)
Parepectolin, Susp. (Rorer)
W/Kaolin, pectin, bismuth subsalicylate, zinc sulfocarbonate.
W/Milk of bismuth, kaolin & pectin.
See: Mul-Sed, Liq. (Webcon)
W/Pectin & kaolin.
See: Parepectolin, Susp. (Rorer)
W/Zinc sulfocarbolate, phenyl salicylate, bismuth subsalicylate, & pepsin.
See: C M with Paregoric, Liq. (Beecham Labs)
Corrective Mixture with Paregoric (Beecham Labs)
PARELIXIR LIQUID. (Purdue Frederick) Tincture of opium and pectin. Bot. 6 fl. oz.
Use: Antidiarrheal.
PARENABOL. Boldenone undecylenate.
PAREPECTOLIN. (Rorer) Paregoric (equivalent) 3.7 ml., pectin 162 mg., kaolin 5.5 Gm./fl. oz. Susp., Bot. 4 fl. oz., 8 fl. oz.
Use: Nonspecific diarrheas.
- **PAREPTIDE SULFATE.** USAN.
Use: Antiparkinsonian.
PAR ESTRO. (Parmed) Conjugated estrogens 1.25 mg./Tab. Bot. 100s.
Use: Conjugated estrogen therapy.
PARETHOXYCAINE HCI.
W/Zirconium oxide, calamine.
See: Zotox, Spray, Cream (Commerce)
PAR-F. (Pharmics) Iron 66 mg., calcium 200 mg., Vit. C 75 mg., A 8000 I.U., D 400 I.U., B-1 5 mg., B-2 2 mg., B-12 2.5 mcg., B-6 5 mg. niacinamide 15 mg., iodine 0.15 mg., manganese 0.5 mg., copper 0.25 mg., zinc 0.5 mg., sodium fluoride 1.1 mg./Cap. Bot. 100s, 1000s.
Use: Vitamin and mineral supplementation.
PARGYLINE. B.A.N. N-Benzyl-N-methylprop-2-ynylamine.
Use: Hypotensive.

See: Eutonyl (hydrochloride)
• **PARGYLINE HYDROCHLORIDE,** U.S.P. XXI. Tab., U.S.P. XXI. N-Methyl-N-2-propynybenzylamine hydrochloride.
Use: Antihypertensive.
See: Eutonyl, Filmtab (Abbott)
W/Methyclothiazide.
See: Eutron Filmtab. (Abbott)
PARKELP. (Phillip R. Park) Pacific sea kelp. **Tab.:** Bot. 100s, 200s, 500s, 800s. **Gran.:** Bot. 2 oz., 7 oz., lb., 3 lb.
Use: Iodine source.
■ **PARKINSONISM.** Parasympatholytic agents.
See: Akineton, Tab., Amp. (Knoll)
Artane, Elix., Tab., Sequels (Lederle)
Caramiphen HCl
Cogentin Sinemet, Tab., Amp. (Merck Sharp & Dohme)
Disipal, Tab. (Riker)
Kemadrin, Tab. (Burroughs Wellcome)
Levodopa, Cap., Tab. (Various Mfr.)
Levsin, Tab., Elix., Inj., Drops (Kremers-Urban)
Levsinex Timecaps, Cap., Syr. (Kremers-Urban)
Pagitane HCl, Tab. (Lilly)
Parsidol HCl, Tab. (Warner-Chilcott)
Phenoxene, Tab. (Merrell Dow)
Symmetrel, Cap., Syr. (Du Pont)
Trihexyphenidyl HCl (Various Mfr.)
PARLAX SYRUP. (Robinson) Docusate sodium 20 mg./5 cc. Bot. 8 oz.
PARLAX. (Parmed) Danthron 75 mg. & calcium pantothenate 25 mg./Tab. Bot. 100s, 1000s.
Use: Laxative.
PARLAX W/CASANTHRANOL. (Robinson) Docusate sodium 100 mg., casanthranol 50 mg./Cap. Docusate sodium 50 mg., casanthranol 25 mg./Cap. Bot. 100s, 1000s.
PARLODEL. (Sandoz) Bromocriptine maleate. **Tab.:** 2.5 mg./Tab. Bot. 30s. **Cap.:** 5 mg./Cap. Bot. 30s, 100s.
Use: Short term treatment of amenorrhea and galactorrhea, prevention of physiological lactation, Parkinson's disease.
PAR-MAG. (Parmed) Magnesium oxide 140 mg./Cap. Bot. 100s.
PARMETH. (Parmed) Promethazine HCl 50 mg./Cap. Bot. 100s, 1000s.
Use: Allergy and motion sickness.
PARMINE. (Parmed) Phentermine HCl 30 mg./Cap. Bot. 100s, 1000s.
Use: Exogenous obesity.
PARMINYL. W/Salicylamide, phenacetin, caffeine, acetaminophen.
See: Dolopar, Tab. (O'Neal)
PAR-NATAL-FA. (Parmed) Vit. A 4000 I.U., D 400 I.U., thiamine HCl 2 mg., riboflavin 2 mg., pyridoxine HCl 0.8 mg., ascorbic acid 50 mg., niacinamide 10 mg., iodine 0.15 mg., folic acid 0.1 mg., cobalamin concentrate 2 mcg., iron 50 mg., calcium 240 mg./Cap. Bot. 100s, 1000s.
Use: Vitamin & mineral supplement in pregnancy & lactation.

PAR-NATAL-RX. (Parmed) Vit. A 6000 I.U., D 400 I.U., thiamine mononitrate 1.1 mg., riboflavin 1.8 mg., pyridoxine HCl 2.5 mg., vit B-12 8 mcg., folic acid 1 mg., iron 65 mg., calcium 125 mg., ascorbic acid 60 mg., niacinamide 15 mg./Tab. Bot. 100s, 1000s.
Use: Dietary supplement during pregnancy & lactation.
PARNATE. (SmithKline) Tranylcypromine sulfate 10 mg./Tab. Bot. 100s, 1000s.
Use: Antidepressant; MAO inhibitor.
PARODONTAX DENTAL CREAM. (Edward J. Moore) Sodium dicarbonate plus five natural herbs. Tube 60 Gm.
Use: Hygenic dentifrice and aid in prevention of periodontosis & caries.
PARODYNE.
See: Antipyrine (Various Mfr.)
PAROLEINE.
See: Petrolatum Liquid (Various Mfr.)
PAROMOMYCIN. B.A.N. An antibiotic substance obtained from cultures of certain *Streptomyces* species, one of which is *Streptomyces rimosus.*
Use: Antiamoebic.
• **PAROMOMYCIN SULFATE,** U.S.P XX. Caps., Syr., U.S.P. XXI.
Use: Antiamebic.
PAROTHYL. (Interstate) Meprobamate 400 mg., tridihexethyl Cl. 25 mg./Tab. Bot. 100s.
Use: Treatment of G.I. tract disorders associated with anxiety and tension.
PAROXYL.
See: Acetarsone (Var. Mfr.)
PARPANIT.
See: Caramiphen Hydrochloride (Var. Mfr.)
PARPANIT HYDROCHLORIDE. Caramiphen, B.A.N.
PARSIDOL HCl. (Parke-Davis) Ethopropazine HCl. Profenamine HCl, Lysivane, 10-(Diethylamino-1-propyl) Phenothiazine HCl. Tab. 10 mg., 50 mg., Bot. 100s.
Use: Parkinsonism.
PARSLEY CONCENTRATE.
W/Garlic conc.
See: Allimin, Tab. (Mosso)
PAR-Supp. (Parmed) Estrone 0.2 mg., lactose 50 mg./Vag. Supp. pkg. 12s.
Use: Vaginitis.
PARTEN. (Parmed) Acetaminophen 10 gr./Tab. Bot. 100s, 1000s.
Use: Antipyretic & analgesic.
PARTIAL ECLIPSE LOTION. (Dorsey) Padimate 0. SPF 15. Bot. 4 oz.
Use: Sunscreen.
PARTREX. (Parmed) Tetracycline 250 mg./Cap. Bot. 100s, 1000s.
Use: Antibacterial.
• **PARTRICIN.** USAN. Antibiotic produced by *Streptomyces aureofaciens.*
Use: Antifungal, antiprotozoal.
PARTUSS. (Parmed) Dextromethorphan hydrobromide 60 mg., pot. guaiacol sulfonate 8 gr., chlorpheniramine maleate 6 mg., ammonium Cl. 8

gr., tartar emetic ¹⁄₁₂ gr., chloroform 2 min./30 cc.
Bot. Gal., pt., 4 oz.
Use: cough mixture.
PARTUSS "A". (Parmed) Acetaminophen 5 gr.,
Salicylamide 2 gr., caffeine ½ gr., atropine sulfate
0.12 mg., guaifenesin 100 mg.,
phenylpropanolamine HCl 25 mg./Tab. Bot. 1000s.
Use: Decongestant, analgesic, & expectorant.
PARTUSS A.C. (Parmed) Guaifenesin 100 mg.,
pheniramine maleate 7.5 mg., codeine phosphate
10.0 mg., alcohol 3.5%/5 cc. Bot 4 oz.
Use: cough suppressant and expectorant.
PARTUSS T.D. (Parmed) Acetaminophen 300 mg.,
salicylamide 300 mg., phenylpropanolamine HCl 60
mg., chlorpheniramine maleate 4 mg./Tab. Bot.
100s, 1000s.
Use: Decongestant.
PAR VAG SUPPOSITORY. (Parmed) Aminacrine HCl
14 mg., sulfanilamide 1.05 Gm., allantoin 140
mg./Suppository.
Use: Vaginitis treatment
PARZONE. (Mallinckrodt) Brand of dihydrocodeine
bitartrate. ⅛ oz., 1 oz., 5 oz.
P.A.S. ACID. (Kasar) Para-aminosalicylic acid 500
mg./Tab. Bot. 1000s.
Use: Tuberculosis.
PAS-C. (Hellwig) Pascorbic. p-aminosalicylic acid 0.5
Gm. with vit. C/Tab. Bot. 1000s.
Use: Tuberculosis therapy.
PASDIUM. (Kasar) Sod. aminosalicylate 0.5 Gm., 1
Gm./Tab. Bot. 1000s.
Use: Tuberculosis.
PASIBAR. (Jenkins) Acetylsalicylic acid 3½ gr.,
acetophenetidin 2½ gr., caffeine alkaloids ¼ gr.,
phenobarbital ¼ gr./Tab. Bot. 1000s. Available in
blue and pink.
Use: Analgesic.
PASIJEN. (Jenkins) Passiflora 1 gr., valerian 1 gr.,
ext. henbane ⅛ gr. (total alkaloids 0.00019 gr.),
phenobarbital ¼ gr./Tab. Bot. 1000s.
Use: Sedative, antispasmodic.
PASKALIUM. (Glenwood) Potassium amino-salicylate.
Envules 3 Gm. envelopes, boxes 100s. **Tab.** 0.5
Gm. Bot. 1000s. **Pow.** Bot. 100 Gm.
Use: Tuberculosis.
PASSIFLORA. Dried flowering & fruiting tops of
Passiflora incarnata.
W/Phenobarbital, ext. hyoscyamus.
See: Somlyn w/Pb, Cap. (Scrip)
W/Phenobarbital, jamaica dogwood.
See: Sominol, Phenobarbital, Tab. (O'Neal)
W/Phenobarbital, valerian, hyoscyamus.
See: Aluro, Tab. (Foy)
PASTEURELLA TULARENSIS ANTIGEN. 10,000
million organisms/cc.
(Lederle)—Vial 5 cc., 20 cc.
Use: Diagnostic use for tularemia.
PATH. (Parker) Buffered neutral formalin sol. 10%.
Bot. 4 oz., 1 gal., 5 gal. Jar 4 oz.
Use: Tissue specimen fixative.
PATHIBAMATE 200. (Lederle) Meprobamate 200
mg., tridihexethyl chloride 25 mg./Tab. Bot. 100s, &
1000s.

PATHIBAMATE-400. (Lederle) Meprobamate 400 mg.,
tridihexethyl chloride 25 mg./Tab. Bot. 100s, 1000s.
Drum 5000s.
Use: Treatment of G.I. tract disorders associated
with anxiety and tension.
PATHILON CHLORIDE. (Lederle) Tridihexethyl
chloride 25 mg./Tab. Bot. 100s, 1000s.
Use: Anticholinergic in the treatment of peptic
ulcer.
W/Meprobamate.
See: Pathibamate 200 & 400, Tabs. (Lederle)
W/Phenobarbital. Pathilon 25 mg., phenobarbital 15
mg./Tab. Bot. 100s, 1000s. (Lederle)
Use: Anticholinergic with sedative in the treatment
of peptic ulcer.
PATHOCIL. (Wyeth) Sodium dicloxacillin
monohydrate. Monohydrate sodium salt of 6[3-(2,6-
dichlorophenyl)-5-methyl-4-isoxazolyl]penicillin. 250
mg./Cap. Bot. 100s. 500 mg./Cap. Bot. 50s. Pow.
for oral susp. 62.5 mg./5 ml. Bot. to make 100 ml.
Use: Staphylococcal infection.
• **PAULOMYCIN.** USAN.
PAVABID. (Marion) Papaverine HCl 150 mg./Cap.
Bot. 100s, 250s, 1000s, 5000s. Unit Dose Paks
100s. Uni-Rx Paks of 60s, 100s. Ctn. 12 × 60. Uni-Rx
12 × 100.
Use: Vasodilator.
PAVABID HP. (Marion) Papaverine HCl 300
mg./Caplet. Uni-Rx Paks 60s.
Use: Vasodilator.
PAVACAP. (Reid-Provident) Papaverine HCl 150
mg./Unicelle. Bot. 100s, 1000s.
Use: Relief of cerebral and peripheral ischemia.
PAVACAPS. (Freeport) Papaverine HCl. 150 mg./T.R.
Cap. Bot. 1000s.
Use: Relief of cerebral and peripheral eschemia.
PAVACEN CENULES. (Central) Papaverine HCl 150
mg./Cap. Bot. 100s, 1000s.
Use: Cerebral vasodilator.
PAVACLOR. (Pasadena Research) Papaverine HCl
150 mg. Cap. Bot. 100s.
PAVACRON CHRONCAPS. (Cenci) Papaverine HCl
150 mg./Cap. Bot. 100s, 1000s.
PAVADEL. (Canright) Papaverine HCl 150 mg./Cap.
Bot. 100s, 1000s.
Use: Relief of cerebral and peripheral ischemia.
PAVADEL PB. (Canright) Papaverine HCl 150 mg.,
phenobarbital 45 mg./Cap. Bot. 100s.
Use: Relief of cerebral and peripheral ischemia.
PAVADON ELIXIR. (Coastal) Codeine phosphate
64.8 mg., acetaminophen 11 gr., alcohol 10%/fl.
oz. Bot. 4 oz., pt.
Use: Analgesic.
PAVADUR. (Century) Papaverine HC1 150 mg./Cap.
Bot. 100s, 1000s.
Use: Vasodilator, smooth muscle relaxant.
PAVADYL. (Bock) Papaverine HCl 150 mg./Cap. Bot.
100s.
Use: Relief of cerebral and peripheral ischemia.
PAVAKEY S.A. (Key) Papaverine HCl 150
mg./Sustained Action Cap. Bot. 100s, 1000s.
Use: Vasodilator.

PAVA-LYN. (Lynwood) Papaverine HCl 150 mg./Cap.
Bot. 100s.
Use: Smooth muscle relaxant.
PAVA-PAR. (Parmed) Papaverine HCl 150 mg./Cap.
Bot. 100s, 1000s.
Use: For the relief of cerebral and peripheral
ischemia.
PAVA-RX. (Blaine) Papaverine HCl 150 mg./Timed
Cap. Bot. 100s.
Use: Vasodilator.
PAVASED. (Mallard) Papaverine HCl 150 mg./Cap.
Bot. 100s, 500s.
PAVASPAN. (Jamieson-McKames) Ethaverine HCl 150
mg./T.R. Cap. Bot. 100s.
Use: Relief of cerebral and peripheral ischemia.
PAVASULE. (Misemer) Papaverine HCl 150 mg./T.D.
Cap. Bot.
Use: Relief of cerebral & peripheral ischemia.
PAVATEST. (Fellows) Papaverine HCl 150 mg./T.D.
Cap. Bot. 100s, 1000s.
Use: Vasodilator.
PAVATIME. (Rocky Mtn.) Papaverine HCl 150
mg./Cap. Bot. 100s.
Use: Vasodilator.
PAVATYM. (Everett) Papaverine HCl 150 mg./T.R.
Cap. Bot. 100s, 1000s., unit dose 100s.
Use: Vasodilatior.
PAVA-WOL. (Wolins) Papaverine HCl 150 mg./Cap.
Bot. 100s, 250s, 1000s.
Use: Relief of cerebral and peripheral ischemia.
PAVERINE SPANCAP. (Vortech) Papaverine HCl 150
mg./Cap. Bot. 100s,
1000s.
Use: Vasodilator.
PAVEROLAN. (Lannett) Papaverine 150
mg./Lanacap. Bot. 100s, 1000s.
Use: Muscle relaxant.
PAVEX. (Xttrium) Papaverine HCl 150 mg./Cap. Bot.
100s.
Use: Smooth muscle relaxant.
PAVRIN-T.D. (Kenyon) Papaverine HCl 150 mg./Cap.
Bot. 100s, 1000s.
Use: Vasodilator.
PAVULON. (Organon) Pancuronium bromide. 2
mg./ml. Amp. 2 ml., 5 ml. Box 25s. 1 mg./ml. Vial
10 ml. Box 25s.
Use: Muscle relaxant (surgical).
PAX-400. (Kenyon) Meprobamate 400 mg./Tab. Bot.
100s, 1000s.
Use: Tranquilizer.
PAXAREL. (Circle) Acetylcarbromal 250 mg./Tab.
Bot. 100s.
Use: Sedative.
PAXIPAM. (Schering) Halazepam 20 mg. or 40
mg./Tab. Bot. 100s, 500s. Unit dose 100s.
Use: Anxiety disorders.
PAYZONE HCl. Nitrovin, B.A.N.
PAZO OINTMENT. (Bristol-Myers) Benzocaine 0.8%,
zinc oxide 4%, ephedrine sulfate 0.2%, camphor
2.18%, Ointment. Tubes: 1 oz., 2 oz.
Use: Hemorrhoid medication.
PAZO SUPPOSITORY. (Bristol-Myers) Benzocaine

15.44 mg., ephedrine sulfate 3.86 mg., zinc oxide 77.2
mg., camphor 42.0/supp.
Boxes: 12s, 24s.
Use: Hemorrhoid medication.
• **PAZOXIDE.** USAN.
Use: Antihypertensive.
PB 100. (Schlicksup) Phenobarbital 1½ gr./Tab. Bot.
1000s.
P.B.N. (Jenkins) Bacitracin 400 u., neomycin sulfate 5
mg., polymyxin B sulfate 5000 u./Gm. Tube ½ oz.
Use: Antibiotic ointment.
PBZ-SR. (Geigy) Tripelennamine HCl 100 mg./Tab. Sus-
tained release. Bot. 100s.
Use: Antihistamine.
PCMX.
See: Para Chloro Meta Xylenol.
PDM. (Century) Phendimetrazine tartrate 35 mg./Tab.
Bot. 1000s.
Use: Anorexic.
PEACOCK'S BROMIDES. (Natcon) **Liq.** Pot. bromide
6 gr., sod. bromide 6 gr., ammonium bromide 3
gr./5 ml. Bot. 8 oz. **Tab.** Pot. bromide 3 gr., sod.
bromide 3 gr., ammonium bromide 1½ gr./Tab.
Bot. 100s.
Use: Sedative.
• **PEANUT OIL,** N.F. XVI.
Use: Pharm. aid. (solvent, oleaginous vehicle).
PECAZINE.   B.A.N.   10-(1-Methyl-3-piperidylmethyl)-
phenothiazine.
Use: Tranquilizer.
See: Pacatal (hydrochloride or acetate)
PECILOCIN. B.A.N. An antibiotic produced by
Paecilomyces variotin banier (var. antibioticus). 1-
(8-Hydroxy-6-methyldodeca-trans trans cis-2,4,6-tri-
enoyl)-2-pyrrolidone.
See: Variotin
PECTAMOL. (British Drug House)
Diethylaminoethoxyethyl-a,a-diethylphenylacetate ci-
trate. Bot. 4, 16, 80, 160 fl. oz.
Use: Non-narcotic antitussive.
• **PECTIN,** U.S.P. XXI. (Various Mfr.)
Use: Protectant, pharmaceutic aid (suspending
agent).
PECTIN W/COMBINATIONS.
See: Amogel, Tab. (Vortech)
Baropectin Susp. (Barry-Martin)
Bismuth, Pectin & Paregoric (Lemmon)
Cholactabs, Tab. (Philips Roxane)
Diastay, Tab. (Elder)
Diatrol, Tab. (Otis Clapp)
DIA-Quel, Liq. (Inter. Pharm.)
Donnagel Susp. (Robins)
Donnagel-PG, Susp. (Robins)
Dua-Pred, Inj. (Reid-Provident)
Duosorb, Liq. (Reid-Provident)
Ekrised, Tab. (Mallard)
Furoxone, Liq., Tab. (Eaton)
Infantol Pink, Liq. (Scherer)
Kamabel, Liq. (Towne)
Kao-Con, Liq. (Upjohn)
Kaolin-Bismuth Pectin Compound
Kaoparin, Susp. (McKesson)
Kaopectate, Liq. (Upjohn)

Kao-pectin, Tab. (Wolins)
Kapigam, Liq. (Reid-Provident)
Kapinal, Tab. (Jenkins)
Kenpectin prods., Susp. (Kenwood)
Keotin, Liq. (Blue Line)
KBP/O, Cap. (Cole)
Metropectin, Tab. (Pennwalt)
Mul-Sed, Susp. (Webcon)
Opecto, Elix. (Bowman)
Parelixir, Liq. (Purdue Frederick)
Parepectolin, Susp. (Rorer)
Pectocel, Liq. (Lilly)
Pectocomp, Liq. (Lannett)
Pecto-Kalin, Susp. (Lemmon)
Pectokay, Liq. (Bowman)
Pektamalt, Liq. (Warren-Teed)
Polymagma Plain Tablets (Wyeth)
Wescola Antidiarrheal-Stomach Upset (Western Research)

PECTOCOMP. (Lannett) Pectin 4 gr., kaolin 90 gr., zinc phenolsulfonate 1⅛ gr./Fl. oz. Bot. pt., gal.
Use: A supportive treatment for diarrhea and other intestinal inflammations.

PECTOKAY MIXTURE. (Bowman) Kaolin and pectin mixture. Bot. pt., gal.
Use: Anti-diarrheal.

PEDAMETH. (O'Neal, Jones & Feldman) Racemethionine. Cap.: 200 mg./Cap. Bot. 50s, 500s. Liq.: 75 mg./5 ml. Bot. pt.
Use: Control of diaper rash.

PE-DE-EM. (Bowman) Phendimetrazine tartrate 35 mg./Tab.
Use: Anorexiant.

PEDENEX. (Approved) Caprylic acid, zinc undecylenate, sod. propionate. Tube 1½ oz. Foot powd. spray 5 oz.
Use: Athlete's foot.

PEDIACOF SYRUP. (Winthrop-Breon) Codeine phos. 5.0 mg., phenylephrine HCl 2.5 mg., chlorpheniramine maleate 0.75 mg., potassium iodide 75.0 mg./5 ml. w/sodium benzoate 0.2%, alcohol 5%. Bot. 16 fl. oz.
Use: Antitussive for coughs due to colds & other upper respiratory infections.

PEDIACON. (CMC) Thiamine HCl 10 mg., B-12 crystalline 25 mg./5 cc. Bot. 4 oz., pt., gal. Same formula W/Elemental iron 30 mg./5 cc. Bot. 4 oz., pt., gal.
Use: Dietary supplement.

PEDIAFLOR FLUORIDE DROPS. (Ross) Sod. Fluoride. 0.5 mg./ml. Bot. 50 ml.
Use: Fluoride supplement, prevention of dental caries.

PEDIALYTE. (Ross) Sod. 30 mEq, pot. 20 mEq, Calcium 4 mEq, Mg 4 mEq, chloride 30 mEq, citrate 28 mEq, dextrose 50 mEq/Liter. Nursing Bot. w/nipple 8 oz. Cans 32 oz. 6s. 6.2 calories/fl. oz.
Use: Oral electrolyte infant formula.

PEDIAMYCIN DROPS. (Ross) Erythromycin ethylsuccinate for oral suspension 100 mg./2.5 ml. Bot. 50 ml. (Dropper enclosed)
Use: Antibiotic.

PEDIAMYCIN 400. (Ross) Erythromycin ethylsuccinate oral suspension 400 mg./5 ml. Bot. pt.
Use: Antibiotic.

PEDIAMYCIN LIQUID. (Ross) Erythromycin ethylsuccinate oral suspension 200 ml./5 ml. Bot. pt.
Use: Antibiotic.

PEDIAMYCIN SUSPENSION. (Ross) Erythromycin ethylsuccinate for oral suspension 200 mg./5 ml., Bot., 100 ml., 150 ml.
Use: Antibiotic.

PEDIATRIC COUGH SYRUP. (Weeks & Leo) Ammonium Cl. 300 mg., sodium citrate 600 mg./oz. Bot. 4 oz.
Use: Cough relief for infants age 3 months and older.

PEDIATROL (B13). (Kenyon) Vit. B-12 25 mcg., B-1 10 mg./5 cc. Bot. pt., gal.

PEDIAZOLE SUSPENSION. (Ross) Erythromycin ethylsuccinate 200 mg., sulfisoxazole acetyl 600 mg./ 5 ml. Bot. Granules reconstituted to 100 ml., 150 ml., 200 ml.
Use: Acute otitis media caused by susceptible strain of *hemophilus influenzae* in children.

PEDI-BATH. (Pedinol) Collodial sulfur, Balsam peru. Bot. 6 oz.
Use: Foot bath and soak.

PEDI-BOOT MIST KIT. (Pedinol) Cetyl pyridinium Cl., triacetin, chloroxylenol. Bot. 2 oz.
Use: Fungicide, sanitizer, deodorizer for foot apparel.

PEDI-BORO SOAK PAKS. (Pedinol) Astringent wet dressing. Box 12s, 100s.
Use: Astringent solution for minor skin irritations.

PEDI-CORT V CREME. (Pedinol) Clioquinol 3%; hydrocortisone 1%, Tube 20 Gm.
Use: Antibacterial, antifungal, antipruritic agent.

PEDICRAN WITH IRON. (Scherer) Vit. B-12 (cryst.) 25 mcg., ferric pyrophosphate, soluble (elemental iron 30 mg.) 250 mg., thiamine mononitrate 10 mg., nicotinamide 10 mg., alcohol 1%/5 cc. Bot. 4 oz., pt.
Use: Iron deficiency anemias.

■ **PEDICULICIDES.**
See: A-200 Pyrinate (Norcliff Thayer)
Benzyl Benzoate, Preps. (Various Mfr.)
Chlorophenothane (Various Mfr.)
Cuprex, Liq. (Calgon Consumer Prods.)
DDT (Various Mfr.)
Kwell, Preps. (Reed & Carnrick)

PEDI-DENT CV. (Stanlabs) Sod. fluoride 2.21 mg., Vit. A 500 I.U., D-2 500 I.U., B-1 3 mg., B-2 2.5 mg., B-6 1 mg., B-12 1 mcg., C 75 mg., niacinamide 2.5 mg./Chewable Tab. Bot. 100s.
Use: Aid in reducing dental caries, vitamin supplement.

PEDI-DRI FOOT POWDER. (Pedinol) Aluminum chlorohydroxide complex, zinc undecylenate, menthol, formaldehyde. Pkg. 2 oz.
Use: Antiperspirant, deodorant, fungicidal foot powder.

PEDI-TOT. (Blue Cross) Bromorphan 5 mg., glyceryl guaiacolate 12.5 mg., ammonium Cl. 60 mg., sodium citrate 40 mg./5 ml. Bot. 4 oz.
Use: Cough syrup.

PEDITUSS. (Sutliff & Case) N-Acetyl-p-amino-phenol 64.5 mg., sod. salicylate 129 mg., phenylephrine 2 mg., guaifenesin 20 mg./5 cc. Bot. 3 oz., 1 pt., 1 gal.
Use: Analgesic, expectorant.

PEDI-VIT A CREME. (Pedinol) Vitamin A 100,000 units/oz. Jar 2 oz., 16 oz., 5 lb.
Use: Skin conditioner.

PEDOLATUM. (King) Salicylic acid w/sod. salicylate oint. Pkg. ½ oz.

PEDO-SOL. (Bock) Butabarbital sodium 30 mg., chlorpheniramine maleate 1.5 mg., hyoscine hydrobromide 0.1 mg./Tab. Tab. Bot. 100s.
Use: Sedative.

PEDRIC ELIXIR. (Vale) Acetaminophen 120 mg./5ml. w/alcohol 10%. Bot. pt., gal.
Use: Analgesic.

PEDRIC SENIOR. (Vale) Acetaminophen 320 mg.
Use: Analgesic

PEDRIC WAFERS. (Vale) Acetaminophen 120 mg./Wafer. Bot. 100s, 500s, 1000s.
Use: Analgesic.

• **PEFLOXACIN.** USAN.
Use: Antibacterial.

PEGANONE. (Abbott) Ethotoin. 3-Ethyl-5-phenyl-hydantoin. Tab. 250 mg. Bot. 100s, 500 mg. Bot. 100s.
Use: Orally, anticonvulsant in the control of grand mal seizures.

PEGLICOL 5 OLEATE. USAN.
Use: Emulsifying agent.

P.E.G. OINTMENT. (Medco Lab) Polyethylene glycol. Jar 16 oz.
Use: Water soluble ointment base.

• **PEGOTERATE.** USAN.
Use: Suspending agent.

• **PEGOXOL 7 STEARATE.** USAN.
Use: Emulsifying agent.

PEKTAMALT. (Adria) Kaolin 6.5 Gm., pectin 0.6 Gm., pot. gluconate, sodium citrate/oz. Bot. 1 pt.
Use: Intestinal distress; antidiarrheal.

PELENTAN. Ethyl Biscoumacetate. (No Mfr. currently lists)

• **PELIOMYCIN.** USAN. An antibiotic derived from *Streptomycin luteogriseus.*
Use: Antineoplastic agent.

• **PEMERID NITRATE.** USAN. 4-[3-(Di-methylimino)-propoxy]-1,2,2,6,6-pentamethylpiperidine dinitrate.
Use: Antitussive.

• **PEMOLINE.** USAN. 2-amino-5-phenyl-4-azolin-4-one.
Use: Childhood attention-defecit syndrome (hyperkinetic syndrome).
See: Cylert Prods. (Abbott)

PEMPIDINE. B.A.N. 1,2,2,6,6-Pentamethylpiperidine.
Use: Hypotensive.
See: Perolysen Tenormal (hydrogen tartrate)

PENAGEN-VK. (Grafton) Penicillin V 250 mg./Tab. Bot. 100s. Powder 250 mg./100 cc.
Use: Antibiotic.

PENAMECILLIN. B.A.N. Acetoxymethyl 6-phenyl-acetamidopenicillanate.
Use: Antibiotic.
See: Havapen

PENAMP "250", "500". (Lannett) 250 mg., 500 mg./Cap. Bot. 100s.

PENAPAR VK. (Parke-Davis) Potassium phenoxymethyl penicillin. **Tab.** 250 mg., Bot. 100s, 1000s, Unit dose 100s; 500 mg. Bot. 100s, 500s.
For oral solution (buffered): 125 mg./5 ml. or 250 mg./5 ml. Bot. 100 ml., 200 ml.
Use: Antibiotic.

• **PENBUTOLOL.** USAN.(−)-1-tert-Butylamino-3-(2-cy-clopentylphenoxy)propan-2-ol.
Use: Beta adrenergic blocking agent.

PENDECAMAINE. B.A.N. NN-Dimethyl-(3-palmitamido-propyl)glycine betaine.
Use: Surface active agent.

PENDIOMID. (Ciba) Azamethonium bromide. B.A.N.

PENETHAMATE HI.
See: Benzylpenicillin 2-diethylaminoethyl ester HI.

PENETHAMATE HYDRIODIDE. B.A.N. 2-Diethylamino-ethyl 6-phenylacetamidopenicillanate hydriodide.
Benzylpenicillin 2-diethylaminoethyl ester hydriodide.
Use: Treatment of respiratory tract infections.
See: Estopen

• **PENFLURIDOL.** USAN. 1-[4,4-bis(p-Flurophenyl)-butyl]-4-(4-chloro-α,α,α-trifluoro-m-tolyl)-4-piperidi-nol. 4-(4-Chloro-3-trifluoromethylphenyl)-1-[4,4-di-(4-fluorophenyl)butyl]piperidin-4-ol.
Use: Tranquilizer.

PENFONYLIN.
See: Pentid, Prods. (Squibb)

PENGUIN FOOT TREAT CREAM. (DeWitt) Bot. 4 oz.

• **PENICILLAMINE,** U.S.P. XXI. Caps., Tab., U.S.P. XXI. (Merck Sharp & Dohme) D-3-Mercaptovaline. Cu-primine.
Use: Metal complexing agent.
See: Cuprimine, Caps. (Merck Sharp & Dohme) Depen, Tab. (Wallace)

PENICILLIN. Unless clarified, it means an antibiotic substance or substances produced by growth of the molds *Penicillium notatum* or *P. chrysogenum.*
Use: Antibiotic.

PENICILLIN ALUMINUM. Aluminum 3,3-dimethyl-7-oxo-6-(2-phenylacetamido)-4-thia-1-azabicyclo-[3.2.0]-heptane-2-carboxylate.
Use: Antibiotic.

PENICILLIN CALCIUM. Calcium 3,3-dimethyl-7-oxo-6-(2-phenylacetamido)-4-thia-1-azabicyclo-[3.2.0]-heptane-2-carboxylate. U.S.P. XIII.

PENICILLIN, DIMETHOXY-PHENYL. Methicillin So-dium.
Use: Antibiotic.
See: Staphcillin, Vial (Bristol)

• **PENICILLIN G. BENZATHINE,** U.S.P. XXI. Sterile Susp., Oral Susp., Sterile, Tab. U.S.P. XXI.
Benzathine penicillin G.
Use: Antibiotic.
See: Permapen, Aq. Susp. (Pfizer Laboratories)

• **PENICILLIN S BENZATHINE AND PENICILLIN G PROCAINE SUSPENSION, STERILE,** U.S.P. XXI.

Use: Antibiotic.

• **PENICILLIN G, POTASSIUM,** U.S.P. XXI. Cap., Inj., for Oral Soln., Sterile, Tab., Tab. for Oral Soln., U.S.P. XXI. (Potassium Penicillin, Benzyl Penicillin Pot.)
Use: Antibiotic.
See: Arcocillin, Prep. (Arcum)
Biotic-T-500, Tab. (Scrip)
Cryspen 400, Tab. (Knight)
Deltapen, Syr., Tab. (Trimen)
G-Recillin-T, Tab. (Reid-Provident)
Hyasorb, Tab. (Key Pharm.)
K-Cillin, Prods. (Mayrand)
K-Pen, Tab. (Kay)
Lanacillin, Pow. (Lannett)
Palocillin-S, Powder (Hauck)
Palocillin-5, Tab. (Hauck)
Parcillin, Tab. (Parmed)
Pensorb, Tab. (Kenyon)
Pentids, Syr., Tab. (Squibb)
Pfizerpen, Tab., Syr. (Pfipharmecs)
Pfizerpen, Inj. (Pfizer Laboratories)
SK-Penicillin G, Tab., Sol. (SmithKline)

PENICILLIN G POTASSIUM W/COMBINATIONS.
See: Lanacillin "200,000", "400,000" (Lannett)
Pentid, Prods. (Squibb)

• **PENICILLIN G, PROCAINE, STERILE,** U.S.P. XXI. (Procaine Penicillin) Sterile Susp. U.S.P. XXI.
Use: Antibiotic.
Parenteral, aq. susp., (Procaine Penicillin, for Aq. Inj.,) Procaine Penicillin and buffered Pen. for aqueous, Inj.
See: Crysticillin A.S., Vial (Squibb)
Diurnal-Panicillin (Upjohn)
Duracillin A.S., Prep. (Lilly)
Pfizerpen-AS (Pfizer Laboratories)
Tu-Cillin, Inj. (Reid-Provident)
Wycillin, Susp. (Wyeth)
Parenteral, in oil w/aluminum monostearate.
Penicillin Procaine in Oil Inj.

PENICILLIN G PROCAINE COMBINATIONS
See: Bicillin All-Purpose, Vial (Wyeth)
Bicillin C-R, Tubex (Wyeth)
Bicillin C-R 900/300 Inj. (Wyeth)
Duracillin F.A., Amp. (Lilly)
Duracillin Fortified, Vial (Lilly)

• **PENICILLIN G SODIUM FOR INJECTION,** U.S.P. XXI. (Various Mfr.) Sodium Benzylpenicillin.
Use: Antibiotic.

• **PENICILLIN G SODIUM, STERILE,** U.S.P. XXI.
Use: Antibiotic.

• **PENICILLIN G PROCAINE W/ALUMINUM STEARATE SUSPENSION, STERILE,** U.S.P. XXI.
Use: Antibiotic.

PENICILLIN HYDRABAMINE PHENOXYMETHYL.
3,3-Dimethyl-7-oxo-6-(2-phenoxyacetamido)-4-thia-1-azabicyclo[3.2.0]heptane-2-carboxylic acid compound with N,N'-bis[(1,2,3,4,-4a,9,10,10a-octahydro-7-isopropyl-1,4a-dimethyl-1-phenanthryl)methyl]ethylenediamine.
Use: Antibiotic.

PENICILLIN N. Adicillin, B.A.N.

Use: Antibiotic.

PENICILLIN O CHLOROPROCAINE. 6-[2-(Allylthio)acetamido]-3-3-dimethyl-7-oxo-4-thia-1-azabicyclo-[3.2.0]heptane-2-carboxylic acid compound with 2-(diethylamino)ethyl 4-amino-2-chlorbenzoate (1:1).
Use: Antibiotic.

PENICILLIN O, SODIUM. Allylmercaptomethyl penicillin.
Use: Antibiotic.

PENICILLIN, PHENOXYETHYL.
Use: Antibiotic.
See: Phenethicillin, Penicillin pot. 152

PENICILLIN PHENOXYMETHYL BENZATHINE.
Use: Antibiotic.
See: Penicillin V Benzathine

PENICILLIN PHENOXYMETHYL HYDRABAMINE.
Use: Antibiotic.
See: Penicillin V Hydrabamine

• **PENICILLIN V,** U.S.P. XX for Oral Susp., Tab. U.S.P. XXI. Phenoxymethyl penicillin. A biosynthetic penicillin formed by fermentation, with suitable precursors of *Penicillin notatum.*
Use: Antibiotic.
See: Biotic pow. (Scrip)
Compocillin-V., Water, Susp. (Ross)
Ledercillin VK(Lederle)
Penagen-VK, Tab., Pow. (Gafton)
Pfizerpen VK (Pfipharmecs)
Robicillin-VK (Robins)
SK-Penicillin VK (SmithKline)
Uticillin VK (Upjohn)
V-Cillin, Preps. (Lilly)
V-Pen, Tab. (Century)

• **PENICILLIN V BENZATHINE,** U.S.P. XXI.
Use: Antibiotic.
See: Pen-Vee, Prods. (Wyeth)

PENICILLIN V HYDRABAMINE. Hydrabamine phenoxymethyl penicillin.
Use: Antibiotic.
See: Compocillin-V Hydrabamine, Oral Susp. (Ross)

• **PENICILLIN V POTASSIUM,** U.S.P. XXI. Oral Soln., Tab., U.S.P. XXI.
Use: Antibiotic.
See: Beepen VK, Tab., Syrup (Beecham Labs)
Betapen VK., Sol., Tab. (Bristol)
Biotic-V-Powder (Scrip)
Bopen, V-K, Tab. (Boyd)
Cocillin V-K, Tab. (Coastal)
Dowpen VK, Tab. (Merrell Dow)
Lanacillin VK, Tab., Pow. (Lannett)
Ledercillin VK, Oral, Sol., Tab. (Lederle)
LV, Tabs. (Elder)
Penapar VK, Tabs. or For Oral Sol'n. (Parke-Davis)
Pen-Vee-K, Sol., Tab. (Wyeth)
Pfizerpen VK, Pow., Tab. (Pfipharmecs)
Phenethicillin Pot.
Repen-VK, Tab., Oral Susp. (Reid-Provident)
Robicillin VK, Tab., Sol. (Robins)
Ro-Cillin VK, Sol., Tab. (Rowell)
Saropen-VK (Saron)
SK-Penicillin VK, Sol., Tab. (SmithKline)

Suspen, Liq. (Circle)
Uticillin VK, Tab., Sol. (Upjohn)
V-Cillin K, Tab., Oral Sol. (Lilly)
Veetids, Solution and Tabs. (Squibb)

PENICILLINASE. B.A.N. An enzyme that hydrolyzes penicillin, obtained from several strains of bacteria *(B. cereus).* Vial (1,000 u.) 20 cc. Clinical lab use only.

PENIDURAL.
Use: Antibiotic.
See: Benazthine Penicillin B.A.N.

PENNATE. (Robinson) Pentaerythritol tetranitrate. **"10":** 10 mg./Tab. Bot. 100s, 1000s. **"20":** 20 mg./Tab. Bot. 100s, 1000s. **"30":** 30 mg./Timed-caps. Bot. 100s, 500s, 1000s.
Use: Vasodilator.

PENNPHENO. (Robinson) Phenobarbital ¼ gr., pentaerythritol 10 mg. or 20 mg./Tab. Bot. 100s, 1000s.
Use: Vasodilator.

PENOTAL. (Coastal) Phenobarbital sod. ⅜ gr., pentobarbital sod. ⅜ gr./Cap. Bot. 100s, 500s.
Use: Mild sedative.

PENOTAL ELIXIR. (Coastal) Phenobarbital sod. ⅛ gr., pentobarbital sod. ⅛ gr./5 cc., alcohol 10%. Bot. 4 oz., pt., gal.
Use: Sedative.

PENSORB. (Kenyon) Crystalline penicillin G potassium 250,000 u., buffered w. Ca carbonate/Tab. Bot. 100s, 1000s.
Use: Antibiotic.

PENSTREP. (MSD AGVET) Penicillin-dihydro-streptomycin injection and suspension. Procaine penicillin G 200,000 u., dihydrostreptomycin 0.25 Gm./cc.
Use: Antibiotic, veterinary medicine.

• **PENTABAMATE.** USAN. 3-Methyl-2,4-pentanediol dicarbamate.
Use: Tranquilizer.

PENTA-CAP #1. (Kenyon) Pentaerythritol tetranitrate 30 mg./Cap. Bot. 90s, 100s, 1000s.
Use: Vasodilator.

PENTA-CAP PLUS. (Kenyon) Pentaerythritol tetranitrate 30 mg., amobarbital 50 mg./Cap. Bot. 100s, 1000s.
Use: Vasodilator.

PENTACHLOROPHENATE SODIUM.
See: Podosan, Pow. (Doak)

PENTACOSACTRIDE. D-Ser¹-Nle⁴-(Val-NH₂)²⁵⁻ β¹ ²⁵ corticotrophin.
Use: Corticotrophic peptide.
See: Norleusactide (I.N.N.)

PENTACYNIUM METHYLSULPHATE. B.A.N. 4-2-[(5-Cyano-5,5-diphenylpentyl)dimethylammonio]ethyl-4-methylmorpholinium di(methylsulfate).
Use: Hypotensive.
See: Presidal

PENTAERYTHRITOL TETRANITRATE, DILUTED, U.S.P. XXI.
Use: Vasodilator.

• **PENTAERYTHRITOL TETRANITRATE,** U.S.P. XXI.

Diluted, U.S.P. XXI.
Use: Vasodilator.
See: Angijen Green, Tab. (Jenkins)
Arcotrate Nos. 1 & 2, Tab. (Arcum)
Baritrate, Tab. (Barry-Martin)
Dilac-80, Cap. (Ascher)
Duotrate, Cap. (Marion)
Duotrate-45, Cap. (Marion)
Kortrate, Cap. (Amid)
Maso-Trol, Tab. (Mason)
Metranil, Cap. (Meyer)
Naptrate, Prep. (Vortech)
Nitrin, Tab. (Vale)
Penta-Cap No. 1, Cap. (Kenyon)
Penta-E., Tab. (Recsei)
Pentafin, Granucap, Tab. (Reid-Provident)
Pentaforte-T, Tab. (Sutliff & Case)
Penta-Tal No. 1&2, Tab. (Kenyon)
Pentestan-80, Cap. (Standex)
Pentetra, Tab. (Paddock)
Pentrate T.D., Cap. (Galen)
Pentritol, Tempule. (Armour)
Pentryate, Cap., Tab. (Fellows-Testagar)
Pentryate Stronger, Cap. (Fellows-Testagar)
Pent-T-80, Cap. (Rocky Mtn.)
Pentylan, Tab. (Lannett)
Pentylan w/Phenobarbital, Tab. (Lannett)
Peritrate, Tab. (Parke-Davis)
Petro-20 mg., Tab. (Foy)
P-T-T, Cap. (La Crosse)
Rate, Cap., Tab. (Scrip)
Reithritol, Tab. (Bowman)
Tentrate, Tab. (Tennessee Pharm.)
Tetracap-30, Cap. (Freeport)
Tetracap-80, Cap. (Freeport)
Tetratab, Tab. (Freeport)
Tetratab No. 1, Tab. (Freeport)
Tranite, Cap., Tab. (Westerfield)
Vasolate, Cap. (Parmed)
Vasolate-80, Cap. (Parmed)

PENTAERYTHRITOL TETRANITRATE W/COMBINATIONS.
See: Angijen No. 3, Tab. (Jenkins)
Angijen S.C., Tab. (Jenkins)
Angitab, Tab. (Moore Kirk)
Antora-B, Cap. (Mayrand)
Arcotrate No. 3, Tab. (Arcum)
Bitrate, Tab. (Arco)
Cartrax, Tab. (Roerig)
Covap, Tab. (Blue Line)
Dimycor, Tab. (Standard Drug)
Equanitrate, Tab. (Wyeth)
Kortrate Plus, Cap. (Amid)
Maso-Trol w/Phenobarbital, Tab. (Mason)
Miltrate, Tab. (Wallace)
Papavatral, Tab. and L.A. Tab. (Kenwood)
Peaton, Tab. (O'Neal)
Penta-Cap Plus. Cap. (Kenyon)
Penta-Tal No. 3&4, Tab. (Kenyon)
Pentetra w/Phenobarbital, Tab. (Paddock)
Pentylan W/Phenobarbital, Tab. (Lannett)
Perbuzem, Tab. (Zemmer)

Peritrate W/Nitroglycerin, Tab.
(Parke-Davis)
Peritrate W/Phenobarbital S.A., Tab.
(Parke-Davis)
Petn Plus, Tab. (Saron)
Rate-10 & P.B. (Scrip)
Rate-20 & P.B. (Scrip)
Respet, Tab. (Westerfield)
Robam-Petn, Tab. (Robinson)
Tetrabarb Tab. (Blaine)
Tetratab No. 2, Tab. (Freeport)
Vasobarb, Cap. (Reid-Provident)
• **PENTAFILCON A.** USAN.
PENTAFORT-T TABLETS. (Sutliff & Case) Pentaery-thritol tetranitrate 10 mg., 20 mg./Tab. Bot. 100s, 1000s.
Use: Vasodilator.
• **PENTAGASTRIN.** USAN. N-t-Butyloxy-carbonyl-β-alanyl-L-tryptophyl-L-methionyl-L-aspartyl-L-phenylalanine amide.
Use: Gastric acid secretion stimulant.
See: Peptavlon, Amp. (Ayerst)
PENTALAMIDE. B.A.N. 2-Pentyloxybenzamide.
Use: Treatment of fungal infections.
See: O-Pentylsalicylamide
• **PENTALYTE.** USAN.
Use: Electrolyte combination.
PENTAMETHONIUM BROMIDE. B.A.N.
Pentamethylenedi(trimethylammonium bromide).
Use: Hypotensive.
See: Lytensium
PENTAMETHONIUM IODIDE. B.A.N.
Pentamethylenedi(trimethylammonium iodide).
Use: Hypotensive.
See: Antilusin
PENTAMIDINE. B.A.N. 4,4'-(Pentamethylenedioxy)-dibenzamidine.
Use: Treatment of trypanosomiasis.
PENTAMETHYLENETETRAZOL.
See: Pentylenetetrazol U.S.P. (Various Mfr.)
PENTAMOXANE HCl. 2-Isoamylamino-methyl-1,4-ben-zodioxane HCl.
Use: Tranquilizing agent.
• **PENTAMUSTINE.** USAN.
Use: Antineoplastic.
1,4-PENTANEDIAMINE,N⁴-(6-CHLORO-2-METHOXY-9-ACRIDINYL)-N',N'-DIETHYL-,DIHYDROCHLO-RIDE, DIHYDRATE. Quinacrine Hydrochloride, U.S.P. XXI.
1,4-PENTANEDIAMINE,N⁴-(7-CHLORO-4-QUINOLIN-YL)-N¹,N¹-DIETHYL-. Chloroquine, U.S.P. XXI.
1,4-PENTANEDIAMINE, N⁴-(6-METHOXY-8-QUINO-LINYL)-,PHOSPHATE (1:2). Primaquine Phosphate, U.S.P. XXI.
PENTANOIC ACID, 4-OXO-, CALCIUM SALT (2:1), DIHYDRATE. Calcium Levulinate, U.S.P. XXI.
PENTAPHONATE. Dodecyltriphenylphosphonium pentachlorophenolate.
Use: Antibacterial.
PENTAPIPERIDE. B.A.N. 1-Methyl-4-(3-methyl-2-phe-nylvaleryloxy)piperidine.
Use: Anticholinergic.

See: Quilene (methylsulfate)
PENTAPIPERIDE METHYLSULFATE. 4'-(1'-Methyl-piperidyl)-2-phenyl-3-methyl-valerate dimethylsulfate.
Valpipamate Methylsulfate
Use: Anticholinergic.
• **PENTAPIPERIUM METHYLSULFATE.** USAN.
Use: Anticholinergic.
PENTAPYRROLIDINIUM BITARTRATE.
See: Pentolinium Tartrate.
PENTAQUINE. B.A.N. 8-(5-Isopropylaminopentyl-ami-no)-6-methoxyquinoline.
Use: Antimalarial.
PENTAQUINE PHOSPHATE. 8-[[5-(Isopropyl-amino)-pentyl]amino]-6-methoxyquinoline phosphate.
PENTARCORT. (Dalin) Hydrocortisone alcohol ½%, soln. coal tar 2%, clioquinol 3%, diperodone HCl ¼%, Vit. A 850 I.U., D 85 I.U./Gm. Tubes: 15 Gm.
Use: Dermatoses.
PENTASODIUM BIS [4,5-DIHYDROXY-M-BEN-ZENEDISULFONATO(4-)]ANTIMONATE(5-)HEPTA-HYDRATE. Stibophen.
PENTASODIUM COLISTINMETHANESULFONATE.
Sterile Colistimethate Sodium, U.S.P. XXI.
PENTA-STRESS. (Penta) Vit. A 10,000 I.U., D 500 I.U., B-1 10 mg., B-2 10 mg., B-6 1 mg., cal. pantothenate 5 mg., niacinamide 50 mg., C 100 mg., E 2 I.U., B-12 3.3 mcg./Cap. Bot. 90s, 1000s. Jar 250s.
Use: Dietary supplement.
PENTA-TAL. (Kenyon) Pentaerythritol tetranitrate 10 mg., 20 mg./Tab. Bot. 100s, 1000s.
PENTA-TAL #3, #4. (Kenyon) Pentaerythritol tetrani-trate 10 mg., 20 mg., phenobarbital 15 mg. Tab. Bot. 100s, 1000s.
PENTAVALENT GAS GANGRENE. Antitoxin.
PENTA-VIRON. (Penta) Cal. carbonate 500 mg., ferrous fumarate 100 mg., C 50 mg., D 167 I.U., A 3.333 I.U., B-1 3.3 mg., B-2 3.3 mg., B-6 2 mg., cal. pantothe-nate 1.6 mg., niacinamide 16.7 mg., E 2 I.U./Cap. Bot. 100s, 1000s. Jar 250s.
Use: Supplement.
PENTAZINE. (Century) Promethazine expectorant. Bot. 4 oz., 16 oz., gal.
PENTAZINE W/CODEINE. (Century) Promethazine expectorant. Bot. 4 oz., 16 oz., gal.
PENTAZINE INJ. (Century) Promethazine 50 mg./cc. Inj. vial 10 cc.
• **PENTAZOCINE,** U.S.P. XXI. 2,6-Methano-3-benzazo-cin-8-ol, 1,2,3,4,5,6-hexahydro-6,11-dimethyl-3-(3-methyl-2-butenyl)-1,2,3,-4,5,6-Hexahydro-cis-6,11-dimethyl-3-(3-methyl-2-butenyl)-2,6-methano-2-benz-azocin-8-ol.
Use: Analgesic.
• **PENTAZOCINE HYDROCHLORIDE,** U.S.P. XXI. Tab., U.S.P. XXI.
Use: Analgesic.
W/ Acetaminophen.
See: Talacen, Cap. (Winthrop-Breon)
• **PENTAZOCINE HYDROCHLORIDE AND ASPIRIN TABLETS,** U.S.P. XXI.
Use: Analgesic.
See: Talwin Compound, Tab. (Winthrop-Breon)
• **PENTAZOCINE LACTATE INJECTION,** U.S.P. XXI.

Use: Analgesic.
See: Talwin Injection, Inj. (Winthrop-Breon)
PENTESTAN 10. (Standex) Pentaerythritol tetranitrate 10 mg./Tab. Bot. 100s.
PENTESTAN 10-P. (Standex) Pentaerythritol tetranitrate 10 mg., phenobarbital 15 mg./Tab. Bot. 100s.
PENTESTAN-80. (Standex) Pentaerythritol tetranitrate 80 mg./Cap. Bot. 100s.
Use: Angina.
• **PENTETATE CALCIUM TRISODIUM.** USAN.
Use: Chelating agent.
• **PENTETATE CALCIUM TRISODIUM Yb 169.** USAN.
Use: Radioactive agent.
• **PENTETATE INDIUM DISODIUM IN 111.** USAN.
Use: Diagnostic aid, radioactive agent.
• **PENTETIC ACID.** USAN.
Use: Diagnostic aid.
PENTETRA-PARACOTE. (Paddock) Pentaerythritol tetranitrate 80 mg./Cap. Bot. 100s, 500s, 1000s. Also 30 mg./Cap., same sizes.
Use: Angina pectoris.
PENTETRAZOL. Analucin. Pentylenetetrazol
Use: Geriatric stimulant, analeptic.
PENTHIENATE. B.A.N. 2-Diethylaminoethyl α-cyclopentyl-α-(2-thienyl).
Use: Antispasmodic.
See: Monodral (methobromide)
PENTHIENATE BROMIDE. Diethyl (2-Hydroxyethyl) methylammonium bromide α-cyclopentyl-2-thiopheneglycolate.
PENTHRANE. (Abbott) Methoxyflurane; 2,2-dichloro-1, 1-difluoroethyl methyl ether. Bot. 15 ml., 125 ml.
Use: Anesthetic for obstetrics and surgery.
PENTHRICHLORAL. B.A.N. 5,5-Di(hydroxymethyl)-2-trichloromethyl-1,3-dioxan.
Use: Hypnotic; sedative.
PENTIDS. (Squibb) Potassium Penicillin G buffered with calcium carbonate.**Tab.:** 125 mg. (200,000 u.)/Tab. Bot. 100s. **Syrup:** 125 mg. (200,000 u)/5ml. Bot. 100 ml., 200 ml.
Use: Antibiotic
PENTIDS 400. (Squibb) Potassium Penicillin G buffered with calcium carbonate. **Tab.:** 250 mg. (400,000 u.)/Tab. Bot. 16s, 100s. Unimatic 100s. **Syrup:** 240 mg. (400,000 u.)/5 ml. Bot. 100 ml., 200 ml.
Use: Antibiotic.
PENTIDS 800. (Squibb) Potassium Penicillin G 500 mg. (800,000 u.)/Tab. buffered with calcium carbonate. Bot. 30s, 100s.
Use: Antibiotic.
PENTIFYLLINE. B.A.N. 1-Hexyl-3,7-dimethyl-xanthine.
Use: Vasodilator.
See: Cosaldon
PENTINA. (Freeport) Rauwolfia serpentina, 100 mg./Tab. Bot. 1000s.
Use: Antihypertensive.
• **PENTISOMICIN.** USAN.
Use: Anti-infective.
• **PENTIZIDONE SODIUM.** USAN.

Use: Antibacterial.
• **PENTOBARITAL,** U.S.P. XXI. Elixir, U.S.P. XXI. (Various Mfr.) 5-Ethyl-5-(1-methylbutyl) barbituric acid.
See: Nembutal, Elix., Gradumets (Abbott) Penta, Tab. (Dunhall)
W/Secobarbital, butabarbital, & phenobarbital.
See: Qui-A-Zone, Tab. (Walker)
PENTOBARBITAL COMBINATIONS.
See: Cafergot-PB, Supp., Tab. (Sandoz)
Dainite, Tab. (Mallinckrodt)
Matropinal Forte, Inserts, Tab. (Comatic)
Matropinal Inserts, Elix., Tab. (Comatic)
Nembutal, Prep. (Abbott)
Neoquess, Tabs. (O'Neal)
Nipirin, Cap. (Elder)
Penotal, Cap., Elix. (Coastal)
Quad-Set, Tab. (Kenyon)
Qui-A-Zone, Tab. (Walker)
Quiess, Tab. (O'Neal)
Spasmasorb, Tab. (Hauck)
Stopp, Supp. (Keene)
• **PENTOBARBITAL, SODIUM,** U.S.P. XXI. Cap. Elixir, Inj.: U.S.P. XXI. 2,4,6,(1H,3H,5H)-Pyrimidinetrione, 5-ethyl-5-(1-methyl-butyl)-, monosodium salt. Sod. 5-Ethyl-5-(1-methylbutyl) barbiturate. Embutal.
Use: Hypnotic, sedative.
See: Maso-Pent, Tab. (Mason)
Nembutal Sodium, Prep. (Abbott)
Night-Caps, Cap. (Bowman)
Penital, Cap., Inj. (Kay)
W/Acetaminophen, salicylamide, codeine phosphate.
See: Tega-Code, Cap. (Ortega)
W/Adiphenine HCl, phamasorb, aluminum hydroxide.
See: Spasmasorb, Tab. (Hauck)
W/Atropine sulfate, hyoscine HBr, hyoscyamine sulfate.
See: Eldonal, Elix., Tab., Cap. (Canright)
W/Carbromal.
See: Carbropent, Tab. (Blue Line)
W/Ephedrine.
See: Ephedrine and Nembutal-25, Cap. (Abbott)
W/Ergotamine tartrate, caffeine alkaloid, bellafoline.
See: Cafergot-P.B., Tab. (Sandoz)
W/Homatropine methylbromide, dehydrocholic acid, ox bile extract.
See: Homachol, Tab. (Lemmon)
W/Phenobarbital sodium.
See: Penotal, Cap., Elix. (Coastal)
W/Pyrilamine maleate.
See: A-N-R, Rectorette (Hauck)
W/Seco-, buta-, phenobarbital.
See: Quadrabarb, Tab. (Vortech)
W/Vitamin compounds, d-methamphetamine HCl.
See: Fetamin, Tab. (Mission)
PENTOBARBITAL, SOLUBLE.
See: Pentobarbital Sodium, U.S.P.
PENTOBEE W/B-12. (Vitarine) Vit. B-1 3 mg., B-2 3 mg., B-6 0.3 mg., B-12 3 mcg., niacinamide 10 mg., cal. pantothenate 3 mg./Cap. Bot. 100s, 250s.
Use: Supplement.

PENTOLINIUM TARTRATE, Pentamethylene-1:5-bis (1'-methylpyrrolidinium bitartrate). N,N'-Pentame-thylenedi-(1-methylpyrrolidinium hydrogen tartrate. Pentapyrrolidinium Bitartrate.
Use: Hypotensive.

• **PENTOMONE.** USAN.
Use: Prostate growth inhibitor.

• **PENTOSTATIN.** USAN.
Use: Potentiator.

PENTOTHAL. (Abbott) Thiopental sodium 500 mg. fliptop vial w/20 ml. water diluent; 1 Gm. fliptop vial w/50 ml. water diluent; 250 mg., 400 mg., and 500 mg. syringes; 5 Gm. in 250 ml. and 10 Gm. in 500 ml. Multi-Dose cont.; kits: 1 Gm./2.5%, 2.5 Gm./2.5%, 5 Gm./2.5%, 2.5 Gm./2.0%, and 5 Gm./2.0%. Penthothal Rectal-susp. in AbboSert. Syr. Single-dose syringe 250 mg., 400 mg., or 500 mg.
Use: Ultra-short-acting anesthetic.

• **PENTOXIFYLLINE.** USAN. Oxpentifylline, B.A.N.
Use: Oral hemorrheologic agent for peripheral vascular disease.
See: Trental (Hoechst)

PENTRASAPAN. (Vitarine) Pentaerythritol tetranitrate 80 mg./timed rel. Cap.
Use: Relief of angina.

PENTRATE T.D. (Galen) Pentaerythritol tetranitrate 30 mg./Cap. Bot. 100s.
Use: Coronary vasodilator. Sustained release.

PENTRAX SHAMPOO. (CooperCare) Tar extract 8.75% w/detergents and conditioning agents. Bot. 4 oz., 8 oz.
Use: Seborrhea, psoriasis, eczematous dermatoses of scalp.

• **PENTRINITROL.** USAN.
Use: Vasodilator.

PENTRITOL TEMPULES. (USV Labs.) Pentaerythritol tetranitrate. Timed Release Cap. 30 mg., Bot. 100s, 250s, 60 mg., Bot. 60s, 250s.
Use: Antianginal used for pain of coronary artery disease.

PENTRYATE TABLETS. (Fellows) Pentaerythritol tetranitrate 10 mg./Tab. Bot. 1000s, 5000s. 20 mg./Tab. Bot. 1000s.

PENTRYATE TIMED CAPSULE. (Fellows) Pentaerythritol tetranitrate 30 mg./Cap. Bot. 30s, 100s, 1000s.

PENTRYATE STRONGER. (Fellows) Pentaerythritol tetranitrate 80 mg./Cap. (timed relaise). Bot. 30s, 100s, 1000s.
Use: Angina pectoris.

PENT-T-80. (Rocky Mtn.) Pentaerythritol tetranitrate 80 mg./Time Cap. Bot. 50s.
Use: Relief of angina pectoris.

PENT-T-80. (Mericon) Pentaerythritol tetranitrate 80 mg./T.D. Cap. Bot. 100s, 1000s.

PENTYLAN. (Lannett) Pentaerythritol tetranitrate 10 mg./Tab. Bot. 500s, 1000s. 20 mg./Tab. Bot. 100s, 1000s.

PENTYLAN W/PHENOBARBITAL. (Lannett) Pentaerythritol tetranitrate 10 mg., phenobarbital ¼ gr./Tab. Bot. 100s, 500s, 1000s. **No. 2:** Pentaerythritol tetranitrate 20 mg., phenobarbital 15 mg./Tab. Bot. 100s, 500s, 1000s.

PENTYLENETETRAZOL. 6,7,8,9-Tetrahydro-5-H-tet-razoloazepine. Leptazol.
Use: Geriatric stimulant, analeptic.
See: Cardiazol, Tab. (Knoll)
Cenalene-M, Tab., Elix. (Central)
Metrazol, Elix., Tab. Pow. (Knoll)
Nelex-100, Tab. (Mallard)
Nioric Modified, Tab., Elix. (Ascher)

PENTYLENETETRAZOL W/COMBINATIONS.
See: Aminobrain P-T, Liq. (Med Prod. Panamericana)
Analeptone, Elix. (Reed & Carnrick)
Cerebro-Nicin, Cap. (Brown)
D-Vaso prods. (Dunhall)
Geriatrazole, Vial (Kenyon)
Gerren Tab. (Wren)
Gevizol (Saron)
Menic, Tab. (Geriatric)
Mentalert, Tab., Elix. (Keene Pharm.)
Neo-Gerastan, Tab. (Standex)
Nialex, Tab. (Mallard)
Niapent, Tab., Elix. (Ferndale)
Nicozol, Elix., Cap. (Hyrex)
Norozol, Tab. (Vortech)
Senilex, Tab. (O'Neal)
Senoral, Liq. (Kay)
Thedrazol prods. (Kenyon)
Tinaplex, Elix. (Blaine)
Tinazole, Elix. (Blaine)
Vasostim, Cap. (Dunhall)
Vita-Metrazol, Elix., Tab. (Knoll)

PEN-VEE-K. (Wyeth) Pot. phenoxymethyl penicillin.
Tab.: 125 mg./Tab. Bot. 36s; **250 mg.**/Tab. Bot. 100s, 500s. Redipak 100s; **500 mg.**/Tab. Bot. 100s, 500s. Redipak 100s.
Use: Penicillin susceptible organisms.

PEN-VEE K FOR ORAL SOLUTION. (Wyeth) Penicillin V potassium **250 mg.**/5 ml. Bot. 100 ml., 150 ml., 200 ml. Redipak Ctn. 20s. **125 mg.**/5 ml. Bot. 100 ml., 200 ml.
Use: Antibiotic.

• **PEPLOMYCIN SULFATE.** USAN.
Use: Antineoplastic.

• **PEPPERMINT,** N.F. XVI. Oil, Water, N.F. XVI.
Use: Pharmaceutic aid (flavor), antitussive, expectorant, nasal decongestant.
See: Vicks Prods. (Vicks)

• **PEPPERMINT OIL,** N.F. XVI.
Use: Pharmaceutic aid (flavor).

• **PEPPERMINT SPIRIT,** U.S.P. XXI.
Use: Digestive aid.

• **PEPPERMINT WATER,** N.F. XVI.
Use: Vehicle.

PEPSAMAR ESP LIQUID. (Winthrop Products) Aluminum hydroxide, glycerin.
Use: Antacid, demulcent, spasmolytic.

PEPSAMAR ESP TABLETS. (Winthrop Products) Aluminum hydroxide, magnesium hydroxide, manitol powder.
Use: Antacid, demulcent, spasmolytic.

PEPSAMAR COMP. TABLETS. (Winthrop Products) Aluminum hydroxide, magnesium hydroxide.
Use: Antacid.

PEPSAMAR HM TABLETS. (Winthrop Products)
Aluminum hydroxide, starch.
Use: Antacid.
PEPSAMAR LIQUID. (Winthrop Products) Aluminum
hydroxide.
Use: Antacid.
PEPSAMAR SUSPENSION. (Winthrop Products)
Aluminum hydroxide magnesium hydroxide, sorbitol.
Use: Antacid, demulcent, spasmolytic.
PEPSAMAR TABLETS. (Winthrop Products)
Aluminum hydroxide.
Use: Antacid.
PEPSATAL. (Kenyon) Pepsin 200 mg., pancreatin
200 mg., bile salts 100 mg., dehydrocholic acid 30
mg., desoxycholic acid 30 mg./Tab. Bot. 100s, 1000s.
PEPSICONE GEL. (Winthrop Products) Aluminum
hydroxide, magnesium hydroxide, simethicone.
Use: Antacid, antiflatulent.
PEPSICONE TABLET. (Winthrop Products) Aluminum
hydroxide, magnesium hydroxide, simethicone.
Use: Antacid, antiflatulent.
PEPSIN.
Use: Digestive aid.
See: Lactopepsinum, Elix. (Noyes)
PEPSIN W/COMBINATIONS.
See: Biloric, Cap. (Arcum)
Bocresin, Liq. (Scrip)
Diethylstilbestrol Digestive Formula, Tab. (Wolins)
Digesplen, Tab., Elix., Drops (Med Prod.
Panamericana)
Digestozyme, Tab. (Wolins)
Donnazyme, Tab. (Robins)
Entozyme, Tab. (Robins)
Enzobile, Tab. (Mallard)
Enzylax, Tab. (Kay)
Enzymet, Tab. (Westerfield)
Foy-Nux, Tab. (Foy)
Gastroenterase, Tab. (Wallace)
Glutasyn, Cap. (Brunswick)
Gourmase, Cap. (Rowell)
Gourmase-PB, Cap. (Rowell)
Kanulase, Tab. (Dorsey)
Konzyme, Tab. (Brunswick Lab.)
Leber Taurine, Liq. (Paddock)
Maso-Gestive, Tab. (Mason)
Normacid, Tab. (Stuart)
Nu'Leven, Tab. (Lemmon)
Nu'Leven Plus, Tab. (Lemmon)
Pepsatal, Tab. (Kenyon)
Pepsin Essence
Ro-Bile, Tab. (Rowell)
Sto-Zyme, Tab. (Jalco)
Zypan, Tab. (Standard Process)
PEPSIN LACTATED, ELIXIR.
See: Peptalac, Liq. (Bowman)
PEPSIN-PAPAIN COMPLEX.
W/Pancreas, malt diastase, glycyrrhiza ext., charcoal.
See: Pepsocoll, Tabs. (Western Research Labs.)
• **PEPSTATIN.** USAN.
Use: Enzyme inhibitor.
PEPTAVLON. (Ayerst) Pentagastrin. 0.25 mg. w/sod.
chloride/ml. Amp. 2 ml. Ctn. 10s.
Use: Evaluation of gastric acid secretion.

PEPTENZYME. (Reed & Carrick) Alcohol 16%.
Pleasantly aromatic. Bot. 1 pt.
Use: Pharmaceutical vehicle.
PEPTO-BISMOL LIQUID. (Procter & Gamble) Bismuth
subsalicylate, Bot. 4 oz., 8 oz., 12 oz., 16 oz.
Use: Indigestion, nausea, diarrhea, upset stomach.
PEPTO-BISMOL TABLETS. (Procter & Gamble) Bis-
muth subsalicylate. Pkg. 24s, 42s, 60s.
Use: Indigestion, nausea, diarrhea, upset stomach.
PEPTO-MANGAN. (Medtech) Liquid 11 oz. Tab. Bot.
50s.
Use: Vitamin tonic with iron.
PERANDREN PHENYLACETATE. (Ciba)
Testosterone phenylacetate.
PERATIZOLE.   B.A.N.   1-[-(2,4-Dimethylthiazol-5-yl)-
butyl]-4-(4-methylthiazol-2-yl)piperazine.
Use: Antihypertensive agent.
PERBUZEM. (Zemmer) Pentaerythritol tetranitrate 10
mg., butabarbital sodium 15 mg./Tab. Bot. 100s,
1000s.
Use: Angina pectoris, hypertension.
PERCAINE.
See: Dibucaine Hydrochloride (Nupercaine HCl.
Ciba)
PERCHLORACAP CAPS. (Mallinckrodt) Potassium
perchlorate, 200 mg./Cap. Bot. 100s.
Use: Radiodiagnostic adjunct.
PERCHLORETHYLENE.
See: Tetrachlorethylene, U.S.P. XXI.
PERCHLORPERAZINE.
See: Compazine, Prep. (SmithKline)
PERCOCET-5. (Du Pont) Oxycodone HCl 5 mg.,
acetaminophen 325 mg./Tab. Bot. 100s, 500s. Unit
dose 250s.
Use: Analgesic.
PERCODAN. (Du Pont) Oxycodone HCl 4.50 mg.,
oxycodone terephthalate 0.38 mg., aspirin 325
mg./Tab. Bot. 100s, 500s, 1000s. Unit dose 250s,
1000s.
Use: Narcotic analgesic.
W/Hexobarbital.
See: Percobarb, Cap. (Du Pont)
PERCODAN-DEMI. (Du Pont) Oxycodone HCl 2.25 mg.,
oxycodone terephthalate 0.19 mg., aspirin 325
mg./Tab. Bot. 100s, 500s, 1000s.
Use: Prompt, prolonged relief from pain.
PERCOGESIC. (Vicks) Acetaminophen 325 mg.
phenyltoloxamine citrate 30 mg./Tab. Pkg. 24s.
Bot. 100s. Hospital Pack Box 960s.
Use: Analgesic.
PERCOMORPH LIVER OIL. (May be blended with
50% other fish liver oils; each Gm. contains 60,000
I.U. Vit. A & 8500 I.U. Vit. D.)
See: Oleum Percomorphum
PERCORTEN ACETATE. (Ciba) Desoxycorticosterone
acetate. Vial (5 mg./ml. in oil w/chlorobutanol
0.5%) Pellets 125 mg. 1s.
Use: I.M., implantation & orally; adrenal cortex
replacement therapy.
PERCORTEN PIVALATE. (Ciba)
Desoxycorticosterone Pivalate. Vial (25 mg./ml.);
also contains methylcellulose 10.5 mg., sod.
carboxymethylcellulose 3 mg., polysorbate 80

1 mg., sod. chloride 8 mg., thimerosal 0.002%. Bot. 4 ml.
Use: I.M.; adrenocortical insufficiency.

PERCY MEDICINE. (Merrick Medicine) Bismuth subnitrate 959.0 mg., calcium hydroxide 21.9 mg./10 ml. w/alcohol 5%
Use: Relief of simple diarrhea & excess acid conditions of the stomach.

PERDIEM. (Rorer) Blend of 82% psyllium & 18% senna as active ingredients in granular form. Sodium content 1.7 mg./rounded tsp. (6 Gm.). Canister 100 Gm., 250 Gm.
Use: Relief of constipation.

PERDIEM PLAIN. (Rorer) Psyllium 100% as active ingredient in granular form. Sodium content 1.8 mg./rounded tsp. (6 Gm.) Canisters 100 Gm. or 250 Gm.
Use: Relief of constipation.

PERDILATAL HYDROCHLORIDE. Buphenin, B.A.N.

PERESTAN. (Interstate) Docusate sodium 100 mg., casanthranol 30 mg./Cap. Bot. 100s, 1000s.
Use: Laxative.

• **PERFILCON A.** USAN.
Use: Contact lens material.
See: Permalens (CooperVision)

PERGALEN.
See: Sodium Apolate

PERGONAL (MENOTROPINS). (Serono) Follicle stimulating hormone (FSH) 75 I.U. and lutenizing hormone (LH) 75 I.U. Unit contains 1 Amp. product and 1 Amp. NaCl diluent.
Use: Replacement of FSH and LH in women or men in hypogonadotropic conditions.

PERGRAVA. (Arcum) Vit. A 2000 I.U., D 300 I.U., B-1 2 mg., B-2 2 mg., nicotinamide 10 mg., B-6 2 mg., B-12 5 mcg., C 60 mg./cal. 40 mg./Cap. Bot. 100s, 1000s.
Use: Pregnancy.

PERGRAVA NO. 2. (Arcum) Vit. A 2000 I.U., D 300 I.U., B-1 2 mg., B-2 2 mg., nicotinamide 10 mg., B-6 2 mg., C 60 mg., cal. lactate monohydrate 200 mg., ferrous gluconate 31 mg., folic acid 0.1 mg./Cap. Bot. 100s, 1000s.
Use: Pregnancy.

• **PERHEXILINE.** USAN. 2-(2,2-Dicyclohexylethyl)-piperidine.
Use: Treatment of angina pectoris.

• **PERHEXILINE MALEATE.** USAN. 2-(2,2-Dicyclohexylethyl) piperidine maleate.
Use: Cardiovascular agent.

PERHYDROL.
See: Hydrogen Peroxide 30% (Var. Mfr.)

PERIACTIN. (Merck Sharp & Dohme) Cyproheptadine HCl 4 mg./Tab. Bot. 100s.
Use: Antipruritic, antihistaminic.

PERIACTIN SYRUP. (Merck Sharp & Dohme) Cyproheptadine HCl 2 mg./5 ml. w/alcohol 5%, sorbic acid 0.1%. Bot. 473 ml.
Use: Antipruritic, antihistaminic.

PERI-CARE. (Sween) Jar/2 oz., 8 oz.
Use: Skin care ointment. Unit dose 100s.

PERI-COLACE. (Mead Johnson) **Cap.:** Docusate so-

dium 100 mg., casanthranol 30 mg./Cap. Bot. 30s, 60s, 250s, 1000s. Unit dose 100s. **Syrup:** Docusate sodium 60 mg., casanthranol 30 mg./15 cc.; ethyl alcohol 10%. Bot. 8 oz., pt.
Use: Fecal softener and laxative.

PERICOLEAST. (Eastwood) Cap. Bot. 100s.

PERI-CONATE. (Cenci) Docusate sodium 100 mg., casanthranol 30 mg./Cap. Bot. 100s, 1000s.
Use: Constipation.

PERICYAZINE. B.A.N. 2-Cyano-10-[3-(4-hydroxy-piperidino)propyl]phenothiazine. Neulactil.
Use: Tranquilizer.

PERIDIN-C. (Beutlich) Hesperidin methyl chalcone 50 mg., hesperidin complex 150 mg., ascorbic acid 200 mg./Tab. Bot. 100s and 500s.
Use: In capillary fragility.

PERIES. (Xttrium) Medicated pads, w/witch hazel and glycerin. Jar 40 pads.
Use: Hygienic wipe and local compress.

PERIFOAM. (Rowell) Benzalkonium chloride 0.1%, pramoxine HCl 1.0%, allantoin 0.3%, methylparaben 0.15%, propylparaben 0.05%, witch hazel 35%, solubilized lanolin, alcohol (approx. 5%), water q.s. to 100%. Aerosol 1.5 oz.
Use: Dermatologic, antipruritic, fungistatic, bacteriostatic cream.

• **PERGOLIDE MESYLATE.** USAN.
Use: Dopamine agonist.

PERIHEMIN. (Lederle) Vit. B-12 5 mcg., intrinsic factor conc. 25 mg., ferrous fumarate 168 mg., folic acid 0.33 mg., ascorbic acid 50 mg./Cap. Bot. 100s.
Use: Orally; anemias.

PERIMYCIN. (Warner-Lambert) An antibiotic of the heptaene type elaborated by *Streptomyces coelicolor* variety *aminophilus.*
Use: Antifungal antibiotic.

PERIODIC CAPSULES. (Towne) Cinnamyl ephedrine HCl 15 mg., acetaminophen 180 mg., caffeine 60 mg., homatropine methylbromide 0.25 mg./Cap. Bot. 16s.

PERI SOFCAP. (Alton) Docusate sodium with peristim. Bot. 100s, 1000s.
Use: Stool softener.

PERISTOMAL COVERING.
See: Stomahesive, Wafers (Squibb)

PERITIME-80. (Kenyon; Werner) Pentaerythritol tetra nitrate 80 mg./Cap. Bot. 100s.

PERITINIC. (Lederle) Elemental iron 100 mg., docusate sodium 100 mg., B-1 7.5 mg., B-2 7.5 mg., B-6 7.5 mg., B-12 50 mcg., C 200 mg., niacinamide 30 mg., folic acid 0.05 mg., pantothenic acid 15 mg./Tab. Bot. 60s.
Use: Hematinic-vitamin.

PERITRATE. (Parke-Davis) Pentaerythritol tetranitrate. **Tab. 10 mg.:** Bot. 100s, 1000s. **Tab. 20 mg.:** Bot. 100s, 1000s. Unit dose 100s. **Tab. 40 mg.:** Bot. 100s. **S.A. Tab. 80 mg.** Bot. 100s, 1000s.
Use: Coronary vasodilator used in angina pectoris.

PERITRATE S.A.. (Parke-Davis) Pentaerythritol tetranitrate 80 mg. (20 mg. in immediate release layer, 60 mg. in sustained release base)/Tab. Bot. 100s, 1000s. Unit dose 100s.

PERI-WASH. (Sween) Bot. 8 oz., gal.
Use: Skin deodorizer.

• **PERLAPINE.** USAN. 6-(4-Methyl-1-piperazinyl) morphanthridine.
Use: Hypnotic.

PERLATAN.
See: Estrone (Various Mfr.)

PERMANGANIC ACID, POTASSIUM SALT.
Potassium Permanganate, U.S.P. XXI.

PERMAPEN. (Pfipharmecs) Benzathine penicillin G 1,200,000 u./cc. Disp. syringe 2 cc.
Use: Antibiotic.

PERMITIL. (Schering) Fluphenazine HCl 0.25 mg., 2.5 mg. or 5 mg./Tab. Bot. 100s; 10 mg. Tabs., Bot. 1000s
Use: Tranquilizer.

PERMITIL ORAL CONCENTRATE. (Schering) Fluphenazine HCl, 5 mg./ml. Bot. 120 ml. w. calibrated dropper. Hospital use.
Use: Tranquilizer.

PERNAVIT 1000. (Ferndale) Vit. B-12 1000 mcg./cc. Vial 10 cc., 30 cc.
Use: Hematopoietic agent.

PERNOX LOTION. (Westwood) Microfine granules of polyethylene 20%, sulfur 2%, salicylic acid in a combination of soapless cleansers & wetting agents. Bot. 6 oz.
Use: Treatment of oily skin & acne.

PERNOX MEDICATED LATHERING SCRUB CLEANSER. (Westwood) Polyethylene granules 26%, sulfur 2%, salicylic acid 1.5%. w/soapless surface active cleansers and wetting agents. Regular or lemon. Tube 2 oz., 4 oz.
Use: Therapeutic cleanser for oily skin and acne.

PERNOX SHAMPOO. (Westwood) Sodium laureth sulfate, water, lauramide DEA, quaternium 22, PEG-75 lanolin/hydrolyzed animal protein, fragrance, sodium chloride, lactic acid, sorbic acid, disodium EDTA, FD&C yellow No. 6 and blue No. 1. Bot. 8 oz.
Use: Cleanser and conditioner for oily hair.

PEROXIDASE. W/Glucose oxidase, pot, iodide.
See: Diastix Reagent Strips (Ames)

PEROXIDE, DIBENZOYL. Benzoyl Peroxide, Hydrous.

■ **PEROXIDES.**
See: Hydrogen Peroxide (Var. Mfr.)
Urea Peroxide
Zinc Peroxide

PEROXYL MOUTHRINSE. (Hoyt) Hydrogen peroxide 1.5% in mint flavored base w/ alcohol 6%. Bot. 8 oz.
Use: Mouthrinse.

• **PERPHENAZINE,** U.S.P. XXI. Inj., Oral Sol., Syrup, Tab., U.S.P. XXI. 2-Chloro-10-[3-[4-(2-hydroxyethyl)-piperazinyl]-phenothiazine. 4-(3-(2-Chloro-phenothiazin-1-yl)propyl)-1-piperazine-ethanol.
Use: Antiemetic, tranquilizer.
See: Trilafon, Prod. (Schering)
W/Amitriptyline HCl.

See: Etrafon, Prod. (Schering)
Triavil, Tab. (Merck Sharp & Dohme)

PERSADOX. (Owen) Benzoyl peroxide 5% in a base of cetyl alcohol, propylene glycol, sod. lauryl sulfate, purified water. Stearyl alcohol in cream only. **Cream** Jar 1 oz., **Lotion** Plastic Bot. 1 oz.
Use: Treatment of acne, fair or normal skin.

PERSADOX HP CREAM. (Owen) Benzoyl peroxide 10% in cetaphil base w/same ingredients as Persadox. **Cream** Jar 1 oz., **Lotion** plastic Bot. 1 oz.
Use: Treatment of acne and oily skin conditions.

PERSA-GEL. (Ortho) Benzoyl peroxide 5% and 10%. Tube 1.5 oz., or 3 oz.
Use: Acne vulgaris treatment.

PERSA-GEL W. (Ortho) Benzoyl peroxide in water-base 5% and 10%. Tube 1.5 oz., 3 oz.
Use: Topical treatment of acne vulgaris.

PERSANGUE. (Arcum) Ferrous gluconate 192 mg., C 150 mg., B-1 3 mg., B-2 3 mg., B-12 50 mcg./Cap. Bot. 100s, 500s.
Use: Iron deficiency anemias.

PERSANTIN. Dipyridamole, B.A.N.

PERSANTINE. (Boehringer Ingelheim) Dipyridamole 25 mg., 50 mg. or 75 mg./Tab. **25 mg.:** Bot. 100s, 1000s. Unit Dose 100s. Unit of Use 90s. **50 mg.:** Bot. 100s, 1000s. Unit Dose 100s. **75 mg.:** Bot. 100s.
Use: Treatment of angina pectoris.

• **PERSIC OIL,** N.F. XVI.
Use: Vehicle.

PERSISTIN. (Fisons) Aspirin 2½ gr., salicylsalicylic acid 7½ gr./Tab. Bot. 50s, 500s.
Use: Anti-inflammatory.

PERTECHNETIC ACID, SODIUM SALT. Sodium Pertechnetate Tc 99 m Solution.

PERTOFRANE. (USV Labs.) Desipramine hydrochloride 25 mg./Cap. Bot. 100s, 1000s. 50 mg./Cap. Bot. 100s, 1000s.
Use: Antidepressant.

PERTROPIN. (Lannett) Linolenic acid 7 min./Cap. Bot. 100s.
Use: Dietary supplement.

PERTSCAN-99m. (Abbott) Inj. Tc-99m.
Use: Radiodiagnostic.

PERTUSSIN COMPLEX D. (Chesebrough-Pond's) Dextromethorphan HBr 10 mg., chlorpheniramine maleate 2 mg., phenylproanolamine, HCl 12.5 mg./5 ml. w/alcohol 9.5%. Bot. 3 oz., 6 oz.
Use: Antitussive, antihistamine, decongestant.

PERTUSSIN 8-HOUR COUGH FORMULA. (Chesebrough-Pond's) Dextromethorphan HBr /5 mg./5 ml. w/alcohol 9.5%. Bot. 3 oz., 6 oz.
Use: Antitussive.

PERTUSSIN WILD BERRY COUGH SYR. (Chesebrough-Pond's) Dextromethorphan HBr 3.5 mg., guaifenesin 25 mg./5 ml. w/alcohol 8.5%. Bot. 3 oz., 6 oz.
Use: Antitussive.

• **PERTUSSIS IMMUNE GLOBULIN.** U.S.P. XXI. (Cutter) A 16.5% solution of the gamma globulin

fraction of blood from healthy, adult human donors hyperimmunized with pertussis vaccine. Vial 1.25 ml.
Use: Passive prevention and treatment of whooping cough.
See: Hypertussis, Vial (Cutter)
• **PERTUSSIS VACCINE,** U.S.P. XXI. (Various Mfr.)
Use: Active immunization against whooping cough.
• **PERTUSSIS VACCINE, ADSORBED,** U.S.P. XXI.
Vial 7.5 cc.
Use: Active immunizing agent.
PERTUSSIS VACCINE AND DIPHTHERIA AND TETANUS TOXOIDS, COMBINED.
Use: Active immunizing agent.
See: Tri-Immunol, Vial (Lederle)
Triple Antigen, Vial (Wyeth)
Tri-Solgen, Vial, Hyporet (Lilly)
PERUVIAN BALSAM
Use: Local protectant, rubefacient.
W/Benzocaine, zinc oxide, bismuth subgallate, boric acid.
See: Anocaine, Supp. (Mallard)
W/Benzocaine, zinc oxide, 8-hydroxyquinoline benzoate, menthol. Unit of Use 90s. 50mg.: Bot. 100s, 1000s. Unit Dose 100s. 75mg.: Bot. 100s.
See: Hemorrhoidal Oint. (Towne)
W/Ephedrine sulfate, ext. belladonna, zinc oxide, boric acid, bismuth oxyiodide and subcarbonate.
See: Wyanoids, Preps. (Wyeth)
W/Lidocaine, bismuth subgallate, Zn oxide, Al subacetate.
See: Xylocaine, Supp. (Astra)
W/Oxyquinoline sulfate, pramoxine HCl, zinc oxide.
See: Zyanoid, Oint. (Elder)
PESON. Sodium Lyapolate. Polyethenesulfonate sodium.
Use: Anticoagulant.
PET-A-VITE. (Vortech) Liver protein 0.5 Gm., Fe 6 mg., iodine 0.068 mg., Vit. A 1000 I.U., D 100 I.U., B-1 mg., B-2 1 mg., B-6 0.1 mg., niacinamide 10 mg., B-12 0.2 mcg., E 2 I.U., dicalcium phosphate anhydrous 340 mg./Tab. Bot. 100s.
Use: Multiple vitamin.
PETERSON'S OINTMENT. (Peterson) Carbolic acid, camphor, tannic acid, zinc oxide. Tube w/pipe 1 oz. Jar 16 oz. Can 1.4 oz., 3 oz.
Use: Rectal irritation and hemorrhoids.
PETHADOL TABLETS. (Blue Cross) Merperidine HCl 50 mg. or 100 mg./Tab. Bot. 100s, 1000s.
Use: Analgesic.
PETHIDINE HYDROCHLORIDE.
See: Meperidine Hydrochloride, U.S.P. XXI.
PETN.
See: Pentaerythritol tetranitrate.
PETRAZOLE. (Kenyon) Pentylenetetrazol 100 mg./cc. Vial 30 cc.
PETRICHLORAL. Pentaerythritol chloral. 1,1′,1″,1‴-(Neopentanetetrayl-tetraoxy)tetrakis [2,2,2-trichloroethanol].
Use: Sedative.
PETRO-20. (Foy) Pentaerythritol tetranitrate 20 mg./Tab. Bot. 100s, 1000s.

PETROGALAR. (Wyeth) Aqueous susp. of mineral oil 65%, plain. Bot. pt.
PETROGALAR, PHENOLPHTHALEIN. (Wyeth)
Mineral oil 65%, phenolphthalein 0.3%. Bot. pt.
• **PETROLATUM,** U.S.P. XXI.
Use: Ointment base.
See: Lipkote, Stick (Plough)
• **PETROLATUM GAUZE,** U.S.P. XXI.
Use: Surgical aid.
• **PETROLATUM, HYDROPHILIC,** U.S.P. XXI.
Use: Absorbent ointment base; topical protectant.
See: Lipkote, (Plough)
PETROLATUM, LIQUID. Mineral Oil, U.S.P. XXI. Light Mineral Oil, U.S.P. XXI. Adepsine Oil, Glymol, Liquid Paraffin, Parolein, White Mineral Oil, Heavy Liquid Petrolatum.
Use: Laxative.
See: Clyserol Oil Retention Enema (Fuller Labs)
Fleet Mineral Oil Enema (Fleet)
Mineral Oil (Various Mfr.)
Nujol, Liq. (Plough)
Saxol (Var. Mfr.)
PETROLATUM, LIQUID, EMULSION.
Use: Lubricant cathartic.
See: Milkinol, Liq. (Kremers-Urban)
W/Agar-Gel.
See: Agoral Plain, Liq. (Parke-Davis)
Petrogalar, Prep. (Wyeth)
W/Cascara.
See: Petrogalar w/Cascara, Emul. (Wyeth)
W/Docusate sodium.
See: Milkinol, Liq. (Kremers-Urban)
W/Irish moss, casanthranol.
See: Neo-Kondremul (Fisons)
W/Milk of magnesia.
See: Haley's M.O., Liq. (Winthrop Products)
Magoleum, Liq. (Blue Line)
W/Phenolphthalein.
See: Agoral, Emul. (Parke-Davis)
Petrogalar w/Phenolph., Emul. (Wyeth)
Petro-Mul-Phen, Emulsion (Mallinckrodt)
Phenolphthalein in liquid Petrolatum Emulsion.
PETROLATUM, RED VETERINARIAN. (Elder) Also known as RVP.
See: Rubrapet, Oint. (Medco)
W/Micasorb.
See: RV Plus, Oint. (Elder)
W/N-diethyl metatoluamide.
See: RV Pellent, Oint. (Elder)
W/Zinc oxide, 2-ethoxyethyl p-methoxycinnamate.
See: RV Paque, Oint. (Elder)
• **PETROLATUM, WHITE,** U.S.P. XXI.
Use: An oleagenous ointment base, topical protectant.
See: Moroline, Oint. (Plough)
PETRO-PHYLIC SOAP. (Doak) Hydrophilic Petrolatum cake 4 oz.
Use: Dry skin & infections.
PFIZER-E. (Pfipharmecs) Erythromycin stearate 250 mg./Tab. Bot. 100s.
Use: Upper and lower respiratory, skin, and soft tissue infections.

PFIZERPEN A. (Pfipharmecs) Ampicillin. **Cap.:** 500 mg./Cap. Bot. 100s. **Oral Susp.:** 125 mg./5 cc. Bot. 100 cc., 200 cc.
Use: Antibiotic.
PFIZERPEN-AS. (Pfipharmecs) Procaine penicillin G. 3,000,000 u. in aqueous susp./Vial. Carton 5s. Multi-Vial Pack, Carton 100s.
PFIZERPEN G. (Pfipharmecs) Potassium penicillin G. **Tab.:** 200,000 u./Tab. Bot. 500s. 250,000 u./Tab. Bot. 100s. 400,000 u./Tab. Bot. 100s, 1000s.
Use: Antibiotic.
PFIZERPEN FOR INJECTION. (Pfipharmecs) Potassium penicillin G, buffered. Multi-Vial Pack: 1,000,000 u., 5,000,000 u./Vial. Carton 10s, 100s; Individual Vial: 20,000,000 u./Vial. 1s, 10s.
PFIZERPEN VK FOR ORAL SUSPENSION. (Pfipharmecs) Penicillin V potassium 125 mg./5 ml. Bot. 200 ml. 250 mg./5 ml. Bot. 100 ml., 200 ml.
Use: Antibiotic.
PFIZERPEN VK TABLETS. (Pfipharmecs) Penicillin V potassium 250 mg., 500 mg. (400,000 u., 800,000 u.)/Tab. **250 mg.** Bot. 100s, 1000s. **500 mg.** Bot. 100s.
Use: Antibiotic.
PGA. See: Folic Acid, U.S.P. XXI.
P.H. TABS. (Scrip) Glycine 180 mg., cal. carbonate 420 mg./Tab. Bot. 100s.
PHacid. (Baker/Cummins) Bot. 8 oz.
Use: Shampoo.
PHANODORM. Cyclobarbitone, B.A.N.
PHANQUINONE (I.N.N.). Phanquone, B.A.N.
PHANQUONE. B.A.N. 4,7-Phenanthroline-5,6-quinone. Phanquinone (I.N.N.)
Use: Treatment of amebiasis.
See: Entobex
PHARMAC-CORT. (Purepac) Hydrocortisone acetate cream 0.5%. Bot. 0.75 oz.
Use: Antipruritic.
PHARMALGEN. (Pharmacia) Freezedried hymenopteria venom/venom protein from honey bee, yellow jacket, yellow hornet white-faced hornet, wasp, mixed vespid. Diagnostic kit: 5 × 1 ml. Vial. Treatment kit: 6 × 1 ml. vial or 1 × 1.1 mg. multiple dose vial. Starter Kit: 6 × 1 ml., prediluted 0.01 mcg. to 100 mcg./ml.
Use: Diagnosis and treatment of hymenoptera sting allergy.
PHARMALGEN RAST STANDARDIZED ALLERGENIC EXTRACTS-POLLENS. (Pharmacia) 100,000 allergenic units/Vial. Box 5 x 1 ml.
Use: Diagnosis & treatment of pollen allergy.
PHASPHORONE. (Metro Med) Bot. 8 oz.
Use: Oral antiseptic.
PHAZYME. (Reed & Carnrick) Simethicone 60 mg./Core Tab. Bot. 50s, 100s, 1000s.
Use: Digestant and antiflatulent.
PHAZYME-95. (Reed & Carnrick) Simethicone 95 mg./Core Tab. Bot. 100s.
Use: Digestant, antiflatulant.
PHAZYME PB. (Reed & Carnrick) Simethicone 60 mg., phenobarbital 15 mg./Core Tab. Bot. 100s, 1000s.
Use: Antiflatulent, sedative, enzyme combination.

PHEDIMETRAZINE TARTRATE.
Use: Sedative.
See: Melfiat Unicelles (Reid-Provident)
PHEDRAL. (Vortech) Phenobarbital 8 mg., theophylline 129 mg., ephedrine 24 mg./Tab. Bot. 1000s.
Use: Anti-asthmatic.
PHEMERIDE. Benzethonium Chloride, B.A.N.
• **PHEMFILCON A.** USAN.
Use: Contact lens material.
PHEMITHYN. (Davis & Sly) Benzethonium chloride monohydrate 3.17% Bot. W/measuring cap. 4 oz.
Use: Vaginal douche.
• **PHENACAINE HYDROCHLORIDE,** U.S.P. XXI. N,N′-Bis(p-ethoxy-phenyl)acetamidine HCl, monohydrate.
Use: Local anesthetic (ophthalmic).
W/Atropine, phenol, nut gall & zinc oxide.
See: Tanicaine, Oint. & Supp. (Upjohn)
W/Cod liver oil.
See: Morusan Ointment (Beecham Labs)
W/Ephedrine. (Upjohn) Phenocaine HCl 1%, epinephrine 1:25,000. Ophth. oint. Tube 1 dr.
W/Mercarbolide. (Upjohn) Holocaine HCl 2% & mercarbolide 1:3000. Ophth. oint., Tube w/applicator tip, 1 dr.
• **PHENACEMIDE,** U.S.P. XXI. Tab., U.S.P. XXI. Phenylacetylurea.
Use: Anticonvulsant.
See: Phenurone, Tab. (Abbott)
PHENACETIN. Acetophenetidin. Ethoxyacetanilide.
Use: Antipyretic, analgesic.
NOTE: The F.D.A. is currently reviewing this drug for possible withdrawal from the market due to liver and kidney toxicity. As a result, many manufacturers have already voluntarily removed this drug from their product lines. This drug is no longer official in the U.S.P.
PHENACETOPHEN. (Wolins) Aspirin 2½ gr., phenacetin 3 gr., phenobarbital ¼ gr./Cap. Bot. 1000s.
PHENACETYLCARBAMIDE.
See: Phenurone, Tab. (Abbott)
PHENACETYLUREA.
See: Phenurone, Tab. (Abbott)
PHENACRIDANE. (9(p-Hexloxphenyl)-10-methyl-acridinium chloride.
See: Micridium (Johnson & Johnson)
PHENACTROPINIUM CHLORIDE. B.A.N. N-Phenacyl-homatropinium chloride. Trophenium.
Use: Hypotensive.
PHENACYL HOMATROPHINIUM HCl. Not available.
PHENADOXONE. B.A.N. 6-Morpholino-4,4-diphenyl-heptan-3-one. Heptalgin hydrochloride.
Use: Analgesic; hypnotic.
PHENAGESIC. (Dalin) Phenylephrine HCl 10 mg., phenylpropanolamine HCl 50 mg., pyrilamine maleate 25 mg., pheniramine maleate 25 mg., acetyl-p-aminophenol 300 mg./Tab. or 5 ml. **Tab.** Bot. 50. **Syrup** without acetaminophen. Bot. 6 oz., pt.
Use: Treatment for the common cold.
PHENAGLYCODOL. B.A.N. 2-p-Chlorophenyl-3-methyl-2,3-butanediol. 2-(4-Chlorophenyl)-3-methylbutane-2,3-diol.

Use: Central nervous system depressant.
See: Ultran, Pulvule, Tab. (Lilly)
W/Acetylsalicylic acid, dextro-propoxyphene.
See: Darvo-Tran, Pulvule. (Lilly)
PHENAHIST. (Robinson) Phenylephrine HCl 5 mg., chlorpheniramine maleate 2 mg., salicylamide 200 mg., caffeine 15 mg., C 20 mg., citrus bioflavonoids 10 mg./Cap. Bot. 100s, 1000s. Vials 20s, Bulk Pack 5000s.
Use: Cold and hay fever symptoms.
PHENAHIST INJECTABLE. (T. E. Williams) Atropine sulfate 0.2 mg., phenylpropanolamine HCl 12.5 mg., chlorpheniramine maleate 5 mg./ml. Vial 10 cc.
Use: Decongestant/antihistamine.
PHENAHIST-TR CAPSULES. (T. E. Williams) Phenylephrine HCl 10 mg., phenylpropanolamine HCl 40 mg., Chlorpheniramine maleate 12 mg./Cap. Bot. 100s.
Use: Decongestant, antihistamine.
PHENALZINE DIHYDROGEN SULFATE.
See: Nardil, Tab. (Parke-Davis)
PHENAMAZOLINE HCl. 2-(Anilinomethyl)-2-imidazoline HCl.
Use: Vasoconstrictor.
PHENAMINE ELIXIR. (Scrip) Diphenhydramine HCl 10 mg./4 cc. Bot. pt.
PHENAMPROMIDE. B.A.N. N-(1-Methyl-2-piperidinoethyl)propionanilide.
Use: Analgesic.
PHENANTOIN. Mephenytoin. N-Methyl-5,5-phenylethylhydantoin.
See: Mesantoin, Tab. (Sandoz)
PHENAPHEN. (Robins) Acetaminophen 325 mg./Cap. Bot. 100s, 1000s.
Use: Analgesic, antipyretic.
PHENAPHEN WITH CODEINE. (Robins) **No. 2:** Acetaminophen 325 mg., codeine 15 mg./Cap.; **No. 3:** Acetaminophen 325 mg., codeine 30 mg./Cap.; **No. 4:** Acetaminophen 325 mg., codeine 60 mg./Cap. Bot. 100s, 500s. Dis-Co packs 4 × 25s.
Use: Analgesic.
PHENAPHEN-650 WITH CODEINE. (Robins) Codeine phosphate 30 mg., acetaminophen 650 mg./Tab. Bot. 50s. Dis-Co packs 4 × 25s.
Use: Analgesic.
PHENAPHTHAZINE. Sod. dinitro phenylazonaphthol disulfonate.
See: Nitrazine paper, Roll (Squibb)
PHENARSONE SULFOXYLATE. (5-Arsono-2-hydroxyanilino)methanesulfinic acid disodium salt.
Use: Antiamebic.
PHENASPIRIN COMPOUND CAPSULES. (Lannett) Aspirin 3½ gr., phenobarbital ¼ gr./Cap. Bot. 1000s, 5000s.
PHENASPIRIN COMPOUND. (Davis & Sly) Phenobarbital ¼ gr., aspirin 3½ gr./Cap. Bot. 1000s.
PHENATIN. (Jenkins) Acetophenetidin 0.2 Gm., acid acetylsalicylic 0.25 Gm., caffeine 30 mg., camphor monobromated 0.1 Gm./Tab. Bot. 1000s.
Use: Analgesic, anodyne.
PHENATIN TD CAPSULE. (Jenkins) Phenylpropanol-

amine HCl 50 mg., chlorpheniramine maleate 1 mg., pheniramine maleate 12.5 mg., atropine sulfate 0.025 mg., scopolamine HBr 0.014 mg., belladonna alkaloids (total) 0.16 mg., hyoscyamine sulfate 0.122 mg./Cap. Bot. 1000s.
PHENATUSS. (Dalin) Codeine phosphate 10 mg., chlorpheniramine maleate 2 mg., phenylephrine HCl 5 mg., guaifenesin 100 mg., 1-menthol 1 mg./5 cc. Bot. 4 oz., pt., gal.
Use: Antitussive.
PHENAZINE. (Jenkins) Phendimetrazine bitartrate 50 mg./cc. Vial 10 cc.
Use: Anorexic.
PHENAZINE. (Keene) Promethazine HCl 25 mg. or 50 mg. Vial 10 ml.
Use: Antihistaminic, antiemetic, sedative.
PHENAZOCINE. B.A.N. 1,2,3,4,5,6-Hexahydro-6,11-dimethyl-3-phenethyl-2,6-methano-3-benzazocin-8-ol.
Use: Analgesic; antipyretic.
See: Narphen hydrobromide.
PHENAZOCINE HBr. 1,2,3,4,5,6-Hexahydro-8-hydroxy-6,11-dimethyl-3-phenethyl-2,6-methano-3-benzazocine HBr.
Use: Analgesic.
PHENAZODINE. (Lannett) Phenylazodiamine-pyridine HCl 0.1 Gm./Tab. Bot. 100s, 500s, 1000s.
Use: Urinary antiseptic.
PHENAZONE.
See: Antipyrine. (Various Mfr.)
PHENAZOPYRIDINE. B.A.N. 2,6-Diamino-3-phenylazopyridine. Gastrotest.
Use: Analgesic.
See: Pyridium (hydrochloride).
W/Azo-sulfisoxazole.
See: Azo-Sulfisoxazole, Tab. (Fellows-Testagar)
W/Sulfisoxazole.
See: Azocet, Tab. (O'Neal)
Azo-Urizole, Tab. (Jenkins)
G-Sox-Azo, Tab. (Scrip)
• **PHENAZOPYRIDINE HCl,** U.S.P. XXI. Tab., U.S.P. XXI. 2,6-Diamino-3-phenylazopyridine HCl.
Use: Analgesic (urinary tract).
See: Azodine, Tab. (Vortech)
Azogesic, Tab. (Century)
Azo-Pyridon, Tab. (Reid-Provident)
Azo-Standard, Tab. (Webcon)
Azo-Sulfizin (Reid-Provident)
Baridium, Tab. (Barry Martin)
Diridone, Tab. (Premo)
Phen-Azo, Tab. (Vanguard)
Phenazodine, Tab. (Lannett)
Phenyl-Idium Prods. (Columbia)
Pyridium, Tab. (Parke-Davis)
Uri-Pak (Westerfield)
Urodine, Tab. (Saron)
PHENAZOPYRIDINE HCl W/COMBINATIONS.
See: Azo-Cyst, Tab. (Moore Kirk)
Azo Gantanol, Tab. (Roche)
Azo Gantrisin, Tab. (Roche)
Azolate, Tab. (Amfre-Grant)
Azo-Mandelamine, Tab. (Parke-Davis)

Azo-Methalate, Tab. (Vortech)
Azosoxazole, Tab. (Columbia)
Azosul, Tab. (Reid-Provident)
Azosulfisoxazole (Var. Mfr.)
Azo-Sulfstat, Tab. (Saron)
Azotrex, Cap. (Bristol Labs.)
Azox, Tab. (Elder)
Buren, Tab. (Ascher)
G-Sox-Azo, Tab. (Scrip)
Mandalay A.P., Tab. (Beutlich)
Prov-U-Sep Forte, Tab. (Reid-Provident)
Pyridium Plus, Tab. (Parke-Davis)
Rosoxol-Azo, Tab. (Robinson)
Soxazo, Tab. (Sutliff & Case)
Suladyne, Tab. (Stuart)
Suldiazo, Tab. (Kay)
Sulfasol Plus, Tab. (Hyrex)
Thiosulfil-A, Tab. (Ayerst)
Thiosulfil-A Forte, Tab. (Ayerst)
Triurisul, Tab. (Sheryl)
Uridium, Tab. (Ferndale; Pharmex)
Uri-Pak, Tab. (Westerfield)
Urisan-P, Tab. (Sandia)
Uritral, Cap. (Central)
Urobiotic, Cap. (Pfizer)
Urochron, Tab. (Saron)
Urogesic, Tab. (Edwards)
Uropeutic, Tab. (Circle)
Urotrol, Tab. (Mills)
Urseptic, Tab. (Century)
PHENBENICILLIN. B.A.N. 6-(α-Phenoxyphenyl-acetamido)pencillanic acid. α-Phenoxybenzylpenicillin.
Use: Antibiotic.
See: Penspek [potassium salt].
• **PHENBUTAZONE SODIUM GLYCERATE.** USAN.
4-Butyl-3-hydroxy-1,2-diphenyl-3-pyrazolin-5-one sodium salt compound with glycerol.
Use: Anti-inflammatory.
PHENBUTRAZATE. B.A.N. 2-(3-Methyl-2-phenylmorpholino)ethyl 2-phenylbutryate.
Use: Appetite suppressant.
PHENCAP. (Jenkins) Phenylpropanolamine HCl 50 mg., chlorpheniramine maleate 8 mg., atropine sulfate 1/180 gr./Cap. Bot. 1000s.
• **PHENCARBAMIDE.** USAN. S-2-Diethyl-ammoethyl diphenylthiocarbamate.
Use: Spasmolytic agent.
See: Escorpal (Farben-Fabriken)
PHENCEN-50. (Central) Promethazine HCl 50 mg., disodium edetate 0.1 mg. calcium Cl. 0.04 mg., phenol 5 mg., /ml. Vial 10 ml. Box 12s.
Use: Antihistaminic, anti-emetic.
PHENCHLOR-EIGHT. (Freeport) Chlorpheniramine maleate 8 mg./T.R. Cap. Bot. 1000s.
Use: Antihistaminic.
PHENCHLOR-TWELVE. (Freeport) Chlorpheniramine maleate 12 mg./T.R. Cap. Bot. 1000s.
Use: Antihistaminic.
PHENCYCLIDINE. B.A.N. 1-(1-Phenylcyclohexyl)piperidine.
Use: Anticholinergic.

• **PHENCYCLIDINE HYDROCHLORIDE.** USAN. 1-(1-Phenylcyclohexyl)piperidine HCl.
Use: Anticholinergic.
PHENDIMETRAZINE. B.A.N. (+)-3,4-Dimethyl-2-phenylmorpholine.
Use: Appetite suppressant.
See: Plegine [tartrate].
• **PHENDIMETRAZINE TARTRATE,** U.S.P. XXI. Cap., Tab., U.S.P. XXI. d-3,4-Dimethyl-2-phenylmorpholine bitartrate.
Use: Anorexic.
See: Adipost, Cap. (Ascher)
Adphen, Tab. (Ferndale)
Anorex, Cap., Tab. (Dunhall)
Bacarate, Tab. (Reid-Provident)
B.O.F. (Saron)
Bontril PDM, Tab. (Carnrick)
Delcozine, Tab. (Delco)
Di-Ap-Trol, Tab. (Foy)
Di-Metrex, Tab. (Fellows-Testagar)
Elphemet, Tab. (Canright)
Ex-Obese, Tab. (Kay)
Limit, Tab. (Bock)
Melfiat, Tab. (Reid-Provident)
Melfiat 105, Cap. (Reid-Provident)
Minus, Tab. (Amfre-Grant)
Obacin, Tab. (Kenyon)
Obalan, Tab. (Lannett)
Obepar, Tabs. (Parmed)
Obe-Tite, Tab. (Scott/Cord)
Obezine, Tab. (Western Research)
Phenazine, Inj. (Jenkins)
Phendorex, Tab. (Wolins)
Phen-70, Tab. (Parmed)
Phentazine, Tab. (Sutliff & Case)
Phenzine, Tab. (Mallard)
Prelu-2, Cap. (Boehringer Ingelheim)
Reducto, Tab. (Arcum)
Robese "P", Tabs., Vial (Rocky Mtn.)
Ropledge, Tab. (Robinson)
Slim-Tabs, Tab. (Wesley)
SPRX 1, 2 & 3 (Reid-Provident)
Statobex, Prods. (Lemmon)
Stodex, Tab., Cap. (Jalco)
Trimtabs, Tab. (Mayrand)
Weightrol, Prep., Tab. (Vortech)
PHENDOREX. (Wolins) Phendimetrazine tartrate 35 mg./Tab. Bot. 1000s.
PHENELZINE. B.A.N. Phenethylhydrazine.
Use: Antidepressant.
See: Nardil [hydrogen sulfate].
• **PHENELZINE SULFATE,** U.S.P. XXI. Tab., U.S.P. XXI. Phenethylhydrazine sulfate. Monoamine oxidase inhibitor, betaphenylethyl-hydrazine dihydrogen sulfate.
Use: Antidepressant.
See: Nardil, Tab. (Parke-Davis)
PHENEREX. (Tunex) Promethazine HCl 50 mg./ml. Vial 10cc.
Use: Management of motion sickness, nausea, vomiting associated with pregnancy.
PHENERGAN COMPOUND. (Wyeth) Promethazine

HCl 6.25 mg., pseudoephedrine HCl 60 mg., aspirin 600 mg./Tab. Bot. 50s.
Use: Symptomatic relief of minor aches and pains and fever.
PHENERGAN-D. (Wyeth) Promethazine HCl 6.25 mg., pseudoephedrine HCl 60 mg./Tab. Bot. 100s.
Use: Antihistaminic/decongestant.
PHENERGAN. (Wyeth) Promethazine HCl.
Expectorant: 5 mg./5 ml. w/ipecac fl. ext. 0.17 min., pot. guaiacolsulfonate 44 mg., citric acid 60 mg., sod. citrate 197 mg., alcohol 7%/5 ml. Bot. 4 oz., 6 oz., 8 oz., pt., gal.; **Expt. w/codeine phosphate** 5 mg./5 ml. w/ipecac, potassium guaiacolsulfonate, citric acid, sodium citrate and alcohol 7%. Bot. 4 oz., 6 oz., 8 oz., pt., gal. **Inj.:** 25 mg. & 50 mg. w/disodium edetate 0.1 mg., calcium chloride 0.04 mg., sod. metabisulfite 0.25 mg., phenol 5 mg., sod. acetate-acetic acid buffer/cc. Amp. 1 cc., 5s, 25s, 25 mg. 5s. **Injection:** 25 mg. or 50 mg./ml. w/disodium edetate 0.1 mg., Ca chloride 0.04 mg., Na metabisulfite 0.025 mg., phenol 5 mg., Na acetate-acetic acid buffer. Amp. 1 cc, 5 cc, Box 25s; 25 mg. Box 5s. **Syrup:** (w/alcohol 1.5%) 6.25 mg./5 cc. Bot. pt. **Syrup Fortis:** 25 mg./5 cc. Bot. pt. **Supp:** 12.5 mg., 25 mg., 50 mg. w/ascorbyl palmitate, silicon dioxide, white wax, cocoa butter. 12.5 mg.: Bot. 1000s, Redipak 100s; 25 mg.: Bot. 100s, 1000s. Redipak 25s, 100s; 50 mg.: Bot. 100s. **Tabs:** 12.5 mg., Bot. 100s, 1000s. Redipak 100s. 25 mg., Bot. 100s, 1000s. Redipak 25s, 100s. 50 mg. Bot. 100s.
PHENERGAN PEDIATRIC. (Wyeth) Dextromethorphan HBr 7.5 mg., promethazine HCl 5.0 mg., fl. ext. ipecac 0.17 min., pot. guaiacolsulfonate 44 mg., citric acid 60 mg., sod. citrate 197 mg., alcohol 7%/5 cc. Bot. 4 oz., 6 oz., pt. gal.
Use: Antitussive.
PHENERGAN VC EXPECTORANT. (Wyeth) **Plain:** Promethazine HCl 5 mg., phenylephrine HCl 5 mg., fl. ext. ipecac 0.17 min., potassium guaiacolsulfonate 44 mg., citric acid 60 mg., sodium citrate 197 mg.,/5 ml. w/alcohol 7%/5 ml. Bot. 4 oz., 6 oz., 8 oz., pt., gal. **W/Codeine** Above formula with codeine phosphate 10 mg./5 ml. Bot. 4 oz., 6 oz., 8 oz., pt., gal.
Use: Decongestant, antihistamine, topical anesthetic & sedative.
PHENERHIST. (Rocky Mtn.) Promethazine HCl 25 mg., 50 mg./cc. Vial 10 cc.
Use: Antihistamine.
PHENERIDINE. 1-(β-Phenyl-b-ethyl)-4-carbethoxy-4-phenylpiperidine. Ethyl 1-phenethyl-4-phenyl-isonipecotate.
Use: Analgesic.
PHENETHICILLIN. B.A.N. 6-(α-Phenoxypropion-amido)penicillanic acid. Broxil [potassium salt].
Use: Antibiotic.
PHENETHICILLIN POTASSIUM. Alpha-phenoxyethyl penicillin pot. Penicillin-152 pot.
Use: Antibiotic.
See: Chemipen

PHENETHYL ALCOHOL. B.A.N. 2-Phenylethanol.
Use: Antiseptic.
I-PHENETHYLBIGUANIDE MONOHYDROCHLORIDE. Phenformin Hydrochloride.
PHENETRON. (Lannett) Chlorpheniramine maleate 8 mg., or 12 mg./Lanacap or Lanatab. Bot. 100s, 1000s. Tabs. 4 mg., Bot. 500s, 1000s.
Use: Antihistaminic.
PHENETRON COMPOUND TABLETS. (Lannett) Salicylamide 3½ gr., phenacetin 2½ gr., caffeine ½ gr., chlorprophenpyridamine maleate 2 mg./Tab. Bot. 100s, 1000s.
PHENETRON INJECTABLE. (Lannett) Chlorpheniramine maleate Amp. (10 mg./cc.) 1 cc. 25s, 100s, Vial 30 cc. (100 mg./cc.) Vial 5 cc.
PHENETRON SYRUP. (Lannett) Chlorpheniramine maleate 2 mg./4 cc. Bot. pt., gal.
PHENETSAL.
PHENETURIDE. B.A.N. (2-Phenylbutyryl)urea. Ethylphenacemide (I.N.N.) Benuride.
Use: Anticonvulsant.
PHENFORMIN. B.A.N. 1-Phenethylbiguanide.
Use: Oral hypoglycemic agent.
Note: Drug recalled from market 10-23-77.
PHENFORMIN HCl. Imidodicarbonimidic diamide, nN-(2-phenylethyl)-monohydrochloride. N¹-β-Phenethyl-biguanide HCl.
Use: Hypoglycemic.
Note: Withdrawn from market in 1978.
PHENGLUTARIMIDE. B.A.N. 2-(2-Diethylaminoethyl)-2-phenylglutarimide. Aturbane hydrochloride.
Use: Treatment of the Parkinsonian syndrome.
PHENIFORM.
See: Phenformin HCl
PHENILAR. (Blue Cross) Dextromethorphan HBr 15 mg., guaifenesin 50 mg., chlorpheniramine maleate 2 mg., phenylephrine HCl 5 mg., acetaminophen 120 mg./10 ml. Bot. 4 oz.
Use: Cough syrup.
PHENINDAMINE. B.A.N. 1,2,3,4-Tetrahydro-2-methyl-9-phenyl-2-azafluorene. 2,3,4,9-Tetrahydro-2-methyl-9-phenyl-1H-indeno-[2,1-c]pyridine. Thephorin [hydrogentartrate].
Use: Antihistamine.
PHENINDAMINE TARTRATE. 2,3,4,9-Tetrahydro-2-methyl-9 phenyl-1 H-indeno-[2,1-c] pyridine bitartrate. 2,3,4,9-Tetrahydro-2-methyl-9-phenyl-lH-indeno-(2,1-c)pyridine Tartrate (1:1).
Use: Antihistaminic.
See: Nolahist, Tab. (Carnrick)
　Thephorin, Tab. (Roche)
W/Chlorpheniramine maleate, phenylpropanolamine HCl.
See: Nolamine, Tab. (Carnrick)
W/Codeine phosphate, phenylephrine HCl, fl. ext. ipecac, pot. guaiacolsulfonate, sodium citrate, citric acid.
See: Cerose, Liq. (Ives)
W/Dextromethorphan HBr, phenylephrine, fl. ext. ipecac, pot. guaiacolsulfonate, sod. citrate, citric acid.
See: Cerose DM, Elix. (Ives)
W/Phenylephrine HCl, aspirin, caffeine, aluminum

hydroxide, magnesium carbonate.
See: Dristan, Tab. (Whitehall)
W/Phenylephrine hydrochloride, caramiphen
ethanedisulfonate.
See: Dondril, Tab. (Whitehall)
W/Phenylephrine HCl, chlorpheniramine maleate,
drytane.
See: Comhist, Tab., Elix. (Baylor)
W/Phenylephrine HCl, chlorpheniramine maleate,
belladonna alkaloids.
See: Comhist L.A., Caps. (Baylor Labs.)
W/Phenylephrine HCl, pyrilamine maleate,
chlorpheniramine maleate, dextromethorphan HBr.
See: Histalet, Histalet-DM, Histalet-Forte, Syr. (Reid-
Provident)
• **PHENINDIONE,** U.S.P. XXI. Tab., U.S.P. XXI. (2-Phe-
nylindane-1,3-Dione; 2-Phenyl-1,3-indandione; Phe-
nylindanedion, Dindevan)
Use: Anticoagulant.
See: Eridione, Tab. (Eric, Kirk & Gary)
Hedulin, Tab. (Merrell Dow)
PHEN-IODINE NO. 2. (Sutliff & Case) Iodine 0.4%, tan-
nic acid 1.1%, phenol 5%. Ext. of witch hazel,
glycerin q.s. Bot., pt., gal.
Use: Antiseptic.
PHENIODOL.
See: Iodoalphionic Acid (Var. Mfr.)
PHENIPRAZINE. B.A.N. α-Methylphenethylhydrazine.
Cavodil [hydrochloride].
Use: Monoamine oxidase inhibitor.
PHENIPRAZINE HCl. (α-Methyl-phenethyl)-hydrazine
monohydrochloride.
Use: Antihypertensive.
PHENIRAMINE. B.A.N. 1-Phenyl-1-(2-pyridyl)-3-dime-
thylaminopropane. ($\pm$)-3-Phenyl-3-(2-pyridyl)propyl-
dimethylamine. Daneral 4-amino-salicylate; Trimeton
[maleate].
Use: Antihistamine.
PHENIRAMINE MALEATE. 2-[a-[2-(Dimethyl-
amino)ethyl]benzyl]-pyridine bimaleate. Prophen-
pyridamine.
Use: Antihist.
See: Inhiston, Tab. (Plough)
W/Combinations:
Allerstat, Cap. (Lemmon)
Chexit, Tab. (Dorsey)
Citra Forte, Cap., Syr. (Boyle)
Corizahist, Tab. (Mason)
Decobel, Cap. (Lannett)
Dri-Hist No. 2 Meta-Kaps (Sutliff & Case)
Fiogesic, Tab. (Sandoz)
Fitacol Stankaps (Standex)
Flavihist, Cap. (American Labs.)
Incorpohist, Tab. (Blue Line)
Kenahist-S.A., Tab. (Kenyon)
Klix Kernal Kaps, Cap. (Bowman)
Koldeze, Cap. (Scrip)
MSC Triaminic, Tab. (Dorsey)
Naso-Dex, Cap. (Commerce)
Partuss AC (Parmed)
Phenagesic, Tab., Syr. (Dalin)
Phenaphen Plus, Tab. (Robins)
Poly-Histine Caps., Elix., Lipospan (Bock)

Propahist, Cap., Tab., Syr. (Blue Line)
Pyma, Cap. (Fellows-Testagar)
Robitussin-AC, Syr. (Robins)
S.A.C., Cold Caps. (Towne)
Symptrol, Syr., Cap., Inj. (Saron)
T.A.C., Caps. (Towne)
Thor, Caps. (Towne)
Triaminic, Preps. (Dorsey)
Triaminicol, Syr. (Dorsey)
Trigelamine, Oint. (Edward J. Moore)
Tritussin, Syr. (Towne)
Triwol, Tab. (Wolins)
Tussagesic, Tab., Susp. (Dorsey)
Tussar-2, Syr. (Armour)
Ursinus, Tab. (Dorsey)
Ventilade, Syr. (Warren-Teed)
Woltac, Cap. (Wolins)
PHENISTIX REAGENT STRIPS. (Ames) Ferric and
magnesium salts with cyclohexylsulfamic acid. Dip-
and-test for phenylketonuria. Bot. 50s, 100s. Foil
wrapped 3s.
Use: Test urine for phenylketone.
PHEN-LETS. (Jenkins) Phenylpropanolamine HCl 100
mg./Tab. Bot. 1000s.
PHENMETRAZINE. B.A.N. ($\pm$)-trans-Tetrahydro-3-
methyl-2-phenyl-1,4-oxazine. 3-Methyl-2-phenyl-mor-
pholine. Preludin hydrochloride.
Use: Appetite suppressant.
• **PHENMETRAZINE HCl,** U.S.P. XXI. Tab., U.S.P.
XXI. 3-Methyl-2-phenylmorpholine hydrochloride.
Use: Anorexic.
See: Melfiat, Tab. (Reid-Provident)
Preludin, Tab., Endurets (Boehringer Ingelheim)
• **PHENOBARBITAL,** U.S.P. XXI. Elixir, Tab., U.S.P.
XXI. 2,4,6(1H,3H,%H) Pyrimidinetrione, 5-ethyl-5-
phenyl. 5-Ethyl-5-phenylbarbituric acid. Phenylethyl-
barbituric acid, phenylethylmalonylurea, Barbenyl,
Dormiral, Duneryl, Neurobarb, Numol, Phenonyl,
Somonal.
Use: Anticonvulsant, hypnotic, sedative.
See: Bar Elix., (Scrip)
Barbipil, Pill (Vortech)
Barbita, Pill (Vortech)
Henomint, Elix. (Bowman)
Hypnette, Supp., Tab. (Fleming)
Luminal, Ovoids (Winthrop-Breon)
Orprine, Liq. (Pennwalt)
Pheno-Square, Tab. (Mallard)
Sedadrops, Liq. (Merrell Dow)
SK-Phenobarbital, Tab. (SmithKline)
Solu-barb, Tab. (Fellows-Testagar)
PHENOBARBITAL W/AMINOPHYLLINE.
See: Aminophylline (Var. Mfr.)
PHENOBARBITAL W/ATROPINE SULFATE.
See: Atropine Sulfate (Var. Mfr.) P.A., Tab. (Scrip)
PHENOBARBITAL W/BELLADONNA.
See: Belladonna Products and Phenobarbital
Combinations.
**PHENOBARBITAL WITH CENTRAL NERVOUS
SYSTEM STIMULANTS.**
See: Amodrine, Tab. (Searle)
Arcotrate No. 3, Tab. (Arcum)
Asminyl, Tab. (Cole)

Belkatal, Tab. (Ferndale)
Bellophen, Tab. (Richlyn)
Bowdrin, Tab. (Bowman)
Bronkolixir, Elix. (Winthrop-Breon)
Bronkotab, Tab. (Winthrop-Breon)
Dainite, Night, Tab. (Mallinckrodt)
Duovent, Tab. (Riker)
Ephenyllin, Tab. (CMC)
Isuprel Compound, Elix. (Winthrop-Breon)
Luasmin, Cap. (Cooper)
Luftodil, Tab. (Mallinckrodt)
Peritrate w/Phenobarbital, Tab. (Parke-Davis)
Phelantin, Cap. (Parke-Davis)
Phyldrox, Tab. (Lemmon)
Quadrinal, Susp., Tab. (Knoll)
Sedamine, Tab. (Dunhall)
Sedatromine, Tab. (Sutliff & Case)
Spabelin, Elix., Tab. (Arcum)
Synophedal, Tab. (Central)
T.E.P., Tab. (Kirkman)
T-E-P Compound, Tab. (Stanlabs)
PHENOBARBITAL COMBINATIONS.
See: Aminophylline W/Phenobarbital, Combinations
Aspirin-Barbiturate, Combinations
Atropine-Hyoscine-Hyoscyamine Combinations
Atropine Sulfate w/Phenobarbital
Belladonna Ext. Combinations
Belladonna Products & Phenobarbital
Combinations
Homatropine Methylbromide & Phenobarbital
Combinations
Hyoscyamus Products & Phenobarbital
Combinations.
Mannitol Hexanitrate w/Phenobarbital
Combinations
Mephenesin & Barbiturates Combinations
Phenobarbital W/Central Nervous System
Stimulants
Secobarbital Combinations
Sodium Nitrite Combinations
Theobromine W/Phenobarbital Combinations
Theophylline W/Phenobarbital Combinations
Veratrum Viride W/Phenobarbital Combinations
**PHENOBARBITAL W/HOMATROPINE
METHYLBROMIDE.**
See: Homatropine Methylbromide & Phenobarbital
Combinations
PHENOBARBITAL W/HYOSCYAMUS.
See: Hyoscyamus Products & Phenobarbital
Combinations
PHENOBARBITAL W/MANNITOL HEXANITRATE.
Use: Anticonvulsant, hypnotic, sedative.
See: Mannitol Hexanitrate w/Phenobarbital
Combinations
• **PHENOBARBITAL SODIUM,** U.S.P. XXI. Inj., Sterile,
Tab., U.S.P. XXI. Sodium 5-ethyl-5-phenylbarbiturate.
2,4,6(1H,3H,5H)-Pyrimidinetrione, 5-ethyl-5 phenyl,
monosodium salt. (Sod. Phenylethylbarbiturate,
Soluble Phenobarbital). (Various Mfr.)
Use: Anticonvulsant, hypnotic, sedative.
See: Luminal Sod., Sol. (Winthrop-Breon)

**PHENOBARBITAL SODIUM IN PROPYLENE
GLYCOL.** Vitarine-Amp. (0.13 Gm.) 1 cc., Box 25s,
100s. (2 gr.) 1 cc., Box 25s, 100s.
Use: Anticonvulsant, hypnotic, sedative.
**PHENOBARBITAL & THEOBROMINE
COMBINATIONS.**
See: Theobromine w/Phenobarbital Combinations
PHENOBARBITAL W/THEOPHYLLINE.
See: Theophylline w/Phenobarbital Combinations
PHENOBARBITAL W/VERATRUM VIRIDE.
See: Veratrum Viride w/Phenobarbital
Combinations
PHEN-O-BEL-T. (Coastal) Phenobarbital 50 mg., hyos-
cyamine sulfate 0.311 mg., atropine sulfate 0.0582
mg., hyoscine HBr 0.0195 mg./T.R. Cap. Bot. 100s,
1000s.
Use: Sedative.
PHENOBUTIODIL. B.A.N. w-(2,4,6-Triiodophenoxy)-
butyric acid. Vesipaque (Warner-Lambert)
Use: Radio-opaque substance.
See: Biliodyl.
PHENOCTIDE. Octaphonium Chloride, B.A.N.
PHENODODECINIUM BROMIDE. Domiphen bromide,
B.A.N.
PHENODYNE. (Blue Line) Aspirin 3½ gr.,
acetophenetidin 2½ gr., caffeine ½ gr.,
phenolphthalein ¼ gr./Cap. Bot. 100s, 1000s.
Use: Orally, analgesic & antipyretic w/laxative.
PHENODYNE W/CODEINE PHOS. (Blue Line) Aspirin
3½ gr., phenacetin 2½ gr., phenolphthalein ¼ gr.,
caffeine (hydrous) ½ gr., codeine phosphate ¼
gr./Cap. Bot. 1000s. ½ gr./Cap. Bot. 100s, 1000s.
Use: Analgesic-antipyretic.
PHENOGESIC. (Wolins) Acetaminophen 325 mg.,
phenyltoloxamine 30 mg./Tab. Bot. 100s, 1000s.
PHENOJECT. (Mayrand) Promethazine HCl 25 mg.,
50 mg./ml. Vial 10 ml.
• **PHENOL,** U.S.P. XXI. Liq., U.S.P. XXI. (Various Mfr.)
Carbolic acid.
Use: Pharm. aid (preservative), topical antipruritic.
W/Aluminum hydroxide, zinc oxide, camphor,
eucalyptol, ichthammol, thyme oil.
See: Almophen, Oint. (Bowman)
W/Benzocaine, ichthammol, balsam peru, alum exsic.,
oil cade, oil eucalyptus, carbolic oil.
See: Alucaine, Oint. (Jenkins)
W/Benzocaine, triclosan,
See: Solarcaine Pump Spray (Plough)
W/Dextromethorphan
See: Chloraseptic DM Lozenges (Eaton)
W/Resorcinol.
See: Black & White Ointment (Plough)
W/Resorcinol, boric acid, basic fuchsin, acetone.
See: Castellani's Paint, Liq. (Various Mfr.)
• **PHENOLATE SODIUM.** USAN.
Use: Disinfectant.
PHENOLAX. (Upjohn) Phenolphthalein 64.8
mg./Wafer. Bot. 100s.
Use: Mild laxative.
• **PHENOL, LIQUEFIED,** U.S.P. XXI.
Use: Topical antipruritic.
• **PHENOLPHTHALEIN,** U.S.P. XXI. Tab., U.S.P. XXI.

(Various Mfr.) 3,3-Bis(p-hydroxyphenyl)phthalide.
Pkg. 1 oz., ¼ lb., 1 lb.
Use: Cathartic.
See: Alophen, Pill (Parke-Davis)
Espotabs, Tab. (Combe)
Evac-U-Lax, Wafer. (Mallard)
Evasof, Tab. (Lemmon)
Ex-Lax Preps. (Ex-Lax)
Feen-A-Mint, Tab. & Gum (Plough)
Phenolax, Wafers (Upjohn)

PHENOLPHTHALEIN W/COMBINATIONS.
See: Amlax, Tab. (Vortech)
Bicholate, Tab. (Blue Line)
Bilocomp, Tab. (Lannett)
Bilstan (Standex)
Correctol, Tab. (Plough)
Dibolans, Tab. (Noyes)
Disolan, Cap. (Lannett)
Evac-Q-Kit, Tab., Supp. (Warren-Teed)
Evac-U-Gen, Tab. (Walker)
Dual Formula Feen-A-Mint Pills. (Plough)
Feen-A-Mint, Gum, Mint, Pills (Plough)
Formula No. 3656, Tab. (Blue Line)
4-Way Cold Tabs. (Bristol-Myers)
Glycols, Tab. (Bowman)
Lanothal Pills (Lannett)
Laxogen, Tab. (Vortech)
Novalax, Cap. (Coastal)
Oxiphen, Tab. (Webcon)
Petrogalar W/Phenolphthalein, Liq. (Wyeth)
Petrolatum, Liq.
Phenodyne, Cap., Tab. (Blue Line)
Sarolax, Cap. (Saron)
Taurocolate, Tab. (Vortech)
Torocol, Tab. (Plessner)
Torocol Compound, Tab. (Plessner)
Tripalax, Cap. (Redford)

PHENOLPHTHALEIN IN LIQUID PETROLATUM EMULSION. (Various Mfr.)
See: Petrolatum, Liq.

PHENOL RED.
See: Phenolsulfonphthalein

PHENOLSULFONATES.
See: Sulfocarbolates

PHENOLSULFONIC ACID. Sulfocarbolic acid.
Note use in Sulphodine, Tab. (Strasenburgh)

• **PHENOLSULFONPHTHALEIN**, U.S.P. XXI. Inj.,
U.S.P. XXI. α-Hydroxy-α,α-bis(p-hydroxyphenyl)-o-
toluene-sulfonic acid)sulfone. 4,4'-(3H-2,1-Benzoxa-
thiol-3-ylidene)-diphenol S,S-dioxide. (Various Mfr.)
Use: I.M., & I.V.; diagnostic aid. Also for renal function.

PHENOLTETRABROMOPHTHALEIN. Disulfonate Disodium.
See: Sulfobromophthalein Sodium, U.S.P. XXI.

PHENOLZINE SULFATE. β-Phenylethylhydrazine hydrogen sulfate.

PHENOMORPHAN. B.A.N. 3-Hydroxy-N-phenethylmor-
phinan.
Use: Narcotic analgesic.

PHENOPERIDINE. B.A.N. Ethyl 1-(3-hydroxy-3-phenyl-

propyl)-4-phenylpiperidine-4-carboxylate. Operidine
hydrochloride.
Use: Narcotic analgesic.

PHENOTHIATAL ELIXIR. (Fellows) Phenobarbital ¼
gr., B-1 5 mg., hyoscine HBr 0.0065 mg., atropine
sulfate 0.0194 mg., hyoscyamine 0.1037 mg./5 cc.
Bot. pts., gal.

PHENOTHIAZINE. Thiodiphenylamine.

PHENOTURIC. (Truett) Phenobarbital 40 mg./Tsp.
Elixir, Bot. 1 pt., gals.
Use: Sedative.

PHENOXYBENZAMINE. B.A.N. 2-(N-Benzyl-2-chloroe-
thylamino)-1-phenoxypropane. N-(2-Chloroethyl)-N-
(1-methyl-2-phenoxyethyl)benzylamine. Dibenyline;
Dibenzyline hydrochloride.
Use: Adrenaline antagonist.

• **PHENOXYBENZAMINE HCl**, U.S.P. XXI. Cap.,
U.S.P. XXI. N-Phenoxyisopropyl-N-benzyl-beta-chlo-
rethylamine HCl. N-(2-Chloroethyl)-N-(1-methyl-2-
phenoxy-ethyl)benzylamine HCl.
Use: Antihypertensive.
See: Dibenzyline, Cap. (SmithKline)

8-PHENOXYETHANOL.
See: Tridenol, Liq. (Spirt)

PHENOXYMETHYL PENICILLIN.
See: Penicillin V.

PHENOXYMETHYL PENICILLIN POTASSIUM.
See: Penicillin V potassium.

PHENOXYNATE. Mixture of phenylphenols 17-18%,
octyl and related alkylphenols 2-3%.
See: Surtenol, Liq. (Guardian Chem.)

PHENOXYPROPAZINE. B.A.N. (1-Methyl-2-phenoxye-
thyl)hydrazine. Drazine hydrogen maleate.
Use: Monoamine oxidase inhibitor.

PHENPROBAMATE. B.A.N. 3-Phenylpropyl carbamate.
Gamaquil.
Use: Skeletal muscle relaxant.

• **PHENPROCOUMON**, U.S.P. XXI. Tab., U.S.P. XXI.
3-(α-Ethylbenzyl)-4-hydroxycoumarin. 4-Hydroxy-3-
(1-phenylpropyl)coumarin. Marcoumar.
Use: Anticoagulant.
See: Liquamar, Tab. (Organon)

PHEN-70. (Parmed) Phendimetrazine Tartrate 70
mg./Tab. Bot. 100s, 1000s.
Use: Anorexiant.

• **PHENSUXIMIDE**, U.S.P. XXI. Cap., U.S.P. XXI. N-
Methyl-2-phenylsuccinimide.
Use: Anticonvulsant.
See: Milontin, Preps. (Parke-Davis)

PHENTAL. (Geneva) Belladonna alkaloids
w/phenobarbital ¼ gr./Tab. Bot. 1000s.

PHENTAZINE. (Sutliff & Case) Phendimetrazine
tartrate 35 mg./Tab. Bot. 100s, 1000s.

• **PHENTERMINE.** USAN. α,α-Dimethylphenethyla-
mine. Phenyl-tertiarybutylamine. Duromine (an ion-
exchange resin complex)
Use: Anorexiant.
See: Adipex, Tab. (Lemmon)
Adipex-8 C.T., Cap. (Lemmon)
Adipex-P, Cap. (Lemmon)
Fastin, Cap. (Beecham Labs)
Parmine, Cap. (Parmed)

Phentrol, Tab. (Vortech)
Rolaphent, Tab. (Robinson)
Tora, Tab. (Reid-Provident)
Unifast Unicelles, Cap. (Reid-Provident)
Wilpowr, Cap. (Foy)
PHENTERMINE AS RESIN COMPLEX.
See: Ionamin, Cap. (Pennwalt)
• **PHENTERMINE HYDROCHLORIDE,** U.S.P. XXI.
Cap., Nasal Jelly, Tab., U.S.P. XXI.
Benzeneethanamine, α,α-dimethyl-, hydrochloride.
Use: Anorexiant.
PHENTETIOTHALEIN SODIUM. Iso-Iodeikon.
Use: Radiopaque medium for cholecystography &
for liver function test.
PHENTOLAMINE. B.A.N. 2-N-(3-Hydroxyphenyl)-p-
toluidinomethyl-2-imidazoline. [Rogitine hydrochlo-
ride or mesylate].
Use: Adrenaline antagonist.
PHENTOLAMINE HYDROCHLORIDE. m-[n-(2-Imi-
dazolin-2-ylmethyl)-p-toluidino]phenol hydrochloride.
Use: Anti-adrenergic.
See: Regitine Hydrochloride, Tab. (Ciba)
• **PHENTOLAMINE MESYLATE.** U.S.P. XXI. For Inj.,
U.S.P. XXI. Phenol, 3-[[(4,5-dihydro-1H-imidazol-2-
yl)methyl]-(4-methyl-phenyl)amino]-, monomethane-
sulfonate (salt). m-[N-(2-Imidazolin-2-ylmethyl)-p-
toluidino]-phenol methanesulfonate.
Use: Anti-adrenergic.
See: Phentolamine methansulfonate
PHENTOLAMINE METHANESULFONATE.
Phentolamine mesylate, U.S.P. XXI.
PHENTOLOX w/APAP. (Richlyn) Phenyltoloxamine
citrate 30 mg., acetaminophen 325 mg./Tab. Bot.
1000s.
Use: Antihistaminic, analgesic.
PHENTOX COMPOUND SYRUP. (Bay)
Phenylpropanolamine HCl 20 mg., phenylephrine
HCl 5 mg., phenytoloxamine citrate 7.5 mg.,
chlorpheniramine maleate 2.5 mg./5 ml. Bot. pt.
gal.
Use: Decongestant, antihistaminic.
PHENTRIDE-8. (Western Research) Phentermine HCl
8 mg./Tab. Handicount 28 (36 bags of 28s)
Use: Anorexic.
PHENTROL. (Vortech) Phentermine HCl 8 mg./Tab.
Bot. 1000s.
Use: Anorexiant.
PHENTROL NO. 2. (Vortech) Phenteramine HCl 30
mg./Cap. Bot. 100s, 1000s.
Use: Anorexiant.
PHENTROL NO. 4 and NO. 5. (Vortech)
Phenteramine HCl 30 mg./Cap. Bot. 100s, 1000s.
Use: Anorexiant.
PHENTYDRONE. 1,2,3,4-Tetrahydrofluoren-9-one.
Use: Systemic fungicide.
PHENURONE. (Abbott) (Phenacemide,
Phenacetylcarbamide, Phenacetylurea) Tab. 0.5
Gm., Bot. 100s.
Use: Psychomotor epilepsy, grand mal & petit mal
epilepsies.
N-PHENYLACETAMIDE.
See: Acetanilid (Var. Mfr.)

• **PHENYLAMINOSALICYLATE.** USAN. Phenyl 4
aminosalicylate. Fenamisal (I.N.N.) PhenyPAS
Tebamin.
Use: Tuberculostatic.
PHENYLACETYLUREA.
See: Phenurone, Tab. (Abbott)
• **PHENYLALANINE,** U.S.P. XXI. $C_9H_{11}NO_2$ as
L-phenylalanine.
See: Phenylketonuria therapy.
**l-PHENYLALANINE, 4-[BIS(2-CHLOROETHYL)-
AMINO-]** Melphalan, U.S.P. XXI.
PHENYLALANINE MUSTARD.
See: Melphalan, U.S.P. XXI.
**PHENYLAZO-DIAMINOPYRIDINE HYDROCHLO-
RIDE.**
See: Rodine, Tab. (Paddock)
PHENYLAZO SULFISOXAZOLE. (A.P.C.)
Sulfisoxazole 0.5 Gm., phenylazopyridine 50
mg./Tab. Bot. 1000s.
PHENYLAZO TABLETS. (APC) Phenylazodiamino-pyri-
dine HCl 1½ gr./Tab. Bot. 1000s.
Use: Urinary analgesic and antiseptic.
PHENYLAZO-DIAMINO-PYRIDINE.
See: Phenazopyridine (Var. Mfr.)
PHENYLAZO-DIAMINO-PYRIDINE HCl or HBr.
See: Phenazopyridine HCl or HBr (Var. Mfr.)
• **PHENYLBUTAZONE,** U.S.P. XXI. Cap., Tab. U.S.P.
XXI. 3,5-Pyrazolidinedione, 4-butyl-1,2-diphenyl-. 4-
Butyl-1,2-diphenyl-3,5-pyrazolidinedione. 4-Butyl-1,2-
diphenylpyrazolidine-3,5-dione. Benzone; Butacote;
Butaphen; Butazone; Flexaz IA-But; Tetnor.
Use: Anti-inflammatory.
See: Azolid, Tab. (USV)
     Butazolidin, Tab. (Geigy)
W/Aluminum hydroxide dried gel, magnesium
trisilicate.
See: Azolid-A, Cap. (USV)
W/Aluminum hydroxide, mag. trisilicate.
See: Butazolidin Alka, Cap. (Geigy)
PHENYL-1-BUTYL-NORSUPRIFEN.
See: Arlidin, Tab. (USV Pharm.)
PHENYLCARBINOL.
See: Benzyl Alcohol, N.F. XVI.
PHENYLCINCHONINIC ACID. Name used for
cinchophen.
PHENYLEPHRINE. B.A.N. (−)-1-(3-Hydroxyphenyl)-
2-methylaminoethanol. Fenox; Neophryn; Neosy-
nephrine hydrochloride.
Use: Vasoconstrictor; hypotensive.
See: Duo-Medihaler, Vial (Riker)
• **PHENYLEPHRINE HYDROCHLORIDE,** U.S.P. XXI.
Inj., Nasal Soln., Ophth. Soln., U.S.P. XXI.
Benzenemethanol, 3-hydroxy-α-[(methylamino)-me-
thyl]-, hydrochloride (S)-. l-m-Hydroxy-a-[(me-
thylamino)methyl]-benzyl alcohol hydrochloride.
(Neophryn).
Use: Sympathomimetic agent, vasoconstrictor &
mydriatic.
See: Alcon-Efrin, Sol. (Webcon)
     Allerest Nasal Spray (Pharmacraft)
     Coricidin Decongestant Nasal Mist (Schering)
     Ephrine, Spray (Walgreen)

Neo-Synephrine HCl, Prep. (Winthrop Products)
Prefrin Liquifilm Ophth. Soln (Allergan)
Pyracort-D, spray (Lemmon)
Sinarest, Nasal Spray (Pharmacraft)
Super-Anahist Nasal Spray (Warner-Lambert)
W/Combinations:
See: Acotus, Liq. (Whorton)
Anodynos Forte, Tab. (Buffington)
Bellafedrol A-H, Tab. (Lannett)
Bur-Tuss Expectorant (Burlington)
C.D.M. Expect. Liq. (Lannett)
Cenahist, Cap. (Century)
Cenaid, Tab. (Century)
Chlor-Trimeton Expect. (Schering)
Chlor-Trimeton Expt. w/Codeine (Scherring)
Clistin-D, Tab. (McNeil)
Col-Decon, Tab. (Columbia)
Conar, Susp., Expt. (Beecham Labs)
Conar-A, Tab., Susp. (Beecham Labs)
Congespirin, Tab. (Bristol-Myers)
Coricidin Demilets (Schering)
Covanamine Tablets (Mallinckrodt)
Dallergy, Syr., Cap., Tab., Inj. (Laser)
Demazin, Syrup (Schering)
Dimetane Decongestant, Tab., Elixir (Robins)
Dimetane Expectorant, Liq. (Robins)
Dimetane Expectorant-DC, Liq. (Robins)
Dimetapp, Elix. Extentabs (Robins)
Doktors, Drops, Spray (Scherer)
Dri-Drip, Liq. (Coastal)
Drinus-M, Cap. (Amfre-Grant)
Eldatapp, Tab., Liq. (Elder)
Emagrin Forte, Tab. (Clapp)
Entex, Prods. (Norwich Eaton)
Expectico Ped. Cough Syr. (Coastal)
Eye-Gene, Sol. (Pearson)
4 Way Tab., Spray (Bristol-Myers)
Furacin Nasal Sol. (Eaton)
Histabid, Cap. (Meyer)
Histapp Prods. (Upsher-Smith)
Histospan-D, Cap. (USV)
Histospan-Plus, Cap. (USV)
Mydfrin Ophthalmic, Liq. (Alcon)
Naal, Timesule (Haag)
Na-Co-Al, Tab. (High)
Nasahist, Cap. (Keene)
Noraphen-Plus Spancap. (Vortech)
Pediacof, Syr. (Winthrop-Breon)
Phenoptic, Sol. (Muro)
Phenylzin Drops, Ophth. Sol. (CooperVision)
Prefrin-A Ophth. Soln. (Allergan)
Prefrin-Z Ophth. Soln. (Allergan)
Pyraphed, Sol. (Lemmon)
Pyristan Cap., Elix. (Arcum)
Queledrine, Syr. (Abbott)
Rhinall, Liq. (Scherer)
Rhinex DM, Tab. (Lemmon)
Rymed, Prods. (Edwards)
Sinex, Nasal Spray (Vicks)
Singlet, Tab. (Merrell Dow)
Spectab, Tab. (Reid-Provident)
Spec-T Sore Throat-Decongestant Loz. (Squibb)

Sucrets Cold Decongestant Lozenge (Calgon)
Tearefrin, Liq. (CooperVision)
Trind, Liq. (Mead Johnson)
Trind-DM, Liq. (Mead Johnson)
Tri-Ophtho, Soln. (Maurry)
T-Spray (Saron)
Turbilixir, liq. (Burlington)
Turbispan Leisurecaps, Cap. (Burlington)
Tympagesic, Liq. (Adria)
Vacon, Liq. (Scherer)
Valihist, Cap. (Clapp)
Vasocidin, Ophth. Soln. (CooperVision)
Vasosulf, Ophth. Soln. (CooperVision)
PHENYLEPHRINE TANNATE.
W/Carbetapentane tannate, chlorpheniramine
tannate, ephedrine tannate.
See: Rynatuss, Tabule (Mallinckrodt)
W/Chlorpheniramine tannate, pyrilamine tannate.
See: Rynatan, Tabules, Susp. (Mallinckrodt)
• **PHENYLETHYL ALCOHOL,** U.S.P. XXI.
Betaphenylethanol. Benzylcarbinol. (Various Mfr.)
Phenethyl Alcohol.
Use: Antibacterial; preservative (ophthalmic).
beta-PHENYL-ETHYL-HYDRAZINE. Phenalzine dihy-
drogen sulfate.
See: Nardil, Tab. (Parke-Davis)
PHENYLETHYLMALONYLUREA.
See: Phenobarbital (Various Mfr.)
PHENYLIC ACID.
See: Phenol, U.S.P. XXI.
PHENYL-IDIUM TABLETS. (Columbia) Phenazopyri-
dine HCl 100 mg./Tab. Bot. 100s, 1000s.
Use: Urinary tract analgesic.
PHENYL-IDIUM 200. (Columbia) Phenazopyridine HCl
200 mg./Tab. Bot. 100s, 1000s.
Use: Urinary tract analgesic.
PHENYLINDANEDIONE. Phenindione, B.A.N.
PHENYLKETONURIA THERAPY.
See: Lofenalac, Powd. (Mead Johnson)
Phenistix Reagent Strips (Ames)
• **PHENYLMERCURIC ACETATE,** N.F. XVI. (Various
Mfr.) (Acetato)phenylmercury. Bot. 1 lb., 5 lb., 10 lb.
Use: Preservative (bacteriostatic).
W/9-Aminoacridine HCl, sodium lauryl sulfate, succinic
acid.
See: Vagiserts w/inserts, Supp. (Vortech)
W/9-Aminoacridine HCl, tyrothricin, urea, lactose.
See: Trinalis, Vag. Supp. (Webcon)
W/Benzocaine, chlorothymol, resorcin.
See: Lanacane Creme (Combe)
W/Boric acid, polyoxyethylenenonylphenol or
oxyquinoline benzoate.
See: Koromex, Prep. (Holland-Rantos)
W/Methylbenzethonium chloride.
See: Norforms, Aer., Supp. (Norwich)
PHENYLMERCURIC BORATE. (F. W. Berk) Pkg.
Custom packed.
W/Benzyl alcohol, benzocaine & butyl p-aminobenzo-
ate.
See: Dermathyn, Oint. (Davis & Sly)
PHENYLMERCURIC CHLORIDE.
Chlorophenylmercury.

• **PHENYLMERCURIC NITRATE,** N.F. XVI.
(Merphenyl Nitrate, Phenmerzyl Nitrate) A.P.L.—
Oint. 1:1500, 1 oz., 4 oz., 1 lb. Chicago Pharm.—
Loz. w/benzocaine. Bot. 100s, 1000s. Ophth. Oint.,
1:3000, Tube ⅛ oz. Sol. 1:20,000, Bot. 1 pt., 1 gal.
Vaginal supp., 1:5000, Box 12s.
Use: Bacteriostatic.
See: Preparation H, Oint., Supp. (Whitehall)
W/Amyl & phenylphenol complex.
See: Lubraseptic Jelly (Guardian)
W/Undecylenic acid.
See: Bridex, Oint. (Briar)
PHENYLMERCURIC PICRATE.
Use: Germicide.
o-PHENYLPHENOL.
W/Amyl complex, phenylmercuric nitrate.
See: Lubraseptic Jelly. (Guardian)
PHENYLPROPANOLAMINE. B.A.N. 2-Amino-1-phenyl-
propan-1-ol. Propadrine.
Use: Sympathomimetic.
• **PHENYLPROPANOLAMINE HYDROCHLORIDE,**
U.S.P. XXI. (±)-Norephedrine Hydrochloride. 2-
Amino-1-phenyl-1-propanol (Mydriatine)
Use: Sympathomimetic.
See: Dietac Pre-Meal Diet Aid Drops (Menley &
James)
Dietac Pre-Meal Diet Aid Tab. (Menley & James)
Obestat, Cap. (Lemmon)
Obestat 150, Cap. (Lemmon)
Propadrine Hydrochloride, Preps. (Merck Sharp &
Dohme)
Propagest, Tab., Syr. (Carnrick)
PHENYLPROPANOLAMINE HCl W/COMBINATIONS.
See: Alclear Anti-allergy Tab. (Walgreen)
Alcon Decongestant, Tab. Liq. (Webcon)
Algecol, Tab. (Winston)
Algetuss, Liq. (Winston)
Allerest Prods. (Pharmacraft)
Allergesic, Tab. (Vitarine)
Allerstat, Cap. (Lemmon)
Amaril "D" Spancap (Vortech)
A.R.M., Tab. (Menley & James)
Bayer Prods. (Glenbrook)
Bifed, Cap. (Alto)
Blu-Hist, Cap. (Bluco)
Bowman Decongestant Compound, Inj.
(Bowman)
BQ Cold Tablets (Bristol-Myers)
Breacol cough Medication, Liq. (Glenbrook)
Bur-Tuss Expectorant (Burlington)
Chexit, Tabs. (Dorsey)
Comtrex, Cap., Liq., Tab. (Bristol-Myers)
Congespirin, Liq., Tab. (Bristol-Myers)
Contac, Cap. (Menley & James)
Contac Jr., Liq. (Menley & James)
Cophene No. 2, Cap. (Dunhall)
Coricidin Children's Cough Syrup. (Schering)
Coricidin Cough Formula (Schering)
Coricidin "D" Decongestant Tablets (Schering)
Coricidin Sinus Headache Tablets (Schering)
Corzone, Syr. (Xttrium)
Covanamine Tablets (Mallinckrodt)

Dalca, Tab. (Ascher)
Daycare, Liq. (Vicks)
Decobel, Cap. (Lannett)
Decongestant, Inj. (Century)
Decongestcaps TDC, Caps. (Ulmer)
Desa-Hist Antitussive Syrup (Pharmics)
Desa-Hist AT, Tab. (Pharmics)
Desa-Hist PF, Cap. (Pharmics)
Dex-A-Diet, Prods. (O'Connor)
Dezest, Cap. (Geneva Drugs)
Dietac 12 Hour Diet Aid Cap. (Menley & James)
Dimetane Expectorant, Liq. (Robins)
Dimetane Expectorant-DC, Liq. (Robins)
Dimetapp, Elix., Extentabs (Robins)
Dorcol Pediatric Cough Syr. (Dorsey)
Dri-Drip, Cap., Liq. (Coastal)
Drinophen, Cap. (Lannett)
Eldatapp, Tab., Liq. (Elder)
Entex, Caps. (Norwich Eaton)
Entex, Liq. (Norwich Eaton)
Entex LA, Tab. (Norwich Eaton)
Fiogesic, Tab. (Sandoz)
Formula 44D Decongestant Cough Mixture, Syr.
(Vicks)
4-Way Nasal Spray (Bristol-Myers)
Ginsopan, Tab., Cap. (O'Neal)
Halls Mentho-Lyptus Cough Formula, Liq. (Warner-
Lambert)
Histalet Forte T.D., Tab. (Reid-Provident)
Histapp Prods. (Upsher-Smith)
Hista-Vadrin, Syr., Tab., Cap. (Scherer)
Kleer Compound, Tab. (Scrip)
Klix Kernel, Cap. (Bowman)
Koryza Tab. (Fellows-Testagar)
Leder, Prods. (Lederle)
Meditussin, Syr. (Hauck)
Meditussin-X Liquid. (Hauck)
Na-Co-Al, Tab. (High)
Naldecon, Drop, Syr., Tab. (Bristol)
Nasahist, Cap., Inj. (Keene)
Nolamine, Tab. (Carnrick)
Novahistine, Prods. (Merrell Dow)
Opasal, Cap. (Elder)
Oraminic, Prods. (Vortech)
Ornacol, Cap., Liq. (Menley & James)
Ornade, Cap. (SmithKline)
Ornex, Cap. (Menley & James)
Panadyl, Tab., Cap. (Misemer)
Partuss-A, Tab. (Parmed)
Partuss T.D., Tab. (Parmed)
Propahist, Tab., Syr., Cap., Inj. (Blue Line)
Pyristan, Cap., Elix. (Arcum)
Rhinex DM, Liq. (Lemmon)
Rohist-D, Cap., Vial (Rocky Mtn.)
Rolanade, Cap. (Robinson)
Rymed, Prods. (Edwards)
Ryna-Tussadine, Tab., Liq. (Mallinckrodt)
Sanhist TD, Tab., Vial (Sandia)
Santussin, Cap., Susp. (Sandia)
Sine-Aid, Tab. (McNeil)
Sine-Off, Tab. (Menley & James)
Sinarest, Tab (Pharmcraft)

Sinubid, Tabs. (Warner-Lambert)
Sinulin, Tab. (Carnrick)
Sinutab, Prods. (Warner-Lambert)
Spec-T Sore Throat-Decongestant Loz. (Squibb)
St. Joseph Cold Tablets for Children (Plough)
Sto-Caps, Cap (Jalco)
Sucrets Cold Decongestant Lozenge (Calgon)
Super-Anahist Tablets (Warner-Lambert)
Symptomax, Liq. (Reid-Provident)
Teragen, Tab. (O'Neal)
Triaminic, Preps. (Dorsey)
Triaminicin, Tab., Chewable, (Dorsey)
Triaminicol, Syr. (Dorsey)
Turbilixir, Liq. (Burlington)
Turbispan Leisurecaps, Cap. (Burlington)
Tusquelin, Syr. (Circle)
Tussagesic, Susp., Tab. (Dorsey)
Tusscaps, Cap. (Martin-Phillips)
Tuss-Ornade, Cap. (SmithKline)
Tusstrol, Liq. (Reid-Provident)
U.R.I., Cap., Liq. (ICN)
Vernate, Inj., Cap., Tab. (Reid-Provident)
Vicks Daycare, Liq. (Vicks)
Vicks Formula 44D Decongestant Cough Mixture,
Syr. (Vicks)
**PHENYLPROPYLMETHYLAMINE HYDROCHLO-
RIDE.** Vonedrine HCl.
PHENYL SALICYLATE. Salol.
W/Atropine sulfate, hyoscyamine, methenamine,
methylene blue, gelsemium, benzoic acid.
See: Lanased, Tab. (Lannett)
Renalgin, Tab. (Meyer)
U-Tract, Tab. (Bowman)
W/Euphorbia ext. & various oils.
See: Rayderm Ointment (Velvet Pharmacal)
W/Methenamine, methylene blue, benzoic acid,
hyoscyamine alkaloid, atropine sulfate.
See: Cystrea, Tab. (Moore Kirk)
Urised, Tab. (Webcon)
UTA, Tab. (ICN)
W/Methenamine, sodium biphosphate, methylene
blue, hyoscyamine, alkaloid.
See: Urostat Forte, Tab. (Elder)
W/Methylene blue, belladonna alkaloids,
methenamine, sod. benzoate.
See: Urilief, Tab. (Mallinckrodt)
PHENYL-TERT-BUTYLAMINE.
See: Phentermine
PHENYLTHILONE. 2-Ethyl-2-phenyl-3,5-thiomorpho-
linedione.
Use: Anticonvulsant.
PHENYLTOLOXAMINE. o-Benzylphenyl-2-dimethyl-
aminoethyl ether.
PHENYLTOLOXAMINE. B.A.N. N-2-(2-Benzylphen-
oxy)ethyldimethylamine.
Use: Antihistamine.
PHENYLTOLOXAMINE CITRATE. N,N-Dimethyl-2-[(al-
pha-phenyl-o-tolyl)oxy]ethylamine citrate.
See: Volaxin Modified, Tab. (Elder)
**PHENYLTOLOXAMINE CITRATE
W/COMBINATIONS.**
See: Col-Decon, Tab. (Columbia)

Conex, Liq. (Westerfield)
Conex-DA, Dual Action Tab. (Westerfield)
Conex Plus, Tab. (Westerfield)
Corzone, Syr. (Xttrium)
Dengesic, Tab. (Scott-Alison)
Euphenex, Tab. (Westerfield)
Hyptran, Tab. (Wallace)
Medache, Tab. (Organon)
Meditussin, Liq. (Hauck)
Meditussin-X, Liq. (Hauck)
Myocalm, Tab. (Parmed)
Naldecon, Prep. (Bristol)
Naldetuss, Syr. (Bristol)
Neotuss-PT, Liq. (Westerfield)
Neo-Vadrin Sinus Headache Formula, Tab.
(Scherer)
Percogesic, Tab. (Du Pont)
Percogesic-C, Tab. (Du Pont)
Poly-histine Prods. (Bock)
Quadrahist, Tab. (Harvey-Pharmex)
S.A.C. Sinus, Tab. (Towne)
Scotgesic, Elix., Cap. (Scott/Cord)
Sinutab, Tab. (Warner-Lambert)
Sinutab Extra Strength, Tab. (Warner-Lambert)
Teragen, Tab. (O'Neal)
Trilamine, Cap. (Lemmon)
Tri-Synar, Tab. (Forrest)
Volaxin, Tab. (Elder)
Volaxin-A, Tab. (Elder)
PHENYLTOLOXAMINE RESIN W/COMBINATIONS.
See: Tussionex, Cap., Liq., Tab. (Pennwalt)
PHENYLZIN. (CooperVision) Zinc sulfate 0.25%,
phenylephrine HCl 0.12%/Lacrivial 15 cc.
Use: Ophthalmic astringent decongestant.
PHENYRAMIDOL. B.A.N. 1-Phenyl-2-(2-pyridylamino)-
ethanol. Analexin hydrochloride.
Use: Analgesic.
• **PHENYRAMIDOL HCL.** USAN. 2(β-Hydroxyphen-
ethylamino)pyridine HCl. α-[2-Pyridylamino)-
methyl]-benzyl alcohol hydrochloride.
Use: Analgesic.
PHENYTHILONE. 2-Ethyl-2-phenyl-3, 5-thiamorpho-
linedione.
• **PHENYTOIN,** U.S.P. XXI. Oral Susp., Tab., U.S.P.
XXI. 2,4-Imidazolidinedione, 5,5-diphenyl-. 5,5-Di-
phenylhydantoin. Diphenylhydantoin.
Use: Anticonvulsant.
See: Dihycon, Caps. (CMC)
Dilantin Prods. (Parke-Davis)
Di-phenyl, T.R. Cap. (Drug. Ind.)
Ekko, Cap. (Fleming)
Toin, Unicelles (Reid-Provident)
• **PHENYTOIN SODIUM.** U.S.P. XXI. Extended Cap.,
Inj., Prompt Cap., Sterile, U.S.P. XXI. 2,4-Imidazoli-
dinedione, 5,5-diphenyl-, monosodium salt. 5,5-Di-
phenylhydantoin sodium salt. Diphenylhydantoin
sodium. Alepsin, Dihydan soluble, Diphentoin,
Silantin Sod., Epanutin, Eptoin, Phenytoin soluble,
Solantoin, Solantyl, Denyl Sod., Soluble Phenytoin
(5,5-diphenyl-hydantoinate Sod.)
Use: Anticonvulsant, cardiac depressant (anti-arr-
hythmic).

See: Dihycon, Cap. (CMC)
Dilantin Sod., Prep. (Parke-Davis)
Di-Phen, Cap. (Vortech)
Diphenylan Sod., Cap. (Lannett)
Ekko Jr. & Sr., Cap. (Fleming)
PHENZINE. (Mallard) Phendimetrazine tartrate 35 mg./Tab. Bot. 1000s.
PHERAZINE EXPECTORANT. (Blue Cross) Promethazine HCl 5 mg. ipecac 0.17 min., potassium guaiacolsulfonate 44 mg., citric acid 60 mg., sodium citrate 197 mg./5 ml. w/alcohol 7%. Bot. Pt., gal.
Use: Expectorant, antihistaminic.
PHERAZINE EXPECTORANT WITH CODEINE. (Blue Cross) Codeine phosphate 10 mg., promethazine HCl 5 mg., ipecac 0.17 min., potassium guaiacolsulfonate 44 mg., citric acid 60 mg., sodium citrate 197 mg./5 ml. w/alcohol 7%. Bot. Pt., gal.
Use: Expectorant, antitussive, antihistaminic.
PHERAZINE EXPECTORANT WITH DEXTROMETHORPHAN. (Blue Cross) Dextromethorphan HBr 7.5 mg., promethazine HCl 5 mg., ipecac 0.17 min., potassium gualocolsulfonate 44 mg., citric acid 60 mg., sodium acid 197 mg./5 ml. w/alcohol 7%. Bot. Pt., gal.
Use: Expectorant, antihistaminic.
PHERAZINE VC EXPECTORANT. (Blue Cross) Promethazine HCl 5 mg., phenylephrine HCl 5 mg., ipecac 0.17 min., potassium guaiacolsulfonate 44 mg., citric acid 60 mg., sodium citrate 197 mg./5 ml. w/alcohol 7%. Bot. Pt., gal.
Use: Expectorant, antihistaminic, decongestant.
PHERAZINE VC EXPECTORANT WITH CODEINE. (Blue Cross) Codeine phosphate 10 mg., promethazine HCl 5 mg., phenylephrine HCl 5 mg., ipecac 0.17 min., potassium guaiacolsulfonate 44 mg., citric acid 60 mg., sodium citrate 197 mg./5 ml. Bot. Pt., gal.
Use: Expectorant, antitussive, antihistaminic, decongestant.
PHERMINE. (Fellows) Phentermine HCl 8 mg./Tab. Bot. 100s, 1000s.
PHETABAR SPACECAP. (Moore Kirk) Amobarbital 90 mg., dextroamphetamine sulfate 15 mg./timed disintegration Cap. Bot. 1000s.
Use: Combat depression; ease tension; as adjunct to diet in obesity.
PHETHARBITAL. 5,5-Diethyl-1-phenylbarbituric acid.
PHETHENYLATE. 5-Phenyl-5-(2-thienyl)hydantoinate. Also sod. salt.
PHILJECT INJECTION. (Fellows) Procaine base 75 mg., butyl-amino-benzoate 300 mg., benzyl alcohol 250 mg./5 cc. in peanut oil. Vial 5 cc.
PHILLIPS' MILK OF MAGNESIA. (Glenbrook) Magnesium hydroxide. Reg. & Mint bot. 4 oz., 12 oz., 26 oz.; Tab. 30s, 100s, 200s.
Use: Laxative, antacid.
PHILLIPS OINTMENT. (Fellows) Bismuth tribromophenate 5%. Base 1 oz., 1 lb., 5 lb.
pHisoAc-BP. (Winthrop Products) Benzoyl peroxide 10% in cream base. Tube 1 oz.

Use: Topical anti-acne agent.
pHisoDan SHAMPOO. (Winthrop Products) Sulfur 5%, sodium salicylate 0.5% w/lanolin cholesterols, entsufon sodium, petrolatum. Bot. 5 oz.
Use: Seborrhea of scalp.
pHisoDerm. (Winthrop Products) Sod. Octoxynol-3 Sulfonate, white petrolatum, water, lanolin, lanolin alcohol, sodium benzoate, Octoxynol-1, methylcellulose and lactic acid. **Regular:** Bot. 5 oz., 9 oz., 16 oz. **Dry type:** Bot. 5 oz., pt. Wall dispenser pt. **Oily type:** Bot. 5 oz., 16 oz. **Fresh Scent:** Bot. 5oz.
Use: Skin cleanser & conditioner.
PHISOHEX. (Cook-Waite) A colloidal dispersion of hexachlorophene 3% (w/w), entsufon sodium, petrolatum, lanolin cholesterols, methylcellulose, polyethylene glycol, polyethylene glycol monostearate, lauryl myristyl diethanolamide, sodium benzoate, & water. pH is adjusted with HCl acid. Bot. gal.
Use: Antiseptic detergent.
pHisoHex. (Winthrop-Breon) Entsufon sodium, hexachlorophene 3%, petrolatum, lanolin cholesterols, methylcellulose, polyethylene glycol, polyethylene glycol monostearate, lauryl myristyl diethanolamide, sod. benzoate, water, pH adjusted with hydrochloric acid. Emulsion, Bot. 5 oz., pt., gal. Wall dispensers pt. Unit packets ¼ oz. Box 50s, Pedal operated dispenser 30 oz.
Use: Surgical scrub & antibacterial cleanser.
pHisoScrub. (Winthrop-Breon) Scrub brush sponge impregnated with pHisoHex. Case of 4 dispensers, 36 u./Disp.
Use: Surgical scrub.
PHISTOL. (Kenyon) Vit. A 10,000 I.U., D 1000 I.U., B-1 5 mg., B-2 3 mg., B-6 1 mg., C 100 mg., calcium pantothenate 5 mg., niacinamide 25 mg./Cap. Bot. 100s, 1000s.
PHOLEDRINE. B.A.N. 4-(2-Methylaminopropyl)-phenol. Veritain; Veritol.
Use: Sympathomimetic.
PHOSCOLIC ACID. 2,2'-Phosphinicodilacetic acid.
Use: Adjuvant.
PHOS-FLUR ORAL RINSE SUPPLEMENT. (Hoyt) Acidulated phosphate sodium fluoride 0.05%. 1 ml fluoride/Tsp. Bot. 250 ml., 500 ml.
Use: Prevent dental caries
PHOSPHACAL-D. (Lannett) Dicalcium phosphate anh. 330 mg., Vit. D 333 I.U./Cap. Bot. 500s, 1000s.
pHOS-pHAID. (Guardian) Ammonium biphosphate 190 mg., sodium biphosphate 200 mg., sodium acid pyrophosphate 110 mg./0.5 Gm. Tab. regular or enteric coated. Bot. 90s, 500s. Also 0.25 Gm., 150s.
Use: Urinary acidifier.
PHOSPHALJEL. (Wyeth) Aluminum phosphate gel 700 mg./15 ml. Bot. 12 oz.
PHOSPHENTASIDE. Adenosine-5-monophosphate. Adenylic acid.
W/Vit. B-12, niacin.
See: Denylex Gel, Vial (Westerfield)
W/Vit. B-12, niacin, B-1.
See: Adenolin, Vial (Lincoln)

PHOSPHOCOL P 32. (Mallinckrodt) Chromic phosphate P 32.

PHOSPHOLINE IODIDE. (Ayerst) Echothiophate Iodide for Ophthalmic Solution. Sterile echothiophate iodide powder w/potassium acetate 40 mg., diluent: chlorobutanol 0.5%, mannitol 1.2%, boric acid 0.06%, sod. phosphate exsic. 0.026% for preparing 0.03%, 0.06%, 0.125%, and 0.25% potencies/5 ml. of sterile eyedrops.
Package: 1.5 mg. for 0.03%; 3.0 mg. for 0.06%; 6.25 mg. for 0.125%; 12.5 mg. for 0.25%.
Use: Glaucoma & accommodative esotropia.

PHOSPHOLIPIDS SOY.
See: Granulestin Conc., Granules (Associated Concentrates)

PHOSPHORATED CARBOHYDRATE SOLUTION.
See: Emetrol, Liq. (Rorer)

• **PHOSPHORIC ACID,** N.F. XVI.
Use: Solvent

• **PHOSPHORIC ACID, DILUTED,** N.F. XVI.

PHOSPHOROFLUORIDIC ACID, BIS(I-METHYL-ETHYL)-, ESTER. Isofluorophate, U.S.P. XXI.
Use: Solvent.

PHOSPHO-SODA. (Fleet) Sod. biphosphate 48 Gm., Sod. phosphate 18 Gm./100 cc. Bot. 1.5 oz., 3 oz., 8 oz. Flavored and unflavored.
Use: A mild saline laxative.

PHOSPHOTEC. (Squibb) Technetium Tc 99m pyrophosphate kit. 10 vials/kit.
Use: Radiodiagnostic.

PHOXIN. B.A.N. α-Diethoxyphosphinothioyloxyimino-α-phenylacetonitrile.
Use: Insecticide; anthelmintic, veterinary medicine.

PHRENILIN FORTE CAPSULES. (Carnrick) Acetaminophen 650 mg., butalbital 50 mg./Cap. Bot. 100s.
Use: Barbiturate-analgesic for tension headache.

PHRENILIN TABLETS. (Carnrick) Butalbital 50 mg., acetaminophen 325 mg./Tab. Bot. 100s.
Use: Barbiturate-analgesic for relief of the symptom complex of tension headache.

PHRENILIN WITH CODEINE #3. (Carnrick) Acetaminophen 325 mg., butalbital 50 mg., codeine phosphate 30 mg./Cap. Bot. 100s.
Use: Analgesic.

PHRENOTROPIN. Prothipendyl, B.A.N.

PHRESH 3.5 FINNISH CLEANSING LIQUIDE. (3M Products) Water, cocamidopropyl betaine, lactic acid, polyoxyethylene disodium stearate, polyoxyethylene monostearate, hydroxyethyl cellulose, sodium phosphate, methylparaben. Bot. 6 oz.
Use: Soapless cleansing agent.

pH SKIN CLEANSING LOTION. (Walgreen) Alcohol 28%, boric acid 1.75%, benzoic acid 0.25% w/thymol, eucalyptol, thyme oil, 0.035% each. Bot. 16. oz.
Use: Astringent & cleanser.

PHTHALAMAQUIN. (Penick) Quinetolate.
Use: Antiasthmatic.

PHTHALAZINE, I-HYDRAZINO-, MONOHYDRO-CHLORIDE. Hydralazine Hydrochloride, U.S.P. XXI.

• **PHTHALOFYNE.** USAN. Mono(l-ethyl-l-methyl-2-propynyl)phthalate.

PHTHALYLSULFACETAMIDE. 4′-(Acetylsulfamoyl) phthalanilic acid. Enterosulfon.

PHTHALYLSULFATHIAZOLE. 4′-(2 Thiazolylsulfamoyl) phthalanilic acid.
Use: Antibacterial (intestinal).
See: Sulfathalidine, Tab. (Merck Sharp & Dohme)

PHYLCARDIN.
See: Aminophylline (Various Mfr.)

PHYLLINDON.
See: Aminophylline (Various Mfr.)

PHYLLOCONTIN. (Purdue Frederick) Aminophylline 225 mg./Controlled Release Tab. Bot. 100s.
Use: Relief and/or prevention of symptoms of asthma & reversible bronchospasm associated with chronic bronchitis & emphysema.

PHYLLOQUINONE. 2-Methyl-3-phytyl-1,4-naphthoquinine, Vit. K.
See: Phytonadione, U.S.P., Inj., Tab. (Var. Mfr.)
Vit. K-1 (Various Mfr.)

PHYSEPTONE. Methadone, B.A.N.

PHYSIOSOL IRRIGATION. (Abbott) Bot. 250 ml., 500 ml., 1000 ml. glass or Aqualite (semi-rigid) containers.
Use: Irrigating solution.

• **PHYSOSTIGMINE,** U.S.P. XXI. Pyrrolo [2,3-b] indol-5-ol methylcarbamate (ester), (3as-cis). 1,2,3a β,8,8a β-Hexahydro-1,3a,8-trimethyl-pyrrolo[2,3-b]-indol-5yl-methylcarbamate. An alkaloid.
Use: Parasympathomimetic agent.

• **PHYSOSTIGMINE SALICYLATE,** U.S.P. XXI. Inj., Ophth. Soln., U.S.P. XXI. Pyrrolo[2,3-b]indol-5-ol, 1,2,3,3a,8,8a-hexahydro-1,3a,8-trimethyl-, methylcarbamate (ester), (3aS-cis)-, mono(2-hydroxybenzoate). Physostigmine monosalicylate. Eserine salicylate. (O'Neal, Jones & Feldman)—Pow., Tube 1 gr., 5 gr., 15 gr.
Use: Parasympathomimetic agent.
See: Antilirium, Amp. (O'Neal, Jones & Feldman)
Isopto-Eserine, Ophth., Sol. (Alcon)
Miocel, Ophth. Sol. (Softcon)
W/Atropine sulfate.
See: Atrophysine, Inj. (Lannett)
W/I-Hyoscyamine HBr.
See: Phyatromine-H, Amp., Vial (Kremers-Urban)
W/Pilocarpine, methylcellulose.
See: Isopto P-ES, Soln. (Alcon)
Miocel, Sol. (Softcon)

• **PHYSOSTIGMINE SULFATE,** U.S.P. XXI. Ophth. Oint., U.S.P. XXI. Pyrrolo[2,3-b]indol-5-ol, 1,2,3,3a, 8,8a-hexahydro-1,3a,8-trimethyl-, methylcarbamate (ester), (3aS-cis)-,sulfate (2:1).
Use: Cholinergic (ophthalmic)

• **PHYTATE PERSODIUM.** USAN.
Use: Pharmaceutic aid.

• **PHYTATE SODIUM.** USAN. Sod. salt of inositolhexaphosphoric acid.

PHYTIC ACID. Inositol hexophosphoric acid.

PHYTOMENADIONE. B.A.N. 2-Methyl-3-phytyl-1,4-naphthaquinone. Vitamin K Konakion; Mephyton.
Use: Antidote to anticoagulants.

See: Phytonadione, U.S.P. (Var. Mfr.)
PHYTONADIOL SODIUM DIPHOSPHATE. Disodium salt of 2-methyl-2-phytyl-1,4-naphthohydroquinone-$0^1,0^4$-diphosphoric acid.
• **PHYTONADIONE,** U.S.P. XXI. Inj., Tabs., U.S.P. XXI. Vit. K 1,4-Naphthalenedione, 2-methyl-3-(3,7,11,-15-tetramethyl-2-hexadecenyl)-,[R-[R*,R*-(E)]]-. Phylloquinone.   2-Methyl-3-phytyl-1,4-naphthoquinone.
   Use: Prothrombogenic.
   See: Aquamephyton, Inj. (Merck Sharp & Dohme)
      Konakion, Amp. (Roche)
      Mephyton, Tab. (Merck Sharp & Dohme)
• **PICENADOL HYDROCHLORIDE.** USAN.
   Use: Analgesic
PICLOXYDINE. B.A.N. NN'-Di-(p-Chlorophenyl-guanidinoformimidoyl)-piperazine. 1,4-Di-(4-chlorophenylguanidinoformimidoyl)piperazine.
   Use: Bactericide; fungicide.
• **PICOTRIN DIOLAMINE.** USAN.
   Use: Keratolytic
PICRIC ACID, TRINITROPHENOL.
   See: Butesyn Picrate Ointment (Abbott)
      Silver Salts (Various Prods.)
PICROTOXIN. Cocculin
   Use: Respiratory stimulant.
P.I.D.
   See: Phenindione (Var. Mfr.)
PIFARNINE. USAN.
   Use: Anti-ulcerative.
PIFENATE. B.A.N. Ethyl 2,2-diphenyl-3-(2-piperidyl)propionate.
   Use: Analgesic.
PIL-DIGIS. (Key) Ground, milled whole leaf of *Digitalis purpurea* 100 mg./Tab. Bot. 100s, 1000s.
   Use: Treatment of congestive heart failure.
PILE-GON. (Edward J. Moore) Bismuth subgallate, balsam of peru, Zn oxide, cod liver oil in petrolatum base./Tube 1¼ oz.
   Use: Rectal ointment.
PILOCAR. (CooperVision) Pilocarpine HCl 0.5%, 1%, 2%, 3%, 4%, 6%. Bot. 15 ml.; Twinpack 2 × 15 ml. 0.5%, 1%, 2%, 4%, 6%; 1 ml. Dropperettes 1%, 2%, 4%. Box 12s.
   Use: Miotic for treatment of glaucoma.
• **PILOCARPINE,** U.S.P. XXI. Ocular system U.S.P. XXI.
   Use: Ophthalmic cholinergic, miotic.
   See: Ocusert Pilo-20 and Pilo-40 (Ciba)
• **PILOCARPINE HYDROCHLORIDE,** U.S.P. XXI. Ophth. Soln., U.S.P. XXI. (Various Mfr.) Pilocarpine muriate.
   Use: 0.5 to 2.0% sol. topically as a miotic.
   (Maurry) 1%, 2%, 3%, 4%, 6%. Dropper Bot. 15 ml. (Mesco) 1%, 2%, 4%. Bot. 3.5 Gm.
   See: Almocarpine (Ayerst)
      Isopto-Carpine, Ophth. (Alcon)
      Mi-Pilo, Sol. (Barnes-Hind)
      Pilocar, Sol. (CooperVision)
      Pilocel, Sol. (Softcon)
      Pilomiotin, Sol. (CooperVision)
      Piloptic, Soln. (Muro)

W/Epinephrine HCl.
   See: E-Carpine, Inj. (Alcon)
      Epicar, Ophth. Sol. (Barnes-Hind)
W/Epinephrine bitartrate, mannitol, benzalkonium chloride.
   See: E-Pilo, Sol. (CooperVision)
W/Eserine salicylate, methylcellulose.
   See: Isopto P-ES, Soln. (Alcon)
W/Physostigmine salicylate.
   See: Miocel, Sol. (Softcon)
• **PILOCARPINE NITRATE,** U.S.P. XXI. Ophth. Soln., U.S.P. XXI. (Various Mfr.) Pow., Bot. 15 gr., ⅛ oz., 1 oz. (Mesco) 1%, 2%. Bot. 3.5 Gm.
   See: P.V. Carpine (Allergan)
W/Phenylephrine HCl.
   Use: Parasympathomimetic agent.
   See: Pilofrin Liquifilm, Ophthalmic (Allergan)
PILOCEL. (Softcon) Pilocarpine HCl ¼, ½, 1, 2, 3, 4 & 6%, buffered in methylcellulose base w/benzalkonium chloride, boric acid, sod. citrate, & pot. chloride. Bot. w/dropper 15 cc. 1%, 2%, & 4%. Also avail. in 30 cc.
   Use: Ophthalmic therapy, miotic.
PIMAFUCIN. Natamycin, B.A.N.
PIMARICIN. Natamycin, B.A.N.
PIMA SYRUP. (Fleming) Potassium iodide 5 gr./5 cc. Bot. pt., gal.
   Use: Expectorant.
• **PIMETINE HYDROCHLORIDE.** USAN. 4-Benzyl-1-(2-dimethylaminoethyl)piperidine hydrochloride.
   Use: Cardiovascular drug (anticholesteremic).
PIMINODINE. B.A.N. 1-(3-Phenylaminopropyl-4-phenyl-piperidine-4-carboxylic acid ethyl ester. Ethyl 4-phenyl-1-(3-phenylaminopropyl)piperidine-4-carboxylate.
   Use: Narcotic analgesic.
PIMINODINE ESYLATE. Ethyl 1-(30 anilinopropyl)-4-phenylisonipecotate monoethanesulfaonte.
   Use: Analgesic.
PIMINODINE ETHANESULFONATE. Ethyl-4-phenyl-1-[3-(phenylamino)propyl]-piperidine-4-carboxylate ethanesulfonate.
   Use: Narcotic analgesic.
• **PIMOZIDE.** USAN. 1-[1-[4,4-bis(p-Fluorophenyl)butyl]-4-piperidyl]-2-benzimidazoline. Orap.
   Use: Tranquilizer.
P-I-N. (Lannett) Isoniazid 50 mg., Vit. B-6 1 mg./Tab. Bot. 100s, 500s, 1000s. Forte-isoniazid 100 mg., Vit. B-6 5 mg./Tab. Bot. 100s, 500s, 1000s.
   Use: Treatment of tuberculosis.
• **PINACIDIL.** USAN.
• **PINDOLOL.** USAN. 1-(Indol-4-yloxy)-3-isopropyl-amino)-2-propanol.
   Use: Hypertension, angina, pectoris, cardiac arrhythmia.
   See: Visken (Sandoz).
P-I-N FORTE SYRUP. (Lannett) Isoniazid 10 mg., pyridoxine HCl 0.5 mg./cc. Bot. pt.
• **PINE NEEDLE OIL,** N.F. XVI.
   Use: Perfume; flavor.
• **PINE TAR,** U.S.P. XXI.
   Use: Local antieczematic; rubefacient.
PINEX CONCENTRATE COUGH SYRUP. (Last)

Dextromethorphan HBr 7.5 mg./5 ml. (after diluting 3 oz. concentrate to make 16 oz. solution).
Bot. 3 oz.
Use: Antitussive.
PINEX COUGH SYRUP. (Last) Dextromethorphan HBr. 7.5 mg./5 ml. Bot. 3 oz., 6 oz.
Use: Antitussive.
PINEX REGULAR. (Pinex) Pot. guaiacolsulfonate, oil of pine & eucalyptus, ext. grindelia, alcohol 3%/30 ml. Syr. 3 oz., 8 oz. Also cherry flavored 3 oz. Super and conc. 3 oz.
Use: Antitussive.
• **PINOXEPIN HCl.** USAN.
Use: Tranquilizer.
PIOXOL. Pemoline, B.A.N.
PIPADONE HYDROCHLORIDE. Dipipanone, B.A.N.
PIPAMAZINE. B.A.N. 1-[3-(2-Chlorophenothiazin-10-yl)-propyl] isonipecotramide. 10-[3-(4-Carbamoyl-piperidino)propyl]-2-chlorophenothiazine. Mornidine.
Use: Antiemetic.
• **PIPAMPERONE.** USAN. 1'-[3-(p-Fluorobenzoyl)-propyl][1,4'-bipiperidine]-4'-carboxamide. Under study.
Use: Tranquilizer.
PIPANOL HYDROCHLORIDE. Benzhexol, B.A.N.
• **PIPAZETHATE.** USAN 2-(2-Piperidinoethoxy)-ethyl pyrido[3,2-b][1,4]benzothiazine-10-carboxylate. Selvigon hydrochloride.
Use: Cough suppressant.
PIPAZETHATE HYDROCHLORIDE. 2-(2-Piperidinoethoxy)ethyl-10-H-pyrido [3,2-b]-[1,4]benzothiazine-10-carboxylate hydrochloride.
Use: Antitussive agent.
PIPENZOLATE BROMIDE. B.A.N. 1-Ethyl-3-piperidyl benzilate methylbromide. 3-Benziloyloxy-1-ethyl-1-methylpiperidinium bromide.
Use: Anticholinergic.
• **PIPERACETAZINE,** U.S.P. XXI. Tab., U.S.P. XXI. 10-{3-[4-(2-Hydroxyethyl)piperidino]propyl} phenothiazin-2-yl methyl ketone.
Use: Tranquilizer; antipsychotic agent.
See: Quide, Tab., (Merrell Dow)
• **PIPERACILLIN SODIUM, STERILE.** U.S.P. XXI.
Use: Antibacterial.
• **PIPERAMIDE MALEATE.** USAN. 4'-[4-[3-(Dimethylamino)propyl]-1-piperazinyl]acetanilide dimaleate.
Use: Antiparasitic.
• **PIPERAZINE,** U.S.P. XXI.
Use: Anthelmintic.
PIPERAZINE CALCIUM EDETATE. B.A.N. [Dihydrogen)ethylenedinitrilo)tetraacetato]-calcium piperazine salt. Perin.
Use: Anthelmintic.
• **PIPERAZINE CITRATE,** U.S.P. XXI. Syrup, Tab., U.S.P. XXI. Piperazine, 2-hydroxy-1,2,3-propanetricarboxylate (3:2) hydrate. Piperazine citrate (3:2) hydrate. Piperazine Citrate Telra Hydrous Tripiperazine Dicitrate.
Use: Anthelmintic.
See: Antepar, Tab., Syr. (Burroughs Wellcome)
Bryrel, Syr. (Winthrop Products)

Multifuge Citrate, Tab., Syr. (Blue Line)
Pin-Tega Tabs., Syr. (Ortega)
Pipril, Liq. (Kenyon)
Ta-Verm, Syr., Tab. (Table Rock)
Vermago, Syr. (Westerfield)
• **PIPERAZINE EDETATE CALCIUM.** USAN.
Dihydrogen
[(ethylenedinitrilo)tetraacetato]calciate(2-) compound with piperazine (1:1). Perin.
Use: Anthelmintic.
PIPERAZINE ESTRONE SULFATE.
See: Estropipate
PIPERAZINE HEXAHYDRATE. Tivazine.
PIPERAZINE PHOSPHATE.
Use: Anthelmintic (intestinal roundworms and trematodes).
PIPERAZINE TARTRATE.
See: Razine Tartrate, Tab. (Paddock)
PIPERIDINE PHOSPHATE.
Use: Psychiatric drug.
PIPERIDINOETHYL BENZILATE HCl. No products listed.
PIPERIDOLATE. B.A.N. 1-Ethyl-3-piperidyl diphenylacetate.
Use: Parasympatholytic.
PIPERIDOLATE HYDROCHLORIDE. 1-Ethyl-3-piperidyl diphenylacetate HCl.
Use: Anticholinergic.
PIPEROCAINE. B.A.N. 3-(2-Methylpiperidino)-propyl benzoate.
Use: Local anesthetic.
PIPEROCAINE HYDROCHLORIDE. 3-Benzoxy-1-(2-methylpiperidino) propane HCl.
PIPERONYL BUTOXIDE. B.A.N. 5-[2-(2-Butoxy-ethoxy)ethoxymethyl]-6-propyl-1,3-benzodioxole.
Use: Acaricide, veterinary medicine.
PIPEROXAN. B.A.N. 2-Piperidinomethyl-1,4-benzodioxan.
Use: Adrenergic blocking agent.
PIPEROXAN HYDROCHLORIDE. 2-(1-Piperidylmethyl)-1,4-benzodioxan HCl. Fourneau 933. Benzodioxane.
Use: Diagnosis of hypertension.
PIPERPHENIDOL HCl. 5-Methyl-4-phenyl-1-(1-piperidyl)-3-hexanol HCl.
PIPETHANATE HCl. 2-Piperidinoethyl benzilate HCl.
Use: Tranquilizer.
• **PIPOBROMAN,** U.S.P. XXI. Tab., U.S.P. XXI. 1,4-Bis(3-bromopropionyl)piperazine. Δ2,a-thiazolidine-acetate.
Use: Antineoplastic.
See: Vercyte, Tab. (Abbott)
• **PIPOSULFAN.** USAN. 1,4-Dihydracryloylpiperazine dimethanesulfonate.
Use: Antineoplastic agent.
PIPOTHIAZINE. B.A.N. 2-Dimethylsulfamoyl-10-3-[4-(2-hydroxyethyl)piperidino]propyl phenothiazine.
Use: Neuroleptic.
• **PIPOTIAZINE PALMITATE.** USAN.
Use: Antipsychotic.
See: Piportil (Ives)

PIPOXOLAN. B.A.N. 5,5-Diphenyl-2-(2-piperidinoethyl)-1,3-dioxolan-4-one.
Use: Antispasmodic.
• **PIPOXOLAN HCl.** USAN. 5,5-Diphenyl-2-(2-piperidinoethyl)-1,3-dioxolan-4-one HCl. Rowapraxin.
Use: Muscle relaxant.
PIPRACIL. (Lederle) Piperacillin sodium 2 Gm, 3 Gm. or 4 Gm./Vial; 3 Gm. or 4 Gm./Infusion Bottle.
Use: Broad spectrum antibiotic.
PIPRADOL. B.A.N. α-2-Piperidylbenzhydrol.
Use: Central nervous system stimulant.
PIPRIL. (Kenyon) Piperazine citrate 0.5 Gm./5 cc. Bot. pt., gal.
Use: Anthelmintic.
PIPRINHYDRINATE. B.A.N. Diphenylpyraline salt of 8-chlorotheophylline. 4-Benzhydryloxy-1-methylpiperidine salt of 8-chlorotheophylline. Kolton; Mepedyl.
Use: Antihistamine.
• **PIPROZOLIN.** USAN. Ethyl 3-ethyl-4-oxo-5-piperidino Δ², alpha-thiazolidineacetate.
Use: Choleretic.
• **PIQUIZIL HCl.** USAN. Isobutyl 4-(6,7-dimethoxy-4-quinazolinyl)-1-piperazinecarboxylate monohydrochloride.
Use: Bronchodilator.
• **PIRACETAM.** USAN. 2-Oxopyrrolidin-1-ylacetamide. Nootropyl.
Use: Cerebral stimulant.
• **PIRANDAMINE HYDROCHLORIDE.** USAN.
Use: Anti-depressant.
• **PIRAZOLAC.** USAN.
Use: Antirheumatic.
• **PIRBENICILLIN SODIUM.** USAN.
Use: Antibacterial.
PIRBUTEROL. B.A.N. 2-tert-Butylamino-1-(5-hydroxy-6-hydroxymethyl-2-pyridyl)ethanol.
Use: Bronchodilator.
• **PIRBUTEROL ACETATE.** USAN.
Use: Bronchodilator.
• **PIRBUTEROL HYDROCHLORIDE.** USAN.
Use: Bronchodilator.
• **PIRENPERONE.** USAN.
Use: Tranquilizer.
• **PIRETANIDE.** USAN.
Use: Diuretic.
Arlix Prods. (Hoechst)
• **PIRFENIDONE.** USAN.
Use: Anti-inflammatory; antipyretic.
PIRIDAZOL.
See: Sulfapyridine, Tab. (Various Mfr.)
• **PIRIDICILLIN SODIUM.** USAN.
Use: Antibacterial.
PIRIDOCAINE HCl. Beta-(2-Piperidyl) ethyl-o-aminobenzoate.
PIRIDOXILATE. B.A.N. The reciprocal salt of (5-hydroxy-4-hydroxymethyl-6-methyl-3-pyridyl)-methoxyglycolic acid with [4,5-bis(hydroxymethyl)-2-methyl-3-pyridyl] oxyglycolic acid (1:1). GLYO-6.
Use: Treatment of angina.
PIRIN-C. (Scrip) Salicylamide 450 mg., Vit. C 30 mg./Tab. Bot. 100s.
PIRITON.
See: Chlorpheniramine (Var. Mfr.)

PIRITRAMIDE. B.A.N. 4-(4-Carbamoyl-4-piperidinopiperidino)-2,2-diphenylbutyronitrile. Dipodolor.
Use: Analgesic.
• **PIRLIMYCIN HYDROCHLORIDE.** USAN.
Use: Antibacterial.
• **PIRMENOL HYDROCHLORIDE.** USAN.
Use: Cardiac depressant.
• **PIRNABINE.** USAN.
Use: Antiglaucoma agent.
• **PIROCTONE.** USAN.
Use: Antiseborrheic.
• **PIROCTONE OLAMINE.** USAN.
Use: Antiseborrheic.
• **PIROGLIRIDE TARTRATE.** USAN.
Use: Antidiabetic.
• **PIROLATE.** USAN.
Use: Anti-asthmatic.
• **PIROLAZAMIDE.** USAN.
Use: Cardiac depressant.
PIROTHESIN HYDROCHLORIDE. Aptocaine, B.A.N.
• **PIROXICAM.** USAN. N-pyridyl-methyl-hydroxy-(benzothiazine-1 idioxide)carboxamide.
Use: Anti-inflammatory.
See: Feldene, Cap (Pfizer)
• **PIRPROFEN.** USAN.
Use: Anti-inflammatory.
See: Rengasil (Geigy)
• **PIRQUINOZOL.** USAN.
Use: Anti-allergic.
PIRSEAL. (Fellows) Acetylsalicylic acid 5 gr., 10 gr./Tab. Bot. 100s, 1000s.
PISO's. (Pinex) Ipecac, ammonium chloride, menthol in syrup base. Bot. 3 oz., 5 oz.
Use: Cough due to colds.
PITAYINE.
See: Quinidine, Preps. (Various Mfr.)
PITOCIN. (Parke-Davis) Oxytocin w/chlorobutanol 0.5%, acetic acid to adjust pH. Amp. (5 u.) 0.5 ml. (10 u.) 1 ml. Box 10s, Steri-dose syringe (10 u.) 1 ml. 10s.
Use: Oxytocic.
PITRESSIN. (Parke-Davis) Vasopressin w/chlorobutanol 0.5%, pH adjusted with acetic acid. Amp. 0.5 ml. (10 pressor u.) & 1 ml. (20 pressor u.) Box 10s.
Use: Prevention & control of abdominal distention.
PITRESSIN TANNATE IN OIL. (Parke-Davis) Vasopressin Tannate in peanut oil. Amp. (5 pressor u.) 1 ml. Box 10s.
Use: Where long-continued action of Pitressin is desired; treatment of diabetes insipidus.
PITTS CARMINATIVE. (Commerce) Bot. 2 oz.
Use: Gas and colic relief.
PITUITARY, ANTERIOR. The anterior lobe of the pituitary gland supplies protein hormones classified under following headings.
See preparation of:
Corticotropin, Preps. (Var. Mfr.)
Gonadotropin, Preps. (Var. Mfr.)
Growth Hormone
Thyrotropic Principle
PITUITARY, POSTERIOR. Pituitary Extract, (Armour) Posterior. Caps ⅔ gr. Bot. 100s.

• **PITUITARY, POSTERIOR, INJECTION,** U.S.P. XXI.
See: Pituitrin, Obstetrical, Amp. (Parke-Davis)
Pituitrin, Surgical, Amp. (Parke-Davis)
PITUITARY, POSTERIOR, HORMONES.
(a) Vasopressin. Pressor principle, β-hypophamine,
postlobin-V.
See: Pitressin, Amp. (Parke-Davis)
Pitressin Tannate, Amp. (Parke-Davis)
(b) Oxytocin. Oxytocic principle. α-hypophamine,
postiobin-O.
See: Oxytocin, Inj.
Pitocin, Amp. (Var. Mfr.)
Syntocin, Amp. (Sandoza)
PITUITRIN-S. (Parke-Davis) Pituitary, posterior ext. 20
units/ml. Amp. 1 ml., Box 10s.
Use: Obstetrical, to stimulate uterine contraction.
Surgical, prevention & control of abdominal
distention.
PIVAMPICILLIN. B.A.N. Pivaloyloxymethyl 6-[D(−)-α-
aminophenylacetamido]penicillinate. Pondocillin
[hydrochloride.]
Use: Antibiotic.
• **PIVAMPICILLIN HYDROCHLORIDE..** USAN.
Use: Antibacterial
• **PIVAMPICILLIN PAMOATE.** USAN.
Use: Antibacterial.
• **PIVAMPICILLIN PROBENATE.** USAN.
Use: Antibacterial.
PIVAZIDE. N-Benzyl-N'-pivaloylhydrazine. Tersavid.
PIVHYDRAZINE. B.A.N. 1-Benzyl-2-pivaloyl-hydrazine.
Use: Monoamine oxidase inhibitor.
PIVMECILLINAM. B.A.N. Pivaloyloxymethyl
(2S,5R,6R)-6-(perhydroazepin-1-ylmethyleneamino)-
penicillanate.
Use: Antibiotic.
PIXACOL. (Pixacol) Liquid ext. of coal tar, modified
by addition of salicylic acid 1%, methylsalicylate
5%, Bot. 1 oz., 4 oz., 8 oz.
Use: Psoriasis.
PIXACREME. (Pixacol) White ointment containing
ammoniated mercury 5%, phenol 2%. Jar 4 oz.
Use: Psoriasis.
PIX CARBONIS.
See: Coal Tar, Prep. (Var. Mfr.)
PIX JUNIPERI.
See: Juniper Tar, Comp. (Var. Mfr.)
Use: Sunscreen, moisturizer.
PIZOTIFEN. B.A.N. 4-(9,10-Dihydrobenzo[4,5]-cy-
clohepta]1,2-b]thien-4-ylidene)-1-methyl-piperi-
dine.
Use: Prophylaxis of migraine.
• **PIZOTYLINE.** USAN. 4-(9,10-Dihydro-4H-benzo[4,5]-
cyclohepta]1,2-b]thien-4-ylidene)-1-methyl-piperidine
Use: Anabolic, antidepressant; migraine
prophylactic.
PLACEBO CAPSULES. (Cowley) No. 3 orange red;
No. 4 yellow, No. 0 clear. Bot. 100s.
Use: Placebo.
PLACEBO TABLETS. (Cowley) 1 gr. white; 2 gr.
white; 3 gr. white, red or yellow, pink, orange; 4 gr.
white; 5 gr. white. Bot. 1000s.
Use: Placebo.

PLACENTA.
See: Gonadotropins, Chorionic, Inj. (Var. Mfr.)
PLACENTEX. (Roche) A latex agglutination-inhibition
tube test for pregnancy sensitive to 1.01.U. of HCG
per ml. of urine.
PLACIDYL. (Abbott) Ethchlorvynol. 100 mg., 200
mg./Cap. Bot. 100s. 500 mg./Cap. Bot. 100s, 500s.
750 mg./Cap. Bot. 100s. Unit dose 100s. (Abbo-Pac
500 mg., 750 mg.)
Use: Nonbarbiturate sedative or hypnotic.
• **PLAGUE VACCINE,** U.S.P. XXI. (Cutter) 2000
million killed *Pasteurella pestis*/ml. Vial 2 ml., 20
ml.
Use: S.C. vaccination, active immunizing agent.
PLANOCAINE.
See: Procaine Hydrochloride, Preps. (Var. Mfr.)
PLANOCHROME.
See: Merbromin, Sol. (Var. Mfr.)
PLANTAGO, OVATA COATING.
See: Effersyllium, Prods. (Stuart)
Konsyl, Pow. (Burton, Parsons)
L.A. Formula, Pow. (Burton, Parsons)
Metamucil, Pow. (Searle)
Mucilose, Preps. (Winthrop Products)
W/Psyllium seed, gum karaya, Brewer's yeast.
See: Plantamucin, Granules (Elder)
W/Vit. B-1.
See: Siblin, Granules (Parke-Davis)
• **PLANTAGO SEED,** U.S.P. XXI. Psyllium Seed,
Plantain Seed.
Use: Fecal softener.
PLANT PROTEASE CONCENTRATE.
See: Ananase, Tab. (Rorer)
PLAQUENIL SULFATE. (Winthrop-Breon) Hydroxy-
chloroquine sulf. 200 mg./Tab. Bot. 100s.
Use: Lupus erythematosus, rheumatoid arthritis &
malaria.
PLAQENIL TABLET. (Winthrop Products)
Hydroxycholorquine sulfate.
Use: Malaria, amebiasis.
PLASBUMIN-5. (Cutter) Normal serum albumin
(Human) 5% U.S.P. fractionated from normal serum
plasma, heat treated against hepatitis virus.
Albumin 12.5 Gm./250 ml. Vial 50 ml. Bot. with set
250 ml., 500 ml.
Use: Blood volume supporter, albumin replacement.
PLASBUMIN-25. (Cutter) Normal serum albumin
(Human) 25% U.S.P. fractionated from normal
serum plasma, heat treated against hepatitis virus.
Albumin 12.5 Gm./50 ml. Vial 20 ml. Bot. with set
50 ml., 100 ml.
Use: Blood volume supporter, albumin replacement.
PLASMA.
See: Normal Human Plasma (Var. Mfr.)
PLASMA EXPANDERS OR SUBSTITUTES.
See: Dextran 6% & LMD 10% (Abbott)
Macrodex, Sol. (Pharmacia)
PLASMA-LYTE A INJECTION. (Travenol) Sodium
140, potassium 5, magnesium 3, chloride 98,
acetate 27, gluconate 23 mEq./L w/pH adjusted to
7.4. Bot. 500 ml., 1000 ml.
Use: Fluid & electrolyte replenisher.
PLASMA-LYTE INJECTION. (Travenol) Sodium 140,

potassium 10, calcium 5, magnesium 3, chloride 103, acetate 47, lactate 8 mEq./L. Bot. 500 ml., 1000 ml.
Use: Fluid & electrolyte replenisher.
PLASMA-LYTE 148 INJECTION. (Travenol) Sodium 140, potassium 5, magnesium 3, Cl 98, acetate 27, gluconate 23 mEq./L. Bot. 500 ml., 1000 ml.
Use: Fluid & electrolyte replenisher.
PLASMA-LYTE and 5% DEXTROSE INJECTION. (Travenol) Sodium 40 meq., potassium 16, calcium 5, magnesium 3, Cl 40, acetate 12, lactate 12 mEq./L. Bot. 500 ml., 1000 ml.
Use: Fluid & electrolyte replenisher.
PLASMA-LYTE and 5% DEXTROSE INJECTION. (Travenol) Sodium 140, potassium 10, calcium 5 magnesium 3, Cl 103, acetate 47, lactate 8 mEq/L. Bot. 500 ml., 1000 ml.
Use: Fluid & electrolyte replenisher.
PLASMA-LYTE and 10% TRAVERT. (Travenol) Sodium 140, potassium 10, calcium 5, magnesium 3, Cl 103, acetate 47, lactate 8 mEq/L. Bot. 1000 ml. in glass.
Use: Fluid & electrolyte replenisher.
PLASMA-LYTE 56 and 5% DEXTROSE. (Travenol) Sodium 40, potassium 13, magnesium 3, Cl 40, acetate 16 mEq/L. Bot. 500 ml., 1000 ml.
Use: Fluid & electrolyte replenisher.
PLASMA-LYTE 148 and 5% INJECTION. (Travenol) Sodium 140, potassium 5, magnesium 3, Cl 98, acetate 27, gluconate 23 mEq./L. Bot. 500 ml., 1000 ml.
Use: Fluid & electrolyte replenisher.
PLASMA-LYTE 56 IN WATER. (Travenol) Sodium 40, potassium 13, magnesium 3, Cl 40, acetate 16/L. Bot. 500 ml., 1000 ml.
Use: Fluid & electrolyte replenisher.
PLASMANATE. (Cutter) Plasma protein fraction (Human) 5%. U.S.P. Vial 50 ml. Bot. 250 ml., 500 ml. with set.
Use: Shock. Hypoproteinemia.
PLASMA PLEX. (Armour) Plasma protein fraction (human) in 5% heat treated solution. Bot. 50 ml., 250 ml., 500 ml.
Use: I.V. use for treatment of shock, burns, & hypoproteinemia.
• **PLASMA PROTEIN FRACTION,** U.S.P. XXI. (Hyland) For the plasma protein preparation obtained from human plasma using the Cohn fractionation technic. Bot. 250 ml.
Use: Blood-volume supporter.
See: Plasmanate, Sol. (Cutter)
  Plasma-Plex, Sol. (Armour)
  Plasmatein (Abbott)
PLASMIN. B.A.N. The proteolytic enzyme derived from the activation of plasminogen. Actase is Plasmin (Human).
PLASMINOGEN. B.A.N. The specific substance derived from plasma which, when activated, has the property of lysing fibrinogen, fibrin, and some other proteins.
PLASMOCHIN NAPHTHOATE. Pamaquine naphthoate.

Use: Malaria.
PLASMOSAN. Povidone, B.A.N.
• **PLATELET CONCENTRATE,** U.S.P. XXI.
Use: Platelet replenisher.
PLATELET FACTOR 4. (Abbott) Test kit 100s.
Use: Radioimmunoassay for quantitative measurement of total PF4 levels in plasma.
PLATINOL. (Bristol) Cisplatin 10 mg./Vial, 50 mg./Vial.
Use: Antineoplastic agent.
• **PLAURACIN.** USAN.
Use: Growth stimulant.
PLEGINE. (Ayerst) Phendimetrazine tartrate 35 mg./Tab. Bot. 100s, 1000s.
Use: Anorexiant.
PLEGISOL. (Abbott) Plegisol, cardioplegic solution. Single Dose Container 1000 ml. without sodium bicarbonate.
Use: Installation into cardiac vasculature after buffering w/sodium bicarbonate.
PLEWIN TABLETS. (Winthrop Products) Glycobiarsol, chloroquine phosphate.
Use: Intestinal amebicide.
PLEXOLAN CREAM. (Last) Zinc oxide, lanolin. Tube 1.25 oz., 3 oz. Jar 16 oz.
Use: Protective for rough skin.
PLEXON. (Sig) Testosterone 10 mg., estrone 1 mg., liver 2 mcg., pyridoxine HCl 10 mg., panthenol 10 mg., inositol 20 mg., choline Cl 20 mg., Vit. B-12 100 mcg., procaine HCl 1%, niacinamide 100 mg., Vit. B-2 2 mg./ml. Vials 10 ml.
Use: Preventive geriatrics and nutritional deficiency.
PLIAGEL. (CooperVision) Poloxamer 407, preserved with sorbic acid 0.25%, edetate trisodium 0.5%. Bot. 25 ml.
Use: Soft contact lens cleaning solution.
• **PLICAMYCIN,** U.S.P. XXI. Inj. U.S.P.XXI. Antibiotic derived from *Streptomyces agrillaceus* & *S. tanashiensis.*
Use: Antineoplastic, antibiotic.
See: Mithracin, Pwd. (Miles Pharm)
PLOVA. (Washington Ethical) Psyllium mucilloid. Pow. Flavored 12 oz. Plain 10 ½ oz.
Use: Bowel regulator, laxative.
PLURAVIT DROPS. (Winthrop Products) Multivitamin.
Use: Dietary supplement.
PLURAXIN. (Winthrop Products) Vit. A, ergocalciferol, thiamin mononitrate, riboflavin, pyridoxine HCl, cyanocobalamin, calcium panthothenate, niacinamide, ascorbic acid.
Use: High potency multivitamin.
PLURI-B. (Pasadena Research) Vit. B-1 50 mg., B-2 5.0 mg., B-6 10 mg., panthenol 10 mg., niacinamide 50 mg./cc. Vial 10 cc., 30 cc. Also w/procaine HCl 1%. Vial 30 cc.
Use: Vitamin supplement, Inj.
PLURI-BEX. (Pasadena Research) Vit. B-1 100 mg., B-2 1 mg., B-6 10 mg., d-panthenol 10 mg., niacinamide 150 mg./cc. Vial 10 cc., 30 cc.
Use: Vitamin supplement.
PLUS-FACTOR TABLETS. (Sutliff & Case) Cal. carbonate 625 mg., docusate sodium 60 mg., Vit. C 50

mg., A 5000 I.U., D 400 I.U., B-1 3 mg., B-2 2 mg., B-6 2 mg., B-12 2 mcg., cal. pantothenate 5 mg., niacinamide 10 mg., iron 30 mg., Mn 1 mg., Mg 5 mg., Cu 1 mg., Zn 1.5 mg., iodine 0.15 mg./Tabs. Bot. 100s, 1000s.
Use: Pregnancy and lactation.

PMB 200. (Ayerst) Premarin (Conjugated Estrogens, U.S.P.) 0.45 mg., meprobamate 200 mg./Tab. Bot. 60s.
Use: Treatment of moderate to severe vasomotor symptoms associated with the menopause with emotional symptoms (anxiety, tension).

PMB 400. (Ayerst) Premarin (Conjugated Estrogens, U.S.P.) 0.45 mg., meprobamate 400 mg./Tab. Bot. 60s.
Use: Treatment of moderate to severe vasomotor symptoms associated with the menopause with emotional symptoms (anxiety, tension).

P-MEDRATE-P.A. (Reid-Provident) Medroxyprogesterone acetate 100 mg./ml. Inj. 5 ml.

P.M.P. COMPOUND. (Mericon) Chlorpheniramine maleate 4 mg., phenylephrine HCl 15 mg., salicylamide 300 mg., scopolamine methylnitrate 0.8 mg./Tab. Bot. 100s, 1000s.

PMP EXPECTORANT. (Mericon) Codeine phosphate 10 mg., phenylephrine HCl 10 mg., guaifenesin 40 mg., chlorpheniramine maleate 2 mg./5 cc. Bot. gal.

P-M-Z HCl EXPECTORANT. (Sutliff & Case) Promethazine HCl 5 mg., ipecac fl. ext. 0.17 min., K guaiacolsulfonate 44 mg., citric acid anhydrous 60 mg., sod. citrate 197 mg./5 cc., alcohol 7% Bot. 4 oz., pt., gal.
W/Codeine phosphate 10 mg./5 cc. Bot. 4 oz., pt., gal.

PNEUMOCOCCAL VACCINE, POLYVALENT PNU-IMUNE 23. (Lederle) Purified capsular polysaccharides from 23 penumococcal types.
Use: Vacination against pneumococcal types.

PNEUMOCOCCI.
W/Haemophilus influenzae, Neisseria catarrhalis, streptococci, Klebsiella pneumoniae, staphylococci, pneumococci, killed.
See: Mixed Vaccine No. 4 w/H. Influenzae, Inj. (Lilly)

PNEUMONIA VACCINE, KILLED DIPLOCOCCUS.
W/Neisseria catarrhalis, Klebsiella pneumoniae, streptococci, staphylococci.
See: Combined Vaccine No. 4 w/Catarrhalis, Inj. (Lilly)

PNEUMONIAE VACCINE, KILLED KLEBSIELLA.
W/Neisseria catarrhalis, Diplococcus pneumoniae, streptococci, staphylococci.
See: Combined Vaccine No. 4 w/Catarrhalis, Inj. (Lilly)

PNEUMOVAX. (Merck Sharp & Dohme) Pneumococcal vaccine polyvalent 0.5 ml./dose. Vials: 5 dose, 1 dose × 5s. Prefilled syringes 0.5ml. Box 5s.
Use: Immunization against pneumonia.

PNS UNNA BOOT. (Pedinol) Non-sterile gauze bandage 10 yds × 3". Box 12s.

Use: Ambulatory procedure in treatment of leg ulcers and varicosities.

PNU-IMUNE 23. (Lederle) Pneumococcal vaccine 0.5 ml. dose. Vial 5 dose. Lederject disposable syringe 5 × 1 dose.
Use: Vaccine against pneumococcal pneumonia.

POCHLORIN. Prophyrinic and chlorophyllic compound.
Use: Anti-hypercholesteremic agent.

PODIASPRAY. (Dalin) Undecylenic acid, salicylic acid, dichlorophene. Spray-on pow. 6 oz.
Use: Fungicide-germicide.

PODIODINE. (A.V.P.) Germicidal surgical scrub and solution.

POD-BEN-25. (C & M Pharmacal) Podophyllin 25% in tincture benzoin. Bot. 1 oz.
Use: Wart removal.

PODOBEN. (Maurry) Resin podophyllum 25%, benzoin comp. 10%; isopropyl alcohol 69-72%. Bot. 5 cc.
Use: Wart therapy.

• **PODOPHYLLUM,** U.S.P. XXI.
Use: Caustic.
W/Cascara sagrada, bile salts, phenolphthalein.
See: Bilstan (Standex)
W/Oxgall, cascara sagrada, dandelion root, tr. nux vomica.
See: Oxachol, Liq. (Philips Roxane)

• **PODOPHYLLUM RESIN,** U.S.P. XXI. Topical Sol., U.S.P. XXI. (Var. Mfr.) podophyllin. Pkg. 1 oz., ¼ lb., 1 lb.
Use: Caustic.
See: Podoben, Liq. (Maurry)
W/Salicylic acid.
See: Ver-Var, Sol. (Owen)

POINT-TWO MOUTHRINSE. (Hoyt) Sodium fluoride 0.2% in a flavored neutral liquid. Bot. 120 ml.
Use: Prevention of dental caries.

POISON ANTIDOTE KIT. (Bowman) Charcoal suspension. Bot. 1½ oz., 4s. Ipecac syrup, Bot. ½ oz., 2/Kit.

POISON IVY EXTRACT. (Parke-Davis) Extract from leaves of Rhus toxicodendron dissolved in sterile almond oil. Single dose 0.1 ml vial.
Use: Prevention of Rhus dermatitis.

• **POISON IVY EXTRACT, ALUM PRECIPITATED.**
USAN. An aqueous suspension of a pyridine extract of poison ivy which is precipitated with alum and adjusted to standard concentrations.
See: Aqua Ivy, Inj. (Miles Pharm)
Poisonivi, Ext. (Cutter)
Poisonok, Ext. (Cutter)

POISON IVY, OAK & SUMAC (RHUS-ALL). (Barry) Triple antigen in oil 0.2 mg./cc. Vial 5 cc.
Use: Prophylactic for hyposensitization.

POISON IVY, OAK AND SUMAC EXT.
See: Allergenic Ext., Vial (Barry)

POISONOAK EXTRACT. USAN.
Use: Anti-allergic.

POISON OAK-IVY EXTRACT. (Hollister-Stier) Poison ivy ext. & poison oak, Vial, Dropper Bot. 15 cc.
See: Ivyol, Vial (Merck Sharp & Dohme)

POLACRILLIN

480

- **POLACRILLIN.** USAN. Methacrylic acid with divinylbenzene. A synthetic ion-exchange resin, supplied in the hydrogen or free acid form. Amberlite IRP-64 (Rohm and Haas).
Use: Pharmaceutic aid.
- **POLACRILLIN POTASSIUM,** N.F.XVI. A synthetic ion-exchange resin, prepared through the polymerization of methacrylic acid and divinylbenzene, further neutralized with potassium hydroxide to form the potassium salt of methacrylic acid and divinylbenzene. Supplied as a pharmaceutical-grade ion-exchange resin in a particle size of 100- to 500-mesh.
Use: Pharmaceutic aid.
See: Amberlite IRP-88 (Rohm and Haas)
POLAMETHENE RESIN CAPRYLATE. The physico-chemical complex of the acid-binding ion exchange resin, polyamine-methylene resin and caprylic acid.
POLARAMINE. (Schering) Dexchlorpheniramine maleate (d-isomer of Chlor-Trimeton). **Repetab:** 4 mg./Tab. Bot. 100s; 6 mg./Tab. Bot. 100s, 1000s. **Syrup:** 2 mg./5 ml. Bot. 16 oz.
Use: Antihistaminic.
POLARAMINE EXPECTORANT. (Schering) Dexchlorpheniramine maleate 2 mg., pseudoephedrine sulfate 20 mg., guaifenesin 100 mg., alcohol 7.2%/5 ml. Bot. 16 oz.
Use: Antihistaminic, decongestant, antitussive.
POLDEMAN AD SUSPENSION. (Winthrop Products) Kaolin.
Use: Antidiarrheal agent.
POLDEMAN SUSPENSION. (Winthrop Products) Kaolin.
Use: Antidiarrheal agent.
POLDEMICINA SUSPENSION. (Winthrop Products) Kaolin.
Use: Antidiarrheal agent.
POLDINE METHYLSULFATE. 2-(Hydroxymethyl)-1,1-dimethyl-pyrrolidinium methylsulfate benzilate. 2-Benziloyloxymethyl-1,1-dimethylpyrrolidinium methylsulfate.
Use: Anticholinergic.
- **POLICAPRAM.** USAN.
Use: Pharmaceutic aid.
POLIDENT DENTU-GRIP. (Block) Carboxymethylcellulose gum, ethylene oxide polymer. Pkg. 0.675 oz., 1.75 oz., 3.55 oz.
POLIDEXIDE. B.A.N. Dextran cross-linked with epichlorhydrin and 0-substituted with 2-diethylaminoethyl groups, some of them quaternized with diethylaminoethyl chloride. Secholex hydrochloride.
Use: Antihypercholesterolemic agent.
- **POLIGEENAN.** USAN. 3,6-Anhydro-4-O-β-D-galactopyranosyl-α-D-galactopyranose 2,4'-bis(potassium/sodium sulfate)-(1-3')-polysaccharide. Polysaccharide produced by limited hydrolysis of carragheen from red algae.
Use: Enzyme inhibitor.
- **POLIGNATE SODIUM.** USAN.
Use: Enzyme inhibitor.

POLI-GRIP. (Block) Karaya gum, magnesium oxide in petrolatum mineral oil base, peppermint and spearmint flavor. Tube 0.75, 1.5. 2.5 oz.
Use: Denture adhesive cream.
POLIOMYELITIS IMMUNE GLOBULIN (HUMAN). (Var. Mfr.) Prep. of gamma globulin primarily assayed for content of poliomyelitis antibodies in accordance with standard procedures licensed by National Institutes of Health.
POLIOMYELITIS VACCINE. (Purified, Salk Type IPV) (Squibb-Connaught) Amp. 5 x 1 ml. Vial 10 dose.
Use: Active immunizing for prevention of poliomyelitis.
- **POLIOMYELITIS VACCINE INACTIVATED,** U.S.P. XXI.
Use: Active immunizing agent.
- **POLIOVIRUS VACCINE LIVE ORAL,** U.S.P. XXI. Poliovirus vaccine, live, oral, type I, II, or III. Poliovirus vaccine, live, oral, trivalent.
Use: Active immunizing agent.
See: Orimune Trivalent I, II & III, Vial (Lederle)
POLIOVIRUS VACCINE, LIVE, ORAL, TRIVALENT.
Use: Immunization against polio strains 1, 2 & 3.
See; Orimune (Lederle)
POLIOMYELITIS VACCINE, PURIFIED. (Squibb-Connaught) Amp. 1 ml. Box 5s. Vial. 10 dose.
Use: S.C.; an active immunizing agent for the prevention of poliomyelitis.
- **POLIPROPENE 25.** USAN.
Use: Pharmaceutic aid.
POLISHED AMBERS DERMANESSE SKIN TONING CREAM. (Revlon) Hydroquinone 2%, padimate 0, oxybenzone in cream base.
Use: Skin bleaching.
POLLEN ANTIGEN, ORAL.
POLORIS POULTICES. (Block) Benzocaine, capsicum. Pkg. 5 and 12 unit.
Use: Dental pain.
- **POLOXALENE.** USAN. Liquid nonionic surfactant polymer of polyoxypropylene polyoxyethylene type.
Use: Surfactant.
POLOXALKOL. B.A.N. A polymer of ethylene oxide, propylene oxide, and propylene glycol.
Use: Surface active agent.
POLOXALKOL. Polyoxyethylene polyoxypropylene polymer.
See: Magcyl, Caps. (Elder)
W/Casanthrol.
See: Casakol, Cap. (Upjohn)
W/Phenylephrine HCl, dextrose sol.
See: Isohalent, Sol. (Elder)
- **POLOXAMER,** N.F. XVI.
Use: Surfactant.
- **POLOXAMER 182 D.** USAN.
Use: Pharmaceutic aid (suxfactant).
- **POLOXAMER 182 LF.** USAN.
Use: Food additive; pharmaceutic aid.
- **POLOXAMER 188.** USAN.
Use: Cathartic.
- **POLOXAMER 188 LF.** USAN.
Use: Pharmaceutic aid (surfactant).

• **POLOXAMER 331.** USAN.
Use: Food additive (surfactant).
POLOXAMER-IODINE.
See: Prepodyne, Sol. (West)
POLOXYL LANOLIN. B.A.N. A polyoxyethylene condensation-product of anhydrous lanolin. Aqualose.
Use: Emollient.
POLYAMINE-METHYLENE RESIN.
See: Exorbin (Var. Mfr.)
POLYAMINE RESIN.
See: Polyamine-Methylene Resin (Var. Mfr.)
POLYANETHOL SULFONATE, SODIUM.
See: Grobax, Vial (Roche Diagnostics)
POLYANHYDROGLUCOSE. Polyanhydroglucuronic acid.
See: Dextran, Inj., Sol. (Var. Mfr.)
POLYBASE. (Paddock) Preblended polyethylene glycol suppository base for incorporation of medications where a water soluble base is indicated. Jar 1 lb., 5 lb.
Use: Suppository base.
POLYBENZARSOL. Benzarsol.
POLY-BON DROPS. (Barrows) Vit. A 3000 I.U., D 400 I.U., C 60 mg., B-1 1 mg., B-2 1.2 mg., niacinamide 8 mg./0.6 cc. Bot. 50 cc.
POLYBRENE. Hexadimethrine Bromide, B.A.N.
• **POLYBUTILATE.** USAN.
Use: Surgical aid.
POLYCARBOPHIL. A synthetic, loosely crosslinked, hydrophilic resin of the polycarboxylic type. Sorboquel.
Use: Absorbent (gastrointestinal).
POLYCILLIN. (Bristol) Ampicillin trihydrate. Cap.: **250 mg.**/Cap. Bot. 100s, 500s. 1000s. **Cap.: 500 mg.** /Cap. Bot. 16s, 100s, 500s. DosaTrol 250 mg., 500 mg. Bot. 100s. **Pediatric Drops:** 100 mg./ml. Dropper Bot. 20 ml.
Use: Antibiotic.
POLYCILLIN-N. (Bristol) Sodium ampicillin 125 mg., 250 mg., 500 mg., 1 Gm., 2 Gm./Vial Pkg. 1s, 10s. Piggyback vials 500 mg., 1 Gm., 2 Gm. Bulk vial 10 Gm.
Use: Antibiotic.
POLYCILLIN ORAL SUSPENSION. (Bristol) Ampicillin trihydrate. **125 mg.**/5 ml. Bot. 80 ml., 100 ml., 150 ml., 200 ml.; **250 mg.**/5 ml. Bot. 80 ml., 100 ml., 150 ml., 200 ml.; **500 mg.**/5 ml. Bot. 100 ml. 100 mg./1 ml. Bot. 20 ml. Pediatric Drops.
Use: Broad spectrum antibacterial agent.
POLYCILLIN-PRB ORAL SUSPENSION. (Bristol) Ampicillin trihydrate 3.5 Gm., probenecid 1 Gm./Bot.
Use: Treatment of uncomplicated urethral, cervical, rectal or pharyngeal infections caused by N. gonorrheae in men and women.
POLYCITRA-K SYRUP. (Willen) Potassium citrate monohydrate 1100 mg., citric acid monohydrate 334 mg., potassium ion 10 mEq./5 ml. Bot. 4 oz., pt.
Use: Systemic alkalizer sodium free.
POLYCITRA-LC. (Willen) Potassium citrate monohydrate 550 mg., sodium citrate dihydrate 500

mg., citric acid monohydrate 334 mg., potassium ion 5 mEq., sodium ion 5 mEq./5 ml. Bot. 4 oz., pt.
Use: Systemic alkalizer sugar free.
POLYCITRA SYRUP. (Willen) Potassium citrate monohydrate 550 mg., sodium citrate dihydrate 500 mg., citric acid monohydrate 334 mg., potassium ion 5 mEq., sodium ion 5 mEq./5 ml. Bot. 4 oz. pt.
Use: Systemic alkalizer.
POLYCOSE. (Ross) Pow.: Glucose polymers derived from controlled hydrolysis of corn starch. KCal. 380, carbohydrate 94.5 Gm., moisture 6.0 Gm., ash 0.5 Gm./100 Gm. Na 115 mg. K 39 mg., chloride 213 mg., Ca 60 mg., P 13 mg./100 Gm. Can 14 oz. **Liq.:** KCal. 200, carbohydrate 50 Gm., moisture 70 Gm., ash 0.25 Gm./100 ml. Na 58 mg., K 20 mg., chloride 107 mg., Ca 30 mg., P 6 mg./100 ml. Bot. 4 oz.
Use: Source of calories solely from carbohydrate.
POLYCYCLINE INTRAVENOUS.
See: Bristacycline, Cap., Vial (Bristol)
• **POLYDEXTROSE.** USAN.
Use: Food additive.
POLYDINE OINTMENT. (Century) Povidone iodine in ointment base. Jar. 1 oz., 4 oz., lb.
Use: Topical anti-infective.
POLYDINE SCRUB. (Century) Povidone iodine in scrub solution. Bot. 1 oz., 4 oz., 8 oz., pt., gal.
Use: Antiseptic scrub solution.
POLYDINE SOLUTION. (Century) Povidone iodine solution. Bot. 1 oz., 4 oz., 8 oz., pt., gal.
Use: Topical anti-infective.
• **POLYDIOXANONE.** USAN.
Use: Surgical aid.
POLYECTIN. (Amid)
See: Am-Tuss Elixir
POLYESTRADIOL PHOSPHATE.
See: Estradurin, Amp. (Ayerst)
• **POLYETHADENE.** USAN. 1,2:3,4-Diepoxybutane polymer with ethylenimine. Erythritol anhydride polyethyleneimine polymer.
Use: Antacid.
• **POLYETHYLENE GLYCOL 300, 400, 600, 1500, 1540, 4000 & 6000,** N.F. XVI. Oint., N.F. XVI.
Use: Water-soluble ointment and suppository base; tablet excipient.
See: Carbowax (Doak Pharmacal)
P.E.G. Lotion (Medco)
• **POLYFEROSE.** USAN. An iron carbohydrate chelate containing approximately 45% of iron in which the metallic (Fe) ion is sequestered within a polymerized carbohydrate derived from sucrose.
Use: Hematinic.
POLYGELINE. B.A.N. A polymer of urea and polypeptides derived from denatured gelatin.
Use: Restoration of blood volume.
• **POLYGLACTIN 370 & 910.** USAN. Lactic acid polyester with glycolic acid.
Use: Synthetic absorbable suture.
• **POLYGLYCOLIC ACID.** USAN. Poly-(oxycarbonylmethylene).
Use: Surgical aid.
See: Dexon Sterile Suture (David & Geck)

• **POLYGLYCONATE.** USAN.

POLYHEXANIDE. B.A.N. Poly-(1-hexamethylene-biguanide hydrochloride).
Use: Antibacterial, veterinary medicine.

POLY-HISTINE CAPSULES. (Bock) Phenyltoloxamine citrate 25 mg., pyrilamine maleate 25 mg., pheniramine maleate 25mg./Cap. Bot. 100s, 500s.
Use: Antihistamine.

POLY-HISTINE-D CAPSULES. (Bock) Phenylpropanolamine HCl 50 mg., phenyltoloxamine citrate 16 mg., pyrilamine maleate 16 mg., pheniramine maleate 16 mg./Cap. Bot. 100s, 1000s.
Use: Decongestant, antihistamine.

POLY-HISTINE-D ELIXIR. (Bock) Phenylpropanolamine HCl 12.5 mg., phenyltoloxamine citrate 4 mg., pyrilamine maleate 4 mg., pheniramine 4 mg./5 ml. w/alcohol 4%. Bot. pt., gal.
Use: Antihistaminic, decongestant.

POLY-HISTINE-DX CAPSULES. (Bock) Pseudoephedrine HCl 120 mg., brompheniramine maleate 12 mg./Cap. Bot. 100s, 1000s.
Use: Decongestant, antihistaminic.

POLY-HISTINE-DX SYRUP. (Bock) Pseudoephedrine HCl 30 mg., brompheniramine maleate 4 mg./5 ml. Bot. pt., gal.
Use: Decongestant, antihistaminic.

POLY-HISTINE ELIXIR. (Bock) Phenyltoloxamine citrate 4 mg., pyrilamine maleate 4 mg., pheniramine maleate 4 mg., thenylpyramine mg./5 ml. w/ alcohol 4%, Elix. Bot. pint, gal.
Use: Contact, inhalant and food allergies.

POLY-HISTINE EXPECTORANT. (Bock) Brompheniramine maleate 2 mg., phenylpropanolamine HCl 12.5 mg., potassium guaiacolsulfonate 100 mg., codeine phosphate 10 mg./5 ml. Bot. pt., gal.
Use: Expectorant.

• **POLYMACON.** USAN. Poly(2-hydroxyethyl methacrylate).
Use: Contact lens material.

POLYMAGMA PLAIN TABLETS. (Wyeth) Activated attapulgite 500 mg., pectin 45 mg./Tab. Bot. 50s.

• **POLYMETAPHOSPHATE P-32.** USAN.
Use: Radioactive agent.

POLYMETHINE BLUE DYE. (3,3′-Diethylhiadicarbocyanine iodide).

POLYMONINE. A formaldehyde polymer of N-methyl-monoanisylamine.

POLYMOX. (Bristol) Amoxicillin. **Cap.:** 250 mg., 500 mg./Cap. Bot. 50s, 100s, 500s Dosatrol 250 mg. or 500 mg./Cap. **Oral Susp.:** 125 mg., 250 mg./5 ml. Bot. 80 ml., 150 ml. Dosatrol 125 or 250 mg./Bot. **Ped. Drops:** 50 mg./ml. Bot. 15 ml.
Use: Anti-infective.

POLYMYXIN. B.A.N. Generic term for antibiotics obtained from fermentations of various media by strains of *Bacillus polymyxa.*
Use: Polymyxins A, B & D active against susceptible gram-negative bacteria.

POLYMYXIN B. (Various Mfr.) (No Pharmaceutical Form Available) Antimicrobial substances produced by *Bacillus polymyxa.*

W/Bacitracin zinc, neomycin sulf., benzalkonium chloride.
See: Biotres, Oint. (Central)

• **POLYMYXIN B SULFATE.** U.S.P. XXI. Otic Soln., Sterile, U.S.P. XXI.
See: Aerosporin, Pow., Sol. (Burroughs Wellcome)

• **POLYMIXIN B SULFATE AND HYDROCORTISONE OTIC SOLUTION,** U.S.P. XXI.
Use: Antibiotic, anti-inflammatory.

POLYMYXIN B SULFATE STERILE. (Pfipharmecs) Polymyxin B sulfate 500,000 u./Vial for reconstitution.

POLYMYXIN B SULFATE W/COMBINATIONS.
See: Aural Acute, Drops (Saron)
Baximin, Oint. (Columbia)
Biotic-O, Oint. (Scrip)
Bro-Parin Otic, Susp. (Riker)
Coracin, Oint. (Mallard)
Cortisporin, Preps. (Burroughs Wellcome)
Epimycin A, Oint. (Delta)
Florotic, Liq. (Squibb)
Lidosporin, Otic Soln. (Burroughs Wellcome)
Maxitrol, Oint., Susp. (Alcon)
Mity-Mycin, Oint. (Reid-Provident)
Mycitracin, Oint., Ophth. Oint. (Upjohn)
My-Cort-Otic, Liq. (Scrip)
My-Cort-Otic #1, Drops (Scrip)
Neomixin, Oint. (Mallard)
Neo-Polycin, Oint., Ophth. Oint., Ophth. Sol. (Merrell Dow)
Neosporin, Preps. (Burroughs Wellcome)
Neosporin-G, Cream (Burroughs Wellcome)
Neosporin G.U. Irrigant, Amp. (Burroughs Wellcome)
Neotal, Oint. (Mallard)
Neo-Thrycex, Oint. (Commerce)
Ophthel, Oint. (Elder)
Ophthocort, Oint. (Parke-Davis)
Otobiotic, Soln. (Schering)
Otoreid-HC, Liq. (Reid-Provident)
P.B.N., Oint. (Jenkins)
Polysporin, Oint., Ophth. Oint. (Burroughs Wellcome)
Pyocidin-Otic Soln. (Berlex)
Statrol, Liq. (Alcon)
Statrol Sterile Ophthalmic Ointment (Alcon)
Terra-Cortril, Aerosol (Pfizer)
Terramycin, Preps. W/Polymyxin (Pfizer)
Tigo, Oint. (Burlington)
Tri-Bow, Oint. (Bowman)
Tribotic, Oint. (Burgin-Arden)
Trimixin, Oint. (Hance)
Triple Antibiotic Ointment (Kenyon)

POLYMYXIN-NEOMYCIN-BACITRACIN OINTMENT. (Various Mfr.)
Use: Antibiotic for treatment of gram-positive and gram-negative organisms.

POLY-NEO-CORT. (Robinson) Ear drops. Bot. 12.5 cc.
Use: Antibiotic ear drops.

POLYNOXYLIN. B.A.N. Poly[methylenedi(hydroxymethyl)urea]Anaflex; Ponoxylan.

Use: Antibacterial; anti-inflammatory.
POLYNOXYLIN.
Poly[methylenedi(hydroxymethyl)urea]. Anaflex.
POLYOXYETHYLENE 8 STEARATE. Myrj 45. (ICI
U.S.)., Polyoxyl 8 Stearate.
**POLYOXYETHYLENE (20) SORBITAN MONOLE-
ATE.**
See: Polysorbate 80, U.S.P. XXI. (Var. Mfr.)
POLYOXYETHYLENE 20 SORBITAN TRIOLEATE.
Tween 85. (ICI U.S.)., Polysorbate 85.
**POLYOXYETHYLENE 20 SORBITAN TRISTEAR-
ATE.** Tween 65. (ICI U.S.)., Polysorbate 65.
POLYOXYETHYLENE 40 MONOSTEARATE.
Polyoxyl 40 Stearate
See: Myrj 52 & Myrj 52S (ICI U.S.)
• **POLYOXYETHYLENE 50 STEARATE,** N.F. XVI.
Use: Surfactant; emulsifying agent.
POLYOXYETHYLENEONYLPHENOL.
W/Alkyldimethylbenzylammonium chloride,
methylrosaniline chloride, polyethylene glycol tert-
dodecylthioether.
See: Hyva, Vag. Tab. (Holland-Rantos)
POLYOXYETHYLENE SORBITAN MONOLAURATE.
Polysorbate 20, N.F. XVI.
W/Ferrous gluconate.
See: Simron, Cap. (Merrell Dow)
W/Ferrous gluconate, vitamins.
See: Simron Plus, Cap. (Merrell Dow)
POLYOXYETHYLENE LAURYL ETHER.
W/Benzoyl peroxide, ethyl alcohol.
See: Benzagel, Gel (Dermik)
Desquam-X, Prep. (Westwood)
W/Hydrocortisone, sulfur.
See: Fostril HC, Lot. (Westwood)
W/Sulfur.
See: Fostril, Lot. (Westwood)
Proseca, Oint. (Westwood)
POLYOXYETHYLENE NONYL PHENOL
W/Sodium edetate, docusate sodium, 9-aminoacridine
HCl.
See: Vagisec Plus, Supp. (Schmid)
• **POLYOXYL 8 STEARATE.** USAN. Polyoxyethylene
8 stearate.
Use: Surfactant.
See: Myrj 45 (Atlas)
• **POLYOXYL 10 OLEYL ETHER,** N.F. XVI.
Use: Pharmaceutic aid (surfactant).
• **POLYOXYL 20 CETOSTEARYL ETHER,** N.F. XVI.
Use: Pharmaceutic aid (surfactant).
• **POLYOXYL 35 CASTOR OIL,** N.F.XVI.
• **POLYOXYL 40 HYDROGENATED CASTOR OIL,**
N.F. XVI.
• **POLYOXYL 40 STEARATE,** N.F. XVI. Macrogic
Stearate 2000 (I.N.N.) Polyoxyethylene 40
monostearate.
Use: Hydrophilic oint., surfactant; surface-active
agent.
See: Myrj 52. (Atlas)
Myrj 52S. (Atlas)
W/Polyethylene glycol, chlorobutanol.
See: Blink-N-Clean (Allergan)
POLY-PRED LIQUIFILM. (Allergan) Prednisolone ace-

tate 0.5%, neopmycin sulfate 0.35%, polymyxin B
sulfate 10,000 u./ml. with polyvinyl alcohol 1.4%.
Bot. 5 ml. dropper bot.
Use: Treatment of nonpurulent bacterial infections
of the eye.
• **POLYPROPYLENE GLYCOL,** N.F. XVI. An addition
polymer of propylene oxide and water.
POLYSEPT. (Dalin) Polymyxin B sulfate 5000 u.,
bacitracin 400 u., neomycin sulfate 5 mg.,
diperodon HCl 10 mg./Gm. Tubes: ½ oz.
Use: Topical antibacterial therapy.
POLYSONIC LOTION. (Parker) Multi-purpose ul-
trasound lotion with coupling efficiency. Bot. 8.5
oz., gal.
Use: For Diagnostic & therapeutic medical
ultrasound.
POLYSORB HYDRATE CREAM. (Fougera) Tube 2
oz., Jar 16 oz.
• **POLYSORBATE 20,** N.F. XVI. (Atlas) Tween 20.
Polyoxyethlene 20 sorbitan monolaurate.
Use: Surface-active agent.
• **POLYSORBATE 40,** N.F. XVI. (Atlas) Tween 40.
Polyoxyethylene 20 sorbitan monopalmitate.
Use: Surface-active agent.
• **POLYSORBATE 60,** N.F. XVI. (Atlas) Tween 60.
Polyoxyethylene 20 sorbitan monostearate.
Use: Surface-active agent.
• **POLYSORBATE 65.** USAN. (Atlas) Tween 65.
Polyoxyethylene 20 sorbitan tristearate.
Use: Surface-active agent.
• **POLYSORBATE 80,** N.F. XVI. Polyoxyethylene (20)
Sorbitan Monooleate.
Use: Surfactant.
• **POLYSORBATE 85.** USAN. (Atlas) Polyoxyethylene
20 sorbitan trioleate. Tween 85.
Use: Surface-active agent.
POLYSPORIN OINTMENT. (Burroughs Wellcome)
Polymyxin B sulfate 10,000 u., bacitracin zinc 500
u. in special white petrolatum base/Gm. Tube ½ &
1 oz. Foil packet ¹⁄₃₂ oz. 144s. Ophth. Tube ⅛ oz.
Use: Active against gram-negative & gram-positive or-
ganisms.
POLY-STRESS THERAPEUTIC. (Xttrium) Vit. A 12,500
I.U., D 400 I.U., C 150 mg., B-1 7.5 mg., B-2 5 mg.,
niacinamide 75 mg., B-6 1.5 mg., B-12 3 mcg., Ca
pantothenate 10 mg., Vit. E 5 I.U., phosphate 182
mg., Ca 55 mg., P 40 mg., Fe 7 mg., iodine 0.07
mg., K 2.5 mg., Cu 0.5 mg., Mn 0.5 mg., Mg 3 mg.,
Zn 0.7 mg./Tab. Bot. 100s, 500s.
Use: Vitamin therapy.
POLYSULFIDES. Polythionate.
POLYTAR BATH. (Stiefel) A 25% polytar blend of
four different vegetable & mineral tars. Bot. 8 fl. oz.
Use: Psoriasis treatment.
POLYTAR SHAMPOO. (Stiefel) A neutral soap
containing 1% Polytar in a surfactant shampoo.
Buffered. Plastic Bot. 6 fl. oz., 12 fl. oz., gal.
Use: Treatment of psoriasis and other scalp
conditions.
POLYTAR SOAP. (Stiefel) A neutral soap containing
1% Polytar. Cake 4 oz.

Use: Treatment of eczema and other skin conditions.

POLYTEF. (Ethicon) Poly(tetrafluoroethylene). PTFE.
Use: Prosthetic aid.

• **POLYTHIAZIDE,** U.S.P. XXI. Tab., U.S.P. XXI. 2-Methyl-3,4-dihydro-3,(2,2,2-Trifluoroethylthiomethyl)-6-chloro-7-sulfamyl-1,2,4-benzothiadiazine, 1,1-dioxide.
6-Chloro-3,4-dihydro-2-methyl-3-[[(2,2,2,-trifluoroethyl)thio]-methyl]-2H-1,2,4-Benzothiadiazine-7-sulfonamide 1,1-dioxide.
Use: Diuretic; antihypertensive.
See: Renese Tab. (Pfizer Laboratories)
W/Prazosin.
See: Minizide, Cap. (Pfizer Laboratories)
W/Reserpine
See: Renese-R, Tab. (Pfizer Laboratories)

POLYTINIC. (Pharmics) B-12 7.5 mcg., iron, elemental 100 mg., C 300 mg., B-1 5 mg., folic acid 1 mg., liver 75 mg., stomach 75 mg., intrinsic factor $^1\!/_{20}$ u./Tab. Bot. 100s. Liq. Bot. 4 oz., 16 oz.
Use: Dietary supplement.

POLYTUSS-DM. (Rhode) Dextromethorphan HBr 15 mg., chlorpheniramine maleate 1 mg., guaifenesin 25 mg./5 ml. Bot. 4 oz., 16 oz.
Use: Cough preparation.

• **POLYURETHANE FOAM.** USAN.
Use: Prosthetic aid.

POLYVIDONE.
See: Polyvinylpyrrolidone

POLY-VI-FLOR 0.5 mg. CHEWABLE TABS. (Mead Johnson) Vit. A 2500 I.U., D 400 I.U., E 15 I.U., C 60 mg., B-1 1.05 mg., B-2 1.2 mg., niacin 13.5 mg., B-6 1.05 mg., B-12 4.5 mcg., fluoride 0.5 mg., folic acid 0.3 mg. Chewable Tab. Bot. 100s. **With Iron:** Above formula plus iron 12 mg., Cu 1 mg., Zn 10 mg./Tab. Bot. 100s.
Use: Caries prophylaxis and diet supplementation.

POLY-VI-FLOR 1 mg. CHEWABLE TABLETS. (Mead Johnson) Vit. A 2500 I.U., D 400 I.U., E 15 I.U., C 60 mg., B-1 1.05 mg., B-2 1.2 mg., niacin 13.5 mg., B-6 1.05 mg., B-12 4.5 mcg., fluoride 1 mg., folic acid 0.3 mg. Chewable Tab. Bot. 100s, 1000s. **With Iron:** Above formula plus iron 12 mg., Cu 1 mg., Zn 10 mg.
Use: Caries prophylaxis and diet supplementation.

POLY-VI-FLOR 0.25 mg. DROPS. (Mead Johnson) Vit. A 1500 I.U., D 400 I.U., E 5 I.U., C 35 mg., B-1 0.5, B-2 0.6 mg., B-6 0.4 mg., niacin 8 mg., B-12 2 mcg., fluoride 0.25 mg./1.0 ml. Drop. Bot. 50 ml.
Use: Caries prophylaxis and dietary supplement.

POLY-VI-FLOR 0.5 mg. DROPS. (Mead Johnson) Vit. A 1500 I.U., D 400 I.U., E 5 I.U., C 35 mg., B-1 0.5 mg., B-2 0.6 mg., B-6 0.4 mg., niacin 8 mg., B-12 2 mcg., fluoride 0.5 mg./1.0 ml. Drops, Bot. 30 ml., 50 ml.

POLY-VI-FLOR 0.5 mg. W/IRON DROPS. (Mead Johnson) Vit. A 1500 I.U., D 400 I.U., E 5 I.U., C 35 mg., B-1 0.5 mg., B-2 0.6 mg., B-6 0.4 mg., niacin 8 mg., fluoride 0.5 mg., iron 10 mg./1.0 ml. Drops. Bot. 50 ml.
Use: Caries prophylaxis and diet supplementation.

POLY-VI-FLOR w/IRON DROPS. (Mead Johnson) Vit.

A 1500 I.U., D 400 I.U., E 5 I.U., C 35 mg., B-1 0.5 mg., B-2 0.6 mg., B-6 0.4 mg., niacin 8 mg., fluoride 0.25 mg., iron 10 mg./1.0 ml. Bot. 50 ml.
Use: Caries prophylaxis, diet supplementation.

POLYVINOX. B.A.N. Poly(butyl vinyl ether). Shostakovsky Balsam.
Use: Skin application.

• **POLYVINYL ACETATE PHTHALATE,** N.F. XVI.

• **POLYVINYL ALCOHOL,** U.S.P. XXI. Ethenol, homopolymer.
Use: Viscosity-increasing agent; pharm. necessity for ophthalmic solution dosage form.
See: Liquifilm Forte (Allergan)
Liquifilm Tears (Allergan)
W/Hydroxypropyl methylcellulose
See: Liquifilm Wetting Soln. (Allergan)

POLYVINYLPYRROLIDONE-IODINE COMPLEX.
POLYVINYLPYRROLIDONE, POLYVIDONE, POVIDONE.
W/Acetrizoate Sod.
See: Salpix, Vial (Ortho)

POLYVINYLPYRROLIDONE VINYLACETATE COPOLYMERS.
See: Ivy-Rid, Spray (Mallard)
W/Benzalkonium.
See: Ivy-Chex, Aerosol (Bowman)

POLY-VI-SOL CHEWABLE TABS. (Mead Johnson) Vit. A 2500 I.U., E 15 I.U., D 400 I.U., C 60 mg., B-1 1.05 mg., B-2 1.2 mg., niacin 13.5 mg., Vit. B-6 1.05 mg., B-12 4.5 mcg., folic acid 0.3 mg./Chewable Tab. Tab. Bot. 100s, 1000s. Circus Shape Tab. Bot. 24s, 100s. **With Iron:** Above formula plus iron 12 mg., Zn 8 mg./Tab. Bot. 100s, 1000s. Circus shape Tab. **With Iron and Zinc:** Bot. 100s
Use: Multivitamin and mineral supplement.

POLY-VI-SOL DROPS. (Mead Johnson) Vit. A 1500 I.U., D 400 I.U., C 35 mg., B-1 0.5 mg., B-2 0.6 mg., Vit. E 5 I.U., B-6 0.4 mg., niacin 8 mg., B-12 2 mcg./1.0 ml. Bot. 30 & 50 ml. with calibrated "Safti-Dropper."
Use: Multivitamin supplement.

POLY-VI-SOL W/IRON DROPS. (Mead Johnson) Vit. A 1500 I.U., D 400 I.U., E 5 I.U., C 35 mg., B-1 0.5 mg., B-2 0.6 mg., B-6 0.4 mg., niacin 8 mg., iron 10 mg./1.0 ml. Bot. 50 ml.
Use: Multivitamin with iron supplement.

POLYVITAMIN DROPS. . (Vitarine) Vit. A 3000 I.U., D 400 I.U., C 60 mg., B-1 1 mg., B-2 1.2 mg., niacinamide 8 mg./0.6 ml. Bot. 50 ml. w/separate dropper.

POLYVITAMINS.
See: Vitamin preparations.

PONARIS. (Jamol) Nasal emollient of mucosal lubricating and moisturizing botanical oils. Cajeput, eucalyptus, peppermint in iodized cottonseed oil. Bot. 1 oz. w/dropper.
Use: Nasal irritations.

PONDERAX HYDROCHLORIDE. Fenfluramine, B.A.N.

PONDIMIN. (Robins) Fenfluramine HCl 20 mg./Tab. Bot. 100s, 500s.
Use: Anorectic.

PONDOCILLIN HYDROCHLORIDE. Pivampicillin, B.A.N.

PONOXYLAN. Polynoxylin, B.A.N.
PONSTAN. B.A.N. Mefenamic acid.
PONSTEL KAPSEALS. (Parke-Davis) Mefenamic acid 250 mg./Cap. Bot. 100s.
Use: Analgesic.
PONTALIN. Chlorbetamide, B.A.N.
PONTOCAINE 2% AQUEOUS SOLUTION.
(Winthrop-Breon) Tetracaine hydrochloride 20 mg., chlorobutanol 4 mg./ml. of 2% solution. Bot. 30 ml. Box 12s. Bot. 118 ml. Box 6s.
Use: Surface anesthesia of the nose and throat.
PONTOCAINE CREAM. (Winthrop-Breon) Tetracaine hydrochloride, equivalent to 1% tetracaine hydrochloride base, in a bland, water-miscible cream with methylparaben and sodium bisulfite as preservatives. Tube 1 oz. Pkg. 6s.
Use: Temporary relief of pain, burning and itching in skin burns and ulcers, sunburn, insect bites and hemorrhoids.
PONTOCAINE EYE OINTMENT. (Winthrop-Breon) Tetracaine 0.5% in a base of white petrolatum and light mineral oil. Tube 1/8 oz. Pkg. 12s.
Use: Short-term surface anesthesia of the eye.
PONTOCAINE HYDROCHLORIDE. (Winthrop-Breon) Niphanoid (instantly soluble) form consisting of a network of extremely fine, highly purified particles, resembling snow. Amp. 20 mg. Box 100s. 1% isotonic, isobaric solution: 10 mg. tetracaine hydrochloride, 6.7 mg. sodium chloride, and not more than 2 mg. acetone sodium bisulfite/ml. Amp. 2 ml. Box 25s.
Use: Spinal anesthesia.
PONTOCAINE HYDROCHLORIDE IN DEXTROSE (Hyperbaric) SOLUTIONS. (Winthrop-Breon) **0.2%:** Tetracaine hydrochloride 2 mg./ml. in a sterile solution containing 6% dextrose. Amp. 2 ml. 10s.
Use: saddle block (spinal anesthesia).**0.3%:** Tetracaine hydrochloride 3 mg/ml in a sterile solution containing 6% dextrose. Amp. 5 ml 10s.
Use: Spinal anesthesia (high, median and low).
PONTOCAINE OINTMENT. (Winthrop-Breon) Tetracaine 0.5% and menthol in an ointment consisting of white petrolatum and white wax. Tube 1 oz.
Use: Temporary relief of pain, burning and itching in hemorrhoids, skin burns and ulcers, scalds, wounds, bruises, abrasions, sunburn, ivy and other plant poisoning and insect bites.
PONTOCAINE 0.5% SOLUTION FOR OPHTHALMOLOGY. (Winthrop-Breon) Tetracaine HCl 5 mg., sodium chloride 7.5 mg., chlorobutanol 4 mg./ml. of 0.5% solution. Bot. 15 ml. Pkg. 12s. Bot. 59 ml. Pkg. 6s.
Use: Short-term surface anesthesia of the eye.
POPPY-SEED OIL, the ethyl ester of the fatty acids w/iodine.
See: Lipiodol, Ascendant & Lafay, Amps., Vial (Savage)
PORCELANA SKIN BLEACHING AGENT. (Jeffrey Martin) **Regular:** Hydroquinone 2%. Jar 2 oz., 4 oz. **Sunscreen:** Hydroquinone 2%, octyl dimethyl PABA 2.5%. Jar 4 oz.

Use: Fading dark patches on skin.
• **PORFIROMYCIN.** USAN.
Use: Antibacterial; antineoplastic.
PORK THYROID, DEFATTED.
See: Tuloidin, Tab. (Reid-Provident)
• **POROFOCON A.** USAN.
Use: Contact lens material.
• **POROFOCON B.** USAN.
Use: Cabcurve lens (soft lenses).
PORTABIDAY. (Washington Ethical) Concentrated soln. of alkylamine lauryl sulfate, a mild detergent with pH approx. 6 for use with Portabiday Vaginal Cleansing Kit. Bot. 3 oz.
Use: Vaginal cleansing.
PORTAGEN. (Mead Johnson) A nutritionally complete dietary powder containing as a % of the calories 14%, protein as caseinate, 41% fat (86% medium chain triglycerides, 14% corn oil), 45% carbohydrate as corn syrup solids and sucrose. Vit. A 5000 I.U., D 500 I.U., E 20 I.U., C 52 mg., B-1 1 mg., B-2 1.2 mg., B-6 1.3 mg., B-12 4 mcg., niacin 13 mg., folic acid 0.1 mg., choline 85 mg., biotin 0.05 mg., Ca 600 mg., P 450 mg., Mg 130 mg., Fe 12 mg., iodine 45 mcg., Cu 1 mg., Zn 6 mg., Mn 2 mg., Cl 550 mg., Na 300 mg., K 800 mg., pantothenic acid 6.7 mg., Vit. K-1 0.1 mg./Qt. 20Kcal/Fl. oz. Can 1 lb.
Use: Nutritionally complete dietary powder containing medium chain triglycerides as its major source of fat and lactose free for use in the nutritional management of infants, children, and adults who do not efficiently digest conventional food fats or absorb long chain fatty acids.
POSKINE. B.A.N. O-Propionylhyoscine. Proscopine hydrobromide.
Use: Central nervous system depressant.
POSTACNE LOTION. (Dermik) Sulfur 2%, S.D. alcohol 29% in flesh-tinted base. Bot. 2 oz.
Use: Antiseptic, antiseborrheic.
POSTAFENE.
See: Bonamine, Tab. (Pfizer)
• **POSTERIOR PITUITARY INJECTION,** U.S.P. XXI.
See: Pituitary, Posterior, Preps. (Various Mfr.)
POSTERISAN. (Kenwood) Sterilized E. coli vaccine with approximately 660 million coliform bacteria, liquefied phenol 6.67 mg., 2-ethylmercuriothio-s-benzoxazol carboxylic acid 0.33 mg./suppository in PEG base.
Use: Hemorrhoid, pruritis ani.
POSTLOBIN-O.
See: Pituitary, Post, Hormone (b)
POSTLOBIN-V.
See: Pituitary, Post., Hormone (a)
POTABA. (Glenwood) Pot. p-aminobenzoate. **Cap.** 0.5 Gm. Bot. 250s, 1000s. **Pow.** 100 Gm., 1 lb., 5 lb. **Tab.** 0.5 Gm., Bot. 100s, 1000s. **Envule.** 2 Gm. Box 50s.
Use: Scleroderma Peyronie's dis., rheumatoid arthritis.
POTABA PLUS 6. (Glenwood) Potassium p-aminobenzoate 0.5 Gm., Vit. B-6 1 mg./Tab. or Cap. **Caps.** Bot. 240s, 1000s. **Tabs.** Bot. 120s, 1000s.
Use: Antifibrosis therapy.

POTABLE-AQUA IODINE. (Wisconsin) Tab. Bot. 50s.
Use: Water purification.

POTABLE AQUA KIT. (Wisconsin) Tab. Bot. 50s with
collapsible gallon container.
Use: Water purification.

POTACHLOR 10%. (Bay) Potassium Cl 20 meq./15
ml. w/alcohol 5%. Bot. pt., gal.
Use: Potassium supplement.

POTACHLOR 20%. (Bay) Potassium Cl 40 meq./15
ml. Bot. pt., gal.
Use: Potassium supplement.

POTASALAN ELIXIR. (Lannett) Potassium chloride
10%. Bot. pt., gal.

• **POTASH, SULFURATED,** U.S.P. XXI.
Use: Pharmaceutic aid (source of sulfide).

POTASSIC SALINE LACTATED INJECTION.
Use: Fluid and electrolyte replenisher.

POTASSINE. (Recsei) Potassium chloride 20
mEq./15 ml. Bot. pt., gal.
Use: Potassium deficiency.

• **POTASSIUM ACETATE,** U.S.P. XXI. Inj., U.S.P. XXI.
Acetic acid, potassium salt. (Various Mfr.) **Inj.:**
(Abbott) 40 mEq., 20 ml. in 50 ml. Vial.
Use: Electrolyte replenisher; to avoid chloride when
high concentration of pot. is needed.

POTASSIUM ACID PHOSPHATE.
See: K-Phos., Tab. (Beach)
Uro-K Tab. (Star)

POTASSIUM p-AMINOBENZOATE.
See: Potaba, Preps. (Glenwood)
W/Potassium salicylate.
See: Pabalate-SF, Tab. (Robins)
W/Pyridoxine.
See: Potaba Plus 6, Caps. or Tabs. (Glenwood)

POTASSIUM AMINOSALICYLATE.
See: Aminosalicylate potassium.

POTASSIUM p-AMINOSALICYLATE.
See: Paskalium, Preps. (Glenwood)
Teebacin Kalium, Preps. (CMC)

• **POTASSIUM ASPARTATE AND MAGNESIUM
ASPARATE.** USAN.
Use: Nutrient.

• **POTASSIUM BICARBONATE,** U.S.P. XXI.
Use: Electrolyte replenisher.

• **POTASSIUM BICARBONATE EFFERVESCENT
TABLETS FOR ORAL SOLUTION,** U.S.P. XXI.

• **POTASSIUM BICARBONATE AND POTASSIUM
CHLORIDE FOR EFFERVESCENT ORAL
SOLUTION,** U.S.P. XXI.
Use: Potassium supplement.

• **POTASSIUM BICARBONATE AND POTASSIUM
CHLORIDE FOR EFFERVESCENT ORAL
SOLUTION,** U.S.P. XXI.
Use: Potassium supplement.

• **POTASSIUM BICARBONATE AND POTASSIUM
CHLORIDE EFFERVESCENT TABLETS FOR
ORAL SOLUTION,** U.S.P. XXI.
Use: Potassium supplement.

POTASSIUM BITARTRATE.
Use: Cathartic.

POTASSIUM BROMIDE. (Mallinckrodt) Granule, Bot.
1 oz., Pow., Pkg. 1 lb., 5 lb.
W/Aspirin, caffeine, sodium bromide.

See: Lanabac, Tab. (Lannett)
W/Sodium bromide, strontium bromide, ammonium
bromide.
See: Lanabrom, Elix. (Lannett)

• **POTASSIUM CHLORIDE,** U.S.P. XXI. Elixir,
Extended-Release Cap., Extended-Release Tab., In
Dextrose Inj., Inj., Oral Soln., For Oral Soln., U.S.P.
XXI.
Use: Potassium deficiency, hypopotassemia.
Ampules:
(Abbott) **Ampules:** 20 mEq., 10 ml.; 40 mEq.,
20 ml. **Pintop Vials:** 10 mEq., 5 ml. in 10 ml.;
20 mEq., 10 ml. in 20 ml.; 30 mEq., 12.5 ml. in
30 ml.; 40 mEq., 12.5 ml. in 30 ml. **Fliptop
Vials:** 20 mEq., 10 ml. in 20 ml.; 40 mEq., 20
ml. in 50 ml. **Univ. Add. Syr.:** 5 mEq./5 ml.,
20 mEq./10 ml., 30 mEq./20 ml., 40 mEq./20
ml. (Lilly) Amp. (40 mEq.) 20 ml., 6s, 25s.
Capsules:
See: Micro-K Extencaps, Cap. (Robins)
Liquid:
See: Cena-K, Liq. (Century)
Choice 10 and 20, Sol. (Whiteworth)
Kaochlor, Preps. (Adria)
Kaon-C1 20%, Liq. (Adria)
Kay Ciel, Elix. (Berlex)
Klor-10%, Liq. (Upsher-Smith)
Klor-Con, Liq. (Upsher-Smith)
Kloride, Eliz. (Fed. Pharm.)
Klorvess Liquid (Dorsey)
Klotrix, Tab. (Mead Johnson)
Klowess (Dorsey)
K-Lyte/C1, Tab. (Mead Johnson)
Pan-Kloride, Liq. (US. Products)
Potassine, Liq. (Recsei)
SK-Potassium Chloride, Sol. (SmithKline)
Taside, Liq. (Reid-Provident)
Powder:
See: Kaochlor-Eff, Gran. (Adria)
Kato Powder (Ingram)
Kay Ciel, Pow. (Berlex)
K-Lor, Pow. (Abbott)
K-Lyte/C1, Pow. (Mead Johnson)
Potage, Pow. (Lemmon)
Tablets:
See: Kaon Tablets, Tab. (Adria)
Kaon Controlled Release Tab. (Adria)
Klorvess Effervescent Tablets (Dorsey)
K-Tab, Tab. (Abbott)
Micro-K Extencaps (Robins)
Slow-K, Tab. (Ciba)

• **POTASSIUM CHLORIDE K 42.** USAN.
Use: Radioactive agent.

POTASSIUM CHLORIDE LIQUID. (Roxane)
Potassium chloride oral solution: 5%, 20 mEq./30
ml. Bot. pt., gal. 10%, 40 mEq./30 ml. Bot. 6 oz.,
pt., gal. 20%, 80 mEq./30 ml. Bot. pt., gal.
Pow: 20 mEq./4 Gm. Pkt. 30s, 100s.
Use: Hypopotassemia.

POTASSIUM CHLORIDE SOLUTION. (Lederle)
Potassium chloride 10%, 20%. Sugar free. Bot. 16
oz., gal.
Use: Hypopotassemia.

POTASSIUM CHLORIDE WITH POTASSIUM GLUCONATE.
See: Kolyum, Prod. (Pennwalt)
• **POTASSIUM CITRATE,** U.S.P. XXI. Tripotassium Citrate.
Use: Systemic alkalizer.
W/Sod. citrate.
See: Bicitra, Liq. (Willen)
W/Sod. citrate, citric acid.
See: Polycitra-K, Liq. (Willen)
Polycitra-LC, Liq. (Willen)
• **POTASSIUM CITRATE AND CITRIC ACID ORAL SOLUTION,** U.S.P. XXI.
POTASSIUM ESTRONE SULFATE.
W/Estrone.
See: Dura-Keelin, Vial (Pharmex)
Estro Plus, Inj. (Rocky Mtn.)
Ferntheelin, Vial (Ferndale)
Mer-Estrone, Inj. (Keene Pharm.)
Sodestrin, Inj. (Reid-Provident)
Spanestrin, Vial (Savage)
W/Estrone.
See: Gynlin R P. (Tunex)
W/Estrone, estradiol.
See: R.I.P. Estrone, Inj. (Vortech)
Tri-Oraphn (Standex)
W/Micro crystalline estrone.
See: Estrones Duo-Action, Vial (Med. Chem.)
• **POTASSIUM GLUCALDRATE.** USAN.
Use: Antacid.
• **POTASSIUM GLUCONATE,** U.S.P. XXI. Elixir, Tab., U.S.P. XXI. Monopotassium D-gluconate.
Use: Electrolyte replenisher.
See: Kalinate, Elix. (Bock)
Kaon, Elixir, Tab. (Warren-Teed)
POTASSIUM GLUCONATE ELIXIR. (Mills) Elemental potassium as potassium gluconate 20 mEq, base w/sorbitol soln./Tbs. Bot. 8 oz.
POTASSIUM GLUCONATE ELIXIR. (Philips Roxane, Lederle) Potassium 40 mEq. provided by potassium gluconate 9.36 Gm., alcohol 5%/30 ml. Bot. pt., Patient-Cup 15 ml.
Use: Replacement therapy.
POTASSIUM GLUTAMATE. The monopotassium salt of l-glutamic acid.
POTASSIUM G PENICILLIN.
See: Penicillin G Potassium, U.S.P. XXI.
• **POTASSIUM GUAIACOLSULFONATE,** U.S.P. XXI.
Sulfoguaiacol. Potassium Hydroxymethoxybenzenesulfonate. Used in many cough preps.
See: Conex, Liq. (Westerfield)
Pinex Regular, Syr. (Pinex)
POTASSIUM GUAIACOLSULFONATE W/COMBINATIONS.
See: Cerose, Liq. (Ives)
Cerose-DM, Liq. (Ives)
Cervo, Liq. (Sutliff & Case)
Cetro-Cirose, Liq. (Ives)
Cheralin Syrup, Syr. (Lannett)
Cherralex, Syr. (Barre)
Cidicol, Liq. (Upjohn)
Clistin, Expect., Liq. (McNeil)

Codel, Expect. (Elder)
Codimal DH Syr. (Central)
Codimal, DM Elix., Syr. (Central)
Codimal, PH Syr. (Central)
Coditrate, Syr., Tab. (Central)
DeWitt's Cough Control Medicine, Syr. (DeWitt)
Doverlyn Children, CT Choc., Tab. (Scrip)
Efricon Expect. (Lannett)
Eucapine Syrup, Syr. (Lannett)
Formadrin, Liq. (Kenyon)
Four Red, Liq. (Mallard)
Ganerphen, Preps. (Mason)
Gomahist, Inj. (Burgin-Arden)
Gomenol, Vial (Pharmex)
Guahist, Vial (Hickam)
Guaiadol Aqueous, Inj. (Med. Chem./Bush)
Guaicohist, Vial (Pharmex)
Guaiodol-Plus, Vial (Kenyon)
Guialyn, Preps. (Scrip)
Mallergan, Liq. (Mallard)
Palodyne, Cap. (Mallard)
Para-Hist DM, Tab. (Pharmics)
Para-Hist Antitussive, Syr. (Pharmics)
Partuss, Liq. (Parmed)
Phenergan, Prods. (Wyeth)
P-M-Z HCl, Expect. (Sutliff & Case)
Proclan, Preps. (Cenci)
Pro-Expectorant, Liq. (Scrip)
Special Cough Formula S.F. 17750 (Upjohn)
Turpoin, Tab. (Mallard)
Tusquelin, Syr. (Circle)
POTASSIUM HETACILLIN.
See: Versapen K, Inj., Cap. (Bristol)
• **POTASSIUM HYDROXIDE,** N.F. XVI.
Use: Pharm. aid (alkalinizing agent).
• **POTASSIUM IODIDE,** U.S.P. XXI. Tab., Oral Soln., U.S.P. XXI.
Use: Expectorant; antifungal; source of iodine.
See: KI-N, Tab. (Mallinckrodt)
Pima, Syr., Expect. (Fleming)
SSKI, Liq. (Upsher-Smith)
POTASSIUM IODIDE W/COMBINATIONS
See: Diastix, Reagent Strips (Ames)
Elixophyllin-KI, Elix. (Berlex)
Entex K.I., Tab. (Baylor Labs.)
Heliogen, Tab. (Brown)
Iodized Lime, Tab. (Elder)
Iodo-Niacin, Tab. (Cole)
Isuprel Compound, Elix. (Winthrop-Breon)
KIE, Syr., Tab. (Laser)
Kiophyllin, Tab. (Rorer)
L.S. Mixture, Liq. (Paddock)
Mudrane, Tab. (Plythress)
Mudrane-2, Tab. (Poythress)
Neo-Asmasan, Cap. (Recsei)
Quadrinal, Tab., Susp. (Knoll)
Ricor, Tab. (Vortech)
Theokin, Elix., Tab. (Knoll)
T.P.K.I., Tab. (Wendt-Bristol)
TSG Croup Liquid (Elder)
TSG-KI, Elix. (Elder)
POTASSIUM IODIDE AND NIACINAMIDE.
See: Iodo-Niacin, Tab. (Cole)

POTASSIUM MENAPHTHOSULPHATE. B.A.N.
Dipotassium   2-methyl-1,4-disulpnatonaphthalene.
Vikastab [dihydrate]
Use: Vitamin K analogue.
• **POTASSIUM METAPHOSPHATE,** N.F. XVI.
Use: Buffering agent.
POTASSIUM PENICILLIN G .
Use: Antibiotic.
See: Penicillin G, Potassium U.S.P. XXI.
POTASSIUM PENICILLIN V.
Use: Antibiotic.
See: Phenoxymethyl Penicillin Potassium, U.S.P. XXI.
POTASSIUM PERCHLORATE.
See: Perchloracap, Cap. (Mallinckrodt)
• **POTASSIUM PERMANGANATE,** U.S.P. XXI. Tab.
for Topical Soln., U.S.P. XXI. Permanganic acid,
potassium salt.
Use: Topical anti-infective.
POTASSIUM PHENETHICILLIN. Phenethicillin
Potassium, U.S.P. XXI.
Use: Antibiotic.
POTASSIUM PHENOXYMETHYL PENICILLIN.
Use: Antibiotic.
See: Penicillin V Potassium, U.S.P. XXI.
• **POTASSIUM PHOSPHATE, DIBASIC,** U.S.P. XXI.
Inj., U.S.P. XXI.
Use: Calcium regulator.
• **POTASSIUM PHOSPHATE, MONOBASIC,** N.F. XVI.
Dipotassium hydrogen phosphate. Solution by
Various Mfr. **Inj.:** (Abbott) 15 mM, 5 ml. in 10 ml.
Vial; 45m M, 15 ml. in 20 ml. Vial.
Use: Buffering agent, source of potassium.
POTASSIUM-REMOVING RESINS.
See: Kayexalate, Pow. (Winthrop-Breon)
POTASSIUM RHODANATE.
See: Pot. Thiocyanate
POTASSIUM SALICYLATE.
See: Neocylate, Tab. (Central)
W/Mephenesin, colchicine alkaloid.
W/Potassium bromide, methapyrilene HCl, vitamins.
See: Alva-Tranquil, Cap., Tab. & T.D. Tab. (Al-
va/Amco)
W/Potassium p-aminobenzoate.
See: Pabalate-SF, Tab. (Robins)
Pabasal N.S., Tab. (Wolins)
POTASSIUM SALT.
See: Potassium Sorbate, N.F. XVI.
• **POTASSIUM SODIUM TARTRATE,** U.S.P. XXI.
Use: Cathartic.
• **POTASSIUM SORBATE,** N.F. XVI. 2,4-Hexadienoic
Acid, Potassium Salt.
Use: Preservative (antimicrobial).
POTASSIUM SULFOCYANATE. Pot. Rhodanate.
See: Pot. Thiocyanate (Var. Mfr.)
POTASSIUM THERAPY.
See: Kaon, Elixir, Tab. (Warren-Teed)
Potassium Chloride, Preps. (Various Mfr.)
POTASSIUM THIOCYANATE. Pot. sulfocyanate, Pot.
Rhodanate.
POTASSIUM THIPHENCILLIN. Potassium 6-(phenyl-
mercaptoacetamido)penicillanate.
Use: Antibiotic.

POTASSIUM TROCLOSENE. (Monsanto) Potassium
dichloroisocyanurate. Dichloro-s-triazine-
2,4,6(1H,3H,5H)trione Potassium derivative.
Use: Local anti-infective.
• **POTASSIUM, WARFARIN,** U.S.P. XXI. Tab., U.S.P.
XXI. Potassium 3-(α-acetonylbenzyl)-4-hydrox-
ycoumarin, Potassium Salt. Athrombin-K.
Use: Anticoagulant.
See: Athrombin-K, Tab. (Purdue-Frederick)
POVAN TABLETS. (Parke-Davis) Pyrvinium pamoate
50 mg./Tab. Bot. 50s.
Use: Control of pinworm infections.
POVIDERM OINTMENT. (Vortech) Povidone-Iodide
10% in ointment base. Tube 1 oz. Jar 1 lb.
Use: Antiseptic ointment.
POVIDERM SOLUTION. (Vortech) Povidone-Iodide 7.-
5%, in liquid base. Bot. pt., Gal.
Use: Antiseptic solution.
POVIDERM SURGICAL SCRUB. (Vortech) Povidone-
Iodine 5% in liquid base. Bot. 16 oz., Gal.
Use: Antiseptic scrub solution.
• **POVIDONE,** U.S.P. XXI. 2-Pyrrolidinone, 1-ethyl,
homopolymer.
Use: Dispersing & suspending agent.
• **POVIDONE I-125.** USAN.
Use: Pharmaceutic aid.
• **POVIDONE I-131.** USAN.
Use: Radioactive agent.
• **POVIDONE-IODINE,** U.S.P. XXI., Topical Aerosol
Soln., Oint., Cleansing Sol., Topical Soln., U.S.P. XXI.
Poly(1-(2-oxo-1-pyrrolidinyl)-ethylene) Iodine Com-
plex.
Use: Local anti-infective.
See: Betadine, Preps. (Purdue-Fredrick)
BPS, Preps. (AVP)
Efo-Dine (Fougera)
Femidine, Liq. (AVP)
Isodine, Preps. (Blair)
POVIDONE-IODINE COMPLEX.
See: Betadine, Prep. (Purdue-Frederick)
Isodine, Preps. (Blair)
POVI-DOUCHE. (Vortech) Povidone-iodine 7.5%
solution. Bot. 240 ml.
Use: Cleansing douche.
POWERS' ASTHMA RELIEF. (Guild) Bot. 4 oz.
POXY COMPOUND-65. (Sutliff & Case) Propoxyphene
HCl 65 mg., aspirin 227 mg., phenacetin 162 mg.,
caffeine 32.5 mg./Cap. Bot. 100s, 1000s.
POYALIVER STRONGER. (Fellows) Liver inj. (eqv. 10
mcg. B-12) Vit. B-12 100 mcg., folic acid 10 mcg.,
niacinamide 1%/cc. Vial 10 cc.
POYAMIN. (Fellows) Vit. B-12 1000 mcg./cc. Vial 10 cc.,
30 cc.
Use: Hematopoietic.
POYAMIN JEL INJECTION. (Fellows)
Cyanocobalamin 1000 mcg./cc. Vial 10 cc.
POYAPLEX. (Fellows) Vit. B-1 100 mg., niacinamide
100 mg., B-6 10 mg., B-2 1 mg., panthenol 10 mg.,
B-12 5 mcg./cc. Vial 10 cc. & 30 cc.
P.P.D. TUBERCULIN.
See: Tuberculin, Purified Protein Derivative, U.S.P.
(Various Mfr.)

P.P. FACTOR (PELLAGRA PREVENTIVE FACTOR).
See: Nicotinic Acid, Preps. (Var. Mfr.)
• **PPG-15 STEARYL ETHER.** USAN.
Use: Pharmaceutic aid (surfactant).
P.R. (Faraday) Acetyl-p-aminophenol 5 gr./Tab. Bot.
30s.
Use: Pain relief.
• **PRACTOLOL.** USAN. 4'-[2-Hydroxy-3-(iso-
propylamino)propoxy]acetanilide.
Use: Antiadrenergic (β-receptors).
PRAENITRONA. Trolnitrate Phosphate, B.A.N.
PRAGMATAR. (Menley & James) Cetyl alcohol-coal tar
distillate 4%, precipitated sulfur 3%, salicylic acid
3% in oil-in-water type emulsion base. Tube 1 oz.
Use: Skin disorders.
PRAJMALIUM BITARTRATE. B.A.N. N-Propylaj-
malinium hydrogen tartrate.
Use: Treatment of heart arrhythmias.
PRALIDOXIME. B.A.N. 2-Hydroxyiminomethyl-1-me-
thylpyridinium.
Use: Antagonist to cholinesterase inhibitors.
• **PRALIDOXIME CHLORIDE,** U.S.P. XXI. Sterile,
Tabs: U.S.P. XXI. Pyridinium, 2-[(hydroxyimino)me-
thyl]-1-methyl-,chloride. 2-Formyl-1-methylpyridinium
Chloride Oxime. Pam.
Use: Anticholinergic.
See: Protopam Chloride, Tab., Vial (Ayerst)
• **PRALIDOXIME IODIDE.** USAN. 2-Pyridine aldoxime
methiodide.
Use: Cholinesterase reactivator.
See: Protopam Iodide (Ayerst)
• **PRALIDOXIME MESYLATE.** USAN.
Use: Cholinesterase reactivator.
PRALIDOXIME METHIODIDE.
See: Pralidoxime Iodide (Var. Mfr.)
PRAMET FA. (Ross) Vit. A 4000 I.U., D-2 400 I.U., C 100
mg., B-1 3 mg., B-2 2 mg., B-6 5 mg., B-12 3 mcg., B-
3 10 mg., d-Calcium pantothenate 0.92 mg., iodine
100 mcg., calcium 250 mg., copper 0.15 mg., Iron
60 mg., Folic acid 1 mg./Gradumet. Bot. 100s.
Use: Prenatal vitamin/mineral supplement & for
treatment of megaloblastic anemias of pregnancy.
PRAMILET FA. (Ross) Vit. A 4000 I.U.; B-1 3 mg.;
B-2 2 mg.; B-6 3 mg.; B-12 3 mcg.; C 60 mg.; D
400 I.U.; Ca panthothenate 1 mg.; niacinamide 10
mg.; Ca 250 mg.; Cu 0.15 mg.; iodine 0.1 mg.; Fe
40 mg.; Mg 10 mg.; Zn 0.085 mg.; folic acid 1.0
mg./Filmtab. Bot. 100s.
Use: Prenatal vitamin/mineral supplement & for
treatment of megaloblastic anemias of pregnancy.
PRAMINIL. Imipramine, B.A.N.
PRAMIVERINE. B.A.N. 4,4-Diphenyl-N-isopropylcy-
clohexylamine.
Use: Spasmolytic.
PRAMOCAINE (I.N.N.). Pramoxine, B.A.N.
Use: Allergic dermatitis.
PRAMOSONE CREAM 0.5%. (Ferndale)
Hydrocortisone acetate 0.5%, pramoxine HCl 1% in
cream base. Tube 1 oz., Jar 1 lb.
Use: Anti-inflammatory, anti-pruritic.
PRAMOSONE CREAM 1%. (Ferndale)

Hydrocortisone acetate 1%, pramoxine HCl 1% in
cream base. Tube 1 oz. Jar. 1 lb.
Use: Anti-inflammatory, anti-pruritic.
PRAMOSONE CREAM 2.5%. (Ferndale)
Hydrocortisone acetate 2.5%, pramoxine HCl 1% in
cream base. Tubes 1 oz., 4 oz. Jar 1 lb.
Use: Anti-inflammatory, anti-pruritic.
PRAMOSONE LOTION 0.5%. (Ferndale)
Hydrocortisone acetate 0.5%, pramoxine HCl 1% in
lotion base. Bot. 1.5 oz., 4 oz., 8 oz., gal.
Use: Anti-inflammatory, anti-pruritic.
PRAMOSONE LOTION 1%. (Ferndale)
Hydrocortisone acetate 1%, pramoxine HCl 1% in
lotion base. Bot. 1.25 oz., 4 oz., 8 oz.
Use: Anti-pruritic.
PRAMOSONE LOTION 2.5%. (Ferndale)
Hydrocortisone acetate 2.5%, pramoxine HCl 1% in
lotion base. Bot 2 oz., gal.
Use: Anti-inflammatory, anti-pruritic.
PRAMOSONE OINTMENT 1%. (Ferndale)
Hydrocortisone acetate 1%, pramoxine HCl 1% in
ointment base. Tube 1 oz., Jar 1 lb.
Use: Anti-inflammatory, anti-pruritic.
PRAMOXINE. B.A.N. 4-[3-(4-Butoxyphenoxy)-propyl]-
morpholine. Pramocaine (I.N.N.)
Use: Local anesthetic.
• **PRAMOXINE HYDROCHLORIDE,** U.S.P. XXI.
Cream, Jelly, U.S.P. XXI. 4-[3-(p-Butoxyphenoxy)-
propyl]morpholine HCl.
Use: Local anesthetic.
See: Prax, Lotion (Ferndale)
Proctofoam, Aero. (Reed & Carnrick)
Tronothane HCl, Cream, Jel (Abbott)
oil, citric acid, natural & artificial flavors, mono
PRAMOXINE HCl W/COMBINATIONS
See: Anti-Itch, Lot. (Towne)
Anugesic, Oint., Supp. (Parke-Davis)
Dermarex, Cream (Hyrex)
Drotic No. 2, Drops (Ascher)
Gentz, Jelly, Wipes (Philips Roxane)
My Cort Otic #2, Ear Drops (Scrip)
1 + 1 Creme, 1 + 1-F Creme (Dunhall)
Orlex HC, Otic (Baylor)
Otocalm-H Ear Drops (Parmed)
Oto Drops (Reid-Provident)
Perifoam, Aerosol (Rowell Labs.)
Proctofoam-HC, Aerosol (Reed-Carnrick)
Quada-Creme, Cream (Sutliff & Case)
Quinsone, Cream (Sutliff & Case)
Sherform-HC, Oint. (Sheryl)
Steraform Creme (Mayrand)
Steramine Otic, Drops (Mayrand)
V-Cort, Cream (Scrip)
PRAMPINE. B.A.N. O-Propionylatropine, PAMN me-
thonitrate.
Use: Treatment of peptic ulcer.
• **PRANOLIUM CHLORIDE.** USAN.
Use: Cardiac depressant.
PRANTAL. (Schering) Diphemanil methylsulfate 100
mg./Tab. Bot. 100s.
Use: Anticholinergic.

PRAX CREAM. (Ferndale) Pramoxine HCl 1% in cream base. Tubes 1 oz. Jars 4 oz., 1 lb.
Use: Anti-pruritic.
PRAX LOTION. (Ferndale) Pramoxine HCl 1.0%. Bot. 15 ml., 120 ml.
Use: Anti-pruritic.
PRAXILENE OXALATE. Naftidrofuryl, B.A.N.
• **PRAZEPAM,** U.S.P. XXI. Cap., Tab. U.S.P. XXI. 7-Chloro-1-(cyclopropylmethyl)-1,2-dihydro-5-phenyl-2H-1, 4-benzodiazepin-2-one.
Use: Muscle relaxant.
See: Centrax, Cap. (Parke-Davis)
Vestran, Cap. (Parke-Davis)
• **PRAZIQUANTEL.** USAN. 2-Cyclohexylcarbonyl-1,3,4,6,7,11b-hexahydro-2H-pyrazino[2,1-a]-isoquinolin-4-one.
Use: Anthelmintic.
PRAZITONE. B.A.N. 5-Phenyl-5-(2-piperidyl)-methylbarbituric acid.
Use: Antidepressant.
PRAZOSIN. B.A.N. 1-(4-Amino-6,7-dimethoxy-quinazolin-2-yl)-4-(2-furyol)piperazine.
Use: Antihypertensive.
W/Polythiazide.
See: Minizide, Cap, (Pfizer Laboratories)
• **PRAZOSIN HYDROCHLORIDE,** U.S.P. XXI. Cap., U.S.P. XXI. 1-(4-Amino-6,7-dimethoxy-2-quinazoliny)-4-(2-furoyl)piperazine monohydrochloride.
Use: Antihypertensive.
See: Minipress, Cap. (Pfizer Laboratories)
PRE-17. (Standex) Vit. A 4,000 I.U., D 400 I.U., B-1 1.5 mg., B-2 2 mg., B-6 2 mg., B-12 2 mcg., C 50 mg., niacinamide 10 mg., Ca pantothenate 5 mg., Folic acid 8 mg., Fe 40 mg., calcium carbonate 240 mg./Tab. Bot. 100s.
PRECISION HIGH NITROGEN DIET. (Doyle) Citrus Fruit Flavor: Maltodextrin, pasteurized egg white solids, sucrose, natural & artificial flavors, medium chain triglycerides, citric acid, partially hydrogenated soybean oil, polysorbate 80, mono & diglycerides, FD& C Yellow No. 5 and No. 6, vitamins & minerals. Powder 2.93 oz. Packets.
Use: Total or supplemental feeding, oral or tube.
PRECISION ISOTONIC DIET. (Doyle) Vanilla Flavor: Maltelextrin egg white solids, sucrose, partially hydrogenated soybean oil with BHA, natural and artificial flavor, sodium caseinate, citric acid, carrageenan, mono and diglycerides, vitamins and minerals. Individual Packets, 2.06 oz.
Use: Total or supplemental feeding, oral or tube.
PRECISION LR DIET. (Doyle) Orange Flavor: Maltodextrin, pasteurized egg white solids, sucrose, medium chain triglycerides, partially hydrogenated soybean oil with BHA, citric acid, natural and artificial flavors, mono and diglycerides, polysorbate 80, FD & C Yellow No.5 and No. 6, vitamins and minerals. Powder in 3 oz. packets.
Use: Total or supplemental feedings, oral or tube.
PRECORTISYL. Prednisolone, B.A.N.
PRED-5. (Saron) Prednisone 5 mg./Tab. Bot. 100s, 1000s.

PRED-A 50. (Tunex) Prednisolone acetate 50 mg./ml. Vial 10cc.
Use: Intra-articular inj.; adrenocortical insufficiency.
PRED-A 100. (Tunex) Prednisolone acetate 100 mg./ml. Vial 10cc.
Use: Intra-articular inj.; adrenocortical insufficiency.
PREDAJECT. (Mayrand) Prednisolone acetate 50 mg./ml. Vial 10 ml.
Use: Longacting anti-inflammatory, corticosteroid.
PREDALONE R.P. (O'Neal, Jones & Feldman) Prednisolone sodium phosphate 20 mg., prednisolone acetate 80 mg./ml. Vial 5 ml.
PREDALONE T.B.A. (O'Neal, Jones & Feldman) Prednisolone tebutate 20 mg./ml. in aqueous suspension. Vial 5 ml.
PREDAMIDE OPHTHALMIC. (Maurry) Sodium sulfacetamide 10%, prednisolone acetate 0.5%, hydroxyethylcellulose, polysobate 80, sodium thiosulfate, sodium phosphate, edetate disodium, benzalkonium Cl 0.025%. Bot. 5 ml.
Use: Anti-inflammatory, anti-bacterial.
PRED-FORTE. (Allergan) Prednisolone acetate 1%, w/benzalkonium Cl, polysorbate 80, boric acid, sod. citrate, sod. bisulfite, NaCl, edetate disodium, hydroxypropyl methylcellulose, purified water. Plastic Dropper Bot. 5 ml., 10 ml., 15 ml.
Use: Ocular anti-inflammatory.
PREDICORT-50. (Dunhall) Prednisolone acetate 50 mg./ml. Vial 10 ml.
Use: Anti-inflammatory, steroid.
PREDICORT-AP. (Dunhall) Prednisolone sodium phosphate 20 mg., prednisolone acetate 80 mg./ml. Vial 10 ml.
Use: Anti-inflammatory, steroid.
PREDICORT-RP. (Dunhall) Prednisolone sodium phosphate equivalent to prednisolone phosphate 20 mg., niacinamide 25 mg./ml. Vial 10 ml.
Use: Short-acting steroid.
PRED MILD. (Allergan) Prednisolone acetate 0.12% w/benzalkonium Cl, polysorbate 80, boric acid, sodium citrate, sodium bisulfite, NaCl, edetate disodium, hydroxypropyl methylcellulose, purified water. Bot. 5 ml., 10 ml.
Use: Ocular anti-inflammatory.
• **PREDNAZATE.** USAN.
Use: Anti-inflammatory.
PREDNELAN ACETATE. Prednisolone, B.A.N.
• **PREDNICARBATE.** USAN.
Use: Glucocorticoid.
PREDNICEN-M. (Central) Prednisone 5 mg./Tab. Bot. 100s, 1000s.
• **PREDNIMUSTINE.** USAN.
Use: Antineoplastic.
PREDNISOLAMATE. B.A.N. Prednisolone 21-diethylaminoacetate. Deltacortril DA hydrochloride.
Use: Corticosteroid.
• **PREDNISOLONE,** U.S.P. XXI. Cream, Tab., U.S.P. XXI. Pregna-1,4-diene-3,20-dione, 11,17,21-trihydroxy-, (11β)- 11β,17,21-Trihydroxypregna-1,4-diene-3,20 dione. Metacortandralone.
Use: Adrenocortical steroid (anti-inflammatory).

See: Cordrol, Tabs. (Vita Elixir)
Delta-Cortef, Tab. (Upjohn)
Fernisolone, Tab., Inj. (Ferndale)
Orasone, Tab. (Rowell)
Orasone 50, Tab. (Rowell)
Panisolone, Tab. (Panray)
Prednis, Tab. (USV Labs.)
Ster 5, Tab. (Scrip)
Sterane Injection, Vial (Pfizer Laboratories)
Sterane Tablets, Tab. (Pfipharmecs)
Ulacort, Tab. (Fellows-Testagar)
W/Aluminum hydroxide gel, dried.
See: Predoxide, Tab. (Mallard)
W/Aspirin.
See: Sarogesic, Tab. (Saron)
W/Chloramphenicol.
See: Chloroptic-P, Ophth. Oint. (Allergan)
W/Hydroxyzine HCl.
W/Neomycin sulfate.
Neo-Deltef, Drops (Upjohn)
W/Sulfacetamide sodium, methylcellulose.
See: Isopto Cetapred, Susp. (Alcon)
W/Sulfacetamide sodium.
See: Cetapred Ophthalmic Oint. (Alcon)
• **PREDNISOLONE ACETATE,** U.S.P. XXI. Sterile
Susp., U.S.P. XXI. Pregna-1,4-diene-3,20-dione, 21-
(acetyloxy)-11,17-dihydroxy-,(11β)-
Use: Adrenocortical steroid (anti-inflammatory).
Durapred Injection (Amfre-Grant)
Econopred, Susp. (Alcon)
Key-Pred, Inj. (Hyrex)
Nisolone, Vial (Ascher)
Pred-A 50, Inj. (Tunex)
Pred-A 100, Inj. (Tunex)
Predicort, Amp. (Dunhall)
Pred Preps. (Allergan)
Pred-Forte, Ophth. Susp. (Allergan)
Savacort-50, 100, Vial (Savage)
Sigpred, Inj. (Sig)
Steraject, Vial (Mayrand)
Sterane, Inj. (Pfizer Laboratories)
Ulacort, Inj. (Fellows-Testagar)
PREDNISOLONE ACETATE W/COMBINATIONS
See: Blephamide Liquifilm, Sol. (Allergan)
Blephamide S.O.P., Ophth, Oint. (Allergan)
Cetapred Opth. Oint. (Alcon)
Dua-Pred, Inj. (Reid-Provident)
Metimyd, Ophth. Susp., Oint. (Schering)
Neo-Delta-Cortef, Preps. (Upjohn)
Panacort R-P, Vial (Ferndale)
Prednefrin, Mild, Susp. (Allergan)
Predulose Bufopto, Sol. (Softcon)
Sulfapred, Susp. (Softcon)
Tri-Ophtho, Ophth. (Maurry)
Vasocidin Preps. (CooperVision)
PREDNISOLONE BUTYLACETATE. 1,4-Pregnadiene-
3,20-dione-11β,17α,21-triol-tert-butyl-acetate.
See: Hydeltra-T.B.A., Vial (Merck Sharp & Dohme)
PREDNISOLONE CYCLOPENTYLPROPIONATE.
d^1,4-Pregnadiene-3,20-dione-11, 17a-diol-21-cy-
clopentylpropionate(prednisolone-21-cyclopentylpro-
pionate).

• **PREDNISOLONE HEMISUCCINATE,** U.S.P. XXI.
Pregna-1,4-diene-3,20-dione,   21-(3-carboxy-1-oxo-
propoxy)-11, 17-dihydroxy-, (11β) −.
Use: Adrenocortical steroid (anti-inflammatory).
• **PREDNISOLONE SODIUM PHOSPHATE,** U.S.P.
XXI. Inj., Ophth. Sol.: U.S.P. XXI. Pregna-1,4-diene-
3,20-dione, 11,17-dihydroxy-21-(phosphonoxy)-,
disodium salt, (11)-.
Use: Adrenocortical steroid (anti-inflammatory).
See: Alto-Pred Soluble, Vial (Alto)
Hydeltrasol, Ophth. Sol., Ophth. Oint., Inj. (Merck
Sharp & Dohme)
Hydeltrone (MSD AGVET)
Hydrosol, Inj. (Rocky Mtn.)
Inflamase Forte Ophthalmic Solution
(CooperVision)
Inflamase Ophth. Solution (CooperVision)
Key-Pred SP, Inj. (Hyrex)
Liquid Pred, Inj. (Muro)
Metreton, Ophth. Sol. Sterile (Schering)
Nor-Preds, Inj. (Vortech)
P.S.P. IV (Four), Inj. (Reid-Provident)
Savacort-S, Inj. (Savage)
Sodasone, Inj. (Fellows Testagar)
Sol-Pred, Inj. (Amfre-Grant)
W/Neomycin sulf.
See: Neo-Hydeltrasol, Ophth. Sol., Ophth. Oint.
(Merck Sharp & Dohme)
W/Niacinamide, disodium edetate, sodium bisulfite,
phenol.
See: P.S.P. IV, Inj. (Reid-Provident)
W/Prednisolone acetate.
See: Panacort R-P, Vial (Ferndale)
Solu-Pred, Vial (Kenyon)
W/Sodium Sulfacetamide.
See: Optimyd, Sol. (Schering)
Vasocidin, Liq. (CooperVision)
• **PREDINISOLONE SODIUM SUCCINATE FOR
INJECTION,** U.S.P. XXI. Pregna-1,4-diene-3-20-
dione,21-(3-carboxy-1-oxopropoxy)-11,17-dihydroxy-
monosodium salt, (11β)−. A hemisuccinate.
Use: Adrenocortical steroid (anti-inflammatory).
PREDNISOLONE TERTIARY-BUTYLACETATE.
See: Prednisolone Tebutate, U.S.P. XXI.
PREDNISOL T.B.A.. (Pasadena Research; Medwick)
Prednisolone tertiary butylacetate 20 mg./ml. Vial
10 cc.
• **PREDNISOLONE TEBUTATE SUSPENSION,
STERILE,** U.S.P. XXI. Pregna-1,4-diene-3,20-dione,
11,17-dihydroxy-21-(3,3-dimethyl-1-oxobutyl)oxy-,
(11β)−.
Use: Adrenocorticol steroid.
See: Durapred T.B.A. Injection (Amfre-Grant)
Hydeltra-T.B.A., Vial (Merck Sharp & Dohme)
Hydeltrone—T.B.A. (MSD AGVET)
Metalone, Vial (Foy)
Rodelta T.B.A., Inj. (Rocky Mtn.)
• **PREDNISONE,** U.S.P. XXI. Tabs., U.S.P. XXI.
Pregna-1,4-diene-3,11,20-trione, 17,21-dihydroxy-. Δ
1,4-Pregnadiene-17α,21-diol-3,11-20-trione. 1-Dehy-
dro-cortisone, Metacortandracin. 17,21-Dihydroxy-
pregna-1,4-diene-3,11,20-trione.

Use: Adrenocortical steroid (anti-inflammatory)
See: Delta-Dome Tab.(Miles Pharm)
  Deltasone, Tab. (Upjohn)
  Keysone, Tab. (Hyrex)
  Lisacort, Tab. (Fellows-Testagar)
  Meticorten, Tab. (Schering)
  Maso-Pred, Tab. (Mason)
  Orasone, Tab. (Rowell)
  Pan-Sone, Tab. (Panray)
  Pred-5 (Saron)
  Ropred, Tab. (Robinson)
  Sarogesic, Tab. (Saron)
  SK-Prednisone, Tab. (SmithKline)
  Sterapred, Tab. (Mayrand)
W/Chlorpheniramine maleate.
  See: Histone, Tab. (Blaine)
W/Phenylephrine HCl.
  See: Prednefrin-S, Sol. (Allergan)
• **PREDNIVAL.** USAN. 11 beta, 17, 21-Trihydroxypregna-1,4-diene-3,20-dione 17 valerate. Under study.
Use: Topical anti-inflammatory.
PREDNYLIDENE. B.A.N. $11\beta,17\alpha,21$-Trihydroxy-16-methylenepregna-1,4-diene-3,20-dione. Dacortilene; Decortilen.
Use: Corticosteroid.
PREDSOL DISODIUM PHOSPHATE. Prednisolone, B.A.N.
PREDULOSE. (Softcon) Prednisolone acetate 0.25%, phenylephrine HCl 0.125%, w/methyl-cellulose, methylparaben 0.04%, propylparaben 0.02%, propylene glycol, monobasic sod. phosphate, dibasic sod. phosphate, sod. thiosulfate, & polysorbate 80. Bot. 5 cc.
Use: Mild allergic & non-infectious inflammatory eye disorders.
PREFLEX. (Alcon) Isotonic, aqueous sol. of sodium phosphates, sodium chloride tyloxapol, hydroxyethylcellulose, polyvinyl alcohol. Bot. 1.5 oz.
Use: Soft contact lenses cleaning sol.
PREFRIN LIQUIFILM. (Allergan) Phenylephrine HCl 0.12%, polyvinyl alcohol 1.4%. Bot. 0.7 fl. oz.
Use: Ocular decongestant.
PREFRIN-A. (Allergan) Phenylephrine 0.12%, pyrilamine maleate 0.1%, antipyrine 0.1% w/benzalkonium chloride, sodium bisulfite, sodium citrate, boric acid, edetate disodium, purified water. Dropper Bot. 15 ml.
Use: Ocular antihistamine, decongestant.
PREFRIN-Z LIQUIFILM. (Allergan) Zinc sulfate 0.25%, phenylephrine HCl 0.12%. polyvinyl alcohol 1.4%. Bot. 0.5 fl. oz.
Use: Astringent; decongestant ophthalmic solution.
PREGESTIMIL. (Mead Johnson) Protein hydrolysate formula supplies 640 calories/qt. w/18 Gm. protein, 26 Gm. fat, 86 Gm. carbohydrate, vitamins and minerals. (Vit. A 2000 I.U., D 400 I.U., E 15 I.U., C 52 mg., folic acid 100 mcg., thiamine 0.5 mg., riboflavin 0.6 mg., niacin 8 mg., B-6 0.4 mg., B-12 2 mcg., biotin 0.05 mg., pantothenic acid 3 mg., K-1 100 mcg., choline 85 mg., inositol 30 mg., Ca 600 mg., P 400 mg., iodine 45 mcg., Fe 12 mg., Mg 70 mg.,

Cu 0.6 mg., Zn 4 mg., Mn 0.2 mg., chloride 550 mg., K 700 mg., Na 300 mg.)/Qt. (20 kcal/fl. oz.); Powder, cans 1 lb.
Use: Complete nutritionally balanced lactose-free hypoallergenic infant diet with readily digestible sources of protein, fat, and carbohydrate.
PREGNENINOLONE.
See: Ethisterone.
• **PREGNENOLONE.** F.D.A. 3-beta-Hydroxypregn-5-en-20-one. Synthetic steroid intermediate. 3-Hydroxy-20-keto-pregene-5.
Use: Treatment of rheumatoid arthritis.
• **PREGNENOLONE SUCCINATE.** USAN. 3-Hydroxy-5-pregnen-20-one, hydrogen succinate.
Use: Glucocorticoid.
PREGNOSIS SLIDE TEST. (Roche) Two-minute indirect test for pregnancy. 10, 50 tests.
PREGNYL. (Organon) Human chorionic gonadatrophin. Vial 10,000 I.U./Vial w/diluent. Vial 10 ml.
Use: I.M., crytorchidism, induction of ovulation & pregnancy in anovulatory women.
PRE-INE. (Kay) Chorionic gonadotropin 10,000 I.U./Vial to be prepared. Multiple dose vial 10 cc. w/diluent.
PREJECT PREINJECTION TOPICAL ANESTHETIC. (Hoyt) Benzocaine 20% in polyethelyne glycol base. Jar 2 oz.
Use: Avoid discomfort of oral injection.
PRELAN. (Lannett) Vit. A 4000 I.U., B-1 0.5 mg., B-2 2 mg., niacin 10 mg., B-6 3 mg., B-12 2 mcg., D 400 I.U., C 50 mg., Ca 200 mg., Fe 30 mg./Tab. Bot. 100s.
Use: Prenatal Vitamin-mineral supplementation.
PRELAN F.A. TABLETS. (Lannett) Vit. A 4,000 I.U., B-1 0.5 mg., B-2 2.0 mg., niacin 10.0 mg., B-6 3.0 mg., B-12 2.0 mcg., D 400 I.U., C 50 mg., calcium 200 mg., iron 30 mg., folic acid 1 mg./Tab. Bot. 100s.
Use: Prenatal vitamin and mineral supplement.
PRELESTRIN. (Pasadena Research) Conjugated estrogens 0.625 mg., 1.25 mg./Tab. Bot. 100s, 1000s.
PRELMYCIN. (Pasadena Research) Tetracycline HCl 250 mg./Cap. Bot. 16s, 25s.
PRELTRON. (Pasadena Research) Sodium glucuronate 200 mg., 500 mg./2 cc. Amp. 25s, 100s.
PRELTRON-ORAL. (Pasadena Research) Glucuronolactone 335 mg./Tab. Bot. 100s, 1000s.
PRELU-2. (Boehringer Ingelheim) Phendimetrazine tartrate 105 mg./Cap. Bot. 100s.
Use: Anorexiant.
PRELUDIN. (Boehringer Ingelheim) Phenmetrazine HCl. **Tab.** 25 mg., Bot. 100s. **Endurets** 75 mg. Bot. 100s.
Use: Anorexiant.
PRELUS ELIXIR. (Winthrop Products) Isoproterenol HCl.
Use: Bronchodilator.
PREMARIN. (Ayerst) Conjugated Estrogens Tablets. Water-soluble conjugated estrogens derived from natural sources. 0.3 mg., 0.625 mg., 0.9 mg., 1.25

mg., or 2.5 mg./Tab. Bot. 100s, 1000s. 0.625 mg.,
1.25 mg. Unit Dose 100s. Cycle packs 21s.
Use: Moderate to severe vasomotor symptoms,
atropohic vaginitis, kraurosis vulvae, female
hypogonadism, etc.
PREMARIN INTRAVENOUS. (Ayerst) Conjugated
Estrogens U.S.P., for Injection. Vial 25 mg./5 ml.
w/diluent. (Vial also contains lactose 200 mg., sod.
citrate 12.5 mg., simethicone 0.2 mg. Diluent
contains benzyl alcohol 2%, Water for Injection,
U.S.P.
Use: Treatment of abnormal uterine bleeding due
to hormonal imbalance in absence of organic
pathology.
PREMARIN VAGINAL CREAM. (Ayerst) Conjugated
Estrogens, U.S.P. 0.625 mg./1 Gm. w/cetyl esters
wax, cetyl alcohol, white wax, glyceryl
monostearate, propylene glycol monostearate,
methyl stearate, phenylethyl alcohol, sod. lauryl
sulfate, glycerin, mineral oil. Tube w/applicator 1½
oz. (42.5 Gm.). Tube refill.
Use: Treatment of atrophic vaginitis & kraurosis
vulvae.
PREMARIN W/MEPROBAMATE.
See: PMB-200 & 400, Tab. (Ayerst)
PREMARIN W/METHYLTESTOSTERONE. (Ayerst)
Premarin (Conjugated Estrogens, U.S.P.) 1.25 mg.,
methyltestosterone 10 mg./Yellow Tab. Premarin
0.625 mg., methyltestosterone 5 mg./Red Tab. Bot.
100s, 1000s.
Use: Moderate to severe vasomotor symptoms
associated with menopause in those patients not
improved by estrogens alone, postpartum breast
engorgement.
W/Methyltestosterone, methamphetamine HCl &
vitamins.
See: Mediatric, Cap., Liq., Tab. (Ayerst)
■ **PREMENSTRUAL TENSION.**
See: Motion Sickness
Pamabrom (Various Mfr.)
Pyranisamine Bromotheophyllinate (Various Mfr.)
PREMESYN PMS. (Chattem Labs.) Pamabrom 25
mg., acetaminophen 500 mg., pyrilamine maleate
15 mg./Cap. Bot. 16s, 32s.
Use: Treatment of menstrual and premenstrual
symptoms.
• **PRENALTEROL HYDROCHLORIDE.** USAN.
Use: Adrenergic.
PRENATAL. (Kenyon) Vit. A 100 I.U., D 500 I.U., B-1
1 mg., C 25 mg., B-2 1 mg., niacinamide 3 mg., Fe
39 mg., Ca 140 mg., P 62 mg., pot. iodide 0.065
mg., Cu sulfate 1 mg., Co sulfate 1 mg., Mg oxide
10 mg., Mn sulfate 14 mg., K sulfate 11 mg., Na
sulfate 0.40 mg., Zn oxide 0.40 mg., fluoride 1
mg./Tab. Bot. 100s, 1000s.
Use: Vitamin supplement.
PRENATAL NO. 2. (Kenyon) Vit. A 4000 I.U., B-1 2 mg.,
B-2 2 mg., B-6 0.8 mg., C 50 mg., niacinamide 10 mg.,
iodide 0.15 mg., folic acid 0.1 mg., B-12 conc. 2 mcg.,
iron 50 mg., calcium 240 mg./Cap. Bot. 100s, 1000s.
Use: Vitamin supplement.
PRENATE 90. (Bock) Vit. A 8000 I.U., D 400 I.U., E

30 I.U., C 120 mg., folic acid 1 mg., B-1 3 mg., B-2
3.4 mg., B-6 12 mg., B-12 12 mcg. niacinamide 20
mg., docusate sodium 50 mg., Ca 250 mg., iodine
0.15 mg., Fe 90 mg., Mg 100 mg., Cu 2 mg., Zn 15
mg./Film Coated Tab. Bot. 100s, 1000s.
Use: Multivitamin, multimineral.
PRENEX. (Coastal) Vit. A 500 I.U., D 400 I.U., B-1 3 mg.,
B-2 3 mg., B-6 10 mg., B-12 3 mcg., niacinamide 20
mg., d-calcium panthothenate 3.3 mg., Fe 42 mg., Ca
350 mg., Mn 0.33 mg., Zn 0.1 mg., Mg 0.67 mg., K
1.67 mg./Tab.
Use: Vitamin and mineral supplement.
PRENISTAT. (Pharmex) Prednisolone sod. phosphate
20 mg., niacinamide 25 mg./cc. Vial 10 cc.
• **PRENYLAMINE.** USAN. N-(3,3-Diphenylpropyl)-α-me-
thylphenethylamine. Segontin; Synadrin lactate.
Use: Coronary vasodilator.
PREPARATION H. (Whitehall) Phenylmercuric nitrate
1:10,000, live yeast cell derivative 2000 u. skin
respiratory factor, shark liver oil 3%. Oint. Tube 1
oz., 2 oz. Supp. 12s, 24s, 48s.
Use: Hemorrhoids.
PREPCORT CREAM. (Whitehall) Hydrocortisone
0.5%. Tube ½ oz., 1 oz.
Use: Topical corticosteroid.
PRE-PEN. (Rorer) Benzylpenicilloylpolylysine in phos-
phate buffer w/sod. chloride. Amp. 0.25 ml. Single
dose, sufficient for scratch and intra-dermal testing
only, 5s.
Use: Skin test reagent for the detection of
penicilloyl reagin associated with penicillin allergy.
PREPODYNE. (West) Titratable iodine. **Solution:** 1%.
Bot. pt., gal. **Scrub:** 0.75%. Bot. 6 oz., gal.
Swabs: Saturated with sol. Pkt. 1s, Box 100s.
Swabsticks: Saturated with sol. Pkt. 1s, Box 50s.
Pkt. 3s, Box 75s.
Use: Topical antiseptic.
PRESALIN. (Mallard) Aspirin 260 mg., salicylamide
120 mg., acetaminophen 120 mg., aluminum
hydroxide gel dried 100 mg./Tab. Bot. 50s.
PRE-SERT. (Allergan) Polyvinyl alcohol 3%, benzalk-
onium Cl. Bot. 0.5 fl. oz.
Use: Hard contact lens cushioning and rewetting
solution.
PRESIDAL. Pentacynium Methylsulfate, B.A.N.
PRESSOR AGENTS.
See: Sympathomimetic agents
PRESSOROL. (Travenol) Metaraminol bitartrate. Vials
10 ml. (10 mg./cc.)
Use: Vasopressor.
PRESUN 4 CREAMY. (Westwood) Octyl dimethyl
PABA. Bot. 4 oz.
Use: Moderate sunscreen protection, resists wash-
off.
PRESUN 8 CREAMY. (Westwood) Octyl dimethyl
PABA, oxybenzone. Bot. 4 oz.
Use: Sunscreen, moisturizer, resists wash-off.
PRESUN 15 CREAMY. (Westwood) Octyl dimethyl
PABA, oxybenzone. Bot. 4 oz.
Use: Ultra sunscreen protection, resists wash-off.
PRESUN 8 GEL. (Westwood) PABA 5%, alcohol 55%

(w/w), water, animal protein derivative, hydroxyethyl cellulose. Tube 3 oz.
Use: Sunscreen, moisturizer.
PRESUN 15 LIP PROTECTOR. (Westwood) Octyl dimethyl PABA 8%, oxybenzone 3%, mineral oil, ozokerite, petrolatum, PEG-4 dilurate, lanoline oil, propylparaben. Stick 15 oz.
Use: Sunscreen and moisturizer for lips.
PRESUN 8 LOTION. (Westwood) PABA, 55% SD alcohol 40. Bot. 4 oz., 7 oz.
Use: Moisturizer; prevention of sunburn.
PRESUN 15 LOTION. (Westwood) PABA, octyl dimethyl PABA, oxybenzone, 58% SD alcohol 40. Bot. 4 oz.
Use: Ultra sunscreen protection.
PRESUREN. Hydroxydione Sodium Succinate, B.A.N.
PRETAMAZIUM IODIDE. B.A.N. 4-(Biphenyl-4-yl)-3-ethyl-2-[4-(pyrrolidin-1-yl)styryl]thiazolium iodide.
Use: Treatment of enterobiasis.
PRETEND-U-ATE. (Vitalax) Enriched candy-appetite pacifier. Pkg. 20s.
PRETHCAMIDE. Mix. of crotethamide & cropropamide. Microen (Geigy)
PRETTY FEET & HANDS. (Norcliff Thayer) Lotion 3 fl. oz.
Use: Rough skin remover.
PREVIDENT DISCLOSING DROPS. (Hoyt) Erythrosine sodium 1%. Bot. 1 oz.
Use: Disclosing dental plaque.
PREVIDENT DISCLOSING TABLET. (Hoyt) Erythrosine sodium 1%/Tab. Unit dose strip 1000s.
Use: Disclosing dental plaque.
PREVIDENT PROPHYLAXIS PASTE. (Hoyt) Sodium fluoride containing 1.2% fluoride ion w/pumice and alumina abrasives. Cups 2 Gm. Box 200s. Jars 9 oz.
Use: Clean and polish teeth.
PREVISION. Mestranol, U.S.P. XXI.
PREXONATE TABLETS. (Tennessee Pharm.) Vit. A acetate 5000 I.U., D 500 I.U., B-6 2 mg., B-1 5 mg., B-2 2 mg., C 100 mg., B-12 2.5 mcg., Ca pantothenate 1 mg., niacinamide 15 mg., folic acid 1 mg., Fe 45 mg., Ca 500 mg., intrinsic factor 3 mg./Tab. Bot. 100s, 1000s.
Use: Vitamin supplement.
• **PRIDEFINE HYDROCHLORIDE.** USAN.
Use: Antidepressant.
PRILOCAINE. B.A.N. N-(2-Propylaminopropionyl)-o-toluidine. 2-Propylamino-o-propionotoluidide. Citanest hydrochloride.
Use: Local anesthetic.
• **PRILOCAINE HYDROCHLORIDE,** U.S.P. XXI. Inj., U.S.P. XXI. 2-(Propylamino)-o-propionotolidide HCl.
Use: Local anesthetic.
See: Citanest Hydrochloride, Vial, Amp. (Astra)
PRIMACAINE. 2′-Diethylamino-ethyl-2-butoxy-3-amino-benzoate HCl.
Use: Dental local anesthesia.
PRIMAQUINE. B.A.N. 8-(4-Amino-1-methylbutyl-amino)-6-methoxyquinoline.
Use: Antimalarial.

• **PRIMAQUINE PHOSPHATE,** U.S.P. XXI. Tab., U.S.P. XXI. 1,4-Pentanediamine, N-(6-methoxy-8-quinolinyl)-, phosphate (1:2). (Winthrop-Breon) 8-(4-Amino-1-methylbutylamino)-6-methoxyquinoline diphosphate. Tab. 26.3 mg., Bot. 100s.
Use: Prevents relapses in nearly all cases of vivax malaria.
PRIMAR. (Amfre-Grant) Ferrous fumarate 200 mg., ascorbic acid 75 mg., folic acid 0.33 mg., pyridoxine HCl 25 mg./Tab. Bot. 100s, 1000s, 5000s.
Use: Vitamin therapy.
PRIMATENE MIST. (Whitehall) Epinephrine 0.5% w/w alcohol 34%. Bot. ½ oz., ¾ oz.
Use: Bronchodilator.
PRIMATENE MIST SUSPENSION. (Whitehall) Epinephrine bitartrate 0.3 mg., epinephrine bitartrate 7.0 mg./cc. Bot. ⅓ oz., ½ oz.
Use: Bronchodilator.
PRIMATENE M. TABLETS. (Whitehall) Theophylline 130 mg., ephedrine HCl 24.3 mg., pyrilamine maleate 16.6 mg./Tab. Bot. 24s, 60s.
Use: Oral bronchodilator.
PRIMATENE P TABLETS. (Whitehall) Theophylline 130 mg., ephedrine HCl 24 mg., phenobarbital 8 mg./Tab. Bot. 24s, 60s.
Use: Oral bronchodilator.
• **PRIMIDOLOL.** USAN.
Use: Anti-anginal; cardiac depressant.
• **PRIMIDONE,** U.S.P. XXI. Tab., Oral Susp., U.S.P. XXI. 4,6(1H,5H)-Pyrimidinedione, 5-ethyldihydro-5-phenyl-. 5-Ethyldihydro-5-phenyl-4,6(1H,5H)-pyrimidinedione. Tab. 250 mg. Bot. 100s, 1000s.
Use: Anticonvulsant.
PRIMOBOLAN ACETATE. Methenolone, B.A.N.
PRIMOLUT DEPOT HEXANOATE. Hydroxyprogesterone, B.A.N.
PRIMOSTRUM. A prep. of primiparous colostrum.
PRIMPERAN HYDROCHLORIDE. Metoclopramide, B.A.N.
PRINALGIN. Alclofenac, B.A.N.
PRINCIPEN '125' FOR ORAL SUSPENSION. (Squibb). Ampicillin trihydrate 125 mg./5 cc. Reconstitution to 80, 100, 150, 200 cc. Unimatic 125 mg./5 cc. Ctn. 25s, 100s.
Use: Broad spectrum antibiotic.
PRINCIPEN '250' FOR ORAL SUSPENSION. (Squibb). Ampicillin trihydrate 250 mg./5 cc. Reconstitution to 80, 100, 150, 200 cc.; Unimatic 5 cc./Bot. 25s. Ctn. 100s.
Use: Broad spectrum antibiotic.
PRINCIPEN '250' CAPSULES. (Squibb) Ampicillin 250 mg./Cap. Bot. 100s, 500s. Unimatic 100s.
Use: Broad spectrum antibiotic.
PRINCIPEN '500' CAPSULES. (Squibb). Ampicillin trihydrate 500 mg./Cap. Bot. 100s, 500s. Unimatic Pack 100s, 500s.
Use: Broad spectrum antibiotic.
PRINCIPEN WITH PROBENECID. (Squibb) Ampicillin 389 mg., probenecid 111 mg./Cap. Bot. 9s.
Use: Treatment of uncomplicated urethral, cervical, rectal, or pharyngeal infections caused by *N. gonorrhoeae* in men & women.

PRINN ½. (Scrip) Conjugated estrogen 0.625 mg./Tab. Bot. 100s.

PRIODERM LOTION. (Purdue Frederick) Malathion 0.5% Bot. 2 oz.
Use: Treatment of head lice & ova.

PRIORA. (Xttrium) Folic acid 0.3 mg., Vit. A 6000 I.U., D 400 I.U., B-1 1.5 mg., B-2 2.5 mg., B-6 3 mg., niacinamide 15 mg., Ca. pantothenate 5 mg., Vit. B-12 2 mcg., iron 40 mg., calcium 250 mg./Tab. Bot. 100s.
Use: Phosphorus-free prenatal dietary supplement.

PRIORA P.F. W/FOLIC ACID. (Xttrium) Calcium 85 mg., Vit. A 2000 I.U., D 400 I.U., C 35 mg., B-1 2 mg., B-2 2 mg., B-6 2 mg., niacinamide 7 mg., folic acid 1 mg., iron 6 mg., Mn 0.12 mg./Tab. Bot. 100s, 1000s.
Use: Phosphorus-free prenatal dietary supplement.

PRISCOLINE. (Ciba) Tolazoline Hydrochloride 25 mg./ml.; w/sod. citrate 0.65%, tartaric a acid 0.65%, chlorobutanol 0.5%. Vial 10 ml. Packages 1s.
Use: Relieves pain, promotes healing & increases blood supply to extremities.

PRISILIDENE HYDROCHLORIDE.
See: Alphaprodine HCl (Var. Mfr.)

PRISTINAMYCIN. B.A.N. An antibiotic produced by Streptomyces pristina spiralis.

PRIVADORN.
See: Bromisovalum (Var. Mfr.)

PRIVINE HYDROCHLORIDE. (Ciba) Naphazoline HCl.
Nasal Sol.: 0.05%, Bot. 0.66 fl. oz. (20 ml.) w/dropper, 16 fl. oz. (473 ml.). **Nasal Spray** 0.05%, plastic squeeze bot. 0.5 fl. oz. (15 ml.).
Use: Vasoconstrictor.

• **PRIZIDILOL HYDROCHLORIDE.** USAN.
Use: Antihypertensive.

PRO-50. (Dunhall) Promethazine HCl 50 mg./ml. Vial 10 ml.
Use: Antihistaminic, sedative.

PRO-ACET DOUCHE CONCENTRATE. (Pro-Acet) Lactic, citric, & acetic acids, sod. lauryl sulfate, lactose, dextrose & sod. acetate. Pkg. polyethylene envelope 10 cc. Contents of 1 envelope to be diluted with 2 quarts of water.
Use: Douche 6 oz., 12 oz. Travel Packets, 10 cc.

• **PROADIFEN HYDROCHLORIDE.** USAN. 2-(Diethylamino)ethyl 2,2-diphenyl-valerate hydrochloride.
Use: Drug potentiator.

PRO-AMID. (T. E. Williams) Protoveratrine A 0.2 mg./Tab. Bot. 100s, 1000s.
Use: Mild to moderate hypertension.

PROAQUA. (Reid-Provident) Benzthiazide 50 mg./Tab. Bot. 100s, 500s.
Use: Diuretic.

PROBALAN. (Lannett) Probenecid 0.5 Gm./Tab. Bot. 100s, 1000s.

PROBAMPACIN. (Robinson) Ampicillin trihydrate 3.5 Gm., probenecid 1 Gm./Unit dose Bottle.
Use: Antibiotic, gonorrhea.

PRO-BANTHINE. (Searle) Propantheline Br. **7.5** mg./Tab. Bot. 100s. **15** mg./Tab. Bot. 100s, 500s. Unit dose 100s.
Use: Anticholinergic for adjunctive therapy in treatment of peptic ulcer.

PRO-BANTHINE W/PHENOBARBITAL. (Searle) Propantheline Br 15 mg., phenobarbital 15 mg./Tab. Bot. 100s. Unit dose 100s.
Use: Treatment of duodenal ulcer and irritable bowel syndrome.

PROBARBITAL SODIUM. 5-Ethyl-5-isopropylbarbiturate sod.

PROBATE. (Vita Elixir) Meprobamate 400 mg./Tab.
Use: Antianxiety & muscle relaxant.

PROBEC-T. (Stuart) Vit. B-1 15 mg., B-2 10 mg., B-3 100 mg., B-6 5 mg., B-12 5 mcg., C 600 mg., Ca pantothenate 20 mg.
Use: Therapeutic supplement in stress situations.

PROBEN. (Richlyn) Probenecid 500 mg., colchicine 0.5 mg./Tab. Bot. 1000s.
Use: Uricosuric.

• **PROBENECID,** U.S.P. XXI. Tabs. U.S.P. XXI. Benzoic acid, 4-[(dipropylamino)sulfonyl)]- p-(Dipropylsulfamoyl) benzoic acid.
Use: Uricosuric.
See: Benacen, Tab. (Cenci)
     Benemid, Tab. (Merck Sharp & Dohme)
     Benn, Tab. (Scrip)
     Probalan, Tab. (Lannett)
     Robenecid, Tab. (Robinson)
     SK Probenecid, Tab. (SmithKline)
W/Ampicillin.
See: Amcill-GC, Oral Susp. (Parke-Davis)
     Polycillin-PRB, Liq. (Bristol)
     Principen W/Probenecid, Cap. (Squibb)
W/Ampicillin trihydrate.
See: Probampacin (Biocraft)

• **PROBENECID AND COLCHICINE CAPSULES,** U.S.P. XXI.
Use: Uricosuric combination for chronic gouty arthritis.
See: Benn-C, Tab. (Scrip)
     Colbenemid, Tab. (Merck Sharp & Dohme)
     Robenecid w/colchicine, Tab. (Robinson)
     Robenecol, Tab. (Robinson)

PROBENZAMIDE. 0-Propoxybenzamide. (Warner-Lambert)

• **PROBICROMIL CALCIUM.** USAN.
Use: Anti-allergenic.

• **PROBUCOL.** USAN. (1) Acetone bis(3,5-di-tertbutyl-4-hydroxyphenyl) mercaptole; (2) 4,4'-(isopropylidenedithio)-bis[2,6-di-tert-butylphenol].
Use: Anticholesteremic.
See: Lorelco, Tab. (Merrell Dow)

PROCAINAMIDE. B.A.N. 4-Amino-N-(2-diethylaminoethyl)benzamide Pronestyl.
Use: Myocardial depressant.

PROCAINAMIDE HCl. (Columbia) Procainamide hydrochloride 250 mg., 500 mg./Cap. Bot. 100s, 1000s.
Use: Cardiac arrhythmia.

• **PROCAINAMIDE HYDROCHLORIDE,** U.S.P. XXI. Cap., Inj., U.S.P. XXI. Benzamide, 4-amino-N-[2-(diethylamino)ethyl]-HCl. p-Amino-N-[2-(diethylaminoethyl]benzamide HCl.

Use: Cardiac depressant in arrhythmias.
See: Procan SR, Tab. (Parke-Davis)
  Procapan, Cap. (Panray)
  Pronestyl, Cap. Vial. (Squibb)
PROCAINE ASCORBATE.
PROCAINE BASE.
W/Benzyl alcohol & propyl-p-aminobenzoate.
Use: Local anesthetic.
See: Durathesia, Inj. (Vortech)
  Rectocaine, Vial (Moore-Kirk)
W/Butyl-p-aminobenzoate, benzyl alcohol, in sweet almond oil.
See: Anucaine, Amp. (Calvin)
PROCAINE BORATE. No products listed.
PROCAINE BUTYRATE. p-Aminobenzoyl-diethylaminoethanol butyrate.
• **PROCAINE HYDROCHLORIDE,** U.S.P. XXI. Inj., Sterile, U.S.P. XXI. Benzoic acid, 4-amino-, 2-(diethylamino)-ethyl ester, HCl. Tab. N.F. XI. 2-Diethylaminoethyl p-aminobenzoate HCl. Allocaine, Bernocaine, Chlorocaine, Ethocaine, Irocaine, Kerocaine, Syncaine. (Abbott) 1% or 2% solution. Multiple-dose Vial 30 ml.
Use: Local anesthetic.
See: Anucaine, Amp. (Calvin)
  Novocain, Amp., Sol. (Winthrop-Breon)
  Unicaine, Vial (Kay)
W/Tetracaine and Nordefrin Hydrochlorides, Inj.
PROCAINE HYDROCHLORIDE AND LEVONORDEFRIN INJECTION.
Use: Local anesthetic.
• **PROCAINE PENICILLIN G SUSPENSION, STERILE,** U.S.P. XXI.
Use: Antibiotic.
See: Crysticillin, Vial (Squibb)
  Penicillin G, Procaine (Various Mfr.)
  Pfizerpen For Injection (Pfipharmecs)
• **PROCAINE, PENICILLIN G W/ALUMINUM STEARATE SUSPENSION, STERILE.,** U.S.P. XXI.
Use: Antibiotic.
See: Penicillin G Procaine with Aluminum Stearate, Sterile, U.S.P. XXI.
• **PROCAINE HYDROCHLORIDE AND EPINEPHRINE INJECTION,** U.S.P. XXI.
Use: Local anesthetic.
• **PROCAINE AND PHENYLEPHRINE HYDROCHLORIDES INJECTION,** U.S.P. XXI.
Use: Local anesthetic (dental).
• **PROCAINE AND TETRACAINE HYDROCHLORIDES AND LEVONORDEFRIN INJECTION,** U.S.P. XXI.
Use: Local anesthetic (dental).
PROCAINE, TETRACAINE AND NORDEFRIN HYDROCHLORIDES INJECTION.
Use: Local anesthetic.
PROCAINE, TETRACAINE AND PHENYLEPHRINE HYDROCHLORIDES INJECTION.
Use: Anesthetic.
PROCALAMINE INJECTION. (American McGaw) Injection of amino acid 3%, and glycerin 3% with electrolytes. Bot. 1000 ml.
Use: Amino acids.

PRO-CAL-THRON. (Vangard) Docusate calcium 60 mg., danthron 50 mg./Cap. Bot. 100s, 1000s.
Use: Stool Softener, laxative.
PROCAMIDE. (Amfre-Grant) Procainamide HCl 250 mg./Cap. Bot. 100s, 1000s.
Use: Anti-arrhythmic.
PROCAN SR. (Parke-Davis) Procainamide HCl sustained release 250 mg. 500 mg. or 750 mg./Tab. Bot. 100s. Unit dose 100s.
Use: Treatment of premature ventricular contractions, ventricular tachycardia, atrial fibrillation, paroxysmal atrial tachycardia.
PRO-CAP 65. (Foy) Propoxyphene HCl 65 mg., aspirin 227 mg., phenacetin 162 mg., caffeine 32.4 mg./Cap. Bot. 500s.
Use: Analgesic.
PROCAPAN. (Panray) Procainamide HCl 0.25 mg./Cap. Bot. 100s, 1000s.
Use: Antiarrythmic.
PROCARBAZINE. B.A.N. N-4-Isopropylcarbamoylbenzyl-N'-methylhydrazine. Natulan hydrochloride.
Use: Treatment of Hodgkin's disease.
• **PROCARBAZINE HCl,** U.S.P. XXI. Cap.: U.S.P. XXI. Benzamide, N-(1-methylethyl)-4-[(2-methyl-hydrazino)methyl]-HCl. (Roche) Natulan.
Use: Cytostatic, Antineoplastic.
See: Matulane, Caps. (Roche)
PROCARDIA. (Pfizer Laboratories) Nifedipine 10 mg./Cap. Bot. 100s. 300s. Unit Dose 100s.
Use: Treatment of angina.
• **PROCATEROL HYDROCHLORIDE.** USAN.
Use: Bronchodilator.
PROCEPTION SPERM NUTRIENT DOUCHE. (Milex) Ringer type glucose douche. Bot. ample for 10 douches.
Use: Precoital douche to promote conception.
• **PROCHLORPERAZINE,** U.S.P. XXI. Suppos., U.S.P. XXI. 10H-Phenothiazine, 2-chloro-10-[3-(4-methyl-1-piperazinyl)propyl]-.
Use: Antiemetic.
See: Compazine, Preps. (SmithKline)
W/Isopropamide.
See: Iso-Perazine, Cap. (Lemmon)
• **PROCHLORPERAZINE EDISYLATE,** U.S.P. XXI. Inj., Oral Sol., Syr., U.S.P. XXI. 10H-Phenothiazine, 2-chloro-10-[3-(4-methyl-1-piperazinyl)propyl]-1,2-ethanedisulfonate (1:1).
Use: Tranquilizer, antiemetic.
See: Compazine, Preps. (SmithKline)
PROCHLORPERAZINE ETHANEDISULFONATE. Prochlorperazine Edisylate, U.S.P. XXI.
Use: Tranquilizing agent.
• **PROCHLORPERAZINE MALEATE,** U.S.P. XXI. Tabs. U.S.P. XXI. 10H-Phenothiazine, 2-chloro-10-[3-(4-methyl-1-piperazinyl)-propyl]-(Z)-2-butenedioate (1:2).
Use: Antiemetic, tranquilizer.
See: Compazine, Preps (SmithKline)
• **PROCINONIDE.** USAN.
Use: Adrenocortical steroid.
PROCLAN EXPECTORANT WITH CODEINE. (Cenci)

Promethazine HCl, codeine phosphate, ipecac, potassium guaiacolsulfonate/5 cc. Bot.

PROCLAN VC EXPECTORANT WITH CODEINE. (Cenci) Codeine phosphate 10 mg., promethazine HCl 5 mg., phenylephrine HCl 5 mg., fl. ext. ipecac 0.17 min., potassium guaiacolsulfonate 44 mg., citric acid anhydrous 60 mg., sod. citrate 197 mg./5 cc., alcohol 7%. Bot.

• **PROCLONOL.** USAN. Bis(p-chlorophenyl)-cyclopropylmethanol. Under study.
Use: Acaricide, fungicide.

PRO COMFORT ATHLETE'S FOOT SPRAY. (Scholl) Tolnaftate 1%. Aerosol Can 4 oz.
Use: Anti-fungal.

PROCOMP-65. (Merchant) Propoxyphene HCl 65 mg., aspirin 227 mg., phenacetin 162 mg., caffeine 32.5 mg./Cap. Bot. 100s, 500s.
Use: Analgesic.

PRO CORT. (Barnes-Hind) Hydrocortisone alcohol 0.5% in cream base. Tube 1 oz.
Use: Relief of minor skin irritations.

PRO CORT M. (Barnes-Hind) Hydrocortisone alcohol 0.5% with menthol in cream base. Tube 1 oz.
Use: Relief of minor skin irritations.

PROCTALME. (Meyer) Benzocaine, chlorbutanol, neomycin, thymol iodide, ointment w/rectal applicator. Tube 1 oz.
Use: Hemorrhoids.

PROCTOCORT. (Rowell) Hydrocortisone 1% in a water-miscible base w/stearyl alcohol, polyoxyethylene 40 stearate, dibasic sodium phosphate, cetyl alcohol, isopropyl palmitate, citric acid, propylene glycol, benzyl alcohol and buffered to a pH of 5.0. Cream 30 gm. w/fingercots and rectal applicator.
Use: Treatment of severe anorectal inflammation.

PROCTOFOAM N.S. (Reed & Carnrick) Pramoxine HCl 1%. Aerosol Bot. 10 Gm. w/applicator.
Use: Inflammatory anorectal disorders.

PROCTOFOAM-HC. (Reed & Carnrick) Hydrocortisone acetate 1% and pramoxine HCl 1% in hydrophilic base of propylene glycol, ethoxylated cetyl and stearyl alcohol, polyoxyethylene-10-stearyl ether, cetyl alcohol, propyl paraben, methyl paraben, trolamine, purified water and inert propellants. Bot. aerosol container Rectal foam 10 Gm.
Use: Inflammatory anorectal disorders.

PROCTOFORM. (Fellows) Bismuth subiodide 0.125 gr., zinc oxide 2.5 gr., bismuth subcarbonate 0.9 gr., boric acid 4 gr., isobutyl-propyl-para-aminobenzoic acid 1 gr./Supp. Box 12s.
Use: Antiseptic & analgesic.

PRO CUTE CREAM. (Ferndale) Silicone, hexachlorophene, lanolin. 2 oz., 1 lb.
Use: Emollient, protective, bacteriostatic.

PROCUTE LOTION. (Ferndale) Hexachlorophene, Silicone, Lanolin. Bot. 8 oz.
Use: Emollient, protective, bacteriostatic.

PROCYCLIDINE. B.A.N. 1-Cyclohexyl-1-phenyl-3-(pyrrolidin-1-yl)propan-1-ol.
Use: Treatment of the Parkinsonian syndrome.

• **PROCYCLIDINE HCl,** U.S.P. XXI. Tab., U.S.P. XXI. α-Cyclohexyl-α-phenyl-1-pyrrolidinepropanol HCl.

Use: Skeletal muscle relaxant.
See: Kemadrin, Tab. (Burroughs Wellcome)

PRO-DEPO. (Vortech) Hydroxyprogesterone caproate 250 mg., benzyl benzoate 46%, benzyl alcohol 2%, castor oil/cc. Vial 5 ml.
Use: Long acting progestational agent.

PRODERM TOPICAL DRESSING. (Hickam) Aerosol topical. Each .82 cc contains castor oil 650 mg., peruvian balsam 72.5 mg. Aerosol 4 oz.
Use: Prevention of decubiti.

• **PRODILIDINE HCl.** USAN. (1,2-Di-methyl-3-phenyl-3-pyrrolidyl propionate HCl.
Use: Analgesic.

• **PRODOLIC ACID.** USAN.
Use: Anti-inflammatory.

PRO-EST. (Burgin-Arden) Progesterone 25 mg., estrogenic substance 25,000 I.U., sodium carboxymethylcellulose 1 mg., sodium cl 0.9% benzalkonium Cl 1:10,000 sodium phosphate dibasic 0.1% in water.

PRO-ESTRONE. (Pharmex) Estradiol benzoate 2.5 mg., progesterone 12.5 mg./cc. Vial 10 cc.

PROESTRONE. (Rocky Mtn.) Progesterone 25 mg., estrone 2.5 mg./cc. Vial 10 cc.

PROFAC-O. (Kay) Progesterone 100 mg., alcohol 20%. Vial 10 ml.
Use: Amenorrhea, abnormal uterine bleeding.

PROFADOL. B.A.N. 1-Methyl-3-propyl-3-(3-hydroxyphenyl)pyrrolidine.
Use: Analgesic; antitussive.

• **PROFADOL HCl.** USAN. m-(1-Methyl-3-propyl-3-pyrrolidinyl)phenol HCl.
Use: Analgesic.

PROFAMINA.
See: Amphetamine (Various Mfr.)

PROFASI HP. (Serono) Chorionic gonadotropin 5,000 U./Vial and 10,000 U./Vial. Ctn. contains 1 vial product and 1 vial diluent (benzyl alcohol 0.9% w/water for injection).
Use: Gonad-stimulating principle.

PROFERDEX. (Fisons) Ferric hydroxide & dextran in 0.9% sodium Cl. sol. for inj. sol. equiv. 50 mg. elem. iron/ml. Amp. 2 ml., 5 ml., or 10 ml.
Use: Iron deficiency anemia by I.M. or I.V. route.

PROFENAMINE HCl. Ethopropazine HCl, B.A.N.
See: Parsidol, Tab. (Parke-Davis)

PROFESSIONAL CARE LOTION, EXTRA STRENGTH. (Walgreen) Zinc oxide in a lotion base. Bot. 16 oz.
Use: Dry skin care.

PROFLAVINE.
Use: Topically; antiseptic.

PROFLAVINE DIHYDROCHLORIDE. 3,6-Diaminoacridine dihydrochloride.

PROFLAVINE SULFATE. 3,6-Diaminoacridine sulfate.

PROGELAN. (Lannett) Progesterone 25 mg., 50 mg., 100 mg./cc. in oil. Vials 10 cc.

PROGELAN AQUEOUS. (Lannett) Progesterone 25 mg., 50 mg., aq. susp./cc. Vials 10 cc.

PROGEST-50. (Tunex) Progesterone 50 mg./ml. w/benzyl alcohol 10% as preservative in sesame oil. Vial 10cc.

Use: Hormonal imbalances.

PROGESTAJECT-50. (Mayrand) Progesterone 50 mg./ml. in oil. Vial 10 ml.
Use: Progesterone agent.

• **PROGESTERONE,** U.S.P. XXI. Inj., Sterile Susp. U.S.P. XXI. 4-Pregnene-3,20-dione. Corpus luteum hormone. Flavolutan, Luteogan, Luteosan, Lutren.
Use: Progestin.

Aq. Susp.
See: Gesterol, Aqueous, Vial (Fellows-Testagar)
Progelan Aq., Vial (Lannett)
Prorone, Inj. (Sig)

In oil
See: Femotrone Injection (Bluco)
Gesterol, Inj. (Fellows-Testagar)
Lipo-Lutin, Amp. (Parke-Davis)
Progelan, Vials (Lannett)
Progest-50, Inj. (Tunex)
Progestin, Vial (Var. Mfr.)
Prorone, Inj. (Sig)

Tab., sublingual.
W/Estradiol benzoate.
See: Pro-Estrone, Vial (Pharmex)
W/Estradiol, testosterone, procaine HCl, procaine base.
See: Hormo-Triad, Vial (Bell)
W/Estrogenic substance.
See: Profoygen Aqueous (Foy)
Progex, Inj. (Pasadena Research)
W/Estrone.
See: Proestrone, Inj. (Rocky Mtn.)

PROGESTERONE INTRAUTERINE CONTRACEPTIVE SYSTEM, U.S.P. XXI.
Use: Contraceptive.

PROGESTERONE-LIKE.
See: Haloprogesterone
Norethynodrel

PROGESTIN. Progesterone. (Various Mfr.)

PRO-GESTIVE. (Nutrition) Pepsin 200 mg., pancreatin 200 mg., bile salts 100 mg., dehydrocholic acid 30 mg./Tab. Bot. 60s.
Use: Relief of digestive disturbances.

PROGESTIVE TABLETS. (NCP) Dehydrocholic acid 25 mg., bile salts 150 mg., pepsine 250 mg., pancreatin 300 mg./Tab. Bot. 60s.

PROGIATRIC. (Nutrition) Ca. L-glutamate 3 Gm., l-lysine 25 mg., C 30 mg., calcium 300 mg., iron 10 mg., vit. A 4000 I.U., B-1 1 mg., B-2 1.2 mg., B-6 1 mg., B-12 5 mcg., folic acid 25 mcg., Ca pantothenate 1 mg., niacin 50 mg./2 Tab. Bot. 90s.
Use: Dietary supplement.

• **PROGLUMIDE.** USAN. $(\pm)$-4-Benzamido-N,N-dipropylglutaramic acid. Nulsa (Wallace).
Use: Anticholinergic.

PROGLYCEM CAPSULES. (Schering) Diazoxide 50 mg., 100 mg./Cap. Bot. 100s.
Use: Management of hypoglycemia due to hyperinsulinism.

PROGLYCEM ORAL SUSPENSION. (Schering) Diazoxide 50 mg./ml. Bot. 30 ml. w/calibrated dropper.

Use: Management of hypoglycemia due to hyperinsulinism.

PROGUANIL HYDROCHLORIDE.
See: Chloroguanide Hydrochloride
Paludrine, Tab. (Ayerst)

PROHEPTAZINE. B.A.N. Hexahydro-1,3-dimethyl-4-phenyl-1H-azepin-4-ol propionate (ester).
Use: Analgesic.

PRO-HYDRO. (Mills) Protein hydrolysates (45% amino acids) 50 gr., iron 46 mg., l-lysine HCl 600 mg., dl-methione 75 mg., niacinamide 30 mg., Vit. B-1 3 mg., B-2 2 mg., B-6 2 mg., B-12 3 mcg., C 60 mg., calcium pantothenate 12 mg./6 Tab. Bot. 168s.
W/O Iron. Same formula as above without iron.
W/Vit. E. Same formula with Vit. E 30 I.U.
Use: Vitamin therapy.

PRO-ISO. (Zenith) Prochlorperazine 10 mg., isopropamide 5 mg./Cap.
Use: Treatment of gastrointestinal disorders.

PROKETAZINE DIMALEATE. Carphenazine, B.A.N.
Use: Tranquilizer.

PROKLAR. (O'Neal, Jones & Feldman) Sulfamethizole 500 mg./Tab. Bot. 100s, 1000s.
Susp. 500 mg./5 ml. Bot. 8 oz.

PROKLAR SYRUP. (O'Neal, Jones & Feldman) Methenamine mandelate 250 mg., sulfacetamide 250 mg., alcohol 10%/5 cc. Bot. 8 fl. oz.
Use: Urinary tract infection.

PROLACTIN RIA. (Abbott) Test units 50s, 100s.
Use: Quantitative measurement of total circulating human prolactin.

PROLADONE PECTINATE. Oxycodone, B.A.N.

PROLADYL. Pyrrobutamine. 1-Pyrrolidyl-3-phenyl-4-(p-chlorophenyl)-2-butene phosphate.
Use: Antihistaminic.

PROLAMINE. (Thompson Medical) Phenylpropanolamine HCl 37½ mg./Tab.
Use: Appetite suppressant.

PROLASE. Proteolytic enzyme from *Carica papaya.*
See: Papain
W/Mylase, cellase, calcium carbonate, magnesium glycinate.
See: Zylase, Tabs. (Vitarine)
W/Mylase-100, dehydrocholic acid, hyoscine HBr, atropine sulfate.
See: Almezyme, Cap. (Meyer)

PRO-LAX. (Vangard) Natural product consisting of equal parts refined psyllium mucilloid, dextrose. Powder. Bot. 16 oz.
Use: Laxative.

PROLENE. (Ethicon) Surgical suture, nonabsorbable.

PROLENS. (Ketchum) Bot. 2 oz.
Use: Contact lens wetting and cleaning solution.

• **PROLINE,** U.S.P. XXI. $C_5H_9NO_2$ as L-proline.
Use: Amino acid.

PROLINTANE. B.A.N. 1-(α-Propylphenethyl)-pyrrolidine. 1-Phenyl-2-(pyrrolidin-1-yl)pentane. Villescon.
Use: Tonic.

• **PROLINTANE HYDROCHLORIDE.** USAN.
Use: Antidepressant.

PRO-LITE. (Devlin) Predigested liquid protein. 1 oz.

equals 20% to 25% minimum daily requirement.
Bot. 16 oz., 32 oz.
Use: Diet supplement.
PROLIXIN. (Squibb) Fluphenazine hydrochloride.
Tabs. 1 mg., 2.5 mg. or 5 mg./Tab. Bot. 50s, 500s.
Unit dose 100s. **Elixir** 0.5 mg./ml. w/alcohol 14%.
Dropper Bot. 60 ml. Bot. pt. **Inj.:** 2.5 mg./ml. Vial 5
cc., 10 cc. Unimatic syringe 1 cc. Single dose syr.
25 mg./cc. 10s.
Use: The management of manifestations of
psychotic disorders, schizophrenia.
PROLIXIN DECANOATE. (Squibb) Fluphenazine
decanoate 25 mg./ml. Syringe 1 ml. Vial 5 ml.
Use: Schizophrenia treatment.
PROLIXIN ENANTHATE. (Squibb) Fluphenazine
enanthate 25 mg./ml. Vial 5 ml.
Use: Schizophrenia treatment.
PROLOID. (Parke-Davis) Thyroid globulin ext. Tab. ¼
gr., ½ gr., 1 gr. 1½ gr., 3 gr. Bot. 100s, 1000s. 2
gr., Bot. 100s.
Use: Myxedema, cretinism & hypothyroid states.
PROLOPRIM. (Burroughs Wellcome) Trimethoprim
100 mg. or 200 mg./Tab. Bot. 100s, Unit Dose
Pack 100s.
Use: Urinary tract infections.
PROMACHLOR. (Geneva) Chlorpromazine HCl 10
mg., 25 mg., 50 mg., 100 mg., 200 mg./Tab. Bot.
100s, 1000s. 100 mg./Tab. Bot. 100s.
PROMAPAR TABLETS. (Parke-Davis) Chlorproma-
zine HCl 10 mg., 25 mg., 50 mg., 100 mg., 200
mg./Tab. Bot. 100s, 1000s. Unit dose 100s.
PROMAZ. (Keene) Chlorpromazine HCl 25 mg./ml.
Inj. Vial 10 ml.
PROMAZINE. B.A.N. 10-(3-Dimethylaminopropyl)-
phenothiazine. Sparine embonate or hydrochloride.
Use: Tranquilizer.
• **PROMAZINE HCl,** U.S.P. XXI. Inj., Oral Soln., Syrup,
Tab., U.S.P. XXI. 10-(α-Dimethylamino-n-propyl)
phenothiazine HCl. 10-[3-(Dimethylamino)propyl]-
phenothiazine monohydrochloride.
See: Sparine, Tab., Vial, Syr. (Wyeth)
PROMENSIN. (Gotham) Progesterone 12.5 mg.,
Estradiol 2.5 mg./cc. in oil. Vial 5 cc.
PROMENSIN-F. (Gotham) Estradiol 2.5 mg., progester-
one 12.5 mg./cc. Vial 10 cc.
PROMETH-50. (Seatrace) Promethazine HCl 50
mg./ml. Vial 10 cc.
PROMETH EXPECTORANT. (Medwick) With or
without codeine. Bot. 4 oz., pt., gal.
W/Dextromethorphan. Bot. 4 oz., pt., gal.
PROMETH EXPECTORANT VC. (Medwick) With or
without codeine. Bot. 4 oz., pt., gal.
PROMETHASTAN. (Standex) Promethazine 25 or 50
mg./cc. Vial 10 cc.
PROMETHAZINE. B.A.N. 10(2-Dimethylamino-propyl)-
phenothiazine. Phenergan hydrochloride.
Use: Antihistamine; antiemetic, sedative.
PROMETHAZINE-50. (Kenyon) Promethazine HCl 50
mg., sod. formaldehyde sulfoxylate 0.75 mg., sod.
methabisulfite 0.25 mg., disodium EDTA 0.1 mg.,
calcium chloride 0.04 mg., phenol 5 mg., buffered
with sod. acetate/cc. Vial 10 cc.

PROMETHAZINE CHLOROTHEOPHYLLINATE.
See: Promethazine Theoclate, B.A.N.
PROMETHAZINE EXPECTORANT. (Columbia)
Promethazine HCl 5 mg., fl. ext. ipecac 0.17
min., pot. guaiacolsulfonate 44 mg., citric acid 60
mg., sodium citrate 197 mg., alcohol 7%. Pt., gal.
• **PROMETHAZINE HYDROCHLORIDE,** U.S.P. XXI.
Tab., Syr., Inj., U.S.P. XXI. 10H-Phenothiazine-10-
ethanamine, N,N-trimethyl-, HCl. 10-(2-Dime-
thylaminopropyl)phenothiazine hydrochloride.
Use: Antihistamine, antiemetic, sedative.
See: Fellozine, Inj. (Fellows-Testagar)
K-Phen, Inj. (Kay)
Methazine, Vial (Pharmex)
Pentazine, Expect., Vial (Century)
Phenerex, Inj. (Tunex)
Phenergan, Prep. (Wyeth)
Phenerhist, Inj. (Rocky Mtn.)
Phenerject, Vial (Mayrand)
Prorex, Vial, Amp. (Hyrex)
Provigan, Inj. (Reid-Provident)
Remsed, Tab. (Du Pont)
Rolamethazine Prods. (Robinson)
Sigazine, Inj. (Sig)
Synalgos, Cap. (Ives)
PROMETHAZINE HCl W/COMBINATIONS.
Use: Antihistaminic; antiemetic.
See: Mallergan, Liq. (Mallard)
Maxigesic, Cap. (W. F. Merchant)
Mepergan, Vial, Cap. (Wyeth)
Phenergan Comp., Tab. (Wyeth)
Phenergan-D, Tab. (Wyeth)
Phenergan Pediatric, Liq. (Wyeth)
Phenergan VC Expectorant (Wyeth)
P-M-Z HCl Expectorant (Sutliff & Case)
Promethazine-50, Vial (Kenyon)
Promethazine Expectorant, Syr. (Columbia)
Rolamethazine Prods. (Robinson)
Synalgos, Cap. (Ives)
Synalgos-DC, Cap. (Ives)
PROMETHAZINE THEOCLATE. Promethazine salt of
8-chlorotheophylline. Promethazine chlorotheophylli-
nate. Avomine.
Use: Antihistamine; antiemetic; sedative.
PROMETHESTROL. B.A.N. 3,4-Di-(4-hydroxy- 3-me-
thylphenyl)hexane. Methestrol (I.N.N.)
Use: Estrogen.
PROMETHESTROL DIPROPIONATE.
Use: Estrogen deficiency.
See: Meprane Dipropionate, Tab. (Reed & Carnrick)
W/Phenobarbital.
See: Meprane-Phenobarbital, Tab. (Reed & Carnrick)
PROMETOL. (Viobin) Concentrated wheat germ oil. 3
min./Cap. Bot. 100s, 250s. 10 min./Cap. Bot. 100s.
PROMINAL.
See: Mebaral, Tab. (Winthrop-Breon)
PROMINTIC. Methyridine, B.A.N.
PRO-MIN-VITE. (Drug Industries) Vit. A 10,000 I.U., D
1000 I.U., E 3 I.U., C 100 mg., B-1 10 mg., B-2 3 mg.,
B-6 2 mg., citrus bioflavonoids 25 mg., cal. pantothe-
nate 10 mg., niacin 20 mg., B-12 2 mcg., biotin 0.1
mg., l-lysine 25 mg., iron 20 mg., Cu 0.5 mg., Mn 2 mg.,

molybdenum 0.5 mg., Zn 1 mg., pot. 5 mg., Mg 5 mg., iodine 0.1 mg./Tab. Bot. 100s, 500s.
Use: Geriatric dietary supplement.

PROMISE TOOTHPASTE. (Block) Potassium nitrate 5%, sodium monofluorophosphate 0.76% W/glycerin, dicalcium phosphate, dihydrate, sorbitol, sodium lauryl sulfate, hydroxyethylcellulose, silica, sodium saccharin, methyl and propyl parabens. Tube 1.0 oz., 1.6 oz., 3.0 oz.
Use: Anticaries dentifrice for sensative teeth.

PROMOX. (Suppositoria) Pramoxine HCl 1% in suppository base. Box 12s, 100s.
Use: Antihemorrhoidal.

PROMOXALAN. B.A.N. 2,2-Diisopropyl-1,3-dioxolane-4-methanol. 4-Hydroxymethyl-2,2-di-isopropyl-1,3-dioxolan.
Use: Skeletal muscle relaxant.

PROMPT. (DePree) **Spray:** Benzocaine 1.5%, parachlorometaxylenol 0.5%. Can 5 oz. **Lot.:** Benzocaine 1%, triclosan 0.2%. Bot. 4 oz. **Tab.:** Acetaminophen 5 gr., Bot. 50s, 100s, 200s.
Use: Pain relief.

PROMPT. (Searle) Psyllium hydrophilic mucilloid and sennosides.
Use: Overnight laxative.

PROMPT BENZOCAINE CREAM. (Eckerd) Benzocaine, resorcin, chlorothymol Bot. 1½ oz., 4 oz.
Use: Local anesthetic.

PRO-NASYL. (Progonasyl Co.) o-Iodobenzoic Acid ½%, triethanolamine 5½% in a special neutral hydrophilic base compounded from oleic acid, mineral oil and vegetable oil. Bot. 15 cc., 60 cc.
Use: Treatment of sinusitis.

PRONDOL HYDROCHLORIDE. Iprindole, B.A.N.

PRONEMIA. (Lederle) Vit. B-12 15 mcg., intrinsic factor conc. 75 mg., ferrous fumarate 350 mg., ascorbic acid 150 mg., folic acid 1 mg./Cap. Bot. 100s.
Use: Hematinic.

PRONESTYL. (Squibb) Procainamide HCl. **Cap.** 0.25 Gm./Cap. Bot. 100s, 1000s. Unit dose Unimatic 100s. 375 mg./Cap. Bot. 100s. Unimatic 100s. 0.5 Gm./Cap. Bot. 100s, 1000s. Unit dose Unimatic 100s. **Inj.:** 100 mg./cc. w/benzyl alcohol 0.9%, sod. bisulfite 0.09%, sod. hydroxide or HCl. Vial 10 cc. 500 mg./cc. w/methylparaben 0.1%, propylparaben 0.2%, sod. hydroxide or HCl. Vial 2 cc. **Tab.:** 250 mg./Tab. Bot. 100s, 1000s. 375 mg./Tab. Bot. 100s. Unit dose Unimatic 100s. 500 mg./Tab. Bot. 100s, 1000s.
Use: Treatment of ventricular arrhythmias & related cardiac conditions.

PRONESTYL-SR. (Squibb) Procainamide HCl 500 mg./Tab. Bot. 100s. Unit dose 100s.
Use: Sustained release preparation for cardiac arrhythmias.

PRONETHALOL. B.A.N. 2-Isopropylamino-1-(2-naph-thyl)-ethanol. Alderlin hydrochloride.
Use: Adrenergic beta-receptor blocking agent.

PRONETHELOL (I.C.I.) Adrenergic beta-receptor antagonist; pending release.

PRONTO-GEL. (Commerce) Tube 2 oz.
Use: Analgesic jelly.

PROPACIL TABLETS. (Columbia) Propylthiouracil 50 mg./Tab. Bot. 1000s.

PROPADERM 17,21-DIPROPIONATE. Beclomethasone, B.A.N.

PROPADRINE. (Merck Sharp & Dohme) Phenylpropanolamine HCl 25 mg./Cap. Bot. 100s, 500s. 50 mg. Bot. 100s.
Use: Nasal decongestant.

PROPAESIN. Propyl p-Aminobenzoate. (Various Mfr.)

PROPAGEST SYRUP. (Carnrick) Phenylpropanolamine HCl 12.5 mg./5 ml. Bot. 16 oz., 4 oz.
Use: Nasal decongestant.

PROPAGEST TABLETS. (Carnrick) Phenylpropanolamine HCl 25 mg./Tab. Bot. 100s.
Use: Nasal decongestant.

PROPAGON-S. (Spanner) Estrone 2 mg./cc., 5 mg./cc. Vial 10 cc.

PROPAHIST. (Blue Line) **Tabs:** Phenylpropanolamine HCl 25 mg., pyrilamine maleate, pheniramine maleate in ratio 2:2:1/Tab. Bot. 100s, 1000s. **Syrup:** Dosage equal to one-half Tab./5 cc. Bot. pt., gal.
Use: Improve ventilation; for hay fever, nasal congestion, etc.

PROPAHIST INJ. (Blue Line) Atropine sulfate 0.2 mg., chlorpheniramine maleate 5 mg., phenylpropanolamine HCl 12.5 mg., chlorobutanol 0.5%/cc. Vial 10 cc.

PROPAHIST COMPOUND CAPSULES. (Blue Line) Phenylpropanolamine HCl 25 mg., pyrilamine maleate 10 mg., pheniramine maleate 5 mg., acetaminophen 325 mg., caffeine 30 mg./Cap. Bot. 100s, 1000s.

PROPAHIST-DM SYRUP. (Blue Line) Dextromethorphan HBr 15 mg., phenylpropanolamine HCl 12.5 mg., Incorpohist antihistamines (Pyrilamine maleate, & pheniramine maleate) 12.5 mg./5 cc. Bot. 2 oz., pt., gal.

PROPAMIDINE. B.A.N. 1,3-Di-(4-amidinophenoxy)-propane. Brolene isethionate.
Use: Bactericide; fungicide.

• **PROPANE,** N.F. XVI.

PROPANEDIOL DIACETATE, 1,2.
See: VoSol, Liq. (Wampole)

1,2,3-PROPANETRIOL, TRINITRATE. Nitroglycerin Tablets, U.S.P. XXI.

• **PROPANIDID.** USAN. [4- | (Diethylcarbamoyl)-methoxy | -3-methoxyphenyl] acetic acid propyl ester. Propyl 4-diethylcarbamoylmethoxy-3-methoxyphenylacetate. Epontol.
Use: Systemic anesthetic.

PROPANOLOL. 1-Isopropylamino-3-(l-napthyloxy)-propan-2-ol. Propranolol.

l-PROPANONE,2-METHYL-1,2-DI-3-PYRIDINYL-. Metyrapone, U.S.P. XXI.

PROPANTHELINE. (Wolins) Propantheline Br 15 mg., phenobarbital 15 mg./Tab. Bot. 100s, 1000s.

• **PROPANTHELINE BROMIDE,** U.S.P. XXI. Sterile, Tabs., U.S.P. XXI. 2-Propanaminium, N-methyl-N-(1-methylethyl)-N-[2-](9H-xanthen-9-ylcarbonyl)oxy[ethyl]-, Br.
Use: Anticholinergic.
See: Norpanth, Tab. (Vortech)
    Pro-Banthine, Prep. (Searle)
    Robantaline, Tab. (Robinson)
    SK-Propantheline Bromide Tab. (SmithKline)
    Spastil, Tab. (Kenyon)
W/Phenobarbital.
See: Probital, Tab. (Searle)
    Propantheline, Tab. (Wolins)
    Robantaline with Phenobarbital (Robinson)
W/Thiopropazate dihydrochloride.
See: Pro-Banthine W/Dartal, Tab. (Searle)
PROPANYL. (Kay) Phenylpropanolamine HCl 75 mg., benzyl alcohol 2% Vial multiple dose.
Use: Nasal decongestant.
PROPA P.H. ACNE COVER-UP STICK. (Commerce) Benzoyl peroxide 10%. Stick 0.05 oz.
Use: Skin tinted acne treatment.
PROPA P.H. ACNE PADS. (Commerce) Benzoyl peroxide 5%. 60 pads/Jar.
Use: Acne medication.
PROPA PH POROX 7. (Commerce) Benzoyl peroxide 7.0%. Tube 1 oz.
Use: Pimple and acne medication.
PROPA P.H. LIQUID ACNE SOAP. (Commerce) Benzoyl peroxide 10%. Bot 4 oz.
Use: Face & body acne medication.
PROPA P.H. SUPER CLEANSER ACNE MEDICATION. (Commerce) Benzethonium Cl. 0.50%. Bot. 6 oz., 10 oz., 16 oz.
Use: Kills acne bacteria, clean clogged pores.
• **PROPARACAINE HCl,** U.S.P. XXI. Ophth. Soln., U.S.P. XXI. Benzoic acid, 3-amino-4-propoxy-, 2-(diethylamino)ethyl ester, HCl. Proxymetacaine, B.A.N.
Use: Anesthetic (topical, ophthalmic).
See: Alcaine Ophth. Soln. (Alcon)
    Ophthaine HCl, Sol. (Squibb)
    Ophthetic, Ophth. Sol. (Allergan)
• **PROPATYL NITRATE.** USAN. 2-Ethyl-2-hydroxymethyl-1,3-propanediol trinitrate. Ettriol Trinitrate. 1,-1,1-Trisnitratomethylpropane. Etrynit; Gina. Invest. drug in U.S. but available in England.
Use: Coronary vasodilator.
PROPAZOLAMIDE. 2-Propionylamino-1,3,4-thiadiazole-5-sulfonamide. Ionaze (Lilly).
p-PROPENYLANISOLE. Anethole, N.F. XVI.
• **PROPENZOLATE HYDROCHLORIDE.** USAN. 1-Methyl-3-piperidyl-α-phenylcyclohexaneglycolate HCl.
Use: Anticholinergic.
PROPERIDINE. B.A.N. Isopropyl 1-methyl-4-phenylpiperidine-4-carboxylate.
Use: Narcotic analgesic.
PROPESIN. Name used for Risocaine.
PROPHENPYRIDAMINE.
See: Pheniramine (Var. Mfr.)
PROPHENPYRIDAMINE MALEATE.
See: Pheniramine Maleate

PROPHENPYRIDAMINE MALEATE W/COMBINATIONS.
See: Amaril-D-Spancap, Cap. (Vortech)
    Four Antihistamines, Tab. (Wolins)
    Histjen, Cap. (Jenkins)
    Hist-Span No. 2, Cap. (Kenyon)
    Nylamine, Tab. (Reid-Provident)
    Panadyl, Tab., Cap. (Misemer)
    Polyectin, Liq. (Amid)
    Pyma, Cap. (Fellows-Testagar)
    Trihistapacq Tabules, Tab. (Horton & Converse)
    Tri-Hist-Cap., Cap. (Burgin-Arden)
    Trimahist Elixir, Liq. (Tennessee)
    Vasotus, Liq. (Sheryl)
    Zerominic, Liq. (Amid)
PROPHENPYRIDAMINE TANNATE W/Phenylephrine tannate, pyrilamine tannate.
See: Rynatan, Susp., Tab. (Mallinckrodt)
PROPHYLLIN. (Rystan) **Powder:** Sodium propionate 1%. Box 12 packets 2.3 Gm. pwd./packet for preparation of 8 fl. oz. Jar 4 oz. bulk powder. **Oint.** Sodium propionate 5%. Tube 1 oz.
Use: Fungistatic wet dressing.
PROPICILLIN. B.A.N. 6-(α-Phenoxybutyramido)-penicillanic acid(1-Phenoxypropyl)penicillin. Brocillin & Ultrapen are the potassium salt.
Use: Antibiotic.
• **PROPIKACIN.** USAN.
Use: Antibacterial.
PROPINE OPTHALMIC. (Allergan) Dipivefrin HCl 0.1% Bot. 5 ml., 10 ml., 15 ml.
Use: Control intraoccular pressure in chronic open-angle glaucoma.
PROPIODAL.
See: Entodon
• **PROPIOLACTONE.** USAN. 2-Oxetanone; beta-propiolactone, Betaprone. Hydracrylic acid, β-lactone.
Use: Sterilization of vaccines and tissue grafts.
• **PROPIOMAZINE.** USAN. 1-[10-(2-Dimethylaminopropyl)-phenothiazine-2-yl]-1-propanone. Dorevane; Indorm.
Use: Sedative.
See: Largon, Amp. (Wyeth)
• **PROPIOMAZINE HYDROCHLORIDE,** U.S.P. XXI. Inj., U.S.P. XXI. 1-[10-[2-(Dimethylamino)propyl]-phenothiazin-2-yl]-1-propanone HCl.
Use: Sedative.
See: Largon, Inj. (Wyeth)
• **PROPIONIC ACID,** N.F. XVI.
W/Sod. propionate, docusate sodium, salicylic acid.
See: Prosal, Liq. (Gordon)
    Propionate-Caprylate Mixtures.
PROPIONATE-CAPRYLATE MIXTURES.
See: Sopronol, Oint., Pow., Sol. (Wyeth)
PROPIONATE COMPOUND.
See: Propion Gel (Wyeth)
PROPIONATE SALTS.
See: Copper
    Potassium
    Sodium
    Zinc

PROPIONYL ERYTHROMYCIN LAURYL SULFATE.
See: Erythromycin Propionate Lauryl Sulfate
PROPIRAM. B.A.N. N-(1-Methyl-2-piperidinoethyl)-N-(2-pyridyl)propionamide.
Use: Analgesic.
• **PROPIRAM FUMARATE.** USAN. N-(1-Methyl-2-piperidinoethyl)-N-(2-pyridyl) propionamide fumarate. 1:1.
Use: Analgesic.
PROPISAMINE.
See: Amphetamine (Various Mfr.)
PROPITOCAINE. Prilocaine.
See: Citanest, Sol., Vial, Amp. (Astra)
PROPLEX. (Hyland) Factor IX Complex (Human), clotting Factor II (prothrombin), VII (proconvertin), IX (PTC, antihemophilic factor B) & X (Stuart-Prower factor) all dried & concentrated. Vial 30 ml. w/Diluent.
Use: Deficiency of factors II, VII, IX, & X.
PROPLEX SX. (Hyland) Factor IX complex, 300–1200 IU/Vial. Vial 30 ml.
Use: Treatment of points with factor IX deficiency (Hemophilia B, Christmas disease).
• **PROPOFOL.** USAN.
PROPONADE CAPSULES. (Blue Cross) Chlorpheniramine maleate 8 mg., phenylpropanolamine HCl 50 mg., isopropamide 2.5 mg./Cap. Bot. 100s.
Use: Antihistaminic, decongestant.
PROPONESIN HYDROCHLORIDE. Tolpronine, B.A.N.
PROPOQUIN. Amopyroquin HCl.
Use: Antimalarial.
PRO-POWER. (Galen) Protein hydrolysates 8.33 gr., 1-lysine HCl 100 mg., dl-methionine 12.5 mg., Vit. E 5 I.U., B-3 5 mg., B-1 0.5 mg., B-2 0.33 mg., B-5 2 mg., B-6 0.33 mg., B-12 0.5 mcg., C 10 mg.,/Cap. Bot. 90s.
Use: Vitamin supplement.
PROPOXAMIDE. o-Propoxybenzamide.
• **PROPOXYCAINE HYDROCHLORIDE,** U.S.P. XXI. 2-(Diethylamino)ethyl-4-amino-2-propoxybenzoate HCl.
Use: Local anesthetic.
• **PROPOXYCAINE AND PROCAINE HYDROCHLORIDES AND LEVONORDEFRIN INJECTION,** U.S.P. XXI.
Use: Local anesthetic (dental).
PROPOXYCAINE AND PROCAINE HYDROCHLORIDES AND NOREPINEPHRINE BITARTRATE INJECTION, U.S.P. XXI.
Use: Local anesthetic (dental).
See: Ravocaine Cartridge (Cook-Waite)
PROPOXYCHLORINOL. Toloxychlorinol.
• **PROPOXYPHENE HCl,** U.S.P. XXI. Caps. U.S.P. XXI. Benzenethanol, α[2-(dimethylamino)-1-methylethyl]-α-phenyl, propanoate (ester), HCl.
Use: Analgesic.
See: Darvon, Pulv. (Lilly)
Dolene, Cap. (Lederle)
Harmar, Cap. (Zemmer)
Myospaz, Improved, Cap. (Vortech)
Progesic, Cap. (Ulmer)
Pro-Pox 65, Cap. (Kenyon)

Ropoxy, Cap. (Robinson)
SK-65, Cap. (SmithKline)
PROPOXYPHENE HCl W/COMBINATIONS.
Use: Analgesic.
See: Bexophene, Cap. (Mallard)
Darvon Compound, Pulvule (Lilly)
Darvon Compound-65, Cap. (Lilly)
Darvon With A.S.A., Cap. (Lilly)
Dolene, AP-65, Tab. (Lederle)
Dolene Compound-65, Cap. (Lederle)
Doraphen-Comp.-65, Cap. (Cenci)
Myospaz, Cap. (Vortech)
PC-65, Cap. (Archer)
Procomp-65, Cap. (W.F. Merchant)
Pro-Pox Plus, Cap. (Kenyon)
Propoxyphene Compound 65, Cap. (Caribe, Wayne, Wolins)
Ropoxy Compound-65, Cap. (Robinson)
SK-65 APAP, Tab. (SmithKline)
SK-65 Compound, Cap. (SmithKline)
S-Pain-CPD-65, Cap. (Saron)
Stogesic, Cap. (Jalco)
Wygesic, Tab. (Wyeth)
• **PROPOXYPHENE HCl AND ACETAMINOPHEN TABLETS,** U.S.P. XXI.
Use: Analgesic.
PROPOXYPHENE HCl AND APC CAPSULES.
Use: Analgesic.
See: Darvon Compound, Cap. (Lilly)
Darvon Compound-65, Cap. (Lilly)
• **PROPOXYPHENE HCl, ASPIRIN AND CAFEEINE CAPSULES,** U.S.P. XXI.
Use: Analgesic.
• **PROPOXYPHENE NAPSYLATE,** U.S.P. XXI. Oral Susp., Tab., U.S.P. XXI.
Use: Analgesic.
See: Darvocet-N (Lilly)
Darvon-N, Tab. (Lilly)
W/Acetaminophen.
Use: Analgesic.
See: Darvocet-N, Tab. (Lilly)
• **PROPOXYPHENE NAPSYLATE AND ACETAMINOPHEN TABLETS,** U.S.P. XXI.
Use: Analgesic.
• **PROPOXYPHENE NAPSYLATE AND ASPIRIN TABLETS,** U.S.P. XXI.
Use: Analgesic.
PROPRANOLOL. B.A.N. 1-Isopropylamino-3-(1-naphthyloxy)propan-2-ol. Propanol.
Use: Beta adrenergic blocking agent.
• **PROPRANOLOL HYDROCHLORIDE,** U.S.P. XXI. Inj., Tab., U.S.P. XXI. 2-Propanol, 1-[(1-methylethyl)amino]-3-(1-naphthalenyloxy)-, HCl. Propanolol HCl.
Use: Antiarrhythmic agent.
See: Inderal, Tab., Inj. (Ayerst)
W/Hydrochlorthiazide.
See: Inderide, Tab. (Ayerst)
PROPYL p-AMINOBENZOATE. (Various Mfr.) Propaesin.
Use: Local anesthetic.
W/Procaine base, benzyl alcohol, phenol.

See: Durathesia, Inj. (Vortech)
Rectocaine, Vial (Moore-Kirk)
• **PROPYL GALLATE,** N.F. XVI.
Use: Pharmaceutic aid (antioxidant).
PROPYLDOCETRIZOATE. B.A.N. Propyl 3-diacetylami-
no-2,4,6-tri-iodobenzoate. Pulmidol.
Use: Radio-opaque substance.
• **PROPYLENE CARBONATE,** N.F. XVI.
Use: Pharmaceutic aid (gelling agent).
• **PROPYLENE GLYCOL,** U.S.P. XXI. 1-2-Propanediol.
Use: Pharm. aid (humectant, solvent).
• **PROPYLENE GLYCOL DIACETATE,** N.F. XVI.
PROPYLENE GLYCOL MONOSTEARATE, N.F. XVI.
1,2-Propanediol monostearate.
Use: Emulsifying agent.
• **PROPYLHEXEDRINE,** U.S.P. XXI. Inhalant, U.S.P.
XXI. N,α-Dimethylcyclohexaneethylamine. Evetin
HCl.
Use: Adrenergic (vasoconstrictor), appetite
suppressant, antihistamine.
See: Benzedrex, Inhalant (Menley & James)
• **PROPYLIODONE,** U.S.P. XXI. Sterile Oil Susp.,
U.S.P. XXI. 1(4H)-Pyridineacetic acid, 3,5-diiodo-4-
oxo-, propyl ester. Sterile oil Susp. (peanut oil). Sterile
water susp. Propyl 3,5-di-iodo-4-oxopyridine-1-ylace-
tate.   3,5-Di-iodo-1-propoxycarbonylmethyl-4-pyri-
done. Dionosil.
Use: Radio-opaque substance.
iso-PROPYLNORADRENALINE.
See: Isoproterenol.
• **PROPYLPARABEN,** N.F. XVI. Propyl p-hydroxybenzo-
ate. Propyl Chemosept (Chemo Puro)
Use: Pharm. aid (antifungal preservative).
• **PROPYLTHIOURACIL,** U.S.P. XXI. Tab. U.S.P. XXI.
4(1H)-Pyrimidinone, 2,3-dihydro-6-propyl-2-thioxo. -
propyl. (Abbott) Tabs. 50 mg. Bot. 100s, 1000s.
(Lilly) Tabs. 50 mg. Bot. 100s, 1000s. (Lederle)
Tabs. 50 mg. Bot. 100s, 1000s. Tabs. 50 mg. Bot.
100s, 1000s, Unit dose 100s.
Use: Thyroid inhibitor.
See: Propacil Tablets (Columbia)
PROPYPHENAZONE. B.A.N. 4-Isopropyl-2,3-dimethyl-
1-phenyl-5-pyrazolone.
Use: Analgesic.
PROQUAMEZINE. B.A.N. 10-(2,3-Bisdimethyl-amino-
propyl)phenothiazine. Aminopromazine (I.N.N.)
Myspamol.
Use: Bronchial spasmolytic.
• **PROQUAZONE.** USAN. 1-Isopropyl-7-methyl-4-phe-
nyl-2 (1H)-quinazolinone.
Use: Anti-inflammatory.
• **PROQUINOLATE.** USAN.
Use: Coccidiostat.
• **PRORENOATE POTASSIUM.** USAN.
Use: Aldosterone antagonist.
PROREX. (Hyrex) Promethazine HCl, 25 or 50
mg./ml. Vial 10 ml.
Use: Antihistamine, antiemetic, sedative.
PRORONE. (Sig) Progesterone 25 mg./ml. Aq. or oil
susp. Vial 10 ml.
Use: Hormone therapy.
• **PROROXAN HYDROCHLORIDE.** USAN.

Use: Anti-adrenergic.
• **PROSCILLARIDIN.** USAN. 3β, 14β-Dihydroxy-bufa-
4,20,22-trienolide 3-rhamnoside. Talusin, Tradenal.
Use: Cardiac glycoside.
PROSCOPINE HYDROBROMIDE. Poskine, B.A.N.
PROSED. (Star) Atropine sulfate 0.03 mg.,
hyoscyamine sulfate 0.03 mg., methenamine 40.8
mg., methylene blue 5.4 mg., phenylsalicylate 18.1
mg., benzoic acid 4.5 mg./Tab. Bot. 100s, 1000s.
Use: Urinary antispasmodic, anticholinergic,
antibacterial.
PROSOBEE. (Mead Johnson) Milk free formula
supplies 640 cal./qt. w/ 19.2 Gm. protein, 34 Gm.
fat, 64 Gm. carbohydrate, vitamins and minerals.
Vit. A 2000 I.U., D 400 I.U., E 20 I.U., C 52 mg.,
folic acid 100 mcg., B-1 0.5 mg., B-2 0.6 mg.,
niacin 8 mg., B-6 0.4 mg., B-12 2 mcg., biotin 50
mg., pantothenic acid 3 mg., K-1 100 mcg., choline
50 mg., Inositol 30 mg., Ca 600 mg., P 475 mg.,
Iodine 65 mcg., Fe 12 mg., Mg 70 mg., Cu 0.6 mg.,
Zn 5 mg., Mn 0.2 mg., chloride 520 mg., K 740
mg., Na 275 mg./Qt. (20 Kcal./fl. oz.) Concentrated
liq. can 13 fl. oz.; Ready-to-use liq. can 8, 32 fl. oz.
Powder, cans 14 oz.
Use: Infant food, hypoallergenic formula, lactose
and sucrose free.
PRO-SOF SG 100. (Vangard) Docusate sodium 100
mg./Cap. Bot. 100s, 1000s. Unit dose 10×10s.
Use: Stool softener.
PRO-SOF SG 200. (Vangard) Docusate sodium 250
mg./Cap. Bot. 100s, 500s. Unit dose pkg. 10×10s.
Use: Laxative.
PRO-SOF SYRUP. (Vangard) Docusate sodium 20
mg./5 ml. Bot. pt.
Use: Laxative.
PRO-SOF w/CASANTHRANOL SG. (Vangard) Can-
santhranol 30 mg., docusate sodium 100 mg./Cap.
Bot. 100s, 1000s.
Use: Laxative.
PROSTAGLANDIN E. Dinoprostone, B.A.N.
Use: Prostaglandin.
PROSTAGLANDIN F. Dinoprost, B.A.N.
Use: Prostaglandin.
• **PROSTALENE.** USAN.
Use: Prostaglandin.
PROSTAPHLIN CAPSULES. (Bristol) Sodium oxacillin
250 mg. and 500 mg./Cap. Bot. 48s, 100s.; 250
mg., 500 mg. Dosatrol Pack 100s.
Use: Staphylococcal infections.
PROSTAPHLIN FOR INJECTION. (Bristol) Crystalline
oxacillin sodium 250 mg., 500 mg., 1 Gm., 2 Gm., 4
Gm./dry filled Vial. Piggyback vials 1 Gm., 2 Gm., 4
Gm. Bulk vial 10 Gm.
Use: Treatment of infections.
PROSTAPHLIN ORAL SOLUTION. (Bristol) Sod.
oxacillin reconstitute for oral soln. 250 mg./5 ml.
Bot. 100 ml. Dosa-Trol Pack 25s.
Use: Orally, staphylococcal infections.
PROTOSTAT. (Ortho) Metronidazole 250 mg. or 500
mg./Tab. 250 mg./Tab. Bot. 100s. 500 mg./Tab.
Bot. 50s.
Use: Treatment of trichomoniasis, antiprotozoal.

PROSTIGMIN BROMIDE. (Roche) Neostigmine bromide. **Tab.** 15 mg., Bot. 100s, 1000s.
Use: Parasympathetic stimulant.
PROSTIGMIN METHYLSULFATE. (Roche) Injectable Neostigmine Methylsulfate, U.S.P. Amp 1:2000 w/methyl and propyl parabens 0.2%, sod. hydroxide 1 ml. Box 10s. 1:4000 w/methyl and propyl parabens 0.2%, sod. hydroxide 1 ml. Box 10s. Vial (1:1000, 1:2000 w/phenol 0.45%, sod. acetate 0.2 mg., acetic acid, sod. hydroxide) 10 ml.
Use: Parasympathetic stimulant.
PROSTIN E2. Dinoprostone, B.A.N.
PROSTIN F2 ALPHA. (Upjohn) Dinoprost tromethamine 5 mg./ml. Amp. 4 ml., 8 ml.
Use: Oxytocic.
PROSTIN VR PEDIATRIC. (Upjohn) Alprostadil 500 mcg./ml. Amp. 1 ml. Box 5s.
Use: Palliatative therapy to maintain patency of the ductus arteriosus in neonates with congenital heart defects.
PROTABOLIN. (Pasadena Research) Methandriol dipropionate 50 mg./cc. Vial 10 cc.
• **PROTAMINE SULFATE,** U.S.P. XXI. Inj., for inj., U.S.P. XXI. (Lilly)-Amp. 1%, 5 cc.; 1s, 25s; 25 cc. 6s. (Upjohn)—Vial 50 mg. w/sod. chloride 45 mg., w/ph adjusted 1s, 5s, 25s; 250 mg./Vial.
Use: I.V.; heparin overdosage.
• **PROTAMINE ZINC INSULIN SUSPENSION,** U.S.P. XXI.
Use: Insulin.
See: Iletin (Insulin, Lilly)
  Insulin, Protamine Zinc, Susp. (Squibb)
PROTARGIN MILD.
See: Silver Protein, Mild (Various Mfr.)
PROTARGOL. (Sterwin) Strong silver protein. Pow., Bot. 25 Gm.
Use: Topically; silver antiseptic.
PROTASE. (Kenyon) Standardized amount of ext. of proteolytic enzymes from *Carica papaya* with 10,000 u. of activity/Tab. Bot. 100s, 1000s.
PROTEASE.
W/Amylase, lipase, cellase, hyoscine HBr.
See: Am-Zyme, Tab. (Vortech)
W/Pancreatin, amylase.
See: Dizymes, Caps. (Recsei)
W/Vit. B-1, B-12.
See: Arcoret, Tab. (Arco)
W/Vit. B-1, B-12, iron.
See: Arcoret W/Iron, Tab. (Arco)
PROTECTOL MEDICATED POWDER. (Daniels) Calcium undecyclenate 15%. Bot. 2 oz.
Use: Diaper rash, chafing.
• **PROTEIN HYDROLYSATE INJ.,** U.S.P. XXI.
Use: Fluid and nutrient replenisher.
See: Amigen, Inj. (Baxter Lab.)
  Aminogen, Amp., Vial (Christina)
  Lacotein, Vial (Christina)
  Travamin, Inj. (Travenol)
  Virex, Inj. (Burgin-Arden)
PROTEIN HYDROLYSATES ORAL.
Use: Nutrient.
See: Lofenalac, Pow. (Mead Johnson)

Nutramigen, Pow. (Mead Johnson)
Pregestimil, Pow. (Mead Johnson)
Stuart Amino Acids, Pow. (Stuart)
W/Lysine HCl, methionine, niacinamide, Ca pantothenate, Vit. B complex, Vit. C, iron.
See: Pro-Hydro, Tab. (Mills)
W/Vitamin B-12.
See: Stuart Amino Acids and B-12, Tab. (Stuart)
■ **PROTEIN, NONSPECIFIC THERAPY.**
See: Lacotein, Vial (Christina)
  Mucusol, Amp., Vial (Kremers-Urban)
PROTENATE. (Hyland) Plasma protein fraction (Human) 5% in buffered stabilized saline diluent. Sod. acetyltryptophanate 0.004M, sod. caprylate 0.004M, pH adjusted to neutral w/sod. bicarbonate. Vial 250 ml. and 500 ml. w/administration set.
Use: Plasma expander. Increase plasma protein & volume.
PROTENIUM. (Pasadena Research) Hydrolized gelatin w/di-tryptophane.
Caps. Bot 300s.
Use: Nutritional supplement.
PROTEOLYTIC ENZYMES.
See: Dornavac (Merck Animal Health)
  Papase, Tab. (Parke-Davis)
  Vardase, Prod. (Lederle)
W/Amylolytic enzyme, cellulolytic enzyme, lipolytic enzyme.
See: Arco-Lase, Tab. (Arco)
  Kutrase, Cap. (Kremmers-Urban)
  Kuzyme, Cap. (Kremmers-Urban)
  Zymme, Cap. (Scrip)
W/Amylolytic enzyme, lipolytic enzyme, cellulolytic enzyme, belladonna ext.
See: Mallenzyme, Tab. (Mallard)
W/Amylolytic, cellulolytic enzymes, lipase, phenobarbital, hyoscyamine sulf., atropine sulf.
See: Arco-Lipase Plus, Tab. (Arco)
W/Amylolytic, cellulolytic enzymes.
See: Trienzyme, Tabs. (Fellows-Testagar)
W/Amylolytic enzyme, homatropine methylbromide, d-sorbitol. (Papain.)
See: Converzyme, Liq. (Ascher)
W/Calcium carbonate, glycine, amylolytic and cellulolytic enzymes.
See: Co-Gel, Tab. (Arco)
W/Combinations
See: Butibel-zyme Tabs. (McNeil)
W/Neomycin palmitrate, hydrocortisone acetate, water-miscible base.
See: Biozyme Oint. (Armour)
W/Protease, lipase, simethicone.
See: Tri-Cone, Cap. (Meyer)
W/*Sus scrofa* Linne var. Domesticus.
See: Saromide Injection, Vial, 1.3 ml. (Saron)
PROTHAZINE. (Vortech) Promethazine HCl 25 mg., sod. formaldehyde sulfoxylate 0.75 mg., sod. metabisulfite 0.25 mg., Ca chloride 0.04 mg., phenol 5 mg./cc. Ampule 1 ml., Vial 10 ml.
Use: Antihistamine, antiemetic, sedative.
PROTHAZINE WITH CODEINE. (Vortech) Promethazine HCl 5 mg., ipecac fluid ext. 0.17 min.,

potassium guaiasulfonate 44 mg., citric acid 60 mg., sod. citrate 197 mg., alcohol 7%, codeine 10 mg./5 ml. Bot. 4 oz., gal.
Use: Antitussive, antihistaminic.

PROTHAZINE EXPECTORANT. (Vortech) Bot. 4 oz., gal.
Use: Antihistaminic, expectorant.

PROTHAZINE PEDIATRIC. (Vortech) Bot. 4 oz., gal.
Use: Antitussive, antihistaminic.

PROTHIADEN HYDROCHLORIDE. Dothiepen, B.A.N.

PROTHIDIUM. Pyrithidium bromide, B.A.N.

PROTHIONAMIDE. B.A.N. 2-Propylisonicotinthioamide.
Use: Treatment of tuberculosis.
See: Trevintix

PROTHIPENDYL. B.A.N. 10-(3-Dimethylaminopropyl)-pyrido[3,2-b][1,4]benzothiazine.
Use: Tranquilizer; antiemetic.
See: Phrenotropin
Tolnate [hydrochloride]

PROTHIPENDYL HCl. [(4-Dimethyl-aminopropyl-pyrido(3,2B)Benzothiazine)] HCl-monohydrate.
Use: Sedative.

PROTICULEEN. (Spanner) Vit. B-12 activity 10 mcg., folic acid 10 mg., B-12 crystalline 50 mcg., niacinamide 75 mg./cc. Multiple dose vial 10 cc. I.M. inj.

• **PROTIRELIN.** USAN. 1-[N-(5-Oxo-L-prolyl)-L-histidyl]--prolinamide. 5-oxo-L-histidyl-L-proline amide.
Use: Thyrotrophin releasing hormone.
See: Thypinone, Inj. (Abbott)

PROTOKYLOL. B.A.N. 1-(3,4-Dihydroxyphenyl)-2-(α-methyl-3,4-methylene-dioxyphenethylamino)-ethanol.
Use: Sympathomimetic.
See: Caytine [hydrochloride]

PROTOKYLOL HCl. 3,4-Dihydroxy-α-[[[α-methyl-3,4-(methylenedioxy) phenethyl]-amino]methyl]-benzyl alcohol HCl.
Use: Adrenergic (bronchodilator).

PROTOPAM CHLORIDE. (Ayerst) Pralidoxime chloride 500 mg./Tab. Bot. 100s.; Vial 1 Gm./20 ml. **Emergency Kit:** One 1 Gm./20 ml. vial of sterile Protopam Chloride porous cake, one 20 ml. vial of sterile water for injection, U.S.P. without preservative, to be used as diluent; sterile disposable 20 ml. syringe. **Hospital package:** Six 20 ml. vials of 1 Gm. each of sterile Protopam Chloride powder, without diluent or syringe.
Use: Antidote for poisoning due to organophosphate pesticides.

PROTOSAN. (Recsei) Protein 87.5%, lactose 0.5%, fat 1.3%, ash 3.5%, sodium 0.02%. Jar 1 lb., 5 lb.
Use: Dietary supplement.

PROT-O-SEA. (Barth's) Protein 90%, containing amino acids and minerals. Bot. 100s, 500s.

PROTOTABS. (Vortech) Leucine 8.4%, lysine 6%, phenylalanine 5.8%, threonine 4%, methionine 2.1%, arginine 8.2%, isoleucine 5.8%, valine 5.8%, histidine 2.6%, tryptophan 1.1%/Tab. Bot. 100s, 1000s.
Use: Dietary supplement.

PROTOVERATRINE A.
See: Pro-Amid, Tab. (Amid)

PROTOVERATRINES A & B MALEATE.

PROTRAN PLUS. (Vangard) Meprobamate 150 mg., ethoheptazine citrate 75 mg., aspirin 250 mg./ Tab. Bot. 100s. 500s.
Use: Anti-anxiety pain reliever.

PROTRIPTYLINE. B.A.N. 7-(3-Methylaminopropyl)-1,2:-5,6-dibenzocycloheptatriene. Concordin HCl.
Use: Antidepressant.

• **PROTRIPTYLINE HYDROCHLORIDE,** U.S.P. XXI. Tab., U.S.P. XXI. N-methyl-5H-dibenzo [a,d]cycloheptene-5-propylamine HCl.
Use: Antidepressant.
See: Vivactil, Tab. (Merck Sharp & Dohme)

PROVAL #3. (Reid-Provident) Acetaminophen 325 mg., codeine phosphate 30 mg./Tab. Bot. 100s, 500s.
Use: Analgesic.

PROVENTIL INHALER. (Schering) Metered dose aerosol unit containing albuterol in propellants. Each actuation delivers 90 mcg. of albuterol. Canister 17.0 Gm. with oral adapter. Box 1s.
Use: Bronchodilator.

PROVENTIL. (Schering) Albuterol sulfate 2 mg. or 4 mg./Tab. Bot. 100s, 500s.
Use: Relief of bronchospasm in patients with reversible obstructive airway disease.

PROVERA. (Upjohn) Medroxyprogesterone acetate 2.5 mg./Tab. Bot. 25s; 10 mg./Tab. Bot. 25s, 100s. Dosepak of 10s.
Use: Secondary amenorrhea; abnormal uterine bleeding due to hormonal imbalance.

PROVIGAN INJECTION. (Reid-Provident) Promethazine HCl 25 or 50 mg./ml. Vial 10 ml.
Use: Antihistaminic.

• **PROXAZOLE.** USAN. 5-[(2-Diethyl-amino)ethyl]-3-(α-ethyl-benzyl)-1,2,4-oxadiazole.
Use: Antispasmodic, analgesic, anti-inflammatory.

• **PROXAZOLE CITRATE.** USAN.
Use: Relaxant, analgesic, anti-inflammatory.

PROXENE. (Bowman) Propoxyphene HCl 65 mg./Cap.
Use: Analgesic.

• **PROXICROMIL.** USAN.
Use: Anti-allergic.

PROXIGEL. (Reed & Carnrick) Formerly Oxygel. Carbamide peroxide 11% in a water free gel base. Tube 1.2 oz.
Use: Oral antiseptic and cleanser.

• **PROXORPHAN TARTRATE.** USAN.
Use: Analgesic; antitussive.

PROXYMETACAINE. B.A.N. 2-Diethylaminoethyl 3-amino-4-propoxybenzoate.
Use: Local anesthetic.
See: Proparacaine
Ophthalne [hydrochloride]

PROXYPHYLLINE. B.A.N. 7-(2-Hydroxypropyl)-theophylline.
Use: Bronchodilator.
See: Brontyl
Thean

PROZINE-50. (Hauck) Promazine HCl 50 mg./ml. Vial 10 ml.

Use: Management tension, anxiety & anti-emetic.

PRUDENTS. (Bariatric) Acetylphenylisatin 5 mg./Tab. Bot. 30s, 100s. Chewable Protein & Amino Acid
Use: Laxative.

PRULET LIQUITAB. (Mission) Phenolphthalein Liquitab. Film strip 50s.
Use: Fruit-flavored chewable laxative.

PRUNE CONCENTRATE. W/cascarin.
See: Prucara, Tab. (ICN)
W/Docusate sodium, guar gum.
See: D-S-S Compound, Cap. (Wolins)

PRUNE POWDER CONCENTRATED DEHYDRATED.
See: Diacetyldihydroxyphenylisatin
W/Cascara fl. ext. aromatic & psyllium husk pow.
See: Casyllium, Pow. (Upjohn)

PRUNE PREPS.
See: Casyllium, Granules (Upjohn)

PRUN-EVAC. (Pharmex) Bot. 30s.
Use: Laxative.

PRUNICODEINE. (Lilly) Codeine sulfate 60 mg., prunus virginiana 1.58 Gm., pinus strobus 1.05 Gm., sanguinaria 262 mg., terpin hydrate 175 mg., alcohol 25%/30 ml. Bot. 16 fl. oz.
Use: Orally; cough.

PRURILO. (Whorton) Menthol ¼%, phenol ¼%, calamine lotion in special lubricating base. Bot. 4 oz., 8 oz.
Use: Relief of pruritus.

PRURITOL OINTMENT. (Blue Line) Tannic acid 45 gr., zinc oxide 45 gr., balsam peru 15 gr., thymol iodide 3 gr., menthol 2 gr./oz. Tube w/rectal pipe 1¼ oz.

P & S LIQUID. (Baker/Cummins) Liquid paraffin oil, sodium chloride, phenol (less than 1%) Bot. 4 oz., 8 oz.
Use: Antiseborrheic shampoo.

P & S SHAMPOO. (Baker/Cummins) Salicylic acid 2%, lactic acid 0.5% Bot. 4 oz.
Use: Antiseborrheic shampoo.

PSEUDODINE C EXPECTORANT. (Bay) Triprolidine HCl 2 mg., pseudoephedrine HCl 30 mg., codeine phosphate 10 mg., guiafenesin 100 mg./5 ml. Bot. 4 oz., pt., gal.
Use: Expectorant, antitussive, decongestant.

PSEUDODINE SYRUP. (Bay) Triprolidine HCl 1.25 mg., pseudoephedrine HCl 30 mg./5 ml. Bot. 4 oz., pt., gal.
Use: Treatment common cold, allergic rhinitis.

• **PSEUDOEPHEDRINE HYDROCHLORIDE,** U.S.P. XXI. Syrup, Tab., U.S.P. XXI. Isoephedrine HCl. α(1-Methylamino)-ethyl benzyl alcohol HCl. (+)-Pseudoephedrine HCl.
Use: Adrenergic.
See: Cenafed, Syr., Tab. (Century)
D-Feda, Cap., Syr. (Dooner)
Novafed, Cap., Liq. (Merrell Dow)
Ro-Fedrin, Tab., Syr. (Robinson)
Sinufed, Cap. (Hauck)
Sudafed, Tab., Syr. (Burroughs Wellcome)
Sudafed S.A., Cap. (Burroughs Wellcome)

PSEUDOEPHEDRINE HCl W/COMBINATIONS
See: Actifed, Tab., Sry. (Burroughs Wellcome)
Actified-C Expectorant, Syr. (Burroughs Wellcome)

Ambenyl-D, Liq. (Marion)
Asmadil Unicelles (Reid-Provident)
Asthmaspan, T.D. Cap. (Wolins)
Atridine, Tab. (Interstate)
Ayr, Liq. (Ascher)
Ayrcap, Cap. (Ascher)
Brexin, Cap., Liq. (Savage)
Bronchobid, Cap. (Meyer)
Cotrol-D, Tab. (Beecham Labs)
Co Tylenol, Tab. (McNeil)
Co Tylenol Liquid Cold Formula (McNeil)
Deconamine, Cap., Tab., Elix., Syrup (Berlex)
Dimacol, Cap., Liq. (Robins)
Eldafed, Tab., Liq. (Elder)
Fedahist, Prods. (Dooner)
Fedrazil, Tab. (Burroughs Wellcome)
Historal, Cap., Liq. (W. F. Merchant)
Isoclor, Preps. (American Critical Care)
Kronofed-A, Cap. (Ferndale)
Novafed A, Liq., Cap. (Merrell Dow)
Novahistine Sinus Tablets, Tab. (Merrell Dow)
Phenergan Comp., Tab. (Wyeth)
Phenergan-D, Tab. (Wyeth)
Rhinosyn, Cap., Liq. (Comatic)
Robitussin-DAC, Liq. (Robins)
Robitussin-PE, Liq. (Robins)
Rondec D, Drops; C, Tab.; S, Syr.; T, Filmtab (Ross)
Rondec DM, Drops, Syr. (Ross)
Ryna, Liq. (Mallinckrodt)
Ryna-Cx, Liq. (Mallinckrodt)
Sinacon, Tab. (Glaxo)
Sudafed Plus, Tab., Syr. (Burroughs Wellcome)
Sudahist, Tab. (Upsher-Smith)
Suda-Proll Tab., Cap., Syr. (Columbia)
Triafed, Tab. (Wolins)
Triphed Tablets (Lemmon)
Triphedrine, Tab. (Redford)
Tussafed Exp. Liq. (Cavital)
Wal-Phed, Syrup, Tab. (Walgreens)

• **PSEUDOEPHEDRINE SULFATE.** U.S.P. XXI.
Use: Nasal decongestant.
See: Afrinol Repetabs (Schering)
W/Chlorpheniramine maleate.
See: Chlor-trimeton Decongestant, Tab. (Schering)
W/Dexbrompheniramine.
See: Disophrol Chronotabs, Tab. (Schering)
Drixoral S.A., Tab. (Schering)
W/Dexchlorpheniramine.
See: Polaramine Expt. (Schering)

PSEUDOMONAS POLYSACCHARIDE.
See: Piromen, Vial (Flint)

"PSEUDO-PHEDRINE". (Whiteworth) Pseudoephedrine HCl 30 mg./Tab. Bot. 100s, 1000s.
Use: Nasal decongestant.

PSEUDO PLUS. (Weeks & Leo) Pseudoephedrine HCl 60 mg., chlorpheniramine maleate 4 mg./Tab. Bot. 40s.
Use: Decongestant.

PSEUDO-PROL SYRUP. (Columbia) Tripolidine HCl 1.25 mg., pseudoephedrine HCl 30 mg./5 ml. Bot. Pts., Gal.
Use: Antihistamine, decongestant.

PSEUDO-PROL TABLETS. (Columbia) Triprolidine HCl 2.5 mg., pseudoephedrine HCl 60 mg./Tab. Bot. 100s, 1000s.
Use: Antihistaminic, decongestant.

PSILOCYBIN. B.A.N. (Sandoz) 3-(2-Dimethylaminoethyl)indol-4-yl dihydrogen phosphate.
Use: Psychotogenic agent.
See: Indocybin

PSORANIDE CREAM. (Elder) Fluocinolone acetonide 0.025% in water washable cream base. Tube 0.5 oz., 2 oz.
Use: Relief of inflammatory and pruritic dermatoses.

PSORIASIS LOTION. (Wolins) Coal tar sol 3%, salicylic acid 1% in a greaseless lotion base. Bot. 8 oz.
Use: Psoriasis.

PSORIGEL. (Owen) Coal tar sol. 7.5%, 33% alcohol in hydroalcoholic gel vehicle Tubes 4 oz.
Use: Eczema, psoriasis, & other coal tar-responsive dermatoses.

P.S.P. IV (Four). (Reid-Provident) Prednisolone sodium phosphate (equivalent to prednisolone phosphate 20 mg.), niacinamide 25 mg., EDTA disodium 0.5 mg., sod. bisulfite 1 mg., phenol 5 mg./cc. pH adjusted w/HCl acid and/or sod. hydroxide. Vial 10 cc. for IM, IV, IA or IB use.

PSYCHOTHERAPEUTIC DRUGS.
See: Ataraxic Agents

PSYLLIUM GRANULES.
Use: Bulk producing laxative.
W/Dextrose.
See: Muci-lax, Granules (Med. Chem.)
W/Senna.
See: Perdiem, Granules (Rorer)

• **PSYLLIUM HUSK,** U.S.P. XXI.
Use: Cathartic
W/Cascara fl. ext. aromatic & prune pow.
Use: Cathartic.
See: Casyllium, Pow. (Upjohn)

PSYLLIUM HYDROCOLLOID.
Use: Bulk producing laxative.
See: Effersyllium, Pow. (Stuart)

PSYLLIUM HYDROPHILIC MUCILLOID.
Use: Bulk producing laxative.
See: Aquamucil, Liq. (Cenci)
Konsyl, Powder (Lafayette)
Mucillium, Powder (Whiteworth)
W/Dextrose.
See: Hydrocil Plain (Rowell)
Konsyl-D Powder (Lafayette)
V-lax, Powder (Century)
W/Dextrose, casanthranol.
See: Hydrocil Fortified (Rowell)
W/Docusate sodium.
See: Sof-Cil, Pow. (Zemmer)
W/Oxyphenisatin acetate.
See: Plova Pow. (WEL)
W/Standardized senna concentrate.
See: Senokot w/Psyllium Powder (Purdue Frederick)

PSYLLIUM SEED GEL.
Use: Bulk producing laxative.
W/Planta Ovata, gum Karaya, Brewer's yeast.

See: Plantamucin, Granules (Elder)

2,4,7-PTERIDINETRIAMINE, 6-PHENYL-. Triamterene, U.S.P. XXI.

PTEROIC ACID. The compound formed by the linkage of carbon 6 of 2-amine-4-hydroxypteridine by means of a methylene group with the nitrogen of p-aminobenzoic acid.

PTEROYLGLUTAMIC ACID.
See: Folic Acid, Prep. (Var. Mfr.)

PTEROYLMONOGLUTAMIC ACID. Pteroylglutamic acid.
See: Folic acid, Prep. (Var. Mfr.)

PTEROYLTRIGLUTAMATE SOD.

PTFE. (Ethicon) Polytef.

PTHALOX. (Sutliff & Case) Cal. ricinoleate 65 mg., phenolphthalein 32.5 mg., sod. glycocholate 32.5 mg., sod. taurocholate 16 mg., cascara sagrada ext. 32.5 mg., aloin 8 mg./Tab. Bot. 100s, 1000s.
Use: Laxative.

PULMIDOL. Propyl Docetrizoate, B.A.N.

PULMOSIN. (Spanner) Guaiacol 0.10 Gm., eucalyptol 0.08 Gm., camphor 0.05 Gm., iodoform 0.02 Gm./2 cc. Multiple dose vial 30 cc. Inj. I.M.

PULMOTOL. (D'Franssia)
Use: Cough syrup.

• **PUMICE,** U.S.P. XXI.
Use: Abrasive (dental).

PURA. (D'Franssia) High potency Vit. E cream.
Use: For rough dry skin.

PUREBROM COMPOUND ELIXIR. (Purepac) Brompheniramine maleate 4 mg./5 ml. w/phenylephrine HCl, phenylpropanolamine HCl, alcohol. Bot. pts., gal.
Use: Antihistaminic, vasoconstrictor.

PUREBROM COMPOUND TABLETS. (Purepac) Brompheniramine maleate 12 mg./Tab. w/phenylephrine HCl, phenylpropanolamine HCl/Tab. Bot. 100s, 1000s.
Use: Antihistaminic, vasoconstrictor.

PURETANE. (Purepac) Brompheniramine maleate 2 mg., guaifenesin 100 mg., phenylephrine HCl 5 mg., phenylpropanolamine HCl 5 mg. Bot. pt.
Use: Antihistaminic, expectorant, vasoconstrictor.

PURGE. (Fleming) Castor oil Bot. 2 oz.
Use: Laxative.

PURGE EVACUANT. (Fleming) Castor oil 95%. Bot. 2 oz.
Use: Bowel evacuant.

PURIFIED OXGALL.
See: Bile Extract, Ox (Various Mfr.)

PURIFIED PROTEIN DERIVATIVE OF TUBERCULIN.
Use: Mantoux TB test.
See: Tuberculin, Old, Vial (Parke-Davis)

1H-PURINE-2,6-DIONE,8-CHLORO-3,7-DIHYDRO-1,3 -DIMETHYL-, COMPOUND WITH 2-(DIPHENYLME-THOXY)-N,N-DIMETHYLETHANAMINE (1:1).
Dimenhydrinate, U.S.P. XXI.

1H-PURINE-2,6-DIONE,3,7-DIHYDRO-1,3-DIMETH-YL-, MONOHYDRATE. Theophylline, U.S.P. XXI.

1H-PURINE-2,6-DIONE,3,7-DIHYDRO-1,3-DIMETHYL -, COMPOUND WITH 1,2-ETHANEDIAMINE (2:1).
Aminophylline, U.S.P. XXI.

1H-PURINE-2,6-DIONE,3,7-DIHYDRO-1,3,7-TRIMETH-YL-. Caffeine, U.S.P. XXI.

1H-PURINE, 6-[(1-METHYL-4-NITRO-1H-IMIDAZOL-5-YL)THIO]-. Azathioprine, U.S.P. XXI.

PURINE-6-THIOL MONOHYDRATE. Mercaptopurine, U.S.P. XXI.

6H-PURINE-6-THIONE, MONOHYDRATE. Mercaptopurine, U.S.P. XXI.

6H-PURINE-6-THIONE, 2-AMINO-1,7-DIHYDRO-. Thioguanine, U.S.P. XXI.

PURINETHOL. (Burroughs Wellcome) Mercaptopurine, Tab. (50 mg.) Bot. 25s, 250s.
Use: Acute leukemia & chronic myelogenous leukemia.

PURODIGIN. (Wyeth) Digitoxin, Crystalline, **Tab.:** 0.1 mg., 0.2 mg./Tab. Bot. 100s, 500s.
Use: Cardiac decompensation & congestive heart failure.

• **PUROMYCIN.** USAN. 3′-(L-α-Amino-p-methoxhydrocinnamamido)-3′-deoxy-N,N-dimethyladenosine.
Use: Antibiotic.

• **PUROMYCIN HYDROCHLORIDE.** USAN.
Use: Antineoplastic; antiprotozoal.

PURPLE FOXGLOVE.
See: Digitalis, Preps. (Various Mfr.)

PURPOSE DRY SKIN CREAM. (Ortho) Water, white petrolatum, propylene glycol, glyceryl stearate, almond oil, sodium lactate, steareth-20, cetyl alcohol, mineral oil, ethyl esters wax, xanthan gum, steareth-2, sorbic acid, lactic acid, & fragrance. Tube 3 oz.
Use: Treatment of dry skin.

PURPOSE SHAMPOO. (Ortho) Water, amphoteric-19, PEG-44 sorbitan laurate, PEG-150 distearate, sorbitan laurate, boric acid, fragrance, & benzyl alcohol. Bot. 8 oz.
Use: Shampoo.

PURPOSE SOAP. (Ortho) Sodium and pot. salts of fatty acids, glycerin, fragrance. Bar 3.6 oz.

PURSETTES PREMENSTRUAL TABLETS. (Jeffrey Martin) Acetaminophen 500 mg., pamabrom 25 mg., pyrilamine maleate 15 mg./Tab. Bot. 24s.
Use: Relief of premenstural period associated symptoms.

P.V. CARPINE LIQUIFILM. (Allergan) Polyvinyl alcohol 1.4%, sodium acetate, sodium chloride, citric acid, menthol, camphor, phenol, eucalyptol, chlorobutanol 0.5% and purified water w/ pilocarpine nitrate ½%, 1%, 2%, or 4%. Dropper Bot. 15 ml.
Use: Miotic, control of intraocular pressure in glaucoma.

PVP-I OINTMENT. (Day-Baldwin) Povidoneiodine. Tube 1 oz., Jar 1 lb., Foilpac 1.5 Gm.

P-V-TUSSIN. (Reid-Provident) Hydrocodone bitartrate 2.5 mg., phenylephrine HCl 5 mg., ammonium chloride 50 mg., pyrilamine maleate 6 mg., chlorpheniramine maleate 2 mg., phenindamine tartrate 5 mg./5 cc. Bot. pt., gal.
Use: Antitussive, antihistaminic, decongestant, expectorant.

P-V TUSSIN TABLETS. (Reid-Provident) Hydrocodone

bitartrate 5 mg., phenindamine tartrate 25 mg., guaifenesin 200 mg./Tab. Bot. 100s.
Use: Antitussive, decongestant, expectorant.

PYCAZIDE. Isoniazid, B.A.N.

PY-CO-PAY TOOTH POWDER. (Block) Sodium chloride, sodium bicarbonate, calcium carbonate, magnesium carbonate, tricalcium phosphate, eugenol and methyl salicylate. Can 7 oz.
Use: Dentifrice.

PYGMAL. (CMC) Tartaric acid, boric acid, Burrow's sol., glycerin, starch, talc & bentonite. Oint., Tube 1½ oz.
Use: Antiseptic skin preparation.

PYLODATE. (Kenyon) Phenylazodiaminopyridine HCl 100 mg., methenamine mandelate 500 mg./Tab. Bot. 100s, 1000s.
Use: Urinary antiseptic.

PYLORA. (Hyrex) **No. 1:** Phenobarbital 16.2 mg., hyoscyamine sulfate 0.1037 mg., atropine sulfate 0.0194 mg., scopolamine HBr 0.0065 mg./Tab. Bot. 100s, 1000s.
Use: Antispasmodic-sedative.

PYMA. (Fellows) **Cap.:** Pyrilamine maleate 50 mg., chlorpheniramine maleate 6 mg., pheniramine maleate 20 mg., phenylephrine HCl 15 mg./Timed Cap. Bot. 30s, 100s, 1000s. **Inj.:** Chlorpheniramine maleate 5 mg., phenylpropanolamine HCl 12.5 mg., atropine sulfate 0.2 mg./cc. Vial 10 cc.

PYOCIDIN-OTIC SOLUTION. (Berlex) Hydrocortisone 5 mg., polymyxin B sulfate 10,000 USP units/ml in a vehicle containing water and propylene glycol. Bot. 10 ml. w/sterile dropper.
Use: Antibiotic & anti-inflammatory for otic use.

PYOPEN. (Beecham Labs). Carbenicillin disodium. 1 Gm., 2 Gm., 5 Gm./Vial. 10s; Piggyback Vials 2 Gm., 5 Gm. in 25s.; Bulk pharm pkg. 10 Gm., 20 Gm. in 25s.
Use: Antibiotic.

• **PYRABROM.** USAN. Pyrilamine 8-bromotheophyllinate. Glybrom.
Use: Antihistaminic.

PYRACOL. (Davis & Sly) Pyrathyn HCl 0.08 Gm., ammonium chloride 0.778 Gm., citric acid 0.52 Gm., menthol 0.006 Gm./fl. oz. Bot. pt.

PYRACOMP COLD TABLETS. (Barry-Martin) Pyrilamine maleate 25 mg., salicylamide 3½ gr., phenacetin 2½ gr., caffeine ½ gr./Tab. Bot. 100s, 1000s.

PYRADIN. (Jenkins) Acetophenetidin 4 gr., antipyrine 1 gr., caffeine ⅛ gr., tinct. hyoscyamus 8 min. (total alkaloids .00032 gr.), tinct. gelsemium 4 min./Tab. Bot. 1000s.
Use: Analgesic, anodyne.

PYRADONE.
See: Aminopyrine (Various Mfr.)

PYRA-MALEATE. (Mallinckrodt) Pyrilamine maleate.
Use: Antihistamine.

PYRAMINYL.
See: Pyrilamine Maleate (Var. Mfr.)

PYRANEURIN INJ. (Nutrition) Vitamin B-1 100 mg., & B-6 100 mg./cc., w/benzyl alcohol 1.5%. Vial. 10 cc.

Use: B-Vitamin Inj.
PYRANILAMINE MALEATE.
See: Pyrilamine Maleate, Preps. (Var. Mfr.)
PYRANISAMINE BROMOTHEOPHYLLINATE.
See: Pyrabrom (Var. Mfr.)
PYRANISAMINE MALEATE.
See: Pyrilamine Maleate, Preps. (Var. Mfr.)
PYRANISTAN. (Standex) Chlorprophenpyridamine 60 mg./10 cc.
PYRANISTAN COMPOUND. (Standex) Chlorpheniramine maleate 2 mg., salicylamide 3½ gr., phenacetin 2½ gr., caffeine ½ gr./Tab. Bot. 100s.
PYRANISTAN CREME. (Standex) Coal tar ext. 5%, pyrilamine maleate 1%, benzocaine 2½%, benzalkonium chloride 1%. Jar 1 oz.
PYRANISTAN STANKAPS. (Standex) Chlorpheniramine maleate 12 mg./Cap. Bot. 100s.
PYRANISTAN SYRUP. (Standex) d-Methorphan HBr 30 mg., guaifenesin 75 mg., sodium citrate 150 mg., chlorpheniramine maleate 3 mg./fl. oz. Bot. pt.
PYRANISTAN TAB. (Standex) Chlorpheniramine maleate 4 mg./Tab. Bot. 100s.
4H-PYRANO 2,3-b 1,4 BENZODIOXIN-4-ONE, DECAHYDRO-4a,7,9-TRIHYDROXY-2-METHYL-6,8 -BIS(METHYLAMINO)-,DI-HYDROCHLORIDE, PENTAHYDRATE. Sterile Spectinomycin HCl, U.S.P. XXI.
PYRANTEL. B.A.N. 1,4,5,6-Tetrahydro-1-methyl-2-[trans-2-(2-thienyl)vinyl]pyrimidine. Combantrin embonate.
Use: Anthelmintic.
• **PYRANTEL PAMOATE,** U.S.P. XXI. Oral Susp., U.S.P. XXI.
Use: Anthelmintic.
See: Antiminth, Oral Susp. (Roerig)
• **PYRANTEL TARTRATE.** USAN. 1,4,5,6-Tetrahydro-1-methyl-2-[trans-2-(2-thienyl)vinyl]-pyrimidine Tartrate.
Use: Anthelmintic.
PYRATHIAZINE HYDROCHLORIDE. (N-(2-Pyrrolidinoethyl)-phenothiazine.
• **PYRAZINAMIDE,** U.S.P. XXI. Tabs., U.S.P. XXI.
Pyrazinecarboxamide. 2-Carbamyl pyrazine.
Pyrazinecarboxamide. Aldinamide, Zinamide.
Pyrazinoic acid 0.5 Gm./Tab. Bot. 500s. Lederle-500 mg./Tab. Bot. 500s.
Use: Antibacterial (tuberculostatic).
PYRAZINECARBOXAMIDE. Pyrazinamide, U.S.P. XXI.
PYRAZODINE. (Cenci) Phenazopyridine HCl 100 mg./Cap. Bot. 100s, 1000s.
Use: Urinary tract analgesic.
• **PYRAZOFURIN.** USAN.
Use: Antineoplastic.
PYRAZOLE. Under study.
Use: Antitumor.
IH-PYRAZOLE-3-ETHANAMINE, DIHYDROCHLORIDE. Betazole HCl, U.S.P. XXI.
3,5-PYRAZOLIDINEDIONE, 4-BUTYL-1,2-DIPHENYL. Phenylbutazone, U.S.P. XXI.

3,5-PYRAZOLIDINEDIONE, 1,2-DIPHENYL-4-2-(PHE-NYLSULFINYL)ETHYL-. Sulfinpyrazone, U.S.P. XXI.
PYRAZOLINE.
See: Antipyrine (Various Mfr.)
IH-PYRAZOLO[3,4-d]PYRIMIDIN-4-OL. Allopurinol, U.S.P. XXI.
PYRBENZINDOLE.
See: Benzindopyrine hydrochloride (Var. Mfr.)
PYRIBENZAMINE.
See: PBZ, Prods. (Geigy)
PYRICAIN. (Jenkins) Cetylpyridium chloride 4 mg., sod. propionate 10 mg., benzocaine 5 mg./Tab. Bot. 1000s.
PYRICARDYL.
See: Nikethamide, Inj. (Various Mfr.)
PYRIDAMIDE. (Galen) Phenylazo-diamine pyridine HCl 50 mg., sulfacetamide 250 mg./Tab. Bot. 100s, 500s, 1000s.
Use: Urinary antiseptic.
PYRIDENE. (Approved) Phenylazo-diaminopyridine HCl 100 mg./Tab. Bot. 24s, 100s, 1000s.
Use: Urinary tract analgesic.
I(4H)-PYRIDINEACETIC ACID, 3,5-DIIODO-4-OXO-, PROPYLESTER. Propyliodone, U.S.P. XXI.
4-PYRIDINECARBOTHIOAMIDE, 2-ETHYL-. Ethionamide, U.S.P. XXI.
3-PYRIDINECARBOXAMIDE. Niacinamide, U.S.P. XXI.
PYRIDINE-3-CARBOXYLIC ACID.
See: Nicotinic Acid, Preps. (Var. Mfr.)
4-PYRIDINECARBOXYLIC ACID, HYDRAZIDE. Isoniazid, U.S.P. XXI.
PYRIDINE-BETA-CARBOXYLIC ACID DIETHYL AMIDE.
See: Nikethamide, Inj. (Various Mfr.)
3,4-PYRIDINEDIMETHANOL, 5-HYDROXY-6-METH-YL-, HCL. Pyridoxine HCl, U.S.P. XXI.
3-PYRIDINEMETHANOL.
See: Roniacol, Prep. (Roche)
2-PYRIDINEPROPANAMINE, gamma-(4-CHLORO-PHENYL)-N,N-DIMETHYL-,(Z)-2-BUTENEDIOATE (1:1). Chlorpheniramine Maleate, U.S.P. XXI.
PYRIDINIUM,3-//(DIMETHYLAMINO)CARBONYL/ OXY-1-METHYL-, BROMIDE. Pyridostigmine Bromide, U.S.P. XXI.
PYRIDINIUM,2-/(HYDROXYIMINO)METHYL/-1-METHYL-, CHLORIDE. Pralidoxime Chloride, U.S.P. XXI.
PYRIDIUM. (Parke-Davis) Phenazopyridine HCl 100 mg. or 200 mg./Tab. Bot. 100s, 1000s. Unit dose 100s.
Use: Urinary analgesic/anti-infectant.
W/Hyoscyamine HBr & butabarbital.
See: Pyridium Plus, Tab. (Parke-Davis)
PYRIDIUM PLUS. (Parke-Davis) Formerly Dolonil. Phenazopyridine HCl 150 mg., hyoscyamine HBr. 0.3 mg., butabarbital 15 mg./Tab. Bot. 100s.
Use: Urinary analgesic, antispasmodic.
• **PYRIDOSTIGMINE BROMIDE,** U.S.P. XXI. Syr., Tabs. U.S.P. XXI. Pyridinium 3-[[(dimethylamino)carbonyl]oxy]-1-methyl-, bromide. Dimethyl carbamic ester of 3-hydroxy-1-methylpyridinium bromide.
Use: Cholinergic.

See: Mestinon, Tab., Syr., Amp. (Roche)
Regonal (Organon)
PYRIDOX. (Oxford) **No. 1:** Pyridoxine HCl 100 mg./Tab. **No. 2:** Pyridoxine HCl 200 mg./Tab. Bot. 100s.
Use: Vitamin B-6 supplement.
PYRIDOXAL. Vit. B-6 3-Hydroxy-4-formyl-5-hydroxymethyl-2-methylpyridine.
Use: Cholinergic.
PYRIDOXAMINE. Vit. B-6. 3-Hydroxy-4-aminomethyl-5-hydroxymethyl-2-methylpyridine.
• **PYRIDOXINE HYDROCHLORIDE,** U.S.P. XXI. Inj., Tab. U.S.P. XXI. Vit. B-6. 3,4-Pyridinedimethanol, 5-hydroxy-6-methyl-, hydrochloride. Pyridoxol hydrochloride.
Use: Enzyme co-factor vitamin.
See: Beesix, Vial (Fellows-Testagar)
HexaBetalin, Amp., Tab., Vial (Lilly)
Hexavibex, Vial (Parke-Davis)
Pan B-6, Tab. (Panray)
PYRIDOXINE HCl, HEXA-BETALIN. (Lilly) Pyridoxine HCl. Vial 10 mg./ml. 10 ml.
Use: Vitamin B-6 therapy.
PYRIDOXOL. 3-Hydroxy-4,5-hydroxymethyl-2-methylpyridine.
See: Pyridoxine, Vit. B-6.
PYRIDYL CARBINOL.
See: Roniacol, El. & Tab. (Roche)
4,4'-(2-PYRIDYLMETHYLENE)DIPHENOL DIACETATE (ESTER). Bisacodyl, U.S.P. XXI.
N¹-2-PYRIDYLSULFANILAMIDE. Sulfapyridine, U.S.P. XXI.
PYRIHIST JR. (Evron) Same formula as Pyrihist Cough Syrup but cherry flavor. Bot. 4 fl. oz., gal.
PYRILAMINE BROMOTHEOPHYLLINATE.
See: Pyrabrom
W/2-amino-2-methyl-1-propanol.
See: Bromaleate
• **PYRILAMINE MALEATE,** U.S.P. XX. Tab., U.S.P. XXI. 2-[[2-(Dimethylamino)ethyl](p-methoxy-benzyl)-amino]-pyridine maleate (1:1). Pyranisamine, Pyranilamine, Pyraminyl, Anisopyradamine.
Available: Cap. sustained action, Cream, Ophth. Sol., Syrup, Tablets.
Use: Antihistamine.
See: Pyma, Cap., Vial (Fellows-Testagar)
Pyristan, Cap., Elix. (Arcum)
W/Combinations.
See: Allergine, Cap. (Wolins)
Antihistamine Cream (Towne)
Anti-Itch Cream (Towne)
Cardui, Tab. (Chattem Labs.)
Corizahist, Tab. (Mason)
Coton, Syr., Tab. (Reid-Provident)
Covanamine Tablets (Mallinckrodt)
C.P.C. Cough Syrup (Coastal)
Femicin, Tab. (Norcliff Thayer)
Four Antihistamines, Tab. (Wolins)
Histjen, Cap. (Jenkins)
Hist-Span No. 2, Cap. (Kenyon)
Kenahist S.A., Tab. (Kenyon)
Miles Nervine, Tab. (Miles)

MSC Triaminic, Tab. (Dorsey)
Nasal Spray (Penta)
Prefrin-A Ophth. Sol. (Allergan)
Triwol, Tab. (Wolins)
PYRILAMINE TANNATE.
W/Chlorpheniramine tannate, d-amphetamine tannate.
See: Nalertan, Tab. (Mallinckrodt)
• **PYRIMETHAMINE,** U.S.P. XXI. Tabs. U.S.P. XXI. 2,4-Pyrimidinediamine, 5-(4-chlorophenyl) 6-ethyl-.2,4-Diamino-5-(p-chlorophenyl)-6-ethyl-pyrimidine. Daraprim.
Use: Antimalarial.
See: Daraprim, Tab. (Burroughs Wellcome)
W/Sulfadoxine
See: Fansidar, Tab. (Roche)
2,4-PYRIMIDINEDIAMINE, 5-(4-CHLORO-PHENYL)-6-ETHYL. Pyrimethamine, U.S.P. XXI.
4,6(1H,5H)-PYRIMIDINEDIONE, 5-ETHYL-DIHYDRO-5-(1-METHYLBUTYL)-2-THIOXO-, MONOSODIUM SALT. Thiopental Sodium, U.S.P. XXI.
4,6(1H,5H)-PYRIMIDINEDIONE, 5-ETHYL-DIHYDRO-5-PHENYL-. Primidone, U.S.P. XXI.
2,4(1H,3H)-PYRIMIDINEDIONE, 5-FLUORO-. Fluorouracil, U.S.P. XXI.
2,4,6(1H,3H,5H)-PYRIMIDINETRIONE, 5-ETHYL-5(1)METHYLBUTYL], MONOSODIUM SALT. Pentobarbital Sodium, U.S.P. XXI.
2,4,6(1H,3H,5H)-PYRIMIDINETRIONE, 5-ETHYL-5-(3-METHYLBUTYL)-, MONOSODIUM SALT. Amobarbital Sodium, U.S.P. XXI.
2,4,6,(1H,3H,5H)-PYRIMIDINETRIONE, 5-ETHYL-5PHENYL. Phenobarbital, U.S.P. XXI.
2,4,6,(1H,3H,5H)-PYRIMIDINETRIONE, 1-METHYL-5-(1-METHYL-2-PENTYNYL)-5-(2-PROPENYL)-, (±), Monosodium salt. Methohexital Sodium for Injection, U.S.P. XXI.
2(1H)-PYRIMIDINONE, 4-AMINO-1β-D-ARABINOFURANOSYL-. Cytarabine, U.S.P. XXI.
4(1H)-PYRIMIDINONE, 2,3-DIHYDRO-6-PROPYL-2-THIOXO-. Propylthiouracil, U.S.P. XXI.
N'-2-PYRIMIDINYLSULFANILAMIDE. Sulfadiazine, U.S.P. XXI.
PYRIMITHATE. B.A.N. 0-2-Dimethylamino-6-methyl-pyrimidin-4-y100-diethyl phosphorothioate.
Use: Insecticide, veterinary medicine.
See: Diothyl.
PYRIN-AID LIQUID. (Columbia) Pyrethrins 0.2%, piperonyl butoxide 2.0%, deodorized kerosene 0.8%. Bot. 2 oz.
Use: Kills head, body & crab lice & their eggs.
• **PYRINOLINE.** USAN.
Use: Cardiac depressant.
See: Surexin (McNeilab)
PYRISTAN. (Arcum) Phenylephrine HCl 8 mg., phenylpropanolamine HCl 15 mg., chlorpheniramine maleate 3 mg., pyrilamine maleate 10 mg./Cap. Bot. 50s, 500s. Elixir Bot. 4 oz., pt., gal.
Use: Decongestant and antihistaminic.
PYRISUL. (Kenyon) Sulfamethylthiadiazole 250 mg., phenylazodiamine pyridine 50 mg./Tab. Bot. 100s, 1000s.
PYRISUL-FORTE. (Kenyon) Sulfamethylthiadiazole 500

mg., phenylazodiamine pyridine 50 mg./Tab. Bot. 100s, 1000s.

PYRISUL PLUS. (Kenyon) Sulfamethylthiadiazole 250 mg., methenamine mandelate 250 mg., phenylazodiamine pyridine 50 mg./Tab. Bot. 100s, 1000s.

PYRITHEN.
See: Chlorothen Citrate. (Var. Mfr.)

PYRITHIDIUM BROMIDE. B.A.N. 3-Amino-8-(2-amino-1,6-dimethylpyrimidinium-4-ylamino)-6-(4-aminophen-yl)-5-methylphenanthridinium dibromide.
Use: Antiprotozoan, veterinary medicine.
See: Prothidium

PYRI-THIME INJ. (Ortega) Thiamine HCl 100 mg., pyridoxine HCl 100 mg./ml. Vial 10 ml.
Use: Nausea of pregnancy, seborrheic dermatitis, thiouracil-induced granulopenia, hyperemesis gravidarum.

• **PYRITHIONE ZINC.** USAN. Bis [1-hydroxy-2-(1H)-pyridinethionato]zinc. Zinc bis(pyridine-2-thiol 1-oxide. Zinc Omadine.
Use: Treatment of seborrhea.
See: Danex Shampoo (Herbert)
     Zincon Shampoo (Lederle)

PYRITINOL. B.A.N. Di(5-hydroxy-4-hydroxy-methyl-6-methyl-3-pyridylmethyl) disulfide.
Use: Cerebral neuroactivator which increases vigilance and increases or normalizes cerebral metabolism and blood flow.
See: Encephabol (Merck Sharp & Dohme)

PYRODYN. (Fellows) Dipyrone 0.5 Gm./cc. Vials 30 cc.

PYROGALLIC ACID OINTMENT. (Gordon) Pyrogallic acid 25% w/chlorobutanol. Jar 1 oz., 2 oz., 1 lb.
Use: Verruca therapy.

PYROGALLOL. Pyrogallic acid.

PYROPHENINDANE. 1-(1-Methyl-3-pyrroli-dylmethyl)-3-phenylindane. (Mead Johnson)

• **PYROVALERONE HCl.** USAN. 4'-Methyl-2-(1-pyr-rolidinyl)valerophenone HCl.
Use: Central stimulant.

• **PYROXAMINE MALEATE.** USAN.
Use: Antihistaminic.

• **PYROXYLIN,** U.S.P. XXI. Soluble guncotton.
Cellulose nitrate.
Use: Pharm. necessity for Collodion.

PYRRALAN COMPOUND CAPSULES. (Lannett) Thenylpyramine fumarate 25 mg., acetylsalicylic acid 3¼ gr., phenacetin 2½ gr., caffeine ¼ gr./Cap. Bot. 100s, 500s, 1000s.
Use: Analgesic w/antihistamine.

PYRRALAN EXPECTORANT. (Lannett) Thenyl-pyramine fumarate 80 mg., ephedrine HCl 30 mg., ammonium chloride 500 mg./fl. oz. Bot. pt., gal.

PYRRALAN EXPECTORANT "DM." (Lannett) Same formula as Pyrralan Expect. w/d-methorphan HBr 10 mg./5 cc. Bot. pt., gal.
Use: Antitussive, antihistaminic, expect.

PYRROBUTAMINE. B.A.N. 1-[4-(4-Chlorophenyl)-3-phe-nylbut-2-enyl]pyrrolidine.
Use: Antihistamine.
See: Pyronil phosphate.

• **PYRROBUTAMINE PHOSPHATE,** U.S.P. XXI. 1-[4-(p-Chlorophenyl)-3-phenyl-2-butenyl]pyrrolidine diphosphate. 1-[α-(p-Chlorobenzyl)cin-namyl]pyrrolidine phosphate (1:2).
Use: Antihistaminic.
W/Clopane HCl, Histadyl.
See: Co-Pyronil, Preps. (Lilly)

• **PYRROCAINE.** USAN. 1-Pyrrolidine-aceto-2',6'-xyli-dide. Endocaine.
Use: Local anesthetic.

PYRROCAINE HYDROCHLORIDE. 1-Pyr-rolidineaceto-2',6'-xylidide HCl.
Use: Local anesthetic (dental).

PYRROCAINE HYDROCHLORIDE AND EPINEPHRINE INJ.
Use: Local anesthetic (dental).

1-PYRROLIDINEACETO-2',6'-XYLIDIDE MONOHY-DROCHLORIDE. Pyrrocaine HCl.

2,5-PYRROLIDINEDIONE, 3-ETHYL-3-METHYL-. Ethosuximide, U.S.P. XXI.

N-(PYRROLIDINOMETHYL)TETRACYCLINE. Pyr-rolidinomethyl.
See: Rolitetracycline, Inj.

2-PYRROLIDINONE, 1-ETHENYL-,HOMOPOLYMER. Povidone, U.S.P. XXI.

• **PYRROLIPHENE HYDROCHLORIDE.** USAN. d-α-Benzyl-β-methyl-α-phenyl-1-pyrrolidine-propanol ac-etate HCl. α-d-2-Acetoxy-1,2-dephenyl-3-methyl-4-pyrrolidinobutane HCl.
Use: Analgesic.

• **PYRROLNITRIN.** USAN. 3-Chloro-4-(3-chloro-2-nitro-phenyl)pyrrole. Under study.
Use: Antifungal.

PYRROLO[2,3-b]INDOL-5-OL, 1,2,3,3a,8,8a-HEXA-HYDRO-1,3a,8-TRIMETHYL-, METHYLCARBA-MATE (ESTER), (3aS-cis). Physostigmine, U.S.P. XXI.

PYRROXATE. (Upjohn) Chlorpheniramine maleate 4 mg., phenylpropanolamine HCl 25 mg., acetaminophen 500 mg./Cap. Blister pkg. 24s. Bot. 500s.
Use: Relief for colds, allergies and sinus congestion.

• **PYRVINIUM PAMOATE,** U.S.P. XXI. Tab., Oral Susp.: U.S.P. XXI. Quinolinium, 6-(dimethyl-amino-2-[2-(2,5-dimethyl-1-phenyl-1H-pyrrol-3-yl)ethenyl]-1-methyl-, salt with 4,4'-methyl-enebis[3-hydroxy-2-naphthalenecarboxylic]
Use: Anthelmintic.

PYTOSIN LIQUID. (Blue Line) Benzoic acid 52 gr., salicylic acid 26 gr., benzocaine 5 gr./oz., alcohol 77% Bot. 1 oz., 1 pt., 1 gal.
Use: Topical; fungicide & desquamative.

Q

Q.S. DIET AID. (Western Research) Potassium bicarbonate 70 mg., alginic acid 200 mg., methylcellulose 100 mg./Tab. Bot. 100s.
Use: Diet aid.

QT QUICK TANNING LOTION. (Plough) Padimate O,

dihydroxyacetone (SPF 2). Tube 2 oz., Bot. 4 oz., 8 oz.
Use: Artificial tanner, ultraviolet sunscreen.

Q-U. (Eastwood) Cough syrup. Bot. 1 pt. With codeine Bot. 1 pt.

QUA-BID. (Quaker City Pharmacal) Papaverine HCl 150 mg./timed disintegrating Cap. Bot. 100s, 1000s.
Use: Smooth muscle relaxant.

QUADA-CREAM. (Sutliff & Case) Pramoxine HCl 1%, cetyl dimethylethyl ammonium bromide 2%, pyrilamine maleate 1%, allantoin 0.4%. Tube 1 oz., Jar 1 lb.
Use: Antihistamine, anesthetic and antiseptic.

QUADRABARB. (Harvey) Secobarbital sod. 3/8 gr., penobarbital sod. 3/8 gr., butabarbital sod. 3/8 gr., phenobarbital 3/8 gr./Tab. Bot. 1000s.
Use: Sedative, hypnotic.

QUADRAHIST. (Harvey; Pharmex; Kenyon) Pyrilamine maleate, phenyltoloxamine dihydrogen citrate, prophenpyridamine maleate/Tab. (Harvey) Bot. 1000s. (Pharmex) Bot. 40s, 1000s. (Kenyon) Bot. 100s, 1000s.
Use: Antihistamine.

QUADRINAL. (Knoll) Ephedrine HCl 24 mg., phenobarbital 24 mg., theophylline calcium salicylate 130 mg., pot. iodide 320 mg./Tab. Bot. 100s, 1000s.
Use: Asthma & related allergic respiratory conditions.

QUADRINAL SUSPENSION. (Knoll) Ephedrine HCl 12 mg., phenobarbital 12 mg., theophylline calcium salicylate 65 mg., potassium iodide 160 mg./5 cc. Bot. pts.
Use: Bronchospasm and wheezing.

QUADRODIDE.
See: Quadrinal, Susp., Tab. (Knoll)

QUADRUPLE SULFONAMIDES.
See: Sulfonamides

QUAD-SET. (Kenyon) Secobarbital 25 mg., pentobarbital 25 mg., butabarbital 25 mg., phenobarbital 25 mg./Tab. Bot. 100s, 1000s.
Use: Sedative.

QUANTRIL. Benzquinamide.
Use: CNS depressant.

QUARTETS. (Eckerd) Phenylpropanolamine HCl 25 mg., chlorpheniramine maleate 2 mg., dextromethorphan HBr 15 mg., ascorbic acid 25 mg./Cap. Bot. 24s.
Use: Antihistaminic, decongestant, antitussive.

QUARZAN. (Roche) Clidinium Bromide 2.5 mg., 5 mg./Cap. Bot. 100s.
Use: Peptic ulcer disease.

• **QUAZEPAM.** USAN.
Use: Sedative; hypnotic.

• **QUAZODINE.** USAN.
Use: Cardiotonic; bronchodilator.

Q-U-CORT. (Eastwood) Cream 1/4% 1/2%, or 1%. Tube 1 oz., or 4 oz.

QUELICIN. (Abbott) Succinylcholine chloride. 50 mg./ml., 10 ml. ampul; 100 mg./ml., 10 ml. ampul; 20 mg./ml., 10 ml. fliptop vial; Quelicin-1000, 10 ml. in

20 ml. fliptop vial; Quelicin-500, 5 ml. in 10 ml. pintop vial; Quelicin-1000, 10 ml. in 20 ml. pintop vial; and 20 mg./ml. 5 ml. Abboject Syringe..
Use: Short-acting muscle relaxant.

QUELIDRINE SYRUP. (Abbott) Dextromethorphan HBr 10 mg., chlorpheniramine maleate 2 mg., ephedrine HCl 5 mg., phenylephrine HCl 5 mg., ammonium Cl 40 mg., ipecac fluid extract 0.005 cc., ethyl alcohol 2%/5 ml. Bot. 4 oz., 1 pt., 1 gal.
Use: Allergic disorders.

QUELLADA. Gamma Benzene Hexachloride, B.A.N.

QUELLS. (Stanlabs) Meclizine hydrochloride 25 mg./Chewable Tab. Box 24s.
Use: Antihistaminic.

QUELTUSS. (O'Neal, Jones & Feldman) Dextromethorphan HBr 15 mg., guaifenesin 100 mg./Tab. or 5 ml. of Syr. **Syr.:** Bot. 4 oz., pt. **Tab.:** Bot. 100s.
Use: Cough control.

QUERCETIN. Active constituent of rutin. Quertine.

QUERTINE. Quercetin. 3,3',4',5,7-Pentahydroxy-flavone.
Use: Treatment of capillary fragility.

QUESTRAN. (Mead Johnson) Cholestyramine resin 4 Gm. active ingredient/9 Gm. Powder Packet. Boxes 50 packets. Can 378 Gm.
Use: Antipruritic for pruritis related to biliary obstruction; Primary Type II hyperlipoproteinemia.

QUIBRON. (Mead Johnson) Theophylline (anhydrous) 150 mg., guaifenesin 90 mg./Cap. or 15 ml. Liquid. **Cap.:** Bot. 100's, 1000's, Box 100's individually wrapped. **Liquid:** Bot. pt., gal.
Use: Bronchodilator for symptomatic treatment of bronchospasm.

QUIBRON-300. (Mead Johnson) Theophylline anhydrous 300 mg., guaifenesin 180 mg./Cap. Bot. 100s.
Use: Bronchodilator for symptomatic treatment of bronchospasm.

QUIBRON PLUS. (Mead Johnson) Ephedrine HCl 25 mg., theophylline (anhydrous) 150 mg., butabarbital 20 mg., guaifenesin 100 mg./Cap. or 15 ml. Elixir. **Cap.:** Bot. 100s. **Elixir:** 15% alcohol. Bot. pt., gal.
Use: Bronchodilator for symptomatic treatment of bronchospasm.

QUIBRON-T DIVIDOSE TABLETS. (Mead Johnson) Theophylline anhydrous 300 mg./Tab. Dividose design breakable into 100 mg., 150 or 200 mg. portions. Immediate release. Bot. 100s.
Use: Bronchodilator for symptomatic treatment of bronchospasm.

QUIBRON-T/SR DIVIDOSE TABLETS. (Mead Johnson) Theophylline anhydrous 300 mg./Tab. Dividose design breakable into 100 mg., 150 mg., or 200 mg. portions. Sustained release. Bot. 100s.
Use: Bronchodilator for symptomatic treatment of bronchospasm.

QUICK-K. (Western Research) Potassium bicarbonate 650 mg. (6.01 mEq.) potassium/Tab. for sol. Bot. 30s, 1000s.
Use: Supplement.

QUIDE. (Merrell Dow) Piperacetazine 10 mg. and 25 mg./Tab. Bot. 100s.
Use: Treatment of psychoses.
QUIEBAR. (Nevin) Butabarbital sodium **Spantab:** 1½ gr./Timed Release Spantab. Bot. 50s, 500s. **Elixir** 30 mg./5 cc. Bot. pt., gal. **Tab.** 15 mg. Bot. 100s, 1000s. 30 mg. Bot. 1000s. **A.C. Cap.** Bot. 100s, 500s.
Use: Hypnotic, sedative.
QUIEBEL. (Nevin) Butabarbital sod. 15 mg., ext. belladonna 15 mg./Cap. Bot. 100s, 1000s. Elixir, pt., gal.
Use: Antispasmodic-sedative.
QUIECOF. (Nevin) Dextromethorphan HBr 7.5 mg., chlorpheniramine maleate 0.75 mg., guaiacol glyceryl ether 25.0 mg. Bot. 4 oz., pt., gal.
Use: Sugarless cough syrup.
QUIESS (O'Neal, Jones & Feldman) Hydroxyzine HCl 25 mg./ml. Vial 10 ml.
QUIET WORLD. (Whitehall) Acetaminophen 2.5 gr., aspirin 3.5 gr., pyrilamine maleate 25 mg./Tab. Bot. 12s, 30s.
Use: Analgesic.
QUIK-CEPT. (Laboratory Diagnostics) Slide test for pregnancy, rapid latex inhibition test. Kits: 25s, 50s, 100s.
Use: For pregnancy testing.
QUIK-CULT. (Laboratory Diagnostics) Slide test for fecal occult blood. Kits. 150s, 200s, 300s, and tape test.
Use: Rapid, convenient method for testing fecal specimens for occult blood.
QUILATE. (Wolins) Theophylline (anhydrous) 150 mg., guaifenesin 90 mg./Cap. Bot. 100s, 1000s.
QUINACILLIN. B.A.N. 6-(3)Carboxyquinoxaline-2-carboxamideo)penicillanic acid.
Use: Antibiotic.
• **QUINACRINE HYDROCHLORIDE,** U.S.P. XXI. Tab., U.S.P. XXI. 1,4-Pentanediamine,N⁴-(6-chloro-2-methoxy-9-acridinyl)-N¹,N¹-diethyl-, dihydrochloride, dihydrate. Mepacrine HCl, 6-Chloro-9- [4-(diethylamino)-1-methyl-butyl]amino -2-methoxyacridine dihydrochloride. 3-Chloro-7-methoxy-9-(1-methyl-4-diethylamino-butylamino)-acridine di-HCl dihydrate.
Use: Anthelmintic.
See: Atabrine HCl, Tab. (Winthrop-Breon)
QUINAGLUTE DURA-TABS. (Berlex) Quinidine gluconate 324 mg./Tab. Bot. 100s, 250s, 500s. Unit dose 100s. Unit of use 90s, 120s.
Use: Cardiac arrhythmias.
QUINALBARBITONE SODIUM. B.A.N. Monosodium derivative of 5-allyl-5-(1-methylbutyl)-barbituric acid.
Use: Hypnotic; sedative.
See: Secobarbital Sodium
    Seconal Sodium
• **QUINALDINE BLUE.** USAN. 1-Ethyl-2-[3-(1-ethyl-2(1H) quinolylidene) propenyl]-quinolinium chloride. Vernitest reagent. (Fuller)
Use: Diagnostic agent (obstetrics).
QUINAMM. (Merrell Dow) Quinine sulf. 260 mg./Tab. Bot. 100s.

Use: Prevention and treatment of nocturnal recumbency leg muscle cramps.
• **QUINAZOSIN HYDROCHLORIDE.** USAN. 2-(4-Allyl-1 piperazinyl)-4-amino-6,7-dimethoxy-quinazoline dihydrochloride.
Use: Hypotensive.
• **QUINBOLONE.** USAN. 17-beta-(1-Cyclo-penten-1-yloxy)-androsta-1,4-dien-3-one.
Use: Anabolic agent.
• **QUINDECAMINE ACETATE.** USAN. 4,4'-(Decamethylenediimino) diquinaldine diacetate dihydrate.
Use: Topical anti-infective.
• **QUINDONIUM BROMIDE.** USAN. 2,3-3α,5,6,11,12,12 α-Octahydro-8-hydroxy-1H-benzo-[α]-cyclopenta[f]-quinolizinium bromide.
Use: Cardiovascular agent.
QUINDOXIN. B.A.N. Quinoxaline 1,4-dioxide.
Use: Growth promoter, veterinary medicine.
See: Grofas
QUINE. (Rowell) Quinine sulfate 200 mg., 300 mg. 200 mg./Cap. Bot. 100s. 300 mg./Cap. Bot. 100s. Unit dose 100s.
Use: Antimalarial.
QUINESTRADOL. B.A.N. 3-Cyclopentyloxyestra-1,3,-5(10)-triene-16α,17β-diol.
Use: Estrogen.
See: Pentovis
• **QUINESTROL,** U.S.P. XXI. Tab., U.S.P. XXI. 3-(Cyclopentyloxy)-19-nor-17-α-pregna-1,3,5(10)-triene-20-yn-1-ol.
Use: Estrogen.
See: Estrovia, Tab. (Parke-Davis)
• **QUINETHAZONE,** U.S.P. XXI. Tab., U.S.P. XXI. 7-Chloro-2-ethyl-6-sulfamyl-1,2,3,4-tetra-hydro-4-quinazolinone. 7-Chloro-2-ethyl-1,2,3,4-tetrahydro-4-oxo-6-quinazolinesulfonamide. Aquamox.
Use: Diuretic.
See: Hydromox, Tab. (Lederle)
W/Reserpine.
See: Hydromox R, Tab. (Lederle)
• **QUINETOLATE.** USAN. 6-(Diethylcarbamoyl)-3-cyclohexene-1-carboxylic acid comp. with 4-((2-(dime-thylamino) ethyl)amino)6-methoxy-quinoline (2:1) Phthalamaquin (Penick).
Use: Antiasthmatic.
• **QUINFAMIDE.** USAN.
Use: Anti-amebic.
QUINGESTANOL. B.A.N. 3-Cyclopentyloxy-19-nor-17α-pregna-3,5-diene-20-yn-17-ol.
Use: Progestational steroid.
• **QUINGESTANOL ACETATE.** USAN. 3-(Cyclopentyloxy)-19-nor-17α-pregna-3,5-dien-20-yn-17-ol acetate. Under study.
Use: Progestational agent.
• **QUINGESTRONE.** USAN. 3-(Cyclopentyloxy)pregna-3,5-dien-20-one.
Use: Progestational agent.
QUINIDEX EXTENTABS. (Robins) Quinidine sulf. 300 mg./Tab. Bot. 100s, 250s. Dis-co pack of 100s.
Use: Cardiac arrhythmias.
QUINIDEX L-A.
See: Quinidex Extentabs (Robins)

- **QUINIDINE GLUCONATE,** U.S.P. XXI., Inj., U.S.P.
  XXI. Cinchonan-9-ol, 6'-methoxy-,(9s)-, mono-D-glu-
  conate (salt). (Lilly) Amp. (80 mg./cc.) 10 cc.
  Use: Quinidine therapy; cardiac depressant.
  See: Duraquin, Tab. (Parke-Davis)
  Quinaglute, Dura-Tabs. (Berlex)
- **QUINIDINE POLYGALACTURONATE.**
  See: Cardioquin Tab. (Purdue Frederick Co.)
- **QUINIDINE SULFATE,** U.S.P. XXI., Cap., Tab.,
  U.S.P. XXI. Cinchonan-9-ol, 6'-methoxy-,(9s)-, sulfate
  (2:1) (salt), dihydrate.
  Use: Cardiac depressant.
  See: Cin-Quin (Rowell)
  Maso-Quin, Tab. (Mason)
  Quinidex Extentabs (Robins)
  Quinora, Tab. (Key)
  SK-Quinidine Sulfate, Tab. (SmithKline)
- **QUININE ASCORBATE.** USAN.
  Use: Deterrent to smoking.
- **QUININE BISULFATE.**
  Use: Orally; analgesic & antipyretic & antimalarial.
- **QUININE DIHYDROCHLORIDE.**
  Use: I.M., I.V.; antimalarial therapy.
- **QUININE ETHYLCARBONATE.**
  See: Euquinine (Various Mfr.)
- **QUININE GLYCEROPHOSPHATE.** Quinine
  compound with glycerol phosphate.
- **QUININE SULFATE,** U.S.P. XXI. Cap., Tab., U.S.P.
  XXI. Cinchonan-9-ol, 6'-methoxy-, (8α,9R)-, sulfate
  (2:1) (salt) dihydrate.
  Use: Antimalarial.
  See: Quinamm, Tab. (Merrell Dow)
  Quine, Cap. (Rowell)
  W/Aminophylline.
  See: Quinite, Tab. (Reid-Provident)
  Strema, Cap. (Foy)
  W/Atropine sulf., emetine HCl, aconitine, camphor
  monobromate.
  See: Coryza, Tab. (Bowman)
  W/Niacin, Vit. E.
  See: Myodyne, Tab. (Paddock)
  W/Strychnine sulf., cinchonine sulf., cinchonidine sulf.,
  alcohol.
  See: Hospital Bitters, Liq. (Noyes)
- **QUININE AND UREA HYDROCHLORIDE.**
  Use: Sclerosing agent.
- **QUINISOCAINE (I.N.N.).** Dimethisoquin, B.A.N.
- **QUINITE.** (Reid-Provident) Quinine sulfate 260
  mg./Tab. Bot. 100s.
  Use: Uricosuric.
- **QUINNONE CREAM.** (Dermohr Pharmacal)
  Hydroquinone 4% in creamy base. Tube 1 oz.
  Use: Temporary bleaching of darkened areas of
  skin.
- **QUINOLINIUM,6-(DIMETHYLAMINO)-2-[2-(2,5-DIME-
  THYL-1-PHENYL-1H-PYRROL-3-YL)ETHENYL]-
  1-METHYL-, SALT WITH 4,4'-METHYLENEBIS[3-
  HYDROXY-2-NAPHTHALENECARBOXYLIC
  ACID](2:1).** Pyrvinium Pamoate, U.S.P. XXI.
- **8-QUINOLINOL, 5,7-DIIODO-.** Diiodohydroxyquin,
  Iodoquinol, U.S.P. XXI.

- **QUINOPHAN.**
  See: Cinchophen (Various Mfr.)
- **QUINORA.** (Key) Quinidine sulfate 3 gr., 5 gr./Tab.
  Bot. 100s, 1000s. Unit dose 100s.
  Use: Cardiac depressant.
- **QUINOXYL.**
  See: Chiniofon
- **QUINPRENALINE.** Quinterenol Sulfate.
- **QUINSONE.** (Sutliff & Case) Clioquinol 30 mg.,
  hydrocortisone acetate 10 mg., pramoxine HCl 5
  mg. in base of sulfonated and polyethoxylated fatty
  alcohols, free fatty alcohols, water/Gm. Oint. Tubes
  ½ oz.
  Use: Dermatologic.
- **QUINTERENOL SULFATE.** USAN. 8-Hydroxy-alpha-
  [(isopropylamino)methyl]-5-quinoline-methanol [sul-
  fate (2:1).
  Use: Bronchodilator.
- **QUINTIOFOS.** B.A.N. O-Ethyl 0-8-quinolyl phenyl-phos-
  phonothioate.
  Use: Insecticide, veterinary medicine.
  See: Bacdip
- **QUINUCLIUM BROMIDE.** USAN.
  Use: Antihypertensive.
- **QUIPAZINE MALEATE.** USAN. 2-(1-Piperazinyl)
  quinoline maleate.
  Use: Oxytocic.
- **QUIPENYL NAPHTHOATE.**
  See: Pamaquine naphthoate; Plasmochin
  naphthoate.
- **QUIT.** (Guild) Bot. ½ oz. w/applicator.
  Use: For nail biting.
- **QUIXALIN.** Halquinol, B.A.N.
- **Q-U-OPH.** (Eastwood) Cough syrup. Bot. Pt. With
  codeine Pt. Cap. Bot. 100s.

R

- **R-3 SCREEN TEST.** (Wampole) A three-minute latex-
  eosin slide test for the detection of rheumatoid
  factor activity in serum. Kit 100s.
  Use: An aid in the diagnosis of rheumatoid arthritis.
- **RABIES IMMUNE GLOBULIN,** U.S.P. XXI.
  Use: Immunizing agent (passive).
- **RABIES VACCINE.** U.S.P. XXI. (Lilly) 1 dose vial.
  1.1 ml. The suspending fluid consists of 0.1%
  cysteine HCl, 5% lactose, 0.2% gelatin and 0.25%
  dibasic potassium phosphate. Vaccine preserved
  w/thimerosal 1:10,000. (Lederle) 1,000 units/vial.
  Antirabies Serum.
  Use: Immunizing agent (active).
- **RABRO TABLETS.** (Orbar) Licorice root ext., light
  magnesium carbonate, bismuth subnitrate, sodium
  bicarbonate, small amounts of frangula and
  calamus. Boxes 30s, 60s.
  Use: Stomach distress, heartburn, indigestion.
- **RACEMETHIONINE,** U.S.P. XXI. Cap., Tab., U.S.P.
  XXI. Dl-2-Amino-4-(methylthio)butyric acid.
  Use: Acidifier (urinary).
  See: Amurex, Cap. (Reid-Provident)
  Odonil, Cap. (Kenyon)

Odor-Scrip, Cap. (Scrip)
Oradash, Cap. (Lambda)
Pedameth. Cap., Liq. (O'Nèal, Jones & Feldman)
Uranap, Cap. (Vortech)
RACEMETHIONINE W/COMBINATIONS.
See: Aminomin, Vial (Pharmex)
Aminovit, Vial (Hickam)
Amodin, Inj. (Vortech)
Ardiatric, Tab. (Burgin-Arden)
Azolate, Tab. (Amfre-Grant)
Cho-Meth Vial (Kenyon)
Geriatrazole, Vial (Kenyon)
Geriatro-B, Vial (Kenyon)
Hi-Pro Wafers, Tab. (Mills)
Licoplex, Tab. (Mills)
Limvic, Tab. (Briar)
Lipo-K, Cap. (Marcen)
Lychol-B, Inj. (Burgin-Arden)
Minoplex, Vial (Savage)
Norimex-Plus, Cap. (Vortech)
Pro-Hydro, Tab. (Mills)
Vio-Geric, Tab. (Rowell)
Vio-Geric-H, Tab. (Rowell)
Vi-Testrogen, Vial (Pharmex)
RACEMETHORPHAN. B.A.N. (+)-3-Methoxy-N-methylmorphinan
Use: Narcotic analgesic.
See: Dromoran (Roche)
RACEMIC CALCIUM PANTOTHENATE.
See: Calcium Pantothenate, Racemic.
RACEMIC DESOXY-NOR-EPHEDRINE.
See: Amphetamine (Various Mfr.)
RACEMIC EPHEDRINE HCl. Racephedrine HCl.
RACEMIC PANTOTHENIC ACID.
See: Vitamin, Preparations
RACEMORAMIDE. B.A.N. (+)-1-(3-Methyl-4-morpholino-2,2-diphenylbutyryl)pyrrolidine.
Use: Narcotic analgesic.
RACEMORPHAN HBr. B.A.N. (+)-3-Hydroxy-N-methylmorphinan.
Use: Narcotic analgesic.
RACEPHEDRINE HYDROCHLORIDE. (Upjohn) dl-a-[1-(Methylamino)ethyl]benzyl alcohol hydrochloride.
Cap. (⅜ gr.) Bot. 40s, 250s, 1000s. Sol. (1%) Bot. 1 fl. oz., 1 pt., 1 gal.
Use: Vasoconstrictor & nasal decongestant.
See: Ephedrine Combinations
W/Aminophylline & phenobarbital.
See: Amodrine, Tab. (Searle)
W/Theophylline sod. glycinate, phenobarbital.
See: Synophedal, Tab. (Central)
• **RACEPHENICOL.** USAN.
Use: Antibacterial.
RACET CREAM. (Lemmon) Clioquinol 3%, hydrocortisone 0.5%. W/stearic acid, cetyl alcohol, petrolatum, polyoxyl 40 stearate, sorbitol, propylene glycol, methylparaben, propylparaben, heather aroma. Tube 15 Gm., 30 Gm.
Use: Dermatologic.
RACET-1% CREAM. (Lemmon) Clioquinol 3%, hydrocortisone 1% w/steric acid cetyl alcohol, petrolatum, polyoxyl 40 stearate, sorbitol, propylene

glycol, methyl paraben, propylparaben, heather aroma, water. Tube 15 Gm.
Use: Dermatologic.
RACET LCD CREAM. (Lemmon) Clioquinol 3%, hydrocortisone 1%, coal tar sol. 5% w/stearic acid, cetyl alcohol, petrolatum, polyoxyl 40 stearate, sorbitol, propylene glycol, methylparaben, propylparaben, heather aroma, rose oil, purified water. Tube 30 Gm.
Use: Dermatoses, eczema.
RACET SE. (Lemmon) Hydrocortisone 0.5 and 1.0% w/cetyl alcohol, petrolatum, polyoxyl 40 stearate, propylene glycol, sorbic acid, potassium sorbate, & purified water. Tube 15 Gm.
Use: Topical anti-inflammatory antipruritic.
RADIOACTIVE ISOTOPES.
See: Medotope, Prods. (Squibb)
Radio-Gold, Sol.
Radio-Iodinated Serum Albumin (Human)
Sodium Radio-Chromate, Inj.
Sodium Radio-Iodide, Sol.
Sodium Radio Phosphate, Sol.
RADIOACTIVE ISOTOPES. (Mallincrodt).
See: Aggregated Radioiodinated Albumin, Human I-131
Chlormerodrin Hg-197, Inj.
Chlormerodrin Hg-203, Inj.
Cyanocobalamin Co-57, Cap.
Cyanocobalamin Co-60, Cap.
Gold Au-198, Inj.
Phosphocol P32 (Mallinckrodt)
Radiodinated Serum Albumin, Human I-125
Radiodinated Serum Albuminia, Human I-131
Selenomethionine Se-75, Inj.
Sodium Chromate Cr-51, Inj.
Sodium Iodide I-125, Sol., Cap.
Sodium Iodide I-131, Sol., Cap.
Sodium Phosphate P-32, Cap., Inj.
Sodium Rose Bengal I-131, Inj.
Strontium Nitrate Sr-85, Inj.
Technetium Tc-99m, Kit., Inj.
Triolein I-131, Cap., Sol.
Xenon Xe-133, Inj.
RADIOGOLD (^{198} Au), SOLUTION. Gold Au-198 Injection, U.S.P. XXI.
Use: Irradiation therapy.
See: Auretope, Vial (Squibb)
RADIO-IODIDE (^{131}I), SODIUM.
Use: Radioactive isotopes.
See: Iodotope (Squibb)
Radiocaps (Abbott)
RADIO-IODINATED (^{131}I) SERUM ALBUMIN.(Human), Iodinated I-131 Albumin Injection, U.S.P. XXI.
RADIO-IODINATED SERUM ALBUMIN (Human),(^{125}I).
See: Albumotope (^{125}I) (Squibb)
RADIO-PHOSPHATE (^{32}P), SODIUM.
Use: Radioactive isotopes.
RADIOSELENOMETHIONINE 75 Se.
Selenomethionine Se 75.
RADIOTOLPOVIDONE I-131. Tolpovidone I-131.

See: Raovin (Abbott)
RAFLUOR. (Pascal Co.) Acidulated, phosphated, 1.23% sodium fluoride prep. Gel 8 oz, 16 oz., 1 qt., 1 gal. Solution 8 oz, 16 oz.
Use: Topical application by dentist to reduce tooth decay.
• **RAFOXANIDE.** USAN.
Use: Anthelminic.
RAGUS. (Miller) Mg. 27 mg., C 100 mg., cal. 580 mg., phosphorus 450 mg., l-lysine 25 mg., dl-methionine 50 mg., lemon bioflavonoid complex 30 mg., A 5000 I.U., D 400 I.U., E 10 mg., B-1 20 mg., B-2 3 mg., B-6 5 mg., B-12 9 mcg., niacinamide 80 mg., pantothenic acid 5 mg., Fe 20 mg., Cu 1 mg., Mn 2 mg., K 10 mg., Zn 2 mg., Iodine 0.1 mg./3 Tabs. Bot. 100s.
Use: Dietary supplement.
RALGRO. (Commercial Solvents) Zeranol.
R A LOTION. (Medco Lab) Resorcinol 3%, calamine 6%, starch 6%, sodium borate 1.3%, alcohol 43%. Pl. bot. 4 oz., 8 oz., 16 oz.
Use: Skin medication for oily skin and acne.
RALS BENZOIN SPRAY. (Rals) Benzoin spray. Can 12 oz.
Use: Topical skin antiseptic.
RAMETIN. Naphthalophos, B.A.N.
RAMSES BENDEX. (Schmid) Flexible cushioned diaphragm; arc-ing spring. 65-90 mm. Pkg. w/Ramses Vaginal Jelly Tube 1 oz., 3 oz.
Use: Contraceptive.
RAMSES DIAPHRAGM. (Schmid) Flexible cushioned diaphragm. 50-95 mm. Pkg. diaphragm, tube of Ramses Vaginal Jelly. Pkg. diaphragm alone.
Use: Contraceptive.
RAMSES JELLY. (Schmid) Dodecoethylene glycol monolaurate 5%, boric acid 1%, glycerin, tragacanth, carboxymethylcellulose & preservative. Tube w/applicator 3 oz. Refill 3 oz., 5 oz.
Use: Contraceptive.
RANDOLECTIL. (Farbenfabriken Bayer) Butaperazine.
Use: Psychotropic agent.
R & C SPRAY III. (Reed & Carnrick) Spray containing pyrethroid (sumethrin) 0.382%, other isomers 0.018%, petroleum distillate 4.255%, Aerosol Container. 5 oz.
Use: An insecticide for use on inanimate objects infested with lice. Not for use on humans or animals.
RANESTOL. Triclofenol piperazine.
Use: Anthelmintic.
• **RANIMYCIN.** USAN.
Use: Antibacterial.
• **RANITIDINE.** USAN.
Use: Antagonist to histamine H-2 receptors.
RANTEX. (Holland-Rantos) Wipes 14s, 36s.
RAPIDAL CALCIUM SALT. Cyclobarbitone, B.A.N.
RASP. (Commerce) Bot. 3 oz.
Use: Children's cough syrup.
RASPBERRY JUICE.
Use: Flavored vehicle.
RASTINON. Tolbutamide, U.S.P. XXI.

RATIO. (Adria) Calcium carbonate 400 mg., magnesium carbonate 50 mg./Tab. Bot. 100s.
Use: Antacid.
RATIODRINE. (Metro Med) Tabs. Bot. 100s, 1000s.
Use: Obesity control.
RATTLESNAKE BITE THERAPY.
See: Antivenin, Snake Polyvalent (Wyeth)
RAUDILAN PB TABLETS. (Lannett) Rauwolfia serpentina root 50 mg., phenobarbital 15 mg./Tab. Bot. 100s, 500s, 1000s.
RAUDIXIN. (Squibb) Rauwolfia whole root. Tab. 50 mg. & 100 mg. Bot. 100s, 1000s. 100 mg. Unimatic single dose carton 100s.
Use: Hypotensive & tranquilizing agent.
W/Benzydroflumethiazide, potassium chloride.
See: Rautrax-N, Tabs. (Squibb)
Rautrax-N, Modified, Tab. (Squibb)
W/Flumethiazide, pot. chloride.
See: Rautrax, Tab. (Squibb)
RAUDOLFIN. (Premo) Rauwolfia serpentina 50 mg., 100 mg./Tab. Bot. 1000s.
Use: Hypotensive agent.
RAUJA. (Table Rock) Whole root Rauwolfia serpentina 50 mg. and 100 mg./Tab. Bot. 100s, 500s.
Use: Treatment of hypertension.
RAUNEED. (Hanlon) Rauwolfia 50 mg., 100 mg./Tab. Bot. 100s.
Use: Tranquilizer.
RAUNESCINE. (Penick) An alkaloid of Rauwolfia serpentina. Under study.
Use: Tranquilizing agent.
RAUNORMINE. (Penick) 11-Desmethoxy reserpine.
RAURINE. (Westerfield) Reserpine. **Tab.** (0.1 mg., 0.25 mg.) Bot. 100s. **Delayed Action:** 0.5 mg./Cap. Bot. 100s.
Use: Orally, sedative & tranquilizing agent.
W/Pentaerythritol tetranitrate.
See: Respet, Tab. (Westerfield)
RAUSERFIA. (New Eng. Phr. Co.) Rauwolfia serpentina 50 mg. or 100 mg./Tab. Bot. 100s.
RAUSERPIN. (Ferndale) Reserpine serpentina 100 mg./Tab. Bot. 100s, 1000s.
Use: Tranquilizer.
RAUTINA. (Fellows) Rauwolfia serpentina whole root 50 & 100 mg./Tab. Bot. 1000s.
Use: Antihypertensive agent.
RAUTRAX. (Squibb) Raudixin 50 mg., flumethiazide 400 mg., pot. chloride 400 mg./Tab. Bot. 100s.
Use: Hypertension.
RAUTRAX-N. (Squibb) Standardized whole root Rauwolfia serpentina (Raudixin) 50 mg., bendroflumethiazide 4 mg., potassium chloride 400 mg./Cap-shaped Tab. Bot. 100s, 1000s.
Use: Hypertension.
RAUTRAX-N MODIFIED. (Squibb) Raudixin 50 mg., bendroflumethiazide 2 mg., KCl 400 mg./Tab. Bot. 100s.
Use: Hypertension.
RAUVAL. (Vale) Rauwolfia serpentina whole root 50 mg. or 100 mg./Tab. Bot. 100s, 500s, 1000s.
Use: Antihypertensive & tranquilizing agent.

RAUVERAT. (Kenyon) Rauwolfia serpentina whole root powder 50 mg., veratrum viride ext. eq. to total alkaloids 1.1 mg./Tab. Bot. 100s, 1000s.
Use: Hypertension.
RAUVERID. (O'Neal, Jones & Feldman) Rauwolfia serpentina pwd. whole root 50 mg./Tab. Bot. 100s.
Use: Hypertension.
RAU-VER-TIN. (Kenyon) Rauwolfia serpentina 40 mg., veratrum viride 25 mg., rutin 20 mg., mannitol hexanitrate 30 mg./Tab. Bot. 100s, 1000s.
Use: Hypertension.
RAUWILOID. (Riker) Alseroxylon fraction of Rauwolfia serpentina. Tab. (2 mg.) Bot. 100s, 1000s.
Use: Hypertension.
W/Hexamethonium. (Riker) Rauwiloid 1 mg., hexamethonium 250 mg./Tab. Bot. 100s.
Use: Hypertension.
RAUWOLFIA CANESCENS ALKALOID.
See: Harmonyl, Tab. (Abbott)
RAUWOLFIA SERPENTINA ACTIVE PRINCIPLES (ALKALOIDS). Deserpidine, Rescinnamine.
See: Reserpine, Inj. (Var. Mfr.)
RAUWOLFIA SERPENTINA ALKALOIDAL EXTRACT.
See: Alseroxylon (Var. Mfr.)
• **RAUWOLFIA SERPENTINA,** U.S.P. XXI. Powder, Tab., U.S.P. XXI.
Use: Antihypertensive.
See: Hyper-Rauw, Tab. (Sutliff & Case)
Rau, Tab. (Scrip)
Raudixin, Tab. (Squibb)
Rauja, Tab. (Table Rock)
Raumason, Tab. (Mason)
Rauneed, Tab. (Hanlon)
Rautina, Tab. (Fellows-Testagar)
Rauval, Tab. (Vale)
Rawfola, Tab. (Foy)
Serfia, Tab. (Westerfield)
Serfolia, Tab. (Mallard)
T-Rau, Tab. (Tennessee Pharm.)
Wolfina, Tab. (Westerfield)
W/Bendroflumethiazide.
See: Rautrax-N, Tab. (Squibb)
Rauzide, Tab. (Squibb)
W/Bendroflumethiazide, pot. chloride (400).
See: Rautrax, Tab. (Squibb)
W/Mannitol hexanitrate, rutin.
See: Maxitate W/Rauwolfia, Tab. (Pennwalt)
W/Phenobarbital.
See: Raudilan PB, Tab. (Lannett)
RAUWOLSCINE. An alkaloid of Rauwolfia canescens. Under study.
Use: Tranquilizing agent.
RAUZIDE. (Squibb) Rauwolfia serpentina (pow.) 50 mg., bendroflumethiazide 4 mg./Tab. Bot. 100s, 1000s.
Use: Antihypertensive.
RAVOCAINE. (Cook-Waite) Propoxycaine HCl 4 mg., procaine 20 mg., levonordefrin 0.05 mg., NaCl 3 mg., acetone sodium bisulfite not more than 2 mg.; propoxycaine HCl 4 mg., procaine 20 mg., norepinephrine bitartrate equivalent to 0.033 mg.

levophed base, NaCl 3 mg., acetone sodium bisulfite not more than 2 mg.; Cartridge 1.8 ml.
Use: Local anesthetic (dental).
RAWFOLA. (Foy) Rauwolfia serpentina 50 mg./Tab. Bot. 1000s.
Use: Hypotensive agent.
RAWL VITE. (Rawl) Vit. A 10,000 I.U., D 500 I.U., B-1 10 mg., B-2 5 mg., B-6 1 mg., Ca pantothenate 5 mg., nicotinamide 50 mg., C 125 mg., E 2.5 I.U./Tab. Bot. 100s.
Use: Multiple vitamin tablets.
RAWL WHOLE LIVER VITAMIN B COMPLEX. (Rawl) Whole liver 500 mg. and amino acids found in the whole liver, B-1 1 mg., B-2 2 mg., niacinamide 5 mg., choline chloride 12 mg., B-6 0.2 mg., cal. pantothenate 0.2 mg., inositol 5 mg., biotin 0.6 mcg., B-12 0.3 mcg./Cap. Bot. 100s, 500s.
Use: Deficiency of Vitamin B complex.
RAY BLOCK. (Del-Ray) Bot. 4 oz.
Use: Sunscreen.
RAY-D. (Nion) Vit. D 400 I.U., Thiamin mononitrate 1 mg. riboflavin 2 mg., niacin 10 mg., iodine 0.1 mg., calcium 375 mg., phosphorus 300 mg.,/6 Tab. Bot. 100s, 500s.
Use: Dietary supplement.
RAYDERM OINTMENT. (Velvet Pharmacal) euphorbia ext., phenyl salicylate, neatsfoot oil, olive oil, lanolin in emulsion base preserved with methyl & propylparabens Tubes 1½ oz, Jar 1 lb.
Use: Radiation burns.
RAY-NOX. (Torch) Para-aminobenzoic acid 9.6% in a non-greasy, hydrophilic cream base. Jar 2 oz., 1 lb.
Use: Skin protection from ultraviolet rays.
• **RAYON, PURIFIED,** U.S.P. XXI.
Use: Surgical aid.
RAYTHESIN. (Raymer)
See: Propyl p-Aminobenzoate.
RAZOXANE. B.A.N. 1,2-Bis(3,5-dioxopiperazin-1-yl)propane.
Use: Antineoplastic.
RCF. (Ross) Carbohydrate free soy protein formula base—concentrated liquid, carbohydrate must be added. "as fed" 12 cal/fl oz; per liter: protein 20.0 g, fat 36.0 g, Ca 0.70 g, P 0.50 g, Na 0.30 g, K 0.71 g, Cl 0.53 g, Mg 50 mg, Zn 5.0 mg, Cu 0.50 mg, Fe 12 mg, I 0.10 mg, Mn 0.20 mg, Vit. A 2500 IU, Vit. D 400 IU, Vit. E 20 IU, Vit. C 55 mg, thiamine 0.40 mg, riboflavin 0.60 mg, Vitamin B-6 0.40 mg, niacin 9.0 (mg eq), folic acid 0.10 mg, Vit. B-12 3.0 mcg, pantothenic acid 5.0 mg, biotin 30 mcg, Vit. K-1 0.15 mg per liter.
Use: in management of infants unable to tolerate the amount or type of carbohydrate in conventional formulas. Carbohydrate to be added at levels appropriate for the individual infant.
REA-LO. (Whorton) Urea in water soluble moisturizing oil base. **Lotion:** 15%. Bot. 4 oz., pt. **Cream:** 30%. Jar 2 oz., 16 oz.
Use: Treatment of hyperkeratosis, dry skin conditions.
REALPHENE.
See: Acetarsone, Tab. (City Chem.)

RECINDAL. (Winthrop Products) Dextromethorphan HBr.
Use: Antitussive, decongestant.

RECINDAL-PC. (Winthrop Products) Dextromethorphan HBr, phenylpropanolamine HCl, chlorpheniramine maleate, alcohol.
Use: Decongestant, antitussive.

RECORTEX. (Fellows) Adrenal cortex inj. equiv. to 100 mcg. of hydrocortisone/cc. Aqueous and lyophilized. Vial 10 cc., 50 cc.
Use: Treatment of adrenal insufficiency.

RECORTEX 2XX. (Fellows) 200 mcg./cc. Aqueous and lyophilized. Vial 10 cc., 50 cc.

RECORTEX 10X IN OIL. (Fellows) 1000 mcg./cc. Vial 10 cc.

RECOVER. (Commerce) Bot. 2.25 oz.
Use: Skin discoloration cover-up cream.

RECTACORT. (Century) Hydrocortisone acetate 10 mg., ext. belladonna 0.5%, ephedrine sulfate 0.1%, zinc oxide, boric acid, bismuth subcarbonate, balsam peru, cocoa butter. Supp. Pkg. 12s. Supp. Pkg. 12s.

RECTAL MEDICONE. (Medicone) Benzocaine 2 gr., balsam Peru 1 gr., oxyquinoline sulfate ¼ gr., menthol ½ gr., zinc oxide 3 gr./Supp. Box 12s, 24s.
Use: Antiseptic & local anesthetic.

RECTAL MEDICONE-HC Suppos. (Medicone) Benzocaine 2 gr., balsam Peru 1 gr., oxyquinoline sulfate ¼ gr., menthol ½ gr., zinc oxide 3 gr., hydrocortisone acetate 10 mg., cocoa butter, veg. and petrolatum oil base q.s./Supp. Box 12s.
Use: Severe anorectal inflammation.

RECTAL MEDICONE UNGUENT. (Medicone) Benzocaine 20 mg., oxyquinoline sulfate 5 mg., menthol 4 mg., zinc oxide 100 mg., balsam peru 12.5 mg., petrolatum 625 mg., lanolin 210 mg./Gm. Tubes 1½ oz.
Use: Anorectal disorders.

RECTAL OINTMENT. (Vortech) Tube. ¼ oz. w/applicator
Use: Antihemorrhoidal.

RECTOCAINE. (Moore Kirk) Phenol 1%, propyl-p-aminobenzoate 7%, benzyl alcohol 7%, procaine 0.5%. Amp. 5 cc.
Use: Rectally; local anesthetic.

RECTULES. (Fellows) Chloral hydrate 10 & 20 gr. Supp. in water-soluble base. Pkg. 12s.
Use: Sedative, hypnotic.

• **RED BLOOD CELLS,** U.S.P. XXI. Human red blood cells given by IV infusion.
Use: Blood replenisher.

RED CELL TAGGING SOLUTION.
See: A-C-D Solution (Squibb)

REDCEL TABLETS. (Morton) Docusate sodium 100 mg., Fe 100 mg./Tab. Bot. 100s.

RED CROSS TOOTHACHE DROPS. (Mentholatum) Eugenol 85%, alcohol 15%. Bot. ⅛ fl. oz.
Use: Topical anesthetic.

RED CROSS TOOTHACHE KIT. (Mentholatum) Complete kit containing toothache drops w/cotton pellets and tweezers.
Use: Topical anesthetic.

• **RED FERRIC OXIDE,** N.F. XVI.
Use: Pharmaceutic aid (color).

RED MERCURIC IODIDE.
Used in: Auralcaine, Liq. (Truett)

REDIPAK. (Wyeth) A special type of packaging which includes the following drugs:
A.P.C. Tablets
Aspirin, U.S.P. 300 mg./Tab. 300 mg. or 600 mg./Suppos.
Ativan. Lorazepam 0.5 mg., 1 mg. or 2 mg./Tab.
Chloral Hydrate 500 mg./Cap.
Codeine Sulfate Tablets. 15 mg., 30 mg., or 60 mg./Tab.
Equagesic. Meprobamate w/aspirin.
Equanil. Meprobamate 200 mg., or 400 mg./Tab.
Meperidine HCl. 50 mg./Tab.
Omnipen. Ampicillin 250 mg. or 500 mg./Cap. 250 mg./5 ml. Susp.
Penicillin G, Potassium U.S.P. 250 mg./Tab.
Pentobarbital Sod. U.S.P. 100 mg./Cap.
Pen-Vee K. Soln. Phenoxymethyl penicillin 250 mg./5 ml.
Pen-Vee K Tablets. Phenoxymethyl penicillin 250 mg., 500 mg./Tab.
Phenergan. Promethazine HCl 12.5 mg. or 25 mg./Tab.; 25 mg. or 50 mg./Suppos.
Phenobarbital. 15 mg., 30 mg., 60 mg., or 100 mg./Tab.
Secobarbital Sod. U.S.P. 100 mg./Cap.
Serax. Oxazepam 10 mg., 15 mg., 30 mg./Cap.
Unipen. Sodium nafcillin 250 mg./Cap.
Wyanoids. Suppositories.
Wygesic. Tablets.
Zactirin Compound-100. Ethoheptazine citrate w/aspirin, phenacetin and caffeine, Tabs.

REDISOL. (Merck Sharp & Dohme) Vit. B-12 (Cyanocobalamin), **Inj.:** 1000 mcg./ml. w/sod. chloride 0.83%, water q.s., methylparaben 0.15%, propylparaben 0.02%. Vial 10 ml. **Tab.:** 50 mcg. Bot. 100s. 500 mcg. Bot. 50s.
Use: Vitamin B-12 therapy (hematopoietic).
See also Alpha Redisol.

REDITEMP-C. (Wyeth) Ammonium nitrate, water and special additives. Pkg. large and small sizes. 4 × 10s.
Use: For short-term topical cold application.

REDODERLEIN. (Fellows) Doederlein's bacillus (*Lactobacillus vaginalis* and *Lactobacillus crassus*) 200,000/Vials (lyophilized) 5 cc. 5s.
Use: Vaginitis therapy.

REDUCTO, IMPROVED. (Arcum) Phendimetrazine bitartrate 35 mg./Tab. Bot. 100s, 1000s.

REFRESH'N. (Stanlabs) Caffeine 500 mg./Tab. Pkg. 75s.
Use: Awakener, stimulant.

REFUIN. (Roche) Under study.
Use: Antineoplastic.

REGITINE. (Ciba) Phentolamine methanesulfonate or HCl. **Hydrochloride:** Tab. (50 mg.) Bot. 100s.
Methanesulfonate (mesylate): Phentolamine mesylate 5 mg., lactose 5 mg./Amp. w/1 ml. Amp. Sterile water for inj. Pkg. 1s, 6s.

Use: Diagnostic test for pheochromocytoma.
REGLAN. (Robins) Metoclopramide HCl **Inj.:** 10 mg./2 ml. Amp. 2 ml. Box 5s, 25s; 50 mg./10 ml. Box 25s. **Syrup:** 5 mg. (as base)/5 ml. Bot. pt. Dis Co Packs 10×10s. **Tab.:** 10 mg./Tab. Bot. 100s, 500s. Dis-co Paks 100s.
Use: Pro-motility agent for diabetic gastroparesis, prevention of nausea in emitogenic cancer chemotherapy.
REGONOL. (Organon) Pyridostigmine bromide 5 mg./ml. Amp. 2 ml. Vial 5 ml. Box 25s.
Use: Reversal agent for non-depolarizing surgical muscle relaxants.
REGROTON. (USV Labs.) Chlorthalidone 50 mg., reserpine 0.25 mg./Tab. Bot. 100s, 1000s.
Use: Antihypertensive.
REGUL-AID. (Columbia) **Liquid:** Docusate sodium 20 mg./5 cc. Bot. pt. **Caps.** 100 mg./Cap. Bot. 100s, 1000s.
Use: Laxative.
REGUTOL. (Plough) Docusate sodium 100 mg./Tab. Box 30s, 60s, 90s.
Use: Stool softener.
REHYZIDE. (Whiteworth) Hydralazine HCl, hydrochlorthiazide, reserpine; 25 mg./15 mg./1 mg./Tab. Bot. 100s, 1000s.
Use: Treatment hypertension.
REIDAMINE INJ. (Reid-Provident) Dimenhydrinate 50 mg./cc. Vial 1 ml., 10 ml.
RELA. (Schering) Carisoprodol 350 mg./Tab. Bot. 100s.
Use: Muscle relaxant.
RELAXIN. A purified ovarian hormone of pregnancy (obtained from sows) responsible for pubic relaxation or separation of the symphysis pubis in mammals.
See: Lutrexin, Tab. (Hynson, Westcott & Dunning)
RELEFACT TRH. (Hoechst) Protirelin 0.5 mg./ml. Amp. 1 ml. Box 5s.
Use: Diagnosis of thyroid function.
RE-LIEVE. (Faraday) Analgesic. Cap. 30s.
• **RELOMYCIN.** USAN. A basic macrolide antibiotic produced by a variant strain of *Streptomyces hygroscopicus.*
Use: Antibacterial antibiotic.
REM COUGH MEDICINE. (Last) Dextromethorphan HBr 5 mg./5 ml. Bot. 3 oz., 6 oz.
Use: Antitussive.
REMEFLIN. Dimefline Hydrochloride, B.A.N.
REMIVOX. (Janssen) Lorcainide HCl.
Use: Cardiac anti-rhythmic.
REMOVING CREAM. (O'Leary) Specially formulated to remove Covermark. Bot. 4 oz., 7½ oz.
REMSED. (Du Pont) Promethazine HCl 50 mg./Tab. Bot. 100s.
Use: Non-barbituate sleeping agent.
RENACIDIN. (Guardian) Antilithiatic agent composed of lactones, anhydrides and acid salts of edible, multivalent organic acids including gluconic and citric. Bot. 25 Gm. 6s; 300 Gm.
Use: Bladder irrigation to aid removal of stones

composed of calcium and magnesium phosphate, indwelling catheter irrigation.
RENALGIN. (Glaxo) Atropine sulfate 0.03 mg., hyoscyamine 0.03 mg., methenamine 41 mg., salol 18 mg., benzoic acid 4.5 mg., methylene blue 5.4 mg./Tab. Bot. 100s, 1000s.
Use: Urinary antibacterial; antispasmodic; analgesic.
RENALTABS-S.C. (Fellows) Methenamine 40.8 mg., benzoic acid 4.5 mg., phenyl salicylate 18.1 mg., hyoscyamine sulfate ½₀₀₀ gr., atropine sulfate 0.03 mg., methylene blue 5.4 mg., gelsemium 6.1 mg./Tab. Bot. 1000s.
RENAMIN. (Travenol) Sterile hypertonic solution of essential non-essential amino acids. Bot. 250 ml., 500 ml.
Use: Nutritional support.
RENANOLONE. 3α-Hydroxypregnane-11,20-dione.
Use: Steroid anesthetic.
RENBU. (Wren) Butabarbital sod. 32.4 mg./Tab. Bot. 100s, 1000s.
RENELATE. (Fellows) Methenamine mandelate 1 Gm./E.C. Tab. Bot. 100s, 500s, 5000s.
Use: Urinary antiseptic.
RENESE. (Pfizer Laboratories) Polythiazide 1 mg., 2 mg., 4 mg./Tab. Bot. 100s, 1000s.
Use: Diuretic.
RENESE-R TABLETS. (Pfizer Laboratories) Polythiazide 2 mg., reserpine 0.25 mg./Tab. Bot. 100s, 1000s.
Use: Hypertension.
RENGASIL. (Geigy) Pirprofen. Pending release.
Use: Anti-inflammatory.
RENNIN. Milk-curdling enzyme obtained from the fourth stomach of the calf.
RENOFORM.
See: Epinephrine, Preps. (Var. Mfr.)
RENOGRAFIN-60,-76. (Squibb) **-60:** Meglumine diatrizoate 52%, sod. diatrizoate 8%. Vial 10 ml., 100 ml., 10s; 30 ml., 50 ml., 25s. **-76:** Meglumine diatrizoate 66%, sod. diatrizoate 10%. Vial 20 ml., 50 ml., 25s; 100 ml., 200 ml., 10s.
Use: Contrast medium.
RENO-M-DIP. (Squibb) Meglumine diatrizoate Inj. 30% for drip infusion pyelography. Bot. 300 cc. Also w/soln. admin. sets. (Formerly Renografin-Dip)
Use: Drip infusion pyelography.
RENO-M-30. (Squibb) Meglumine diatrizoate 30%. Vial 50 cc., 100 cc. Box 25s.
Use: Retrograde pyelography.
RENO-M-60. (Squibb) Meglumine diatrizoate 60%. Vial 10 ml., 30 ml., 50 ml., 100 ml. 150 ml. Box 25s.
Use: Radiopaque contrast agent.
RENOQUID. (Glenwood) Sulfacytine 250 mg./Tab. Bot. 100s. Therapy paks 41s. Unit dose 100s.
Use: Sulfonamide therapy for urinary infection.
REN-O-SAL. (Salsbury) 3-Nitro-4-hydroxyphenylarsonic acidroxarsone 36 mg./Tab. Bot. 100s, 250s, 1000s, 10,000s.
Use: Growth promotant and coccidiosis treatment.
RENO-SED. (Vita Elixir) Methenamine 2 gr., salol ½ gr., methylene blue ⅒ gr., benzoic acid ⅛ gr.,

atropine sulfate $^1/_{1000}$ gr., hyoscyamine sulfate $^1/_{2000}$ gr./Tab.
Use: Genito-urinary antisepsis & sedation.
RENOVIST INJ. (Squibb) Diatrizoate methylglucamine 34.3%, sodium diatrizoate 35%, equivalent to 59.7% base which contains 62% iodine, sol. contains 37% firmly bound iodine. Vial 50 ml. Box 25s.
Use: Radiopaque medium.
RENOVIST II. (Squibb) Sodium diatrizoate 29.1%, meglumine diatrizoate 28.5%. Inj. Vial 30 cc., 60 cc. Box 25s.
Use: Radiopaque medium.
RENOVUE-65. (Squibb) Iodamide meglumide 65%, organically bound iodine 30% w/edetate disodium. Vial 50 ml.
Use: Radiopaque urographic contrast agent.
RENOVUE-DIP. (Squibb) Iodamide meglumide 24%. Infusion Bot. 300 ml.
Use: Radiopaque contrast agent for drip infusion pyelography.
RENPAP. (Wren) Acetaminophen 4 gr., salicylamide 3 gr., caffeine $^2/_3$ gr., allylisobutylbarbituric acid ¾ gr./Tab. Bot. 100s, 1000s.
RENTUSS. (Wren) Dextromethorphan HBr 10 mg., guaifenesin 100 mg., phenylephrine HCl 5 mg., phenylpropanolamine HCl 25 mg., chlorpheniramine maleate 2 mg., acetaminophen 300 mg./Tab. Bot. 100s, 500s, 1000s. Syr: same except guaifenesin 50 mg., acetaminophen 120 mg./5 cc. pt., gal.
REPAN. (Everett) Butalbital 50 mg., caffeine 40 mg., acetaminophen 325 mg./Tab. Bot. 100s.
REPEL. (Wisconsin) Lotion 2 oz. Non-aerosol Spray 4 oz.
Use: Insect repellent.
REPENDO. (Standex) Ascorbic acid 100 mg., menadione 0.1 mg./Cap. Bot. 100s.
Use: Treatment of capillary wall permeability.
REPEN-VK. (Reid-Provident) Penicillin V potassium 250 mg. Tab. Bot. 100s, 500s.
Use: Antibiotic.
REPODRAL SOLUTION. (Winthrop Products) Stibophen.
Use: Antibilharziasis.
REP-PRED 40. (Central) Methylprednisolone acetate 40 mg. polyethylene glycol 4000 29 mg., sodium chloride 8.7 mg./ml. Vial 5 ml.
REP-PRED 80. (Central) Methylprednisolone acetate 80 mg., polyethylene glycol 4000 28 mg., sodium chloride 8.5 mg./ml. Vial 5 ml.
REPRIEVE. (Mayer) Caffeine, alk. 32 mg., salicylamide 225 mg., B-1 50 mg., homatropine methylbromide 0.5 mg./Tab. Bot. 8s, 16s.
Use: Analgesic.
• **REPROMICIN.** USAN.
Use: Antibacterial.
• **REPROTEROL HYDROCHLORIDE.** USAN.
Use: Bronchodilator.
REPTILASE-R. (Abbott) Reptilase-R coagulation test system. Tests 10/Vial. Box 3 Vials
Use: Investigation of fibrin formation & disturbances in fibrin formation.

REQUA'S CHARCOAL TABLETS. (Requa) Wood charcoal 10 gr./Tab. Pkg. 50s. Can 125s.
Use: Flatulence, diarrhea.
RESA. (Vita Elixir) Reserpine 0.25 mg./Tab.
Use: Tranquilizing & antihypertensive agent.
RESCINNAMINE. Methyl 18β-Hydroxy-11,17 α-dimethoxy-3β20α-yohimban-16β-carboxylate 3,4,5-Trimeth-oxycinnamate (Ester). Methyl 0-(3,4,5-trimethoxy-cinnamoyl)reserpate.
Use: Tranquilizer; hypotensive.
See: Anaprel.
 Cinnasil, Graduals (Amfre-Grant)
 Moderil, Tab. (Pfizer Laboratories)
RESCON CAPSULES. (Ion) Methscopolamine nitrate 2.5 mg., chlorpheniramine maleate 8 mg., phenylpropanolamine 50 mg./T.R. Cap. Bot. 100s.
Use: Drying agent for excessive secretions, antihistaminic.
RESCON LIQUID. (Ion) Phenylpropanolamine HCl 12.5 mg., chlorpheniramine maleate 2 mg./5 ml. Bot. 4 oz.
Use: Decongestant, antihistaminic.
RESERJEN. (Jenkins) Reserpine 0.25 mg./Tab. Bot. 1000s.
RESERPANEED. (Hanlon) Reserpine 0.25 mg./Tab. Bot. 100s, 1000s.
Use: Tranquilizer.
• **RESERPINE,** U.S.P. XXI. Elixir, Inj. Tab., U.S.P. XXI. Yohimban-16-carboxylic acid, 11,17-dimethoxy-18-[(3,4,5-trimethoxybenzyol)oxy]-, methyl ester. Pure alkaloid from Rauwolfia serpentina.
Use: Antihypertensive.
See: Arcum R-S, Tab. (Arcum)
 Broserpine, Tab. (Brothers)
 De Serpa, Tabs. (De Leon)
 Elserpine, Tab. (Canright)
 Hyperine, Tab. (Sutliff & Case)
 Maso-Serpine, Tab. (Mason)
 Rauloydin, Tab. (Reid-Provident)
 Raurine, Tab. (Westerfield)
 Rauserpin, Tab. (Ferndale)
 Reserjen, Tab. (Jenkins)
 Reserpaneed, Tab. (Hanlon)
 Sandril, Tab., Inj. (Lilly)
 Serpalan, Tab. (Lannett)
 Serpanray, Tab., Amp. (Panray)
 Serpasil Preps. (Ciba)
 Serpate, Tab. (Vale)
 Serpena, Tab. (Haag)
 Sertabs, Tab. (Table Rock)
 Sertina, Tab. (Fellows-Testagar)
 SK-Reserpine, Tab. (SmithKline)
 Tensin (Standex)
 T-Serp, Tab. (Tennessee)
 Vio-Serpine, Tab. (Rowell)
 Zepine, Tab. (Foy)
RESERPINE W/COMBINATIONS
See: Aquapres-R, Tab. (Coastal)
 Demi-Regroton, Tab. (USV Labs.)
 Diupres, Tab. (Merck Sharp & Dohme)
 Diutensen-R, Tab. (Mallinckrodt)
 Dralserp, Tab. (Lemmon)

Harbolin, Tab. (Arcum)
Hyd-Res-Ine, Tab. (Columbia)
Hydromox R, Tab. (Lederle)
Hydropres-25 or -50, Tab. (Merck Sharp & Dohme)
Hydroserp, Tab. (Zenith)
Hydroserpine, Tab. (Geneva)
Hydroserpine Plus, Tab. (Zenith)
Hydroserpine No. 1, Tab. (Zenith)
Hydroserpine No. 2,3,4, Tab. (Zenith)
Hydrotensin-Plus, Tab. (Mayrand)
Hydrotensin-50, Tab. (Mayrand)
Hyperserp, Tab. (Elder)
Mallopress, Tab. (Mallard)
Metatensin, Tab. (Merrell Dow)
Naquival, Tab. (Schering)
Regroton, Tab. (USV Labs.)
Renese-R, Tab. (Pfizer Laboratories)
Salutensin, Tab. (Bristol)
Ser-Ap-Es, Tab. (Ciba)
Serapine, Tab. (Cenci)
Serpahyde TM, Tab. (Wolins)
Serpasil-Apresoline, Tab. (Ciba)
Serpasil-Esidrix, Tab. (Ciba)
Thia-Serp-25, Tab. (Robinson)
Thia-Serp-50, Tab. (Robinson)
Thia-Serpa-Zine, Tab. (Robinson)
Unipres, Tab. (Reid-Provident)
• **RESERPINE AND HYDROCHLOROTHIAZIDE TABLETS.** U.S.P. XXI.
Use: Antihypertensive.
• **RESERPINE, HYDRALAZINE HCl and HYDROCHLORTHIAZIDE,** U.S.P. XXI.
Use: Antihypertensive.
RESINOL MEDICINAL OINTMENT. (Mentholatum) Zinc oxide 12%, calamine 6%, resorcinol 2% in a lanolin and petrolatum base. Jar 3½ oz., 1¼ oz.
Use: Skin protectant, analgesic.
RESIN UPTAKE KIT WITH LIOTHYRONINE I-125 BUFFER SOLUTION.
See: Thyrostat-3 (Squibb)
■ **RESINS, ANTACID.**
See: Polyamine methylene Resins.
RESISTON-C. (CMC) Vit. B-1 1.5 mg., B-6 0.1 mg., cal. pantothenate 1 mg., B-2 2 mg., yeast 155 mg., niacinamide 10 mg./Cap. Bot. 100s, 250s, 1000s.
RESOCHIN. Chloroquine Phosphate, B.A.N.
RESONIUM-A. (Winthrop Products) Sodium polystyrene sulfonate.
Use: Hyperkalemia.
RESORCIN.
See: Resorcinol (Var. Mfr.)
• **RESORCINOL,** U.S.P. XXI. Compound Ointment, U.S.P. XXI. 1,3-Benzenediol.
Use: Local antifungal; keratolytic.
• **RESORCINOL AND SULFUR LOTION.** U.S.P. XXI.
Use: Scabicide, parasiticide, antifungal.
RESORCINOL W/COMBINATIONS
See: Acne-Aid Cream (Steifel)
Acnomel, Cake, Cream. (Menley & James)
Bicozene, Cream (Ex-Lax)
Biscolan, Supp. (Lannett)
Black and White Ointment, (Plough)

Castaderm, Prep. (Lannett)
Cenac Lotion (Central)
Clearasil, Stick (Vicks)
Derma-Cover, Liq. (Scrip)
Derma-Cover-Hc, Liq. (Scrip)
Doctient, Supp. (Suppositoria)
Doctient HC, Supp. (Suppositoria)
Exzit, Creme & Lotion (Miles Pharm)
Fusinol, Liq. (Westerfield)
Hydro Surco, Lot. (Alma)
Komed, Lot. (Barnes-Hind)
Lanacane Creme (Combe)
Mazon, Oint. (Thayer)
Mild Komed, Lot. (Barnes-Hind)
RA Lotion (Medco)
Rezamid Lotion (Dermick)
Resulin, Oint., Lot. (Almay)
Resulin-F, Cream (Almay)
Serp, Preps. (Scrip)
Tackle, Gel (Colgate-Palmolive)
Thera-Blem, Cream (Noxell)
Therac, Lot. (C & M Pharm.)
Vegoil W/Isocaine, Oint. (Philips Roxane)
Zinc Boric Lotion, Liq. (Emerson)
• **RESORCINOL MONOACETATE,** U.S.P. XXI. (Various Mfr.) Resorcin acetate.
Use: Antiseborrheic; keratolytic.
See: Euresol, Liq. (Knoll)
W/Salicylic acid, ethyl alcohol, castor oil.
See: Resorcitate w/oil, Lot. (Almay)
W/Salicylic acid, LCD, betanaphthol, castor oil, isopropyl alcohol.
See: Neomark, Liq. (C&M Pharm.)
RESORCINOLPHTHALEIN SODIUM.
See: Fluorescein Sodium, U.S.P. XXI. (Var. Mfr.)
W/Oil. Resorcinol monoacetate 1.5%, salicylic acid 1.5% castor oil 1.5%, ethyl alcohol 81%. Bot. 8 fl. oz.
Use: Scalp lotion.
RESOTREN. Cloquinate, B.A.N.
RESPAIRE-60. (Laser) Pseudoephedrine HCl 60 mg. guaifenesin 200 mg./S.R. Cap. Bot. 100s, 1000s.
Use: Decongestant, expectorant.
RESPAIRE-SR-120. (Laser) Pseudoephedrine HCl 120 mg., guaifenesin 250 mg./S.R. Cap. Bot. 100s, 1000s.
Use: Adrenergic, expectorant.
RESPBID. (Boehringer Ingelheim) Theophylline anhydrous 250 mg. or 500 mg./Tab. Bot. 100s.
Use: Bronchodilator.
RESPENYL. Guaiphenesin, B.A.N.
RESPIHALER DECADRON PHOSPHATE. (Merck Sharp & Dohme)
See: Decadron phosphate, respihaler (Merck Sharp & Dohme)
RESPINOL G CAPSULES. (Misemer) Bot. 100s.
RESPINOL-G TABLETS. (Misemer) Phenylephrine HCl 5 mg., phenylpropanolamine HCl 45 mg., guaifenesin 200 mg./Tab.
Use: Temporary relief of nasal congestion, respiratory allergies.
RESPINOL LA CAPSULES. (Misemer)

Phenylpropanolamine HCl 75 mg., phenylephrine HCl 10 mg., guaifenesin 300 mg./L.A. Cap.
Use: Relief of symptoms of bronchitis, bronchial asthma, emphysema, sinusitis.

RESPIRATORY VACCINE. (Various Mfr.) Cold Vaccines.

RES-Q. (Boyle) Activated charcoal 50%, magnesium hydroxide 25%, tannic acid 25% (Universal antidote). Pkg. ½ oz.
Use: Universal antidote for accidental poisoning.

REST EASY. (Walgreen) Acetaminophen, 600 mg., ephedrine sulfate, 8 mg., d-methorphan HBr, 15 mg., doxylamine succinate 75 mg./30 ml. Bot. 6 oz.
Use: Decongestant, antihistamine, analgesic, antitussive.

RESTIME. (Stanlabs) Bot. 14s.

RESTORA. (Circle) Methyltestosterone 2.0 mg., ethinyl estradiol 0.01 mg., Vit. A 5000 I.U., D 400 I.U., E 10 I.U., B-1 2 mg., B-2 2 mg., B-6 0.3 mg., B-12 1 mcg., C30 mg., nicotinamide 20 mg., Ca panothenate 3 mg., iron 10 mg., Cu 0.2 mg., Mo 0.3 mg., Zn, Mg 5 mg., K 2 mg., iodine 0.15 mg./Cap. Bot. 100s.
Use: Vitamin, mineral supplement.

RESTORIL. (Sandoz) Temazepam 15 mg. or 30 mg./Cap. Bot. 100s, 500s. ControlPak 25s. SandoPak (unit dose) 100s.
Use: Hypnotic, sedative.

RETADIAMONE. (Rocky Mtn.) Testosterone enanthate 90 mg., estradiol valerate 4 mg./cc. Vial 10 cc. In sesame oil. Also available in double strength. Vial 5 cc.
Use: Androgen & estrogen therapy.

RETANDROS. (Rocky Mtn.) Testosterone enanthate 200 mg./cc. in sesame oil. Vial 10 cc.
Use: Androgen therapy.

RETCIN. Erythromycin, B.A.N.

RETENEMA 17-VALERATE. Betamethasone, B.A.N.

RETESTRIN. (Rocky Mtn.) Estradiol-17 valerate in sesame oil 10 mg., 40 mg./cc. Vial 10 cc.
Use: Amenorrhea, menopausal syndrome.

RETET. (Reid-Provident) Tetracycline HCl 250 mg./Cap. Bot. 100s, 1000s.
Use: Broad-spectrum antibiotic.

RETET-500. (Reid-Provident) Tetracycline HCl 500 mg./Cap. Bot. 100s.
Use: Broad-spectrum antibiotic.

RETICULEX. (Lilly) Vit. B-12 10 mcg., C 50 mg., folic acid 0.3 mg., ferrous sulfate 75 mg., liver-stomach concentrate 222 mg./Pulvule. Bot. 100s.
Use: Orally, anemias.

RETICULOGEN. (Lilly) Vit. B-1 5 mg., B-12 20 mcg./1 ml. Also sod. bisulfite 0.1%, phenol 0.5%. **Vial.** 5 ml. **Fortified:** Vit. B-1 5 mg., B-12 40 mcg./ml. Vial 5 ml.
Use: I.M.; anemias.

RETIN-A CREAM. (Ortho) Tretinoin 0.1% or 0.05% with isopropyl myristate, polyoxyl 40 stearate, stearyl alcohol, stearic acid, xanthan gum, sorbic acid, butylated hydroxytoluene. Tube 20 Gm., 45 Gm.
Use: Acne treatment.

RETIN-A GEL. (Ortho) Tretinoin 0.01% or 0.025% hy-

droxypropyl cellulose, butylated hydroxytoluene, alcohol 90% w/w. Tube 15 Gm., 45 Gm.
Use: Acne treatment.

RETIN-A LIQUID. (Ortho) Tretinoin (retinoic acid, Vitamin A acid) 0.05%, polyethylene glycol 400, butylated hydroxytoluene, and alcohol 55%. Bot. 28 ml.
Use: Acne treatment.

RETINOIC ACID. Tretinoin, U.S.P. XXI.
Use: Keralotytic.
See: Retin A Prods. (Ortho)

ALL TRANS-RETINOIC ACID. Tretinoin, U.S.P. XXI.

RETINOL. B.A.N. 3,7-Dimethyl-9-(2,6,6-trimethyl-cyclohex-1-enyl)nona-2,4,6,8-all-trans-tetraen-1-ol.
See: Vitamin A alcohol.

REVAC SUPPRETTES. (Webcon) Docusate sodium 100 mg. in neocera base/Supp. Jar 12s.
Use: Constipation.

REVONAL. Methaqualone, B.A.N.

REVS CAFFEINE T.D. CAPSULES. (Vitarine) Caffeine 250 mg./Cap. Bot. 15s.
Use: Combat drowsiness, fatigue, restore mental alertness.

REXAHISTINE. (Econo-Rx) Phenylephrine HCl 5 mg., chlorpheniramine maleate 1 mg., menthol 1 mg., sodium bisulfite 0.1%, alcohol 5%/5 ml. Bot. Gal.
Use: Decongestant.

REXAHISTINE DH. (Econo-Rx) Codeine phosphate 10 mg., phenylephrine HCl 10 mg., chlorpheniramine maleate 2 mg., menthol 1 mg., alcohol 5%/5 ml. Bot. Gal.
Use: Relief of coughs due to cold and allergy.

REXAHISTINE EXPECTORANT. (Econo-Rx) Codeine phosphate 10 mg., phenylephrine HCl 10 mg., chlorpheniramine maleate 2 mg., guaifenesin 100 mg., menthol 1 mg., alcohol 5%/5 ml. Bot. Gal.
Use: Expectorant.

REXIGEN. (Ion) Amobarbital 60 mg., dextroamphetamine sulfate 15 mg. Tab. Bot. 100s.
Use: Anorexiant.

REXOLATE. (Hyrex) Sod. thiosalicylate 50 mg./cc. Vial 30 cc.
Use: Antipyretic, analgesic.

REZAMID LOTION. (Dermik) Sulfur 5%, resorcinol 2%, parachlorometaxylenol 0.5% w/alcohol 28.5% in flesh-tinted base. Bot. 2 oz.
Use: Acne, oily skin.

REZIDE. (Edwards) Reserpine 0.1 mg., hydralazine HCl 25 mg., hydrochlorothiazide 15 mg./Tab. Bot. 100s, 1000s.
Use: Diuretic, antihypertensive.

RF LATEX TEST. (Laboratory Diagnostics) Latex slide test for rheumatoid factor. Kit. 100s.
Use: Rapid latex agglutination test for the qualitative screening and semi-quantitative determination of rheumatoid factor.

R-GEN. (Owen) Purified water, amphoteric 2, hydrolyzed animal protein, lauramine oxide, methylparaben, benzalkonium chloride, tetrasodium, EDTA, propylparaben, fragrance. Bot. 8 oz.
Use: Protein hair repair shampoo.

R-GENE 10. (Cutter) Arginine HCl 10 Gm./100 ml. in 300 I.V. flasks.
Use: Diagnostic for human growth hormone stimulation.

R-HCTZ-H. (Lederle) Reserpine 0.1 mg., hydrochlorothiazide 15 mg., hydralazine HCl 25 mg./Tab. Bot. 100s, 500s.
Use: Hypertension treatment.

RHEABAN. (Leeming) **Tabs.:** Colloidal activated attapulgite 600 mg./Tab. Blister 12s. **Liquid:** Colloidal activated attapulgite 4.2 Gm./oz. Bot. 5.5 oz.
Use: Diarrhea treatment.

RHEOMACRODEX. (Pharmacia) Dextran 40. A 10% solution in normal saline or in 5% dextrose in water. Bot. 500 ml.
Use: Plasma expander, adjunctive therapy in shock, prophylaxis therapy against venous thrombosis and pulmonary embolism.

RHEUMASAL. (Jenkins) Sod. salicylate 5 gr., potassium iodide 1 gr., ext. gelsemium ¼ gr., ext. cimicifuga ⅛ gr./Tab. Bot. 1000s.

RHEUMATEX. (Wampole) A latex agglutination test for the qualitative detection and quantitative determination of rheumatoid factor in serum.. Kit 100s.
Use: An aid in the diagnosis of rheumatoid arthritis.

RHEUMATON. (Wampole) A two-minute hemagglutination slide test for the qualitative and quantitative determination of rheumatoid factor in serum or synovial fluid. Test Kits 20s, 50s, 150s.
Use: Diagnostic agent for rheumatoid arthritis.

RHINALL DROPS. (Scherer) Phenylephrine HCl 0.25%. Bot. 1 oz.
Use: Nasal decongestant.

RHINALL SPRAY. (Scherer) Phenylephrine HCl 0.25%. Bot. 1 oz.
Use: Nasal decongestant.

RHINALL 10. (Scherer) Phenylephrine HCl 0.2%. Drop. Bot. 1 oz.
Use: Nasal decongestant.

RHINDECON. (McGregor) Phenylpropanolamine HCl 75 mg./Sustained release Cap. Bot. 60s.
Use: Decongestant, bronchodilator.

RHINEX D-LAY. (Lemmon) Acetaminophen 300 mg., salicylamide 300 mg., phenylpropanolamine HCl 60 mg., chlorpheniramine maleate 4 mg./Tab. Bot. 100s, 1000s.

RHINIHAB JR. (BOWMAN) Phenyelephrine HCl 2.5 mg., chlorpheniramine maleate 1 mg./Tab. Bot. 100s, 1000s.
Use: Nasal decongestant, antihistaminic.

RHINOCAPS. (Ferndale) Aspirin 162 mg., acetaminophen 162 mg., phenylpropanolamine HCl 20 mg./Cap. Bot. 100s.
Use: Analgesic, decongestant and antipyretic.

RHINOGESIC. (Vale) Phenylephrine HCl 5 mg., chlorpheniramine maleate 2 mg., salicylamide 250 mg., acetaminophen 150 mg./Tab. Bot. 100s, 500s, 1000s.

RHINOGESIC-GG. (Vale) Phenylephrine HCl 5 mg., chlorpheniramine maleate 2 mg., salicylamide 250

mg., acetaminophen 150 mg., guaifenesin 100 mg./Tab. Bot. 100s, 500s, 1000s.

RHINOGESIC JUNIOR. (Vale) Phenylephrine HCl 2 mg., Chrlorpheniramine maleate 1 mg., Salicylamide 90 mg., acetaminophen 60 mg./Tab. Bot. 100s, 500s.

RHINOLAR. (McGregor) Phenylpropanolamine HCl 75 mg., chlorpheniramine maleate 8 mg., methscopalamine nitrate 2.5 mg./Cap. Bot. 60s. Sustained release.
Use: Antihistaminic, decongestant, antisecretory.

RHINOLAR-EX. (McGregor) Phenylpropanolamine HCl 75 mg., chlorpheniramine maleate 8 mg./Cap. Bot. 60s.
Use: Antihistamine, decongestant, sustained release.

RHINOLAR-EX 12. (McGregor) Phenylpropanolamine HCl 75 mg., chlorpheniramine maleate 12 mg./Cap. Bot. 60s.
Use: Antihistaminic, decongestant, sustained release.

RHINOSYN. (Comatic) Pseudoephedrine HCl 120 mg., chlorpheniramine maleate 10 mg./Sust. Released Cap. Bot. 100s.
Use: Antihistamine, decongestant.

RHINOSYN-DM. (Comatic) Dextromethorphan HBr 15 mg., pseudoephedrine HCl 30 mg., chlorpheniramine maleate 2 mg./5 ml. w/alcohol 1.4%. Bot. 4 oz.
Use: Antitussive, decongestant, antihistamine.

RHINOSYN-PD. (Comatic) Chlorpheniramine maleate 2 mg., pseudoephedrine HCl 30 mg./5 ml. w/alcohol 1.2%. Bot. 4 oz.
Use: Antihistamine, decongestant.

RHINOSYN SYRUP. (Comatic) Pseudoephedrine HCl 60 mg., chlorpheniramine maleate 4 mg. /5 ml. No artificial additives. Bot. Pt.
Use: Antihistamine, decongestant.

RHINOSYN-X. (Comatic) Guaifenesin 100 mg., dextromethorphan HBr 10 mg., pseudoephedrine HCl 30 mg./5 ml. w/ alcohol 7.5%. Bot. 4 oz.
Use: Expectorant, antitussive, decongestant.

RHODANATE.
See: Potassium Thiocyanate

RHODANIDE. More commonly rhodanate, same as thiocyanate.
See: Potassium thiocyanate.

RhoGAM. (Ortho Diagnostic) Rho (D) immune globulin (human). Pkg. of single dose vials in 25s, 72s. Single Dose Vials, Pkg. 6s.
Use: Prevention of Rh hemolytic disease of the newborn.

• **RHO (D) IMMUNE GLOBULIN,** U.S.P. XXI.
See: Gamulin Rh, Vial (Parke-Davis)

RHUBAMINT ELIXIR. (Blue Line) Glycerinated, alkaline, aqueous ext. fl. rhubarb and hydrastis, spirits of cinnamon and peppermint w/potassium bicarbonate, alcohol 3%. pt., gal.

RHUBARB AND SODA MIXTURE. (Lannett) Bot. pt., gal.

RHUBARB AND SODA TABLETS. (Lannett) Tr. nux vomica 5 min., pow. rhubarb 2 gr., sod. bicarb. 5

gr., pow. ipecac ¼ gr., oil peppermint qs./Tab. Bot. 1000s, 5000s.
RHUEX. (Kay) Zirconium oxide 4.5%, calamine 6%, zinc oxide 4%, Actamer 0.1%. Bot. 4 oz., 16 oz., gal.
Use: Itching, discomfort due to poison ivy, oak or sumac; insect bites, sunburn, and minor skin irritations.
RHULICAINE. (Lederle) Benzocaine, triclosan, menthol w/alcohol 32% and isopropyl alcohol 9%. Spray can 4 oz.
Use: Sunburn & minor skin irritations.
RHULICORT. (Lederle) Hydrocortisone 0.5%. **Cream:** Tube 20 Gm. **Lotion:** Bot. 60 ml.
Use: Anti-inflammatory, topically.
RHULICREAM. (Lederle) Benzocaine 1%, zirconium oxide 1%, menthol 0.7%, camphor 0.3%, w/Methylparaben 0.08%, propylparaben 0.02%, isopropyl alcohol 8.8% in cream base. Tube. 2 oz.
Use: Topically; local anesthetic.
RHULIGEL. (Lederle) Phenylcarbinol 2%, menthol 0.3%, camphor 0.3%, alcohol 31%. Tube 2 oz.
Use: Analgesic-anesthetic gel.
RHULISPRAY. (Lederle) Phenylcarbinol 0.674%, benzocaine 1.153%, menthol 0.025%, camphor 0.253%, calamine 4.717% w/isopropyl alcohol 28.767%. Aerosol can 2 oz., 4 oz.
Use: Topically, analgesic, anesthetic for treatment of minor skin irritations.
RHUS-ALL. (Barry) Triple antigen against poison ivy, oak or sumac. Multiple dose vial 5 cc.
RHUS TOX ANTIGEN. (Lemmon) Poison ivy extract 40 mg./ml. Vial 1 ml. Box 4s.
Use: Antigen against poison ivy.
RHUTOX LOTION. (Blue Line) Lead acetate, grindelia, echinacea in alcohol. Bot. 4 oz., 1 pt., 1 gal.
Use: Antiseptic skin preparation.
• **RIBAMINOL.** USAN. Ribonucleic acid compd. w/2-(diethylamino)-ethanole. Under study.
Use: Learning and memory enhancer.
RIBOCEE CAPSULES. (Key) Vit. B-2 25 mg., C 250 mg., B-1 25 mg., niacinamide 50 mg., B-6 3 mg., cal. pantothenate 10 mg./Cap. Bot. 100s, 1000s.
Use: Pre- and postoperatively and as a diet supplement.
• **RIBOFLAVIN,** U.S.P. XXI. Inj., Tab. U.S.P. XXI. Vit. B-2, Vit. G, yellow enzyme, Lactoflavin.
W/Nicotinamide. (Lilly) Riboflavin 5 mg., nicotinamide 200 mg./cc. Amp. 1 cc., Box 100s.
Use: I.M., I.V.; Vitamin B therapy.
W/Vitamins.
See: Vitamin Preparations
• **RIBOFLAVIN-5'-PHOSPHATE SODIUM,** U.S.P. XXI.
RIBOFLAVIN, METHYLOL.
• **RIBOPRINE.** USAN. N-(3-Methyl-2-butenyl) adrenosin.
Use: Antineoplastic.
RIBOTEX. (Pasadena Research) Vit. B-1 100 mg., B-2 10 mg., B-6 10 mg., niacinamide 75 mg./cc. Vial 10 cc.

RIBOZYME INJECTION. (Fellows) Riboflavin-5-Phosphate Sodium 50 mg./cc. Vial 10 cc.
RICINOLEATE, CALCIUM.
See: Pthalox, Tab. (Sutliff & Case)
RICINOLEATE SODIUM.
See: Preceptin, Gel. (Ortho)
RICOLON SOLUTION. (Winthrop Products) Ricolon concentrate.
Use: Leucocytotic preparation.
RID. (Pfipharmecs) Piperonyl butoxide 3.0%, pyrethrins 0.3%, petroleum distillate 1.2%, benzyl alcohol 2.4%. Bot. 2 oz., 4 oz., 64 oz.
Use: Pediculicide.
RID-A-COL. (Panray) Chlorpheniramine maleate 2 mg., aspirin 390 mg., caffeine 30 mg./Tab. Bot. 100s, 1000s.
Use: Antihistamine, analgesic.
RID-A-COL "D". (Panray) Chlorapheniramine 2 mg., aspirin 288.8 mg., caffeine 32.4 mg., phenylephrine 10 mg./Tab. Bot. 1000s.
Use: Antihistamine.
RID-A-COLD. (Panray) Chlorpheniramine maleate 2 mg., asprin 388.8 mg., caffeine 32.4 mg./Tab. Bot. 1000s.
Use: Antihistaminic.
RIFADIN. (Merrell Dow) Rifampin 150 mg. /Cap. Bot. 30s. 300 mg./Cap. Bot. 30s, 60s, 100s.
Use: Antibiotic for treatment of pulmonary tuberculosis and meningococcal carriers.
RIFAMATE. (Merrell Dow) Rifampin 300 mg., isoniazid 150 mg./Cap. Bot. 60s.
Use: Pulmonary tuberculosis treatment.
• **RIFAMIDE.** USAN.
Use: Antibacterial.
RIFAMPICIN. B.A.N. 3-(4-Methylpiperazin-1-yliminomethyl)rifamycin SV.
Use: Antibiotic.
See: Rifadin.
Rimactane.
• **RIFAMPIN,** U.S.P. XXI. Cap., U.S.P. XXI. Hydrazone 3-(4-Methyl-piperazinylimino-methyl rifamycin SV.
Use: Antibacterial (tuberculostatic).
See: Rifadin, Cap. (Merrell Dow)
Rifomycin (Var. Mfr.)
Rimactane, Cap. (Ciba)
• **RIFAMPIN AND ISONIAZID CAPSULES.** U.S.P. XXI.
RIFAMYCIN. B.A.N. Rifamycin SV, an antibiotic produced by certain strains of *Streptomyces mediterranei.* 3-[[(4-Methyl-1-piperazinyl)imino]-methyl]-.
See: Rifampin, U.S.P. XXI.
RIFOCIN-M. Rifamide, B.A.N.
RIL-SWEET. (Plough) Sodium saccharin sodium 3.3%. Bot. 4 oz.
Use: Artificial sweetener.
RIMACTANE. (Ciba) Rifampin 300 mg./Cap. Bot. 30s, 60s, 100s.
Use: Pulmonary tuberculosis.
RIMACTANE/INH. (Ciba) Dual pack: 60 Rimactane 300 mg./Cap. & 30 Isoniazid 300 mg./Tab.
Use: Treatment of tuberculosis.

• **RIMANTADINE HCl.** USAN. Alpha-methyl-1-adamantanemethylamine HCl.
Use: Antiviral.

RIMIFON. Isoniazid, B.A.N.

RIMITEROL. B.A.N. erythro-3,4-Dihydroxy-α-(2-piperidyl)benzyl alcohol.
Use: Bronchodilator.

• **RIMITEROL HYDROBROMIDE.** USAN. α-(3,4-Dihydroxy-phenyl)-2-piperidinemethanol HBr.
Use: Bronchodilator.

RIMSO-50. (Research Industries) Dimethyl sulfoxide 50%, water 50%. Bot. 50 ml.
Use: Interstitial cystitis intravesical instillation.

RINADE. (Econo Med) Chlorpheniramine maleate 8 mg., phenylephrine HCl 20 mg., methscopolamine nitrate 2.5 mg./Cap. Bot. 120s.
Use: Common cold therapy.

RINADE B.I.D. (Econo Med) Chlorpheniramine maleate 8 mg., d- isoephedrine HCl 120 mg./Sus. Rel. Cap. Bot. 100s.
Use: Relief upper respiratory congestion.

RINALGIN. (Meyer) Atropine sulfate 0.03 mg., hyoscyamine 0.03 mg., gelesmium 6 mg., methenamine 41 mg., salol 18 mg., benzoic acid 4.5 mg., methylene blue 5.4 mg./Tab. Bot. 100s, 1000s.
Use: Urinary tract infections.

• **RINGER'S INJECTION,** U.S.P. XXI. Lactated, U.S.P. XXI. (Abbott) 250 ml., 500 ml., 1000 ml. (Invenex), 250 ml., 500 ml., 1000 ml. Abbo-Vac glass or flexible containers, Vial 50 ml. Pkg. 25s. (Lilly) Amp. 20 ml. Pkg. 6s. (Cutter) Bot. 500 ml., 1000 ml.
Use: Fluid and electrolyte replenisher, irrigating solution.
W/Dextrose. (Cutter) 5% solution. Bot. 1000 ml.

RINGER'S INJECTION, ACETATED. (Cutter) Bot. 1000 ml.
Use: Water, electrolyte and calorie source.

• **RINGER'S INJECTION, LACTATED,** U.S.P. XXI.
Use: Fluid and electrolyte replenisher.

• **RINGER'S IRRIGATION,** U.S.P. XXI. (Abbott) 500 ml., 1000 ml.
Use: Irrigation solution.

RINOCIDIN CAPSULES. (Cenci) Phenylephrine HCl 10 mg., chlorpheniramine maleate 1 mg., pyrilamine maleate 1.5 mg., Vit. C 50 mg., caffeine 30 mg., acetophenetidin 130 mg., salicylamide 200 mg./Cap. Bot. 48s.
Use: Analgesic, antipyretic, decongestant.

RINOCIDIN EXPECTORANT. (Cenci) Codeine phosphate 10.08 mg., phenylephrine HCl 10 mg., chlorpheniramine maleate 2 mg., pyrilamine maleate 6.25 mg., ammonium chloride 60 mg., sodium citrate 85 mg./5 cc. Bot. pts., gals.
Also avail. (plain) without codeine. Bot. 1 pt., gal.
Use: Antitussive, antihistaminic, decongestant, expectorant.

RIOBIN. (Pasadena Research) Riboflavin 5′ phosphate sod. 50 mg./cc. Vial 10 cc.

RIO-DOPA. (D.D.R. Pharm.) Levodopa 500 mg./Cap. Bot. 100s.

Use: Anti-Parkinson agent.

RIOPAN. (Ayerst) Magaldrate. **Tab.**: Magaldrate 480 mg., sodium 0.1 mg./Tab. (Chew or Swallow). Pkg. 60s, 100s. Single rollpacks of 12s. **Susp.** Magaldrate 540 mg., sodium 0.1 mg. (0.004 m Eq)/5 ml. Bot. 12 oz. Individual Cups 30 ml. ea. 10 cups/Tray. 10 Trays/Packer
Use: Antacid & G.I. disturbances.

RIOPAN PLUS. (Ayerst) **Chew Tab.**: Magaldrate 480 mg., simethicone 20 mg., sodium 0.1 mg. (0.004 m Eq)/Chew Tab. Bot. 60s. **Susp.**: Magaldrate 540 mg., simethicone 20 mg., sodium 0.1 mg. (0.004 m Eq)/5 ml. Bot. 12 oz. Individual Cups 30 ml. each. 10 cups/Tray. 10 Trays/Packer
Use: Antacid, antiflatulent.

• **RIOPROSTIL.** USAN.
Use: Gastric antisecretory.

• **RIPAZEPAM.** USAN.
Use: Tranquilizer (minor).

• **RISOCAINE.** USAN.
Use: Anesthetic (local).

RISTOCETIN. B.A.N. An antibiotic from species of *Actinomycetes Norcardia lurida.*

RITALIN HYDROCHLORIDE. (Ciba) Methylphenidate HCl Tab. 5 mg., 10 mg., Bot. 100s, 500s, 1000s. Tab. 20 mg., Bot. 100s, 1000s. 10 mg. Accu-Pak 100s.
Use: Psychomotor stimulant.

RITE-DIET. (Edward J. Moore) Methylcellulose, benzocaine, Vit. A, D, B-1, B-2, C plus iron, calcium, potassium, niacinamide/Cap. Bot. 42s.

• **RITODRINE.** USAN. Erythro-p-Hydroxy-α-[1-[(p-hydroxyphenethyl)amino]ethyl] benzyl alcohol
Use: Smooth muscle relaxant.
See: Prempar hydrochloride.
Yutopar, Tab., Inj. (Astra)

• **RITODRINE HYDROCHLORIDE,** U.S.P. XXI. Inj., Tab., U.S.P. XXI.
Use: Relaxant (smooth muscle).

RIVOTRIL. Clonazepam, B.A.N.

RMS SUPPOSITORIES. (Upsher-Smith) Morphine sulfate 5 mg., 10 mg., or 20 mg./Supp. Box 12s.
Use: Narcotic analgesic.

ROAMPICILLIN. (Robinson) Ampicillin 250 mg./Tab. Bot. 100s.
Use: Antibiotic.

ROAMPICILLIN POWDER. (Robinson) Ampicillin powder 125 mg. or 250 mg./5 cc. Vials 80cc, 100cc, 150cc, 200cc.
Use: Antibiotic.

ROBAMATE. (Robinson) Meprobamate 200 mg./Tab. Bot. 100s, 400 mg./Tab. Bot. 1000s.

ROBAMOL. (Cenci) Methocarbamol 750 mg./Tab. Bot. 100s, 1000s.
Use: Musculoskeletal conditions.

ROBAM-PETN. (Robinson) Meprobamatepentaerythritol tetranitrate, Tab. Bot. 100s, 1000s.
Use: Tranquilizer-coronary vasodilator.

ROBANTALINE. (Robinson) Propantheline Bromide 15 mg./Tab. Bot. 100s, 500s, 1000s.
Use: Anticholinergic.

ROBANTALINE WITH PHENOBARBITAL. (Robinson) Propantheline bromide with

phenobarbital Tab. Bot. 100s, 500s, 1000s.
Use: Anticholinergic.
ROBANUL.
See: Robinul, Preps. (Robins)
ROBARB. (Robinson) Amobarbital ¼ gr., ½ gr., and
1 gr./Cap. Bot. 100s.
ROBAXIN. (Robins) Methocarbamol. **Tab.** 500 mg.,
Bot. 100s, 500s; Dis-Co Paks 100s. **Inj.:** 1 Gm./10
cc. of a 50% aqueous solution of polyethylene
glycol 300. Single Dose Vial 10 cc. Pkg. 5s, 25s.
Use: Skeletal muscle relaxant.
ROBAXIN-750. (Robins) Methocarbamol 750 mg./Tab.
Tab. Bot. 100s, 500s; Dis-Co Paks 100s.
Use: Skeletal muscle relaxant.
ROBAXISAL. (Robins) Methocarbamol (Robaxin) 400
mg., aspirin 325 mg./Tab. Bot. 100s, 500s. Dis-Co
pack 100s.
Use: Muscle relaxant/analgesic.
ROBENECID. (Robinson) Probenecid 0.5 Gm./Tab.
Bot. 100s, 1000s.
Use: Uricosuric.
ROBENECID WITH COLCHICINE. (Robinson)
Colchicine 0.5 mg., probenecid 500 mg./Tab. Bot.
100s.
ROBENECOL. (Robinson) Probenecid with colchicine
Tab. Bot. 100s, 1000s.
Use: Uricosuric.
ROBENIDINE. B.A.N. 1,3-Bis(4-chlorobenzyl-ideneami-
no)guanidine.
Use: Antiprotozoam, veterinary medicine.
See: Cycostat.
• **ROBENIDINE HYDROCHLORIDE.** USAN.
Use: Coccidiostat.
ROBESE. (Rocky Mtn.) Dextroamphetamine sulfate 5
mg./Tab. Bot. 100s, 1000s.
Use: Weight control.
ROBESE C. CAP NON-AMPHETAMINE W.C. (Rocky
Mtn.) Carboxymethylcellulose 500 mg., benzocaine
9 mg., Vit. A 5000 I.U., D 400 I.U., B-1 2 mg.,- B-2
2.5 mg., niacinamide 20 mg., ascorbic acid 50 mg.,
B-6 1 mg., calcium pantothenate 1 mg., iron 15
mg./3 Caps. Bot. 48s, 96s.
ROBESE C. INJ. NON-AMPHETAMINE W.C. (Rocky
Mtn.) Caffeine 250 mg., sodium benzoate 250
mg./2 cc. Vial 30 cc.
Use: Weight control.
ROBESE FORTE. (Rocky Mtn.) d-Amphetamine HCl 20
mg., sod. carboxymethylcellulose 2 mg., benzyl
alcohol 1.5%/cc. Vial 30 cc. d-Amphetamine sulfate
15 mg., atropine sulfate 0.36 mg., aloin 16.2 mg.,
phenobarbital 16.2 mg./T.R. Tab. Bot. 100s.
Use: Weight control.
ROBESE "P" INJ. (Rocky Mtn.) Phenyl-propanolamine
HCl 75 mg., protein hydrolysate containing amino
acid 100 ml., leucine 0.415 Gm., valine 0.30 Gm.,
lysine 0.35 Gm., isoleucine 0.24 Gm., phenylalanine
0.28 Gm., arginine 0.15 Gm., threonine 0.18 Gm.,
methionine 0.22 Gm., histidine 0.12 Gm.,
tryptophan 0.05 Gm./cc. Vial 10 cc.
ROBESE "P" TABLETS. (Rocky Mtn.)
Phendimetrazine tartrate 35 mg./Tab. Bot. 100s,
1000s.
ROBICILLIN VK. (Robins) Penicillin V Potassium 250

mg. (400,000 u.)/Tab. Bot. 100s, 1000s. 500 mg.
(800,000 u.)/Tab. Bot. 100s, 500s. Oral 125 mg.
(200,000 u.)/5 ml. 250 mg. (400,000 u.)/5 ml. Bot.
100 ml., 200 ml.
Use: Antibiotic.
RO-BILE. (Rowell) Pepsin 260 mg., pancreatic enzyme
conc. 75 mg., ox bile ext. 100 mg., dehydrocholic
acid 30 mg.; belladonna ext. 8 mg./Tab. Bot. 100s.
Use: Digestant.
ROBIMYCIN. (Robins) Erythromycin 250 mg./Tab.
Bot. 100s, 500s.
Use: Antibiotic.
ROBINUL. (Robins) Glycopyrrolate. 1 mg./Tab. Bot.
100s, 500s.
Use: Anticholinergic.
ROBINUL-FORTE TABLETS. (Robins) Glycopyrrolate
2 mg./Tab. Bot. 100s, 500s.
Use: Anticholinergic.
ROBINUL INJECTABLE. (Robins) Glycopyrrolate 0.2
mg., benzyl alcohol (preservative) 0.9%. Vial 1 ml.
Box 5s, 25s; 2 ml. Box 25s; 5 ml. Box, 25s; 20 ml.
1s.
Use: Anticholinergic.
ROBITET. (Robins) Tetracycline HCl. **Caps.** 250
mg./Cap. Bot. 100s, 1000s; 500 mg./Cap. Bot.
100s, 500s.
Use: Antibiotic.
ROBITUSSIN. (Robins) Guaifenesin 100 mg./5 ml.
w/alcohol 3.5% Bot 1 oz. (4 x 25s), 4 oz., 8 oz., 1
pt., 1 gal. Dis-Co Unit Dose 5 ml., 10 ml., 15 ml. 10 x
10s.
Use: Expectorant.
ROBITUSSIN A-C. (Robins) Guaifenesin 100 mg., co-
deine phosphate 10 mg./5 cc. w/alcohol 3.5%.
Bot. 2 oz., 4 oz., pt., gal.
Use: Expectorant, antitussive.
ROBITUSSIN-CF. (Robins) Guaifenesin 100 mg., phe-
nylpropanolamine HCL 12.5 mg., dextromethorphan
HBr 10 mg./5 ml. w/alcohol 4.75%. Bot. 4 oz., 8
oz., pt.
Use: Antitussive, nasal decongestant, expectorant.
ROBITUSSIN-DAC. (Robins) Guaifenesin 100 mg.,
pseudoephedrine HCl 30 mg., codeine phosphate
10 mg/5 ml. w/alcohol 1.4%. Bot. pt.
Use: Antitussive, nasal decongestant, expectorant.
ROBITUSSIN DIS-CO unit dose pack. (Robins) Guai-
fenesin 100 mg., alcohol 3.5%/5 cc. Syr. unit dose
packs 5 cc., 10 cc. 15cc. (10 x 10s).
Use: Antitussive and expectorant.
ROBITUSSIN-DM. (Robins) Guaifenesin 100 mg., dex-
tromethorphan HBr 15 mg./5 ml. w/alcohol 1.4%.
Bot. 4 oz., 8 oz., pt., gal. Dis-Co Paks 5 ml., 10 ml.
(10 x 10s).
Use: Antitussive, expectorant.
ROBITUSSIN-DM COUGH CALMERS. (Robins) Dex-
tromethorphan HBr 7.5 mg., guaifenesin 50
mg./Loz. Box 16s.
Use: Antitussive, expectorant.
ROBITUSSIN NIGHT RELIEF. (Robins)
Acetaminophen 1,000 mg., phenylephrine HCl 10
mg., pyrilamine maleate 50 mg., dextromethorphan
HBr. 30 mg./oz. w/alcohol 25% Bot. 4 oz., 8 oz.
Use: Adult strength for relief of all cold symptoms.

ROBITUSSIN-PE. (Robins) Guaifenesin 100 mg., pseudoephedrine HCl 30 mg./5 ml. w/alcohol 1.4%. Bot. 4 oz., 8 oz., pt.
Use: Decongestant, expectorant.
ROBOLIC. (Rocky Mtn.) Methandriol dipropionate 50 mg./cc. Vial 10 cc.
ROCAINE. (Rocky Mtn.) Lidocaine HCl 1%, 2%. Vial 50 cc.
Use: Local anesthetic.
ROCALOSAN. (Rocky Mtn.) Calcium glycerophosphate 1%, calcium levulinate 1.5%. Vial 30 cc.
ROCALTROL. (Roche) Calcitriol 0.25 mcg. and 0.5 mcg./Cap. 0.25 mcg./Cap. Bot. 100s, Pak 30s; 0.5 mcg./Cap. Bot. 100s.
Use: Management of hypocalcemia in patients undergoing chronic renal dialysis.
ROCCAL. Benzalkonium Chloride, B.A.N.
ROCHE DIAGNOSTICS. (Roche) Roche laboratories markets the following line of diagnostic products:
Amylochrome
CPK-CS
Isomune-LD
Isomune-CK
Isomune-CK Substrate
Cardiotrol-CK Control
Placentex
Pregnosis
Sensi-Tex
Sensi-Slide
Pregnancy Test Controls
Enterotube II
Oxi/Ferm Tube
V-P Reagent
Liquoid Blood Culture Bottle
Grobax
Fluram
ROCHE DIAGNOSTIC PRODUCTS. (Roche)
Abuscreen. An immunological assay.
Use: Detecting morphine and morphine glucuronide in nanogram levels. Under study.
Amylochrome. Complete reagent system including a chemical standard for the colorimetric assay of human serum (or urine) amylase activity. Tests: 60.
Bact-Chek. For Quality control of bacteriology. Set, Vials 8, Discs 30, or 10 free with 20 discs.
Enterobacter cloacae. Vial: 1 containing 30 discs.
Escherichia coli. Vial: 1 containing 30 discs.
Proteus vulgaris. Vial: 1 containing 30 discs.
Pseudomonas aeruginosa. Vial: 1 containing 30 discs.
Salmonella typhimurium. Vial: 1 containing 30 discs.
Staphylococcus aureus. Vial: 1 containing 30 discs.
Staphylococcus epidermidis. Vial: 1 containing 30 discs.
Streptococcus pyogenes. Vial: 1 containing 30 discs.
Carcindex. Utilizes a ^{125}I labeled antigen in the radioimmunoassay procedure for the detection of carcinoembryonic antigen. Under study.
Enterotube. Biochemical differentiation of the

enterobacteriaceae isolated from biologic specimens. Tubes: 25.
Grobax. Sterile 5% aqueous solution of sodium polyanethol sulfonate. Vials: 4 × 10 ml.
Use: Blood culture bottles.
Liquoid Blood Culture Bottle. Sodium polyanethol sulfonate & tryptic soy broth. Bot.: 12 × 45 ml., 1-4 u., 5-8 u., 9 or more u.
Use: Detection of bacteria from circulating blood.
Pregnosis Slide Test. A 2-minute indirect test for pregnancy. Tests: 50.
ROCHLOMETHIAZIDE. (Robinson) Trichlormethiazide 4 mg./Tab. Bot. 100s, 500s.
Use: Diuretic, antihypertensive.
ROCHORIC. (Rocky Mtn.) Chorionic gonadotropin 10,000 I.U./10 cc. Univial 10 cc.
RO-CHLOROZIDE. (Robinson) Chlorothiazide 250 or 500 mg./Tab. Bot. 100s, 1000s.
Use: Treatment of edema.
ROCKY MOUNTAIN SPOTTED FEVER VACCINE.
Use: Active immunizing agent.
ROCORT LOTION. (Rocky Mtn.) Hydrocortisone 0.5%. Bot. 4 oz.
ROCYCLO INJECTION. (Robinson) Dicyclomine HCl 10 mg./cc. Vial 10cc.
ROCYCLO-PHEN. (Robinson) Dicyclomine HCl w/phenobarbital. Tab. Bot. 100s, 500s.
Use: Anticholinergic, sedative.
ROCYCLO-10. (Robinson) Dicyclomine HCl 10 mg./Cap. Bot. 100s, 500s.
Use: Anticholinergic.
ROCYCLO-20. (Robinson) Dicyclomine HCl 20 mg./Tab. Bot. 100s, 500s.
Use: Anticholinergic.
RODELTA T.B.A. (Rocky Mtn.) Prednisolone tertiary butylacetate 20 mg./10 cc. Vial 10 cc.
RODESINE. (Rocky Mtn.) Adenosine 5 monophosphoric acid 25 mg., sod. nicotinate 20 mg., B-12 cryst. 75 mcg., benzyl alcohol 1.5%/cc. Vial 10 cc.
Use: Anti-inflammatory.
RO-DIET. (Robinson) Diethylpropion HCl 25 mg./Tab. Bot. 100s, 1000s.
Use: Anorexigenic.
RO-DIET TIMED. (Robinson) Diethylpropion HCl (time disintegration) 75 mg./Tab. Bot. 100s, 1000s.
Use: Anorexigenic.
• **RODOCAINE.** USAN.
Use: Local anesthetic.
RODOX. (Rocky Mtn.) Docusate sodium 100 mg. or 250 mg./Cap. Bot. 100s.
Use: Stool softener.
RODOX/W. (Rocky Mtn.) Docusate sodium 100 mg., casanthranol 75 mg./Cap. Bot. 100s, 1000s.
Use: Fecal softener and laxative.
RODRYL. (Rocky Mtn.) Diphenhydramine HCl 10 mg./cc. Vial 30 cc.
RODRYL-50. (Rocky Mtn.) Diphenhydramine HCl 50 mg./cc. Vial 10 cc.
Use: Antihistamine.
ROENTGENOGRAPHY.
See: Iodine Products, Diagnostic

RO-FEDRIN. (Robinson) Pseudoephedrine HCl 60 mg./Tab. Bot. 100s, 1000s.
Use: Respiratory decongestant.
RO-FEDRINE SYRUP. (Robinson) Pseudoephedrine HCl 30 mg./5 cc. Bot. pt.
Use: Respiratory decongestant.
• **ROFLURANE.** USAN. 2-Bromo-1, 1,2-trifluoroethyl methyl ether.
Use: General inhalation anesthetic.
ROGENIC. (O'Neal, Jones & Feldman) **S.C. Tab.:** Iron 60 mg., Vit. C 100 mg., B-6 6 mg., B-12 25 mcg., desiccated liver/S.C. Tab.
Use: Multivitamin.
Dual release Tab. First release: Ferrous fumarate 40 mg., ferrous sulfate 20 mg., ferrous gluconate 7 mg., Vit. C 50 mg., cobalamin 25 mcg., B-6 5 mg., desic. liver 15 mg.; second release: ferrous fumarate 10 mg., ferrous sulfate 10 mg., ferrous gluconate 3 mg., Vit. C 20 mg., cobalamin 25 mcg., B-6 5 mg., desic. liver 15 mg./Tab. Bot. 100s. **Inj.** B-12 500 mcg., peptonized iron 20 mg., liver 10 mcg./cc. Vial 10 cc.
Use: Treatment of iron deficiency anemias.
ROGITINE. Phentolamine, B.A.N.
RO-HYDRAZIDE. (Robinson) Hydrochlorothiazide 25, 50, 100 mg./Tab. Bot. 100s, 500s, 1000s.
Use: Diuretic.
ROHIST. (Rocky Mtn.) Chlorpheniramine 12 mg./T.D. Tab. Bot. 100s.
ROHIST C. (Rocky Mtn.) Chlorpheniramine 100 mg./cc. Vial 10 cc.
RO-HIST. (Robinson) Tripelennamine HCl 50 mg./Tab. Bot. 100s, 1000s.
ROHIST-D. (Rocky Mtn.) Chlorpheniramine 5 mg., phenylpropanolamine HCl 12.5 mg., atropine sulfate 0.2 mg., Vit. C 100 mg./Cap. Bot. 100s. Vial 10 cc.
Use: Decongestant.
ROHIST PLUS. (Rocky Mtn.) Chlorpheniramine 12 mg., d-desoxyephedrine HCl 8 mg./T.R. Tab. Bot. 100s.
Use: Antihistamine plus stimulant, decongestant.
RO HONEY PROTEIN. (Rocky Mtn.) Protein 70%. Bot. 250s.
Use: Protein supplement.
ROHYDRA. (Robinson) **Capsules:** Diphendydramine HCl 25, 50 mg./Cap. Bot. 100s, 1000s. **Elixir:** Diphenhydramine HCl 80 mg., ammonium chloride 12 gr., sod. citrate 5 gr., menthol 0.1 gr./fl. oz. Bot. pts. gal.
Use: Allergy therapy.
ROHYDRA EXPECTORANT. (Robinson) Diphenydramine HCl. Bot. pts., gal.
Use: Allergy therapy.
RO-HYDRAZIDE. (Robinson) Hydrochlorothiazide 100 mg./Tab. Bot. 100s, 1000s.
Use: Treatment of edema.
ROLA-BEE. (Robinson) Vit. B-1 15 mg., B-2 10 mg., niacinamide 50 mg., cal. pantothenate 10 mg., C 250 mg., B-6 5 mg./Cap. Bot. 100s.
Use: Supplement.
ROLABROMOPHEN. (Robinson) Brompehniramine maleate 4 mg./Tab. Bot. 100s, 5000s.
Use: Antihistaminic.

ROLABROMOPHEN DECONGESTANT ELIXIR. (Robinson) Brompheniramine maleate 4 mg., phenylephrine HCl 5 mg., phenylpropanolamine HCl 5 mg., alcohol 2.3%/5 ml. Bot. Pt., Gal.
Use: Rhinitis treatment.
ROLABROMOPHEN ELIXIR. (Robinson) Brompheniramine maleate 2 mg., alcohol 3%/5 ml. Bot. Pts., Gal.
Use: Antihistiminic.
ROLABROMOPHEN EXPECTORANT. (Robinson) Brompheniramine maleate 2 mg., phenylephrine HCl 5 mg., phenylpropanolamine HCl 5 mg., guaifenesin 100 mg., alcohol 3.5%/5 ml. Bot. Pt., Gal.
Use: Decongestant and expectorant.
ROLABROMOPHEN FORTE. (Robinson) Brompheniramine maleate-forte extended. Bot. 100s, 500s, 1000s.
ROLABROMOPHEN INJECTION. (Robinson) Bropheniramine maleate injection. 10 mg./cc. Vial 30 cc.; 100 mg./cc. Vial 10 cc.
Use: Antihistaminic.
ROLABROMOPHEN TIMED. (Robinson) Bropheniramine maleate time disintegration 8 mg., 12 mg./Tab. Bot. 100s, 1000s.
Use: Antihistamine.
ROLAIDS ANTACID TABLETS. (Warner-Lambert) Dihydroxy aluminum sodium carbonate 334 mg./Tab. Regular, wintergreen and spearmint flavors. Roll 12s. Bot. 75s, 150s.
Use: Antacid.
ROLA-METHAZINE. (Robinson) Promethazine HCl 12.5 mg., 25 mg., 50 mg./Tab. Bot. 100s, 500s, 1000s.
Use: Antihistamine, antiemetic, sedative.
ROLA-METHAZINE EXPECTORANT PLAIN. (Robinson) Promethazine with expectorant plain. Bot. pt., gal.
ROLAMETHAZINE INJECTION. (Robinson) Promethazine HCl injection 25 mg./cc. Vial 10 cc.
Use: Antiemetic, antihistamine.
ROLA-METHAZINE PEDIATRIC LIQUID. (Robinson) Promethazine pediatric liq. Bot. pt., gal.
Use: Antihistamine.
ROLA-METHAZINE VC EXPECTORANT. (Robinson) Promethazine VC Expectorant. Bot. pt., gal.
Use: Antihistamine, decongestant, expectorant.
ROLA-METHAZINE VC EXPECTORANT WITH CODEINE. (Robinson) Promethazine VC expectorant with codeine. Bot. Pts., gal.
ROLA-METHAZINE WITH CODEINE. (Robinson) Promethazine expectorant with codeine. Bot. pt., gal.
Use: Antihistamine, expectorant, antitussive.
ROLAPHENT. (Robinson) Phentermine 8 mg./Tab. Bot. 100s.
Use: Anorexiant.
ROLATHIMIDE. (Robinson) Glutethimide 0.5 Gm./Tab. Bot. 100s, 500s.
Use: Hypnotic.
ROLANADE. (Robinson) Chlorpheniramine maleate 8

mg., phenylpropanolamine HCl 50 mg., atropine sulfate 1/180 Gr./Cap. Bot. 100s, 500s, 1000s.
Use: Cold capsules.

ROLAZID. (Robinson) Isonicotinic acid hydrazide 100 mg., 300 mg./Tab. Bot. 100s, 1000s.
Use: Antibacterial (Tuberculostatic).

ROLAZINE. (Robinson) Hydralazine HCl 25 mg. or 50 mg./Tab. Bot. 100s, 500s, 1000s.
Use: Hypotensive agent.

ROLCEDIN. (Robinson) Chlorpheniramine maleate 2 mg., salicylamide 3½ gr., acetophenetidin 2½ gr., caffeine ½ gr./Tab. Bot. 100s, 1000s.
Use: Cold symptoms.

ROLECITHIN. (Robinson) **Capsules:** Soya lecithin 259.2 mg., soy bean oil 170.2 mg., D 150 u./Cap. **Tablets:** Soya lecithin 7 gr./Tab. Bot. 100s, 250s, 1000s.

• **ROLETAMIDE.** USAN. 3′,4′,5′-Trimethoxy-3-(3-pyrrolin-1-yl) acrylophenone.
Use: Hypnotic.

ROLICAP. (Arcum) Vits. A acetate 5,000 I.U., D-2 400 I.U., B-1 3.0 mg., B-2 2.5 mg., B-6 10 mg., C 50 mg., niacinamide 20 mg., B-12 1.0 mcg./Chewable Tab. Bot. 100s, 1000s.
Use: Multiple vitamin.

ROLICTON. Amisometradine, B.A.N.

ROLICYPRAM. B.A.N. (+)-5-Oxo-N-(trans-2-phenylcyclopropyl)-L-pyrrolidine-2-carboxamide.
Use: Antidepressant.

• **ROLICYPRINE.** USAN. (+)-5-Oxo-N-(trans-2-phenyl-cyclopropyl)-L-2-pyrrolidinecarboxamide.
Use: Antidepressant.

ROLIDIOL. (Robinson) Ethinyl estradiol 0.02, 0.05 mg./Tab. Bot. 100s, 1000s.
Use: Estrogen therapy.

ROLIDRIN-6. (Robinson) Nylidrin HCl 6 mg./Tab. Bot. 100s, 1000s.
Use: Peripheral vasodilator.

ROLIDRIN-12. (Robinson) Nylidrin HCl 12 mg./Tab. Bot. 100s, 1000s.
Use: Peripheral vasodilator.

RO-LINOIL. (Robinson) Linolenic acid 51%, linoleic acid 17%, oleic acid 23%, stearic acid 2%, palmitic acid 7%. Cap. 200 min. Bot. 100s, 500s.
Use: Unsaturated free fatty acid diet.

• **ROLIPRAM.** USAN.
Use: Tranquilizer.

ROLISOX-10. (Robinson) Isoxsuprine HCl 10 mg./Tab. Bot. 100s.
Use: Vasodilator.

ROLISOX-20. (Robinson) Isoxsuprine HCl 20 mg./Tab. Bot. 100s.
Use: Vasodilator.

• **ROLITETRACYCLINE, STERILE,** U.S.P. XXI. Inj., U.S.P. XXI. N-(Pyrrolidinomethyl) tetracycline. 4-(Dimethylamino)-1,4,4a,5,5a,6,11,12a-octahydro-3,6,-10,12,12a-pentahydroxy-6-methyl-1,11-dioxo-N-(1-pyrrolidinylmethyl)-2-naphthacenecarboxamide. Tetrex PMT nitrate Inj. Syntetrin Inj. (Bristol) Velacycline (Squibb)
Use: Antibacterial.

• **ROLITETRACYCLINE NITRATE.** USAN. Tetrim.

Use: Antibacterial.

• **ROLODINE.** USAN. 4-(Benzylamino)-2-methyl-7H-pyrrolo-[2,3-d]-pyrimidine.
Use: Muscle relaxant.

ROLOX. (Purepac) Magnesium hydroxide, aluminum hydroxide gel. Bot. 12 oz., gal.
Use: Antacid.

ROLSERP. (Robinson) Reserpine. **Tablets:** 0.1 mg., 0.25 mg., 0.5 mg./Tab. Bot. 100s, 1000s. **Vial:** 5 mg./cc. Vial 10 cc. **Timedcaps:** 0.25 mg., 0.5 mg. or 0.75 mg./Cap. Bot. 100s, 500s, 1000s, Bulk Pack 5000s. **Elixir:** 0.25 mg./5 cc. Bot. 16 oz.

ROLUTIN. (Rocky Mtn.) Hydroxyprogesterone caproate in oil 125 mg./10 cc. Vial 10 cc.

ROLUTIN 2X. (Rocky Mtn.) Hydroxyprogesterone caproate in oil 125 mg./5 cc. Vial 5 cc.

ROLZYME. (Robinson) Pepsin 250 mg., pancreatin 200 mg., bile salts 150 mg., dehydrocholic acid 25 mg./Tab. Bot. 100s, 1000s.

ROMAPHED. (Robinson) Aminophylline, ephedrine, amobarbital. Tab. Bot. 100s, 500s, 1000s.
Use: Smooth muscle relaxant (bronchodilator).

ROMETHOCARB. (Robinson) Methocarbamol 500 mg., 750 mg./Tab. Bot. 100s, 500s.
Use: Skeletal muscle relaxant.

ROMEX COUGH & COLD CAPSULES. (APC) Guaifenesin 65 mg., dextromethorphan HBr 10 mg., chlorpheniramine maleate 1.5 mg., pyrilamine maleate 12.5 mg., phenylephrine HCl 5 mg., acetaminophen 160 mg./Cap. Bot. 21s.
Use: Decongestant.

ROMEX COUGH & COLD TABLETS. (APC) Dextromethorphan HBr 7.5 mg., phenylephrine HCl 2.5 mg., ascorbic acid 30 mg. Box 15s.
Use: Relief of cold symptoms, cough.

ROMEX TROCHES & LIQUID. (A.P.C.) **Troche:** Polymyxin B sulfate 1000 u., benzocaine 5 mg., cetalkonium chloride 2.5 mg., gramicidin 100 mcg., chlorpheniramine maleate 0.5 mg., tyrothricin 2 mg./Troche. Pkg. 10s. **Liq.** Guaifenesin 200 mg., dextromethorphan HBr 60 mg., chlorpheniramine maleate 12 mg., phenylephrine HCl 30 mg./fl. oz. Bot. 4 oz.
Use: Minor throat and mouth irritations.

ROMICIL. Oleandomycin, B.A.N.

ROMILAR III. (Block) Dextromethorphan HBr,5.0 mg., phenylpropanolamine HCl, alcohol 20%. Bot. 3 oz., 5 oz.
Use: Decongestant cough syrup.

ROMILAR CF. (Block) Dextromethorphan HBr 5.0 mg., w/alcohol 20%, Bot. 1.75 oz., 3 oz., 5 oz.
Use: Cough suppressant.

ROMILAR, Children's Cough Syrup. (Block) Dextromethorphan HBr 2.5 mg.,. Bot. 3 oz., 6 oz.
Use: Cough therapy.

ROMINAL W/C. (Robinson) Vit. B-1 25 mg., B-2 12.5 mg., nicotinamide 75 mg., B-6 3 mg., cal. pantothenate 10 mg., C 250 mg., B-12 3 mcg./Cap. Bot. 100s.
Use: Vitamin supplement therapy.

ROMINE. (Rocky Mtn.) Dimenhydrinate 50 mg. w/propylene glycol/cc. Vial 10 cc.

ROMOTAL HYDROCHLORIDE. Tacrine, B.A.N.

ROMPUN. Xylazine, B.A.N.
RONDASE. Hyaluronidase, B.A.N.
RONDEC DROPS. (Ross) Carbinoxamine maleate 2 mg., pseudoephedrine HCl 25 mg./ml. Bot. 30 ml. with dropper.
Use: Decongestant for infants 1 to 17 months.
RONDEC DM DROPS. (Ross) Carbinoxamine maleate 2 mg., pseudoephedrine HCl 25 mg., dextromethorphan HBr 4 mg./ml., alcohol 0.6%. Bot. w/dropper 30 ml.
Use: Non-narcotic cough mixture.
RONDEC DM SYRUP. (Ross) Carbinoxamine maleate 4 mg., pseudoephedrine HCl 60 mg., dextromethorphan HBr 15 mg./5 ml. w/alcohol 0.6%. Bot. pt., 4 oz.
Use: Non-narcotic cough mixture.
RONDEC SYRUP. (Ross) Carbinoxamine maleate 4 mg., pseudoephedrine HCl 60 mg./5 ml. Syrup. Bot. 4 oz., pt.
Use: Decongestant for children 18 mo. and older.
RONDEC TABLET. (Ross) Carbinoxamine maleate 4 mg., pseudoephedrine HCl 60 mg./Tab. Bot. 100s, 500s.
Use: Relief of respiratory tract congestion.
RONDEC TR. (Ross) Carbinoxamine 8 mg., pseudoephedrine HCl 120 mg./S.R. Tab.
Use: Antihistaminic, decongestant for 12 hour dosing.
RONDEC WITH HYDROCODONE SYRUP. (Ross) Carbinoxamine maleate 4 mg., pseudoephedrine HCl 60 mg., hydrocodone bitartrate 5 mg./5cc. Bot. 16 fl. oz.
Use: Narcotic antitussive, decongestant.
RONDOMYCIN. (Wallace) Methacycline HCl. 150 mg. or 300 mg./Cap. **150 mg.:** Bot. 100s. **300 mg.:** Bot. 50s.
Use: Antibiotic.
RONIACOL. (Roche) Nicotinyl alcohol. **Elixir** (50 mg./5 ml.) Bot. 1 pt. **Tab.** (50 mg.) Bot. 100s, 500s.
Use: Treatment of peripheral vascular disease.
RONIACOL TIMESPAN TABS. (Roche) Nicotinyl tartrate 150 mg./Tab. Bot. 100s, 500s.
Use: Impaired peripheral circulation.
RONICOTIN. (Rocky Mtn.) Nicotinic acid 500 mg./Tab. Bot. 100s, 1000s.
Use: Vasodilator.
• **RONIDAZOLE.** USAN.
Use: Antiprotozoal.
RONIL. (Rocky Mtn.) Milk sugar 3 gr./T.D. Tab. Bot. 100s.
Use: Placebo.
RONIUM. (Pasadena Research) Iron 90 mg., Vit. C 75 mg./Cap. Bot. 100s, 1000s.
Use: Hematinic.
• **RONNEL.** USAN. Fenchlorphos.
Use: Insecticide (systemic)
See: Korlan (Dow)
Trolene (Dow)
RONTYL. Hydroflumethiazide, B.A.N.
RONVET. (Geneva) Erythromycin stearate. 250 mg./Tab. Bot. 100s.

RONYL. Pemoline, B.A.N.
RO OPTHO. (Rocky Mtn.) Sodium sulfacetamide 100 mg., prednisolone 5 mg., phenylephrine HCl 0.12%/cc. Bot. 5 cc.
Use: Therapeutic eye drops.
RO-PAPAV. (Robinson) Papaverine HCl time disintegration 150 mg./Tab. Bot. 100s, 250s, 1000s.
Use: Smooth muscle relaxant.
RO-PHYLLINE. (Robinson) Theophylline 80 mg./15 ml. w/alcohol 20% in a fruit-flavored, sugar-free solution. Bot. pt., gal.
Use: Diuretic.
• **ROPITOIN HYDROCHLORIDE.** USAN.
Use: Cardiac depressant.
• **ROPIZINE.** USAN.
Use: Anticonvulsant.
ROPLEDGE. (Robinson) Phendimetrazine tartrate 35 mg./Tab. Bot. 100s, 1000s.
Use: Anorexiant.
ROPOXY. (Robinson) Propoxyphene HCl 65 mg./Cap. Bot. 100s, 500s, 1000s.
Use: Analgesic.
ROPOXY COMPOUND-65. (Robinson) Propoxyphene compound. Cap. Bot. 100s, 500s.
Use: Analgesic.
ROPRED. (Robinson) Prednisone 1.0 mg., 2.5 mg., 5.0 mg., 20 mg./Tab. Bot. 100s, 500s, 1000s.
Use: Adrenocortical steroid.
RO-PRENATE. (Robinson) Prenatal vitamin and mineral. Tab. Bot. 100s, 1000s.
Use: Prenatal vitamin.
ROPREDLONE. (Robinson) Prednisolone. **Tablets:** 1 mg., 5 mg./Tab. Bot. 100s, 500s, 1000s. **Vial:** 25 mg., 50 mg., 100 mg./cc. Vial 10 cc.
Use: Adrenocortical steroid.
ROQUINE. (Robinson) Chloroquine phosphate 0.25 Gm./Tab. Bot. 100s, 500s, 1000s.
ROSA GALLICAL.
See: Estivin, Sol. (Alcon)
ROSANILINE DYES.
See: Fuchsin, Basic (Var. Mfr.)
Methylrosaniline Chloride Sol., Inj. (Var Mfr.)
• **ROSARAMICIN.** USAN.
Use: Antibacterial.
• **ROSARAMICIN BUTYRATE.** USAN.
Use: Antibacterial.
• **ROSARAMICIN PROPIONATE.** USAN.
Use: Antibacterial.
• **ROSARAMICIN SODIUM PHOSPHATE.** USAN.
Use: Antibacterial.
• **ROSARAMICIN STEARATE.** USAN.
Use: Antibacterial.
ROSCORB 5. (Rocky Mtn.) Vit. C 500 mg./Tab. Bot. 100s, 1000s.
Use: Vitamin supplement.
ROSE BENGAL.
See: Robengatope (Squibb)
• **ROSE BENGAL SODIUM I-125.** USAN.
Use: Radioactive agent.
• **ROSE BENGAL SODIUM I-131 INJECTION,** U.S.P. XXI. Sodium 4,5,6,7-Tetrachloro-2',-4',5',7'-tetraiodo-fluorescein.

Use: Diagnostic aid (hepatic function determination).

ROSE BENGAL STRIPS. (Barnes-Hind) Strips 1.3 mg. Box 100 strips.
Use: Diagnostic agent for disclosing corneal injury and pathology.

ROSE-C LIQUID. (Barth's) Vit. C 300 mg., rose hip extract/Tsp. Dropper Bot. 2 oz., Bot. 8 oz.

ROSE HIPS. (Burgin-Arden) Vitamin C 300 mg., in base of sorbitol. Bot. 4 oz., 8 oz.
Use: Vitamin C supplement.

ROSE HIPS C. (Columbia) Vit. C 500 mg./Tab. Bot. 100s.
Use: Vitamin C therapy.

ROSE HIPS VITAMIN C. (Kirkman) Vit. C 100 mg./Tab. Bot. 100s, 250s. Vit. C 250 mg., 500 mg./Tab. Bot. 100s, 250s, 500s.
Use: Vitamin C therapy.

• **ROSE OIL,** N.F. XVI.
Use: Perfume.

• **ROSE WATER, STRONGER,** N.F. XVI.
Use: Perfume.

• **ROSE WATER OINTMENT,** U.S.P. XXI.
Use: Emollient; ointment base.

• **ROSIN,** U.S.P. XXI.
Use: Stiffening agent; Pharm. necessity for Zinc-Eugenol cement.

• **ROSOXACIN.** USAN.
Use: Antibacterial.

ROSOXOL TABLETS. (Robinson) Sulfisoxazole 500 mg./Tab. Bot. 100s, 1000s.
Use: Sulfonamide, anti-infective.

ROSOXOL-AZO. (Robinson) Sulfisoxazole, phenazopyridine HCl./Tab. Bot. 100s, 1000s.
Use: Sulfonamide, anti-infective.

RO-SULFIRAM-500. (Robinson) Disulfiram 500 mg./Tab. Bot. 50s, 500s.
Use: Treatment of alcoholism.

RO-SUPER-B TABLETS. (Robinson) Vit. B-1 50 mg., B-2 20 mg., B-6 5 mg., B-12 15 mcg., C 300 mg., liver desic. 100 mg., dried yeast 100 mg., niacinamide 25 mg., Ca pantothenate 5 mg., iron 10 mg./Tab. Bot. 100s, 250s, 1000s.
Use: Therapeutic B-complex.

ROTAZYME. (Abbott) Test kit 50s.
Use: Qualitative enzyme immunoassay for detection of rotavirus antigen in human fecal material.

ROTENSE. (Robinson) Aspirin, phenacetin, & caffeine w/allybarbituric acid/Tab. Bot. 100s, 1000s.
Use: Analgesic, sedative.

ROTERSEPT DIGLUCONATE. Chlorhexidine, B.A.N.

ROTHERAMIN. (Robinson) Vit. A 25,000 I.U., D 1000 I.U., B-1 10 mg., B-2 5 mg., niacinamide 100 mg., B-6 1 mg., B-12 5 mcg., C 150 mg., Ca 103.6 mg., phosphorus 80.2 mg., iron 10 mg., Mg 5.5 mg., Mn 1 mg., K 5 mg., Zn 1.4 mg./Cap. or Tab. Bot. 100s, 250s, 1000s.
Use: Vitamin-mineral therapy.

RO-THYRONINE. (Robinson) Liothyronine sodium 25 mcg., or 50 mcg./Tab. Bot. 100s, 500s, 1000s.
Use: Thyroid therapy.

RO-THYROXINE. (Robinson) L-thyroxine sodium 0.1 mg., 0.2 mg./Tab. Bot. 100s, 500s, 1000s.
Use: Hypothyroidism.

• **ROTOXAMINE TARTRATE.** USAN. (−)-2-[p-Chloro-α-[2-(dimethylamino)ethoxy]-benzyl pyridine tartrate (1:1).
Use: Antihistaminic.

RO-TRAN. (Robinson) Salicylamide 250 mg., powd. ext. valerian 15 mg., pwd. ext. passiflora 15 mg./Tab. Bot. 100s.
Use: Minor tensions and anxiety.

ROTRILATE. (Robinson) Trimethylcyclohexyl mandelate 200 mg./Tab. Bot. 100s, 1000s.

RO TRIM. (Rocky Mtn.) d-Amphetamine sulfate 15 mg., atropine sulfate 1/100 gr., aloin 1/4 gr., phenobarbital 1/4 gr./Cap. Bot. 100s.
Use: Weight reduction.

ROTRIM T. (Rocky Mtn.) Thyroid 3 gr./T.R. Tab. Bot. 100s.
Use: Thyroid supplement.

ROTYL HCl. (Rocky Mtn.) Dicylomine HCl 10 mg./cc. Vial 10 cc.
Use: Smooth muscle relaxant and antispasmodic.

ROVAMYCIN. Spiramycin, B.A.N.

ROVIMINS T.F.. (Rocky Mtn.) Zinc sulfate 50 mg., magnesium sulfate 50 mg., Vit. A 25,000 I.U., D 400 I.U., B-1 20 mg., B-2 30 mg., B-6 3 mg., B-12 25 mcg., Ca pantothenate 30 mg., niacinamide 100 mg., C 400 mg., E 2 I.U., managanese 3 mg., potassium sulfate 5 mg., copper oxide 1 mg., iodine 0.15 mg./Pill. Bot. 100s, 1000s.
Use: Therapeutic and stress vitamin and mineral formula.

ROXANOL ORAL SOLUTION. (Roxane) Morphine sulfate oral sol. 20 mg./ml. Bot. 30 ml. calibrated dropper.
Use: Narcotic analgesic.

• **ROXARSONE.** USAN. 3-Nitro-4-hydroxy-phenylarsonic acid.
Use: Coccidiostat and antibacterial.

ROXYN. (Rocky Mtn.) d-Desoxyephedrine HCl 15 mg./Tab. Bot. 100s.
Use: Weight reduction.

ROZINC. (Rocky Mtn.) Zinc sulfate 220 mg./Cap. Bot. 100s, 1000s.

RP-MYCIN. (Reid-Provident) Erythromycin, E.C. Tabs. 250 mg./Tab. Bot. 100s.
Use: Antibacterial.

R-S LOTION. (Hill) **No. 2:** Sulfur 8%, resorcinol monoacetate 4%. Bot. 2 oz.
Use: Drying medication.

RUBACELL II DIAGNOSTIC TEST. (Abbott) Passive hemagglutination procedure for the detection of antibody to rubella virus. 100 & 1000 test units.
Use: Qualitative & quantitative detection of antibody to Rubella virus in serum or reclacified plasma.

RUBA-TECT. (Abbott) Rubella diagnosis test system. 100s.
Use: Hemagglutination inhibition test for the detection & quantitation of rubella antibody in serum.

RUBAZYME. (Abbott) Test kit 100s, 1000s.

Use: Enzyme immunoassay for IgG antibody to rubella virus.

RUBAZYME-M. (Abbott) Test kit 50s.
Use: Enzyme immunoassay for IgM antibody to rubella virus.

• **RUBELLA & MUMPS VIRUS VACCINE, LIVE.** U.S.P. XXI.
Use: Active immunizing agent.
See: Biavax, Disp. Syringe. (Merck Sharp & Dohme)

• **RUBELLA VIRUS VACCINE, LIVE,** U.S.P. XXI.
Use: Active immunizing agent.
See: Cendevax, Inj. (SmithKline)
Meruvax, Vial (Merck Sharp & Dohme)
W/Measles vaccine.
See: M-R-Vax, Inj. (Merck Sharp & Dohme)
W/Measles vaccine, mumps vaccine.
See: M-M-R, Vial (Merck Sharp & Dohme)

RUBELLA VIRUS VACCINE, LIVE ATTENUATED.
Live attenuated strain of rubella virus HPV-77.
Use: Active immunizing agent.
W/Measles vaccine.
See: Lirubel, Vial (Merrell Dow)
W/Measles vaccine, mumps vaccine.
See: Lirutrin, Vial (Merrell Dow)

RUBESOL-1000. (Central) Cyanocobalamin U.S.P. 1000 mcg./ml. Vial 10 ml., 30 ml. Box 12s.

RUBICAPS. (Stanlabs) Vit. A 10,000 I.U., D 1000 I.U., B-1 16 mg., B-2 8 mg., C 100 mg., B-6 0.5 mg., B-12 6 mcg., E 1.25 I.U., niacinamide 10 mg., Ca pantothenate 5 mg., inositol 30 mg., choline bitartrate 62 mg., dl-methionine 30 mg., ferrous gluconate 30 mg., Ca 58 mg., P 45 mg., potassium iodide 0.15 mg., magnesium sulfate dried 7.2 mg., copper sulfate dried 5 mg., manganese sulfate 3.4 mg., potassium chloride 1.3 mg., liver desic. 100 mg., yeast dried 100 mg./Tab. Cartons 50s, 100s; apothecary 250s.

RUBICAPS B COMPLEX W/C. (Stanlabs) Vit. B-1 15 mg., B-2 10 mg., B-6 5 mg., C 300 mg., niacinamide 50 mg., Ca pantothenate 10 mg./Cap. Bot. 100s.
Use: Therapeutic B complex.

RUBICAPS SUPER M. (Stanlabs) Vit. A 50,000 I.U., D 1500 I.U., B-1 16 mg., B-2 10 mg., B-6 2 mg., B-12 12 mcg., C 150 mg., E 5 I.U., Ca pantothenate 10 mg., niacinamide 100 mg., rutin 10 mg., hesperidin 15 mg., biotin 20 mcg., betaine HCl 10 mg., para-aminobenzoic acid 20 mg., choline bitartrate 50 mg., inositol 20 mg., dl-methionine 20 mg., Fe 25 mg., iodine 0.15 mg., Cu 2.5 mg., Mn 2 mg., Zn 3 mg., Mg 6 mg., Ca 58 mg., P 45 mg., K 5 mg., liver desic. 100 mg./Geltab. Bot. 100s.
Use: Therapeutic Vitamin Supplement.

• **RUBIDIUM CHLORIDE Rb 86.** USAN.
Use: Radioactive agent.

RUBRAMIN PC. (Squibb) Vit. B-12 U.S.P. (cyanocobalamin) w/benzyl alcohol 1%, sod. chloride, sod. hydroxide or HCl acid. (100 mcg./cc.; cobalt content 4 mcg./ml.) Vial 10 cc. (1000 mcg./cc.; cobalt content 40 mcg./ml.) Vial 1, 10 cc. Unimatic: 100 mcg./cc. 1 dose syringe 1s, 10s. 1,000 mcg./cc. 1 dose syringe 1s, 10s.
Use: Vitamin for various anemias.

RUBRAPET OINTMENT. (Medco Lab) Red veterinary petrolatum for light protection Jar. 16 oz.

RUBRAPLEX. (Lannett) Vitamins B-1 2.5 mg., B-2 2 mg., B-6 0.5 mg., B-12 5 mcg., cal. pantothenate 1 mg., niacinamide 20 mg./Cap. Bot. 100s, 1000s.

RUBRATOPE-57. (Squibb) Cyanocobalamin Co 57 Capsules; Solution U.S.P.

RUBRAVITE LIQUID. (Lannett) Vit. B-1 10 mg., B-12 25 mcg./5 cc. Bot. pt.

RUELENE. Crufomate, B.A.N.

RUFEN. (Boots) Ibuprofen 400 mg. or 600 mg./Tab. Bot. 100s, 500s.
Use: Relief of mind to moderate pain in rheumatoid arthritis, osteoarthritis, dysmenorrhea.

RUFOCROMOMYCIN. B.A.N. An antibiotic produced by *Streptomyces rufochromogenus.*

RUFOLEX. (Lannett) Vit. B-1 1.5 mg., B-2 1.5 mg., B-61 mg., B-12 5 mcg., C 50 mg., niacinamide 10 mg., ferrous fumarate 200 mg., d-sorbitol 200 mg., folic acid 0.25 mg./Cap. Bot. 100s.
Use: Iron & vitamin deficiencies.

RUM-K-SYRUP. (Fleming) Potassium chloride 10 mEq/5 u. in butter/rum flavored base. Bot. pt., gal.
Use: Potassium supplement.

RUPHENAMIN. (Lannett) Aminophylline 100 mg., phenobarbital 15 mg., rutin 20 mg./Cap. Bot. 1000s.
Use: Cardiovascular disorders.

RUSCORB. (Robinson) 20/100: Rutin 20 mg., C 100 mg./Tab. 50/300: Rutin 50 mg., C 300 mg./Tab. Bot. 100s, 1000s.

RUST INHIBITOR.
See: Anti-Rust, Tab. (Winthrop Labs.)
Sodium Nitrite, Tab. (Var. Mfr.)

• **RUTAMYCIN.** USAN. From strain of *Streptomyces rutgersensis.* Under study.
Use: Antifungal antibiotic.

RUTGERS 612.
See: Ethohexadiol. (Var. Mfr.)

RUTIN. 3-Rhamnoglucoside of 5,7,3',4'-tetrahydroxyflavonol. Eldrin, globulariacitrin, myrticalorin, oxyritin, phytomelin, rutoside, sophorin. Various Mfr.—Tab. (20, 50, 60 & 100 mg.)
Use: Vascular disorders.

RUTIN COMBINATIONS
See: Hexarutan, Tab. (Westerfield)
Hyrunal, Tab. (Kenyon)
Vio-Geric-H, Tab. (Rowell)

RUTOSIDE.
See: Rutin, Tab. (Var. Mfr.)

RU-TUSS EXPECTORANT. (Boots) Bot. Pts.
Use: Expectorant, antitussive, antihistaminic, nasal decongestant.

RU-TUSS PLAIN. (Boots) Bot. Pt.
Use: Relief of symptoms of hayfever, allergies, nasal congestion.

RU-TUSS TABLETS. (Boots) Bot. 100s, 500s.
Use: Decongestant, antisecretory.

RU-TUSS w/HYDROCODONE. (Boots) Bot. pt.
Use: Relief of symptoms of hay fever, allergies, nasal congestion & cough.

RU-VERT M. (Reid-Provident) Meclizine HCl 25 mg./Tab. Bot. 100s.
Use: Antihistamine.
RUVITE 1000. (Savage) Vit. B-12 1000 mcg./cc. Vial 10 cc.
Use: Hematinic.
RVP. (Elder) Red petrolatum, paraben & lanolin-free sunscreen. Oint. Tube 2 oz.
Use: Topical sunscreen ointment.
RVPaba. (Elder) p-Aminobenzoic acid 5% in neutral red petrolatum-wax base/Lipstick. Stick 4.4 Gm.
RV PAQUE. (Elder) Red petrolatum, zinc oxide, 2-ethoxyethyl p-methoxycinnamate in water-resistant base. Tube 0.5 oz., 1.25 oz.
Use: Opaque sunblock.
RYMED. (Edwards) Phenylephrine HC1 5 mg., phenylpropanolamine HC1 45 mg., guaifenesin 200 mg./Cap. Bot. 100s.
Use: Decongestion, expectorant.
RYMED-JR. (Edwards) Phenylephrine HC1 2.5 mg., phenylpropanolamine HC1 22.5 mg., guaifenesin 100 mg./Cap. Bot. 100s.
Use: Decongestion, expectorant.
RYMED LIQUID. (Edwards) Phenylephrine HC1 5 mg., phenylpropanolamine HC1 20 mg., guaifenesin 100 mg./5cc. w/alcohol 5%. Bot. pt.
Use: Decongestant, expectorant.
RYMED-TR. (Edwards) Phenylephrine HCl 10 mg., phenylpropanolamine HCl 75 mg., guaifenesin 300 mg./Cap. Bot. 100s.
Use: Decongestion, expectorant.
RYNA. (Wallace) Chlorpheniramine 2 mg., pseudoephedrine HCl 30 mg./5 ml. Bot. 4 oz., pt.
Use: Antihistaminic, nasal decongestant.
RYNA-C. (Wallace) Codeine phosphate 10 mg., pseudoephedrine HCl 30 mg., chlorpheniramine maleate 2 mg./5 ml. Bot. 4 oz., pt.
Use: Excessive coughs.
RYNA-CX. (Wallace) Guaifenesin 100 mg., pseudoephedrine HCl 30 mg., codeine phosphate 10 mg./5 cc. Bot. 4 oz., pt.
Use: Dry unproductive cough.
RYNAL. (Blaine) dl-Desoxyephedrine HCl 0.22%, antipyrine 0.28%, pyrilamine maleate 0.01%, methyldodecylbenzyltrimethylammonium chloride 0.02%, glycerine dehydrated 1.50%/20 cc.
Use: Nasal decongestion.
RYNATAN. (Wallace) **Tab.:** Phenylephrine tannate 25.0 mg., chlorpheniramine tannate 8 mg., pyrilamine tannate 25 mg./Tab. Bot. 100s, 500s.
Pediatric Susp. Phenylephrine tannate 5 mg., chlorpheniramine tannate 2 mg., pyrilamine tannate 12.5 mg./5 ml. Bot. pt., gal.
Use: Upper respiratory congestion resulting from colds, sinusitis, allergic rhinitis.
RYNATAPP. (General Pharm.) Brompheniramine maleate 4 mg., phenylephrine HCl 5 mg., phenylpropanolamine HCl 5 mg., alcohol 2.3%/5 ml. Bot. Pts.
Use: Rhinitis treatment.
RYNATUSS. (Wallace) Carbetapentane tannate 60 mg., chlorpheniramine tannate 5 mg., ephedrine

tannate 10 mg., phenylephrine tannate 10 mg./Tab. Bot. 100s, 500s.
Use: Treatment of cough associated with common cold.
RYNATUSS PEDIATRIC SUSPENSION. (Wallace) Carbetapentane tannate 30 mg., chlorpheniramine tannate 4 mg., ephedrine tannate 5 mg., phenylephrine tannate 5 mg./5 ml. Susp. Bot. 8 oz., pt.
Use: Treatment of cough associated with common cold.
RYTHMOL. 2,6-bis(1-Piperidylmethyl)-4-(α,α-di-methyl-benzyl)phenol dihydrobromide.
Use: Treatment of cardiac arrhythmias.
RHTHMODAN. Disopyramide, B.A.N.
RYTHROSITE. (Xttrium) Vit. B-12 12.5 mcg., intrinsic factor concentrate 10 mg., dried ferrous sulfate 200 mg., folic acid 2 mg., Vit. C 100 mg., liver desic. 50 mg./Tab. Bot. 100s, 1000s.
Use: Hematinic and vitamin supplement.

S

S-2 INHALANT & NEBULIZERS. (Nephron) Racemic epinephrine HCl 2.25%. Bot. 1 oz., ½ oz., ¼ oz.
Use: Inhalant for bronchial asthma.
SAC-500. (Western Research) Vitamin C 500 mg./Timed Release Cap. Bot. 1000s.
Use: Vitamin supplement.
S.A.C. COLD CAPSULES. (Towne) Pheniramine maleate 5 mg., pyrilamine maleate 10 mg., atropine sulfate 0.1 mg., salicylamide 250 mg., caffeine 30 mg./Cap. Bot. 18s, 50s.
S.A.C. COLD CAPSULES W/PHENYLEPHRINE. (Towne) Pheniramine maleate 5 mg., pyrilamine maleate 10 mg., phenylephrine HCl 5 mg., salicylamide 250 mg., caffeine 30 mg./Cap. Bot. 18s, 50s.
S.A.C. COUGH FORMULA. (Towne) Guaifenesin 100 mg., dextromethorphan HBr 15 mg./5 cc. Bot. 4 oz.
S.A.C. EAR DROPS. (Towne) Propylene glycol 79.7%, anhydrous glycerin 20.0%, methylparaben 0.16%, urea 0.10%, propylparaben 0.02%, butylparaben 0.02%. Bot. ½ fl. oz.
S.A.C. NASAL SPRAY. (Towne) Benzalkonium chloride 0.02%, phenylephrine HCl 0.5%. Bot. ⅔ fl. oz.
Use: Nasal decongestant.
S.A.C. SINUS TABS. (Towne) Acetaminophen 150 mg., salicylamide 150 mg., phenylpropanolamine HCl 25 mg., phenyltoloxamine citrate 22 mg./Tab. Bot. 30s, 100s.
S-A-C TABLETS. (Lannett) Salicylamide 230 mg., acetominophen 150 mg., caffeine 30 mg./Tab. Bot. 36s, 100s, 1000s, 5000s.
Use: Muscular aches.
S.A.C. THROAT LOZENGES. (Towne) Benzocaine 10 mg., terpin hydrate 100 mg., phenylpropanolamine HCl 10 mg., cetylpyridinium chloride 1:1500/Loz. Bot. 12s.

SACCHARIN

534

• **SACCHARIN,** N.F. XVI. 1,2-Benzisothiazolin-3-one-1, 1-dioxide.
(Mallinckrodt)-Pkg. 1 oz., ¼ lb., 1 lb.
(Merck)—Pkg. 1 oz., ¼ lb., 1 lb.
(Squibb) Tabs. ¼, ½ gr. Bot. 500s, 1000s; 1 gr. Bot. 1000s.
Use: Sweetening agent when sugar is contraindicated.
See: Necta Sweet, Tab. (Norwich Eaton)
• **SACCHARIN CALCIUM,** U.S.P. XXI. 1,2-Benziso-thiazolin-3-one 1, 1-dioxide calcium salt hydrate (2:7)
Use: Non-nutritive sweetener.
• **SACCHARIN SODIUM,** U.S.P. XXI. Oral Soln., Tab., U.S.P. XXI. (Mallinckrodt) (Benzosulfimide Sod., Soluble Gluside, Soluble Saccharine) Pow., Bot. 1 oz., ¼ lb., 1 lb. Tab. usual sizes. (Various Mfr.)
Use: Sweetening agent & test for circulation time of blood.
See: Crystallose, Crystals, Liq. (Jamieson)
Ril Sweet, Liq. (Plough)
Sucaryl, Liq., Tab. (Abbott)
SACCHARIN SOLUBLE.
See: Saccharin Sodium, Tab., Pow. (Var. Mfr.)
SACO. (Jenkins) B-12 activity 20 mcg., B-1 10 mg./Tab. Bot. 100s.
Use: Hematinic.
SACO JR. (Jenkins) B-12 activity 20 mcg., B-1 10 mg./Tab. Bot. 100s.
Use: Nutritional supplement hematinic.
SAFAPRYN. Paracetamol, B.A.N.
SAFESKIN. (C & M Pharmacal) A dermatologically acceptable detergent for patients who are sensitive to ordinary detergents. No whiteners, brighteners or other irritants. Bot. Qt.
Use: Laundry detergent for sensitive skin.
SAFE SUDS. (Ar-Ex) Hypoallergenic, all-purpose detergent for patients whose hands or respiratory membranes are irritated by soaps or detergents. pH 6.8. No enzymes, phosphates, lanolin, fillers, bleaches. Bot. 22 oz.
SAFETY-COATED ARTHRITIS PAIN FORMULA. (Whitehall) Entericcoated aspirin 500 mg./Tab. Bot. 24s, 60s.
Use: Arthris pain.
SAFFLOWER OIL.
See: Safflower Oil Caps. (Various Mfr.)
W/Choline bitartrate, soybean lecithin, inositol, natural tocopherols, B-6, B-12, & panthenol.
See: Nutricol, Cap., Vial (Nutrition)
SAFROLE. 4-Allyl-1,2-(methylenedioxy) benzene.
SAF-T-COIL. (Schmid) Intrauterine device. Sizes 33-S, 32-S, 25-S. 1s, 6s.
Use: Contraceptive.
SAFTIVAC. (Cutter) Vacuum Bot., evacuated flask. Bot. 150, 250, 500, 1000, 2000 ml.
Use: IV compounding aid.
SALACETIN.
See: Acetylsalicylic Acid (Var. Mfr.)
SALACID 25%. (Gordon) Salicylic acid 25% In ointment base. Jar 2 oz.
Use: Keratolytic.

SALACID 60%. (Gordon) Salicylic acid 60% in ointment base. Jar 2 oz.
Use: Keratolytic.
SALACTIC FILM. (Pedinol) Salicylic acid 16.7%, lactic acid 16.7% in flexible collodian w/color.
Use: Topical removal of verrucae.
• **SALANTEL.** USAN.
Use: Anthelmintic.
SALATAR CREAM. (Lannett) Coal tar solution 5%, salicylic acid 3%. Jar 4 oz., 1 lb.
SALAZOPYRIN. Sulphasalazine, B.A.N.
SALAZOSULFAPYRIDINE (I.N.N.). Sulphasalazine, B.A.N.
SALAZOSULPHADIMIDINE. B.A.N. 4'-(4,6-Dimethyl-pyrimidin-2-ylsulphamoyl)-4-hydroxyazo-benzene-3-carboxylic acid.
Use: Sulfonamide.
See: Azudimidine
SALBUTAMOL. B.A.N. 1-(4-Hydroxy-3-hydroxy-methyl-phenyl)-2-(t-butylamino)ethanol.
Use: Bronchodilator.
See: Ventolin
SALCATONIN. B.A.N. A component of natural salmon calcitonin.
Use: Treatment of hypercalcemia and Paget's disease.
SALCEGEL. (Apco) Sodium salicylate 5 gr., calcium ascorbate 25 mg., calcium carbonate 1.0 gr., dried aluminum hydroxide gel 2.0 gr./Tab. Bot. 100s.
Use: Arthritis, rheumatoid involvements.
• **SALCOLEX.** USAN.
Use: Analgesic, anti-inflammatory.
SAL-DEX. (Scrip) Undecylenic acid 10%, salicylic acid 15%, Isopropyl alcohol 40%, propylene glycol. Bot. 15 cc.
SAL DEX BORO. (Scrip) Tannic acid 46 mg., boric acid 29 mg., salicylic acid 8 mg., isoprpyl alcohol 56%/cc. 15 cc.
SALETIN.
See: Acetylsalicylic Acid (Var. Mfr.)
• **SALETHAMIDE MALEATE.** USAN. N-[2-Di-ethyl-(amino)ethyl]-salicylamide maleate. Under study.
Use: Analgesic.
SALETO. (Mallard) Aspirin 210 mg., acetaminophen 115 mg., salicylamide 65 mg./caffeine anhydrous 16 mg./Tab. Bot. 50s, 100s, 1000s.
Use: Analgesic.
SALETO-D. (Mallard) Acetaminophen 240 mg., salicyla-mide 120 mg., caffeine 16 mg., phenylpropanolamine HCl 20 mg./Cap. Bot. 50s.
SALFURIDE.
See: Nifursol, B.A.N.
SALIBAR Jr. (Jenkins) Aspirin 2 gr., phenobarbital ⅛ gr./Tab. Bot. 1000s.
Use: Analgesic and sedative.
• **SALICYL ALCOHOL.** USAN.
Use: Local anesthetic.
SALICYLAMIDE. B.A.N. (Bryant) o-Hydroxybenzamide. Salimed
Use: Analgesic; antipyretic.
See: Amid-Sal, Tab. (Glenwood)
Doldram, Tab. (Dram)

Os-Cal-Gesic (Marion)
Salamide, Tab. (Philips Roxane)
Salrin, Tab. (Warren-Teed)
SALICYLAMIDE W/COMBINATIONS
See: A.C.A. #5, Tab. (Scrip)
A.C.D., Tab. (Philips Roxane)
Akes-N-Pain, Cap. (Edward J. Moore)
Aludine C.T. Lav., Tab. (Scrip)
Anodynos, Tab. (Buffington)
Anodynos Forte, Tab. (Buffington)
APC W/Antihistamine, Tab. (Sutliff & Case)
Arthol, Tab. (Towne)
Asco, Cap., Tab. (Sutliff & Case)
Bancaps (Westerfield)
Bancaps-C (Westerfield)
Banesin-Forte, Tab. (Westerfield)
Calm Caps, Cap. (Edward J. Moore)
Calsuxaphen, Cap., Tab. (Lannett)
Cenaid, Tab. (Century)
Centuss, MLT Tab. (Century)
Children's Cold Tab. (Towne)
Chlorphen, Tab. (Wolins)
Chlorphenwol, Cap. (Wolins)
Codalan, 1,2,3, Tab. (Lannett)
Colchek, Tab. (Creomulsion)
Coriforte, Cap. (Schering)
Dapco, Tab. (Mericon)
Decohist, Cap. (Towne)
Dengesic, Tab. (Scott-Alison)
Dodamin, Tab. (Reid-Provident)
Dolopar, Tab. (O'Neal)
Dovamide, Cap. (Philips Roxane)
Du-Min Chewable, Tab. (Scrip)
Duoprin, Tab. (Dunhall)
Duo-3X, Tab. (Med Spec)
Duramid, Tab. (O'Neal)
Emagrin, Tab. (Otis Clapp)
Emagrin Forte, Tab. (Otis Clapp)
Emersal, Liq. (Medco)
Enz-Cold, Cap. (Edward J. Moore)
Excedrin P.M., Tab. (Bristol-Myers)
F.C.A.H., Cap. (Scherer)
Femicin, Tab. (Norcliff Thayer)
Guaiamine, Cap. (Sutliff & Case)
Her-Caps, Cap. (Edward J. Moore)
Hista-Derfule, Cap. (Cole)
Hista-Compound #5 Tab. (Vortech)
Histalets, Tab., (Columbia)
Histalets, Tab. (Edward J. Moore)
Hi-Temp (Saron)
Hycoff Cold, Caps. (Saron)
Kiddisan, Tab. (O'Neal)
Kleer Compound, Tab. (Scrip)
Medache, Tab. (Organon)
Medigesic, Tab. (Medics)
Metrogesic, Tab. (Metro Med)
Midran, Tab. (Columbia)
Myocalm, Tab. (Parmed)
Neo-Pyranistan (Standex)
Nokane, Tab. (Wren)
Nosalco, Cap. (Noyes)
Nytol, Tab., Cap. (Block)

Orastin, Tab. (Commerce)
Ornex, Cap. (SmithKline)
Os-Cal-Gesic, Tab. (Marion)
Panritis, Tab. (Pan Amer.)
Parba-KS, Tab. (Elder)
Parbocyl, Tab. (Elder)
Partuss-A, Tab. (Parmed)
Partuss T.D., Tab. (Parmed)
Phenatrohist, Cap. (O'Neal)
Phenetron Compound, Tab. (Lannett)
Pirin-C, Tab. (Scrip)
P.M.P. Compound, Tab. (Mericon)
Presalin, Tab. (Mallard)
Pyradyne, Tab. (Lemmon)
Pyradyne Comp., Tab. (Lemmon)
Pyranistan Compound (Standex)
Renpap, Tab. (Wren)
Rhinex, Tab. (Lemmon)
Rinocidin, Cap. (Cenci)
S-A-C, Tab. (Lannett)
S.A.C., Preps. (Towne)
Saleto, Preps. (Mallard)
Salimeph-Forte, Tab. (Kremers-Urban)
Salipap, Tab. (Freeport)
Salocol, Tab. (Mallard)
Salphenyl, Liq., Cap. (Mallard)
Sanger Special, Tab. (Edward J. Moore)
Scotgesic, Cap., Elix. (Scott/Cord)
Sedacane, Cap. (Edward J. Moore)
Sedagesic, Tab. (Kay)
Sedalgesic, Tab. (Table Rock)
Sedragesic, Tab. (Lannett)
Sino-Comp., Tab. (Bio-Factor)
Sinulin, Tab. (Reed & Carnrick)
Sleep, Tab. (Towne)
Sominex, Cap., Tab. (J.B. Williams)
S.P.C., Prep. (Vortech)
Statomin Maleate, Tab. (Bowman)
Stopain, Tab. (Columbia)
Sure-Sleep, Tab. (Amer. Lab.)
Tega-code Caps (Ortega)
Teragen, Tab. (O'Neal)
Thor, Cap (Towne)
Triaprin-DC, Cap. (Dunhall)
Tri-Hist-Cap, Cap. (Burgin-Arden)
Tripac, Tab. (Person & Covey)
Tussapap, Tab. (Sutliff & Case)
Volaxin, Tab. (Elder)
Volaxin-A, Tab. (Elder)
SALICYLANILIDE. N-Phenyl salicylamide.
Use: Antifungal agent.
SALICYLATED BILE EXTRACT. Chologestin.
• **SALICYLATE MEGLUMINE.** USAN.
Use: Antirheumatic, analgesic.
SALICYLAZOSULFAPYRIDINE.
See: Sulfasalazine, U.S.P. XXI.
• **SALICYLIC ACID,** U.S.P. XXI. Collodion, Plaster,
Gel, U.S.P. XXI. Benzoic acid, 2-hydroxy. Orthohy-
droxybenzoic acid Cryst., Pkg. 1 oz., ¼ lb., 1 lb.
Pow., Pkg. ¼ lb., 1 lb.
Use: Keratolytic agent.
See: Calicylic, Creme (Gordon)

Listrex Scrub, Lig. (Warner-Lambert)
Salonil, Cream (Torch)
Sebulex, Cream (Westwood)

SALICYLIC ACID COMBINATIONS

See: Acnaveen, Bar (Cooper)
Acno (Cummins)
Akne Drying Lotion, Liq. (Alto)
Aromatic Foot Pow. (Gordon)
Barseb Thera-spray, aerosol (Barnes-Hind)Alt
Cuticura (Purex)
D.D.D. Prescription, Regular (Campana)
Derma-Cover, Liq. (Scrip)
Domerine Medicated Shampoo (Miles Pharm)
Duofilm, Liq. (Stiefel)
Duo-WR, Sol. (Whorton)
Estercol, Emulsion (Torch)
Exzit Cleanser (Miles Pharm)
Fibrodon, Oint. (Gordon)
Fomac Foam (Dermik)
Fostex, Cream, Liq. (Westwood)
Fostril, Cream (Westwood)
Foursalco, Tab. (Jenkins)
Fungicidal, Oint. (Gordon)
Furol Cream (Torch)
Gets-It, Liq. (Plough)
Ionax, Liq. (Owen)
Ionil, Liq. (Owen)
Ionil T, Liq. (Owen)
Keralyt, Gel (Westwood)
Klaron, Lot. (Dermik)
Komed, Lot. (Barnes-Hind)
Komed HC, Lot. (Barnes-Hind)
Lasan Pomade, Cream (Stiefel)
Lasan 2, Cream (Stiefel)
Lasan 4, Cream (Stiefel)
Maseda Foot Powder, Pow. (Elder)
Mild Komed, Lot. (Banres-Hind)
Neutrogena Disposables (Neutrogena)
NP-27 Prod. (Norwich)
Onycho-Phytex, Liq. (Unimed)
Pernox, Lot. (Westwood)
Pixacol, Bot. (Pixacol)
Podiaspray, Aerosol Pow. (Dalin)
Pragmatar, Oint. (Menley & James)
Prosal, Liq. (Gordon)
Prosol, Emulsion (Torch)
Pytosin, Liq. (Blue Line)
Resorcitate, Lot. (Almay)
Rezamid, Liq. (Dermik)
Salatar, Cream (Lannett)
Sal-Dex, Liq. (Scrip)
Salicide, Oint. (Gordon Labs.)
Salicylic Acid Soap (Stiefel)
Saligel, Gel (Stiefel)
Salsprin, Tab. (Seatrace)
Sal-Su-Tar, Oint. (ulmer)
Sebaveen, Shampoo (Cooper)
Sebucare, Liq. (Westwood)
Sebulex Shampoo, Liq. (Westwood)
Skaylos, Cream, Lot. (Ambix)
Tan-Bar-Sal, Liq. (Gordon)
Therac, Lot. (C&M Pharm.)

Therapads, Pads (Fuller)
Tinver, Lot. (Barnes-Hind)
Vanseb, Dandruff Shampoo (Herbert)
Vanseb-T Tar Shampoo (Herbert)
Verdefam, Cream, Sol. (Owen)
Vericin, Oint. (Gordon)
Ver-Var, Sol. (Owen)
Zemacol, Lotion (Norwich)

SALICYLIC ACID CREAM. (Durel) Salicylic acid 5%,
in Duromantel cream.
Use: Superficial fungus infections, psoriasis,
hyperkeratosis of palms and soles.

SALICYLIC ACID SOAP. (Stiefel) Neutral soap
containing salicylic acid 3.5%. Cake 4 oz.
Use: Softens rough skin.

SALICYLIC ACID & SULFUR SOAP. (Stiefel)
Salicylic acid 3%, sulfur 10% in neutral soap bar.
Cake 4.1 oz.
Use: Anti-fungal cleansing.

• **SALICYLIC ACID TOPICAL FOAM,** U.S.P. XXI.

SALICYLSALICYLIC ACID.
Use: Analgesic.
See: Arcylate, Tab. (Hauck)
Disalcid, Tab. (Riker)
W/Aspirin.
See: Causalin, Tab. (Amfre-Grant)
Duragesic, Tab. (Meyer)
Persistin, Tab. (Fisons)

SALICYLSULPHONIC ACID. Sulfosalicylic acid.
Dextrotest (Ames).

SALIGEL. (Stiefel) 5% salicylic acid in a special
hydroalcoholic gel base. Tube. 2 oz.
Use: Acne therapy.

SALIGENIN. (City Chem.) Salicyl alcohol. Bot. 25
Gm., 100 Gm.
W/Merodicein.
See: Thantis, Loz. (Hyson, Westcott & Dunning)

SALIMED. Salicylamide, B.A.N.

SALINAZID. B.A.N. 2'-Salicylideneisonicotinohydrazide.
Use: Treatment of tuberculosis.
See: Nupa-sal

SALINEX NASAL MIST. (Muro) Buffered isotonic
saline nasal mist. Bot. 50 ml.
Use: Allergy therapy.

SALIPAP. (Freeport) Salicylamide 5 gr.,
acetaminophen 5 gr./Tab. Bot. 1000s.
Use: Relief of minor aches and pains.

SALIPRAL. (Kenyon) Allylisobutyl-barbituric acid ¾ gr.,
aspirin 3 gr., phenacetin 2 gr., caffeine ⅔ gr./Tab.
Bot. 1000s.

SALIPRAL-C. (Kenyon) Same formula as above w/Vit.
C/Cap. Bot. 100s, 1000s.
Use: Sedative-analgesic.

SALITHOL LIQUID. (Madland) Balm of methyl
salicylate, menthol and camphor. Bot. pt., gal. Also
ointment, jar 1 & 5 lbs.
Use: Liquid analgesic balm.

SALIVART. (Westport) Carbooxymethylcellulose
sodium 1 gr., sorbitol 3 gr., sodium Cl 0.084 gr.,
potassium Cl 0.12 gr., Ca Cl 0.015 gr., magnesium
Cl 0.005 gr., potassium monohydrogen phosphate
0.034 gr./100 ml. Bot. 50 ml. aerosol spray cans.

Use: Synthetic saliva.
SALMEFAMOL. B.A.N. 1-(4-Hydroxy-3-hydroxy-methyl-phenyl)-2-(4-methoxy-α-methylphenethylamino)etha-nol.
Use: Bronchodilator.
SALOCOL. (Mallard) Aspirin 210 mg., acetaminophen 115 mg., salicylamide 65 mg., caffeine anhydrous 16 mg./Tab. Bot. 100s.
SALONIL. (Torch) Salicylic acid 40%, in lanolin. Jar. 1 lb.
Use: Treat hyperkeratotic plaques & callosites.
SALPABA W/COLCHICINE. (Madland) Sodium salicylate 0.25 Gm., para-aminobenzoic acid 0.25 Gm., Vit. C 20 mg., colchicine 0.25 mg./Tab. Bot. 100s, 1000s.
Use: Gout and gouty arthritis.
SALPHENYL. (Mallard) Salicylamide 200 mg., acetaminophen 130 mg., chlorpheniramine maleate 2 mg., phenylephrine HCl 10 mg./Cap. Bot. 100s.
Use: Analgesic, antipyretic, nasal decongestant.
SAL-RUB. (Mallard) Triethanolamine salicylate 10% in nongreasy base. Tube 2 oz.
Use: External rubbing creme.
• **SALSALATE.** USAN.
Use: Antiarthritic.
See: Disalcid, tab. (Riker)
SALTEN. (Wren) Salicylamide 10 gr./Tab. Bot. 100s, 1000s.
▪ **SALT SUBSTITUTES.**
Use: Sodium free seasoning agent.
See: Diasal Salt (Savage)
Neocurtasal Granules (Winthrop Products)
NoSalt (Norcliff Thayer)
SALT TABLETS. (Cross) Sodium chloride 650 mg./Tab. Dispensers 500s.
Use: Replace salt lost from perspiration.
SALT TABLETS. (Walgreen) Sodium Cl 7 gr., dextrose 3 gr./Tab. Bot. 100s.
Use: Salt supplement.
SALUPRES. Hydrochlorothiazide, B.A.N.
SALURIC. Chlorothiazide, B.A.N.
SALURON. (Bristol) Hydroflumethiazide 50 mg./Tab. Bot. 100s.
Use: Diuretic.
SALUTENSIN. (Bristol) Hydroflumethiazide 50 mg., reserpine 0.125 mg./Tab. Bot. 100s, 1000s.
Use: Antihypertensive.
SALUTENSIN-DEMI. (Bristol) Hydroflumethiazide 25 mg., reserpine 0.125 mg./Tab. Bot. 100s.
Use: Antihypertensive.
SALVARSAN.
Use: Antisyphilitic.
See: Arsphenamine (Various Mfr.)
SALVITE-B. (Faraday) Sodium chloride 7 gr., dextrose 3 gr., B-1 1 mg./Tab. Bot. 100s, 1000s.
SALYRGAN.
See: Mersalyl (Various Mfr.)
SAMORIN HCl. Isometamidium, B.A.N.
SANAMYCIN. B.A.N. Actinomycin.
Use: Antineoplastic agent.
SANCHIA SILICONE PROTECTIVE CREAM. (Otis

Clapp) Silicones and lanolin in greaseless cream base. Tubes ¾ oz., 3 oz. Jars 16 oz.
Use: Protective coating against industrial and medicinal chemicals.
• **SANCYCLINE.** USAN. 6-Demethyl-6-deoxytetracy-cline. Formerly Norcycline.
Use: Antibiotic.
See: Bonomycin
SANDIMMUNE. (Sandoz) Cyclosporine. **Oral soln.:** 100 mg./ml. Bot. 50 ml. **Inj.:** 50 mg./ml. Amp. 5 ml. Box 10s.
Use: Prevention of rejection in kidney, liver, heart for transplants.
SANDOGLOBULIN. (Sandoz) Immune globulin 1 Gm./33 ml. reconstitution fluid; 3 Gm./100 ml. reconstitution fluid; 6 Gm./200 ml. reconstitution fluid.
Use: Immunodeficiency.
SANDOPTAL. Isobutyl allylbarbituric acid.
See: Butalbital
W/Caffeine, aspirin, phenacetin.
See: Fiorinal, Tab., Cap. (Sandoz)
W/Caffeine, aspirin, phenacetin, codeine phosphate.
See: Fiorinal w/codeine, Cap. (Sandoz)
SANDOPTAL SODIUM.
W/Sodium diethylbarbiturate, sod. phenylethylbarbiturate, scopolamine HBr, dihydroergotamine methanesulfonate.
See: Plexonal (Sandoz)
SANDOSTEN TARTRATE. Thenalidine, B.A.N.
SANDRIL. (Lilly) **Inj.:** Reserpine 2.5 mg./ml. Vial 10 ml.
Use: Hypertension treatment.
SANESTRO. (Sandia) Estrone 0.7 mg., estradiol 0.35 mg., estriol 0.14 mg./Tab. Bot. 100s, 1000s.
SANGER HER CAPS. (Edward J. Moore) Acetaminophen 227 mg., aspirin 227 mg., caffeine arh. 32.4 mg./Cap. Bot. 18s.
Use: Menstrual pain and cramps.
SANGER SPECIAL C-12. (Edward J. Moore) Salicyla-mide, Co. colocynth ext., dried ferrous sulf., blue cohosh./Tab. Bot. 24s.
SANGER VAGINAL ITCH CREAM. (Edward J. Moore) Benzocaine, dibucaine, tetracaine. Tube 1¼ oz.
Use: Relief of vaginal itch.
SANGUIS. (Sig) Liver 10 mcg., B-12 100 mcg., folic acid 1 mcg./ml. Vial 10 ml.
SANHIST T.D. 5. (Sandia) Phenylpropanolamine HCl 50 mg., chlorpheniramine maleate 5 mg., ascorbic acid 100 mg./Tab. Bot. 100s, 1000s.
SANHIST T.D. 12. (Sandia) Phenylpropanolamine HCl 50 mg., chlorpheniramine maleate 12 mg., ascorbic acid 100 mg., methscopalamine nitrate 4 mg./Tab. Bot. 100s, 1000s.
SANILENS. (Ketchum) Bot. 4 oz.
Use: Contact lens soaking solution.
SANI-VESS. (Fellows) Papain, sodium bicarbonate, ci-tric acid, tartaric acid, lactose, thymol, aromatics. Pkg. 6 oz.
SANLUOL.
See: Arsphenamine (Various Mfr.)

SANMETTO. (Medtech) Saw palmetto, sandalwood, corn silk & alcohol. Bot. 5½ fl. oz.
Use: Urinary sedative.

SANOREX. (Sandoz) Mazindol 1 mg., 2 mg./Tab. Bot. 100s.
Use: Treatment & control of obesity.

SANSERT. (Sandoz) Methysergide maleate 2 mg./Tab. Bot. 100s.
Use: Vascular headaches.

SANSPRIN. (Wolins) Acetaminophen 5 gr./Tab. Bot. 100s, 1000s.
Use: Analgesic.

SANSTRESS. (Sandia) Vit. A 25,000 I.U., Vit. D 400 I.U., B-1 10 mg., B-2 5 mg., niacinamide 100 mg., B-6 1 mg., B-12 5 mcg., C 150 mg., calcium 103 mg., phosphorus 80 mg., iron 10 mg., copper 1 mg., iodine 0.1 mg., magnesium 5.5 mg., manganese 1 mg., potassium 5 mg., zinc 1.4 mg./Cap. Bot. 100s, 1000s.
Use: Therapeutic vitamin & mineral preparation.

SANTISEPTIC LOTION. (Santiseptic) Menthol, phenol, benzocaine, zinc oxide, calamine. Bot. 4 oz.
Use: Itching and burning of eczema, hives, etc.

SANTONIN. (Mallinckrodt) Cryst. & Pow. Bot. ⅛ oz., 1 oz.
Use: Anthelmintic.

SANTOPHEN 1. (Monsanto) Septiphene. 4-Chloro-al-pha-phenyl-o-cresol.
Use: Disinfectant.

SANTUSSIN ADULT SUSPENSION. (Sandia) Noscapine 10 mg., phenylpropanolamine HCl 12.5 mg., chlorpheniramine maleate 1.5 mg., acetaminophen (APAP) 60 mg., guiachlor compound (alcohol 12% by volume) 75 mg., guaifenesin 5 mg., ammonium chloride 70 mg./5 cc. Bot. 16 oz., gal.

SANTUSSIN CAPSULES. (Sandia) Noscapine 10 mg., phenylpropanolamine HCl 12.5 mg., chlorpheniramine maleate 1.5 mg., acetaminophen 120 mg., guaifenesin 100 mg./Cap. Bot. 100s, 1000s.

SANTUSSIN PEDIATRIC SUSPENSION. (Sandia) Noscapine 5 mg., phenylpropanolamine HCl 6.25 mg., chlorpheniramine maleate 0.75 mg., acetaminophen (APAP) 30 mg., guiachlor compound (alcohol 12% by volume) 37.5 mg./5 cc. Bot. 16 oz., gal.

SANTYL. (Knoll) Proteolytic enzyme derived from *Clostridium histolyticum.* 250 u./Gm. Oint. Tube 15 Gm., 30 Gm.
Use: Debriding dermal ulcers.

SAPONATED CRESOL SOLUTION.
See: Cresol (Var. Mfr.)

SAPONINS, WATER SOLUBLE.

• **SARALASIN ACETATE.** USAN.
Use: Antihypertensive.

SARAPIN. (High) An aqueous distillate of *Sarracenia purpurea,* pitcher plant, prepared for parenteral administration. Amps. 10 cc. 12s. Multidose Vials 50 cc.
Use: Relief of pain of neuromuscular or neuralgic origin.

SARATOGA OINTMENT. (Blair) Boric acid, zinc oxide, eucalyptol, servum preparatum & white petrolatum. Tube 1 oz., 2 oz.
Use: Relief of minor skin irritations.

L-SARCOLYSIN. Melphalan, U.S.P. XXI.

SARDO BATH OIL CONCENTRATE. (Plough) Mineral oil, isopropyl palmitate. Bot. 4 oz., 8 oz., 16 oz.
Use: Dry skin treatment.

SARDOETTES MOISTURIZING TOWELETTES. (Plough) Mineral oil, isopropyl palmitate, impregnated towelling material. Individual packets. Box 25s.
Use: Dry skin treatment.

SARENIN. (Norwich Eaton) Saralasin acetate 18 mg./30 ml. Amp.
Use: Detection of angiotensin II dependent hypertension.

SARISOL NO. 2. (Blue Cross) Sodium butabarbital 30 mg./Tab. Bot. 1000s.
Use: Sedative and hypnotic.

• **SARMOXICILLIN.** USAN.
Use: Antibacterial.

SARNA LOTION. (Stiefel) Camphor 0.5%, menthol 0.5%, phenol 0.5% in a soothing emollient base. Bot. 8 oz.
Use: Lotion for dry, itching skin.

SAROCYCLINE CAPSULES. (Saron) Tetracycline HCl. 250 mg./Cap. Bot. 100s.
Use: Antibiotic.

SARODANT. (Saron) Nitrofurantoin 50 mg./Tab. Bot. 100s, 1000s.
Use: Urinary tract antibacterial agent.

SAROFLEX. (Saron) Chlorzoxazone 250 mg., acetaminophen 300 mg./Cap.
Use: Muscle relaxant, analgesic

SAROLAX. (Saron) Docusate sodium 200 mg., phenolphthalein yellow 15 mg., dehydrocholic acid 20mg./Cap. Bot. 100s.
Use: Laxative

SAROTEN HYDROCHLORIDE. Amitriptyline, B.A.N.

• **SARPICILLIN.** USAN.
Use: Antibacterial.

S.A.S.P. (Zenith) Salicylazosulapyridine 500 mg./Tab. Bot. 100s, 500s.
Use: Ulcerative colitis.

SASTID PLAIN. (Stiefel) Sulfur 1.6%, salicylic acid 1.6%, in a surfactant cream base. Tube 2.5 oz.
Use: Cleanser; keratolytic & antiseborrheic, in management of acne.

SASTID (AL). (Stiefel) Sulfur 1.6%, Salicylic acid 1.6% w/20% aluminum oxide particles. Tube 2.9 oz.
Use: Keratolytic & antiseborrheic in management of acne.

SASTID SOAP. (Stiefel) Sulfur 10%, salicylic acid 3% in a richly lathering soap base. Bar 4.1 oz.
Use: Cleanser & drying aid for acne treatment.

SATRIC. (Savage) Metronidazole. **250** mg./Tab. Bot. 100s, 250s. **500** mg./Tab. Bot. 60s.
Use: Anti-infective therapy for trichomoniasis and anaerobic bacterial infections.

SAUREX. (Enzyme Process) P 30 mg. pepsin

1:10,000 equal to 100 mg. pepesin 1:3000, betaine HCl 125 mg./Tab. Bot. 100s, 250s.
Use: Digestive aid.
SAVACORT D. (Savage) Dexamethasone sodium phosphate 4 mg./ml. Vial 5 ml.
Use: Anti-inflammatory.
SAVACORT-50. (Savage) Prednisolone acetate 50 mg./cc. Vial 10 cc.
SAVACORT-100. (Savage) Prednisolone acetate 100 mg./cc. Vial 10 cc.
SAXOL.
See: Petrolatum Liquid (Various Mfr.)
S.B.P. (Lemmon) Sodium secobarbital 50 mg., sodium butabarbital 30 mg., phenobarbital 15 mg./Tab. Bot. 1000s.
Use: Hypnotic; sedative.
SCABENE LOTION. (Stiefel) Lindane 1% in lotion base. Bot. 2 oz., 16 oz.
Use: Scabies & pediculosis treatment.
SCABENE SHAMPOO. (Stiefel) Lindane 1% in shampoo base. Bot. 2 oz., 16 oz.
Use: Treatment of pediculus capitis, phithirus pubis.
SCABICIDES.
See: Benzyl Benzoate (Var. Mfr.)
  Cuprex, Liq. (Calgon)
  Eurax, Cream, Lot. (Geigy)
  Kwell, Lot., Cream, Shampoo (Reed & Carnrick)
SCADAN SCALP LOTION. (Miles Pharm) Cetyl trimethyl ammonium bromide (cetab) 1%, stearyl dimethyl benzyl ammonium chloride 0.1% in a nonalcoholic, nongreasy, pleasantly scented vehicle. Bot. plastic 4 oz.
SCAN. (Parker) Water soluble gel for ultrasound B scan procedures. Bot. 8 oz., gal.
Use: Ultrasound B scan procedures.
SCARLET RED. (Lilly) Oint. 5%. Tube 1 oz.
SCHAMBERG'S LOTION. (C & M Pharmacal) Menthol 0.15%, phenol 1.0%, zinc oxide, peanut oil, dispersant. Bot. pt., gal.
Use: Pruritic type eczema.
• **SCHICK TEST CONTROL,** U.S.P. XXI.
Use: Diagnostic aid (dermal reactivity indicator).
See: Diphtheria Toxin, Diagnostic, Inactiv., (Var. Mfr.)
SCHIRMER TEAR TEST. (CooperVision) 10 envelopes of 5 sets.
Use: In vitro diagnostic.
SCHLESINGER'S SOLUTION.
See: Morphine HCl (Var. Mfr.)
SCLAVO BIOLOGICALS. (Sclavo) A wide variety of generic forms of biological products.
SCLAVOTEST-PPD. (Sclavo) Tuberculin purified protein derivative (PPD) multiple puncture device. 5 T.U. Box 20s, 250s.
Use: Tuberculin PPD screening.
SCLEREX. (Miller) Inositol 2 Gm., glutamic acid magnesium complex 19 mg., magnesium gluconate 7.5 mg., vit. C 100 mg., calcium succinate 25 mg., vit. A 2500 I.U., D 200 I.U., E 61.U., B-1 5 mg., B-2 2 mg., B-6 4 mg., B-12 3 mcg., niacin 5 mg., niacinamide 30 mg., Ca pantothenate 7.5 mg., Fe 10 mg., Cu 1 mg., Mn 1 mg., Zn 3 mg., Iodine 0.10 mg./3 Tab. Bot. 100s.

Use: Dietary supplement.
SCLEROSING AGENTS.
See: Glucose, Liq. (Var. Mfr.)
  Invert Sugar (Various Mfr.)
  Quinine & Urea HCl
  Sodium Morrhuate, Inj. (Various Mfr.)
  Sotradecol Sod., Vial (Elkins-Sinn)
SCOLINE. Suxamethonium Chloride, B.A.N.
• **SCOPAFUNGIN.** USAN.
Use: Antifungal, antibacterial.
SCOPETTES. (Birchwood) **Swabs:** 16″
Protosigmoidoscopic Swabs. Case 12s, 500s.
Junior: 8″ throat or vaginal swab. case 12s, 500s.
Sterile Junior: Same as Junior and sterile.
SCOPINE CHRONCAP. (Cenci) Scopolamine HBr 0.0195 mg., atropine sulfate 0.0582 mg., hyoscyamine sulfate 0.311 mg., phenobarbital 50.0 mg./Cap. Bot. 100s.
Use: Antispasmodic, sedative.
SCOPODEX. (CMC) Scopolamine aminoxide HBr, genoscopolamine HBr. Pellet 0.5 mg., Bot. 100s.
Use: Motion sickness.
SCOPOLAMINE. Hyoscine, l-Scopolamine, Epoxytropine tropate.
See: Hyoscine Preps. (Various Mfr.)
SCOPOLAMINE AMINOXIDE HBr.
See: Genoscopolamine, Pellets (CMC)
W/Acetylcarbromal and bromisovalum.
See: Tranquinal, Tab. (Barnes-Hind)
• **SCOPOLAMINE HYDROBROMIDE,** U.S.P. XXI. Inj., Ophth. Oint., Ophth. Soln., Tab., U.S.P. XXI.
Benzeneacetic acid, α-(hydroxymethyl)-, 9-methyl-3-oxa-9-azatricyclo [3.3.1.02,4]non-7-yl ester, hydrobromide, trihydrate. 6β, 7β-Epoxy-lαH,5αH-tropan-3α-ol(−)-tropate(ester)hydrobromide   trihydrate. Hyoscine HBr.
Use: Hypnotic & sedative, anticholinergic, mydriatic and cyclopegic.
W/Atropine sulf., ammonium benzoate, methenamine, salol.
See: Cystorrhoids W/Atropine, Tab. (Noyes)
W/Atropine and hyoscyamine.
See: Atropine sulfate table
  Belladonna alkaloids
W/Butabarbital, chlorpheniramine maleate.
See: Pedo-Sol, Elix., Tab. (Warren)
W/Homatropine methylbromide, atropine sulfate, butabarbital, hyoscyamine sulfate.
See: Butabell HMB, Elix., Tabs. (Saron)
W/Hydroxypropyl methylcellulose.
See: Isopto HBr, Sol. (Alcon)
W/Hyoscyamine sulfate, atropine sulfate, phenobarbital.
See: Bar-Cy-Amine, Elix. (Sutliff & Case)
  Bar-Cy, Tabs. (Sutliff & Case)
  DeTal, Eliz., Tab. (DeLeon)
  Donnacin, Elix., Tab. (Pharmex)
  Fenatron, Prep. (Panray)
  Hyonal C.T., Tab. (Paddock)
  Hytrona, Tab. (Webcon)
  Nilspasm, Tab. (Parmed)
  Peece Kaps (Scrip)
  Peece TC, Cap. (Scrip)

Scopine, Cap. (Cenci)
Sedamine, Tab. (Dunhall)
Sedapar, Tab. (Parmed)
Setamine, Tab. (Reid-Provident)
Spasaid, Cap. (Century)
Spasidon, Tab. (Haag)
Spasmolin, Tab. (Wolins)
Stannitol (Standex)
W/Pamabrom, pyrilamine maleate, homatropine methylbromide, hyoscyamine sulfate, methamphetamine HCl.
See: Aridol, Tabs. (MPL)
W/Phenylephrine, phenylpropanolamine, atropine sulfate, chlorpheniramine maleate, acetaminophen, hyoscyamine HBr.
See: Koryza Tab. (Fellows-Testagar)

SCOPOLAMINE HYDROBROMIDE COMBINATIONS.
See: Belladonna Products
Hyoscione HBr. (Var. Mfr.)

SCOPOLAMINE METHOBROMIDE.
See: Methscopolamine Bromide, Preps. (Var. Mfr.)

SCOPOLAMINE METHYLBROMIDE.
See: Methscopolamine Bromide, Preps. (Var. Mfr.)

SCOPOLAMINE METHYL NITRATE.
See: Methscopolamine Nitrate, Prep. (Var. Mfr.)

SCOPOLAMINE SALTS.
See: Belladonna Products
Hyoscine salts

SCORBEX/12. (Pasadena Research) Vit. B-1 20 mg., B-2 3 mg., B-6 5 mg., d-panthenol 75 mg., B-12 1000 mcg., C 100 mg./cc. Vial 10 cc.
Use: Vitamin supplement.

SCOTAVITE. (Scott/Cord) Vit. A 25,000 I.U., D 400 I.U., B-1 10 mg., B-2 10 mg., B-6 5 mg., B-12 5 mcg., niacinamide 100 mg., Ca pantothenate 20 mg., C 200 mg., d-alpha tocopheryl 15 I.U., acid succinate iodine 0.15 mg./Tab. Bot. 100s, 500s.
Use: Vitamin & mineral supplement.

SCOTCIL. (Scott/Cord) **Tab.:** Potassium penicillin 400,000 u. w/calcium carbonate/Tab. Bot. 100s, 500s. **Pow.** 80 cc., 150 cc.
Use: Antibiotic.

SCOTCOF. (Scott/Cord) Dextromethorphan HBr 6.85 mg., chlorpheniramine maleate 1.8 mg., phenylephrine HCl 4.4 mg., guaifenesin 66.00 mg., ammonium chloride 30.00 mg., chloroform 0.125 mg., alcohol 4.10%/5 cc. Bot. 4 oz., pt., gal.

SCOTGESIC. (Scott/Cord) **Cap.** Acetaminophen 240 mg., salicylamide 100 mg., phenyltoloxamine dihydrogen citrate 30 mg., butabarbital ⅛ gr./Cap. Bot. 100s, 500s, 1000s. **Liq.** Butabarbital 12.15 mg., acetaminophen 300 mg., salicylamide 60 mg., phenyltoloxamine citrate 30 mg./15 cc. Bot. 4 oz., pt.
Use: Analgesic.

SCOTNORD. (Scott/Cord) Chlorpheniramine maleate 8 mg., phenylephrine HCl 20 mg., methscopolamine nitrate 2.5 mg./Cap. Bot. 100s, 500s.

SCOTONIC. (Scott/Cord) Vit. B-1 10 mg., B-2 5 mg., B-6 1 mg., niacinamide 50 mg., choline chloride 100 mg., inositol 100 mg., B-12 25 mcg., calcium 19 mg., iron 50 mg., folic acid 0.15 mg., alcohol 15%, sodium benzoate 0.1%/45 cc. Bot. pt., gal.

SCOTRATE. (Robinson) Scopolamine methyl nitrate 0.5 mg./cc. Multiple dose vial 30 cc.

SCOTREX. (Scott/Cord) Tetracycline 250 mg./Cap. or 5 ml. Bot. 16s, 100s, 500s. Syr.: 2 oz., pt.

SCOTT'S EMULSION. (Beecham Products) Vit. A 5000 U., Vit. D 400 U./4 tsp. Bot. 6¼ oz., 12½ oz.
Use: Vitamin A & D supplement.

SCOT-TUSSIN DC SUGAR-FREE. (Scot-Tussin) Dextromethorphan HBr 15 mg., chlorpheniramine maleate 2 mg./5 ml. Bot. 4 oz., 8 oz., 16 oz., gal.
Use: Cough cold medicine for diabetics, thyroid, high blood pressure, and heart disease patients.

SCOT-TUSSIN SUGAR-FREE. (Scot-Tussin) Phenylephrine HCl 4.17 mg., pheniramine maleate 13.33 mg., sodium citrate 83.33 mg., sodium salicylate 83.33 mg., caffeine citrate 25 mg./5 ml. Non-narcotic, non-alcoholic. Bot. 4 oz., 8 oz., 16 oz., gal.
Use: Coughs, colds, allergies.

SCOT-TUSSIN WITH SUGAR. (Scot-Tussin) Phenylephrine HCl 4.17 mg., pheniramine maleate 13.3 mg., sodium citrate 83.33 mg., sodium salicylate 83.33 mg., caffeine citrate 25 mg./5 ml. Bot. 4 oz., 8 oz., 16 oz. gal.
Use: Colds, coughs, allergies.

SCOT-TUSSIN SYRUP. (Scot-Tussin) Phenylephrine HCl 25 mg., sodium citrate 500 mg., caffeine citrate 150 mg., pheniramine maleate 80 mg., sodium salicylate 500 mg./30 cc. Bot. 4 oz., 8 oz., 16 oz., gal. Regular and sugar free.
Use: Cough and colds.

SCOTUSS. (Scott/Cord) d-Methorphan 15 mg., chlorpheniramine maleate 1 mg., phenylephrine HCl 5 mg., phenylpropanolamine HCl 5 mg., N-acetyl-P-aminophenol 120 mg., guaifenesin 100 mg., alcohol 8.2%/5 cc. Bot. 4 oz., pt., gal.
Use: Cough due to colds.

SCOTUSS PEDIATRIC COUGH SYRUP. (Scott/Cord) Dextromethorphan HBr 7.5 mg., guaifenesin 50 mg., chlorpheniramine maleate 0.5 mg., phenylephrine HCl 2.5 mg., acetaminophen 60 mg., phenylpropanolamine HCl 2.5 mg., methylparaben 0.15%, propylparaben 0.05%/5 cc. Bot. 4 oz., pt.

SC-PLUS. (Western Research) Sodium carboxymethylcellulose 500 mg., docusate sodium 100 mg./Tab. Bot. 1000s.
Use: Bulk laxative.

SCRIP-DRI. (Scrip) Formalin soln., formaldehyde in perfumed aqueous base. Bot. 2 oz.

SCRIP SUPER DRI. (Scrip) Formalin soln. in perfumed aqueous base. Bot. 2 oz.

SCRIP-ZINC. (Scrip) Zinc sulfate 220 mg./Cap. Bot. 100s.

SCURENALINE.
See: Epinephrine, Prep. (Various Mfr.)

SCUROFORME.
See: Butyl Aminobenzoate (Various Mfr.)

S-DSS. (Western Research) Senna 175 mg., docusate sodium 50 mg./Tab. Bot. 1000s.
Use: Laxative.

SEA GREENS. (Modern) Iodine 0.25 mg./Tab. Bot. 220s, 460s.

SEALE'S LOTION-MODIFIED. (C & M Pharmacal)

Sulfur 6.4%, sodium borate, zinc oxide, acetone, bentonite, purified water. Bot. pt., gal.
Use: Acne therapy.

SEA MASTER. (Barth's) Vit. A 10,000 u., D 400 u./Cap Bot. 100s, 500s.

SEATRA-GESIC. (Seatrace) Aspirin 325 mg., phenyltoloxamine 20 mg./Tab. Bot. 100s, 1000s, 5000s.
Use: Analgesic, antihistaminic.

SEBACIDE. (Paddock) Coconut oil, pine oil, castor oil, lanolin, cholesterols, lecithin, parachlorometaxylenol. Bot. 4 oz., pt., gal.
Use: Bactericidal sudsing skin cleanser.

SEBACLEN HYDROCHLORIDE. Xenysalate, B.A.N.

SEBA-LO. (Whorton) Acetone-alcohol cleanser. Bot. 4 oz.
Use: Oily skin cleanser.

SEBANA SHAMPOO. (Myers) Salicylic acid 2%. Bot. 4 oz., 8 oz., pt., qt., ½ gal.
Use: Sebhorrhea, dandruff, oily skin.

SEBANATAR SHAMPOO. (Myers) Salicylic acid 2%, liquor carbonis detergens 3%. Bot. 4 oz., 8 oz., pt., qt., ½ gal., gal.
Use: Sebhorrhea, dandruff.

SEBA-NIL CLEANSER. (Owen) Cleansing mixture of alcohol 49.7%, acetone, polysorbate 20, purified water and fragrance. Bot. 8 oz., 16 oz. Towelettes, Pkg. 24s.
Use: Oily skin cleanser for acne.

SEBA-NIL CLEANSING MASK. (Owen) Astringent face mask containing water, bentonite, polyethylene, SD alcohol-40, sulfated castor oil, titanium dioxide, kaolin, chromium oxide, methylparaben, fragrance. Tubes 3.5 oz.
Use: Cleanser for pimples, blackheads and oily skin.

SEBAQUIN SHAMPOO. (Summers) Iodoquinol 3% in a neutral, soapless detergent, lathering base. Bot. 4 oz.
Use: Antiseborrheic shampoo.

SEBASORB. (Summers) Activated attapulgite 10%, hexachlorophene 1%, polysorbate 80 1%, colloidal sulfur 2%, salicylic acid 2%, propylene glycol. Plas. Bot. 2 oz. w/dispenser top.

SEBASUM. (Summers) Polysorbate 80 1.25%, acetone 14%, isopropanol 50%. Bot. 4 oz., pt.
Use: Skin cleanser.

SEBAVEEN SHAMPOO. (CooperCare) Aveeno colloidal oatmeal 5%, sulfur 2%, salicylic acid 2%, emollients 4% in soap-free base. Plastic bottle 4 oz.
Use: Antiseborrheic.

SEBISOL. (C & M Pharmacal) Salicylic acid 2%, o-benzyl-p-chlorophenol 0.1%, betanaphthol 1% in surfactant base. Shampoo bot. 4 oz., pt., gal.
Use: Antiseborrheic.

SEBIZON LOTION. (Schering) Sulfacetamide sod. 100 mg., methylparaben 1 mg. w/trisodium edetate, sod. thiosulfate, propylene glycol, isopropyl myristate, propylene glycol monostearate, polyethylene glycol 400 monostearate & water. Tube 3 oz., plastic squeeze.
Use: Scaling dermatoses, antibacterial.

SEBUCARE SCALP LOTION. (Westwood) Laureth-

4, salicylic acid 1.5%, alcohol 61%, water, PPG 40 butyl ether, dihydroabietyl alcohol, fragrance. Bot. 4 oz.
Use: Treatment of dandruff, seborrhea capitis.

SEBULEX CREAM SHAMPOO. (Westwood) Same formula as Sebulex in a cream shampoo. Tube 4 oz.

SEBULEX SHAMPOO. (Westwood) Sulfur 2%, salicylic acid 2% in sebulytic brand of surface-active cleansers and wetting agents. Plastic bot. 4 oz., 8 oz.
Use: Therapeutic shampoo for dandruff and seborrheic dermatitis.

SEBULEX CONDITIONING SHAMPOO WITH PROTEIN. (Westwood) Sulfur 2%, salicylic acid 2%, water, sodium octoxynol-3 sulfonate, sodium lauryl sulfate, lauramide DEA, acetamide MEA, amphoteric-2, hydrolyzed animal protein, magnesium aluminum silicate, propylene glycol, methylcellulose, PEG-14 M, fragrance, disodium EDTA, docusate sodium, FD&C blue 1, D & C yellow. Bot. 4 oz., 8 oz.
Use: Therapeutic and conditioning shampoo for dandruff, seborrheic dermatitis.

SEBUTONE CREAM SHAMPOO. (Westwood) Tar equivalent to Coal Tar USP 5%, sulfur 2%, salicylic acid 2%, in sebulytic type surface-active soapless cleansers & wetting agents. Tubes 4 oz.
Use: Therapeutic shampoo for stubborn dandruff and psoriasis.

SEBUTONE THERAPEUTIC TAR SHAMPOO. (Westwood) Tar equivalent to Coal Tar USP 0.5%, sulfur 2%, salicylic acid 2%, in Sebulytic type of surface-active soapless cleansers and wetting agents. Plastic bot. 4 oz. 8 oz.
Use: Therapeutic shampoo for stubborn dandruff and psoriasis.

SECBUTOBARBITONE. B.A.N. 5-sec-Butyl-5-ethylbarbituric acid. Butabarbitone.
Use: Hypnotic; sedative.

SECHOLEX HCl. Polidexide, B.A.N.

• **SECOBARBITAL,** U.S.P. XXI. Elixir U.S.P. XXI. 5-Allyl-5-(methylbutyl)-barbituric acid. Pow., Bot. ⅛ oz., 1 oz.
Use: Hypnotic.
See: Seco-8, Cap. (Fleming)

SECOBARBITAL COMBINATIONS.
 See: Amoseco, Cap. (Robinson)
   Buffadyne w/Barbiturates, Tabs. (Lemmon)
   Butseco, S.C.T., Tab. (Bowman)
   Corovas, Preps. (Amfre-Grant)
   Dusotal, Cap. (Harvey)
   Efed, Syr., Tab. (Alto)
   Gaysal, Tab. (Geriatric)
   Monosyl, Tab. (Arcum)
   Naus-A-Tories, Supp. (Table Rock)
   Quad-Set, Tab. (Kenyon)
   Secophen, Tab. (Mallard)
   Sedalgesic, Tab. (Table Rock)
   Stim 15/60, Cap. (Scrip)

SECOBARBITAL ELIXIR.
 See: Seconal Elixir. (Lilly)

• **SECOBARBITAL SODIUM,** U.S.P. XXI. Cap., Inj., Sterile, U.S.P. XXI. Sod. 5-allyl-5-(1-methyl-butyl)-barbiturate. Quinalbarbitone Sodium, B.A.N.

Use: Hypnotic, sedative.
Generic Products:
(Bowman) Secobarbital sodium 1½ gr./Tab.
(CMC)—50 mg./cc. Vial 30 cc.
(Hance)—Cap. 1½ gr., Bot. 100s, 1000s.
(Lannett)—Cap. ¾ gr., 1½ gr., Bot. 100s, 500s.
(Parke-Davis)—Cap. 1½ gr. Bot. Unit dose 100s.
(Robinson) Cap. ¾ gr., 1½ gr., Pow. 1 oz.
See: Seco-8, Cap. (Fleming)
Seconal Sodium, Prep. (Lilly)
• SECOBARBITAL SODIUM AND AMOBARBITAL
SODIUM CAPSULES, U.S.P. XXI.
Use: Hypnotic, sedative.
See: Tuinal, Caps. (Lilly)
9,10-SECOCHOLESTA-5,7,10(19)-TRIEN-3-OL.
Cholecalciferol, U.S.P. XXI.
9,10-SECOERGOSTA-5,7,10(19),22-TETRAEN-3-OL,
(3 beta)-. Ergocalciferol, U.S.P. XXI.
SECONAL SODIUM. (Lilly)
Vial: 50 mg./ml. Vial. 20 ml. Pulvules: 50 mg. Bot.
100s, 500s. Blister pkg. 10 x 10s; 100 mg. Bot.
100s, 500s. Blister pkg. 10 x 10s. Dispenser rolls
40 x 25s unit dose pkg. Supp.: 30 mg., 60 mg.,
120 mg., 200 mg. Pkg. 12s.
Use: Hypnotic & sedative.
W/Amytal Sod.
See: Tuinal, Cap. (Lilly)
W/Ephedrine sulfate.
See: Ephedrine & Seconal Sodium, Pulvule (Lilly)
SECRAN. (Scherer) Vit. B-12 (cryst.) 25 mcg., thiamine
mononitrate 10 mg., niacinamide 10 mg., alcohol
17%/5 cc. Bot. pt.
Use: B-Vitamin deficiencies.
SECRAN/FE ELIXIR. (Scherer) Vit. B-12 (cryst.) 25
mcg., ferric pyrophosphate, soluble (elemental iron
30 mg.), thiamine mononitrate 15 mg., nicotinamide
10 mg./5 cc., alcohol 1%. Bot. pt.
Use: Iron deficiency anemia.
SECRAN PRENATAL TABS. (Scherer) Vit. A acetate
8000 u., D-2 400 I.U., E acetate 30 I.U., C 60 mg.,
Niacinamide 20 mg., B-2 2 mg., B-1 1.7 mg., B-6 2.5
mg., B-12 8 mcg., folic acid 1.0 mg., calcium 250 mg.,
magnesium 25 mg., elemental zinc 20 mg., iron 60
mg./Tab. Bot. 100s, 240s.
Use: Nutritional supplement.
SECRETIN. B.A.N. A hormone obtained from
duodenal mucosa.
Use: Diagnostic aid.
SECRETIN-BOOTS. (Adria) Hormone from porcine
duodenal mucosa, freeze dried sterile powder, 100
units.
Use: Diagnostic for pancreatic dysfunction.
SECRETIN-KABI. (Pharmacia) Secretin 75 cu/Vial. Box
5 x 10 ml.
Use: Diagnosis of pancreatic dysfunction.
SEDACANE. (Edward J. Moore) Acetaminophen 120
mg., salicylamide 210 mg., caffeine 30 mg., Ca
gluconate 60 mg./Cap. Bot. 12.
Use: Analgesic.
SEDAFORM.
See: Chlorobutanol (Various Mfr.)
SEDAGESIC. (Kay) Isobutylallyl barbituric acid ¾ gr.,

aspirin 3 gr., acetophenetidin 2 gr., caffeine ⅔
gr./Tab. Bot. 100s, 1000s.
Use: Sedative, analgesic.
SEDAJEN. (Jenkins) Phenobarbital 5/16 gr., passiflora
1½ gr., hyoscyamus ¾ gr. (total alkaloids 0.0003
gr.)/Tab. Bot. 1000s.
Use: Sedative & antispasmodic.
SEDALGESIC INSERTS. (Table Rock) Aspirin 195
mg., secobarbital 30 mg./Insert. Box 12s.
Use: Sedative, analgesic; antipyretic.
SEDALGESIC TABLETS. (Table Rock) Bromisovalum
150 mg., acetaminophen 100 mg., salicylamide 100
mg./Tab. Bot. 100s, 500s.
Use: Analgesic-sedative.
SEDAMINE. (Approved) Phosphorated carbohydrate
sol. Bot. 4 oz.
Use: Anti-nausea.
SEDAMINE. (Dunhall) Hyoscyamine sulfate 0.1037
mg., atropine sulfate 0.0194 mg., hyoscine HBr
0.0065 mg., phenobarbital 16.2 mg./Tab. Bot. 100s,
1000s.
Use: Antispasmodic.
SEDAPAP-10 TABLETS. (Mayrand) Acetominophen
10 gr., butabarbital 16 mg./Tab. Bot. 100s, 500s.
Use: Analgesic, sedative.
SEDAPAR. (Parmed) Atropine sulfate 0.0195 mg.,
hyoscine HBr 0.0065 mg., hyoscyamine sulfate
0.1040 mg., phenobarbital ¼ gr./Tab. Bot. 1000s.
Use: Sedative & antispasmodic.
SEDAQUIN. Methaqualone, B.A.N.
SEDATANS TABLETS. (Lannett) Tab. Bot. 100s,
1000s.
■ SEDATIVE/HYPNOTIC AGENTS.
See: Bromides (Var. Mfr.)
Barbiturates (Var. Mfr.)
Butisol Sodium (McNeil)
Carbamide (Urea) Compounds (Var. Mfr.)
Chloral Hydrate Preparations (Var. Mfr.)
Chlorobutanol (Var. Mfr.)
Dalmane, Caps. (Roche)
Intasedol, Elix. (Elder)
Largon, Inj. (Wyeth)
Lotusate, Cap. (Winthrop-Breon)
Noludar, Tab., Cap. (Roche)
Paraldehyde, Preps. (Var. Mfr.)
Phenergan HCl, Preps. (Wyeth)
Placidyl, Cap. (Abbott)
Plexonal, Tab. (Sandoz)
Quaalude, Tab. (Rorer)
Restoril, Cap. (Sandoz)
Valmid, Tab. (Lilly)
Vingesic, Cap. (Amid)
SEDATROMINE TABLETS. (Sutliff & Case)
Phenobarbital ¼ gr., hyoscyamus 1/48 gr.,
belladonna 1/20 gr., atropine sulfate 1/300 gr.,
hyoscyamine sulfate 1/1200gr., hyoscine HBr 1/2400
gr./Tab. Bot. 100s, 1000s.
Use: Antispasmodic, sedative.
SEDEVAL.
See: Barbital (Various Mfr.)
SEDRAGESIC TABLETS. (Lannett) Acetaminophen
0.325 Gm., salicylamide 0.195 Gm., d-amphetamine

sulfate 2.5 mg., hexobarbital 8 mg., secobarbital sod. 2.7 mg., butabarbital sod. 2.7 mg., phenobarbital 2.7 mg./Tab. Bot. 100s, 1000s.
Use: Sedative.

SEDRAL. (Vita Elixir) Phenobarbital ⅛ gr., theophylline 2 gr., ephedrine ⅜ gr./Tab.
Use: Treatment of bronchial asthma, hay fever.

SEDRALEX. (Kay) **Liq.** Phenobarbital 16.0 mg., hyoscyamine sulfate 0.1037 mg., atropine sulfate 0.0194 mg., scopolamine HBr 0.0065 mg./5 ml. Bot. 4 oz., 16 oz., gal.; **Tabs.** Bot. 1000s.
Use: Antispasmodic sedative.

SEDS. (Pasadena Research) Phenobarbital 16 mg., hyoscyamine HBr 0.128 mg., hyoscine HBr 0.0072 mg., atropine sulfate 0.024 mg./Tab. Bot. 100s, 1000s.

• **SEELAZONE.** USAN.
Use: Anti-inflammatory, uricosuric.

SEGO LIQUID. (Pet Milk Co.) Protein 77 Gm., carbohydrate 103 Gm., fat 20 Gm., Vit. A 5000 I.U., D 400 I.U., C 100 mg., B-1 2 mg., B-2 3 mg., niacinamide 15 mg., B-6 2 mg., Ca pantothenate 10 mg., Iodine 150 mcg., K 3.5 Gm., Na 0.9 Gm., Mn 2 mg., Zn 5 mg./4 cans. Can 10 oz., Powd. Inst. mix 1 oz.
Use: Liquid diet food.

SELAN CREAM, PLAIN. (Noyes) Cetyl alcohol 12%, glyceryl stearate 2%, lanolin 0.5%, glycerin 10%, Na lauryl sulfate 1%, methyl and butyl parabens as preservatives. Jar 2 oz., 4 oz., 1 lb.
Use: Skin irritations.

SELAN WITH SILICONE. (Noyes) Cetyl alcohol 12%, glyceryl stearate 2%, lanolin anhyd. 0.5%, S-F-96 2.5%, sorbo 10%, Na lauryl sulfate 1% w/methyl, propyl, butyl parabens as preservatives. **Cream:** Jar 2 oz., 4 oz., 1 lb. **Lotion:** 8 oz., pt., gal.

SELENICEL. (Pasadena Research) Selenium yeast complex 200 mcg., Vit. C 100 mg., E 100 mg./Cap. Bot. 90s.
Use: Dietary supplement.

SELENITRACE. (Armour) Selenious acid injection containing selenium 40 mcg./1 ml. Vial 10 ml. Box 25s.
Use: Supplement to I.V. solutions for selenium deficiency.

SELENIUM. (Nion) Selenium 50 mcg./Tab. Bot. 100s.
Use: Dietary supplement.

SELENIUM DISULFIDE.
See: Selenium Sulfide, Deterg. Susp. (Var. Mfr.)

• **SELENIUM SULFIDE,** U.S.P. XXI. Lot. U.S.P. XXI.
Use: Treatment of dandruff; antifungal, antiseborrheic.
See: Exsel Lotion (Herbert)
      Iosel 250, Liq. (Owen)
      Selsun, Susp. (Abbott)

• **SELENOMETHIONINE Se 75 INJECTION,** U.S.P. XXI. 2-Amino-4-(methylselenyl) butyric acid (⁷⁵Se)
Use: Diagnostic aid (pancreas function determination).
See: Sethotope, Inj. (Squibb)

SELESTOJECT. (Mayrand) Betamethasone sodium phosphate 4 mg./ml. Vial 5 ml.

Use: Glucocorticoid.

SELSUN BLUE. (Abbott Prods) Selenium sulfide 1% in lotion base. Bot. 4 oz., 7 oz., 11 oz. Dry, Oily, Normal formulas.
Use: Anti-dandruff shampoo.

SELSUN SUSPENSION. (Abbott) Selenium sulfide 2½%. Bot. 4 fl. oz.
Use: Seborrheic dermatitis of scalp and tinea versicolor.

SELVIGON HYDROCHLORIDE. Pipazethate, B.A.N.

SEMETS. (Beecham Labs) Cetylpyridinium chloride 1:1500, benzocaine 3 mg./Loz. Pkg. Bot. 450s.
Use: Infections of throat & mouth.

SEMICID. (Whitehall) Nonoxynol-9 100 mg./Suppos. Box 10s, 20s.
Use: Contraceptive.

SEMILENTE INSULIN.
See: Iletin, Vial (Lilly)

• **SEMUSTINE.** USAN.
Use: Antineoplastic.

SENAGRADA TABLETS. (Blue Line) Phenolphthalein 1 gr., senna 2½ gr., cascarin bitterless ⅛ gr./Tab. Bot. 100s, 1000s.

SENATHALIN WAFERS. (Blue Line) Phenolphthalein 1 gr., senna 2½ gr., cascarin, bitterless ⅛ gr./Wafer. 100s, 1000s.

SENILAVITE. (Defco) Vit. A 5000 I.U., C 100 mg., B-1 2.5 mg., B-2 2 mg., nicotinamide 10 mg., B-6 1 mg., Ca pantothenate 5 mg., B-12 w/intrinsic factor conc. 0.133 I.U., ferrous fumarate 150 mg., glutamic acid HCl 150 mg., docusate sodium 50 mg./Cap. Bot. 100s.
Use: Nutritional supplement.

SENILEZOL ELIXIR. (Edwards) Vit. B-1 2.5 mg., B-2 2.5 mg., B-6 1 mg., B-12 5mcg., dexpanthenol 5 mg., niacin 10 mg., ferric pyrophosphate 20 mg. 130 ml. w/ alcohol 15% Bot. pt.
Use: Vitamin and mineral supplement.

• **SENNA,** U.S.P. XXI. Fluidextract, Syrup, U.S.P. XXI. Alexandrian.
Use: Cathartic.
See: Casafru, Liq. (Key)

SENNA CONC., STANDARDIZED.
Use: Cathartic.
See: Senokot, Gran., Tab., Supp. (Purdue Frederick)
      X-Prep. Pow. (Gray)
W/Docusate sodium.
See: Gentlax S. Tab. (Blair)
      Senokap-DSS, Cap. (Purdue Frederick)
      Senokot S. Tab. (Purdue Frederick)
W/Guar gum.
See: Gentlax B Tab., Granules (Blair)
W/Psyllium.
See: Perdiem, Granules (Rorer)
      Senokot W/Psyllium Powder (Purdue Frederick)

SENNA FRUIT EXTRACT, STANDARDIZED.
Use: Cathartic.
See: Senokot Syrup (Purdue Frederick)
      X-Prep, Liq. (Gray)

SENNA POWDER COMPOUND. (Penick) Comp. licorice pow. Bot. ¼ lb., 1 lb.

Use: Mild cathartic.

• **SENNOSIDES,** U.S.P. XXI. Tab., U.S.P. XXI.
Use: Laxative, stool softener.

SENOKAP-DSS CAPSULES. (Purdue Frederick) Docusate sodium (dioctyl sodium sulfosuccinate) 50 mg., standardized senna conc. 163 mg./Cap. Bot. 30s, 60s.
Use: Laxative, stool softener.

SENOKOT TABLETS and GRANULES. (Purdue Frederick) **Granules:** Standardized senna concentrate. Canister 2 oz., 6 oz., 12 oz. **Tabs.:** Bot. 50s, 100s, 1000s. Unit Strip Pack 100s. Box 20s.
Use: Laxative.

SENOKOT W/PSYLLIUM POWDER. (Purdue Frederick) Standardized senna conc. w/psyllium. Canister 5.5 oz.
Use: Management of constipation.

SENOKOT S TABLETS. (Purdue Frederick) Standardized senna concentrate w/docusate sodium. Tab. Bot. 30s, 60s, 1000s.
Use: Laxative, stool softener.

SENOKOT SUPPOSITORIES. (Purdue Frederick) Standardized senna concentrate. Pkg. 6s, 48s, 500s.
Use: Rectal laxative.

SENOKOT SYRUP. (Purdue Frederick) Standardized ext. senna fruit. Bot. 2 oz., 8 oz.
Use: Relief of constipation.

SENORAL-M. (Kay) Pentylenetetrazol 100 mg., B-1 1.67 mg., B-6 7.5 mg., cyanocobalamin 2.5 mcg. w/alcohol 15%. 5 cc. Bot. pt., gal.
Use: Analeptic in patients with mental confusion, apathy and memory defects.

SENSI-SLIDE. (Roche) Latex agglutination inhibition slide test for pregnancy (0.8IU/ml HCG) requiring only two minutes for clear-cut results. Clinical studies show 98.4 percent accuracy of test. 25 and 50 test kits.

SENSI-TEX. (Roche) Latex agglutination-inhibition tube test for pregnancy employing a latex bound beta-human chorionic gonadotropin antigen. Vial 2.5 ml.
Use: Pregnancy test.

SENSITIVE EYES SALINE SOLUTION. (Bausch & Lomb) Sterile, preserved solution for cleaning, rinsing, heat disinfection & storing soft contact lens. Bot. 8 oz.
Use: Solution for soft contact lens.

SENSODYNE TOOTHPASTE. (Block) Glycerin, sorbitol, sodium methyl cocoyl taurate, PEG-40 stearate, strontium chloride hexahydrate 10%, methyl and propylparabens, tint. Tubes 2.1, 4.0 oz.
Use: Sensitive teeth.

SENSORCAINE. (Astra) Bupivacaine HCl 0.25%, 0.50% or 0.75%. Amp. 30 ml.
Use: Local anesthetic.

• **SEPAZONIUM CHLORIDE.** USAN.
Use: Anti-infective, topical.

• **SEPERIDOL HCl.** USAN. 4-[4-(4-Chloro-α,α,α-trifluoro-m-tolyl)-4-hydroxypiperidino]-4'-fluorobutyrophenone HCl. Under study.
Use: Neuroleptic.

SEPO. (Otis Clapp) Benzocaine. Loz. Bot. 80s. Safety pack 1000s.
Use: Salt free anesthetic for sore throat relief.

SEPP. (Marion) Isopropyl alcohol 70%, acetone 10%, iodine tincture 2%, PVP iodine sol. 10%, green soap tincture, benzoin tincture. Carton 200 applicators.
Use: Antiseptic for skin preparation.

SEPTA. (Circle) Bacitracin 400 units, neomycin sulfate 5 mg., polymixin B sulfate 5,000 units/Gm. in ointment base. Tube 1 oz.
Use: Antibiotic.

SEPTI-CHEK. (Roche) Blood culture and simultaneous sub-culture system with four media to support clinically significant pathogens. Quick and easy assembly forms a closed system to protect sub-cultures from contamination. Clinical studies show differentiation selectivity in 76 percent of positives.

SEPTILINE SOLUBLE. (Noyes) NaCl, Na borate (formed), eucalyptol, Me salicylate, thymol, menthol, chlorothymol. Wafers 100s, 1000s.

SEPTIPHENE. 4-Chloro-α-phenyl-o-cresol. Santophen 1. (Monsanto).
Use: Disinfectant.

SEPTO. (Vita Elixir) Methylbenzethonium Cl., ethanol 2%, menthol.
Use: Germicidal & antiseptic liquid.

SEPTRA. (Burroughs Wellcome) Sulfamethoxazole 400 mg., trimethoprim 80 mg./Tab. Tab. Bot. 100s, 500s. Unit dose 100s.
Use: Urinary infections, *Pneumocystis Carinii pneumonitis,* otitis media, bronchitis.

SEPTRA DS. (Burroughs Wellcome) Trimethoprim 160 mg., sulfamethoxazole 800 mg./Tab. Bot. 60s. Compliance Pak 20s.
Use: Urinary infections, *Pneumocystis Carinii pneumonitis,* otitis media, bronchitis.

SEPTRA I.V. (Burroughs Wellcome) Trimethoprim 80 mg., sulfamethoxazole 400 mg./5 ml. amp. Box 10s. Multiple Dose Vials 10 ml., 20 ml.
Use: Urinary tract infection, shigellosis, *Pneumocystis Carinii pneumonitis.*

SEPTRA SUSPENSION. (Burroughs Wellcome) Trimethoprim 40 mg., sulfamethoxazole 200 mg./5 ml. Bot. 100 ml., 473 ml.
Use: Urinary tract infections , *Pneumocystis Carinii pneumonitis* and otitis media.

SEPTRIN. Co-trimoxazole, B.A.N.

SEQUENS. Mestranol, B.A.N.

• **SERACTIDE ACETATE.** USAN. Ala[26]-Gly[27]-SER[31]α[1]-[39] corticotrophin acetate.
Use: Corticotrophic peptide.
See: Acthar Gel (Armour)

SER-AP-ES. (Ciba) Reserpine 0.1 mg., hydralazine HCl 25 mg., hydrochlorothiazide 15 mg./Tab. Bot. 100s, 1000s; Consumer Packs of 100s; Accu-Pak 100s.
Use: Hypertension.

SERAPINE TABLETS. (Cenci) Hydralazine HCl 25 mg., hydrochlorothiazide 15 mg., reserpine 0.1 mg./Tab. Bot. 100s, 1000s.

SERAX. (Wyeth) Oxazepam. **Caps.** 10 mg., 15 mg., 30 mg. Bot. 100s, 500s. 10 mg. Redipak 25s. 15

and 30 mg. Redipak 25s, 100s. **Tabs.** 15 mg., Bot. 100s.
Use: Psychotropic.
SERBIO. (Metro Med) Capsules Bot. 100s, 1000s.
Use: Hypertension.
SERC DIHYDROCHLORIDE. Betahistine, B.A.N.
SEREEN. (Foy) Chlordiazepoxide HCl 5 mg., 10 mg./Cap. Bot. 500s, 1000s.
Use: Antianxeity, sedative.
SERENACE. Haloperidol, B.A.N.
SERENE. (Approved) Salicylamide 2 gr., scopolamine aminoxide HBr 0.2 mg./Cap. Bot. 24s, 60s.
Use: Tranquilizer.
SERENSIL. Ethchlorvynol, B.A.N.
SERENTIL. (Boehringer Ingelheim) Mesoridazine besylate. **Inj.** 25 mg./ml. (w/disodium edetate 0.5 mg., sod. chloride 7.2 mg., carbon dioxide gas q.s.) Amp. 20s, 100s. **Tab.** 10, 25, 50, 100 mg. Bot. 100s, 5000s. **Oral Concentrate** 25 mg./cc. Grad. dropper Bot. 4 oz.
Use: Antipsychotic.
SERFOLIA. (Mallard) Rauwolfia serpentina 100 mg./Tab. Bot. 1000s.
Use: Hypotensive agent.
SERICINASE. A proteolytic enzyme.
• **SERINE**, U.S.P. XXI. $C_3H_7NO_3$ as L-serine.
Use: Amino acid.
• **SERMETACIN.** USAN.
Use: Anti-inflammatory.
SERNYLAN. Phencyclidine., B.A.N. 1-(1-Phenycyclohexyl)-piperidine HCl.
Use: Anesthetic.
SERODEN. Thiacetazone, B.A.N.
SEROMYCIN. (Lilly) Cycloserine 250 mg./Pulvule. Bot. 40s.
Use: Pulmonary tuberculosis.
SEROPHENE. (Serono) Clomiphene citrate 50 mg./Tab. Box 30s.
Use: Induction of ovulation in selected anovulatory women.
SERPAHYDE. (Wolins) Reserpine 0.1 mg., hydralazine HCl 25 mg., hydrochlorothiazide 15 mg./Tab. Bot. 100s, 1000s.
SERPALAN TABLETS. (Lannett) Reserpine alkaloid 0.1 mg., 0.25 mg., 1.0 mg./Tab. Bot. 100s, 500s, 1000s.
SERPANRAY. (Panray) Reserpine 0.25 mg., 1 mg./Tab. Bot. 100s, 1000s.
SERPASIL. (Ciba) Reserpine. **Tab.:** 0.25 mg./Tab. Bot. 100s, 500s, 1000s. Consumer Packs of 100s; 0.1 mg./Tab. Bot. 100s, 1000s. **Amp.:** (2.5 mg./ml.) w/dimethylacetamide 0.1 ml., adipic acid 10 mg., versene 0.1 mg., benzyl alcohol 0.01 ml., polyethylene glycol 0.05 ml., ascorbic acid 0.5 ml., sod. sulfite 0.1 mg./ml. 2 ml., 5s.
Use: Antihypertensive & tranquilizing agent.
SERPASIL-APRESOLINE. (Ciba) #1: Reserpine 0.1 mg., hydralazine HCl 25 mg./Tab. Bot. 100s. #2: Reserpine 0.2 mg., hydralazine HCl 50 mg./Tab. Bot. 100s.
Use: Hypertensive disorders.
SERPASIL-ESIDRIX. (Ciba) # 1: Reserpine 0.1 mg., hy-

drochlorothiazide 25 mg./Tab. #2: Reserpine 0.1 mg., hydrochlorothiazide 50 mg./Tab. Bot. 100s, 1000s.
Use: Mild-to-moderate hypertension.
SERPATE. (Vale) Reserpine 0.1 mg. or 0.25 mg./Tab. Bot. 100s, 500s, 1000s.
Use: Antihypertensive & tranquilizing agent.
SERPENA. (Haag) Reserpine 0.25 mg./Tab. Bot. 100s, 500s, 1000s.
SERTABS. (Table Rock) Reserpine 0.25 mg., 0.5 mg./Tab. Bot. 100s, 500s.
Use: Tranquilizer and antihypertensive.
SERTINA. (Fellows) Reserpine 0.25 mg./Tab. Bot. 1000s, 5000s.
Use: Antihypertensive and ataraxic.
• **SERTRALINE HYDROCHLORIDE.** USAN.
Use: Antidepressant.
SERUM, ALBUMIN, NORMAL HUMAN.
See: Albumin Human, U.S.P. XXI. (Var. Mfr.)
SERUM, ALBUMIN, HUMAN, RADIOIODINATED.
See: Iodinated. I-125
   Albumin Injection, U.S.P. XXI.
SERUM, ANTIHEMOPHILUS INFLUENZAE TYPE B (RABBIT). Antihaemophilus (influenzae Type B Serum, Rabbit). (Squibb)
SERUM, GLOBULIN (HUMAN), IMMUNE.
See: Globulin Immune Serum (Human), (Var. Mfr.)
SERUM, MEASLES IMMUNE, HUMAN.
See: Measles Virus Vaccine Live, U.S.P. XXI.
SERUM PERTUSSIS IMMUNE, HUMAN.
See: Pertussis Vaccine Adsorbed, U.S.P. XXI.
SERUTAN. (Beecham Products) Vegetable hemicellulose from Plantago Ovata. **Gran.:** Pkg. 7 oz., 18 oz. **Pow.:** 3½ oz., 7 oz., 14 oz., 21 oz. Fruit flavored: 6 oz., 12 oz., 18 oz.
Use: Laxative.
• **SESAME OIL,** N.F. XVI.
Use: Pharm. aid (solvent).
SESTRON. N-Ethyl-3,3'-diphenyl-dipropylamine. Profenil. (Smith, Miller & Patch)
SETHADIL. Sulphaethidole, B.A.N.
SETHOTOPE. (Squibb) Selenomethionine Se 75; available as 0.25, 1.0 m C i.
SEVEN-FIFTY. (Freeport) Acetylsalicylic acid 7.5 gr./Tab. Bot. 1000s.
Use: Relief of minor aches and pains.
SEVIN. Carbaryl, B.A.N.
• **SEVOFLURANE.** USAN. Fluoromethyl 2,2,2-trifluoro-1-(trifluoromethyl)ethyl ether.
Use: Anesthetic (inhalation).
SEXOVID. Cyclofenil, B.A.N.
SHADE SUNSCREEN LOTION. (Plough) Homosalate, oxybenzone, SPF 6. Bot. 4 oz., 8 oz.
Use: Ultraviolet sunscreen.
SHAMPOO-ETS TRAVEL PACKET. (Matthew) Caps. 20s.
SHAPE AID. (Wolins) Benzocaine 3 mg., sodium carboxymethylcellulose 167 mg., Vit. A 1667 I.U., D2 133 I.U., B-1 0.67 mg., C 16.67 mg., B-2 0.833 mg., B-6 0.334 mg., niacinamide 6.67 mg., iron 5 mg., D-calcium pantothenate 0.334 mg./Cap. Bot. 100s, 1000s.

• **SHELLAC,** N.F.XVI.
Use: Pharmaceutic aid (tablet coating agent).
SHEPARD'S CREAM LOTION. (Dermik) Creamy lotion with no lanolin or mineral oil, for entire body. Scented or unscented. Bot. 8 oz., 16 oz.
Use: Skin dryness.
SHEPARD'S MOISTURIZING SOAP. (Dermik) Mildly scented, superfatted with lanolin. Bar 4 oz.
SHEPARD'S SKIN CREAM. (Dermik) Scented or unscented, w/no lanolin or mineral oil. Jar 4 oz.
Use: Lubricant and emollient.
SHERAMIN ELIXIR. (Blue Line) Thiamine hydrochloride, detannated sherry wine, sugar, citric acid, 0.1% w/v benzoic acid as preservative, alcohol 14%. Standardized to supply 8 mg., Vit. B-1 per fl. oz. or 27 mg. per 100 cc. Bot. pt., gal.
SHERFORM-HC CREME. (Sheryl) Hydrocortisone 1%, pramoxine HCl 0.5%, clioquinol 3%. Oint. tube ½ oz.
Use: Skin disorders.
SHERHIST. (Sheryl) Phenylphrine HCl, pyrilamine maleate/Tab. 100s. Liq. 1 pt.
Use: Relief of sinusitis.
SHERNATAL TABLETS. (Sheryl) Phosphorus free calcium, non-irritating iron, trace minerals and essential vitamins. Tab. 100s.
Use: Prenatal vitamin and mineral supplement.
SHERRY-JEN TONIC. (Jenkins) Vit. B-1 8 mg., B-2 4 mg., cyanocobalamin 4 mcg., nicotinamide 20 mg., Ca pantothenate 5 mg., B-6 1 mg., inositol 30 mg., choline bitartrate 60 mg., ferric ammonium citrate 60 mg., alcohol 9%/fl. oz. Bot. 4 oz., 8 oz., gal.
SHERTUS LIQUID. (Sheryl) Dextromethorphan HBr, chlorpheniramine maleate, phenylephrine HCl, ammonium chloride. Liq. 1 pt.
Use: Relief of cough and respiratory congestion.
SHIELD. (Birchwood) Pkg. 1 shield.
Use: Anorectical protective garmet.
SHOHL'S SOLUTION. Sodium Citrate and Citric Acid Oral Solution, U.S.P. XXI.
Use: Systemic alkalizer.
SHOSTAKOVSKY BALSAM. Polyvinox, B.A.N.
SHUR SEAL GEL. (Milex) Nonoxynol-9 6 Gm./5 oz. pre-measured pak. Box 24s.
Use: Contraceptive jelly for use with diaphragm.
SIALCO. (Foy) Chlorpheniramine maleate 4 mg., salicylamide 150 mg., acetaminophen 125 mg., phenylephrine HCl 5 mg./Tab. Bot. 100s, 500s, 1000s.
Use: Antihistaminic, analgesic, nasal decongestant.
SIBELIUM. (Janssen) Flunarizine HCl.
Use: Vasodilator.
SIBLIN. (Parke-Davis) Water-absorbent material from plantago/Tsp. Box 4 oz., 1 lb.
Use: Bulk laxative.
SIDEROL. (Doral) Chelated iron ammonium citrate 720 mg., folic acid 400 mcg., B-12 25 mcg., B-1 50 mg., B-6 1 mg., niacin 60 mg., panthenol 10 mg., PABA 6 mg., 1-lysine HCl 100 mg., inositol 10 mg., choline citrate 50 mg., methionine 6.25 mg., trace minerals: Cu, Zn, Mn., K, Mg., in base with sorbitol, liver fraction no. 1, & beef peptone/cc. Bot. 6 oz.

Use: Prevention & treatment of iron, vit. B complex, folic acide deficiencies.
SIGAMINE. (Sig) Cyanocobalamin injection 1000 mcg./cc. Vial 10 ml., 30 ml. Also Sigamine L.A. Vial 10 ml.
Use: Vit. B-12 deficiency.
SIGAZINE. (Sig) Promethazine HCl 50 mg./ml. Vial 10 ml.
Use: Antihistamine.
SIGESIC. (Rand) Cap. Bot. 100s, 1000s.
Use: Analgesic and sedative.
SIGNA CREME. (Parker) Conductive cosmetic quality electrolyte cream.
Use: High conductive electrode cream for ECG, EEG, defibrillation.
SIGNA GEL. (Parker) Conductive saline electrode gel.
Use: Defibrillation, ECG, EMG, electrosurgery.
SIGNA PAD. (Parker) Pre-moistened electrode pads.
Use: Defibrillation, ECG, EMG, electrosurgery.
SIGNATAL C. (Sig) Calcium 230 mg., iron 49.3 mg., Vit. A 4000 I.U., D 400 I.U., B-1 2 mg., B-2 2 mg., B-6 1 mg., B-12 2 mcg., folic acid 0.1 mg., niacinamide 10 mg., Vit. C 50 mg., iodine 0.15 mg./S.C. Tab. Bot. 100s, 1000s.
Use: Pre-and postnatal dietary supplement.
SIGNATE. (Sig) Dimenhydrinate 50 mg. propylene glycol 50%, benzyl alcohol 5%/ml. Vial 10 ml.
Use: Prophylaxis and treatment of motion sickness.
SIGNEF "SUPPS". (Fellows) Hydrocortisone 15 mg./Supp. 12s. w or w/out appl.
Use: Vaginal treatment.
SIGPRED. (Sig) Prednisolone acetate. Vial 10 ml.
SIGTAB. (Upjohn) Vit. A 5000 I.U., D 400 I.U., B-1 10.3 mg., B-2 10 mg., C 333 mg., niacin 100 mg., B-6 6 mg., pantothenic acid 20 mg., folic acid 0.4 mg., B-12 18 mcg., Vit. E 15 I.U./Tab. Bot. 30s, 90s, 500s.
Use: Vitamin supplement.
• **SILAFILCON A.** USAN.
Use: Contact lens material.
• **SILAFOCON A.** USAN.
Use: Contact lens material.
SILAIN. (Robins) Simethicone (activated methylpolysiloxane). Tab. 50 mg. Bot. 100s.
Use: Antiflatulant.
SILAIN-GEL. (Robins) Simethicone 25 mg., aluminum hydroxide 282 mg., magnesium hydroxide 285 mg./5 ml. Bot. 12 oz.
Use: Antiflatulant, antacid.
• **SILANDRONE.** USAN. 17 β-(Trimethylsioloxy)-androst-4-en-3-one.
Use: Androgen.
SILBEPHYLLINE. Diprophylline, B.A.N.
SILEXIN SYRUP. (Otis Clapp) Dextromethorphan HBr and guaifenesin in sugar, salt and alcohol free vehicle. Bot. 1 oz. (12s), 4 oz., 16 oz.
Use: Antitussive, expectorant cough syrup.
SILEXIN TABS. (Otis Clapp) Dextromethorphan HBr, benzocaine/Tab. Safety Pack 400s.
Use: Sore throat relief, cough suppressant, anesthetic.
• **SILICA GEL,** N.F. XVI.

Use: Pharm. aid (suspending agent; anticaking agent; disintegrating agent;.
• **SILICEOUS EARTH, PURIFIED,** N.F. XVI.
Use: Filtering medium.
SILICONE. (Dow Chemicals) Dimethicone. Liq., Bot. 1 oz. Bulk Pkg. Oint.
See also: Simethicone (Var. Mfr.)
W/Lanolin.
See: Sanchia Silicone Protective Cream (Otis Clapp)
W/Nitro-Cellulose & castor oil.
See: Covicone, Cream (Abbott)
W/Triethylene glycol & mineral oil.
See: Allergex, Liq., Spray (Hollister-Stier)
• **SILICONE DIOXIDE, COLLOIDAL,** N.F. XVI.
Use: Tablet diluent, suspending & thickening agent.
SILICONE OINTMENT. Dimethicone Dimethyl polysiloxane.
See: Covicone Cream (Abbott)
SILICONE OINTMENT #2. (C & M Pharmacal) 10% high viscosity silicone in a blend of petrolatum and hydrophobic starch. Jar 2 oz., 1 lb.
Use: Protective ointment.
SILICONE POWDER. (Gordon) Talc with silicone.
Pkg. 4 oz., 1 lb., 5 lb.
Use: Dusting powder to prevent tape from adhering to clothing.
SILMAGEL. (Lannett) Aluminum hydroxide 2.5 gr., magnesium trisilicate 3.85 gr./Tab. Bot. 1000s, 5000s.
Use: Protective antacid.
• **SILODRATE** USAN. Mag. aluminosilicate hydrate.
Use: Antacid.
SILTEX. (Edward J. Moore) Camphor, menthol, allantoin, tinct. benzoin in lanolin-petrolatum base. Tube ¼ oz.
Use: Chapped lips, cold sores, fever blisters.
SILVADENE. (Marion) Silver sulfadiazine (10 mg./1Gm.) 1%, base w/white petrolatum, stearyl alcohol, isopropyl myristate, sorbitan monooleate, polyoxyl 40 stearate, propylene glycol, water, methylparaben 0.3%. Cream Jar 50 Gm., 400 Gm., 1000 Gm. Tube 20 Gm.
Use: Anti-infective.
SILVER COMPOUNDS.
See: Silver Iodide, Colloidal
Silver Nitrate, Preps. (Various Mfr.)
Silver Picrate (City Chem.)
Silver Protein, Mild (Various Mfr.)
Silver Protein, Strong (Various Mfr.)
• **SILVER NITRATE,** U.S.P. XXI. Ophth. Soln., Toughened, U.S.P. XXI. Nitric acid silver.
Use: Astringent, caustic & antiseptic.
• **SILVER NITRATE OPHTHALMIC SOLUTION,** U.S.P. XXI. (Wax Amp.)
Use: Astringent, anti-infective.
Generic Products:
(Lilly)—Amp. 1%, 100s.
(Parke-Davis)—Cap. 1%, 100s.
• **SILVER NITRATE, TOUGHENED,** U.S.P. XXI. Silver nitrate plus 4% silver chloride.
Use: Caustic.

SILVER PICRATE. (City Chem.) 1 oz.
Use: Antiseptic.
SILVER PROTEIN, MILD. Argentum Vitellinum, Cargentos, Mucleinate Mild, Protargin Mild
See: Argyrol Prods. (CooperVision)
SILVER PROTEIN, STRONG.
See: Protargol, Pow. (Sterling)
• **SILVER SULFADIAZINE.** USAN.
Use: Topical anti-infective.
See: Silvadene, Oint. (Marion)
SILVER SULFADIAZINE CREAM. (Flint) Silver sulfadiazine 1% in opaque, water-miscible cream base. Jar. 50 Gm., 400 Gm.
Use: Topical antibacterial.
SIMECO. (Wyeth) Aluminum hydroxide 365 mg., magnesium hydroxide 300 mg., simethicone 30 mg./ 5 ml. Bot. 12 oz.
Use: Antacid, antiflatulant.
• **SIMETHICONE,** U.S.P. XX, Emulsion, Oral Susp., Tab., U.S.P. XXI. Mixture of liquid dimethyl polysiloxanes with silica aerogel.
Use: Antiflatulent; pharmaceutic aid (release agent).
See: Mylicon, Tab. & Liq. (Stuart)
Mylicon-80, Tab. (Stuart)
Silain, Tab. (Robins)
Ingredients of:
Mylanta, Tab., Liq. (Stuart)
Phazyme, Tab. (Reed & Carnick)
W/Aluminum hydroxide & magnesium hydroxide
See: Di-Gel, Liq. Tab. (Plough)
Mylanta, Mylanta II, Tab. & Liq. (Stuart)
Silain-Gel, Liq. (Robins)
Simeco, Liq. (Wyeth)
Simethox, Liq. (Columbia)
W/Enzymes.
See: Phazyme, Tabs. (Reed & Carnrick)
Tri-Cone, Cap. (Glaxo)
W/Hyoscyamine sulfate, atropine sulfate, hyoscine HBr, butabarbital sod.
See: Sidonna, Tab. (Reed & Carnrick)
W/Hyoscyamine sulfate, atropine sulfate, scopolamine HBr & phenobarbital.
See: Kinesed, Chewable Tab. (Stuart)
W/Magnesium aluminum hydroxide
See: Maalox Plus, Susp. (Rorer)
W/Magnesium carbonate.
See: Di-Gel, Tab. & Liq. (Plough)
W/Magnesium hydroxide.
See: Laxsil, Liq. (Reed & Carnrick)
W/Magnesium hydroxide & dried aluminum hydroxide gel.
See: Maalox Plus, Tab. (Rorer)
W/Pancreatin.
See: Phazyme, Tab. (Reed & Carnrick)
Phazyme-95, Tab. (Reed & Carnrick)
W/Pancreatin, phenobarbital.
See: Phazyme-PB, Tab. (Reed & Carnrick)
SIMETHOX. (Columbia) Aluminum hydroxide 400 mg., magnesium hydroxide 400 mg., simethicone 30 mg./5 cc. Bot. 12 oz.
Use: Antacid, antiflatulent.

SIMILAC 13/SIMILAC 13 WITH IRON. (Ross) milk-based formula ready-to-feed. Each liter contains: protein 11.9 g, fat 23.2 g, carbohydrate 46.0 g, Ca 0.41 g, P 0.31 g, Na 0.22 g, K 0.58 g, Cl 0.41 g, Mg 32 mg, Fe 7.8 mg. (1.0 mg. in Similac 13), Zn 3.3 mg., Cu 0.39 mg., iodine 65 mcg., Mn 22 mcg., Vit. A 1625 IU, D 260 IU, E 13 IU, C 36 mg., B-1 0.42 mg., B-2 0.65 mg., niacin 4.6 mg. Eq., B-6 0.26 mg., folic acid 65 mcg., B-12 1.0 mcg., pantothenic acid 2.0 mg. Bot. 4 fl. oz.
Use: For infants requiring a dilute feeding.

SIMILAC 20/SIMILAC 20 WITH IRON. (Ross) Milk-based formula, ready-to-feed (20 cal. fl. oz.). Each liter contains: protein 15.5 g, fat 36.1 g, carbohydrate 72.3 g, Ca 0.51 g, P 0.39 g, Na 0.25 g, K 0.78 g, Cl 0.53 g, Mg 41 mg., Zn 5.0 mg., Cu 0.60 mg., iron 12.0 mg. (1.5 mg. in Similac 20 regular), iodine 0.10 mg., Mn 34 mcg., Vit. A 2500 IU, D 400 IU, E 20 IU, C 55 mg., B-1 0.65 mg., B-2 1.0 mg., niacin 7.0 (mg. Eq), B-6 0.40 mg., folic acid 100 mcg., B-12 1.5 mcg., pantothenic acid 3 mg. Bot. 4 fl oz; 8 fl oz; 32 fl oz;
Use: When a formula of standard dilution is desired for an infant.

SIMILAC 24 LBW. (Ross) Milk-based medium chain triglyceride low osmolar formula, ready-to-feed (24 cal./fl. oz.) Each liter contains: protein 22.0 g, fat 44.9 g, carbohydrate 84.9 g, Ca 0.73 g, P 0.56 g, Na 0.36 g, K 1.22 g, Cl 0.89 g, Mg 80 mg., Fe 3.0 mg., Zn 8.0 mg., Cu 0.80 mg., iodine 0.12 mg., Mn 41 mcg., Vit. A 3000 IU, D 480 IU, E 24 IU, C 100 mg., B-1 1.0 mg., B-2 1.2 mg., niacin 8.4 mg. Eq, B-6 0.50 mg., folic acid 100 mcg., B-12 2.0 mcg., pantothenic acid 3.6 mg. Bot. 4 fl. oz.
Use: For low-birth-weight infants who need a low osmolar concentrated feeding containing medium chain triglycerides.

SIMILAC 24/SIMILAC 24 WITH IRON. (Ross) Milk-based formula ready-to-feed (24 cal./fl. oz.). Each liter contains: protein 22.0 g, fat 42.8 g, carbohydrate 84.9 g, Ca 0.73 g, P 0.56 g, Na 0.33 g, K 1.07 g, Cl 0.74 g, Mg 55 mg., Fe 15 mg. (1.8 mg in Similac 24 Regular), Zn 6.0 mg., Cu 0.72 mg., iodine 0.120 mg., Mn 41 mcg., Vit. A 3000 IU, D 480 IU, E 24 IU, C 66 mg., B-1 0.78 mg., B-2 1.2 mg., niacin 8.4 mg. Eq, B-6 0.48 mg., folic acid 120 mcg., B-12 1.8 mcg., pantothenic acid 3.6 mg. Bot. 4 fl. oz.
Use: For infants who need a concentrated feeding.

SIMILAC 27. (Ross) Milk-based ready-to-feed formula (27 cal./fl. oz.). Each liter contains: protein 24.7 g, fat 48.1 g, carbohydrate 95.5 g, Ca 0.81 g, P 0.62 g, Na 0.39 g, K 1.2 g, Cl 0.81 g, Mg 61 mg., Fe 2.0 mg., Zn 6.8 mg., Cu 0.81 mg., iodine 0.14 mg., Mn 46 mcg., Vit. A 3375 IU, D 540 IU, E 27 IU, C 74 mg., B-1 0.88 mg., B-2 1.4 mg., niacin 9.4 mg. Eq, Vit. B-6 0.54 mg., folic acid 140 mcg., Vit. B-12 2.0 mcg., pantothenic acid 4.0 mg. Bot. 4 fl. oz.
Use: For low-birth-weight infants requiring a concentrated feeding.

SIMILAC 60/40 POWDER. (Ross) Milk-based formula powdered. Each liter contains (as fed 20 cal./fl. oz.): protein 15.7 g, fat 35.4 g, carbohydrate 75.7 g,

Ca 0.40 g, P 0.20 g, Na 0.16 g, K 0.58 g, Cl 0.45 g, Mg 42 mg., Fe 2.6 mg., Zn 4.0 mg., Cu 0.40 mg., iodine 40 mcg., Mn 34 mcg., Vit. A 2500 IU, D 400 IU, E 15 IU, C 55 mg., B-1 0.65 mg., B-2 1.0, Niacin mg. Eq. 7.3, B-6 0.30 mg., folic acid 50 mcg., Vit. B-12 1.5 mcg., pantothenic acid 3.0 mg., Vit. K-1 27 mcg. Cans 1 lb.
Use: For infants requiring low electrolyte formula.

SIMILAC Concentrated Liquid/SIMILAC Concentrated Liquid With Iron. (Ross) 13 fl. oz. diluted 1:1 to give 20 Cal/fl. oz. See SIMILAC 20/SIMILAC 20 With Iron for composition on "as fed" 20 cal./fl. oz. basis.

SIMILAC POWDER/SIMILAC POWDER WITH IRON. (Ross) Milk-based formula, "as" fed (20 cal./fl. oz.). Each liter contains: protein 15.5 g, fat 36.1 g, carbohydrate 72.3 g, Ca 0.51 g, P 0.39 g, Na 0.30 g, K 1.1 g, Cl 0.49 g, Mg 41 mg., Fe 12.0 mg., Zn 5.0 mg., Cu 0.60 mg., iodine 0.10 mg., Mn 34 mcg., Vit. A 2500 IU, D 400 IU, E 15 IU, C 55 mg., B-1 0.65 mg., B-2 1.0 mg., niacin 7.0 mg. Eq., B-6 0.40 mg., folic acid 100 mcg., B-12 1.5 mcg., K-1 27 mcg., pantothenic acid 3.0 mg. Cans 1 lb.
Use: For infants requiring standard dilution formula or one with an increased concentration.

SIMILAC SPECIAL CARE 20. (Ross) Infant Formula ready-to-feed (20 Cal./fl. oz.). Milk-based formula with 60:40 protein:casein ratio and containing medium chain triglycerides. Each liter contains: protein 18.3 g, fat 36.7 g, carbohydrate 71.7 g, Ca 1200 mg., P 600 mg., Na 290 mg., potassium 830 mg., Cl 540 mg., Mg 83 mg., Fe 2.5 mg., Zn 10.0 mg., Cu 1.7 mg., Mn 0.17 mg., iodine 0.125 mg., Vit. A 4580 IU, D 1000 IU, E 25 IU, C 250 mg., B-1 1.7 mg., B-2 4.2 mg., niacin 34 mg. Eq., pantothenic acid 12.5 mg., B-6 1.7 mg., folic acid 0.25 mg., biotin 0.25 mg., B-12 3.7 mcg., choline 67 mg., inositol 37 mg., K-1 83 mcg. Bot. 4 fl. oz.
Use: For growing low-birth-weight infants who require only a 20 cal./fl. oz. formula.

SIMILAC SPECIAL CARE 24. (Ross) Infant Formula ready-to-feed (24 Cal./fl. oz.) Milk-based low osmolar formula with 60:40 protein:casein ratio and containing medium chain triglycerides. Each liter contains: protein 22.0 g, fat 44.0 g, carbohydrate 86.0 g, Ca 1440 mg., P 720 mg., Na 350, K 1000 mg., Cl 650 mg., Mg 100 mg., Fe 3.0 mg., Zn 12 mg., Cu 2.0 mg., iodine 0.150 mg., Mn 0.20 mg., Vit. A 5500 I.U., D 1200 I.U., E 30 mg., C 300 mg., B-1 2.0 mg., B-2 5.0 mg., niacin 40 mg., B-6 2.0 mg., folic acid 0.3 mg., B-12 4.5 mcg., K-1 100 mcg., pantothenic acid 15 mg., choline 80 mg., inositol 45 mg. Bot. 4 fl. oz.
Use: For growing low-birth-weight infants.

SIMRON. (Merrell Dow) Iron (supplied as ferrous gluconate) 10 mg./Cap. Bot. 100s.
Use: Prevention and treatment of iron deficiency and iron deficiency anemia.

SIMRON PLUS. (Merrell Dow) Iron 10 mg. (supplied as ferrous gluconate), Vit. B-12 3.33 mcg., ascorbic acid 50 mg., B-6 1 mg., folic 0.1 mg./Cap. Bot. 100s.
Use: Prevention and treatment of iron deficiency and iron deficiency anemia.

• **SIMTRAZENE.** USAN. 1,4-Dimethyl-1,4-diphenyl-2-tetrazene.
Use: Antineoplastic.
SINAC. (Marin) Phenacetin 150 mg., acetaminophen 150 mg., phenylpropanolamine HCl 25 mg., phenyltoloxamine citrate 22 mg./Tab. Bot. 30s, 100s.
Use: Relief sinus headache and common cold symptoms.
SINAPREL. (Pasadena Research) Chlorpheniramine maleate 8 mg., phenylephrine HCl 20 mg., methscopolamine nitrate 2.5 mg./Cap. Bot. 100s, 1000s. Box 30s.
SINAREST. (Pharmacraft) Acetaminophen 325 mg., chlorpheniramine maleate 2 mg., phenylpropanolamine HCl 18.7 mg./Tab. Sleeve Pack 20s, 40s. Bot. 80s.
Use: Sinus headache, congestion.
SINAREST DECONGESTANT NASAL SPRAY. (Pharmacraft) Phenylephrine HCl 0.5%. Bot. 0.5 oz.
Use: Nasal decongestant.
SINAREST, EXTRA-STRENGTH. (Pharmacraft) Acetaminophen 500 mg., chlorpheniramine maleate 2 mg., phenylpropanolamine HCl 18.7 mg./Tab. Sleeve Pack 24s.
Use: Sinus headache, congestion.
SINASCOL. (Vitarine) Chlorpheniramine maleate 8 mg., phenylephrine HCl 20 mg., methscopolamine nitrate 2.5 mg./Cap.
Use: Antihistaminic and decongestant.
SINAXAR. Styramate, B.A.N.
• **SINCALIDE.** USAN.
Use: Choleretic.
SINE-AID TABLETS. (McNeil Prods) Acetaminophen 325 mg., phenylpropanolamine HCl 25 mg./Tab. Bot. 24s, 50s, 100s.
Use: Sinus headache pain and pressure.
SINECOD CITRATE. Butamyrate, B.A.N.
• **SINEFUNGIN.** USAN.
Use: Antifungal.
SINEMET 10/100. (Merck Sharp & Dohme) Carbidopa 10 mg., Levodopa 100 mg./Tab. Bot. 100s. Unit dose 100s. Unit-of-use Bot. 100s.
Use: Treatment of Parkinson's disease.
SINEMET 25-100. (Merck Sharp & Dohme) Carbidopa 25 mg., levodopa 100 mg./Tab. Bot. 100s. Unit dose 100s. Unit-of-use Bot. 100s.
Use: Treatment of Parkinson's disease.
SINEMET 25/250. (Merck Sharp & Dohme) Carbidopa 25 mg., levodopa 250 mg./Tab. Bot. 100s. Unit dose 100s. Unit-of-use Bot. 100s.
Use: Treatment of Parkinson's disease.
SINE-OFF CAPSULES WITH ACETAMINOPHEN. (Menley & James) Chlorpheniramine maleate 2.0 mg., phenylpropanolamine HCl 18.75 mg., acetaminophen 500 mg./Cap. Pkg. 20s.
Use: Sinus headache and congestion.
SINE-OFF CAPSULES, NO DROWSINESS FORMULA. (Menley & James) Phenylpropanolamine HCl 18.75 mg., acetaminophen 500 mg./Cap. Pkg. 20s.
Use: Sinus headache and congestion relief when drowsiness is a problem.

SINE-OFF TABLETS. (Menley & James) Chlorpheniramine maleate 2.0 mg., phenylpropanolamine HCl 18.75 mg., aspirin 325 mg. Tab. Pkg. 24s, 48s, 100s.
Use: Sinus headache & congestion.
SINE-OFF TABLETS WITH ACETAMINOPHEN. (Menley & James) Chlorpheniramine maleate 2.0 mg., phenylpropanolamine HCl 18.75 mg., acetaminophen 500 mg./Tab. Pk. 4s, 20s, 24s.
Use: Sinus headache and congestion.
SINEQUAN. (Roerig) Doxepin HCl **Cap.** 10 mg./Cap. Bot. 100s, 1000s. Unit dose 100s; 25 mg., 50 mg./Cap. Bot. 100s, 1000s, 5000s. Unit dose 100s; 75 mg./Cap. Bot. 100s, 1000s; Unit Dose 100s; 100 mg./Cap. Bot. 100s, 1000s. Unit Dose 100s; 150 mg./Cap. Bot. 50, 500s. **Oral Concentrate** 10 mg./ml. Bot. 120 ml.
Use: Psychotherapeutic drug.
SINEX. (Vicks) Phenylephrine HCl 0.5%, cetylpyridinium chloride 0.04%, camphor, menthol, eucalyptol, methyl salicylate w/thimersal 0.0001% preservative. Nasal Spray. Plastic Squeeze Bot. 0.5 oz., 1 oz.
Use: Nasal decongestant spray.
SINEXIN. (Bowman) Acetaminophen 324 mg., phenylehrine HCl 5 mg., chlorpheniramine maleate 2 mg., caffeine 32.4 mg./Cap.
Use: Analgesic, decongestant, antihistaminic.
SINEX LONG ACTING. (Vicks) Oxymetazoline HCl 0.05% in aqueous soln. with mentholated vapors and thimerosal 0.001% Nasal spray. Bot. 0.5 oz., 1 oz.
Use: Nasal decongestant.
SINGLET. (Merrell Dow) Phenylephrine HCl 40 mg., chlorpheniramine maleate 8 mg., acetaminophen 500 mg./Tab. Bot. 100s.
Use: Decongestant, analgesic, antihistamine.
SINO-COMP. (Bio-Factor) Salicylamide 3½ gr., caffeine 10 mg., phenylephrine HCl 5 mg., Vit. C 20 mg., chlorprophenpyridamine maleate 2 mg./Tab. Bot. 1000s.
Use: Decongestant & analgesic.
SINOCON TR. (Vangard) Phenylpropanolamine HCl 20 mg., phenylephrine HCl 5 mg., phenyltoloxamine citrate 7.5 mg., chlorpheniramine maleate 2.5 mg./Tab. Bot. 100s, 1000s.
Use: Antihistamine, decongestant.
SINODEC. (Primedics) Chlorpheniramine maleate 8 mg., phenylephrine HCl 20 mg., methscopolamine nitrate 2.5 mg./Cap. Bot. 100s, 500s.
Use: Antihistaminic.
SINO-EZE MLT. (Richlyn) Salicylamide 3½ gr., acetaminophen 100 mg., phenylephrine HCl 5 mg., chlorpheniramine maleate 2 mg./Tab. Bot. 1000s.
Use: Sinus, colds.
SINOGRAFIN. (Squibb) Meglumine diatrizoate 40% and meglumine iodipamide 20%. Vial 10 cc.
Use: Diagnostic.
SINOPHEN. (Kay) Phenylephrine HCl 1% in buffered isotonic sol., sodium bisulfite 0.2%. Methylparaben 0.02%, propyparaben 0.01%. Bot. Pts.
Use: Nasal decongestant.
SINO-TUSSIN MLT. (Richlyn) Dextromethorphan HBr 10 mg., salicylamide 3½ gr., acetaminophen 100

mg., phenylephrine HCl 5 mg., chlorpheniramine maleate 2 mg./Tab. Bot. 1000s.
Use: Cold therapy.

SINOVAN TIMED. (Drug Industries) Chlorpheniramine maleate 8 mg., phenylephrine HCl 20 mg., methscopolamine nitrate 2.5 mg./Cap. Bot. 100s, 1000s.
Use: Cold, hay fever, allergies.

SINTHROME. Nicoumalone, B.A.N.

SINTISONE L-STEAROYLGYLCOLATE. Prednisolone, B.A.N.

SINUADE. (Kay) Chlorpheniramine maleate 8 mg., phenylpropanolamine HCl 50 mg./Timed Release Cap. Bot. 100s, 1000s.

SINUBID. (Parke-Davis) Acetaminophen 600 mg., phenylpropanolamine HCl 100 mg., phenyltoloxamine 66 mg./Tab. Bot. 100s.
Use: Relief of common cold.

SINUCOL. (Tennessee Pharm.) Chlorpheniramine maleate 8 mg., phenylephrine HCl 20 mg., methscopolamine nitrate 2.5 mg./Cap. Bot. 100s, 500s. Parenteral. Vial 10 cc.
Use: Respiratory congestion and hypersecretion.

SINUDRAIN. (Wolins) Phenylephrine 5 mg., phenindamine 10 mg., aspirin, caffeine, aluminum hydroxide magnesium carbonate, co-dried gel/Tab. Bot. 100s, 1000s.

SINUESE. (Jenkins) Pot. guaiacolsulfonate 40 mg., sod. iodide 50 mg., menthol, camphor, guaiacol, eucalyptol/cc. Vial 30 cc., 12s.

SINUFED TIMECELLE. (Hauck) Pseudoephedrine HCl 60 mg., guaifenesin 300 mg./Cap. Bot. 100s.
Use: Nasal decongestant.

SINUGESIC. (Vortech) Bot. 1000s.
Use: Antihistaminic, decongestant.

SINU-LETS. (Columbia) Acetaminophen 325 mg., phenylpropanolamine HCl 25 mg., phenyltoloxamine citrate 25 mg./Tab. Vials 36s. Bot. 100s, 1000s.
Use: Sinus headaches.

SINULIN TABLETS. (Carnrick) Phenylpropanolamine HCl 37.5 mg., chlorpheniramine maleate 2 mg., acetaminophen 325 mg., salicylamide 250 mg., homatropine methylbromide 0.75 mg./Tab. Bot. 20s, 100s. Blisters of 24s.
Use: Sinus congestion, headache.

SINUPAN. (Ion) Phenylephrine HCl 40 mg., guaifenesin 200 mg./S.R. Cap. Bot. 100s.
Use: Decongestant.

SINUS. (Zenith) Phenacetin 150 mg., acetaminophen 150 mg., phenylpropanolamine HCl 25 mg., phenyltoloxamine citrate 22 mg./Tab. Bot. 1000s.
Use: Antihistamine, decongestant.

SINUS HEADACHE TABLETS. (Eckerd)
Phenylpropanolamine HCl 12.5 mg., acetaminophen 325 mg./Tab. Bot. 24s, 48s.
Use: Analgesic, decongestant.

SINUS TABLETS. (Kenyon) Phenacetin 150 mg., acetaminophen 150 mg., phenyltoloxamine dihydrogen citrate 22 mg./Tab. Bot. 100s, 1000s.

SINUS TABLETS. (Walgreen) Acetaminophen 325 mg., phenylpropanolamine 25 mg., phenyltoloxamine citrate 22 mg./Tab. Bot. 30s.

Use: Analgesic, decongestant, antihistamine.

SINUS TABLETS #2. (Vitarine) Acetaminophen 325 mg., phenylpropanolamine HCl 25 mg./Tab.
Use: Temporary relief of sinus headache & congestion.

SINUSTAT. (Vitarine) Acetaminophen 325 mg., phenylpropanolamine HCl 25 mg., phenyltoloxamine citrate 22 mg./Tab. Bot. 50s.
Use: Relief from the pain of sinus headaches and the common cold.

SINUTAB. (Warner-Lambert) Acetaminophen 325 mg., pseudoephedrine HCl 30 mg., chlorpheniramine HCl 2 mg./Tab. Bot. 100s. Blister pack 12s, 30s.
Use: Analgesic, decongestant, antihistaminic.

SINUTAB MAXIMUM STRENGTH. (Warner-Lambert) Acetaminophen 500 mg., pseudoephedrine HCl 30 mg., chlorpheniramine maleate 2 mg./Tab. or Cap. Blister pack 24s.
Use: Analgesic, decongestant, antihistaminic.

SINUTAB II MAXIMUM STRENGTH NO DROWSINESS FORMULA. (Warner-Lambert) Acetaminophen 500 mg. pseudoephedrine HCl 30 mg./Tab. or Cap. Pack 24s.
Use: Analgesic, decongestant.

SINUTROL. (Weeks & Leo) Phenylpropanolamine HCl 25 mg., phenyltoloxamine citrate 22 mg., acetaminophen 325 mg./Tab. Bot. 40s, 90s.
Use: Sinus headache.

SINU-WOL. (Wolins) Acetaminophen 150 mg., phen-acetin 150 mg., phenylpropanolamine HCl 25 mg., phenyltoloxamine citrate 22 mg./Tab. Bot. 100s, 1000s.
Use: Analgesic, decongestant, antihistaminic.

SINU-WOL II. (Wolins) Acetaminophen 150 mg., phen-acetin 150 mg., phenylpropanolamine HCl 25 mg./Tab. Bot. 100s, 1000s.
Use: Analgesic, decongestant.

SIROIL. (Siroil) Mercuric oleate, cresol, vegetable & mineral oil. Emulsion, Bot. 8 oz.
Use: Antiseptic skin therapy.

SIR-O-LENE. (Siroil) Tube 4 oz.
Use: Skin softener.

• **SISOMICIN.** USAN.
Use: Antibacterial.

• **SISOMICIN SULFATE,** U.S.P. XXI. Inj., U.S.P. XXI.
Use: Antibacterial.

SISTOMETRIL. Mestranol, B.A.N.

SITABS. (Canright) Lobeline Sulf. 1.5 mg., benzocaine 2 mg., aluminum hydroxide—magnesium carbonate co-dried gel 150 mg./Loz. Bot. 100s.
Use: Discourage smoking.

• **SITOGLUSIDE.** USAN.
Use: Antiprostatic hypertrophy.

SITOSTEROLS. A mixture of 80 to 90% beta-sitosterol and 10 to 20% dihydro-beta-sitosterol.
See: Cytellin, Susp. (Lilly)

SIXAMEEN. (Spanner) Vit. B-1 100 mg., B-6 100 mg./cc. Vial 10 cc.
Use: B vitamin therapy.

SK-65. (SmithKline) Propoxyphene HCl 65 mg./Cap. Bot. 100s, 500s.
Use: Analgesic.

SK-65 APAP. (SmithKline) Propoxyphene HCl 65 mg., Acetaminophen 650 mg./Tab. Bot. 100s, 500s.
Use: Pain relief.
SK-65 COMPOUND. (SmithKline) Propoxyphene HCl 65 mg., aspirin 389 mg., caffeine 32.4 mg./Cap. Bot. 100s, 500s.
Use: Analgesic.
SK-AMITRIPTYLINE. (SmithKline) Amitriptyline HCl 10 mg., 25 mg., 50 mg./Tab. Bot. 100s, 1000s. 75 mg., 100 mg., 150 mg./Tab. Bot. 100s.
Use: Relief of depression, anxiety symptoms.
SK-AMPICILLIN. (SmithKline) Ampicillin **Cap.** 250, 500 mg./Cap. Bot. 24s, 100s, 500s. **Oral Susp.** 100 mg./ml. Bot. 20 ml.; 125, 250 mg./5 ml. Bot. 100 ml., 150 ml., 200 ml.
Use: Treatment of infections.
SK-AMPICILLIN-N. (SmithKline) Ampicillin sodium 500 mg./Vial. Box 1s.
Use: Treatment of infections.
SK-APAP W/CODEINE. (SmithKline) Acetaminophen 300 mg., codeine phosphate 15 mg./Tab. Bot. 100s. Acetaminophen 300 mg., codeine phosphate 30 mg./Tab. Bot. 100s, 1000s. Acetaminophen 300 mg., codeine phosphate 60 mg./Tab. Bot. 100s, 500s.
Use: Pain Relief.
SK-BAMATE. (SmithKline) Meprobamate 200 mg., 400 mg./Tab. Bot. 100s. 400 mg. Bot. 1000s.
Use: Relief of anxiety and tension.
SK-CHLORAL HYDRATE. (SmithKline) Chloral Hydrate 500 mg./Cap. Bot. 100s.
Use: Hypnotic.
SK-CHLOROTHIAZIDE. (SmithKline) Chlorothiazide 250 mg., 500 mg./Tab. Bot. 100s, 1000s.
Use: Edema, hypertension.
SK-DEXAMETHASONE. (SmithKline) Dexamethasone 0.5 mg., 0.75 mg., 1.5 mg./Tab. Bot. 100s.
Use: Anti-inflammatory.
SK-DIPHENOXYLATE. (SmithKline) Diphenoxylate HCl 2.5 mg., atropine sulfate 0.025 mg. Bot. 100s, 1000s.
Use: Adjunctive therapy in diarrhea.
SKELAXIN. (Robins) Metaxalone 400 mg./Tab. Bot. 100s.
Use: Skeletal muscle relaxant.
■**SKELETAL MUSCLE RELAXANTS.**
See: Anectine, Sol., Pow. (Burroughs Wellcome)
Mephenesin (Var. Mfr.)
Metubine Iodide, Vial (Lilly)
Neostig, Tab. (Freeport)
Paraflex, Tab. (McNeil)
Parafon Forte, Tab. (McNeil)
Quelicin, Fliptop & pintop vials, Syringe w/lancet, Ampules. (Abbott)
Rela, Tab. (Schering)
Robaxin, Tab., Inj. (Robins)
Skelaxin, Tab. (Robins)
Soma, Preps. (Wallace)
Sucostrin, Vial, Amp. (Squibb)
Syncurine, Vial (Burroughs Wellcome)
Trancopal, Cap. (Winthrop-Breon)
d-Tubocurarine Chloride (Var. Mfr.)

SK-ERYTHROMYCIN. (SmithKline) Erythromycin Stearate 250 mg./Film Coated Tab. Bot. 100s, 500s. 500 mg./Tab. Bot. 100s.
Use: Antibiotic.
SK-FUROSEMIDE. (SmithKline) Furosemide 20 or 40 mg./Tab. Bot. 100s, 500s.
Use: Diuretic.
SK-HYDROCHLOROTHIAZIDE. (SmithKline) Hydrochlorothiazide 25 mg. or 50 mg./Tab. Bot. 100s, 1000s.
Use: Treatment of edema, hypertension.
SKIN CARE. (Sween) Bot. unit-dose 2 oz., 9 oz.
Use: Cream for irritated skin.
SKIN DEGREASER. (Aeroceuticals) Freon 100%. Bot. 2 oz., 4 oz.
Use: Presurgical skin degreaser.
SKIN SHIELD LIQUID BANDAGE. (Commerce) Dyclonine HCl benzethonium Cl. Bot. 0.45 oz.
Use: Protection for cuts, bruises & scrapes.
SK-LYGEN. (SmithKline) Chlordiazepoxide HCl 5 mg., 10 mg., 25 mg./Cap. Bot. 100s, 500s.
Use: Relief of anxiety, tensions.
SK-OXYCODONE w/ACETAMINOPHEN. (SmithKline) Oxycodone HCl 5 mg., acetaminophen 325 mg./Tab. Bot 100s, 500s.
Use: Relief of moderate to moderately severe pain.
SK-OXYCODONE w/ASPIRIN. (SmithKline) Oxycodone HCl 4.5 mg., oxycodone terephthalate 0.38 mg., aspirin 325 mg./Tab. Bot. 100s.
Use: Relief of moderate to moderately severe pain.
SK-PENICILLIN G. (SmithKline) Penicillin G Potassium 400,000 u./Tab. Bot. 100s, 1000s. 800,000 u./Tab. Bot. 100s.
Use: Infections.
SK-PENICILLIN VK. (SmithKline) Penicillin V potassium. **Oral Sol.:** 125 mg., 250 mg./5 ml. Bot. 100 ml., 200 ml.; **Tab.:** 250 mg. Bot. 100s, 500s, 1000s; 500 mg. Bot. 100s.
Use: Infections.
SK-PHENOBARBITAL. (SmithKline) Phenobarbital 15, 30 mg./Tab. Bot. 1000s.
Use: Sedative, hypnotic.
SK-POTASSIUM CHLORIDE. (SmithKline) Potassium chloride. 10%: Each 30 ml. contains 40 mEq. potassium chloride, alcohol 5%. **20%:** Each 30 ml. contains 80 mEq. potassium chloride, 5% alcohol. Bot. 16 oz..
Use: Treatment of hypopotassemia.
SK-PRAMINE. (SmithKline) Imipramine HCl 10 mg./Tab. Bot. 100s; 25 mg./Tab. Bot. 100s, 1000s; 50 mg./Tab. Bot. 100s, 1000s.
Use: Antidepressant.
SK-PREDNISONE. (SmithKline) Prednisone 5 mg./Tab. Bot. 100s, 1000s.
Use: Adrenocortical Steroid (antiinflammatory).
SK-PROBENECID. (SmithKline) Probenecid 500 mg./Tab. Bot. 100s, 1000s.
Use: Treatment of hyperuicemia associated with gout.
SK-PROPANTHELINE BROMIDE. (SmithKline) Propantheline bromide 15 mg./Tab. Bot. 100s, 1000s.

Use: Adjunctive ulcer therapy for treatment of peptic ulcer.

SK-QUINIDINE SULFATE. (SmithKline) Quinidine Sulfate 200 mg./Tab. Bot. 100s, 500s, 1000s.
Use: Anti-arrhythmic.

SK-RESERPINE. (SmithKline) Reserpine 0.25 mg./Tab. Bot. 1000s.
Use: Antihypertensive.

SK-SOXAZOLE. (SmithKline) Sulfisoxazole 500 mg./Tab. Bot. 100s.
Use: Urinary tract infections.

SK-TERPIN HYDRATE AND CODEINE ELIXIR. (Smith-Kline) Terpin hydrate 85 mg., codeine 10 mg./5 ml. Bot. 4 oz., 16 oz.
Use: Antitussive.

SK-TETRACYCLINE CAPSULES. (SmithKline) Tetracycline HCl 250 mg./Cap. Bot. 100s, 1000s. 500 mg./Cap. Bot. 100s.
Use: Antibiotic.

SK-TETRACYCLINE SYRUP. (SmithKline) Tetracycline 125 mg./5 ml. w/methylparaben 0.12%, propylparaben 0.03%/5 ml. w/alcohol 1%. Bot. pt.
Use: Antibiotic.

SK-THIORIDAZINE HCL. (SmithKline) Thioridazine HCl 10, 25, or 50 mg./Tab. Bot. 100s, 1000s.
Use: Antipsychotic, sedative.

SK-TOLBUTAMIDE. (SmithKline) Tolbutamide 500 mg./Tab. Bot. 100s, 1000s.
Use: Antidiabetic.

SLEEP II. (Walgreen) Diphenhydramine HCl 25 mg./Tab. Bot. 16s, 32s, 72s.
Use: Sleep aid.

SLEEP AID. (Burgin-Arden) Scopolamine aminoxide 0.50 mg./Cap. Bot. 100s.

SLEEP CAP. (Weeks & Leo) Diphenhydramine HCl 50 mg./Cap. Vials 25s, 50s.
Use: Induce relaxed sleep.

SLEEP-EZE TABLETS. (Whitehall) Diphenhydramine HCl 25 mg./Tab. Pkg. 12s, 26s, 52s.
Use: Mild sedative, soporific.

SLEEP TABS. (Towne) Scopolamine aminoxide HBr 0.2 mg., salicylamide 250 mg./Tab. Bot. 36s, 90s.
Use: Sleep aid.

SLEEP TABLET. (Walgreen) Pyrilamine maleate 25 mg./Tab. Bot 32s, 72s, 16s.
Use: Sleep aid.

SLENDER. (Carnation) Skim milk, veg. oils, caseinates, vitamins, minerals. **Liquid:** 220 cal./ 10 oz. Can. **Powder:** 173 or 200 cal. mixed w/6 oz. skim or low fat milk. Pkg 1 oz.
Use: Diet food.

SLENDER-X. (Progressive Drugs) Phenylpropanolamine, methylcellulose, caffeine, vitamins/Tab. Pkg. 21s, 42s, 84s. Gum 20s, 60s.

SLIMETTES. (Blue Cross) Phenylpropanolamine HCl 35 mg., caffeine 140 mg./Cap. Box 20s.
Use: Appetite depressant.

SLIM-FAST. (Thompson Medical) Meal replacement powder mixed with milk to replace 1, 2 or 3 meals a day.

SLIM-LINE. (Thompson Medical) Benzocaine, dextrose/Chewing gum. Box 36s, 60s.

SLIM PLAN PLUS. (Whitworth) Phenylpropanolamine HCl 75 mg., caffeine 200 mg./Tab. Box 40s.
Use: Appetite control.

SLIM-TABS. (Wesley) Phendimetrazine tartrate 35 mg./Tab. Bot. 1000s.

SLOAN'S LINIMENT. (Warner-Lambert) Capsicum oleoresin 0.62%, methyl salicylate 2.66%, oil of camphor 3.35%, turpentine oil 46.76%, oil of pine 6.74%. Bot. 2 oz., 7 oz.
Use: Counterirritant, rubefacient.

SLO-BID GYROCAPS. (Rorer) Theophylline anhydrous 50 mg., 100 mg., 200 mg., or 300 mg./Timed Release Cap. Bot. 100s, 1000s. Unit dose.
Use: Bronchodilator.

SLO-PHYLLIN 80 SYRUP. (Rorer) Theophylline 80 mg./15 ml. Nonalcoholic. Bot. 4 oz., pt., gal., Unit dose 15 ml.
Use: Bronchodilator.

SLO-PHYLLIN GG. (Rorer) Theophylline 150 mg., guaifenesin 90 mg./Cap. or 15 ml. syrup. **Cap.** Bot. 100s. **Syr.** Bot. pt.

SLO-PHYLLIN GYROCAPS. (Rorer) Theophylline anhydrous 60 mg., 125 mg. or 250 mg./T.R. Cap. Bot. 100s, 1000s. Unit dose.
Use: Bronchodilator.

SLO-PHYLLIN TABLETS. (Rorer) Theophylline anhydrous 100 mg. or 200 mg./Tab. Bot. 100s, 1000s. Unit dose.
Use: Bronchodilator.

SLOW-K. (Ciba) Potassium Chloride Bot. 100s, 1000s. Accu-Pak units of 100. Consumer Packs 100s.
Use: Potassium supplement.

SLOW FE. (Ciba) Dried ferrous sulfate 160 mg./Tab. Bot. 30s.
Use: Iron deficiency anemia.

SLT. (Western Research) Sodium levo-thyroxine 0.1 mg., 0.2 mg. or 0.3 mg. /Tab. Bot. 1000s.
Use: Hyprothyroidism treatment.

SLYN-LL. (Edwards) Phendimetrazine tartrate 105 mg./T.R. Cap. Bot. 100s.
Use: Appetite suppressant.

S-M-A FORMULA. (Wyeth) **Liquid.** The 40:60 casein: whey protein ratio is like that of human milk. Iron (as ferrous sulfate) 12 mg./qt. Liquid, Ready-to-feed 8 oz., 32 fl. oz. **Concentrated Liquid.** Can 13 fl. oz. **Powder** Can 1 lb.
Use: For infant feeding.

SMALL FRY CHEWABLE TABS. (Approved) Vit. A 5000 I.U., D 1000 I.U., B-12 5 mcg., B-1 3 mg., B-2 2.5 mg., B-6 1 mg., C 50 mg., niacinamide 20 mg., Cal. pantothenate 1 mg., E 1 I.U., l-lysine 15 mg., biotin 10 mg./Tab. Bot. 100s, 250s, 365s.

• **SMALLPOX VACCINE,** U.S.P. XXI. (Lederle, Avianized)—Tube 1s, 5s, 10s, vaccinations. 1 vaccination and needle in glass capillary tube. (Wyeth)—Tube 1s, 5s, 10s, vaccinations. Vaccinia Immune Globulin (Human), Inj. (Hyland) W/Brilliant Green 1s, 10s.

Use: Active immuniziing agent.
SMURF. (Mead Johnson) Multivitamin. Bot. 60s
Use: Multivitamin
SMURF WITH IRON & ZINC. (Mead Johnson) Multivitamin with iron and zinc. Bot. 60s.
Use: Multivitamin and mineral supplement.
SN-13, 272.
See: Primaquine Phos., U.S.P. XXI. (Var. Mfr.)
SNAKE VENOM.
Use: S.C., I.M. & orally; trypanosomiasis.
See: Antivenin. (Wyeth)
SNAP PAK ASPIRIN. (DeWitt) Aspirin 325 mg./Tab. Pak 16 Tabs.
Use: Analgesic.
SOACLENS. (Alcon) Thiomerosal 0.004%, EDTA 0.1%. Bot. 5 cc., 4 oz.
Use: Contact lens soaking and wetting solution.
SOAKARE. (Allergan) Benzalkonium chloride 0.01%, edetate disodium, buffer and purified water. Bot. 4 fl. oz.
Use: Hard contact lens soaking solution.
■ **SOAPS, GERMICIDAL.**
See: Dial, Preps. (Armour)
  Fostex, Cake, Cream, Liq. (Westward)
  pHisoHex, Liq. (Winthrop-Breon)
  Thylox, Shampoo, Soap (Dent)
■ **SOAP SUBSTITUTES.**
See: Acne-Dome, Cleanser (Miles Pharm)
  Domerine, Shampoo (Miles Pharm)
  Lowila, Cleanser (Westwood)
  pHisoDerm, Preps. (Winthrop Products)
SOCYLATE. (Tunex) Sodium thiosalicylate 50 mg./ml. w/benzyl alcohol 2% as preservative. In water for injection. Vial 30cc.
Use: Analgesic, antipyretic.
• **SODA LIME,** N.F. XVI.
Use: Carbon dioxide absorbant.
SODA MINT. (Bowman) Sodium bicarbonate 5 gr., oil peppermint q.s./Tab. Bot. 100s, 1000s.
SODA MINT TABLETS. (Lilly) Sodium bicarbonate 5 gr., oil peppermint q.s./Tab. Bot. 100s.
SODASONE. (Fellows) Prednisolone sod. phosphate 20 mg., niacinamide 25 mg./ml. Vial 10 ml.
Use: Adrenocortical hormone therapy.
• **SODIUM ACETATE,** U.S.P. XXI. Inj., Soln., U.S.P. XXI. Acetic acid, sodium salt, trihydrate. (Abbott) 40 mEq., 20 ml. in 50 ml. Fliptop Vial.
Use: Alkalizer; pharmaceutic acid (in solution for hemodialysis & peritoneal dialysis.)
SODIUM ACETATE & THEOPHYLLINE.
• **SODIUM ACETAZOLAMIDE.** Acetazolamide Sodium, U.S.P. XXI.
Use: Carbonic anhydrase inhibitor.
SODIUM ACETOSULFONE. Sodium 2-N-acetylsulfamyl-4,4′-diaminodiphenylsulfone.
Use: Leprostatic agent.
See: Promacetin, Tab. (Parke-Davis)
SODIUM ACETRIZOATE INJECTION, B.A.N. Sodium 3-acetamino-2,4,6-triiodobenzoate, Diaginol.
Use: Radio-opaque substance.
See: Salpix, Vial (Ortho)

SODIUM ACID PHOSPHATE.
See: Sodium Biphosphate (Various Mfr.)
SODIUM ACTINOQUINOL. 8-Ethoxy-5-quinoline sulfonic acid sodium salt.
Use: Treatment of flash burns (ophthalmic).
See: Uviban
SODIUM ALGINATE, N.F. XVI.
Use: Suspending agent.
See: Algin
  Kelgin (Kelco)
SODIUM AMINOBENZOATE. Sodium p-aminobenzoate.
Use: Dermatomyositis and scleroderma.
SODIUM AMINOPTERIN. Aminopterin Sod.
SODIUM AMINOSALICYLATE.
See: Aminosalicylate Sodium, U.S.P. XXI.
SODIUM AMOBARBITAL. Amobarbital Sodium, U.S.P. XXI.
• **SODIUM AMYLOSULFATE.** USAN. Sod. salt of potato amylopectin. Depepsin.
Use: Peptic ulcer.
SODIUM ANAZOLENE. 4-[(4-Anilino-5-sulfo-1-naphthyl)azo]-5-hydroxy-2,7-naphthalene disulfonic acid trisodium salt.
Use: Diagnostic aid for blood volume and cardiac output.
SODIUM ANOXYNAPHTHONATE. B.A.N. Sodium 4′-anilino-8-hydroxy-1,1′-azonaphthalene-3,-5′,6-trisulfonate.
Use: Investigation of cardiac disease.
See: Anazolene Sodium (I.N.N.)
  Coomassie Blue
SODIUM ANTIMONYLGLUCONATE. B.A.N. Sodium salt of a trivalent antimony derivative of gluconic acid.
Use: Treatment of schistosomiasis.
See: Triostam
SODIUM APOLATE. B.A.N. (Lloyd Bros.) Sodium ethenesulfonate polymer.
Use: Anticoagulant.
See: Pergalen
  Peson (Hoechst)
  Sod. Lyapolate
• **SODIUM ARSENATE AS 74.** USAN.
Use: Radioactive agent.
• **SODIUM ASCORBATE,** U.S.P. XXI. Monosodium L-ascorbate.
Use: Pharmaceutic necessity for Ascorbic acid Injection.
See: Cenolate, Inj. (Abbott)
  Liqui-Cee, Bot. (Arnar-Stone)
  Sodascorbate, Tab. (Mosso)
  Vitac Injection, Vial (Hickman)
SODIUM AUROTHIOMALATE.
See: Gold Sodium Thiosulfate, U.S.P. XXI.
• **SODIUM BENZOATE,** N.F. XVI.
Use: Pharm. aid (antifungal agent, preservative).
SODIUM BENZYLPENICILLIN. Penicillin G Sodium, U.S.P. XXI. Sodium Penicillin G.
Use: Antibiotic.
• **SODIUM BICARBONATE,** U.S.P. XXI. Inj., Oral Powder, Tabs, U.S.P. XXI. (Abbott) Injection. **4.2%:**

(5 mEq) Infant 10 ml. Syringe (21 G × 1.5 in. needle). **7.5%:** (44.6 mEq) 50 ml. Syringe (18 G x 1.5 in. needle) or 50 ml. Amp. **8.4%:** (10 mEq) Pediatric 10 ml. Syringe (21 G × 1.5 in. needle) or (50 mEq) 50 ml. Syringe (18 G × 1.5 in. needle) or 50 ml. Vial.
Use: Antacid, electrolyte replenisher systemical alkalizer.
W/Bismuth subcarbonate and Magnesia.
See: Anachloric A, Tab. (Upjohn)
W/Sodium Bitartrate.
See: Ceo-Two, Supp. (Beutlich)
Col-Evac, Supp. (Fellows)
W/Sodium carboxymethylcellulose, alginic acid.
See: Pretts, Tabs. (Marion)
SODIUM BIPHOSPHATE.
Use: Cathartic.
See: Sodium Phosphate Monobasic, U.S.P. XXI.
SODIUM BISMUTH TARTRATE.
See: Bismuth Sod. Tartrate, Preps.
SODIUM BISULFITE. Sulfurous acid, monosodium salt. Monosodium sulfite.
Use: Antioxidant.
• **SODIUM BORATE,** N.F. XVI.
Use: Pharm. aid (alkalizing agent).
SODIUM BUTABARBITAL.
See: Butabarbital Sodium, U.S.P. XXI.
SODIUM CALCIUMEDETATE. B.A.N. Calcium chelate of the disodium salt of ethylenediamine-NNN'-N'-tetra-acetic acid.
Use: Treatment of lead poisoning.
See: Calcium Disodium Versenate.
SODIUM CALCIUM EDETATE.
See: Calcium Disodium Versenate, Amp., Tab. (Riker)
• **SODIUM CARBONATE,** N.F. XVI.
Use: Pharm aid (alkalizing agent).
SODIUM CARBOXYMETHYLCELLULOSE.
Carboxymethylcellulose Sodium, U.S.P. XXI. CMC. Cellulose Gum.
SODIUM CELLULOSE GLYCOLATE.
See: Carboxymethylcellulose, Sod. (Various Mfr.)
SODIUM CEPHALOTHIN. Cephalothin Sodium, U.S.P. XXI.
Use: Antibiotic.
• **SODIUM CHLORIDE,** U.S.P. XXI. Inhalation Soln., Inj., Bacteriostatic for Inj., Irrigation, Ophth. Soln., Tab., Tab. for Soln., U.S.P. XXI.
Use: Fluid and Irrigation, electrolyte replenisher, isotonic vehicle.
• **SODIUM CHLORIDE AND DEXTROSE TABLETS,** U.S.P. XXI.
Use: Electrolyte and nutrient replenisher.
• **SODIUM CHLORIDE INJECTION,** U.S.P. XXI.
(Abbott) - Normal Saline 0.9% available in 150 ml., 250 ml., 500 ml. and 1,000 ml. cont.; **Partial-fills:** 50 ml. in 200 ml., 50 ml. in 300 ml., and 100 ml. in 300 ml.; **fliptop vials:** 10 ml., 20 ml., 50 ml. and 100 ml.,; **Bacteriostatic vials:** 10 ml., 20 ml. and 30 ml.; 50 mEq, 20 ml. in 50 ml. fliptop or pintop vial; 100 mEq, 40 ml. in 50 ml. fliptop vial; 50 mEq, 20 ml. univ. add. syr.; Sod. Chl. 0.45%, 500 ml. and

1,000 ml.; Sod. Chl. 5%, 500 ml.; Sodium Chloride Irrigating Sol., 250 ml., 500 ml., 1,000 ml., 3,000 ml.; (Upjohn) Sodium chloride 9 mg./ml. w/benzyl alcohol 9.45 mg. Vial 20 ml. (Winthrop-Breon) **Carpuject:** 2 ml. fill cartridge, 22 gague 1 1/4 inch needle or 25 gauge 5/8 inch needle.
Use: Fluid and irrigation, electrolyte replenisher, isotonic vehicle.
• **SODIUM CHLORIDE Na 22.** USAN.
Use: Radioactive agent.
SODIUM CHLORIDE SUBSTITUTES.
See: Salt substitutes.
SODIUM CHLORIDE TABLETS, U.S.P. XXI.
(Parke-Davis) Sodium chloride 15 1/2 gr./Tab. Bot. 1000s.
Use: Preparation of normal saline solution.
SODIUM CHLORIDE THERAPY.
See: Thermolene, Tab. (Lannett)
Thermotabs., Tab. (Calgon)
SODIUM CHLOROTHIAZIDE, FOR INJECTION.
Chlorothiazide Sodium For Injection, U.S.P. XXI.
Use: Diuretic.
SODIUM CHOLATE. (City Chem.) Sodium cholate Bot. 100 Gm.
• **SODIUM CHROMATE Cr 51 INJ.,** U.S.P. XXI.
Use: Diagnostic aid (blood volume determination).
See: Radio Chromate Cr 51 Sodium
• **SODIUM CITRATE,** U.S.P. XXI. 1,2,3-Propanetricarboxylic acid, 2-hy-droxy-, trisodium salt. Trisodium citrate. Trisodium citrate dihydrate.
Use: Anticoagulant.
See: Anticoagulant Citrate Dextrose Solution, U.S.P. XXI.
Anticoagulant Citrate Phosphate Dextrose Solution, U.S.P. XXI.
• **SODIUM CITRATE AND CITRIC ACID ORAL SOLUTION,** U.S.P. XXI. Shohl's Solution.
Use: Systemic alkalizer.
SODIUM CLOXACILLIN.
See: Cloxacillin Sodium, U.S.P. XXI.
SODIUM COLISTIMETHATE. Colistimethane Sodium, Sterile, U.S.P. XXI. Antibiotic produced by Aerobacillus colistinus.
SODIUM COLISTIN METHANESULFONATE.
Colistimethane Sodium, U.S.P. XXI. The sodium methanesulfonate salt of an antibiotic substance elaborated by Aerobacillus colistinus.
Use: Antibiotic.
• **SODIUM DEHYDROACETATE,** N.F. XVI.
Use: Pharmaceutic aid (antimicrobial preservative).
SODIUM DEXTROTHYROXINE. Sodium D-3,3',5,5'-tetraiodothyronine. Sodium D-3-(4-(4-Hydroxy-3,5-diiodophenoxy)-3,5-diiodophenyl)-alanine.
Use: Anticholesteremic.
SODIUM DIATRIZOATE. Diatrizoate Sodium, U.S.P. XXI.
Use: Radiopaque medium.
SODIUM DIBUNATE. B.A.N. Sodium 2,7-di-t-butylnaphthalene-1-sulfonate.
Use: Cough suppressant.
See: Becantyl

SODIUM[2,3-DICHLORO-4-(2-METHYLENEBUTYRYL)-PHENOXY]ACETATE. Ethacrynate Sodium for Injection, U.S.P. XXI.
SODIUM DICLOXACILLIN. Dicloxacillin Sodium, U.S.P. XXI.
Use: Antibiotic.
SODIUM DICLOXACILLIN MONOHYDRATE.
Use: Antibiotic.
See: Pathocil, Prep. (Wyeth)
SODIUM DIHYDROGEN PHOSPHATE. Sodium Biphosphate U.S.P. XXI.
SODIUM DIMETHOXYPHENYL PENICILLIN.
See: Methicillin Sodium (Var. Mfr.)
SODIUM DIOCTYL SULFOSUCCINATE.
See: Docusate Sodium U.S.P. XXI.
SODIUM DIPHENYLHYDANTOIN. Phenytoin Sodium, U.S.P. XXI. Diphenylhydantoin Sodium.
Use: Anticonvulsant.
SODIUM DIPROTRIZOATE, B.A.N. Sodium 3,5-dipropionamide-2,4,6-triiodobenzoate.
SODIUM DIURIL INTRAVENOUS. (Merck Sharp & Dohme) Chlorothiazide sodium equiv. to 0.5Gm. chlorothiazide w/mannitol 0.25 Gm., sod. hydroxide, thimerosal 0.4 mg./vial.
Use: Diuretic, antihypertensive.
SODIUM EDECRIN INTRAVENOUS. (Merck Sharp & Dohme) Ethacrynate sod. equiv. to 50 mg. ethacrynic acid w/mannitol 62.5 mg., thimerosal 0.1 mg./Vial (50 mg.)
Use: Diuretic.
SODIUM EDETATE, Edetate Disodium, U.S.P. XXI. Tetrasodium ethylenediaminetetraacetate.
Use: Chelating agents.
See: Vagisec products (Julius Schmid)
SODIUM ETHACRYNATE For INJ. Ethacrynate Sodium for Injection, U.S.P. XXI.
Use: Diuretic.
• **SODIUM ETHASULFATE.** USAN.
Use: Detergent.
SODIUM 6-(2-ETHOXY-1-NAPHTHAMIDO)-PENICILLANATE. Nafcillin Sodium, U.S.P. XXI.
SODIUM ETHYL-MERCURI-THIO-SALICYLATE.
See: Thimerosal, (Var. Mfr.)
    Merthiolate, Prep. (Lilly)
SODIUM FEREDETATE (I.N.N.). Sodium Ironedetate, B.A.N.
SODIUM FLUORESCEIN, Fluorescein Sodium U.S.P. XXI. Resorcinolphthalein sodium.
Use: Diagnostic aid (corneal trauma indicator).
• **SODIUM FLUORIDE,** U.S.P. XXI. Oral Soln, Tab, U.S.P. XXI.
Use: Prophylactic dental caries.
See: Dentafluor, Tab., Drops (Saron)
    Flura Drops, Drops (Kirkman)
    Flura-Loz, Lozenge (Kirkman)
    Karidium, Liq., Tab. (Lorvic)
    Kari-Rinse, Liq. (Lorvic)
    Luride, Tab. (Davies, Rose-Hoyt)
    NaFeen, Tab., Liq. (Pacemaker)
    Pediaflor, Drop (Ross)
    Solu-Flur, Tab. (Robinson)
    T-Fluoride, Tab. (Tennessee Pharm.)

W/Vitamins.
See: Fluorac, Tab. (USV)
    Luride, Tab. & Drops (Davies, Rose-Hoyt)
    Mulvidren-F, Tab. (Stuart)
    So-Flo, Tab., Drop (Professional Pharm.)
W/Vit. A, D, C.
See: Cari-Tab, Softab. (Stuart)
    Tri-Vi-Flor, Drops, Tab. (Mead Johnson)
SODIUM FLUORIDE SOLUTION PEDIATRIC DROPS
. (Moyco) 1.0 ml. once/day 0–3 yrs. 2.0 ml. once/day over 3 yrs. Bot. 50 ml.
Use: Aid in the prevention of dental caries.
• **SODIUM FLUORIDE AND PHOSPHORIC ACID GEL,** U.S.P. XXI.
• **SODIUM FLUORIDE AND PHOSPHORIC ACID TOPICAL SOLUTION,** U.S.P. XXI.
SODIUM FOLATE. Monosodium folate.
Use: Water-soluble, hematopoietic vitamin.
SODIUM FORMALDEHYDE SULFOXYLATE, N.F. XVI. (Various Mfr.) $H_2C(OH)SO_2Na$.
Use: Reducing agent; preservative.
SODIUM-FREE SALT.
See: Co-Salt, Bot. (USV Pharm.)
    Diasal, Prep. (Savage)
    Neocurtasal, Prep. (Winthrop Products)
SODIUM GAMMA-HYDROXYBUTYRIC ACID. Under study.
Use: Anesthetic adjuvant.
SODIUM GENTISATE.
See: Gentisate, Sod.
SODIUM GLUCALDRATE. B.A.N. Sodium gluconatodihydroxyaluminate.
Use: Treatment of gastric hyperacidity.
See: Glymaxil
SODIUM GLUCASPALDRATE, B.A.N. Octasodium tetrakis (gluconato)-bis (salicylato), μ-diacetatodialuminate(III) dihydrate.
Use: Analgesic.
SODIUM GLUCOSULFONE INJ. Disodium 1,1'-[Sulfonylbis(p-phenyleneimino)]bis-[D-gluco-2,3,4,5,6-pentahydroxy-1-hexanesulfonate].
Use: Leprostatic.
SODIUM GLUTAMATE.
See: Glutamate
SODIUM GLYCEROPHOSPHATE. Glycerol phosphate sodium salt.
Use: Pharmaceutic necessity.
SODIUM GLYCOCHOLATE, A BILE SALT.
See: Bile Salts.
W/Phenolphthalein, cascara sagrada ext., sodium taurocholate, aloin.
See: Oxiphen, Tab. (Webcon)
W/Sod. nitrite, blue flag.
See: So-Nitri-Nacea, Cap. (Scrip)
W/Sod. taurocholate, sod. salicylate, phenolphthalein, bile ext., cascara sagrada ext.
See: Glycols, Tab. (Bowman)
SODIUM HEPARIN. Heparin Sodium, U.S.P. XXI.
Use: Anticoagulant.
SODIUM HEXACYCLONATE. Sodium 1-hydroxymethylcyclohexaneacetate.

SODIUM HEXOBARBITAL. Sodium 5-(1-cyclohexen-1-yl)-1,5-dimethylbarbiturate.
Use: Intravenous general anesthetic.
SODIUM HYDROGEN CITRATE. (Various Mfr.)
• **SODIUM HYDROXIDE,** N.F. XVI. Caustic Soda.
Use: Pharm. aid (alkalizing agent).
SODIUM HYDROXYDIONE SUCCINATE. Sodium 21-hydroxypregnane-3,20-dione succinate.
• **SODIUM HYPOCHLORITE SOLUTION,** U.S.P. XXI.
Use: Local anti-infective; disinfectant.
See: Antiformin
Dakin's Soln.
Hyclorite
SODIUM HYPOPHOSPHITE. Sodium phosphinate.
Use: Pharmaceutic necessity.
SODIUM HYPOSULFITE.
See: Sodium Thiosulfate (Var. Mfr.)
SODIUM INDIGOTINDISULFONATE.
Indigotindisulfonate Sodium, U.S.P. XXI. Indigo Carmine.
Use: I.V., I.M., diagnostic aid for renal function determination.
• **SODIUM IODIDE,** U.S.P. XXI. Soln., U.S.P. XXI.
Use: Iodine therapy; Pharm. necessity for Iodine Tincture.
See: Guaiadol Aqueous Sol., Vial (Medical Chem.)
Prodide (Hickam)
W/Foreign protein, benzyl alcohol, phenol.
See: I-pro, Inj. (Century)
W/Iodinated peptone.
W/Potassium guaiacolsufonate.
See: Guaiadol Aqueous, Vial (Medical Chem.)
W/Potassium guaiacolsulfonate, chlorpheniramine maleate, sodium bisulfite.
See: Gomahist, Inj. (Burgin-Arden)
W/Sulfur, sod. citrate, phenol, benzyl alcohol.
See: Sulfo-Iodide, Inj. (Marcen)
• **SODIUM IODIDE I-125 SOLUTION,** U.S.P. XXI.
Use: Diagnostic aid (thyroid function determination).
• **SODIUM IODIDE I-131 CAPSULES & SOLUTION,** U.S.P. XXI.
Use: Diagnostic aid (thyroid function determination); antineoplastic; thyroid inhibitor.
See: Iodotope I-131 (Squibb)
Oriodide (Abbott)
Radiocaps (R)-131 (Abbott)
Theriodide (R)-131 (Abbott)
SODIUM IODIPAMIDE. Disodium 3,3'-(Adipoyl-diimino) bis-[2,4,6-triiodobenzoate].
Use: Radiopaque medium.
SODIUM ortho-IODOHIPPURATE. Iodohippurate Sodium, I-131 Injection, U.S.P. XXI.
See: Hippuran, Pow. (Mallinckrodt)
Hipputope (Squibb)
SODIUM IODOMETHAMATE. Disodium 1,4-dihydro-3,5-diiodo-1-methyl-4-oxo-2,6-pyridine dicarboxylate. (Iodoxyl, Pyelecton, Uropac)
SODIUM IODOMETHANE SULFONATE. Methiodal Sodium, U.S.P. XXI.
SODIUM IOTHALAMATE. Iothalmate Sodium Injection, U.S.P. XXI.
Use: Radiopaque medium.

See: Angio-Conray, Vial (Mallinckrodt)
W/Meglumine iothalamate.
See: Vascoray, Vial (Mallinckrodt)
SODIUM IOTHIOURACIL. Sod. 5-iodo-2-thiouracil.
SODIUM IPODATE. Ipodate Sodium, U.S.P. XXI.
Use: Radiopaque.
See: Biloptin
Oragrafin Sodium, Cap. (Squibb)
SODIUM IRONEDETATE. B.A.N. Iron chelate of the monosodium salt of ethylenediamine-NNN′N′-tetra-acetic acid.
Use: Treatment of iron-deficiency anemia.
See: Sodium Feredetate (I.N.N.)
Sytron
SODIUM ISOAMYLETHYLBARBITURATE.
See: Amytal Sodium, Prep. (Lilly)
• **SODIUM LACTATE INJECTION,** U.S.P. XXI.
Propanoic acid, 2-hydroxy-, monosodium salt. Monosodium lactate. (Abbott) 1/6 Molar, 250 ml., 500 ml., and 1,000 ml.; 50 mEq, 10 ml. in 20 ml. fliptop vial.
Use: Fluid and electrolyte replenisher.
• **SODIUM LACTATE SOLUTION,** U.S.P. XXI.
• **SODIUM LAURYL SULFATE,** N.F. XVI. Sulfuric acid monododecyl ester sodium salt. Sodium monododecyl sulfate.
Use: Pharm aid (Surfactant).
See: Duponol
W/Aluminum ammonium sulfate, boracic acid, citric acid, menthol.
See: Femid Green Label, Pow. (Cenci)
W/9-Aminoacridine HCl, phenylmercuric acetate, succinic acid.
See: Vagiserts W/Inserts, Tab. (Vortech)
W/Hydrocortisone.
See: Nutracort, Cream, Lot. (Owen)
W/Danthron.
See: Alu-Scop, Cap., Susp. (Westerfield)
W/Iodoquinol, phenylmercuric acetate, lactose, pot. alum., papain.
See: Baculin, Tab. (Amfre-Grant)
SODIUM LEVOTHYROXINE. Levothyroxine Sodium, U.S.P. XXI.
SODIUM LIOTHYRONINE. Liothyronine Sodium, U.S.P. XXI.
Use: Thyroid hormone.
SODIUM LYAPOLATE. Polyethylene sulfonate sodium. Peson (Hoechst). Sodium Apolate, B.A.N.
Use: Anticoagulant.
SODIUM MALONYLUREA.
See: Barbital Sod. (Various Mfr.)
SODIUM MERALEIN. (Hynson, Westcott & Dunning) Mono-sodium salt of 2,7-diiodo-4-hydroxy-mercuriresorcinsulfonphthalein. Merodicein.
Use: Local anti-infective.
SODIUM MERCAPTOMERIN. Mercaptomerin Sodium, U.S.P. XXI.
Use: Diuretic.
• **SODIUM METABISULFITE,** N.F. XVI.
SODIUM METHIODAL. Methiodal Sodium, U.S.P. XXI. Sodium monoiodomethanesulfonate. Sodium Iodomethanesulfonate, Inj.

Use: Radiopaque medium.
SODIUM METHOHEXITAL FOR INJECTION.
Methohexital Sodium for Injection, U.S.P. XXI.
Use: General anesthetic.
See: Brevital Sod., Pow. (Lilly)
SODIUM METHOXYCELLULOSE. Mixture of
methylcellulose and sod. CMC
SODIUM METRIZOATE, B.A.N. Sodium 3-acetamido-
2,4,6-triiodo-5-(N-methyl-acetamido) benzoate.
Use: Contrast medium.
See: Triosil
• **SODIUM MONOFLUOROPHOSPHATE,** U.S.P.
XXI.
SODIUM MORRHUATE, INJ. Morrhuate Sodium Inj.,
U.S.P. XXI.
Use: Sclerosing agent.
SODIUM NAFCILLIN. Nafcillin Sodium, U.S.P. XXI.
Use: Antibacterial.
SODIUM NICOTINATE. Sod. pyridine-3-carboxylate
(Various Mfr.)
W/Adenosine 5 monophosphoric acid.
Use: I.V., nicotinic acid therapy.
See: Rodesine, Inj. (Rocky Mtn.)
SODIUM NITRATE. (Var. Mfr.) Granules, Pkg. 1 lb.
W/Sod. nitrite, ox bile & exhinacea.
See: Hyper-Zem, Tab. (Zemmer)
• **SODIUM NITRITE,** U.S.P. XXI. Inj., U.S.P. XXI.
(Various Mfr.) Gran., Bot. ¼ lb., 1 lb.
See: Anti-Rust, Tabs. (Winthrop-Breon)
W/Sodium Thiosulfate, amyl nitrite.
Use: Vasodilator and antidote to cyanide poisoning.
See: Cyanide Antidote Pkg. (Lilly)
SODIUM NITRATE COMBINATIONS.
See: Hyperlon, Tab. (Kenyon)
Hyper-Zem, Tab. (Zemmer)
Veraphen, Tab. (Davis and Sly)
Veratrum, Tab. (Vortech)
• **SODIUM NITROPRUSSIDE,** U.S.P. XXI. Sterile,
U.S.P. XXI.
Use: Hypotensive agent
See: Keto-Diastix (Ames)
Nipride, Vial (Roche)
Nitropress, Vial (Abbott)
**SODIUM NORAMIDOPYRINE
METHANESULFONATE.** Dipyrone, B.A.N.
SODIUM NOVOBIOCIN. Sodium salt of antibacterial
substance produced by *Streptomyces niveus.*
Novobiocin monosodium salt.
Use: Antibiotic.
See: Albamycin, Cap., Syr., Vial (Upjohn)
• **SODIUM OXYBATE.** USAN. Sodium 4-hydroxybuty-
rate.
Use: Adjunct to anesthesia.
SODIUM PANTOTHENATE.
Use: Orally, dietary supplement.
SODIUM PARA-AMINOBENZOATE.
See: p-Aminobenzoate, Sod. (Various Mfr.)
SODIUM PARAAMINOHIPPURATE INJECTION.
Use: I.V., to determine kidney tubular excretion
function.
SODIUM PARA-AMINOSALICYLATE.
See: p-Aminosalicylate, Sod. (Various Mfr.)

SODIUM PENICILLIN G. Penicillin G Sodium, Sterile,
U.S.P. XXI. Sodium benzylpenicillin.
SODIUM PENICILLIN O. Sodium-6-[2-(allylthio)-
acetamido]-3,3-dimethyl-7-oxo-4-thia-1-azabicyclo-
[3.2.0]heptane-2-carboxylate.
**SODIUM 3,3-PENTAMETHYLENE-4-HYDROXYBUTY-
RATE.** Hexacyclonate Sodium. Under study.
SODIUM PENTOBARBITAL. Pentobarbital Sodium,
U.S.P. XXI.
Use: Hypnotic.
SODIUM PERBORATE. Sodium Peroxyborate.
Sodium peroxyhydrate.
SODIUM PEROXYBORATE.
See: Sod. Perborate. (Var. Mfr.)
SODIUM PEROXYHYDRATE.
See: Sodium Perborate (Var. Mfr.)
• **SODIUM PERTECHNETATE Tc 99 m INJECTION,**
U.S.P. XXI. Pertechnetic acid, sodium salt.
Use: Diagnostic aid (brain scanning; thyroid
scanning.)
See: Minitec (Squibb)
SODIUM PHENOBARBITAL. Phenobarbital Sodium,
U.S.P. XXI.
Use: Anticonvulsant, hypnotic.
SODIUM PHENYLETHYLBARBITURATE.
Phenobarbital Sodium, U.S.P. XXI.
• **SODIUM PHOSPHATE,** U.S.P. XXI. Dired,
Effervescent, Inj., U.S.P. XXI. Disodium hydrogen
phosphate. (Abbott) 45 mM P, 15 ml. in 30 ml.
fliptop vial.
Use: Cathartic, buffering agent, source of
phosphate.
W/Gentamicin sulfate, monosodium phosphate,
sodium chloride, benzalkonium chloride.
See: Garamycin Ophthalmic Sol. (Schering)
W/Sod. biphosphate.
See: Enemeez, Enema (Armour)
Fleet Enema (Fleet)
Phospho-Soda, Liq. (Fleet)
Saf-tip, Enemas (Fuller)
• **SODIUM PHOSPHATE, DIBASIC,** U.S.P. XXI.
• **SODIUM PHOSPHATE, DRIED,** U.S.P. XXI.
Use: Cathartic.
• **SODIUM PHOSPHATE, MONOBASIC,** U.S.P. XXI.
Monosodium Phosphate. Sod. Acid Phosphate,
Sod. Dihydrogen Phosphate, Sodium Biphosphate.
Use: Cathartic.
See: Travad, Enema (Flint)
W/Gentamicin sulfate, disodium phosphate, sodium
chloride, benzalkonium chloride.
See: Garamycin Ophthalmic Sol. (Schering)
W/Methenamine.
See: Uro-Phosphate, Tab. (Poythress)
W/Methenamine mandelate, levo-hyoscyamine sulfate.
See: Levo-Uroquid, Tab. (Beach)
W/Methenamine, phenyl salicylate, methylene blue,
hyoscyamine, alkaloid.
See: Urostat Forte, Tab. (Elder)
W/Sod. acid pyrophos, sodium bicarbonate.
See: Vacuetts, Supp. (Dorsey)
W/Sod. phosphate.
See: Enemeez Enema (Armour)

Fleet Enema (Fleet)
Phospho-Soda, Liq. (Fleet)
Saf-tip Enemas (Fuller)
• **SODIUM PHOSPHATES ENEMA,** U.S.P. XXI.
Use: Cathartic.
• **SODIUM PHOSPHATES ORAL SOLUTION,** U.S.P.
XXI.
Use: Cathartic.
• **SODIUM PHOSPHATE P32 SOLUTION,** U.S.P. XXI.
Phosphoric -32P acid, disodium salt. Disodium phosphate -32P.
Use: Antineoplastic, antipolycythemic. Diagnostic.
aid (ocular tumor localization.).
SODIUM PHYTATE. Nonasodium phytate: Sod.
cyclohexanehexyl (hexaphosphate).
Use: Chelating agent.
SODIUM PICOSULPHATE. B.A.N. diSodium 4,4'-(2-
pyridyl)methylenedi(phenyl sulfate).
Use: Laxative.
See: Laxoberal
• **SODIUM POLYPHOSPHATE.** USAN.
Use: Pharmaceutic aid.
• **SODIUM POLYSTYRENE SULFONATE,** U.S.P. XXI.
Benzene, ethenyl-, homopolymer, sulfonated, sodium
salt. Styrene polymer, sulfonated, sodium salt.
Use: Ion exchange resin (potassium).
See: Kayexalate, Pow. (Winthrop-Breon)
• **SODIUM PROPIONATE,** N.F. XVI. 5% Soln. Eye
drops (Crookes-Barnes) Lacrivial 15 cc.
Use: Preservative.
W/Chlorophyll 'a'
See: Prophyllin, Pwd., Oint. (Rystan)
W/Neomycin sulfate.
See: Otobiotic, Ear Drops (Schering)
W/Propionic acid, docusate sodium, salicylic acid.
See: Prosal, Liq. (Gordon)
W/Sod. caprylate, propionic acid & undecylenic acid.
See: Sopronol, Pwd. (Wyeth)
W/Sod. caprylate, zinc caprylate, dioctyl sod.
sulfosuccinate, propionic acid.
See: Sopronol, Oint., Sol. (Wyeth)
W/Sodium chloride, methylene blue.
SODIUM PSYLLIATE.
Use: Sclerosing agent.
• **SODIUM PYROPHOSPHATE.** USAN.
Use: Pharmaceutic aid.
SODIUM RADIO CHROMATE INJ. Sod. Chromate Cr
51 Inj., U.S.P. XXI.
SODIUM RADIO IODIDE SOLUTION. Sodium Iodide
I-131 Solution, U.S.P. XXI.
Use: Thyroid tumors, hyperthyroidism & cardiac
dysfunction.
SODIUM RADIO-PHOSPHATE, P-32 Soln. Radio-
Phosphate P32 Solution. Sodium phosphate P-32 So-
lution, U.S.P. XXI.
SODIUM REMOVING RESINS.
See: Resins
SODIUM RHODANATE.
See: Sodium Thiocyanate
SODIUM RHODANIDE.
See: Sodium Thiocyanate
SODIUM SACCHARIN. Saccharin Sodium, U.S.P. XXI.

Use: Noncaloric sweetener.
• **SODIUM SALICYLATE,** U.S.P. XXI. Tab., U.S.P.
XXI.
Use: Analgesic.
See: Uracel, Tab. (Vortech)
W/Iodide. (Various Mfr.)
Use: Intravenous injection.
W/Iodide & cholchicine. (Various Mfr.)
Use: I.V., gout.
SODIUM SALICYLATE, NATURAL.
Use: Analgesic.
See: Alysine, Elixir (Merrell Dow)
SODIUM SALICYLATE COMBINATIONS.
See: Apcogesic, Tabs. (Apco)
Bisalate, Tab. (Allison)
Bufosal, Gran. (Table Rock)
Colsalide, Tab. (Vortech)
Corilin, Liq. (Schering)
Dibolans, Tab. (Noyes)
Gaysal-S, Tab. (Geriatric)
Glycols, Tab. (Bowman)
Laxogen, Tab. (Vortech)
Nucorsal, Tab. (Westerfield)
Pabalate, Tab. (Robins)
pHisoDan, Liq. (Winthrop Products)
Pedituss, Syr. (Sutliff & Case)
Ruphon, Tab. (Elder)
Ricor, Tab. (Vortech)
Salcoce, Tab. (Cole)
Thi-Cin, Cap. (Warren-Teed)
Thymaxol, Tab. (Noyes)
SODIUM SECOBARBITAL. Secobarbital Sodium,
U.S.P. XXI.
Use: Hypnotic.
**SODIUM SECOBARBITAL AND SODIUM
AMOBARBITAL CAPSULES.**
Use: Sedative.
See: Tuinal, Cap. (Lilly)
• **SODIUM STARCH GLYCOLATE,** N.F. XVI.
• **SODIUM STEARATE,** N.F. XVI. Octadecanoic acid,
sodium salt.
Use: Emulsifying and stiffening agent.
SODIUM STIBOGLUCONATE. B.A.N. Sodium salt of
a pentavalent antimony derivative of gluconic acid.
Use: Treatment of leishmaniasis.
See: Pentostam
SODIUM SUCCINATE.
Use: Alkalinize urine & awaken patients following
barbiturate anesthesia.
Sodium SULAMYD Ophthalmic Oint. 10% Sterile.
(Schering) Sulfacetamide sod. 10%. (100 mg.)
W/Methylparaben, propylparaben, benzalkonium Cl,
sorbitan monolaurate and water. Tube ⅛ oz.
Use: Ophthalmic Anti-infective.
Sodium SULAMYD Ophthalmic Sol. 10% Sterile.
(Schering) Sulfacetamide sodium 10% W/V
solution with methylcellulose, sod. thiosulfate,
methylparaben, propylparaben, sod. dihydrogen
phosphate. Bot. 5 ml. Box 25s. 15 ml. Box 1s.
Use: Ophthalmic Anti-infective.
**Sodium SULAMYD Ophthalmic Solution 30%
Sterile.** (Schering) Sulfacetamide sod. 30% W/V

w/sod. thiosulfate 1.5 mg., methylparaben 0.5 mg., propylparaben 0.1 mg. as preservative, sod. dihydrogen phosphate as buffer./ml. Bot. 15 ml. Box 1s.
Use: Ophthalmic Anti-infective.
SODIUM SULFABROMOMETHAZINE. Sodium N¹-(5-Bromo-4,6-dimethyl-2-pyrimidinyl) sulfanilamide.
Use: Antibacterial.
SODIUM SULFACETAMIDE.
See: Sulfacetamide Sodium Preps. (Various Mfr.)
SODIUM SULFADIAZINE.
See: Sulfadiazine Sodium Preps. (Various Mfr.)
SODIUM SULFAMERAZINE.
See: Sulfamerazine Sodium Preps. (Various Mfr.)
SODIUM SULFAPYRIDINE.
See: Sulfapyridine Sodium Pow. (Pfaltz & Bauer)
• **SODIUM SULFATE,** U.S.P. XXI. Inj., U.S.P. XXI.
Use: Cathartic.
• **SODIUM SULFATE S 35.** USAN.
Use: Radioactive agent.
SODIUM SULFATHIAZOLE.
Use: Antibacterial.
See: Sulfathiazole Sodium, Inj. (Various Mfr.)
SODIUM SULFOACETATE. W/Sod. alkyl aryl polyether sulfonate, docusate sodium, kerohydric, sulfur, salicylic acid, hexachlorophene.
See: Sebulex, Liq., Cream (Westwood)
SODIUM SULFOBROMOPHTHALEIN.
Sulfobromophthalein Sodium, U.S.P. XXI.
Use: Diagnostic aid (hepatic function determination).
SODIUM SULFOCYANATE.
See: Sodium Thiocyanate. (Var. Mfr.)
SODIUM SULFOXONE. Sulfoxone Sodium, U.S.P. XXI. Disodium sulfonylbis (p-phenyleneimino)dimethanesulfonate.
See: Diasone Sodium, Tab. (Abbott)
SODIUM SURAMIN.
See: Suramin Sodium
SODIUM TAUROCHOLATE, A BILE SALT.
See: Bile Salts.
W/Phenolphthalein, cascara sagrada ext. sodium glycocholate, aloin.
See: Oxiphen, Tab. (Webcon)
SODIUM TETRADECYL SULFATE.
See: Sotradecol, Inj. (Elkins-Sinn)
SODIUM TETRAIODOPHENOLPHTHALEIN.
See: Iodophthalein Sod. (Var. Mfr.)
SODIUM THIACETPHENARSAMIDE. The trivalent organic arsenical p-[bis-(carboxymethylmercapto)-arsino] benzamide. Ceparsolate Sodium (Abbott)
SODIUM THIAMYLAL FOR INJECTION. Thiamylal Sodium For Injection, U.S.P. XXI.
Use: General anesthetic.
See: Surital, Inj. (Parke-Davis)
SODIUM THIOCYANATE. Sodium Sulfocyanate. Sod. Rhodanide.
SODIUM THIOPENTAL.
See: Thiopental Sodium, U.S.P. XXI.
SODIUM THIOSALICYLATE.
See: Arthrolate, I.M. (Reid-Provident)
Osteolate, Vial (Fellows-Testagar)

Rexolate, Vial (Hyrex)
Socylate, Inj. (Tunex)
Thiodyne, Vial (Savage Lab.)
Thiolate (Hickam; Pharmex)
Thiosal, Inj. (Keene)
Th-Sal, Vial (Foy)
• **SODIUM THIOSULFATE,** U.S.P. XXI. Inj., U.S.P. XXI. Sod. hyposulfite. "Hypo." Thiosulfuric acid, disodium salt, pentahydrate. Disodium thiosulfate pentahydrate.
Use: For argyria, cyanide & iodine poisoning, arsphenamine reactions; prevention of spread of ringworm of feet.
W/Salicylic acid, hydrocortisone acetate, alcohol.
See: Komed HC, Lot. (Barnes-Hind)
W/Salicylic acid, isopropyl alcohol.
See: Tinver, Lotion (Barnes-Hind)
W/Salicylic acid, resorcinol, alcohol.
See: Mild Komed, Lot. (Barnes-Hind)
Komed, Lot. (Barnes-Hind)
W/Sodium nitrite, amyl nitrite.
See: Cyanide Antidote Pkg. (Lilly)
SODIUM L-THYROXINE.
See: Letter, Tab. (Armour)
Levoid, Inj., Tab. (Nutrition Control)
Roxstan, Tab. (Reid-Provident)
Synthroid, Tab., Inj. (Flint)
SODIUM TOLBUTAMIDE. Tolbutamide Sodium, U.S.P. XXI.
Use: Diagnostic aid (diabetes).
SODIUM TRICLOFOS. Sodium trichloroethylphosphate.
Use: Sedative, hypnotic.
• **SODIUM TRIMETAPHOSPHATE.** USAN.
Use: Pharmaceutic aid.
SODIUM TYROPANOATE, B.A.N. Sodium 3-butyramido-α-ethyl-2,4,6-triiodohydrocinnamate. Radiopaque.
Use: Cholecystographic agent.
See: Bilopaque, Cap. (Winthrop-Breon)
SODIUM VERSENATE. (Riker) Disodium Edetate Inj., U.S.P. 1 Gm./5 cc. 20% Amp. 15 ml. Box 5s.
See: Edathamil
Use: (I.V. infusions) Hypercalcemia.
SODIUM VINBARBITAL INJECTION.
Use: Sedative.
SODIUM WARFARIN. Warfarin Sodium, U.S.P. XXI.
Use: Anticoagulant.
SOD-LATE 10. (Schlicksup) Sodium salicylate 10 gr./Tab. Bot. 1000s.
Use: Analgesic.
SODUBEN. (Arcum) Butabarbital sodium 30 mg./Tab. Bot. 100s, 1000s.
Use: Sedative.
SOFCAPS. (Alton) Docusate sodium 100 mg., or 250 mg./Cap. Bot. 100s, 1000s.
Use: Stool softener.
SOF-CIL. (Zemmer) Psyllium mucilloid, plantago ovata, dextrose, docusate sodium 10 mg./rounded teaspoonful. Pkg. 2 oz., 6 oz., 12 oz.
Use: Treatment of constipation.
SOFENOL 5. (C & M Pharmacal) Collagen, allantoin, and dimethicone. Bot. 8 oz.

Use: Hand & body moisturizer.

SOFLENS ENZYMATIC CONTACT LENS CLEANER.
(Allergan) Stabilized papain tablets for solution.
W/Vials 12s, 24s, 48s. Refill 24s, 36s.
Use: Enzymatic cleansing agent for soft contact
lenses.

SOFT-B-M CAPSULE. (Morton) Docusate sodium 100
mg. or 250 mg./Cap. Bot. 100s.
Use: Stool softener.

SOFT-CARE STERILE DISINFECTING SOL.
(Barnes-Hind) Aqueous isotonic sol. of sodium Cl,
povidone, octylphenoxy ethanols w/ borate buffer.
Bot. 12 oz.
Use: Soft contact lens care.

SOFT'N SOOTHE. (Ascher) Benzocaine, menthol,
moisturizers. Tube 50 Gm.
Use: Dry, itchy skin.

SOFTOL CUTICLE REMOVER. (Guild) Bot. ½ oz.

SOFTON. (Stanlabs) Docusate sodium 100 mg., 250
mg./Cap. Bot. 100s.
Use: Laxative, constipation aid.

SOFT MATE COMFORT DROPS. (Barnes-Hind) Sterile,
aqueous, isotonic, buffered, lubricating & rewetting
solution w/edetate disodium 0.1%.
Use: Soft contact lens care.

SOFT-MATE SALINE SOLUTION. (Barnes-Hind) Ster-
ile aqueous isotonic solution of sodium chloride.
Bot. 8 oz., 12 oz.
Use: Soft contact lens care.

SOFT MATE WEEKLY CLEANING SOLUTION.
(Barnes-Hind) Non enzymatic surfactant cleaning so-
lution.
Use: Soft contact lens weekly cleaner.

SOLACEN. Tybamate, B.A.N.

SOLAGEST. (Canright) Pancreatin 10½ gr.,
hyoscyamine sulf. 0.072 mg., atropine sulf. 0.013
mg., hyoscine HBr 0.0047 mg., pentobarbital sod.
10.8 mg./Tab. Bot. 100s, 1000s.
Use: Antispasmodic, digestant formula.

SOLANEED. (Hanlon) Vit. A 25,000 u./Cap. Bot.
100s.

SOLAPSONE. B.A.N. Tetrasodium salt of bis-[4-(3-
phenyl-1,3-disulfopropylamino)phenyl]sulfone.
Use: Antileprotic.
See: Solasulfone (I.N.N.)
    Sulphetrone

SOLAQUIN. (Elder) Hydroquinone 2%, ethyl
dihydroxypropyl PABA 5%, dioxybenzone 3%,
oxybenzone 2%. Tube 1 oz.
Use: Skin bleaching agent with sunscreen.

SOLAQUIN FORTE CREAM. (Elder) Hydroquinone
4%, ethyl dihydroxypropyl PABA 5%, dioxybenzone
3%, oxybenzone 2% in a vanishing cream base.
Tube 1 oz.
Use: Skin bleaching agent with sunscreen.

SOLAQUIN FORTE GEL. (Elder) Hydroquinone 4%,
ethyl dihydroxypropyl-p-amino benzoate 5%, dioxybenzone 3% in hydroalcoholic base. Tubes 0.5 oz.,
1 oz.
Use: Skin bleaching agent with sunscreen.

SOLARCAINE. (Plough)
Cream: Benzocaine 1%, triclosan. Tube 0.5 oz., 1
oz., 2 oz.

Lotion: Benzocaine 0.5%, triclosan. Bot. 3 oz., 6
oz.
Spray (aerosol): Benzocaine 9.4%, triclosan
0.18%, isopropyl alcohol 24%. Can 3 oz, 5 oz.
Use: Sunburn remedy.

SOLAR CREAM. (Doak) PABA, titanium dioxide &
magnesium stearate in a flesh-colored, water-repellent base. Tube 1 oz.
Use: Protection from ultraviolet rays.

SOLARGENTUM.
See: Mild silver protein (Various Mfr.)

SOLATENE. (Roche) Beta-carotene 30 mg./cap. Bot.
100s.
Use: Ameliorate photosensitivity.

SOLBAR CREAM. (Person & Covey) Oxybenzone
3%, dioxybenzone 3%. Cream 1 oz., 2.5 oz.
Use: Ultraviolet protection.

SOLBAR PF. (Person & Covey) Oxybenzone 5%,
dioxybenzone 2% sunscreen. SP 10. Tube 2.5 oz.
Use: PABA free sunscreen.

SOLBAR PLUS 15. (Person & Covey) Oxybenzone
6%, octyl dimethyl PABA 6%. Tube 4 oz.
Use: Sunscreen (SPF 15).

SOLFOTON. (Poythress) Phenobarbital 16 mg.,
dispersed on colloidal bentonite./Tab. or Cap. Bot.
100s, 500s. Tabs. 100s, 500s.
Use: Orally, mild sedation.

SOLFOTON S/C TABS. (Poythress) Phenobarbital 16
mg., bensulfoid 65 mg./sugar coated Tab. Bot.
100s.
Use: Mild sedation.

SOLGANAL. (Schering) Aurothioglucose, 50 mg., /ml.
in sesame oil. Vial 10 ml.; Box 1s.
Use: I.M., gold therapy, antiarthritic.

SOLIWAX. Docusate Sodium, U.S.P. XXI. Docusate
Sodium, Solasulfone (I.N.N.).

SOLPADEINE TABLETS. (Winthrop Products)
Paracetamol.
Use: Analgesic.

SOL-PRED. (Amfre-Grant) Prednisolone sodium phosphate 20 mg./ml. Vial 10 ml.
Use: Hormone supplement.

SOLTEX. (C & M Pharmacal) Alkylaryl surfactant,
polyethylene glycol, alkanolamid conditioners,
orthobenzylparachlorophenol 0.1%. Bot. pt.
Use: Dermatologic shampoo.

SOLTICE HIGH THERM. (Chattem Labs.) Menthol,
methyl salicylate, camphor, eucalyptus oil. Tube
1¼ oz.
Use: Topical analgesic balm.

SOLTICE QUICK-RUB. (Chattem Labs.) Methyl salicylate, camphor, menthol, eucalyptol. Cream. 1½, 3¾
oz.
Use: Chest rub.

SOLU-BARB 0.25 TABLETS. (Fellows) Phenobarbital
¼ gr./Tab. Bot. 24s.

SOLUCAP C. (Jamieson-McKames) Vit. C 1000
mg./Capsulet. Bot. 100s.

SOLUCAP E. (Jamieson-McKames) Vit. E 100 I.U., 400
I.U., or 1000 I.U./Cap. Bot. 100s.

SOLU-CORTEF. (Upjohn) **100 mg.:** Hydrocortisone sodium succinate 100mg., sodium biphosphate 0.8
mg., sodium phosphate 8.73 mg./2 ml. Vial w/or

w/out ampoule bacteriostatic water for injection and benzyl alcohol 0.9% w/v. Vials 5s, 25s; Hydrocortisone sodium succinate 100 mg., sodium biphosphate 0.8 mg., sodium phosphate 8.76 mg., benzyl alcohol 18.1 mg. Mix-O-Vial 5s, 25s. **250 mg.:** Hydrocortisone sodium succinate 250 mg., sodium biphosphate 2 mg., sodium phosphate 21.8 mg., benzyl alcohol 16.4 mg./2 ml. Mix-O-Vial 1s, 5s, 25s. **500 mg.:** Hydrocortisone sodium succinate 500 mg., sodium biphosphate 4 mg., sodium phosphate 44 mg., benzyl alcohol 33.4 mg./4 ml. Mix-O-Vial 1s, 5s, 25s. **1000 mg.:** Hydrocortisone sodium succinate 1000 mg., sodium biphosphate 8 mg., sodium phosphate 88 mg., benzyl alcohol 66.9 mg./8 ml. Mix-O-Vial 1s, 5s, 10s.
Use: (I.V.) Treatment of acute adrenal cortical insufficiency.

SOLU-EXE. (O'Neal, Jones & Feldman) Hydroxyquinoline 0.12%, carbitol acetate 12.10%. Bot. 3 oz.

SOLU-FLUR. (Robinson) Sodium fluoride 2.21 mg./Tab. Bot. 100s, 1000s.
Use: Prophylactic dental caries.

SOLUJECT. (Mayrand) Prednisolone acetate 80 mg., prednisolone sodium phosphate 20 mg./ml. Vial 10 ml.
Use: Longacting/short acting anti-inflammatory.

SOLU-MEDROL. (Upjohn) **40 mg.:** Methylprednisolone sodium succinate 40 mg., lactose 25 mg., sodium biphosphate 1.6 mg., sodium phosphate 17.46 mg., benzyl alcohol 8.8 mg., water for injection q.s. 1 ml. Mix-O-Vial 1s, 5s, 25s, 50s, 100s; Mix-O-Vial 40 mg./1 ml. Pack 25s, 50s, 100s. **125 mg.:** Methylprednisolone sodium succinate 125 mg., sodium biphosphate 1.6 mg., sodium phosphate 17.4 mg., benzyl alcohol 17.6 mg., water for injection q.s. 2 ml. Mix-O-Vial 1s, 5s, 25s, 50s, 100s; Mix-O-Vial 125 mg./2 ml. Pack 25s, 50s, 100s. **500 mg.:** Methylprednisolone sodium succinate 500 mg., sodium biphosphate 6.4 mg., sodium phosphate 69.6 mg., benzyl alcohol 70.2 mg./Vial w ampoule bacteriostatic water for injection 8 ml., benzyl alcohol 9.45 mg./ml. Vials 1s, 5s, 25s. **1000 mg.:** Methylprednisolone sodium succinate 1000 mg., sodium biphosphate 12.8 mg., sodium phosphate 139.2 mg., benzyl alcohol 141 mg./Vial w ampoule bacteriostatic water for injection 16 ml., benzyl alcohol 9.45 mg./ml. Vials 1s, 5s, 25s; Vial 1000 mg. w/I.V. Administration set. Pack 1s, 5s, 25s. Vials without diluent 500 mg., 1000 mg.
Use: Treatment of emergency hypersensitivity.

SOLUMOL. (C & M Pharmacal) Petrolatum, mineral oil, cetyl-steryl alcohol, sodium lauryl sulfate, glycerin, propylene glycol, sorbic acid. Jars 1 lb.
Use: Washable ointment base.

SOLU-PRED. (Kenyon) Prednisolone sod. phosphate equiv. to prednisolone phosphate 20 mg., niacinamide 25 mg., disodium edetate 0.5 mg., sod. bisulfite 1 mg., phenol 5 mg./cc. Vial 10 cc.

SOLU PREDALONE. (O'Neal, Jones & Feldman) Prednisolone sodium phosphate 20 mg./ml. Vial 5 ml.

SOLUVITE-F. (Pharmics) Vit. A 3000 I.U., D 400 I.U., C 100 mg., fluoride 0.25 mg./0.6 cc. Bot. 57 cc.
Use: Fluoride therapy with vitamins.

SOLUREX. (Hyrex) Dexamethasone sodium phosphate 4 mg./ml. Vial 5 ml., 10 ml., 30 ml.
Use: Adrenocortical steroid therapy.

SOLUREX L A. (Hyrex) Dexamethasone acetate suspension 8 mg./ml. Vial 5 ml.
Use: Adrenocortical steroid therapy.

SOLU-SONE R.P. (Seatrace) Prednisolone sodium phosphate 20 mg., prednisolone acetate 80 mg./ml. Vial 10 cc.

SOLVISYN-A. (Towne) Water soluble Vit. A 10,000 u./Cap. 25,000 u./Cap. 50,000 u./Cap. Bot. 100s, 1000s.

• **SOLYPERTINE TARTRATE.** USAN. 7- 2-[4-(o-Me-thoxy-phenyl)-1-piperazinyl]ethyl 5H-1,3-dioxolo[4,5-f]indole tartrate.
Use: Anti-adrenergic.

SOMA. (Wallace) Carisoprodol 350 mg./Tab. Bot. 100s, 500s, 500s Unit dose.
Use: Musculoskeletal agent for acute muscle spasms, pain & stiffness.

SOMA COMPOUND TABS. (Wallace) Carisoprodol 200 mg., phenacetin 160 mg., caffeine 32 mg./Tab. Bot. 100s, 500s. Unit dose 500s.
Use: Analgesic with musculoskeletal agent for acute muscle spasms, pain & stiffness.

SOMA COMPOUND W/CODEINE. (Wallace) Carisoprodol 200 mg., phenacetin 160 mg., caffeine 32 mg., codeine phosphate 16 mg./Tab. Bot. 100s.
Use: Analgesic with musculoskeletal agent for muscle spasms, pain & stiffness.

• **SOMANTADINE HYDROCHORIDE.** USAN.

• **SOMATROPIN.** USAN. Growth hormone derived from the anterior pituitary gland.
Use: Growth stimulant.

SOMILAN. Chloral Betaine, B.A.N.

SOMINEX 2. (Beecham Products) Diphenhydramine HCl 25 mg./Tab. Blister packs 16s, 32s, 72s.
Use: Mild sedative.

SOMNATABS. (Thurston) Pow. ext. Passiflora incarnata 3 gr., pow. ext. Piscidia erythrina 2 gr., pow. ext. Viburnum opulus 1 gr., pow. ext. hyoscyamus ⅛ gr./Tab. Bot. 50s, 100s, 500s.

SOMNESIN. Methylpentynol, B.A.N.

SOMOPHYLLIN-CRT. (Fisons) Anhydrous theophylline 100 mg., 200 mg., 250 mg., or 300 mg./Sust. Release Cap. Bot. 100s, 500s. Unit dose 100s.
Use: Bronchodilator.

SOMOPHYLLIN-DF ORAL LIQUID. (Fisons) Aminophylline 105 mg./5 ml. that provides 90 mg. theophylline base/5 ml. Dye Free. Bot. 8 oz.
Use: Bronchodilator.

SOMOPHYLLIN ORAL LIQUID. (Fisons) Aminophylline 105 mg./5 ml. that provides 90 mg. theophylline base/5 ml. w/dye. Bot. 8 oz., 32 oz.
Use: Bronchodilator.

SOMOPHYLLIN RECTAL SOLUTION. (Fisons) Aminophylline 300 mg./5 ml. Bot. 3 oz. W/18 rectal tips; Bot. 5 oz. W/30 rectal tips.

Use: Rectally administered bronchodilator.
SOMOPHYLLIN-T CAPSULES. (Fisons) Theophylline 50 mg., 100 mg., 200 mg., 250 mg./Cap. Bot. 100s.
Use: Bronchodilator.
SONACIDE. (Ayerst) Potentiated acid glutaraldehyde. Bot. 1 gal., 5 gal.,
Use: Sterilizing & disinfecting.
SONDRATE ELIXIR. (Kenyon) Chloral hydrate 1.6 Gm./Fl. oz. Bot. 4 oz., pt., gal.
SONEKAP. (Eastwood) Cap. Bot. 100s.
SONERYL.
See: Butethal (Var. Mfr.)
SONIPHEN. (O'Neal, Jones & Feldman) Phenobarbital 16 mg., sodium nitrite 65 mg./Tab. Bot. 100s.
SOOTHE. (Walgreen) Bismuth subsalicylate 100 mg./Tsp. Bot. 9 oz.
Use: Upset stomach, nausea, simple diarrhea.
SOOTHE. (Alcon) Camphor 0.01%, phenylephrine HCl 0.15%, thiomerosal 0.002%/cc. Bot. 15 cc.
Use: Eye decongestant.
SOPRONOL OINTMENT. (Wyeth) Sod. propionate, sodium caprylate, zinc caprylate in ointment base. Tube 1 oz.
Use: Dermatophytosis (Athlete's foot).
SOPRONOL POWDER. (Wyeth) Sod. propionate, sodium caprylate, zinc propionate. Can 2 oz.
Use: Prophylactic fungicide.
SOPRONOL SOLUTION. (Wyeth) Sodium propionate, sodium caprylate, docusate sodium, n-propyl alcohol. Bot. 2 fl. oz.
Use: Dermatophytosis.
SOQUETTE. (Barnes-Hind) Alkyl dimethyl benzyl ammonium chloride 0.01%, disodium salt of ethylenediamine tetraacetic acid 0.20%, polyvinyl alcohol. Bot. 4 fl. oz.
Use: Soaking and storing hard contact lenses.
SORBASE COUGH SYRUP. (Fort David) Dextromethorphan HBr 10 mg., guaifenesin 100 mg./5 cc. in sorbitol base. Bot. 4 oz., pt., gal.
SORBASE II COUGH SYRUP. (Fort David) Hydrocodone bitartrate 5 mg., guaifenesin 100 mg./5 cc.
• **SORBIC ACID,** N.F. XVI.
Use: Preservative (antimicrobial).
SORBIDE T.D. (Mayrand) Isosorbide dinitrate 40 mg./T.R. Cap. Bot. 100s.
Use: Coronary vasodilator.
SORBIDE NITRATE. B.A.N. 1,4:3,6-Dianhydrosorbitol 2,5-dinitrate. Isosorbide Dinitrate (I.N.N.)
Use: Coronary vasodilator.
See: Cedocard
    Vascardin
SORBIDON HYDRATE. (Gordon) Water-in-oil ointment. Jar 2 oz., ½ oz., 1 lb., 5 lb.
Use: Treatment of dry skin.
SORBIMACROGOL OLEATE 300.
See Polysorbate 80.
• **SORBINIL.** USAN.
Use: Enzyme inhibitor.
• **SORBITAN MONOLAURATE.** N.F. XVI. Mixture of laurate esters of sorbitol and its anhydrides.

Use: Surface-active agent; emulsifying agent.
See: Span 20 (ICI U.S.)
• **SORBITAN MONOOLEATE,** N.F. XVI. Mixture of oleate esters of sorbitol and its anhydrides.
Use: Surface-active agent.
See: Span 80 (ICI U.S.)
SORBITAN MONOOLEATE POLYOXYETHYLENE DERIVATIVES.
See: Polysorbate 80, N.F. XVI.
• **SORBITAN MONOPALMITATE,** N.F. XVI. Mixture of palmitate esters of sorbitol and its anhydrides.
Use: Surface-active agent.
See: Span 40 (ICI U.S.)
• **SORBITAN MONOSTEARATE,** N.F. XVI. Mixture of stearate esters of sorbitol and its anhydrides.
Use: Surface-active agent.
See: Span 60 (ICI U.S.)
• **SORBITAN SESQUIOLEATE.** USAN. Sorbitan mono-oleate and sorbitan dioleate.
Use: Surfactant.
See: Arlacel C (ICI U.S.)
• **SORBITAN TRIOLEATE.** USAN.
Use: Surfactant.
See: Span 85 (ICI U.S.)
• **SORBITAN TRISTEARATE.** USAN.
See: Span 65 (ICI U.S.)
SORBITANS.
See: Polysorbate 80, U.S.P.
• **SORBITOL,** N.F. XVI. Solution, U.S.P. XXI.
Use: Diuretic; dehydrating agent; humectant; pharmaceutic aid (sweetening agent, tablet excipient).
See: Sorbo (ICI U.S.)
W/Homatropine methylbromide.
See: Probilagol Liquid (Purdue Frederick)
W/Mannitol.
See: Sorbitol-mannitol Irrigation (Abbott)
SORBITON. (Kenyon) Vit. B-12 5 mcg., folic acid 0.1 mg., ferrous fumarate 100 mg., D-sorbitol 500 mg./Tab. Bot. 100s, 1000s.
Use: Hematinic.
SORBITRATE. (Stuart) Isosorbide dinitrate. **Oral Tab.:** 5 mg. Bot. 100s, 500s. Unit dose 100s; 10 mg. Bot. 100s, 500s. Unit Dose 100s; 20 mg, 30 mg., 40 mg. Bot. 100s. Unit Dose 100s. **Sustained Action Tab.** 40 mg. Bot. 100s. Unit Dose 100s; **Sublingual Tab.** 2.5 mg., 5 mg. Bot. 100s, 500s. Unit Dose 100s; 10 mg. Bot. 100s. Unit dose 100s.**Chewable Tab.** 5 mg. Bot. 100s, 500s. Unit Dose 100s. 10 mg. Bot. 100s. Unit Dose 100s.
Use: Prevention and treatment of angina pectoris.
SORBO. (ICI Americas) Sorbitol Solution, U.S.P. XXI.
SORBUTUSS. (Dalin) d-Methorphan HBr 10 mg., guaifenesin 100 mg., ipecac fl. ext. 0.05 min., potassium citrate 85 mg., citric acid 35 mg./5 cc. Bot. 3 oz., pt.
Use: For coughs.
SORDINOL. Clopenthixol, B.A.N.
Use: Tranquilizer.
SORETHYTAN (20) MONO-OLEATE.
See: Polysorbate 80, (Var. Mfr.)
SORETTS LOZENGES. (Lannett) Benzocaine ½ gr.,

ext. licorice ⅛ gr., menthol ½₂₀₀ gr./Loz. Bot. 500s,
1000s.
Use: Antiseptic throat lozenges.
SORMODREN. Bornaprine, B.A.N.
SOSEGON SOLUTION. (Winthrop Products)
Pentazocine
Use: Analgesic.
SOSEGON SUSPENSION. (Winthrop Products)
Pentazocine.
Use: Analgesic.
SOSEGON TABLETS. (Winthrop Products)
Pentazocine
Use: Analgesic.
S.O.S. FIRST AID CREAM. (Columbia) Benzalkonium
Cl, diperodon HCl 0.5%, allantoin 0.2% in base
w/eucalyptol & benzyl alcohol. Tube 1½ oz.
Use: Antiseptic & anesthetic.
SOTACOR HCl. Sotalol, B.A.N.
SOTALOL. B.A.N. (±)-4'-(1-Hydroxy-2-isopropylamino-
ethyl)methanesulf-onanilide.
Use: Beta adrenergic blocking agent.
See: Beta-Cardone
    Sotacor (hydrochloride)
• **SOTALOL HYDROCHLORIDE.** USAN. 4'-[1-Hydroxy-
2-(isopropylamino)-ethyl]methanesulfonanilide hydro-
chloride. Under study.
Use: Adrenergic β-receptor antagonist.
• **SOTERENOL HYDROCHLORIDE.** USAN.
Use: Adrenergic (bronchodilator).
SORADECOL. (Elkins-Sinn) Sodium tetradecyl sulfate
1% or 3%. Amp. 2 ml.
Use: Sclerosant for varicose veins.
SOVENTOL. Bamipine, B.A.N.
SOXA-FORTE. (Vita Elixir) Sulfisoxazole 0.5 Gm.,
phenazopyridine 50 mg./Tab.
Use: Sulfa therapy.
SOXA TABLETS. (Vita Elixir) Sulfisoxazole 0.5
Gm./Tab. Bot. 100s, 1000s.
Use: Treatment of infections due to hemolytic
streptococci, staphylococci, gonococci.
SOXAZO TABLETS. (Sutliff & Case) Sulfisoxazole
500 mg., phenazopyridine HCl 50 mg./Tab. Bot.
100s, 1000s.
SOXO TABLETS. (Sutliff & Case) Sulfonamides 500
mg. Bot. 100s.
SOYALAC. (Loma Linda) Infant formula based on an
extract from whole soybeans containing all
essential nutrients. **Ready to Serve Liquid:** Cans
32 fl. oz. **Double Strength Concentrate:** Cans 13
fl. oz. **Powder:** Cans 14 oz.
Use: Alternative and supplement to breast milk for
infants, for adults and infants sensitive to animal
milk
SOYALAC-i. (Loma Linda) Soy protein isolate formula
containing no corn derivatives and a negligible
amount of soy carbohydrates. Contains all essential
nutrients in various forms. **Ready to Serve Liquid:**
Cans 32 fl. oz. **Double Strength Concentrate:**
Cans 13 fl. oz.
Use: Breast milk supplement for infant feeding, for
individuals senstitive to animal milk or corn
products.

SOYA LECITHIN. Soybean extract. 100s.
Use: Phosphorus therapy.
See: Neo-Vedrin (Scherer)
SOYBEAN LECITHIN.
W/Safflower oil, choline bitartrate, whole liver,
inositol, methionine, natural tocopherols, B-6, B-12,
panthenol.
See: Nutricol, Cap., Vial (Nutrition Control)
• **SOYBEAN OIL,** U.S.P. XXI.
SOY-DOME CLEANSER. (Miles Pharm) Hexachloro-
phene 3%, polyvinylpyrrolidone 1%, colloidal soy
bean complex, in a bland lotion base. Squeeze Bot.
w/applicator 6 oz.
Use: Antiseptic skin lotion.
SPABELIN No. 1. (Arcum) Phenobarbital 15 mg.,
belladonna pow. ext. ⅛ gr./Tab. Bot. 100s, 1000s.
SPABELIN NO. 2. (Arcum) Phenobarbital 30 mg.,
belladonna pow. ext. ⅛ gr./Tab. Bot. 100s, 1000s.
SPABELIN ELIXIR. (Arcum) Hyoscyamine sulfate 81
mcg., atropine sulfate 15 mcg., scopolamine HBr 5
mcg., phenobarbital 16.2 mg./5 cc. Bot. 16 oz., 1
gal.
SPAN 20. (ICI Americas) Sorbitan Monolaurate, N.F.
XVI.
SPAN 40. (ICI Americas) Sorbitan Monopalmitate,
N.F. XVI.
SPAN 60. (ICI Americas) Sorbitan Monostearate, N.F.
XVI.
SPAN 65. (ICI Americas) Sorbitan tristearate. Mixture
of stearate esters of sorbitol and its anhydrides.
Use: Surface active agent.
SPAN 80. (ICI Americas) Sorbitan Monooleate, N.F.
XVI.
SPAN 85. (ICI Americas) Sorbitan trioleate. Mixture of
oleate esters of sorbitol and its anhydrides.
Use: Surface active agent.
SPAN-AC. (Stanlabs) Box 12s.
Use: Timed release cold capsule.
SPANCAP #1. (Vortech) Dextroamphetamine sulfate
15 mg./Cap. Bot. 100s, 1000s.
Use: Central stimulant.
SPANCAP C. (Vortech) Sodium ascorbate 500
mg./Cap. Bot. 50s, 100s, 1000s.
Use: Timed Vitamin C therapy.
SPAN-FF. (Metro Med) Ferrous fumarate 5 gr./Sus-
tained release Cap. Bot. 60s, 500s.
SPAN-NIACIN. (Scrip) Nicotinic acid 150 mg./Tab. Bot.
100s.
SPAN-RD. (Metro Med) d-Methamphetamine HCl 12
mg., dl-methamphetamine HCl 6 mg., butabarbital 30
mg./Tab. Bot. 100s, 1000s.
SPANTAC. (Vortech) Phenylpropanolamine HCl 50
mg., belladonna alkaloids 0.2 mg., chlorpheniramine
maleate 4 mg./Cap. Bot. 12s, 100s, 1000s.
Use: Common cold & hay fever symptoms.
SPANTRAN. (Hauck) Meprobamate 400 mg./Tab.
Bot. 100s.
Use: Management of anxiety and tension.
SPANTUSS LIQUID. (Arco) d-Methorphan HBr 15 mg.,
chlorpheniramine maleate 4 mg., phenylephrine HCl
5 mg., acetaminophen 120 mg./5 cc. Bot. 4 oz., 1
pt.

Use: Relief from cough and congestion.
SPANTUSS TABLET. (Arco) Chlorpheniramine maleate 8 mg., phenylephrine HCl 25 mg., dextromethorphan HBr 5 mg./Tab. Bot. 60s.
Use: Antihistamine, decongestant antitussive.
• **SPARFOSATE SODIUM.** USAN.
Use: Antineoplastic.
SPARINE EMBONATE, Promazine, B.A.N.
SPARINE. (Wyeth) Promazine hydrochloride.**Tab.** 10 mg., 25 mg., 50 mg., or 100 mg./Tab. Bot. 50s, 500s. 10 mg. Bot. 50s only. **Inj.** 25 mg./cc. Vial 10 cc. Tubex 1 cc., 50 mg./cc. Vial 2 cc., 10 cc. Tubex 1 cc., 2 cc. **Syrup** 10 mg./5 cc. Bot. 4 oz. **Concentrate** 30 mg./cc., dropper Bot. 4 oz.
Use: Ataraxic.
• **SPARSOMYCIN.** USAN.
Use: Antineoplastic.
• **SPARTEINE SULFATE.** USAN.
Use: Oxytocic.
W/Sod. chloride.
See: Tocosamine sulfate, Amp. (Trent)
SPARTUS. (Lederle) Vit. A 5000 I.U., E 30 I.U., C 300 mg., folic acid 400 mcg., B-1 7.5 mg., B-2 8.5 mg., niacinamide 100 mg., B-6 10 mg., B-12 30 mcg., D 400 I.U., biotin 45 mcg., pantothenic acid 50 mg., magnesium 100 mg., iodine 150 mcg., copper 3 mg., chromium 15 mcg., molybdenium 15 mcg., selenium 15 mcg., manganese 5 mg., potassium 15 mg., chloride 13.6 mg., zinc 22.5 mg./Tab. Bot. 60s.
Use: High potency vitamin, mineral & electrolyte supplement.
SPARTUS PLUS IRON. (Lederle) Vit. A 5000 I.U., E 30 I.U., C 300 mg., folic acid 400 mcg., B-1 7.5 mg., B-2 8.5 mg., niacinamide 100 mg., B-6 10 mg., B-12 30 mcg., D 400 I.U., biotin 45 mcg., pantothenic acid 50 mg., iodine 150 mcg., iron 27 mg., magnesium 100 mg., copper 3 mg., chromium 15 mcg., molybdenium 15 mcg., selenium 15 mcg., manganese 6 mg., potassium 15 mg., chloride 13.6 mg., zinc 22.5 mg./Tab. Bot. 60s.
Use: High potency vitamin, mineral & electrolyte supplement.
SPASAID. (Century) Hyoscyamine sulfate 0.30 mg., atropine sulfate 0.06 mg., hyoscine HBr 0.02 mg., phenobarbital ¾ gr./Cap. Bot. 100s, 1000s.
SPASASED. (Wolins) Sodium phenobarbital ¼ gr., scopolamine HBr ¹/₁₀₀₀ gr., magnesium carbonate 5 gr./Tab. Bot. 1000s.
SPASDEL CAPSULES. (Marlop) Atropine sulfate 0.0582 mg., hyoscine HBr 0.0195 mg., hyoscyamine sulfate 0.311 mg., phenobarbital 50 mg./T.R. Cap. Bot. 100s.
Use: Antispasmodic, sedative.
SPASIDON. (Haag) Phenobarbital ¼ gr., hyoscyamine sulfate 0.1037 mg., atropine sulfate 0.0194 mg., hyoscine hydrobromide 0.0065 mg./Tab. Bot. 100s, 500s, 1000s.
SPASLIN. (Blaine) Phenobarbital 16.2 mg., hyoscyamine sulfate 0.1040 mg., atropine sulfate. 0.0195 mg., scopolamine HBr 0.0065 mg./Tab. Bot. 100s, 1000s.

Use: Antispasmodic and sedative.
SPASLOIDS. (Harvey) Hyoscyamine sulfate 0.1040 mg., atropine sulfate 0.0195 mg., hyoscine HBr 0.0065 mg., phenobarbital ¼ gr./Tab. Bot. 1000s.
Use: Antispasmodic & sedative.
SPASMATOL. (Pharmed) Homatropine MeBr 3 mg., pentobarbital 12 mg., mephobarbital 8 mg./Tab. Bot. 100s, 1000s.
Use: Antispasmodic.
SPASMED. (Jenkins) Hyoscyamine HBr 0.1037 mg., atropine sulfate 0.0194 mg., hyoscine HBr 0.0065 mg., tri-bar (⅓ each sod. butabarb., sod. pentobarb., sod. phenobarb.) 16.2 mg./Tab. or 5 ml. **Tab.:** Bot. 1000s. **Elixir:** Bot. 4 oz., pt., gal. Alcohol 15%.
Use: Sedative and antispasmodic.
SPASMED JR. (Jenkins) Homatropine methylbromide ¹/₉₆ gr., phenobarbital sod. ⅛ gr., lactose, special mint flavor/Tab. Bot. 1000s.
Use: Sedative.
SPASMID. (Dalin) Methscopolamine nitrate 2.5 mg., phenobarbital 8.0 ᵐg./Tab. or 5 cc. **Elix.:** Bot. 4 oz., pt. **Tab.:** Bot. 50s, 100s.
Use: Antispasmodic, anticholinergic.
SPASMOBARB. (Wolins) Hyoscyamine HBr 0.128 mg., hyoscine HBr 0.007 mg., atropine sulfate 0.024 mg., butabarbital sodium/Tab. Bot. 1000s.
Use: Sedative and antispasmodic.
SPASMODINE. (Noyes) Alcohol 4%, emulsion of infused oils lobelia, stillingia, cajeput, lavender, cassia, eucalyptol. Mixture 3 oz., pt., gal.
Use: Sugar free expectorant.
SPASMOJECT. (Mayrand) Dicyclomine HCl 10 mg./ml. Vial 10 ml.
Use: Antispasmodic for G.I. spasms.
SPASMOLIN. (Richlyn) Phenobarbital 16.2 mg., hyoscyamine sulfate 0.1037 mg., atropine sulfate 0.0194 mg., hyoscine HBr 0.0065 mg./Tab. Bot. 1000s
Use: Sedative and antispasmotic.
SPASMOLIN. (Wolins) Hyoscyamine sulfate 0.1037 mg., hyoscyamine HBr 0.0065 mg., atropine sulfate 0.0194 mg., phenobarbital 16.2 mg./Tab., Cap. Bot. 1000s, 5000s.
Use: Sedative and antispasmodic.
SPASMOLIN NO. 3 OR NO. 4 (Wolins) Phenobarbital 16.2 mg., hyoscyamine sulfate 0.1040 mg., atropine sulfate 0.0195 mg., hyoscine HBr 0.0065 mg./Cap. Bot. 1000s.
Use: Sedative and antispasmodic.
SPASMOLIN TDC. (Wolins) Hyoscyamine sulfate 0.311 mg., hyoscyamine HBr 0.0195 mg., atropine sulfate 0.0582 mg., phenobarbital 50 mg./Cap. Bot. 1000s, 5000s.
Use: Antispasmodic and sedative.
SPASMOLYN. (Heun) Mephenesin 0.5 Gm./Tab. Bot. 100s.
SPASMOLYTIC AGENTS.
See: Antispasmodics
SPASMOPHEN. (Lannett) Phenobarbital 15 mg., hyoscyamine sulf. 0.1037 mg., atropine sulf. 0.0194 mg., hyoscine HBr 0.0065 mg./Tab. or 5 cc. **Tabs.** Bot. 500s, 1000s. **Liq.** Bot. pt., gal.

Use: Antispasmodic-sedative.
SPASNIL. (Rhode) Phenobarbital 15 mg., hyoscyamine sulfate 0.1037 mg., atropine sulfate 0.0194 mg., hyoscine 0.0065 mg./Tab. Bot. 100s.
Use: GI antispasmodic & sedative.
SPASNO-LIX. (Freeport) Phenobarbital 16.2 mg., hyoscyamine sulfate 0.1037 mg., atropine sulfate 0.0194 mg., hyoscine HBr. 0.0065 mg., alcohol 21-23 %/5 cc. Bot. 4 oz.
Use: Sedative, antispasmodic.
SPASODIL. (Rand) Ethaverine HCl 50 mg. & 100 mg./Tab. Bot. 100s & 1000s.
Use: Antispasmodic, vasodilator.
SPASTIL. (Kenyon) Propantheline Br 15 mg./Tab. Bot. 100s, 1000s.
Use: Antispasmodic.
SPASTOLATE. (Barry-Martin) Phenobarbital 16.2 mg., hyoscyamine sulf. 0.1037 mg., atropine sulf. 0.0194 mg., hyoscine HBr. 0.0065 mg./Tab. or 5 cc. **Tab.** Bot. 1000s. **Elix.** qt., gal.
Use: Antispasmodic w/sedative.
SPASTOSED. (Vortech) Calcium carbonate 226 mg., magnesium carbonate 162 mg./Tab. Bot. 1000s.
Use: Antacid.
SPASTYL. (Pharmex) Dicyclomine HCl 10 mg./cc. Vial 10 cc.
S.P.B. TABLET. (Sheryl) Therapeutic B complex formula with 300 mg. of ascorbic acid. Tabs. 100s.
Use: To replace stress-depleted vitamin reserves.
SPD. (A.P.C.) Methyl salicylate, methyl nicotinate, dipropyleneglycol salicylate, oleoresin capsicum, camphor, menthol. Cream Bot. 4 oz., Tube 1½ oz.
Use: Relief of arthritis, rheumatism, neuralgia.
• **SPEARMINT,** N.F. XVI.
Use: Flavor.
• **SPEARMINT OIL,** N.F. XVI.
Use: Flavor.
SPECIAL FORMULA OINTMENT "RF". (Lannett) Zinc oxide 10%, boric acid 4%, starch 10%, camphor 1%, menthol ½% in a petrolatum-aquaphor base. Jar 1 lb.
Use: Dermatological.
SPECTAZOLE. (Ortho) Pegoxol 7 stearate, peglicol 5 oleate, mineral oil, benzoic acid, butylated hydroxyanisole. Tube 15 Gm., 30 Gm., 85 Gm.
Use: Antifungal, candidal agent.
SPECTINOMYCIN. Formerly Actinospectocin. An antibiotic isolated from broth cultures of *Streptomyces spectabilis.*
Use: Antibacterial.
See: Trobicin, Vial, Amp. (Upjohn)
• **SPECTINOMYCIN HYDROCHLORIDE, STERILE,** U.S.P. XXI. An antibiotic produced by *Streptomyces spectabilis.*
Use: Antibacterial.
SPECTRA 360. (Parker) Electrode contact medium gel with no salts. Tube 8 oz.
Use: T.E.N.S. application.
SPECTRA PAD FOR T.E.N.S. (Parker) Pre-moistened salt-free pads.
Use: Transcutaneous electrical nerve stimulation.
SPECTROBID POWDER FOR ORAL SUSPENSION.

(Roerig) Bacampicillin powder 125 mg./5 ml.
Use: Antibacterial.
SPECTROBID TABLETS. (Roerig) Bacampicillin HCl 400 mg./Tab. Bot. 100s.
Use: Antibacterial.
SPECTRO-BIOTIC. (A.P.C.) Bacitracin 400 u., neomycin sulfate 5 mg., polymyxin B sulfate 5000 u./Gm. Oint. ½ oz., 1 oz.
Use: Infection in cuts, wounds, etc.
SPECTROCIN. (Squibb) Neomycin sulfate equivalent to 2.5 mg. neomycin base, gramicidin 0.25 mg./Gm. Tube 0.5 oz., 1 oz.
SPECTRO-JEL. (Recsei) glycol polysiloxane. cetylpyridinium chloride, 15% v/v isopropylalcohol in methylcellulose base jelly. Bot. 4 oz., pts., gal.
Use: Degerming cleansing agent in acne, diaper rash and pyodermas.
SPEC-T SORE THROAT ANESTHETIC LOZENGES. (Squibb) Benzocaine 10 mg./Loz. Box 10s.
Use: Topical oral antibacterial.
SPEC-T SORE THROAT/COUGH SUPPRESSANT LOZENGES. (Squibb) Benzocaine 10 mg., dextromethorphan HBr 10 mg.
Use: Local anesthetic & cough suppresant.
SPEC-T SORE THROAT/DECONGESTANT LOZENGES. (Squibb) Benzocaine 10 mg., phenylephrine HCl 5 mg., phenylpropranolamine HCl 10.5 mg./Loz. Pkg. 10s.
Use: Local anesthetic & decongestant.
SPEEDRIN. (Columbia) Buffered aspirin 5 gr. Bot. 100s, 1000s.
SPERMACETI.
Use: Stiffening agent; pharm. necessity for Cold Cream.
SPERMINE. Diaminopropyltetramethylene.
SPEROTABS—C.T. (Fellows) Amobarbital 4 mg., atropine sulfate 0.064 mg., magnesium hydroxyaminoacetate 100 mg., magnesium oxide, heavy 150 mg., aluminum hydroxide, dense 150 mg., methylcellulose 100 mg., magnesium trisilicate 150 mg., chlorophyllin, water soluble, 2 mg., benzocaine 4 mg./Tab. Bot. 1000s, 5000s.
SPERTI OINTMENT. (Whitehall) Live yeast cell derivative supplying 2,000 u. skin respiratory factor/oz. w/shark liver oil 3.0%, phenylmercuric nitrate 1:10,000. Tube 1 oz.
Use: Healing ointment.
SPHERULIN. (Berkeley Biologicals) Coccidioidin: Sterile filtrate prepared from spherules of *Coccidioides immitis.* Vial 1 ml., 1:100 equivalent. 0.5 ml., 1:10 equivalent.
Use: Skin test.
SPIDER-BITE ANTIVENIN.
See: Antivenin Crotalidae and Micrurus, U.S.P. XXI.
• **SPIPERONE.** USAN. 8-[3-(p-Fluorobenzoyl)-propyl]-1-phenyl-1,3,8-triazaspiro-[4.5]decan-4-one.
Use: Tranquilizer.
• **SPIRAMYCIN.** USAN. (Ives) Antibiotic substance from cultures of *Streptomyces ambofaciens.* Rovamycin.
Use: Antibiotic.

SPIRILENE. B.A.N. 8-[4-(4-Fluorophenyl)pent-3-enyl]-1-phenyl-1,3,8-triazaspiro[4,5]decan-4-one.
Use: Tranquilizer.

SPIROBARBITAL SODIUM. 1-Ethyl-2,4-dimethyl-8-thio-7,9-diazaspiro[4.5]decane-6,8,10-trione sodium salt.

• **SPIROGERMANIUM HYDROCHLORIDE.** USAN.
Use: Antineoplastic.

• **SPIROMUSTINE.** USAN. Formerly spirohydantoin mustard.
Use: Anti-neoplastic.

• **SPIRONOLACTONE,** U.S.P. XXI. Tab. U.S.P. XXI. 17-Hydroxy-7α-mercapto-3-oxo-17α-pregn-4-ene-21-carboxylic acid γ-lactone 7-acetate: 3-(3-oxo-7 α-acetylthio-17β-hydroxy-4-androsten-17   α-yl)   propionic
acid γ-lactone.
Use: Diuretic.
See: Aldactone, Tab. (Searle)
W/Hydrochlorothiazide.
See: Aldactazide, Tab. (Searle)

SPIROPITAN. (Janssen) Spiperone
Use: Antipsychotic.

• **SPIROPLATIN.** USAN.
Use: Antineoplastic.

SPIROTRIAZINE HCl. 2,4-Diamino-5(p-chlorophenyl)-9-methyl-1,3,5-triazaspiro [5.5]undeca-1,3-diene HCl.
Use: Anthelmintic.

• **SPIROXASONE.** USAN.
Use: Diuretic.

• **SPONGE, ABSORBABLE GELATIN,** U.S.P. XXI.
Use: Local hemostatic.

SPRAY SKIN PROTECTANT. (Morton) Isopropyl alcohol, polyvinylpyrolidine, vinyl alcohol, plasticizer & propellant. Aerosol can 6 oz.
Use: Protective skin coating.

SPREADING FACTOR.
See: Hyaluronidase (Various Mfr.)

SPRX-1. (Reid-Provident) Phendimetrazine tartrate 35 mg./Tab. Bot. 100s.
Use: Anorexic.

SPRX-3. (Reid-Provident) Phendimetrazine tartrate 35 mg./Cap. Bot. 100s.
Use: Anorexic.

SPRX 105 CAPSULES. (Reid-Provident) Phendimetrazine tartrate 105 mg./S.R. Cap. Bot. 28s, 500s.
Use: Anorexic.

S-P-T. (Fleming) Pork thyroid, desiccated. 1,2,3,5 gr./Cap. Bot. 100s, 1000s.
Use: Hypothyroidism.

S.Q. (MSD AGVET) Sulfaquinoxaline: 40% medicated feed. Solution 20%.
Use: Sulfonamide, veterinary medicine.

SQUIBB GOLDEN BOUNTY PRODUCTS. (Squibb)
B Complex with C Capsules. Bot. 90s.
Use: Vitamins B & C.
Brewers Yeast Tablets. Yeast 7.5 gr./Tab. Bot. 500s.
Use: Vitamin.
Cod Liver Oil Capsules. Cod liver oil 0.6 ml./Cap. Bot. 100s.
Use: Vitamin A & D.

Vitamin A Capsules. Vit. A 10,000 I.U./Cap. Bot. 100s.
Use: Vitamin A supplement.
Vitamin C. Vitamin C from rose hips 250 mg., 500 mg./Tab. Bot. 100s, 250 mg.; 90s for 500 mg.
Vitamin E. Vit. E 100 I.U., 200 I.U., 400 I.U./Cap. Bot. 100s for 100 I.U. & 200 I.U.; 60s, 90s for 400 u.
Use: Vitamine E supplement.

SRC EXPECTORANT. (Edwards) Hydrodone bitartrate 5 mg., pseudoephedrine HCl 60 mg., guaifenesin 200 mg. w/alcohol 12.5%. Bot. pt.
Use: Decongestant, expectorant, anti-tussive.

SSKI. (Upsher-Smith) Potassium iodide oral solution 300 mg./0.3 cc. Dropper Bot. 1 oz., 8 oz.
Use: Chronic pulmonary diseases.

S-SPAS. (Southern States) Pentobarbital 16.2 mg., atropine sulfate 0.0194 mg., hyoscyamine sulfate 0.1037 mg., hyoscine HBr 0.0065 mg./Tab. or 5 cc.
Liq. Bot. pt. **Tab.** Bot. 100s, 1000s.
Use: Sedative & antispasmodic.

S.T. 37. (Beecham Products) Hexylresorcinol 0.1% in glycerin aqueous solution. Bot. 5 oz., 12 oz.
Use: General antiseptic.

STABINOL. Isobuzole, B.A.N.

STABL-PLEX W/VITAMIN C. (Morton) Vit. B-1 25 mg., B-2 7.13 mg., B-6 5 mg., panthenol 5 mg., niacinamide 50 mg., Vit. C 50 mg., gentisic acid ethanolamine 2.5%, polyethylene glycol 300 10%, benzyl alcohol 2%/cc. Vial 30 cc.

STADOL. (Bristol) Butorphanol tartrate 1 mg./ml. Vial 1 ml. 2 mg./ml. disposable syringe. Vial 1 ml., 2 ml., 10 ml.
Use: Analgesic.

STAFTABS. (Modern) Fine bone flour containing calcium, phosphorus, iron, iodine, Vit. D, magnesium Tab. Bot. 85s, 160s.

STAINLESS IODIZED OINTMENT. (Day-Baldwin) Jar 1 lb.

STAINLESS IODIZED OINTMENT WITH METHYL SALICYLATE 5%. (Day-Baldwin) Jar 1 lb.

STALL. (Cenci) o-Hydroxybenzoic acid ½ %, thymol ½ %, ethyl alcohol S.D. 70%. Bot. ½, 2 oz. w/dropper.
Use: Earache and ear infections.

• **STALLIMYCIN HYDROCHLORIDE.** USAN.
Use: Antibacterial.

STAMYL TABLETS. (Winthrop Products) Pancreatin.
Use: Pancreatic deficiency, dyspepsia.

STANACAINE. (Standex) Lidocaine HCl 2% Bot. 50 cc.

STANACILLIN. (Standex) Buffered penicillin 250,000 u./Tab. 500,000 u./Tab. Bot. 100s.

STANACILLIN PO. (Standex) Buffered penicillin Pow. 250,000 u. Bot. 60 cc. 500,000 u. Bot. 80 cc.

STAN-APAP. (Stanlabs) Acetaminophen 500 mg./Cap. Bot. 50s.
Use: Analgesic.

STAN A SYN. (Standex) Vit A palmitate 50,000 I.U./Cap. Bot. 100s.

STAN A SYN CREME. (Standex) Vits. A & D. 1 oz.

STAN A SYN FORTE. (Standex) Vit. A palmitate 10,000 I.U./Cap. Bot. 100s.

STAN A SYN FORTE S. (Standex) Vit. A soluble 10,000 I.U./Cap. Bot. 100s.

STAN A SYN JR. (Standex) Vit. A palmitate 25,000 I.U./Cap. Bot. 100s.

STAN A SYN S. (Standex) Vit. A soluble 50,000 I.U./Cap. Bot. 100s.

STANBACK ANALGESIC POWDERS. (Stanback) Aspirin 650 mg., salicylamide 200 mg., caffeine 15 mg./Powder. Pkgs. 2s, 6s., 24s, 50s.
Use: Analgesic, antipyretic, anti-inflammatory.

STANBACK MAX-EXTRA STRENGTH. (Stanback) Aspirin 850 mg./powder. Pkg. 2s, 4s, & 36s.
Use: Analgesic, antipyretic, anti-inflammatory.

STANCARE. (Block) Stannous fluoride 10 mg./Tab. One tablet in 10 ml. water prepares a 0.1% solution. Box 28s, 46s.
Use: Fluoride mouth rinse.

STANDEX. (Standex) Vit. A 1333 I.U., D 133 I.U., B-1 0.33 mg., B-2 0.40 mg., C 10 mg., niacinamide 3.3 mg., Fe 3.3 mg., Ca 15 mg., P 29 mg., sod. carboxymethylcellulose 100 mg./Cap. Bot. 100s.

STANNITOL ELIXIR. (Standex) Phenobarbital ¼ gr., hyoscyamine sulfate 0.1037 mg., atropine sulfate 0.0194 mg., scopolamine HBr 0.0065 mg., alcohol 23%/5 cc. Bot. pt.

STANNITOL INJ. (Standex) Dicyclomine HCl 10 mg./cc. Vial 10 cc.

STANNITOL TAB. (Standex) Phenobarbital ¼ gr., atropine sulfate 0.0195 mg., hyoscine HBr 0.0065 mg., hyoscyamine sulfate 0.1040 mg./Tab. Bot. 100s.

• **STANNOUS CHLORIDE.** USAN.
Use: Pharmaceutic aid.

• **STANNOUS FLUORIDE,** U.S.P. XXI. Tin fluoride.
Use: Dental caries prophylactic.

STANNOUS FLUORIDE. (City Chem.) Stannous fluoride. Bot. 4 oz., lb.

• **STANNOUS PYROPHOSPHATE.** USAN.
Use: Diagnostic aid (bone imaging).

• **STANNOUS SULFUR COLLOID.** USAN.
Use: Diagnostic aid.

STANOLONE, B.A.N. Androstanolone, dihydrotestosterone, androstane-17(β)-ol-3-one. 17 β-Hydroxy-5 α-androstan-3-one.
See: Anabolex
Anabolic steroid.
Anaprotin

• **STANOZOLOL,** U.S.P. XXI. Tab., U.S.P. XXI. 17 β-Hydroxy-17 α-methylandrostano[3,2-c] pyrazole. 17-Methyl-2′H-5 α-androst-2-eno(3,2-c)pyrazol-17 β-ol. Formerly Androstanazole.
Use: Anabolic agent.
See: Stromba
Winstrol Tab. (Winthrop-Breon)

STANPRO-75. (Standex) Phenylpropanolamine 75 mg./cc. Vial 30 cc.

STANTEEN CAP. (Standex) Vit. A 5000 I.U., D 400 I.U., B-1 3 mg., B-2 2.5 mg., C 50 mg., niacinamide 20 mg., Ca 46 mg., P 35 mg., Fe 1.34 mg., B-6 1 mg., Ca pantothenate 2 mg., B-12 2 mcg., Mg 1 mg., Mn 1.5 mg., K 5 mg., Zn 1.4 mg./Cap. Bot. 100s.

STAPHAGE LYSATE (SPL). (Delmont) Phage-lysed staphylococci 120-180 million/cc. Amp. 1 cc. package 10s for inj.; multidose vials 10 cc. for other methods of administration.
Use: Prophylaxis and treatment of staphylococcal infections.

STAPHCILLIN. (Bristol) Sodium methicillin 1 Gm., equiv. to 900 mg. methicillin activity/Vial. Vial 1 Gm., 4 Gm., 6 Gm.; Piggyback vials. 1 Gm., 4 Gm.
Use: Penicillin therapy.

• **STARCH,** N.F. XVI.
Use: Dusting powder; tablet disintegrant.
See: Mexsana, Pwd. (Plough)

STARCH GLYCERITE.
Use: Emollient.

• **STARCH, PREGELATINIZED,** N.F. XVI.
Use: Pharm. aid (tablet excipient).

• **STARCH, TOPICAL,** U.S.P. XXI.
Use: Dusting powder.

STAR-OTIC. (Star) Burrows sol. 10%, acetic acid 1.0%, boric acid 1.0%. Drop bot. 15 cc.
Use: Treatment of otitis externa, bacterial & fungal infections of ear canal.

STATICIN 1.5%. (Westwood) Erythromycin 15 mg./ml. in clear solution w/alcohol 55%, propyleme glycol, Laureth-4 and fragrance. Bot. 60 ml.
Use: Topical control of acne vulgaris.

STATOBEX. (Lemmon) Phendimetrazine tartrate 35 mg./Tab. or Cap. Bot. 1000s. Green & white.
Use: Exogenous obesity.

STATOBEX-G. (Lemmon) Phendimetrazine tartrate 35 mg./Tab. Bot. 1000s. Green.
Use: Anorexiant.

• **STATOLON.** USAN. Antiviral agent derived from *Penicillium stoloniferum.*
Use: Antiviral agent.

STATOMIN MALEATE II. (Bowman) Chlorpheniramine maleate 2 mg., acetaminophen 324 mg., caffeine 32 mg./Tab. Bot. 1000s.
Use: Decongestant, analgesic, antihistaminic.

STATROL. (Alcon) Polymixin B sulfate 16, 250 u./ml., neomycin 3.5 mg./ml. hydroxypropyl methylcellulose 0.5%. Droptainer 5 ml.
Use: Bacterial infections of the eye.

STATROL STERILE OPHTHALMIC OINTMENT. (Alcon) Polymyxin B sulfate 10,000 U., neomycin 3.5 mg./Gm. Tube 3.5 Gm.
Use: Bacterial infections of the eye.

STA-WAKE DEXTABS. (Approved) Caffeine 1½ gr., dextrose 3 gr./Tab. Bot. 36s, 1000s.
Use: Stimulant.

STAY-ALERT. (Edward J. Moore) Caffeine 250 mg./Cap. Bot. 12s, 18s.

STAY AWAKE. (Towne) Caffeine 200 mg., niacin 10 mg., Vit. B-1 10 mg., dextrose sod. biphosphate, calcium phosphate monobasic, oleoresin capsicum/Tab. Bot. 12s, 30s.

STAYMINS. (Stayner) Vit. A 5000 I.U., D 500 I.U., B-1 1.5 mg., B-2 1.5 mg., niacinamide 10 mg., B-6 0.5 mg., C 50 mg., B-12 2 mcg./5 ml. Bot. 16 oz.
Use: Multivitamin liquid.

STAYMINS TABLETS. (Stayner) Vit. A 5000 I.U., D 500 I.U., E 1 I.U. B-1 2.5 mg., B-2 2.5 mg., B-6 0.5 mg., B-12 2 mcg., C 50 mg., Ca pantothenate 5 mg.,

niacinamide 20 mg., inositol 10 mg., choline bitartrate 10 mg./Tab. Bot. 100s, 1000s.
Use: Multivitamin tablet.

STAYNERAL TABLETS. (Stayner) Vit. A 5000 I.U., D 500 I.U., E 5 I.U., B-1 5 mg., B-2 5 mg., B-6 1 mg., C 100 mg., B-12 2 mcg., niacinamide 25 mg., Ca pantothenate 5 mg., Ca 50 mg., P 40 mg., Fe 10 mg., Mn 0.5 mg., Zn 0.1 mg., Mg 0.5 mg., Iodine 0.2 mg., Cu 0.1 mg./Tab. Bot. 100s, 1000s.
Use: Vitamin-mineral therapy.

STAY-UPS. (Faraday) Tab. Bot. 30s.
Use: To combat fatigue.

STAZE. (Commerce) Tube 1.75 oz., 3.5 oz.
Use: Denture adhesive.

S-T DECONGEST. (Scot-Tussin) Phenylephrine HCl 5 mg., phenylpropanolamine HCl 5 mg., brompheniramine maleate 4 mg./5 ml. w/alcohol 2.3%. Sugar free and dye free. Bot. 8 oz., 16 oz., gal.
Use: Hay fever and allergies.

STEAPSIN.
W/Oxidized bile acids, ox bile, homatropine methylbromide.
See: Oxacholin, Tab. (Philips Roxane)

• **STEARIC ACID,** N.F. XVI. Purified, N.F. XVI. Octadecanoic acid.
Use: Pharm aid (emulsion adjunct, tablet lubricant).

• **STEARYL ALCOHOL,** N.F. XVI.
Use: Pharm aid (emulsion adjunct).

STECSOLIN. Oxytetracycline, B.A.N.

• **STEFFIMYCIN.** USAN.
Use: Antibacterial, antiviral.

STELAZINE. (SmithKline) Trifluoperazine HCl. **Tab.** 1 mg., 2 mg., 5 mg. & 10 mg., Bot. 100s, 1000s. Unit dose 100s. **Vial** 10 ml. (2 mg./ml.) Box 1s, 20s. **Oral Conc.** (10 mg./ml.) Bot. 2 fl. oz. Ctn. 12s.
Use: Tranquilizing agent.

STEMETIL. Prochlorperazine, B.A.N.

STEMULTROLIN. (Lincoln) Chorionic gonadotropin (Human) 500 I.U./cc. Vial 10 cc.
Use: Male senility.

• **STENOBOLONE ACETATE.** USAN. 17-beta-Hydroxy-2-methyl-5-alpha-androst-1-en-3-one acetate.
Use: Inj. anabolic.

STERA-FORM CREME. (Mayrand) Hydrocortisone 1%, clioquinol 3%, pramoxine HCl 0.5%. Pkg. ½ oz.

STERAJECT. (Mayrand) Prednisolone acetate 25 mg., 50 mg./ml. Vial 10 ml.

STERAMINE OTIC. (Mayrand) Pramoxine HCl 1.0%, hydrocortisone 1.0%, parachlorometaxylenol 0.1%, benzalkonium chloride 0.02%, acetic acid 2.0% in a nonaqueous propylene glycol vehicle. Bot. 10 cc.
Use: Antibacterial, antifungal, anti-inflammatory anesthetic.

STERANE TABLETS. (Pfipharmecs) Prednisolone 5 mg./Tab. Bot. 100s, 5000s.
Use: Rheumatoid arthritis, allergies and various inflammatory skin conditions.

STERAPRED TABLETS. (Mayrand) Prednisone 5 mg./Tab. Bot. 100s, 1000s.

Use: Anti-inflammatory steroid.

STERAPRED-UNIPAK. (Mayrand) Prednisone 5 mg./Tab. Dosepak 21 tab.
Use: Anti-inflammatory steroid.

STERCULIA GUM.
See: Karaya Gum (Var. Mfr.)
W/Vit. B-1.
See: Imbicoll W/Vit. B-1 (Upjohn)

STERIBOLIC. (Kay) Methandriol dipropionate 50 mg./cc. Vial 10 cc.
Use: Anabolic steroid.

STERICOL. (Alton) Isopropyl alcohol 91% Bot. 16 oz, 32 oz., Gal.
Antibacterial, topical anti-infective.

• **STERILE AUROTHIOGLUCOSE SUSPENSION,** U.S.P. XXI. Authothioglucose Injection. Gold thioglucose. Gold, (l-thio-D-glucopyranosato)-. (l-Thio-D-glucopyranosato) gold.
Use: Antirheumatic.
See: Solganal, Vial (Schering)

• **STERILE ERYTHROMYCIN GLUCEPTATE,** U.S.P. XXI. Erythromycin monoglucoheptonate (salt). Erythromycin glucoheptonate (1:1) (salt).
Use: Antibacterial.

STERILE THIOPENTAL SODIUM. Thiopental sodium, U.S.P. XXI.
See: Pentothal Sodium, Amp. (Abbott)

STERISIL. Hexetidine, B.A.N.

STERI-UNNA BOOT. (Pedinol) Glycerin, gum acacia, zinc oxide, white petrolatum, amylum in an oil base. 10 Yds. × 3½ in. steralized bandage.
Use: Treatment of leg ulcers, varicosities, sprains, strains & reduce swelling after surgery.

STERNEEDLE TESTING KIT FOR HEAF TUBERCULIN TEST, ALLERGY & SMALLPOX. (Panray) 1 "Sterneedle" device, 100 "Sterneedle" No. 6 cartridge, concentrated tuberculin PPD solution 'Connaught'. Vial 1 cc. Also available w/50 smallpox No. 3 and 50 TB Test cartridges No. 6./Kit. Also mass testing kit.

STEROLOX. (Kenyon) Benzethonium Cl. benzoic acid, salicylic acid, thymol, menthol, isopropyl alcohol 50%. Bot. 2 oz., pt., gal.

STEROXIN. Chlorquinaldol, B.A.N.

S-T EXPECTORANT. (Scot-Tussin) Guaifenesin 100 mg./5 ml. w/alcohol 3.5%. Dye free and sugar free.
Use: Expectorant.

S-T FORTE. (Scot-Tussin) Hydrocodone bitartrate 2.5 mg., phenylephrine HCl 5 mg., phenylpropanolamine HCl 5 mg., pheniramine maleate 13.33 mg., guaifenesin 80 mg./5 ml. Regular or sugar free. Bot. pt. gal.
Use: Cough and cold treatment.

STIBAMINE GLUCOSIDE. B.A.N. Sodium 4-glucosylaminophenylstibonate.
Use: Treatment of leishmaniasis.

STIBOCAPTATE. B.A.N. Antimony(III) sodium meso-2, 3- dimercaptosuccinate.
Use: Treatment of schistosomiasis.
See: Astiban

STILBAMIDINE. B.A.N. 4, 4'-Diamidinostilbene.
Use: Treatment of trypanosomiasis.

STILBAMIDINE ISETHIONATE. 2-Hydroxyethane-sulfonic acid compound with 4, 4′-stilbenedicarboxamidine.
Use: Antiprotozoal.
• **STILBAZIUM IODIDE.** USAN. 1-Ethyl-2, 6-bis(p-1-pyrrolidinyl-styryl)-pyridinium iodide.
Use: Anthelmintic.
See: Monopar
STILBESTROL.
See: Diethylstilbestrol, U.S.P. XXI. (Various Mfr.)
STILBESTRONATE.
See: Diethylstilbestrol Dipropionate (Various Mfr.)
STILBOESTROL.
See: Diethylstilbestrol (Various Mfr.)
STILBOESTROL DP.
See: Diethylstilbestrol Dipropionate (Various Mfr.)
STILLMAN'S. (Stillman) Cream Jar. ⅞ oz., 1⅞ oz., Cream Bella Aurora: ⅞ oz.
• **STILONIUM IODIDE.** USAN.
Use: Antispasmodic.
STILPHOSTROL. (Miles Pharm) Diethylstilbestrol diphosphate. Amp. (250 mg./5 cc.) 5 cc. Box 20s. Tab. 50 mg., Bot. 50s.
Use: Inoperable prostatic carcinoma.
STILRONATE.
See: Diethylstilbestrol Dipropionate (Var. Mfr.)
STIMULAX. (Geriatric) Docusate sodium 250 mg., casathranol 30 mg./Cap. Bot. 30s, 100s, 500s.
Use: Fecal softener & laxative.
STIMURUB. (Otis Clapp) Menthol, methyl salicylate, oleo resin of capsicum, in greaseless base. Tubes 36 × ¼ oz., 1 oz., Jar. 16 oz.
Use: Relief from muscular aches, strains, sprains.
STING-EZE. (Wisconsin) Bot. ½ oz.
Use: After bite treatment.
STINGING INSECT ANTIGEN. (Barry) Polyvalent whole-body insect extract of wasp, hornet, bumblebee, honey bee and yellow jacket antigens/Vial. Set 3 special dilution.
STIRIMAZOLE. B.A.N. 2-(4-Carboxystyryl)-5-nitro-1-vinylimidazole.
Use: Treatment of amebiasis, trichomoniasis, and trypanosomiasis.
• **STIRIPENTOL.** USAN.
Use: Anticonvulsant.
• **STIROFOS.** USAN.
Use: Insecticide (veterinary).
ST. JOSEPH ADULT MAXIMUM STRENGTH ASPIRIN-FREE TABLETS. (Plough) Acetaminophen 500 mg./Tab. Bot. 40s.
Use: Internal analgesic.
ST. JOSEPH ASPIRIN FOR ADULTS. (Plough) Aspirin 5 gr./Tab. Bot. 36s, 100s, 200s.
Use: Internal analgesic.
ST. JOSEPH ASPIRIN FOR CHILDREN. (Plough) Aspirin 1.25 gr./Tab. Bot. 36
Use: Internal analgesic.
ST. JOSEPH ASPIRIN-FREE ELIXIR FOR CHILDREN. (Plough) Acetaminophen 80 mg./2.5 ml. Bot. 2 oz., 4 oz.
Use: Internal analgesic.

ST. JOSEPH ASPIRIN-FREE INFANT DROPS. (Plough) Acetaminophen 80 mg./0.8 ml. dropper. Bot. 0.5 oz.
Use: Internal analgesic.
ST. JOSEPH ASPIRIN-FREE TABLETS FOR CHILDREN. (Plough) Acetaminophen 80 mg./Tab. Bot. 30s.
Use: Internal analgesic.
ST. JOSEPH COLD TABLETS FOR CHILDREN. (Plough) Aspirin 81 mg., phenylpropanolamine HCl 3.125 mg./Tab. Bot. 30s.
Use: Analgesic, antipyretic, antihistaminic.
ST. JOSEPH COUGH SYRUP FOR CHILDREN. (Plough) Dextromethorphan HBr 7.5 mg./5 ml. Bot. 2 oz., 4 oz.
Use: Antitussive.
STO-CAPS. (Misemer) Chlorpheniramine maleate 8 mg., phenylpropanolamine HC1 50 mg., methscopolamine nitrate 2.5 mg./Cap.
Use: Relief of the symptoms of common cold, sinusitis, allergic rhinitis.
STOMACH SUBSTANCE DESICCATED. W/Vit. B-12, cobalt gluconate & ferrous gluconate.
STOMAHESIVE. (ConvaTec) **Peristomal covering** gelatin, pectin, sod. CMC, polyisobutylene. Nonsterile wafers 4″ × 4″. Box 5s; 8 × 8 Box 3s. **Wafer with Surfit flange:** 4 × 4 wafer and one consists of the following flanges: 38 mm. (1½ inch) flange. Box 5s.; 45 mm. (1¾ inch) flange. Box 5s., 57 mm. (2¼ inch) flange. Box 5s.; 70 mm. (2¾ inch) flange. Box 5s. **Surfit drainable pouch.** 10 inch or 12 inch opaque with one of the following flanges: 38 mm. (1½ inch) flange. Box 10s.; 45 mm. (1¾ inch) flange, Box 10s.; 57 mm. (2¼ inch) flange, Box 10s.; 70 mm. (2¾ inch) flange, Box 10s.
Use: To protect skin from contact with exudates from colostomy or ileostomy.
STOMAHESIVE OSTOMY APPLIANCE BELT. (ConvaTec) Adjustable belt to be used with the Surfit ostomy appliance.
STOMAL. (Foy) Phenobarbital 16.2 mg., hyoscyamine sulfate 0.1037 mg., atropine sulfate 0.0194 mg., scopolamine HBr 0.0065 mg./Tab. Bot. 1000s.
Use: Treatment of peptic ulcer.
STOMASEPTINE DOUCHE POWDER. (Berlex) Sodium perborate, sodium bicarbonate, sodium chloride, sodium borate, fragrance. Pow. Bot. 6 oz., 15 oz.
Use: Vaginal douche powder.
STOOL SOFTENER. (Weeks & Leo) Docusate sodium 100 mg. or 250 mg./Cap. Bot. 30s, 100s. Calcium docusate 240 mg./Cap. Bot. 100s.
Use: Stool softener.
STOP. (CooperCare) Stannous fluoride 0.4% in water-free base. Tube 2 oz.
Use: Topical application to aid in prevention of dental caries.
STOPAYNE. (Springbok) Codeine phosphate 30 mg., promethazine HCl 6.25 mg., acetaminophen 357 mg./Cap. Bot. 100s, 500s. Unit dose 100s.
Use: Analgesic.

STOPAYNE SYRUP. (Springbok) Acetaminophen 120 mg., promethazine HCl 6.25 mg., codeine phosphate 5 mg./5 ml. Bot. 4 oz., 16 oz.
Use: Analgesic, antipyretic.
STOP-KOFF. (Stanley) Dextromethorphan HBr 15 mg., benzocaine 3 mg./soft gelatin cap. Bot. 30s.
Use: Commmon cold therapy.
STOP-ZIT. (Purepac) Denatonium benzoate in a clear nailpolish base. Bot. 0.75 oz.
Use: Thumbsucking-nail biting deterrent.
• **STORAX,** U.S.P. XXI.
Use: Pharm, necessity for Compound Benzoin Tincture.
STOVARSOL.
Use: Trichomonas vaginalis vaginitis, amebiasis & Vincent's angina.
See: Acetarsone, Tab.
STOXIL. (SmithKline) Idoxuridine. **Ophthalmic solution:** 0.1%, Thimerosal 1:50,000. 15 ml. Bot. with droppers. **Ophthalmic ointment:** 0.5%, Petrolatum base (5 mg./Gm.) Tube 4 Gm.
Use: Antiviral agent for herpetic keratitis.
STO-ZYME. (Misemer) Pancreatic enzyme 100 mg., ox bile extract 100 mg., cellulase 10 mg./Tab.
Use: Digestive enzymes.
STRAMONIUM. (Penick) Pow., Bot. ¼ lb., 1 lb.
Use: Sedative & antispasmodic.
STREMA. (Foy) Quinine sulfate 260 mg./Cap. Bot. 100s, 500s, 1000s.
STREN-TAB. (Barth's) Vit. C 300 mg., B-1 10 mg., B-2 10 mg., niacin 33 mg., B-6 2 mg., pantothenic acid 20 mg., B-12 4 mcg./Tab. Bot. 100s, 300s, 500s.
STREPTASE I.V. (Hoechst) Streptokinase I.V. infussion. Ctn. 10 vials, 250,000 IU/vial; 10 vials 750,000 IU/vial.
Use: Thrombolytic.
STREPTOCOCCI.
W/*Haemophilus influenzae, Neisseria catarrhalis, Klebsiella pneumoniae, staphylocci, pneumococci,* killed.
See: Mixed Vaccine No. 4 W-H. Influenzae (Lilly)
STREPTOCOCCI VACCINE, KILLED.
W/*Neisseria catarrhalis, Klebsiella pneumoniae, Diplococcus pneumoniae, staphylococci.*
See: Combined Vaccine No. 4 W/Catarrhalis (Lilly)
STREPTODORNASE. B.A.N. An enzyme obtained from cultures of various strains of *Streptococcus hemolyticus.*
See: Streptokinase-Streptodornase
STREPTODUOCIN. B.A.N. A mix. of equal parts of streptomycin & dihydrostreptomycin sulfates.
Use: Antibiotic.
See: Dimycin
Mixtamycin
STREPTOHYDRAZID. Streptomyclidene isonicotinyl hydrazine sulfate. Streptonicozid, B.A.N. Streptomycin isoniazid.
Use: Tuberculosis treatment.
STREPTOKINASE. B.A.N. An enzyme obtained from cultures of various strains of *Streptococcus hemolyticus.*

See: Kabikinase
Streptase, Inj. (Hoechst)
STREPTOLYSIN O TEST. (Laboratory Diagnostics) Reagent 6 × 10 ml., buffer 6 × 40 ml., Control Serum, 6 × 10 ml. or Kit.
Use: Diagnosis of "Group A" Streptococcal infections.
STREPTOMYCIN CALCIUM CHLORIDE.
Streptomycin Calcium Chloride Complex.
STREPTOMYCIN ISONIAZID.
See: Streptohydrazid
• **STREPTOMYCIN SULFATE INJECTION,** U.S.P. XXI. Sterile. U.S.P. XXI. (Various Mfr.)
Use: Antibacterial (tuberculostatic).
W/Dihydrostreptomycin sulfate.
See: Streptoduocin, Inj. (Various Mfr.)
STREPTOMYCYLIDENE ISONICOTINYL HYDRAZINE SULFATE.
See: Streptohydrazid
STREPTONASE-B. (Wampole) A tube test for the quantitative determination of *antideoxyribonuclease-B* (ADNase-B) titers in serum. Kit 10s.
Use: Diagnosis of *Streptoccal A* sequelae.
• **STREPTONICOZID.** USAN. Streptomycylidene isonicotinyl hydrazine sulfate.
Use: Antibiotic.
See: Streptohydrazid
• **STREPTONIGRIN.** USAN. Antibiotic isolated from both filtrates of *Streptomyces flocculus.* 5-Amino-6-(7-amino-5, 8-dihydro-6-methoxy-5, 8-dioxo-2-quinolyl)-4-(2-hydroxy-3, 4-dimethoxyphenyl)-3-methylpicolinic acid.
Use: Antineoplastic agent.
See: Nigrin (Pfizer)
STREPTONIVICIN. Novobiocin, B.A.N. (Various Mfr.)
STREPTOVARICIN. An antibiotic composed of several related components derived from cultures of *Streptomyces variabilis.* Dalacin (Upjohn)
• **STREPTOZOCIN.** USAN.
Use: Antineoplastic.
See: Zanosar, Powder (Upjohn).
STREPTOZYME. (Wampole) Rapid hemagglutination slide test for the qualitative detection and quantitative determination of streptococcal extracellular antigens in serum, plasma and peripheral blood. Kits 15s, 50s, 150s
Use: An aid in the diagnosis of *Streptococcal A* sequelae.
STRESSAIDS. (Vitarine) High potency stress formula with Vit. B & C.
Use: Dietary supplement.
STRESSAIDS 600 W/IRON. (Vitarine) Vit. B-1 15 mg., B-2 15 mg., B-6 25 mg., B-12 12 mcg., C 600 mg., niacinamide 100 mg., E 30 I.U., Ca 20 mg., folic acid 400 mcg., Iron 27 mg./Tab.
Use: Dietary supplement.
STRESSAIDS 600 WITH ZINC. (Vitarine) High potency stress formula with Vit. B, C and E, and zinc.
Use: Dietary supplement.
STRESSCAPS. (Lederle) Vit. B-1 10 mg., B-2 10 mg., niacinamide 100 mg., C 300 mg., B-6 2 mg., B-12

4 mcg., Ca pantothenate 20 mg./Cap. Bot. 30s, 100s.
Use: Vitamin B complex therapy.

STRESS COMPLEX TABLETS. (Eckerd) Vit. C 600 mg., folic acid 0.4 mg., thiamin 25 mg., riboflavin 25 mg., niacin 100 mg., B-6 15 mg., B-12 25 mg., Ca pantothenate 25 mg., Cu 4 mg., Zn 30 mg./Tab. Bot. 40s, 80s.
Use: High potency vitamin supplement.

STRESSTABS 600. (Lederle) Vit. B-1 15 mg., B-2 15 mg., B-6 5 mg., B-12 12 mcg., C 600 mg., niacinamide 100 mg., Vit. E 30 I.U., calcium pantothenate 20 mg./Tab. Bot. 30s, 60s, 500s. Unit dose 100s. Unit of Use Pkg. 50 × 30s, 50 × 60s.
Use: Multivitamin.

STRESSTABS 600 WITH IRON. (Lederle) Stresstab 600 formula with Vit. B-6 25 mg., choline 400 mcg., ferrous fumerate 27 mg./Tab. Bot. 30s, 60s.
Use: Multivitamin with iron.

STRESSTABS 600 WITH ZINC. (Lederle) Vit. B-1 20 mg., B-2 10 mg., B-6 10 mg., B-12 25 mcg., C 600 mg., E 45 I.U., niacinamide 100 mg., pantothenic acid 25 mg., folic acid 400 mcg., Cu 3 mg., zinc 23.9 mg./Tab. Bot. 30s, 60s.
Use: Multavitamin with zinc.

STRESSTEIN. (Doyle) Maltodextrin, medium chain triglycerides, L-leucine, soybean oil, L-isoleucine, L-valine, L-glutamic acid, L-arginine, L-lysine acetate, L-alanine, L-threonine, L-phenylalamine, L-aspartic acid, L-histidine, L-methionine, glycine, polyglycerol esters of fatty acids, L-serine, L-proline, sodium chloride, L-tryptophan, L-cysteine sodium citrate, vitamins and minerals. Powder 3.4 oz. packets.
Use: Tube feeding.

STRESSVICON. (CMC) Vit. B-1 10 mg., B-2 10 mg., C 150 mg., niacinamide 100 mg., B-6 5 mg., cal. pantothenate 25 mg., B-12 10 mcg., liver conc. 50 mg., brewer's yeast 50 mg./Cap. Bot. 30s, 100s, 250s, 500s, 1000s.
Use: Therapeutic vitamins.

STRIATRAN. Emylcamate, B.A.N.

STRI-DEX B.P. (Glenbrook) Benzoyl peroxide 10%. in greaseless, vanishing cream base.
Use: Acne medication.

STERI-DEX LOTION. (Glenbrook) Salicylic acid 0.5%, alcohol 28%, sulfonated alkyl benzenes, citric acid, sodium carbonate, simethicone, water. Bot. 4 oz.
Use: Acne medication.

STRI-DEX PADS. (Glenbrook) Salicylic acid 0.5%, alcohol 28%, sulfonated alkyl benzenes, citric acid, sodium carbonate, simethicone, water. Jar 42 pads, 75 pads.
Use: Acne medication.

STRIP-EASE. (Medtech) Blend of 1,1,1 trichloroethane. **Aerosol Spray:** 8 oz., **Sol.:** Bot. pt., gal.
Use: Adhesive bandage remover.

STROMBA AMPULES. (Winthrop Products) Stanozolol.
Use: Anabolic steroid.

STRONTIUM BROMIDE. Cryst. or Granule, Bot. ¼ lb., 1 lb. Amp. 1 Gm./10 cc.
Use: Sedative & antiepileptic.

W/Bromides of sodium, potassium, ammonium.
See: Lanabrom, Elix. (Lannett)

• **STRONTIUM CHLORIDE Sr 85.** USAN.
Use: Radioactive agent.

STRONTIUM LACTATE TRIHYDRATE.

• **STRONTIUM NITRATE Sr 85.** USAN.
Use: Radioactive agent.

STRONTIUM SR 85 INJECTION.
Use: Diagnostic aid (bone scanning).

STROPHANTHIN. K-strophanthin.

STROPHEN. (Kenyon) Prednisone 0.75 mg., salicylamide 5 gr., alum. hydroxide gel 75 mg., Vit. C 20 mg./Tab. Bot. 100s, 1000s.
Use: Arthritis.

STRYCHNINE. (Various Mfr.) Pow., Bot. ⅛ oz., 1 oz.

STRYCHNINE SULFATE. (Various Mfr.) Cryst., Bot. ⅛ oz., 1 oz. Pow., Bot. ⅛ oz., 5 lb.
W/Thyroid ext., yohimbine HCl.
See: Andro-Medicone (Medicone)

STUART FORMULA. (Stuart) Vit. A 5000 I.U., B-1 1.5 mg., B-2 1.7 mg. niacin 20 mg., B-6 2 mg., B-12 6 mcg., C 60 mg., D 400 I.U., E 15 I.U., Ca 160 mg., Fe 18 mg., magnesium 100 mg., phos. 125 mg., folic acid 0.4 mg., iodine 150 mcg./Tab. Bot. 100s, 250s.
Use: Dietary vitamin & mineral supplement.

STUARTINIC. (Stuart) Vit. B-12 25 mcg.,B-1 6 mg., B-2 6 mg., niacinamide 20 mg., Ca pantothenate 10 mg., Vit. B-6 1 mg., C 500 mg., iron 100 mg./Tab. Bot. 60s.
Use: Hematinic; iron deficiency.

STUARTNATAL 1 + 1. (Stuart) Vit. A 8000 I.U., B-1 2.55 mg., B-2 3 mg. niacin 20 mg., B-6 10 mg., B-12 12 mcg., C 90 mg., D 400 I.U., E 30 I.U., Folic Acid 1 mg. Ca 200 mg., magnesium 100 mg., Iron 65 mg., iodine 150 mcg./Tab. Bot. 100s, 500s.
Use: Vitamin, mineral supplement in pregnancy and lactation.

STUART PRENATAL. (Stuart) Vit. A 8000 I.U., B-1 1.7 mg., B-2 2 mg., B-6 4 mg., B-12 8 mcg., C 60 mg., D 400 I.U., E 30 I.U., Niacin 20 mg., Fe 60 mg., Ca 200 mg., magnesium 100 mg., iodine 150 mcg., Folic Acid 0.8 mg./Tab. Bot. 100s, 500s.
Use: Vitamin & mineral supplement in pregnancy & lactation.

STUGERON. Cinnarizine, B.A.N.

STULEX. (Bowman) Docusate sodium 100 mg. or 250 mg./Tab. Bot. 100s, 1000s.
Use: Nonlaxative fecal softener.

STYE. (Commerce) Tube 0.125 oz.
Use: Minor irritation and infection of eyelid.

STYPTIRENAL.
See: Epinephrine (Various Mfr.)

STYPTO-CAINE SOLUTION. (Pedinol) Hydroxyquinoline sulphate, tetracaine HCl, aluminum Cl, aqueous glycol base. Bot. 2 oz.
Use: Hemostatic solution.

STYRAMATE, B.A.N. 1-Phenyl-1,2-ethanediol 2-carbamate. β-Hydroxyphenethyl carbamate. 2-Hydroxy-2-phenylethyl carbamate.
Use: Skeletal muscle relaxant.
See: Sinaxar

STYRENE POLYMER, SULFONATED, SODIUM SALT. Sodium Polystyrene Sulfonate, U.S.P. XXI.
STYRONATE RESINS. Ammonium and potassium salts of sulfonated styrene polymers.
Use: Conditions requiring sodium restriction.
SUAVITIL HYDROCHLORIDE. Benactyzine, B.A.N.
SUBLIMAZE. (Janssen) Fentanyl 0.05 mg./cc. Amp. 10 ml., 20 ml. Pkg. 5s.
Use: Analgesic.
SUBSTRATE REAGENT. (Roche) Enzyme substrate reagent for the quantitation of creatine kinase. Box 8 × 10 ml.
SUCARYL LIQUID. (Abbott) Saccharin 1.21% (as sodium saccharin), benzoic acid 0.1%, methyl paraben 0.5% as preservative, water. Bot. 6 oz, 12 oz.
Use: Artificial sweetening agent.
SUCARYL TABLETS. (Abbott) Saccharin 12.5 mg. (equivalent to approx. 0.25 gr. sodium saccharin)/Tab. Bot. 1000s.
Use: Artificial sweetning agent.
• **SUCCIMER.** USAN.
Use: Diagnostic aid.
SUCCINATES.
See: Calcium succinate
Sodium succinate
Succinic acid
SUCCINCHLORIMIDE. N-Chlorosuccinimide.
SUCCINIC ACID.
W/9-Aminoacridine HCl, phenyl mercuric acetate, sod. lauryl acetate.
See: Vagiserts W/Inserts, Tab. (Vortech)
W/9-Aminoacridine undecylenate, N-myristyl-3-hydroxybutylamine hydrochloride, methylbenzethonium chloride.
See: Cenasert, Tab. (Central)
• **SUCCINYLCHOLINE CHLORIDE,** U.S.P. XXI. Inj., Sterile, U.S.P. XXI. Ethanaminium, 2,2'-[(1,4-dioxo-1,4-butanediyl)bis(oxy)]bis-N,NN-tri-methyl-, dichloride. Choline chloride succinate (2:1).
Use: Skeletal muscle relaxant.
See: Anectine chloride, Amp. (Burroughs Wellcome)
Quelicin, Amp., Additive Syringes, Fliptop & Pintop Vials (Abbott)
Sucostrin, Amp., Vial (Squibb)
SUCCINYLSULFATHIAZOLE. 4'-(2-Thiazolysulfamoyl)
Use: Intestinal antibacterial.
SUCOSTRIN CHLORIDE. (Squibb) Succinylcholine chloride 20 mg./cc. w/methylparaben 0.1%, propylparaben 0.01%, sodium hydroxide or hydrochloric acid. Vial 10 cc.; For infusion 50 mg./cc. Vial. 10 cc. High potency 100 mg./cc. Vial 10 cc.
Use: Muscle relaxant.
• **SUCRALFATE.** USAN. Beta-D-fructofuranosyl-alpha-D-glucopyranoside octakis (hydrogen sulfate) aluminum hydroxide complex.
Use: Duodenal ulcer therapy.
See: Carafate, Tab. (Marion)
SUCRALOX. B.A.N. A polymerized complex of sucrose and aluminum hydroxide.
Use: Treatment of gastric hyperacidity.

See: Malalox AS
SUCRETS COLD DECONGESTANT LOZENGE. (Beecham Products) Phenylpropanolamine HCl 25 mg./Lozenge. Box 24s.
Use: Decongestant.
SUCRETS COUGH CONTROL LOZENGE. (Beecham Products) Dextromethorphan HBr 7.50 mg./Lozenge. Tin 24s.
Use: Antitussive.
SUCRETS MAXIMUM STRENGTH SORE THROAT LOZENGES. (Beecham Products) Dyclonine HCl 2.4 mg./Lozenge. Tin 24s.
Use: Temporary relief of minor sore throat & mouth irritation.
SUCRETS SORE THROAT LOZENGE. (Beecham Products) Hexylresorcinol 2.4 mg./Loz. Regular: Tin 24s, Bot. 55s; Children's Cherry flavor: Tin 24s; Mentholated: Tin 24s.
Use: Minor throat irritations.
• **SUCROSE,** N.F. XVI. Compressible, Confectioners, N.F. XVI. Saccharose. Sugar. α-D-Glucopyranoside, β-D-fructo-furanosyl-.
Use: I.V.; diuretic & dehydrating agent; pharm. aid (sweetening agent).
• **SUCROSE OCTAACETATE,** N.F. XVI.
Use: Alcohol denaturant.
SUDAFED. (Burroughs Wellcome) Pseudoephedrine HCl **Tab:** 30 mg./Tab. Box 24s, Bot. 100s, 1000s; 60 mg./Tab. Bot. 100s, 1000s. **Syr.** (30 mg./5 cc.) Bot. 4 oz., 1 pt.
Use: Decongestant of respiratory tract mucosa.
W/Chlorcyclizine HCl.
See: Fedrazil, Tab. (Burroughs Wellcome)
W/Codeine phosphate, acetophenetidin, aspirin, caffeine.
See: Emprazil-C, Tabs. (Burroughs Wellcome)
SUDAFED COUGH SYRUP. (Burroughs Wellcome) Pseudoephedrine HCl 30 mg., dextromethorphan HBr 10 mg., guaifenesin 100 mg./5 ml. w/alcohol 2.4%. Bot. 4 oz., 8 oz.
Use: Cough treatment.
SUDAFED PLUS. (Burroughs Wellcome) **Tab.:** Pseudoephedrine HCl 60 mg., chlorpheniramine maleate 4 mg./Tab. Box 24s, 48s. **Syrup:** Pseudoephedarine HCl 30 mg., chlorpheniramine maleate 2 mg./5 ml. Bot. 4 oz.
Use: Sinus & upper respiratory tract decongestant.
SUDAFED S.A. (Burroughs Wellcome) Pseudoephedrine HCl 120 mg./Sustained Action Cap. Bot. 40s, 100s. Box 10s.
Use: Nasal or eustachin tube congestion.
SUDANYL. (Dover) Pseudoephedrine HCl./Tab. Sugar and salt free. Unit dose 500s.
Use: Decongestant.
SUDDEN TAN LOTION. (Plough) Padimate O, dihydroxyacetone, Bot. 4 oz.
Use: Artificial tanning agent, ultraviolet sunscreen, moisturizer.
SUDERMO. Mesulphen, B.A.N.
• **SUDOXICAM.** USAN. 4-Hydroxy-2-methyl-N-thiazol-2-yl-2H-1,2-benzothiazine-3-carboxamide   1,1-dioxide.

Use: Anti-inflammatory.

SUDRIN. (Bowman) Pseudoephedrine HCl 30 mg. or 60 mg./Tab. Bot. 100s, 1000s.
Use: Nasal decongestant.

SUEDA-G. (Hyrex) Guaifenesin 250 mg., pseudoephedrine HCl 120 mg./T.R. Cap. Bot. 100s, 1000s.
Use: Expectorant, decongestant.

SUFAMAL. (Milex) Sulfanilamide 15.0%, aminacrine HCl 0.2%, allantoin 2.0%. Tube 4 oz. w/ or w/o applicator.
Use: Trichomonads, moniliasis, streptococcus pyogenes (Group A), haemophilus vaginalis.

SUFENTA. (Janssen) Sufentanil citrate.
Use: Analgesic.

• **SUFENTANIL.** USAN.
Use: Analgesic.

SUFREX. (Janssen) Ketanserin tarfrate.
Use: Serotonin antagonist.

• **SUGAR, COMPRESSIBLE,** U.S.P. XXI.
Use: Pharm. aid (sweetening agent, tablet excipient).

• **SUGAR, CONFECTIONER'S,** U.S.P. XXI.
Use: Pharm. aid (sweetening agent; tablet excipient).

• **SULAZEPAM.** USAN. 7-Chloro-1,3-dihydro-1-methyl-5-phenyl-2H-1,4-benzodiazepine-2-thione.
Use: Tranquilizer (minor).

SULAZO. (Freeport) Sulfisoxazole 500 mg., phenylazodiaminopyridine HCl 50 mg./Tab. Bot. 1000s.
Use: Urinary tract infections complicated by pain.

• **SULBACTAM BENZATHINE.** USAN.

• **SULBACTAM PIVOXIL.** USAN.
Use: Inhibitor, synergist.

• **SULBENOX.** USAN.
Use: Growth stimulant (veterinary).

SUL-BLUE SHAMPOO. (Columbia) Selenium sulfide 1%. Bot. 4 oz.
Use: Dandruff treatment.

SULCOLON. (Lederle) Sulfasalazine 500 mg./Tab. Bot. 500s.
Use: Anti-infective, ulcerative colitis.

• **SULCONAZOLE NITRATE.** USAN.
Use: Antifungal.

SULDIAZO. (Kay) Sulfisoxazole 0.5 Gm., phenazopyridine HCl 50 mg./Tab. Bot. 100s, 1000s.
Use: Urinary tract infections.

SULF-10. (CooperVision) Na sulfacetamide 10%. Bot. 15 ml.; Dropperette 1 ml. Box 12s.
Use: External bacterial eye infections.

SULF-10 OPHTHALMIC. (Maurry) Sodium sulfacetamide 10%, hydroxyethylcellulose, sodium borate, boric acid, disodium edetate, sodium metabisulfite, sodium thiosulfate 0.2%, chlorobutanol 0.2%, methyl paraben 0.015%. Bot. 15 ml.
Use: Antibacterial.

• **SULFABENZ.** USAN.
Use: Antibacterial, coccidiostat.

• **SULFABENZAMIDE,** U.S.P. XXI. Benzamide, N-(4-aminophenyl) sulfunyl)-N-Sulfanilylbenzamide. Sulfanilylbenzamide, N′ benzoylsulfanilamide.
See: Sultrin, Vag. Tab., Cream (Ortho)

SULFABROMETHAZINE SODIUM.
Use: Antibacterial.

SULFACARBAMIDE (I.N.N.). Sulphaurea, B.A.N.

SULFACEL-15. (Softcon) Sod. sulfacetamide 15%, methylcellulose ¼%, methylparaben 0.05%, propylparaben 0.01%, sod. thiosulfate, monobasic and dibasic sod. phosphate, propylene glycol. Bot. 5 cc., 15 cc.
Use: External ophthalmic bacterial infections.

SULFACET. (Dermik)
See: Sulfacetamide

• **SULFACETAMIDE,** U.S.P. XXI. Acetamide, N-(4-aminophenyl) sulfonyl)-N-Sulfanilylacetamine. N-acetylsulfanilamide.
Use: Antibacterial.
See: Isopto-Cetamide, Ophth. Sol. (Alcon)

SULFACETAMIDE W/COMBINATIONS.
See: Acet-Dia-Mer Sulfonamides
Azosul, Tab. (Reid-Provident)
Cetapred, Oint. (Alcon)
Cetazine, Tab. (Bowman)
Chero-Trisulfa (V), Susp. (Vita Elixir)
Neogel W/Sulfa, Tab. (Vortech)
Sulf-10, Ophth. Soln. (CooperVision)
Sulfa-Plex Vaginal Cream (Rowell)
Sultrin, Tab., Cream (Ortho)
Triosulfon, Tab. (CMC)
Triurisul, Tab. (Sheryl)
Uridium, Tab. (Pharmex)
Urotrol, Tab. (Mills)
Vagi-Plex, Cream (Rowell)

• **SULFACETAMIDE SODIUM,** U.S.P. XXI. Ophth. Oint., Ophth. Sol., U.S.P. XXI. Acetamide, N-[(4-aminophenyl)sulfonyl]-, monosodium salt, monohydrate. N-Sulfanilylacetamide monosodium salt monohydrate.
Use: Antibacterial (Ophthalmic).
See: Bleph 10, Liquifilm (Allergan)
Centamide, Ophth. Oint. (Alcon)
Sebizon Lotion (Schering)
Sodium Sulamyd Opthalmic Ointment 30% (Schering)
Sulf-10, Drops (Maurry)
Sulf-10, Soln. Drops (Smith, Miller & Patch)
W/Methylcellulose.
See: Sodium Sulamyd Ophth. Sol. 10% (Schering)
W/Phenylephrine HCl, methylparaben, propylparaben.
See: Vasosulf, Liq. (CooperVision)
W/Prednisolone.
See: Cetapred Ophthalmic Ointment (Alcon)
Vasocidin, Soln. (CooperVision)
W/Prednisolone acetate.
See: Blephamide S.O.P., Ophth. Oint. (Allergan)
Metimyd, Ophth. Oint. and Susp. (Schering)
W/Prednisolone, methylcellulose.
See: Isopto Cetapred, Susp. (Alcon)
W/Prednisolone acetate, phenylephrine.
See: Blephamide Liquifilm Ophth. Susp. (Allergan)
Tri-Ophtho, Ophth. Drops (Maurry)

W/Prednisolone phosphate.
See: Optimyd Sol., Sterile (Schering)
W/Prednisolone sodium phosphate, phenylephrine, sulfacetamide sodium.
Vasocidia Ophth. Sol. (CooperVision)
W/Sulfur.
See: Sulfacet-R, Lot. (Dermik)
SULFACETAMIDE, SULFADIAZINE, & SULFAMERAZINE ORAL SUSPENSION.
See: Acet-Dia-Mer-Sulfonamides.
SULFACET-R LOTION. (Dermik) Sodium sulfacetamide 10%, sulfur 5%, in flesh-tinted base. Bot. 1 oz.
Use: Treatment of acne and seborrheic dermatitis.
SULFACHLORPYRIDAZINE. B.A.N. N^1-(6-chloro-3-pyridazinyl) sulfanilamide.
See: Cosulid
Nefrosul, Tab. (Riker)
Sonilyn, Tab. (Mallinckrodt)
• **SULFACYTINE.** USAN. 4-(4-Aminobenzene-sulfonamido)-1-ethyl-1,2-dihydropyrimidin-2-one. 1-Ethyl-N-sulfanilylcytosine.
Use: Antibacterial.
See: Renoquid, Tab. (Parke-Davis)
SULFADIASULFONE SODIUM. Acetosulfone sodium.
• **SULFADIAZINE,** U.S.P. XXI.; Tab., U.S.P. XXI. 2-Sulfanilamidopyridine, N'-2-pyrimidinylsulfanilamide. Benzenesulfonamide, 4-amino-N-2-pyrimidi-nyl-.
Use: Antibacterial.
See: Microsulfon, Tab. (Consolid. Mid.)
SULFADIAZINE COMBINATIONS.
See: Acet-Dia-Mer-Sulfonamides. (Various Mfr.)
Amide, Preps. (Scrip)
Benegyn, Vag. Insert, Cream (North Am. Pharm.)
Buffonamide, Liq. (Reid-Provident)
Cetazine, Tab. (Bowman)
Chemozine, Tab., Susp. (Tennessee Pharm.)
Cherasulfa, Liq, Tab. (Cenci)
Chera-Sulfa Improved, Susp. (Sutliff & Case)
Chero-Trisulfa, Susp. (Vita Elixir)
Dia-Mer-Sulfonamides (Various Mfr.)
Dia-Mer-Thia-Sulfonamide (Various Mfr.)
Gynben, Cream, Inserts (ICN)
Gynben Insufflate, Pow. (ICN)
Lantrisul, Tab., Susp. (Lannett)
Meth-Dia-Mer-Sulfonamides (Various Mfr.)
Quadetts, Tab. (Elder)
Quad-Ramoid, Susp. (Elder)
Silvadene (Marion)
Suladyne (Reid-Provident)
Suladyne, Tab. (Stuart)
Sulfajen, Cream. (Jenkins)
Sulfaloid Suspension (Westerfield)
Sul-Trio, Preps. (Kay)
Terfonyl, Liq, Tab. (Squibb)
Triosulf, Tab. (Jenkins)
Triple Sulfa, Tab. (Various Mfr.)
Trisem, Tab., Susp. (Beecham Labs)
Trisuval, Tab. (Jalco)
SULFADIAZINE AND SULFAMERAZINE. Citrasulfas.
See: Dia-Mer-Sulfonamides
• **SULFADIAZINE SODIUM,** U.S.P. XXI. Sterile Inj., U.S.P. XXI. Benzenesulfonamide, 4-amino-N-2-

pyrimidinyl-, monosodium salt. N^1-2-Pyrimidinylsulfanilamide monosodium salt.
Use: Antibacterial.
W/Sod. bicarbonate.
(Pitman-Moore)—Tab. 5 gr., Bot. 1000s; 2½ gr., Bot. 100s, 500s, 1000s.
SULFADIAZINE, SULFAMERAZINE & SULFACETAMIDE SUSPENSION.
See: Acet-Dia-Mer-Sulfonamides
Coco Diazine (Lilly)
SULFADIMETHOXINE. Sulphadi-methoxine, B.A.N. N'-(2,6-Dimethoxy-4-pyrimidinyl) sulfanilamide.
Use: Antibacterial.
SULFADIMETINE. N^1-(2-6-Dimethyl-4-pyrimidyl) sulfanilamide. Sulfisomidine. Elkosin (Ciba)
SULFADIMIDINE
See: Sulfamethazine
SULFADINE.
See: Sulfadimidine
Sulfamethazine
Sulfapyridine, Tab. (Various Mfr.)
• **SULFADOXINE,** U.S.P. XXI. N^1-(5,6-dimethoxy-4-pyrimidinyl) sulfanilamide. 4-(4-Aminobenzene-sulfonamido)-5,6-dimethoxypyrimidine. Fanasil Fanzil (Roche)
Use: Antibacterial sulfonamide.
W/Pyrimethamine.
See: Fansidar, Tab. (Roche)
• **SULFADOXINE AND PYRIMETHAMINE TABLETS,** U.S.P. XXI.
Use: Antibacterial, antimalarial.
SULFAETHIDOLE. Sulphaethicole, B.A.N. Sulfaethylthiadiazole. N^1-(5-ethyl-1,3,4-thiadiazole-2-yl) sulfanilamide. Sulfaethylthiadiazole. Sethadil.
Use: Antibacterial.
SULFAETHYLTHIADIAZOLE.
See: Sulfaethidole.
SULFAFURAZOLE. B.A.N. 5-(4-Aminobenzene-sulphonamido)-3,4-dimethylisoxazole. Gantrisin. Sulphafurazole. Sulfisoxazole
SULFAGAN. (Zenith) Sulfisoxazole 500 mg./Tab. Bot. 100s.
Use: Anti-infective.
SULFAGUANIDINE. (N-Guanylsulfanilamide; Abiguanil; Ganidan; Guamide).
Use: G.I. tract infections.
W/Sulfacetamide, neomycin sulf., atropine methyl nitrate, carob flour.
See: Neogel W/Sulfa, Tab. (Vortech)
W/Sulfamethazine, sulfamerazine & sulfadiazine.
See: Quadetts, Tab. (Elder)
Quad-Ramoid, Susp. (Elder
SULFA-GYN. (Mayrand) Sulfathiazole 3.42%, sulfacetamide 2.86%, sulfabenzamide 3.70%, urea 0.64%. Tube 85 Gm.
Use: Triple sulfa cream.
SULFAJEN CREAM. (Jenkins) Sulfamerazine 0.167 Gm., sulfadiazine 0.167 Gm., sulfamethazine 0.167 Gm./5 cc. Bot. 3 oz., 4 oz., gal.
Use: Triple sulfonamide therapy.
• **SULFALENE.** USAN. N'-(3-Methoxypyrazinyl) sulfanilamide. Sulfametopyrazine, B.A.N.

Use: Antibacterial.
See: Kelfizina (Abbott)
SULFALOID SUSPENSION. (O'Neal, Jones & Feldman) Sulfadiazine 167 mg., sulfamerazine 167 mg., sulfamethazine 167 mg./5 ml. Bot. 2 oz., 3 oz., 4 oz., 16 oz.
Use: Antibacterial.
SULFALOID TABLETS. (O'Neal, Jones & Feldman) Meth-Dia-Mer-Sulfonamides. Tab. 0.5 Gm. (0.167 Gm. each). Bot. 100s.
Use: Antibacterial.
• **SULFAMERAZINE,** U.S.P. XXI. Tab., U.S.P. XXI. Benzenesulfonamide, 4-amino-N-(4-methyl-2-pyrimidinyl)-.   N¹-(4-Methyl-2-pyrimidinyl)-sulfanilamide. (Sumedine)
Use: Infections caused by susceptible bacteria.
SULFAMERAZINE COMBINATIONS.
Use: Antibacterial.
See: Amide, Preps. (Scrip)
   Cetazine, Tab. (Bowman)
   Chemozine Tab., Susp. (Tennessee Pharm.)
   Cherasulfa, Liq, Tab. (Cenci)
   Chera-Sulfa Improved, Susp. (Sutliff & Case)
   Chero-Trisulfa-V, Susp. (Vita Elixir)
   Gelazine, Liq. (Mallard)
   Lantrisol, Tab., Susp. (Lannett)
   Quadetts, Tab. (Elder)
   Quad-Ramoid, Susp. (Elder)
   Sul-Trio, Preps. (Kay)
   Terfonyl, Liq, Tab. (Squibb)
   Triosulfon, Tab. (CMC)
   Triple Sulfa, Tab. (Various Mfr.)
SULFAMERAZINE SODIUM.
Use: Antibacterial.
SULFAMERAZINE & SULFADIAZINE.
See: Dia-Mer-Sulfonamides.
SULFAMERAZINE, SULFADIAZINE & SULFAMETHAZINE.
Use: Antibacterial.
See: Meth-Dia-Mer-Sulfonamides
SULFAMERAZINE, SULFADIAZINE & SULFATHIAZOLE.
Use: Antibacterial.
See: Dia-Mer-Thia-Sulfonamides
• **SULFAMETER.** USAN. N¹(5-methoxy-2-pyrimidinyl)-sulfanilamide. 4-Amino-N-(5-methoxy-2-pyrimidinyl) benzenesulfonamide.
Use: Antibacterial.
See: Sulla, Tab. (Robins)
• **SULFAMETHAZINE,** U.S.P. XXI.
Benzenesulfonamide, 4-amino-N-(4,6-dimethyl-2-pyrimidinyl)-.   4,6-Dimethyl-2-sulfanilamidopyrimidine. NI-(4,6-Dimethyl-2-pyrimidinyl)sulfanilamide.
Use: Antibacterial.
See: Neotrizine, Susp., Tab. (Lilly)
W/Sulfacetamide, sulfadiazine, sulfamerazine.
See: Sulfa-Plex, Vaginal Cream (Rowell)
W/Sulfadiazine, sulfamerazine.
See: Lantrisul, Tab., Susp. (Lannett)
   Sulfaloid, Susp. (Westerfield)
   Terfonyl, Liq, Tab. (Squibb)
   Triple Sulfa, Tab. (Var. Mfr.)

W/Sulfadiazine, sulfamerazine, sodium citrate.
See: Chera-Sulfa, Cab. (Century)
   Cherasulfa, Liq. Tab. (Cenci)
   Triple Sulfa, Susp. (Standex)
• **SULFAMETHIZOLE,** U.S.P. XXI. Oral Susp., Tab., U.S.P. XXI. N'-(5/Methyl-1,3,4-thiadiazole-2-yl)-sulfanilamide. Methisul, Mizol, Uolueosil.
Sulphamethizole.
Use: Antibacterial.
See: Bursul, Tab. (Burlington)
   Microsul, Tab. (Star)
   Proklar-M, Liq., Tab. (Westerfield)
   Sulfasol, Tab. (Hyrex-Key)
   Sulfstat, Forte, Tab. (Saron)
   Sulfurine, Tab. (Table Rock)
   Thiosulfil, Forte, Tab. (Ayerst)
   Uri-Pak (Westerfield)
   Urifon, Tab. (Amid)
SULFAMETHIZOLE W/COMBINATIONS.
Use: Antibacterial.
See: Azosul, Tab. (Reid-Provident)
   Azo Sulfstat, Tab. (Saron)
   Azotrex, Cap. (Bristol)
   Microsul-A, Tab. (Star)
   Signasul Azopak, Tab. (Amer. Urological)
   Sulfasol Plus, Tab. (Hyrex-Key)
   Thiosulfil-A, Tab. (Ayerst)
   Thiosulfil-A Forte, Tab. (Ayerst)
   Triurisul, Tab. (Sheryl)
   Urobiotic, Cap. (Pfizer)
   Uropeutic, Tab. (Circle)
   Urotrol, Tab. (Mills)
SULFAMETHOMIDINE. (Warner-Lambert) N'-(6-methoxy-2-methyl-4-pyrimidinyl)sulfanilamide monohydrate.
Use: Antibacterial sulfonamide.
• **SULFAMETHOXAZOLE,** U.S.P. XXI. Oral Susp., Tab., U.S.P. XXI. Sulphamethoxazole, Methyl sulfanilamidoisoxazole.   5-Methyl-3-sulfanilamido-isoxazole. N'-(5-methyl-3-isoxazolyl) sulfanilamide.
Use: Antibacterial.
See: Gantanol, Prep. (Roche)
W/Trimethoprim.
See: Bactrim, Prods. (Roche)
   Septra, Tab. (Burroughs Wellcome)
   Septra DS, Tab. (Burroughs Wellcome)
SULFAMETHOXAZOLE AND PHENAZOPYRIDINE HCl.
Use: Urinary antibacterial.
See: Azo-Gantanol, Tab. (Roche)
• **SULFAMETHOXAZOLE AND TRIMETHOPRIM ORAL SUSPENSION,** U.S.P. XXI.
Use: Urinary antibacterial.
• **SULFAMETHOXAZOLE AND TRIMETHOPRIM TABLETS,** U.S.P. XXI.
Use: Urinary antibacterial.
SULFAMETHOXYDIAZINE. Sulfameter
Use: Antibacterial.
See: Sulla, Tab. (Robins)
SULFAMETHOXYPYRIDAZINE, B.A.N. N¹-(6-Methoxy-3-pyridazinyl) sulfanilamide. 3-(4-Aminobenzenesulfonamido)-6-methoxypyridazine.

Use: Antibacterial.
See: Kynex.
 Lederkyn.
SULFAMETHOXYPYRIDAZINE ACETYL.
Use: Antibacterial.
SULFAMETHYLTHIADIAZOLE.
Use: Antibacterial.
See: Sulfamethizole, Preps.
SULFAMETIN. N¹-(5-Methoxy-2-pyrimidinyl)sulfanila-
mide. (Formerly sulfamethoxydiazine)
Use: Antibacterial.
See: Sulla, Tab. (Robins)
SULFAMETOPYRAZINE. B.A.N. 2-(4-Aminoben-
zenesulfonamido)-3-methoxypyrazine.
Use: Antibacterial.
See: Sulfalene (I.N.N.)
 Kelfizine.
SULFAMEZANTHENE.
Use: Antibacterial.
See: Sulfamethazine
• **SULFAMONOMETHOXINE.** USAN. N¹-(6-methoxy-
4-pyrimidinyl) sulfanilamide.
Use: Antibacterial sulfonamide.
• **SULFAMOXOLE.** USAN. N′-(4,5-dimethyl-2-oxa-zolyl)
sulfanilamide.
Use: Antibacterial.
See: Nuprin (Upjohn)
p-**SULFAMOYLBENZYLAMINE HCl.** Sulfbenzamide.
SULFAMYLON CREAM. (Winthrop-Breon) Mafenide
acetate equiv. to 85 mg. of base/Gm. W/cetyl
alcohol, stearyl alcohol, cetyl esters wax, polyoxyl
40 stearate, polyoxyl 8 stearate, glycerin, water
w/methylparaben and propylparaben, sodium
bisulfite, edetate disodium. Tube 2 oz., 4 oz. Can
14.5 oz.
Use: Adjunctive therapy in second and third-degree
burns.
SULFANILAMIDE. p-Aminobenzenesulfonamide.
Use: Antibacterial.
SULFANILAMIDE COMBINATIONS.
Use: Antibacterial.
See: AVC/Dienestrol Cream, Supp. (Merrell Dow)
 AVC, Cream, Supp. (Merrell Dow)
 D.I.T.I. Cream (Kenyon)
 Femguard, Vag. Cream (Reid-Provident)
 K.D.C. Vaginal Cream (Kenyon)
 Par Cream (Parmed)
 Sulfem Vag. Cream (Federal Pharm.)
 Tricholan, Vaginal Cream (Spencer-Mead)
 Vagacreme, Cream (Delta)
 Vagisan Creme (Sandia)
 Vagisul, Creme (Sheryl)
 Vagitrol, Cream, Suppos. (Lemmon)
2-**SULFANILAMIDOPYRIDINE.** Sulfadiazine, U.S.P.
XXI.
Use: Antibacterial.
• **SULFANILATE ZINC.** USAN.
Use: Antibacterial.
N-**SULFANILYLACETAMIDE.**
Use: Antibacterial.
See: Sulfacetamide, Tab. (Various Mfr.)

SULFANILYLBENZANIDE.
Use: Antibacterial.
See: Sulfabenzamide
• **SULFANITRAN.** USAN. 4′-[(p-Nitrophenyl) sulfamoyl]-
acetanilide.
Use: Antibacterial.
SULFAPHENAZOLE. Sulphaphenzaole, B.A.N. N′-(1-
phenyl-5-pyrazolyl) sulfanilamide. 5-(4-Aminoben-
zenesulphonamido)-1-phenylpyrazole.
See: Orisulf (Ciba)
SULFAPRED. (Softcon) Prednisolone acetate 0.25%,
sodium sulfacetamide 10%, phenylephrine HCl
0.125%, in a sterile buffered Methulose suspension
w/methylparaben 0.04%, propylparaben 0.02%,
propylene glycol, monobasic and dibasic sod.
phosphate, sod. thiosulfate, polysorbate 80. Plas.
Bot. 5 cc., 15 cc.
Use: Allergic and inflammatory diseases of the eye.
SULFAPYRAZOLE. B.A.N. N¹-(3-Methyl-1-phenyl-
pyrazol-5-yl)sulfanilamide.
Use: Sulphonamide, veterinary medicine.
See: Vesulong.
• **SULFAPYRIDINE,** U.S.P. XXI. Tab., U.S.P. XXI.
Benzenesulfonamide, 4-amino-N-2-pyridinyl-. 2-Sul-
fanilamidopyridine. N′-2-Pyridylsulfanilamide. (Pfaltz
& Bauer) Pow., Bot. 1 lb.
Use: Dermatitic herpetiformis suppressant.
SULFAQUINOXALINE.
See: S.Q. Preps (MSD AGVET)
SULFARSPHENAMINE. Disodium-[arsenobis[6-hy-
droxy-m-phenylene)imino]]-dimethanesulfonate.
• **SULFASALAZINE,** U.S.P. XXI. Tab., U.S.P. XXI. 5-
[[p-(2-Pyridylsulfamoyl)-phenyl]azo]salicylic acid. 4-
Hydroxy-4′-(2-pyridylsulfamoyl)azobenzene-3-car-
boxylic acid. Sulphasalazine, B.A.N.
Use: Antibacterial.
See: Azulfidine, Tab., Susp. (Pharmacia)
 Salazopyrin.
 Salicylazosulfapyridine.
 Salazopyrin.
 S.A.S.P., Tab. (Zenith)
 Sulcolon, Tab. (Lederle)
 Sulfapyridine (I.N.N.)
• **SULFASOMIZOLE.** USAN. 5-(4-Aminobenzenesul-
fonamido)-3-methylisothiazole. N′-(3-methyliso-
thiazolyl)sulfanilamide.
Use: Antibacterial sulfonamide.
See: Bidizole.
SULFASOX. (Bowman) Sulfasoxazole 500 mg./Tab.
Bot. 100s, 1000s.
Use: Treatment of urinary tract infections.
SULFASYMASINE. N′-(4,6-Diethyl-S-triazin-2-yl) sul-
fanilamide.
Use: Antibacterial sulfonamide.
SULFA-TER-TABLETS. (A.P.C.) Trisulfapyrimidines,
U.S.P. Bot. 1000s.
• **SULFATHIAZOLE,** U.S.P. XXI. Benzenesulfonamide,
4-amino-N-2-thiazolyl-N′-2-Thiazolylsulfanilamide. 2-
Sulfanilamidothiazole.
Use: Antibacterial.
W/Chlorophyllin.
See: Thiaphyll Cr. (Lannett)

SULFATHIAZOLE COMBINATIONS.
See: Sultrin, Tab. & Cream (Ortho)
SULFATHIAZOLE CARBAMIDE.
See: Otosmosan, Liq. (Ayerst)
• **SULFATHIAZOLE, SULFACETAMIDE, AND SULFABENZAMIDE VAGINAL CREAM,** U.S.P. XXI.
Use: Antibacterial.
• **SULFATHIAZOLE, SULFACETAMIDE, AND SULFABENZAMIDE VAGINAL TABLETS,** U.S.P. XXI.
Use: Antibacterial.
SULFA TRIPLE NO. 2. (Richlyn) Sulfadiazine 162 mg., sulfamerizine 162 mg., sulfamethazine 162 mg./Tab. Bot. 1000s.
Use: Antibacterial.
• **SULFAZAMET.** USAN. N'-(3-Methyl-1-phenylpyrazol-5-yl) sulfanilamide.
Use: Antibacterial.
See: Vesulong (Ciba)
SULFBENZAMINE HYDROCHLORIDE. Mafenide HCl p-Methylaminophenyl sulfonamide HCl. Pow., Bulk.
Use: Bacteriostatic.
SULFEM VAGINAL CREAM. (Amfre-Grant) Sulfanilamide 15%, 9-aminoacridine HCl 0.2%, allantoin 1.5%. Tube 4 oz. W/applicator.
Use: Antibacterial and antifungal.
SULFHYDRYL ION.
See: Hydrosulphosol (Lientz)
• **SULFINALOL HYDROCHLORIDE.** USAN.
Use: Antihypertensive.
• **SULFINPYRAZONE,** U.S.P. XXI. Caps., Tab., U.S.P. XXI. 1,2-Diphenyl-4-(2-phenylsulphinylethyl)pyrazolidine-3,5-dione. 1,2-Diphenyl-4-(2-phenylsulfinylethyl-3,5-pyrazolidine-dione. Sulphinpyrazone, B.A.N.
Use: Uricosuric.
See: Anturane, Tab., Cap. (Ciba)
SULFISOMIDINE. Sulfadimetine. Sulphasomidine, B.A.N.
SULFISOXAZOLE. (Purepac) Sulfisoxazole 0.5 Gm./Tab. Bot. 100s, 1000s.
Use: Urinary tract infections.
• **SULFISOXAZOLE,** U.S.P. XXI. Tab., U.S.P. XXI. N'-(3,4-Dimethyl-5-isoxazolyl)sulfaniamide.
Use: Anti-infective sulfa.
See: Barazole, Tab. (Barry Martin)
Gantrisin Preps. (Roche)
G-Sox, Tab. (Scrip)
Rosoxol, Tab. (Robinson)
SK-Soxazole, Cap. (SmithKline)
Soxa, Tab. (Vita Elixir)
Sulfagan, Tab. (Zenith)
Sulfisoxazole, Tab. (Purepac)
Sulfium, Ophthalmic, Sol., Oint. (Alcon)
Sulfizin, Tab. (Reid-Provident)
Velmatrol, Tab. (Kenyon)
W/Aminoacridine HCl, allantoin.
See: Vagilia, Cream (Lemmon)
W/Phenazopyridine.
See: Azo-Gantrisin, Tab. (Roche)
Azo-Soxazole, Tab. (Columbia)

Azo-Sulfisoxazole, Tab. (Richlyn; Century)
Azo-Urizole, Tab. (Jenkins)
Barazole-Azo, Tab. (Barry Martin)
Rosoxol-Azo, Tab. (Robinson)
Soxazo, Tab. (Sutliff & Case)
Suldiazo, Tab. (Kay)
W/Phenylazodiaminopyridine HCl.
See: Azo-sulfisoxazole, Tab. (Vortech)
Azo-Sulfizin (Reid-Provident)
Velmatrol-A Tab. (Kenyon)
• **SULFISOXAZOLE, ACETYL,** U.S.P. XXI. Oral Susp., U.S.P. XXI. Acetamide, N-(4-amino-phenyl)sulfonyl-N-(3,4-dimethyl-5-isoxazolyl)-. N-(3,4-Dimethyl-5-isoxazolyl)-N-sulfanilylacetamide.
Use: Antibacterial.
See: Gantrisin Acetyl, Preps. (Roche)
W/Erythromycin Ethylsuccinate.
See: Pediazol, Susp. (Ross)
SULFISOXAZOLE DIETHANOLAMINE. Sulfisoxazole Diolamine.
• **SULFISOXAZOLE DIOLAMINE.** U.S.P. XXI. Inj., Ophth. Oint, Ophth. Sol. U.S.P. XXI. 2,2'-Iminodiethanol salt of N¹-(3,4-Dimethyl-5-isoxazolyl)sulfanilamide compound with 2,2'-iminodiethanol(1:1). Gantrisin diolamine.
Use: Antibacterial.
See: Gantrisin, Ophth. Sol. & Oint. (Roche)
• **SULFOBROMOPHTHALEIN SODIUM,** U.S.P. XXI. Inj., U.S.P. XXI.
Use: Liver function test.
SULFOCARBOLATES. Salts of Phenolsulfonic Acid, Usually Ca, Na, K, Cu, Zn.
SULFOCYANATE.
See: Potassium Thiocyanate.
SULFO-GANIC. (Marcen) Thioglycerol 20 mg., sod. citrate 5 mg., phenol 0.5%, benzyl alcohol 0.5%/cc. Vial 10 cc., 30 cc.
Use: I.M., adjunctive treatment in arthritides due to sulfur metabolism disorders or deficiencies.
SULFOGUAIACOL.
See: Pot. Guaiacolsulfonate
SULFOIL. (C & M Pharmacal) Sulfonated castor oil, water. Bot. pt., Gal.
Use: Soap free cleanser for skin and hair.
SULFO-LO. (Whorton) Sublimed sulfur, freshly precipitated polysulfides of zinc, potassium, sulfate, and calamine in aqueous-alcoholic suspension. **Lotion:** Bot. 4 oz., 8 oz., **Soap:** 3 oz.
Use: Treatment of acne.
SULFOMYL. Mafenide, B.A.N.
• **SULFOMYXIN.** USAN.
Use: Antibacterial.
SULFONAMIDE, DOUBLES.
See: Dia-Mer-Sulfonamides
SULFONAMIDE PREPS.
See: Acet-Dia-Mer (Various Mfr.)
Dia-Mer Sulfonamides (Various Mfr.)
Dia-Mer-Thia (Various Mfr.)
Meth-Dia-Mer, Preps. (Various Mfr.)
SULFONAMIDES, VETERINARY USE.
See: S.Q. (Merck Animal Health)
Sulfabrom (Merck Animal Health)

Sulfastrep w/streptomycin (Merck Animal Health)
Sulfathalidine (Merck Animal Health)
Sul-Thi-Zol (Merck Animal Health)
SULFONAMIDES, QUADRUPLE.
See: Quadetts, Tab. (Elder)
Quad-Ramoid, Susp. (Elder)
SULFONAMIDES, TRIPLE.
See: Acet-Dia-Mer Sulfonamides
Dia-Mer-Thia Sulfonamides
Meth-Dia-Mer Sulfonamides
SULFONES.
See: Avlosulfon, Tab. (Ayerst)
Dapsone
Diasone, Enterabs (Abbott)
Glucosulfone Sodium
Promacetin, Tab. (Parke-Davis)
SULFONETHYLMETHANE. 2,2-Bis-(ethylsulfonyl)butane.
SULFONITHOCHOLYLGLYCINE.
See: S.L.C.G., Kit (Abbott)
SULFONMETHANE. 2,2-Bis(ethylsulfonyl)propane.
SULFONPHTHAL.
See: Phenolsulfonphthalein, Prep. (Various Mfr.)
• **SULFONTEROL HYDROCHLORIDE.** USAN.
Use: Bronchodilator.
4,4'-SULFONYLDIANILINE. Dapsone, U.S.P. XXI.
SULFONYLUREAS.
See: Diabinese, Tab. (Pfizer)
Dymelor, Tab. (Lilly)
Orinase, Tab., Vial (Upjohn)
Tolinase, Tab. (Upjohn)
SULFORCIN LOTION. (Owen) Sulfur 5%, resorcinol 2%, alcohol 11.65%, methylparaben. Bot. 4 oz., 16 oz.
Use: For acne, seborrheic dermatitis & oily skin conditions.
SULFORMETHOXINE. Name used for Sulfadoxine.
SULFORTHOMIDINE. Name used for Sulfadoxine.
SULFOSALICYLATE W/Methenamine
See: Hexalet, Tab. (Webcon)
SULFOSALYCYLIC ACID. Salicylsulphonic acid.
• **SULFOXONE SODIUM,** U.S.P. XXI. Tab., U.S.P. XXI.
SULFOXYL LOTION REGULAR. (Stiefel) Benzoyl peroxide 5%, sulfur 2% Bot. 2 oz.
Use: Acne treatment.
SULFOXYL LOTION STRONG. (Stiefel) Benzoyl peroxide 10%, sulfur 5% Bot. 2 oz.
Use: Acne treatment.
SULFUR-8 HAIR & SCALP CONDITIONER. (Plough) Sulfur 2%, menthol 1%, triclosan 0.1%. Jar 1, 2, 4, 8 oz.
Use: Antiseborrheic.
SULFUR-8 SHAMPOO. (Plough) Triclosan 0.2%. Bot. 6 oz., 12 oz.
Use: Antiseborrheic.
SULFUR, ANTIARTHRITIC.
See: Thiocyl, Amp. (Torigian)
■ **SULFUR COMBINATIONS.**
See: Acnaveen, Bar (Cooper)
Acne-Aid, Cream, Lot. (Stiefel)
Acnederm, Liq. (Lannett)

Akne Oral Kapsulets, Cap. (Alto)
Acnomel, Cake, Cream. (Menley & James)
Acno, Sol., Lot. (Cummins)
Acnotex, Liq. (C&M Pharm.)
Akne, Drying Lot. (Alto)
Antrocol, Tab., Cap. (Poythress)
Aracain Rectal Oint. (Commerce)
Clearasil, Stick (Vicks)
Derma Cover-HC, Liq. (Scrip)
Epi-clear, Lotion (Squibb)
Exzit, Preps. (Miles Pharm)
Fomac, Cream (Dermik)
Fostex, Liq. Cream, Bar (Westwood)
Fostex, Cream, Liq. (Westwood)
Fostex CM, Cream (Westwood)
Fostril, Cream (Westwood)
Furol Cream (Torch)
Hydro Surco, Lot. (Almo)
Klaron, Lot. (Dermik)
Liquimat, Liq. (Owen)
Lotio-P (Alto)
Neutrogena Disposables (Neutrogena)
Pernox, Lot. (Westwood)
pHisoDan, Liq. (Winthrop Products)
Postacne, Lot. (Dermik)
Pragmatar, Oint. (Menley & James)
Proseca, Liq. (Westwood)
Rezamid, Lot. (Dermik)
Sastid Soap (Stiefel)
Sebaveen, Shampoo (Cooper)
Sebulex Shampoo, Liq. (Westwood)
Sulfacet-R, Lot. (Dermik)
Sulfo-lo, Lot. (Wharton)
Sulforcin, Pow., Lot. (Owen)
Sulfur-8, Prods. (Plough)
Teenac, Cream (Elder)
Thera-Blem, Cream (Noxell)
Vanseb, Cream (Herbert)
Vanseb-T Tar Shampoo (Herbert)
Xerac, Oint. (Person & Covey)
• **SULFUR DIOXIDE,** N.F. XVI.
Use: Antixodant, pharmaceutic aid.
• **SULFUR OINTMENT,** U.S.P. XXI.
Use: Scabicide, parasiticide.
• **SULFUR, PRECIPITATED,** U.S.P. XXI.
Use: Scabicide; parasiticide.
See: Bensulfoid, Pow., Lot. (Poythress)
Epi-Clear, Lot. (Squibb)
Ramsdell's Sulfur Cream (Fougera)
Sulfur Soap (Steifel Labs)
SULFUR, SALICYL DIASPORAL. (Doak)
See: Diasporal, Cream (Doak)
SULFUR SOAP. (Stiefel) Sulfur 10%. Cake 4.1 oz.
Use: Acne treatment.
• **SULFUR, SUBLIMED,** U.S.P. XXI. Flowers of Sulfur.
Use: Parasiticide, scabicide.
SULFUR, TOPICAL.
See: Thylox, Liq., Soap (Dent)
• **SULFURATED LIME TOPICAL SOLUTION,** U.S.P. XXI. Vleminckx Lotion.
Use: Scabicide, parasiticide.
• **SULFURIC ACID,** N.F. XVI.

Use: Pharmaceutic aid (acidifying agent).

SULFURINE. (Table Rock) Sulfamethizole 0.5 Gm./Tab. Bot. 100s & 500s.
Use: Treatment of urinary infections.

SULGLYCOTIDE. B.A.N. The sulfuric polyester of a glycopeptide isolated from pig duodenum.
Use: Treatment of peptic ulcer.
See: Gliptide (sodium salt)

• **SULINDAC,** U.S.P. XXI. Tab., U.S.P. XXI.
Use: Anti-inflammatory.
See: Clinoril Tab. (Merck Sharp & Dohme)

• **SULISOBENZONE.** USAN. 5-Benzoyl-4-hydroxy-2-methoxybenzenesulfonic acid.
Use: Sunscreen agent.
See: Uval Lotion (Dorsey)
Uvinul MS-40 (General Aniline & Film)

• **SULMARIN.** USAN.
Use: Hemostatic.

• **SULNIDAZOLE.** USAN.
Use: Antiprotozoal.

SULOCARBILATE. 2-Hydroxyethyl-p-sulfamylcarbanilate.

• **SULOCTIDIL.** USAN.
Use: Vasodilator.

• **SULOXIFEN OXALATE.** USAN.
Use: Bronchodilator.

SULOXYBENZONE. 4-p-Anisoyl-3-hydroxybenzene sulfonic acid. 2-Hydroxy-4'-methoxy-5-sulfobenzophenone. Cyasorb UV 284 (Lederle)

SULPHABENZIDE.
See: Sulfabenzamide

SULPHALOXIC ACID. B.A.N. 4'-[(Hydroxymethylcarbamoyl)sulfamoyl]phthalanilic acid.
See: Enteromide calcium salt.

SULPHAMETHOXYDIAZINE. B.A.N. 2-p-Aminobenzenesulphonamido-5-methoxypyrimidine, 5-Methoxy-2-sulphanilamidopyrimidine Durenate.

SULPHAMOPRINE. B.A.N. 2-(4-Aminobenzenesulfonamido)-4,6-dimethoxypyrimidine.

SULPHAMOXOLE. B.A.N. 2-(4-Aminobenzenesulfonamido)-4,5-dimethyloxazole.
See: Nuprin.

SULPHAN BLUE. B.A.N. Sodium 4-(4-diethylaminobenzylidene)cyclohexa-2,5-dienylidenediethylammonium -α-benzene-2,4-disulfonate.
Use: Investigation of the cardiovascular system.
See: Blue VRS
Disulphine Blue VNS

SULPHAPROXYLINE. B.A.N. N¹-(4-Isopropoxybenzoyl)-4-aminobenzenesulfonamide.

SULPHASOMIDINE. B.A.N. 4-(4-Aminobenzenesulfonamido)-2,6-dimethylpyrimidine.
See: Sulfisomidine (I.N.N.)
Elkosin.

SULPHATHIOUREA. B.A.N. 4-Aminobenzenesulfonylthiourea.
See: Badional.

SULPHATOLAMIDE. B.A.N. 4-Aminobenzenesulphonylthiourea salt of α-amino-p-toluenesulfonamide.
See: Marbadal

SULPHAUREA. B.A.N. 4-Aminobenzesulfonylurea.

See: Euvernil
Sulfacarbamide (I.N.N.)

SULPHETRONE. Solapsone, B.A.N.

SULPHO-LAC CREAM. (Last) Sulfur 5% in cream base. Jars 2 oz., 7 oz., 20 oz.
Use: Acne medication.

SULPHO-LAC SOAP. (Last) Sulfur in soap base. Bar 3 oz.
Use: Acne medication.

SULPHOMYXIN. Penta-(N-sulphomethyl) polymyxin B.

SULPHOMYXIN SODIUM. B.A.N. A mixture of sulfomethylated polymyxin B and sodium bisulfite.
Use: Antibiotic.
See: Thiosporin.

SULPHRIN SUSPENSION. (Muro) Sodium sulfacetamide 100 mg., prednisolone acetate 5 mg., phenylephrine HCl 0.12% Bot. 5 ml.
Use: Ophthalmic.

SULPIK. (Durel) Sulfur 5%, salicylic acid 3%, in Duromantel cream.
Use: Superficial tinea infections, seborrheic dermatitis.

SULPIK T. (Durel) Sulfur 5%, salicylic acid 3%, LCD (coal tar solution) 3%. In Duromantel Cream.
Use: Superficial tinea, infections, non-exudative forms of seborrheic dermatitis.

• **SULPIRIDE.** USAN. (1) N-[(1-ethyl-2-pyrrolidinyl)methyl]-5-sulfamoyl-o-anisamide; (2) N-[(Ethyl-1-pyrrolidinyl-2)-methyl]methoxy-2-sulfamoyl-5-benzamide. Dogmatyl (Laboratories Delagrange, France).
Use: Antidepressant.

• **SULPROSTONE.** USAN.
Use: Prostaglandin.

SULRAY SOAP. (Last) Sulfur soap. Bar 3 oz.
Use: Acne medication.

• **SULTAMICILLIN.** USAN.
Use: Antibacterial.

• **SULTHIAME.** USAN. Formerly Sulphenytame. p-(Tetrahydro-2H-1,2-thiazin-2-yl)-benzenesulfonamide-S,S -dioxide.
Use: Anticonvulsant.

SULTRIN Triple Sulfa Vaginal Tablets. (Ortho) Sulfathiazole 172.5 mg., sulfacetamide 143.75 mg., sulfabenzamide 184 mg./Vag. Tab. Pkg. 20s w/appl.
Use: Treatment of *H. vaginalis* (Gardnerella) vaginitis.

SULTRIN Triple Sulfa Cream. (Ortho) Sulfathiazole 3.42%, sulfacetamide 2.86%, sulfabenzamide 3.7%, urea 0.64%. Tube 78 Gm. with measured dose applicator.
Use: Treatment of *H. vaginalis* (Gardnerella) vaginitis.

SUL-TRIO. (Kay) Sulfadiazine 166 mg., sulfamerazine 166 mg., sulfamethazine 166 mg./5 cc. Bot. pt., gal.

SUL-TRIO MM. (Kay) Sulfadiazine 167 mg., sulfamethazine 167 mg., sulfamerazine 167 mg./Tab. Bot. 1000s.

SULVESOR LOTION. (Durel) Sulfur 2%, resorcinol 1%, neocalamine, talc, titanium dioxide, alcohol 34%. 2 oz., 4 oz., gal.

Use: Antifungal, antibacterial, keratolytic antiseborrheic.

SUMMER'S EVE DISPOSABLE DOUCHE. (Fleet) Single or twin 4.5 oz. disposable units. Regular, herbal, vinegar & water.
Use: Cleansing douche.

SUMMER'S EVE MEDICATED DISPOSABLE DOUCHE. (Fleet) Contains povidone-iodide. Single or twin 4.5 oz. disposable units.
Use: Temporary relief of minor vaginal irritation and itching.

SUMMER'S EVE VAGINAL SUPPOSITORIES. (Fleet) Box 10s w/applicator.
Use: Feminine suppository.

SUMOX. (Reid-Provident) Amoxicillin. **Cap.:** 250 mg. Bot. 100s. **Pow. for oral sus.:** 125 mg./5ml. Bot. 80 cc.; 250 mg./5 ml 80 cc.
Use: Antibiotic.

SUMSCREEN. (Summers) Red petrolatum. Tube 100 Gm.
Use: Sunscreen.

SUMYCIN. (Squibb) Tetracycline HCl. **Cap.** 250 mg./Cap. Bot. 100s, 1000s. Unimatic 100s. 500 mg./Cap. Bot. 100s, 500s. Unimatic 100s. **Syr.** 125 mg., 500 mg./5 ml. Bot. 60 cc., 1 pt. **Tab.** 250 mg./Tab. Bot. 100s, 1000s. 500 mg./Tab. Bot. 100s, 500s.
Use: Antibiotic.

SUNBURN REMEDY.
See: Solarcaine, Prods. (Plough)

• **SUNCILLIN SODIUM.** USAN. 3,3-Dimethyl-7-oxo-6-[2-phenyl-D-2-(sulfoamino)acetamido]-4-thia-1-azabicyclo[3.2.0]heptane-2-carboxylic acid disodium salt.
Use: Antibacterial.

SUNDOWN. (Johnson & Johnson) A series of products marketed under the Sundown name including: **Moderate** (SPF 4) padimate O 3.8%.; **Extra** (SPF 6) padimate O 3.3%, oxybenzone 1.0%; **Maximal** (SPF 8) padimate O 4.75, oxybenzone 1.75%; **Ultra** (SPF 15) padimate O 7%, octyl salicylate 5%, oxybenzone 4%. Bot. 4 oz.
Use: Prevention of sunburn (sunscreen).

SUNGER. (Plough) A series of products is marketed under the Sunger name including Extra Protection Lotion (SPF 6), Lip Protector, Moisturizer, Sunblock Lotion (SPF 15), Suntan Lotion (SPF 4, Sun & Weather Stick (SPF 4), Tanning Stick and Wine Coolers. Most contain homosalate in various oil and lotion bases.
Use: Ultraviolet sunscreen.

SUNICE. (Citroleum) Allantoin 0.25%, menthol 0.25%, methyl salicylate 10%/Cream. 3 oz.
Use: Burn remedy.

SUNRIL. (Emko-Schering) Acetaminophen 300 mg., pamabrom 50 mg., pyrilamine maleate 25 mg./Cap. Bot. 100s.
Use: Premenstrual tension.

SUNSTICK. (CooperCare) Lipand face protectant containing digalloyl trioleate 2.5%in emollient base. Plas. swivel container 0.14 oz.

Use: Prevention & relief of chapping and sunburning of lips.

SUPAC. (Mission) Acetaminophen 160 mg., aspirin 230 mg., caffeine 33 mg., calcium gluconate 60 mg./Tab. Filmstrips 24s, Bot. 100s, 1000s.
Use: Analgesic.

SUPEN AMPICILLIN TRIHYDRATE. (Reid-Provident) Semi-synthetic penicillin derived from the penicillin nucleus. 6-amino-penicillanic acid. **Caps.** 250 mg. Bot. 100s, 500s. 500 mg.: Bot. 100s. **Susp.** 125 mg./5 ml. Bot. 100 ml.; 250 mg./5 ml. Bot. 100 ml.
Use: Antibiotic.

SUPER AFKO-HIST. (APC) Chlorpheniramine maleate 2 mg., aspirin 230 mg., phenacetin 160 mg., caffeine 32 mg./Tab. Bot. 1000s.
Use: Antihistamine, analgesic, antipyretic.

SUPER-ANAHIST. (Warner-Lambert) Acetaminophen 325 mg., pseudoephedrine HCl 30 mg./Tab. Blister Pack 30s.
Use: Decongestant, analgesic.

SUPER AYTINAL TABLETS. (Walgreen) Vit. A 7,000 I.U., B-1 5 mg., B-2 5 mg., B-5 10 mg., B-6 3 mg., B-12 9 mcg., C 90 mg., D400 I.U., E 30 I.U., niacin 30 mg., biotin 55 mcg., folic acid 0.4 mg., iron 30 mg., Ca 162 mg., P 125 mg., iodine 150 mcg., Cu 3 mg., Mn 7.5 mg., Mg 100 mg., K 7.7 mg., Zn 24, Chloride 7 mg., Cr 15 mcg., Se 15 mcg., Mo 15 mcg., choline bitartrate 1000 mcg., inositol 1000 mcg., PABA 1000 mcg., rutin 1000 mcg., yeast 12 mg. Bot. 50s, 100s, 365s.
Use: Multiple vitamins with minerals.

SUPER-B. (Towne) Vit. B-1 50 mg., B-2 20 mg., B-6 5 mg., B-12 15 mcg., C 300 mg., liver desic. 100 mg., dried yeast 100 mg., niacinamide 25 mg., Ca pantothenate 5 mg., iron 10 mg./Captab. Bot. 30s, 50s, 72s, 100s, 250s.

SUPER B KAPSULES. (Pharmex) High potency Vit. B. Cap. Bot. 50s, 100s.

SUPER C-1000. (Pharmex) Vit. C 1000 mg./Tab. Bot. 100s.

SUPERCITIN SUGAR-FREE. (Vitarine) Dextromethorphan HBr 20 mg., chlorpheniramine maleate 2 mg., sod. citrate 100 mg., acetaminophen 120 mg./10 cc. Bot. 4 oz.
Use: Cough syrup.

SUPER D. (Upjohn) Vit. A 10,000 I.U., D 400 I.U./Perle. Bot. 100s.
Use: Vitamin A & D therapy.

SUPER-DECON COLD CAPSULES. (Vitarine) Salicylamide 250 mg., phenylephrine HCl 5 mg., C 50 mg., caffeine 32 mg./Cap. Vial 15s.
Use: Decongestant, antihistaminic, analgesic.

SUPER DOSS. (Ferndale) Brewer's yeast 210 mg., docusate sodium 120 mg./Tab. Bot. 100s, 1000s.
Use: Constipation.

SUPERE-PECT. (Barth's) Alpha tocopherol 400 I.U., apple pectin 100 mg./Cap. Bot. 50s, 100s, 250s.
Use: Vitamin E supplement.

SUPER "HISTA-C" CAPSULES. (Eckerd) Dextromethorphan H Br 10 mg., phenylpropanolamine HCl 12.5 mg., pyrilamine maleate 12.5 mg., acetaminophen 325 mg./Cap. Bot. 24s.

Use: Cough and cold symptoms.

SUPER "HISTA-C" SYRUP. (Eckerd) Dextromethorphan H Br 10 mg., phenylpropanolamine HCl 12.5 mg., acetaminophen 195 mg., chlorpheniramine maleate 0.66 mg./5 ml. Bot. 4 oz., 8 oz.
Use: Treatment of cough and cold symptoms.

SUPER HYDRAMIN PROTEIN POWDER. (Nion) Protein 65%, carbohydrate 21.8%, fat 1% in powder form. Cans 1 lb.
Use: Dietary supplement.

SUPER K-B-T TABLETS. (Columbia) Vit. B-6 50 mg., soya lecithin 1200 mg., kelp 100 mg., dry cider vinegar 240 mg./3 Tabs. Bot. 100s, 250s.

SUPERINONE. Tyloxapol.
See: Triton WR-1339 (Rohm & Haas)

SUPER MANIVIM. (Vitarine) Vit. A 33,000 I.U., D 1600 I.U., E 3.3 I.U., B-1 25 mg., B-2 12 mg., B-6 1.2 mg., B-12 25 mcg., C 150 mg., niacinamide 75 mg., cal. pantothenate 3 mg., biotin 2 mcg., cal. carbonate 100 mg., ferrous gluconate 30 mg., pot. iodide 0.15 mg., Mg sulfate 7.2 mg., Cu sulfate 5 mg., Mn sulfate 3.4 mg., pot. chloride 6.6 mg., Zn sulfate 3.2 mg., amino acids, nutrient, natural and other factors/Cap. Bot. 30s, 100s, 250s.
Use: Diet supplement, convalescence.

SUPER MANIVIM-FORMULA #46. (Vitarine) Multivitamin & multimineral supplement for adults.
Use: Dietary supplement.

SUPER NUTRI-VITES. (Faraday) Vit. A 36,000 I.U., D 400 I.U., B-1 25 mg., B-2 25 mg., B-6 50 mg., B-12 50 mcg., niacinamide 50 mg., Ca pantothenate 12.5 mg., choline bitartrate 150 mg., inositol 150 mg., betaine HCl 25 mg., PABA 15 mg., glutamic acid 25 mg., desic. liver 50 mg., C 150 mg., E 12.5 I.U., Mn gluconate 6.15 mg., bone meal 162 mg., Fe gluconate 50 mg., Cu gluconate 0.25 mg., Zn gluconate 2.2 mg., K iodide 0.1 mg., Ca 53.3 mg., P 24.3 mg., Mg gluconate 7.2 mg./Protein Coated Tab. Bot. 60s, 100s.

SUPER PLENAMINS MULTIPLE VITAMINS AND MINERALS. (Rexall) Vit. A 8000 I.U., D-2 400 I.U., Vit. B-1 2.5 mg., B-2 2.5 mg., C 75 mg., niacinamide 20 mg., B-6 1.0 mg., B-12 3.0 mcg., biotin 20 mcg., E 10 I.U., pantothenic acid 3.0 mg., liver conc. 100 mg., Fe 30 mg., Ca 75 mg., P 58 mg., Iodine 0.15 mg., Cu 0.75 mg., Mn 1.25 mg., Mg 10.0 mg., Zn 1.0 mg./Tab. Bot. 36s, 72s, 144s, 288s, 365s.
Use: Multivitamin with minerals.

SUPER POLI-GRIP/WERNET'S CREAM (Block) Carboxymethylcellulose gum, ethylene oxide polymer, petrolatum-mineral oil base. Tube 0.7, 1.4, 2.4 oz.
Use: Denture adhesive cream.

SUPER SHADE LOTION. (Plough) Padimate O 7%, oxybenzone 3% (SPF 15). Bot. 4 oz. Tube ½ oz.
Use: Ultra-violet sunscreen, sunblock.

SUPER-T. (Towne) Vit. A palmitate 10,000 I.U., D 400 I.U., B-1 10 mg., B-2 10 mg., B-6 1 mg., B-12 6 mcg., C 200 mg., niacinamide 100 mg., Vit. E 15 I.U., Ca 103 mg., P 80 mg., Fe 10 mg., Iodine 0.1 mg., Cu 1 mg., K 5 mg., Mg 5.5 mg., Mn 1 mg., Zn 1.4 mg./Captab. Bot. 30s, 50s, 100s, 250s.

SUPER TETRO. (Wisconsin) Bot. 4 oz., 8 oz., gal.
Use: Cleanser.

SUPER THERA 46. (Faraday) Vit. A 36,000 I.U., essential vitamins, minerals, amino acids w/nutrient factors, digestive enzymes, B-12 25 mcg./Tab. Bot. 100s.

SUPER TROCHE. (Weeks & Leo) Benzocaine 5 mg., cetalkonium Cl 1 mg./Lozenge. Bot. 15s, 30s.
Use: Relief of minor sore throat & irritation.

SUPER TROCHE PLUS. (Weeks & Leo) Benzocaine 10 mg., cetalkonium Cl. 2 mg./Loz. Bot. 12s.
Use: Relief of minor sore throat & irritation.

SUPER WERNET'S POWDER. (Block) Carboxymethylcellulose gum, ethylene oxide polymer. Bot. 0.63, 1.75, 3.55 oz.
Use: Denture adhesive.

SUPER WESVITE. (Western Research) Vit. A 10,000 I.U., B-1 15 mg., B-2 15 mg., B-6 25 mg., B-12 25 mcg., C 100 mg., D 400 I.U., Vit. E 30 I.U., biotin 500 mcg., Ca 100 mg., Ca pantothenate 25 Gm., choline bitartrate 10 mg., lemon bioflavonoids 10 mg., copper 2 mg., pantothenic acid 25 mg., inositol 20 mg., iron 20 mg., magnesium 50 mg., folic acid 400 mcg., hesperidin complex 10 mg., rutin 20 mg., potassium 25 mg., molybdenum 100 mcg., manganese 6 mg., niacin 40 mg., para-aminobenzoic acid 8 mg., phosphorus 52 mg., potassium iodide 0.1 mg., zinc 5 mg., iodine 100 mcg./Tab. Bot. 1000s.
Use: Vitamin-mineral and amino acid supplement.

SUPLEX. (Rocky Mtn.) Vit. B-1 100 mg., B-2 2 mg., B-6 4 mg., niacinamide 100 mg., panthenol 12 mg./cc. Vial 30 cc.

SUPPORT. (Mission) Calcium caseinate, nonfat dry milk, artificial flavors, sodium bicarbonate, salt, sodium saccharin and maltol. Ca 330 mg., P 300 mg., K 244 mg., Na 81 mg., Protein 16 Gm., carbohydrate 8 Gm., Calories 99/oz. Pow. Container 10 oz.
Use: Extra nutritional support.

SUPPORT-500. (Doral) Vit. A 12,500 I.U., D 50 I.U., B-1 10 mg., B-2 5 mg., niacinamide 25 mg., B-6 2 mg., Ca-pantothenate 10 mg., C 500 mg., E 50 I.U., Mg sulfate 70 mg., Mn sulfate 4 mg., Zn 80 mg./Cap.
Use: Vitamin-mineral supplement.

SUPRARENAL. Dried, partially defatted and powdered adrenal gland of cattle, sheep or swine.

SUPRINS. (Towne) Vit. A palmitate 10,000 I.U., D 400 I.U., B-1 25 mg., B-2 10 mg., B-6 5 mg., B-12 25 mcg., C 250 mg., Ca pantothenate 20 mg., niacinamide 100 mg., biotin 25 mcg., Vit. E 15 I.U., Ca 103 mg., P 80 mg., Fe 10 mg., Iodine 0.1 mg., Cu 1.0 mg., Zn 0.5 mg., Mn 1.0 mg./Captab. Bot. 60s, 100s.

• **SUPROFEN.** USAN.
Use: Anti-inflammatory.

SURAMIN SODIUM. Hexa-Sodium bis-(m-amino-benzoyl-m-amino-p-methylbenzoyl-1-naph-thylamino-4,6,-8-trisulfonate) carbamide. (Bayer 205; Germanin).

SURBEX FILMTAB. (Abbott) Thiamine mononitrate 6 mg., B-2 6 mg., nicotinamide 30 mg., B-6 2.5 mg., Ca

pantothenate 10 mg., Vit. B-12 5 mcg., Filmtab. Bot. 100s.
Use: Vit. B-complex therapy.
W/Vit. C. (Abbott) Same as Surbex Filmtab, except Vit. C 250 mg./Filmtab Bot. 100s, 500s.
SURBEX-T FILMTAB. (Abbott) Vit. B-1 15 mg., B-2 10 mg., niacinamide 100 mg., Vit. B-6 5 mg., B-12 10 mcg., Ca pantothenate 20 mg., Vit. C 500 mg./Filmtab. Bot. 50s, 100s, 500s. Abbo-Pac 100s.
Use: Vitamin deficiencies.
SURBEX-750 WITH IRON. (Abbott) Vit. B-1 15 mg., B-2 15 mg. B-6 25 mg., B-12 12 mcg., C 750 mg., Ca pantothenate 20 mg., E 30 I.U., niacinamide 100 mg., iron 27 mg., folic acid 0.4 mg./Tab. Bot. 50s.
Use: Vitamin & mineral supplement.
SURBEX-750 WITH ZINC. (Abbott) B-1 15 mg., B-2 15 mg., B-6 20 mg., B-12 12 mcg., C 750 mg., E 30 I.U., pantothenic acid 20 mg., niacin 100 mg., folic acid 0.4 mg., zinc 22.5 mg./Tab. Bot. 50s.
Use: Vitamin & mineral supplement.
SURFACAINE. (Lilly) Cyclomethycaine sulfate. **Cream** 0.5%, Tube 1 oz. **Jelly** 0.75%, Tube 1 oz., 5 oz. **Oint.** 1%, Tube 1 oz.
SURFACE-ACTIVE AGENTS.
See: Antiseptics, Surface-Active
SURFADIL. (Lilly) Cyclomethycaine and diphenhydramine. **Cream:** Diphenhydramine 2%, cyclomethycaine 0.5%. Tube 1 oz. **Lot:** Diphenhydramine 2 Gm., cyclomethycaine 0.5 Gm., benzyl alcohol 2 Gm., titanium dioxide 5 Gm./100 ml. Plastic Bot. 75 ml.
Use: Dermatitis treatment.
SURFAK. (Hoechst) Docusate calcium 50 mg. or 240 mg./Cap. 50 mg., Bot. 30s, 100s; 240 mg. Bot. 30s, 100s, 500s. Unit Dose Pack 100s.
SURFATHESIN SULFATE. Cyclomethycaine, B.A.N.
SUR-FIT O.R. SET 1. (ConvaTec) Sterile stomahesive wafer with Sur-fit Flange. Sterile standard urostomy pouch. Night drain adapter.
Use: Operating room when urostomy is formed.
SUR-FIT O.R. SET 2. (ConvaTec) Sterile package of stomahesive wafer with Sur-Fit flange and Sur-Fit drainable pouch with tailclip.
Use: In operating room when colostomy or ileosotym is formed.
SUR-FIT UREOSTOMY POUCH. (Squibb) Small & standard sizes.
Use: Receptacles for urine from urostomies.
SURFOL IMMERSION BATH OIL. (Stiefel) Mineral oil, isopropyl myristate, isostearic acid, PEG-40, sorbitan peroleate, Bot. 8 oz.
Use: Post-Immersion bath oil for dry skin.
• **SURFOMER.** USAN.
Use: Hypolipidemic.
SURGASOAP. (Wade) Castile vegetable oils. Bot. qt., gal.
Use: Surgical soap.
SURGEL LIQUID. (Ulmer) Patient lubricant fluid. Bot. 4 oz., 8 oz., pt., gal.
• **SURGIBONE.** USAN. Bone and cartilage obtained from bovine embryos and young calves.
Use: Prosthetic aid (internal bone splint).

See: Unilab Surgibone (Unilab)
SURGICAL SIMPLEX P. (Howmedica) Methyl methacrylate 20 ml. poly 6.7 Gm., methyl methacrylate-styrene copolymer 33.3 Gm. **Powd.** 40 Gm. **Liq.** 20 ml.
Use: Bone cement.
SURGICAL SIMPLEX P RADIOPAQUE. (Howmedica) Methyl methacrylate 20 ml., poly 6 Gm., methyl methacrylate-styrene copolymer 30 Gm. **Powd.** 40 Gm. **Liq.** 20 ml.
Use: Bone cement.
• **SURGICAL SUTURE, ABSORBABLE,** U.S.P. XXI.
Use: Surgical aid.
• **SURGICAL SUTURE, NONABSORBABLE,** U.S.P. XXI.
Use: Surgical aid.
SURGICEL ABSORBABLE HEMOSTAT. (Johnson & Johnson) Sterile absorbable knitted fabric prepared by controlled oxidation of regenerated cellulose. Sterile strips 2″×14″, 4″×8″, 2″×3″, ½″×2″.
Use: Absorbable hemostat.
SURGIDINE. (Continental) Iodine 0.8% in iodine complex. Germicide. Bot. 8 oz., gal. Foot operated dispenser 8 oz., gal.
Use: Antiseptic.
SURGI-KLEEN. (Sween) Methylbenzethonium chloride, refined coconut oil superamides, lanolin derivatives, cleansers, water soluble base. Bot. pt., gal.
Use: Topical anti-bacterial cleanser.
SURGILUBE. (Day-Baldwin) Sterile-bacteriostatic. Foil-pac: 3 Gm., 5 Gm., Tube: 5 Gm., 2 oz., 4½ oz.
Use: Surgical lubricant.
SURGILUBE. (Fougera) Sterile surgical lubricant. Foilpac 3 Gm., 5 Gm.; Tube 5 Gm., 2 oz. 4½ oz.
Use: Sterile surgical lubricant.
SURIN OINTMENT. (McKesson) Tube 1.25 oz.
SURITAL SODIUM. (Parke-Davis) Thiamylal sodium. **Steri-Vial:** 1 Gm., 25s; 5 Gm., 10s; 10 Gm., 10s.
Use: I.V.; short-acting anesthetic.
SURMONTIL. (Ives) Trimipramine maleate 25 mg., 50 mg. or 100 mg./Cap. Bot. 100s. Clinipaks.
Use: Antidepressant.
SUROFENE. Hexachlorophene.
SUSADRIN. (Merrell Dow) Nitroglycerin 1 mg., 2 mg., 3 mg./Transmucosal Tab. Bot. 100s. **Note: Manufacture voluntarily stopped in 1983.**
Use: Prophylaxis, treatment and management of angina pectoris.
SUSANO. (Blue Cross) Phenobarbital ¼ gr., hyoscyamine sulfate 0.1037 mg., atropine sulfate 0.0194 mg., scopolamine HBr 0.0065 mg./Tab. Bot. 1000s.
Use: Sedative, antispasmotic.
SUSANO ELIXIR. (Blue Cross) Phenobarbital ¼ gr., hyoscyamine sulfate 0.1037 mg., atropine sulfate 0.0194 mg., scopalamine HBr 0.0065 mg./5 ml. Bot. 16 oz., gal.
Use: Sedative, antispasmotic.
SUSPEN. (Circle) Penicillin V potassium 250 mg./5 ml. Bot. 100 ml.
Use: Antibiotic.

SUS-PHRINE INJECTION. (Berlex) Epinephrine 1:200 Amp. 0.3 ml., 12s, 25s. Multiple Dose Vial 5 ml., 1s.
Use: Bronchial asthma.

SUS SCROFA LINNE var DOMESTICUS.
W/Proteolytic enzyme, autolyzed.
See: Saromide Injection, Vial (Saron)

SUSTACAL HC. (Mead Johnson) High calorie nutritionally complete food. Protein 16%, fat 34%, carbohydrate 50%. Cans 8 oz. Vanilla or eggnog.
Use: Complete, concentrated oral nutition.

SUSTACAL LIQUID. (Mead Johnson) A vanilla, eggnog or chocolate flavored liquid containing as a % of the calories 24% protein, 21% fat, 55% carbohydrate with appropriate vitamin and mineral levels to meet 100% of the US RDA's. Cans, 8, 12 and 32 fl. oz.
Use: High protein, nutritionally complete, oral nutritional supplement, lactose free.

SUSTACAL POWDER. (Mead Johnson) Caloric distribution and nutritional value when added to milk are similar to that of Sustacal liquid except lactose added. Vanilla: Pow. 1.9 oz. packets 4's, 3.8 lb. can; Chocolate 1.9 oz. packets 4's.
Use: High protein, nutritionally complete, oral nutritional supplement.

SUSTACAL PUDDING. (Mead Johnson) Ready-to-eat fortified pudding containing at least 15% of the US RDA's for protein, vitamins and minerals, in a 240 calorie serving. As a % of the calories protein 11%, fat 36%, carbohydrate 53%. Flavors: chocolate, vanilla, and butterscotch. Tins, 5 oz., 110 oz.
Use: Complete nutritional supplement to help increase patient acceptance of nutritional support.

SUSTAGEN. (Mead Johnson) High calorie, high protein supplement containing as a % of the calories 24% protein, 8% fat, 68% carbohydrate. Contains all known essential vitamins and minerals. Prepared from nonfat milk, corn syrup solids, powdered whole milk, calcium caseinate, and dextrose. Vanilla: Can 1, 2½ & 5 lb. Chocolate: Can 1 lb.
Use: Complete nutrient, nutritional supplement.

SUSTAIRE. (Roerig) Theophylline 100 mg., 300 mg./Sust. Released Tab. Bot. 100s.
Use: Long acting relief of reversible bronchospasm.

• **SUTILAINS,** U.S.P. XXI. Oint., U.S.P. XXI.
Proteolytic enzymes.
Use: Debriding agent.
See: Travase, Oint. (Flint)

SUVAPLEX TABLET. (Tennessee Pharm.) Vit. A 5000 I.U., D 500 I.U., B-1 2.5 mg., B-2 2.5 mg., B-6 0.5 mg., B-12 1 mcg., C 37.5 mg., Ca pantothenate 5 mg., niacinamide 20 mg., folic acid 0.1 mg./Tab. Bot. 100s.
Use: Vitamin supplement.

SUXAMETHONIUM BROMIDE. B.A.N. Bis-2-di-methylaminoethyl succinate bismethobromide 00'-Succinyldi-(2-oxyethyltrimethylammonium bromide).
Use: Neuromuscular blocking agent.
See: Brevidil M

SUXAMETHONIUM CHLORIDE, B.A.N.

See: Anectine
  Brevidil M
  Scoline
  Succinylcholine Chloride, Inj. (Var. Mfr.)

• **SUXEMERID SULFATE.** USAN. Bis-(1,2,2,6,6-pen-tamethyl-4-piperidyl)succinate sulfate.
Use: Antitussive.

SUXETHONIUM BROMIDE. B.A.N. 00'-Succinyldi-[(2-oxyethyl)ethyldimethylammonium bromide].
Use: Neuromuscular blocking agent.
See: Brevidil E

SU-ZOL. (Boots) Pentylenetetrazol 50 mg., 15 ml. w/alcohol 15%. ml. Bot. 16 oz.
Use: Cerebral, respiratory stimulant.

SWAMP ROOT. (Medtech) Compound of various organic roots in an alcohol base. Bot. 4 oz. 8 oz.
Use: Diuretic to the kidney.

SWEEN SKIN CARE. (Sween) Methylbenzethonium chloride, cod liver oil w/Vit. A & D., keratin fraction of lanolin, water-repellent base. Jar 2 oz., 9 oz.
Use: Topical antiseptic.

SWEETA. (Squibb) Saccharin sodium and sorbitol. Bot. 24 ml., 2 oz., 4 oz.
Use: Sweetening Agent

SWEETASTE. (Purepac) Saccharin 0.25 gr., 0.5 gr., 1 gr./Tab. w/Sodium bicarbonate. Bot. 1000s.
Use: Sugar substitute.

■ **SWEETENING AGENTS.**
See: Ril-Sweet (Plough)
  Saccharin, Preps. (Various Mfr.)
  Sucaryl, Preps. (Abbott)
  Sweetaste, Tab. (Purepac)

SWIM EAR. (Fougera) Bot. 1 oz.
Use: Prevention of external otitis.

SWIM 'N CLEAR. (Wisconsin) Swimmers ear drops. Bot. 1¼ oz.
Use: Drops for swimmers ears to dry up excess water.

SWIRL CLEAN. (Alcon) Display carton.
Use: Electric hard contact lens cleaner.

SWISS KRISS. (Modern) Senna leaves, herbs. Coarse cut mixture. Can 1.5 oz., 3.25 oz., Tab. 120s, 250s.
Use: Laxative.

SYLLACT. (Wallace) Psyllium seed husks. Pow. Bot. 10 oz.
Use: Orally, laxative.

• **SYMCLOSENE.** USAN. Trichloroisocyanuric acid.
Use: Local anti-infective.

• **SYMETINE HCl.** USAN. 4,4'-(Ethylenedioxy)-bis-[N-hexyl-N-methylbenzylamine dihydrochloride].
Use: Amebicidal compound.

SYMMETREL. (Du Pont) Amantadine HCl. **Caps.** 100 mg./Cap. Bot. 100s, 500s. Unit Dose 100s. **Syr.** 50 mg./5 ml. Bot. pt.
Use: Antiviral agent, treatment of Parkinson's disease, treatment of drug induced extrapyramidal symptoms.

■ **SYMPATHOLYTIC AGENTS.**
See: Adrenergic-Blocking Agents
  D.H.E. 45, Amp. (Sandoz)
  Dibenzyline, Cap. (SmithKline)

Dihydroergotamine
Ergotamine Tartrate
Gynergen, Amp., Tab. (Sandoz)
■ SYMPATHOMIMETIC AGENTS.
See: Adrenalin (Parke-Davis)
Adrenergic agents
Aerolate Sr. & Jr., Cap. (Fleming)
Aerolone Cpd. (Lilly)
Afrin, Preps. (Schering)
Amesec, Enseal, Pulvule (Lilly)
Aramine, Amp., Vial (Merck Sharp & Dohme)
Arlidin HCl, Tab. (USV Pharm.)
Benzedrine Sulfate, Spansule, Tab. (SmithKline)
Brethine, Amp., Tab (Geigy)
Bronkephrine, Amp., Vial (Winthrop-Breon)
Bronkometer (Winthrop-Breon)
Bronkosol Sol. (Winthrop-Breon)
Delcobese, Tab. (Delco)
Demazin, Tab., Syr. (Schering)
Desoxyn, Gradumet, Tab. (Abbott)
Dexamyl Tab. (SmithKline)
Dexedrine, Elix. Spansule, Tab. (SmithKline)
D-Feda, Cap., Liq. (Dooner)
Didrex, Liq. Tab. (Upjohn)
Dimetapp, Elix., Tab. (Robins)
Drinus Graduals (Amfre-Grant)
Duovent, Tab. (Riker)
Ectasule Minus Sr. & Jr., Cap. (Fleming)
Ectasule III, Cap. (Fleming)
Ephedrine preps.
Epinephrine salts
Extendryl, Cap., Syr., Tab. (Fleming)
Fedrazil, Tab. (Burroughs Wellcome)
Fiogesic, Tab. (Sandoz)
Histabid, Cap., Vial (Meyer)
Isoephedrine HCl
Isuprel HCl, Preps. (Winthrop-Breon)
Levophed Bitartrate, Amp. (Winthrop-Breon)
Metaproterenol Sulfate (Var. Mfr.)
Napril, Cap. (Marion)
Neo-Synephrine HCl, Preps. (Winthrop Products)
Nolamine, Tab. (Carnrick)
Norisodrine Sulfate, Sol. (Abbott)
Obedrin-LA, Tab. (Beecham Labs)
Obetrol, Tab. (Obetrol)
Orthoxine, Orthoxine & Aminophylline (Upjohn)
Orthoxine HCl, Tab., Syr. (Upjohn)
Otrivin, Sol., Spray (Geigy)
Phenylephrine HCl, Preps.
Phenylpropanolamine HCl
Propadrine HCl, Cap., Elix. (Merck Sharp & Dohme)
Pseudoephedrine HCl, Syr., Tab.
Rondec DSC & T (Ross)
Slo-Fedrin & Slo-Fedrin A (Dooner)
Sudafed, Tab., Syr. (Burroughs Wellcome)
Triaminic, Prep. (Dorsey)
Triaminicol, Syr. (Dorsey)
Tussagesic, Susp., Tab. (Dorsey)
Tussaminic, Tab. (Dorsey)
Ursinus, Tab. (Dorsey)
Vasoxyl HCl Amp., Vial (Burroughs Wellcome)
Wyamine Sulfate, Amp., Vial (Wyeth)

SYMPTROL. (Saron) Phenylpropanolamine HCl 50 mg., chlorpheniramine maleate 8 mg./S.R. Cap. Bot. 50s.
Use: Decongestant, antihistaminic.
SYNA-CLEAR. (Pruvo) Decongestant plus Vit. C. 25 mg./Tab. Bot. 12s, 30s.
Use: Decongestant.
SYNACORT. (Syntex) Hydrocortisone cream. **1%:** Tube 15 Gm., 30 Gm., 60 Gm. **2.5%:** Tube 30 Gm.
Use: Topical steroid.
SYNACTHEN. Tetracosactrin, B.A.N. (Ciba) Cosyntropin.
SYNADRIN LACTATE. Prenylamine, B.A.N.
SYNALAR. (Syntex) Fluocinolone acetonide, **Cream: 0.01%** Tube 15 Gm., 45 Gm., 60 Gm. Jar 120 Gm., 425 Gm. **0.025%** Tube 15 Gm., 30 Gm., 60 Gm., Jar 120 Gm., 425 Gm. **Oint.: 0.025%:** Tube 15 Gm., 30 Gm., 60 Gm., 120 Gm. Jar 425 Gm. **Soln. 0.01%:** Bot. 20 ml., 60 ml.
Use: Topical steroid.
SYNALAR-HP. (Syntex) Fluocinolone acetonide 0.2%. **Cream** Tubes 12 Gm.
Use: Topical steroid.
SYNALGOS CAPSULES. (Ives) Aspirin 356.4 mg., caffeine 30 mg./Cap. Bot. 100s, 500s.
Use: Treatment of mild to moderate pain.
SYNALGOS-DC CAPSULES. (Ives) Dihydrocodeine bitartrate 16 mg., aspirin 356.4 mg., caffeine 30 mg./Cap. Bot. 100s, 500s.
Use: Analgesic, relaxant.
SYNANDONE ACETONIDE. Fluocinolone, B.A.N.
SYNAPP-R. (Blue Cross) Acetaminophen 325 mg., phenylpropanolamine HCl 25 mg., phenyltoloxamine citrate 22 mg./Tab. Bot. 40s.
Use: Analgesic, decongestant.
SYNATUSS-ONE. (Freeport) Guaifenesin 100 mg., dextromethorphan HBr. 15 mg., alcohol 1.4%/5 cc. Bot. 4 oz.
Use: Antitussive.
SYNCAINE.
See: Procaine Hydrochloride, Inj., Tab. (Various Mfr.)
SYNCELAX. (Blue Line) Casanthranol 30 mg., docusate sodium 100 mg./Tab. Bot. 100s, 1000s.
Use: Laxative.
SYNCELOSE. (Blue Line) Methylcellulose. Tab. 0.5 Gm., Bot. 100s, 1000s.
Use: Hydrophilic colloid laxative.
SYNCORT.
See: Desoxycorticosterone Acetate, Inj., Pellets (Various Mfr.)
SYNCORTYL.
See: Desoxycorticosterone Acetate, Inj., Pellets (Various Mfr.)
SYNDOLOR CAPSULES. (Knight) Bot. 100s, 1000s.
Use: Analgesic.
SYNEMOL. (Syntex) Fluocinolone acetonide 0.025%. Tube 15 Gm., 30 Gm., 60 Gm., 120 Gm.
Use: Topical steroid.
SYNEPHRICOL. (Winthrop Products) Paracetamol.
Use: Cold treatment.
SYNIODIN. (Blue Line) Iodine 1 gr. combined w/protein/Tab. Bot. 100s.

Use: Iodine therapy.

SYNKAYVITE. (Roche) Menadiol sodium disphosphate. **Amp.:** 5 mg. or 10 mg./1 ml. w/sodium metabisulfite 2 mg., phenol 0.45% NaCl 0.4%. Amp. 1 ml. Box 10s; 75 mg./2 ml. Amp. 2 ml. Box 10s. **Tab.** 5 mg., Bot. 100s.
Use: Synthetic Vitamin K for hemorrhagic tendency.

SYNKONIN.
See: Hydrocodone (Various Mfr.)

SYNOPEN HYDROCHLORIDE. Halopyramine, B.A.N.

SYNOPHYLATE. (Central) Theophylline sodium glycinate. **Elix.:** Theophylline 165 mg./15 ml. w/alcohol 20%. Bot. pt., gal. **Tab.:** Theophylline 165 mg./Tab. Bot. 100s, 1000s.
Use: Vasodilator.

SYNOPHYLATE-GG. (Central) Theophylline sod. glycinate 300 mg., guaifenesin 100 mg./15 ml. or Tab. **Syr.** pt., gal. **Tabs.** Bot. 100s.
Use: Symptomatic treatment of bronchial asthma.

SYNTHALOIDS. (Buffington) Benzocaine, calcium-iodine complex/Lozenge. Bot. 100s, 1000s. Unit boxes 8s, 16s, 24s. Dispens-A-Kit 500s. Aidpaks 100s. Medipaks 200s.
Use: Sore throat relief.

SYNTHOESTRIN.
See: Diethylstilbestrol, Preps. (Various Mfr.)

SYNTHROID. (Flint) Sodium levothyroxine 25 mcg., 50 mcg., 75 mcg., 100 mcg., 125 mcg., 150 mcg., 200 mcg., 300 mcg./Tab. Bot. 100s, 1000s. Unit Dose available in all strengths.
Use: Thyroid deficiencies.

SYNTHROID INJECTION. (Flint) Lyophilized sodium levothyroxine 100 mcg., 200 mcg., 500 mcg. w/mannitol 10 mg and tribasic sodium phosphate anhydrous 0.7 mg. Vial 10 ml.
Use: Thyroid deficiency; myxedema coma.

SYNTHROX. (Vortech) Sod. levothroxine 0.1 mg., 0.2 mg./Tab. Bot. 1000s.
Use: Thyroid deficiencies.

SYNTOCINON AMPULS. (Sandoz) A sterile aqueous sol. of synthetic oxytocin w/sodium acetate 1.0%, chlorobutanol 0.5%, alcohol 0.61%, acetic acid. Amp. (10 I.U./ml.) 1 ml. SandoPak Pkg. 20s, 100s.
Use: Induction, stimulation or management of labor and for prevention and control of postpartum hemorrhage.

SYNTOCINON NASAL SPRAY. (Sandoz) Syn. oxytocin 40 I.U./cc. w/exsic. sodium phosphate, citric acid, sodium chloride, glycerine, sorbitol, methyl & propylparaben, chlorobutanol 0.05% and Purified Water U.S.P. q.s. Squeeze bottle 2 ml. & 5 ml.
Use: Initial milk let-down.

SYNTOPRESSIN. Lypressin, B.A.N.

SYPHILIS (FTA-ABS) FLUORO KIT. (Clinical Sciences)
Use: Test for syphilis.

SYRAJEN. (Jenkins) Codeine phosphate 10.9 mg., chlorpheniramine maleate 2 mg., pot. guaiacolsulfonate 44 mg., citric acid 60 mg., sod. citrate 197 mg./5 cc. Bot. 4 oz., gal.
Use: Expectorant.

SYRCODATE. (Blue Line) Codeine phosphate 1 gr.,

ammonium chloride 8 gr., Sod. benzoate 4 gr., aromatics flavors in sugar syr. Bot. 4 oz., 1 gal.
Use: Sedative expectorant.

SYRIDYL A-F CAPSULES. (Fellows) N-acetyl-p-amino-phenol 0.130 Gm., salicyamide 0.195 Gm., caffeine 32.5 mg., Dover's Pow. 30 mg., ascorbic acid 50 mg., chlorpheniramine maleate 2 mg., phenylephrine HCl 5 mg., opium 3.2 mg., ipecac 3.2 mg./Cap. Bot. 100s, 500s, 1000s.

SYRIDYL A-F COMPOUND. (Fellows) Phenylephrine HCl 5 mg., chlorpheniramine maleate 1.5 mg., pyrilamine maleate 6.25 mg., potassium guaiacolsulfonate 83.3 mg., sodium citrate 166.6 mg., citric acid 53.3 mg., dihydrocodeinone bitartrate 1.67 mg. alcohol 2%/5 cc. Bot. pt., gal.

SYRIDYL D MINTS. (Fellows) Phenylephrine hydrochloride 5 mg., chlorpheniramine maleate 2 mg./Tab. Bot. 100s.

SYRIDYL EXPECTORANT. (Fellows) Pheniramine maleate 7.5 mg., sodium citrate 42 mg., ammonium chloride 104.8 mg., alcohol 6.7%/5 cc. Bot 4 oz., pt., gal.

SYROCOHIST SYRUP. (Blue Line) Codeine phosphate 20 mg., pyrilamine maleate 30 mg., pheniramine maleate 15 mg., ephedrine sulf. 75 mg., in flavored nonalcoholic syrup/30 cc. Bot. pt., gal.

SYROCOHIST EXPECTORANT SYRUP. (Blue Line) Codeine phosphate 60 mg., ephedrine sulf. 75 mg., pyrilamine maleate 30 mg., pheniramine maleate 15 mg., ammonium chloride 600 mg., sod. citrate 1200 mg., alcohol 4.75%/30 cc. Bot. pt., gal.

SYROSINGOPINE. B.A.N. 4-Ethoxy-carbonyl-3,5-dime-thoxybenzoic acid ester of methyl reserpate. Methyl 18β-Hydroxy-11-17α-dimethoxy-3β, 20α-yohimban-16β-carboxylate-4-Hydroxy-3,5-dimethoxybenzoate Ethyl Carbonate (Ester). Methyl O-(4-ethox-ycarbonyloxy-3,5-dimethoxybenzoyl)reserpate.
Use: Hypotensive.
See: Isotense.
W/Hydrochlorothiazide.
Use: Hypotensive.

SYRPALTA. (Emerson) Syr. containing comb. of fruit flavors. Bot. 1 pt., 1 gal.
Use: Vehicle for masking drug taste.

SYRTUSSAR. Dextromethorphan, B.A.N.

• **SYRUP,** N.F. XVI.
Use: Flavored vehicle.

SYTOBEX. (Parke-Davis) Cyanocobalamin 1000 mcg./ml. w/buffer and preservatives. Vial 10 ml.
Use: Vitamin B-12 deficiency.

SYTRON. Sodium Ironedetate, B.A.N.

T

T-3 RIABEAD. (Abbott) Test kit 50s, 100s.
Use: Radioimmunoassay for qualitative measurement of total circulating serum liothyronine.

T-3 SQUIBB. (Squibb) Radioimmune assay kit for T-3. 100 tests/kit.
Use: Radioimmune assay.

T-3 UPTAKE, SQUIBB. (Squibb) Diagnostic kit. 200 tests/kit.
Use: Diagnostic test.

T-4 CLASP-RIA KIT. (Squibb) Solid phase I-125 T-4 assay kit. 200 tests/kit.
Use: Radio assay test.

T-4 RIA (peg). (Abbott) Diagnostic kit 50s, 100s, 500s.
Use: For quantitative measurement of total circulating serum thyroxine.

T-4 SQUIBB. (Squibb) Radioimmune assay kit for T-4. 200 tests./kit.
Use: Radioimmune assay.

T-14. (Freeport) Cyanocobalamin 1000 mcg./ml. w/sodium Cl. 0.5%, benzyl alcohol 1.5%. Vials 30 cc.
Use: Treatment of vitamin B-12 deficiencies.

T-16. (Freeport) Pyridoxine HCl 100 mg., thiamine HCl 100 mg., benzyl alcohol 1.5%/ml. Vials 10 cc.
Use: Treatment of vitamin B-1 and vitamin B-6 deficiencies.

T-38. (Freeport) Testosterone cypionate 100 mg., benzyl alcohol 0.9% in cottonseed oil/cc. Vials 10 cc.
Use: Androgen replacement therapy.

T-81. (Freeport) Estrogenic substance 2 mg., sodium carboxymethylcellulose 2 mg., povidone 2 mg., dried sodium phosphate 2.9 mg., citric acid 2.05 mg., methylparaben 0.9 mg., propylparaben 0.1 mg., benzyl alcohol 1%/ml. Vials 30 cc.
Use: Estrogen replacement therapy.

T-95. (Freeport) Cyanocobalamine 1000 mcg., thiamine HCl 100 mg., sodium Cl. 0.9% benzyl alcohol 1.5%/ml. Vials 10 cc.
Use: Vitamin B-1 and B-12 replacement therapy.

T-100. (Freeport) Testosterone cypionate 100 mg., benzyl alcohol 0.9% in cottonseed oil/cc. Vials 10cc.
Use: Androgen replacement therapy.

T-846 PREDOXIDE-5. (Mallard) Prednisolone 5 mg./Tab. Bot. 1000s.

TA. (Wampole-Zeus) Anti-thyroid antibodies by IFA. Test 48s.
Use: A useful tool in identifying two thyroid autoantibodies in a single test.

TAASA. (Haag) Acetylsalicylic acid 7½ gr./Tab. Bot. 100s, 1000s.

TABALGIN. Paracetamol, B.A.N.

TABASYN. (Freeport) Chlorpheniramine maleate 2 mg., phenylephrine HCl 10 mg., acetaminophen 5 gr., salicylamide 5 gr./Tab. Bot. 1000s.
Use: Relief of muscular aches, headache, nasal congestion due to colds.

TABRON. (Parke-Davis) Ferrous fumarate 304.2 mg. (representing ele. iron 100 mg.), docusate sodium 50 mg., Vit. E 30 I.U., B-1 6 mg., B-2 6 mg., niacinamide 30 mg., cal. pantothenate 10 mg., B-6 5 mg., C 500 mg., folic acid 1 mg., B-12 25 mcg./Filmseal Bot. 100s. Unit dose pkg. 100s.
Use: Nutritional supplement.

TACARYL. (Westwood) Methdilazine HCl **Tab.:** 8 mg./Tab. Bot. 100s. **Syr.** 4 mg./5 ml. Bot. 16 oz.
Use: Antipruritic.

TACARYL CHEWABLE TAB. (Westwood) Methdilazine, 3.6 mg./Tab. Bot. 100s.
Use: Antipruritic.

T.A.C. CAPSULES. (Towne) Pheniramine maleate 12.5 mg., chlorpheniramine maleate 1 mg., belladonna alkaloids 0.16 mg., (atropine sulfate 0.024 mg., scopolamine HBr 0.014 mg., hyoscyamine sulfate 01.22 mg in tristearin) phenylpropanolamine HCl 50 mg./Cap. Bot. 12s, 24s.

TACE. (Merrell Dow) Chlorotrianisene 12 mg., 25 mg., 72 mg./Cap. (12 mg.) Bot. 28s, 100s, 500s; (25 mg.) Bot. 60s. (72 mg.) Pkg. 48s.
Use: Estrogen therapy.

TACHYSTEROL.
See: Dihydrotachysterol, Tab. (Philips Roxane)

TACITIN. (Ciba) Under study. Benzoctamine, B.A.N.

TACKLE. (Colgate) Resorcinol 2%, benzyl alcohol 1%, menthol 0.2%, allantoin 0.2%. Clear gel. Tube 1 oz., 2 oz., 3 oz.
Use: Dermatologic.

• **TACLAMINE HYDROCHLORIDE.** USAN.
Use: Tranquilizer (minor).

TA CREAM. (C & M Pharmacal) Triamcinolone acetonide 0.025% or 0.05%. Jar 2 oz., 8 oz., 1 lb.
Use: Topical anti-inflammatory.

TACRINE. B.A.N. 9-Amino-1,2,3,4-tetrahydroacridine.
Use: Central nervous system stimulant.
See: Romotal hydrochloride.

TAGAMET. (SmithKline) Cimetidine **Tab.:** Cimetidine 200 mg. or 300 mg./Tab. Bot 100s. Single unit pkg. 100s; **Liquid;** Cimetidine HCl 300 mg./5 ml. Bot. 8 oz. **Vials:** Cimetidine HCl 300 mg./2 ml. Vials 2 ml., 8 ml., 10s.
Use: Hydrogen receptor histamine antagonist for treatment of duodenal ulcer and gastrointestinal diseases.

TAGAMET PRE-FILLED SYRINGES. (SmithKline) Cimetidine HCl 300 mg./2 ml. prefilled syringe.
Use: Ulcer therapy.

TAKARA. (Ladco) Aluminum, boric acid, phenol, oil of peppermint/Pow. 120 Gm. 12s. Can 3.75 oz., 8 oz.
Use: Vaginal douche.

TALACEN. (Winthrop-Breon) Pentazocine HCl 25 mg., acetaminophen 650 mg./Caplet. Bot. 100s.
Use: Analgesic.

TALAMPICILLIN. B.A.N. Phthalidyl 6-[D(-)-α-aminophenylacetamido] penicillinate.
Use: Antibiotic.

• **TALAMPICILLIN HYDROCHLORIDE.** USAN.
Use: Antibacterial.

TALATROL. Trometamol, B.A.N.

• **TALBUTAL,** U.S.P. XXI. Tab., U.S.P. XXI. 5-Allyl-5-sec-butylbarbituric acid.
Use: Hypnotic.
See: Lotusate, Cap. (Winthrop-Breon)

• **TALC,** U.S.P. XXI. A native hydrous magnesium silicate.
Use: Dusting powder, pharmaceutical aid.

TALC TABLETS. (U.S. Products) Talc 25 mg., 50 mg., 75 mg. or 100 mg./Tab. Bot. 1000s.
Use: Radioimmunoassay, for laboratory use only.

• **TALERANOL.** USAN.
Use: Enzyme inhibitor.

- **TALISOMYCIN.** USAN.
  Use: Antineoplastic.
- **TALMETACIN.** USAN.
  Use: Analgesic, antipyretic, anti-inflammatory.
- **TALNIFLUMATE.** USAN.
  Use: Anti-inflammatory, analgesic.
TALOIN. (Adria) Methylbenzethonium chloride, zinc oxide, calamine, eucalyptol in a water-repellent base. Oint.: Tube 14oz.
  Use: Skin protective & antiseptic.
- **TALOPRAM HYDROCHLORIDE.** USAN.
  Use: Potentiator.
- **TALOSALATE.** USAN.
  Use: Analgesic, anti-inflammatory.
TALOXIMINE. B.A.N. 4-(2-Dimethylaminoethoxy)-1,2-dihydro-1-hydroxyiminophthalazine.
  Use: Respiratory stimulant.
TALWIN COMPOUND. (Winthrop-Breon) Pentazocine HCl 12.5 mg., asprin 325 mg./Tab. Bot. 100s.
  Use: Analgesic.
TALWIN INJECTION. (Winthrop-Breon) Pentazocine lactate injection. **Ampuls:** Uni-amp: 30 mg./1 ml. 25s; 45 mg./1.5 ml. 25s; 60 mg./2 ml. 25s. **Vial:** 30 mg./10 ml. **Uni-Nest:** 30 mg./ml. Box 25s; 60 mg./2 ml. Box 25s. **Carpuject:** 30 mg./ml. Box 10s; 45 mg./1.5 ml. Box 10s; 60 mg./2 ml. Box 10s.
  Use: Analgesic.
TALWIN NX. (Winthrop-Breon) Pentazocine HCl 50 mg., naloxone 0.5 mg./Tab. Bot. 100s. Dispenser Pkg. 250s, 10 sleeve 25s. Unit dose 100s.
  Use: Analgesic.
- **TAMETRALINE HYDROCHLORIDE.** USAN.
  Use: Antidepressant.
- **TAMOXIFEN CITRATE,** U.S.P. XXI. Tab., U.S.P. XXI. (Z)-(4-(1,2-diphenyl-1-butenyl) phenoxy)-N,N-dime-thylethanamine 2-hydroxy-1,2,3-propanetricarboxy-late (1:1).
  Use: Treatment of mammary carcinoma.
  See: Nolvadex, Tab. (Stuart)
TAMP-R-TEL. (Wyeth) A tamper-resistant package for narcotic drugs which includes the following:
  Codeine phosphate 30 mg., 60 mg./1 cc.
  Hydromorphone HCl 1 mg., 2 mg., 3 mg., 4 mg./Tubex
  Meperidine HCl 25 mg./cc. and **Promethazine HCl** 25 mg./cc. 2 cc.
  Meperidine HCl 25 mg./1 cc., 50 mg./1 cc., 75 mg./1 cc., 100 mg./1 cc.
  Morphine Sulfate 2mg., 4mg., 8 mg., 10 mg., 15 mg./1 cc.
  Pentobarbital, Sodium 50 mg./1 cc., 100 mg./2 cc.
  Phenobarbital, Sodium 30 mg., 60 mg., 130 mg./1 cc.
  Secobarbital, Sodium 50 mg./1 cc., 100 mg./2 cc.
TANAC LIQUID. (Commerce) Benzalkonium Cl, benzocaine, tannic acid in a special base. Bot. 0.45 oz.
  Use: Mouth sores, cold sores, fever blisters.

TANAC ROLL-ON. (Commerce) Tannic acid, benzalkonium Cl, benzocaine. Bot. 0.3 oz.
  Use: Cold sores, fever blister, cracked lips.
TANAC STICK. (Commerce) Benzocaine, tannic acid, octyl dimethyl PABA, allantoin, benzalkonium Cl., emollient core & base. Stick 0.1 oz.
  Use: Cold sores, fever blisters, dry lips.
TANADEX. (Commerce) Bot. 3 oz.
  Use: Throat gargle.
TAN-A-DYNE. (Archer-Taylor) Tannic acid compound w/iodine. Bot. 4 oz., pt., gal.
  Use: Swab and gargle concentrate.
TANBISMUTH.
  See: Bismuth Tannate.
TAN CARE AFTER TANNING LOTION. (Plough) Bot. 6 oz., 10 oz.
  Use: After-sun skin moisturizer
TANCOLIN. Dextromethorphan, B.A.N.
- **TANDAMINE HYDROCHLORIDE.** USAN.
  Use: Antidepressant.
TANDEARIL. (Geigy) Oxyphenbutazone 100 mg./Tab. Bot. 100s, 1000s. Unit Dose 100s.
  Use: Anti-inflammatory, antiarthritic, analgesic, antipyretic.
- **TANNIC ACID.** U.S.P. XXI. Gallotannic acid. Glycerite. Tannin.
  Use: 1 to 20% solution as an astringent.
  See: Amertan, Oint. (Lilly)
  W/Benzocaine, benzyl alcohol, diisobutylphenoxyethoxyethyl dimethyl benzyl ammonium chloride.
    See: Kankex, Liq. (Edward J. Moore)
  W/Benzocaine, phenol, thymol iodide, ephedrine HCl, zinc oxide, peru balsam.
    See: Hemocaine, Oint. (Mallard)
  W/Bisacodyl.
    See: Clysodrast, Packet (Barnes-Hind)
  W/Boric acid, salicylic acid, isopropyl alcohol.
    See: Sal Dex Boro, Liq. (Scrip)
  W/Chlorobutanol, isopropyl alcohol.
    See: Outgro, Sol. (Whitehall)
  W/Cyanocobalamin, zinc acetate, glutathione, phenol.
    See: Depinar, Amp. (Armour)
  W/Merthiolate.
    See: Amertan, Oint. (Lilly)
  W/Phenol, iodine.
    See: Phen-Iodine No. 2, Liq. (Sutliff & Case)
  W/Salicylic acid, boric acid.
    See: Tan-Bor-Sal, Liq. (Gordon)
TANNIC SPRAY. (Gebauer) Tannic acid 4.5%, chlorbutanol 1.3%, menthol less than 1%, benzocaine less than 1%. propylene glycol 33%, ethanol 60.5% Bot. 57 Gm., 114 Gm.
  Use: Relief of sunburn and other minor burns.
TANPHETAMIN.
  See: Dextroamphetamine tannate
TAO. (Roerig) Troleandomycin Bot. 100s. 250 mg./Cap.
  Use: Antibiotic therapy.
TAORYL EDISYLATE. Caramiphen, B.A.N.
TAPAL AMPULS. (Winthrop Products) Dipyrone.
  Use: Analgesic, antipyretic, anti-inflammatory.

TAPAL TABLETS. (Winthrop Products) Dipyrone.
Use: Analgesic, antipyretic, anti-inflammatory.
TAPAR TABLETS. (Parke-Davis) Acetaminophen 325
mg./Tab. Bot. 100s.
Use: Analgesic.
TAPAZOLE. (Lilly) Methimazole. 1-methyl-2-mercap-
toimidazole. Tab. (5 mg. & 10 mg.) Bot. 100s.
Use: Hyperthyroidism.
• **TAPE, ADHESIVE,** U.S.P. XXI.
Use: Surgical aid.
TA-POFF. (Ulmer) Adhesive tape remover. Bot. 1 pt.
Aerosol. Can 6 oz.
TAPULINE. (Wesley) Activated attapulgite 600 mg.,
pectin 60 mg., homatropine methylbromide 0.5
mg./Chewable Tab. Bot. 100s, 1000s.
Use: Diarrhea.
TAR.
See: Coal Tar, Preps.
TARACTAN. (Roche) Trans isomer 2-chloro-9-(3-di-
methyl aminopropylidene) thioxanthene. **Tab.:**
Chlorprothixene 10, 25, 50 or 100 mg./Tab. Bot.
100s, 500s. **Concentrate** 100 mg./5 ml. Bot. 1 pt.
Amp. (w/methyl and propyl parabens 0.2%.) 25
mg./2 ml., 10s.
Use: Tranquilizer.
TAR DISTILLATE. (Doak) Decolorized fractional
distillate of crude coal tar. Each cc. equiv. to 1 Gm.
whole crude coal tar. Bot. 2 oz., 16 oz.
Use: Active ingredient for dermatologic
preparations.
TARLENE LOTION. (Medco Lab) Refined crude coal
tar, salicylic acid, propylene glycol. Plastic
Applicator Bot. 2 oz.
Use: seborrheic dermatitis.
TARPASTE. (Doak) Coal tar, distilled 5% in zinc
paste. Tube 1 oz., Jar 4 oz., w/Hydrocortisone
½%. Tube 1 oz.
Use: Dermatitis.
TAR-QUIN-HC. (Jenkins) Hydrocortisone 0.5%, liquor
carbonis detergens 3.0%, clioquinol 1.0%. Oint.
Tube ½ oz.
TARSUM. (Summers) Coal tar 10%, salicylic acid 5%.
Bot. 4 oz.
Use: Dermatologic, shampoo.
TARTAR EMETIC.
See: Antimony Potassium Tartrate, U.S.P.
• **TARTARIC ACID,** N.F. XVI.
Use: Buffer.
TASHAN, Skin Cream. (Block) Vit. A palmitate, D-2, D-
panthenol, Vit. E. Tube 1 oz.
TAUROCHOLIC ACID.
W/Pancreatin, pepsin.
See: Enzymet, Tabs. (Westerfield)
TAUROLIN. B.A.N. 4,4'-Methylenedi(tetrahydro-1,2,4-
thiadiazine-1-dioxide).
Use: Antibacterial.
See: Tauroflex.
TAUROPHYLLIN. (Vale) Ext. ox bile 32.4 mg.,
phenolphthalein 32.4 mg., ext. cascara sagrada
32.4 mg.,/Tab. Bot. 100s, 1000s, 5000s.
TAURULTAM. B.A.N. Tetrahydro-1,2,4-thiadiazine 1,1-
dioxide.
Use: Antibacterial; antifungal.

TAVEGIL HYDROGEN FUMARATE. Clemastine,
B.A.N.
TA-VERM. (Table Rock) Piperazine citrate 100 mg./cc.
Syr. Bot. 1 pt., 1 gal. Tabs. 500 mg. Bot. 100s,
500s.
Use: Anthelmintic.
TAVILEN PLUS. (Table Rock) Liver solution 1 Gm.,
ferric pyrophosphate soluble 500 mg., Vit. B-12 24
mcg., B-1 6 mg., B-2 7.2 mg., B-6 3 mg., panthenol 3
mg., niacinamide 60 mg., l-lysine HCl 300 mg., 5%
alcohol/cc. Bot. 16 oz., 1 gal.
Use: Hematinic.
TAVIST. (Sandoz) Clemastine fumarate 2.68
mg./Tab. Bot. 100s.
Use: Antihistamine.
TAVIST-1 TABLETS. (Sandoz) Clemastine fumarate
1.34 mg./Tab. Bot. 100s.
Use: Antihistamine.
TAVIST-D. (Sandoz) Clemastine fumarate 1.34 mg.,
phenylpropanolamine HCl 75 mg./Tab. Bot. 100s.
Use: Relief of allergic rhinitis symptoms.
TAXOL. (CMC) Bile Salts 1 gr., aloes ⅔ gr.,
hyoscyamus ext. ¹⁄₁₃ gr., w/pancreas,
duodenum/Tab. Bot. 50s, 500s.
Use: Laxative.
TAYSTRON. (Vale) Elemental iron 15 mg., Vit. B-1 3
mg., C 20 mg., B-12 4 mcg./Tab. Bot. 100s, 500s,
1000s.
Use: Iron and vitamin supplement.
• **TAZOLOL HYDROCHLORIDE.** USAN.
Use: Cardiotonic.
TBA-PRED. (Keene) Prednisolone tebutate 10 mg./ml.
susp. Vial 10 ml.
Use: Corticosteroid for intra-articular and soft tissue
injection.
T-BENZETTES. (Wolins) Benzocaine 5 mg., anise fla-
vor/Loz. Bot. 1000s.
TBZ. (MSD AGVET) Thiabendazole. **Cubes:** 3.3%
thiabendazole; **Paste:** 43% thiabendazole; **Pellets:**
6.6%; **Bolus:** 2 Gm., 15 Gm.; **Suspension:** Various
sizes.
Use: Anthelmintic, veterinary medicine.
TBZ-6. (MSD AGVET) Thiabendazole suspension 6
Gm./oz.
Use: Anthelmintic, veterinary medicine.
T-CAINE 1%. (Tunex) Lidocaine HCl 10 mg./ml. Vial
50cc.
Use: Infiltration & nerve block anesthesia.
T-CAINE 2%. (Tunex) Lidocaine HCl 20 mg./ml. Vial
50cc.
Use: Infiltration & nerve block anesthesia.
T.C.M. 200. (Zenith) Tridihexethyl Cl 25 mg.,
meprobamate 200 mg./Tab.
Use: Tranquilizer.
T.C.M. 400. (Zenith) Tridihexethyl Cl 25 mg.,
meprobamate 400 mg./Tab.
Use: Tranquilizer.
T/DERM. (Neutrogena) Neutar coal tar extract 5% in
oil base. Bot. 4 oz.
Use: Psoriasis treatment.
T-DRYL 10. (Tunex) Diphenhydramine HCl 10 mg./ml.
Vial 30 cc.
Use: Antihistaminic.

T-DRYL 50. (Tunex) Diphenhydramine HCl 50 mg./ml. Vial 10cc.
Use: Antihistaminic.
T.D. THERALS. (Reid-Provident) Vit. A 10,000 I.U., D 400 I.U., E 5 I.U., C 100 mg., B-1 10 mg., B-2 5 mg., B-6 0.5 mg., B-12 5 mcg., niacinamide 50 mg., calcium pantothenate 5 mg., ferrous sulfate 30 mg., pot. iodide 0.13 mg., manganese sulfate 3 mg., pot. sulfate 11 mg., copper sulfate 2.8 mg., zinc sulfate 3.9 mg., magnesium sulfate 10 mg./T.R. Cap. Bot. 100s.
Use: Multiple avitaminosis therapy.
TEAR AID. (Ketchum) Vial 15 cc.
Use: Decongestant-emollient.
TEARISOL. (CooperVision) An isotonic buffered aqueous sol. of hydroxypropyl methylcellulose 0.5%, edetate disodium 0.01%, benzalkonium chloride 0.01%, boric acid, sodium carbonate, potassium chloride Bot. 15 ml.
Use: Artificial tears in many eye conditions.
TEARS NATURALE. (Alcon) Duasorb water soluble polymeric system, benzalkonium chloride 0.01%, disodium edetate 0.05%. Droptainer 15 ml. & 30 ml.
Use: Artificial tear & lubricant for ocular irritation & dry eyes.
TEARS PLUS. (Allergan) Polyvinyl alcohol, povidine. Bot. 0.5 oz., 1 oz.
Use: Artificial tears.
TEATCOTE PLUS. Polyhexanide, B.A.N.
• **TEBUQUINE.** USAN.
Use: Antimalarial.
T.E.C. (Invenex) Zn 1 mg., Cu 0.4 mg., Cr. 4.0 mcg., Mn 0.1 mg. Vial 10 ml.
Use: Trace element additives for TNP therapy.
TECALDRINE. Dextromethorphan, B.A.N.
TECHENESCAN MAA. (Mallinckrodt) Aggregated albumin (human).
Use: Preparation of Tc 99m Aggregated Albumin (Human).
TECHNECOLL KIT. (Mallinckrodt) Technetium Tc 99 m Sulfur Colloid Kit.
TECHNEPLEX. (Squibb) Technetium Tc 99m penetate kit. 10 vials/kit.
Use: Radiodiagnostic.
TECHNESCAN PYP KIT. (Mallinckrodt) Soln. stannous pyrophosphate 15.4 mg.
Use: Radiodiagnostic.
TECHNETIUM.
See: Ultra-TechneKow (Mallinckrodt)
TECHNETIUM 99m-IRON-ASCORBATE-DTPA.
See: Renotec (Squibb)
TECHNETIUM Tc 99m. Neimotec; Ultra-TechneKow Generator (Mallinckrodt).
• **TECHNETIUM Tc-99m ALBUMIN INJECTION,** U.S.P. XXI.
Use: Radioactive agent.
• **TECHNETIUM Tc-99m ALBUMIN AGGREGATED INJECTION,** U.S.P. XXI.
Use: Diagnostic aid (Lung scanning)
• **TECHNETIUM Tc-99m ETIDRONATE INJECTION,** U.S.P. XXI.

TECHNETIUM Tc-99m Generat or Solution. (New England Nuclear) Pertechnetate sodium Tc 99 m.
Use: Radiodiagnostic.
• **TECHNETIUM Tc-99mFERPENTETATE INJECTION,** U.S.P. XXI.
Use: Radioactive agent.
• **TECHNETIUM Tc-99m MEDRONATE INJECTION,** U.S.P. XXI.
• **TECHNETIUM Tc-99m OXIDRONATE INJECTION,** U.S.P. XXI.
• **TECHNETIUM Tc-99m PENTETATE INJECTION,** U.S.P. XXI.
Use: Radioactive agent.
• **TECHNETIUM Tc-99m PYROPHOSPHATE INJECTION,** U.S.P. XXI.
Use: Radioactive agent.
• **TECHNETIUM Tc-99m (Pyro- and trimetra-) PHOSPHATES INJECTION,** U.S.P. XXI.
Use: Radioactive agent.
• **TECHNETIUM Tc-99m SODIUM INJECTION,** U.S.P. XXI.
Use: Radioactive agent.
• **TECHNETIUM Tc-99m SUCCIMER INJECTION,** U.S.P. XXI.
Use: Radioactive agent.
TECHNETIUM Tc-99m SULFUR COLLOID KIT.
Use: Radioactive agent.
See: Technecol Kit (Mallinckrodt)
    Tesuloid (Squibb)
• **TECHNETIUM Tc-99m SULFUR COLLOID INJECTION,** U.S.P. XXI.
Use: Diagnostic aid (liver scanning)
TECLOSINE. Under study.
Use: Amebacide.
TECLOTHIAZIDE. B.A.N. 6-Chloro-3,4-dihydro-3-trichloromethyl-1,2,4-benzothiadiazine-7-sulfonamide 1,1-dioxide.
Use: Diuretic.
See: Deplet potassium derivative.
• **TECLOZAN.** USAN. N,N'-(p-Phenylenedimethylene)-bis]2,2-dichloro-N-(2-ethoxy-ethyl)-acetamide].
Use: Amebicide.
See: Falmonox (Winthrop Products)
TEDRAL. (Parke-Davis) **Tab.:** Theophylline 130 mg., ephedrine HCl 24 mg., phenobarbital 8 mg./Tab. Bot. 24s, 100s, 1000s. Unit dose 100s. **Susp. (Pediatric):** Theophylline 65 mg., ephedrine HCl 12 mg., phenobarbital 4 mg./5 cc. Bot. 8 oz., 16 oz.
Use: Symptomatic relief in asthma.
TEDRAL-25. (Parke-Davis) Identical with Tedral except that butabarbital 25 mg. has been substituted for phenobarbital, 8 mg./Tab. Bot. 100s.
Use: Relief of bronchospasms and bronchial asthma.
TEDRAL ELIXIR. (Parke-Davis) Theophylline 32.5 mg., ephedrine HCl 6 mg., phenobarbital 2 mg./5 cc. Alcohol 15%. Pediatric. Bot. pt.
Use: Bronchospasm of asthma.
TEDRAL EXPECTORANT TABLETS. (Parke-Davis) Theophylline 130 mg., ephedrine HCl 24 mg., phenobarbital 8 mg., guaifenesin 100 mg./Tab. Bot. 100s.

Use: Expectorant.

TEDRAL-SA. (Parke-Davis) Theophylline 180 mg., ephedrine HCl 48 mg., phenobarbital 25 mg./S.A. Tab. Bot. 100s, 1000s. Unit dose 100s.
Use: Prevention of asthmatic attacks.

TEEBACIN. (CMC) Sod. p-aminosalicylate **Tab.** 0.5 Gm. Bot. 500s, 1000s. 1 Gm./Tab. Bot. 500s, 1000s. **Pow.** Bot. 1 lb. Packettes. 4.18 Gm., 5.57 Gm./Packette. 100s.
Use: Tuberculosis.

TEEBACIN ACID BUFFERED. (CMC) p-Aminosalicylic acid 0.5 Gm. with magnesium glycinate & carbonate/Tab. Bot. 500s, 1000s.
Use: Tuberculosis treatment.

TEEBACONIN. (CMC) Isoniazid 100, 300 mg./Tab. Bot. 100s, 250s, 1000s. Pow. 1 lb.
Use: Tuberculosis.

TEEBACONIN W/Vit. B-6. (CMC) Isoniazid 100 mg., and 5, 10 or 50 mg. pyridoxine HCl/Tab. Bot. 100s, 500s, 1000s.
Use: Tuberculosis susceptible to isoniazid therapy.

TEEBAZONE. Tibione. 4-Acetylamino-benzaldehyde thiosemicarbazone. Under study.
Use: Antituberculosis.

TEEPHEN. (Robinson) **Capsules, Tablets:**
Theophylline 2 gr., ephedrine ⅜ gr., phenobarbital ⅛ gr./Cap. or Tab. Bot. 100s, 1000s. Bulk Pack 5000s. **Suppositories:** Same formula as Caps and Tabs. Box 12s. **Suspension:** Theophylline 1 gr., ephedrine HCl ⅕ gr., phenobarbital ¹⁄₁₅ gr./5 cc. Bot. 8 oz.

• **TEFLURANE.** USAN. 2-Bromo-1,1,1,2-tetrafluoroethane.
Use: General inhalation anesthetic.

TEGA-ATRIC ELIXIR. (Ortega) Pentylenetetrazol 100 mg., niacin 50 mg., vit. B-1 30 mg., B-2 30 mg., B-6 10 mg., B-12 100 mcg., choline bitartrate 150 mg., inositol 100 mg./30 ml. w/alcohol 15%. Sherry wine flavor. Bot. pt., gal.
Use: Geriatric therapy.

TEGA-C-CAPS. (Ortega) Ascorbic acid 500 mg./T. R. Cap. Bot. 100s, 1000s.
Use: Dietary supplement.

TEGACID.
See: Glyceryl monostearate.

TEGA-CODE M. (Ortega) Acetaminophen 300 mg., salicylamide 200 mg., codeine phosphate 30 mg./Cap. Bot. 100s, 500s.
Use: Analgesic.

TEGA CORT FORTE 1%. (Ortega) Micronized hydrocortisone alcohol 1% in water washable base. Bot. 2 oz., 4 oz.
Use: Topical lotion for relief of inflammatory dermatoses.

TEGA CORT LOTION 0.5%. (Ortega) Micronized hydrocortisone alcohol 0.5% in water washable base. Bot. 2 oz., 4 oz.
Use: Topical lotion for relief of inflammatory dermatoses.

TEGA-FLEX. (Ortega) Orphenadrine citrate 30 mg./ml. Vial 10 ml.
Use: Musculoskeletal conditions.

• **TEGAFUR.** USAN. (Mead Johnson)
Use: Antineoplastic.

TEGAMIDE. (G&W) Trimethobenzamide HCl 100 mg., or 200 mg./ Supp. Boxes 10s, 50s.
Use: Control of nausea and vomiting.

TEGA OTIC. (Ortega) Hydrocortisone alcohol 1%, pramoxine HCl 1%, parachlorometaxylenol 0.1%, benzalkonium Cl 0.02%, glacia acetic acid 20 mg./ml. Bot. 10 cc.
Use: Bacterial & fungal infection of the ear.

TEGA-PAP. (Ortega) Acetaminophen 120 mg., alcohol 10%/Tab. or 5 cc. Bot. pt., gal. Tab. Bot. 100s, 1000s.
Use: Analgesic, antipyretic.

TEGA VERT. (Ortega) Niacin 50 mg., dimenhydrinate 25 mg./Cap. Bot. 100s, 1000s.
Use: Vertigo, meniers syndrome.

TEGOPEN. (Bristol) Cloxacillin sodium 250 mg./Cap. Bot. 100s. 500 mg./Cap. Bot. 100s. Granules for Soln. 125 mg./5 ml. Bot. 100 ml., 200 ml.
Use: Antibiotic.

TEGRETOL. (Geigy) Carbamazepine 200 mg./Tab. Bot. 100s, 1000s, Unit Dose 100s. Gy-Pak 100s. **Chewable Tab.:** 100mg./Tab. Bot.100s. Unit dose 100s.
Use: Epilepsy; trigeminal neuralgia.

TEGRIN CREAM. (Block) Allantoin 2%, coal tar ext. 5% in cream base. Tube 2 oz., 4.4 oz.
Use: Psoriasis.

TEGRIN SHAMPOO. (Block) Tar extract 5% in cream base shampoo. Tube. 2 oz., 3.2 oz., 5 oz. Bot. 3.75 oz., 6.6 oz. **Cream** Jar 2 oz., 4.4 oz., **Lotion:** Bot. 3.75, 6.6 oz. **Soap** Bar 4.5 oz.
Use: Antiseborrheic, antidandruff.

T.E. IONATE P.A.. (Reid-Provident) Testosterone cypionate 50 mg., estradiol cipionate 2 mg., chlorobutanol 0.5%, in cottonseed oil/cc. Vial 10 cc. 1s, 6s, 12s.

TEK-CHEK. (Ames) Controls for routine urinalysis. Pkg. 4 vials.
Use: For use with Ames urinalysis strips.

TELDRIN MULTI-SYMPTOM ALLERGY RELIEVER. (Menley & James) Chlorpheniramine maleate 2 mg., acetaminophen 325 mg., pseudoephedrine HCl 30 mg./Cap. Pkg. 20s.
Use: Antihistaminic, analgesic, decongestant for hay fever and sinusitis symptoms.

TELDRIN TIMED-RELEASE ALLERGY CAPSULE. (Menley & James) Chlorpheniramine maleate 8 mg. or 12 mg./Spansule. Pkg. 12s, 24s. Bot. 50s, 500s. Single unit pack 100s.
Use: Antihistamine for hay fever and allergy.

TELEFON. (Kenyon) Ferrous sulfate 150 mg./Cap. Bot. 100s, 1000s.

TELEPAQUE. (Winthrop-Breon) Iopanoic acid. 0.5 Gm./Tab. Envelope of 6 Tablets. Box 25 envelopes.
Use: Orally; cholecystographic medium.

TELMID IODIDE. Dithiazanine. B.A.N.

TELODRON. (Norden) Chlorpheniramine maleate.

TELOTREX. Tetracycline, B.A.N.

TEM. Tretamine, B.A.N.

See: Triethylenemelamine, Tab. (Lederle)

TEMARIL. (SmithKline) Trimeprazine tartrate. **Tab.** Trimeprazine tartrate 2.5 mg./Tab. Bot. 100s, 1000s. Single Unit Pak 100s. **Syr.** 2.5 mg./5 ml. w/alcohol 5.7%. Bot. 4 oz. **Spansule** 5 mg. Bot. 50s, Single Unit Pak, 100s.
Use: Antipruritic.

• **TEMAZEPAM.** USAN. 7-Chloro-1,3-dihydro-3-hydroxy-1-methyl-5-phenyl-2H-1,4-benzodiazepin-2-one.
Use: Minor tranquilizer.
See: Restoril, Cap. (Sandoz)

• **TEMEFOS.** USAN.
Use: Ectoparasiticide.

TEMETAN. (Nevin) Acetaminophen 324 mg./Tab. Bot. 100s, 500s. Elixir (324 mg./5 cc.) Bot. pt.
Use: Analgesic.

• **TEMODOX.** USAN.
Use: Growth stimulant.

TEMPO. (Vicks) Calcium carbonate 414 mg., aluminum hydroxide 133 mg., magnesium hydroxide 81 mg., simethicon 20 mg./Tab. Bot. 10s, 30s, 60s.
Use: Antacid, antiflatulant.

TEMPRA. (Mead Johnson) Acetaminophen. **Red drops** 80 mg./0.8 ml. Bot. w/dropper 15 ml. **Red syrup** 160 mg./5 ml. Bot. 4 oz., 1 pt. **Tab.:** 80 mg./Chewable Tab. Grape flavor. Bot 30s.
Use: Relief of fever and pain.

TENDRON. (Amfre-Grant) Dexamethasone sodium phosphate 4 mg./ml. Vial 5 ml.
Use: Hormone supplement.

TENDRON L.A. (Amfre-Grant) Dexamethasone acetate 8 mg./ml. Vial 5 ml.
Use: Hormone.

• **TENIPOSIDE.** USAN.
Use: Antineoplastic.

TENOL. (Vortech) Acetaminophen 5 gr./Tab. Bot. 100s, 1000s.
Use: Analgesic.

TENOL LIQUID. (Vortech) Acetaminophen 120 mg., NAPA alcohol 7%/5 cc. Bot. 3 oz., 4 oz., Gal.
Use: Analgesic.

TENORMAL HYDROGEN TARTRATE. Pempidine, B.A.N.

TENORMIN. (Stuart) Atenolol 50 mg. or 100 mg./Tab. Bot. 100s. Unit dose 100s.
Use: Antihypertensive.

TENSAWAY. (Stanlabs) Vit. B-1, B-2, B-6, niacinamide, ext. passion flower, salicylamide, scopolamine aminoxide HBr, pyrilamine maleate. Tab. Carton 30s.
Use: Nervous tension.

TENSEZE. (A.P.C.) Phenyltoloxamine citrate 88 mg., salicylamide 130 mg./Cap. Bot. 10s.
Use: Nervous tension.

TENSILON. (Roche) Edrophonium chloride. **Vial:** 10 mg./ml., w/phenol 0.45%, sodium sulfite 0.2%, sodium citrate, citric acid. Box 1s; **Amp.** 10 mg./ml., w/sodium sulfite 0.2%, sodium citrate, citric acid 1 ml. Box 10s.
Use: Curare antagonist, muscle stimulant.

TENSIN. (Standex) Reserpine 0.25 mg./Tab. Bot. 100s.

TENSOCAINE TABLETS. (Winthrop Products) Acetominophen.
Use: Analgesic, antipyretic.

TENSOLAX TABLETS. (Winthrop Products) Chlormezanone.
Use: Analgesic, muscle relaxant.

TENSOLATE. (Apco) Phenobarbital ¼ gr., hyoscyamine sulfate 0.1037 mg., atropine sulfate 0.0194 mg., hyoscine HBr 0.0065 mg./Tab. Bot. 100s.
Use: Antispasmodic sedative, for visceral spasm.

TENSOPIN. (Apco) Phenobarbital ¼ gr., homatropine methylbromide 2.5 mg./Tab. Bot. 100s.
Use: Antispasmodic.

TENSOR. (Crystal) Mannitol hexanitrate 30 mg., veratrum viride 100 mg., rutin 20 mg., Rauwolfia serpentina alkaloids 0.75 mg./Tab. Bot. 100s.
Use: Hypertension.

TENSTAN. (Standex) Isobutylallylbarbituric acid ¾ gr., caffeine ⅔ gr., aspirin 3 gr., phenacetin 2 gr./Tab. Bot. 100s.
Use: Analgesic.

TENTRATE. (Tennessee Pharm.) Pentaerythritol tetranitrate 20 mg./Tab. Bot. 100s, 1000s.

TENUATE. (Merrell Dow) Diethylpropion HCl 25 mg./Tab. Bot. 100s.
Use: Anorectic.

TENUATE DOSPAN. (Merrell Dow) Diethylpropion HCl 75 mg./Controlled Release Tab. Bot. 100s, 250s.
Use: Anorectic.

T-E-P COMPOUND. (Stanlabs) Theophylline 2 gr., ephedrine ⅜ gr., phenobarbital ⅛ gr./Tab. Bot. 1000s.
Use: Bronchial antispasmodic.

TEOQUIL. Hedaquinium Chloride, B.A.N.

TEPANIL. (Riker) Diethylpropion HCl. Tab. 25 mg. Bot. 100s.
Use: Treatment and control of obesity.

TEPANIL TEN-TAB. (Riker) Diethylpropion 75 mg./Tab. Bot. 30s, 100s, 250s.
Use: Treatment and control of obesity.

• **TEPROTIDE.** USAN.
Use: Enzyme-inhibitor.

TEQUINOL SODIUM. Name used for Actinoquinol Sodium.

TERALASE. W/Pancreatin, polysorbate-80.
See: Digolase, Cap. (Boyle)

• **TERAZOSIN HYDROCHLORIDE.** USAN.
Use: Antihypertensive.

TERBUTALINE. B.A.N. 1-(3,5-Dihydroxyphenyl)-2-(t-butylamino)ethanol.
Use: Bronchodilator.

• **TERBUTALINE SULFATE,** U.S.P. XXI. Inj., Tab., U.S.P. XXI. a-[(tert-Butylamino)methyl]-3,5-dihydroxybenzyl alcohol sulfate.
Use: Bronchodilator.
See: Brethine, Amp., Tab. (Geigy)

TERCODRYL. (Approved) Codeine phos. ¾ gr., pyrilamine maleate 25 mg./fl. oz. Bot. 4 oz.

Use: Antihistamine.
- **TERCONAZOLE.** USAN.
Use: Antifungal.
- **TERFENADINE.** USAN.
Use: Antihistaminic.
- **TERODILINE HYDROCHLORIDE.** USAN.
Use: Vasodilator (coronary).
TERFONYL SUSPENSION. (Squibb)
Trisulfapyrimidines 500 mg./5 ml. Bot. pt.
Use: Bacterial infections sensitive to sulfonamides.
TERFONYL TABLETS. (Squibb) Trisulfapyramidines
500 mg./Tab. sulfadiazine 0.167 Gm.,
sulfamerazine 0.167 Gm., sulfamethazine 0.167
Gm./Tab. Bot. 100s.
Use: Triple sulfonamide therapy.
See: Meth-Dia-Mer-Sulfonamides
TERG-A-ZYME. (Alconox) Alconox with enzyme action.
Box 4 lb. Ctn. 9×4 lb., 25 lb., 50 lb., 100 lb., 300
lb.
Use: Biodegradeable detergent and wetting agent.
TERIDOL JR. (Approved) Terpin hydrate, cocillana,
pot. guaiacolsulfonate, ammonium chloride. Bot. 3
oz.
Use: Children's cough syrup.
- **TEROXALENE HYDROCHLORIDE.** USAN 1-(3-Chloro-p-tolyl)-4-[6-(p-tert-pentylphenoxy)-hexyl] piperazine
hydrochloride.
Use: Antischistosomal.
- **TEROXIRONE.** USAN.
Use: Antineoplastic.
TERPACOF. (Jenkins) Codeine phosphate 10 mg.,
terpin hydrate 88 mg./5 ml. Bot. 3 oz., gal.
Use: Cough sedative and expectorant.
TERPATE. (Geneva) Pentaerythritol tetranitrate 10
mg., 20 mg./Tab. Bot. 100s.
TERPEX JR. (Approved) d-Methorphan 25 mg., terpin
hydrate, pot. guaiacolsulfonate, cocillana,
ammonium chloride. Bot. 4 oz.
Use: Children's cough syrup.
TERPHAN ELIXIR. (Vale) Terpin hydrate 85 mg.,
dextromethorphan hydrobromide 10 mg., 15ml.
w/alcohol 40% Bot. pt., gal., 3 oz.
Use: Sedative.
- **TERPIN HYDRATE,** U.S.P. XXI. Elixir, with Codeine
Elixir, U.S.P. XXI. cis-p-Menthane-1,8-diol hydrate.
Cryst. & Pow., Pkg. ¼ lb., 4 oz., 1 lb.
Use: Expectorant for chronic cough.
See: Creoterp (Jenkins)
SK-Terpin Hydrate and Codeine, Liq. (SmithKline)
Terp, Liq. (Scrip)
TERPIN HYDRATE W/COMBINATIONS
See: Cerose Comp. Cap. (Ives)
Dicodethal, Elix. (Lannett)
Gylanphen, Tab. (Lannett)
Histogesic, Tab. (Century)
Ipaterp C.T., Tab. (Fellows)
Palodyne, Cap. (Mallard)
Prunicodeine, Liq. (Lilly)
S.A.C. Throat Lozenges (Towne)
Terpichlor, Tab. (Richlyn)
Terpium, Tab. (Scrip)

Toclonol Expectorant, Liq. (Cenci)
Toclonol W/Codeine, Liq. (Cenci)
Turpoin, Tab. (Mallard)
W/Dextromethorphan, phenylephrine HCl,
chloropheniramine maleate, acetaminophen,
ascorbic acid.
See: Cerose Compound, Cap. (Ives)
W/Dextromethorphan, phenylpropanolamine HCl,
pheniramine maleate, pyrilamine maleate.
See: Tussaminic, Tab. (Dorsey)
W/Dextromethorphan, phenylpropanolamine HCl,
pheniramine maleate, pyrilamine maleate,
acetaminophen.
See: Chexit, Tab. (Dorsey)
Tussagesic, Tab., Liq. (Dorsey)
- **TERPIN HYDRATE AND DEXTROMETHORPHAN
HYDROBROMIDE ELIXIR,** U.S.P. XXI.
Use: Expectorant, antitussive.
See: Dicodethal, Elix. (Lannett)
TERRA-CORTRIL. (Pfipharmecs)
Use: Anti-inflammatory, antibiotic.
Topical Oint.: Hydrocortisone 1%, terramycin 3%
in base of mineral oil and petrolatum. Tube ½ oz.
Ophth. Susp.: Hydrocortisone 15 mg. terramycin
HCl 5 mg./cc. Bot. w/dropper 5 cc.
TERRAMYCIN. (Pfipharmecs) Oxytetracycline
Use: Antibiotic.
Caps.: HCl salt 250 mg./Cap. Bot. 16s, 100s, 500s.
Unit-Dose Pak Box 100s.
I.M. Solution: Oxytetracycline 100 mg. or 250
mg./2 cc.w/lidocaine 2%. Amp. 5s, 100s, 50
mg./cc. Vial 10 cc. Pkg. 5s.
I.V.: HCl salt 250 mg. Vial 5s, 500 mg. Vial 5s.
Oint., Ophth. W/Polymyxin B Sulfate:
Oxytetracycline HC1 5 mg.w/Polymyxin B sulfate 1
mg./Gm. Tube 1/8 oz.
Oint., Topical: Oxytetracycline HCl 30 mg.
w/Polymyxin B Sulfate 10,000 u./Gm. Tube ½ oz.,
1 oz. 12s.
Powd. Topical: Oxytetracycline HCl 30 mg.
w/Polymyxin B Sulfate 1 mg./Gm. Bot. 1 oz.
Syrup: Calcium oxytetracycline (125 mg./5 cc.)
Bot. 2 oz., pt.
Tab., Oral: Oxytetracycline HCl 250 mg./Tab. Bot.
100s.
Tab., Vaginal: Oxytetracycline HCl 100 mg.
w/Polymyxin B sulfate 100,000 units/Tab., starch,
sod. carboxymethylcellulose, lactose, Mg stearate,
methyl-paraben 0.3%, propylparaben 0.07%. Box
10s.
W/Hydrocortisone.
See: Terra-Cortril (Pfipharmecs)
TERRASTATIN. (Pfipharmecs) Oxytetracycline 250
mg., nystatin 250,000 units/Cap Bot. 50s
Use: Antibiotic, antifungal.
TERRASYL. (Zenith) Chlorpheniramine maleate
2 mg., aspirin 324 mg., caffeine/Tab. Bot. 100s.
TERSAVID. N¹-pivaloyl-N²-benzyl-hydrazine.
Use: Monoamine oxidase inhibitor.
TERTIARY AMYL ALCOHOL.
See: Amylene Hydrate. (Various Mfr.)

4'-TERT-BUTOXYACETANILIDE.
See: Tromal (Burroughs Wellcome)
6-TERT-BUTYL-3-(2-IMIDAZOLIN-2-YLMETHYL)-2,4-
DIMETHYL-PHENOL   MONO-HYDROCHLORIDE.
Oxymetazoline Hydrochloride, U.S.P. XXI.
TERTROXIN SODIUM DERIVATIVE. Liothyronine,
B.A.N.
TESAMONE. (Dunhall) Testosterone aqueous
suspension.
'25' (25 mg./ml.) Amp. 10 ml.
'50' (50 mg./ml.) Amp. 10 ml.
'100' (100 mg./ml.) Amp. 10 ml.
Use: Androgen therapy.
• **TESICAM.** USAN. 4'-Chloro-1,2,3,4-tetrahydro-1,3-
dioxo-4-isoquinolinecarboxanilide.
Use: Anti-inflammatory.
• **TESIMIDE.** USAN.
Use: Anti-inflammatory.
TESLAC. (Squibb) Testolactone 50 mg./Tab. Bot.
100s.
Use: Antineoplastic agent.
TESOGEN. (Sig) Testosterone 25 mg., estrone 2
mg./ml. Vial 10 ml.
Use: Hormone therapy.
TESOGEN L.A.. (Sig) Testosterone enanthate 180
mg., 90 mg., 50 mg., estradiol valerate 8 mg., 4
mg. and 2 mg. respectively/ml. Vial 10 ml.
Use: Androgen therapy.
TESONE. (Sig) Testosterone 25 mg., 50 mg., 100
mg./ml. Vial 10 ml.
Use: Androgen hormonal therapy.
TESONE L.A. (Sig) Testosterone enanthate 200
mg./ml. Vial 10 ml.
Use: Hormonal therapy.
TESSALON. (Du Pont) Benzonatate 100 mg./Perle
Bot. 100s.
Use: Antitussive.
TESTA-C INJECTABLE. (Vortech) Testosterone cy-
pionate 200 mg., benzyl alcohol 0.9%, benzyl ben-
zoate 20%, cottonseed oil/cc. Vial 10 cc.
Use: Androgen therapy.
TESTADIATE-DEPO. (Kay) Testosterone cypionate 50
mg., estradiol cypionate 2 mg., chlorobutanol 0.5%
in cottonseed oil/cc. Vial 10 cc.
Use: Hormone therapy.
TESTANATE No. 1. (Kenyon) Testosterone
enanthate 100 mg., lipophilic soln. 200 mg./cc. Vial
10 cc.
TESTANATE No. 2. (Kenyon) Testosterone
enanthate 90 mg., estradiol valerate 4 mg./cc. Vial
10 cc.
TESTANATE No. 3. (Kenyon) Testosterone
enanthate 180 mg., estradiol valerate 8 mg./cc.
Vial 10 cc.
TES-TAPE. (Lilly) Diagnostic test for glucose in urine.
Glucose oxidase, glucose peroxidase, orthotolidine.
Single Pkg. 100 tests.
Use: Diagnostic agent.
TESTAQUA. (Kay) Testosterone 25 mg., 50 mg., or
100 mg./cc. Vial 10 cc.
Use: Male hormone therapy.

TESTARR GRANULES, FLAKES, PLAIN &
FORTIFIED. (Fellows) Plantago seed mucilage.
Also available w/thiamine. Pkg. 180 Gm., 390 Gm.
Use: Laxative.
TESTATE. (Savage) Testosterone enanthate 100
mg./cc. Vial 10 cc.
Use: Androgen therapy.
TESTAVOL-S. (Fellows) Vitamin A palmitate. 50,000
u./Cap. Bot. 100s, 1000s.
Use: Vitamin A deficiencies.
TEST-ESTRIN. (Marlyn) **Injection** (aqueous) Multiple
dose vial 10 cc. 1s, 6s, 25s, 100s.
TESTEX. (Pasadena Research) Testosterone
propionate in sesame oil 25 mg., 50 mg., 100
mg./cc. Vial 10 cc.
TESIONATE 100. (Seatrace) Testosterone cypionate
100 mg./ml. Vial 10 cc.
TESIONATE 200. (Seatrace) Testosterone 200
mg./ml. Vial 10 cc.
TEST-IONATE 200. (Tunex) Testosterone cypionate
200 mg./ml. w/benzyl benzoate 20%, benzyl
alcohol 0.9%, cottonseed oil. Vial 10cc.
Use: Androgen therapy.
TESTOJECT. (Mayrand) Testosterone cypionate 100
mg./ml. Vial 10 cc.
Use: Androgenic hormone
TESTOJECT-50. (Mayrand) Testosterone 50 mg./ml.
Vial 10 ml.
Use: Androgenic hormone.
TESTOJECT E.P. (Mayrand) Testosterone enanthate
200 mg., testosterone propianate 25 mg./ml. Vial 1
ml.
Use: Replacement therapy for male hypogonadism.
TESTOJECT LA. (Mayrand) Testosterone cypionate
100 mg./ml. in oil. Vial 10 ml.
Use: Longacting androgenic hormone.
• **TESTOLACTONE,** U.S.P. Sterile Suspension,
Tab., U.S.P. XXI. 13-Hydroxy-3-oxo-13, 17-secoan-
drosta-1,4-dien-17oic acid-8-lactone.
Use: Antineoplastic agent.
See: Teslac, Vial, Tab. (Squibb)
TESTOLIN. (Pasadena Research) Testosterone
suspension 25 mg., 50 mg., 100 mg./cc. Vial 10 cc.
25 mg./cc. Vial 30 cc.
TESTONE L. A. (Vortech) Testosterone enanthate
100 mg., 200 mg., benzyl alcohol 2%/ml. Vial. 10
ml.
Use: Androgen therapy (long acting).
TESTONEX 50. (Tunex) Testosterone 50 mg./ml. Vial
10 cc.
Use: Androgen therapy.
TESTONEX 100. (Tunex) Testosterone 100 mg./ml.
Vial 10 cc.
Use: Androgen therapy.
• **TESTOSTERONE,** U.S.P. XXI. Pellets, Sterile Susp.,
U.S.P. XXI. 17 β-Hydroxyandrost-4-en-3-one.
Use: Androgen.
See: Android-T, Vial (Brown)
Androlan, Vial (Lannett)
Andronaq, Aq. Susp., Vial (Central)
Depotest, Vial (Hyrex)
Dura-Testrone, Vial (Pharmex)

Homogene-S, Inj., Vial (Spanner)
Malotrone Aqueous Injection (Bluco)
Nendron, Inj. (Noyes)
Neo-Hombreol-F, Aq. Susp., Vial (Organon)
Tesone, Inj. (Sig)
Testaqua, Aq. Susp., Vial (Kay)
Testolin, Vial (Pasadena Research)
Testonex 50, Inj. (Tunex)
Textonex 100, Inj. (Tunex)
Testrone, Vial (Pharmex)

TESTOSTERONE W/COMBINATIONS
See: Andesterone, Vial (Lincoln)
Android-G Vial (Brown)
Androne, Vial (Rocky Mtn.)
Anestrol, Inj. (Mallard)
Angen, Vial (Davis & Sly)
Depo-Testadiol, Vial (Upjohn)
Di-Genik, Vial (Savage)
Di-Hormone, Susp. (Paddock)
Di-Steroid, Vial (Kremers-Urban)
Duogen, Inj. (Vortech)
Duogen, Vial (Bel-Mar)
Estrone-Testosterone, Vial (Maurry)
Estrovag-Femogen, Supp. (Fellows-Testagar)
Geramine, Tab., Inj. (Brown)
Geratic Forte, Inj. (Keene Pharm.)
Geriamic, Tab. (Vortech)
Gerihorm, Inj. (Burgin-Arden)
Glutest, Vial (Brown)
Halodrin, Tab. (Upjohn)
Hormo-Triad, Vial (Bell)
Hormox Plus, Tab. (Parmed)
Mal-O-Fem, Aq. Susp., Vial (Fellows)
Terogen, Vial (Pasadena Research)
Tesogen, Inj. (Sig)
Testrolix, Inj. (Vortech)
Testrone, Vial (Pharmex)
Tostestro, Vial (Bowman)
Vi-Testrogen, Vial (Pharmex)

TESTOSTERONE CYCLOPENTANE PROPIONATE.
Testosterone Cypionate, U.S.P. XXI.
• **TESTOSTERONE CYPIONATE,** U.S.P. XXI. Inj.,
U.S.P. XXI. 17-β-Hydroxyandrost-4-en-3-one cyclopentanepropionate. Androst-4-en-3-one, 17-(3-cyclopentyl-1-oxopropoxy)-, (17β-Testosterone cyclopentanepropionate.
Use: Androgen.
See: Andro-Cyp 100, Inj. (Keene)
Andro-Cyp 200, Inj. (Keene)
Androgen-860, Inj. (Blue Line)
Depo-Testosterone, Inj. (Upjohn)
Dep-Test, Inj. (Sig)
Depotest, Vial (Hyrex)
D-Test 100, 200, Inj. (Burgin-Arden)
Durandro, Inj. (Ascher)
Testa-C, Inj. (Vortech)
Testra-C, Inj. (Amfre-Grant)
Test-Ionate 200, Inj. (Tunex)
Testromed-P.A., Vial (Medics)
Testoject, Vial (Mayrand)
T-Ionate-P.A., Vial (Reid-Provident)
W/Combinations.
See: D-Diol, Inj. (Burgin-Arden)

Depotestogen, Vial (Hyrex)
Depo-Testadiol, Sol. (Upjohn)
Dep-Testradiol, Inj. (Rocky Mtn.)
Duo-Cyp (Keene)
Duo-Ionate, Inj. (Tunex)
Duracrine, Inj. (Ascher)
Esangen, Sol. (Blue Line)
Estran-C, Inj. (Amfre-Grant)
Menoject-L.A. Vial (Kay)
Span F. M., Inj. (Scrip)
Spenduo, Inj. (Spencer-Mead)
Testa-C, Inj. (Vortech)
T.E. Ionate P.A., Inj. (Reid-Provident)
Testadiate-Depo, Vial (Kay)

• **TESTOSTERONE ENANTHATE,** U.S.P. XXI. Inj.,
U.S.P. XXI. Androst-4-en-3-one, 17-(1-oxoheptyl)-oxy-(17β)-. Testosterone heptanoate. 17β-Hydroxyandrost-4-en-3-one heptanoate.
Use: Androgen.
See: Andryl, Inj. (Keene)
Arderone 100, 200, Inj. (Burgin-Arden)
Delatest, Inj. (Dunhall)
Delatestryl, Inj. Vial (Squibb)
Dura-Testosterone, Vial (Pharmex)
Everone 200 Mg., Vial (Hyrex)
Repo-Testro Med., Vial (Medics)
Retandros-200, Inj. (Rocky Mtn.)
Span-Test 100 & 200. (Scrip)
Tesone L. A., Inj. (Sig)
Testate, Inj. (Savage)
Testra-E, Inj. (Amfre-Grant)
Testrin-P.A., Inj. (Pasadena Research)
Testone L. A. in Oil, Inj. (Vortech)
W/Chlorobutanol.
See: Anthatest, Vial (Kay)
W/Estradiol valerate.
See: Ardiol 90/4, 180/8, Inj. (Burgin-Arden)
Bi-Nate, Inj. (Tunex)
Deladumone, Vial (Squibb)
Delatestadiol, Vial (Dunhall)
Ditate, Ditate DS, Vial (Savage)
Duoval-P.A., Inj. (Reid-Provident)
Estran-E.V., Inj., (Amfre-Grant)
Repo-Duo Med., Vial (Medics)
Repose-TE. (Paddock)
Retadiamone, Vial (Rocky Mtn.)
Span-Est-Test 4, Inj. (Scrip)
Teev, Preps. (Keene)
Testanate No. 2 & 3, Vial (Kenyon)
Valertest, Amp., Vial (Hyrex)

TESTOSTERONE HEPTANOATE.
Use: Androgen.
See: Testosterone enanthate.

• **TESTOSTERONE KETOLAURATE.** USAN.
Testosterone 3-oxododecanoate.
Use: Androgen.

• **TESTOSTERONE PHENYLACETATE.** USAN.
Perandren phenylacetate.
Use: Androgen.

• **TESTOSTERONE PROPIONATE,** U.S.P. XXI. Tab., Inj.,
U.S.P. XXI. Androst-4-en-3-one, 17-(1-oxopropoxy)-, (17β)-. 17β-Hydroxyandrost-4-en-3-one propionate.
Use: Androgen.

See:Androlan, Vial (Lannett)
  Androlin, Vial (Lincoln)
  Malotrone-P Injection (Bluco)
  Neo-Hombreol, Vial (Organon)
  Testex, Vial (Pasadena Research)
W/Estrone.

TESTOSTROVAL-P.A. (Reid-Provident) Testosterone enanthate 200 mg./cc. In oil. Vial 5 cc. 1s, 6s, 12s.

TESTRA-C. (Amfre-Grant) Testosterone cypionate 100 mg./ml. Vial 10 ml.
  Use: Hormone.

TESTRA-E. (Amfre-Grant) Testosterone enanthate 100 mg./ml. Vial 10 ml.
  Use: Hormone.

TESTRAMONE. (Harvey) Testosterone 12.5 mg., Vit. B-1 10 mg., B-2 2 mg., B-6 5 mg., niacinamide 40 mg., inositol 50 mg., choline chloride 10 mg., methionine 10 mg./cc. Vial 10 ml.
  Use: Androgen therapy with Vitamin B complex.

TESTRIN-P.A. (Pasadena Research) Testosterone enanthate 200 mg., benzyl alcohol 2%/cc. Vial 10 cc.

TESTRED. (ICN) Methyltestosterone 10 mg./Cap. Bot. 100s.
  Use: Androgen therapy.

TESTRONE. (Pharmex) Testosterone 25 mg., estrone 2 mg./cc. Vial 10 cc.
  Use: I.M.; androgen therapy.

TESTRONE L.A. IN OIL. (Vortech) Testosterone enanthate 100 mg., 200 mg., benzyl alcohol 2%/cc. Vial 10 cc.

TESTURIA. (Ayerst) Combination kit containing 5 × 20 sterile dip strips and 5 × 20 culture trays of trypticase soy agar.
  Use: Diagnostic aid.

TESULOID. (Squibb) Technetium Tc 99m sulfur colloid 5 vials/kit.
  Use: Radiodiagnostic.

• **TETANUS ANTITOXIN,** U.S.P. XXI. (Wyeth)—Vial 1500, 3,000, 20,000 & 40,000 u. Tubex Sterile Cartridge Needle Unit 1500, 3000, 5000 u./t.
  Use: Passive immunizing agent.
  See: Homo-Tet, Vial, Syringe (Savage)

TETANUS AND DIPHTHERIA TOXOIDS ADSORBED FOR ADULT USE, U.S.P. XXI.
  Use: Active immunizing agent for persons over 7 yrs. old.
  Generic Products:
  (Squibb-Connaught) Vial 5 ml. for I.M. use.
  (Lederle) Vial 5 ml.

TETANUS-DIPHTHERIA TOXOIDS ADSORBED, ALUMINUM PHOSPHATE ADSORBED. (Wyeth) Vial 5 cc. Tubex 0.5 cc.
  Use: I.M., Primary immunization or maintenance in persons over 10 years old.

TETANUS AND DIPHTHERIA TOXOIDS COMBINED PUROGENATED. (Lederle) Lederject disposable syringe 10 × 0.5 ml. Vial 5 ml. New package.

• **TETANUS IMMUNE GLOBULIN,** U.S.P. XXI. (Hyland) Gamma globulin fraction of the plasma of persons who have been hyperimmunized with tetanus toxoid, 16.5%. Vial 250 u.
  Use: Prophylaxis of injured, against tetanus passive immunizing agent.

See: Gamulin-T, Vial (Merrell Dow)
  Homo-Tet Vial, 1 cc. (Savage)
Hu-Tet, Vial (Hyland)
  Hyper-Tet Injection Vial, 250 u. (Cutter)
  Immu-Tetanus, Vial, Disp. Syr. (Parke-Davis)
  T-I-Gammagee, Disp. Syr. (Merck Sharp & Dohme)

TETANUS IMMUNE GLOBULIN, HUMAN, (Wyeth) 250 u./Tubex, 1 cc. Dissolved in glycine 0.3 M; contains thimerosal 0.01%.
  See: Ar-Tet, Syringe, Vial (Armour)

• **TETANUS TOXOID,** U.S.P. XXI. (Squibb-Connaught)—Vial 7.5 ml. for I.M. or S.C. use. (Lederle)—Vial 0.5 cc., 5 cc. (Wyeth)—Vial 7.5 cc. Tubex 0.5 cc.
  Use: Active immunizing agent against tetanus.

• **TETANUS TOXOID, ADSORBED,** U.S.P. XXI. (Serums and Vaccines of America) 20 Lf purified tetanus toxoid, 0.01% thimerosal as preservative/ml. Box 2 ampuls of 0.5 ml. Vial 5 ml., 7.5 ml., 0.5 ml. Amp. for booster injection. (Squibb-Connaught) Vial 5 ml. for I.M. use (Lederle)—Vial 5 ml. Steri-Dose syringe 0.5 ml. 10s. (Wyeth)—Vial 5 cc. Tubex 0.5 cc.
  Use: Active immunizing agent against tetanus.

TETANUS TOXOID ADSORBED PUROGENATED. (Lederle) Vial 5 cc. Disp. syringe 0.5 cc.
  Use: Active immunizing agent.

• **TETANUS TOXOID, ALUMINUM PHOSPHATE ADSORBED.**
  Use: Active immunizing agent.
  See: (Lederle) Vial 5 cc. 10s. Lederject Disp. Syr. 10 × 0.5 cc.
  (Wyeth) Vial 5 cc. Tubex 0.5 cc.

TETANUS TOXOID, ALUM PRECIPITATED.
  Use: Active immunizing agent.
  See: (Cutter)—Vial 5 cc.
  (Lilly)—Vial 1 & 5 cc. Hyporets 0.5 cc. 10s, 100s.
  (Merck Sharp & Dohme)—Vial 5 cc.

TETANUS TOXOID, FLUID. (Lederle)—Vial 7.5 cc., 0.5 cc. 10s, 100s.
  Use: Active immunizing agent.

TETANUS TOXOID FLUID PUROGENATED. (Lederle) Lederject Disposable syringe 10 × 0.5 ml. Vial 7.5 ml.

TETANUS TOXOID PURIFIED, FLUID. (Wyeth)—Vial 7.5 cc., Tubex 0.5 cc.
  Use: Active immunizing agent.

TET-CY. (Metro Med) Tetracycline HCl 250 mg./Cap. Bot. 100s, 1000s.
  Use: Antibiotic.

TETIOTHALEIN SODIUM.
  See: Iodophthalein Sodium. (Var. Mfr.)

TETNOR. Phenylbutazone, B.A.N.

TETRABEAD-125. (Abbott) T-4 diagnostic kit 100s, 500s.
  Use: Quantitative measurement of total circulating serum thyroxine.

TETRA-C. (Century) Tetracycline HCl 250 mg./Cap. Bot. 100s, 1000s.
  Use: Antibiotic.

TETRABENAZINE. B.A.N. 1,3,4,6,7,11b-Hexahydro-3-isobutyl-9, 10-dimethoxybenzo[a] quinolizin-2-one.
  Use: Tranquilizer.

See: Nitoman

**4,5,6,7-TETRABROMO-3',3"-DISULFOPHENOLPHTH-
ALEIN DISODIUM SALT.** Sulfobromophthalein Sodium, U.S.P. XXI.

• **TETRACAINE,** U.S.P. XXI. Oint., Ophth. Oint.,
U.S.P. XXI. 2-Dimethylaminoethyl p-butyl-aminoben-
zoate.
Use: Local anesthetic.

• **TETRACAINE AND MENTHOL OINTMENT,** U.S.P.
XXI.
Use: Local anesthetic.

• **TETRACAINE HYDROCHLORIDE,** U.S.P. XXI.
Cream, Inj., Ophth. Soln., Topical Soln., Sterile,
U.S.P. XXI. 2-(Dimethyl-amino)-ethyl p-(butylamino)-
benzoate HCl. Benzoic acid, 4-(butylamino)-, 2-(dime-
thylamino)ethyl ester, monohydrochloride.
Use: Local anesthetic, topical anesthetic, spinal
anesthetic.
See: Bristacycline, Cap. (Bristol)
    Pontocaine Hydrochloride Prods. (Winthrop-Breon)
W/Benzocaine, butyl aminobenzoate.
See: Cetacaine, Liq., Oint., Spray (Cetylite)
W/Hexachlorophene, dimethyl polysiloxane, methyl
salicylate, pyrilamine maleate, zinc oxide.
W/Isocaine, benzalkonium Cl.
See: Isotraine Oint. (Philips Roxane)

TETRACAINE HYDROCHLORIDE 0.5%.
(Alcon) 0.5%/1 cc. Drop-Tainer, Ophth. 15 cc. Steri-
Unit, 2 cc. (Cooper Vision) Dropperettes 1 ml. in 10s.

TETRACAP 250. (Circle) Tetracycline hydrochloride
250 mg./Cap. Bot. 100s.
Use: Antibiotic.

TETRACHEL. (Rachelle) Tetracycline HCl 250
mg./Cap. Bot. 1000s. Tetracycline HCl 500
mg./Cap. Bot. 250s.
Use: Antibiotic.

• **TETRACHLORETHYLENE,** U.S.P. XXI. Cap., U.S.P.
XXI. Perchlorethylene, tetrachlorethylene.
Use: Anthelmintic (hookworms and some
trematodes).

**4,5,6,7-TETRACHLORO-2',4',5',7'-TETRAIODOFLUO-
RESCEIN DISODIUM SALT.** Rose Bengal Sodium I-
131 Injection, U.S.P. XXI.

TETRACLOR. (Kenyon) Tetracycline HCl 250
mg./Cap. Bot. 100s, 1000s.

TETRACLOR-L. (Kenyon) Tetracycline HCl 125 mg./5
cc. Bot. pt.

TETRA-CO. (Coastal) Tetracycline HCl 250 mg./Tab.
Bot. 100s, 1000s. Syr. Bot. pt.

TETRA-CO 500 BID. (Coastal) Tetracycline 500
mg./Cap. Bot. 100s, 1000s.

TETRACON. (Professional Pharmacal)
Tetrahydrozoline HCl 0.5 mg., disodium edetate 1.0
mg., boric acid 12 mg., benzalkonium Cl. 0.1 mg.,
sodium Cl. 2.2 mg., sodium borate 0.5 mg./ml.
w/water. Bot. 15 ml.
Use: Minor eye irritation.

TETRACOSACTIDE. (I.N.N.). Tetracosactrin, B.A.N.

TETRACOSACTRIN. B.A.N. β^{1-24}-Corticotrophin.
Use: Corticotrophic peptide.
See: Cortrosyn
    Cosyntropin

Synacthen
    Tetracosactide (I.N.N.)

• **TETRACYCLINE,** U.S.P. XXI. Oral Susp., U.S.P.
XXI. 4-(Dimethylamino)-1,4,4a,
5,5a,6,11,12a-octahydro-3,-6,10,12,12a-penta hy-
droxy-6-methyl-1,11-dioxo-2-naphthacenecarboxami-
de.
Use: Antibiotic.
See: Robitet, Syr. (Robins)
    Sumycin, Syrup (Squibb)
W/N-acetyl-para-amino-phenol, phenyltoloxamine ci-
trate.
Use: Antibacterial; antiamebic; antirickettsial.
See: Paltet, Cap. (Hauck)
    Tetrex, Bid Cap., Cap., Vial (Bristol)

• **TETRACYCLINE AND AMPHOTERICIN B,** U.S.P.
XXI. Cap., Oral Susp., U.S.P. XXI.

• **TETRACYCLINE HYDROCHLORIDE,** U.S.P. XXI.
Cap., Inj., Oint., Ophth Oint., Topical Soln., Ophth.
Susp., Sterile, Tab., U.S.P. XXI.
Use: Antibiotic.
See: Achromycin, Preps. (Lederle)
    Amer-Tet, Tab. (Robinson)
    Amer-Tet Suspension (Robinson)
    Anacel, Sol. (Softcon)
    Bicycline, Caps. (Knight)
    Centet 250, Tab. (Central)
    Cyclopar, Cap. (Parke-Davis)
    Desamycin, Cap. (Pharmics)
    Fed-Mycin, Cap. (Amfre-Grant)
    G-Mycin, Cap. & Syr. (Coast)
    Maso-Cycline, Cap. (Mason)
    Nor-Tet, Cap. (Vortech)
    Partrex, Cap. (Parmed)
    Retet, Cap. (Reid-Provident)
    Robitet, Cap. (Robins)
    Sarocycline, Cap., Inj., Syr. (Saron)
    Scotrex, Caps. (Scott/Cord)
    SK-Tetracycline, Cap., Syr. (SmithKline)
    Sumycin, Cap., Tab., Syr. (Squibb)
    Tet-Cy, Cap. (Metro)
    Tetracap 250, Cap. (Circle)
    Tetra-C, Cap. (Century)
    Tetrachel, Cap. (Rachelle)
    Tetrachor, Tetrachor-L, Cap. Liq. (Kenyon)
    Tetra-Co, Cap. (Coastal)
    Tetracycline HCl, Cap.
    Tetracycline HCl, Preps.
    Tetracyn, Cap., Inj., (Pfipharmecs)
    Tetralan "250", "500", Cap. (Lannett)
    Tetram and Tetram-S, Cap., Syr. (Dunhall)
    Tetramax, Cap. (Rand)
    Topicycline, Liq. (Proctor & Gamble)
    Trexin, Cap. (A.V.P. Pharm.)
W/Citric Acid.
See: Achromycin V, Cap., Drop, Susp., Syr.
    (Lederle)
W/Nystatin.
See: Comycin, Cap. (Upjohn)
    Tetrastatin, Cap. (Pfipharmecs)
W/Sulfamethizole, phenazopyridine HCl.
See: Azotrex, Cap. (Bristol)

• **TETRACYCLINE HYDROCHLORIDE AND
NYSTATIN CAPSULES,** U.S.P. XXI.
Use: Antibiotic, antifungal.
See: Comycin, Cap. (Upjohn) Tetrastatin, Cap.
(Pfipharmecs)
• **TETRACYCLINE ORAL SUSPENSION,** U.S.P. XXI.
Use: Antibiotic.
See: Brand names under Tetracycline.
• **TETRACYCLINE PHOSPHATE COMPLEX,** U.S.P.
XXI. Cap., Inj., Sterile, U.S.P. XXI. A sparingly
soluble complex of sodium metaphosphate and
tetracycline.
Use: Antibiotic.
See: Bristrex
   Tetrex, Cap., Vial (Bristol)
   Tetrex-S, Ped. Drops, Syr. (Bristol)
W/Amphotericin B.
See: Mysteclin F, Cap., Drops & Syr. (Squibb)
TETRACYN. (Pfipharmecs) Tetracycline HCl. 250 mg.
Cap. Bot. 100s, 1000s. 500 mg. Bot. 100s.
Use: Antibiotic.
TETRACYN I.M. (Pfipharmecs) Tetracycline HCl 100
mg./Vial 1 cc., 5s.
TETRAETHYLAMMONIUM BROMIDE (TEAB).
Use: Diagnostic & therapeutic agent in peripheral
vascular disorders. Diagnostic in hypertension.
TETRAETHYLAMMONIUM CHLORIDE.
Use: Ganglionic blocking agent.
TETRAETHYLTHIURAM DISULFIDE.
See: Disulfiram
• **TETRAFILCON A.** USAN.
Use: Contact lens material.
TETRAGEN. Tetracycline, B.A.N.
**2-(1,2,3,4-TETRAHYDRO-1-NAPHTHYL)-2-IMIDAZOL-
INE MONOHYDROCHLORIDE.** Tetrahydrozoline Hy-
drochloride, U.S.P. XXI.
TETRAHYDROPHENOBARBITAL CALCIUM.
See: Cyclobarbital Calcium, Prep.
TETRAHYDROXYQUINONE. Name used for
Tetroquinone.
TETRAHYDROZOLINE. B.A.N. 2-(1,2,3,4-Tetrahydro-
1-naphthyl)-2-imidazoline.
Use: Vasoconstrictor.
See: Tetryzoline (I.N.N.)
   Tyzanol hydrochloride.
• **TETRAHYDROZOLINE HYDROCHLORIDE,** U.S.P.
XXI. Nasal Sol., Ophth. Sol. U.S.P. XXI. 2-(1,2,3,4-
Tetrahydro-1-naphthyl)-2-imidazoline HCl.
Use: Adrenergic.
See: Murine Plus (Abbott)
Tyzine, Sol. (Key)
Visine, Sol. (Leeming)
**2′,4′,5′,7′-TETRAIODOFLUORESCEIN DISODIUM
SALT MONOHYDRATE.** Erythrosine Sodium, U.S.P.
XXI.
TETRAIODOPHENOLPHTHALEIN SODIUM.
See: Iodophthalein Sodium.
TETRAIODOPHTHALEIN SODIUM.
See: Iodophthalein Sodium.
1-3,5,3′,5′-TETRAIODOTHYRONINE SODIUM. Levo-
thyroxine Sodium U.S.P. XXI.

TETRALAN "250". (Lannett) Tetracycline HCl 250
mg./Cap. Bot. 100s, 1000s.
TETRALAN "500". (Lannett) Tetracycline HCl 500
mg./Cap. Bot. 100s, 1000s.
TETRALYSAL. Lymecycline, B.A.N.
TETRAM. (Dunhall) Tetracycline 250 mg./Cap. Bot.
100s.
Use: Antibiotic.
TETRAMAX. (Rand) Tetracycline HCl 250 mg./Cap.
Bot. 100s, 1000s.
Use: Antibacterial & antirickettsial.
TETRAMETHYLENE DIMETHANESULFONATE.
See: Busulfan, U.S.P. XXI.
**1,2,2,6-TETRAMETHYL-4-PIPERIDYL MANDELATE
HYDROCHLORIDE.** Eucatropine Hydrochloride,
U.S.P. XXI.
TETRAMETHYLTHIURAM DISULFIDE. Thiram.
Use: Antibacterial & antifungal agent.
See: Rezifilm, Aerosol (Squibb)
TETRAMISOLE. B.A.N. (±)-2,3,5,6-Tetrahydro-6-
phenylimidazo[2,1-b]thiazole.
Use: Anthelmintic, veterinary medicine.
See: Nilverm hydrochloride.
• **TETRAMISOLE HYDROCHLORIDE.** USAN. ±
2,3,5,6-Tetrahydro-6-phenylimidazo   [2,1-b]-thiazole
HCl.
Use: Anthelmintic.
See: Ripercol (American Cyanamid)
TETRANEED. (Hanlon) Pentaerythritol tetranitrate 80
mg./Time Cap. Bot. 100s.
TETRANTOIN. 7,8-Benzo-1,3-diazaspiro(4,5)-decane-
2,4-dione. 3′,4′-Dihydrospiro-[imidazolidine-4,2′(1′H)-
naphthalene]-2,5-dione.
Use: Anticonvulsant.
TETRATAB. (Freeport) Pentaerythritol tetranitrate 10
mg./Tab. Bot. 1000s.
Use: Management, prophylaxis and treatment of
angina attacks.
TETRATAB NO. 1. (Freeport) Pentaerythritol
tetranitrate 20 mg./Tab. Bot. 1000s.
Use: Management, prophylaxis, & treatment of
angina attacks.
TETRATAB NO. 2. (Freeport) Pentaerythritol
tetranitrate 10 mg., phenobarbital ¼ gr./Tab. Bot.
1000s.
Use: Prophylactic treatment of angina.
TETRATE. (Pasadena Research) Pentaerythritol
tetranitrate 30, or 80 mg./Cap. Bot. 100s, 1000s.
Use: Coronary vasodilator.
TETRAZYME. (Abbott) Test kit 100s, 500s.
Use: Enzyme immunoassay for quantitative
measurement of total circulating serum thyroxine
(free and protein bound).
TE TREE OIL. (Metabolic Prod.) Australian oil of
Melaleuca alternifolia 100% pure. Bot. 1, 4, 8, 16
oz. **Cream** Bot. 8 oz. **Oint.** Tube 1 oz., 3 oz.
Use: Antiseptic, fungistatic.
TETREX. (Bristol) Tetracycline phosphate complex
equivalent to 250 mg. tetracycline HCl/Cap. Bot.
100s.
W/Sulfamethizole and phenylazo-diaminopyridine HCl.
See: Azotrex, Cap. (Bristol)

TETREX bid CAPS. (Bristol) Tetracycline phosphate complex equivalent to 500 mg., tetracycline HCl/Cap. Bot. 50s, 100s.
TETREX PMT NITRATE. Rolitetracycline, B.A.N.
• **TETROQUINONE.** USAN. Tetrahydroxy-p-benzoquinone.
Use: Treat keloids, keratolytic.
See: Kelox (Elder)
• **TETRYDAMINE.** USAN. 4,5,6,7-Tetrahydro-2-methyl-3-(methylamino)-tetrahydroindazole.
Use: Analgesic, anti-inflammatory.
TETRYZOLINE (I.N.N.). Tetrahydrozoline, B.A.N.
TETTERINE. (Shuptrine) **Oint.:** Antifungal agents in green petrolatum base. Tin 1 oz., Tube 1 oz. **Pow.:** Fungicide, germicide formula powder for heat and diaper rash. Can 2.5 oz. **Soap:** Bar 3¼ oz.
Use: Treatment ringworm, athlete's foot, diaper rash and other skin conditions.
TEXACORT SCALP LOTION. (CooperCare) Hydrocortisone alcohol 1%, benzalkonium chloride, alcohol 33%, propylene glycol, polysorbate 20, purified water. Dropper Bot. 1 fl. oz.
Use: Corticosteroid.
T-FLUORIDE. (Tennessee) Sodium fluoride 2.21 mg./Tab. Bot. 100s, 1000s.
Use: Dental caries and prophylactic.
T-GESIC CAPSULE. (Tennessee) Acetyl para-amino phenol 200 mg., phenacetin 2½ gr., hyoscyamine sulfate 0.031 mg., pentobarbital ¼ gr./Cap. Bot. 100s.
Use: Analgesic.
THALFED. (Beecham Labs) Theophylline, hydrous 0.12 Gm., ephedrine HCl 25 mg., phenobarbital 8 mg./Tab. Tab. Bot. 100s.
Use: Asthma.
• **THALIDOMIDE.** USAN. a-(N-Phthalimido)glutarimide. 2-Phthalimidoglutarimide.
Use: Hypnotic, sedative.
See: Kevadon (Merrell-National)
THALITONE. (Boehringer Ingelheim) Chlorthalidone 25 mg./Tab. Bot. 100s.
Use: Diuretic.
THALLIUM 201. (Squibb) Thallous chloride Tl 201. 2.2, 6.6 nmCi/vial.
Use: Radiodiagnostic.
• **THALLOUS CHLORIDE TL-201 INJECTION,** U.S.P. XXI.
Use: Diagnostic aid (radioactive agent).
THAM SOLUTION. (Abbott) Tromethamine 18 Gm., acetic acid 2.5 Gm., in water for inj. Single-dose container.
Use: For prevention and correction of severe systemic acidosis.
THAM-E. (Abbott) Tromethamine 36 Gm., sodium Cl. 1.75 Gm., potassium Cl. 0.37 Gm./150 ml. powder. Vial for reconstitution.
Use: Systemic acidosis in life-threatening situations.
THANTIS LOZENGES. (Hynson, Westcott & Dunning) Merodicein ⅛ gr., saligenin 1 gr./Loz. Display carton 12 × 12s.
Use: Antiseptic, anesthetic lozenge.
THEAMIN. Monoethanolamine salt of theophylline

See: Monotheamin, Supp. (Lilly)
W/Amobarbital.
See: Monotheamin and Amytal, Pulvule (Lilly)
THEAN. Proxyphylline, B.A.N.
THEBACON. B.A.N. O⁶-Acetyl-O³-methyl-Δ⁶-morphine.
Use: Narcotic analgesic; cough suppressant.
See: Acetyldihydrocodeinone
THEDRAZOL. (Kenyon) Pentylenetetrazol 100 mg., nicotinic acid 50 mg./Tab. Bot. 100s, 1000s.
Use: Hypertension.
THEDRAZOL-L. (Kenyon) Pentylenetetrazol 100 mg., niacin 50 mg./5 cc. Bot. 4 oz., pt., gal.
THEELIN AQUEOUS SUSPENSION. (Parke-Davis) A suspension of estrone in isotonic sodium chloride solution for I.M. adm. **Steri**-Vial: 2 mg. (20,000 I.U.)/ml. Vial 10 ml.
Use: For treating symptoms associated with menopause.
THEELIN INJECTION. (Morton) Estrone suspension 2 mg. or 5 mg./ml. Vial 10 ml. For I.M. administration.
Use: Estrogen.
THEELIN IN OIL. (Morton) Natural estrogenic substance 2 mg./ml. (20,000 I.U./ml.) in oil. Vial 30 cc.
Use: Estrogen.
THEMALON. Diethylthiambutene, B.A.N.
THENALIDINE. B.A.N. 1-Methyl-4-N-(2-thenyl)-anilinopiperidine.
Use: Antihistamine.
See: Sandosten (tartrate)
THENALIDINE TARTRATE. 1-Methyl-4-(N-2-thenylanilino) piperidine tartrate.
Use: Antihistaminic; antipruritic.
THENDELATE. (Blue Line) Methenamine mandelate 0.5 gr./Tab. Bot. 100s, 1000s.
THENFADIL. Thenyldiamine, B.A.N.
• **THENIUM CLOSYLATE.** USAN. N,N-Dimethyl, N2-phenoxy-ethyl-N-2-thenylammonium p-chlorobenzenesulfonate.
Use: Canine hookworm.
See: Bancari (Burroughs Wellcome)
THENYLDIAMINE. B.A.N. 2-(N-2-Pyridyl-N-2-thenyl-amino)ethyldimethylamine.
Use: Antihistamine.
See: Thenfadil (hydrochloride)
THENYLDIAMINE HYDROCHLORIDE. 2-[(2-Dimethylaminoethyl)-3-thenyl-amino] pyridine HCl, thenyl-dramine chloride. Dethylandiomine.
W/Phenylephrine HCl, isoetharine methanesulfonate, Freon propellant.
See: Bronko-meter, Aerosol (Winthrop-Breon)
Bronkosol, Sol. (Winthrop-Breon)
THENYLPYRAMINE.
See: Methapyrilene Hydrochloride, Preps.
THEO-24. (Searle) Theophylline anhydrous 100 mg., 200 mg., or 300 mg./Controlled- Release Cap. Bot. 100s. Unit Dose 100s.
Use: Bronchodilator, antiasthmatic.
THEOBID. (Glaxo) Theophylline 260 mg./Timed Cap. Bot. 60s, 500s. Unit dose 100s.
Use: Bronchial asthma, chronic obstructive pulmonary disease.

THEOBID JR DURACAP. (Glaxo) Anhydrous theophylline 130 mg./Cap. Sustained release. Bot 60s, 500s.
Use: Bronchial asthma, chronic obstructive disease.

THEOBROMA OIL. Cocoa Butter, N.F. XVI.
Use: Suppository base.

THEOBROMINE WITH PHENOBARBITAL COMBINATIONS.
See: Harbolin, Tab. (Arcum)
Theocardone, Tab. (Lemmon)
T.P. KI, Tab. (Wendt-Bristol)

THEOBROMINE CALCIUM GLUCONATE.
(Bates)—Tab., Bot. 100s, 1000s. Also available w/phenobarbital.
(Grant)—Tab., Bot. 100s, 500s, 1000s.

THEOBROMINE MAGNESIUM OLEATE.
W/Magnesium nicotinate.
See: Athemol-N, Tab. (Glaxo)

THEOBROMINE SODIUM ACETATE. Theobromine calcium salt mixture with calcium salicylate.
Use: Diuretic; smooth muscle relaxant.

THEOBROMINE SODIUM SALICYLATE.
See: Doan's Pills (Purex)
W/Cal. lactate, Phenobarbital.
See: Theolaphen, Tab. (Elder)

THEOBRON SR. (Upsher-Smith) Theophyllin anhydrous 125 mg. or 250 mg./S.R. Cap. Bot. 100s, 1000s. Unit dose 100s.
Use: Bronchodilator.

THEOCALBITAL. (Forrest) Cal. lactate 1 gr., phenobarbital sod. ¼ gr., theobromine 3½ gr./Tab. Bot. 100s.
Use: Diuretic with sedative.

THEOCAP. (Glaxo) Theophylline anhydrous 200 mg./Cap. Bot. 60s, 500s.
Use: Bronchial asthma, obstructive pulmonary disease.

THEOCLEAR 80 SYRUP. (Central) Theophylline 80 mg./15 ml. Bot. Pt., Gal.
Use: Bronchodilator

THEOCLEAR-100 TABLETS. (Central) Theophylline anhydrous 100 mg./Tab. Bot. 100s.
Use: Bronchodilator

THEOCLEAR-200 TABLETS. (Central) Theophylline anhydrous 200 mg./Tab. Bot. 100s.
Use: Bronchodilator

THEOCLEAR L.A.-130 (Central) Theophylline 130 mg./Cenule. Bot. 100s, 1000s.
Use: Bronchodilator

THEOCLEAR L.A.-260 (Central) Theophylline 260 mg./Cenule Bot. 100s, 1000s.
Use: Bronchodilator

THEO-COL. (Columbia) Theophylline 150 mg., guaifenesin 90 mg./ 15 ml. Elix. w/alcohol 15%. Cap. Bot. 100s, 1000s, Elix. Bot. pt., gal.

THEOCOLATE LIQUID. (Bay) Theophylline 150 mg., guaifenesin 90 mg./15 cc. Bot. pt., gal.
Use: Bronchodilator, expectorant for treatment of bronchospasm.

THEOCOMP CAPSULES. (Barry-Martin) Aminophylline 2 gr., ephedrine sulfate ⅜ gr., amobarbital ⅜ gr./Cap. Bot. 1000s.

THEODRENALINE. B.A.N. 7-[2-(3,4,β-Trihydroxy-phenethylamino)ethyl]theophylline.
Use: Analeptic.

THEO-DROX. (Columbia) Ephedrine sulfate 25 mg., theophylline 130 mg., hydroxyzine HCl 10 mg./Tab. Bot. 100s, 500s.
Use: Bronchodilator.

THEO-DUR SPRINKLE (Key) Anhydrous theophylline 50 mg., 75 mg., 125 mg. or 200 mg./Sust. Action Cap. Bot. 100s.
Use: Bronchodilator.

THEO-DUR TABLETS. (Key) Anhydrous theophylline 100 mg., 200 mg., 300 mg./Sust. Action Tab. Bot. 100s, 500s, 1000s, 5000s. Unit dose 100s.
Use: Bronchodilator.

THEOFED. (Sutliff & Case) Phenobarbital 8 mg., theophylline 130 mg., ephedrine HCl 24 mg., atropine sulfate ⅟₃₀₀ gr., pyrilamine maleate 25 mg., magnesium trisilicate 130 mg., guaifenesin 50 mg./Tab. Bot. 100s, 1000s.
Use: Diuretic, antispasmodic, sedative, bronchodilator and antihistamine.

THEOFEDRAL FORMULA. (Wolins) Phenobarbital ⅛ gr., theophylline 2 gr., ephedrine HCl ⅜ gr./Tab. Bot. 100s, 1000s, 5000s.

THEOFENAL. (Cumberland) Theophylline 130 mg., ephedrine HCl 24 mg., phenobarbital 8 mg./ Tab. Bot. 100s.
Use: Symptomatic relief in asthma.

• **THEOFIBRATE.** USAN.
Use: Antihyperlipoproteinemic.

THEOFORT. (Amfre-Grant) Theophylline sod. glycinate 320 mg./15 cc. Bot. pt., gal.
Use: Bronchial dilator.

THEOGEN. (Sig) Conjugated estrogens 2 mg./ml. Vial 10 cc., 30 cc.
Use: Menopausal syndrome.

THEOGEN I.P. (Sig) Estrone 2 mg., potassium estrone sulfate 1 mg./ml. Vial 10 ml.
Use: Estrogen therapy.

THEO-GUAIA. (Sutliff & Case) **Liq.:** Theophylline 50 mg., guaifenesin 35 mg., alcohol 20%/5 cc. Bot. pts., gals.
Use: Asthmatic disorders.

THEOLAIR. (Riker) Anhydrous theophylline 125 mg./Tab. Boxes 250s foil sealed. Bot. 100s.
Use: Relief of bronchospasm.

THEOLAIR 250. (Riker) Theophylline anhydrous 250 mg./Tab. Bot. 100s. Box 250s foil sealed.
Use: Bronchial dilator.

THEOLAIR LIQUID. (Riker) Theophylline anhydrous 80 mg./15 ml. Bot. pt.
Use: Bronchdilator.

THEOLAIR PLUS LIQUID. (Riker) Theophylline 80 mg., guaifenesin /15 ml. Bot. Pt.
Use: Relief of acute bronchial asthma.

THEOLAIR PLUS TABLETS. (Riker) **125:** Theophylline 125 mg., guaifenesin 100 mg./Tab. Bot. 100s. **250:** Theophylline 250 mg., guaifenesin 200 mg./Tab. Bot. 100s.
Use: Relief of acute bronchial asthma.

THEOLAIR-SR 200. (Riker) Theophylline anhydrous 200 mg./Tab. (slow release). Bot. 100s, 250s.
Use: Bronchial dilator.

THEOLAIR-SR 250. (Riker) Theophylline anhydrous 250 mg./Tab. (slow release). Bot. 100s, 250s.
Use: Bronchial dilator.

THEOLAIR-SR 300. (Riker) Theophylline anhydrous 300 mg./Tab. (slow release). Bot. 100s, 250s.
Use: Bronchial dilator.

THEOLAIR-SR 500. (Riker) Theophylline anhydrous 500 mg./Tab. (slow release). Bot. 100s, 250s.
Use: Bronchial dilator.

THEO-LIX. (Freeport) Theophylline 80 mg., alcohol 19-20% per 15 cc. Bot. pt.
Use: Treatment of bronchial asthma, bronchitis, and cardiac dyspnea.

THEO-LIX. (Vale) Theophylline 80 mg.,/15ml. w/alcohol 20%. Bot. pt., gal.
Use: Spasmolytic, bronchodilator.

THEOLIXIR. (Panray) Theophylline 80 mg., alcohol 20%/15 cc. Bot. 4 oz., 8 oz., pt., gal.
Use: Bronchodilator.

THEOLIXIR LIQUID. (Ulmer) Theophylline 80 mg., alcohol 20%. Bot. pt.
Use: Bronchodilator.

THEOMER INJECTION. (Fellows) Sod. mersalyl 100 mg., theophylline 50 mg./cc. Vial 10 cc.

THEON. (Bock) Theophylline 150 mg./15 cc. w/alcohol 10%. Bot. pt., gal
Use: Bronchodilator.

THEON-300. (Bock) Theophylline (anhydrous) 300 mg./Cap. Bot. 100s, 1000s.
Use: Bronchial asthma treatment.

THEO-NAR 100. (Key) Noscapine 15 mg., theophylline 100 mg./Delayed-action Tab. Bot. 100s, 500s.
Use: Bronchial asthma and emphysema.

THEO-NAR 200. (Key) Noscapine 30 mg., theophylline 200 mg./Sustained Action Tab. Bot. 100s, 500s.
Use: Bronchodilator for asthma and emphysema.

THEO-ORGANIDIN. (Wallace) Theophylline anhydrous 120 mg., iodinated glycerol 30 mg./15 cc. w/alcohol 15%. Bot. pt., gal.
Use: Bronchodilator, mucolytic-expectorant combination.

THEOPHYL-225. (McNeil Pharm) Anhydrous theophylline. **Tab.:** 225 mg./Tab. Bot. 100s. **Elixir:** 225 mg./30 ml. Bot. pt.
Use: Bronchodilator.

THEOPHYL CHEWABLE TABLETS. (McNeil Pharm) Anhydrous theophylline 100 mg./Chewable Tab. Bot. 100s.
Use: Bronchodilator.

THEOPHYL-SR. (McNeil Pharm) Anhydrous theophylline 125 mg. or 250 mg./SR Cap. Bot. 100s.
Use: Bronchodilator.

• **THEOPHYLLINE,** Cap., U.S.P. XXI. Tab., U.S.P. XXI. 1,3-Dimethylxanthine. 1H-Purine-2,6-dione,3,-7-dihydro-1,3-dimethyl-, monohydrate.
Use: Coronary vasodilator & diuretic; pharm necessity for Aminophylline Injection.
See: Accurbron, Liq. (Merrell Dow)
Aerolate, Cap., Elix. (Fleming)

Aquaphyllin, Syr. (Ferndale)
Bronkodyl, Cap., Elix. (Winthrop-Breon)
Duraphyl, Tab. (McNeil Pharm)
Elixicon, Susp. (Berlex)
Elixophyllin, Elix., Cap. (Berlex)
Elixophyllin SR, Cap. (Berlex)
Lanophyllin, Elix. (Lannett)
Lodrane, Cap. (Poythress)
Optiphyllin, Elix. (Fougera)
Oralphyllin, Liq. (Consol. Midland)
Quibron-T Dividose, Tab. (Mead Johnson)
Quibron-T/SR Dividose, Tab. (Mead Johnson)
Slo-bid, Caps. (Rorer)
Slo-Phyllin, Cap., Syr., Tab. (Dooner)
Somophyllin, Cap. (Fisons)
Sustaire, Tab. (Roerig)
Theo-II, Elix. (Fleming)
Theobid, Cap. (Glaxo)
Theobid Jr, Cap. (Glaxo)
Theobron, Cap. (Upsher-Smith)
Theocap, Cap. (Glaxo)
Theoclear 80, Liq. (Central)
Theoclear L.A., Cenule (Central)
Theo-Dur, Tab. (Key)
Theolair, Tab., Liq. (Riker)
Theolair SR, Tab. (Riker)
Theolix, Elix. (Vale)
Theolixir, Elix. (Panray)
Theolixir (Ulmer)
Theon, Cap., Elix. (Bock)
Theospan, Cap. (Laser)
Theostat, Prods. (Laser)
Theovent Long-Acting, Cap. (Schering)

THEOPHYLLINE W/COMBINATIONS
See: Airet Y, Tab., Elix. (Baylor)
Anti-Asthma, Tab. (Panray)
Asmabar, Tab. (Blue Line)
Asma-lief, Tab., Susp. (Columbia)
Asma Syrup (Coastal)
Asthmaspan, Cap. (Wolins)
Ayrcap, Cap. (Ascher)
B.A. Prods. (Federal)
Broncholate, Cap., Elix. (Bock)
Bronkaid, Tab. (Brew)
Co-Xan, Liq. (Central)
Elixophyllin-Kl, Elix. (Berlex)
Emphysal Cap. (Douglas)
Eponal, Tab. (Cenci)
Fedrelen, Tab. (Scrip)
Foyuretic, Vial (Foy)
Isophed, Tab. (Jamieson-McKames)
Lardet, Tab. (Standex)
Lardet Expectorant, Tab. (Standex)
Liquophylline, Liq. (Paddock)
Marax DF, Syr. (Roerig)
Marax, Tab. (Roerig)
Maso-Thyllin, Tab. (Mason)
Meprophyl, Vial (Lemmon)
Mernephria, Inj. (Paddock)
Mersaline, Inj. (Standex)
Mersaphyllin, Vial (Pharmex)
Phedral, Tab. (Vortech)

Pheno-Fed, Tab. (Wendt-Bristol)
Phyllicin, Pow. (Knoll)
Quibron, Cap., Liq.(Mead Johnson)
Quibron-300, Cap. (Mead Johnson)
Quibron Plus, Cap. (Mead Johnson)
Quilate, Cap. (Wolins)
Slo-Phyllin Gg, Cap. Syr. (Dooner)
Synate-M, Tab. (Central)
Synophylate, Liq. (Central)
Tedral SA, Tab. (Parke-Davis)
Theobid, Cap. (Glaxo)
Theocol, Cap. Liq. (Columbia)
Theofed, Tab. (Sutliff & Case)
Theofedral Formula, Tab. (Wolins)
Theofenal, Tab. (Cumberland)
Theolair Plus, Tab., Liq. (Riker)
Theo-Organidin, Elix. (Wampole)
Thephecon, Improved, Cap. (Marsh-Emory)
Theophylline-KI Elixir (G & W Labs)

THEOPHYLLINE WITH PHENOBARBITAL COMBINATIONS.
See: Aqualin-Plus, Supp. (Webcon)
  Asma-Lief, Tab., Susp. (Columbia)
  Asminyl, Tab. (Cole)
  Bronkolixir, Elix. (Winthrop-Breon)
  Bronkotab, Tab. (Winthrop-Breon)
  Ceepa, Tab. (Geneva)
  Chlorphen, Tab., Cap., Vial (Truxton)
  Emfaseen, Cap. (Saron)
  For-Az-Ma, Syr. (Vitarine)
  Iso-Asminyl, Tab. (Cole)
  Isuprel Compound, Elix. (Winthrop-Breon)
  Luftodil, Tab. (Mallinckrodt)
  Synophedal, Tab. (Central)
  Synophylate w/Phenobarbital, Tab., (Central)
  T-E-P Compound, Tab. (Stanlabs)
  Thephecon Improved, Cap. (Marsh-Emory)
  Thymodyne, Tab. (Noyes)
  Vitaphen, Tab. (Vitarine)

THEOPHYLLINE AMINOISOBUTANOL. Theophylline
  w/2-amino-2-methyl-1-propanol.
  See: Butaphyllamine (Var. Mfr.)
THEOPHYLLINE, 8-BROMO, AMINOISOBUTANOL.
  See: Pamabrom
THEOPHYLLINE, 8-BROMO, PYRILAMINE.
  See: Pyrabrom
THEOPHYLLINE-CALCIUM SALICYLATE.
W/Ephedrine HCl, phenobarbital, pot. iodide.
  See: Quadrinal, Tab., Susp. (Knoll)
W/Phenobarbital, ephedrine HCl, guaifenesin.
  See: Verequad, Tab., Susp. (Knoll)
W/Potassium iodide.
  See: Theokin, Tab., Elix. (Knoll)
THEOPHYLLINE, 8-CHLORO, DIPHENHYDRAMINE.
Dimenhydrinate, U.S.P. XXI.
  See: Dramamine, Prep. (Searle)
THEOPHYLLINE CHOLINE SALT.
  See: Choledyl, Tab., Elix. (Warner-Chilcott)
• **THEOPHYLLINE, EPHEDRINE HYDROCHLORIDE, AND PHENOBARBITAL TABLETS,** U.S.P. XXI.
  Use: Bronchodilator, sedative.

THEOPHYLLINE ETHYLENEDIAMINE.
  See: Aminophylline, Prep., (Var. Mfr.)
• **THEOPHYLLINE AND GUAIFENESIN CAPSULES,**
  U.S.P. XXI.
  Use: Smooth muscle relaxant, expectorant.
THEOPHYLLINE MONOETHANOLAMINE.
  See: Fleet Brand, Rectal (Fleet)
    Monotheamin, Supp. (Lilly)
THEOPHYLLINE OLAMINE. Theophylline compound
  with 2-amino-ethanol (1:1).
  Use: Smooth muscle relaxant.
• **THEOPHYLLINE SODIUM GLYCINATE,** U.S.P. XXI.
  Elixir, Tab., U.S.P. XXI.
  Use: Smooth muscle relaxant.
  See: Bronchobid, Cap. (Glaxo)
    Synophylate, Elix., Tab. (Central)
    Theofort, Elix. (Federal Pharm.)
W/Guaifenesin.
  See: Asbron G, Tab., Elix. (Dorsey)
    Synophylate-GG, Tab., Syr. (Central)
W/Phenobarbital.
  See: Synophylate w/Phenobarbital, Tab. (Central)
W/Potassium iodide.
  See: TSG-KI, Elix. (Elder)
W/Potassium iodide, ephedrine HCl, codeine
  phosphate.
  See: TSG Croup Liquid. (Elder)
W/Racephedrine & phenobarbital.
  See: Synophedal, Tab. (Central)
THEOSPAN-SR 130. (Laser) Theophylline anhydrous
  130 mg./Cap. Bot. 100s, 1000s.
  Use: Bronchodilator.
THEOSPAN-SR 260. (Laser) Theophylline anhydrous
  260 mg./Cap. Bot. 100s, 1000s.
  Use: Bronchodilator.
THEOSTAT 80 SYRUP. (Laser) Theophylline
  anhydrous 80 mg./15 ml. Bot. Pts., Gal.
  Use: Bronchodilator.
THEO-SYL-R. (Kay) Sodium mersalyl 100 mg., theop-
  hylline 50 mg./cc. Vial 10 cc.
  Use: Mercury diuretic.
THEOTABS. (Panray) Theophylline 130 mg.,
  ephedrine HCl 25 mg., phenobarbital 8 mg./Tab.
  Bot. 100s, 1000s.
  Use: Anti-asthmatic.
THEOVENT LONG-ACTING. (Schering) Theophylline
  anhydrous 125 mg. or 250 mg./Cap. Bot. 100s,
  500s.
  Use: Bronchial dilator.
THEPHECON IMPROVED CAPSULES. (Marsh-Emory)
  Theophylline 260 mg., pseudoephedrine
  hydrochloride 50 mg., butabarbital 15 mg./Cap.
  Bot. 100s, 1000s.
  Use: Bronchial dilatation.
THERA. (Zenith) Multiple vitamin tablet. Bot. 100s.
THERA-9. (Columbia) Vit. A 10,000 I.U., D 400 I.U., C
  200 mg., B-1 10 mg., B-2 10 mg., B-6 2 mg., B-12 5
  mcg., niacinamide 100 mg., calcium pantothenate
  20 mg./Tab. Jar 100s. Tin 1000s.
  Use: Therapeutic formula vitamin.
THERA-9M. (Columbia) Vit. A 10,000 I.U., D 400 I.U., C
  200 mg., B-1 10 mg., B-2 10 mg., B-6 5 mg., B-12 5

mcg., niacinamide 100 mg., Ca pantothenate 20 mg., Vit. E 5 I.U., Iodine 0.15 mg., Fe 12 mg., Cu 2 mg., Mn 1 mg., Mg 65 mg., Zn 1.5 mg./Tab. Jar 100s. Tin 1000s.
Use: Therapeutic vitamins and minerals.

THERA BEE CEE. (Reid-Provident) Vit. B-1 15 mg., B-2 10 mg., B-6 5 mg., niacinamide 50 mg., calcium pantothenate 10 mg., Vit. C 300 mg./Cap. Bot. 100s.
Use: Vitamin supplement.

THERABID. (Mission) Vit. C 500 mg., B-1 15 mg., B-2 10 mg., niacinamide 100 mg., Ca pantothenate 20 mg., B-6 10 mg., B-12 5 mcg., Vit. A acetate 25,000 I.U., Vit. D-2 200 I.U., E 30 I.U./Tab. Bot. 100s.

THERABLOAT. (Norden) Poloxalene.

THERABRAND. (Approved) Vit. A 25,000 I.U., D 1000 I.U., B-1 10 mg., B-2 10 mg., niacinamide 100 mg., C 200 mg., B-6 5 mg., cal. pantothenate 20 mg., B-12 5 mcg./Cap. Bot. 100s, 1000s.
Use: Vitamin therapy.

THERABRAND-M. (Approved) Vit. A 25,000 I.U., D 1000 I.U., C 200 mg., B-1 10 mg., B-2 10 mg., B-6 5 mg., niacinamide 100 mg., cal. pantothenate 20 mg., E 5 I.U., B-12 5 mcg., iodine 0.15 mg., iron 15 mg., Cu 1 mg., Ca 125 mg., Mn 1 mg., Mg 6 mg., Zn 1.5 mg./Cap. Bot. 100s, 1000s.
Use: Vitamin, mineral therapy.

THERAC. (C & M Pharmacal) Colloidal sulfur 4.0%, salicylic acid 2.35%, in an aqueous base. Bot. 2 oz., pt.
Use: Vanishing anti-acne lotion.

THERACAP. (Arcum) Vit. A 10,000 I.U., D 400 I.U., B-1 10 mg., B-2 5 mg., niacinamide 150 mg., C 150 mg./Cap. Bot. 100s, 1000s.
Use: Dietary supplement.

THERACAPS. (Alton) Bot. 100s 1000s.
Use: Dietary supplement.

THERACAPS M. (Alton) Bot. 100s, 1000s.
Use: Dietary supplement with minerals.

THERACEBRIN. (Lilly) Vit. A 25,000 I.U., D 1500 I.U., B-12 10 mcg., B-1 15 mg., B-2 10 mg., B-6 2.5 mg., niacinamide 150 mg., C 150 mg., pantothenic acid 20 mg., E 18.5 I.U./Pulvule. Bot. 100s.
Use: Multiple vitamin deficiencies.

THERACORT. (C & M Pharmacal) Hydrocortisone 0.25%, colloidal sulfur 4%, salicylic acid 2.35%, magnesium aluminum silicate, acacia, propylene glycol, purified water. Lot. Bot. 2 oz.
Use: Vanishing anti-acne lotion.

THERADAN. (Danbury) Vit. A 8,333 I.U., D 133 I.U., B-1 3.30 mg., B-2 3.30 mg., Ca pantothenate 11.70 mg., E 5 I.U., Cu 0.67 mg., Mg 41.70 mg., Fe 66.70 mg., B-12 50 mcg., folic acid 0.33 mg., C 100 mg./Tab. Bot. 100s, 1000s.
Use: Anemia treatment.

THERA-FLUR. (Hoyt) Acidulated fluoride phosphate. Fluoride ion 0.5% (from sod. fluoride 1.1%). Gel-Drops. Bot. 24 ml.
Use: Protection dental caries.

THERA-FLUR-N. (Hoyt) Neutral sodium fluoride 1.1% Bot. 24 ml., 60 ml.

Use: Protection against dental caries.

THERAFORMS. (Horton & Converse) Vit. A 25,000 I.U., D 1000 I.U., C 150 mg., B-1 10 mg., B-2 10 mg., B-6 1 mg., B-12 5 mcg., niacinamide 100 mg., cal. pantothenate 5 mg., Vit. E 5 I.U. w/minerals/Tab. Bot. 100s, 250s, 500s.
Use: Vitamin-mineral deficiencies.

THERA FORMULA. (Zenith) Vit. A 10,000 I.U., D 400 I.U., B-1 10 mg., B-2 10 mg., B-6 5 mg., B-12 5 mcg., niacinamide 100 mg., Ca pantothenate 20 mg., Vit. C 200 mg., E 15 I.U./Tab. Bot. 100s.

THERAFORTIS. (General Vitamin) Vit. A 12,500 I.U., D 1000 I.U., B-1 5 mg., B-2 5 mg., B-6 1 mg., B-12 3 mcg., niacinamide 50 mg., pantothenic acid salt 10 mg. Vit. C 150 mg., folic acid 0.5 mg./Cap. Bot. 100s, 1000s.
Use: Multivitamin therapy.

THERAGARDS M. (Eckerd) Vit. A 10,000 I.U., D 400 I.U., B-1 10 mg., B-2 10 mg., B-6 5 mg., B-12 5 mcg., niacinamide 100 mg., cal. pantothenate 20 mg., C 200 mg., E 15 I.U., w/iodine, Fe, Cu, Mn, Mg, Zn/Tab. Bot. 100s, 200s.
Use: Vitamin, mineral dietary supplement.

THERAGRAN. (Squibb) Vit. A 5,500 I.U., C 120 mg., B-1 3 mg., B-2 3.4 mg., niacin 30 mg., B-6 3 mg., B-12 9 mcg., D 400 I.U. pantothenic acid 10 mg., folic acid 0.4 mg., biotin 15.5 mcg./Tab. Bot. 30s, 60s, 100s. 180s, 1000s. Unimatic 100s. **Liquid:** 1 teaspoonful of liquid is equiv. to 1 tablet. Bot. 4 oz. Unimatic 5 cc. 100s.
Use: Multiple vitamin.

THERAGRAN HEMATINIC. (Squibb) Theragran formula with minerals: Iodine 150 mcg., iron 27 mg., Mg. 100 mg., Cu 2 mg., Zn 15 mg., Mn 5 mg., Cr 15 mcg., Se 10 mcg., Mb 15 mcg., K 7.5 mg., Cc 7.5 mg./Tab. Bot. 90s.
Use: Multiple vitamin with minerals.

THERAGRAN-M. (Squibb) Vit. A 10,000 I.U., D 400 I.U., C 200 mg., B-1 10 mg., B-2 10 mg., niacinamide 100 mg., Cal. pantothenate 20 mg., Vit. B-6 5 mg., E 15 I.U., B-12 5 mcg., w/Ca, Iodine 150 mcg., Fe 12 mg., Mg 65 mg., Cu 2 mg., Zn 1.5 mg., Mn 1 mg./Tab. Bot. 30s, 60s, 100s, 180s, 1000s, Unimatic 100s.
Use: Multivitamin therapy.

THERAGRAN-Z. (Squibb) Vit. A 10,000 I.U., D 400 I.U., E 15 I.U., C 200 mg., thiamine moninitrate 10 mg., riboflavin 10 mg., niacinamide 100 mg., pyridoxine HCl 5 mg., B-12 5 mcg., Ca pantothenate 20 mg., iodine 150 mcg., iron 12 mg., Cu 2 mg., Mn 1 mg., zinc 22.5 mg./Cap.
Use: Vitamin and mineral supplement.

THERA-HEXAMIN. (Galen) Vit. A 25,000 I.U., D 400 I.U., B-1 10 mg., B-2 5 mg., niacinamide 100 mg., C 150 mg./Cap. Bot. 100s.
Use: Multiple vitamin deficiencies.

THERALAX. (Beecham Labs) **Tabs:** Bisacodyl 5 mg./Tab. Bot. 100s, 1000s, unit dose 10 × 10; **Supp.:** Bisacodyl 10 mg./supp. 50s.
Use: Laxative.

THERALETS. (Panray) Vit. A 10,000 IU., D 400 IU., E 15 IU., C 200 IU., B-1 10 mg., B-2 10 mg., Niacinamide

100 mg., pyridoxine HCl 5 mg., B-12 5 mcg., Ca pantothenate 20 mg./Cap.
Use: Vitamin supplement.

THERMODENT. (Mentholatum) Strontium Cl. 10%. Tubes.
Use: Toothpaste for sensitive teeth.

THERALETS M. (Panray) A 10,000 IU., D 400 IU., E 15 IU., C 200 mg., B-1 10 mg., B-2 10 mg., niacinamide 100 mg., B-6 5 mg., B-12 5 mcg., Ca pantothenate 20 mg., Ca 125 mg., Iodine 150 mcg., iron 12 mg., magnesium 65 mg., manganese 1 mg., Cu 2 mg., Zn 1.5 mg./Cap.
Use: Vitamin & mineral supplement.

THERALETS S.C.. (Panray) Vit. A 25,000 I.U., D 400 I.U., B-1 10 mg., B-2 5 mg., niacinamide 150 mg., C 150 mg./Tab. Bot. 1000s.
Use: Vitamin therapy.

THERAMIN. (Arcum) Vit. A 10,000 I.U., D 400 I.U., B-1 10 mg., B-2 5 mg., niacinamide 100 mg., B-6 5 mg., B-12 10 mcg., C 150 mg., cal. pantothenate 15 mg., Ca 103.6 mg., Iodine 0.1 mg., Fe 15 mg., P 80 mg., Mg 6 mg./Tab. Bot. 30s, 100s, 1000s.

THERAMIN CAPSULES. (VRC Vitamin Research) Vit. A 25,000 I.U., D 1000 I.U., B-1 10 mg., B-2 5 mg., B-6 1 mg., B-12 5 mcg., C 150 mg., niacinamide 100 mg., Ca 103.6 mg., P 80.2 mg., Fe 10 mg., Mn 0.954 mg., K 4.93 mg., Zn 1.4 mg., Mg 5.56 mg./Cap. Bot. 100s.

THERANEED. (Hanlon) Vit. A 16,000 I.U., B-1 10 mg., B-2 10 mg., B-6 2 mg., C 300 mg., Ca pantothenate 10 mg., niacinamide 10 mg., B-12 10 mcg./Cap. Bot. 100s.

THERAPALS. (Faraday) Vit. A 25,000 I.U., D 400 I.U., B-1 10 mg., B-2 5 mg., niacinamide 150 mg., B-6 0.5 mg., E 5 I.U., C 150 mg., B-12 10 mcg., Ca 103 mg., Co 0.1 mg., Cu 1 mg., Vit. K 0.15 mg., Mg 6 mg., Mn 1 mg., molybdenum 0.2 mg., P 80 mg., K 5 mg., Zn 1.2 mg./Tab. Bot. 100s, 250s, 1000s.

THERAPEUTIC B COMPLEX W/ASCORBIC ACID. (Horton & Converse) Vit. C 300 mg., niacinamide 100 mg., B-1 10 mg., B-2 6 mg., B-6 40 mg., cal. pantothenate 40 mg., Vit. B-12 activity 4 mcg./2 Caps. Bot. 100s.

THERAPEUTIC LIQUID. (Kenwood) Vit. A 10,000 I.U., D 400 I.U., E 4.5 I.U., C 150 mg., B-1 6 mg., B-2 3 mg., B-6 1 mg., niacinamide 60 mg., calcium pantothenate 6 mg., calcium 38 mg., phosphorus 29 mg., magnesium 6 mg., manganese 1 mg., potassium 5 mg./15 cc. Bot. 12 oz.
Use: High potency vitamin and mineral.

THERAPEUTIC M. (Stanlabs) Vit. A 10,000 I.U., D 400 I.U., B-1 10 mg., B-2 10 mg., B-6 5 mg., B-12 5 mcg., C 200 mg., E 15 I.U., Ca pantothenate 20 mg., niacinamide 100 mg., Cu 2 mg., Mn 1 mg., Zn 1.5 mg., Mg 65 mg., Fe 12 mg., Iodine 0.15 mg./Cap. Bot. 100s.
Use: Dietary supplement.

THERAPEUTIC VITAMIN CAPSULES. (Lannett) Vit. A 25,000 I.U., D 1000 I.U., B-1 10 mg., B-2 5 mg., niacinamide 150 mg., C 150 mg./Cap. Bot. 100s, 500s, 1000s. Tab. Bot. 1000s.
Use: Vitamin supplement.

THERAPEUTIC VITAMIN CAPSULES AND TABLETS—IMPROVED FORMULA. (Lannett) Vit. A 25,000 I.U., D 1000 I.U., thiamine mononitrate 12.5 mg., B-2 12.5 mg., niacinamide 100 mg., B-6 5 mg., B-12 5 mcg., calcium pantothenate 25 mg., C 200 mg./Cap. Caps. 100s, 500s, 1000s. Tab. Bot. 1000s.
Use: Vitamin supplement.

THERAPEUTIC VITAMIN FORMULA W/MINERALS. (Towne) Vit. A palmitate 10,000 I.U., D 400 I.U., B-1 15 mg., B-2 10 mg., B-6 5 mg., B-12 12 mcg., C 200 mg., niacinamide 100 mg., Ca pantothenate 20 mg., Vit. E 15 I.U., Ca 103 mg., Fe 10 mg., Mn 1 mg., K 5 mg., Zn 1.5 mg., Mg 6 mg./Cap. Bot. 30s, 60s, 100s, 250s.

THERAPEUTIC VITAMIN FORMULA W/MINERALS. (Towne) Vit. A palmitate 25,000 I.U., D 1000 I.U., B-1 10 mg., B-2 5 mg., B-6 1 mg., B-12 5 mcg., C 150 mg., niacinamide 100 mg., Ca 103 mg., P 80 mg., Fe 10 mg., Iodine 0.1 mg., Mn 1 mg., K 5 mg., Cu 1 mg., Zn 1.4 mg., Mg 5.5 mg./Cap. Bot. 100s, 1000s.

THERAPEUTIC VITAMIN TABLET. (Vortech) Vit. A 10,000 I.U., D 400 I.U., B-1 10 mg., B-2 10 mg., niacinamide 100 mg., C 200 mg., B-6 5 mg., d-calcium pantothenate 20 mg., B-12 5 mcg., E 15 I.U./Tab. Bot. 100s.
Use: Multiple vitamin.

THERAPHON. (Approved) Vit. A 25,000 I.U., D 1000 I.U., B-1 10 mg., B-2 5 mg., C 150 mg., niacinamide 150 mg./Cap. Bot. 100s, 1000s.

THERAPLEX. (Kenyon) Vit. A 25,000 I.U., D 1000 I.U., B-1 10 mg., B-2 10 mg., niacinamide 150 mg., B-12 5 mcg./Tab. Bot. 100s, 1000s.

THERAPLEX-PLUS. (Kenyon) Vit. A palmitate 25,000 I.U., D 1000 I.U., B-1 10 mg., B-2 5 mg., B-6 1 mg., B-12 5 mcg., C 150 mg., niacinamide 100 mg., dical. phosphate 360 mg., Ca 106 mg., P 82 mg., ferrous sulfate 34 mg., Mn sulfate 3 mg., pot. sulfate 11 mg., Zn sulfate 3.9 mg., Mg sulfate 40 mg./Cap. Bot. 100s, 1000s.

THERA-STAY. (Stayner) Vit. A 25,000 I.U., D 1000 I.U., B-1 12.5 mg., B-2 12.5 mg., niacinamide 100 mg., B-6 5 mg., cal. pantothenate 25 mg., B-12 5 mcg., C 200 mg./Cap. Bot. 100s.
Use: Vitamin therapy.

THERA-STAY "M". (Stayner) Vit. A 25,000 I.U., D 1000 I.U., B-1 10 mg., B-2 5 mg., B-6 1 mg., B-12 5 mcg., C 150 mg., niacinamide 100 mg., Ca 104 mg., P 80 mg., Fe 10 mg., Iodine 0.1 mg., Mn 1 mg., K 5 mg., Cu 1 mg., Zn 1.4 mg., Mg 5.5 mg., E 2 I.U./Cap. Bot. 100s, 500s.
Use: Vitamin-mineral therapy.

THERATINIC. (Jamieson-McKames) Vit. B-12 5 mcg., fortified iron 59 mg., niacin 50 mg., pyridoxine 0.3 mg., cyanocobalamin 2 mcg., folic acid 2 mg./2 cc. w/sod. citrate 1%, phenol 0.5%, procaine HCl 1%.
Use: Hypochromic and hematopoietic anemia.

THERAVEE HEMATINIC VITAMIN. (Vangard) Vit A 2.5 mg., D 3.3 mcg., thiamine 3.3 mg., riboflavin 3.3 mg., pyridoxine HCl 3.3 mg., niacinamide 33.3 mg., calcium pantothenate 11.7 mg., Vit. E 5 mg.,

copper 0.67 mg., magnesium 41.7 mg., iron 66.7 mg., B-12 50 mcg., folic acid 0.33 mcg., C 100 mg./Tab. Bot. 100s. Unit dose 10×10s.
Use: Dietary supplement.

THERAVEE M VITAMIN. (Vangard) Vit A 3 mg., D 10 mcg., E 15 mg., C 200 mg., thiamine 10.3 mg., riboflav 10 mg., niacin 100 mg., B-6 4.1 mg., B-12 5 mcg., pantothenic acid 18.4 mg., iodine 150 mcg., iron 12 mg., magnesium 65 mg., copper 2 mg., zinc 1.5 mg., manganese 1 mg./Tab. Bot. 100s, 1000s. Unit dose 10×10s
Use: Dietary supplement.

THERAVEE VITAMIN. (Vangard) Vit. A 10,000 I.U., D 400 I.U., E 14 I.U., C 200 mg., Thiamine 10.3 mg., riboflavin 10 mg., niacin 100 mg., B-6 4 .1 mg., B-12 5 mcg., pantothenic acid 18.4 mg./Tab. Bot. 100s. Unit dose Pkg. 250s.
Use: Dietary supplement.

THERAVILAN CAPSULES. (Lannett) Vit. A 25,000 I.U., D 1000 I.U., B-1 10 mg., B-2 5 mg., B-6 1 mg., C 150 mg., B-12 5 mcg., niacinamide 100 mg., dicalcium phosphate anhyd. 360 mg., ferrous sulfate dried 34 mg., potassium iodide 0.133 mg., manganese sulfate dried 3 mg., cobalt sulfate 0.49 mg., potassium sulfate 11 mg., sodium molybdate 0.45 mg., copper sulfate monohydrate 2.8 mg., zinc sulfate dried 3.9 mg., magnesium sulfate dried 40 mg./Cap., Tab. Caps. Bot. 100s, 500s, 1000s. Tab. Bot. 100s, 1000s.
Use: Multivitamin with minerals.

THERAVIM CAPSULES. (Robinson) Vit. A 25,000 I.U., D 400 I.U., B-1 10 mg., B-2 5 mg., C 150 mg., niacinamide 150 mg./Cap. Bot. 50s, 100s, 500s, 1000s. Bulk Pack 5000s. W/Vit. B-12 5 mcg./Cap. Bot. 100s, 250s, 1000s.
Use: Therapeutic standard formula vitamin capsules.

THERAVIM HI-PO. (Robinson) Vit. A 25,000 I.U., D 400 I.U., B-1 10 mg., B-2 10 mg., B-6 5 mg., B-12 5 mcg., C 200 mg., E 15 I.U., niacinamide 100 mg., calcium pantothenate 20 mg./Cap. or Tab. Bot. 100s, 1000s.
Use: Therapeutic high potency vitamins.

THER-CO-MIN. (Coastal) Vit. B-1 15 mg., B-2 2 mg., B-6 2 mg., pantothenic acid (Ca pantothenate racemic) 10 mg., niacinamide 100 mg., B-12 7.5 mcg., C 150 mg., E 5 I.U., A 25,000 I.U., D 1000 I.U., Cu 1 mg., Fe 15 mg., Mn 1 mg., Zn 1.5 mg., Iodine 0.015 mg./Cap. Bot. 100s.
Use: Multivitamin with minerals.

THEREL. (La Crosse) Triethanolamine lauryl sulfate w/diglycol laurate. Bot. 8 oz., 0.5 gal.
Use: Soapless non-allergenic shampoo.

THEREVAC. (Bowman) Docusate potassium 283 mg., benzocaine/20 mg./Tube capsule w/soft soap in PEG 400 and glycerin base. , Unit 4cc., packages 4s, 12s, 50s.
Use: Disposable enema.

THEREX NO. 1. (Blue Cross) Vit A 10,000 I.U., D 400 I.U., E 15 I.U., C 200 mg., B-1 10 mg., B-2 10 mg., niacinamide 100 mg., B-6 5 mg., B-12 5 mcg., calcium pantothenate 20 mg./Tab. Bot. 100s.
Use: High potency vitamin supplement for adults.

THEREX-M. (Blue Cross) Vit. A 10,000 I.U., D 400 I.U., E 15 I.U., C 200 mg., B-1 10 mg., B-2 10 mg., niacinamide 100 mg., B-6 5 mg., B-12 5 mcg., calcium pantothenate 20 mg., iodine 150 mcg., iron 12 mg., Mg 65 mg., Cu 2 mg., zinc 1.5 mg., Mn 1 mg./Tab. Bot. 100s.
Use: Vitamin and mineral supplement.

THEREX-Z. (Blue Cross) Vit. A 10,000 I.U., D 400 I.U., E 15 I.U., C 200 mg., B-1 10 mg., B-2 10 mg., niacinamide 100 mg., B-12 5 mcg., B-6 5 mg., Ca pantothenate 20 mg., iodine 150 mcg., Cu 2 mg., iron 12 mg., Zn 22.5 mg./Tab. Bot. 100s.
Use: Vitamin, mineral supplement.

THERMA-KOOL. (Nortech) Compresses in following sizes: 3″ × 5″, 4″ × 9″, 8½″ × 10½″.
Use: Cold or hot compress.

THERMOLENE. (Lannett) Sodium chloride 7 gr., dextrose 3 gr., Vit. B-1 1 mg./Tab. Bot. 1000s.

THERMOLOID. (Mills) Thyroid 1 gr., 2 gr., 3 gr., 4 gr., 5 gr./Tab. Bot. 100s.
Use: Thyroid therapy.

THERMOTABS. (Beecham Products) Sod. chloride 0.45 Gm., pot. chloride 30 mg., cal. carb. 18 mg., dextrose 0.2 Gm./Tab. Bot. 100s.
Use: Heat fatigue.

THEROAL. (Vangard) Theophylline 24 mg., ephedrine HCl 24 mg., phenobarbital 8 mg./Tab. Bot. 100s, 1000s.
Use: Antiasthmatic.

THERUHISTIN. Isothipendyl, B.A.N.

THEX FORTE CAPSULES. (Medtech) Vit. C 500 mg., B-1 25 mg., B-2 15 mg., B-6 5 mg., niacinamide 100 mg., Ca pantothenate 10 mg./Cap. Bot. 60s, 100s.
Use: Saturation vitamin therapy, vitamin supplement.

THEX MULTI VITAMINS/MINERALS. (Medtech) Cap. Bot. 60s.
Use: Dietary supplement.

THEX VITAMIN C. (Medtech) Vit. C 500 mg./T.R. Cap. Bot. 100s.
Use: Dietary supplement.

THEX VITAMIN E. (Medtech) Vitamin E 400 I.U./Cap. Bot. 100s.
Use: Dietary supplement.

THIA. (Sig) Thiamine HCl 100 mg./ml. Vial 30 ml.
Use: Thiamine deficiency.

• **THIABENDAZOLE,** U.S.P. XXI. Oral Susp., Tab. U.S.P. XXI. 1H-Benzimidazole,2-(4-thiazolyl)-2-(4-Thiazolyl)-benzimidazole.
Use: Anthelmintic.
See: Mintezol, Tab., Susp. (Merck Sharp & Dohme)

THIABENDAZOLE, VETERINARY USE. 2-(4-Thiazolyl)-1H-benzimidazole
See: Equizole (MSD AGVET)
Equizole A w/piperazine (MSD AGVET)
Equizole B w/trichlorfon (MSD AGVET)
Omnizole (MSD AGVET)
TBZ (MSD AGVET)
Thibenzole (MSD AGVET)

THIACETARSAMIDE SODIUM. Sodium mercaptoacetate S,S-diester with p-carbamoyldithiobenzenearsonous acid.

Use: Antitrichomonal.
THIACETAZONE, B.A.N. p-Acetylaminobenzaldehyde thiosemicarbamazone.
Use: Treatment of tuberculosis and leprosy.
See: Berculon A
    Neustab
    Seroden
    Thioparamizone
THIACIDE. (Beach) Methenamine mandelate 500 mg., pot. acid phosphate 250 mg./Tab. Bot. 100s, 500s.
Use: Control of urinary infection.
THIA-DIA-MER-SULFONAMIDES. Sulfadiazine w/sulfamerazine & sulfathiazole.
See: Trionamide, Tab. (O'Neal)
THIADOX. (Barry-Martin) Thiamine HCl 100 mg., pyridoxine HCl 100 mg./cc. Vials 10 cc.
THIAHEP INJECTION. (Lannett) Liver ext. (derived from 10 U.S.P. Units injectable) 100 mg., liver ext. (derived from 10 U.S.P. Units crude liver) 100 mg., iron peptonate 20 mg., niacinamide 50 mg., pyridoxine HCl 0.3 mg., riboflavin 3 mg./2 cc. Multiple dose vial 300 cc.
THIALBARBITAL.
See: Kemithal
THIALBARBITONE. B.A.N. 5-Allyl-5-(cyclohex-2-enyl)-2-thiobarbituric acid.
Use: Anesthetic.
See: Kemithal (sodium salt)
THIAMAZOLE (I.N.N.). Methimazole, B.A.N.
THIAMBUTOSINE. B.A.N. 1-(4-Butoxyphenyl)-3-(4-dimethylaminophenyl)thiourea.
Use: Treatment of leprosy.
• **THIAMINE HYDROCHLORIDE,** U.S.P. XXI. Elixir, Inj., Tab., U.S.P. XXI. 3-[(4-amino-2-methyl-5-pyrimidinyl)-methyl]-5-(2-hydroxyethyl)-4-methyl-, chloride, monohydrochloride. Aneurine HCl, thiamine chloride, Vit. B-1 HCl. Thiazolium,
Use: Enzyme co-factor vitamin.
See: Apatate Drops (Kenwood)
    Betalin S, Amp., Elixir, Tab. (Lilly)
    Thia, Vial (Sig)
• **THIAMINE MONONITRATE,** U.S.P. XXI. Elixir, U.S.P. XXI. Thiazolium, 3-[(4-amino-2-methyl-5-pyrimidinyl)-methyl]-5-(2-hydroxyethyl)-4-methyl-, nitrate (salt). (Various Mfr.) Thiamine nitrate.
Use: Enzyme CD Factor Vitamin.
W/Sodium salicylate, colchicine.
See: Sodsylate, Tab. (Durst)
• **THIAMIPRINE.** USAN. 2-Amino-6-[(1-methyl-4-nitroimidazol-5-yl)thio] purine.
Use: Antileukemic.
• **THIAMPHENICOL.** USAN.
Use: Antibacterial.
• **THIAMYLAL SODIUM, FOR INJECTION,** U.S.P. XXI. Sodium 5-allyl-5-(1-methylbutyl)-2-thiobarbiturate.
Use: Anesthetic (systemic).
See: Surital Sodium, Prep. (Parke-Davis)
THIAPHYLL CREAM. (Lannett) Sulfathiazole 5%, chlorophyllin 1%. Jar 4 oz. & 1 lb.
Use: Topically to promote healing.

THIA-SERP-25. (Robinson) Hydrochlorothiazide 25 mg., reserpine alkaloid 0.125 mg./Tab. Bot. 100s, 1000s.
Use: Hypertensive disorders.
THIA-SERP-50. (Robinson) Hydrochlorothiazide 50 mg., reserpine alkaloid 0.125 mg./Tab. Bot. 100s, 1000s.
Use: Hypertensive disorders.
THIA-SERPA-ZINE. (Robinson) Reserpine alkaloid, hydrochlorothiazide, hydralazine HCl. Tab. Bot. 100s, 1000s.
Use: Hypertensive disorders.
THIA-TWELVE. (Rocky Mtn.) B-12 cryst. 1000 mcg., B-1 100 mg./cc. Vial 10 cc.
Use: Nutritional supplement.
• **THIAZESIM.** USAN. 5-(2-Dimethylaminoethyl) 2,3-dihydro-2-phenyl-1,5-benzothiazepin-4-one.
Use: Antidepressant.
THIAZESIM HCl. 5-[2-(Dimethylamino)-ethyl]-2,3-dihydro-2-phenylbenzo-1,5-thiazepin-4-(5H)-one hydrochloride.
Use: Antidepressant.
• **THIAZINAMINIUM CHLORIDE.** USAN.
Use: Antiallergic.
THIAZOLIUM, 3-[(4-AMINO-2-METHYL-5-PYRIMIDINYL)METHYL]-5-(2-HYDROXYETHYL)-4-ME-THY-L-, CHLORIDE, MONOHYDROCHLORIDE. Thiamine Hydrochloride, U.S.P. XXI.
2-(4-THIAZOLYL)BENZIMIDAZOLE. Thiabendazole, U.S.P. XXI.
THIBENZOLE "100". (MSD AGVET) Thiabendazole medicated feed: 100 Gm./lb.
Use: Anthelmintic, veterinary medicine.
THIBENZOLE "200". (MSD AGVET) Medicated feed. 200 Gm./lb.
Use: Anthelmintic, veterinary medicine.
THIENO[1',2':1,2]THIENO[3,4-d]IMIDAZOL-5-IUM, DECAHYDRO-2-OXO-1,3-BIS-(PHENYLMETHYL)-, SALT WITH (+)-7,7-DIMETHYL-2-OXOBICY-CLO[2.2.1]HEPTANE-1-METHANESULFONIC ACID (1:1). Trimethaphan Camsylate, U.S.P. XXI.
7-(2-THIENYL ACETAMIDO) CEPHALOSPORANIC ACID, SOD. SALT. Cephalothin Sodium, U.S.P. XXI.
THIETHANOMELAMINE.
See: Tretamine, B.A.N.
THIETHYLENE THIOPHOSPHORAMIDE.
See: Thiotepa, B.A.N.
• **THIETHYLPERAZINE.** USAN. 2-Ethylthio-10-[3-(4-methylpiperazin-1-yl)propyl]phenothiazine.
Use: Central nervous system depressant.
See: Torecan
• **THIETHYLPERAZINE MALEATE,** U.S.P. XXI. Inj., Suppos., Tab., U.S.P. XXI. Torecan, 2-Ethyl-mercapto-10-[3'-(1"-methyl-piperazinyl-4")propyl-1"]phenothiazine maleate. 2-(Ethylthio)-10-[3-(4-methyl-1-piperazinyl)propyl]phenothiazine maleate (1:2).
Use: Antiemetic.
See: Torecan, Amp., Supp., Tab. (Boehringer Ingelheim)
THIHEXINOL METHYLBROMIDE. alpha-Dithienyl-(4-dimethylamino-cyclohexyl)-carbinolmethbromide. [4-

THIMERFONATE SODIUM

606

(Hydroxydi-2-thienylmethyl)cyclohexyl] trimethylammonium Bromide.
Use: Anticholinergic.
• **THIMERFONATE SODIUM.** USAN. Ethyl(hydrogen p-mercaptobenzenesulfonato)mercury sodium salt; Sodium p-[(ethylmercuri)-thio] benzenesulfonate. Sulfo-Merthiolate (Lilly).
Use: Topical anti-infective.
• **THIMEROSAL,** U.S.P. XXI. Topical Aerosol, Topical Soln., Tr., U.S.P. XXI. Sod. Ethylmercurithiosalicylate. Sodium Ethyl (Sodium o-mercaptobenzoate)mercury.
Use: Local anti-infective; pharmaceutical aid (preservative).
See: Aeroaid, Aerosol (Aeroceuticals)
Merphol Tincture 1:1000, Liq. (Bowman)
Mersol, Liq. (Century)
Merthiolate, Prep. (Lilly)
2,2-THIOBIS (4,6-dichlorophenol).
See: Bithionol.
THIOCARBANIDIN. Under study.
Use: Tuberculosis.
THIOCARLIDE. B.A.N. 1,3-Di-(4-isopentyloxyphenyl)-thiourea.
Use: Treatment of tuberculosis.
See: Isoxyl
THIOCYANATE SODIUM. Sodium thiocyanate.
Use: Hypotensive.
THIOCYL. (Torigian) Sodium thiosalicylate 100 mg./2 ml. Amp. 2 cc. Box 25s, 100s.
Use: I.M. Rheumatism.
THIODINONE. Name used for Nifuratel.
THIODIPHENYLAMINE.
See: Phenothiazine.
THIODRIL. Carboxymethylcysteine, B.A.N.
THIODYNE. (Savage) Sodium thiosalicylate 50 mg., benzyl alcohol 2.0%/cc. Vial 30 cc.
Use: Rheumatoid arthritis.
THIOFURADENE. 1[(5-Nitrofurfurylidene)-amino]-2-imidazolidinethione.
THIOGLYCEROL.
W/Sod. citrate, phenol, benzyl alcohol.
See: Sulfo-ganic, Vial (Marcen)
• **THIOGUANINE,** U.S.P. XXI. Tab. U.S.P. XXI. 6H-Purine-6-thione,2-amino-1,7-dihydro-.2-Amino-purine-6-thiol, hemihydrate. Tabloid (Burroughs Wellcome) 40 mg., Bot. 25s.
Use: Antineoplastic agent.
THIOHEXAMIDE. N-(p-Methyl-mercaptophenylsulfonyl)-N′-cyclohexylurea.
Use: Blood sugar lowering compound.
THIOISONICOTINAMIDE. Under study.
Use: Antituberculosis drug.
THIOLATE. (Hickman; Pharmex) Sod. thiosalicylate 50 mg./cc. Vial 30 cc.
THIOMERSAL. B.A.N. Sodium salt of (2-carboxyphenyl-thio)ethylmercury.
Sodium ethylmercurithiosalicylate
Thiomerosal
Thiomersalate
Use: Antiseptic; preservative.
See: Merthiolate
THIOMESTERONE. B.A.N. 1α,7α-Bis-(acetylthio)-17β-hydroxy-17α-methylandrost-4-en-3-one.

Use: Anabolic steroid.
See: Emdabol
THIOPARAMIZONE. Thiacetazone, B.A.N.
• **THIOPENTAL SODIUM,** U.S.P. XXI.; Inj., U.S.P. XXI. Sodium 5-ethyl-5-(1-methylbutyl)-2-thiobarbiturate. Thiopentone sodium.
Use: Anesthetic (intravenous), anticonvulsant.
See: Pentothal Sodium, Amp. (Abbott)
THIOPHOSPHORAMIDE.
See: Thio-Tepa, Vial (Lederle)
THIOPROPAZATE. B.A.N. 10-{3-[4-(2-Acetoxy-ethyl)-piperazin-1-yl]propyl}-2-chlorophenothiazine.
Use: Tranquilizer.
See: Dartalan [hydrochloride]
• **THIOPROPAZATE HYDROCHLORIDE.** 2-Chloro-10-{3-[(2-acetoxyethyl)-4-piperazinyl]-propyl} phenothiazine dihydrochloride.4-[3-(2-Chlorophenothiazine-10-yl)propyl]-1-piperazine ethanol Acetate Dihydrochloride.
Use: Tranquilizer.
THIOPROPERAZINE. B.A.N. 2-Dimethylsulfamoyl-10-[3-(4-methylpiperazin-1-yl)propyl]phenothiazine.
Use: Tranquilizer; antiemetic.
See: Majeptil (mesylate)
THIOPROPERAZINE MESYLATE. N,N-Dimethyl-10-[3-(4-methyl-1-piperazinyl)propyl] phenothiazine-2-sulfonamide dimethanesulfonate.
Use: Central depressant; antiemetic.
• **THIORIDAZINE,** U.S.P. XXI. Oral Susp., U.S.P. XXI. 10-[2-(1-Methyl-2-piperidyl)ethyl]-2-methylthiophenothiazine.
Use: Tranquilizer.
See: Mellaril, Susp. (Sandoz)
• **THIORIDAZINE HCl,** U.S.P. XXI. Oral Soln., Tab., U.S.P. XXI. 10-[2-(1-Methyl-2-piperidyl)-ethyl]-2-(methylthio) phenothiazine hydrochloride. 10H-Phenothiazine, 10-[2-(1-methyl-2-piperidinyl)-ethyl]-2-(methylthio)-, monohydrochloride.
Use: Tranquilizer.
See: Mellaril, Tabs., Soln., (Sandoz)
THIOSAL. (Keene) Sodium thiosalicylate 50 mg./ml. Inj.
Vial 30 ml.
• **THIOSALAN.** USAN. 3,4′,5-Tribromo-2-mercaptobenzanilide. Under study.
Use: Germicide.
THIOSALICYLIC ACID SALT.
THIOSTAN. (Standex) Sodium thiosalicylate 50 mg./30 cc. Bot. 1 oz.
THIOSUL. (Vortech) Thiosalicylic acid as sodium salt 50 mg., benzyl alcohol 2%/cc. Vial 30 ml.
Use: Analgesic, antipyretic.
THIOSULFIL-A. (Ayerst) Sulfamethizole 0.25 Gm., phenazopyridine HCl 50 mg./Tab. Bot. 100s, 1000s.
Use: Urinary tract infections, analgesic.
THIOSULFIL-A FORTE. (Ayerst) Sulfamethizole 0.5 Gm., phenazopyridine HCl 50 mg./Tab. Bot. 100s, 1000s.
Use: Urinary tract infections, analgesic.
THIOSULFIL DUO-PAK. (Ayerst) Combination package w. 1 bottle, Thiosulfil Forte, 32 white tablets and 1 bottle, Thiosulfil-A Forte, 24 yellow tablets.

Use: Initial management of urinary tract infection.

THIOSULFIL FORTE. (Ayerst) Sulfamethizole 0.5 Gm./Tab. Bot. 100s.
Use: Treatment urinary tract infections.

• **THIOTEPA,** U.S.P. XXI. For Inj., U.S.P. XXI. Thiophosphoramide. N, Tris(1-Aziridinyl phosphine sulfide. (Lederle) Triethylenethiophosphoramide 15 mg./Vial.
Use: Antineoplastic.

THIOTEPA. (Lederle) The ethylenimine-type N, N; N''-Triethylene thiophosphoramide. Powder for reconstitution: Thiotepa powder 15 mg., Na chloride 80 mg., Na bicarbonate 50 mg./Vial. Vial 15 mg.
Use: A polyfunctional alkylating agent used in the chemotherapy of certain neoplastic diseases.

• **THIOTHIXENE,** U.S.P. XXI. Cap., U.S.P. XXI. N,N,-Dimethyl-9-(3-(4-methyl-1-piperazinyl)propylidene)thioxanthene-2-sulfonamide. As HCl salt.
Use: Psychotherapeutic agent.
See: Navane, Cap., Vial (Roerig)
    Navane Concentrate Solution (Roerig)

• **THIOTHIXENE HCl,** U.S.P. XXI. Inj., Oral Soln., U.S.P. XXI.
Use: Antipsychotic.
See: Navane Hydrochloride (Pfizer)

THIOURACIL. 2-Thiouracil.
Use: Treatment of hyperthyroidism, angina pectoris, congestive heart failure.

THIOUREA. (City Chem.) Pow., Bot., 1 lb.
Use: The same as thiouracil and to stimulate granulating tissue.

THIOXANTHENE DERIVATIVE.
See: Taractan, Prep. (Roche)

THIOXOLONE. B.A.N. 6-Hydroxy-1,3-benzoxathiol-2-one.
Use: Keratolytic agent.
See: Camyna

THIPHENAMIL. F.D.A. S-[2-(Diethylamino)-ethyl]-diphenylthioacetate.

• **THIPHENAMIL HYDROCHLORIDE.** USAN. S-[2-(Diethylamino)ethyl] diphenylthioacetate HCl.
Use: Anticholenergic.
See: Trocinate, Tab. (Poythress)

• **THIPENCILLIN POTASSIUM.** USAN. (1) Potassium 3,3-dimethyl-7-oxo-6-[2-(phenylthio)acetamido]-4-thia-1-azabicyclo[3.2.0] heptane-2-carboxylate; (2) Potassium 6-(phenylmercaptoacetamido)-penicillanate.
Use: Antibacterial.

THIPYRI-12. (Sig) Vit. B-1 1000 mg., B-6 1000 mg., cyanocobalamin (B-12) 10,000 mcg., sod. chloride 0.5%, sod. bisulfite 0.1%, benzyl alcohol (as preservative) 0.9%. Univial 10 ml.

• **THIRAM.** USAN. Bis(dimethylthiocarbamoyl) disulfide.
Use: Antifungal.

THIURETIC TABLETS. (Parke-Davis) Hydrochlorothiazide Tabs. 25 mg./Tab. Bot. 100s. 50 mg./Tab. Bot. 100s, 1000s. Unit dose 10 × 10.
Use: Diuretic, antihypertensive.

THIXO-FLUR TOPICAL GEL. (Hoyt) Acidulated phosphate sodium fluoride in gel base 1.2%. Bot. 32 oz. 8 oz., 4 oz.
Use: Dental caries prevention.

• **THONZONIUM BROMIDE,** U.S.P. XXI. Hexadecyl { 2-[(p-methoxybenzyl)-2-pyrimidinylamino]ethyl} dimethylammonium bromide.
Use: Detergent.
W/Colistin base, neomycin base, hydrocortisone acetate, polysorbate 80, acetic acid, sodium acetate.
See: Coly-Mycin-S, Otic, Liq. (Warner-Chilcott)
W/Isoproterenol.
See: Nebair, Aerosol (Warner-Chilcott)
W/Neomycin sulfate, gramicidin, thonzylamine HCl, phenylephrine HCl.
See: Biomydrin, Spray, Drops (Warner-Chilcott)

THONZYLAMINE. B.A.N. 2-[N-p-Anisyl-N-(pyrimidin-2-yl)amino]ethyldimethylamine.
Use: Antihistamine.
See: Neohetramine

THONZYLAMINE HYDROCHLORIDE. 2[[2-(Dimethylamino)ethyl](p-methoxybenzyl)amino]pyrimidine monohydrochloride.
Use: Antihistamine.

THOR CAPSULES. (Towne) Dextromethorphan HBr 5 mg., phenylephrine HCl 5 mg., chlorpheniramine maleate 0.5 mg., pheniramine maleate 5 mg., caffeine 30 mg., salicylamide 200 mg./Cap. Bot. 15s.

THOR SYRUP. (Towne) Dextromethorphan HBr 90 mg., pyrilamine maleate 22.5 mg., phenylephrine HCl 10 mg., ephedrine sulfate 15 mg., sod. citrate 325 mg., ammon. chloride 650 mg., guaifenesin 50 mg.,/fl. oz. Bot. 4 oz.

THORADEX HCl. (Cenci) Chlorpromazine 10 mg., 25 mg., 50 mg., 100 mg./Tab. Bot. 100s, 1000s.

THORAGOL. Bibenzonium Bromide, B.A.N.

THORAZINE. (SmithKline) Chlorpromazine HCl, **Tab.:** (10, 25, 50, 100, 200 mg.) Bot. 100s, 1000s. Single unit pkg. 100s. **Amp.:** (25 mg. w/ascorbic acid 2 mg., sodium bisulfite 1 mg., sodium sulfite 1 mg., NaCl 6 mg./1 ml.), 1 ml., 2 ml. Box 10s, 100s, 500s. Vial: 10 ml. Box 1s, 20s, 100s. **Spansule:** 30, 75, 150 & 200 mg. Bot. 50s, 100s (S.U.P.), 500s. 300 mg. Bot. 50s, 100s (S.U.P.). **Syr.:** (10 mg./5 ml.) Bot. 4 oz. **Supp.:** Chlorpromazine base, w/glycerin, glyceryl monopalmitate, glyceryl monostearate, hydrogenated cocoanut oil fatty acids, hydrogenated palm kernel oil fatty acids. (25, 100 mg.) Box 12. **Conc:** (30 mg./ml.) Bot. 4 oz., 1 gal. (100 mg./ml.) Bot. 8 oz.
Use: Antiemetic. Neuropsychiatric disorders.

THORETS. (Buffington) Benzocaine 18.9 mg./lozenge. Dispens-A-Kits 500s.
Use: Sugar free sore throat relief.

THORPHAN. (Vitarine) Dextromethorphan HBr 15 mg., chlorpheniramine maleate 2 mg., phenylephrine HCl 5 mg., acetyl-p-aminophenol 120 mg., ascorbic acid 30 mg./10 cc. Bot. 4 oz.
Use: Treatment of common cold.

THORZETTES LOZENGES. (Towne) Dextromethorphan HBr 3 mg., cetylpyridinum chloride 1.5 mg., benzocaine 5 mg./Lozenge. Bot. 15s.

• **THOZALINONE.** USAN. 2-Dimethylamino-5-phenyl-2-oxazolin-4-one.
Use: Antidepressant.
See: Stimsen (Lederle)

THREACON EXPECTORANT. (CMC) Pheniramine maleate, phenylephrine HCl, guaifenesin, sod. citrate, citric acid in mentholate humectant syrup base. Bot. pt., gal.

THREE AMINE TD. (Vitarine) Phenylpropanolamine HBr 50 mg., pheniramine maleate 25 mg., pyrilamine maleate 25 mg./Time Rel. Cap.
Use: Antihistamine and decongestant.

• **THREONINE,** U.S.P. XXI. $C_4H_9NO_3$ as L-threonine.
Use: Amino acid.

THROAT DISCS. (Marion) Formerly Parke, Davis Capsicum, peppermint, anise, cubeb, glycyrrhiza, linseed. Box 60s.

THROAT DISCS. (Wolins) Benzocaine 5 mg., sodium propionate 10 mg./Tab. Bot. 1000s.

THROAT-EZE. (Faraday) Cetylpyridinium chloride 1:3000, cetyl dimethyl benzyl ammonium chloride 1:3000, benzocaine 10 mg./Wafer. Loz., foil wrapped. Vial 15.
Use: Anesthetic lozenge.

• **THROMBIN,** U.S.P. XXI. Thrombin, topical, mammalian origin.
(Parke-Davis)—Thrombin, Topical (Bovine).
(Upjohn)—Vial (1000 u.) 30 ml.
Use: Local hemostatic.

THROMBINAR. (Armour) Thrombin topical. Vial 1000, 5000, 10,000, 50,000 U.S. Standard Units.
Use: Topical hemostat.

THROMBOPLASTIN.
Use: Diagnostic aid (prothrombin estimation).

THROMBOSTAT. (Parke-Davis) Prothrombin is activated by tissue thromboplastin in the presence of calcium chloride. **1000** U.S. (N.I.H.) units. Vial 10 ml. **5000** U.S. units. Vial 10 ml. and 5 ml. diluent. **10,000** U.S. units. Vial 20 ml. and 10 ml. diluent. **20,000** U.S. units. Vial 30 ml. and 20 ml. diluent.
Use: Local hemostatic.

TH SAL. (Foy) Sodium thiosalicylate 50 mg. Vial 30 ml.
Use: Antipyretic.

THURFYL NICOTINATE. B.A.N. Tetrahydrofurfuryl nicotinate. Trafuril.
Use: Topical vasodilator.

THYCAL. (Mills) Thermoloid (thyroid) 2 gr., iodized calcium 2 gr., peptone 1 gr./Tab. Bot. 1000s.

THYLIN. Nifenazone, B.A.N.

THYLOX. (C.S. Dent) Medicated shampoo & soap, contains absorbable sulfur. Bot. 6 oz. Bar 3⅜ oz.
Use: Seborrheic dermatitis, Dandruff Control. Bot. 6 oz.

• **THYMOL,** N.F. XVI. Phenol, 5-methyl-2-(1-methyle-thyl)- p-Cymen-3-ol. (Var. Mfr.) ¼ lb., 1 lb.
Use: Antifungal, anti-infective local anesthetic, antitussive, nasal decongestant.
See: Vicks Regular & Wild Cherry Medicated Cough Drops (Vicks)
Vicks Vaporub, Oint. (Vicks)

W/Combinations.
See: Listerine Antiseptic, Sol. (Warner-Lambert)

THYMOL IODIDE.
Use: Antifungal; anti-infective.

THYMOLIDINE. (Blue Line) Phenol 0.5%, iodine, camphor, thymol in mineral oil. Liq. 1 pt., 1 gal.
Use: Topically; antiseptic.

• **THYMOPENTIN.** USAN. Formerly thymopoietin
Use: Immunoregulator.

THYMOXAMINE. B.A.N. 4-(2-Dimethylamino-ethoxy)-5-isopropyl-2-methylphenyl acetate. Moxisylyte (I.N.N.) Opilon [hydrochloride].
Use: Peripheral vasodilator.

THYODATIL. Name used for Nifuratel.

THYPINONE. (Abbott) Protirelin 500 mcg./1 ml. Amp.
Use: Adjunctive agent in the diagnostic assessment of thyroid function.

THYRAR. (USV Labs.) Bovine thyroid preparation. ½, 1, 2 gr./Tab. Bot. 100s.
Use: Hypothyroid states.

THYROBROM. (Mills) Brominated thyroid. Tab. or S.C. Tab. (1 gr. & 2 gr., 3 gr., 4 gr.) Bot. 1000s.
Use: Thyroid therapy.

THYROCALCITONIN. Calcitonin, B.A.N.

• **THYROGLOBULIN,** U.S.P. XXI. Tab., U.S.P. XXI. Substance obtained by fractionation of thyroid glands from hog, *Sus scrofa* Linne' var. domesticus Gray (Fam. Suidae), containing not less than 0.7% iodine.
Use: Thyroid hormone.
See: Proloid, Tab. (Parke-Davis)
Thyrar, Tab. (Armour)

• **THYROID,** U.S.P. XXI.; Tab., U.S.P. XXI.
Use: Thyroid hormone.
See: Arco Thyroid, Tab. (Arco)
Armour Thyroid, Tab. (USV Labs.)
Dathroid 0.05 & 3, Tab. (Scrip)
Delcoid, Tab. (Delco)
S-P-T., Cap. (Fleming)
Thermoloid, Tab. (Mills)
Thyrocrine, Tab. (Lemmon)
Thyroid Strong, Tab. (Marion)
Thyro-Teric, Tab. (Mallard))

THYROID COMBINATIONS.
See: Andro-Medicone, Tab. (Medicone)
Foyaloid-B, Tab. (Foy)
Geramine, Vial (Brown)
Hemocrine, Tab. (Mallard)
Henydin, Prep. (Arcum)
Lotone, Tab. (Westerfield)
Thycal, Tab. (Mills)

THYROID BROMINATED.
See: Thyrobrom, Tab. (Mills)

THYROID HORMONES.
See: Liothyronine Sod.
Synthroid, Inj., Tab. (Flint)
Thyroxin (Var. Mfr.)

THYROID PREPARATIONS.
See: Proloid, Tab. (Parke-Davis)
Thyrar, Tab. (USV Labs.)
Thyrobrom, Tab. (Mills)
Thyroxin, Prep. (Var. Mfr.)

THYROID STRONG, COATED. (Marion) Thyroid

hormone 0.5 gr., 2 gr., 3 gr./Tab. Bot. 100s; 1 gr./Tab. Bot. 100s, 1000s.
Use: Thyroid replacement.

THYROID STRONG, UNCOATED. (Marion) Thyroid 0.5 gr., 1 gr., or 2 gr. Bot. 100s, 1000s.
Use: Thyroid replacement.

THYROLAR. (USV Labs.) Liotrix. ¼ gr./Tab. Bot. 100s; ½ gr., 1 gr., 2 gr., 3 gr./Tab. Bot. 100s, 1000s.
Use: Thyroid deficiency.

• **THYROMEDAN HYDROCHLORIDE.** USAN. 2-(Diethylamino)ethyl [3,5-diiodo-4-(3-iodo-4-methoxyphenoxy) phenyl] acetate hydrochloride.
Use: Thyromimetic.

THYROPROPIC ACID. 4-(4-Hydroxy-3-iodophenoxy)-3,5-diiodohydrocinnamic acid. Triopron (Warner Chilcott)
Use: Anticholesteremic.

THYRO-TERIC. (Mallard) Thyroid 1 gr./Tab. Bot. 1000s.

THYROTROPHIN. B.A.N. Thyrotrophic hormone. Thytropar; Thyrophin.

THYROTROPIC PRINCIPLE OF BOVINE ANTERIOR PITUITARY GLANDS.
See: Thytropar, Vial (Armour Labs.)

• **THYROXINE I-125.** USAN.
Use: Radioactive agent.

• **THYROXINE I-131.** USAN.
Use: Radioactive agent.

L-THYROXINE, SODIUM.
See: Levoid, Vial (Pharmex)
Synthroid, Tab., Inj. (Flint)

THYTROPAR. (Armour) Thyrotropic principle of bovine anterior pituitary glands. Thyrotropin, B.A.N. Vial 10 IU.
Use: Thyroid myxedema due to pituitary insufficiency.

THYTROPHIN. Thyrotrophin, B.A.N.

THYROZYME-II A. (Abbott) T-4 diagnostic kit. 100 & 500 test units.
Use: Quantitative measurement of unsaturated thyroxine binding globulin in serum.

• **TIAMENIDINE HYDROCHLORIDE.** USAN.
Use: Antihypertensive.

• **TIAMULIN.** USAN.
Use: Antibacterial.

• **TIAMULIN FUMARATE.** USAN.
Use: Antibacterial.

• **TIARAMIDE HYDROCHLORIDE.** USAN.
Use: Anti-asthmatic.

• **TIAZOFURIN.** USAN.
Use: Poultry coccidiostat.

• **TIAZURIL.** USAN.
Use: Coccidiostat.

• **TIBOLONE.** USAN. (1) 17-Hydroxy-7α-methyl-19-nor-17α-pregn-5(10)-en-20-yn-3-one; (2) 17α-Ethynyl-17-hydroxy-7α-methyl-5 (10)-estren-3-one.
Use: Anabolic.

• **TIBRIC ACID.** USAN. 2-Chloro-5-(cis-3,5-dimethyl-piperidinosulfonyl)benzoic acid.
Use: Treatment of hyperlipemia.

• **TIBROFAN.** USAN. 4,4′,5-Tribromo-2-thiophenecarboxanilide. Under study.
Use: Disinfectant.

• **TICABESONE PROPIONATE.** USAN.
Use: Glucocorticoid.

TICAR. (Beecham Labs) Ticarcillin disodium. 1 Gm., 3 Gm., 6 Gm./Vial in 10s. Piggyback vials 3 Gm. in 25s.
Use: Antibiotic.

• **TICARBODINE,** USAN. α,α,α-Trifluoro-2,6-dimethylthio-1-piperidinecarboxy-m-toluidide. 2,6-Dimethylpiperidino-3′-(trifluoromethyl)thioformanilide.
Use: Anthelmintic.

• **TICARCILLIN CRESYL SODIUM.** USAN.
Use: Antibacterial.

• **TICARCILLIN DISODIUM, STERILE,** U.S.P. XXI. 6-[2-Carboxy-2-(3-thienyl)-acetamido]penicillanic acid.
Use: Antibiotic.
See: Ticar, inj. (Beecham Labs.)

• **TICLATONE.** USAN. 6-Chloro-1,2-benzisothiazolin-3-one.
Use: Antibacterial, antifungal.
See: Landromil (Dosey).

• **TICLOPIDINE HYDROCHLORIDE.** USAN.
Use: Inhibitor (platelet).

TICON. (Hauck) Trimethobenzamide HCl 100 mg./ml. Vial 20 ml.
Use: Treatment postoperative nausea & vomiting.

• **TICRYNAFEN.** USAN.
Use: Diuretic, uricosuric, antihypertensive.

TIDEX. (Allison) Dextroamphetamine sulfate, 5 mg./Tab. Bot. 100s, 1000s.
Use: Obesity control.

TIDEXSOL TABLETS. (Winthrop Products) Acetominophen.
Use: Analgesic, antipyretic.

TIEMONIUM IODIDE. B.A.N. 4-[3-Hydroxy-3-phenyl-3-(2-thienyl)propyl]-4-methylmorpholinium iodide.
Use: Antispasmodic; anticholinergic.

TIGAN. (Beecham Labs) Trimethobenzamide hydrochloride.**Cap.** 100 mg. Bot. 100s, 250 mg. Bot. 100s, 500s. **Amp.** (100 mg./ml.) 2 ml. Box 10s. Vial 20 cc. **Thera-Ject** (100 mg./ml.) 2 ml. Box 25s. **Supp.** 200 mg. Box 10s, 50s. **Pediatric Supp.** 100 mg. Box 10s.
Use: Nausea and vomiting.

• **TIGESTOL.** USAN. (1) 19-Nor-17α-pregn-5(10)-en-20-yn-17-ol; (2) 17-α-Ethynyl-5(10)-estren-17-ol. Under study.
Use: Progestin.

TIGLOIDINE. B.A.N. Tiglylpseudotropeine. Tiglyssin [hydrobromide]
Use: Treatment of the Parkinsonian syndrome.

TIGLYSSIN HYDROBROMIDE. Tigloidine, B.A.N.

TIGO. (Burlington) Polymixin B sulfate 5,000 u., zinc bacitracin 400 u., neomycin sulfate 5 mg./Gm. Oint. Tube ½ oz.
Use: Triple antibiotic.

TIHIST-DP. (Vita Elixir) d-methorphan HBr 10 mg., pyrilamine maleate 16 mg., sodium citrate 3.3 gr./5 cc
Use: Cough syrup.

TIHIST NASAL DROPS. (Vita Elixir) Pyrilamine maleate 0.1%, phenylephrine HCl 0.25%, sodium

bisulfite 0.2%, methylparaben 0.02%, propylparaben 0.01%/30cc.
Use: Nasal decongestant.

TIJA TABLETS. (Vita Elixir) Oxytetracycline HCl 250 mg./Tab.
Use: Antibiotic.

TIJA SYRUP. (Vita Elixir) Oxytetracycline HCl 125 mg./5 cc.
Use: Antibiotic.

TIJECT-20. (Mayrand) Trimethobenzamide HCl 100 mg./ml. Vials 20 ml.
Use: Anti-emetic.

• **TILETAMINE HCl,** USAN. 2-(Ethylamino)-2-(2-thienyl)cyclohexanone HCl.
Use: Anesthetic; anticonvulsant.

TILIDATE. B.A.N. Ethyl 2-dimethylamino-1-phenylcyclohex-3-ene-1-carboxylate.
Use: Analgesic.

• **TILIDINE HCl.** USAN. ($\pm$)-Ethyl trans-2-(dimethylamino)-1-phenyl-3-cyclohexene-1-carboxylate HCl.
Use: Analgesic.

• **TILORONE HCl.** USAN. 2,7-Bis[2-(diethylamino)ethoxy]fluoren-9-one dihydrochloride.
Use: Antiviral.

TIME CAPS. (Weeks & Leo) Phenylpropanolamine HCl 50 mg., chlorpheniramine 4 mg., atropine sulfate 0.024 mg., scopolamine HBr 0.014 mg., hyoscyamine sulfate 0.122 mg.,/T.R. Cap. Bot. 14s, 28s.
Use: Decongestant, drying agent for colds and hay fever.

TIMED REDUCING AIDS-CAFFEINE FREE. (Weeks & Leo) Phenylpropanolamine HCl 75 mg./T.R. Cap. Bot. 28s, 56s.
Use: Reducing aid.

• **TIMEFURONE.** USAN.

• **TIMOBESONE ACETATE.** USAN.

TIMOLIDE. (Merck Sharp & Dohme) Timolol maleate 10 mg., hydrochlorothiazide 25 mg./Tab. Bot. 100s. Unit dose 100s.
Use: Antihypertensive.

• **TIMOLOL MALEATE,** U.S.P. XXI. Ophth. Sol., Tab., U.S.P. XXI. (S)-1-[Cl, 1-dimethyl-ethyl) amino]-3-[[4-(4 morpholinyl)-1,2,5-thiadiazol-3-yl]oxy]-2-propanol, (Z)-butenedioate (1:1) salt.
Use: Treatment of chronic open angle, aphakic and secondary glaucoma.
See: Blocadren, Tab. (Merck Sharp & Dohme)

• **TIMOLOL MALEATE AND HYDROCHLORO-THIA-ZIDE TABLETS,** U.S.P. XXI.
Use: Antihypertensive.
See: Timolide, Tab. (Merck Sharp & Dohme)

TIMOPTIC. (Merck Sharp & Dohme) Timolol maleate 0.25% and 0.5% solution. Dispenser Bot. 5 ml., 10 ml., 15 ml.
Use: Treatment of chronic open angle, aphakic and secondary glaucoma; patients with elevated IOP at risk to require lowering of ocular pressure.

• **TINABINOL.** USAN.
Use: Antihypertensive.

TINACTIN. (Schering) **Soln. 1%:** Tolnaftate (10

mg./ml.) w/butylated hydroxytoluene, in nonaqueous homogeneous PEG 400. Plastic squeeze bot. 10 ml. **Cream 1%:** Tolnaftate (10 mg./Gm.) in homogeneous, nonaqueous vehicle of PEG-400, propylene glycol, carboxypolymethylene, monoamylamine, titanium dioxide and butylated hydroxytoluene. Tube 15 Gm. **Powder 1%:** Tolnaftate w/corn starch, talc. Plastic container 45 Gm. **Powd. Aerosol 1%:** Tolnaftate w/butylated hydroxytoluene, talc. polyethylene-polypropylene glycol monobutyl ether, denatured alcohol and inert propellant of isobutane. Spray can 100 Gm.
Use: Topical fungicidal agent.

TINADERM. Tolnaftate, B.A.N.

TINASTAT. (Vita Elixir) Sodium hyposulfite, benzethonium Cl./2 oz.
Use: Keratolytic lotion.

TINDAL. (Schering) Acetophenazine maleate 20 mg./Tab. Bot. 100s.
Use: Tranquilizer.

TINE TEST, OLD TUBERCULIN, Rosenthal. (Lederle)
See: Tuberculin Tine Test (Lederle)

TINE TEST, PURIFIED PROTEIN DERIVATIVE. (Lederle)
See: Tuberculin Tine Test (Lederle)

TIN FLUORIDE. Stannous Fluoride, U.S.P. XXI.

TING. (Pharmacraft) **Cream:** Benzoic acid, boric acid, zinc oxide, zinc stearate, alcohol 16%. Tube 0.9 oz., 1.8 oz. **Powder:** Boric acid, benzoic acid, zinc stearate, zinc oxide. Can 2.5 oz. **Soap:** Undecylenic acid 2%. Cake 3.25 oz. **Aerosol (hydrocarbon):** Undecylenic acid 2%, zinc undecylenate 20%. Can 2.7 oz.
Use: Fungus infections, athlete's foot.

• **TINIDAZOLE.** USAN. 1-[2-(Ethylsulfonyl)-ethyl]-2-methyl-5-nitroimidazole.
Use: Antiprotozoal.
See: Fasigyn (Pfizer)
    Simplotan (Pfizer)

TINSET. (Janssen) Oxatomide.
Use: Anti-allergenic, anti-asthmatic.

TINVER LOTION. (Barnes-Hind) Sodium thiosulfate 25%, salicylic acid 1%, isopropyl alcohol 10%, propylene glycol, menthol, disodium edetate, colloidal alumina.
Plastic Bot. 6 oz.
Use: Specific for tinea versicolor.

• **TIOCONAZOLE.** USAN.
Use: Antifungal.

• **TIODAZOSIN.** USAN.
Use: Antihypertensive.

• **TIODONIUM CHLORIDE.** USAN.
Use: Antibacterial.

T-IONATE-P.A. (Reid-Provident) Testosterone cypionate 200 mg., benzyl benzoate 20%, benzyl alcohol 0.9%, in cottonseed oil/ml. Vial 10 ml. 1s, 6s, 12s.

• **TIOPERIDONE HYDROCHLORIDE.** USAN.
Use: Antipsychotic.

TIOPHYLL. (Schaffer Lab) Iodine 0.71%, boric acid 0.61%, phenol 0.60%, viscarin 0.48%, chlorophyll 0.45%. Liq. Bot. pt. gal.

Use: Minor urinary tract infections.
- **TIOPINAC.** USAN.
  Use: Anti-inflammatory, analgesic.
- **TIOTIDINE.** USAN.
  Use: Antagonist.
- **TIOXIDAZOLE.** USAN.
  Use: Anthelmintic.
TIP-A-LIP. (Eckerd) Metahomomethyl salicylate, allantoin, lanolin derivative, silicone, camphor, menthol, white petrolatum, mineral oil, white beeswax. Bot. ⅜ oz.
  Use: Lip protectant.
TIPRENOLOL. B.A.N. 3-Isopropylamino-1-[2-(methylthio)phenoxy]propan-2-ol.
  Use: Beta adrenergic receptor blocking agent.
- **TIPRENOLOL HCl.** USAN. (±)-1-(Isopropylamino)-3-[o-(methylthio)-phenoxy]-2-propanol HCl.
  Use: Anti-adrenergic (β-receptor).
- **TIPRINAST MEGLUMIDE.** USAN. A Mead Johnson investigative drug.
  Use: Anti-allergenic agent.
- **TIPRINAST MEGLUMINE.** USAN.
- **TIPROPIDIL HYDROCHLORIDE.** USAN.
  Use: Vasodilator.
- **TIQUINAMIDE HYDROCHLORIDE.** USAN.
  Use: Anticholingeric.
TIREND. (Norcliff Thayer) Caffeine 100 mg./Tab. Bot. 12s, 25s, 50s.
  Use: Stimulant.
TISSUE FIXATIVE AND WASH SOLUTION. (Wampole-Zeus) A modified Michel's tissue fixative and buffered wash solution.
  Use: To facilitate the transport and processing of fresh tissue biopsies.
TIS-U-SOL. (Travenol) NaCl 800 mg., KCl 40 mg., Mg sulf. 20 mg., sod. phosphate 8.75 mg., pot. phosphate 6.25 mg., dextrose 100 mg./100 mg. Bot. 250 ml., 1000 ml.
  Use: Physiologic irrigating solution.
TITAN. (Barnes-Hind) Benzalkonium chloride, EDTA, nonionic cleaner buffers. Bot. 1 oz., 2 oz.
  Use: Hard contact lens cleaning solution.
TITAN II WEEKLY CLEANING SOLUTION. (Barnes-Hind) Non-enzymatic surfactant cleaning solution.
  Use: Hard contact lens weekly cleaner.
- **TITANIUM DIOXIDE,** U.S.P. XXI.
  Use: Solar ray protectant.
TITICUM RIPENS.
  W/Oxyquinoline sulfate, charcoal.
  See: Triticoll, Tabs. (Western Research)
TITRALAC. (3M Products) **Tab.:** Cal. carb. 0.42 Gm./Tab. Bot. 9s, 40s, 60s, 100s, 500s, 1000s. **Liq.:** Cal. carb. 1.0 0.30 Gm./5 ml. Bot. 12 fl. oz.
  Use: Gastric antacid.
- **TIXANOX.** USAN.
  Use: Anti-allergic.
T-MATINIC. (Tennessee) Iron 100 mg., liver desic. 200 mg., stomach pwd. 100 mg., Vit. B-12 10 mcg., C 50 mg., folic acid 1 mg./Cap. Bot. 100s, 1000s. Vial 30 cc.
TOBAVIM. (Blue Cross) Vit. A 2500 I.U., D 400 I.U. C 60 mg., E 15 I.U., B-1 1.05 mg., B-2 1.2 mg., niacin

13.5 mg., B-6 1.05 mg., B-12 4.5 mcg./5 ml.
  Use: Vitamin supplement for children 4 years old to adults.
- **TOBRAMYCIN,** U.S.P. XXI. Opth. Oint., Ophth. Soln., U.S.P. XXI. An antibiotic obtained from cultures of *Streptomyces tenebrarius.*
  Use: Antibiotic.
  See: Tobrex, Soln., Oint. (Alcon)
- **TOBRAMYCIN SULFATE INJECTION,** U.S.P. XXI.
  See: Nebcin, Amp., Hyporet. (Lilly)
TOBREX OPHTHALMIC OINTMENT. (Alcon) Tobramycin 0.3% in sterile ointment base. Tube 3.5 Gm.
  Use: External opthalmic bacterial infections.
TOBREX SOLUTION. (Alcon) Tobramycin 0.3%. ophthalmic solution. Bot. 5 ml. w/dropper.
  Use: Topical ophthalmic anti-infective.
TOCAINIDE. USAN.
  Use: Cardiac depressant.
- **TOCAMPHYL.** USAN. 1-p, α-Dimethyl-benzyl camphorate 1:1 salt with 2,2'-iminodiethanol.
  Use: Choleretic.
  See: Gallogen, Tab. (Beecham-Massengill)
TOCE. Diethadione, B.A.N.
TOCLONOL EXPECTORANT. (Cenci) Carbetapentane citrate 7.25 mg., terpin hydrate 16.65 mg., menthol 0.83 mg., alcohol 7.2%, sodium citrate 66.15 mg., citric acid 6.65 mg., glycerin 45 min./5 cc. Bot. 3 oz., 6 oz., 16 oz.
  Use: Cough.
TOCLONOL W/CODEINE ELIXIR. (Cenci) Same as Toclonol Expectorant plus codeine 10 mg./5 cc. Bot. pt., gal.
TOCOPHER. (Columbia) Vit. E (from d-alpha tocopheryl acetate conc.) 100 I.U./Cap. Bot. 100s, 1000s.
TOCOPHER-400. (Columbia) Vit. E (d-alpha tocopheryl acetate conc.) 400 I.U./Cap. Bot. 100s, 1000s.
TOCOPHER-M. (Columbia) Vit. E (from mixed tocopheryls conc.) 1000 I.U./Cap. Bot. 50s, 100s.
TOCOPHER-PLUS. (Columbia) Vit. E(d-alpha tocopheryl acetate conc.) 200 I.U./Cap. Bot. 100s, 1000s.
TOCOPHEROL-DL-ALPHA. Vitamin E, U.S.P. XXI. 5,-7,8-Trimethyltocol, alpha-Tocopherol, dl-alpha-tocopherol, vit. E, wheat germ oil. dl-2,5,7,8-Tetramethyl-2-(4',8',12'-trimethyltridecyl)-6-chromanol.
  Cap. & Tab.:
    Denamone, Cap. (3 min., 10 min.) wheat germ oil (Vio-Bin)
    Ecofrol, Cap. (O'Neal)
    Eprolin, Gelseal (Lilly)
    Epsilan M, Cap. (Warren-Teed)
    Lib-E, Cap. (AVP)
  Oint.:
    Myopone (Drug Prods.)
  Sol.:
    Aquasol E, Sol. (USV Pharm.)
- **TOCOPHERSOLAN.** USAN. (+)-α-Toco-pheryl polyethylene glycol 1000 succinate.
  Use: Vitamin E supplement.
TOCOPHERYL ACETATE-d-ALPHA. Vitamin E, U.S.P. XXI.
  See: Aquasol E, Prods. (USV Labs.)

E-Ferol, Prep. (Fellows)
Epsilan-M, Cap. (Warren-Teed)
Lib-E-400, Cap. (AVP)
Tocopher, Cap. (Columbia)
Tokols, Cap. (Ulmer)
Vit. E. (Var. Mfr.)
TOCOPHERYL ACETATES, CONC. D-ALPHA. Vitamin E, U.S.P. XXI. d-alpha-Toco-pheryl acetate.
Use: Treatment of habitual & threatened abortion.
TOCOPHERYL ACID SUCCINATED D-ALPHA. Vitamin E, U.S.P. XXI.
See: E-Ferol Succinate, Tab., Cap. (Fellows)
Vit. E (Var. Mfr.)
TOCOSAMINE. (Trent) Sparteine sulfate 150 mg., sod. chl. 4.5 mg./cc. Amps. 1 cc. Box 12s, 100s.
Use: I.M. Oxytocic.
TODAY VAGINAL CONTRACEPTIVE SPONGE. (VLI) Nonoxynol-9, citric, sorbic, benzoic acid, sodium dihydrogen, citrate, sodium metabisulfite, polyurethane foam sponge. 3/pk.
Use: Contraceptive.
TODRAZOLINE. B.A.N. Ethyl 3-phthalazin-1-ylcarbazate. Binazine.
Use: Antihypertensive.
TOFENACIN. B.A.N. N-Methyl-2-(2-methyl-benzhydryloxy)ethylamine. Elamol hydrochloride
Use: Treatment of the Parkinsonian syndrome.
• **TOFENACIN HCl.** USAN. N-Methyl-2-[(o-methyl-α-phenyl-benzyl)oxy]-ethylamine HCl.
Use: Anticholinergic.
TOFRANAZINE. (Geigy) Combination of imipramine and promazine. Pending release.
TOFRANIL. (Geigy) Imipramine HCl **Tab.** 10 mg. Bot. 100s, 1000s; 25 mg. & 50 mg. Bot. 100s, 1000s. Unit Dose 100s. Gy-Pak 100s, 1 unit (12×100); 6 units (72×100). **Amps.** 25 mg./2 cc. w/ascorbic acid 2 mg., sod. bisulfite 1 mg., sod. sulfite 1 mg. Box 10s.
Use: Antidepressant, antienuretic.
TOFRANIL-PM. (Geigy) Imipramine pamoate 75 mg., 100 mg. , 125 mg. or 150 mg./Cap. Bot. 30s, 100s. 75 mg./Cap. Bot. 1000s. Unit dose 75 mg. and 150 mg. in 100s.
Use: Antidepressant.
• **TOLAMOLOL.** USAN. 4-[2-(2-Hydroxy-3-o-tolyloxypropylamino)ethoxy]benzamide.
Use: Beta adrenergic receptor blocking agent.
TOLANASE. Tolazamide, B.A.N.
• **TOLAZAMIDE,** U.S.P. XXI. Tabs., U.S.P. XXI. (Upjohn) 1-(Hexahydro-1-azepinyl)-3-(p-tolylsulfonyl)urea. 1-Perhydroazepin-yl-3-toluene-p-sulphonylurea. Tolanase. Benzenesulfonamide, N-[[(hexahydro-1H-azepin-1-yl)amino]carbonyl]-4-methyl-. 1-(Hexahydro-1H-azepin-1-yl)-3-(p-tolylsulfonyl)urea.
Use: Hypoglycemic agent.
See: Tolinase, Tab. (Upjohn)
• **TOLAZOLINE HYDROCHLORIDE,** U.S.P. XXI. Inj., Tab., U.S.P. XXI. Benzazoline HCl, 2-Benzyl-2-imidazoline HCl. Vasimid, Vasodil.
Use: Anti-adrenergic.
See: Priscoline, Prep. (Ciba)

Tazol, Tab. (Durst)
Toloxan, Tab. (Kenyon)
Tolzol, Tab. (Robinson)
• **TOLBUTAMIDE,** U.S.P. XXI. Tab. U.S.P. XXI. N-Butyl-N'-toluene-p-sulfonylurea. Benzenesulfonamide, N-[(butylamino)carbonyl]-4-methyl-. 1-Butyl-3-(p-tolylsulfonyl)urea.
Use: Hypoglycemic.
See: Orinase, Prep. (Upjohn)
SK-Tolbutamide, Tab. (SmithKline)
TOLBUTAMIDE SODIUM.
Use: Diagnostic aid (diabetes).
See: Orinase Diagnostic (Upjohn)
• **TOLCICLATE.** USAN.
Use: Antifungal.
TOLDIMFOS. B.A.N. 4-Dimethylamino-o-tolylphosphinic acid. Tonophosphan (sodium salt)
Use: Phosphorus source, veterinary medicine.
TOLECTIN. (McNeil Pharm) Tolmetin sodium 200 mg./Tab. Bot. 100s, 500s.
Use: Anti-inflammatory.
TOLECTIN DS. (McNeil Pharm) Tolmetin sodium 400 mg./Cap Bot. 100s.
Use: Anti-inflammatory.
• **TOLFAMIDE.** USAN.
Use: Enzyme inhibitor.
TOLFRINIC. (Ascher) Ferrous fumarate 600 mg., Vit. B-12 25 mcg., Vit. C 100 mg./Tab. Bot. 100s.
Use: Hemopoietic.
• **TOLIMIDONE.** USAN.
Use: Antiulcerative.
TOLINASE. (Upjohn) Tolazamide. **100 mg.**/Tab. Unit of use 100s. **250 mg.**/Tab. Unit of use 100s, 200s, 1000s. Unit Dose 100s. **500 mg.**/Tab. Unit of use 100s.
Use: Hypoglycemic agent.
• **TOLINDATE.** USAN.
Use: Antifungal.
See: Dalnate (USV Pharm.)
• **TOLIODIUM CHLORIDE.** USAN.
Use: Food additive.
• **TOLMETIN.** USAN.
Use: Anti-inflammatory.
• **TOLMETIN SODIUM,** U.S.P. XXI. Cap., Tab., U.S.P. XXI. Sodium 1-Methyl-5-p-toluoylpyrrole-2-acetic acid.
Use: Anti-inflammatory.
See: Tolectin, Tab. (McNeil).
Tolectin DS, Cap. (McNeil)
• **TOLNAFTATE,** U.S.P. XXI. Topical Aerosol Powder, Cream, Gel, Powder, Topical Soln., U.S.P. XXI. o-2-Naphthyl m,N-dimethyl-thiocarbanilate. Naphthmate-T; Tinaderm. Carbamothoic acid, methyl(3-methylphenyl)-, 0-2-naphthalenyl ester.
Use: Topical antifungal agent.
See: Aftate, Prods. (Plough)
Tinactin, Sol., Cream, Pow., Pow. Aer. (Schering)
TOLNATE HYDROCHLORIDE. Prothipendyl, B.A.N.
TOLONIUM CHLORIDE. 3-Amino-7-dimethyl-amino-2-methyl-phenazathionium. Blutene Chloride
TOLOXAN. (Kenyon) Tolazoline HCl 25 mg./Tab. Bot. 100s, 1000s.

TOLOXYCHLORINAL. 1,1'-[[(o-Tolyloxy)-methyl]ethy-
lenedioxy]bis[2,2,2-trichloro-ethanol].1,1'-[3-o-Tolylo-
xypropylenedioxy]bis (2,2,2-trichloroethanol. Propoxychlorinol
Use: Sedative.

3-o-TOLOXY-1,2-PROPANEDIOL.
See: Mephenesin, Prep. (Var.Mfr.)

TOLPENTAMIDE. B.A.N. 1-Cyclopentyl-3-toluene-p-
sulfonylurea.
Use: Hypoglycemic agent.

TOLPERISONE. B.A.N. 2-Methyl-3-piperidino-1-p-tolyl-
propan-1-one. Mydocalm
Use: Muscle relaxant.

TOLPIPRAZOLE. B.A.N. 5-Methyl-3-[2-(4-m-tolylpiper-
azin-1-yl)ethyl]pyrazole.
Use: Tranquilizer.

• **TOLPOVIDONE I-131.** USAN. ω-(p-Iodobenzyl)-po-
ly[1-(2-oxo-1-pyrrolidinyl)ethylene]-[131]I.
Use: Differential diagnosis of source of
hypoalbuminemia.
See: Raovin (Abbott)

TOLPRONINE. B.A.N. 1-(1,2,3,6-Tetrahydro-1-pyridyl)-
3-o-tolyloxypropan-2-ol. Proponesin [hydrochloride]
Use: Analgesic.

TOLPROPAMINE. B.A.N. NN-Dimethyl-3-phenyl-3-p-
tolypropylamine. Tylagel [hydrochloride]
Use: Antipruritic.

• **TOLPYRRAMIDE.** USAN. N-p-tolylsulfonyl-1-pyr-
rolidinecarboxamide.   1-Tetramethylene-3-p-tolysul-
fonylurea.
Use: Oral hypogiycemic

TOLSERAM CARBAMATE. Mephenesin, B.A.N.

• **TOLU BALSAM,** U.S.P. XXI.
Use: Pharm. necessity for Compound Benzoin
Tincture, expectorant.
See: Vicks Regular & Wild Cherry Medicated Cough
Drops (Vicks)

• **TOLU BALSAM SYRUP,** N.F. XVI. (Lilly) Bot. 16 fl.
oz.
Use: Vehicle.

• **TOLU BALSAM TINCTURE,** N.F. XVI.
Use: Flavor.

TOLUIDINE BLUE O CHLORIDE.
See: Blutene Chloride

TOLU-SED (No Sugar). (Scherer) Codeine phosphate
10 mg., guaifenesin 100 mg./5 ml. w/alcohol 10%.
Bot. 4 oz., pt.
Use: Temporary relief of coughs due to colds, and
minor throat irritations.

TOLU-SED DM (No Sugar). (Scherer) d-Methorphan
HBr. 10 mg., guaifenesin 100 mg./5 ml. w/alcohol
10%. Bot. 4 oz., pt.
Use: Temporary relief of cough due to the common
cold.

TOLYCAINE. B.A.N. Methyl 2-diethylaminoacetamido-
m-toluate. Baycain [hydrochloride]
Use: Local anesthetic.

TOLYD. (Galen) Mephenesin 325 mg., hyoscyamine
HBr 0.1105 mg., hyoscine HBr 0.013 mg.,
homatropine methyl bromide 0.039 mg., sodium
phenobarbital 8.1 mg./Tab. Bot. 100s, 1000s.
Use: Antispasmodic, muscle relaxant.

TOLZOL. (Robinson) Tolazoline HCl 25 mg./Tab. Bot.
100s, 1000s. Bulk pack 5000.

• **TOMOXETINE HYDROCHLORIDE.** USAN.

TONACON. (CMC) Vit. B-1 5 mg., B-2 5 mg., B-12 3
mcg., B-6 1 mg., niacinamide 100 mg., panthenol 4
mg., methionine 100 mg., choline 100 mg., iron 100
mg./fl. oz. Bot. pt., gal.
Use: Dietary supplement.

TONAMINE. (Kenyon) Liver, B-12 equiv. 1 mcg., ferrous
gluconate 44 mg., Vit. B-2 0.5 mg., folic acid 2 mg., d-
panthenol 2.5 mg., dl-methionine 10 mg., niacinamide
100 mg., procaine HCl 2%/2 cc. Vial 30 cc.

TONAVITE. (Apco) Vit. B-1 2 mg., niacinamide 5 mg.,
strychnine sulfate 1/60 gr., arsenous acid 1/60 gr.,
protochloride of mercury 1/50 gr., ex. gentian 1 gr.,
dried iron sulfate 2.5 gr./Tab. Bot. 100s.
Use: Tonic.

• **TONAZOCIN MESYLATE.** USAN.
Use: Analgesic.

TONBEC TABLETS. (A.V.P.) Vit. B-1 15 mg., B-2 10
mg., B-6 5 mg., nicotinamide 50 mg., Ca pantothenate
10 mg., ascorbic acid 300 mg./Tab. Bot. 60s.
Use: Therapeutic vitamin B and C supplement.

TONECOL. (A.V.P.) Promethazine w/expectorant and
vasoconstrictor. Bot. pt.
Use: Cough medicine.

TONECOL COUGH SYRUP. (A.V.P.) Dextromethorphan HBr 10 mg., phenylephrine HCl 5 mg.,
chlorpheniramine maleate 1 mg., sodium citrate 15
mg., guaifenesin 25 mg./5 ml. w/alcohol 7%. Bot.
1 pt.
Use: Treatment of cold symptoms, expectorant.

TONELAX TABLETS. (A.V.P.) Danthron 75 mg.,
calcium pantothenate 25 mg./Tab. Bot. 100s,
1000s.
Use: Peristaltic stimulant, laxative.

TONEX. (Vitarine) Vit. A 10,000 I.U., D 400 I.U., B-1 10
mg., B-2 5 mg., B-6 2 mg., pantothenic acid 10 mg.,
niacinamide 30 mg., cobalamin conc. 3 mcg., C
100 mg., alpha tocopherol 5 I.U., Fe 15 mg., Cu 1
mg., Iodine 0.15 mg., Mn 1 mg., Mg 5 mg., Zn 1.5
mg./Tab. Bot. 100s.

TONEX T. (Vitarine) Vit. A 10,000 I.U., D 400 I.U., B-1
15 mg., B-2 10 mg., B-6 2 mg., pantothenic acid 10
mg., niacinamide 100 mg., B-12 7.5 mcg., C 150
mg., E 5 I.U., Fe 15 mg., Cu 1 mg., Iodine 0.15
mg., Mn 1 mg., Mg 5 mg., Zn 1.5 mg./Tab. Bot.
100s.

TONOCO. (Sutliff & Case) Strychnine sulfate 0.8 mg.,
thyroid 4 mg., zinc phosphide 4 mg., iron 65 mg.,
calcium gluconate 97 mg./Tab. Bot. 1000s.
Use: Systemic stimulant and tonic.

TONOPHOSPHAN SODIUM SALT. Toldimfos, B.A.N.

TOOTHACHE DROPS. (DeWitt) Oil of cloves 10%,
Benzocaine 5%, creosote 4.8%, alcohol 20%,
ether 207 grains/oz. Bot. 0.25 oz.
Use: Temporary relief of pain from toothache.

TOP 20. (Eckerd) Benzocaine 20%, para-chlorometax-
ylenol 1% Tube 1½ oz.

TOP BRASS ZP-11. (Revlon) Zinc pyrithione 0.5% in
cream base.
Use: Anti-dandruff hairdress.

TOPEX. (Vicks Prods) Benzoyl peroxide 10%. Bot. 1 oz.
Use: Acne clearing lotion.

TOP-FORM. (Hoyt) Topical formfitting gel applicators.
Disposible trays for topical fluoride office
treatments, plus permanent trays for topical fluoride
home self treatments. Box 100s.
Use: Topical fluoride applications in home or office.

TOPIC. (Syntex) 5% benzyl alcohol in greaseless gel
base containing camphor, menthol, w/30%
isopropyl alcohol. Tube 2 oz.
Use: Antipruritic.

TOPICAL FLUORIDE. (Pacemaker). Acidulated
phosphate fluoride. Flavors: orange, bubblegum,
lime, raspberry, grape cinnamon. Liq. Bot. 4 oz., pt.

TOPICORT. (Hoechst) Desoximetasone 0.25%
emollient cream consisting of isopropyl myristate,
cetylstearyl alcohol, white petrolatum, mineral oil,
lanolin alcohol and purified water. Tubes 15 Gm.,
60 Gm.
Use: Synthetic corticosteroid for relief of
dermatoses.

TOPICORT LP. (Hoechst) Desoximetasone 0.05%.
Tubes 15 Gm, 60 Gm.
Use: Synthetic corticosteroid for relief of
dermatoses.

TOPICYCLINE. (Norwich Eaton) Tetracycline HCl 2.2
mg./ml. w/4-epitetracycline HCl, sodium bisulfite.
Bot. 70 ml.
Use: Topical treatment of acne vulgaris.

TOPILAR. Fluclorolone Acetonide, B.A.N.

TOPOCAINE.
See: Surfacaine (Lilly)

TOPSYN GEL. (Syntex) Fluocinonide 0.05% in gel
base of propylene glycol, propyl gallate, edetate
disodium, carbomer 940. Tube 15 Gm., 30 Gm., 60
Gm., 120 Gm.
Use: Topical corticosteroid.

• **TOPTERONE.** USAN.
Use: Anti-androgen.

• **TOQUIZINE.** USAN.
Use: Anticholinergic.

TORA. (Reid-Provident) Phentermine HCl 8 mg./Tab.
Bot. 1000s.

TORECAN. (Boehringer Ingelheim) Thiethylperazine
maleate **Tab.** 10 mg. Bot. 100s; **Amp.** 10 mg./2 cc.
(w/sod. metabisulfite 0.5 mg., ascorbic acid 2 mg.
sorbitol 40 mg., carbon dioxide) Box 20s, 100s.
Supp. 10 mg. (w/theobroma oil) Box 12s.
Use: Antiemetic and antinauseant.

TORNALATE TABLETS. (Winthrop Products)
Bitolterol mesylate.
Use: Bronchodilator.

TOROFOR. (Torch) Clioquinol 3% in hydrophilic
vehicle. Jar 2 oz., 1 lb.
Use: Cream anti-eczematous, antibacterial, anti-fungal, antipruritic.

TORULA YEAST, DRIED, Obtained by growing
Candida (torulopsis) utilis yeast on wood pulp
wastes (Nutritional Labs.) Conc. 100 lb. drums.
Use: Natural source of protein & Vitamin B-complex
vitamins.

• **TOSIFEN.** USAN.
Use: Anti-anginal.

TOSMILEN. Demecarium Bromide, B.A.N.

TOTACILLIN. (Beecham Labs) Ampicillin trihydrate
equivalent to:**Cap.** 250 mg./Cap. Bot. 100s, 500s.
500 mg./Cap. Bot. 50s, 500s. **Susp.:** 125 mg. 15
cc. Bot. 100 ml., 150 ml., 200 ml. 250 mg./5 cc.
Bot. 80 ml., 100 ml., 150 ml., 200 ml.

TOTACILLIN-N. (Beecham Labs) Ampicillin sodium 125
mg., 250 mg., 500 mg., 1 Gm., 2 Gm./Vial in 10s;
Piggyback vials 500 mg., 1 Gm., 2 Gm., in 25s;
Bulk pharm. pkg. 10 Gm. in 25s.
Use: Antibiotic.

TOTAL. (Allergan) Polyvinyl alcohol, edetate disodium
and benzalkonium chloride in a sterile buffered,
isotonic solution. Bot: 2 fl. oz., 4 fl. oz.
Use: Hard contact lens all purpose solution.

TOTAL ECLIPSE ALCOHOL BASE LOTION.
(Dorsey) Oxybenzone, padimate 0, glyceryl PABA.
SPF 15. Bot. 4 oz.
Use: Sunscreen.

TOTAL ECLIPSE MOISTURIZING BASE LOTION.
(Dorsey) Padimate 0, octyl salicylate, oxybenzone.
SPF 15. Bot. 4 oz., 6 oz.
Use: Sunscreen.

TOTAQUINE, Alkaloids from Cinchona bark, 7 to
12% quinine anhydr., 70% to 80% total alkaloids
(cinchonidine, cinchonine, quinidine & quinine).

TOTOMYCIN HYDROCHLORIDE. Tetracycline, U.S.P.
XXI.

TOXICODENDRON QUERCIFOLIUM EXTRACT.

TOXIFERINE. (Roche) Skeletal muscle relaxant;
pending release.

• **TOXIN, DIPHTHERIA FOR SCHICK TEST,** U.S.P.
XXI.

TOXO. (Wampole-Zeus) Toxoplasma antibody test system. Tests 120s.
Use: An IFA test system for the detection of
antibodies to toxoplasma gondii.

• **TOXOID, DIPHTHERIA,** U.S.P. XXI.
See: Diphtheria Toxoid, Aluminum Hydroxide,
Adsorbed

• **TOXOID, TETANUS ADSORBED,** U.S.P. XXI.

TOXOID MIXTURE.
See: Tri-Solgen, Vial (Lilly)

T.P.L. TROCHES. (Kasdenol) Triamite. Loz. 5 Gm.
15s.

TPM-TEST. (Wampole) Indirect hemagglutination test
for the qualitative and quantitative determination of
antibodies to *Toxoplasma gondii* in serum. Kits
120s.
Use: An aid in the diagnosis of toxoplasmosis.

TPN ELECTROLYTES. (Abbott) multiple electrolyte
additive: 321 mg sodium chloride, 331 mg calcium
chloride, 1491 mg potassium chloride, 508 mg
magnesium chloride, 2420 mg. sodium acetate; 20
ml in 50 ml fliptop or pintop vial or 20 ml Univ.
Add. Syr.
Use: Provides electrolytes during total parenteral
nutrition.

TP TROCHES. (Edward J. Moore) Triamite. Jars
500s, Box 15s.

Use: Temporary relief of minor sore throat & mouth.

• **TRACAZOLATE.** USAN.
  Use: Sedative.

TRAC TABS. (Hyrex) Atropine sulfate 0.03 mg., hyoscyamine 0.03 mg., methenamine 40.8 mg., methylene blue 5.4 mg., phenyl salicylate 18.1 mg., gelsemium 6.1 mg., benzoic acid 4.5 mg./Tab. Bot. 100s, 1000s.
  Use: Urinary tract infections.

TRAC TABS 2X. (Hyrex) Atropine sulfate 0.06 mg., hyoscyamine 0.06 mg., methenamine 81.6 mg., methylene blue 10.8 mg., phenyl salicylate 36.2 mg., gelsemium 12.2 mg., benzoic acid 9.0 mg./Tab. Bot. 100s, 1000s.
  Use: Urinary tract infections.

TRACE. (Lorvic) Erythrosine conc. sol. Squeeze Bot. 30 ml., 60 ml. Dispenser Packets 200s.
  Use: Plaque dye sol.

TRACEPLEX. (Enzyme Process) Iron 30 mg., iodine 0.1 mg., Cu 0.5 mg., Mg 40 mg., zinc 10 mg., B-12 5 mcg./4 Tabs. Bot. 100s, 250s.
  Use: Mineral supplement.

TRACILON. (Savage) Triamcinolone diacetate 40 mg./ml suspension. Vial 5 ml.
  Use: Corticosteroid.

TRACO-DISCS. (Neoco; Nion) Mag. trisilicate 3 gr., Cal. carb. 7 gr./Disc. Bot. 100s.
  Use: Antacid, adsorbent.

TRACRIUM INJECTION. (Burroughs Wellcome) Atracurium besylate 10 mg./ml. Amp. 5 ml. Box 10s.
  Use: Surgical muscle relaxant.

TRAFURIL. Thurfyl Nicotinate, B.A.N.

• **TRAGACANTH,** N.F. XVI.
  Use: Pharmaceutical aid (suspending agent).

TRAL FILMTABS. (Abbott) Hexocyclium methylsulfate 25 mg./Tab. Bot. 100s.
  Use: Anticholinergic agent.

TRAL GRADUMETS. (Abbott) Hexocyclium methylsulfate 50 mg./Gradumet. Bot. 100s.
  Use: Anticholinergic agent in sustained release form.

TRALMAG. (O'Neal, Jones & Feldman) Dihydroxyaluminum aminoacetate 200 mg., magnesium hydroxide 150 mg., aluminum hydroxide gel 150 mg./5 ml. Bot. 12 oz.
  Use: Antacid.

• **TRALONIDE.** USAN.
  Use: Glucocorticoid.

• **TRAMADOL HYDROCHLORIDE.** USAN.
  Use: Analgesic.

• **TRAMAZOLINE,** USAN. 2-[(5,6,7,8-Tetrahydro-1-naphthyl)amino]-2-imidazoline.
  Use: Adrenergic.

TRANCAPS. (Seatrace) Brompheniramine maleate 12 mg., phenylephrine HCl 15 mg., phenylpropanolamine HCl 15 mg./Cap. Bot. 100s, 1000s.
  Use: Antihistaminic, nasal decongestant.

TRANCIN. Fluphenazine.
  Use: Treat anxiety and tension.

TRANCOGESICO TABLETS. (Winthrop Products) Dipyrone, chlormezanone.
  Use: Analgesic, antipyretic, muscle relaxant.

TRANCOPAL. (Winthrop-Breon) Chlormezanone 100 mg./Cap. Bot. 100s. 200 mg./Cap. Bot. 100s, 1000s.
  Use: Relaxant and tranquilizer for mild anxiety and tension states.

• **TRANEXAMIC ACID.** USAN. Trans-4-(Aminornethyl) cyclohexanecarboxylic acid. Amstat. (lederle) Amikapron.
  Use: Hemostatic.

TRANMEP. (Reid-Provident) Meprobamate 400 mg./Tab. Bot. 100s, 1000s.
  Use: Relief of anxiety and tension.

TRANQUIL. (Kenyon) Mephenesin 400 mg., mephobarbital 10 mg., hyoscine HBr 0.25 mg./Tab. Bot. 1000s.

TRANQUIL CAPSULES. (Vortech) Pyrilamine maleate 25 mg./Cap. Bot. 42s, 1000s.
  Use: Mild relaxant.

■ **TRANQUILIZERS.**
  See: A-poxide, Cap. (Abbott)
    Atarax, Prep. (Roerig)
    Centrax, Cap. (Parke-Davis)
    Compazine, Prep. (SmithKline)
    Equanil, Tab., Susp. (Wyeth)
    Equanil L.A., Cap. (Wyeth)
    Fenarol, Tab. (Winthrop Products)
    Haldol, Tab., Inj., Conc. Sol. (McNeil)
    Harmonyl, Tab. (Abbott)
    Librium, Cap., Ing. (Roche)
    Loxitane, Prod. (Lederle)
    Mellaril, Tab., Sol. (Sandoz)
    Meprobamate (Various Mfr.)
    Miltown, Prep. (Wallace)
    Permitil, Prep. (Schering)
    Proketazine Maleate, Prep. (Wyeth)
    Prolixin, Prep. (Squibb)
    Sparine HCl, Prep. (Wyeth)
    Stelazine, Prep. (SmithKline)
    Taractan, Prep. (Roche)
    Thorazine HCl, Prep. (SmithKline)
    Tindal, Tab. (Schering)
    Trancopal, Cap. (Winthrop-Breon)
    Tranxene, Cap. (Abbott)
    Trilafon, Prep. (Schering)
    Tybatran, Cap. (Robins)
    Ultran, Prep. (Lilly)
    Valium, Prep. (Roche)
    Vesprin, Prep. (Squibb)
    Vistaril, Prep. (Pfizer)

TRANQUILS CAPSULES. (Blue Cross) Pyrilamine maleate 25 mg./Cap. Bot. 30s.
  Use: Night time sleep aid.

TRANQUILS TABLETS. (Blue Cross) Acetaminophen 300 mg., pyrilamine maleate 25 mg./Tab. Bot. 30s.
  Use: Analgesic & night time sleep aid.

TRANSACT. (Westwood) Laureth-4 6%, sulfur 2%, alcohol 37%, in greaseless gel base. Tube 1 oz.
  Use: Drying & peeling of acne skin.

TRANSCLOMIPHENE. (E)-2-[p-(2-Chloro-1, 2-di-phenylvinyl) phenoxy] triethylamine.
TRANSDERM-NITRO. (Ciba) Nitroglycerin 2.5 mg., 5 mg., 10 mg. or 15 mg. **2.5 mg.:** 2.5 mg./24 hr. Pkg. 30s. **5 mg.:** 5 mg./24 hr. Pkg. 7s, 30s. **10 mg.:** 10 mg./24 hr. Pkg. 30s. **15 mg.:** 15 mg./24 hr. Pkg. 30s.
Use: Prevention and treatment of angina pectoris due to coronary artery disease.
TRANSDERM-SCOP. (Ciba) Scopolamine 0.5 mg. per 2-unit blister pkg. (programmed delivery over 3 day period).
Use: Antiemetic, antinauseant.
TRANSITHAL. Buthalitone Sodium, B.A.N.
TRANSTHYRETIN EIA. (Abbott) Test kits 100s.
Use: Enzyme immunoassay for the quantitative determination of transthyretin in human serum or plasma.
TRANXENE CAPSULES. (Abbott) Clorazepate dipotassium 3.75 mg., 7.5 mg., 15 mg./Cap. Bot. 30s, 100s, 500s. Abbo-Pac 100s.
Use: Minor tranquilizer.
TRANXENE TABLETS. (Abbott) Chlorazepate dipotassium tab. 3.75 mg., 7.5 mg or 15 mg./Tab. Bot. 100s.
Use: Mild Tranquilizer.
TRANXENE-SD. (Abbott) Chlorazepate dipotassium 22.5 mg./Tab. Bot. 100s.
Use: Minor tranquilizer.
TRANXENE-SD HALF STRENGTH TABLETS. (Abbott) Chlorazepate dipotassium 11.25 mg./Tab. Bot. 100s.
Use: Minor tranquilizer.
TRANYLCYPROMINE. B.A.N. (+)trans-2-Phenylcyclo-propylamine. Parnate (sulfate).
Use: Monoamine oxidase inhibitor; antidepressant.
• **TRANYLCYPROMINE SULFATE,** U.S.P. XXI. Tab., U.S.P. XXI. Trans-dl-2-phenylcyclopropylamine sul-fate (+)-trans-2-phenylcyclopropylamine sulfate (2:-1).
Use: Antidepressant.
See: Parnate, Tab. (SmithKline)
TRAPENS. (Mills) Triticum 4 gr., oxyquinoline sulf. 1/20 gr., pow. charcoal ½ gr./Tab., Bot. 100s.
TRASICOR. (Ciba) Oxprenolol HCl, B.A.N.
TRATES. (Reid-Provident) Nitroglycerin 2.5 mg. or 6.5 mg./Granucap. Bot. 100s.
TRAUMACAL. (Mead Johnson) Nutritionally complete formula for traumatized patients. Cans 8 oz. Vanilla flavor.
Use: Specific for nitrogen and energy needs in a limited volume for multiple trauma and major burns.
TRAUM-AID HBC. (American McGaw) Advanced high branched chain amino acids diet.
Use: For trauma & sepsis patients.
T-RAU TABLET. (Tennessee Pharm.) Rauwolfia ser-pentina 50 mg. or 100 mg./Tab. Bot. 100s, 1000s.
Use: Hypotensive, tranquilizer.
TRAVAMIN. (Travenol) Protein Hydrolysate (Injection). 5% w/5% dextrose. Bot. 1000 ml. 5% w/12.5% fructose, 2.4% alcohol. Bot. 1000 ml. 10% Bot. 500 ml.

TRAV-AREX. (Columbia) Dimenhydrinate 50 mg./Cap. Bot. 24s, 100s, 1000s.
Use: Motion sickness.
TRAVASE. (Flint) Proteolytic enzyme ointment, from bacillus subtilis; 82,000 casein units of proteolytic activity/ Gm. Tube 14.2 Gm.
Use: Debriding agent.
TRAVASOL. (Travenol) Crystalline L-Amino acids injection 5.5%, 8.5% (with or without electrolytes). IV Bot. 500 ml.
Use: Parenteral nutrition.
TRAVASOL 3.5% M INJECTION WITH ELECTROLYTE #48. (Travenol) Crystalline L-Amino acids 3.5% Sol. Bot. I.V. 500 ml., 1000 ml.
Use: Parenteral nutrition.
TRAVEL AIDS. (Faraday) Dimenhydrinate 50 mg./Tab. Bot. 30s.
Use: Motion sickness.
TRAVEL-EZE. (Approved) Pyrilamine maleate 25 mg., hyoscine hydrobromide 0.325 mg./Tab. Pkg. 20s.
Use: Motion sickness.
TRAVEL SICKNESS. (Walgreen) Dimenhydrinate 50 mg./Tab. Bot. 24s.
Use: Nausea, dizziness, vomiting.
TRAVELTABS. (Geneva) Dimenhydrinate 50 mg./Tab. Bot. 100s.
Use: Motion sickness.
TRAVERT. (Travenol) Invert sugar. Sol (5%) water or saline 50 mg./cc., Bot. 1000 cc. Water or saline 100 mg./cc., Bot.1000 cc. In 0.9% NaCl Bot. 1000 cc. In 0.3% KCL and 0.45% NaCl Bot. 1000 cc. W/electrolyte No. 1 Bot. 1000 cc. W/electrolyte No. 2 Bot. 500 cc., 1000 cc., W/electrolyte No. 3 Bot. 1000 cc. W/electrolyte No. 4 Bot. 250, 500 cc. Sol. (10%)
• **TRAZODONE HYDROCHLORIDE,** USAN. 2-[3-[4-(m-Chlorophenyl)-1-piperazinyl]propyl]-1,2,4-triazolo[-4,3-a]pyridin-3(2H)-one monohydrochloride.
Use: Antidepressant.
See: Desyrel, Tab. (Mead Johnson)
TREATS PLUS IRON. (Eckerd) Vit. A 5000 I.U., D 400 I.U., E 15 I.U., C 75 mg., folic acid 0.4 mg., thiamin 1.9 mg., riboflavin 2.1 mg., niacin 25 mg., B-6 2.5 mg., B-12 7.5 mcg. iron 22.5 mg./Cap. Bot. 100s.
Use: Vitamin supplement with iron.
• **TREBENZOMINE HYDROCHLORIDE,** USAN.
Use: Antidepressant.
TRECATOR S.C. (Ives) Ethionamide. 2-Ethyl thi-oisonicotinamide. 250 mg./Tab. Bot. 100s.
Use: Anti-tubercular agent.
• **TRELOXINATE,** USAN.
Use: Antihyperlipoproteinemic.
TREMONIL HYDROCHLORIDE. Methixene, B.A.N.
TRENBOLONE. B.A.N. 17β-Hydroxyoestra-4,9,11-trien-3-one. Finajet (acetate).
Use: Anabolic steroid, veterinary medicine.
• **TRENBOLONE ACETATE,** USAN.
Use: Anabolic steroid.
TRENDAR. (Whitehall) Acetaminophen 325 mg., pamabrom 25 mg./Tab. Bot. 24s, 50s.

Use: Menstrual pain.
TRENIMON. Triaziquone, B.A.N.
TRENTADIL HYDROCHLORIDE. Bamifylline, B.A.N.
TRENTAL. (Hoechst) Pentoxifylline.
Use: Oral hemorrheologic agent for peripheral vascular disease.
TREOSULFAN. B.A.N.L-Threitol 1,4-dimethane-sulphonate.
• **TREPIPAM MALEATE.** USAN.
Use: Sedative.
• **TRESTOLONE ACETATE.** USAN.
Use: Antineoplastic, androgen.
TRESADERM. (MSD AGVET) Thiabendazole 40 mg., dexamethasone 1 mg., neomycin 3.2 mg./ml. solution.
Use: Dermatologic solution, veterinary medicine.
TRESCATYL. Ethionamide, B.A.N.
TRETAMINE. B.A.N. 2,4,6-Tri(aziridin-1-yl)-1,3,5-triazine. Triethanomelamine; Triethylene Melamine; TEM.
Use: Antineoplastic agent.
TRETHINIUM TOSYLATE. B.A.N. 2-Ethyl-1,2,3,4-tetrahydro-2-methylisoquinolinium toluene-p-sulfonate.
Use: Hypotensive.
TRETHOCANOIC ACID. 3-Hydroxy-3,7,11-trimethyldodecanoic acid.
Use: Anticholesteremic.
• **TRETINOIN,** U.S.P. XXI. Cream, Gel, Topical Soln., U.S.P. XXI. 3,7-Dimethyl-9-(2,6,6-trimethylcyclohex-1-enyl)nona-2,4,6,8-all-transtetraenoic acid. All trans-Retinoic acid. Vit. A acid.
Use: Keratolytic.
See: Retin-A, Cream, Gel, Sol. (Ortho)
TREVINTIX. Prothionamide, B.A.N.
TREXIN. (A.V.P.) Tetracycline HCl 250 mg./Cap. Bot. 100s.
Use: Antibiotic.
TRIACET CREAM. (Lemmon) Triamcinolone acetonide 0.025%, 0.1%, 0.5%. **0.025%:** Tube 15 Gm., 80 Gm.; **0.1%:** Tube 15 Gm., 80 Gm.; **0.5%:** Tube 15 Gm.
Use: Topical anti-inflammatory steroid.
• **TRIACETIN,** U.S.P. XXI. Glyceryl triacetate.
Use: Topical antifungal.
See: Enzactin, Preps. (Ayerst)
Fungacetin, Oint. (Blair)
TRIACETYLOLEANDOMYCIN. Troleandomycin.
Use: Antibiotic.
TRIACORT. (Kay) Triamcinolone deacetate 40 mg./ml. Vial 5 ml.
Use: Anti-inflammatory.
TRIACT LIQUID. (Winthrop Products) Aluminum, magnesium hydroxide, simethicone.
Use: Antacid, antiflatulent.
TRIACT TABLETS. (Winthrop Products) Aluminum, magnesium hydroxide, simethicone.
Use: Antacid, antiflatulent.
TRIAFED. (Wolins) Triprolidine HCl 2.5 mg., pseudoephedrine 60 mg./Tab. Bot. 100s, 1000s.
• **TRIAFUNGIN.** USAN.
Use: Antifungal.
• **TRIAMCINOLONE,** U.S.P. XXI. Tabs., U.S.P. XXI. 9-

Alpha fluoro-16-alpha hydroxy-prednisolone. 9-Fluoro-11β, 16α,17,21-tetrahydroxypregna-1,4-diene-3, 20-dione.
Use: Adrenocortical steroid (anti-inflammatory).
See: Aristocort, Tab., Syr. (Lederle)
Aristoderm, Foam (Lederle)
Aristospan, Parenteral (Lederle)
Kenacort, Tab., Syr. (Squibb)
SK-Triamcinolone, Tab. (SmithKline)
• **TRIAMCINOLONE ACETONIDE,** U.S.P. XXI. Topical Aerosol, Cream, Oint., Dental Paste, Lotion, Sterile Susp., U.S.P. XXI. 9-α-fluoro-16-α-17-α-isopropylidenedioxy-Δ' hydrocortisone. Pregna-1,4-diene-3,20-dione,8-fluoro-11,21-dihydroxy-16-17-[(1-methylethylidene)bis(oxy)]-,(11β,16α)-. 9-Fluoro-11β,16α,17,21-tetrahydroxypregna-1,4-diene-3,20-dione cyclic 16,-17-acetal with acetone.
Use: Glucocorticoid, topical anti-inflammatory.
See: Aristocort, Cream, Oint (Lederle)
Aristoderm Foam (Lederle)
Aristogel, Gel (Lederle)
Kenalog Preps. (Squibb)
Triacet, Cream (Lemmon)
Tramacin, Cream (Johnson & Johnson)
Tri-Kort, Inj. (Keene)
W/Neomycin, gramicidin, Nystatin.
See: Mycolog, Preps. (Squibb)
• **TRIAMCINOLONE ACETONIDE SODIUM PHOSPHATE.** USAN.
Use: Glucocorticoid.
See: Aristosol (Lederle)
• **TRIAMCINOLONE DIACETATE,** U.S.P. XXI. Sterile Susp., Syrup, U.S.P. XXI. 9-Alpha-fluoro-16-alpha-hydroxyprednisolone diacetate. 9-Fluoro-11β, 16α, 17,21-tetrahydroxy-pregna-1,4-diene-3,20-dione-16,2-1-diacetate.
Use: Glucocorticoid.
See: Amcort, Inj. (Keene)
Aristocort Diacetate Forte (Lederle)
Aristocort Diacetate Intralesional, Inj. (Lederle)
Cinex-40, Inj. (Tunex)
Kenacort, Syr. (Squibb)
Tracilon, Susp. (Savage)
Triam-Forte, Inj. (Hyrex)
• **TRIAMCINOLONE HEXACETONIDE,** U.S.P. XXI. Sterile Susp., U.S.P. XXI. 9-Fluoro-11β,16α,17,21-tetra hyroxypregna-1,-4-diene-3,20-dione cyclic 16, 17-acetal with acetone, 21-(3,3-dimethylbutyrate).
Use: Injectable glucocorticoid.
See: Aristospan, Prep. (Lederle)
TRIAM-FORTE. (Hyrex) Triamcinolone diacetate 40 mg./ml. Vial 5 ml.
Use: Adrenocortical steroid therapy.
TRIAMINIC. (Dorsey) Pyrilamine maleate 25 mg., pheniramine maleate 25 mg., phenylpropanolamine HCl 50 mg./Timed-release Tab. Bot. 100s, 250s.
Use: Antihistaminic.
W/Dormethan, terpin hydrate.
See: Tussaminic, Tab. (Dorsey)
TRIAMINIC ALLERGY TABLETS. (Dorsey) Phenylpropanolamine HCl 25 mg., chlorpheniramine maleate 4 mg./Tab. Blister pk. 12×24s.

Use: Decongestant, antihistamine.

TRIAMINIC CHEWABLES. (Dorsey) Phenylpropanolamine HCl 6.25 mg., chlorpheniramine maleate 0.5 mg./Tab. Bot. 24s.
Use: Chewable decongestant for children.

TRIAMINIC COLD SYRUP. (Dorsey) Phenylpropanolamine HCl 12.5 mg., chlorpheniramine maleate 2 mg./5 ml. Bot. 4 oz., 8 oz., 1 pt., 1 gal.
Use: Decongestant in colds and allergies.

TRIAMINIC COLD TABLETS. (Dorsey) Phenylpropanolamine HCl 12.5 mg., chlorpheniramine maleate 2 mg./Tab. Bot. 24s, 48s.
Use: Temporary relief of cold, flu, hay fever, sinusitis symptoms.

TRIAMINIC-DM COUGH FORMULA. (Dorsey) Phenylpropamolamine HCl 12.5 mg., dextromethorphan HBr 10 mg./5 ml. Bot. 4 oz., 8 oz.
Use: Antitussive, decongestant.

TRIAMINIC EXPECTORANT. (Dorsey) Phenylpropanolamine HCl 12.5 mg., guaifenesin 100 mg./5 ml. w/alcohol 5%.. Bot. 4 oz., 8 oz., 1 pt.
Use: Decongestant-expectorant.

TRIAMINIC EXPECTORANT W/CODEINE. (Dorsey) Phenylpropanolamine HCl 12.5 mg., codeine phosphate 10 mg., guaifenesin 100 mg./5 ml. w/alcohol 5%. Bot. 4 oz., pt.

TRIAMINIC EXPECTORANT DH. (Dorsey) Guaifenesin 100 mg., phenylpropanolamine HCl 12.5 mg., pheniramine maleate 6.25 mg., pyrilamine maleate 6.25 mg., hydrocodone bitartrate 1.67 mg./5 ml. w/alcohol 5%. Bot. 1 pt.
Use: Treatment of cough.

TRIAMINIC JUVELETS. (Dorsey) Phenylpropanolamine HCl 25 mg., pyrilamine maleate 12.5 mg., pheniramine maleate 12.5 mg./Tab. Bot. 50s.
Use: Decongestant in common cold.

TRIAMINIC ORAL INFANT DROPS. (Dorsey) Phenylpropanolamine HCl 20 mg., pheniramine maleate 10 mg., pyrilamine maleate 10 mg./ml. Dropper bot. 15 ml.
Use: Decongestant and antihistaminic action.

TRIAMINIC-12 TABLETS. (Dorsey) Phenylpropanolamine HCl 75 mg., chlorpheniramine maleate 12 mg./S.R. tab. Pkg. 10s, 20s.
Use: Decongestant, antihistaminic.

TRIAMINIC TR TABLETS. (Dorsey) Phenylpropanolamine HCl 50 mg., pheniramine maleate 25 mg., pyrilamine maleate 25 mg./T.R. Tab.
Use: Decongestant, antihistaminic.

TRIAMINICIN TABLETS. (Dorsey) Phenylpropanolamine HCl 25 mg., aspirin 450 mg., caffeine 30 mg., chlorpheniramine maleate 2 mg./Tab. Pkg. 2s, 12s, 24s, 48s, 100s.
Use: Treatment of the common cold.

TRIAMINICOL MULTI SYMPTOM COLD SYRUP. (Dorsey) Phenylpropanolamine HCl 12.5 mg., pyrilamine maleate 6.25 mg., chlorpheniramine

maleate 2 mg., dextromethorphan HBr 10 mg./5 ml. (cough syr.) Bot. 4 oz., 8 oz.
Use: Cough depressant & decongestant.

TRIAMINICOL MULTI-SYMPTOM COLD TABLET. (Dorsey) Phenylpropanolamine HCl 12.5 mg., chlorpheniramine maleate 2 mg., dextromethorphan HBr 10 mg./Tab. Bot. 24s, 48s.
Use: Temporary relief of nasal congesion, cold, flu, bronchial irritation.

TRIAMINILONE-16,17-ACETONIDE.
See: Triamcinolone acetonide.

2,4,7-TRIAMINO-6-PHENYLPTERIDINE. Triamterene, U.S.P. XXI.

TRIAMOLONE 40. (O'Neal, Jones & Feldman) Triamcinolone diacetate 40 mg./ml. Vial 5 ml.

TRIAMONIDE 40. (O'Neal, Jones & Feldman) Triamcinolone acetonide 40 mg./ml. Vial 5 ml.

• **TRIAMPYZINE SULFATE.** USAN. 2-(Dimethylamino)-3,5,6-trimethylpyrazine sulfate.
Use: Anticholinergic.

• **TRIAMTERENE,** U.S.P. XXI. Caps., U.S.P. XXI. (SmithKline) 2,4,7-Triamino-6-phenyl-pteridine. 2,4,7-Pteridinetriamine,6-phenyl-Dytac.
Use: Diuretic.
See: Dyrenium, Cap. (SmithKline)
W/Hydrochlorothiazide.
Use: Diuretic.
See: Dyazide, Cap. (SmithKline)

TRIANIDE. (Seatrace) Triamcinolone acetonide 40 mg./ml. Vial 5 cc.

TRIAPRIN. (Dunhall) Acetaminophen 250 mg., salicylamide 250 mg., pentobarbital 25 mg./Caps. Bot. 100s, 500s.
Use: Analgesic, sedative.

TRIAPRIN-DC. (Dunhall) Acetaminophen 250 mg., salicylamide 250 mg., dihydrocodeine bitartrate 20 mg./Cap. Bot. 100s, 500s.
Use: Analgesic, antitussive.

TRIASYN B. (Panray) Vit. B-1 2 mg., niacinamide 20 mg., B-2 3 mg./Tab. Bot. 1000s.
Use: Nutritional supplement.

TRIATROPHENE. (Lannett) Magnesium trisilicate 7½ gr., phenobarbital ⅛ gr., atropine sulfate ¹/₁₀₀₀ gr./Tab. Bot. 1000s.
Use: G.I. sedative.

TRIAVIL. (Merck Sharp & Dohme) Perphenazine 4 mg., amitriptyline HCl 10 mg./salmon-colored Tab.; perphenazine 2 mg., amitriptyline HCl 25 mg./orange Tab.; perphenazine 4 mg., amitriptyline 25 mg./yellow Tab.; perphenazine 2 mg., amitriptyline HCl 10 mg./blue Tab. Bot. 100s, 500s. Unit dose 100s. Perphenazine 4 mg., amitryptyline 50 mg./orange Tab. Bot. 60s, 100s. Unit dose 100s.
Use: Tranquilizer, antidepressant.

TRIAZIQUONE. B.A.N. Tri(aziridin-1-yl)-1,4-benzoquinone. Trenimon
Use: Antineoplastic agent.

• **TRIAZOLAM.** USAN.
Use: Sedative, hypnotic.
See: Halcion, Tab. (Upjohn).

TRI-BAY-FLOR DROPS. (Bay) Vit. A 1500 I.U., D 400 I.U., C 35 mg., fluoride 0.5 mg./1 ml. Bot. 50 ml.
Use: Multivitamin with fluoride.
TRIBARB. (Lannett) Cap. Bot. 100s, 1000s.
• **TRIBENOSIDE.** USAN. Ethyl 3,5,6-tri-O-benzyl-D-glucofuranoside. Glyvenol Not available in U.S.
Use: Venoprotective agent.
TRI-BIOCIN. (Approved) Bacitracin 400 u., polymyxin B sulfate 5000 u., neomycin 5 mg./Gm. Tube ½ oz.
Use: Topical antibiotic.
TRI-BIOTIC OINTMENT. (Standex) Polymyxin B sulfate 5,000 u., bacitracin 400 u., neomycin sulfate 5 mg./Gm. Tube ½ oz.
TRIBROMOETHANOL. 2,2,2-Tribromoethanol.
Use: Anesthetic (inhalation).
TRIBROMOMETHANE. Bromoform.
• **TRIBROMSALAN.** USAN. 3,4′,5-Tribromosalicylanilide. Hilomid.
Use: Germicide.
See: Diaphene (or ASC-4) (Stecker)
    Tuasol 100 (Merrell Dow)
TRI-CALSATE. (Paxton) Tri-cal. phosphate 35.5%, tri-sod. phosphate 12.5%, sod. citrate 52%. Aq. susp., Bot. 4½ oz., 18 oz.
Use: Antacid.
• **TRICETAMIDE.** USAN. 3,4,5-Trimethoxybenzoylglycine diethylamide.
Use: Sedative.
TRI-CHLOR. (Gordon) Trichloracetic acid 80%. Bot. 15 cc.
Use: Topical, as a caustic verruca cauterant.
TRICHLORAN.
See: Trichloroethylene
• **TRICHLORMETHIAZIDE,** U.S.P. XXI. Tab., U.S.P. XXI. 3-Dichloromethyl-6-chloro-7-sulfamyl-3,4-dihydro-1,2,4-benzothiadiazine-1,1-dioxide. 6-Chloro-3-(dichloromethyl)-3,4-dihydro-2H-1,2,4-benzothiadiazine-7-sulfonamide-1,1-Dioxide.
Use: Diuretic; antihypertensive.
See: Aquex, Tab. (Lannett)
    Metahydrin, Tab. (Merrell Dow)
    Naqua, Tab. (Schering)
    Rochlomethiazide, Tab. (Robinson)
W/Reserpine.
See: Metatensin, Tab. (Merrell Dow)
    Naquival, Tab. (Schering)
TRICHLORMETHINE (I.N.N.).
See: Trimustine, B.A.N.
• **TRICHLOROACETIC ACID,** U.S.P. XXI. Acetic acid, trichloro.
Use: Topical, as a caustic.
TRICHLOROBUTYL ALCOHOL.
See: Chlorobutanol
TRICHLOROCARBANILIDE. W/Salicylic acid, sulfur.
1,1,1-TRICHLORO-2-METHYL-2-PROPANOL. Chlorobutanol, N.F. XVI.
Use: Analgesic (inhalation).
• **TRICHLOROMONOFLUOROMETHANE,** N.F. XVI.
Use: Aerosol propellant.
TRICHLORPHON. Metriphonate, B.A.N.
TRICHOLINE CITRATE.
See: Choline citrate

TRICHOMYCIN. Hachimycin, B.A.N.
TRICHORAD. Acinitrazole, B.A.N.
TRICHOTINE. (Reed & Carnrick) **Powd.** Sodium lauryl sulf., sod. perborate, chloride, aromatics. Pkg. 5, 12, 20 oz. **Liq.** Sodium lauryl sulfate, sodium borate, ethyl alcohol 8%, aromatics. Bot. 4 oz., 8 oz.
Use: Vaginal douche.
TRICIDIN. (Amlab) Neomycin sulf. 3.5 mg., gramicidin 0.25 mg., polymyxin B sulf. 2000 u., benzocaine 1%/Gm. Oint. Tube ½ oz.
Use: Topically, antibiotic and anesthetic ointment.
• **TRICIRIBINE PHOSPHATE.** USAN.
Use: Antineoplastic.
• **TRICITRATES ORAL SOLUTION,** U.S.P. XXI.
TRICLOBISONIUM. Triburon, Oint. (Roche)
TRICLOBISONIUM CHLORIDE. Hexamethylenebis[dimethyl[1-methyl-3-(2,2,6-trimethylcyclohexyl)propyl]-ammonium] Dichloride.
Use: Topical anti-infective.
• **TRICLOCARBAN.** USAN. 3,4,4′-Trichloro-carbanilide.
Use: Germicide.
See: Artra Beauty Ban (Plough)
W/Clofulcarban.
See: Safeguard Bar Soap, (P & G)
• **TRICLOFENOL PIPERAZINE.** USAN. Piperazine (1:2) with (2,4,5-trichlorophenol).
Use: Anthelmintic (nematodes).
TRICLOFOS. B.A.N. 2,2,2-Trichloroethyl dihydrogen phosphate. Tricloryl (mono-sodium salt)
Use: Hypnotic.
• **TRICLOFOS SODIUM.** USAN.
Use: Hypnotic; sedative.
See: Triclos, Tab., Liq. (Merrell Dow)
• **TRICLONIDE.** USAN.
Use: Anti-inflammatory.
TRICLORYL MONO-SODIUM SALT. Triclofos, B.A.N.
• **TRICLOSAN.** USAN. 5-Chloro-2-(2,4-dichlorophenoxy)phenol.
Use: Antibacterial
See: Clearasil Soap (Vicks)
TRI-CONE. (Glaxo) Amylase 10 mg., Prolase 10 mg., lipase 10 mg., simethicone 40 mg./Cap. Bot. 60s, 500s.
Use: Aid digestion, relieve gaseousness.
TRI-CONE PLUS. (Glaxo) Amylase 10 mg., prolase 10 mg., lipase 10 mg., simethicone 40 mg., hyoscyamine sulfate 0.025 mg./Tab. Bot. 60s, 500s.
Use: Digestion aid, antiflatulant.
TRICONOL VAGINAL CREAM. (Coastal) Sulfanilamide 15%, 9-aminoacridine HCl 0.2%, allantoin 2.0%. Tab. Bot. 100s.
Use: Vaginal infections.
TRICYCLAMOL CHLORIDE, B.A.N. 1-(3-Cyclohexyl-3-hydroxy-3-phenylpropyl)-1-methylpyrroidinium chloride. Elorine Chloride; Lergine.
Use: Anticholinergic.
TRICYLATATE HCI. 1-Methyl-3-pyrrolidylmethyl benzilate HCl.

TRIDESILON CREAM. (Miles Pharm) Desonide 0.05% in vehicle buffered to the pH range of normal skin w/glycerin, methyl paraben, sodium lauryl sulfate, aluminum acetate, cetyl stearyl alcohol, synthetic bees-wax, white petrolatum, mineral oil. Tube 15 Gm., 60 Gm. Plastic Jar 5 Gm., lb.
Use: Corticosteroid therapy.

TRIDESILON OTIC. (Miles Pharm) Desonide 0.05%, acetic acid 2% in vehicle. Bot. 10 ml.
Use: Otitis externa treatment.

TRIDEX TAB., TIMED TRIDEX CAP., TIMED TRIDEX JR. CAP. (Fellows) Changed to Daro Tab., Daro Timed Cap., Daro Jr. Timed Cap.

TRI-DIAZOLE LIQUID. (Coastal) Sulfamethazine 2.5 gr., sulfadiazine 2.5 gr., sulfamerazine 2.5 gr., sod. citrate 0.75 gr./Tsp. Bot. 16 oz.

• **TRIDIHEXETHYL CHLORIDE,** U.S.P. XXI. Inj., Tab., U.S.P. XXI. (3-Cyclohexyl-3-hydroxy-3-phenylpropyl)-tri-ethylammonium chloride.
Use: Anticholinergic.
W/Meprobamate.
See: Milpath, Tab. (Wallace)
Pathibamate, Tab. (Lederle)
W/Phenobarbital.
See: Pathilon w/Phenobarbital Tab., Cap. (Lederle)

TRIDIL 0.5 mg./ml. (American Critical Care) Nitroglycerin 0.5 mg./ml. w/alcohol 10%, water for injection, buffered with sodium phosphate. Amp. 10 ml. Box 20s.
Use: Vasodilator; anti-anginal, hypotensive.

TRIDIL 5 mg./ml. (American Critical Care) Nitroglycerin 5 mg./ml. w/alcohol 30%, propylene glycol 30%, water for injection. Amp. 5 ml., 10 ml. Vial 5 ml., 10 ml. Box 20s. Special administration set w/10 ml.Amp.
Use: Vasodilator; anti-anginal, hypotensive.

TRIDIONE. (Abbott) Trimethadione. (Troxidone). Cap. 300 mg., Bot. 100s. Dulcet Tab. 150 mg., Bot. 100s. Sol. 1.2 Gm./fl. oz., Bot. 1 pt.
Use: Epilepsy.

TRIDRATE BOWEL EVACUATION KIT. (Mallinckrodt) Each kit contains: Tridrate solution, magnesium citrate solution Bot. 10 oz.; 3 Tridrate tablets, bisacodyl 5 mg./Tab.; Tridrate suppository, bisacodyl 10 mg./supp.
Use: Bowel evacuant.

TRIENZYME. (Fellows) Amylolytic 30 mg., proteolytic 10 mg., celluloytic 3 mg./Tab. Bot. 1000s.
Use: Relief of functional digestive disorders.

TRI-ERGONE. (Columbia) **0.5 mg. Tab.:** Hydrogenated ergot alkaloids as dihydroergocornine 0.167 mg., dihydroergokryptine 0.167 mg., dihydroergocristine 0.167 mg./Sublingual tab. Bot: 100s, 1000s. **1.0 mg. Tab.:** Hydrogenated ergot alkaloids as dihydroergocornine 0.334 mg., dihydroergokryptine 0.334 mg., dihydroergocristine 0.334 mg./Sublingual Tab. Bot. 100s, 1000s.
Use: Selected symptoms in elderly patients.

TRI-ESTROGEN. (Rocky Mtn.) Potassium estrone sulfate 1 mg., estrone 2 mg., estradiol 0.2 mg./10 cc. Vial 10 cc.

TRIETHANOLAMINE,
See: Trolamine, N.F. XVI.

TRIETHANOLAMINE POLYPEPTIDE OLEATE CONDENSATE.
See: Cerumenex, Drops (Purdue Frederick)

TRIETHANOLAMINE SALICYLATE.
See: Aspercreme, Cream (Sperti)
Aspergel, Oint. (LaCrosse)
Myoflex, Cream (Warren-Teed)

TRIETHANOLAMINE TRINITRATE BIPHOSPHATE.
Trolnitrate Phosphate.

TRIETHYLENEMELAMINE. Tretamine TEM. 2,4,6-Tris(1-aziridinyl)-5-triazine.
Use: Antineopolastic.

• **TRIFLOCIN.** USAN. 4-(α,α,α-Trifluoro-m-toluidino) nicotinic acid.
Use: Diuretic.

• **TRIFLUBAZAM.** USAN.
Use: Tranquilizer.

• **TRIFLUMIDATE.** USAN. Ethyl m-benzoyl-N-[(tri-fluoromethyl)sulfonyl]carbanilate.
Use: Anti-inflammatory.

• **TRIFLUPERIDOL.** USAN.
Use: Antipsychotic.

TRIFLUOMEPRAZINE. B.A.N. NN-Dimethyl-2-(2-tri-fluoromethylphenothiazin-10ylmethyl) propylamine. Nortran.
Use: Tranquilizer, veterinary medicine.

TRIFLUOPERAZINE. B.A.N. 10-[3-(4-Methyl-piperazin-1-yl)propyl]-2-trifluoromethylphenothiazine.
Use: Tranquilizer; antiemetic.

• **TRIFLUOPERAZINE HCL,** U.S.P. XXI. Inj., Syrup, Tab., U.S.P. XXI. 10-[3-(1-Methyl-4-piperazinyl)-propyl]-2-trifluoromethyl phenothiazine HCl. 10-(3-(4-Methyl-1-piperazinyl)propyl)-2-(trifluoromethyl)phe-nothiazine dihydrochloride.
Use: Tranquilizer.
See: Stelazine Inj., Liq., Tab. (SmithKline)

2,2,2-TRIFLUOROETHYL ETHER.
See: Indoklon

4-[3-[2-(TRIFLUOROMETHYL)PHENOTHIAZIN-10-YL]PROPYL]-1-PIPERAZINEETHANOL. Fluphena-zine Enanthate, U.S.P. XXI.

• **TRIFLUPROMAZINE,** U.S.P. XXI. Oral Susp., XXI.
Use: Tranquilizer, antipsychotic agent.

• **TRIFLUPROMAZINE HCl,** U.S.P. XXI. Inj., Tab., U.S.P. XXI. 10-[3-Di-methylamino)propyl]-2-(tri-fluoromethyl)phenothiazine HCl. Fluopromazine, B.A.N.
Use: Tranquilizer, antipsychotic agent.
See: Vesprin, Prep. (Squibb)

• **TRIFLURIDINE.** USAN.
Use: Antiviral used to treat herpes simplex eye infections.
See: Viroptic (Burroughs Wellcome)
See: Viroptic Ophthalmic Soln., (Burroughs Wellcome)

TRIGELAMINE. (Edward J. Moore) Pyrilamine maleate, pheniramine maleate, chlorpheniramine maleate, benzalkonium Cl, menthol. Tube. 1¼ oz.
Use: Triple antihistamine gel.

TRIGESIC. (Squibb) Acetyl-p-aminophenol 2 gr., aspirin 3½ gr., caffeine ½ gr./Tab. Bot. 100s.
Use: Analgesic.

TRI-GRAIN. (Pharmex) Isometheptene tartrate. **Inj.** 100 mg./cc. Vial 10 cc. **Tab.** Bot. 24s, 100s.

TRIHEMIC-600. (Lederle) Vit. C 600 mg., B-12 25 mcg., intrinsic factor conc. 75 mg., folic acid 1 mg., Vit. E 30 I.U., ferrous fumarate 350 mg., dioctyl sod. succinate 50 mg./Tab. Bot. 30s, 500s.
Use: Anemias.

• **TRIHEXYPHENIDYL HYDROCHLORIDE,** U.S.P. XXI. Elix., Tab. U.S.P. XXI. α-Cyclohexyl-α-phenyl-1-
piperidinepropanol HCl. 1-Piperidine-propanol, α-cyclohexyl-α-phenyl-, HCl. Benzhexol, B.A.N.
Use: Anticholinergic, antiparkinsonian.
See: Artane, Elixir & Tab. (Lederle)
Hexyphen-2, Tab. (Robinson)
Hexyphen-5, Tab. (Robinson)

TRIHISTAPACQ TABULES. (Horton & Converse) Prophenpyridamine maleate 6 mg., pyrilamine maleate 8 mg., phenylpropanolamine HCl 15 mg., salicylamide 3 gr., phenacetin 2 gr., caffeine citrate ½ gr., ascorbic acid 100 mg., hesperidin 100 mg./Tab. Bot. 18s.
Use: Relief of headache, muscular aches and fever due to common colds.

TRI-HIST-CAP. (Burgin-Arden) Prophenpyridamine maleate 6.25 mg., methapyrilene HCl 8.33 mg., pyrilamine maleate 8.33 mg., lemon bioflavonoid 25 mg., hesperidin 25 mg., ascorbic acid 50 mg., ephedrine sulfate 10 mg., salicylamide 3.5 gr., caffeine alkaloid 0.5 gr., atropine sulfate ⅟₆₀₀ gr./Cap. Bot. 20s.

TRI-HISTIN. (Recsei) **25 mg. Tab.**: Pyrilamine maleate 10 mg., chlorpheniramine maleate 1 mg. **50 mg. Tab.**: Pyrilamine maleate 20 mg., methapyrilene HCl 15 mg., chlorpheniramine maleate 2 mg. **100 mg. S.A. Cap.**: Pyrilamine maleate 40 mg., pheniramine maleate 25 mg. **Expectorant:** Pyrilamine maleate 5 mg., chlorpheniramine maleate 0.5 mg., guaifenesin 20 mg., phenylpropanolamine 7.5 mg., phenylephrine HCl 2.5 mg., sod. citrate 100 mg./5 cc. Bot. pt. gal. **Liquid:** Pyrilamine maleate 5 mg., chlorpheniramine maleate 0.5 mg./5 cc. Bot. pt. gal. **Tab.** Bot. 100s, 500s 1000s. 50 mg. Bot. 1000s.**Cap.** Bot. 100s, 500s, 1000s.
Use: Triple antihistamine therapy.
W/Benzyl alcohol, chlorobutanol & isopropyl alcohol.
See: Derma-Pax, Liq. (Recsei)
W/Codeine phosphate, guaifenesin, phenylpropanolamine, phenylephrine HCl, sodium citrate.
See: Trihista-Cod., Liq. (Recsei)
W/Ephedrine HCl, aminophylline, mephobarbital.
See: Asmasan, Tab. (Recsei)

TRIHYDROXYESTRINE. Trihydroxyestrin.

TRIHYDROXYETHYLAMINE. Triethanolamine.

11β,17,21-TRIHYDROXY-6-α-METHYLPREGNA-1,4-DIENE-3,20-DIONE 21-ACETATE. Methylprednisolone Acetate, U.S.P. XXI.

11β,17,21-TRIHYDROXYPREGNA-1,4-DIENE-3,20-DIONE (ANHYDROUS). Prednisolone, U.S.P. XXI.

TRI-IMMUNOL. (Lederle) Diphtheria & tetanus toxoids & pertussis vaccine combined, aluminum phosphate-adsorbed purogenated. Vial 7.5 cc.
Use: I.M., Immunization.

TRIIODOMETHANE.
See: Iodoform. (Various Mfr.)

L-TRIIODOTHYRONINE SOD.
See: Cytomel, Tab. (SmithKline)
Liothyronine Sod.

dl-TRIIODOTHYRONINE SODIUM.

3,7,12-TRIKETOCHOLANIC ACID.
See: Dehydrocholic Acid (Various Mfr.)

TRI-K. (Century) Potassium acetate 0.5 Gm., potassium bicarbonate 0.5 Gm., potassium citrate 0.5 Gm./fl. oz. Bot. pt., gal.

• **TRIKATES ORAL SOLUTION,** U.S.P. XXI.
Use: Potassium deficiency.

TRIKATES ORAL SOLUTION. (Lilly) Potassium 15 mEq. from pot. acetate, pot. bicarbonate and pot. citrate/5 ml. Bot. 16 fl. oz., gal.
Use: Potassium deficiency.

TRI-KORT. (Keene) Triamcinalone acetonide suspension 40 mg./ml. Vial 5 ml.
Use: Anti-inflammatory.

TRILAFON. (Schering) Perphenazine. **Tab.** 2, 4, 8 mg., & 16 mg. Bot. 100s, 500s. **Inj:** 5 mg./ml., w/disodium citrate 24.6 mg., sod. bisulfite 2 mg., and water for injection/ml. Amp. 1 ml. Box 100s. **Repetabs** 8 mg., Bot. 100s. **Concentrate** 16 mg./5 ml. Bot. 4 oz. w/dropper.
Use: Tranquilizer.

TRILAX. (Drug Industries) Docusate sodium 200 mg., yellow phenolphthalein 30 mg., dehydrocholic acid 20 mg./Cap. Bot. 100s, 500s.
Use: Laxative, fecal softener, choleretic.

TRILISATE LIQUID. (Purdue Frederick) Choline magnesium trisalicylate from choline salicylate 293 mg., magnesium salicylate 362 mg./ tsp. to provide 500 mg. salicylate/tsp. Bot. 8 oz.
Use: Non-steroidal anti-inflammatory, anti-arthritic.

TRILISATE TABLETS. (Purdue Frederick) Choline magnesium trisalicylate **500 mg./Tab.** of salicylate from choline salicylate 293 mg., magnesium salicylate 362 mg./Tab. Bot. 100s. **750 mg./Tab.** of salicylate from choline salicylate 400 mg. and magnesium salicylate 544 mg. Bot. 100s.
Use: Non-steroidal anti-inflammatory, anti-arthritic.

TRILLEKAMIN HYDROCHLORIDE. Trimustine, B.A.N.

TRILOG. (Hauck) Triamcinolone acetonide 40 mg./ml. Vial 5 ml.
Use: Steroid therapy.

TRILONE. (Century) Triamcinalone diacetate susp. Amp. 10cc.
Use: Corticosteroid.

TRILONE. (Hauck) Triamcinolone diacetate 40 mg./ml. Vial 5 ml.
Use: Steroid therapy.

• **TRILOSTANE.** USAN.
Use: Adrenocortical suppressant.

TRILOX. (Blue Line) **Susp.,** Mag. trisilicate 75 gr., aluminum hydroxide gel 90 gr., alcohol 1%/fl. oz. Bot. 14 oz. **Tab.,** Mag. trisilicate 7½ gr., aluminum hydroxide gel, dried 5 gr./Tab. Bot. 100s, 500s, 1000s.
Use: Gastric antacid.

TRIMAGEL TABLETS. (Columbia) Magnesium trisilicate 0.5 Gm., dried aluminum hydroxide gel 0.25 Gm./Tab. Bot. 100s, 500s.
Use: Gastric hyperacidity.

TRIMAHIST ELIXIR. (Tennessee Pharm.) Phenylephrine HCl 5 mg., prophenpyridamine maleate 12.5 mg., l-menthol 1 mg., alcohol 5%/5 cc. Bot. pt., gal.
Use: Antihistaminic elixir.

TRIM-AID CAPSULES. (Wolins) Sodium carboxymethylcellulose 134 mg., benzocaine 5 mg., Vit. A 1,500 I.U., D 200 I.U., B-1 1 mg., B-2 1.2 mg., niacinamide 5 mg., C 30 mg., calcium 45 mg., phosphorus 23 mg./Cap. Bot. 18s, 60s, 1000s.

TRIMAX GEL. (Winthrop Products) Aluminum, magnesium hydroxide, simethicone.
Use: Antacid, antiflatulent.

TRIMAX TABLET. (Winthrop Products) Aluminum, magnesium hydroxide, simethicone.
Use: Antacid, antiflatulent.

TRIMAZINOL. α-{[(4,6-Diaminos-triazin-2-yl)-aminol]-methyl} benzyl alcohol.
Use: Anti-inflammatory agent.

• **TRIMAZOSIN HYDROCHLORIDE.** USAN.
Use: Antihypertensive.

TRIMCAPS. (Mayrand) Phendimetrazine tartrate 105 mg./Slow-rel. Cap. Bot. 30s, 100s.
Use: Anorectic.

TRIMELARSAN. Melarsonyl Potassium, B.A.N.

TRIMEPERIDINE. B.A.N. 1,2,5-Trimethyl-4-phenyl-4-piperidyl propionate.
Use: Narcotic analgesic.

TRIMEPRAZINE. B.A.N. 10-(3-Dimethylamino-2-methylpropyl)phenothiazine. Alimemazine (I.N.N.) Vallergan.
Use: Tranquilizer; antihistamine.

TRIMEPRAZINE TARTRATE, U.S.P. XXI. Syrup, Tab., U.S.P. XXI. ($\pm$)-10-(3-Dimethylamino-2-methylpropyl)-phenothiazine tartrate (2:1) 10H-Phenothiazine-10-propanamine N,N,β-trimethyl-2,3-dihydroxybutanedioate (2:1).
Use: Anti-pruritic.
See: Temaril, Prep. (SmithKline)

TRIMETAMIDE. Trimethamide.

TRIMETAPHAN CAMSYLATE. B.A.N. 1,3-Dibenzyldecahydro-2-oxoimidazo[4,5-c]thieno[1,2-a]-thiolium(+)-camphor-10-sulfonate.
Use: Hypotensive.
See: Arfonad.

TRIMETAZIDINE. B.A.N. 1-(2,3,4-Trimethoxybenzyl)-piperazine.
Use: Vasodilator.
See: Vastarel dihydrochloride.

• **TRIMETHADIONE,** U.S.P. XXI. Cap., Oral Soln., Tab., U.S.P. XXI. 3,5,5-Trimethyl-2,4-oxazolidinedione.
Use: Anticonvulsant.

See: Tridione, Prep. (Abbott)

TRIMETHADIONE (I.N.N.). Troxidone, B.A.N.

TRIMETHAMIDE. N-[(2-Amino-6-methyl-3-pyridyl)methyl]3,4,5-trimethoxybenzamide.
Use: Antihypertensive agent.

TRIMETHAPHAN CAMPHORSULFONATE. Trimethaphan Camsylate, U.S.P. XXI.

• **TRIMETHAPHAN CAMSYLATE,** U.S.P. XXI. Inj., U.S.P. XXI. d-3,4-(1',3'-Dibenzyl-2'-ketoimidazolido)-1,2-trimethylenethiophanium d-camphorsulfonate. Trimethaphan camphorsulfonate. (+)-1,3-Dibenzyldecahydro-2-oxoimidazo[4,5-c]thieno-[1,2-α]-thiolium 2-oxo-10-bornanesulfonate.
Use: Antihypertensive.
See: Arfonad, Amp. (Roche)

TRIMETHIDINIUM METHOSULFATE, B.A.N. d-(N-methyl-N-(gamma-trimethyl-ammonium-propyl))-1-methyl-8,8-di-methyl-3-azabicyclo-(3,2,1) octane dimethosulfate. 1,3,8,8-Tetramethyl-3-(3-(trimethylammonio)propyl)-3-azoniabicyclo(3.2.1)octane. Tab.
Use: Antihypertensive.

• **TRIMETHOBENZAMIDE HCl,** U.S.P. XXI. Cap., Inj., U.S.P. XXI. N- {p-[2-(Dimethylamino) ethoxy]-benzyl} -3,4,5-trimethoxybenzamide HCl.
Use: Antiemetic.
See: Tegamide, Suppos. (G & W)
Tigan, Preps. (Beecham Labs.)

TRIMETHOBENZAMIDE HYDROCHLORIDE AND BENZOCAINE SUPPOSITORIES.
Use: Antiemetic.

• **TRIMETHOPRIM,** U.S.P. XXI. Tab., U.S.P. XXI. 2,4-Diamino-5-(3,4,5-trimethoxybenzyl)pyrimidine. Syraprim.
Use: Antibacterial agent.
See: Proloprim, Tab. (Burroughs Wellcome)
Trimpex, Tab. (Roche)
W/Sulfamethoxazole.
See: Bactrim, Oral Susp. Ped. Susp., Tab. (Roche)
Septra, Tab. (Burroughs Wellcome)
Septra DS, Tab. (Burroughs Wellcome)

• **TRIMETHOPRIM SULFATE.** USAN.

2,5,9-TRIMETHYL-7H-FURO[3,2-g][1]BENZOPYRAN-7-ONE. Trioxsalen, U.S.P. XXI.

3,5,5-TRIMETHYL-2,4-OXAZOLIDINEDIONE. Trimethadione, U.S.P. XXI.

2,4,6-TRIMETHYL-s-TRIOXANE. Paraldehyde, U.S.P. XXI.

1,3,7-TRIMETHYLXANTHINE. Caffeine.

TRIMETHYLENE. Cyclopropane, U.S.P. XXI.

TRIMETON. Pheniramine, B.A.N.

• **TRIMETOZINE.** USAN.
Use: Sedative.

• **TRIMETREXATE.** USAN.
Use: Antineoplastic.

TRIMETTE. (Wesley) Phenobarbital ¼ gr., atropine sulf. 2/300 gr., dextroamphetamine sulf., 15 mg., aloin ¼ gr./Cap. or Tab. Bot. 1000s.

TRIMEX. (Mills) Dextroamphetamine sulf. 15 mg., amobarbital 60 mg., thyroid 3 gr./Cap. Bot. 50s.
No. 2: dextroamphetamine sulf. 10 mg., amobarbital 60 mg., thyroid 2 gr./Cap. Bot. 50s.

- **TRIMIPRAMINE.** USAN. 5-[3-(Dimethylamino)-2-methylpropyl]-10,11-dihydro-5H-dibenz[b,f]-aze-pine.
  Use: Antidepres
  See: Surmontil (Ives)
- **TRIMIPRAMINE MALEATE.** USAN. 5-[3-(Di-methylamino)-2-methylpropyl]-10,11-dihydro-5H-dibenz[b,f]azepine maleate (1:1).
  Use: Antidepressant.
  See: Surmontil Maleate (Ives)

TRIMIXIN. (Hance) Bacitracin 200 u., polymyxin B sulfate 4000 u., neomycin sulfate 3 mg./Gm. Oint., Tube ½ oz.
  Use: Topically, antibiotic therapy.

- **TRIMOPROSTIL.** USAN.
  Use: Gastric antisecretory.

TRIMO-SAN. (Milex) Oxyquinoline sulfate, sodium lauryl sulfate 0.0084%, boric acid 1.0%, borax 0.70%. Tube 4 oz. w/boilable nylon jel Jector; 4 oz. refill tube.
  Use: Restore and maintain vaginal acidity.

TRIMOX. (Squibb) **Cap.:** Amoxicillin trihydrate 250 mg./Cap. Bot. 100s, 500s. Unit Dose 100s; 500 mg./Cap. Bot. 50s, 500s. Unit Dose 100s. **Oral Susp.:** 125 mg./5 ml. Bot. 80 ml., 100 ml., 150 ml. Unimatic Bot. 5 ml., Ctn. 4 × 25s. 250 mg./5 ml. Bot. 80 ml., 100 ml., 150 ml. Unimatic Bot. 5 ml., Ctn. 4 × 25s.
  Use: Antibiotic.

- **TRIMOXAMINE HYDROCHLORIDE.** USAN. α-Allyl-3,4,5-trimethoxy-N-methylphenethylamine HCl.
  Use: Antihypertensive.

TRIMPEX. (Roche) Trimethoprim 100 mg./Tab. Bot. 100s; Tel-E-Dose 100s; Prescription paks 20s.
  Use: Treatment of initial episodes of uncomplicated urinary tract infections.

- **TRIMOPROSTIL.** USAN.

TRIMSTAT. (Laser) Phendimetrazine tartrate 35 mg./Tab. Bot. 100s, 1000s.
  Use: Anorexiant.

TRIMTABS. (Mayrand) Phendimetrazine tartrate 35 mg./Tab. Bot. 100s, 500s.
  Use: Management of obesity.

TRIMUSTINE. B.A.N. Tri-(2-chloroethyl)amine. Trichlomethine (I.N.N.) Trillekamin hydrochloride.
  Use: Antineoplastic agent.

TRIMYCIN OINTMENT. (Blue Cross) Polymyxin B sulfate 5000 units, bacitracin 400 units, neomycin 5 mg., diperodon HCl 10 mg./Gm. Tube 0.5 oz.
  Use: Antibiotic.

TRINALIN REPETABS. (Schering) Azatadine maleate 1 mg., pseudoephedrine sulfate 120 mg./Tab. Bot 100s.
  Use: Long-acting antihistamine, decongestant.

TRIND. (Mead Johnson) Phenylpropanolamine HCl 12.5 mg., chlorpheniramine maleate 2 mg./5 ml. w/alcohol 5%. Bot. 5 oz.
  Use: Relief of cold symptoms.

TRIND DM. (Mead Johnson) Phenylpropanolamine HCl 12.5 mg., dextromethorphan HBr 7.5 mg., Chlorpheniramine maleate 2 mg./5 ml. w/alcohol 5%. Bot. 5 oz.
  Use: Relief of cough and cold symptoms.

TRINIAD. (Kasar) Isoniazid 300 mg./Tab. Bot. 30s, 100s, 1000s.
  Use: Treatment of tuberculosis.

TRINIAD PLUS 30. (Kasar) Isoniazid 300 mg., pyridoxine HCl 30 mg./Tab. Bot. 30s, 100s, 1000s.

TRINITRIN TABLETS.
  See: Nitroglycerin Tablets, U.S.P. XXI.

TRINITROPHENOL. Picric acid. 2,4,6-Trinitrophenol.
  See: Picric Acid (Var. Mfr.)

TRINOL HYDROCHLORIDE. Benzhexol, B.A.N.

TRINOTIC. (Fellows) Secobarbital 65 mg., amobarbital 40 mg., phenobarbital 25 mg./Tab. Bot. 1000s.
  Use: Hypnotic.

TRINSITRATE. (Columbia) Desic. liver 350 mg., B-12 activity 25 mcg., ferrous sulfate exsic. 800 mg., C 150 mg./2 Caps. Bot. 100s, 1000s.
  Use: Hematinic formula.

TRIO-BAR. (Jenkins) Butabarbital sod. 33⅓%, phenobarbital sod. 33⅓%, phenobarbital sod. 33⅓%. Total barbituates ¼ gr., ¾ gr. or 1½ gr./Tab. Bot. 1000s.
  Use: Sedative.

TRIOBEAD-125. (Abbott) T3 diagnostic kit. Test units 50s, 100s, 500s.
  Use: Quantitative measure of thyroid functioning.

TRIOCIL.
  See: Hexetidine

- **TRIOLEIN I-125.** USAN.
  Use: Radioactive agent.
- **TRIOLEIN I-131.** USAN.
  Use: Radioactive agent.

TRI-ORAPIN. (Standex) Estrone 2 mg., estradiol 0.2 mg., potassium estrone 1 mg./10 cc.

TRIOSIL. Sodium Metrizoate, B.A.N.

TRIOSTAM. Sodium Antimonylgluconate, B.A.N.

TRIOSULF. (Jenkins) Sulfadiazine 2.5 Gr., sulfamerazine 2.5 gr., sulfamethazine 2.5 gr./Tab. Bot. 1000s.

TRIOSULFON. (CMC) Sulfacetamide 0.166 Gm., sulfamethazine 0.166 Gm., sulfamerazine 0.166 Gm./Tab. Bot. 30s, 100s, 1000s.
  Use: Sulfonamide therapy.

TRIOSULFON DMM. (CMC) Tab. Bot. 100s, 250s, 1000s.

TRIOXANE.
  See: Trioxymethylene (Var. Mfr.)

1,3,5-TRIOXANE,2,4,6-TRIMETHYL-. Paraldehyde, U.S.P. XXI.

- **TRIOXIFEN MESYLATE.** USAN.
  Use: Anti-estrogen.

- **TRIOXSALEN,** U.S.P. XXI. Tab., U.S.P. XXI. 6-Hydroxy-β,2,7-trimethyl-5-benzofuranacrylic acid,δ-lactone; 4,5,-8-trimethylpsoralen. 2,5,9-Trimethyl-7H-furo-(3,2-g)(1)benzopyran-7-one. 7H-Furo[3,2-g][1]benzopyran-7-one, 2,5,9-trimethyl-.
  Use: Pigmenting and phototherapeutic agent.
  See: Trisoralen, Tab. (Elder)

TRIOXYMETHYLENE. Name is incorrectly used to denote paraformaldehyde in some pharmaceuticals.
  See: Paraformaldehyde (Various Mfr.)
  W/Sod. oleate, triethanolamine, docusate sodium, stearic acid & aluminum silicate.

See: Cooper Creme (Whittaker)
• **TRIPAMIDE.** USAN.
Use: Antihypertensive, diuretic.
TRIPARANOL. B.A.N. 2-(p-Chlorophenyl)-1-[p-[2-(die-thylamino)ethoxy]phenyl]-1-p-tolylethanol.
Use: Blood lipid lowering agent.
TRIPELENNAMINE. B.A.N. 2-(N-Benzyl-N-2-pyridyl)e-thyldimethylamine.
Use: Antihistamine.
See: Pyribenzamine citrate or hydrochloride. (Geigy)
• **TRIPELENNAMINE CITRATE,** U.S.P. XXI. Elixir U.S.P. XXI. 2-(Benzyl[2-dimethylamino-ethyl]-amino) pyridine dihydrogen citrate. 1,2-Ethanediamine, N,N-dimethyl-N′-(phenylmethyl)-N′-2-pyridinyl-,2-hydroxy-1,2,3-propanetricarboxylate (1:1).
Use: Antihistaminic.
• **TRIPELENNAMINE HYDROCHLORIDE,** U.S.P. XXI. Tab. U.S.P. XXI.
Use: Antihistaminic.
See: Pyribenzamine hydrochloride, Preps. (Geigy)
Ro-Hist, Tab. (Robinson)
TRIPHED. (Lemmon) Triprolidine HCl 2.5 mg., pseudoephedrine HCl 60 mg./Tab. Bot. 100s, 1000s. Unit dose 100s.
Use: Allergic rhinitis, common cold symptoms.
TRI-PHEN ELIXIR. (Bay) Brompheniramine maleate 4 mg., phenylephrine HCl 5 mg., phenylpropanolamine HCl 5 mg./5 ml. w/alcohol 2.3% Bot. 4 oz., pt., gal.
Use: Antihistaminic, decongestant.
TRI-PHEN EXPECTORANT. (Bay) Brompheniramine maleate 2 mg., phenylephrine HCl 5 mg., phenylpropanolamine HCl 5 mg., guaifenesin 100 mg./5 ml. w/alcohol 3.5%. Bot. 4 oz., pt., gal.
Use: Antihistaminic, decongestant, expectorant.
TRI-PHEN EXPECTORANT D.C. (Bay) Codeine phosphate 10 mg., brompheniramine maleate 2 mg., phenylephrine HCl 5 mg., phenylpropanolamine HCl 5 mg., guaifenesin 100 mg./5 ml. Bot. 4 oz., pt., gal.
Use: Antitussive, antihistaminic, decongestant, expectorant.
TRIPHENYLMETHANE DYES.
See: Fuchsin
Methylrosaniline Chloride
TRIPHENYLTETRAZOLIUM CHLORIDE. TTC.
See: Uroscreen (Pfizer)
TRIPHEX CAPSULES. (Tennessee Pharm.) Dextroamphetamine sulfate 15 mg., amobarbital 100 mg./Cap. Bot. 100s.
TRIPIPERAZINE DICITITRATE, HYDROUS.
See: Piperazine Citrate, U.S.P. XXI.
TRIPIRIN. (CMC) Multi-layered aspirin 7.5 gr./Tab. Bot. 24s, 100s, 1000s.
TRIPLAN-D. (Eastwood) Antibiotic ointment. Tube 0.5 oz. Jar 4 oz.
TRIPLE ANTIBIOTIC OINTMENT. (Century) Bacitracin, Neomycin and Polymixin-B in ointment base.
Use: Antibacterial ointment.
TRIPLE ANTIBIOTIC OINTMENT. (Vortech) Bacitracin 400 u., neomycin sulfate 5 mg., polymyxin B sulfate 5000 u./Tube ½ oz.

Use: Antibacterial ointment.
TRIPLE ANTIBIOTIC OINTMENT. (Walgreen) Bacitracin 400 u., polymyxin-B sulfate 5000 u., neomycin sulfate 5.0 mg./Gm. Tube 0.5 oz., 1 oz.
Use: Antibiotic ointment
TRIPLE ANTI-B OINTMENT. (Eckerd) Bacitracin 400 U., neomycin sulfate 5 mg., polymixin B sulfate 5000 U./Gm.
Use: Topical antibacterial.
TRIPLE ANTIGEN. (Wyeth) H. pertussis 30 billion/cc. w/alum-precipitated diphtheria & tetanus toxoids. Vial 7.5 cc. Ultrafined Tubex 0.5 cc.
Use: I.M. & S.C.; protection against diphtheria, tetanus & whooping cough.
TRIPLE BARBITURATE ELIXIR. (CMC) Phenobarbital ¼ gr., butabarbital ⅛ gr., pentobarbital ⅛ gr./5 cc. Bot. pt., gal.
Use: Pediatric sedative.
TRIPLE BROMIDES, EFFERVESCENT TABLETS. W/Phenobarbital.
See: Palagren, Liq. (Westerfield)
TRIPLE DYE. (Kerr) Gentian violet, proflavine, hemisulfate, brilliant green in water. Dispensing Bot. 15 ml.
Use: Umbilical area antiseptic.
TRIPLE DYE. (Xttrium) Brilliant green 2.29 mg., proflavine hemisulfate 1.14 mg., gentian violet 2.29 mg./ml. Bot. 30 ml.
Use: Umbilical area disinfectant.
TRIPLEN. (Interstate) Tripelennamine HCl 50 mg./Tab. Bot. 100s, 1000s.
Use: Antihistamine.
TRIPLE PASTE. (Torch) Burow's sol. 1 part, absorption base 2 parts, Lassar's zinc oxide paste 3 parts. Jar 2 oz., 1 lb.
Use: Eczemas.
TRIPLE SULFA. (Sutliff & Case) Sulfadiazine 2½ gr., sulfamethazine 2½ gr., sulfamerazine 2½ gr./Tab. Bot. 100s, 1000s.
Use: Antibacterial, sulfonamide therapy.
TRIPLE SULFA. (Standex; Kenyon) Sulfadiazine 2½ gr., sulfamethazine 2½ gr., sulfamerazine 2½ gr./Tab. Bot. 100s. (Kenyon) Bot. 100s, 1000s.
Use: Antibacterial, sulfonamide therapy.
TRIPLE SULFA LIQUID. (Vortech) Bot. 4 oz., Gal.
Use: Triple sulfonamide therapy.
TRIPLE SULFA SUSPENSION. (Standex) Sulfamethazine 2.5 gr., sulfadiazine 2.5 gr., sulfamerazine 2.5 gr., sodium citrate 0.75 gr./5 cc. Bot. pt.
Use: Antibacterial, sulfonamide therapy.
TRIPLE SULFA SUSPENSION. (CMC) Sulfadiazine 0.166 Gm., sulfamethazine 0.166 Gm., sulfamerazine 0.166 Gm./5 cc. Bot. pt., gal.
Use: Antibacterial, sulfonamide therapy.
TRIPLE SULFA SUSPENSION, NO. 2. (Fellows) Sulfamethazine 2.5 gr., sulfadiazine 2.5 gr., sulfamerazine 2.5 gr., sod. citrate 7.5 gr./Tsp. Bot. gal.
Use: Antibacterial, sulfonamide therapy.
TRIPLE SULFA TABLETS. (Century; Stanlabs)

Sulfadiazine 2½ gr., sulfamerazine 2½ gr., sulfamethazine 2½ gr./Tab. Bot. 100s, 1000s.
Use: Antibacterial, sulfonamide therapy.

TRIPLE SULFA TABLETS #2-C.T. (Wolins) Sulfadiazine 166 mg., sulfamerazine 166 mg., sulfamethazine 166 mg./Tab. Bot. 100s, 1000s.
Use: Antibacterial, sulfonamide therapy.

TRIPLE SULFOID. (Vale) Sulfadiazine 167 mg., sulfamerazine 167 mg., sulfamethazine 167 mg./5 ml. or Tab. Bot. pt., 2 oz. 12s. Tab. Bot. 100s, 1000s.
Use: Sulfonamide therapy.

TRIPLE SULFONAMIDE. Dia-Mer-Thia Sulfonamides. Meth-Dia-Mer Sulfonamides.
Use: Sulfonamide therapy.

TRIPLE X. (Youngs Drug) Pyrethrins 0.3%, piperonyl butoxide 3.0%, petroleum distilate 1.2%, benzyl alcohol 2.4% Bot. 2 oz, 4 oz.
Use: Pediculocide for human use, head body & pubic lice.

TRIPOLE-F. (Spanner) Testosterone 25 mg., estrone 6 mg., progesterone 25 mg./cc. Vial 10 cc.

TRIPOSED SYRUP. (Blue Cross) Triprolidine HCl 1.25 mg., pseudoephedrine HCl 30 mg./5 ml. Bot. pt., gal.
Use: Antihistaminic, decongestant.

TRIPOSED TABLETS. (Blue Cross) Triprolidine HCl 2.5 mg., pseudoephedrine HCl 60 mg./Tab. Bot. 100s, 1000s.
Use: Antihistaminic, decongestant.

TRIPOTASSIUM CITRATE.
See: Potassium Citrate, U.S.P. XXI.

TRIPROFED. (Robinson) Tiprolidine HCl w/pseudoephedrine. Bot. 100s, 1000s.
Use: Antihistamine, nasal decongestant.

TRIPROFED EXPECTORANT WITH CODEINE.
(Robinson) Triprolidine HCl w/pseudoephedrine, codeine, expt., Bot. pt., gal.
Use: Antitussive, antihistaminic.

TRIPROFED SYRUP. (Robinson) Triprolidine HCl w/pseudoephedrine syrup. Bot. pts., gal.
Use: Antihistaminic, nasal decongestant.

TRIPROLIDINE. B.A.N. trans 1-(2-Pyridyl)-3-(pyrrolidin-1-yl)-1-p-tolylprop-1-ene.
Use: Antihistamine.
See: Actidil hydrochloride.

• **TRIPROLIDINE HCl,** U.S.P. XXI. Syrup, Tab., U.S.P. XXI. Trans 1-4-methylphenyl)-1-(2-pyridyl)-3-pyrrolidino-prop-1-ene HCl. Trans-2-[3-(1-pyrrolidinyl)-1-(p-tolyl)-propenyl]pyri-dine hydrochloride. (E)-2-(3-(1-Pyrrolidinyl)-1-p-tolypropenyl)pyridine monohydrochloride monohydrate.
Use: Antihistiminic.
See: Actidil, Syr. (Burroughs Wellcome)
W/Codeine phosphate, pseudoephedrine HCl, guaifenesin.
See: Actifed-C Syr. (Burroughs Wellcome)

• **TRIPROLIDINE AND PSEUDOEPHEDRINE HYDROCHLORIDE SYRUP,** U.S.P. XXI.
Use: Antihistaminic, decongestant.

• **TRIPROLIDINE AND PSEUDOEPHEDRINE HYDROCHLORIDE TABLETS,** U.S.P. XXI.
Use: Antihistaminic, decongestant.
W/Pseudoephedrine.
See: Actifed, Tab., Syr. (Burroughs Wellcome)
Atridine, Tab. (Interstate)
Sudahist, Tab. (Upsher-Smith)
Suda-Prol, Tab., Cap. (Columbia)
Triafed, Tab. (Wolins)
Triphed, Tab. (Lemmon)
Triphedrine, Tab. (Redford)
Triprofed Preps. (Robinson)

TRIPTONE. (Commerce) Scopolamine hydrobromide 0.25 mg./Cap. Bot. 12s.
Use: Motion sickness relief.

2,4,6-TRIS(1-AZIRIDINYL)-S-TRIAZINE. Triethylenemelamine.

TRI-SOF. (Vangard) Docusate potassium 100 mg., casanthranol 30 mg./Cap. Bot. 100s, 500s.
Use: Stool softener, laxative.

TRISOL. (Buffington) Berberine HCl, borax, sodium Cl, boric acid. Irrigator Bot. 1 oz., 4 oz.
Use: Eye wash, tear substitute.

TRISORALEN. (Elder) Trioxsalen 5 mg./Tab. Bot. 28s, 100s.
Use: Repigmentation of idiopathic vitiligo; increasing tolerance to sunlight; enhancing pigmentation.

TRISTOJECT. (Mayrand) Triamcinolone diacetate 40 mg./ml. Vial 5 ml.
Use: Anti-inflammatory corticosteroid.

TRISULFAPYRIMIDINES. Oral Susp., Tab., U.S.P. XXI.
Use: Antibacterial.
See: Meth-Dia-Mer Sulfonamides (Various Mfr.)
Neotrizine, Prep. (Lilly)
Terfonyl, Liq. Tab. (Squibb)

TRI-SYNAR. (Forrest) Belladonna ext. 4.1 mg., phenyltoloxamine 20 mg., ethaverine HCl 20 mg./Tab. Bot. 100s.
Use: Antispasmodic.

TRI-SYNAR PLUS. (Forrest) Belladonna pow. ext. 4.1 mg., phenyltoloxamine 20 mg., ethaverine HCl 12.5 mg., phenobarbital 2.03 mg., butabarbital sod. 2.025 mg., pentobarbital sod. 6.075 mg., secobarbital sod. 6.075 mg./Tab. Bot. 100s.
Use: Sedatives w/antispasmodic.

TRITANE. (Econo-Rx) Brompheniramine maleate 2 mg., guaifenesin 100 mg., phenylephrine HCl 5 mg., phenylpropanolamine HCl 5 mg., alcohol 3.5%/5 ml. Bot. Gal.
Use: Expectorant.

TRITANE DC. (Econo-Rx) Brompheniramine maleate 2 mg., guaifenesin 100 mg., phenylephrine HCl 5 mg., phenylpropanolamine HCl 5 mg., alcohol 3.5%, codeine phosphate 10 mg./5 ml. Bot. Gal.
Use: Expectorant and antitussive.

TRITHEON. Acinitrazole, B.A.N.

TRITHION. Carbophenothion, B.A.N.

• **TRITIATED WATER.** USAN.
Use: Radioactive agent.
See: Tritiotope (Squibb)

TRITICOLL. (Western Research) P.E. triticum repens

4 gr., oxyquinoline sulf. 1/20 gr., charcoal 1/2 gr./Tab. Bot. 1000s.
Use: Diuretic.

TRI-TINIC. (Vortech) Liver desic. 75 mg., stomach 75 mg., Vit. B-12 15 mcg., Fe 110 mg., folic acid 1 mg., ascorbic acid 75 mg./Cap. Bot. 30s, 100s, 1000s.
Use: Hematinic.

TRITON WR-1339. (Rohm & Haas) Oxyethylated tertiary octyl-phenol-formaldehyde polymer.

TRITUSSIN COUGH SYRUP. (Towne) Pyrilamine maleate 40 mg., pheniramine maleate 10 mg., citric acid 100 mg., ammonium chloride 520 mg., potassium giaiacolsulfonate 520 mg., codeine phosphate 58 mg./fl. oz. Bot. 4 oz.

TRIURISUL. (Sheryl) Sulfacetamide 250 mg., sulfamethizole 250 mg., phenazopyridine HCl 50 mg./Tab. Bot. 100s.
Use: Urinary Antiseptic-analgesic.

TRIVA. (Boyle) Alkyl aryl sulfonate 35%, sod. sulfate 52.5%, oxyquinoline sulfate 2%, lactose 9.67% and disodium ethylene hydrated silica 0.5% EDTA .33% Packet 3 Gm., 24s.
Use: Douche for trichomonal and monilial infections.

TRI-VAC. (Rhode) Docusate sodium 100 mg., casanthranol 30 mg., sodium carboxymethylcellulose 400 mg./Cap. Bot. 30s, 100s.
Use: Laxative.

TRIVA-COMBINATION. (Boyle) Oxyquinoline benzoate and sulfate, alkly aryl sulfonate, disodium ethylenediamine-tetra-acetate, 9-aminoacridine HCl, copper sulfate./3 Gm. Douche Packet 24s and Jel tube 85 Gm. w/applicator.
Use: Therapeutic vaginal douche and jelly.

TRIVA JEL. (Boyle) Oxyquinoline benzoate 7.5 mg., alkyl aryl sulfonate 62.5 mg., disodium ethylenediamine tetra-acetate 2.5 mg., 9-aminoacridine HCl 10 mg., copper sulfate 0.063 mg., sodium sulfate 6.9 mg./5 Gm w/tragacanth, Irish moss, lanolin, glycerin, sod. bicarb, methyl-, propyl-, and butyl-parahydroxybenzoate. Tubes 85 Gm.
Use: Vulvovaginitis, monilia, trichomonas.

TRI-VERT. (T.E. Williams) Dimenhydrinate 25 mg., niacin 50 mg., pentylenetetrazol 25 mg./Cap. Bot. 100s.
Use: Motion sickness treatment.

TRI VIDA F. (Pharmics) Vit. A 3000 I.U., D 400 I.U., C 100 mg., fluoride 0.25 mg., B-6 1 mg./0.6 cc. Bot. 57 cc.
Use: Dietary supplement.

TRI-VI-FLOR 0.5 mg. DROPS. (Mead Johnson) Fluoride 0.5 mg., Vit. A 1500 I.U., D 400 I.U., C 35 mg./1.0 ml. Bot. 30, 50 ml.
Use: Caries prophylaxis and diet supplementation.

TRI-VI-FLOR 0.25 mg. DROPS. (Mead Johnson) Fluoride 0.25 mg., Vit. A 1500 I.U., D 400 I.U., C 35 mg./1.0 ml. Drop. Bot. 50 ml.
Use: Caries prophylaxis, dietary supplement.

TRI-VI-FLOR 0.25 mg. WITH IRON DROPS. (Mead Johnson) Fluoride 0.25 mg., Vit. A. 1500 I.U., D. 400 I.U., C 35 mg., iron 10 mg./1.0 ml. Drop. Bot. 50 ml.
Use: Caries prophylaxis, dietary supplement with iron.

TRI-VI-FLOR 1.0 mg. CHEWABLE TABLETS. (Mead Johnson) Fluoride 1 mg., Vit. A 2500 I.U. D 400 I.U., Vit. C 60 mg./Tab. Bot. 100s, 1000s.
Use: Carries prophylaxis and diet supplementation.

TRI-VI-SOL. (Mead Johnson) Vitamin A 2500 I.U., D 400 I.U., C 60 mg./Chewable tab. or Vit. A 1500 I.U., D 400 I.U., C 35 mg./1.0 ml.**Drops.** Bot. 30, 50 ml. with calibrated 'Safti-dropper.'**Chewable tab.** Bot. 100s.
Use: Vitamin A, C and D supplement.

TRI-VI-SOL WITH IRON DROPS. (Mead Johnson) Vit. A 1500 I.U., C 35 mg., D 400 I.U., iron 10 mg./1.0 ml. Bot. 50 ml.
Use: Vitamin A, C and D with iron supplement.

TRI-VITE. (Foy) Thiamine HCl 100 mg., pyridoxine HCl 100 mg., cyanocobalamine 1000 mcg./ml. Vial 10 ml.
Use: B vitamin therapy.

TRIZMA. Trometamol, B.A.N.

TROBICIN. (Upjohn) Spectinomycin HCl equivalent to spectinomycin activity: **2 Gm.**/Vial w/Ampoule of diluent containing bacteriostatic water for injection 3.2 ml., benzyl alcohol 0.945% in ampoule. **4 Gm.**/Vial w/Ampoule of diluent containing bacteriostatic water for injection 6.2 ml., benzyl alcohol 0.945%.
Use: Treatment of gonorrhea.

TROCAINE LOZENGES. (Vortech) Benzocaine 5 mg./Tab. Bot. 1000s.
Use: Anesthetic throat lozenge.

TROCINATE. (Poythress) Thiphenamil HCl. Tab. 100 mg., Bot. 100s, 500s. 400 mg./Tab. Bot. 25s, 100s.
Use: Antispasmodic.

• **TROCLOSENE POTASSIUM.** USAN. (1) 1,3-Dichloro-s-triazine-2,4,6 (1H,3H,5H)trione potassium salt; (2) Potassium dichloroisocyanurate.
Use: Topical anti-infective.

TRODAX EGLUMINE SALT. Nitroxynil, B.A.N.

TROFAN. (Upsher-Smith) L-Tryptophan 0.5 Gm./Tab. Bot. 30s, 100s.
Use: Dietary supplement.

TROKETTES. (Vitarine) Cetylpyridinium chloride 1:3000, cetyldimethylbenzylammonium chloride 1:3000, benzocaine 10 mg./Troche. Pkg. 10s, Jar 15s, 1000s.
Use: Throat and mouth irritations.

• **TROLAMINE,** N.F. XVI. 2,2″,2″-Nitrilotriethanol Ethanol, 2,2′,2″-nitrilotris-. Triethanolamine.
Use: Pharmaceutic aid (alkalizing agent).
W/Ortho-iodobenzoic.
   See: Progonasyl (Saron)

• **TROLEANDOMYCIN,** U.S.P. XXI Cap., Oral Susp., U.S.P. XXI. Triacetyloleandomycin.
Use: Antibiotic.
   See: Tao (Roerig)

TROLENE. Fenchlorphos, B.A.N.

TROLNITRATE PHOSPHATE, B.A.N. Di[tri-(2-nitratoethyl)ammonium]hydrogen phosphate. Praenitrona.
Use: Vasodilator.
   See: Nitretamin (Squibb)

TROMAL. Butacetin. 4′-tert-Butoxyacetanilide.
Use: Analgesic antidepressant agent.

TROMETAMOL. B.A.N. 2-Amino-2-hydroxymethyl-propane-1,3-diol. Tromethamine, Talatrol, Trizma.
Use: Treatment of gastric hyperacidity.
• **TROMETHAMINE,** U.S.P. XXI. For Inj., U.S.P. XXI. 2-Amino-2(hydroxymethyl)-1,3-propanediol. Trometamol, B.A.N.
Use: Alkalizer.
TRONOLANE CREAM. (Abbott Prods) Pramoxine HCl 1% in cream base. Tubes 1 oz., 2 oz.
Use: Anesthetic hemorrhoidal cream.
TRONOLANE SUPPOSITORIES. (Abbott Prods) Pramoxine HCl 1% in a lubricating suppository base. Pkg. 10s, 20s.
Use: Anesthetic hemorrhoidal suppository.
TRONOTHANE HYDROCHLORIDE. (Abbott) Pramoxine HCl Jelly (1%) Tube 1 oz. Cream (1%) Tube 1 oz.
Use: Local anesthetic.
1αH,3αH-TROPAN-3α-OL MANDELATE (ESTER) HYDROBROMIDE. Homatropine Hydrobromide, U.S.P. XXI.
1αH, 5αH-TROPAN-3-α-OL ($\pm$)-TROPATE (ESTER), SULFATE (2:1)(SALT) MONOHYDRATE. Atropine Sulfate, U.S.P. XXI.
TROPHENIUM. Phenactropinium Chloride, B.A.N.
TROPH-IRON. (Menley & James) Vit. B-12 25 mcg., B-1 10 mg., iron 30 mg./5 cc. Bot. 4 fl. oz.
Use: Vitamin B, B-1, B-12 and iron supplement.
TROPHITE. (Menley & James) Vitamin B-12 25 mcg., B-1 10 mg./5 cc. or Tab.**Elixir,** Bot. 4 oz., **Tab.** Bot. 50s.
Use: Vitamin B supplement.
TROPICAL BLEND. (Plough) A series of products is marketed under the Tropical Blend name including After Sun Lotion, Dark Tanning Butter (SPF 2), Dark Tanning Lotion (SPF 2), Lite Formula Oil (SPF 2), and Sunscreen Lotion (SPF 4). Most contain homosalate in various oil and lotion bases.
• **TROPICAMIDE,** U.S.P. XXI. Ophth. Soln., U.S.P. XXI. N-Ethyl-2-phenyl-N-(4-pyridylmethyl)hydracrylamide. Benzeneacetamide, N-ethyl-α-(hydroxymethyl)-N-(4-pyridinylmethyl)-. Formerly Bis-Tropamide.
Use: Anticholinergic, ophthalmic.
See: Mydriacyl, Drops. (Alcon)
TROPIGLINE. B.A.N. Tiglytropeine.
Use: Treatment of the Parkinsonian syndrome.
TROPINE BENZOHYDRYL ESTER METHANE-SULFONATE. (also named benztropine methane-sulfonate).
TROVIT. (Sig) Vit. B-2 0.3 mg., B-6 1 mg., choline Cl 25 mg., panthenol 2 mg., dl-methionine 10 mg., inositol 20 mg., niacinamide 50 mg., Vit. B-12 10 mg./ml. Vial 30 ml.
Use: B-complex deficiency.
TROXERUTIN. B.A.N. 3′,4′,7-Tri-[0-(2-hydroxyethyl)]rutin.
Use: Treatment of venous disorders.
TROXIDONE. B.A.N. 3,5,5-Trimethyloxazolidine-2,4-dione.
Use: Anticonvulsant.
See: Trimethadione (I.N.N.) Tridione.
TROXONIUM TOSYLATE. B.A.N. Triethyl-2-(3:4:5-trimethoxybenzoyloxy)ethylammonium toxylate

(Tosylic acid is the trivial name for p-toluenesulfonic acid).
Use: Hypotensive.
TROXYPYRROLIUM TOSYLATE. B.A.N. N-Ethyl-N-2-(3:4:5-trimethyoxybenzoyloxy)-ethyl-pyrrolidinium toxylate (Tosylic acid is the trivial name for p-toluene-sulphonic acid).
Use: Hypotensive.
TRYMEX. (Savage) Triamincinolone acetonide.
Cream: 0.025% Tube. 15 Gm., Jar 80 Gm., 1 lb.; 0.1% Tube 15 Gm., Jar 80 Gm., 1 lb.; 0.5% Tube. 15 Gm. **Ointment:** 0.025% Tube. 15 Gm. Jar 80 Gm.; 0.1% 15 Tube. Jar 80 Gm.
Use: Anti-inflammatory, anti-pruritic, topical steroid.
TRYPARSAMIDE. Monosodium N-(Carbamoyl-methyl)arsanilate.
TRYPSIN, CRYSTALLIZED, U.S.P. XXI. For Inhalation Aerosol, U.S.P. XXI.
Use: Proteolytic enzyme.
W/Castor oil.
See: Granulex (Hickam)
W/Chymotrypsin.
See: Chymolase, Tab. (Warren-Teed)
Chymoral, Tab. (Armour)
Orenzyme, Tab. (Merrell Dow)
TRYPTIZOL HYDROCHLORIDE. Amitriptyline HCl, U.S.P XXI.
• **TRYPTOPHAN,** U.S.P. XXI. $C_{11}H_{12}N_2O_2$ as L-tryptophan.
Use: Amino acid.
TRYSUL. (Savage) Sulfathiazole 3.42%, sulfacetamide 2.86%m sulfabenzamide 3.70%, urea 0.64%. Tube 78 Gm.
Use: Vaginits treatment.
T-SERP TABLET. (Tennessee Pharm.) Reserpine alkaloid 0.25 mg./Tab. Bot. 100s, 1000s.
Use: Hypotensive and tranquilizer.
TSH-SQUIBB. (Squibb) Radioimmune kit for thyroid-stimulating hormone. 100 tests/kit.
Use: Radioimmune kit.
T-STAT. (Westwood) Erythromycin 20 mg./ml. w/alcohol 71.2%. Bot. 60 ml.
Use: Acne vulgaris treatment.
TTC. Triphenyltetrazolium Chloride.
See: Uroscreen, Tube (Pfizer)
T.T.P. (Webcon) Trinalis HC Supprettes 6/Jar, Trinalis Supprettes (with applicator) 14/Jar. Treatment package HC Supprettes 1 Jar; Supprette w/applic. 2 Jars.
Use: Vaginal infections.
• **TUAMINOHEPTANE,** U.S.P XXI. Inhalant, U.S.P. XXI.
Use: Adrenergic.
TUAMINOHEPTANE SULFATE. 1-Methylhexylamine sulfate (2:1).
Use: Adrenergic (vasoconstrictor)
TUBERCULIN, MONO-VACC TEST. (Lincoln) Mono-Vacc test is a sterile, disposable multiple puncture scarifier with liquid Old Tuberculin on the points. Box 25 tests.
Use: Diagnostic.
• **TUBERCULIN.** U.S.P. XXI.
Use: Diagnostic aid (dermal reactivity indicator).

TUBERCULIN PPD, STABILIZED. (Panray) Stabilized solution in sterile isotonic phosphate-buffered saline w/phenol 0.3% and Tween 80 0.0005%. 1st strength, Vial 1.0 cc.; Intermediate strength Vial 1.0 cc., 5.0 cc.; 2nd strength, concentr. Vial 1 cc.

TUBERCULIN PURIFIED PROTEIN DERIVATIVE. (Squibb-Connaught) A concentrated solution for multiple puncture testing. Vial 1 ml.
Use: For screening tuberculin activity.

TUBERCULIN PURIFIED PROTEIN DERIVATIVE. See: Tubersol, Inj. (Squibb-Connaught)

TUBERCULIN TINE TEST. (Lederle) **Old Tuberculin (OT):** Each disposable test unit consists of a stainless steel disc, with four tines (or prongs) 2 millimeters long, attached to a plastic handle. The tines have been dip-dried with antigenic material. The entire unit is sterilized by ethylene oxide gas. The test has been standardized by comparative studies, utilizing 0.05 mg. U.S. Standard Old Tuberculin (5 International Units) or 0.0001 mg. U.S. Standard (5 International Units) by the Mantoux technique. The reliability appears to be comparable to the standard Mantoux. 100s, 500s, 1000s. **Purified Protein Derivative (PPD):** Equivalent to or more potent than 5 TU PPD Mantoux test. Tests in a jar, 25s or 100s.

TUBERLATE. (Heun) Sod. p-aminosalicylate 12 gr., succinic acid 4 gr./Tab. Bot. 500s.
Use: Tuberculosis treatment.

TUBERSOL. (Squibb-Connaught) Tuberculin purified protein derivative (Mantoux) 1TU, 5 TU, or 250 TU.
Use: For the detection of tuberculosis infection.

TUBEX. (Wyeth) The following drugs are available in various Tubex sizes:
Ativan
Bicillin C-R
Bicillian C-R 900/300
Bicillin Long-Acting
Chlorpromazine HCl
Codeine Phosphate
Cyanocobalamin
Dexamethasone Sodium Phosphate
Digoxin
Dimenhydrinate
Diphenhydramine HCl
Diphtheria and Tetanus Toxoids Adsorbed (Pediatric)
Epinephrine
Furosemide
Heparin Lock Flush.
Heparin Sodium Solution
Hydromorphone HCl
Hydroxyzine HCl
Immune Serum Globulin (Human)
Influenza Virus Vaccine, Trivalent
Largon
Lidocaine HCL
Mepergan
Meperidine HCl
Morphine Sulfate
Oxytocin

Pentobarbital Sodium
Phenergan
Phenobarbital Sodium
Prochlorperazine Edisylate
Secobarbital Sodium
Sodium Chloride
Sparine
Tetanus and Diphtheria Toxoids Adsorbed Human
Tetanus Immune Globulin (Human)
Tetanus Toxoid Alum. Phos. Ad.
Thiamine Hydrochloride
Triple Antigen
Wyamine Sulfate
Wycillin

• **TUBOCURARINE CHLORIDE,** U.S.P. XXI. Inj., U.S.P. XXI. Tubocuraranium, 7',12'-dihydroxy-6,6'-dimethoxy-2,2',2'-trimethyl-, chloride, hydrochloride, pentahydrate. d-Tubocurarine chloride. Various mfr. Metubine Iodide (Lilly) 3 mg./ml. Amp. 10 ml. (Abbott) 3 mg./ml. in 10 ml fliptop vials; 15 mg. in 5 ml. Abboject Syringe.
Use: Skeletal muscle relaxant.

TUBOCURARINE CHLORIDE, DIMETHYL. Dimethyl ether of d-tubocurarine chloride.

(+)-TUBOCURARINE CHLORIDE HYDROCHLORIDE PENTAHYDRATE. Tubocurarine Chloride, U.S.P. XXI.

TUBOCURARINE IODIDE, DIMETHYL. Dimethyl ether of d-tubocurarine iodide.
Use: Skeletal muscle relaxant.
See: Metubine, Vial (Lilly)

TUBOMEL. Isoniazid, B.A.N.

TU-CILLIN-4. (Reid-Provident) Penicillin G potassium 400,000 u. when prepared/5 cc. Bot. 80 cc.
Use: Antibiotic.

TUCKS. (Parke-Davis) Pads saturated with solution of witch hazel 50%, glycerin 10%, methylparaben 0.1%, benzalkonium Cl 0.003% Jar 40s, 100s.
Use: Proctologic & dermatologic disorders.

TUCKS OINTMENT AND CREAM. (Parke-Davis) Witch hazel 50% in cream or ointment base. Tube 40 Gm. w/rectal applicator.
Use: Astringent.

TUCKS TAKE-ALONGS. (Parke-Davis) Non-woven wipes saturated with solution of witch hazel 50%, glycerine 10% w/purified water, methylparaben 0.1%, benzalkonium chloride 0.003%. Box 12s.

TUGON. Metriphonate, B.A.N.

TUINAL. (Lilly) Equai parts Seconal Sod. & Amytal Sod. Pulvule **50 mg.** Bot. 100s; **100 mg.** Bot. 100s, 1000s. Blister Pkg. 10 × 10s. Dispenser rolls, 40 × 25s; **200 mg.** Bot. 100s, 1000s. Blister Pkg. 10 × 10s.
Use: Sedative & hypnotic.

TUMS. (Norcliff Thayer) Calcium carbonate 500 mg./Tab. Available in peppermint and assorted flavors in various package sizes. Rolls singles, 3-roll wraps. Bot. 75s, 150s.
Use: Antacid.

TUR-BI-KAL NASAL DROPS. (Emerson) Phenylephrine HCl in a salin solution. Dropper Bot. 1 oz., 12s.

Use: Nasal decongestant.

TURBILIXIR. (Burlington) Chlorpheniramine maleate 2 mg., phenylephrine HCl 5 mg., phenylpropanolamine HCl 5 mg./5 ml. Bot. Pts., gal.
Use: Antihistamine, decongestant.

TURBINAIRE.
See: Decadron Phosphate, Preps. (Merck Sharp & Dohme)

TURBISPAN LEISURECAPS. (Burlington) Chlorpheniramine maleate 12 mg., 1-phenylephrine HCl 15 mg., phenylpropanolamine HCl 15 mg./Sus. Rel. Cap. Bot. 30s.
Use: Antihistamine, decongestant.

TURGASEPT AEROSOL. (Ayerst) Ethyl alcohol 44.25%, essential oils 0.90%, n-alkyl (50% C-14, 40% C-12, 10% C-16) dimethyl benzylammonium Cl 0.33%, o-phenylphenol 0.25% w/propellant. Spray can 11.5 oz. in bouquet, fresh lemon, leather, citrus blossom scents.
Use: Spray disinfectant, air deodorant.

TURGEX. (Xttrium) Hexachlorophene 3% w/emulsifying agents. Aerosol Foam 6 oz. Liq. 5 oz., gal.
Use: Antibacterial.

TURPENTINE OIL W/COMBINATIONS.
See: Sloan's Liniment, Liq. (Warner-Lambert)

TUSAL. (Hauck) Sodium thiosalicylate 50 mg./ml. Vial 30 ml.
Use: Relief of muscular pains, acute gout, arthritis, rheumatic fever.

TUSANA. Dextromethorphan, B.A.N.

TUS-F. (Orbit) Dextromethorphan HBr 10 mg./5 ml. Bot. 4 oz., Pts.
Use: Antitussive, decongestant.

TUSILAN. Dextromethorphan HBr.

TUS-ORAMINIC. (Vortech) Bot. 100s, 1000s.
Use: Antitussive, decongestant.

TUSQUELIN. (Circle) Dextromethorphan HBr 15 mg., chlorpheniramine maleate 2 mg., phenylpropanolamine 5 mg., phenylephrine HCl 5 mg., fl. ext. ipecac 0.17 min., potassium guaiacolsulfonate 44 mg.,/5 ml., alcohol 5% Syrup, pt.
Use: Antitussive w/expectorant; antihistamine.

TUSREN. (Wren) Guaifenesin 200 mg./Tab. Bot. 100s, 1000s.

TUSSABAR. (Tennessee) Acetaminophen 400 mg., salicylamide 500 mg., potassium guaiacolsulfonate 120 mg., pyrilamine maleate 30 mg., ammonium chloride 500 mg., sodium citrate 500 mg., phenylephrine HCl 30 mg./oz. Bot. pt., gal.
Use: Analgesic, antipyretic, decongestant and expectorant.

TUSSACOL. (Jenkins) Dextromethorphan HBr 7.5 mg., pyrilamine maleate 8.0 mg., chlorpheniramine maleate 0.3 mg., phenylephrine HCl 5.0 mg., acetaminophen 100.0 mg., guaifenesin 50 mg./Tab. Bot. 1000s.

TUSSAFED DROPS. (Everett) Carbinoxamine maleate 2 mg., pseodoephedrine HCl 25 mg., dextromethorphan HBr 9 mg./1 ml. Bot. 30 ml. with calibrated dropper.

Use: Temporary relief of cough, nasal congestion, runny nose.

TUSSAFED SYRUP. (Everett) Dextromethorphan HBr 15 mg., pseudoephedrine HCl 60 mg., carbinoxamine maleate 4 mg./5 ml. Bot. 4 oz., 16 oz.
Use: Antitussive, decongestant, antihistamine.

TUSSAFED EXPECTORANT. (Calvital) Chlorpheniramine maleate 2 mg., pseudoephedrine HCl 30 mg., guaifenesin 100 mg./5 cc. Bot. pt., gal.
Use: Cough relief.

TUSSAGESIC TABLETS. (Dorsey) Phenylpropanolamine HCl 25 mg., pheniramine maleate 12.5 mg., pyrilamine maleate 12.5 mg., dextromethorphan HBr 30 mg., terpin hydrate 180 mg., acetaminophen 325 mg./T.R. Tab. Bot. 100s.
Use: Common cold symptoms.

TUSSAGESIC SUSPENSION. (Dorsey) Phenylpropanolamine HCl 12.5 mg., pheniramine maleate 6.25 mg., pyrilamine maleate 6.25 mg., dextromethorphan HBr 15 mg., terpin hydrate 90 mg., acetaminophen 120 mg./5 ml. Liq. Bot. pt.
Use: Common cold symptoms.

TUSSAHIST. (Defco) Codeine phosphate 10 mg., phenylpropanolamine HCl 12.5 mg., chlorpheniramine maleate 2 mg., pyrilamine maleate 7.5 mg., guaifenesin 100 mg./5 cc. Bot. 4 oz. pt., gal.
Use: Treatment of coughs.

TUSSANIL. (Misemer) **Tab.:** Phenylephrine HCl 20 mg., chlorpheniramine maleate 2 mg., phenylpropanolamine HCl 10 mg., pyrilamine maleate 6 mg./Tab. Bot. 100s.
Syrup: Phenylephrine HCl 10 mg., chlorpheniramine maleate 1.66 mg., phenylpropanolamine HCl 5 mg., pyrilamine maleate 3.33 mg., menthol 0.166 mg./5 cc. Bot. pt.
Use: Treatment of colds, sinus and allergic rhinitis.

TUSSANIL DH. (Misemer) Same as Tussanil Syrup w/dihydrocodeinone bitartrate 1.66 mg./5 cc. Bot. pt.

TUSSANIL PLAIN SYRUP. (Misemer) Phenylephrine HCl 10 mg., phenylpropanolamine HCl 5 mg., pyrilamine maleate 3.33 mg., chlorpheniramine maleate 1.66 mg./5 ml.
Use: Symptomatic relief of colds, sinus, & allergic rhinitis.

TUSSANOL. (Tyler) Pyrilamine maleate ¾ gr., codeine phosphate 1 gr., ammonium chloride 7½ gr., sodium citrate 5 gr., menthol 1/10 gr./fl. oz. Bot. 4 fl. oz., pt., gal.
Use: Antihistamine, antitussive.

TUSSANOL with EPHEDRINE. (Tyler) Ephedrine sulfate 2 gr., pyrilamine maleate ¾ gr., codeine phosphate 1 gr., ammonium chloride 7½ gr., sodium citrate 5 gr., menthol 1/10 gr./30 cc. Bot. 16 fl. oz.
Use: Cough syrup. Bronchodilator, decongestant, antihistaminic.

TUSSAPAP. (Sutliff & Case) N-Acetyl-p-amino-phenol 195 mg., aspirin 130 mg., phenylephrine HCl 5 mg.,

noscapine 5 mg., caffeine 32.5 mg., pyrilamine maleate 12.5 mg./Tab. Bot. 100s, 1000s.
Use: Treatment of common cold.

TUSSAR-2 SYRUP. (USV Labs.) Codeine phosphate 10 mg., carbetapentane citrate 7.5 mg., chlorpheniramine maleate 2 mg., guaifenesin 50 mg., sod. citrate 130 mg., citric acid 20 mg./5 ml. w/alcohol 5%, methyl paraben 0.1%. Bot. pt.
Use: Cough suppressant.

TUSSAR DM. (USV Labs.) Dextromethorphan HBr 15 mg., chlorpheniramine maleate 2 mg., phenylephrine HCl 5 mg./5 ml. w/methylparaben 0.1% Bot. pt.
Use: Antitussive, Antihistaminic, decongestant.

TUSSAR SF. (USV Labs.) Codeine phosphate 10 mg., carbetapentane citrate 7.5 mg., chlorpheniramine maleate 2 mg., guaifenesin 50 mg., sod. citrate 130 mg., citric acid 20 mg./5 ml., methylparaben 0.1%, alcohol 12%. Bot. pt.
Use: Coughs.

TUSSCAPINE TABLETS. (Fisons) Noscapine 15 mg./Chewable Tab. Box 24s.
Use: Antitussive.

TUSSCAPS. (Martin-Philips) Chlorpheniramine maleate 8 mg., phenylpropanolamine 50 mg., dextromethorphan 20 mg., atropine sulfate 0.25 mg./Cap. Bot. 100s.
Use: Common cold.

TUSS-CHLORPHENADE. (Wolins) Chlorpheniramine maleate 8 mg., phenylpropanolamine HCl 50 mg., dextromethorphan 20 mg., atropine sulfate 0.36 mg./Cap. Bot. 100s, 1000s.

TUSSCIDIN EXPECTORANT. (Cenci) Guaifenesin 100 mg./5 cc. Bot. 4 oz., pt., gal.

TUSSCIDIN EXPECTORANT-D. (Cenci) Dextromethorphan HBr 15 mg., guaifenesin 100 mg./5 cc. Bot. 4 oz., pt., gal.

TUSSEND EXPECTORANT. (Merrell Dow) Pseudoephedrine HCl 60 mg., hydrocordone bitartrate 5 mg., guaifenesin 200 mg./5ml. w/ alcohol 12.5%. Bot. Pt.
Use: Antitussive, decongestant, expectorant.

TUSSEND LIQUID. (Merrell Dow) Hydrocodone bitartrate 5 mg., pseudoephedrine HCl 60 mg./5 ml. w/alcohol 5%. Bot. pt.
Use: Antitussive-decongestant.

TUSSEND TABLETS. (Merrell Dow) Hydrocodone bitartrate 5 mg., pseudoephedrine HCl 60 mg./Tab. Bot. 100s.
Use: Antitussive, decongestant.

TUSSIDRAM. (Dram) d-Methorphan 10 mg., phenylpropanolamine 12.5 mg., guaifenesin 50 mg., chlorpheniramine maleate 2 mg./5 cc. Bot. pt.
Use: Nasal decongestion and coughs.

TUSSILEX. Dropropizine, B.A.N.

TUSSIONEX. (Pennwalt) Hydrocodone (as resin complex) 5 mg., phenyltoloxamine 10 mg. as the resin complex/Tab. Cap., 5 cc. **Tab.:** Bot. 100s, **Liq.:** Bot. 1 pt., 900 ml. **Cap.:** Bot. 50s.
Use: Antitussive.

TUSSI-ORGANIDIN LIQUID. (Wallace) Codeine phos-

phate 10 mg.; Organidin 30 mg.; chlorpheniramine maleate 2 mg.; alcohol 15%/5 ml. Bot. 16 fl. oz., gal.
Use: Antitussive and expectorant combination.

TUSSI-ORGANIDIN DM LIQUID. (Wallace) Dextromethorphan HBr 10 mg., Organidin 30 mg., chlorpheniramine maleate 2 mg., alcohol 15%/5 ml. Bot. pt., gal.
Use: Antitussive and expectorant combination.

TUSSIREX WITH CODEINE. (Scot-Tussin) Codeine phosphate 10 mg., pheniramine maleate 13.33 mg., phenylephrine HCl 4.17 mg., sodium citrate 83.33 mg., sodium salicylate 83.33 mg., caffeine citrate 25 mg./5 ml. With and without sugar. Bot. Pts., gal.
Use: Coughs, colds.

TUSS-ORNADE LIQUID. (SmithKline) Caramiphen edisylate 6.7 mg., phenylpropanolamine HCl 12.5 mg./5 ml. w/alcohol 5%. Bot. pt.
Use: Antitussive/decongestant.

TUSS-ORNADE SPANSULE. (SmithKline) Caramiphen edisylate 40 mg., phenylpropanolamine HCl 75 mg./Cap. Bot. 50s, 500s.
Use: Decongestant.

TUSS-ORAMINIC. (Vortech) Chlorpheniramine maleate 8 mg., phenylpropanolamine HCl 50 mg., atropine sulfate 1/180 gr., dextromethorphan HBr 20 mg./Spancap. Bot. 100s, 1000s.
Use: Antihistaminic, decongestant, antitussive.

TUSSTAT EXPECTORANT. (Century) Diphenhydramine HCl 80 mg., ammonium chloride 12 gr., sodium citrate 5 gr., menthol ¹⁄₁₀ gr., alcohol 5%/oz. Bot. 4 fl. oz., pt., gal.

T.V.M. (Vitarine) Vit. A 10,000 I.U., D 400 I.U., B-1 10 mg., B-2 10 mg., niacinamide 100 mg., B-6 5 mg., B-12 5 mcg., C 200 mg., d-calcium pantothenate 20 mg., E 15 I.U., Fe 12 mg., Mn 1 mg., Mg 65 mg., Iodine 0.15 mg., Cu 2 mg., Zn 1.5 mg./Captab. Bot. 100s, 250s, 1000s.

TWEEN 20, 40, 60, 80. (ICI Americas) Polysorbates, N.F. XVI.
Use: Surface active agents.

TWENDEX PB. (Allison) Dextroamphetamine sulfate 20 mg., phenobarbital 1 gr./Tab. Bot. 30s, 100s.
Use: Obesity and mood stimulant.

TWENTISEC. (Schmid) Twenty second pregnancy test. 20 tests/Kit.

TWENTY EIGHTS. (Faraday) Tab. Bot. 28s.
Use: Relief of menstrual pain.

TWIN-K. (Boots) Potassium ions 20 mEq./15 ml. Bot. Pt.
Use: Treatment of hypokalemia.

TWIN-K-CL. (Boots) Potassium 15 mEq., chloride 4 mEq./15 ml. Bot. 16 oz.
Use: Oral potassium therapy.

TWO-CAL IM. (Fellows) Calcium glycerophosphate 10 mg., calcium levulinate 15 mg./ml. Vial 100 ml.
Use: Hypocalcemia.

2-24 COLD AND HAY FEVER TIME CAPSULE. (Walgreen) Belladonna alkaloids 0.2 mg., phenylpropanolamine HCl 50 mg., chlorpheniramine maleate 4 mg./Cap. Bot. 10s.
Use: Cold and hayfever.

TWO-DYNE CAPSULES. (Hyrex) Butalbital 50 mg.,

caffeine 40 mg., acetaminophen 325 mg./Cap. Bot. 100s, 1000s.
Use: Pain, nervous tension.

• **TYBAMATE.** USAN. 2-Methyl-2-propyl-trimethylene butylcarbamate carbamate. 2-(Hydroxymethyl)-2-methylpentyl butylcarbamate carbamate. 2-Carbamoyloxymethyl-2-methylpentyl butylcarbamate. Benvil; Solacen.
Use: Tranquilizer.

TYCOPAN. (Lilly) Vit. A 20,000 I.U., D 1000 I.U., B-1 10 mg., B-2 8 mg., B-6 10 mg., pantothenic acid 60 mg., niacinamide 60 mg., Vit. B-12 15 mcg., C 200 mg., E 22 I.U., biotin 0.16 mg., folic acid 0.45 mg., aminobenzoic acid 33 mg., inositol 160 mg., lipoic acid 0.3 mg., choline bitartrate 160 mg./3 Caps. Bot. 100s.
Use: Chronic alcoholism.

TYFORMIN. B.A.N. 4-Guanidinobutyramide.
Use: Oral hypoglycemic agent.
See: Augmentin hydrochloride.

TYLAGEL HYDROCHLORIDE. Tolpropamine, B.A.N.
TYLAN. Tylosin, B.A.N.

TYLENOL CHILDREN'S CHEWABLE TABLETS. (McNeil Prods) Acetaminophen 80 mg./Tab. Pkg. 30s.
Use: Analgesic, antipyretic.

TYLENOL CHILDREN'S ELIXIR. (McNeil Prods) Acetaminophen 160 mg./5 ml. Bot. 2 oz., 4 oz., pt., gal. Unit Dose 100 × 5 ml., 100 × 10 ml.
Use: Analgesic, antipyretic.

TYLENOL EXTRA-STRENGTH ADULT LIQUID. (McNeil Prods) Acetaminophen 1000 mg./30 ml. Bot. 8 oz. Unit Dose 100 × 20 ml., 100 × 30 ml.
Use: Analgesic, antipyretic.

TYLENOL EXTRA STRENGTH. (McNeil Prods) **Tab.:** Acetaminophen 500 mg./Tab. Bot. 30s, 60s, 100s, 200s. Vial 12s. **Caps.:** Bot. 24s, 50s, 100s, 165s. Hospital Sizes: Bot. 500s. Unit dose 200 × 2, 5 × 100.
Use: Analgesic, antipyretic.

TYLENOL INFANTS' DROPS. (McNeil Prods) Acetaminophen 80 mg./0.8 ml. Bot. w/dropper 15 ml.
Use: Analgesic, antipyretic.

TYLENOL MAXIMUM STRENGTH. (McNeil Prods) Acetaminophen 500 mg., pseudoephedrine HCl 30 mg./Cap. Bot. 20s, 24s.
Use: Temporary relief of the pain and congestion caused by sinusitis and colds.

TYLENOL REGULAR STRENGTH. (McNeil Prods) Acetaminophen. **Tabs:** 325 mg. Tin 12s. Vial 12s. Bot. 24s, 50s, 100s, 200s, 1000s. Unit dose 1000s, 200 × 2, 250 ×2. Hospital Sizes: Bot. 1000s, 5000s. Drum 25,000. Unit dose 2500 ×2, 5 × 1000. **Cap.:** 325 mg. Bot. 24s, 50s, 100s.
Use: Analgesic, antipyretic.

W/Carbinoxamine, phenylephrine HCl.
See: Clistin-D, Tab. (McNeil)
W/Chlorpheniramine maleate & pseudoephedrine HCl.
See: Cotylenol Cold Formula, Liq., Tab. (McNeil)
W/Chlorzoxazone.
See: Parafon Forte, Tab. (McNeil)

TYLENOL WITH CODEINE. (McNeil Pharm) **Tab.:** Acetaminophen 300 mg. **No. 1:** codeine phosphate 7.5 mg. Bot. 100s. **No. 2:** codeine phosphate 15 mg. Bot. 100s, 500s. Unit dose 100s. **No. 3:** codeine phosphate 30 mg. Bot. 100s, 500s, 1000s. Unit dose 100s. **No. 4:** codeine phosphate 60 mg. Bot. 100s, 500s. Unit dose 100s. **Cap.:** Acetaminophen 300 mg., **No. 3:** codeine phosphate 30 mg./Cap. Bot. 100s. Unit dose 100s. **No. 4:** codeine phosphate 60 mg./Cap. Bot. 100s. Unit dose 100s.
Use: Analgesic, antipyretic.

TYLENOL WITH CODEINE ELIXIR. (McNeil Pharm) Acetaminophen 120 mg., codeine phosphate 12 mg./5 ml. w/alcohol 7% Bot. Pts.
Use: Analgesic, antipyretic.

TYLOSIN. B.A.N. An antibiotic derived from an actinomycete resembling Streptomyces fradie. Tylan.
Use: Antibiotic, veterinary medicine.

TYLOX. (McNeil Pharm) Oxycodone HCl 4.5 mg., oxycodone terephthalate 0.38 mg., acetaminophen 500 mg./Cap. Bot. 100s unit dose 4 × 25s.
Use: Relief of moderate to severe pain.

• **TYLOXAPOL.** U.S.P. XXI. p-(1,1,3,3-Tetramethylbutyl) phenol polymer with formaldehyde and ethylene oxide.
Use: Detergent.

TYMATRO THROAT TROCHES. (Bowman) Cetylpyridinium Cl 1.5 mg., benzocaine 5 mg./Lozenge.
Use: Throat anesthetic.

TYMAZOLINE. B.A.N. 2-(5-Isopropyl-2-methylphenoxymethyl)-2-imidazoline. Pernazene hydrochloride.
Use: Vasoconstrictor.

TYMPAGESIC. (Adria) Phenylephrine HCl 0.25%, antipyrine 5%, benzocaine 5%, in propylene glycol. Liq., Bot. w/dropper 13 cc.
Use: Antihistaminic & analgesic ear drops.

TYMTRAN. (Adria) Ceruletide diethylamine salt equiv to 40 mcg., sodium thiomalate 2.2 mg./2 cc.
Use: Aid in oral cholecystography.

• **TYPHOID VACCINE,** U.S.P. XXI. (Wyeth)—Vial 5 cc., 10 cc., 20 cc.
Use: Active immunizing agent.

TYPHUS VACCINE.
Use: Active immunizing agent.

TYRIMIDE. Isopropamide Iodide, B.A.N.

TYROBENZ. (Mallard) Benzocaine 5 mg., cetalkonium chloride 2.5 mg., aromatics qs./Troche. Bot. 500s.
Use: Sore throat.

TYROHIST NASAL SPRAY. (Columbia) Pyrilamine maleate, desoxyephedrine HCl, cetalkonium chloride. Bot. 20 cc.
Use: Antihistamine, antibacterial, decongestant.

TYRO-LOZ. (Kenyon) Tyrothricin 2 mg., benzocaine 5 mg./Loz. Bot. 100s, 1000s.
Use: Sore throat.

• **TYROPANOATE SODIUM,** U.S.P. XXI. Cap, U.S.P. XXI. Sodium 3-butyramido-α-ethyl-2,4,6-triiodohydrocinnamate.

Use: Diagnostic aid (radiopaque medium-cholecysto-graphic).
See: Bilopaque (Winthrop-Breon)
TYROPAQUE CAPS. (Winthrop Products)
Tyropanoate sodium.
Use: Oral cholecystographic medium.
• **TYROSINE,** U.S.P. XXI. L-Tyrosine.
Use: Amino acid.
L-TYROSINE, 3-HYDROXY- Levodopa, U.S.P. XXI.
LEVO-TYROSINE, 3-HYDROXY-α-METHYL-, ETHYL ESTER HYDROCHLORIDE. Methyldopate Hydro-chloride, U.S.P. XXI.
L-TYROSINE,3-HYDROXY-α-METHYL-, SESQUIHY-DRATE. Methyldopa, U.S.P. XXI.
L-TYROSINE, O-(4-HYDROXY-3,5-DIIODOPHENYL)-3,5-DIIODO-MONOSODIUM SALT, HYDRATE. Levothyroxine Sodium, U.S.P. XXI.
L-TYROSINE, O-(4-HYDROXY-3-IODO-PHENYL-3,5-DIIODO-, MONOSODIUM SALT. Liothyronine So-dium, U.S.P. XXI.
TYROSUM. (Summers) Isopropanol 50%, polysorbate 80 & acetone. Bot. 4 oz., 1 pt. Pkg. 24s, 50s. w/3 cc. pad. Packetts 25s, 30s.
Use: Skin cleaner.
• **TYROTHRICIN,** U.S.P. XXI. Spray. Sol., Troches: An antibiotic from *Bacillus brevis.* Tyrodac; Tyroderm.
TYROTHRICIN COMBINATIONS.
TYZANOL HYDROCHLORIDE. Tetrahydrozoline, B.A.N.
TYZINE NASAL SOLUTION. (Key) Tetrahydrozoline HCl 0.1% Bot. pt., oz.
Use: Nasal decongestant.
TYZINE NASAL SPRAY. (Key) Tetrahydrozoline HCl 0.17. Bot. 0.5 oz.
Use: Nasal decongestant.
TYZINE PEDIATRIC NASAL DROPS. (Key) Tetrahydrozoline HCl 0.05%. Bot. 0.5 oz.
Use: Nasal decongestant.

U

UAA. (Econo Med) Methenamine 40.8 mg., phenyl salicylate 18.1 mg., methylene blue 5.4 mg., benzoic acid 4.5 mg., atropine sulfate 0.03 mg., hyoscyamine 0.03 mg./Tab. Bot. 100s.
Use: Antispasmodic and urinary antiseptic.
UBRETID. Distigmine Bromide, B.A.N.
UCG-BETA SLIDE MONOCLONAL. (Wampole) Two-minute latex agglutination inhibition slide test for the qualitative detection of B-hCG/hCG sensitivity 0.5 I.U. hCG/ml. in urine. Kits 50s, 100s, 300s.
Use: Aid in the diagnosis of pregnancy.
UCG-BETA STAT. (Wampole) One-hour passive hemagglutination inhibition tube test for the qualitative detection and quantitative determination of B-hCG/hCG sensitivity 0.2 I.U. hCG/ml. in urine. Kits 50s, 300s.
Use: Aid in the diagnosis of pregnancy.
UCG-LYPHOTEST. (Wampole) One-hour passive hemagglutination inhibition tube test for qualitative or quantitative the determination of human

chorionic gonadotropin (sensitivity 0.5-1.0 I.U. hCG/ml.) in urine. Kits 10s, 50s, 300s.
Use: Aid in the diagnosis of pregnancy.
UCG-SLIDE TEST. (Wampole) Rapid latex agglutination inhibition slide test for the qualitative detection of human chorionic gonadotropin (Sensitivity: 2 I.U. hCG/ml) in urine. Kits 30s, 100s, 300s, 1000s.
Use: Aid in the diagnosis of pregnancy.
UCG-TEST. (Wampole) Two-hour hemagglutination in-hibition tube test for the determination of human chorionic gonadotropin (sensitivity 0.5 I.U. hCG/ml undiluted specimen). 1.5 I.U. hCG/ml. 1:3 diluted specimen) in urine and serum. Kits 10s, 25s, 100s, 300s.
Use: Aid in the diagnosis of pregnancy.
UCG-TITRATION SET. (Wampole) A two-hour hemag-glutination inhibition tube test for the determination of human chorionic gonadotropin (Sensitivity 1 I.U. hCG/ml.) in urine or serum. Kit 45s.
Use: Aid in the diagnosis of pregnancy.
ULACORT. (Fellows) Prednisolone 5 mg./Tab. Bot. 1000s.
Use: Rheumatoid arthritis.
ULACORT (AQUASPENSION INJECTIONS). (Fellows) Prednisolone acetate 25 mg. or 50 mg./cc. Vial 10 cc.
ULBREVAL. Buthalitone Sodium, B.A.N.
ULCERIN P TABLETS. (Winthrop Products) Aluminum hydroxide.
Use: Antacid.
ULCERIN TABLETS. (Winthrop Products) Aluminum hydroxide.
Use: Antacid.
■ **ULCER THERAPY.**
See: Antacids
Anticholinergic Agents
ULCIMINS. (Miller) Glutamic acid magnesium complex 100 mg., magnesium oxide 100 mg., N-acetyl-p-aminophenol 64 mg., dl-methionine 25 mg., dl-α-tocopheryl acetate 5 I.U., glycine 150 mg., soybean flour/Tab. Bot. 100s.
Use: Antacid.
ULCORT CREAM. (Ulmer) Hydrocortisone in cream base. **0.5%:** Tube 1 oz. **1%:** Tube 1 oz. Jar 1 lb.
Use: Topical anti-inflammatory.
ULCORT LOTION. (Ulmer) Hydrocortisone in lotion base. **0.5%:** Bot. 2 oz., 4 oz.; **1%:** Bot. 2 oz., 4 oz.
Use: Topical anti-inflammatory.
ULO. (Riker) SL 501, Bayer B 186, Detigon. Chlophedianol HCl. alpha-(2-Dimethylaminoethyl)-o-chlorobenzhydrol HCl. Syr. (25 mg./5 ml.) Bot. 12 fl. oz.
Use: Acute cough associated with various respiratory infections, inflammations.
ULTANDREN. Fluoxymesterone, B.A.N.
ULTAR, CREAM. (Ulmer) Tar Extract 1% in a mentholated vanishing cream base. Jars 1 oz., 1 lb.
Use: Anti-eczematic cream.
ULTIMA II SCIENTIFIC SUN PRODUCTS. (Revlon) Padimate O, oxybenzone in lotion, oil, & stick.
Use: Sunburn prevention.
ULTRABEX. (Approved) Vit. B-1 20 mg., C 50 mg., B-

2 2 mg., B-6 0.5 mg., niacinamide 35 mg., cal. pantothenate 0.5 mg., wheat germ oil 30 mg., B-12 20 mcg., liver desic. 150 mg., Fe 11.58 mg., Ca 29 mg., P 23 mg., dicalcium phos. 100 mg., Mg 1.11 mg., Mn 1.30 mg., K 2.24 mg., Zn 0.68 mg., choline 25 mg., inositol 25 mg., pepsin 32.5 mg., diastase 32.5 mg., hesperidin 25 mg., biotin 20 mcg., hydrol. yeast 81.25 mg., protein digest 47.04 mg., amino acids 34.21 mg./Cap. Bot. 50s, 100s, 1000s.
Use: Dietary supplement.

ULTRACAIN HCI. Carticaine, B.A.N.

ULTRACAINE INJECTION. (Ulmer) Lidocaine HCl, Inj. 1%. Vial 50 ml.

ULTRA CAP. (Weeks & Leo) Acetaminophen 300 mg., guaifenesin 50 mg., chlorpheniramine maleate 4 mg., phenylephrine HCl 10 mg., dextromethorphan HBr. 6 mg./Cap. Vial 18s.
Use: Cold & flu relief.

ULTRACEF CAPSULES. (Bristol) Cefadroxil 500 mg./Cap. Bot. 50s, 100s.
Use: Antibiotic, antibacterial.

ULTRACEF ORAL SUSPENSION. (Bristol) Cefadroxil 125 mg. or 250 mg./5 ml. Bot. 50 ml., 100 ml.
Use: Antibiotic, antibacterial.

ULTRACEF TABLETS. (Bristol) Cefadroxil 1 Gm./Tab. Bot. 24s.
Use: Antibiotic, antibacterial.

ULTRACORTENOL. Prednisone, B.A.N.

ULTRACORTINOL. (Ciba) Agent to suppress over-active adrenal glands. Pending release.

ULTRA-DERM BATH LOTION. (Baker/Cummins) Mineral oil, lanolin derivatives, cetyl alcohol, glycerine, emulsifiers, perfume, preservatives and water. Bot. 8 oz.
Use: Medicament vehicle & emollient.

ULTRA-DERM BATH OIL. (Baker/Cummins) Mineral oil, lanolin derivatives, isopropyl myristate, emulsifier & perfume. Bot. 8 oz.
Use: Skin moisturizer.

ULTRA-DEW. (La Crosse) Therapeutic bath oil. Bot. 8 oz., 0.5 gal.
Use: Dry skin care.

ULTRALANUM 21-HEXANOATE. Fluocortolone, B.A.N.

ULTRALENTE INSULIN.
See: Iletin (Lilly)

ULTRA MIDE 25. (Baker/Cummins) Urea 25% Bot. 8 oz.
Use: Moisturizer lotion.

ULTRAN. Phenaglycodol, B.A.N.

ULTRAPAQUE- C. (Lafayette) Barium sulfate 96%. Containers 100 lbs.
Use: Alimentary tract radiography.

ULTRAPEN POTASSIUM SALT.
See: Propicillin, B.A.N.

ULTRASONE. (Gordon) Ultrasonic contact cream. Bot. qt., gal. Plastic Bot. 8 oz.

ULTRA TEARS. (Alcon) Hydroxypropyl methylcellulose 1%, benzalkonium chloride 0.01%/15 cc. Drop-tainer disp. 15 cc.
Use: Artificial tears.

ULTRA-TECHNEKOW. (Mallinckrodt) Technetium 99m.
Use: Radiopharmaceutical-diagnostic.

ULTRAZINE. (Vortech) Prochlorperazine 5 mg./ml. w/preservative & buffer. Vial 10 ml.
Use: I.M. or I.V. as antiemetic, tranquilizer.

10-UNDECENOIC ACID. Undecylenic Acid, U.S.P. XXI.

10-UNDECENOIC ACID, ZINC (2+) SALT. Zinc Undecylenate, U.S.P. XXI.

UNDECOYLIUM CHLORIDE-IODINE. 1-[[(2-Hydroxyethyl) carbamoyl]methyl]-pyridimium chloride alkanoates compound with I_2 (1:1). Virac, Prep. (Ruson)
Use: Topical anti-infective.

• **UNDECYLENIC ACID.** U.S.P. XXI. Compound Oint. U.S.P. XXI. 10-Undecenoic acid. (Lannett) Cap. 0.44 Gm., Bot. 100s, 500s, 1000s. Oint. comp. N.F.
Use: Topical antifungal.
See: Desenex Soap (Pharmacraft)
Ting Soap (Pharmacraft)
W/Benzethonium chloride, benzalkonium chloride, tannic acid, isopropyl alcohol.
See: Tulvex, Liq. (Commerce)
W/Dichlorophene.
See: Fungicidal Talc. (Gordon)
Onychomycetin, Liq. (Gordon)
W/Salicylic acid.
See: Sal-Dex, Liq. (Scrip)
W/Salicylic acid, benzoic acid, sulfur, dichlorophene.
See: Fungicidal Oint. (Gordon)
W/Salicylic acid, dichlorophene, hexachlorophene.
See: Podiaspray, Aerosol Pow. (Dalin)
W/Sod. propionate, sod. caprylate, propionic acid, salicylic acid, copper undecylenate.
See: Verdefam, Sol. (Texas)
W/Zinc undecylenate.
See: Desenex, Prep. (Pharmacraft)
Ting, Aerosol (Pharmacraft)
Undoguent, Cream (Torch)

UNDECYLENIC ACID SALTS. Calcium, Copper, Zinc.

UNDE-JEN. (Jenkins) Undecylenic acid 5%, zinc undecylenate 20%. Tube 1 oz., lb.

UNDEX CREAM. (Durel) Undecylenic acid 5%, zinc undecylenate 5% in Duromantel cream.
Use: Treatment and prevention of superficial dermatomycoses.

UNDOGUENT. (Torch) Undecylenic acid 5%, zinc undecylenate 20% in a non-greasy, water-washable cream base. Jar. 2 oz., 1 lb.
Use: Antifungal, antiseptic cream.

UNDULANT FEVER DIAGNOSIS. Brucella Abortus Antigen. Brucellergen.

UNGUENTINE OINTMENT "ORIGINAL FORMULA". (Procter & Gamble) Phenol 1% in ointment base. Tube 1 oz.
Use: Antiseptic, anesthetic for pain relief of minor burns.

UNGUENTINE PLUS FIRST AID CREAM. (Procter & Gamble) Parachlorometaxylenol 2%, lidocaine HCl 2%, phenol 0.5% in a moisturizing cream base. Tube 1 oz.

Use: Antiseptic, anesthetic for sunburn, minor burns, cuts and insect bites.

UNGUENTINE SPRAY. (Procter & Gamble) Benzocaine, alcohol. Can 5 oz.
Use: Sunburn, minor burns, itch, cuts and scrapes.

UNGUENTUM BOSSI. (Doak) Ammoniated mercury 5%, hexamethylene tetramine sulfosalicylic acid 2%, tar distillate "Doak" 5%, Doak oil 40%, nonionic emulsifiers 5%, unguentum "Doak" 48%. Tube 2 oz. Jar 16 oz.
Use: Psoriasis.

UNIAD. (Kasar) Isoniazid 100 mg./Tab. Bot. 100s, 1000s.
Use: Tuberculosis.

UNIAD-PLUS. (Kasar) Isoniazid 100 mg. pyridoxine HCl 5 mg. or 10 mg./Tab. Bot. 1000s.
Use: Tuberculosis.

UNIBASE. (Parke-Davis) Water-absorbing oint. base. Jar 1 lb.
Use: Ointment base.

UNICAP. (Upjohn) Vit. A 5000 I.U., D 400 I.U., E 15 I.U., C 60 mg., folic acid 400 mcg., B-1 1.5 mg., B-2 1.7 mg., niacin 20 mg., B-6 2 mg., B-12 6 mcg./Tab. or Cap. Tab.: Bot. 90s; Cap. Bot. 90s, 240s, 1000s.
Use: Multivitamin.

UNICAP CHEWABLE. (Upjohn) Vit. A 5000 I.U., D 400 I.U., E 15 I.U., C 60 mg., folic acid 400 mcg., B-1 1.5 mg., B-2 1.7 mg., niacin 20 mg., B-6 2 mg., B-12 6 mcg./Tab. Bot. 90s.
Use: Multivitamin.

UNICAP M. (Upjohn) Vit A 5000 I.U., D 400 I.U., E 15 I.U., C 60 mg., folic acid 400 mcg. B-1 1.5 mg., B-2 1.7 mg., niacin 20 mg., B-6 2 mg., B-12 6 mcg., pantothenic acid 10 mg., iodine 150 mcg., Fe 18 mg., Cu 2 mg., Zn 15 mg., Mn 1 mg., K 5 mg./Tab. Bot. 30s, 90s, 120s, 180s, 500s.
Use: Multiple vitamins with mineral supplement.

UNICAP PLUS IRON. (Upjohn) Vit. A 5000 I.U., D 400 I.U., E 15 I.U., C 60 mg., folic acid 400 mcg., B-1 1.5 mg., B-2 1.7 mg., niacin 20 mg., B-6 2 mg., B-12 6 mcg., pantothenic acid 10 mg., iron 18 mg./Tab. Bot. 90s.
Use: Vitamin supplement with iron.

UNICAP SENIOR. (Upjohn) Vit. A 5000 I.U., E 15 I.U., C 60 mg., folic acid 400 mcg., B-1 1.2 mg., B-2 1.7 mg., niacin 14 mg., B-6 2 mg., B-12 6 mcg., pantothenic acid 10 mg., iodine 150 mcg., Fe 10 mg., Cu 2 mg., Zn 15 mg., Mn 1 mg., K 5 mg./Tab. Bot. 90s.
Use: Supplement to the often deficient diet.

UNICAP T. (Upjohn) Vit. A 5000 I.U., D 400 I.U., E 15 I.U., C 300 mg., folic acid 400 mcg., B-1 10 mg., B-2 10 mg., niacin 100 mg., B-6 6 mg., B-12 8 mcg., pantothenic acid 10 mg., iodine 150 mcg., Fe 18 mg., Cu 2 mg., Zn 15 mg., Mn 1 mg., K 5 mg./Tab. Bot. 30s, 60s, 500s.
Use: Nutritional deficiencies.

UNIFAST UNICELLES. (Reid-Provident) Phentermine HCl 30 mg./Cap. Bot. 100s.
Use: Appetite suppressant.

UNIGEN IN OIL. (Vortech) Natural estrogen in sesame oil 20,000 I.U./cc. Vial 30 ml.

Use: Estrogen therapy.

UNILAX. (Ascher) Danthron 75 mg., docusate sodium 150 mg./Tab. Pkg. 10s, 20s. Bot. 60s, 100s.
Use: Laxative, stool softener.

UNIMYCIN DIHYDRATE. Oxytetracycline, B.A.N.

UNIPEN. (Wyeth) Sodium nafcillin **Cap.** 250 mg. Bot. 100s. Redipak 100s. **Tab.** 500 mg. Bot. 50s. Cap. and Tab. buffered w/calcium carbonate. **Inj.** 500 mg./Vial, 10s. Buffered to make 2 cc. 1 Gm., 2 Gm. **Vial:** Piggyback Vials 1 Gm., 1.5 Gm., 2 Gm., 4 Gm. Bulk vial 10 Gm. **Oral Sol.** w/alcohol 2% 250 mg./5 cc. Bot. to make 100 cc.
Use: Treatment of infections.

UNIPRES. (Reid-Provident) Hydralazine HCl 25 mg., hydrochlorothiazide 15 mg., reserpine 0.1 mg./Tab. Bot. 100s, 1000s.
Use: Anti-hypertension.

UNISOL. (CooperVision) Sterile, preservative-free saline solution. Vials 15 ml. Box 10s, 25s.
Use: Rinsing after cleaning heat disinfection and storage of soft contact lenses.

UNISOL 4. (CooperVision) Sterile saline sol. for all soft lenses. Bot. 4 oz. Box 2s.
Use: Rinsing, heat disinfection & storage of soft lenses.

UNISOM. (Leeming) Doxylamine succcinate 25 mg./Tab. Blister 8s, 16s, 32s.
Use: Sleep aid.

UNNA'S BOOT.
See: Zinc Gelatin, U.S.P. XXI.

UNPROCO CAPSULES. (Reid-Provident) Dextromethorphan HBr 30 mg., guaifenesin 200 mg./Cap. Bot. 100s.
Use: Antitussive, expectorant.

■ **UNSATURATED ACIDS.**
See: Fatty acids, unsaturated; fats, unsaturated.

UPLEX. (Arcum) Vit. A 5000 I.U., D 400 I.U., B-1 3 mg., B-2 3 mg., B-6 1 mg., B-12 2.5 mcg., nicotinamide 20 mg., calcium pantothenate 5 mg., Vit. C 50 mg./Cap. Bot. 100s, 1000s.
Use: Dietary supplement.

UPLEX NO. 2. (Arcum) Vit. A palmitate 10,000 I.U., D 400 I.U., B-1 5 mg., B-2 5 mg., C 100 mg., B-6 2 mg., B-12 3 mcg., E 2.5 I.U., niacinamide 25 mg., ca pantothenate 5 mg./Cap. Bot. 100s, 1000s.
Use: Dietary supplement.

URACEL. (Vortech) Sod. salicylate 324 mg./Tab. Bot. 1000s.
Use: Analgesic.

URACID. (Wesley) dl-Methionine 0.2 Gm./Cap. Bot. 100s, 1000s.
Use: Diaper Rash.

• **URACIL MUSTARD,** U.S.P. XXI. Cap., U.S.P. XXI. 5-[Bis(2-Chloroethyl)amino]uracil. (Upjohn) 1.0 mg./Cap. Bot. 50s.
Use: Antineoplastic.

URADAL.
See: Carbromal (Various Mfr.)

URALENE TABLETS. (Sutliff & Case) Methenamine 40.8 mg., atropine sulfate 0.03 mg., hyoscyamine sulfate 0.03 mg., salol 18.1 mg., benzoic acid 4.5 mg., methylene blue 5.4 mg./Tab. Bot. 1000s.
Use: Urinary antiseptic.

URAMINE. (Kay) Atropine sulfate 0.03 mg., hyoscyamine 0.03 mg., methenamine 40.8 mg., methylene blue 5 4 mg., phenyl salicylate 18.1 mg., benzoic acid 4.5 mg./Tab. Bot. 1000s.
Use: Urinary antiseptic.
URAMUSTINE. B.A.N. 5-Di-(2-chloroethyl) aminouracil.
Use: Antineoplastic agent.
URANAP. (Vortech) dl-Methionine 0.2 Gm./Cap. Bot. 100s.
Use: Control of diaper rash.
URANTOIN. Nitrofurantoin, B.A.N.
URDEX. (Pharmex) Phenylpropanolamine 12.5 mg., atropine sulfate 0.2 mg., chlorpheniramine 5 mg./cc. Vial 10 cc.
• **UREA,** U.S.P. XXI. Sterile U.S.P. XXI. Carbamide (Various Mfr.)
Use: Topically for dry skin.
See: Aquacare, Cream, Lot. (Herbert)
  Aqucare-HP, Cream, Lot. (Herbert)
  Artra Ashy Skin Cream (Plough)
  Calmurid, Cream (Pharmacia)
  Carmol, Cream (Ingram)
  Carmol Ten Lotion (Ingram)
  Elaqua 10% or 20%, Cream (Elder)
  Gormel Cream (Gordon)
  Nutraplus, Cream, Lot. (Owen)
  Rea-lo, Lot. (Whorton)
W/Benzocaine, benzyl alcohol, p-chloro-m-xylenol, propylene glycol.
See: 20-Cain Burn Relief, Bot. (Alto)
W/Hydrocortisone acetate
See: Carmol-HC, Cream (Ingram)
W/Glycerin.
See: Kerid Ear Drops, Liq. (Blair)
W/Sulfur colloidal, red mercuric sulfide.
See: Teenac Cream, Oint. (Elder)
W/Zinc oxide, sulfur, salicylic acid, benzalkonium chloride, isopropyl alcohol.
See: Akne Drying Lotion, Bot. (Alto)
UREACIN-10 LOTION. (Pedinol) Urea 10%. Bot. 8 oz.
Use: Moisturizing and softening lotion for dry, hard, rough, hardened skin.
UREACIN-20 CREME. (Pedinol) Urea 20%. Jars 2.5 oz.
Use: Moisturizing and softening cream for dry, hard skin when extra penetration needed.
UREACIN-40 CREME. (Pedinol) Urea 40%. Jar 1 oz.
Use: Nail destruction and dissolution.
UREA PEROXIDE.
UREAPHIL. (Abbott) Sterile urea 40 Gm., citric acid 1 mg./150 ml. Bot. 150 ml.
Use: Osmotic dehydrating agent.
URECHOLINE. (Merck Sharp & Dohme) Bethanechol Chloride Inj., 5 mg./ml., Vial 1 ml. 6s. Tab. 5 mg., 10 mg., 25 mg., 50 mg. Bot. 100s. Unit Dose Pkg. 100s.
Use: Parasympathomimetic.
• **UREDEPA.** USAN. Ethyl[bis(1-aziridinyl)-phos-phinyl]-carbamate.
Use: Anti-neoplastic.
See: Avinar (Armour)
p-UREIDOBENZENEARSONIC ACID.
See: Carbarsone, U.S.P. XXI.
• **UREDOFOS.** USAN.

Use: Anthelmintic.
See: Sansalid (Beecham)
URELIEF. (Rocky Mtn.) Methenamine 2 gr., salol ½ gr., methylene blue ¹⁄₁₀ gr., benzoic acid ⅛ gr., hyoscyamine sulfate ¹⁄₂₀₀₀ gr., atropine sulfate ¹⁄₁₀₀₀ gr./Tab. Bot. 100s.
Use: Urinary anti-infective.
URELIM. Ethebenecid, B.A.N.
UREMIDE. (Mallard) Phenylazodiaminopyridine HCl 50 mg., sulfamethazole 250 mg./Tab. Bot. 50s.
Use: Analgesic, antibacterial, antispasmodic.
URESE. (Roerig)
See: Benzthianide.
URETHAN. Ethyl Carbamate, Ethyl Urethan, Urethane.
Use: Antineoplastic.
UREX TABLETS. (Riker) Methenamine hippurate 1 Gm./Tab. Bot. 100s, 500s.
Use: Urinary anti-infective.
URICOSURIC AGENTS.
See: Anturane, Tab., Cap. (Geigy)
  Benemid, Tab. (Merck Sharp & Dohme)
U.R.I. (Sig) Atropine sulfate 0.2 mg., chlorpheniramine maleate 5 mg., phenylpropanolamine HCl 12.5 mg./ml. Vial 10 ml.
Use: Symptomatic relief of colds.
URIDINAL. (Crystal) Phenylazodiamino pyridine HCl 1.5 gr./Tab. Bot. 100s.
Use: Urinary antiseptic.
URIDINAL-S. (Crystal) Tab. Bot. 100s.
4-[3-[2-(TRIFLUOROMETHYL)PHENOTHIAZIN-10-YL]PROPYL]-1-PIPERAZINEETHANOL. Fluphenazine or Enanthate Hydrochloride.
URIDINE, 2-DEOXY-5-IODO-. Idoxuridine, U.S.P. XXI.
URIDIUM. (Ferndale; Pharmex) Phenylazodiamine pyridine HCl 75 mg., sulfacetamide 250 mg./Tab. Bot. 30s, 100s, 1000s. (Ferndale) 100s.
Use: Urinary antiseptic.
URIFON. (T.E. Williams) Sulfamethizole 500 mg./Tab. Bot. 100s, 1000s.
URIFON-FORTE. (T.E. Williams) Sulfamethizole 450 mg., phenazopyridine HCl 50 mg./Cap. Bot. 100s, 1000s.
URIGEN. (Fellows) Calcium mandelate 0.2 Gm., methenamine 0.2 Gm., phenazopyridine HCl 50 mg., sodium phosphate 80 mg./Cap. Bot. 100s, 1000s.
URILENE. (Crystal) Tab. Bot. 100s.
URINARY ANTISEPTIC #2 S.C.T. (Lemmon) Atropine sulfate 0.03 mg., hyoscyamine 0.03 mg., methenamine 40.8 mg., methylene blue 5.4 mg., phenyl salicylate 18.1 mg., benzoic acid 4.5 mg./Tab. Bot. 100s, 1000s.
Use: Urinary antiseptic.
URINE.
See: Diagnostic agents
URINE SUGAR TEST.
See: Clinistix (Ames)
URIN-TEK. (Ames) Tubes, plastic caps, adhesive labels, collection cups, and disposable tube holder. Package 100×5.
URI-PAK. (O'Neal, Jones & Feldman) Sulfamethizole 500 mg./blue Tab. phenazopyridine HCl 200 mg./red Tab. 58 blue Tabs. 15 red Tabs.

Use: Urinary anti-infective.

URIPREL. (Pasadena Research) Methenamine 40.8 mg., atropine sulfate 0.03 mg., hyoscyamine sulfate 0.03 mg., salol 18.1 mg., benzoic acid 4.5 mg., methylene blue 5.4 mg., gelsemium 6.1 mg./Tab. Bot. 100s, 1000s.

URISAN-P. (Sandia) Atropine sulfate 0.03 mg., hyoscyamine 0.03 mg., gelsemium 6.1 mg., methenamine 40.8 mg., salol 18.1 mg., benzoic acid 4.5 mg., methylene blue 5.4 mg., phenylazodiaminopyridine HCl 100 mg./Tab. Bot. 100s, 1000s.
Use: Urinary antiseptic, analgesic.

URISED. (Webcon) Atropine sulfate 0.03 mg., hyoscyamine 0.03 mg., methenamine 40.8 mg., methylene blue 5.4 mg., benzoic acid 4.5 mg., phenyl salicylate 18.1 mg./Tab. Bot. 100s, 500s, 1000s.
Use: Relief of pain in urinary infections.

URISEDAMINE. (Webcon) Methenamine mandelate 500 mg., l-hyoscyamine 0.15 mg./Tab. Bot. 100s.
Use: G.U. antiseptic & antispasmodic.

URISEPT. (Robinson) Urinary antiseptic Tab. Bot. 100s, 1000s.

URISPAS. (SmithKline) Flavoxate HCl 100 mg./Tab. Bot. 100s. Unit Dose 100s.
Use: Urinary antispasmodic.

URISTIX. (Ames) Firm paper two-test strip. Proteinuria: Yellow tip-tetrabromphenol blue. Glycosuria: Red tip-glucose oxidase. Bot. 100s.
Use: Dip and read test for protein and glucose in urine.

URITABS. (Vortech) Atropine sulfate 0.03 mg., hyoscyamine 0.03 mg., methenamine 40.8 mg., salol 18.1 mg., benzoic acid 4.5 mg., methylene blue 5.4 mg./Tab. Bot. 100s, 1000s.
Use: Urinary tract antiseptic.

URITHOL. (O'Neal, Jones & Feldman) Methenamine 40.8 mg., Methylene blue 5.4 mg., benzoic acid 4.5 mg., atropine sulfate 0.03 mg., hyoscyamine 0.03 mg., salol 18.1 mg./Tab. Bot. 100s.
Use: Cystitis, pyelitis, urethritis.

URITIN. (Richlyn) **Purple:** Methenamine 40.8 mg., atropine sulfate 0.03 mg., hyoscyamine sulfate 0.03 mg., salol 18.1 mg., benzoic acid 4.5 mg., methylene blue 5.4 mg., gelsemium 6.1 mg./Tab. Bot. 1000s.

URITIN FORMULA. (Vangard) Atropine sulfate 0.03 mg., hyoscyamine 0.03 mg., methenamine 40.8 mg., methylene blue 5.4 mg., phenyl salicylate 18.1 mg., benzoic acid 4.5 mg./Tab. Bot. 1000s.
Use: Urinary antiseptic.

URITIN MODIFIED FORMULA. (Wolins) Methenamine 40.8 mg., atropine sulfate 0.03 mg., hyoscyamine sulfate 0.03 mg., salol 18.1 mg., benzoic acid 4.5 mg., methylene blue 5.4 mg./Tab. Bot. 1000s.

URITROL. (Kenyon) Atropine sulfate 0.03 mg., hyoscyamine 0.03 mg., gelsemium 6.1 mg., methenamine 40.8 mg., salol 18.1 mg., benzoic acid 4.5 mg., methylene blue 5.4 mg./Tab. Bot. 100s, 1000s. Double Strength Tabs. Bot. 100s, 1000s.

URIZOLE. (Jenkins) Sulfisoxazole 7.7 gr./Tab. Bot. 1000s.

UROBILISTIX. (Ames) p-Dimethylaminobenzaldehyde in an acid buffer. Bot. 50s, strips.
Use: Dip and read test for urine urobilinogen.

UROBIOTIC. (Roerig) Oxytetracycline as the HCl equiv. to 250 mg. oxytetracycline, sulfamethizole 250 mg., phenylazodiaminopyridine HCl 50 mg./Cap. Bot. 50s. Unit-dose pack. Box 100s.
Use: Urinary tract infections.

URODINE. (Interstate) Phenazo pyridine HCl 100 mg./Tab. Bot. 1000s.
Use: Urinary analgesic and antiseptic.

URODINE. (Kenyon) Phenylazodiaminopyridine HCl 100 mg./Tab. Bot. 100s, 1000s.
Use: Urinary analgesic and antiseptic.

URODINE. (Robinson) Phenylazo-diamino-pyridine HCl 1½ gr./Tab. Bot. 100s, 1000s.
Use: Urinary antiseptic.

UROGESIC. (Edwards) Phenazopyridine HCl 100 mg., hyoscyamine HBr 0.12 mg., atropine sulfate 0.08 mg., scopolamine HBr 0.003 mg./Tab. Bot. 100s, 500s.
Use: Analgesic for urinary tract disturbances.

■**UROGRAPHY AGENTS.**
See: Diodrast
Iodohippurate Sodium, Inj.
Iodopyracet
Iodopyracet Compound
Methiodal, Inj.
Renografin (Squibb)
Renovist (Squibb)
Renovue (Squibb)
Sodium Acetrizoate, Inj.
Sodium Iodomethamate, Inj.

• **UROKINASE.** USAN. Plasminogen activator isolated from human kidney tissue.
Use: Plasminogen activator.

URO-KP-NEUTRAL. (Star) Sodium (as dibasic sodium phosphate) 1361 mg., potassium 298.6 mg., phosphorous (as dibasic potassium phosphate) 1037 mg./6 Tabs. Bot. 100s.
Use: Treatment of oxalate renal calculi.

UROLENE BLUE. (Star) Methylene blue 65 mg./Tab. Bot. 100s, 1000s.
Use: Urinary antiseptic & stimulant to mucous membrane surfaces.

UROLOGIC SOL G. (Abbott) Bot. 1000 ml.
Use: Irrigating solution.

UROLUCOSIL. Sulphamethizole, B.A.N.
See: Thiosulfi, Preps. (Ayerst)

URO-MAG. (Blaine) Magnesium oxide 140 mg./Cap. Bot. 100s, 1000s.
Use: Antacid; calcium oxalate urinary stone prevention.

UROMIDE. (Edwards) Salicylamide 0.667 Gm./Tab. Bot. 100s, 500s.
Use: Prevention of calcium-containing urinary calculi.

URONAL.
See: Barbital (Various Mfr.)

URO-PHOSPHATE. (Poythress) Sod. acid phosphate

500 mg., methenamine 300 mg./S.C. Tab. Bot. 100s, 1000s.
Use: Urinary antiseptic.
UROQID-ACID. (Beach) Methenamine mandelate 350 mg., sodium acid phosphate 200 mg./Tab. Bot. 100s, 500s.
Use: Urinary acidifier, antibacterial.
UROQID-ACID NO. 2. (Beach) Methenamine mandelate 500 mg., sodium acid phosphate 500 mg./Tab. Bot. 100s, 500s.
Use: Urinary acidifier, antiseptic.
UROSCREEN. (Warner-Lambert) 2,3,5, Triphenyltetrazolium chloride. Individual test tubes containing dry, buffered tetrazolium reagent for in-vitro testing of urine. Each tube is calibrated at the 2 cc. level. Boxes 12s, 50s.
Use: Diagnostic agent for urinary infection.
UROTROL. (Mills) Sulfacetamide 250 mg., sulfamethizole 250 mg., phenazopyridine HCl 50 mg./Tab. Bot. 100s.
Use: Urinary tract infection and pain.
UROTROPIN NEW. Methenamine Anhydromethylene Citrate (Various Mfr.)
UROVIST CYSTO. (Berlex) Diatrizoate meglumine 300 mg., edetate calcium disodium 0.05 mg./ml. Bot.: 500 ml. dilution bot. w/300 ml. soln.
Use: Diagnostic radiopaque medium intended for instillation.
UROVIST CYSTO PEDIATRIC. (Berlex) Diatrizoate meglumine 300 mg., edetate calcium disodium 0.05 mg./ml. Bot.: 300 ml. dilution bot. w/100 ml. soln.
Use: Diagnostic radiopaque medium intended for instillation.
UROVIST MEGLUMINE DIU/CT. (Berlex) Diatrizoate meglumine 300 mg., edetate calcium disodium 0.05 mg./ml. Bot. 300 ml. Ctn. 10s.
Use: Diagnostic radiopaque medium for parenteral use.
UROVIST SODIUM 300. (Berlex) Diatrizoate sodium 500 mg., edetate calcium disodium 0.1 mg./ml. Vial 50 ml. Box 10s.
Use: Diagnostic radiopaque medium for parenteral use.
URSINUS INLAY-TABS. (Dorsey) Calcium carbaspirin (equivalent to aspirin 300 mg.), phenylpropanolamine HCl 25 mg., pheniramine maleate 12.5 mg. pyrilamine maleate 12.5 mg./Tab. Bot. 24s, 100s.
Use: Analgesic, decongestant.
URSULFADINE NO. 1. (Kenyon) Phenylazodiaminopyridine HCl 50 mg., sulfacetamide 250 mg./Tab. Bot. 100s, 1000s.
UTEN CAPSULES. Papaveroline, B.A.N.
UTICILLIN VK. (Upjohn) Penicillin V Potassium 250 mg./Tab. Bot. 1000s, 500 mg./Tab. Bot. 100s.
Use: Penicillin susceptible infections.
UTICORT GEL. (Parke-Davis) Betamethasone benzoate 0.025% in solubilized gel base. Tubes 15 Gm., 60 Gm.
Use: Relief of inflammatory manifestations of corticosteroid responsive dermatoses.

UTICORT CREAM. (Parke-Davis) Betamethasone benzoate 0.025%. Tube 15 Gm., 60 Gm.
Use: Relief of inflammatory manifestations of corticosteroid responsive dermatoses.
UTICORT LOTION. (Parke-Davis) Betamethasone benzoate 0.025%. Bot. 15 ml., 60 ml.
Use: Relief of inflammatory manifestations of corticosteroid responsive dermatoses.
UTICORT OINTMENT. (Parke-Davis) Betamethasone benzoate 0.025%. Tube 15 Gm., 60 Gm.
Use: Relief of inflammatory manifestations of corticosteroid responsive dermatoses.
UTIMOX, (Parke-Davis) Amoxicillin trihydrate **Cap.:** 250 mg., or 500mg./Cap. Bot. 100s, 500s. Unit dose 100s. **Oral susp.:** 125 mg. or 250 mg./5 ml. Bot. 80 ml, 100 ml., 150 ml., 200 ml.
Use: Antibiotic.
U-TRACT. (Bowman) Atropine sulfate 0.03 mg., hyoscyamine sulfate 0.03 mg., methenamine 40.8 mg., methylene blue 5.4 mg., phenylsalicylate 18.1 mg., benzoic acid 4.5 mg./Tab. Bot. 100s, 1000s.
Use: Treatment urinary tract infections.
U-TRAN. (Scruggs) Atropine sulfate 0.03 mg., hyoscyamine 0.03 mg., methenamine 40.80 mg., benzoic acid 4.50 mg., salol 18.10 mg., methylene blue 5.40 mg./Tab. Bot. 100s, 1000s.
U-TRI SPEC FORMULA. (U-Tri) Oint. Tube 4 oz., 8 oz. Jar 4 oz., 8 oz.
Use: Athletics, muscular aches and pains, colds.
UVALERAL.
See: Bromisovalum.
UVA URSI. Leaves. (Sherwood Labs.) Fluid ext. Bot. pt., gal.
W/Buchu leaves, corn silk, juniper, caffeine.
See: Diuretane #1, Tab. (Wolins)
UVIBAN. Sodium Actinoquinol.
Use: Treatment of flash burns. (ophthalmic)
UVINUL MS-40. (General Aniline & Film)
See: Sulisobenzone.
UVISTAT. Mexenone, B.A.N.

V

VABRA ASPIRATOR. (CooperVision) Sterile uterine curette, diameter 3 mm., Disposable.
Use: Endometrial screening.
VACCINE, MUMPS. Mumps Virus Vaccine Live, U.S.P. XXI.
• **VACCINE, PERTUSSIS.** Pertussis Vaccine, U.S.P. XXI.
Use: Active immunizing agent.
• **VACCINE, PERTUSSIS, ADSORBED.** Pertussis Vaccine Adsorbed, U.S.P. XXI.
Use: Active immunizing agent.
See: Pertussis Vaccine, Aluminum Hydroxide Adsorbed
• **VACCINE, PERTUSSIS, ALUM PRECIPITATED.**
Use: Active immunizing agent.
See: Pertussis Vaccine, Alum Precipitated (Various Mfr.)

• **VACCINE, POLIOMYELITIS.** Poliovirus Vaccine Inactivated, U.S.P. XXI.
Use: Active immunizing agent.

• **VACCINE, RABIES (DUCK EMBRYO),** Rabies Vaccine U.S.P. XXI.
Use: Active immunizing agent.

• **VACCINE, SMALLPOX.** Smallpox Vaccine, U.S.P. XXI.
Use: Active immunizing agent.

VACCINE, WHOOPING COUGH. Pertussis Vaccine, U.S.P. XXI.
Use: Active immunizing agent.

• **VACCINIA IMMUNE GLOBULIN,** U.S.P. XXI. (Hyland) Gamma globulin fraction of serum of healthy adults recently immunized w/vaccinia virus 16.5%. Vial 5 ml.
Use: Prevention or modification of smallpox or vaccinia infections; passive immunizing agent.

VACOCIN. Under study.
Use: Antibiotic.

VACON. (Scherer) Phenylephrine HCl 0.20% with benzalkonium chloride. Nasal solution, Bot. 1 oz. Drops 1 oz.
Use: Nasal decongestant.

VAGACREME. (Delta) Sulfanilamide 12%, sulfacetamide 3%, 9-aminoacridine HCl 0.2%, allantoin 1.5%. Tube 4 oz. w/appl.
Use: Vaginitis.

VAGICREAM. (Vortech) Sulfanilamide 15%, 9-aminocridine HCl 0.2%, allantoin 1.5%. Tube 4 oz.
Use: Vaginitis and non-specific vaginal infections.

VAGILIA CREAM. (Lemmon) Sulfisoxazole 10%, aminacrine HCl 0.2%, allantoin 2% in a water-miscible base w/stearic acid, mineral oil, polysorbate 60, sorbitan monostearate, sorbitol, methylparaben, propylparaben, purified water. Cream, Tube 90 Gm.
Use: Treatment of vaginitis and cervicitis.

VAGILLA SUPPOSITORIES. (Lemmon) Sulfisoxazole 600 mg., aminacrine HCl 12 mg., allantoin 120 mg./Supp. Box 16s.
Use: Treatment of vaginitis, cervicitis.

VAGINEX CREME. (Schmidt) Benzocaine and resorcinol in cream base.
Use: Antipruritic for feminine itching.

VAGISAN CREME. (Sandia) Sulfanilamide 15%, 9-aminoacridine HCl 0.2%, allantoin 1.5%. In a dispersible base. Tube 4 oz. w/applicator.

VAGISEC. (Schmid) Polyoxyethylene nonyl phenol, sodium ethylenediaminetetraacetate, docusate sodium. Plastic Bot. 4 oz. Liquid, Packettes, 12s.
Use: Trichomonacide.

VAGISEC PLUS SUPPOSITORIES. (Schmid) Polyoxyethylene nonyl phenol 0.175%, sodium edetate 0.022%, docusate sodium 0.0024%, 9-aminoacridine HCl 0.2%, in a polyethylene glycol base w/glycerin and citric acid. Box 28s.

VAGISUL CREME. (Sheryl) Sulfanilamide 15%, aminoacridine 0.2%, allantoin 1.5%. Tube 4 oz.
Use: Vaginitis, cervicitis and post-cauterization therapy.

VAGITROL. (Lemmon) **Cream:** Sulfanilamide 15%, aminacrine HCl 0.2%, allantoin 2%. w/lactose,

stearic acid, cetyl alcohol, triethanolamine, sod. lauryl sulfate, glycerin, methylparaben and propylparaben as preservatives, buffered w/lactic acid to a pH of approximately 4.5. Tube 4 oz. **Suppos:** Sulfanilamide 1.05 Gm., allantoin 0.14 Gm., aminacrine HCl 0.014 Gm./Suppos. in a water miscible base w/lactose, polyethylene glycol 400, polysorbate 80, polyethylene glycol 4000, glycerin, lactic acid and coloring, methylparaben and propylparaben as preservatives. Supp. equiv. to applicatorful of Vagitrol Cream. Blister Pkg. 16s.
Use: Vaginitis treatment.

VALACET. (Vale) Hyoscyamus 10.8 mg., aspirin 259.2 mg., caffeine anhydrous 16.2 mg., gelsemium ext. 0.6 mg./Tab. or Cap. Bot. 100s, 1000s, 5000s.

VALADOL. (Squibb) Acetaminophen. **Tabs.:** 5 gr. Bot. 100s, 500s. **Liq.:** (w/alcohol 9%) 120 mg./5 cc. Bot. 4 oz.
Use: Aspirin substitute.

VALAX. (Vale) Danthron 37.5 mg., docusate sodium 100 mg./Tab. Bot. 100s, 1000s.
Use: Laxative, fecal softener.

VALCAPS. (Roche) Diazepam 2 mg., 5 mg., 10 mg./Cap. Box 100s. Limited marketing.
Use: Anxiety disorders; tension, anxiety, apprehension and fatigue associated with psychoneurotic states; acute alcohol withdrawl; skeletal muscle spasms; etc.

VALDRENE. (Vale) Diphenhydramine HCl 50 mg./Tab. Bot. 100s, 1000s, 5000s.
Use: Antihistamine.

VALDRENE EXPECTORANT. (Vale) Diphenhydramine HCl 80 mg., ammonium chloride 778 mg., sod. citrate 324 mg., menthol 6.5 mg./30 ml. w/alcohol 5%. Syr. Bot. 3 oz., pt., gal.
Use: Antitussive.

VALERGEN. (Hyrex) Estradiol valerate 10 mg., 20 mg., 40 mg./ml. Vial 10 ml.

VALERIAN. (Lilly) Tincture, alcohol 68%. Bot. 4 fl. oz., 16 fl. oz.
W/Phenobarbital, passiflora, hyoscyamus.
See: Aluro, Tab. (Foy)

VALERTEST. (Hyrex) **No. 1:** Estradiol valerate 4 mg., testosterone enanthate 90 mg./cc. Vial 10 cc. **No. 2:** Double strength. Vial 10 cc. Amp. 2 cc., 10s.
Use: Combined estrogen and androgen therapy.

• **VALETHAMATE BROMIDE,** 2-Diethylaminoethyl 3-methyl-2-phenylvalerate methylbromide. Di-ethyl(2-hydroxyethyl)methyl-ammonium bromide 3-methyl-2-phenylvalerate. Murel.
Use: Anticholinergic.

VALIHIST. (Otis Clapp) Phenylephrine HCl, chlorpheniramine maleate, caffeine, acetaminophen/Tab. Sugar and salt free. Safety paks 400s.
Use: Decongestant, antihistaminic and analgesic for cold sinus amd hay fever relief.

• **VALINE,** U.S.P. XXI. $C_5H_{11}NO_2$ as L-valine.
Use: Amino acid.

d-VALINE, 3-MERCAPTO-. Penicillamine, U.S.P. XXI.

VALISONE. (Schering) Betamethasone valerate. **Cream:** 1 mg./Gm. Hydrophilic cream of water,

mineral oil, petrolatum, polyethylene glycol 1000 monocetyl ether, cetostearyl alcohol, monobasic sod. phosphate, phosphoric acid, 4-chloro-m-cresol as preservative. Tube 15 Gm., 45 Gm., 110 Gm.
Oint.: 1 mg./Gm. Base of liquid and white petrolatum and hydrogenated lanolin. Tube 15 Gm., 45 Gm. **Lotion:** 1 mg./Gm. w/isopropyl alcohol 47.5%, water slightly thickened w/carboxy vinyl polymer, pH adjusted w/sod. hydroxide. Bot. 20 ml., 60 ml. **Reduced Strength Cream 0.01%:** Hydrophilic cream of water, mineral oil, petrolatum, polyethylene glycol 1000 monocetyl ether, cetostearyl alcohol, monobasic sod. phosphate, phosphoric acid, 4-chloro-m-cresol as preservative. Tubes 15 Gm. 60 Gm.
Use: Anti-inflammatory dermatological.
VALIUM TABLETS. (Roche) Diazepam. 2 mg., 5 mg., or 10 mg./Tab. Bot. 100s, 500s. Tel-E-Dose 100s (10 ×10), (4×25) RPN (Reverse Numbered Packages); Prescription Paks 50s, 500s.
Use: Anxiety disorders; tension, anxiety, apprehension and fatigue associated with psychoneurotic states; acute alcohol withdrawl; skeletal muscle spasms; etc.
VALIUM INJECTABLE. (Roche) Diazepam 5 mg./ml. w/propylene glycol 40%, ethyl alcohol 10%, sodium benzoate, benzoic acid 5%, benzyl alcohol 1.5%. Amps. 2 ml. 10s. Vial 10 ml. Box 1s; Tel-E-Ject (Disposable syringes) 2 ml., Box 10s.
Use: Anxiety disorders; tension, anxiety, apprehension and fatigue associated with psychoneurotic states; acute alcohol withdrawl; skeletal muscle spasms; etc.
VALLERGAN. Trimeprazine, B.A.N.
VALLERGINE.
See: Promethazine HCl, U.S.P. XXI.
VALMID. (Dista) Ethinamate. Pulvule 500 mg. Bot. 100s.
Use: Nonbarbiturate sedative.
VALMIDATE. Ethinamate, B.A.N.
• **VALNOCTAMIDE.** USAN.
Use: Tranquilizer.
See: Axiquel (McNeil)
VALOID HYDROCHLORIDE. Cyclizine, B.A.N.
VALORIN. (Otis Clapp) Acetaminophen 325 mg./Tab. Sugar and salt free. Safety packs 500s. Aidpacks 100s.
Use: Analgesic, antipyretic.
VALORIN EXTRA. (Otis Clapp) Acetaminophen 500 mg./Tab. Sugar and salt free. Safety packs 500s. Aidpacks 100s.
Use: Extra strength non-aspirin analgesic, antipyretic.
VALPIN 50. (Du Pont) Anisotropine methyl-bromide 50 mg./Tab. Bot. 100s, 1000s.
Use: Antispasmodic, anticholinergic.
VALPIN 50-PB. (Du Pont) Anisotropine methylbromide 50 mg. with phenobarbital 15 mg./Tab. Bot. 100s, 1000s.
Use: Anticholinergic.
VALPIPAMATE METHYLSULFATE.
See: Pentapiperide Methylsulfate.

• **VALPROATE SODIUM.** USAN.
Use: Anticonvulsant.
• **VALPROIC ACID.** USAN. 2-Propylpentanoic acid.
Use: Anticonvulsant.
See: Depakene, Cap. Liq. (Abbott)
VALRELEASE. (Roche) Diazepam 15 mg./S.R. Cap. Pk 30s, Bot. 100s.
Use: Relief of anxiety.
VALUMIN. (Towne) Vit. A acetate 10,000 I.U., D 400 I.U., B-1 15 mg., B-2 10 mg., B-6 0.5 mg., B-12 10 mcg., C 100 mg., niacinamide 25 mg., Ca pantothenate 5 mg., Vit. E 15 I.U., choline bitartrate 25 mg., inositol 25 mg., dried yeast pow. 75 mg., liver desic. 75 mg., Ca 105 mg., Fe 10 mg., Iodine 0.05 mg., Mn 1 mg., Zn 1.5 mg., Mg 6 mg., K 5 mg./Captab. Bot. 72s, 100s.
VANADRYX TR. (Vangard) Dexbrompheniramine maleate 6 mg., psuedoephedrine sulfate 120 mg./Tab. Bot. 100s, 500s.
Use: Antihistamine, decongestant.
VANCENASE NASAL INHALER. (Schering) Metered-dose aerosol unit containing beclomethasone dipropionate in propellants. Each actuation delivers 42 mcg. Canister 16.8 Gm.w/nasal adapter.
Use: Treatment of seasonal or perennial rhinitis.
VANCERIL INHALER. (Schering) Metered-dose aerosol unit of beclomethasone dipropionate in propellants. Each actuation delivers 42 mcg. of beclomethasone dipropionate. Canister 16.8 Gm. w/oral adapter. Box 1s.
Use: Treatment of chronic bronchial asthma.
VANCOCIN HCl. (Lilly) Vancomycin HCl Vial: 500 mg./10 ml. Rubber-stoppered Vial. 10 ml. Pow. Bot. 10 Gm.
Use: Severe resistant infections.
• **VANCOMYCIN HCl,** U.S.P. XXI. For Oral Soln., Sterile, U.S.P. XXI. An antibiotic from *Streptomyces orientalis.*
Use: (I.V.) Gram-positive (staph.) infection; antibacterial.
See: Vancocin HCl, Preps. (Lilly)
VANDID. Ethamivan, B.A.N.
• **VANILLA.** N.F. XVI. Tinct. N.F. XVI.
Use: Pharmaceutic acid (flavor).
VANILLAL.
See: Ethyl Vanillin.
• **VANILLIN,** N.F. XVI. 4-Hydroxy-3-methoxy-benzaldehyde.
Use: Pharmaceutic aid (flavor).
VANIROME.
See: Ethyl Vanillin.
VANOBID. (Merrell Dow) Candicidin. **Oint.** 0.6 mg./Gm., Pkg. 2 tubes. 75 Gm. W/applicators. **Tabs.** 3 mg. w/starch, lactose, magnesium stearate. 28s w/inserter.**Note: Manufacturer voluntarily stopped in 1983.**
Use: Vaginal candidiasis.
VANODONNAL TIMECAPS. (Drug Industries) Phenobarbital 50 mg., atropine sulfate 0.0582 mg., hyoscyamine sulfate 0.311 mg., hyoscine hydrobromide 0.0195 mg./S.R. Cap. Bot. 100s.

Use: Long-acting antispasmodic and sedative.

VANOXIDE. (Dermik) Benzoyl peroxide 5% w/propylene glycol, hydroxy-ethylcellulose, FD & C color, cholesterol-sterol, cetyl alcohol, propylene glycol stearate, polysorbate 20, lanolin alcohol, propylparaben, decyl oleate, purcelline oil syn., antioxidants, vegetable oil, methylparaben, tetrasodium EDTA, buffers, cyclohexanediamine tetraacetic acid, calcium phosphate, silicone emulsion, silica. Bot. 25 Gm., 50 Gm.
Use: Severe, recalcitrant acne.

VANOXIDE-HC. (Dermik) Hydrocortisone alcohol 0.5%, benzoyl peroxide 5%/25 Gm. in lotion w/same ingredients as Vanoxide. Bot. 25 Gm.
Use: Severe, recalcitrant acne.

VANQUIN. Viprynium Embonate, B.A.N.

VANQUISH. (Glenbrook) Aspirin 227 mg., acetaminophen 194 mg., caffeine 33 mg., dried aluminum hydroxide gel, 25 mg., magnesium hydroxide 50 mg./Tab. Capsuleshaped tablets. Bot. 15s, 30s, 60s, 100s.
Use: Relief of headache, muscular aches and pains, neuralgia and neuritic pain, functional menstrual pain, minor pains of arthritis and rheumatism.

VANSEB DANDRUFF SHAMPOO. (Herbert) Sulfur 2%, salicylic acid 1%, surfactants, proteins. **Cream:** Tube 3 oz. **Lotion:** Bot. 4 oz.
Use: Antidandruff, antiseborrheic.

VANSEB-T TAR SHAMPOO. (Herbert) Sulfur 2%, salicylic acid 1%, Coal Tar Solution. U.S.P. 5%, surfactants, protein. **Cream:** Tube 3 oz. **Lotion:** Bot. 4 oz.
Use: Antidandruff, antiseborrheic.

VANSIL. (Pfipharmecs) Oxaminiquine 250 mg./Cap. Bot. 24s.
Use: Schistosomicide.

VAPO-ISO SOLUTION. (Fisons) Isoproterenol HCl 0.5%, sod. chloride, glycerin. Vial 10 cc.
Use: Bronchodilator.

VAPONA. Dichlorvos, B.A.N.

VAPONEFRIN SOLUTION. (Fisons) A 2.25% solution of bioassayed racemic epinephrine as HCl, chlorobutanol 0.5%. Vials 7.5, 15, 30 cc.
Use: Bronchodilator.

VAPORUB. (Vicks)
See: Vicks Vaporub (Vicks)

VAPOSTEAM. (Vicks)
See: Vicks Vaposteam (Vicks)

VARICELLA-ZOSTER IMMUNE GLOBULIN, U.S.P. XXI. A sterile buffered solution of the globulin fraction of human plasma containing 99% immunoglobulin G with traces of immunoglobulins A and M. It is derived from adult human plasma selected for high titers of varicella-zoster antibiodies.
Use: Passive immunizing agent.

VARI-FLAVORS. (Ross) Dextrose, artificial flavoring & coloring (strawberry, cherry, lemon, orange). Dextrose & artificial flavoring (pecan). Packets 1 Gm. 24s/Ctn.
Use: Liquid nutrition flavoring aid.

VARIOTIN. Pecilocin, B.A.N.

VARITOL. (Kenyon) Atropine sulfate 0.03 mg., hyoscyamine 0.03 mg., gelsemium 6.1 mg., methenamine 40.8 mg., salol 18.1 mg., benzoic acid 4.5 mg., methylene blue 5.4 mg./Tab. Bot. 100s, 1000s.

VARITOL-D.S. (Kenyon) Atropine sulfate 0.06 mg., hyoscyamine 0.06 mg., gelsemium 12.2 mg., methenamine 81.6 mg., salol 36.2 mg., benzoic acid 9 mg., methylene blue 10.8 mg./Tab. Bot. 100s, 1000s.

VASCARDIN. Sorbide Nitrate, B.A.N.

VASCORAY SOLUTION. (Mallinckrodt) Iothalamate meglumine 52%, iothalamate sodium 26% Inj. Vial 25 ml. Pkgs. 25s, 50s, 100s; 50 ml. Pkg. 10s, 50s, 100s.
Use: Radiopaque medium.

VASCORIL HYDROGEN MALEATE. Cinepazate, B.A.N.

VASULIT SULPHATE. Bamethan, B.A.N.

VASCUNITOL. (Apco) Mannitol hexanitrate ½ gr./Tab. Bot. 100s.
Use: Vasodilator.

VASCUSED. (Apco) Mannitol hexanitrate ½ gr., phenobarbital ¼ gr./Tab. Bot. 100s.
Use: Vasodilator.

VASELINE DERMATOLOGY FORMULA CREAM. (Chesebrough-Pond's) Petrolatum, mineral oil, dimethicone. Jar 3 oz., 5.25 oz.
Use: Treatment for severe cases of dry skin.

VASELINE DERMATOLOGY FORMULA LOTION. (Chesebrough-Pond's) Petrolatum, mineral oil, dimethicon. Bot. 5.5 oz., 11 oz., 16 oz.
Use: Treatment for severe cases of dry skin.

VASELINE FIRST AID CARBOLATED PETROLEUM JELLY. (Chesebrough-Pond's) Petrolatum, chloroxylenol. Plastic Jar 1.75 oz., 3.75 oz. Plastic Tube 1 oz., 2.5 oz.
Use: Medicated antibacterial.

VASELINE PURE PETROLEUM JELLY SKIN PROTECTANT. (Chesebrough-Pond's) White petrolatum. Tubes 1 oz., 2.5 oz. Jars 1.75 oz., 3.75 oz., 7.75 oz., 13 oz.
Use: Protectant for minor skin irritations.

VASIMID.
See: Tolazoline HCl, U.S.P. XXI.

VASO-80 UNICELLES. (Reid-Provident) Pentaerythritol tetranitrate 80 mg./Cap. Bot. 100s.
Use: To reduce the number of episodes and severity of anginal pain.

VASOCIDIN OPHTHALMIC SOLUTION. (CooperVision) Prednisolone sodium phosphate 0.25% (equiv. to Prednisolone 0.3%), sulfacetamide sod. 10%, thimerosal 0.01%. Plastic dropper-tip squeeze bot. 5 cc., 10 cc., 15 cc.
Use: Anti-inflammatory, anti-bacterial, decongestant.

VASOCLEAR. (CooperVision) Naphazoline HCl 0.02% in Lipiden polymeric system, benzalkonium Cl 0.01%, edetate disodium 0.03%. Bot. 15 ml., 30 ml.
Use: Decongestant eye drops.

VASOCLEAR A. (CooperVision) Naphazoline HCl

0.02%, zinc sulfate 0.25%, polyvinylalcohol 0.25%.
Bot. 15 ml.
Use: Decongestant astringent lubricating eyedrops.
VASOCON-A OPHTHALMIC SOLUTION. (CooperVision) Naphazoline HCl 0.05%, antazoline phosphate 0.5%. Plastic squeeze bot. w/dropper tip 15 cc.
Use: Ocular decongestant and antihistamine.
VASOCON REGULAR. (CooperVision) Naphazoline HCl 0.1%. Bot. plastic squeeze w/dropper tip 15 cc.
Use: Topical ocular vasoconstrictor.
VASOCONSTRICTOR.
See: Epinephrine Prep.
VASODIL.
See: Tolazoline HCl, U.S.P. XXI.
VASODILAN. (Mead Johnson) Isoxsuprine HCl 10 mg./Tab. Bot. 100s, 1000s, 5000s. Unit Dose 100s. 20 mg./Tab. Bot. 100s, 500s, 1000s, 5000s. Unit dose 100s. Amp. 2 ml. (5 mg./cc.) Box 6s.
Use: Arterial insufficiency. Peripheral vascular disease. Cerebrovascular disorders.
■ **VASODILATORS.**
See: Amyl Nitrite
   Apresoline, Tab., Amp. (Ciba)
   Arlidin, Tab. (USV)
   Cardilate, Tab. (Burroughs Wellcome)
   Cyclospasmol, Tab., Cap. (Ives)
   Erythrityl Tetranitrate, Tab.
   Glyceryl Trinitrate, Preps.
   Isordil, Tab. (Ives)
   Kortrate, Cap. (Amid)
   Kortrate Plus, Cap. (Amid)
   Mannitol Hexanitrate
   Metamine, Tab. (Pfizer)
   Nisine, Elix. (Amid)
   Nitroglycerin
   Pentritol, Cap., Tempule (Armour)
   Peritrate, Tab. (Parke-Davis)
   Sodium Nitrite
   Sorbitrate, Tab. (Stuart)
   Vasodilan, Tab., Amp. (Mead Johnson)
■ **VASODILATORS, CORONARY.**
See: Glyceryl Trinitrate, Preps. (Various Mfr.)
   Isordil, Tab. (Ives)
   Khellin (Various Mfr.)
   Papaverine, Inj., Tab. (Various Mfr.)
   Pentaerythritol Tetranitrate, Tab.
   Peritrate, Tab. (Parke-Davis)
   Roniacol Elix., Tab. (Roche)
   Sorbitrate, Tab. (Stuart)
VASODISTAL HYDROGEN MALEATE. Cinepazide, B.A.N.
VASOFLO. (Hauck) Papaverine HCl 150 mg./Cap. Bot 100s.
Use: Cerebral and peripheral ischemia.
VASOLATE. (Parmed) Pentaerythritol tetranitrate 30 mg./Cap. Bot. 100s, 1000s.
Use: Relief of angina pectoris.
VASOLATE-80. (Parmed) Pentaerythritol tetranitrate 80 mg./Cap. Bot. 100s, 1000s.
Use: Relief of angina pectoris.

VASOMIDE TABLETS. (Lannett) Niacin 50 mg., salicylamide 300 mg., ascorbic acid 15 mg., Vit. B-1 3 mg., dl-desoxyephedrine HCl 2.5 mg., B-12 3 mcg./Tab. Bot. 100s, 1000s.
VASOMINIC-T.D. (A.V.P.) Phenylpropanolamine HCl 50 mg., chlorpheniramine 25 mg., pyrilamine maleate 25 mg./T.R. Tab. Bot. 100s.
Use: Antihistaminic, decongestant.
• **VASOPRESSIN INJECTION.** U.S.P. XXI. beta-Hypophamine. Post. pituitary pressor hormone.
Use: Posterior pituitary hormone (antidiuretic).
See: Pitressin, Amp. (Parke-Davis)
VASOPRESSIN TANNATE INJECTION. beta-Hypophamine tannate.
See: Pitressin Tannate, Amp. (Parke-Davis)
VAS-O-SPAN. (Scrip) Papaverine 150 mg./Cap. Bot. 100s.
VASOSPAN. (Ulmer) Papaverine HCl 150 mg./Cap. Bot. 100s, 500s.
Use: Smooth muscle relaxant.
VASOSTIM. (Dunhall) Niacin acid 100 mg., pnetylenetetrazol 100 mg./Cap. Bot. 100s, 1000s.
Use: Cerebral stimulant.
VASOSULF. (CooperVision) Sulfacetamide sodium 15%, phenylphrine HCl 0.125%, methylparaben 0.02%, propylparaben 0.005%. Bot. 5 cc., 15 cc.
Use: Ophthalmic antibacterial/decongestant.
VASO T.D. CAPSULES. (Knight) Bot. 100s, 1000s.
VASOTHERM INJ. (Pharmex) Niacin as sod. salt 100 mg., benzyl alcohol 1.5%/cc. Vial 30 cc.
Use: Vasodilator.
VASOTRAN HYDROCHLORIDE. Isoxsuprine, B.A.N.
VASOTUS LIQUID. (Sheryl) Codeine phosphate ⅛ gr., phenylephrine HCl, prophenpyridamine maleate. Liq. 1 pt.
Use: Cough and respiratory congestion.
VASOXINE. Methoxamine, B.A.N.
VASOXYL INJECTION. (Burroughs Wellcome) Methoxamine HCl 20 mg./ml. w/citric acid anhydrous 0.3%, sodium citrate 0.3%. Vial 1 ml.
Use: Supporting, restoring, maintaining blood pressure during anesthesia.
VASTAREL DIHYDROCHLORIDE. Trimetazidine, B.A.N.
VASYLOX HYDROCHLORIDE. Methoxamine, B.A.N.
VATENSOL. Guanoclor sulfate, B.A.N.
Use: Adrenergic neuron blocking agent.
VA-TRO-NOL. (Vicks)
See: Vicks Va-Tro-Nol (Vicks)
VAZADRINE. Isoniazid, B.A.N.
VAZOSAN. (Sandia) Papaverine HCl 150 mg./Tab. Bot. 100s, 1000s.
VB-6 DOUBLE STRENGTH. (O'Connor) Kelp, lecithin, cider vinegar, Vit. B-6. Bot. 90 Cap.
Use: Dietary supplement.
V-CILLIN-K. (Lilly) Penicillin V potassium. **125 mg.**/Tab. Bot. 50s, 100s; **250 mg.**/Tab. Bot. 24s, 100s, 500s. **500 mg.**/Tab. Bot. 24s, 100s, 500s.
Use: Orally, penicillin therapy.
V-CILLIN-K FOR ORAL SOLUTION. (Lilly) Penicillin V potassium. 125 mg./5 ml. Bot. 5 ml. Pkg. 100s.

Bot. 40, 100, 150, 200 ml. 250 mg./5 ml. Bot. 5 ml.
Pkg. 100s. Bot. 100 ml., 150 ml., 200 ml.
Use: Orally, penicillin therapy.

V-COMP TABLETS. (Eckerd) Acetaminophen 325 mg.,
pseudoephedrine HCl 15 mg., d-Methorphan HBr 10
mg., chlorpheniramine maleate 2 mg., guaifenesin
50 mg./Tab. Bot. 24s.
Use: Relieves cold and flu virus symptoms.

V-CORT. (Scrip) Hydrocortisone 1%, clioquinol 3%, pramoxine HCl 0.5% in a washable base. Tube 1 oz.

VDRL ANTIGEN. (Laboratory Diagnostics) VDRL
antigen with buffered saline. **Vial:** Sufficient for 500
tests. **Amp.:** 10 × 0.5 ml. sufficient for 500 tests.
Use: Blood test in diagnosis of syphilis.

VDRL SLIDE TEST. (Laboratory Diagnostics) VDRL
antigen. Vial 5 ml. Complete kit, reactive control,
nonreactive control, 5 ml.
Use: Slide flocculation and spinal fluid test for
syphilis.

VE-400. (Western Research) Vitamine E 400
I.U./Caps. Bot. 100s.
Use: Vitamin supplement.

VE-T4. (Western Research) dl-Alpha tocopheryl
acetate 400 I.U./Tab. Bot. 100s.
Use: Vitamin E therapy.

• **VECURONIUM BROMIDE.** USAN.

VEETIDS. (Squibb) Penicillin-V potassium. **Solution** 125
mg. or 250 mg./5 ml. Bot. 100 ml., 200 ml. **Tab.**
250 mg. or 500 mg./Tab. Bot. 100s, 1000s.
Unimatic 100s.

• **VEGETABLE OIL, HYDROGENATED,** U.S.P. XXI.
Use: Pharm. aid (tablet lubricant).

VEGOLYSEN. Hexamethonium Bromide, B.A.N.

VEINAMINE. (Cutter) 8% amino acids injection. Bot.
1000 ml. containing 500 ml. of 8% soln.; Kit, Bot.
1000 ml. containing 500 ml. of 8% soln., transfer
set, additive cap, label.
Use: Amino acid source.

VELACYCLINE. N-Pyrrolidinomethyl tetracycline.
Use: Antibiotic.

VELBAN. (Lilly) Ext. from Vinca rosea Linn.
Vinblastine sulfate, lyophilized Vial 10 mg./10 ml.
Box 10s.
Use: Antineoplastic.

VELBE SULPHATE. Vinblastine, B.A.N.

VELDOPA. Levodopa, B.A.N.

VELLADA TABLETS. (Fellows) Phenobarbital ¼ gr.,
ext. hyoscyamus ⅛ gr., ext. passiflora ¼ gr., ext.
valerian ¼ gr./Tab. Bot. 1000s.

VELMATROL. (Kenyon) Sulfisoxazole 500 mg./Tab.
Bot. 100s, 1000s.

VELMATROL-A. (Kenyon) Sulfisoxazole 500 mg.,
phenylazodiaminopyridine HCl 50 mg./Tab. Bot.
100s, 1000s.
Use: Urinary antibiotic, antiseptic.

VELOSEF. (Squibb) Cephradine. **Oral Susp.:** 125 mg.,
or 250 mg./5 ml. Bot. 100 ml., 200 ml.**Cap.:** 250
mg., or 500 mg./Cap. Bot. 24s, 100s. Unit dose
Unimatic 100s. **Inj.** (w/anhydrous sod. carbonate.
Sodium equiv. to 136 mg./Gm. of cephradine) 250
mg., 500 mg., 1 Gm./Vial 2 Gm., 4 Gm./100 ml.; 2
Gm. sodium free for infusion. Bot. 200 ml.

Use: Antibiotic.

VELOSULIN. (Nordisk) Purified pork insulin injection
100 I.U./ml.
Use: Diabetes care (IDDM).

VELTANE. (Lannett) Brompheniramine maleate 4
mg./Tab. Bot. 1000s.
Use: Antihistamine.

VELTAP. (Lannett) Brompheniramine maleate 4 mg.,
phenylephrine HCl 5 mg., phenylpropanolamine HCl
5 mg., alcohol 2.3%/5 ml. Bot. pts., gal.
Use: Upper respiratory infections.

VELVACHOL. (Owen) Hydrophilic ointment base
petrolatum, mineral oil, cetyl alcohol, cholesterol,
parabens, stearyl alcohol, purified water, sodium
lauryl sulfate. Jar 1 lb.
Use: Hydrophilic ointment base.

VELVEDERM CLEANSER. (Torch) Sulfonated
detergent with a stable emulsion of vegetable oil.
Bot. 8 oz.
Use: Cleansing lotion.

VELVEDERM-HANDORA NORMALIZER. (Torch)
Glycerine, fatty alcohols, fatty acid in hydrophilic
base w/pH of 5.0 to 5.5. Cream 4 oz., 8 oz. jar.
Lotion 8 oz. Bot.
Use: Emollient skin cream and lotion.

VELVEDERM MOISTURIZER. (Torch) Mineral oil,
emulsifiers, fatty alcohol, propylene glycol,
hydroxymethylcellulose and water. Bot. 4 oz.
Use: Lubricating skin lotion, vehicle for common
dermatologicals.

VENESETIC.
See: Amobarbital Sodium, Preps. (Various Mfr.)

VENETHENE. No mfr. listed.

VENOMIL. (Hollister-Stier) Diagnostic 1 mcg./ml.
Maintenence 100 mcg./ml. Individual patient kits.
Use: Hymenoptera (stinging insect) sensitive
patients.

VENSTAT. (Seatrace) Atropine sulfate 0.2 mg.,
chlorpheniramine maleate 5 mg./ml. Vial 10 cc.

VENTABS. (Seatrace) Acetaminophen 325 mg.,
phenylpropanolamine HCl 18 mg., atropine sulfate
0.15 mg./Tab. Bot. 100s, 1000s.
Use: Nasal decongestant, analgesic, anti-pyretic.

VENTHERA. (Amfre-Grant) Vit. A acetate 25,000 I.U.,
D-2 1000 I.U., B-1 12.5 mg., B-2 12.5 mg.,
niacinamide 100 mg., C 200 mg., B-6 5 mg., d-calcium
pantothenate 20 mg., B-12 5 mcg., E acetate 5
I.U., biotin 1 mcg., Ca 105 mg., P 80 mg., Iodine
0.15 mg., Fe 15 mg., potassium sulfate 5 mg.,
copper sulfate 1 mg., manganese sulfate 1 mg.,
mag. oxide 6 mg., zinc sulfate 1.5 mg./Tab. Bot.
100s.
Use: Treatment of deficiencies of essential vitamins
and minerals.

VENTOLIN. Salbutamol, B.A.N.

VENTOLIN INHALER. (Glaxo) Albuterol 90
mcg./actuation. Aerosol cannister 17 Gm.
containing 200 metered inhalations. Cannister 17
Gm. w/oral adapter.

VENTROMIL. Orphenadrine, B.A.N.

VEPESID. (Bristol) Etoposide inj. 100 mg. Vial
Use: Antineoplastic agent.

VERACOLATE. (C-D Consumer Products) Bile salts 1.07 gr., phenolphthalein ½ gr., capsicum oleoresin 0.05 min., cascara ext. 1 gr./Tab. Bot. 100s.
Use: Laxative.
VERACTIL. Methotrimeprazine, B.A.N.
• **VERADOLINE HYDROCHLORIDE.** USAN.
Use: Analgesic.
• **VERAPAMIL.** USAN. 5-[3,4-Di-methoxyphenethyl)methylamino]-2-(3,4-dimethoxyphenyl)-2-isopropylvaleronitrile. Isoptin. Cordilox hydrochloride.
Use: Coronary vasodilator.
• **VERAPAMIL HYDROCHLORIDE.** USAN.
Use: Coronary vasodilator.
VERAPHEN. (Davis & Sly) Phenobarbital ¼ gr., veratrum viride ¾ gr., sodium nitrite 1 gr./Tab. Bot. 1000s.
VERATRUM ALBA.
See: Protoveratrines A & B. (Various Mfr.)
VERATRUM VIRIDE. Approx. 1 gr. equals 4 craw units.
Use: Hypertension treatment.
See: Cryptenamine
Gartrone, Vials (Eric, Kirk & Gary)
Unitensen, Tab. & Vial (Mallinckrodt)
W/Sod. nitrite, aconite, nitroglycerin & pot. nitrate.
See: Nyomin, Tab. (Elder)
VERATRUM VIRIDE WITH PHENOBARBITAL COMBINATIONS.
See: Hyperlon, Tab. (Kenyon)
Hyrunal, Tab. (Kenyon)
Verabar, Tab. (Bowman)
VERATRUM VIRIDE UNIT.
See: C.S.R. Unit
VERAZEPTOL. (Femco) Chlorothymol, eucalyptol, menthol, phenol, boric acid & zinc sulfate. Pow., Bot. 3 oz., 6 oz., 10 oz.
Use: Vaginal douche.
VERAZIDE. B.A.N. 2'-Veratrylideneisonicotino-hydrazide.
Use: Treatment of tuberculosis.
VERAZINC. (O'Neal, Jones & Feldman) Zinc sulfate 220 mg./Cap. Bot. 100s, 1000s.
Use: Astringent.
VERCYTE. (Abbott) Pipobroman 25 mg./Tab. Bot. 100s.
Use: Antineoplastic.
VERDEFAM CREAM. (Owen) Sodium propionate 1%, sodium caprylate 1%, propionic acid 3%, salicylic acid 3%, undecylenic acid 2%, copper undecylenate 0.5%, vanishing cream base. Tube 1 oz.
Use: Treatment of fungal infections.
VERDEFAM SOLUTION. (Owen) Sod. propionate 2%, sod. caprylate 2%, propionic acid 3%, undecylenic acid 5%, salicylic acid 5%, copper undecylenate 0.5%, docusate sodium 0.1%, purified water, isopropyl alcohol 59%. Sol. Bot. 2 oz.
Use: Fungus infections.
VERGO OINT. (Daywell) Cal. pantothenate 8%, ascorbic acid 2%, starch. Tube ½ oz.
Use: Treatment of warts.
• **VERILOPAM HYDROCHLORIDE.** USAN.

Use: Analgesic.
VERIN. (Verex) Aspirin 650 mg./Time Release Tab. Bot. 100s.
Use: Treatment of arthritis.
VERI-STAPH. (Wampole-Zeus) Latex agglutination slide test for Staphlococclus aurens. Tests 120s.
Use: Rapid detection of both clumping factors and protein A seen in staphylococcus aureus cultures.
VERITAIN. Pholedrine, B.A.N.
VERITOL. Pholedrine, B.A.N.
VERMANTIN. (Trout) Phenobarbital ¼ gr., veratrum viride pow. ext. ⅖ gr., mannitol hexanitrate ½ gr., rutin ⅓ gr./Tab. Bot. 100s, 1000s.
Use: Hypertension.
VERMICIDE. (Pharmex) Tube 2 oz.
Use: Crab lice.
VERMITRATE. (Vortech) Piperazine citrate 100 mg./cc. Bot. pt., gal.
VERMIZINE. (Vortech) Syr. Piperazine citrate 100 mg./cc. Bot. 4 oz., pt., gal; Tab. 250 mg./Tab., Bot. 1000s.
Use: Treatment of pinworms & roundworms.
VERMOX. (Janssen) Mebendazole 100 mg./Tab. Box 12s.
Use: Anthelmintic.
VERNACEL. (Professional Pharmacal) Prophenpyridamine maleate ½%, phenylephrine HCl ⅛% in a methylcellulose solution. Plastic Bot. 15 cc., 30 cc.
Use: Ophthalmic allergic symptoms.
VERNAMYCINS. Under study.
Use: Antibiotic.
VERNOLEPIN. A sesquiterpene dilactone. Under study.
Use: Against Walker carcinosarcoma 256.
• **VEROFYLLINE.** USAN.
Use: Bronchodilator, anti-asthmatic.
VERONAL SODIUM.
See: Barbital Sodium (Various Mfr.)
• **VERR-CANTH.** (C & M Pharmacal) Cantharidin 0.7%, penederm 0.5%. Bot. 7.5 cc w/applicator tip.
Use: Wart removal.
VERREX. (C & M Pharmacal) Salicylic acid 30%, podophyllin 10%, penederm 0.5%. Bot. 7.5cc w/applicator tip.
Use: Wart Removal.
VERRUSOL. (C & M Pharmacal) Salicylic acid 30%, podophyllin 5%, cantharidin 1%, penederm 0.5%. Bot. 7.5 cc. w/applicator tip.
Use: Wart removal.
VERSACAPS. (Seatrace) Brompheniramine maleate 4 mg., pseudoephedrine HCl 60 mg., guaifenesin 300 mg./Cap. Bot. 100s, 1000s.
Use: Antihistaminic, nasal decongestant, antitussive.
VERSAL. (Suppositoria) Bismuth subgallate, Peru balsam, zinc oxide, benzyl benzoate/Supp. Box 12s, 100s, 1000s.
Use: Antihemorrhoidal.
VERSAL HC. (Suppositoria) Hydrocortisone acetate 10 mg./Supp. w/bismuth subgallate, balsam peru, zinc oxide, benzyl benzoate Box 12s, 100s, 1,000s.

Use: Antihemorrhoidal.

VERSAPEN. (Bristol) Hetacillin. **Oral Susp.:** Hetacillin equiv. to 112.5 mg., ampicillin/5 ml. Bot. 100 ml., 225 mg./5 ml. Bot. 100 ml.

VERSAPEN K. (Bristol) Potassium hetacillin equiv. to ampicillin 225/Cap. Bot. 100s.
Use: Antibiotic.

VERSA-QUAT. (Ulmer) Quaternary ammonium one-step cleaner-disinfectant-sanitizer-fungicide-virucide for general housekeeping. Bot. gal., 5 gal., 15 gal. Drum 55 gal.
Use: Cleanser, disinfectant.

VERSENATE, CALCIUM DISODIUM.
See: Calcium Disodium Versenate, Amp. (Riker)

VERSENATE DISODIUM.
See: Disodium Versenate, Amp. (Riker)

VERSENE ACID. Edetic Acid, B.A.N.

VERSIDYNE. Methopholine. 1-(p-Chlorophenethyl)-2-methyl-6,7-dimethoxy-1,2,3,4-tetrahydroisoquinoline.
Use: Analgesic.

VERSTAT. (Saron) Pheniramine maleate 12.5 mg., nicotinic acid 50 mg./Cap.

VERSTRAN. (Parke-Davis) Prazepam.
Use: Muscle relaxant.
See: Centrax, Tab. (Parke-Davis)

VERTON ACETATE. Chlormadinone, B.A.N.

VERV ALERTNESS CAPSULES. (APC) Caffeine 200 mg./Cap. Vial 15.
Use: Maintain physical and mental alertness.

VESICHOLINE. (Star) Bethanechol chloride 25 mg./Tab. Bot. 100s, 1000s.
Use: Non-obstructive urinary retention.

VESIPAQUE. (Warner-Lambert) Phenobutiodil.
Use: Radiopaque diagnostic aid.

VESPRAL. Fluopromazine, B.A.N.

VESPRIN. (Squibb) Triflupromazine. **Inj.** 20 mg./ml. w/benzyl alcohol 1.5%. Single dose syringe 1 cc. 1s. **High Pot. Susp.** 50 mg./5 cc. Bot. 120 cc.
Use: Tranquilizer.

VESULONG. (Ciba) Sulfazamet. Sulfapyrazole, B.A.N.

VETALAR. (Parke-Davis) Ketamine HCl 100 mg./ml. Bot. 10 ml.
Use: Anesthetic for veterinary use.

V-GAN. (Hauck) Promthazine HCl 25 or 50 mg./ml. Vials 10 ml.
Use: Anti-emetic, antihistaminic.

VIACAPS. (Manne) Vit. A (soluble) 45,000 I.U., C 500 mg./Caps. Bot. 60s, 120s, 1000s.
Use: Acne therapy.

VIADRIL. Hydroxydione Sodium Succinate, B.A.N.

VI-AQUA CAPSULES. (Armour) Aqueous multiple vitamins. Bot. 100s.
Use: Dietary supplement.

VI-AQUA FORTE. (Armour) Aqueous multivitamin formula. Bot. 100s.
Use: Dietary supplement.

VI-AQUAMIN FORTE CAPSULES. (Armour) Aqueous vitamins with minerals. Bot. 100s.
Use: Dietary supplement.

VIATRIC. (Pasadena Research) Ethinyl estradiol 0.01 mg., methyltestosterone 2.5 mg., ferrous fumarate 15 mg., l-lysine 50 mg., Vit. A 7500 I.U., D 500 I.U., B-1 7.5 mg., B-2 7.5 mg., B-6 2 mg., niacinamide 50 mg., Ca pantothenate 10 mg., B-12 10 mcg., C 50 mg., rutin 15 mg., choline bitartrate 50 mg., inositol 25 mg., Vit. E 10 I.U., with trace elements/Tab. Bot. 100s, 1000s.
Use: Androgen-estrogen therapy with nutritional vitamin and mineral supplements.

VIBAZINE DIHYDROCHLORIDE. Buclizine, B.A.N.

VIBEDOZ Injection. (Blue Line) Cyanocobalamin 1000 mcg./ml. Benzyl alcohol 1½%. Normal saline, sterile sol. Vial 10 ml.

VIBESATE. Polvinate 9.3%, molrosinol 3.1% with propellant.

VIBRAMYCIN. (Pfizer Laboratories) Doxycycline **Caps.** 50 mg./Cap. Bot. 50s, unit dose pak 100s, X-Pack (10 Caps.) 5s.; 100 mg./Cap. Bot. 50s, 500s; unit dose pak 100s. V-Pak (5 Caps) 5s. Nine-Pak 10s. **Ped. Oral Susp.** 25 mg./5 cc. Bot. 2 oz. **Syrup:** 50 mg./5 cc. Bot. oz., pt.
Use: Antibiotic.

VIBRAMYCIN INTRAVENOUS. (Pfizer Laboratories) Doxycycline hyclate 100 mg., ascorbic acid 480 mg./Vial, 5s; doxycycline hyclate 200 mg., ascorbic acid 960 mg./Vial, 1s.

VIBRA-TABS. (Pfizer Laboratories) Doxycycline hyclate 100 mg./Tab. Bot. 50s, 500s. Unit dose Pack 100s.
Use: Antibiotic.

VICAM-IV. (Keene) B-1 50 mg., B-2 5 mg., B-12 1000 mcg., pyridoxine HCl 5 mg., d-panthenol 6 mg., niacinamide 125 mg., ascorbic acid 50 mg./ml. Vial 10 ml.
Use: Parenteral dietary supplement for I.V. or I.M. injection.

VICAM-R. (Keene) **Sol. #1:** Vit. B-1 3 mg., B-2 3.6 mg., biotin 60 mcg., niacin 40 mg., B-6 4 mg., C 100 mg., pantothenic acid 15 mg./ml. **Sol #2:** Vit. B-12 5 mcg., folic acid 400 mg./ml. Vial multiple dose.
Use: Parenteral dietary supplement for I.M. injection.

VICEF. (Drug Industries) Thiamin HC1 10 mg., pyridoxine HCl 10 mg., Vit B-12 50 mcg., C 100 mg., E 100 I.U., niacinamide 25 mg. folic acid 1.5 mg., ferrous fumarate 45 mg./2 Cap. Bot. 100s.
Use: Vitamin, mineral supplement.

VICHOX. (Vitarine) Vit. A 5000 I.U., D 400 I.U., C 60 mg., B-1 1.5 mg., B-2 1.7 mg., B-6 2 mg., B-12 6 mcg., niacinamide 20 mg., E 15 I.U., folic acid 0.4 mg./Tab. Bot. 100s, 250s. w/iron. Bot. 100s.
Use: Dietary supplement.

VICHOX w/IRON. (Vitarine) Multivitamin supplement w/iron/Chewable Tab.
Use: Dietary supplement.

VICKS BLUE COUGH DROPS. (Vicks) Menthol in a soothing sugar base. Stick-Pack 10s. Bag 23s.
Use: Cough drop.

VICKS COUGH SYRUP. (Vicks) Dextromethorphan hydrobromide 10.5 mg., guaifenesin 75 mg./15 ml. w/alcohol 5%. Bot. 3 oz., 6 oz.
Use: Cough syrup.

VICKS COUGH SILENCERS. (Vicks) Dextromethorphan HBr 2.5 mg., benzocaine 1 mg., Special Vicks Medication (menthol, peppermint oil, anethole) 0.35%/Loz. Box 13s.
Use: Cough medication.

VICKS DAYCARE CAPSULES. (Vicks)
Acetaminophen 325 mg., phenylpropanolamine HCl
12.5 mg., dextromethorphan HBr 10 mg./Cap.
Blister Pack 20's, 36's.
Use: Multi-symptom colds medicine.
VICKS DAYCARE LIQUID. (Vicks) Acetaminophen
650 mg., dextromethorphan HBr 20 mg.,
phenylpropanolamine HCl 25 mg./oz. w/alcohol
10%. Bot. 6 oz., 10 oz.
Use: Multi-symptom colds medicine.
VICKS FORMULA 44 COUGH CONTROL DISCS.
(Vicks) Dextromethorphan (HBr equivalent) 5 mg.,
benzocaine 1.25 mg., Special Vicks Medication
(menthol, peppermint oil, anethole) 0.35%/Disc.
Pkg. 24s.
Use: Cough medication.
VICKS FORMULA 44. (Vicks) Dextromethorphan HBr
15 mg., doxylamine succinate 7.5 mg./10 ml.
w/alcohol 10%. Bot. 3 oz., 6 oz., 8 oz.
Use: Effective strength cough mixture.
VICKS FORMULA 44D. (Vicks) Dextromethorphan
HBr 30 mg., phenylpropanolamine HCl 37.5 mg.,
guaifenesin 300 mg./15 ml. Alcohol 10%. Bot. 3
oz., 6 oz., 8 oz.
Use: Cough mixture and decongestant.
VICKS HEADWAY. (Vicks) Acetaminophen 325 mg.,
phenylpropanolamine HC1 18.72 mg.,
chlorpheniramine maleate 2 mg./Tab. or Cap.**Tab.:**
Bot. 20s, 40s. **Cap.:** Bot. 16s, 36s.
Use: Decongestant, analgesic, antihistaminic.
VICKS INHALER. (Vicks) I-Desoxyephedrine 50 mg.,
Special Vicks Medication (menthol, camphor,
methylsalicylate, bornyl acetate) 150 mg. Inhaler
0.007 oz.
Use: Nasal decongestant.
VICKS LIFESTAGE-CHILDREN'S FORMULA. (Vicks)
Vit. A 5000 I.U., D 400 I.U., E 30 I.U., C 60 mg.,
folic acid 0.4 mg., B-1 1.5 mg., B-2 1.7 mg., niacin 20
mg., B-6 2 mg., B-12 6 mcg., biotin 0.3 mg., panto-
thenic acid 10 mg., iron 9 mg./2 Chewable Tabs.
Bot. 60s.
Use: Vitamin & iron supplement.
VICKS LIFESTAGE-MEN'S FORMULA. (Vicks) Vit. A
10,000 I.U., D 400 I.U., E 50 I.U., C 200 mg., folic
acid 0.4 mg., B-1 10 mg., B-2 10 mg., niacin 100 mg.,
B-6 5 mg., B-12 6 mcg., pantothenic acid 20 mg.,
iodine 150 mcg., iron 18 mg., magnesium 100 mg.,
copper 2 mg., zinc 15 mg., manganese 1.25
mg./Tab. Bot. 30s.
Use: High potency vitamin and mineral supplement.
VICKS LIFESTAGE-STRESS FORMULA FOR MEN.
(Vicks) Vit. E 45 I.U., C 500 mg., folic acid 0.4 mg.,
B-1 20 mg., B-2 10 mg., niacin 100 mg., B-6 10 mg.,
B-12 25 mcg., magnesium 100 mg., zinc 22.5
mg./Tab. Bot. 30s.
Use: High potency vitamin supplement with zinc
and magnesium.
**VICKS LIFESTAGE-STRESS FORMULA FOR
WOMEN.** (Vicks) Vit. E 45 I.U., C 500 mg., folic acid
0.4 mg., B-1 20 mg., B-2 10 mg., niacin 100 mg., B-
6 10 mg., B-12 25 mcg., iron 27 mg., magnesium 100
mg., zinc 22.5 mg./Tab. Bot. 30s.

Use: High potency vitamin supplement with zinc,
magnesium, & iron.
VICKS LIFESTAGE-TEEN'S FORMULA. (Vicks) Vit. A
5000 I.U., D 400 I.U., E 30 I.U., C 100 mg., folic
acid 0.4 mg., B-1 15 mg., B-2 10 mg., niacin 50 mg.,
B-6 7.5 mg. B-12 12.5 mcg., pantothenic acid 10 mg.,
calcium 160 mg., phosphorus 125 mg., iron 18
mg./Tab. Bot. 30s.
Use: Vitamin & mineral supplement.
VICKS LIFESTAGE-WOMEN'S FORMULA. (Vicks) Vit.
A 5000 I.U., D 400 I.U., E 30 I.U., C 100 mg., folic
acid 0.4 mg., B-1 3 mg., B-2 3.4 mg., niacin 40 mg., B-
6 4 mg., B-12 12 mcg., pantothenic acid 10 mg., iodine
150 mcg., iron 27 mg., magnesium 100 mg., copper
2 mg., zinc 15 mg./Tab. Bot. 60s.
Use: Vitamin & mineral supplement with iron.
VICKS NYQUIL. (Vicks) Acetaminophen 1000 mg.,
doxylamine succinate 7.5 mg., pseudoephedrine
HCl 60 mg., dextromethorphan HBr 30 mg./oz.
w/FD&C Yellow #5 tartrazine and alcohol 25%.
Bot. 6 oz., 10 oz., 14 oz.
Use: Nighttime colds medicine.
VICKS ORACIN. (Vicks) Benzocaine 6.25 mg.,
menthol 0.1% (Regular) 0.08% (cherry) in a cooling
sorbitol base/Loz. Regular or Cherry flavor.
Contains FD&C Yellow #5 tartrazine. Pkg. 18s.
Use: Cooling throat lozenge.
VICKS SINEX. (Vicks) Phenylephrine HCl 0.5%,
cetylpyridinium Cl 0.04%, Special Vicks Blend of
Aromatics (menthol, eucalyptol, camphor, methyl
salicylate). w/thimersal 0.0001% preservative.
Nasal Spray. Plastic Squeeze Bot. 0.5 oz., 1 oz.
Use: Nasal decongestant spray.
VICKS SINEX LONG-ACTING. (Vicks) Oxymetazoline
HCl 0.05% in aqueous soln. containing menthol
vapors and thimersal 0.001%.. Nasal Spray. Plastic
Squeeze Bot. 1 oz., 0.5 oz.
Use: Nasal decongestant spray, long acting.
VICKS THROAT DROPS. (Vicks) Menthol in soothing
Vicks sugars base. Regular, wild cherry, lemon
flavor. Box 13s. Bag 30s.
Use: Cough Drop.
VICKS THROAT LOZENGES. (Vicks) Benzocaine 5
mg., cetylpyridinium Cl 1.66 mg., Special Vicks
Medication (menthol, eucalyptus oil, camphor). Loz.
12s.
Use: Sore throat and coughs of colds.
VICKS VAPORUB. (Vicks) Special Vicks Medication
(camphor 4.73%, menthol 2.67%, spirits of
turpentine 4.5%, eucalyptus oil 1.2%) 14%. Jar 1.5
oz., 3 oz. 6 oz.
Use: Decongestant vaporizing ointment.
VICKS VAPOSTEAM. (Vicks) Polyoxyethylene
dodecanol 1.8%, eucalyptus oil 1.7%, camphor
6.2%, tincture of benzoin 5%, w/alcohol 55%. Bot.
4 oz., 6 oz.
Use: Steam medication, decongestant and
antitussive.
VICKS VA-TRO-NOL. (Vicks) Ephedrine sulfate 0.5%,
Special Vicks Aromatic Blend in an aqueous base
(menthol, eucalyptol, camphor, methyl salicylate)
0.06%. Nose Drop Bot. 0.5 oz., 1 oz.
Use: Nasal decongestant, vapor-action.

VICODIN. (Knoll) Hydrocodone bitartrate 5 mg., acetaminophen 500 mg./Tab. Bot. 100s. Hospital pack 100s.
Use: Analgesic, antipyretic.

VICON-C. (Glaxo) Ascorbic acid 300 mg., niacinamide 100 mg., zinc sulfate 80 mg., magnesium sulfate 70 mg., Vit. B-1 20 mg., d-calcium pantothenate 20 mg., B-2 10 mg., B-6 5 mg./Cap. Bot. 60s, 500s. Unit dose 240s.
Use: Therapeutic vitamin-mineral complex.

VICON CHEWABLE TABLETS. (Glaxo) Vit. A 2000 I.U., E 25 I.U., C 75 mg., Zn 10 mg., Mg 35 mg., Niacinamide 12.5 mg., Thiamine 5 mg., Calcium pantothenate 5 mg., Riboflavin 2.5 mg., Mn 2 mg., pyridoxine HCl 1 mg. Bot. 60s, 500s.
Use: Vitamin deficiencies.

VICON FORTE. (Glaxo) Vit. A 8000 I.U., E 50 I.U., C 150 mg., zinc sulf. 80 mg., mag. sulf. 70 mg., niacinamide 25 mg., B-1 10 mg., calcium pantothenate 10 mg., B-2 5 mg., B-6 2 mg., B-12 10 mcg., folic acid 1 mg., manganese Cl 4 mg./Cap. Bot. 60s, 500s. Unit dose 240s.
Use: Therapeutic vitamin-mineral complex.

VICON PLUS. (Glaxo) Vit. A acetate 4000 I.U., E 50 I.U., C 150 mg., zinc sulfate 80 mg., magnesium sulf. 70 mg., niacinamide 25 mg., B-1 10 mg., d-calcium pantothenate 10 mg., .B-2 5 mg., manganese chloride 4 mg., B-6 2 mg./Cap. Bot. 60s, 500s.
Use: Therapeutic vitamin-mineral complex.

VICON WITH IRON. (Glaxo) B-complex with iron, zinc, Vit. C & E. Caps. Bot. 60s, 500s.
Use: Vitamin, mineral supplement.

VICRYL SUTURES. (Ethicon) Polyglactin 910.

VICTORS. (Vicks) Special Vicks Medication (menthol, eucalyptus oil) in a soothing Vicks sugar base. Regular or Cherry flavor drops. Stick-Pack 10s, Bag 30s, 3 pack sticks (30 drops).
Use: Cough drop.

• **VIDARABINE PHOSPHATE.** USAN.
Use: Antiviral.

• **VIDARABINE, STERILE.** U.S.P. XXI., Conc. for Inj., Ophth. Oint., U.S.P. XXI. 9-β-D-Arabinofuranosyladenine.
Use: Antiviral.
See: Vira-A Ophthalmic, Oint. (Parke-Davis)
Vira-A Inj. (Parke-Davis)

• **VIDARABINE SODIUM PHOSPHATE.**
Use: Antiviral.

VI-DAYLIN ADC DROPS. (Ross) Vit. A 1500 I.U.; C 35 mg.; D 400 I.U./1 ml. Bot. 30 ml., 50 ml. Also available w/iron 10 mg./ml. Bot. 50 ml., w/dropper.
Use: Pediatric vitamin supplement.

VI-DAYLIN ADC PLUS IRON. (Ross) Vit. A 1500 I.U.; C 35 mg.; D 400 I.U.; iron 10 mg./1 ml. Bot. 50 ml.
Use: Multivitamin with iron.

VI-DAYLIN CHEWABLE. (Ross) Vit. A 2500 I.U., D 400 I.U., E 15 I.U., C 60 mg., folic acid 0.3 mg., B-1 1.05 mg., B-2 1.2 mg., niacin 13.5 mg., B-6 1.05 mg., B-12 4.5 mcg./Tab. Bot. 100s.
Use: Multivitamin supplement.

VI-DAYLIN CHEWABLE W/FLUORIDE. (Ross) Fluoride 1 mg. B-1 1.05 mg., B-2 1.2 mg., niacinamide 13.5 mg., B-6 1.05 mg., C 60 mg., A 2500 I.U., B-12 4.5 mcg., E 15 I.U., folic acid 0.3 mg., D 400 I.U./Tab. Bot. 100s.
Use: Multivitamin with fluoride supplement.

VI-DAYLIN DROPS. (Ross) Vit. A 1500 I.U., D 400 I.U., E 5 I.U., C 35 mg., B-1 0.5 mg., B-2 0.6 mg., niacin 8 mg., B-6 0.4 mg., B-12 1.5 mcg./1 ml. Bot. 50 ml.
Use: Multivitamin supplement for infants and children under 4 years of age.

VI-DAYLIN/F ADC DROPS. (Ross) Vit. A 1500 I.U., D 400 I.U., C 35 mg., fluoride 0.25 mg./1 ml. Bot. 50 ml.
Use: As an aid in the prevention of dental caries and as prophylaxis of vit. A, D & C deficiencies.

VI-DAYLIN/F ADC PLUS IRON DROPS. (Ross) Vit. A 1500 I.U.; C 35 mg.; D 400 I.U.; iron 10 mg.; fluoride 0.25 mg./1 ml. Bot. 50 ml.
Use: Multivitamin with iron and fluoride supplement.

VI-DAYLIN/F DROPS. (Ross) Vit. A 1500 I.U., D 400 I.U., E 5 I.U., C 35 mg., B-1 0.5 mg., B-2 0.6 mg., niacin 8 mg., B-6 0.4 mg., fluoride 0.25 mg./1 ml. Bot. 50 ml.
Use: Aid in prevention of dental caries and prophylaxis of vitamin deficiencies in infants & children.

VI-DAYLIN/F PLUS IRON DROPS. (Ross) Fluoride 0.25 mg., Vit. A 1500 I.U., D 400 I.U., E 5 I.U., C 35 mg., B-1 0.5 mg., B-2 0.6 mg., niacin 8 mg., B-6 0.4 mg., iron 10 mg./ml. Bot. 50 ml.
Use: Multivitamin with fluoride and iron.

VI-DAYLIN LIQUID. (Ross) Vit. A 2500 I.U.; B-1 1.05 mg.; B-2 1.2 mg.; B-6 1.05 mg.; B-12 4.5 mcg.; C 60 mg.; D 400 I.U.; E 15 I.U., Niacinamide 13.5 mg./5 ml. Bot. 8 oz., pt.
Use: Liquid multivitamin for children.

VI-DAYLIN PLUS IRON CHEWABLE. (Ross) Vit. A 2500 I.U., D 400 I.U., E 15 I.U., C 60 mg., folic acid 0.3 mg., B-1 1.05 mg., B-2 1.2 mg., niacin 13.5 mg., B-6 1.05 mg., B-12 4.5 mcg., iron 12 mg./Tab. Bot. 60s.
Use: Multivitamin with iron.

VI-DAYLIN PLUS IRON DROPS. (Ross) Vit. A 1500 I.U., D 400 I.U., E 15 I.U., C 60 mg., folic acid 0.3 mg., B-1 1.05 mg., B-2 1.2 mg., niacin 13.5 mg., B-6 1.05 mg., B-12 4.5 mcg., iron 12 mg./1 ml. Bot. 50 ml.w/dropper.
Use: Multivitamin with iron for children.

VI-DAYLIN PLUS IRON LIQUID. (Ross) Vit. A 2500 I.U., D 400 I.U., C 60 mg., E 15 I.U., B-1 1.05 mg., B-2 1.2 mg., Niacin 13.5 mg., B-6 1.05 mg., B-12 4.5 mcg., iron 10 mg./tsp. Bot. 8 oz., 16 oz.
Use: Liquid multivitamin & iron supplement for children.

VIDEC. (Pharmics) Vit. A 5000 I.U., D 1000 I.U., C 50 mg., B-1 2 mg., B-2 2 mg., B-6 0.5 mg., d-Ca pantothenate 2 mg., nicotinamide 20 mg., B-12 2 mcg., Fe 15 mg., Iodine 15 mg., Mn 1 mg., K 5 mg., Cu (Cu sulfate) 1 mg., Zn 0.5 mg., Mg 1 mg./Cap. Bot. 100s, 1000s.
Use: Vitamin-mineral supplement.

VIDECON. (Vita Elixir) Vit. D 50,000 units/Cap.

Use: Dietary supplement.

VI-DERM SOAP. (Arthrins) Extract of Amaryllis. 10% Pkg. 1 cake. 3½ oz. bar.
Use: Hypo-allergenic and antipruritic.

VIDES CT W/FLUORIDE. (Pharmics) Vit. A 4000 I.U., D 400 I.U., B-1 1 mg., B-2 1.2 mg., B-6 1.5 mg., B-12 2 mcg., C 60 mg., d-panthenol 2.5 mg., niacinamide 10 mg., E 1 I.U., sod. fluoride 2.2 mg./Tab. Bot. 100s, 1000s.
Use: Dietary supplement.

VIFEX. (Mallard) Liver injection, equiv. in cyanocobalamin activity 10 mcg., cyanocobalamin 100 mcg., folic acid 1 mg./cc.

• **VIFILCON A.** USAN.
Use: Contact lens material.

VIFLUORINEED. (Hanlon) Vit. A 5000 I.U., D 400 I.U., C 75 mg., B-1 2 mg., B-2 3 mg., niacinamide 20 mg., fluoride 1 mg./Chew. Tab. Bot. 100s.
Use: Vitamin supplement.

VIGANIC. (Commerce)
Vit. A: 10,000 I.U./Cap. Bot. 100s.
Vit. B Complex: Bot. 100s.
Vit. B Complex W/C and Iron: Tab. Bot. 100s.
Vit. C: 150 mg., 300 mg., 1000 mg./Tab.; Sugarless 500 mg./Tab. Bot. 100s.
Vit. E: 100, 200, 400, 600, 1000 I.U./Cap. Bot. 100s.
Lecithin: 260 mg., Vit. A & D./Cap. Bot. 100s.

VI-GEROL ELIXIR. (Columbia) Iron 100 mg., Vit. B-1 100 mg., B-2 5 mg., B-6 5 mg., B-12 1 mcg., niacinamide 3 mg., panthenol 100 mg., choline bitartrate 100 mg., alcohol 12%/Fl. oz. Bot. pt.

VIGEROLAN. (Lannett) Geriatric vitamin-mineral capsule with choline, inositol, and methionine. Bot. 100s, 500s, 1000s.

VIGORAMIN THERAPEUTIC. (CMC) High potency vitamin. Cap. Bot. 30s, 100s, 250s, 1000s.

VIGOWAYNE ELIXIR. (Wayne) Bot. pt.

VIGRAN. (Squibb) **Chewable:** Vit. B-1 0.7 mg., B-2 0.8 mg., niacinamide 9 mg., B-6 0.7 mg., C 40 mg., A 2500 I.U., D 400 I.U., E 10 I.U., B-12 3 u., folic acid 0.2 mg./Chewable Tab. Bot. 60s. **Tab.:** Vit. A 5000 I.U., D 400 I.U., E 30 I.U., C 60 mg., folic acid 0.4 mg., B-1 1.5 mg., B-2 1.7 mg., niacin 20 mg., B-6 2 mg., B-12 6 mcg./Cap. Bot. 100s, Pkg. 2 bot. **Plus Iron:** B-1 1.5 mg., B-2 1.7 mg., niacinamide 20 mg., B-6 2 mg., C 60 mg., A 5000 I.U., D 400 I.U., E 30 I.U., B-12 6 mcg., folic 0.4 mg., iron (as ferrous fumarate) 27 mg./Tab. Bot. 90s.
Use: Multivitamin at least 125% of the M.D.R.

VIKASTAB DIHYDRATE. Potassium Menaphthosulphate, B.A.N.

VILEX. (Dunhall) Vit. B-1 100 mg., riboflavin phosphate sodium 1 mg., B-6 10 mg., panthenol 5 mg., niacinamide 100 mg./ml. Amp. 30 ml.
Use: Multiple Vit. B deficiency.

VILIVA. (Vita Elixir) Ferrous fumarate 3 gr.
Use: Iron therapy, anemia.

VILLESCON. Prolintane, B.A.N.

VILOXAZINE. B.A.N. 2-(2-Ethoxyphenoxymethyl)-tetrahydro-1,4-oxazine.
Use: Treatment of mental disease.

See: Vivalan hydrochloride.

• **VILOXAZINE HCL.** USAN.
Use: Antidepressant.

VIMEGA-B/C. (Pasadena Research) Vit. B-1 25 mg., B-2 15 mg., B-6 10 mg., B-12 10 mcg., niacinamide 100 mg., cal. pantothenate 50 mg., Vit. C 750 mg./Tab. Bot. 100s, 1000s, Box 30s.

VIMINAL CAPSULES. (Cenci) Vit. A 5000 I.U., D 400 I.U., B-1 3 mg., B-2 2.5 mg., niacinamide 20 mg., B-6 1.5 mg., Ca pantothenate 5 mg., B-12 2.5 mcg., C 50 mg., E 3 I.U., Ca 215 mg., P 166 mg., Fe 13.4 mg., Mg 7.5 mg., Mn 1.5 mg., K 5 mg., Zn 1.4 mg./Cap. Bot. 30s, 100s, 500s.
Use: Dietary supplement.

VIMINAL G CAPSULES. (Cenci) Vit. A 12,500 I.U., D 400 I.U., B-1 5 mg., B-2 2.5 mg., niacinamide 40 mg., B-6 1 mg., Ca pantothenate 4 mg., B-12 2 mcg., C 75 mg., E 2 I.U., choline bitartrate 31.4 mg., inositol 15 mg., Ca 75 mg., P 58 mg., Fe 30 mg., Mg 3 mg., Mn 0.5 mg., K 2 mg., Zn 0.5 mg./Cap. Bot. 30s, 100s, 500s.
Use: Geriatric vitamin.

VIMINAL T. (Cenci) Vit. A 25,000 I.U., D 400 I.U., B-1 10 mg., B-2 5 mg., niacinamide 100 mg., B-6 1 mg., B-12 5 mcg., C 150 mg., Ca 103.6 mg., P 80.2 mg., Fe 10 mg., Mg 5.5 mg., Mn 1 mg., K 5 mg., Zn 1.4 mg./Cap. Bot. 100s, 500s.
Use: Vitamin deficiencies.

VIMIN-CO. (Jenkins) Vit. A 5000 I.U., D 400 I.U., B-1 3 mg., B-2 2.5 mg., B-6 1 mg., B-12 2 mcg., C 50 mg., niacinamide 20 mg., Ca 46 mg., P 35 mg., Fe 13.4 mg., Ca pantothenate 2 mg., Mg 1 mg., Mn 1.5 mg., K 5 mg., Zn 1.4 mg./Cap. Bot. 1000s.
Use: Vitamin-mineral capsule.

VI-MIN-FOR-ALL. (Barth's) Vit. A 3 mg., D 10 mcg., C 120 mg., B-1 35 mg., B-12 15 mcg., biotin, niacin 2.33 mg., E 30 I.U., B-6, pantothenic acid, Ca 375 mg., P 180 mg., Fe 20 mg., Iodine 0.1 mg., rutin 10 mg., hesperidin-lemon bioflavonoid complex 10 mg., choline, inositol 2.4 mg., Cu 10 mcg., Mn 2 mg., Zn 110 mcg., silicone 210 mcg./Tab. 100s, 500s.
Use: Diet supplement.

VIMMS-38. (Approved) Vit. A 12,500 I.U., D 1200 I.U., B-1 15 mg., B-2 10 mg., C 75 mg., niacinamide 30 mg., Ca pantothenate 2 mg., B-6 0.5 mg., E-5 I.U., Brewer's yeast 10 mg., B-12 15 mcg., Fe 11.58 mg., desic. liver 15 mg., choline bitartrate 30 mg., inositol 30 mg., Ca 59 mg., P 45 mg., Zn 0.68 mg., Fr. dicalcium phos. 200 mg., Mn 1.11 mg., Mg 1 mg., K 0.68 mg., pepsin 16.5 mg., diastase 16.5 mg., yeast 40.63 mg., protein digest 23.52 mg., amino acids 34.22 mg./Cap. Bot. 50s, 100s, 1000s.
Use: Supplement and therapy.

VINACTANE SULFATE. (Ciba) Viomycin Sulfate.

• **VINAFOCON A.** USAN
Use: Contact lens material.

VINBARBITAL. 5-Ethyl-5-(1-methyl-1-butenyl)barbituric acid.
Use: Sedative.

VINBARBITAL SODIUM. 5-Ethyl-5-(1-methylbut-1-enyl)-barbiturate sod.

Use: Sedative.

VINBARBITONE. B.A.N. 5-Ethyl-5-(1-methylbut-1-enyl)barbituric acid.
See: Delvinal
Use: Hypnotic; sedative.

• **VINBLASTINE SULFATE,** U.S.P. XXI. Sterile, U.S.P. XXI. Vincaleukoblastine. Alkaloid extracted from *Vinca rosea* Linn.
Use: Antineoplastic.
See: Velban, Amp., Vial (Lilly)

VINCALEUKOBLASTINE, 22-OXO-, SULFATE (1:1)(SALT). Vincristine Sulfate, U.S.P. XXI.

• **VINCOFOS.** USAN.
Use: Anthelmintic.

• **VINCRISTINE SULFATE,** U.S.P. XXI. Inj., U.S.P. XXI. (Lilly) Vincaleukoblastine, 22-oxo-,sulfate (1:1)(salt) Leurocristine. An alkaloid extracted from Vinca rosea Linn.
Use: Antineoplastic.
See: Oncovin, Amp. (Lilly)

• **VINDESINE.** USAN.
Use: Antineoplastic.

• **VINDESINE SULFATE.** USAN.
Use: Antineoplastic.

• **VINEPIDINE SULFATE.** USAN.

• **VINGLYCINATE SULFATE.** USAN. 4-Deacetylvincaleukoblastine 4-(N,N-dimethylglycinate) (ester) sulfate (1:1½)(salt).
Use: Antineoplastic.

• **VINLEUROSINE SULFATE.** USAN. Sulfate salt of an alkaloid extracted from *Vinca rosea* Linn. Also see Vinblastine.
Use: Antineoplastic.

• **VINPOCETINE.** USAN.
See: Cavinton (Abbott)

• **VINROSIDINE SULFATE.** USAN. Sulfate salt of an alkaloid extracted from *Vinca rosea* Linn. Also see Vinblastine.
Use: Antineoplastic.

VINYLACETATE-POLYVINYLPYRROLIDONE.
See: Ivy-Rid, Spray (Mallard)

VINYL ALCOHOL POLYMER. Polyvinyl Alcohol, U.S.P. XXI.

VINYLBITONE. B.A.N. 5-(1-Methylbutyl)-5-vinyl-barbituric acid.
Use: Hypnotic; sedative.

• **VINYL ETHER,** U.S.P. XXI.
Use: General anesthetic (inhalation.)
See: Vinethene, Liq.

1-VINYL-2-PYRROLIDINONE POLYMER. Povidone, U.S.P. XXI.

VINYZENE. Bromchlorenone.
Use: Fungicide and bactericide.

• **VINZOLIDINE SULFATE.** USAN.
Use: Antineoplastic.

VIO-BEC. (Rowell) Vit. B-1 25 mg., B-2 25 mg., niacinamide 100 mg., Ca pantothenate 40 mg., B-6 25 mg., C 500 mg./Cap. Bot. 100s. Unit-dose 100s.
Use: Vitamin & mineral supplement.

VIO-BEC FORTE. (Rowell) Vit. B-1 25 mg., B-2 25 mg., B-6 25 mg., C 500 mg., calcium pantothenate 40 mg., niacinamide 100 mg., E 30 I.U., B-12 5 mcg., folic acid

0.5 mg., Zn 25 mg., Cu 3 mg./Tab. Bot. 100s. Unit dose 100s.
Use: Vitamin therapy.

VIOFORM. (Ciba) Clioquinol.
Cream: (3%) Tube 1 oz.
Oint.: (3% in petrolatum base) Tube 1 oz.
Use: Antifungal, antibacterial.

VIOFORM-HYDROCORTISONE. (Ciba) **Cream:** Clioquinol 3%, hydrocortisone 1% in water-washable base w/stearyl alcohol, cetyl alcohol, stearic acid, sod. lauryl sulfate, glycerin, petrolatum. Tubes 20 Gm. **Ointment:** Clioquinol 3%, hydrocortisone 1% in petrolatum base. Tubes 20 Gm. **Lotion:** Clioquinol 3%, hydrocortisone 1% in water-washable base w/stearic acid, cetyl alcohol, lanolin, propylene glycol, sorbitan trioleate, polysorbate 60, triethanolamine, methylparaben, propylparaben. Plastic squeeze Bot., 15 ml. **Mild Cream** Clioquinol 3%, hydrocortisone 0.5% w/ingredients included in Cream. Tube ½ oz., 1 oz. **Mild Ointment:** Clioquinol 3%, hydrocortisone 0.5% in petrolatum base. Tube 1 oz.
Use: Antibacterial, antifungal, antipruritic, antiinflammatory.

VIO-HYDROCORT CREAM. (Columbia) Hydrocortisone 10 mg., clioquinol 30 mg./Gm. Tube 5 Gm., 20 Gm.
Use: Antifungal, anti-inflammatory.

VIO-HYDROSONE CREAM. (Vortech) Hydrocortisone 0.1%, clioquinol 3%, pramoxine HCl 0.5%. Tube ½ oz.
Use: Relieves pain and itching associated with dermatologic disorders.

VIOKASE. (Viobin) **Tab.:** Lipase 8000 u., protease 30,000 u., amylase 30,000 u./16,800 mg. Tab. Bot. 100s, 500s. **Powder:** Lipase 16,800 u., protease 70,000 u., amylase 70,000 u./0.7 Gm. (¼ tsp.)
Use: Aid digestion.

VIOMYCIN SULFATE. STERILE, Sulfate salt of antibiotic produced by selected strains of *actinomycete* to which *Streptomyces puniceus* & *Streptomyces floridea* have been applied.
Use: Tuberculostatic, antibacterial.

VIONACTANE PANTOTHENATE-SULPHATE. Viomycin, B.A.N.

VIO-PRAMOSONE CREAM. (Ferndale) Clioquinol 3%, hydrocortisone acetate 0.5%, pramoxine HCl 1.0% in cream. Bot. 1 oz.
Use: Contact or atopic dermatitis, eczema, infectious dermatitis, anti-pruritic.

VIO-PRAMOSONE LOTION. (Ferndale) Clioquinol 3%, hydrocortisone acetate 0.5%, pramoxine HCl 1.0% in lotion. Bot. 1¼ oz.
4 oz.
Use: Contact or atopic dermatitis, eczema, infectious dermatitis, antipruritic.

VIOSTEROL W/HALIBUT LIVER OIL. Vit. A 50,000 I.U., Vit. D 10,000 I.U./Gm.
(Abbott)—Bot. 5 cc., 20 cc., 50 cc. Cap. Vit. A 5000 I.U., D 1000 I.U.
(Ives) Cap. Vit. A 5000 I.U., D 1700 I.U.

VI-PENTA INFANT DROPS. (Roche) Vit. A 5000 I.U., D 400 I.U., C 50 mg., E 2 I.U./0.6 ml. Bot. 50 ml.

Use: Progressive vitamin therapy for specific age groups.

VI-PENTA MULTIVITAMIN DROPS. (Roche) Vit. A 5000 I.U. B-1 1 mg., B-2 1 mg., B-6 1 mg., C 50 mg., D 400 I.U., d-panthenol 10 mg., niacinamide 10 mg. E 2 I.U., d-biotin 30 mcg./0.6 ml. Bot. 50 ml.
Use: Progressive vitamin therapy for specific age groups.

VI-PENTA F CHEWABLES. (Roche) Vit. A acetate 5000 I.U., calciferol 10 mcg., C 60 mg., B-1 1.2 mg., B-2 1.5 mg., B-6 1.2 mg., B-12 3 mcg., d-biotin 40 mcg., niacinamide 10 mg., E 2 I.U., d-calcium pantothenate 10 mg., fluoride 1 mg./chewable Tab. Bot. 100s. Available in 5 fruit flavors with matching colors.
Use: Nutritional support.

VI-PENTA F INFANT DROPS. (Roche) Vit. A 5000 I.U., calciferol 10 mcg., C 50 mg., dl-alpha-tocopheryl acetate 2 mg., fluoride 0.5 mg./0.6 ml. Bot. 30 ml. w/calibrated dropper.
Use: Infant nutritional.

VI-PENTA F MULTIVITAMIN DROPS. (Roche) Vit. A palmitate 5000 I.U., calciferol 10 mcg., C 50 mg., B-1 1 mg., B-2 1 mg., B-6 1 mg., dl-α-tocopheryl acetate 2 I.U., d-biotin 30 mcg., niacinamide 10 mg., d-panthenol 10 mg., fluoride 0.5 mg./0.6 ml. Bot. 30 ml. with a calibrated dropper.
Use: Nutritional supplement.

VIPRYNIUM EMBONATE. B.A.N. 6-Dimethyl-amino-2-[2-(2:5-dimethyl-1-phenyl-3-pyrrolyl)vinyl]-1-methyl-quinolinium embonate. (Embonic acid is adopted as the trivial name for 4:4' methylenebis-(3-hydroxymaphthalene-2-carboxylic acid). Vanquin. Pyrvinium Pamoate.
Use: Anthelmintic.

VIRA-A FOR INFUSION. (Parke-Davis) Vidarabine for infusion 200 mg./ml. Vial 5 ml.
Use: Treatment of Herpes simplex virus encephalitis.

VIRA-A OPHTHALMIC. (Parke-Davis) Vidarabine 3% in a sterile inert base. Tube 3.5 Gm.
Use: Treatment of acute keratoconjunctivitis & recurrent epithelial keratitis due to Herpes Simplex Virus types 1 & 2.

VIRAC. (Ruson) Undecoylium chloride-iodine. Iodine complexed with a cationic detergent. Surgical sol. Bot. 2 oz., 8 oz., 1 gal.
Use: Antiseptic.

VIRACIL. (Approved) Phenylephrine HCl 5 mg., hesperidin 50 mg., thenylene HCl 12½ mg., pyrilamine maleate 12½ mg., C 50 mg., salicylamide 2½ gr., caffeine ½ gr., sod. salicylate 1¼ gr./Cap. Bot. 16s, 36s.
Use: Cold symptoms.

VIRAMISOL. (Seatrace) Adenosine phosphate 25 mg./ml. Vial 10 cc.

VIRANOL. (Americal Dermal) Salicylic acid 16.7%, lactic acid 16.7% in flexible collodion vehicle. Bot. 10 ml.
Use: Removal of warts.

• **VIRIDOFULVIN.** USAN.
Use: Antifungal.

• **VIRGINIAMYCIN.** USAN. An antibiotic produced by *Streptomyces virginie.*

VIRIDIUM. (Vita Elixir) Phenylazodiaminopyridine HCl 100 mg./Tab.
Use: Genito-urinary antisepsis.

VIRILON. (Star) Methyltestosterone 10 mg./Cap. (sustained release) Bot. 100s, 1000s.
Use: Male climacteric, hypogonadal impotence, neurasthenia.

VIROMED LIQUID. (Whitehall) Acetaminophen 10 gr., pseudoephedrine HCl 30 mg., dextromethorphan HBr 20 mg., alcohol 16.63%. Bot. 6 oz.
Use: Antitussive, analgesic.

VIROMED TABLETS. (Whitehall) Aspirin 5 gr., chlorpheniramine maleate 1 mg., pseudoephedrine HCl 15 mg., dextromethorphan HBr 7.5 mg., guaifenesin 50 mg./Tab. Bot. 20s, 48s.
Use: Antitussive, analgesic.

VIROPTIC OPHTHALMIC SOLUTION. (Burroughs Wellcome) Trifluridine 1%. Bot. 7.5 ml.
Use: Herpes simplex eye infection treatment.

• **VIROXIME.** USAN.
Use: Antiviral.

VIROZYME INJECTION. (Marcen) Sodium nucleate 2.5%, phenol 0.5%, protein hydrolysate 2.5%, benzyl alcohol 0.2%. Vial 5 cc., 10 cc.
Use: Promote leukocytosis and phagocytosis.

VIRUGON. Under study. Anhydro bis-(beta-hydroxyethyl) biguanide derivative.
Use: Treatment of influenza, mumps, measles, chickenpox, and shingles.

VISALENS SOAKING & CLEANING SOLUTION. (Leeming) Sterile sol. containing cleaning agents, benzalkonium chloride, buffered sol. Bot. 4 oz.
Use: Soaking & cleaning sol. for hard contact lenses.

VISALENS WETTING SOLUTION. (Leeming) Sterile sol. containing polyvinyl alcohol with hydroxypropyl methylcellulose, edetate disodium, sodium chloride, benzalkonium chloride 1:25,000 Bot. 2 oz.
Use: Wetting agent for hard contact lenses.

VISCARIN W/IODINE, BORIC ACID, PHENOL, CHLOROPHYLL.
See: Triophyll, Liq. (Schaffer)

VISCLAIR HYDROCHLORIDE. Methyl Cysteine, B.A.N.

VISCULOSE. (Softcon) Methylcellulose ½%, 1% w/benzalkonium chloride 1:25,000 Bot. 15 cc.
Use: Substitute for lacrimal secretions, for patients with tear deficiencies.

VISCUM ALBUM, EXTRACT. Visnico.
Use: Vasodilator.

VISIDEX. (Ames) Disposable plastic test strip with two reagent pads. Glucose oxidase reaction. Bot. 25s.
Use: Blood glucose testing using visual interpretation of test results.

VISINE. (Leeming) Tetrahydrozoline HCl 0.05%, NaCl, boric acid, sodium borate, benzalkonium chloride 0.01%, disodium ethylenediamine tetraacetate 0.1%. Dropper Bot. ½ oz.; Plastic bot. ½ oz., ¾ oz., 1 oz.
Use: Eye irritations.

VISINE AC. (Leeming) Tetrahydrozoline HCl 0.05%, zinc sulfate 0.25%, benzalkonium chloride 0.01%, NaCl, boric acid, sodium citrate, ethylene diamine tetraacetate 0.1%. Bot. ½ oz., 1 oz.
Use: Eye irritations accompanied by allergy and colds.

VISKEN. (Sandoz) Pindolol 5 mg. or 10 mg./Tab. Bot. 100s.
Use: Hypertension treatment.

VISNADINE. B.A.N. 10-Acetoxy-9,10-dihydro-8,8-di-methyl-9-α-methylbutyryloxy-2H,8H-benzo-[1,2-b:3,4-b′]dipyran-2-one. Cardine.
Use: Coronary vasodilator.

VISTACON. (Hauck) Hydroxyzine HCl 25 mg./ml. Vial 10 ml. 50 mg/ml. Vial 10 ml. Amp. 1 ml. 100 mg./2 ml. Vial 2 ml. Box. 25s.
Use: Management of tension, anxiety, psychomotor agitation.

VISTAJECT 25 & 50. (Mayrand) Hydroxyzine HCl 25 mg. or 50 mg./ml. Vial 10 ml.
Use: Relief of anxiety and tension.

VISTAREX 50. (Tunex) Hydroxyzine HCl 50 mg./ml. Vial 10cc.
Use: Anxiety, nausea, vomiting.

VISTARIL. (Pfizer Laboratories) Hydroxyzine pamoate equiv. to Hydroxyzine HCl, **Cap.:** 25, 50, 100 mg. Bot. 100s, 500s, Unit Dose 100s. **Oral susp.** 25 mg./5 cc. Bot. 120 ml., pt.
Use: Psychotherapeutic agent.

VISTARIL I.M. (Pfipharmecs) Hydroxyzine HCl 25 mg./ml. & 50 mg./ml. Vial 10 ml. Unit dose 25 mg./ml.; 50 mg./ml.; 75 mg./1.5 ml.; 100 mg./2 ml. Box 10's.
Use: Ataraxic.

VISTARIL ISOJECT I.M. (Pfipharmecs) Hydroxyzine HCl 50 mg./ml. & 100 mg./2 ml. Amp. 1 ml., 2 ml.
Use: Ataraxic.

VISTAZINE 50. (Keene) Hydroxyzine HCl 50 mg./ml. Vial 10 mg./ml.
Use: Psychotherapeutic agent.

VISTRAX 5 & 10. (Pfizer Laboratories) Oxyphencyclimine 5 mg. or 10 mg., hydroxyzine 25 mg./Tab. Bot. 100s.
Use: Anticholinergic.

VITABANK. (Williams) Vit. A 5,000 I.U., E 30 I.U.,C 90 mg., folic acid 400 mcg., B-1 2.25 mg., B-2 2.6 mg., niacinamide 20 mg., B-6 3 mg., B-12 9 mcg., D 400 I.U., biotin 45 mcg., pantothenic acid 10 mg., Ca 170 mg., P 130 mg., iodine 150 mcg., Fe 18 mg., Mg 100 mg., Cu 2 mg., Mn. 2.5 mg., K 7.5 mg., Zn 15 mg., selenium 25 mcg./Tab. Bot. 60s.
Use: Multivitamin with minerals.

VITABEE 1. (CMC) Thiamine **Inj.:** 100 mg./cc. Vial 10 cc., 30 cc. **Tab.:** 10 mg., 25 mg., 50 mg., 100 mg., 250 mg. Bot. 100s, 1000s.

VITABEE 2. (CMC) Riboflavin **Inj.:** 40 mg./cc. Vial 10 cc. **Tab.:** 10 mg., 25 mg., 50 mg. Bot. 100s, 1000s.

VITABEE 6. (CMC) Pyridoxine HCl **Inj.:** 100 mg./cc. Vial 10 cc. **Tab.:** 10 mg., 25 mg., 50 mg., 100 mg., 250 mg. Bot. 100s, 1000s.

VITABIX. (Spanner) Vit. B-1 100 mg., B-2 2 mg., B-6 5 mg., B-12 30 mcg., niacinamide 100 mg., pan-

thenol 10 mg./cc. 10 cc. Multiple dose vial 30 cc. Inj. I.M. or I.V.

V-I TABS. (Kenyon) Vit. A 5000 I.U., D-2 500 mg., B-1 3 mg., B-2 2.5 mg., B-6 1 mg., B-12 1 mg., C 50 mg., niacinamide 20 mg., Ca pantothenate 1 mg., Fe 15 mg./Tab. Bot. 100s, 1000s.

VITA-CEBUS. (Cenci) Vit. A 10,000 I.U., D 1000 I.U., C 100 mg., B-1 5 mg., B-2 5 mg., B-6 1 mg., B-12 1 mcg., niacin and niacinamide 30 mg., Ca pantothenate 5 mg., E 3 mg., yeast 1 gr., liver 1 gr., hesperidin complex 10 mg., Ca 200 mg., Cu 0.75 mg., Mg 5 mg., Mn 1 mg., K 5 mg., Zn 0.3 mg./2 Tabs. Bot. 100s, 250s. Liquid, 4 oz., 8 oz.
Use: Dietary supplement.

VITACEE. (CMC) Vitamin C 100 mg. or 500 mg./2 cc. Amp. 2 cc. 500 mg. Amp. 5 cc. I.M.-I.V. 1000 mg. Amp. 10 cc.

VITACOMP. (Jenkins) Vit. A 5000 I.U., D 400 I.U., B-1 3 mg., B-2 2.5 mg., C 50 mg., B-6 1 mg., B-12 1 mcg., niacinamide 20 mg., pantothenic acid 1 mg./Tab. Bot. 1000s.
Use: Multiple vitamin tablet.

VITACREST. (Nutrition) Vit. A 25,000 I.U., D 400 I.U., E 10 I.U., B-1 25 mg., B-2 12 mg., B-6 10 mg., B-12 10 mcg., biotin 10 mcg., folic acid 0.1 mg., Ca pantothenate 25 mg., niacinamide 50 mg., inositol 25 mg., l-glutamic acid 10 mg., l-lysine HCl 20 mg., p-aminobenzoic acid 25 mg., C 250 mg., wheat germ oil 10 mg., brewers yeast, dried 10 mg., whole liver desic. 10 mg., soybean lecithin 50 mg., iron 10 mg., cal. carbonate 625 mg., Cu 0.2 mg., Zn 0.2 mg., Mg 10 mg., Mn 0.2 mg., K 10 mg./Cap. Bot. 100s.
Use: Therapeutic vitamin-mineral formula.

VITADYE. (Elder) F.D. & C yellow No. 5, D. & C. red. No. 40, F.D. & C. blue No. 1 dyes & dihydroxyacetone 5%. Bot. 0.5 oz., 2 oz.
Use: Cosmetic cover for hypopigmented skin.

VITAFOL. (Everett) Vitamins, folic acid, iron, calcium. Bot. 100s, 1000s.
Use: Dietary supplement

VITA ELIXIR. (Vita Elixir) Alcohol 25%, Vit. A palmitate 5000 U., D-2 500 U., iron 10 mg./45 cc. w/multivitamins & minerals.
Use: Dietary supplement.

VITAFORT. (Kessel) Vit. A 4,000 I.U., D 400 I.U., E 15 I.U., C 70 mg., folic acid 1 mg., B-1 2 mg., B-2 2 mg., niacinamide 20 mg., B-6 2 mg., B 12 5 mcg., Ca-pantothenate 10 mg./Cap. Bot. 60s.
Use: Nutritional supplement

VITAGETTS. (Vortech) Vit. A palmitate 5000 I.U., Vit. D 1000 I.U., B-1 3 mg., B-2 2.5 mg., nicotinamide 20 mg., B-6 1.5 mg., calcium pantothenate 5 mg., B-12 2.5 mcg., C 50 mg., Vit. E 3 I.U., Ca 251 mg., P 166 mg., Fe 13.4 mg., Mg 7.5 mg., Mn 1.5 mg., K 5 mg., Zn 1.4 mg./Tab. Bot. 100s, 1000s.
Use: Vitamin & mineral therapy.

VITA-GLEN. (Glenwood) Pediatric multiple vitamin. Cap. Bot. 100s.

VITA-IRON. (Century) Vit. A 5000 I.U., D 500 I.U., B-1 2 mg., B-2 2.5 mg., C 50 mg., B-6 1 mg., B-12 1 mcg., niacinamide 20 mg., Ca pantothenate 1 mg., iron 15 mg./Tab. Bot. 30s, 100s, 1000s.

Use: Multivitamin with iron.

VITA-IRON FORMULA. (Barth's) Iron 120 mg., B-1 5 mg., B-2 10 mg., C 20 mg., niacin 2 mg., B-12 25 mcg. lysine, desic. liver 200 mg., bromelain/Tab. Bot. 100s, 500s.

VITAJEN. (Jenkins) Vit. B-1 12 mg., B-2 4 mg., B-12 10 mcg., B-6 2 mg., Ca pantothenate 6 mg., nicotinic acid 40 mg./Fl. oz. Bot. 4 oz., gal.
Use: B complex supplement.

VITA-KAPS FILMTABS. (Abbott) Vit. A 5000 I.U., D 400 I.U., B-1 3 mg., B-2 2.5 mg., nicotinamide 20 mg., B-6 1 mg., C 50 mg., B-12 3 mcg./Filmtab. Bot. 100s.
Use: Dietary supplement.

VITAKAPS-M. (Abbott) Vit. A 5000 I.U., D 400 I.U., B-1 3 mg., B-2 2.5 mg., nicotinamide 20 mg., B-6 1 mg., B-12 3 mcg., C 50 mg., Fe 10 mg., Cu 1 mg., Iodine 0.15 mg., Mn 1 mg., Zn 7.5 mg./Filmtab. Bot. 100s.
Use: Multivitamin with minerals.

VITAL. (Ross) Each packet contains: Protein 12.5 Gm., fat 3.25 Gm., carbohydrates 56.5 Gm., Vit. A 1000 I.U., Vit. D 80 I.U., Vit. E 12 I.U., Vit C 18 mg., folic acid 0.08 mg., B-1 0.3 mg., B-2 0.34 mg., B-6 0.44 mg., B-12 1.2 mcg., niacin 4 mg., biotin 0.06 mg., pantothenic acid 2 mg., Vit K-1 56 mcg., choline 40 mg., Ca 200 mg., phosphorus 200 mg., Na 115 mg., potassium 350 mg., Cl 200 mg., Mg 80 mg., iodine 30 mcg., Mn 0.75 mg., Cu 0.4 mg., Zn 3 mg., Fe 3.6 mg./Packet W/glucose oligo- and polysaccharides, enzymatically hydrolyzed proteins (soy, whey and meat), sucrose, corn starch, safflower oil. Packets 2.75-oz (79 Gm.)/Case of 72.
Use: Hydrolyzed, low-residue feeding for patients with impared gastrointestinal function.

VITALAX. (Vitalax) Candy base, gumdrop flavored. Pkg. 20s.
Use: Laxative.

VITALITY E CAPSULES. (Columbia) Wheat germ oil 3 min./Cap. Bot. 100s, 1000s.

VITALITY-E "6" CAPSULES. (Columbia) Wheat germ oil 6 minims/Cap. Bot. 100s, 1000s.

VITALITY-E "14". (Columbia) Wheat germ oil 14 minims/Cap. Bot. 100s, 1000s.

VITALITY-E "20". (Columbia) Wheat germ oil 20 minims/Cap. Bot. 100s, 1000s.
Use: Vitamin supplement.

VITAMEL-M. (Eastwood) Liquid Bot. 16 oz.

VITAMEL WITH IRON. (Eastwood) Drops 50 cc. Chewable Tab. Bot. 100s.

• **VITAMIN A,** U.S.P. XXI. Caps., U.S.P. XXI.
Use: Anti-xerophthalmic vitamin, emollient.
Ampules
　Aquasol A Preps. (USV Pharm.)
Capsules
　Acon (Du Pont)
　Alphalin (Lilly)
　Aquasol A (USV Labs.)
　Vi-Dom-A (Miles Pharm)
Ointment
　Aquasol A (USV Pharm.)
　Retin-A (Johnson & Johnson)

Tablets
　Dispatabs (Person & Covey)
Vials
　Aquasol A (USV Labs.)
VITAMIN A, ALPHALIN. (Lilly) Vit. A. 50,000 I.U./Gelseal. Bot. 100s.
Use: Vitamin A deficiency.
VITAMIN A, WATER MISCIBLE, OR SOLUBLE.
Water Miscible vitamin A.
VITAMIN Bc.
See: Folic acid (Var. Mfr.)
VITAMIN B-1. Thiamine Hydrochloride, U.S.P. XXI.
VITAMIN B-1 & B-12. (Pharmex) Vit. B-1 100 mg., B-12 1000 mcg./cc. Vial 10 cc.
VITAMIN B-1 W/PANCREATIN, OX BILE EXT. PEP-SIN, GLUTAMIC ACID HCl.
See: Maso-Gestive, Tab. (Mason)
VITAMIN B-1 W/THYROID.
See: T & T, Tab. (Mason)
VITAMIN B-2. Riboflavin, U.S.P. XXI.
VITAMIN B-3. Niacinamide, U.S.P. XXI. Nicotinamide.
VITAMIN B-5. Calcium Pantothenate U.S.P. XXI.
VITAMIN B-6. Pyridoxine Hydrochloride, U.S.P. XXI.
See: Hexa-Betalin, Tab. (Lilly)
　Hexavibex, Vial (Parke-Davis)
VITAMIN B-6 & B-1. (Pharmex) Vit. B-6 100 mg., B-1 100 mg./cc. Vial 10 cc.
VITAMIN B-12. Cyanocobalamin, U.S.P. XXI. Cobalamine.
See:
Capsules & Tablets
　Redisol (Merck Sharp & Dohme)
Vials & Ampules
　Bedoce (Lincoln)
　Berubigen (Upjohn)
　Betalin-12 (Lilly)
　Cabadon-M (Reid-Provident)
　Cobadoce Forte (Reid-Provident)
　Crysto-Gel (Reid-Provident)
　Cyano-Gel, Liq. (Maurry)
　Dodex (Organon)
　Poyamin (Fellows)
　Redisol (Merck Sharp & Dohme)
　Rhodavin (Noyes)
　Rubramin (Squibb)
　Ruvite 1000 (Savage)
　Sigamine (Sig)
　Sytobex-H (Parke-Davis)
　Vibedoz, Inj. (Blue Line)
　Vi-Twel, Inj. (Berlex)
W/Ferrous-sulfate, ascorbic acid, folic acid.
　See: Intrin, Cap. (Merit)
W/Folic acid, niacinamide, liver.
　See: Hepfomin 500 Inj. (Keene Pharm.)
W/Thiamine.
　See: Cobalin, Vial (Ulmer)
　Cyamine, Vial (Keene)
W/Thiamine & vitamin B-6.
　See: Orexin, Tab. (Stuart)
VITAMIN B-12a & b.
See: Hydroxocobalamin (Var. Mfr.)

VITAMIN B-15. Pangamic acid, betaglucono-dimethylaminoacetic acid.
Use: Alleged to increase oxygen supply in blood. Not approved by FDA as a vitamin or drug. Illegal to sell Vitamin B-15.

VITAMIN B-17.
See laetril.

VITAMIN B COMPLEX. Conc. ext. of dried brewer's yeast & ext. of corn processed w/*Clostridium acetobutylicum.*
See: Becotin, Pulvule (Lilly)
    Betalin Complex, Amp. (Lilly)
    Savaplex, Vial (Savage)
W/Estrone, testosterone.
See: Amplex, Inj. (Vortech)

VITAMIN B COMPLEX. (Maurry) Vit. B-1 100 mg., B-2, B-6 10 mg., panthenol 5 mg., niacinamide 100 mg., sulfoxylate 0.01%, chlorobutanol 0.35%, benzyl alcohol 2%, sodium formaldehyde. Bot. 30 ml.
Use: Multivitamin.

VITAMIN B COMPLEX CAPSULES, N.J.F. (Columbia) Vit. B-1 2 mg., B-2 3 mg., B-6 1 mg., niacinamide 20 mg., dried yeast 300 mg./Cap. Bot. 100s, 1000s.

VITAMIN B COMPLEX NO. 104. (Century) Vit. B-1 100 mg., B-2 2 mg., B-6 2 mg., d-panthenol 10 mg., niacinamide 125 mg., benzyl alcohol 1%, gentisic acid ethanolamide 2.5%/Vial 30 cc.

VITAMIN B COMPLEX, BETALIN COMPLEX, ELIXIR. (Lilly) Vit. B-1 2.7 mg., B-2 1.35 mg., B-12 3 mcg., B-6 0.555 mg., pantothenic acid 2.7 mg., niacinamide 6.75 mg., liver fraction 500 mg./5 ml. w/alcohol 17%. Bot. 16 oz.
Use: Vitamin B supplement.

VITAMIN B-COMPLEX W/C. (Sutliff & Case) Vit. B-1 2.5 mg., B-2 3 mg., niacinamide 25 mg., calcium pantothenate 5 mg., B-6 2.5 mg., C 100 mg., B-12 2 mcg., brewer's yeast 240 mg./Tab. Bot. 100s, 1000s.

VITAMIN B COMPLEX W/NIACIN & IRON. (Berlex) L-Glutavite Caps.: Vit. B-1 0.96 mg., B-2 1.92 mg., niacin 45 mg., B-6 1 mg., B-12 6 mcg. iron 10.2 mg./6 Caps. Bot. 100s.
Use: Vitamin and mineral supplement.

VITAMIN B COMPLEX W/VITAMIN C. (Century) Vit. B-1 25 mg., B-2 5 mg., B-6 5 mg., niacinamide 50 mg., panthenol 5 mg., calcium 50 mg., propethylene glycol 300 10%, gentisic acid ethanolamide 2.5%, benzyl alcohol 2%/Vial 30 cc.

VITAMIN B COMPOUND, BETALIN COMPOUND. (Lilly) Vit. B-1 1 mg., B-2 2 mg., B-6 0.4 mg., pantothenic acid 3.333 mg., niacinamide 10 mg., Vit. B-12 1 mcg./Pulvule. Bot. 100s, 500s.
Use: Orally, vitamin B complex deficiencies.

VITAMIN C.
See: Ascorbic Acid, Preparations.

VITAMIN C, CEVALIN. (Lilly) Ascorbic acid. **250 mg.**/Tab. Bot. 100s. **500 mg.**/Tab. Bot. 100s, 500s.
Use: Vitamin C deficiency.

VITAMIN C W/COMBINATIONS.
See: Allbee C-800, Prods. (Robins)
    Allbee with C, Cap. (Robins)
    Allbee-T, Tab. (Robins)

Anti-therm, Tab. (Scrip)
Bejectal w/Vit. C (Abbott)
Colrex, Cap. (Rowell)
C.P.C. plus, Tab. (Coastal)
Nialexo-C, Tab. (Mallard)
Thex, Cap. (Ingram)
Thex Forte, Cap. (Ingram)
Vicon-C, Cap. (Glaxo)
Vicon Chewable, Tab. (Glaxo)
Vicon Forte, Cap. (Glaxo)
Vicon Plus, Cap. (Glaxo)
Vi-Zac, Cap. (Glaxo)
Z-BEC, Tab. (Robins)

VITAMIN C SYRUP. (Columbia) Vit. C 500 mg./5 cc. Bot. 4 oz.

VITAMIN D. Cholecalciferol, B.A.N.

VITAMIN D, DELTALIN. (Lilly) Vit. D 2. 50,000 Units (1.25 mg.)/Gelseal. Bot. 100s.
Use: Vitamin D deficiency.

VITAMIN D, SYNTHETIC.
See: Activated 7-Dehydro-cholesterol Calciferol

VITAMIN D-2. Activated ergasterol.
See: Calciferol, Prep. (Various Mfr.)
    Drisdol, Liq. (Winthrop-Breon)
    Viosterol (Various Mfr.)

VITAMIN D-3.
See: Activated 7-dehydrocholesterol
    Calciferol Prep. for related activity

VITAMIN D-3-CHOLESTEROL. Cpd. of crystalline vitamin D-3 & cholesterol.

VITAMIN D-4.
See: Dihydrotachysterol, Prep. (Various Mfr.)

VITAMIN D CAPSULES. (Columbia) Vit. D 50,000 I.U./Cap. Bot. 100s, 1000s.

• **VITAMIN E,** U.S.P. XXI. Preparation, Cap., U.S.P. XXI. (Upjohn) 200 I.U./Cap. Bot. 90s.
See: Aquasol E (USV)
    Eprolin, Gelseal (Lilly)
    E-Vites, Cap. (Columbia)
    Pertropin Caps. (Lannett)
    Solucap E. Cap. (Jamieson-McKames)
    Tega-E-Cream (Ortega)
    Tocopher, Prod. (Columbia)
    Tocopherol, Prep. (Various Mfr.)
    Wheat Germ Oil (Various Mfr.)

VITAMIN E, EPROLIN. (Lilly) Alpha-tocopherol, 50 units/Gelseal. Bot. 100s; 100 units/Gelseal. Bot. 100s.
Use: Vitamin E therapy.

VITAMIN E W/QUININE SULFATE, NIACIN.
See: Myodyne, Tab. (Paddock)

VITAMIN E LOTION. (Vortech) D-alpha tocopherol acetate (natural) 200 I.U., 1000 I.U./oz. in non-greasy emollient residual base. Bot. 1 oz., 2 oz., 4 oz., 16 oz.
Use: Dermatologic.

VITAMIN E SKIN OIL. (Columbia) Pure Vit. E 28,000 I.U. Bot. 1 Oz.
Use: Emollient.

VITAMIN F.
See: Fats, Unsaturated
    Fatty Acids, Unsaturated

VITAMIN G.
See: Riboflavin
VITAMIN K.
See: Hykinone, Amp. (Abbott)
Menadiol, Sodium Diphosphate, Prep.
(Various Mfr.)
Menadione, Prep. (Various Mfr.)
Menadione Sod. Bisulfite, Prep. (Various Mfr.)
VITAMIN K. Phytomenadione, B.A.N.
VITAMIN K-1.
See: Phytonadione, U.S.P. XXI.
VITAMIN K-3.
See: Menadione, U.S.P. XXI.
VITAMIN K OXIDE. Not available, but usually K-1 is desired.
VITAMIN M.
See: Folic Acid, U.S.P. XXI.
VITAMIN P. Citrin.
See: Bio-Flavonoid Cpds. (Various Mfr.)
Hesperidin Preps. (Various Mfr.)
Quercetin (Various Mfr.)
Rutin, Prep. (Various Mfr.)
VITAMIN T. Sesame seed factor, termite factor.
Use: Claimed to aid proper blood coagulation and promote formation of blood platelets. Not approved by FDA as an active vitamin.
VITAMIN U. Present in cabbage juice.
VITAMINS W/ANTIOBESITY AGENTS.
See: Fetamin Tab. (Mission)
Obedrin Cap. or Tab. (Massengill)
VITAMINS W/LIVER & LIPOTROPIC AGENTS.
See: Heptuna, Cap. (Roerig)
Lederplex, Preps. (Lederle)
Livitamin, Preps. (Beecham Labs)
Metheponex, Caps. (Rawl)
Methischol, Caps. (USV Pharm.)
VITAMIN, MAINTENANCE FORMULA.
See: Stuart Formula, Tab & Liq. (Stuart)
Vi-Magna, Cap. (Lederle)
VITA-MINS. (Mills) Vit. A 5000 I.U., D 200 I.U., C 30 mg., B-1 1 mg., B-2 2 mg., B-6 0.1 mg., B-12 1 mcg., d-calcium pantothenate 0.5 mg., niacinamide 20 mg., folic acid 0.1 mg., ferrous gluconate 25 mg., copper gluconate 5 mg., zinc gluconate 5 mg., manganese gluconate 5 mg./Tab. Bot. 100s.
Use: Vitamin and mineral therapy.
VITAMINS: STRESS FORMULA.
See: Cebefortis, Tab. (Upjohn)
Folbesyn, Tab., Vial (Lederle)
Probec-T, Tab. (Stuart)
Stresscaps, Cap. (Lederle)
Stresscaps With Iron (Lederle)
Stresscaps With Zinc (Lederle)
Stresstabs-600 (Lederle)
Thera-combex Kap. (Parke-Davis)
VITA NATAL. (Scot-Tussin) Folic Acid 1 mg./Tab. Bot. 100s.
Use: Vitamin therapy.
VITA NO. ONE. (Freeport) Thiamine monitrate 15 mg., riboflavin 10 mg., pyridoxine HCl 5 mg., nicotinamide 50 mg., calcium pantothenate 10 mg., ascorbic acid 300 mg./Cap. Bot. 100s.

Use: Vit. B-Complex & C deficiencies.
VITAON. (Vita Elixir) Vit. B-12 25 mcg., thiamine HCl 10 mg., ferric pyrophosphate 250 mg./5 cc.
Use: Therapeutic elixir.
VITAPACE. (Miles) Vit. B-6 20 mg., thiamine 15 mg., riboflavin 17 mg., B-12 60 mcg., niacin 100 mg., pantothenic acid 20 mg., C 300 mg./Tab. Bot. 60s.
Use: Supplement for adults.
VITA PLUREX FORTE. (Standex) Vit. B-1 1.5 mg., B-2 2.0 mg., B-6 0.1 mg., Ca pantothenate 1.0 mg., niacinamide 10.0 mg./Tab. Bot. 100s.
VITA PLUREX W/C CAPSULES. (Standex) Vit. B-1 15 mg., B-2 10 mg., B-6 5 mg., niacinamide 50 mg., Ca pantothenate 10 mg., Vit. C 300 mg./Cap. Bot. 100s.
VITA-PLUS B-12. (Scot-Tussin) Vit. B-12 injection 1,000 mcg./ml.
Use: Vitamin B-12 therapy.
VITA-PLUS E. (Scot-Tussin) Vit. E 400 I.U./Cap.
Use: Vitamin E therapy.
VITA-PLUS H CAPSULES. (Scot-Tussin). Bot. 100s.
Use: Hematinic.
VITA-PLUS H LIQUID. (Scot-Tussin) Vit. B-1 10 mg.; l-lysine monohydrochloride 100 mg.; B-12 25 mcg.; B-6 5 mg.; iron pyrophosphate soluble 100 mg./Tsp. Bot. 4 oz., 8 oz. pt., gal.
Use: Hematinic with B vitamins.
VITAREX. (Pasadena Research) Vit. A 25,000 I.U., D 400 I.U., B-1 15 mg., B-2 10 mg., B-6 3 mg., B-12 5 mcg., C 300 mg., niacinamide 100 mg., Ca pantothenate 20 mg., E 10 I.U., Fe 15 mg., Iodine 0.15 mg., Ca 50 mg., P 40 mg., Cu 0.1 mg., Mn 0.1 mg., Mg 5 mg., K 2 mg./Tab. Bot. 30s, 100s, 4000s.
VITA-SED. (Galen) Phenobarbital ½ gr., Vit. B-1 1½ mg., B-2 2 mg., C 20 mg./Tab. Bot. 100s, 1000s.
Use: Sedative, vitamin combination.
VITA-SUP. (Kenyon) Vit. A 12,500 I.U., D 1000 I.U., B-1 5 mg., B-2 2.5 mg., B-6 1 mg., B-12 2 mcg., C 75 mg., niacinamide 40 mg., Ca pantothenate 4 mg., E 3 I.U., dical. phosphate 260 mg., choline bitartrate 31.4 mg., inositol 15 mg., liver protein fraction 25 mg., ferrous sulfate 102 mg., Mn sulfate 1.5 mg., pot. sulfate 4.5 mg., Zn sulfate 1.4 mg., Mg sulfate 21.6 mg./Cap. Bot. 100s, 1000s.
VITATONE DROPS. (Winthrop Products) Multivitamin.
Use: Dietary supplement.
VITAZIN. (Mesmer) Ascorbic acid 300 mg., niacinamide 100 mg., thiamine monoitrate 20 mg., d-Calcium pantothenate 20 mg., riboflavin 10 mg., pyridoxine HCl 5 mg., magnesium sulfate 70 mg., zinc 110 mg./Cap.
Use: Vitamin & mineral supplement.
VI-TESTROGEN. (Pharmex) Testosterone 10 mg., estrogenic substance (natural) 1 mg., Vit. B-1 50 mg., B-2 2 mg., B-6 5 mg., panthenol 10 mg., niacinamide 100 mg., inositol 25 mg., choline chloride 25 mg., d,l-methionine 25 mg./cc, sod. carboxymethylcellulose 0.05%, procaine HCl 1%, benzyl alcohol 2%. Vial 10 cc.
VITEX-C. (Pasadena Research) Vit. B-1 10 mg., riboflavin-5'-phosphate Na 10 mg., B-6 20 mg., panthenol

20 mg., biotin 0.2 mg., C 100 mg., niacinamide 100 mg./2 cc. Amp. 2 cc., 25s, 100s. Vial 10 cc., 30 cc.
Use: Vitamin supplement for IM or IV use.

VITEXIN. (Pasadena Research) Vit. B-1 100 mg., B-2 10 mg., B-6 50 mg., d-panthenol 20 mg., niacinamide 75 mg./cc. Vial 10 cc.

VIT-MIN-I-FACT. (Sutliff & Case) Vit. A 5000 I.U., D 400 I.U., E 2 I.U., B-1 3 mg., B-2 3 mg., B-6 0.5 mg., B-12 1 mcg., niacinamide 25 mg., calcium pantothenate 5 mg., C 75 mg., Cu 1 mg., Mn 3 mg., Mg 6 mg., dicalcium phosphorous anhydrous 200 mg., K 5 mg./Tab. Bot. 100s.

VITORMAINS. (Hauck) Tab. Bot. 100s.

VITRAMONE. (Harvey) Natural estrogenic hormone 1 mg., w/Vit. B-1 10 mg., B-2 2 mg., B-6 5 mg., niacinamide 40 mg., inositol 50 mg., choline chloride 10 mg., methionine 10 mg./cc. 10 ml.
Use: Estrogen therapy w/Vitamin B complex.

VITRON-C. (Fisons) Ferrous fumarate 200 mg., ascorbic acid 125 mg. Tab. Bot. 100s, 1000s.
Use: Iron deficiency anemia.

VITRON-C PLUS TABLETS. (Fisons) Ferrous fumarate 400 mg., Vit. C 250 mg./Tab. Bot. 30s, 100s, 500s.
Use: Iron deficiency anemia.

VITRONIC LIQUID. (Coastal) Vit. B-1 5 mg., B-2 5 mg., B-6 1 mg., B-12 3 mcg., iron 100 mg., nicotinic acid 100 mg., magnesium 5 mg./30 cc., alcohol 15%. Bot. pt.

VI-TWEL INJECTION. (Berlex) Cyanocobalamin (Vit. B-12) 1 mg./ml. w/benzyl alcohol 1.5%, sodium chloride for isotonicity. Multiple Dose Vial 10 ml.
Use: Pernicious anemia.

VIVACTIL. (Merck Sharp & Dohme) Protriptyline HCl. 5 mg./Tab. Bot. 100s, 1000s. 10 mg./Tab. Bot. 100s, 1000s. Unit dose pkg. 100s.
Use: Antidepressant.

VIVALAN HYDROCHLORIDE. Viloxazine, B.A.N.

VIVARIN. (Beecham Products) Caffeine. alkaloid 200 mg./Tab. Bot. 16, 40, 80.
Use: Stimulant.

VIVIKON. (Brown) Vit. B-1 5 mg., B-2 2 mg., B-6 10 mg., d-panthenol 5 mg., niacinamide 10 mg., procaine HCl 2%/cc. 100 cc.

VIVONEX FLAVOR PACKETS. (Norwich Eaton) Orange-pineapple, lemon-lime, strawberry, and vanilla. Pkg. 60s.
Use: Non-nutritive flavoring for Vivonex diets when consumed as the oral feedings.

VIVONEX, HIGH NITROGEN. (Norwich Eaton) Free amino acid/complete enteral nutrition. Ten packets provide 3,000 kilocalories, 20 Gm. available nitrogen, 135 Gm. amino acids, 2.61 Gm. fat, 630 Gm. carbohydrate & full day's balanced nutrition. Calorie: nitrogen ratio is 150:1. Unflavored powder, 80 Gm. packets, Pkg. 10s.
Use: Elemental high nitrogen diet for drinking & enteral catheter feeding.

VIVONEX, STANDARD. (Norwich Eaton) Free amino acid/complete enteral nutrition. Six packets provide 1,800 kilocalories, 5.88 Gm. available nitrogen (37.08 Gm. usable protein), 2.61 Gm. fat, 407 Gm. carbohydrate, and full day's balanced nutrition.

Calorie: nitrogen ratio is 300:1. Unflavored powder, 80 Gm. packets, Pkg. 6s.
Use: Elemental diet for drinking and enteral catheter feeding.

VIVONEX T.E.N. (Norwich Eaton) Elemental diet for total enteral nutrition. Pkg. 80.4 Gm. Ctn. 10s.
Use: Dietary.

VI-ZAC. (Glaxo) Vit. A 5000 I.U., C 500 mg., E 50 I.U., zinc sulfate 80 mg./Cap. Bot. 60s, 500s.
Use: Therapeutic vitamin-mineral complex.

V-LAX. (Century) Psyllium mucilloid (hydrophilic) 50%, dextrose 50%. Powder ¼ lb., 1 lb., 5 lb.
Use: Fecal softener.

VLEMASQUE. (Dermik) Sulfurated lime topical solution 6% (Vleminck's Soln.) w/alcohol 7% in drying clay mask. Jar. 4 oz.
Use: Treatment of acne.

VLEM-DOME. (Miles Pharm) Vleminckx solution in powder form. Calcium polysulfide, calcium thiosulfate, sulfur. 4 cc. container mixed w/1 pt. water. Packets 6s.
Use: Skin conditions (acne).

VLEMINCKX'S SOLUTION. Solution of Sulfurated Lime.
Use: Antiseptic.
See: Ulmer.

VM. (Last) Vit. B-1 6 mg., B-2 4 mg., niacinamide 40 mg., iron 100 mg., calcium 188 mg. phosphorus 188 mg., manganese 4 mg., alcohol 12%. Bot. 16 oz.
Use: Vitamin, mineral supplement.

V-M TAB. (Kenyon) Vit. A palmitate 5000 I.U., D-2 500 I.U., B-1 2.5 mg., B-2 2.5 mg., B-6 0.5 mg., B-12 1 mcg., C 50 mg., niacinamide 15 mg., E 0.5 I.U., d-cal. pantothenate 5 mg., iron 25 mg., Cu 0.375 mg., Mn 0.5 mg., Zn 0.15 mg., K 2.5 mg., Mg 2.5 mg., Iodine 0.05 mg./Tab. Bot. 100s, 1000s.
Use: Multivitamin with minerals.

VOCALZONES. (CMC) Menthol, myrrh, peppermint oil, licorice. Lozenges Tin 1 oz.
Use: Relief of pharyngitis.

• **VOLAZOCINE.** USAN. 3-(Cyclopropylmethyl)-1,2,3,4,-5,6-hexahydro-cis-6,11-dimethyl-2,6-methano-3-benzazocine. Under study.
Use: Analgesic.

VOLIDAN. (British Drug House) Megestrol acetate.

VOLITAL. Pemoline, B.A.N.

VOLITANE. (Trent) Parethoxycaine 0.2%, hexachlorophene 0.025%, dichlorophene 0.025%. Aerosol spray cans 3 oz.
Use: Treatment of minor burns and bites.

VOLTAROL SODIUM SALT. Diclofenac, B.A.N.

VONEDRINE HYDROCHLORIDE. Vonedrine (phenylpropylmethylamine) HCl.
Use: Nasal decongestant.

VONTROL. (SmithKline) Diphenidol 25 mg./Tab. Bot. 100s.
Use: Treatment of vertigo, nausea, & vomiting.

VORTEL. Clorprenaline HCl.
Use: Bronchodilator.

VORGHESA SUN PRODUCTS. (Revlon) Padimate O, oxybenzone in cream and gel base.
Use: Sunburn prevention.

VOSOL OTIC SOLUTION. (Wallace) Propylene glycol diacetate 3%, acetic acid 2%, benzethonium Cl 0.02%, sodium acetate 0.015% in propylene glycol. Multi-Pack 3 × 15 ml., 3 × 30 ml.
Use: Treatment of acute otitis externa.

VOSOL HC OTIC SOLUTION. (Wallace) Propylene glycol diacetate 3%, acetic acid 2%, benzethonium Cl 0.02%, sodium acetate 0.015% in propylene glycol, citric acid 0.2%, hydrocortisone 1%. Multi-Pack 3 × 10 ml.
Use: Treatment of acute otitis externa with inflammation.

V-TUSS EXPECTORANT. (Vangard) Hydrocodone bitartrate 5 mg., pseudoephendrine HCl 60 mg., guaifenesin 200 mg./5 ml. w/alcohol 12.5%.
Use: Decongestant, cough depressant, expectorant.

VULVAELINE. (Scrip) Zinc oxide 10%, boric acid 5%, benzoic acid 2%, carbolic acid 1.5%, salicylic acid 1%. Jar 1 lb.
Use: Dermatologic.

V.V.S. SUPPOSITORIES. (Econo Med) Sulfisoxazole 700 mg., allantoin 140 mg., aminacrine HCl 14 mg./Supp. Box 16s.
Use: Trichomonads, monillasis.

VYTONE CREAM. (Dermik) Hydrocortisone 0.5% or 1%, iodoquinol 1% in a greaseless vehicle w/propylene glycol, glyceryl monostearate, cholesterol and related sterols, isopropyl myristate, polysorbates 20 and 60, cetyl alcohol, sorbitan monostearate, polyoxyl 40 stearate, sorbic acid, purified water. Cream 0.5% or 1% Tube 1 oz.
Use: Dermatologic.

W

WADE GESIC BALM. (Wade) Menthol 3%, methyl salicylate 12%, petrolatum base. Tube 1 oz. Jar 1 lb.
Use: Analgesic.

WADE'S DROPS. Compound Benzoin Tincture.

WAKESPAN. (Weeks & Leo) Caffeine 250 mg./T.R. Cap. Vial 15s.
Use: CNS stimulant for alertness.

WAL-FINATE ALLERGY TABS. (Walgreen) Chlorpheniramine maleate 4 mg./Tab. Bot. 50s.
Use: Antihistamine.

WAL-FINATE DECONGESTANT TABS. (Walgreen) Chlorpheniramine maleate 4 mg., d-isoephedrine sulfate 60 mg./Tab. Bot. 50s.
Use: Antihistaminic, decongestant.

WAL-FORMULA D COUGH SYRUP. (Walgreen) Dextromethorphan HBr 20 mg., phenylpropanolamine HCl 25 mg., guaifenesin 100 mg./10 ml. w/alcohol 10%. Bot. 6 oz.
Use: Nasal decongestant, expectorant, non-narcotic cough suppressant.

WALGREEN ARTIFICIAL TEARS. (Walgreen) Hydroxypropyl methylcellulose 0.5%. Bot. 0.5 oz.
Use: Lubrican for dry eyes.

WALGREEN SODA MINTS. (Walgreen) Sodium bicarbonate 300 mg./Tab. Bot. 100s, 200s,
Use: Antacid.

WAL-MINIC. (Walgreen) Phenylpropanolamine HCl 12.5 mg., guaifenesin 100 mg./5 ml. w/alcohol 5%. Bot. 6 oz.
Use: Expectorant decongestant.

WAL-MINIC COLD RELIEF MEDICINE. (Walgreen) Phenylpropanolamine HCl 12.5 mg., chlorpheniramine maleate 2 mg./5 ml. Bot. 6 oz.
Use: Non-alcoholic antihistamine, decongestant.

WAL-MINIC DM. (Walgreen) Phenylpropanolamine HCl 12.5 mg., dextromethorphan HBr 10 mg./5 ml. Bot. 6 oz.
Use: Non-narcotic non-alcoholic antitussive decongestant.

WAL-PHED PLUS. (Walgreen) Pseudoephedrine HCl 60 mg, chlorpheniramine maleate 4 mg./Tab. Bot. 50s.
Use: Decongestant, antihistamine.

WAL-PHED SYRUP. (Walgreen) Pseudoephedrine HCl 30 mg./5 ml. Bot. 4 oz.
Use: Decongestant.

WAL-PHED TABLETS. (Walgreen) Pseudoephedrine HCl 30 mg./Tab. Bot. 50s, 100s.
Use: Decongestant.

WAL-TUSSIN. (Walgreen) Guaifenesin 100 mg./5 ml. Bot. 4 oz.
Use: Expectorant.

WAL-TUSSIN DM. (Walgreen) Guaifenesin 100 mg., dextromethorphan HBr 15 ml./5 ml. Bot. 4 oz.
Use: Expectorant, cough suppressant.

WANS. (Webcon) Pyrilamine maleate 25 mg., pentobarbital sod. 30 mg./Children's Supp. **No. 1:** pyrilamine maleate 50 mg., pentobarb, sod. 45 mg./Supp. **No. 2:** pyrilamine maleate 50 mg., pentobarb. 100 mg./Supp. Jar 12s.
Use: Nausea.

WARFARIN, B.A.N. (Various Mfr.) Comp. 42. 3-(alpha-Acetonylbenzyl)-4-hydroxycoumarin. 4-Hydroxy-3-(3-oxo-1-phenylbutyl)coumarin.
Use: Rodenticide; anticoagulant.
See: Coumadin
    Marevan (sodium derivative)

• **WARFARIN POTASSIUM,** U.S.P. XXI. Tab., U.S.P. XXI.
Use: Anticoagulant.
See: Athrombin-K, Tabs. (Purdue Frederick)

• **WARFARIN SODIUM,** U.S.P. XXI. For Inj., Tab., U.S.P. XXI. 2H-1-Benzopyran-2-one, 4-hydroxy-3-(3-oxo-1-phenylbutyl)-, sod. salt. 3-(alpha-Acetonyl-benzyl)-4-hydroxycoumarin & its sod. salt athrombin.
Use: Anticoagulant.
See: Coumadin Sodium, Tab., Inj. (Du Pont)
    Panwarfin, Tab. (Abbott)

WART-AWAY. (Eckerd) Salicylic acid 13.13%, glacial acetic acid 1.8%, camphor 1.8%, castor oil 3.12%, pyroxylin 6.88%, acetone 75%. Liq. Bot. ½ oz.
Use: Wart removal.

WART FIX. (Last) Castor oil 100%. Bot. 0.3 fl. oz.
Use: Wart treatment.

WART-OFF. (Pfipharmecs) Salicylic acid in flexible colloidion. Bot. 0.5 oz.
Use: Wart remover.

WARTGON. (Edward J. Moore) Castor oil. Tube ½ oz.

Use: Wart removal.
• **WATER,** U.S.P. XXI is found in the following grades of purity:
Bacteriostatic Water for Injection, U.S.P. XXI.
Purified Water, U.S.P. XXI.
Sterile Water For Inhalation, U.S.P. XXI.
Sterile Water For Injection, U.S.P. XXI.
Sterile Water For Irrigation, U.S.P. XXI.
Water, U.S.P. XXI.
Water For Injection, U.S.P. XXI.
Use: Pharmaceutic aid (Solvent), irrigation therapy, vehicle, fluid.
See: Abbott Lab⁻ for sizes of each available. Upjohn for sizes available.
WATERMELON SEED EXTRACT. Citrin (Table Rock)
WATERMELON SEED EXTRACT W/Phenobarbital & theobromine. Cithal (Table Rock)
WATER-MISCIBLE VITAMIN A.
See: Acon, Cap. (Du Pont)
Aquasol Vit. A, Caps. (USV Labs.)
Testavol-S, Cap. (Fellows)
Vi-Dom-A, Cap. (Miles Pharm)
• **WAX, CARNAUBA,** N.F. XVI.
Use: Pharmaceutic aid (tablet polishing agent).
• **WAX, EMULSIFYING,** N.F. XVI.
Use: Emulsifying agent, stiffening agent.
• **WAX, MICROCRYSTALLINE,** N.F. XVI.
Use: Pharmaceutic aid (stiffening agent).
• **WAX, WHITE,** U.S.P. XVI.
Use: Pharm. aid (stiffening agent)
• **WAX, YELLOW,** N.F. XVI.
Use: Stiffening agent.
WAXSOL. Docusate Sodium, U.S.P. XXI.
WAYDS. (Wayne) Docusate sodium 100 mg./Cap. Bot. 100s.
Use: Relief of constipation.
WAYDS-PLUS CAPSULES. (Wayne) Docusate w/casanthranol. Bot. 50s.
Use: Constipation.
WAYNADE T-D CAPSULES. (Wayne) Antihistamine compound. Bot. 100s.
Use: Relief of nasal congestion, runny nose.
WAYNE-E CAPSULES. (Wayne) Vit. E 100 I.U., 200 I.U./Cap. Bot. 1000s. 400 I.U./Cap. Bot. 100s.
WAYSED TABLETS. (Wayne) Bot. 100s, 1000s.
WAYVITE ELIXIR. (Wayne) Bot. pt.
WEHAMINE. (Hauck) Dimenhydrinate 50 mg./ml. Vial 1 ml., 10 ml. Box. 25s.
Use: Management of nausea, vertigo, vomiting.
WEH-LESS. (Hauck) Phendimetrazine tartrate 35 mg./Cap. Bot. 100s.
Use: Management of exogenous obesity.
WEHLESS-105 TIMECELLES. (Hauck) Phendimetrazine tartrate 105 mg./SA Cap. Bot. 100s.
Use: Anorexic.
WEHVERT. (Hauck) Meclizine HCl 25 mg./Tab. Bot. 100s, 500s.
Use: Management of nausea vomiting, and dizziness.
WEHYDRYL. (Hauck) Diphenhydramine HCl 50 mg./ml. Vials 10 ml.

Use: Antihistaminic.
WEIGHTROL TAB. (Vortech) Phendimetrazine tartrate 35 mg./Tab. Bot. 100s., 1000s.
Use: Anorexiant.
WELDERS EYE LOTION. (Weber) tetracaine, potassium chloride, boric acid, camphor, glycerin. w/disodium edetate, benzal konium chloride as preservatives. Bot. 1 oz.
Use: Relief for "welding flash" and "arc burn."
WELLCOVORIN. (Burroughs Wellcome) Leucovorin calcium 5 mg. or 25 mg./Tab. 5 mg./Tab. Bot. 100s; 25 mg./Tab. Bot. 25s.
Use: Prophylaxis and treatment of the undesired hematopoietic effects of folic acid antagonists.
WELLCOVORIN INJECTION. (Burroughs Wellcome) Leucovorin calcium 5 mg./1 ml. Amp. Box 12s. 25 mg./5 ml. Amp. Box 10s.
Use: Prophylaxis and treatment of the undesired hematopoietic effects of folic acid antagonists.
WELLDORM. Dichloralphenazone, B.A.N.
WERNET'S ADHESIVE CREAM. (Block) Carboxymethlcellulose gum, ethylene oxide polymer, petrolatum in mineral oil base. Tube 1.5 oz.
Use: Denture adhesive cream.
WERNET'S POWDER. (Block) Gum karaya, ethylene oxide polymer. Bot. 0.63, 1.75, 3.55 oz.
Use: Denture adhesive.
WES-B/C. (Western Research) Vit. B-1 15 mg., B-2 10 mg., B-6 5 mg., niacinamide 50 mg., Ca pantothenate 10 mg., Vit. C 300 mg./Cap. Bot. 1000s.
WESCOHEX. (West) Bot. 5 oz., pt., gal.
Use: Antibacterial skin cleanser.
WESMATIC FORTE TABLETS. (Wesley) Phenobarbital ⅛ gr., ephedrine sulfate ¼ gr., chlorpheniramine maleate 2 mg., guaifenesin 100 mg./Tab. Bot. 100s, 1000s.
Use: Treatment of bronchitis and emphysema.
WESTCORT CREAM. (Westwood) Hydrocortisone valerate 0.2% in a hydrophilic base of white petrolatum, stearyl alcohol, propylene glycol, amphoteric-9, carbomer 940, sodium phosphate, sodium lauryl sulfate, sorbic acid, water. Tubes 15 Gm., 45 Gm., 60 Gm., 120 Gm.
Use: Topical anti-inflammatory.
WESTHROID. (Western Research) Thyroid ½ gr., 1 gr., 2 gr., 3 gr. or 4 gr./Tab. 5 gr. S.C. Tab. Handicount 28 (36 bags of 28s).
Use: Treatment of hypothyroidism.
WESTRIM. (Western Research) Phenylpropanolamine HCl 37.5 mg./Tab. Bot. 100s.
Use: Anorectic.
WESTRIM-LA 50. (Western Research) Phenylpropanolamine HCl 50 mg./Timed Release Cap. Bot. 1000s.
Use: Anorectic-decongestant.
WESTRIM-LA 75. (Western Research) Phenylpropancolamine HCl 75 mg./Timed Release Cap. Bot. 100s.
Use: Anorectic-decongestant.
WESVITE. (Western Research) Vit. B-1 10 mg., B-2 5 mg., B-6 2 mg., pantothenic acid 10 mg., niacinamide

30 mg., B-12 3 mcg., C 100 mg., E 5 I.U., Vit. A 10,000 I.U., D 400 I.U., Fe 15 mg., Cu 1 mg., Iodine 0.15 mg., Mn 1 mg., Zn 1.5 mg./Tab. Bot. 1000s.
Use: Vitamin-mineral supplement.

WET-N-SOAK. (Allergan) Polyvinyl alochol, edetate disodium & benzalkonium chloride 1/25,000 in sterile sol. Bot. 4 oz.
Use: Wetting and soaking sol. for hard and Polycon and Paraperm oxygen gas permeable contact lenses.

WETTING SOLUTION. (Barnes-Hind) Hydroxypropyle-thylcellulose 0.5%, polyvinyl alcohol 2%, benzalkonium chloride 0.004%, EDTA 0.02%, sod. chloride. Bot. 35 ml., 2 oz.
Use: Hard contact lens wetting solution.

WHEATACOL. (Eckerd) Iron, B-2, B-1, B-6, B-12, C, E, niacinamide, Ca pantothenate, calcium, phosphorus, Mg., Mn, Zn/Tab. Bot. 40s, 100s, 200s. Elix. Alcohol 12%. Bot. pt.

WHEATACOL TABLET. (Eckerd) Iron 50 mg., Vit. B-1 15 mg., B-2 7.5 mg., B-6 2 mg., B-12 5 mcg., niacinamide 40 mg., pantothenic acid 5 mg., Vit. C 100 mg., E 5 I.U., Ca 60 mg., P 44 mg., Mg 2 mg., Mn 1 mg./Tab. Bot. 100s, 200s.
Use: Vitamin and mineral supplement.

WHEATAVIMS. (Eckerd) Vit. A 10,000 I.U., D 400 I.U., E 50 I.U., C 250 mg., folic acid 0.4 mg., B-1 25 mg., B-2 25 mg., niacinamide 100 mg., B-6 5 mg., B-12 25 mcg., biotin 50 mcg., pantothenic acid 25 mg., Ca 162 mg., P 125 mg., iodine 150 mcg., Fe 27 mg., Mg 100 mg., Cu 3 mg., Zn 22.5 mg., wheatgerm 200 mg./2 Tab. Bot. 60s, 150s.
Use: Vitamin and mineral supplement.

WHEAT GERM OIL. (Viobin) **Liq.:** Bot. 4 oz., 8 oz., pt., qt., **Cap.: 3 min.:** Bot. 100s, 400s; **6 min.:** Bot. 100s, 225s, 400s; **20 min.:** Bot. 100s.

WHEAT GERM OIL. (Various Mfr.)
See: Natural Wheat Germ Oil, Cap., Oint. (Spirt) Natural Viobin Wheat Germ Oil, Liq. (Spirt) Tocopherol Prep. (Various Mfr.)
Use: Vit. E deficiency.

WHEAT GERM OIL CAPSULES. (Robinson) Soft gelatin, oblong, clear 3,6, 14 min./Cap. 100s, 1000s.

WHEAT GERM OIL CONCENTRATE. (Thurston) Perles. 6 min. Bot. 100s.
Use: Heart disorders, heart muscle fatigue.

WHIRL-SOL. (Sween) Lipid-soluble de-waxed fraction of lanolin. Bot. 8 oz., pt.
Use: Emollient, antipruritic.

WHITE IODINE. (Pharmex) Bot. ½ oz.

• **WHITE LOTION,** U.S.P. XXI.
Use: Astringent; topical protectant.
See: Lotioblanc, Lotion (Arnar-Stone)

• **WHITE OINTMENT,** U.S.P. XXI.
Use: Pharmaceutic aid (oleaginous ointment base).

WHITE PRECIPITATE.
See: Ammoniated Mercury, U.S.P. XXI.

WHITFIELD'S OINTMENT. (Various Mfr.) Benzoic acid 12%, salicylic acid 6%. Tube 1 oz., 1½ oz. Jar 1 lb.
Use: Fungicidal.

WHITSPHILL. (Torch) Salicylic acid 6%, benzoic acid 12% in hydrophilic vehicle. Jar 1 lb., 2 oz. Also avail. in half-strength.
Use: Fungus infections.

WHOOPING COUGH VACCINE.
See: Pertussis Vaccine, U.S.P. XXI.

WHORTON'S CALAMINE LOTION. (Whorton) Calamine, zinc oxide, and glycerin (U.S.P. strength) in carboxymethylcellulose lotion vehicle. Bot. 4 oz., gal.

WHORTON'S SKIN CARE CREAM. (Whorton) 5 oz., 16 oz.

WIBI LOTION. (Owen) Purified water, SD alcohol 40, glycerin, PEG-4, PEG-6-32 stearate, PEG-6-32, glycol stearate, carbomer 940, PEG-75, methylparaben, pro-pylparaben, triethanolamine, menthol & fragrance. Bot. 8 oz., 16 oz.
Use: Dry skin lotion.

WIDOW SPIDER SPECIES ANTIVENIN (LATRODECTUS MACTANS). Antivenin, Lactrodectus mactans, U.S.P. XXI.
Use: Passive immunizing agent.

WIGRAINE. (Organon) Ergotamine tartrate 1.0 mg., caffeine 100 mg./Tab. or Supp. **Tab.** Box 20s, 100s. **Supp.** Box 12s.
Use: Migraine, vascular headache.

WIGRETTES. (Organon) Ergotamine tartrate 2 mg./Sublingual Tab. Bot. 24s.
Use: Migraine, vascular headache.

WILD CHERRY.
Use: Flavored vehicle.

WILPOWR. (Foy) Phentermine HCl. 30 mg./Cap. Bot. 100s, 500s, 1000s.
Use: Anorexiant.

WILPOR-CLEAR. (Foy) Phentermine HCl 30 mg./Cap. Bot. 1000s.
Use: Anorexiant.

WINADOL SYRUP. (Winthrop Products) Paracetemol.
Use: Analgesic, antipyretic.

WINADOL TABLETS. (Winthrop Products) Paracetamol.
Use: Analgesic, antipyretic.

WINASMA TABLETS. (Winthrop Products) Theophylline anhydrous, ephedrine sulphate, chlormezanone.
Use: Antiasthmatic.

WINASORB DROPS. (Winthrop Products) Paracetamol.
Use: Analgesic, antipyretic.

WINASORB SUSPENSION. (Winthrop Products) Paracetamol.
Use: Analgesic, antipyretic.

WINASORB SYRUP. (Winthrop Products) Paracetamol.
Use: Analgesic, antipyretic.

WINASORB TABLETS. (Winthrop Products) Paracetamol.
Use: Analgesic, antipyretic.

WINAVIT TABLETS. (Winthrop Products) Stanozolol, vitamins.
Use: Anabolic steroid with vitamins.

WINDOLOR TABLETS. (Winston) Butabarbital 15

mg., acetaminophen 200 mg., phenacetin 120 mg., caffeine 30 mg./Tab. Box. 100s, 1000s.
Use: Analgesic, antitensive.

WINGEL. (Winthrop-Breon) Short polymer, hexitol stabilized aluminum-magnesium hydroxide equiv. to aluminum hydroxide 180 mg. and magnesium hydroxide 160 mg./5 ml. or Tab. **Liq.:** Bot. 6 oz., 12 oz.**Tab.:** Box 50s, 100s.
Use: Antacid.

WINORYLATE SACHET. (Winthrop Products) Benorylate.
Use: Analgesic.

WINOLATE SUSPENSION. (Winthrop Products) Benorylate.
Use: Analgesic.

WINSTEROID TABLETS. (Winthrop Products) Stanozolol.
Use: Anabolic steroid.

WINSTROL. (Winthrop-Breon) Stanozolol 2 mg./Tab. Bot. 100s.
Use: Anabolic steroid.

WINTERGREEN OINTMENT. (Wisconsin) Bot. 2 oz., 1 lb.
Use: Muscle soreness, arthritis pain.

WINTHROCIN SUSPENSION. (Winthrop Products) Erythromycin sterate.
Use: Antibiotic.

WINTHROCIN TABLETS. (Winthrop Products) Erythromycin sterate.
Use: Antibiotic.

WINTODON TABLETS. (Winthrop Products) Glycobiarsol.
Use: Amebicide.

WINTOMYLON CAPS. (Winthrop Products) Nalidixic acid.
Use: Urinary, intestinal infections.

WINTOMYLON SUSPENSION. (Winthrop Products) Nalidixic acid.
Use: Urinary, intestinal infections.

WINTOMYLON TABLETS. (Winthrop Products) Nalidixic acid.
Use: Urinary, intestinal infections.

WINTOSIN COUGH SYRUP. (Winthrop Products) Dextromethorphan HBr.
Use: Antitussive decongestant.

WINTRAMOX CAPSULES. (Winthrop Products) Amoxicillin trihydrate.
Use: Antibiotic.

WINTRAMOX SUSPENSION. (Winthrop Products) Amoxicillin trihydrate
Use: Antibiotic.

WINTREX CAPSULES. (Winthrop Products) Tetracycline HCl.
Use: Antibiotic.

WINTROPLEX TABLETS. (Winthrop Products) Aspirin, chlormezanone.
Use: Analgesic, tranquilizer.

WNS SUPPOSITORIES. (Winthrop Products) Sulfamylon HCl.
Use: Hemorrhoidal preparation.

WOJTAB. (Roxane) Prednisone 20 mg./Tab. Bot. 100s, 500s.

Use: Glucocorticoid.

WOLFINA. (O'Neal, Jones & Feldman) Rauwolfia serpentina 50 or 100 mg./Tab. Bot. 100s.
Use: Antihypertensive, tranquilizing agent.

WOLGRAINE. (Wolins) Aspirin 3 gr., phenacetin 2 gr., caffeine ⅔ gr., isobutyl-allylbarbituric acid ¾ gr./Tab. Bot. 100s, 1000s.

WOL-LAC. (Wolins) Aminoacetic acid (glycine) 0.18 Gm., calcium carbonate 0.42 Gm./Tab. Bot. 1000s.

WOLTAC. (Wolins) Belladonna alkaloids (total 0.16 mg.) atropine sulfate 0.024 mg., scopolamine HBr 0.014 mg., hyoscyamine sulfate 0.122 mg., phenylpropanolamine HCl 50 mg., chlorpheniramine maleate 1 mg., pheniramine maleate 12.5 mg./Cap. Bot. 100s, 1000s.

WONDERFUL DREAM SALVE. (Kondon) Phenylmercuric nitrate 1:5000, oils of tar, turpentine, olive and linseed oil, rosin, burgundy pitch, camphor.

WOOD CHARCOAL TABLETS. (Cowley) 5 gr.: 10 gr./Tab. Bot. 1000s.

WOOD CREOSOTE.
See: Creosote (Various Mfr.)

WORMAL TABLETS. (Salsbury) Phenothiazine 500 mg., piperazine 50 mg., dibutyltin dilaurate 125 mg./Tab. Bot. 100s, 1000s, 10,000s.
Use: Treatment for worming poultry.

WOOL FAT. Lanolin Anhydrous.

W-T LOTION. (Adria) Aromatized M.O. emulsion, lanolin free. Bot. 8 oz.
Use: Professional skin lotion.

WUN-A-VIT. (Blue Cross) Vit. A 5000 I.U., D 400 I.U., E 15 I.U., C 60 mg., folic acid 0.4 mg., B-1 1.5 mg., B-2 1.7 mg., niacin 20 mg., B-6 2 mg., B-12 6 mcg./Tab. Bot. 100s.
Use: Vitamin supplement.

WUN-A-VIT PLUS IRON. (Blue Cross) Vit. A 5000 I.U., D 400 I.U., E 15 I.U., C 60 mg., folic acid 0.4 mg., B-1 1.5 mg., B-2 1.7 mg., niacin 20 mg., B-6 2 mg., B-12 6 mcg., iron 18 mg./Tab. Bot. 100s.
Use: Vitamin supplement with iron.

WUN-TABS. (Columbia) Vit. A 5000 I.U., D 400 I.U., C 50 mg., B-1 2 mg., B-2 2.5 mg., B-6 1 mg., B-12 1 mcg., niacinamide 20 mg., pantothenic acid 1 mg./Cap. Bot. 250s, 1000s. Jar 100s.
Use: Multiple vitamin.

WUN-TABS W/IRON. (Columbia) Vit. A 5000 I.U., D 400 I.U., C 50 mg., B-1 2 mg., B-2 2.5 mg., B-6 1 mg., B-12 1 mcg., niacinamide 20 mg., cal. pantothenate 1 mg., iron 15 mg./Tab. Jar 100s, Bot. 1000s.
Use: Supplement.

WUN-TAB M. (Columbia) Vit. A 5000 I.U., D 500 I.U., C 50 mg., B-1 2.5 mg., B-2 2.5 mg., B-6 0.5 mg., B-12 2 mcg., niacinamide 20 mg., calcium pantothenate 5 mg., Ca 35 mg., Cu 1 mg., Iodine 0.15 mg., Fe 10 mg., Mn 1 mg., Mg 6 mg., K 5 mg./Tab. Bot. 1000s. Jar 100s.
Use: Dietary supplement.

W/W-ANTI-SPAS. (Whiteworth) Antispasmodic compound Bot. 16 oz.
Use: Antispasmodic.

W/W-BROMINE. (Whiteworth) Brompheniramine elixir. Bot. 16 oz., gal.
Use: Expectorant.

W/W-BROMINE DS. (Whiteworth) Brompheniramine DC. Bot. 16 oz.
Use: Expectorant.

W/W-FED LIQUID. (Whiteworth) Triprolidine w/pseudoephedrine in syrup. Bot. 16 oz., gal.
Use: Antihistaminic, decongestant.

W/W-FED TABLETS. (Whiteworth) Triprolidine w/pseudoephedrine. Tab. Bot. 100s, 1000s.
Use: Antihistaminic, decongestant.

W/W FED w/C. (Whiteworth) Triprolidine w/pseudoephedrine, codeine. Bot. 16 oz., gal.
Use: Expectorant.

W/W HISTINE DH. (Whiteworth) Phenylhistine DH elixir. Bot. 16 oz.
Use: Antihistamine.

W/W-HISTINE ELIXIR. (Whiteworth) Phenylhistine elixir. Bot. 16 oz.
Use: Antihistamine.

W/W-HISTINE EXPECTORANT. (Whiteworth) Phenylhistine expectorant. Bot. 16 oz.
Use: Antihistamine.

WYAMINE SULFATE INJECTION. (Wyeth) Mephentermine sulfate 15 mg., sod. acetate, methylparaben 1.8 mg., propylparaben 0.2 mg./cc. Vial 10 cc., Amp. 2 cc., 25s. 30 mg./cc. Vial 10 cc. Tubex 30 mg./Tubex 1 cc.
Use: I.V. or I.M.; in hypotensive states not associated with hemorrhage.

WYAMYCIN-E LIQUID. (Wyeth) Erythromycin ethylsuccinate oral susp. 200 mg., or 400 mg./5 ml. Bot. Pts.
Use: Antibacterial agent.

WYAMYCIN-S TABLETS. (Wyeth) Erythromycin stearate 250 mg./Tab. Bot. 100s, 500s. 500 mg./Tab. Bot. 100s.
Use: Antibacterial agent.

WYANOIDS. (Wyeth) Ephedrine sulfate 3 mg., w/belladonna ext. 15 mg., boric acid, zinc oxide, bismuth oxyiodide & subcarb., balsam peru & cocoa butter./Supp., Box 12s.
Use: Hemorrhoids.

WYANOIDS HC. (Wyeth) Hydrocortisone acetate 10 mg., belladonna ext. 15 mg., ephedrine sulf. 3 mg., zinc oxide 176 mg., boric acid 543 mg., bismuth oxyiodide 30 mg., bismuth subcarbonate 146 mg., Peruvian balsam 30 mg./Supp. Box 12s. Redipak 25s.
Use: Anorectal disorders.

WYCILLIN. (Wyeth) Penicillin G procaine susp. 300,000 u./cc. in a stabilized aqueous suspension w/sod. citrate buffer, w/v lecithin approximately 0.5%, carboxymethylcellulose 0.5%, povidone 0.5%, methylparaben 0.1%, propylparaben 0.01%. Tubex 1 cc. 10s. Vial 600,000 u./cc. Tubex 1 cc. 10s, 50s. 1,200,000 u./Tubex 2 cc. 10s. 2,400,000 u./disposable syringe 4 cc., 10s.

WYCILLIN INJECTION AND PROBENECID TABLETS. (Wyeth) Combination Pkg. containing two disposable syringes of procaine penicillin G 2,400,000 U./4 ml. size and two probenecid tablets 0.5 Gm. each.
Use: Treatment of gonorrhea.

WYDASE LYOPHILIZED. (Wyeth) Hyaluronidase. Vial 150 U.S.P. [TR]u./1 cc. 1500 U.S.P. [TR]u./10 cc.
Use: Spreading factor.

WYDASE STABILIZED SOLUTION. (Wyeth) Hyaluronidase 150 U.S.P. [TR]u. in sterile saline sol. Vial 1 cc., 10 cc. Store below 59°F., stable 3 yrs.
Use: Hypodermoclysis.

WYOVIN HYDROCHLORIDE. Dicyclomine, B.A.N.

WYGESIC. (Wyeth) Propoxyphene HCl 65 mg., acetaminophen 650 mg./Tab. Bot. 100s, 500s. Redipak 100s.
Use: Pain relief.

WYMOX. (Wyeth) Amoxicillin **Cap.:** 250 mg./Cap. Bot. 100s, 500s. 500 mg./Cap. Bot. 50s, 500s. **Oral Susp.:** 125 mg./5 ml. Bot. to make 80 ml., 100 ml., 150 ml.; 250 mg./5 ml. Bot. to make 80 ml, 100 ml., 150 ml.
Use: Ear, nose, throat, G.I. tract infections.

WYTENSIN. (Wyeth) Guanabenz acetate 4 mg. or 8 mg./Tab. Bot. 100s.
Use: Antihypertensive.

WYVAC RABIES VACCINE. (Wyeth) Human diploid-cell strain subvirion antigen. Single dose Amp.
Use: Rabies vaccine.

X

• **XAMOTEROL.** USAN.

XANAX. (Upjohn) Alprazolam 0.25 mg., 0.5 mg. or 1 mg./Tab. Bot. 100s. Unit dose 100s, 500s.
Use: Management of anxiety disorders.

• **XANOXATE SODIUM.** USAN.
Use: Bronchodilator.

• **XANTHAN GUM,** N.F. XVI.
Use: Suspending agent.

XANTHINE DERIVATIVES.
See: Caffeine
Theobromine
Theophylline

XANTHINOL NIACINATE. USAN. 7-{2-Hydroxy-3-[(2-hydroxyethyl))methylamino]-propyl} theophylline compound with nicotinic acid.
Use: Vasodilator.
See: Complamex
Complamin

XANTHIOL HCl. 4-[3-(2-Chlorothioxanthene-9-yl)-propyl]-1-pipera zinepropanol dihydrochloride.
Use: Antinauseant.
See: Daxid (Roerig)

XANTHOCILLIN. B.A.N. Antibiotics obtained from the mycelium of Penicillium notatum (Xanthocillin X is 2:3-Diisocyano 1:4-di(p-hydroxyphenyl) buta-1:3-diene).

XANTHOTOXIN. Methoxsalen.

X-A-PAIN ANALGESIC TABLETS. (Eckerd)

Acetaminophen 325 mg., phenyltoloxamine citrate 30 mg., caffeine 30 mg./Tab.
Use: Analgesic, antihistaminic.
X-DRIN. (Pharmex) **Cap.:** Bot. 72s. **Pellets:** Bot. 144s. **Tab.:** Bot. 21s, 90s.
Use: Dietary.
YELLOW FEVER VACCINE.
See: YF-VAX, Inj. (Squibb-Connaught).
XENEISOL 133. (Mallinckrodt) Xenon Xe 133.
XENEISOL XE 133 INJECTION. (Mallinckrodt) Xenon Xe 133 Injection.
• **XENON XE 133,** U.S.P. XXI. Inj., U.S.P. XXI. Xeneisol (Mallinckrodt)
Use: Radioactive agent.
XENTHIORATE HCl. 2-Diethylaminoethyl-2(4-biphenylyl)thiobutyrate HCl.
XENYSALATE, B.A.N. 2-Diethylaminoethyl 3-phenylsalicylate. Sebaclen is the hydrochloride.
Use: Treatment of seborrhea.
XERAC. (Person & Covey) Isopropyl alcohol 44%, microcrystalline sulfur 4%. Tube 1½ oz.
Use: Acne vulgaris management.
XERAC AC. (Person & Covey) Aluminum Cl hexahydrate 6.25% in anhydrous ethanol. Bot 35 ml., 60 ml.
Use: Antiperspirant.
XERAC BP5. (Person & Covey) Benzoyl peroxide 5% in hydrogel. Tubes 1½ oz., 3 oz.
Use: Aid in management of acne.
XERAC BP10. (Person & Covey) Benzoyl Peroxide 10% in hydrogel. Tubes 1½ oz., 3 oz.
Use: Acne management.
XEROFORM OINTMENT 3%.
(City) Pwder. ¼ lb., 1 lb.
(Consolidated) Jar 1 lb., 5 lb.
(Robinson) Jar. 1 lb., 5 lb.
XERO-LUBE. (Scherer) Potassium phosphate, dibasic potassium phos., magnesium chloride, potassium chloride, calcium chloride, sodium chloride, sodium fluoride, sorbitol sol., sodium carboxymethylcellulose, methyl paraben. Bot. 6 oz.
Use: Moisten & lubricate oral cavity.
YF-VAX. (Squibb-Connaught) Yellow fever vaccine. Vials 1 or 5 dose.
Use: Active immunizing agent against yellow fever.
• **XILOBAM.** USAN.
Use: Relaxant.
• **XIPAMIDE.** USAN.
Use: Antihypertensive, diuretic.
• **XORPHANOL MESYLATE.** USAN.
Use: Analgesic.
X-OTAG. (Reid-Provident) Orphenadrine citrate. **Inj.:** 30 mg./ml. Vial 10 ml.**Tab:** 100 mg./Tab. Bot. 100s.
Use: Skeletal muscle relaxant.
X-PREP BOWEL EVACUANT KIT. (Gray) Kit contains Senokot S tablets.
Use: Pre-radiographic bowel evacuant.
X-PREP BOWEL EVACUANT KIT-2. (Gray) Citrolax granules.
Use: Pre-radiographic bowel evacuant.
X-PREP LIQUID. (Gray) Standardized extract of senna fruit. Bot. 2½ oz.

Use: Pre-radiographic bowel evacuant.
X-RAY CONTRAST MEDIA.
See: Iodine Products, Diagnostic.
X SEB SHAMPOO. (Bake/Cummins) Salicylic acid 4%, coal tar solution 10% in a blend of surface active agents. Bot. 4 oz.
Use: Antiseborrheic shampoo.
Use: Itching scalp.
X SEB T. (Baker/Cummins) Coal tar sol 10%, salicylic acid 4% Bot. 4 oz.
Use: Psoriasis, dandruff, seborrhic dermatitis.
XTRACARE. (Sween) Cream. Bot. 8 oz.
Use: Foot care.
XTRA-VITES. (Barth's) Vit. A 10,000 I.U., D 400 I.U., C 150 mg., B-1 5 mg., B-2 1 mg., niacin 3.33 mg., pantothenic acid 183 mcg., B-6 250 mcg., B-12 215 mg., E 15 I.U., rutin 20 mg., citrus bioflavonoid complex 15 mg., choline 6.67 mg., inositol 10 mg., folic acid 50 mcg., biotin, aminobenzoic acid/Tab. Bot. 30s, 90s, 180s, 360s.
Use: Vitamin supplement.
X-TRO. (Xttrium) Atropine oxide hydrochloride 0.2 mg./Cap. Bot. 100s, 1000s.
W/Phenobarb. 15 mg./Cap. Bot. 100s, 1000s.
Use: Anticholinergic.
X-TROZINE CAPSULES. (Rexar) Phendimetrazine tartrate 35 mg./Cap. Bot. 1000s.
Use: Treatment of obesity.
X-TROZINE S.R. CAPSULES. (Rexar) Phendimetrazine tartrate 105 mg./S.R. Cap. Bot. 100s, 200s, 1000s.
Use: Treatment of obesity.
X-TROZINE TABLETS. (Rexar) Phendimetrazine tartrate 35 mg./Tab. Bot. 1000s.
Use: Treatment of obesity.
X-WAX. (CMC) Bot. 10 ml.
Use: Earwax remover.
• **XYLAMIDINE TOSYLATE.** USAN. N-[2-(m-Methoxyphenoxy)propyl]-2-m-tolylacetamidine mono-p-toluenesulfonate hemihydrate.
Use: Antiserotonin.
XYLAZINE. B.A.N. N-(5,6-Dihydro-4H-1,3-thiazin-2-yl)-2,6-xylidine.
Use: Analgesic, veterinary medicine.
See: Rompun
• **XYLAZINE HYDROCHLORIDE.** USAN.
Use: Analgesic, relaxant (muscle).
XYLOCAINE HYDROCHLORIDE. (Astra) Lidocaine HCl **Amp.** (1%): 2 cc., 10s; 5 cc., 10s; 30 cc., 5s; w/epinephrine 1:200,000 30 cc., 5s. (1.5%): 20 cc., 5s; w/epinephrine 1:200,000 30 cc., 5s. (2%): 2 cc., 10s; 10 cc., 5s; w/epinephrine 1:200,000 20 cc., 5s. (4%): 5 cc., 10s. **Multi. Dose Vials.** (0.5%): 50 cc. w/epinephrine 1:200,000 50 cc. (1%): 20 cc., 50 cc. w/epinephrine 1:100,000 20 cc., 50 cc. (2%): 20 cc., 50 cc.; w/epinephrine 1:100,000 20 cc., 50 cc. **Single dose Vials:** (1%); 30 cc. (1.5%): 20 cc.; w/epinephrine 1:200,000 30 cc. (2%) w/epinephrine 1:200,000 20 cc.
Use: Local anesthetic.
XYLOCAINE HYDROCHLORIDE FOR CARDIAC ARRHYTHMIA. (Astra) **Intravenous:** lidocaine 2% Single inj. 100 mg./5 cc. amp., 10s. Continuous

infusion 1 Gm./25 ml. Vial; 2 Gm./50 ml. Vial. Prefilled syringe 100 mg./5 cc. 12s. Continuous infusion prefilled syringe 1 Gm., 2 Gm. **Intramuscular:** Amp. 10%, 5 ml.
XYLOCAINE HYDROCHLORIDE 4% SOLUTION. (Astra) Retrobulbar and transtracheal injection and topical use. Lidocaine Amp. 5 cc. Box 10s. Topical use only. 50 cc. Screw top Bot.
XYLOCAINE HYDROCHLORIDE FOR SPINAL ANESTHESIA. (Astra) Lidocaine HCl 1.5% & 5%, glucose 7.5%, sod. hydroxide to adjust pH. Specific gravity 1.028-1.034 Amp. 2 cc. Box 10s.
XYLOCAINE JELLY. (Astra) Lidocaine HCl 20 mg., methyl-p-hydroxbenzoate 0.7 mg., propyl-p-hydroxy-benzoate 0.3 mg., sod. hydroxide, sodium carboxyme-thylcellulose and preservatives/Tube 30 cc. Use: Urilogical.
XYLOCAINE OINTMENT. (Astra) 2.5% Lidocaine base OTC. 35 Gm./Tube. 5% Lidocaine base 35 Gm./Tube 5% Lidocaine base flavored 3.5 Gm./Tube, 10s. Jar 35 Gm. Ointment base of polyethylene glycols and propylene glycol. Use: Topical anesthetic.
XYLOCAINE VISCOUS. (Astra) Lidocaine HCl 2%, sodium carboxymethylcellulose, flavoring agents and preservatives. Bot. 20 cc. 25s; 100 cc.; 450 cc. Use: Anesthesia of mouth and pharynx.
• **XYLOMETAZOLINE HCl,** U.S.P. XXI. Nasal Soln., U.S.P. XXI. 2-(4-tert-Butyl-2,6-dimethyl benzyl)-2-imidazoline HCl. Use: Adrenergic (vasoconstrictor).
See: Isohalent L.A., Liq. (Elder)
   Long Acting Neo-Synephrine, Prod. (Winthrop Products)
   Otrivin Spray (Geigy)
   Rhinall L.A., Liq. (First Texas)
   Sine-Off, Spray (Menley & James)
   Vicks Sinex Long Acting, Nasal Spray (Vicks)
XYLO-PFAN. (Adria) D-xylose 25 Gm./Bot. Use: Diagnostic agent for evaluating intestinal absorption.
XYLOPHAN D-XYLOSE TOLERANCE TEST. (Pfan-stiehl) D-xylose 25 Gm./Unit dose bot. Use: Evaluation of intestinal absorption.
• **XYLOSE,** U.S.P. XXI. Use: Diagnostic aid (intestinal function determination).
XYLOTOX. Lignocaine, B.A.N.

Y

YAGER'S LINIMENT. (Yager) Oil of turpentine and Camphor w/clove oil fragrance, emulsifier, emollient and ammonium oleate (less than 0.5% free ammonia) penetrant base. Use: Rubefacient liniment.
YATREN. See: Chiniofon, Tab.
YDP LICE SPRAY. (Youngs Drug) Synthetic pyrethroid in aerosol. Can. 5 oz. Use: Control of lice on inanimate objects.

YEAST ADENYLIC ACID. An isomer of adenosine 5-monophosphate, has been found inactive. See: Adenosine 5-Monophosphate, Preps. for active compounds.
• **YEAST, DRIED.** Use: Protein and Vit. B Complex source.
• **YEAST TABLETS, DRIED.** Use: Supplementary source of B complex vitamins. See: Brewer's Yeast, Tab.
YEAST, TORULA. See: Torula Yeast
YEAST W/IRON. See: Natural Super Iron Yeast Powder (Spirt) (Pharmex) Bot. 200s.
YELLOW ENZYME. See: Riboflavin (Var. Mfr.)
• **YELLOW FERRIC OXIDE,** N.F. XVI.
• **YELLOW FEVER VACCINE,** U.S.P. XXI. Use: Active immunizing agent. See: YF-VAX, Inj. (Squibb-Connaught)
• **YELLOW OINTMENT,** U.S.P. XXI. Use: Pharmaceutic aid (ointment base).
• **YELLOW WAX,** N.F. XVI. Use: Pharmaceutic aid (stiffening agent).
YF-VAX. (Squibb-Connaught) Yellow fever vaccine. Vials 1 dose or 5 dose plus diluent. Use: Active immunizing agent.
• **YITTERBIUM Yb 169 PENTETATE INJECTION,** U.S.P. XXI.
YOCON. (CMC) Yomimbine HCl 5.4 mg./Cap. Bot. 100s, 1000s. Use: Impotency.
YODORA DEODORANT CREAM. (Norcliff Thayer) Jar 2 oz.
YODOXIN. (Glenwood) Iodoquinol 210 mg./Tab. Bot. 25s, 100s, 1000s. Pow. Bot. 25 Gm.
YOHIMBAN-16-CARBOXYLIC ACID, 11, 17-DIME-THOXY-18-[(3,4,5-TRIMETHOXY-BENZOYL)-OXY]-, METHYL ESTER. Reserpine, U.S.P. XXI.
YOHIMBINE. W/Thyroid and strychnine. See: Andro-Medicone, Tab. (Medicone)
YOHIMBINE HCl. W/Methyl testosterone, nux vomica ext. See: Climactic, Tab. (Burgin-Arden)
   Rochor, Tab. (Rocky Mtn.)
W/Thyroid, strychnine sulf. See: Andro-Medicone, Tab. (Medicone)
YOMESAN. (Farbenfabriken Bayer) Niclosamide, B.A.N. Under study. Use: Anthelmintic.
YUTOPAR. (Astra) Ritodrine HCl. **Tab.:** 10 mg./Tab. Bot. 60s. **Inj.:** 10 mg./ml. Amp. 5 ml. Box 12s. Use: Smooth muscle relaxant.

Z

ZACTIPAR. Paracetamol, B.A.N.
ZANIL. Oxyclozanide, B.A.N.
ZANOSAR. (Upjohn) Streptozocin sterile powder 1 Gm./Vial.

Use: Metastatic islet cell carcinoma of the pancreas.

ZANTAC. (Glaxo) Ranitidine HCl 150 mg./Tab. Bot. 60s.
Use: Short term treatment of duodenal ulcer.

ZANTRYL. (Ion) Phentermine HCL 30 mg./S.R. Cap. Bot. 100s.
Use: Exogenous obesity.

ZARONTIN. (Parke-Davis) Ethosuximide. **Cap:** 250 mg./Cap. Bot. 100s. **Syrup:** 250 mg./5 ml. Bot. pt.
Use: Treatment of petit mal epilepsy.

ZAROXOLYN. (Pennwalt) Metolazone 2.5 mg., 5 mg., 10 mg./Tab. Bot. 100s, 500s, 1000s. Strip Pack 100s.
Use: Diuretic, antihypertensive.

Z-BEC. (Robins) Vit. E 45 I.U., C 600 mg., B-1 15 mg., B-2 10.2 mg., niacin 100 mg., B-6 10 mg., B-12 6 mcg., pantothenic acid 25 mg., Zn 22.5 mg./Tab. Bot. 60s, 500s; Dis-Co Packs (tabs) 100s.
Use: Nutritional supplement.

ZEASORB POWDER. (Stiefel) Talc, microporous cellulose, supersorb carbohydrate acrylic copolymer. Sifter-top-Cans 2 oz., 8 oz.
Use: Moisture absorbent.

ZEMACON LOTION. (CMC) Sulfur, zinc oxide, titanium oxide, camphor. Bot. 2 oz., pt., gal.
Use: External treatment of acne.

ZEMACON SKIN CLEANSER. (CMC) Sod. alkylaryl polyether sulfonate, lanolin cholesterols, petrolatum, hexachlorophene 3%. Bot. 4 oz., pt., gal.

ZEMALO. (Barre) Sulfur, ZnO, camphor, titanium oxide. Bot. 4 oz., pt., gal.

ZEMARINE. (Zemmer) Butabarbital sod. 16.2 mg., hyoscine HBr 0.0065 mg., hyoscyamine sulfate 0.1037, atropine sulfate 0.0194/Dr. Tab. or T.R. Cap. Cap. Bot. 100s, 1000s. **Elix.** Bot. 3 oz., pts., gal. **Tab.** Box 100s, 1000s.
Use: Antispasmodic or sedative.

ZEM-HISTINE. (Zemmer) Pyrilamine maleate Tab. 25 mg., Bot. 100s, 1000s.
W/Butacaine. Oint: Methapyrilene HCl 2%, butacaine sulfate 1%, chlorobutanol 0.5%. Tube 1 oz.
W/Codeine. Syrup: Pyrilamine maleate 16 mg., codeine phosphate 10.95 mg./5 ml. Bot. pt., gal.
W/Thenylpyramine HCl 25 mg., pyrilamine maleate 12.5 mg./Cap. Bot. 100s, 1000s.
Use: Antihistaminic.

ZEMO LIQUID. (Plough) Phenol 1.0%, methyl salicylate 0.3%, alcohol 34%. Bot. 7.5 oz.
Use: Anti-pruritic.

ZEMO LIQUID EXTRA STRENGTH. (Plough) Phenol 1.5%, alcohol 40%. Bot. 7.5 oz.
Use: Anti-pruritic.

ZEMO OINTMENT REGULAR AND EXTRA STRENGTH. (Plough) Bismuth subnitrate, methyl salicylate, menthol, triclosan. Regular Strength: Tube 1.125 oz. Extra Strength: Tube 2.5 oz.
Use: Anti-pruritic.

ZENATE. (Reid-Provident) Vit. A 5000 I.U., D 400 I.U., E 30 I.U., C 80 mg., folic acid 1 mg., thiamine 3 mg., riboflavin 3 mg., niacin 20 mg., B-6 10 mg., B-12 12 mcg., Ca 300 mg., iodine 175 mcg., iron 65 mg., magnesium 100 mg., zinc 20 mg./Tab. Bot. 100s.
Use: Dietary supplement for pregnancy and lactation.

• **ZENAZOCINE MESYLATE.** USAN.
Use: Analgesic.

ZENDIUM. (CooperCare) Sodium fluoride 0.22%. Tube 0.9 oz., 2.3 oz.
Use: Toothpaste.

ZENI B W/C. (Zenith) Vit. C 500 mg., B-1 15 mg., B-2 10 mg., B-6 5 mg., niacin 50 mg., calcium pantothenate 10 mg./Tab. Bot. 100s.

ZENIVITES M. (Zenith) Vit. A 4000 I.U., D 400 I.U., B-1 1 mg., B-2 1.2 mg., B-6 2 mg., B-12 2 mcg., Ca pantothenate 5 mg., niacinamide 10 mg., C 30 mg., Ca 100 mg., P 76 mg., Fe 10 mg., Mn 1 mg., Mg 1 mg., Zn 1 mg./Tab. Bot. 100s.

ZENTINIC. (Lilly) Elemental iron (as ferrous fumarate) 100 mg., folic acid 0.05 mg., Vit. B-1 7.5 mg., B-2 7.5 mg., B-6 7.5 mg., B-12 50 mcg., pantothenic acid 15 mg., niacinamide 30 mg., C 200 mg./Pulvule. Bot. 60s.
Use: Treatment of iron deficiency anemia.

ZENTRON. (Lilly) Iron (as ferrous sulfate) 20 mg., Vit. B-1 1 mg., B-2 1 mg., B-6 1 mg., B-12 5 mcg., pantothenic acid 1 mg., niacinamide 5 mg., C 100 mg./5 ml./, alcohol 2%. Bot. 8 fl. oz.
Use: Liquid hematinic.

ZENTRON CHEWABLE. (Lilly) Elemental iron 20 mg., (as ferrous fumarate) B-1 1 mg., B-2 1 mg., B-6 1 mg., B-12 5 mcg., pantothenic acid 1 mg., niacinamide 5 mg., C 100 mg./Chewable tab. Bot. 50s.

ZEPHIRAN CHLORIDE. (Winthrop-Breon) Benzalkonium Chloride **Tinct.** 1:750 tinted (w/alcohol 50%, acetone 10%) Bot. 1 gal.; **Aqueous soln.** 1:750 Bot. 8 oz., 1 gal.; **Spray:** Bot. 1 fl. oz., 6 fl. oz. Use; Antiseptic; **Conc.** 17%, Bot. 4 fl. oz., 1 gal.
Use: Germicide, disinfectant.

ZEPHIRAN TOWELETTES. (Winthrop-Breon) Moist paper towels with solution of zephiran chloride 1:750. Boxes 20s, 100s, 1000s.
Use: Antiseptic skin cleanser.

ZEPINE. (Foy) Reserpine alkaloid 0.25 mg./Tab. Bot. 100s, 500s, 1000s.

• **ZERANOL.** USAN. (1) (3S, 7X)-3,4,5,6,7,8,9,10,11,12-Decahydro-7, 14,16-trihydroxy-3-methyl-1H-2-benzoxacyclotetradecin-1-one; (2) (6X, 10S)-6-(6,-10-dihyroxyundecyl)-β-resorcylic acid lactone. Ralgro (Commercial Solvents).
Use: Anabolic.

ZETAR EMULSION. (Dermik) Colloidal whole coal tar 30% (300 mg./ml.) in polysorbates. Bot. 6 oz.
Use: Generalized recalcitrant dermatoses, for the bath and for prescription compounding.

ZETAR SHAMPOO. (Dermik) Colloidal whole coal tar 1% in a shampoo. 6 oz. Plastic bottles.
Use: Antiseptic, antibacterial, antiseborrheic.

ZIDE. (Reid-Provident) Hydrochlorothiazide 50 mg./Tab. Bot. 30s.

• **ZIDOMETACIN.** USAN.
Use: Anti-inflammatory.

• **ZILANTEL.** USAN.
Use: Anthelmintic.

ZIMCO. (Sterwin) Vanillin.
• ZIMELDINE HYDROCHLORIDE. USAN.
    Use: Antidepressant.
• ZIMELIDINE HYDROCHLORIDE.
    Use: Antidepressant.See: Zimeldine hydrochloride.
ZINACEF. (Glaxo) Cefuroxime sodium 750 mg. or 1.5 Gm./Vial.
    Use: Antibiotic.
ZINAMIDE. Pyrazinamide, B.A.N.
ZINCATE. (Paddock) Zinc sulfate 220 mg./Cap. Bot. 100s, 500s, 1000s.
    Use: Emetic and astringent.
ZINC-220. (Alto) Zinc sulfate/Cap. Bot. 100s, 1000s, 5000s, 10,000s.
    Use: Dietary supplement, zinc deficiency.
• ZINC ACETATE, U.S.P. XXI. Acetic acid, zinc salt, dihydrate.
    Use: Pharm, necessity for Zinc eugenol Cement.
ZINC BACITRACIN. Bacitracin Zinc, U.S.P. XXI.
    Use: Antibiotic.
ZINC BROMIDE. W/Sodium Br., ammonium Br, potassium Br, ext. hyoscyamus, ext. belladonna.
    See: Neurosine, Tab., Liq. (Dios)
• ZINC CHLORIDE, U.S.P. XXI. Inj., U.S.P. XXI.
    Use: Astringent, desensitizer for dentin, replacement therapy.
    See: Zinctrace, Inj. (Armour)
W/Formaldehyde.
    See: Forma Zincol Concentrate (Ingram)
• ZINC CHLORIDE Zn 65. USAN.
    Use: Radioactive agent.
ZINCFRIN. (Alcon) Zinc sulfate ¼%, phenylephrine HCl 0.12% in buffered sol. Droptainer 15 cc.
    Use: Astringent and ocular decongestant.
• ZINC-EUGENOL CEMENT, U.S.P. XXI.
    Use: Dental protectant.
• ZINC GELATIN, U.S.P. XXI. Zinc gelatin boot. Unna's Boot.
    Use: Topical protectant.
• ZINC GELATIN IMPREGNATED GAUZE, U.S.P. XXI.
    Use: Topical protectant.
ZINC-GLENWOOD. (Glenwood) Zinc Sulfate 220 mg./Cap. Bot. 100s.
ZINCHLORUNDESAL. Zincundesal.
ZINC INSULIN.
    See: Insulin Zinc, Prep. (Various Mfr.)
ZINCON SHAMPOO. (Lederle) Pyrithione zinc 1%. w/sodium methyl cocoyltaurate, NaCl MgAl silicate, Na cocoylisethionate, gluthural, water. pH adjusted. Bot. 4 oz., 8 oz.
    Use: Dandruff Shampoo.
• ZINC OXIDE, U.S.P. XXI. Flowers of zinc.
    Use: Mild astringent & antiseptic in skin diseases.
    See: Calamine Preps.
W/Combinations.
    See: Akne, Drying Lotion (Alto)
        Almophen, Oint. (Bowman)
        Anecal, Cream (Lannett)
        Anocaine, Supp. (Mallard)
        Anoids Rectal Supp. (Scrip)
        Anugesic, Oint., Supp. (Parke-Davis)

Anulan, Vial. (Lannett)
Anusol, Oint., Supp. (Parke-Davis)
Anusol-HC, Supp. (Parke-Davis)
Aracain Rectal Oint., Supp. (Commerce)
Biscolan, Supp. (Lannett)
Bonate, Supp. (suppositoria)
Calamatum, Preps. (Blair)
Cala-Zinc-Ol, Liq. (Emerson)
Caldesene, Oint. (Pharmacraft)
Caleate HC Cream, Oint. (Elder)
Caloxide W/Benzocaine, Cream (Blue Line)
Caloxol, Oint. (Bowman)
CZO, Lot. (Elder)
Derma Medicone HC, Supp. (Medicone)
Dermatrol, Oint. (Gordon)
Desitin, Oint. (Leeming)
Diaprex, Oint. (Moss, Belle)
Doctient, Supp. (Suppositoria)
Elder Diaper Rash Oint. (Elder)
Epinephricaine, Oint. (Upjohn)
Ergophene, Oint. (Upjohn)
Hemocaine, Oint. (Mallard)
Hemorrhoidal Oint. (Towne)
Hydro Surco, Lot. (Alma)
Ladd's Paste (Paddock)
Lanaburn, Oint. (Lannett)
Lasan, Oint. (Stiefel)
Medicated Powder (Johnson & Johnson)
Medicated Foot Powder (Upjohn)
Mexsana, Pow. (Plough)
Nullo Foot Cream (DePree)
Obtundia Calamine Cream (Otis Clapp)
Pazo, Oint. & Supp. (Bristol-Myers)
Petrozin Compound Oint. (Bowman)
Pile-Gon, Oint. (Edward J. Moore)
PZM Ointment (Wendt-Bristol)
Rectal Medicone HC, Supp. (Medicone)
Rhuex, Liq. (Kay)
RVPaque, Oint. (Elder)
Saratoga, Oint. (Blair)
Schamberg, Lot. (Paddock)
Sebasorb, Lot. (Summer)
Supertah, Oint. (Purdue Frederick)
Taloin, Tube (Warren-Teed)
Ting, Cream, Pow. (Pharmacraft)
Unguentine Oint. "Original Formula" (Norwich-Eaton)
Versal, Supp. (Suppositoria)
Wyanoids, Preps. (Wyeth)
Xylocaine Supp. (Astra)
Zinc Boric Lotion, Liq. (Emerson)
Zonox Colloidal, Liq. (Scrip)
ZINC OXIDE OINTMENT, U.S.P. XXI. (Norwich Eaton) Tubes 1 oz., 2¼ oz.
    Use: Protective coating for minor skin irritations.
• ZINC OXIDE PASTE, U.S.P. XXI.
    Use: Topical protectant, astringent
• ZINC OXIDE AND SALICYLIC ACID PASTE, U.S.P. XXI.
    Use: Topical protectant; astringent.
ZINC PEROXIDE. (Mallinckrodt) Zinc Superoxide. Bot. 113.4 Gm.

Use: Anti-infective (oxidant).

ZINC PHENOLSULFONATE.
Use: Astringent.
W/Belladonna leaf ext., kaolin, pectin, sodium carboxymethylcellulose.
See: Gelcomul, Liq. (Commerce)
W/Bismuth subgallate, kaolin, pectin, opium pow.
See: Amogel, Tab. (Vortech)
Diastay, Tab. (Elder)
W/Bismuth subsalicylate, salol, methyl salicylate.
See: Pepto-Bismol, Liquid (Norwich Eaton)
W/Kaolin, pectin.
See: Pectocel, Liq. (Lilly)
W/Mag. trisilicate, cal. carb., bis. subcarb., cerium oxalate.
See: Bismosalicate Comp., Liq. (Blue Line)
W/Opium pow., bismuth subgallate, pectin, kaolin.
See: Bismuth, Pectin & Paregoric (Lemmon)
B.K.Z., Tab. (Sutliff & Case)

ZINC PYRITHIONE. Bis-[1-hydroxy-2(1H)-pyridineth-ionato] zinc.
Use: Bactericide, fungicide, antiseborrheic.
See: Breck One, Shampoo (Breck)
Zincon, Shampoo (Lederle)
ZP-11, Liq. (Revlon)

• **ZINC STEARATE,** U.S.P. XXI. Octadecanoic acid, zinc salt.
Use: Dusting powder.
W/Combinations.
See: Ting, Cream, Pow. (Pharmacraft)

ZINC SULFANILATE. Zinc sulfanilate tetrahydrate.
Nizin, Op-Isophrin-Z, Op-Isophrin-Z-M (Broemmel).
Use: Antibacterial.

• **ZINC SULFATE,** U.S.P. XXI. Inj., Ophth. Sol. U.S.P. XXI. Sulfuric acid, zinc salt (1:1), heptahydrate.
Use: Astringent (ophthalmic).
See: Bufopto Zinc Sulfate, Sol. (Softcon)
Medizinc, Tab. (Medics)
Op-Thal-Zin Ophth. (Alcon)
Scrip-Zinc, Cap. (Scrip)
Zinc-Glenwood, Cap. (Glenwood)
Zin-Cora, Caps. (Elder)
W/Boric acid, phenylephrine HCl.
See: Oc-U-Zin, Ophth. Sol. (Blue Line)
Phenylzin Drops, Ophth. Sol. (Smith Miller & Patch)
W/Calcium lactate.
See: Zinc-220, Cap. (Alto)
W/Menthol, methyl salicylate, alum, boric acid, oxyquinoline citrate.
See: Maso pH Powder (Mason)
W/Phenylephrine HCl, polyvinyl alcohol.
See: Prefrin-Z, Liquifilm (Allergan)
W/Piperocaine HCl, boric acid, potassium chloride.
See: M-Z Drops (Smith, Miller & Patch)
W/Sodium Chloride.
See: Bromidrosis Crystals (Gordon)
W/Sulfur, hexachlorophene.
See: Acnederm, Lot. (Lannett)
W/Vitamins.
See: Neovicaps TR, Cap. (Scherer)
Vicon-C, Cap. (Glaxo)

Vicon Chewable, Tab. (Glaxo)
Vicon Forte, Cap. (Glaxo)
Vicon Plus, Cap. (Glaxo)
Vi-Zac, Cap. (Glaxo)
Z-Bec, Tab. (Robins)

ZINC SULFATE BUFOPTO. (Softcon) Zinc sulfate 0.25%, benzalkonium chloride 1:25,000. Bot. 15 cc., 30 cc.
Use: Astringent, antiseptic, bacteriostatic.

ZINC SULFATE COMPOUND. (Lilly) Zinc sulfate 12.5 Gm., salicylic acid 500 mg., phenol, eucalyptol, menthol, and thymol 100 mg., boric acid 86.6 Gm./100 Gm. Bot. 4 oz.

ZINC SULFIDE, LOTION.
See: White Lotion, U.S.P.

ZINC SULFOCARBOLATE.
W/Aluminum hydroxide, pectin, kaolin, bismuth subsalicylate, salol.
See: Wescola Antidiarrheal-Stomach Upset (Western Research)

ZINCTRACE. (Armour) Zinc chloride injection containing zinc 1 mg./1 ml. Vial 10 ml. Box 25s.
Use: Supplement to I.V. solutions for zinc deficiency.

ZINCUNDESAL.
See: Zinchlorundesal

ZINC-10-UNDECENOATE.
See: Zinc Undecylenate, U.S.P. XXI.

• **ZINC UNDECYLENATE,** U.S.P. XXI. 10-Undecenoic acid, zinc (2+) salt. Zinc 10-undecenoate. (Various Mfr.)
Use: Antifungal.
W/Benzocaine, hexachlorophene.
See: Fung-O-Spray (Scrip)
W/Benzocaine, undecylenic acid, menthol.
See: Decyl-Cream LBS (Scrip)
W/Caprylic acid, sodium propionate.
See: Deso-Cream (Columbia)
Deso-Talc, Foot Powder (Columbia)
W/Parachlorometaxyenol.
See: Cruex, Cream (Pharmacraft)
W/Undecylenic acid.
See: Desenex, Prods. (Pharmacraft)
Ting, Aerosol (Pharmacraft)
Quinsana, Med. Oint. (Mennen)

ZINKAPS. (Ortega) Zinc sulfate 220 mg./Cap. Bot. 100s, 1000s.
Use: Zinc supplement.

• **ZINOCANAZOLE HYDROCHLORIDE.** USAN.

• **ZINOSTATIN.** USAN.
Use: Antineoplastic.

• **ZINTEROL HYDROCHLORIDE.** USAN.
Use: Bronchodilator.

• **ZINVIROXIME.** USAN.
Use: Antiviral.

ZIPAN-25/50. (Savage) Promethazine HCl 25 mg., 50 mg./ml. Vial 10 ml. Box 25 × 1.
Use: Antihistaminic, sedative, anti-motion anticholinergic.

ZIRADRYL LOTION. (Parke-Davis) Benadryl HCl 2%, zinc oxide 2%, alcohol 2%. Bot. 6 oz.
Use: Poison ivy and related dermatitis.

665

ZYMOWIN

ZIRCONIUM CARBONATE OR OXIDE.
See: Dermaneed, Lot. (Hanlon)
W/Benzocaine, menthol, camphor.
See: Rhulicream, Oint. (Lederle)
W/Benzocaine, menthol, camphor, calamine, pyrilamine maleate.
See: Ivarest, Cream (Carbisulphoil)
W/Benzocaine, menthol, camphor, calamine, isopropyl alcohol.
See: Rhulispray, Aerosol (Lederle)
W/Benzocaine, pyrilamine maleate, povidone.
See: Poison Ivy Cream (McKesson)
W/Calamine, zinc oxide, pyrilamine maleate.
See: Zircostan, Creme (Standex)
W/Parethoxycaine, calamine.
See: Zotox, Spray, Oint. (Commerce)
ZIRCOSTAN CREME. (Standex) Zirconium oxide 4.5%, calamine 6.0%, zinc oxide 4.0%, pyrilamine maleate 0.5%.
ZNG. (Western Research) Zinc gluconate 35 mg./Tab. Handicount 28 (36 bags of 28 tab.)
Use: Supplement.
Zn-PLUS. (Miller) Zinc in a zinc-protein complex made with isolated soy protein and Torula yeast 5 mg./Tab. Bot. 100s.
Use: Dietary supplement.
ZODEAC-100. (Econo Med) Multivitamin and multi-mineral supplement with 1 mg. folic acid. Bot. 100s.
Use: Dietary supplement.
ZOALENE. Dinitolmide, B.A.N.
ZOAMIX. Dinitolmide, B.A.N.
ZODIEX. (Eckerd) Phenacetin 125 mg., salicylamide, Pamabrom 25 mg., pyrilamine maleate/Tab. Pack 24s.
Use: Premenstrual discomfort.
• **ZOLAMINE HCl.** USAN. 2-[[2-(Dimethylamino)ethyl]-(p-methoxybenzyl)-amino]thiazole monohydrochloride.
Use: Antihistamine and local anesthetic.
W/Eucupin dihycrochloride.
See: Otodyne, Sol. (Schering)
• **ZOLAZEPAM HYDROCHLORIDE.** USAN.
Use: Sedative.
• **ZOLERTINE HYDROCHLORIDE.** USAN. 1-Phenyl-4-[2-(1H-tetrazol-5-yl)ethyl]piperazine HCl.
Use: Antiadrenergic; vasodilator.
ZOLYSE. (Alcon) Lyophilized alpha-chymotrypsin 750 units balanced salt solution 10 cc./Unit pak. 12s.
Use: Cataract surgery.
ZOMAX. (McNeil Pharm) Zomepirac sodium 100 mg./Tab. Bot. 100s.
Use: Relief of mild to moderately severe pain.
• **ZOMEPIRAC SODIUM,** U.S.P. XXI. Tab., U.S.P. XXI.
Sodium 5-(4-chlorobenzoyl)-1, 4-dimethyl-1H-pyrrole-2-acetate dihydrate.
Use: Non-steroidal, anti-inflammatory and analgesic agent.
See: Zomax, Tab. (McNeil)
• **ZOMETAPINE.** USAN.
Use: Antidepressant.
ZONE-A LOTION. (UAD Labs) Hydrocortisone acetate 1%, pramoxine HCl 1%. Bot. 2 oz.

Use: For relief of the inflammatory manifestations of corticosteroid responsive dermatoses.
ZONITE LIQUID DOUCHE CONCENTRATE. (Norcliff Thayer) Benzalkonium chloride 0.1%, propylene glycol, menthol, thymol in buffered solution. Bot. 8 fl. oz., 12 fl. oz.
Use: Vaginal douche.
ZONIUM CHLORIDE. (Lannett) Benzalkonium chloride 12.8%, 17%, 50%. Bot. pt., gal. 12.8%, 17% Bot. 4 oz. Also as 1:1,000, Bot. 1 pt., 1 gal.
Use: Antiseptic.
• **ZORBAMYCIN.** USAN.
Use: Antibacterial.
ZORPRIN. (Boots) Aspirin 800 mg./S.R. Tab. Bot. 100s.
Use: Treatment of rheumatoid arthritis, osteoarthritis.
• **ZORUBICIN HYDROCHLORIDE.** USAN.
Use: Antineoplastic.
ZOVIRAX OINTMENT 5%. (Burroughs Wellcome) Acyclovir 50 mg./Gm Tube 15 Gm.
Use: Management of initial herpes genitalis and mucocutaneous herpes simplex virus infections.
ZOVIRAX STERILE POWDER. (Burroughs Wellcome) Acyclovir sodium 500 mg./Vial. Vial 10 ml. ctn. 25s.
Use: Treatment of initial and recurrent mucosal & cutaneous herpes simplex.
ZOXAPHEN. (Mallard) Chlorzoxazone 250 mg., acetaminophen 300 mg./Tab. Bot. 500s.
Use: Musculoskeletal disorders.
ZOXAZOLAMINE, B.A.N. 2-Amino-5-chlorobenzoxazole. Flexin.
Use: Skeletal muscle relaxant-uricosuric.
Z-PRO-C. (Person & Covey) Elemental zinc 45 mg., ascorbic acid 100 mg./Tab. Bot. 100s.
Use: Zinc and vitamin C therapy.
Z-TEC. (Seatrace) Iron equivalent 50 mg./ml. from iron dextran complex. Vial 10 cc.
• **ZUCLOMIPHENE.** USAN.
ZYLOPRIM. (Burroughs Wellcome) Allopurinol 100 mg./Tab. Bot. 100s, 1000s, unit dose packs 100s; 300 mg./Tab. Bot. 30s, 100s, 500s, unit dose packs 100s.
Use: Antigout.
ZYLORIC. Allopurinol, B.A.N.
ZYMACAP. (Upjohn) Vit. A 5000 I.U., D 400 I.U., E 15 I.U., C 90 mg., folic acid 400 mcg., B-1 2.25 mg., B-2 2.6 mg., niacin 30 mg., B-6 3 mg., B-12 9 mcg., pantothenic acid 15 mg./Cap. Bot. 90s, 240s.
Use: Vitamin deficiencies.
ZYMENOL. (Houser) Brewer's yeast 12%, mineral oil 50%, agar q.s. Bot. 8 oz., 14 oz., Reg. or chocolate.
Use: Bowel management.
ZYMME. (Scrip) Dl-methyl polysiloxane 0.8 mg., ox bile 100 mg., pancreatin 50 mg., cellulase 0.3 mg., betaine HCl 4 gr./Cap. Bot. 100s.
Use: Enzymatic digestive.
ZYMOWIN. (Winston) Amylolytic enzyme 25 mg., proteolytic enzyme 10 mg., cellulolytic enzyme 1 mg., dehydrocholic acid 100 mg., hyoscyamine HBr

0.1 mg., hyoscine HBr 0.0065 mg., atropine sulfate 0.02 mg./Tab. Bot. 100s, 1000s.
Use: Enzyme-antispasmodic in digestive disturbances.

ZYMOZYME TABLETS. (Inwood) Vit. A 25,000 I.U., D 2000 I.U., B-12 10 mcg., B-1 10 mg., B-2 10 mg., niacinamide 150 mg., B-6 1 mg., cal. pantothenate 10 mg., C 150 mg., D 12 I.U., rutin 25 mg., citrus bioflavonoid complex 25 mg., choline bitartrate 50 mg., inositol 25 mg., dl-methionine 25 mg., K 1 mg., nucleic acid 25 mg., yeast enzymatic hydrolysate 25 mg., glutamic acid 12.5 mg., glycine 12.5 mg., cysteine HCl 12.5 mg., iron 20 mg., Mn 1 mg., Cu 0.45 mg., Mg 1 mg., pot. 5 mg., Zn 0.5 mg./Tab. Bot. 100s.
Use: Multivitamin, mineral, lipotopic and phosphorylating therapy.

ZYNOXUN OINTMENT. (Alton) Tube 5 oz. Jar. 1 lb.
Use: Protective ointment.

ZYPAN TABLETS. (Standard Process) Pancreatin 1.5 Gm., pepsin (1:3000) 1.5 Gm., betaine HCl 2.75 Gm., ammonium chloride 0.15 Gm./Tab. Bot. 100s.
Use: Digestive aid.

Word	Abbreviation	Meaning
ana	āā, aa	of each
ante cibum	a.c.	before meals or food
ad	ad	to, up to
aurio dextra	a.d.	right ear
ad libitum	ad lib.	at pleasure
aurio laeva	a.l.	left ear
ante meridiem	A.M.	morning
aqua	aq.	water
aqua destillata	aq. dest.	distilled water
aurio sinister	a.s.	left ear
aures utrae	a.u.	each ear
bis in die	b.i.d.	twice daily
bowel movement	b.m.	bowel movement
blood pressure	b.p.	blood pressure
cong	c.	a gallon
cum	c̄	with
capsula	caps.	capsule
	cc.	cubic centimeter
compositus	comp.	compound
dies	d.	day
dilue	dil.	dilute
dispensa	disp.	dispense
divide	div.	divide
dentur tales doses	d.t.d.	give of such a dose
elixir	el.	elixir
	e.m.p.	as directed
et	et	and
	ex aq.	in water
fac, fiat, fiant	f., ft.	make, let be made
gramma	Gm., g.	gram
granum	gr.	grain
gutta	gtt.	a drop
hora	h.	hour
hora somni	h.s., hor. som.	at bedtime
	i.m., I.M	intramuscular
	i.v.	intravenous
liquor	liq.	a liquor, solution
	mcg.	microgram
	mg.	milligram
	ml.	milliliter
misce	M.	mix
more dictor	m. dict.	as directed
mixtura	mixt.	a mixture
National Formulary	N.F.	National Formulary
numerus	no.	number
nocturnal	noc.	in the night
non repetatur	non. rep.	do not repeat, no refills
octarius	O, Oct.	a pint
oculus dexter	o.d.	right eye
oculus laevus	o.l.	left eye
oculus sinister	o.s.	left eye
oculo uterque	o.u.	each eye
post cibos	p.c., post. cib.	after meals
post meridiem	P.M.	afternoon or evening
per os	p.o.	by mouth
pro re nata	p.r.n.	as needed
pulvis	pulv.	a powder

*The listing of commonly used abbreviations is included as an aid in interpreting medical orders.

Word	Abbreviation	Meaning
	q.d.	every day
quiaque hora	q.h.	every hour
quater in die	q.i.d.	four times a day
	q.o.d.	every other day
quantum sufficiat	q.s.	a sufficient quantity
	q.s. ad	a sufficient quantity to make
quam volueris	q.v.	as much as you wish
recipe	Rx	take, a recipe
repetatur	rep.	let it be repeated
sine	s̄, s	without
secundum artem	s.a.	according to art
sataratus	sat.	saturated
signa	Sig.	label, or let it be printed
solutio	sol.	solution
	solv.	dissolve
semis	s̄s̄., ss	one-half
si opus sit	s.o.s.	if there is need
statim	stat.	at once, immediately
suppositorium	supp.	suppository
syrupus	syr.	syrup
tabella	tab.	tablet
	tal.	such
	tal. dos.	such doses
ter in die	t.i.d.	three times a day
tincture	tr., tinct.	tincture
tritura	trit.	triturate
	tsp.	teaspoonful
unguentum	ung.	ointment
United States Pharmacopeia	U.S.P.	United States Pharmacopeia
ut dictum	ut. dict.	as directed
while awake	w.a.	while awake

555

Weight Equivalents

1 grain	= 1 gr	=	64.8	milligrams
1 gram	= 1 Gm or g	=	15.432	grains
1 kilogram	= 1 Kg	=	2.20	pounds avoirdupois (lb)
1 ounce avoirdupois	= 1 oz	=	28.35	grams
1 ounce apothecary	= 1 ℥	=	31.1	grams
1 pound avoirdupois	= 1 lb	=	454.	grams

Measure Equivalents

1 milliliter	= 1 ml	=	16.23	minims (♏)
1 fluidram†	= 1 f℥	=	3.4	ml
1 teaspoonful†	= 1 tsp	=	5.00	ml
1 tablespoonful	= 1 tbs or tbsp	=	15.	ml
1 fluidounce	= 1 f℥	=	29.57	ml
1 wineglassful	= 2 f℥	=	60.	ml
1 teacupful	= 4 f℥	=	120.	ml
1 tumblerful	= 8 f℥	=	240.	ml
1 pint	= 1 pt or O or Oct	=	473.	ml
1 liter	= 1 L	=	33.8	fluidounces (f℥)
1 gallon	= 1 gal or C or Cong	=	3785.	ml

*The listing of approximate practical equivalents is included to aid the practitioner in calculating and converting dosages among the various systems.

†Note: On prescription a fluidram is assumed to contain a teaspoonful which is 5 ml.

METRIC SYSTEM

Metric Weight

1 microgram†	μg (mcg)	=	0.000,001	g
1 milligram	mg	=	0.001	g
1 centigram	cg	=	0.01	g
1 decigram	dg	=	0.1	g
1 gram	g	=	1.0	g
1 dekagram	Dg	=	10.0	g
1 hectogram	hg	=	100.0	g
1 kilogram	Kg	=	1000.0	g

Metric Liquid Measure

1 microliter	μl	=	0.000,001	L
1 milliliter	ml	=	0.001	L
1 centiliter	cl	=	0.01	L
1 deciliter	dl	=	0.1	L
1 liter	L	=	1.0	L
1 dekaliter	Dl	=	10.0	L
1 hectoliter	hl	=	100.0	L
1 kiloliter	Kl	=	1000.0	L

APOTHECARY SYSTEM

Apothecary Weight

1 grain‡	gr	=	1 gr		
1 scruple	℈	=	20 gr		
1 dram	ʒ	=	60 gr	= 3℈	
1 ounce	℥	=	480 gr	= 8ʒ	
1 pound	℔	=	5760 gr	= 12℥	

Apothecary Liquid Measure

1 minim	♏	=	1♏		
1 fluidram	fʒ	=	60♏		
1 fluidounce	f℥	=	480♏	= 8 fʒ	
1 pint	pt	=	7680♏	= 16f℥	
1 quart	qt	=	15630♏	= 32 fʒ	
1 gallon	gal	=	61440♏	= 8 pt℥	

AVOIRDUPOIS SYSTEM

Avoirdupois Weight

1 ounce = 1 oz	=	437.5 grains (gr)			
1 pound = 1 lb	=	16 ounces (oz)	=	7000 grains (gr)	

*The listing of common systems of weight and measure is included to aid the practitioner in calculating dosages.

†Note: The abbreviation μg or mcg is used for microgram in pharmacy rather than gamma (γ) as in biology.

‡Note: The grain in each of the above systems has the same value, and thus serves as a basis for the interconversion of the other units.

Glossary

Abduction—the act of drawing away from a center.

Abstergent—a cleansing application or medicine.

Acaricide—an agent lethal to mites.

Achlorhydria—the absence of hydrochloric acid from gastric secretions.

Acidifier, systemic—a drug used to lower internal body pH in patients with systemic alkalosis.

Acidifier, urinary—a drug used to lower the pH of the urine.

Acidosis—an accumulation of acid in the body.

Acne—an inflammatory disease of the skin accompanied by the eruption of papules or pustules.

Addison's Disease—a condition caused by adrenal gland destruction.

Adduction—the act of drawing toward a center.

Adenitis—a gland or lymph node inflammation.

Adjuvant—an ingredient added to a prescription which complements or accentuates the action of the primary agent.

Adrenergic—a syapathomimetic drug that activates organs innervated by the sympathetic branch of the autonomic nervous system.

Adrenocorticotropic Hormone—an anterior pituitary hormone that stimulates and regulates secretion of the adrenocortical steroids.

Adrenocortical steroid, anti-inflammatory—an adrenal cortex hormone that participates in regulation of organic metabolism and inhibits the inflammatory response to stress; a glucocorticoid.

Adrenocortical steroid, salt regulating—an adrenal cortex hormone that maintains sodium-potassium electrolyte balance by stimulating and regulating sodium retention and potassium excretion by the kidneys.

Adsorbent—an agent that binds chemicals to its surface; it is useful in reducing the free availability of toxic chemicals.

Alkalizer, systemic—a drug that raises internal body pH in patients with systemic acidosis.

Allergen—a specific substance that causes an unwanted reaction in the body.

Amblyopia—pertaining to a dimness of vision.

Amebiasis—an infection with a pathogenic ameba.

Amenorrhea—an abnormal discontinuation of the menses.

Amphiarthrosis—a joint in which the surfaces are connected by discs of fibrocartilage.

Anabolic—an agent that promotes conversion of simple substance into more complex compounds; a constructive process for the organism.

Analeptic—a potent central nervous system stimulant used to maintain vital functions during severe central nervous system depression.

Analgesic—a drug that selectively suppresses pain perception without inducing unconsciousness.

Ancyclostomiasis—the condition due to the presence of hookworms in the intestine.

Androgen—a hormone that stimulates and maintains male secondary sex characteristics.

Anemia—a deficiency of red blood cells.

Anesthetic, general—a drug that eliminates pain perception by inducing unconsciousness.

Anesthetic, local—a drug that eliminates pain perception in a limited area by local action on sensory nerves; a topical anesthetic.

Angina pectoris—a sharp chest pain starting in the heart, often spreading down the left arm. A symptom of coronary disease.

Angiography—an X-ray of the blood vessels.

Anhydrotic—a drug that checks perspiration flow systemically; an antidiaphoretic.

Anodyne—a drug which act on the sensory nervous system, either centrally or peripherally, to produce relief from pain.

Anorexiant—a drug that suppresses appetite, usually secondary to central stimulation of mood.

Anorexigenic—an agent promoting a dislike or aversion to food.

Antacid—a drug that neutralizes excess gastric acid locally.

Anthelmintic—a drug that kills or inhibits worm infestations such as pinworms and tapeworms (nematodes, cestodes, trematodes).

Antiadrenergic—a drug that prevents response to sympathetic nervous system stimulation and adrenergic drugs; a sympatholytic or sympathoplegic drug.

Antiamebic—a drug that kills or inhibits the pathogenic protozoan.*Endamoeba histolytica,* the causative agent of amebic dysentery.

Antianemic—a drug that stimulates the production of erythrocytes in normal size, number and hemoglobin content; useful in treating anemias, antidoting overdoses of anemia-causing drugs.

Antiasthmatic—an agent that relieves the spasms of asthma.

Antibacterial—a drug that kills or inhibits pathogenic bacteria, the causative agents of many systemic gastrointestinal and superficial infections.

Antibiotic—an agent produced by or derived

from living cells of molds, bacteria or other plants, which destroy or inhibit the growth of microbes.

Anticholesteremic—a drug that lowers blood plasmacholesterol levels.

Anticholinergic—a drug that prevents response to parasympathetic nervous system stimulation and cholinergic drugs; a parasympatholytic or parasympathoplegic drug.

Anticoagulant—a drug that inhibits clotting of circulating blood or prevents clotting of collected blood.

Anticonvulsant—a drug that selectively prevents epileptic seizures; a central depressant used to arrest convulsions by inducing unconsciousness.

Antidepressant—a psychotherapeutic drug that induces mood elevation, useful in treating depressive neuroses and psychoses.

Antidiabetic—a drug used to prevent the development of diabetes.

Antidote—a drug that prevents or counteracts the effects of poisons or drug overdoses, by adsorption in the gastrointestinal tract (general antidotes) or by specific systemic action (specific antidotes).

Antieczematic—a topical drug that aids in the control of exudative inflammatory skin lesions.

Antiemetic—a drug that prevents vomiting, especially that of systemic origin.

Anti-fibrinolytic—an agent (drug) that inhibits liquifaction of fibrin.

Antifilarial—a drug that kills or inhibits pathogenic filarial worms of the superfamily *Filarioidea*, the causative agents of diseases such as loaiasis.

Antiflatulant—an agent inhibiting the excessive formation of gas in the stomach or intestines.

Antifungal—a drug that kills or inhibits pathogenic fungi, the causative agents of systemic, gastrointestinal, and superficial infections.

Antihemophilic—a blood derivative containing the clotting factors absent in the hereditary disease hemophilia.

Antihistaminic—a drug that prevents response to histamine, including histamine released by allergic reactions.

Antihypercholesterolemic—a drug that lowers blood cholesterol levels, especially elevated levels sometimes associated with cardiovascular disease.

Antihypertensive—a drug that lowers blood pressure, especially diastolic blood pressure in hypertensive patients.

Anti-infective, local—a drug that kills a variety of pathogenic microorganisms and is suitable for sterilizing the skin or wounds.

Anti-inflammatory—a drug which counteracts or suppresses inflammation, and produces suppression of the pain, heat, redness and swelling of inflammation.

Antileishmanial—a drug that kills or inhibits pathogenic protozoa of the genus *Leishmania*, the causative agents of diseases such as kala-azar.

Antileprotic—an agent which fights leprosy, a generally chronic skin disease.

Antilipemic—an agent reducing the amount of circulating lipids.

Antimalarial—a drug that kills or inhibits the causative agents of malaria.

Antimetabolite—a substance that competes with or replaces a certain metabolite.

Antimethemoglobinemic—a drug that reduces non-functional methemoglobin (Fe^{+++}) to normal hemoglobin (Fe^{++}).

Antimycotic—an agent inhibiting the growth of fungi.

Antinauseant—a drug that suppresses nausea, especially that due to motion sickness.

Antineoplastic—a drug that is selectively toxic to rapidly multiplying cells and is useful in destroying malignant tumors.

Antioxidant—an agent used to reduce decay or transformation of a material from oxidation.

Antiperiodic—a drug that modifies or prevents the return of malarial fever; an antimalarial.

Antiperistaltic—a drug that inhibits intestinal motility, especially for the treatment of diarrhea.

Antipruritic—a drug that prevents or relieves itching.

Antipyretic—a drug employed to reduce fever temperature of the body; a febrifuge.

Antirheumatic—a drug that alleviates inflammatory symptoms of arthritis and related connective tissue diseases.

Antirickettsial—a drug that kills or inhibits pathogenic microorganisms of the genus Rickettsia, the causative agents of diseases such as typhus. (Chloramphenicol USP)

Antischistosomal—a drug that kills or inhibits pathogenic flukes of the genus *Schistosoma*, the causative agents of schistosomiasis.

Antiseborrheic—a drug that aids in the control of seborrheic dermatitis ("dandruff").

Antiseptic—a substance that will inhibit the growth and development of microorganisms without necessarily destroying them.

Antisialagogue—a drug which diminishes the flow of saliva.

Antispasmodic—an agent used to quiet the spasms of voluntary and involuntary muscles; a calmative or antihysteric.

Anti-syphilitic—a remedy used in the treatment of syphilis.

Antitoxin—a biological drug containing antibodies against the toxic principles of a pathogenic microorganism, used for passive immunization against the associated disease.

Antitrichomonal—a drug that kills or inhibits the pathogenic protozoan *Trichomonas vaginalis*, the causative agent of trichomonal vaginitis.

Antitrypanosomal—a drug that kills or inhibits pathogenic protozoa of the genus *Trypanosoma*, the causative agents of diseases such as West African trypanosomiasis.

Antitussive—a drug that suppresses coughing.

Antivenin—a biological drug containing antibodies against the venom of a poisonous animal, and useful in antidoting the animal's bite.

Anxiety—a feeling of apprehension, uncertainty and fear.

Aperient—a mild laxative.

Aphakic—having no crystalline lens.

Aphasia—the inability to use and/or understand written and spoken words, due to damage of cortical speech centers.

Aphonia—a whisper voice due to disease of the larynx or its innervation.

Apnea—the absence of breathing.

Areola—a pigmented ring on the skin.

Arsenical—having to do with arsenic.

Arteriosclerosis—a hardening of the arteries.

Arthritis—an inflammation of a joint.

Ascariasis—a condition caused by roundworms in the intestine.

Ascaricide—an agent that kills roundworms of the genus *Ascaris*.

Aspergillus—a fungi genus including many types of molds.

Astasia—the ability to stand up without help.

Asthma—a disease characterized by recurring breathing difficulty due to bronchial muscle constriction.

Astringent—a mild protein precipitant suitable for local application to toughen, shrink, blanch, wrinkle and harden tissue, diminish secretions, and coagulate blood.

Ataractic—an agent having a quieting, tranquilizing effect.

Ataxia—incoordination, especially of gait.

Atheroma—a fatty granular degeneration of an artery wall.

Atrophy—a wasting away.

Avitaminosis—a disease caused by lack of one or more vitamins in the diet.

Axilla—armpit.

Bacteriostatic—an agent that inhibits the growth of bacteria.

Basedow's disease—a form of hyperthyroidism, also known as Grave's disease and Parry's disease.

Biliary Colic—a sharp pain in the upper right side of the abdomen due to a gallstone impaction.

Bilirubin—a bile pigment.

Biliuria—the presence of bile in the urine.

Blood Calcium Regulator—a drug that maintains the blood level of ionic calcium, especially by regulating its metabolic disposition elsewhere.

Blood Volume Supporter—an intravenous solution whose solutes are retained in the vascular system to supplement the osmotic activity of plasma proteins.

Bradycardia—a slow heart rate.

Bright's Disease—a disease of the kidneys, including the presence of edema and excessive urine protein formation.

Bromidrosis—foul smelling perspiration.

Bronchitis—an inflammation of the bronchi.

Bronchodilator—a drug which can dilate the lumina of air passages of the lungs.

Bruit—an arterial sound audible with a stethoscope.

Buerger's Disease—a thromboangiitis obliterans inflammation of the walls and surrounding tissue of the veins and arteries.

Bursitis—an inflammation of the bursa.

Callus—a hard bonelike material developing around a fractured bone.

Calmative—a sedative.

Candidiasis—an infection by the yeastlike organism *Candida albicans*.

Carbonic Anhydrase Inhibitor—an enzyme inhibitor, the therapeutic effects of which are diuresis and reduced formation of intraocular fluid.

Carcinoma—a malignant growth.

Cardiac Depressant—a drug that depresses myocardial function so as to supress rhythmic irregularities characterized by fast rate; an antiarrythmic.

Cardiac Stimulant—a drug that increases the contractile force of the myocardium, especially in weakened conditions such as congestive heart failure; a cardiotonic.

Cardiopathy—a disease of the heart.

Caries—decay of the teeth.

Carminative—an aromatic or pungent drug that mildly irritates the gastrointestinal tract and is useful in the treatment of flatulence and colic. Peppermint Water is a common carminative.

Caruncle—a small fleshy projection on the skin.

Cathartic—a drug that promotes defecation, usually by enhancing peristalsis or by softening and lubricating the feces.

Caudal—pertains to the distal end or tail.

Caustic—a topical drug that destroys tissue on contact and is suitable for removal of abnormal skin growths.

Central Depressant—a drug that reduces the functional state of the central nervous system and with increasing dosage induces sedation, hypnosis, and general anesthesia; respiration is depressed.

Central Stimulant—a drug that increases the functional state of the central nervous system and with increasing dosage induces restlessness, insomnia, disorientation, and convulsions; respiration is stimulated.

Cerebral—pertaining to the brain.

Cerumen—earwax.

Chloasma—skin discoloration.

Cholagogue—a drug that stimulates the emptying of the gallbladder and the flow of bile into the duodenum.

Choleciptitis—an inflammation of the gallbladder.

Cholecystokinetic—an agent that promotes emptying of the gallbladder.

Cholelithiasis—the presence of calculi (stones) in the gallbladder.

Choleretic—a drug that increases the production and secretion of dilute bile by the liver.

Chorea—a disorder, usually of childhood, characterized by uncontrolled spasmotic muscle movements; sometimes referred to as St. Vitus' dance.

Chymotrypsin—a proteinase in the gastrointestinal tract; proposed use has been treatment of edema and inflammation.

Claudication—limping.

Climacteric—a time period in women just preceding termination of the reproductive processes.

Clonus—a spasm in which rigidity and relaxation succeed each other.

Coagulant—a drug that replaces a deficient blood factor necessary for coagulation; clotting factor.

Coccidiostat—a drug used in the treatment of coccidal (protozoal) infections in animals, especially birds; used in veterinary medicine.

Colitis—an inflammation of the colon.

Colloid—a disperse system of particles larger than those of true solutions but smaller than those of suspensions (1 to 100 millimicrons in size).

Collyrium—an eyewash.

Colostomy—the surgical formation of a more or less permanent opening into the colon.

Corticoid—a term applied to hormones of the adrenal cortex or any substance, natural or synthetic, having similar activity.

Corticosteroid—a steroid produced by the adrenal cortex.

Coryza—a headcold.

Counterirritant—an agent (irritant) which causes irritation of the part to which it is applied, and draws blood away from a deep seated area.

Cranial—pertaining to the skull.

Crepitation—the grating of a joint.

Cryptitis—an inflammation of a follicle or glandular tubule, usually in the rectum.

Cryptococcus—a genus of fungi which does not produce spores, but reproduces by budding.

Cryptorchidism—the failure of one or both testes to descend.

Cutaneous—pertaining to the skin.

Cyanosis—a blue or purple skin discoloration due to oxygen deficiency.

Cycloplegia—the loss of accommodation.

Cyclopegic—a drug which paralyzes accommodation of the eye.

Cystitis—an inflammation of the bladder.

Cystourethography—the examination by x-ray of the bladder and urethra.

Cytostasis—a slowing of the movement of blood cells at an inflamed area, sometimes causing capillary blockage.

Debridement—the cutting away of dead or excess skin from a wound.

Decongestant—a drug which reduces congestion caused by an accumulation of blood.

Decubitus—the patient's position in bed; the act of lying down.

Demulcent—an agent used generally internally to sooth and protect mucous membranes.

Dermatitis—an inflammation of the skin.

Dermatomycosis—lesions or eruptions caused by fungi on the skin.

Detergent—an emulsifying agent useful for cleansing wounds and ulcers as well as the skin.

Dextrocardia—when the heart is located on the right side of the chest.

Diagnostic Aid—a drug used to determine the functional state of a body organ or the presence of a disease.

Diaphoretic—a drug used to increase perspiration; a hydrotic or sudorfice.

Diarrhea—an abnormal frequency and fluidity of stools.

Digestive Enzyme—an enzyme that promotes digestion by supplementing the naturally occurring counterpart.

Digitalization—the administration of digitalis to obtain a desired tissue level of drug.

Diplopia—double vision.

Disinfectant—an agent that destroys pathogenic microorganisms on contact and is suitable for sterilizing inanimate objects.

Distal—farthest from a point of reference.

Diuretic—a drug that promotes renal excretion of electrolytes and water, thereby increasing urine volume.

Dysarthia—difficulty in speech articulation.

Dysmenorrhea—pertaining to painful menstruation.

Dysphagia—difficulty in swallowing.

Dyspnea—difficult breathing.

Ecbolic—a drug used to stimulate the gravid uterus to the expulsion of the fetus, or to cause uterine contraction; an oxytocic.

Eclampsia—a toxic disorder occurring late in pregnancy involving hypertension, weight gain, edema and renal dysfunction.

Ectasia—pertaining to distension or stretching.Ectopic—out of place.

Ectopic—out of place; not in normal position.

Eczema—an inflammatory disease of the skin with infiltrations, watery discharge, scales and crust.

Effervescent—bubbling; sparkling; giving off gas bubbles.

Embolus—a blood clot in the blood stream lodged in a vessel, thus obstructing circulation.

Emetic—a drug that induces vomiting, either locally by gastrointestinal irritation or systemically by stimulation of receptors in the central nervous system.

Emollient—a topical drug, especially an oil or fat, used to soften the skin and make it more pliable.

Encometrium—the uterine mucous membrane.

Enteralgia—an intestinal pain.

Enterobiasis—a pinworm infestation.

Enuresis—involuntary urination, as in bedwetting.

Epidermis—the outermost layer of the skin.

Episiotomy—a surgical incision of the vulva when deemed necessary during childbirth.

Epistaxis—a nosebleed.

Erythema—redness.

Erythrocyte—a red blood cell.

Escharotic—corrosive.

Estrogen—a hormone that stimulates and maintains female secondary sex characteristics and functions in the menstrual cycle to promote uterine gland proliferation.

Etiology—the cause of a disease.

Euphoria—an exaggerated feeling of well being.

Eutonic—having normal muscular tone.

Exfoliation—a scaling of the skin.

Exophthalmos—a protrusion of the eyeballs.

Expectorant—a drug that increases secretion of respiratory tract fluid, thereby lowering its viscosity and cough-inducing irritancy and promoting its ejection.

Extension—the movement of a joint to move 2 body parts away from each other.

Exteroceptors—receptors on the exterior of the body.

Fasiculations—the visible twitching movements of muscle bundles.

Fibroid—a tumor of fibrous tissue, resembling fibers.

Filariasis—the condition of having round worm parasites reproducing in the body tissues.

Fistula—an abnormal opening leading from a body cavity to the outside of the body or to another cavity.

Flexion—the movement of a joint in which 2 moveable parts are brought toward each other.

Fungistatic—inhibiting the growth of fungi.

Furunculosis—a condition marked by the presence of boils.

Gallop Rhythm—a heart condition where 3 separate beats are heard instead of 2.

Gastralgia—a stomach pain.

Gastritis—inflammation of the stomach lining.

Gastrocele—a hernial protrusion of the stomach.

Gastrodynia—pain in the stomach, a stomach ache.

Geriatrics—a branch of medicine which treats problems peculiar to old age.

Germicidal—an agent that is destructive to pathogenic microorganisms.

Gingivitis—an inflammation of the gums.

Glaucoma—a disease of the eye evidenced by an increase in intraoccular pressure and resulting in hardness of the eye, atrophy of the retina and eventual blindness.

Glossitis—an inflammation of the tongue.

Glucocorticoid—a corticoid which increases gluconeogenesis, thereby raising the concentration of liver glycogen and blood sugar.

Glycosuria—an abnormal quantity of glucose in the urine.

Gout—a disorder which is symptomized by a high uric acid level and sudden onset recurrent arthritis.

Granulation—the formation of small round fleshy granules on a wound in the healing process.

Hematemesis—the vomiting of blood.

Hematinic—a drug that promotes hemoglobin formation by supplying a factor essential for its synthesis.

Hemiplegia—a condition in which one side of the body is paralyzed.

Hematopoietic—a drug that stimulates formation of blood cells, especially by supplying deficient vitamins.

Hemoptysis—bleeding in the lungs.

Histoplasmosis—a lung infection caused by the inhalation of fungus spores, often resulting in pneumonitis.

Hodgkin's Disease—a disease marked by chronic lymph node enlargement sometimes including spleen and liver enlargement.

Hydrocholeresis—putting out a thinner, more watery bile.

Hypercholesterolemia—the condition of having an abnormally large amount of cholesterol in the body cells.

Hemorrhage—copious bleeding.

Hemostatic—a locally acting drug that arrests hemorrhage by promoting clot formation or by serving as a mechanical matrix for a clot.

Hepatitis—an inflammation of the liver.

Hyperemia—an excess of blood in any part of the body.

Hyperesthesia—an increase in sensations.

Hyperglycemic—a drug that elevates blood glucose level, especially for the treatment of hypoglycemic states.

Hypertension—blood pressure above the normally accepted limits, high blood pressure.

Hypertriglyceridemia—an increased level of triglycerides in the blood.

Hypnotic—a central depressant which, with suitable dosage, induces sleep.

Hypodermoclysis—a subcutaneous injection with a solution.

Hypoesthesia—a diminished touch of sensation.

Hypoglycemic—a drug that promotes glucose metabolism and lowers blood glucose level, useful in the control of diabetes mellitus.

Hypokalemia—an abnormally small concentration of potassium ions in the blood.

Hyposensitize—to reduce the sensitivity to an agent, referring to allergies.

Hypotensive—a drug which diminishes tension or pressure, to lower blood pressure.

Ichthyosis—an inherited skin disease characterized by dryness and scales.

Idiopathic—denoting a disease of unknown cause.

Ileostomy—the establishment of an opening from the ileum to the outside of the body.

Immune Serum—a biological drug containing antibodies for a pathogenic microorganism, useful for passive immunization against the associated disease.

Immunizing Agent, active—an antigenic preparation (toxoid or vaccine) used to induce formation of specific antibodies against a pathogenic microorganism, which provides delayed but permanent protection against the associated disease.

Immunizing Agent, passive—a biological preparation (antitoxin, antivenin or immune serum) containing specific antibodies against a pathogenic microorganism, which provides immediate but temporary protection against the associated disease.

Impetigo—an inflammatory skin disease with isolated pustules.

Insulin—one of the hormones that regulate carbohydrate metabolism, used as replacement therapy in diabetes mellitus.

Inversion—a turning inward.

Irrigating solution—a solution for washing body surfaces and/or various body cavities.

Isoniazid—a compound effective in tuberculosis treatment.

Kakidrosis—foul smelling perspiration.

Keratitis—an inflammation of the cornea.

Keratolytic—a topical drug that softens the superficial keratin-containing layer of the skin to promote exfoliation.

Lacrimal—pertaining to tears.

Laxative—a gentle purgative medicine; a mild cathartic.

Leishmaniasis—a number of types of infections transmitted by sandflies.

Leucocytopenia—a decrease in the number of white cells.

Leucocytosis—an increased white cell count.

Leukoderma—an absence of pigment from the skin.

Libido—sexual desire or creative energy.

Leucocyte—a white blood cell.

Lipoma—a fatty tumor.

Lipotropic—a drug, especially one supplementing a dietary factor, that prevents the abnormal accumulation of fat in the liver.

Lochia—a vaginal discharge of mucus, blood and tissue after childbirth.

Lues—a plague; specifically syphilis.

Macrocyte—a large red blood cell.

Malaise—a general felling of illness.

Melasma—a darkening of the skin.

Melena—black feces from altered blood in the higher CIT.

Meninges—the membranes covering the brain and spinal cord.

Metastasis—the shifting of a disease or its symptoms from one part of the body to another.

Mastitis—an inflammation of the breast.

Miotics—agents which constrict the pupil of the eye; a myotic.

Moniliasis—an infection with any of the species of monilia types of fungi (Candida).

Mucolytic—an agent that can destroy or disolve mucous membrane secretions.

Myalgia—a pain in the muscles.

Myasthenia Gravis—a chronic progressive muscular weakness caused by myoneural conduction, usually spreading from the face and throat.

Myelocyte—an immature white blood cell in the bone marrow.

Myelogenous—originating in bone marrow.

Myoclonus—involuntary, sudden and rapid unpredictable jerks; faster than chorea.

Mydriatic—a drug that dilates the pupil of the eye, usually by anticholinergic or adrenergic mechanism.

Myoneural—pertaining to muscle and nerve.

Myopia—nearsightedness.

Narcotic—a drug that produces insensibility or stupor; a class of drug regulated by law.

Neonatal—pertaining to the first four weeks of life.

Neoplasm—an abnormal tissue growing more rapidly than usual showing a lack of structural organization.

Nephritis—an inflammation of the kidney.

Nephrosclerosis—a hardening of the kidney tissue.

Neuralgia—a pain extending along the course of one or more of the nerves.

Neurasthenia—nervous prostration.

Neuroglia—the supporting elements of the nervous system.

Neuroleptic—a substance that acts on the nervous system.

Neurosis—a functional disorder of the nervous system.

Nocturia—urination at night.

Normocytic—pertaining to anemia due to some defect in the blood-forming tissues.

Nuchal—the nape of the neck.

Nystagmus—a rhythmic oscillation of the eyes.

Oleaginous—oily or greasy.

Omphalitis—an inflammation of the navel in a newborn.

Onychomycosis—a ringworm or fungus infection of the nails.

Ophthalmic—pertaining to the eye.

Oral—pertaining to the mouth.

Orthopnea—a discomfort in bleeding in any but the upright sitting or standing positions.

Osmidrosis—foul smelling perspiration.

Ossification—a formation of, or conversion to, bone.

Osteomyelitis—an inflammation of the marrow of the bone.

Osteoporosis—a reduction in bone quantity; skeletal atrophy.

Otalgia—pain in the ear; an earache.

Otitis—inflammation of the ear.

Otomycosis—an ear infection caused by fungus.

Otorrhea—a discharge from the ear.

Oxytocic—a drug that selectively stimulates uterine motility and is useful in obstetrics, especially in the control of postpartum hemorrhage.

Ozochrotia—foul smelling perspiration.

Palpitations—an awareness of one's heart action.

Paget's Disease—a disease characterized by lesions around the nipple and areola found in elderly women.

Pallor—the lack of the normal red color imparted to the skin by the blood of the superficial vessels.

Parasympatholytic—See Anticholinergic.

Parasympathomimetic—See Cholinergic.

Parenteral—pertaining to the administration of a drug by means other than through the alimentary canal; subcutaneous, intramuscular or intravenous administration of drug.

Parkinsonism—a group of neurological disorders marked by hypokinesia, tremor, and muscular rigidity.

Paroxysm—a sudden recurrance of intensification of symptoms.

Pathogenic—giving origin to disease.

Pediatric—pertaining to children's diseases.

Pediculicide—an insecticide suitable for erradicating louse infestations in humans (pediculosis).

Pediculosis—an infestation with lice.

Pellagra—a condition characterized by GI disturbances, mental disorders, and skin redness and scaling.

Pernicious—particularly dangerous or harmful.

Phlebitis—an inflammation of a vein.

Pleurisy—an inflammation of the membrane surrounding the lungs and the thoracic cavity.

Pneumonia—an infection of the lungs.

Poikilocytosis—a condition in which pointed or irregularly shaped red blood cells are found in the blood.

Polydipsia—excessive thirst.

Posology—the science of dosage.

Posterior Pituitary Hormone(s)—a multifunctional hormone with oxytocic-milk ejectory, and antidiuretic-vasopressor fractions.

Progestin—a hormone that functions in the menstrual cycle and during pregnancy to promote uterine gland secretion and to reduce uterine motility.

Pronation—the act of turning the palm downward or backward.

Prophylactic—a remedy that tends to prevent disease.

Protectant—a topical drug that remains on the skin and serves as a physical barrier to the environment.

Proteolytic Enzyme—an enzyme used to liquefy fibrinous or purulent exudates.

Psoriasis—an inflammatory skin disease accompanied with itching.

Psychotherapeutic—a drug that selectively affects the central nervous system to alter emotional state. See Antidepressant; Tranquilizer.

Ptosis—a drooping or sagging of the muscle.

Pulmonary—pertaining to the lungs.

Purulent—containing or forming pus.

Pyelitis—a local inflammation of renal and pelvic cells due to bacterial infection.

Pylorospasm—a spasmodic muscle contraction of a sphincter.

Pyoderma—any skin discharge characterized by pus formation.

Radiopaque Medium—a diagnostic drug, opaque to X rays, whose retention in a body organ or cavity makes X-ray visualization possible.

Reynaud's Phenomenon—spasms of the digital arteries with blanching and numbness of the fingers, usually with another disease.

Reflex Stimulant—a mild irritant suitable for application to the nasopharynx to induce reflex respiratory stimulation.

Rheumatoid—a condition resembling rheumatism.

Rhinitis—an inflammation of the mucous membrane of the nose.

Rubefacient—a topical drug that induces mild skin irritation with erythema, sometimes used to relieve the discomfort of deep-seated inflammation.

Rubeola—a synonym popularly used for both measles and rubella.

Saprophytic—getting nourishment from dead material.

Sarcoma—a malignant tumor derived from connective tissue.

Scabicide—an insecticide suitable for the

erradication of itch mite infestations in humans (scabies).

Schistosomacide—an agent which destroys schistosomes; destructive to the trematodic parasites or flukes.

Schistosomiasis—an infection with *Schistosoma haematobium* involving the urinary tract and causing cystitis and hematuria.

Scintillation—a visual sensation manifested by an emission of sparks.

Sclerosing Agent—an irritant suitable for injection into varicose veins to induce their fibrosis and obliteration.

Scotomata—an area of varying size and shape within the visual field in which vision is absent or depressed.

Seborrhea—a condition arising from an excess secretion of sebum.

Sebum—the secretions of the fatty glands.

Sedative—a central depressant which, in suitable dosage, induces mild relaxation useful in treating tension.

Sinusitis—an inflammation of a sinus.

Skeletal Muscle Relaxant—a drug that inhibits contraction of voluntary muscles, usually by interfering with their innervation.

Smooth Muscle Relaxant—a drug that inhibits contraction of involuntary (e.g., visceral) muscles, usually by action upon their contractile elements.

Sociopath—a psychopathic person who, due to his unaccepted attitudes, is badly adjusted to society.

Spasmolytic—an agent that relieves spasms and involuntary contraction of a muscle; an antispasmodic.

Sputum—mucous spit from the mouth.

Stenosis—the narrowing of the lumen of a blood vessel.

Stomachic—a drug which is used to stimulate the appetite and gastric secretion.

Stomatitis—an inflammation of the mouth.

Subcutaneous—under the skin.

Sudorific—causing perspiration.

Superacidity—an increase of the normal acidity of the gastric secretion; hyperacidity.

Supination—the act of turning the palm forward or upward.

Suppressant—a drug useful in the control, rather than the cure, of a disease.

Surfactant—a surface active agent that decreases the surface tension between two miscible liquids; used to prepare emulsions, act as a cleansing agent, etc.

Synarthrosis (fibrous joint)—a joint in which the bony elements are united by continuous fibrous tissue.

Syncope—fainting.

Synovia—clear fluid which lubricates the joints; joint oil.

Systole—the ventricular contraction phase of a heartbeat.

Tachycardia—a rapid contraction rate of the heart.

Taeniacide—an agent used to kill tapeworms.

Taeniafuge—an agent used to expel tapeworms.

Therapeutic—A remedy for the treatment of disease.

Thoracic—pertaining to the chest.

Thyroid Hormone—a drug containing one or more of the iodinated amino acids that stimulate and regulate the metabolic rate and functional state of body tissues.

Thyroid Inhibitor—a drug that reduces excessive thyroid hormone production, usually by blocking synthesis of iodinated amino acids.

Tics—a repetitive twitching of muscles, often in the face and upper trunk.

Tinea—a fungal infection of the skin.

Tonic—an agent used to stimulate the restoration of tone to muscle tissue.

Tonometry—the measurement of tension in some part of the body.

Topical—the local external application of a drug to a particular place.

Toxoid—a modified bacterial toxin, less toxic than the original form, used to induce active immunity to bacterial pathogens.

Tranquilizer—a psychotherapeutic drug that induces emotional repose without significant sedation, useful in treating certain neuroses and psychoses.

Tremors—involuntary rhythmic tremulous movements.

Trichomoniasis—an infestation with parasitic flagellate protozoa of the genus *Trichomonas*.

Trypanosomiasis—a disease caused by protozoan flagellates in the blood.

Uricosuric—a drug that promotes renal excretion of uric acid, useful in the treatment of gout.

Urolithiasis—a condition marked by the formation of stones in the urinary tract.

Urticaria—a rash of hives generally of systemic origin.

Vaccine—a preparation containing live attenuated or dead pathogenic microorganisms, used to induce active immunity.

Vasoconstrictor—an adrenergic drug used locally in the nose to constrict blood vessels and reduce tissue congestion.

Vasodilator—a drug that relaxes vascular smooth muscles, expecially for the purpose of improving peripheral or coronary blood flow.

Vasopressor—an andrenergic drug used systemically to constrict blood vessels and raise blood pressure.

Verruca—a wart.

Vertigo—dizziness, giddiness.

Vesicant—an agent which when applied to the skin causes blistering and the formation of vesicles; an epispastic.

Visceral—pertaining to the internal organs.

Vitamin—an organic chemical essential in small amounts for normal body metabolism, used therapeutically to supplement the naturally occurring counterpart in foods.

TITLE CHANGES FOR U.S.P. XXI AND THE N.F. XVI MONOGRAPHS

The following official monograph title changes appear in: (1) U.S.P. XXI–N.F. XVI, the official compendia published by the U.S. Pharmacopeial Convention, Inc, together in a single binding, which became official on January 1, 1985. U.S.P. consulted with the U.S. Adopted Names (USAN) Council and also with interested parties from industry and government in deciding upon the announced names.

Among the more significant title changes are diiodohydroxyquin to iodoquinol, dioctyl sodium sulfosuccinate to docusate sodium (and the calcium salt to docusate calcium), gamma benzene hexachloride to lindane, iodochlorhydroxyquin to clioquinol, and levarterenol bitartrate to norepinephrine bitartrate.

The listing of changes in U.S.P. and N.F. titles is added as an aid to the practitioner in identifying drug products.

New Title in U.S.P. XXI[1] or N.F. XVI[2]	Former Official Title
Albumin Human[1]	Normal Human Serum Albumin
Aluminum Acetate Topical Solution[1]	Aluminum Acetate Solution
Aluminum Subacetate Topical Solution[1]	Aluminum Subacetate Solution
Aminobenzoic Acid Topical Solution[1]	Aminobenzoic Acid Solution
Aminosalicylate Calcium[1]	Calcium Aminosalicylate
Aminosalicylate Calcium Capsules[1]	Calcium Aminosalicylate Capsules
Aminosalicylate Calcium Tablets[1]	Calcium Aminosalicylate Tablets
Aminosalicylate Potassium[1]	Potassium Aminosalicylate
Aminosalicylate Potassium Tablets[1]	Potassium Aminosalicylate Tablets
Aminosalicylate Sodium[1]	Sodium Aminosalicylate
Aminosalicylate Sodium Tablets[1]	Sodium Aminosalicylate Tablets
Antihemophilic Factor[1]	Human Antihemophilic Factor
Antipyrine and Benzocaine Otic Solution[1]	Glycerin Otic Solution
Antivenin (Crotalidae) Polyvalent[1]	Polyvalent Crotaline Antivenin
Antivenin (Latrodectus mactans)[1]	Widow Spider Species Antivenin (Latrodectus mactans)
Sterile Aurothioglucose Suspension[1]	Aurothioglucose Injection
Benzethonium Chloride Topical Solution[1]	Benzethonium Chloride Solution
Benzoic and Salicylic Acids Ointment[1]	Benzoic and Salicylic Acid Ointment
Betamethasone Valerate Topical Aerosol[1]	Betamethasone Valerate Aerosol
Blood Grouping Serums Anti-D, Anti-C, Anti-E, Anti-c, Anti-e[1]	Anti-Rh Typing Serums
Blood Group Specific Substances A, B, and AB[1]	Blood Group Specific Substances A and B
Blood Cells, Red[1]	Human Red Blood Cells
Blood, Whole[1]	Whole Human Blood
Bupivacaine and Epinephrine Injection[1]	Bupivacaine Hydrochloride and Epinephrine Injection
Butacaine Sulfate Topical Solution[1]	Butacaine Sulfate Solution
Calcium Hydroxide Topical Solution[1]	Calcium Hydroxide Solution
Candicidin Vaginal Tablets[1]	Candicidin Suppositories
Carbamide Peroxide Topical Solution[1]	Carbamide Peroxide Solution
Carbomer 934 P[2]	Carbomer
Carphenazine Maleate Oral Solution[1]	Carphenazine Maleate Solution
Cefamandole Nafate, Sterile[1]	Cefamandole Nafate
Microcrystalline Cellulose and Carboxymethylcellulose Sodium[2]	Microcrystalline Cellulose and Sodium Carboxymethylcellulose
Cephalothin Sodium, Sterile[1]	Cephalothin Sodium
Cetyl Esters Wax[2]	Synthetic Spermaceti
Cetylpyridinium Chloride Topical Solution[1]	Cetylpyridinium Chloride Solution
Clioquinol[1]	Iodochlorhydroxyquin
Clioquinol Cream[1]	Iodochlorhydroxyquin Cream
Clioquinol Ointment[1]	Iodochlorhydroxyquin Ointment
Compound Clioquinol Powder[1]	Compound Iodochlorhydroxyquin Powder
Clioquinol Tablets[1]	Iodochlorhydroxyquin Tablets
Cloxacillin Sodium for Oral Solution[1]	Cloxacillin Sodium for Solution
Coal Tar Topical Solution[1]	Coal Tar Solution
Cyanocobalamin Co 57 Oral Solution[1]	Cyanocobalamin Co 57 Solution
Cyanocobalamin Co 60 Solution[1]	Cyanocobalamin Co 60 Solution

New Title in U.S.P. XXI[1] or N.F. XVI[2]	Former Official Title
Cyclopentamine Hydrochloride Nasal Solution[1]	Cyclopentamine Hydrochloride Solution
Dehydrocholate Sodium Injection[1]	Sodium Dehydrocholate Injection
Dexamethasone Topical Aerosol[1]	Dexamethasone Aerosol
Diatrizoate Sodium Solution[1]	Diatrizoate Sodium Oral Solution
Diphenoxylate Hydrochloride and Atropine Sulfate Oral Solution[1]	Diphenoxylate Hydrochloride and Atropine Sulfate Oral Solution
Diphtheria Toxoid Adsorbed[1]	Adsorbed Diphtheria Toxoid
Diphtheria and Tetanus Toxoids Adsorbed[1]	Adsorbed Diphtheria and Tetanus Toxoids
Diphtheria and Tetanus Toxoids and Pertussis Vaccine Adsorbed[1]	Adsorbed Diphtheria and Tetanus Toxoids and Pertussis Vaccine
Docusate Calcium[1]	Dioctyl Calcium Sulfosuccinate
Docusate Calcium Capsules[1]	Dioctyl Calcium Sulfosuccinate Capsules
Docusate Sodium[1]	Dioctyl Sodium Sulfosuccinate
Docusate Sodium Capsules[1]	Dioctyl Sodium Sulfosuccinate Capsules
Docusate Sodium Solution[1]	Dioctyl Sodium Sulfosuccinate Solution
Docusate Sodium Syrup[1]	Dioctyl Sodium Sulfosuccinate Syrup
Docusate Sodium Tablets[1]	Dioctyl Sodium Sulfosuccinate Tablets
Dyclonine Hydrochloride Topical Solution[1]	Dyclonine Hydrochloride Solution
Epinephrine Inhalation Solution[1]	Epinephrine Inhalation
Ergocalciferol Oral Solution[1]	Ergocalciferol Solution
Erythrosine Sodium Topical Solution[1]	Erythrosine Sodium Solution
Estropipate[1]	Piperazine Estrone Sulfate
Estropipate Vaginal Cream[1]	Piperazine Estrone Sulfate Vaginal Cream
Estropipate Tablets[1]	Piperazine Estrone Sulfate Tablets
Ethiodized Oil Injection[1]	Ethiodized Oil
Fluorescein Sodium Ophthalmic Strips[1]	Fluorescein Sodium Ophthalmic Strip
Gentian Violet Topical Solution[1]	Gentian Violet Solution
Glucose Enzymatic Test Strip[1]	Glucose Oxidase Reagent Strip
Glycine[1]	Aminoacetic Acid
Glycine Irrigation[1]	Aminoacetic Acid Irrigation
Guaifenesin[1]	Glyceryl Guaiacolate
Guaifenesin Capsules[1]	Glyceryl Guaiacolate Capsules
Guaifenesin Syrup[1]	Glyceryl Guaiacolate Syrup
Guaifenesin Tablets[1]	Glyceryl Guaiacolate Tablets
Haloperidol Oral Solution[1]	Haloperidol Solution
Hexachlorophene Cleansing Emulsion[1]	Hexachlorophene Detergent Lotion
Hexylcaine Hydrochloride Topical Solution[1]	Hexylcaine Hydrochloride Solution
Hydrocortisone[1]	Cortisol
Hydrocortisone Acetate[1]	Cortisol Acetate
Hydrocortisone Acetate Cream[1]	Cortisol Acetate Cream
Hydrocortisone Acetate Ointment[1]	Cortisol Acetate Ointment
Hydrocortisone Acetate Ophthalmic Ointment[1]	Cortisol Acetate Ophthalmic Ointment
Hydrocortisone Acetate Ophthalmic Suspension[1]	Cortisol Acetate Ophthalmic Suspension
Sterile Hydrocortisone Acetate Suspension[1]	Sterile Cortisol Acetate Suspension
Hydrocortisone Cream[1]	Cortisol Cream
Hydrocortisone Cypionate[1]	Cortisol Cypionate
Hydrocortisone Cypionate Oral Suspension[1]	Cortisol Cypionate Oral Suspension
Hydrocortisone Enema[1]	Cortisol Enema
Hydrocortisone Hemisuccinate[1]	Cortisol Hemisuccinate
Hydrocortisone Lotion[1]	Cortisol Lotion
Hydrocortisone Ointment[1]	Cortisol Ointment
Hydrocortisone Sodium Phosphate[1]	Cortisol Sodium Phosphate
Hydrocortisone Sodium Phosphate Injection[1]	Cortisol Sodium Phosphate Injection
Hydrocortisone Sodium Succinate[1]	Cortisol Sodium Succinate
Hydrocortisone Sodium Succinate for Injection[1]	Cortisol Sodium Succinate for Injection
Sterile Hydrocortisone Suspension[1]	Sterile Cortisol Suspension
Hydrocortisone Tablets[1]	Cortisol Tablets
Immune Globulin[1]	Immune Human Serum Globulin
Rh$_0$ (D) Immune Globulin[1]	Rh$_0$ (D) Immune Human Globulin
Hydrogen Peroxide Topical Solution[1]	Hydrogen Peroxide Solution
Hydroquinone Cream[1]	Hydroquinone Ointment

New Title in U.S.P. XXI[1] or N.F. XVI[2]	Former Official Title
Iodine Topical Solution[1]	Iodine Solution
Iodinated I-125 Albumin Injection[1]	Iodinated I-125 Serum Albumin
Iodinated I-131 Albumin Injection[1]	Iodinated I-131 Serum Albumin
Iodinated I-131 Albumin Aggregated Injection[1]	Macroaggregated Iodinated I-131 Serum Albumin
Rose Bengal Sodium I-131 Injection[1]	Sodium Rose Bengal I-131 Injection
Iodoquinol[1]	Diiodohydroxyquin
Iodoquinol Tablets[1]	Diiodohydroxyquin Tablets
Isoetharine Inhalation Solution[1]	Isoetharine Hydrochloride Inhalation
Isoproterenol Inhalation Solution[1]	Isoproterenol Hydrochloride Inhalation
Isoproterenol Sulfate Inhalation Aerosol[1]	Isoproterenol Sulfate Aerosol
Lidocaine Topical Aerosol[1]	Lidocaine Aerosol
Sulfurated Lime Topical Solution[1]	Sulfurated Lime Solution
Lindane[1]	Gamma Benzene Hexachloride
Lindane Cream[1]	Gamma Benzene Hexachloride Cream
Lindane Lotion[1]	Gamma Benzene Hexachloride Lotion
Magnesium Citrate Oral Solution[1]	Magnesium Citrate Solution
Measles Virus Vaccine Live[1]	Live Attenuated Measles Virus Vaccine
Measles, Mumps, and Rubella Virus Vaccine Live[1]	Live Measles, Mumps, and Rubella Virus Vaccine
Measles and Rubella Virus Vaccine Live[1]	Live Measles and Rubella Virus Vaccine
Mepenzolate Bromide Syrup[1]	Mepenzolate Bromide Oral Solution
Methadone Hydrochloride Oral Concentrate[1]	Methadone Hydrochloride Oral Solution
Methenamine and Monobasic Sodium Phosphate Tablets[1]	Methenamine and Sodium Biphosphate Tablets
Methicillin Sodium, Sterile[1]	Methicillin Sodium
Metocurine Iodide[1]	Dimethyl Tubocurarine Iodide
Metocurine Iodide Injection[1]	Dimethyl Tubocurarine Iodide Injection
Minocycline Hydrochloride Oral Suspension[1]	Minocycline Hydrochloride Syrup
Monobasic Sodium Phosphate[1]	Sodium Biphosphate
Mumps Virus Vaccine Live[1]	Live Mumps Virus Vaccine
Neomycin and Polymyxin B Sulfates Solution for Irrigation[1]	Neomycin Sulfate and Polymyxin B Sulfate Solution for Irrigation
Neomycin and Polymyxin B Sulfates and Bacitracin Zinc Ointment[1]	Neomycin Sulfate, Polymyxin B Sulfate, and Bacitracin Zinc Ointment
Neomycin and Polymyxin B Sulfates and Hydrocortisone Otic Solution[1]	Neomycin and Polymyxin B Sulfates and Cortisol Otic Solution
Neomycin and Polymyxin B Sulfates and Hydrocortisone Otic Suspension[1]	Neomycin and Polymyxin B Sulfates and Cortisol Otic Suspension
Nitrofurazone Topical Solution[1]	Nitrofurazone Solution
Nitromersol Topical Solution[1]	Nitromersol Solution
Norepinephrine Bitartrate[1]	Levarterenol Bitartrate
Norepinephrine Bitartrate Injection[1]	Levarterenol Bitartrate Injection
Nortriptyline Hydrochloride Oral Solution[1]	Nortriptyline Hydrochloride Solution
Octoxynol 9[2]	Octoxynol
Penicillin G Potassium Tablets for Oral Solution[1]	Penicillin G Potassium Tablets for Solution
Penicillin G Sodium, Sterile[1]	Penicillin G Sodium
Penicillin G Procaine, Sterile[1]	Penicillin G Procaine
Perphenazine Oral Solution[1]	Perphenazine Solution
Pertussis Immune Globulin[1]	Pertussis Immune Human Globulin
Pertussis Vaccine Adsorbed[1]	Adsorbed Pertussis Vaccine
Plasma Protein Fraction[1]	Human Plasma Protein Fraction
Plicamycin[1]	Mithramycin
Plicamycin for Injection[1]	Mithramycin for Injection
Poliovirus Vaccine Inactivated[1]	Poliomyelitis Vaccine
Poliovirus Vaccine Live Oral[1]	Live Oral Poliovirus Vaccine
Polyoxyl 50 Stearate[2]	Polyoxyethylene 50 Stearate
Potassium Chloride in Dextrose Injection[1]	Dextrose and Potassium Chloride Injection
Potassium Iodide Oral Solution[1]	Potassium Iodide Solution
Potassium Permanganate Tablets for Topical Solution[1]	Potassium Permanganate Tablets for Solution

TITLE CHANGES FOR U.S.P. XXI AND N.F. XVI MONOGRAPHS

684

New Title in U.S.P. XXI[1] or N.F. XVI[2]	Former Official Title
Povidone-Iodine Topical Aerosol Solution[1]	Povidone-Iodine Aerosol
Povidone-Iodine Topical Solution[1]	Povidone-Iodine Solution
Prednisolone Hemisuccinate[1]	Prednisolone Succinate
Prochlorperazine Edisylate Oral Solution[1]	Prochlorperazine Edisylate Solution
Promazine Hydrochloride Oral Solution[1]	Promazine Hydrochloride Solution
Propoxycaine and Procaine Hydrochlorides and Levonordefrin Injection[1]	Procaine and Propoxycaine Hydrochlorides and Levonordefrin Injection
Propoxycaine and Procaine Hydrochlorides and Norepinephrine Bitartrate Injection[1]	Procaine and Propoxycaine Hydrochlorides and Levarterenol Bitartrate Injection
Racemethionine[1]	Methionine
Racemethionine Capsules[1]	Methionine Capsules
Racemethionine Tablets	Methionine Tablets
Ringer's Irrigation[1]	Ringer's Solution
Rolitetracycline, Sterile[1]	Rolitetracycline
Rubella Virus Vaccine Live[1]	Live Rubella Virus Vaccine
Rubella and Mumps Virus Vaccine Live[1]	Live Rubella and Mumps Virus Vaccine
Sennosides[1]	Sennosides A and B
Sennosides Tablets[1]	Sennosides A and B Tablets
Sodium Chloride Inhalation Solution[1]	Sodium Chloride Inhalation
Sodium Citrate and Citric Acid Oral Solution[1]	Sodium Citrate and Citric Acid Solution[3]
Sodium Fluoride Oral Solution[1]	Sodium Fluoride Solution[3]
Sodium Fluoride and Phosphoric Acid Gel[1]	Sodium Fluoride and Orthophosphoric Acid Gel
Sodium Fluoride and Phosphoric Acid Topical Solution[1]	Sodium Fluoride and Orthophosphoric Acid Solution
Sodium Phosphate, Monobasic[1]	Sodium Biphosphate
Sodium Phosphates Enema[1]	Sodium Phosphate and Biphosphate Enema
Sodium Phosphates Oral Solution[1]	Sodium Phosphate and Biphosphate Oral Solution
Technetium Tc 99m Albumin Aggregated Injection[1]	Technetium Tc 99m Aggregated Albumin
Sodium Pertechnetate Tc 99m Injection[1]	Sodium Pertechnetate Tc 99m Solution
Technetium Tc 99m Ferpentetate Injection[1]	Technetium Tc 99m Iron Ascorbate Pentetic Acid Complex Injection
Technetium Tc 99m Pentetate Injection[1]	Technetium Tc 99m Pentetate Sodium Injection
Technetium Tc 99m Gluceptate Injection[1]	Technetium Tc 99m Sodium Gluceptate Injection
Tetanus Immune Globulin[1]	Tetanus Immune Human Globulin
Tetanus Toxoid Adsorbed[1]	Adsorbed Tetanus Toxoid
Tetanus and Diphtheria Toxoids Adsorbed for Adult Use[1]	Adsorbed Tetanus and Diphtheria Toxoids for Adult Use
Theophylline Olamine Enema[1]	Theophylline Olamine Solution
Thimerosal Topical Aerosol[1]	Thimerosal Aerosol
Thimerosal Topical Solution[1]	Thimerosal Solution
Thioridazine Hydrochloride Oral Solution[1]	Thioridazine Hydrochloride Solution
Thiothixene Hydrochloride Oral Solution[1]	Thiothixene Hydrochloride Solution
Tolnaftate Topical Solution[1]	Tolnaftate Solution
Triamcinolone Acetonide Topical Aerosol[1]	Triamcinolone Acetonide Aerosol
Trolamine[2]	Triethanolamine
Crystallized Trypsin[1]	Trypsin Crystallized
Crystallized Trypsin for Inhalation Aerosol[1]	Trypsin Crystallized for Aerosol
Tuaminoheptane Sulfate Nasal Solution[1]	Tuaminoheptane Sulfate Solution
Vaccinia Immune Globulin[1]	Vaccinia Immune Human Globulin
Xylometazoline Hydrochloride Nasal Solution[1]	Xylometazoline Hydrochloride Solution
Zinc Oxide and Salicylic Acid Paste[1]	Zinc Oxide Paste with Salicylic Acid

CONTAINER REQUIREMENTS FOR U.S.P. XXI DRUGS*

Legend:

WC = well closed container	LR = light resistant container
T = tight container	+ = controlled temperature

a = tablets	g = ointment	m = vaginal tablets	t = gel
b = capsules	h = lotion	n = lozenges	v = otic
c = solution	i = suppository	o = powder	w = intraocular solution
d = syrup	j = suspension	p = enema	
e = elixir	k = ophthalmic	r = inhalation	
f = cream	l = aerosol	s = nasal	

Drug (Dosage Form)	WC	T	LR	Drug (Dosage Form)	WC	T	LR
Acetaminophen		X[a b e j]		Aminosalicylate Sodium (tab)		X	X
Acetaminophen and Aspirin (tab)		X		Amitriptyline HCl (tab)	X		
Acetaminophen for Effervescent Oral Soln.		X		Aromatic Ammonia Spirit		X	X
Acetazolamide (tab)	X			Ammonium Chloride (tab)		X	
Acetic Acid Otic Soln.		X		Amobarbital	X[a]	X[e]	
Acetohexamide (tab)	X			Amobarbital Sodium (cap)		X	
Acetophenazine Maleate (tab)		X		Amodiaquine		X	
Acetylcysteine (soln)		X		Amodiaquine HCl (tab)		X	
Acetylcysteine and Isoproterenal HCl Inhalation Soln.		X		Amoxicillin		X[a b +]	
Acrisorcin (cream)		X		Amphetamine Sulfate (tab)		X	
Allupurinol (tab)	X			Amphotericin B	X[g h i]		
Alumina and Magnesia	X[a]	X[+ i]		Ampicillin (all dosage forms)		X	
Alumina and Magnesia and Carbonate	X[a]	X[+ i]		Ampicillin and Probenecid		X[b i j]	
Alumina and Magnesium Trisilicate		X[i]		Amprolium		X[o c]	
Aluminum Acetate Topical Soln.		X		Amyl Nitrate (inhalant)		X	X
Aluminum Hydroxide (gel)	X[a]	X[i]		Anileridine HCl (tab)		X	X
Aluminum Phosphate (gel)	X[a]	X[i]		Anthralin Ointment	X		X
Aluminum Subacetate Topical Solution		X		Antipyrine and Benzo- caine Otic Solution			X
Amantadine Hydrochloride		X[b d]		Apomorphine HCl (tab)		X	
Amcinonide		X[f g]		Ascorbic Acid		X[a c]	X[a c]
Amiloride HCl (tab)	X			Aspirin	X[i +]	X[a b]	
Amiloride HCl and Hydrochloro- thiazide (tab)	X			Atropine Sulfate	X[a]	X[k]	
Aminobenzoic Acid	X[t c]	X[t c]		Azothioprine (tab)			X
Aminobenzoate Potassium	X[b a]	X[c]		Bacampicillin HCl		X[a i]	
Aminocaproic Acid		X[a d]		Bacitracin (ointment)	X		
Aminoglutethimide (tab)	X			Bacitracin Zinc (ointment)	X[+]		
Aminophylline	X[i]	X[a]		Bacitracin Zinc and Polymixin B Sulfate (ointment)	X	X[k]	X
Aminosalicylate Calcium (cap)		X	X	Barium Sulfate	X[i]		

*The listing of container requirements for Compendial drugs is included as an aid to the practitioner in storing and dispensing.

Drug (Dosage Form)	WC	T	LR
Belladonna Extract (tab)		X	X
Belladonna (tincture)		X	X
Bendroflumethiazide (tab)		X	
Benoxinate HCl (opthalmic soln)		X	
Benaethonium Chloride Topical Solution (tincture)		X	X
Benzocaine HCl		X$^{f g}$	X$^{f g}$
Benzocaine Otic Soln		X	X
Benzocaine Topical		X$^{c i +}$	X$^{c +}$
Benzoic and Salicylic Acid (ointment)	X		
Cp. Benzointincture		X	X
Benzonatate (cap)		X	X
Benzoyl Peroxide		X$^{h t}$	
Benzthiazide (tab)		X	
Benztropine Mesylate (tab)	X		
Benzyl Benzoate (lot)		X	X
Benzylpenicilloyl Polylysine Concentrate		X	
Bephenium Hydroxy-naphthoate Oral Suspension		X	
Beta Carotene Caps		X	X
Betaine HCl	X		
Betamethasone	X$^{a d}$	X^{f}	
Betamethasone Benzoate (gel)		X	
Betamethasone Dipropionate	X^{g}	X$^{f h l}$	
Betamethasone Valerate		X$^{f g l}$	X^{h}
Bethanechol Chloride (tab)	X		
Biperiden HCl (tab)	X		
Bisacodyl	X$^{a i +}$		
Bromodiphen Hydramine HCl		X^{b}	X^{e}
Bromocriptine Mesylate		X^{a}	X^{a}
Brompheniramine Maleate	X^{e}	X^{a}	X^{e}
Busulfan (tab)	X		
Butabarbital Sodium	X$^{a b}$	X^{e}	
Calamine (lot)		X	
Calamine, Phenolated (lot)		X	
Calcifedol (cap)		X	X
Calcium Carbonate, Precipitated (tab)	X		
Calcium Carbonate and Magnesia	X^{a}		
Calcium and Magnesium Carbonates	X^{a}		
Calcium Gluconate (tab)	X		
Calcium Hydroxide Topical Soln.		X	
Calcium Lactate (tab)		X	
Calcium Pantothenate (tab)		X	
Calcium Phosphate, dibasic (tab)	X		
Camphor Spirit		X	
Candicidin	X^{g}	X^{m}	
Carbachol Solution		X$^{k w +}$	
Carbamazepine (tab)		X	
Carbamide Peroxide Topical Solution		X	X
Carbenicillin Indanyl Sodium (tab)	X		
Carbidopa and Levodopa	X^{a}		X^{a}
Carbinoxamine Maleate (tab)		X	X
Carbol-Fuchsin Topical Solution		X	X
Carphenazine Maleate Oral Solution		X	X
Carboxymethyl-cellulose Sodium Paste	X^{+}		
Cascara Sagrada Extract		X	X
Cascara Sagrada Fluid Extract		X	X
Cascara (tab)		X	
Cascara, Aromatic Fluid Extract		X^{+}	X
Castor Oil (cap)		X^{+}	
Cefaclor		X$^{b j}$	
Cefadroxil		X$^{a b j}$	
Cephalexin		X$^{a b j}$	
Cephradine		X$^{a b j}$	
Cetylpyridinium Chloride	X^{n}	X^{c}	
Chloral Hydrate		X^{b}	X^{d}
Chlorambucil (tab)	X		X
Chloramphenicol (all dosage forms)		X	
Chloramphenicol Palmitate Oral Suspension		X	X
Chloramphenicol, Polymyxin B Sulfate and Hydrocomsine Acetate Ophthalmic Oint.		X^{+}	

Drug (Dosage Form)	WC	T	LR
Chloramphenicol and Polymixin B Sulfate Ophthalmic Oint.		X+	
Chloramphenicol and Prednisolone Ophthalmic Oint.		X+	
Chlordiazepoxide (tab)		X	X
Chlordiazepoxide and Amitriptyline HCl		X^a	X^a
Chlordiazepoxide HCl (cap)		X	X
Chloroquine Phosphate (tab)	X		
Chlorothiazide	X^a	X^i	
Chlorotrianisene (cap)	X		
Chlorophenoxamine HCl (tab)		X	X
Chlorpheniramine Maleate		X^a	X^d
Chlorpromazine HCl	X$^{a\,i}$	X^d	X$^{a\,i}$
Chlorpropamide (tab)	X		
Chlorprothixene	X^a	X^i	X^a
Chlortetracycline HCl	X^g	X^b	X$^{g\,b}$
Chlorthalidone (tab)	X		
Chlorzoxazone Tabs		X	
Chlorzoxazone and Acetaminophen		X$^{a\,b}$	
Cholestyramine Oral Suspension		X	
Chymotrypsin Opthalmic Solution		X	
Ciclopirox Olamine Cream	X+		
Cinoxacin	X^b		
Cinoxate Lotion		X	X
Clemastine Fumante Tabs		X	X+
Clindinium Bromide (cap)		X	
Clindamycin HCl (cap)		X	
Clindamycin Palmitate HCl Oral Solution		X	
Clindamycin Phosphate Topical Solution		X	
Clioquinol (Iodochlor-hydroxyquin)	X^o	X$^{f\,g}$	X$^{f\,g}$
Clocortolone Pivalate		X^f	X^f
Clofibrate (cap)	X		X
Clomiphene Citrate (tab)	X		X
Clonazepam		X^a	X^a
Clonidine HCl	X^a		
Clonidin HCl and Chlorthalidone (tab)	X		
Clotrimazole		X^m	X$^{c\,f}$
Cloxacillin Sodium		X$^{b\,c}$	
Coal Tar		X$^{c\,g}$	
Colistin and Neomycin Sulfates and Hydrocortisone Acetate Otic Susp.		X	
Cyanocobalamin Co-57	X^b	X^c	X^b
Cyanocobalamin Co-60	X^b		X$^{b\,c}$
Cocaine HCl Tablets for Topical Solution	X		
Cod Liver Oil		X	
Codeine Phosphate (tab)	X		X
Codeine Sulfate (tab)	X		
Colchicine (tab)	X		X
Cold Cream		X	
Colistin Sulfate Oral Suspension		X	X
Collodion		X	
Cortisone Acetate (tab)	X		
Cromolyn Sodium for Inhalation		X	X
Crotamiton (cream)		X	X
Cyclacillin		X$^{a\,i}$	
Cyclizine HCl (tab)		X	X
Cyclobenzapine HCl (tab)	X		
Cyclomethycaine Sulfate	X^i	X$^{f\,g}$	
Cylcopentamine HCl (solution)		X^s	
Cyclopentolate HCl Opthalmic Solution		X	
Cyclophosphamide (tab)		X	
Cycloserine HCl (tab)		X	
Cyclothiazide (tab)	X		
Cyproheptadine HCl	X^a	X^d	
Danazol (cap)	X		
Danthron (tab)	X		
Dapsone (tab)	X		
Decavitamin	X^a	X^b	X^b
Dehydrocholic Acid (tab)	X		
Demecarium Bromide Opthalmic Solution		X	X
Demeclocycline Oral Suspension		X	X
Demeclocycline HCl		X$^{a\,b}$	X$^{a\,b}$
Demeclocycline HCl and Nystatin		X$^{a\,b}$	X$^{a\,b}$

Drug (Dosage Form)	WC	T	LR
Desipramine HCl		X$^{a\,b}$	
Desoximetasone	X$^{f\,t\,+}$	X$^{f\,t\,+}$	X^{f}
Desoxycorticosterone Acetate Pellets		X	
Dexamethasone	X^{a}	X$^{e\,k\,t\,+}$	
Dexamethasone Sodium Phosphate		X$^{f\,r}$	X^{k}
Dexchlorpheniramine Maleate		X^{a}	X^{d}
Dextroamphetamine Sulfate	X^{a}	X$^{e\,b}$	X^{e}
Dextroamphetamine Sulfate	X^{a}	X$^{e\,b}$	X^{e}
Dextromethorphan HBr (syr)		X	X
Dextrothyroxine Sodium (tab)	X		
Diatrizoate Meglumine and Diatrizoate Sodium Solution		X	X
Diatrizoate Sodium (soln)		X	X
Diazepam		X$^{a\,b}$	X$^{a\,b}$
Diazepam Extended Release (cap)		X	X
Diazoxide	X^{b}	X$^{i\,b}$	X$^{i\,b}$
Dibucaine		X$^{f\,g}$	X$^{f\,g}$
Dichlorphenamide (tab)	X		
Dicloxacillin Sodium	X$^{b\,i}$		
Dicumarol	X$^{a\,b}$		
Dicyclomine HCl	X$^{a\,b}$	X^{d}	
Dienestrol (cream)		X	
Diethylcarbamazine Citrate (tab)		X	
Diethylpropion HCl (tab)	X		
Diethylstilbesterol	X^{a}	X^{i}	
Diethyltoluamide Topical Soln.		X	
Diflunisal (tab)	X		
Digitalis		X$^{a\,b}$	
Digitoxin (tab)	X		
Digoxin		X$^{a\,e\,+}$	
Dihydrotachysterol	X$^{b\,a}$	X^{c}	X$^{b\,a\,c}$
Dihydroxyaluminum Aminoacetate	X^{a}		
Dihydroxyaluminum Sodium Carbonate (tab)	X		
Dimenhydrinate	X^{a}	X^{d}	
Dimethisoquin HCl		X^{i}	
Dimethyl Sulfoxide		X^{+}	X
Dioxybenzone (cream)		X	
Diperodon (ointment)		X	
Diphemanil Methyl sulfate (tab)		X	
Diphenhydramine HCl		X^{b}	X^{e}
Diphenoxylate HCl and Atropine Sulfate	X^{a}	X^{i}	X^{a}
Diphenylpyraline HCl (tab)		X	
Dipyridamole Tabs		X	X
Disopyramide Phosphate (cap)	X		
Disulfiram (tab)		X	X
Docusate Calcium (cap)		X	
Docusate Potassium (cap)		X^{+}	
Docusate Sodium	X^{a}	X$^{b\,c}$	X^{d}
Doxepin HCl	X^{b}	X^{c}	X^{c}
Doxycycline for Oral Suspension		X	X
Doxycycline Calcium Oral Susp.		X	X
Doxycycline Hyclate (cap)		X	X
Doxycycline Hyclate (tab)		X	X
Doxylamine Succinate	X^{a}	X^{d}	X^{a}
Dyclonine HCl Topical Solution		X	X
Dyclonine HCl (gel)		X	X
Dydrogesterone (tab)	X		
Dyphylline (tab)		X	
Echothiophate Iodide for Ophthalmic Solution		X^{+}	
Ephedrine Sulfate	X^{a}	X$^{b\,d\,s}$	X$^{b\,d\,s}$
Ephedrine Sulfate and Phenobarbital (cap)	X		
Epinephrine		X$^{k\,r\,s}$	X$^{k\,r\,s}$
Epinephrine Inhalation Aerosol		X	X
Epinephrine Bitartrate		X^{k}	X^{r}
Epinephryl Borate Opthalmic Solution		X	X
Ergocalciferol		X$^{a\,b\,c}$	X$^{a\,b\,c}$
Ergoloid Mesylates		X$^{c\,a}$	X$^{c\,+\,a}$
Ergonovine Maleate (tab)	X		
Ergotamine Tartrate (tab)	X		
Ergotamine Tartrate Inhalation Aerosol		X	X
Ergotamine Tartrate and Caffeine	X^{a}	X^{i}	X^{a}
Erythrityl Tetranitrate (tab)		X	
Erythromycin		X$^{a\,g\,b}$	
Erythromycin Topical Soln.		X	

Drug (Dosage Form)	WC	T	LR	Drug (Dosage Form)	WC	T	LR
Erythromycin				Folic Acid			
Estolate		X[abj]		(tab)	X		
Erythromycin				Furosemide (tab)		X	X
Ethylsuccinate		X[ai]		Gemfibrozil (cap)		X	
Erythromycin				Gentamicin Sulfate		X[fgk]	
Stearate		X[ai]		Gentain Violet		X[cf]	
Erythrosine Sodium		X[ac]	X[ac]	Glutethimide	X[ab]		
Estradiol (tab)		X	X	Glycerin	X[i]	X[ck]	
Estrogens, Con-				Glycobiarsal			
jugated (tab)	X			(tab)	X		X
Estrogens, Esteri-				Glycopyrrolate			
fied (tab)	X			(tab)		X	
Estropipate (Pipera-				Griseofulvin		X[abj]	
zine Estrone				Guaifenesin		X[abd]	
Sulfate) (tab)	X			Guanethidine Mono-			
Ethacrynic Acid				sulfate (tab)	X		
(tab)	X			Guanethidine Sulfate			
Ethambutol HCl				(tab)	X		
(tab)	X			Halazone Tablets			
Ethchlorvynol				for Solution		X	X
(cap)		X	X	Haloperidol		X[ac]	X[ac]
Ethinamate (cap)		X		Haloprogin		X[+f]	X[f]
Ethinyl Estradiol				Haloprogin			
(tab)	X			(topical soln)		X[+]	X
Ethionamide (tab)		X		Hetacillin		X[ai]	
Ethopropazine HCl				Hetacillin Potassium			
(tab)	X		X	(cap)		X	
Ethosuximide				Hexavitamin		X[ab]	X[ab]
(cap)		X		Hexobarbital (tab)	X		
Ethynadiol Diacetate				Hexylcaine HCl			
and Ethinyl Estradiol				Topical Soln.		X	
(tab)	X			Hexylresorcinol			
Ethynadiol Diacetate				(pills)	X		
and Mestranol Tabs	X			Homatropine Hydro-			
Eucatropine HCl				bromide Opthalmic			
Opthalmic Soln.		X		Solution		X	
Fenoprofen Calcium	X[ab]			Homatropine Methyl-			
Ferrous Fumarate				bromide (tab)		X	X
(tab)		X		Hydralazine HCl			
Ferrous Gluconate		X[ae]	X[ae]	(tab)		X	X
Ferrous Sulfate		X[a]	X[c]	Hydrochlorothiazide			
Flucytosine				(tab)	X		
(cap)		X	X	Hydrocodone			
Fluhydrocortisone				Bitartrate (tab)		X	X
Acetate (tab)	X			Hydrocortisone		X[t]	
Flunisolide Nasal				Hydrocortisone			
Soln.		X	X[+]	(Cortisol)	X[ag]	X[fhp]	
Fluocinolone				Hydrocortisone			
Acetonide		X[cfg]		Acetate	X[fg]	X[k]	
Fluocinolone		X[fgt]		Hydrocortisone			
Fluorometholone				Cypionate Oral			
Ophthalmic Susp.		X		Suspension		X	X
Fluorouracil		X[cfc]		Hydrocortisone			
Fluoxymesterone				Acetate Lotion		X	
(tab)	X		X	Hydrocortisone			
Fluphenazine HCl		X[a]	X[ce]	Valerate	X[f]		
Flurandrenolide		X[fgh]	X[fgh]	Hydroflumethiazide			
Flurazepam HCl				(tab)		X	
(cap)		X	X	Hydrogen Peroxide			
				Topical Soln.		X	X

Drug (Dosage Form)	WC	T	LR
Hydromorphone HCl (tab)		X	X
Hydroquinone (cream)	X		X
Hydroquinone (topical soln)		X	X
Hydroxyamphetamine HBr Opthalmic Solution		X	X
Hydroxychloroquin Sulfate (tab)	X		
Hydroxypropyl Methylcellulose Opthalmic Solution		X	
Hydroxyurea (cap)		X	
Hydroxyzine HCl		X[a]	X[d]
Hydroxyzine Pamoate	X[b]	X[j]	X[j]
Hyoscyamine (tab)	X		X
Hyoscyamine Sulfate		X[aec]	X[aec]
Ibuprofen (tab)	X		
Ichthammol (ointment)		X	
Idoxuridine Ophthalmic Soln.		X	X
Imipramine HCl (tab)		X	
Indomethacin (cap)	X		
Iocetamic Acid (tab)		X	
Strong Iodine Tincture		X	X
Iodine Topical Solution		X	X
Iodide, Sodium, I-123 (cap)	X		
Iodide, Sodium, I-125 (cap)	X		
Iodide, Sodium, I-131 (cap)	X		
Iodoquinol (tab)	X		
Iopanoic Acid (tab)		X	X
Ipecac Syrup		X	
Ipodate Calcium for Oral Susp.	X		
Iopodate Sodium (cap)		X	
Isocarboxazide (tab)	X		
Isoetharine Inhalation Solution		X	X
Isoetharine Mesylate Inhalation			X
Isoniazid	X[a]	X[d]	X[a]
Isopropamide Iodide (tab)	X		
Isoproterenol Inhalation (soln)		X	X
Isoproterenol HCl	X[a]	X[r]	X[rl]
Isoproterenol HCl and Phenylephrine Bitartrate Inhalation			X
Isoproterenol Sulfate Inhalation		X[c]	X[cl]
Isoproterenal Sulfate Inhalation (soln)		X	X
Isosorbide Dinitrate (tab)	X		
Isosorbide Oral (soln)		X	
Isoxsuprine HCl (tab)		X	
Kanamycin Sulfate (cap)		X	
Lactolose (syr/conc)		X+	
Levodopa (cap/tab)		X	X
Levopropoxyphene Napsylate		X[b]	X[j]
Levorphanol Tartrate (tab)	X		
Levothyroxine Sodium (tab)		X	X
Lidocaine (ointment)		X	
Lidocaine Oral Topical Soln.		X	
Lidocaine HCl Topical Soln.		X	
Lime, Sulfurated, Topical Soln.		X	
Lincomycin HCl (cap/syrup)		X	
Lindaine (cream/lot)		X	
Liothyronine Sodium (tab)		X	
Liotrix (tab)		X	
Lithium Carbonate (cap/tab)	X		
Loperamide HCl (cap)	X		
Mafenide Acetate (cream)		X	X
Magaldrate	X[a]	X[j]	
Magnesia (tab)	X		
Magnesium Carbonate and Sodium Bicarbonate for Oral Susp.		X	
Magnesium Gluconate (tab)	X		
Magnesium Salicylate (tab)		X	
Maprotiline HCl (tab)	X		
Mazindol (tab)		X+	
Mebendazol (tab)	X		
Mecamylamine HCl (tab)	X		

Drug (Dosage Form)	WC	T	LR
Meclizine HCl (tab)	X		
Meclocycline Sulfosalicylate Cream		X	X
Meclofenamate Sodium (cap)		X	X
Medroxyprogesterone Acetate	X^a		
Medrysone Opthalmic Suspension	X	X	
Megestrol Acetate	X^a o		X^o
Melphalon (tab)	X		
Menadiol Sodium Diphosphate (tab)	X		X
Menpenzolate Bromide	X^a	X^d	X^d
Meperidine HCl	X^a	X^d	X^a
Mephenytoin (tab)	X		
Mephobarbital (tab)	X		
Meprobamate	X^a	X^j	
Mercaptopurine (tab)	X		
Mercury, Ammoniated (ointment)	X		
Mesoridazine Besylate	X^a	X^j	X^j
Methacycline HCl		X^b j	X^b j
Methadone HCl	X^a	X^d	
Methadone HCl Oral Concentrate		X	X^+
Methantheline Bromide (tab)		X	X
Methaqualone (tab)	X		
Metharbital (tab)		X	
Methazolamide (tab)	X		
Methdilazine (tab)		X	X
Methdilazine HCl		X^a d	X^a d
Methenamine	X^a	X^e	
Methenamine and Monobasic Sodium Phosphate (tab)		X	
Methenamine Hippurate (tab)	X		
Methenamine Mandelate	X^a	X^j	
Methenamine Mandelate for Oral Soln.		X	
Methimazole (tab)	X		X
Methocarbamol (tab)	X	X	
Methotrexate (tab)	X		
Methoxsalen Topical Solution		X	X
Methscopolamine Bromide (tab)		X	
Methsuximide (cap)		X	
Methylclothiazide (tab)	X		
Methylbenzethonium Chloride		X^h	
Methylcellulose	X^a	X^c k	X^c
Methyldopa	X^a	X^j	X^j +
Methyldopa and Hydrochlorothiazide (tab)	X		
Methylergonovine Maleate (tab)		X	X
Methylphenidate HCl (tab)		X	
Methylprednisolone (tab)		X	
Methylprednisolone Acetate	X^p	X^f	X^f
Methyltestosterone (tab/cap)	X		
Methyprylon (tab/cap)		X	X
Methysergide Maleate (tab)		X	
Metoprolol Tartrate (tab)		X	X
Metronidazole (tab)	X		X
Metyrapone (tab)		X	X
Metyrosine (cap)	X		
Miconazole Nitrate		X^f	
Mineral Oil Emulsion	X		
Minocycline HCl		X^a b j	X^a b j
Mitotane (tab)	X		X
Monobenzone Ointment		X^+	
Nafcillin Sodium		X^b c	X^a
Nalidixic Acid (tab/oral susp)	X		
Naphazoline HCl		X^k	X^s
Naproxen (tab)	X		
Naproxen Sodium (tab)	X		
Natamycin Ophthalmic Susp.		X	X
Neomycin Sulfate	X^g f +	X^a	X^c
Neomycin Sulfate and Bacitracin		X^g	X^g +
Neomycin Sulfate Bacitracin Zinc	X^g		
Neomycin Sulfate and Dexamethasone Sodium Phosphate		X^f	
Neomycin Sulfate and Dexamethasone Sodium Phosphate Ophthalmic		X^g c +	X^g c +
Neomycin Sulfate and Fluocinolone Acetonide		X^f	
Neomycin Sulfate and Fluorometholone	X^g		

Drug (Dosage Form)	WC	T	LR
Neomycin Sulfate and Flurandrenolide		X[f g]	X[f g]
Neomycin Sulfate and Gramicidin	X[g]		
Neomycin Sulfate and Hydrocortisone	X[f g]		
Neomycin Sulfate and Hydrocortisone Otic Susp.	X		X
Neomycin Sulfate and Hydrocortisone Acetate	X[f g]		
Neomycin Sulfate and Hydrocortisone Acetate Ophthalmic		X[i g]	
Neomycin Sulfate and Methylprednisolone Acetate		X[f]	X[f]
Neomycin Sulfate and Prednisolone Acetate		X[g k]	X[g k]
Neomycin Sulfate and Prednisolone Acetate Ophthalmic Susp.		X	
Neomycin Sulfate and Prednisolone Sodium Phosphate Ophthalmic Oint.		X	
Neomycin Sulfate, Sulfacetamide Sodium and Prednisolone Acetate Ophthalmic		X[g]	
Neomycin Sulfate and Triamcinolone Acetonide Ophthalmic Oint.		X	
Neomycin and Polymyxin B Sulfates Ophthalmic	X[g]	X[g]	
Neomycin and Polymyxin B Sulfate and Bacitracin Zinc	X[g o]	X[k g l]	X[g +]
Neomycin and Polymyxin B Sulfate and Bacitracin Zinc and Hydrocortisone Oint.	X[+]	X[k +]	
Neomycin and Polymyxin B Sulfate and Bacitracin Zinc and Hydrocortisone Acetate Oint.	X[+]		
Neomycin and Polymyxin B Sulfates, Bacitracin and Hydrocortisone Acetate Ointment	X[g k +]		
Neomycin and Polymyxin B Sulfate and Hydrocortisone Otic Soln.		X	X
Neomycin and Polymyxin B Sulfates and Dexamethasone Ophthalmic	X[g]	X[i]	X[i]
Neomycin and Polymyxin B Sulfate and Gramicidin	X[f]	X[c]	
Neomycin and Polymyxin B Sulfate and Gramicidin Ophthalmic Soln.		X	
Neomycin and Polymyxin B Sulfates, Gramicidin and Hydrocortisone Acetate Cream	X		
Neomycin and Polymyxin B Sulfates and Hydrocortisone Ophthalmic Susp.		X	
Neomycin and Polymyxin B Sulfates and Hydrocortisone Acetate Ophthalmic Susp.		X	
Neomycin and Polymyxin B Sulfates and Prednisolone Acetate Ophthalmic Susp.		X	
Neostigmine Bromide (tab)		X	
Niacin (tab)	X		
Niacinamide (tab)		X	
Nifedipine (cap)		X	X[+]
Nitrofurantoin (tab/oral susp)		X	X
Nitrofurazone (cream/ ointment)		X	X
Nitroglycerin		X[a g]	
Nitromersol Topical Solution		X	X
Northindrone (tab)	X		
Norethindrone and Ethinyl Estradiol (tab)	X		
Norethindrone and Mestranol (tab)	X		
Norethindrone Acetate (tab)	X		
Norethindrone Acetate and Ethinyl Estradiol (tab)	X		
Norgestrel (tab)	X		
Norgestrel and Ethinyl Estradiol	X[a]		
Nortriptyline HCl		X[a]	X[c]

Drug (Dosage Form)	WC	T	LR
Novobiocin Calcium Oral Susp.		X	X
Nylidrin HCl (tab)		X	
Nystatin	X^g	X$^{a\,f\,h\,m}$	X$^{a\,j\,m}$
Nystatin Vaginal Supp.		X	X+
Nystatin and Iodochlorhydroxyquin		X^g	X$^{g\,+}$
Nystatin, Neomycin Sulfate, Gramicidin and Triamcinolone Acetonide		X$^{f\,g}$	
Oleovitamin A and D (cap)		X	X
Oxacillin Sodium (cap)		X	
Oxamniquine (cap)		X	
Oxytetracycline and Phenazopyridine Hydrochlorides and Sulfamethizole (cap)		X	X
Oxandrolone (tab)		X	X
Oxazepam (tab/cap)	X		
Oxymetazoline HCl Nasal Soln.		X	
Oxymetholone (tab)	X		
Oxymorphone HCl Suppositories	X		
Oxyphenbutazone (tab)		X	
Oxyphencyclimine HCl (tab)		X	
Oxytetracycline (tab)		X	X
Oxytetracycline Calcium Oral Suspension		X	X
Oxytetracycline and Nystatin		X$^{b\,j}$	X$^{b\,j}$
Oxytetracycline HCl and Hydrocortisone Ointment	X		X
Oxytetracycline HCl and Hydrocortisone Acetate Ophthalmic Susp.		X	X
Oxytetracycline HCl and Polymyxin B Sulfate Ointment	X$^{g\,o\,m}$		X^g
Oxytetracycline HCl and Polymyxin B Ophthalmic Oint.	X+		
Oxytriphylline (cap)		X$^{a\,e}$	X
Pancreatin (tab/cap)		X	
Pancrelipase (tab/cap)		X	
Papain Tablets for Topical Soln.		X	X

Drug (Dosage Form)	WC	T	LR
Papaverine HCl (tab)		X	
Paramethadione		X^b	X^c
Paramethasone Acetate (tab)	X		
Pargyline HCl (tab)	X		
Paromomycin Sulfate (cap)	X		
Penicillamine (tab/cap)		X	
Penicillin G Benzathine		X$^{a\,j}$	
Penicillin G Potassium		X$^{a\,c}$	
Penicillin V		X$^{a\,j}$	
Penicillin V Potassium		X$^{a\,c}$	
Pentaerythritol Tetranitrate		X^a	
Pentazocine HCl (tab)		X	X
Pentazocine HCl (tab)		X	X
Pentazocine HCl and Aspirin (tab)		X	X
Pentobarbital Elixir		X	
Pentobarbital Sodium		X$^{b\,e}$	
Perphenazine	X$^{c\,d}$	X^a	X$^{c\,d}$
Phenacemide (tab)	X		
Phenazopyridine HCl (tab)		X	
Phendimetrazine Tartrate	X^b	X^a	
Phenelzine Sulfate (tab)		X	X
Phenindione (tab)	X		
Phenmetrazine HCl (tab)		X	
Phenobarbital	X^a	X^e	X^e
Phenobarbital Sodium (tab)		X	
Phenolphthalein (tab)		X	
Phenoxybenzamine HCl (cap)	X		
Phenprocoumon (tab)	X		
Phensuximide		X	
Phentermine HCl		X$^{b\,a}$	
Phenylbutazone	X^a	X^b	
Phenylephrine HCl		X$^{k\,s}$	X$^{k\,s}$
Phenylephrine HCl Nasal Jelly		X	
Phenytoin	X^a	X^j	
Phenytoin Sodium, Extended		X^b	
Phenytoin Sodium, Prompt		X^b	
Physostigmine Salicylate Ophthalmic Solution		X	X
Phytonadione (tab)		X	X

Drug (Dosage Form)	WC	T	LR
Pilocarpine HCl Opthalmic Soln		X	X
Pilocarpine Nitrate Ophthalmic		X	X
Piperacetazine (tab)	X		X
Piperazine Citrate (tab/syr)		X	
Pipobroman (tab)	X		
Podophyllum Resin Topical Soln.		X	X
Polymyxin B Sulfate and Hydrocortisone Otic Soln.		X	X
Polythiazide (tab)		X	X
Potassium Bicarbonate Effervescent Tabs for Oral Soln.		X+	
Potassium Bicarbonate and Potassium Chloride for Effervescent Oral Soln.		X+ o a	
Potassium Chloride Elixir		X	Xe
Potassium Chloride Extended Release		Xab +	
Potassium Citrate and Citric Acid Oral Solution		X	
Potassium Gluconate		Xa	Xe
Potassium Iodide		Xa	Xc
Potassium Permanganate Tablets for Topical Solution		X	
Povidone Iodide Topical Soln.		X	
Povidone-Iodine Oint		X	
Povidone-Iodine Cleansing Soln.		X	
Pralidoxime Chloride (tab)	X		
Pramoxine HCl (cream)		X	
Prazepam		Xa b	Xa b
Prazosin HCl (cap)	X		X
Prednisolone	Xa	Xf	
Prednisolone Sodium Phosphate Ophthalmic Solution		X	X
Prednisone (tab)	X		
Primaquine Phosphate (tab)	X		X
Primadone	Xa		Xi
Probenecid (tab)	X		
Probenecid and Colchicine (tab)	X		X
Procainamide HCl (cap)		X	
Procarbazine HCl (cap)		X	X

Drug (Dosage Form)	WC	T	LR
Prochlorperazine Suppositories		X	
Prochlorperazine Edisylate Syr.		X	X
Prochlorperazine Maleate (tab)	X		X
Procyclidine HCl (tab)		X	
Promazine HCl (tab/syr)		X	X
Promazine HCl (tab/syr)		X	X
Promethazine HCl (tab/syr)		X	X
Propantheline Bromide (tab)	X		
Proparacaine HCl Opthalmic Soln.		X	X
Propoxyphene HCl (cap)		X	
Propoxyphene HCl and Acetaminophen		Xa	
Propoxyphene HCl, Aspirin, and Caffeine (cap)		X+	
Propoxyphene Napsylate		Xa	Xi
Propoxyphene Napsylate and Aspirin		Xa	
Propanolol HCl (tab)	X		X
Propylhexedrine Inhalant		X	
Propylthiouracil (tab)	X		
Protriptylene HCl (tab)		X	
Psueodephedrine HCl		Xa	Xd
Pyrantel Pamoate Oral Suspension		X	X
Pyrazinamide (tab)	X		
Pyridostigmine Bromide		Xa	Xd
Pyridoxine HCl (tab)	X		
Pyrilamine Maleate (tab)	X		
Pyrimethamine (tab)		X	X
Pyrvinium Pamoate		Xa i	Xa i
Quinacrine HCl (tab)		X	
Quinestrol (tab)	X		
Quinethazone (tab)		X	
Quinidine Sulfate	Xa	Xb	Xb
Quinine Sulfate	Xa	Xb	
Racemethionine (Methionine) (tab/cap)	X		X
Rauwolfia Serpentina (tab)		X	X
Reserpine (tab/elix)		X	X

Drug (Dosage Form)	WC	T	LR
Reserpine and Hydrochloro-thiazide (tab)		X	X
Reserpine, Hydrala-zine and Hydrochloro-thiazide (tab)		X	X
Resorcinol, Compound (ointment)		X	
Resorcinol and Sulfur (lot)		X	
Riboflavin (tab)		X	X
Rifampin (cap)		X	X
Rifampin and Isonia-zid (cap)		X	X
Ritodrine HCl (tab)		X+	
Rose Water Ointment		X	X
Saccharin Sodium (tab)	X	X[c]	
Salicylic Acid Gel		X+	
Salicylic Acid Topical Foam		X	
Scopolamine HBr (tab)		X	X
Secobarbital Elixir		X	
Secobarbital Sodium (cap)		X	
Senna Syrup		X	
Sennosides (tab)	X		
Silver Nitrate Opthalmic Soln.			X
Simethicone	X[a]		X[j]
Sodium Acetate Soln.		X	
Sodium Bicarbonate (tab)	X		
Sodium Bicarbonate Oral Powder	X		
Sodium Chloride	X[a]	X[k]	
Sodium Chloride and Dextrose	X[a]		
Sodium Citrate and Citric Acid Oral Solution		X	
Sodium Fluoride (tab/oral soln.)		X	
Sodium Iodide		X[c]	
Sodium Phosphate	X[p]	X[c]	
Sodium Salicylate (tab)	X		
Spironolactone (tab)		X	X
Stanozolol (tab)		X	X
Topical Starch	X		
Sulfacetamide Sodium Opthalmic Solution		X	X
Sulfadiazine (tab)	X		X
Sulfadoxine and Pyrimethamine (tab)	X		X
Sulfamerazine (tab)	X		
Sulfamethizole	X[a]	X[j]	X[j]
Sulfamethoxazole	X[a]	X[j]	X[a]
Sulfamethoxazole and Trimethoprim	X[a]	X[j]	X[j]
Sulfapyridine (tab)	X		
Sulfasalazine (tab)	X		
Sulfathiaxole, Sulfacetamide and Sulfabenzamide Vaginal	X[m f]		X[m f]
Sulfinpyrazone (tab/cap)	X		
Sulfisoxazole (tab)	X		X
Sulfisoxazole Acetyl Oral Suspension		X	X
Sulfisoxazole Diola-mine Opthalmic Solution		X	X
Sulfoxone Sodium (tab)		X	X
Sulfur Ointment	X		
Sulindac Tabs	X		
Sutilains Ointment		X	
Talbutal (tab)		X	
Tamoxifen Citrate (tab)	X		X
Terbutaline (tab)		X	
Terpin Hydrate Elixir		X	
Terpin Hydrate and Codeine Elixir		X	
Terpin Hydrate and Dextromethorphan HBr Elixir		X	
Testolactone (tab)		X	
Testosterone (tab)		X	
Tetracaine HCl		X[c k]	X[c k]
Tetracaine and Menthal Oint.	X	X	
Tetrachlorethylene (cap)		X	
Tetracycline Oral Suspension		X	X
Tetracycline and Amphotericin B		X[b j]	X[b j]
Tetracycline HCl (tablet/capsule/Ophtalmic Sus-pension/topical solution)	X[g]+	X	X
Tetracycline HCl and Nystatin		X[b]	X[b]
Tetracycline Phosphate Complex		X[b]	X[b]
Tetrahydrozoline HCl		X[k s]	
Theophylline	X[a b]		

Drug (Dosage Form)	WC	T	LR
Theophylline, Ephedrine HCl and Phenobarbital (tab)		X	
Theophylline and Guaifenesin (cap)		X	
Theophylline Sodium Glycinate	X^a	X^e	
Thiabendazole (oral susp/tab)		X	
Thiamine HCl		X$^{a\,e}$	X$^{a\,e}$
Thiamine Mononitrate Elixir		X	X
Thiethylperazine Maleate (tab)		X	X
Thimerosol Topical Solution		X$^+$	X
Thimerosal Tincture		X$^+$	X
Thioguanine (tab)		X	
Thioridazine Oral Suspension		X	X
Thioridazine HCl	X^a	X^c	X^c
Thiothixene (cap)	X		X
Thiothixene HCl Oral Solution		X	X
Thyroglobulin (tab)		X	
Thyroid (tab)		X	
Timolol Maleate Ophthalmic Soln.	X^a	X	X^a
Timolol Maleate and Hydrochlorothiazide (tab)	X		X
Tobramycin Ophthalmic		X$^{c\,g}$	
Tolazamide (tab)		X	
Tolazoline HCl (tab)	X		
Tolbutamide (tab)	X		
Tolmetin Sodium	X^a	X^b	
Tolnaftate		X$^{c\,f\,t}$	
Tranylcypromine Sulfate (tab)	X		X
Tretinoin		X$^{d\,f\,t}$	X$^{c\,f\,t}$
Triamcinolone (tab)	X		
Triamcinolone Acetonide	X^g	X$^{f\,h}$	
Triamcinolone Diacetate (syr)		X	X
Triamterene (cap)		X	X
Trichlormethiazide (tab)		X	
Tricitrates Oral Solution		X	

Drug (Dosage Form)	WC	T	LR
Tridihexethyl (tab)	X		
Trifluoperazine HCl	X^a	X^d	X^a
Triflupromazine Oral Suspension		X	X
Triflupromazine HCl (tab)	X		X
Trihexyphenidyl HCl		X$^{a\,e}$	
Trikates Oral (soln)		X	X
Trimeprazine Tartrate	X^a	X^d	X^a
Trimethadione		X$^{a\,b\,c}$	
Trimethobenzamide HCl (cap)	X		
Trimethoprim (tab)		X	X
Trioxsalen (tab)	X		X
Tripelennamine HCl (tab)	X		
Tripelennamine Citrate Elixir		X	X
Triprolidine HCl		X$^{a\,d}$	X$^{a\,d}$
Triprolidine and Pseudoephedrine Hydrochlorides		X$^{a\,d}$	X$^{a\,d}$
Trisulfapyrimidines	X^a	X^i	
Troleandomycin		X$^{b\,j\,+}$	
Tropicamide Ophthalmic Soln.		X	
Tyropanoate Sodium (cap)		X	X
Undecylenic Acid, Compound Ointment		X	
Uracil Mustard (cap)		X	
Vancomycin HCl	X^b	X^c	
Vitamin A (cap)		X	X
Vitamin E (cap)		X	X
Warfarin Potassium (tab)		X	X
Warfarin Sodium (tab)		X	X
Xylometazoline HCl Nasal Soln.		X	X
Zinc-Eugenol Cement	X		
Zinc Gelatin		X	
Zinc Oxide (oint/paste)	X$^+$		
Zinc Sulfate Ophthalmic Solution		X	
Zomepirac Sodium (tab)	X		

CONTAINER AND STORAGE REQUIREMENTS FOR STERILE U.S.P. XXI DRUGS*

Legend:

I =containers for sterile solids as described under injections	D =type II or III glass depending on final soln pH
S =single dose	LR =light resistant
M =multiple dose	L =protect from light
U =unspecified	R =refrigerator (2–8C°)
A =type I glass	F =freezer (−4C°)
B =type II glass	H =protect from heat
C =type III glass	RT =controlled room temperature

Drugs	Container	Glass Type	Storage Conditions
Sterile Acetazolamide Sodium	I	C	
Acetic Acid Irrigation	S	A,B	
Acetylcholine for Ophthalmic Soln.	I		
Amikacin Sulfate Inj.	S,M	A,C	
Dehydrated Alcohol Inj.	S	A	
Alcohol and Dextrose Inj.	S	A,B	
Alphaprodine HCl Inj.	S,M	A	
Amikacin Sulfate Inj.	S,M	A,C	
Aminoacetic Acid Irrigation	S	A,B	
Aminocaproic Acid Inj.	S,M	A	
Aminohipurate Sodium Inj.	S,M	A	
Aminophylline Inj.	S	A	CO$_2$ excluded
Amitriptyline HCl Inj.	S,M	A	
Ammonium Chloride Inj.	S,M	A,B	
Ammonium Molybdate Inj.	S,M	A,B	
Sterile Amobarbital Sodium	I	D	
Amphotericin B for Inj.	I		R,L
Sterile Ampicillin	I		
Sterile Ampicillin Sodium	I		R,L
Anileridine Inj.	S,M	A	L
Anticoagulant Sodium Citrate Soln.	S	A,B	
Anticoagulant Heparin Soln.	S	A,B	
Antivenin (Latrodectus mectans)	S		H
Antivenin (Crotalidae) Polyvalent	S		H
Antivenin (Micrurus fulvius)	S		H
Arginine HCl Inj.	S	B	
Antirabies Serum	U		R
Ascorbic Acid Inj.	S	A,B	LR
Atropine Sulfate Inj.	S,M	A	
Sterile Aurothioglucose Susp.	S,M	A	L
Azathioprine Sodium for Inj.	I	C	RT
Sterile Azlocillin Sodium	I		
Sterile Bacitracin	I	D	R
Sterile Bacitracin Zinc	I		R(cool place)
BCG Vaccine	U	A	R
Benztropine Mesylate Inj.	S,M	A	
Benzylpenicilloyl Polylysine Inj.	M		R
Sterile Betamethasone Sodium Phosphate and Betamethasone Acetate (Susp.)	M	A	
Bethanechol Chloride Inj.	S	A	
Biperiden Lactate Inj.	S	A	L
Sterile Bleomycin Sulfate	I	B	
Blood Grouping Serums (All)	U		R
Brompheniramine Maleate Inj.	S,M	A	L
Bupivacaine HCl Inj.	S,M	A	
Bupivacaine and Epinephrine Inj.	S,M	A	
Butorphanol Tartrate Inj.	S,M	A	L
Caffeine and Sodium Benzoate Inj.	S	A	

*The listing of container and storage requirements for sterile Compendial drugs is included as an aid to the practitioner in storing and dispensing.

Drugs	Container	Glass Type	Storage Conditions
Calcium Chloride Inj.	S	A	
Calcium Gluceptate Inj.	S	A,B	
Calcium Gluconate Inj.	S	A	
Calcium Levulinate Inj.	S	A	
Sterile Capreomycin Sulfate	I	B	R
Sterile Carbenicillin Disodium	I	D	
Carboprost Tromethamine Inj.	S,M	A	R
Cefamandole Naftate for Inj.	I	D	
Cefamandole Sodium for Inj.	I		
Sterile Cefamandole Sodium	I		
Sterile Cefazolin Sodium	I	B	
Cefaxolin Sodium Inj.	I		F
Sterile Cefotaxime Sodium	I	B	
Sterile Cefoperezone Sodium	I		
Sterile Cefoxitin Sodium	I	B	
Sterile Ceftizoxime Sodium	I		
Cephalothin Sodium Inj.	I		F
Sterile Cephapirin Sodium	I	D	
Cephradine for Inj.	I		
Sterile Cephradine	I		
Chloramphenicol Inj.	S,M		
Sterile Chloramphenicol	I		
Sterile Chloramphenicol Sodium Succinate	I	B	
Sterile Chlordiazepoxide HCl	I	B	L
Chloroprocaine HCl Inj.	S,M	A	
Chloroquine HCl Inj.	S	A	
Chlorothiazide Sodium for Inj.	I	C	
Chlorphenamine Maleate Inj.	S,M	A	L
Chlorpromazine HCl Inj.	S,M	A	L
Chlorprothixene Inj.	S		L
Sterile Chlortetracycline HCl	I		L
Cholera Vaccine	U		R
Sodium Chromate Cr51 Inj.	S,M		
Chromic Chloride Inj.	S,M	A,B	
Clindamycin Phosphate Inj.	S,M	A	
Sterile Clindamycin Phosphate	I	D	
Codeine Phosphate Inj.	S,M	A	L
Colchicine Inj.	S	A	L
Sterile Colistemethate Sodium	I	D	
Corticotropin Inj.	S,M	A	R
Corticotropin for Inj.	I	B	
Repository Corticotropin Inj.	S,M	A	
Sterile Corticotropin Zinc Hydroxide (Susp.)	S,M	A	RT
Sterile Cortisone Acetate Susp.	S,M	A	
Cupric Chloride Inj.	S,M	A,B	
Cupric Sulfate Inj.	S,M	A,B	
Cyclophosphamide for Inj.	I		RT
Cyanocobalamin Inj.	S,M	A	LR
Cyclizine Lactate Inj.	S	A	
Cyclophosphamide for Inj.	I	B	RT
Cysteine HCl Inj.	S,M	A	
Sterile Cytarabine	I	B	
Dacarbazine for Inj.	S,M, or I	A	L
Dactinomycin for Inj.	I	B	H,LR
Daunorubicin HCl for Inj.	I	B	LR
Digitoxin Inj.	S	A	avoid excessive heat
Dextrose and Sodium Chloride Inj.	S	A,B	
Diatrizoate Meglumine Inj.	S,M	A,C	L

Drugs	Container	Glass Type	Storage Conditions
Diatrizoate Meglumine and Diatrizoate Sodium Inj.	S	A,C	L
Diatrizoate Sodium Inj.	S,M	A,C	L
Diazepam Inj.	S,M	A	L
Diazoxide Inj.	S	A	L
Dibucaine HCl Inj.	S,M	A	L
Sterile Dicloxacillin Sodium	I	D	
Dicyclomine HCl Inj.	S,M	A	
Diethylstilbestrol Inj.	S,M	A	LR
Digitoxin Inj.	S,M	A	L
Digoxin Inj.	S	A	LR,H
Dihydroergotamine Mesylate Inj.	S	A	avoid heat
Dimenhydrinate Inj.	S,M	A,C	
Dimercaprol Inj.	S,M	A,C	
Dimethyl Sulfate Irrigation	S		RT,L
Diphenhydramine HCl Inj.	S,M	A	L
Diphtheria Antitoxin	U		R
Diphtheria Toxoid	U		R
Diphtheria Toxoid Adsorbed	U		R
Diphtheria and Tetanus Toxoids/Adsorbed	U		R
Diphtheria and Tetanus Toxoids and Pertussis Vaccine/Adsorbed	U		R
Dobutamine HCl for Inj.	I	B	RT
Dopamine HCl Inj.	S	A	
Dopamine HCl and Dextrose Inj.	S	A,B	
Doxapram HCl Inj.	S,M	A	
Doxorubicin HCl for Inj.	I		
Doxorubicin HCl for Inj.	I	B	
Doxycycline Hyclate for Inj.	I	B	L
Sterile Doxycycline Hyclate	I		L
Droperidol Inj.	S,M	A	L
Dyphylline Inj.	S,M	A	RT,L
Edetate Calcium Disodium Inj.	S	A	
Edetate Disodium Inj.	S	A	
Edrophonium Chloride Inj.	S,M	A	
Emetine HCl Inj.	S	A	LR
Ephedrine Sulfate Inj.	S,M	A	LR
Epinephrine Inj.	S,M	A	LR
Sterile Epinephrine Oil Susp.	S	A,C	LR
Ergonovine Maleate Inj.	S	A	LR,R
Ergotamine Tartrate Inj.	S	A	LR
Erythromycin Ethylsuccinate Inj.	S,M	A	
Sterile Erythromycin Ethylsuccinate	I		
Sterile Erythromycin Gluceptate	I	D	
Erythromycin Lactobionate for Inj.	I	D	
Sterile Estradiol Suspension	S,M	A	
Estradiol Cypionate Inj.	S,M	A	LR
Estradiol Valerate Inj.	S,M	A,C	LR
Estrone Inj.	S,M	A	
Sterile Estrone Suspension	S,M	A	
Ethacrynate Sodium for Inj.	I	D	
Ethiodized Oil Inj.	S,M		LR
Ethylnorepinephrine HCl Inj.	S,M	A	LR
Evans Blue Inj.	S	A	
Fentanyl Citrate Inj.	S	A	L
Sterile Floxuridine	M	A	L
Fluorexein Sodium Inj.	S	A	
Fluorouracil Inj.	S	A	RT,L
Fluphenazine Enanthate Inj.	S,M	A,C	L

Drugs	Container	Glass Type	Storage Conditions
Fluphenazine HCl Inj.	S,M	A	L
Folic Acid Inj.	S,M	A	
Fructose Inj.	S	A,B	
Fructose and Sodium Chloride Inj.	S	A,B	
Furosemide Inj.	S,M	A	LR
Gallamine Triethiodide Inj.	S,M	A	L
Gallium Citrate Ga67 Inj.	S,M		
Sterile Gallium Citrate Ga67 Inj.	I	D	
Gentamicin Sulfate Inj.	S,M	A	
Anti-Human Globulin Serum	U		R
Glucagon for Inj.	I/S,M w/solvent	A	
Glycine Irrigation	S	A,B	
Glycopyrrolate Inj.	S,M	A	
Gold Sodium Thiomalate Inj.	S,M	A	L
Chorionic Gonadotropin for Inj.	I	D	
Haloperidol Inj.	S,M	A	L
Heparin Sodium Inj.	S,M	A	
Heparin Calcium Inj.	S,M	A	R
Hepatitis B Virus Vaccine Inactivated	U		R
Sterile Hetacillin Potassium	I		
Hexafluorenium Bromide Inj.	S,M	A	L
Histamine Phosphate Inj.	S,M	A	L
Hyaluronidase Inj.	S,M	A	R
Hyaluronidase for Inj.	I	A,C	RT
Hydralazine HCl Inj.	S,M	A	
Sterile Hydrocortisone (Cortisol) Suspension	S,M	A	
Sterile Hydrocortisone (Cortisol) Acetate Suspension	S,M	A	
Hydrocortisone (Cortisol) Sodium Phosphate Inj.	I	C	
Hydrocortisone (Cortisol) Sodium Succinate for Inj.	I	C	
Hydromorphone HCl Inj.	S,M	A	L
Hydroxocobalamin Inj.	S,M	A	L
Hydroxyprogesterone Caproate Inj.	S,M	A,C	
Sterile Hydroxystilbamidine Isethionate	I	D	LR
Hydroxyzine HCl Inj.	S,M		L
Hyoscyamine Sulfate Inj.	S,M	A	
Indium InIII Pentetate Inj.	S		
Imipramine HCl Inj.	S	A	LR
Indigotindisulfonate Sodium Inj.	S	A	LR
Sterile Indocyanine Green	I	B	
Insulin Inj.	M		R
Isophane Insulin Suspension	M		R
Insulin Zinc Suspension	M		R
Extended Insulin Zinc Suspension	M		R
Prompt Insulin Zinc Suspension	M		R
Protamine Zinc Insulin Suspension	M		R
Insulin Human Inj.	M		
Inulin and Sodium Chloride Inj.	S	A,B	
Iodinated I125 Albumin Inj.	S,M		R
Iodinated I131 Albumin Inj.	U		
Iodinated I131 Albumin Aggregated Inj.	S,M		R
Iodohippurate Sodium I131 Inj.	S,M		
Rose Bengal Sodium I131 Inj.			
Iodipamide Inj.	S	A	L
Iodipamide Meglumine Inj.	S	A,C	

Drugs	Container	Glass Type	Storage Conditions
Iophendylate Inj.	S	A	
Iothalamate Meglumine Inj.	S	A	L
Iothalamate Meglumine and Sodium Iothalamate Inj.	S	A	L
Iothalamate Sodium Inj.	S	A	L
Ferrous Citrate Fe54 Inj.	S,M		
Iron Dextran Inj.	S,M	A,B	
Iron Sorbitex Inj.	S	A	
Isobucaine HCl and Epinephrine Inj.	S	A	
Isoniazid Inj.	S,M	A	L
Isoproterenol HCl Inj.	S	A	L
Isoxsuprine HCl Inj.	S,M	A	
Kanamycin Sulfate Inj.	S,M	A,C	
Sterile Kanamycin Sulfate	I		
Ketamine HCl Inj.	S,M	A	L,H
Leucovorin Calcium Inj.	S	A	LR
Levallorphan Tartrate Inj.	S,M	A	
Levorphanol Tartrate Inj.	S,M	A	
Lidocaine HCl Inj.	S,M	A	
Sterile Lidocaine HCl	I		
Lidocaine HCl and Dextrose Inj.	S	A,B	
Lidocaine HCl and Epinephrine Inj.	S,M	A	LR
Lincomycin HCl Inj.	S,M	A	
Sterile Lincomycin HCl	I		
Magnesium Sulfate	S,M	A	
Manganese Chloride Inj.	S,M	A,B	
Manganese Sulfate Inj.	S,M	A,B	
Mannitol Inj.	S	A,B	
Mannitol and Sodium Chloride Inj.	U	D	
Measles Virus Vaccine Live	S,M		LR,R
Measles and Mumps Virus Vaccine Live	S,M		LR,R
Measles, Mumps and Rubella Virus Vaccine Live	S,M		LR,R
Measles and Rubella Virus Vaccine Live	S,M		LR,R
Mechlorethamine HCl for Inj.	I	B	
Sterile Medroxyprogesterone Acetate (Susp.)	S,M	A	
Menadiol Sodium Diphosphate Inj.	S	A	LR
Menadione Inj.	S,M	A	
Meningococcal Polysaccharide Vaccine (Group A)	M		R
Meningococcal Polysaccharide Vaccine (Group C)	M		R
Meningococcal Polysaccharide Vaccine (Groups A and C combined)	M		R
Meperidine HCl Inj.	S,M	A	
Mephentermine Sulfate Inj.	S,M	A	
Mepivacaine HCl Inj.	S,M	A	
Mepivacaine HCl and Levonordefrin Inj.	S,M	A	
Meprobamate Inj.	S	A	
Meprylcaine HCl and Epinephrine Inj.	S	A	L
Mesoridazine Besylate Inj.	S	A	L
Metaraminol Bitartrate Inj.	S,M	A	L
Methadone HCl Inj.	S,M	A	LR
Sterile Methantheline Bromide	I	D	
Methicillin Sodium for Inj.	I		L,RT
Sterile Methicillin Sodium	I		RT
Methiodal Sodium Inj.	S,M	A	
Methocarbamol Inj.	S	A	

Drugs	Container	Glass Type	Storage Conditions
Methohexital Sodium for Inj.	I	C	
Methotrexate Sodium Inj.	S,M	A	L
Methotrimeprazine Inj.	S,M	A	L
Methoxamine HCl Inj.	S,M	A	L
Methscopolamine Bromide Inj.	S,M	A	
Methydopate HCl Inj.	S	A	
Methylene Blue Inj.	S	A	
Methylergonovine Maleate Inj.	S	A	LR
Sterile Methylprednisolone Acetate (Susp.)	S,M	A	
Methylprednisolone Sodium Succinate for inj.	I	C	
Metocurine Iodide Inj.	S,M	A	
Metronidazole Inj.	S	A,B	
Sterile Mezlocillin Sodium	I		
Miconazole Inj.	S	A	RT
Sterile Minocycline HCl	I		L
Mitomycin for Inj.	I	D	L
Morphine Sulfate Inj.	S,M	A	L
Morrhuate Sodium Inj.	S,M	A	
Moxalactam Disodium for Inj.	I		
Mumps Virus Vaccine Live	S,M		LR,R
Nafcillin Sodium for Inj.	I	D	
Sterile Nafcillin Sodium	I		
Naloxone HCl Inj.	S,M	A	L
Nandrolone Decanoate Inj.	S,M	A	L
Nandrolone Phenpropionate Inj.	S,M	A	L
Sterile Neomycin Sulfate	I		
Neostigmine Methylsulfate Inj.	S,M		L
Netilmicin Sulfate Inj.	S,M	A	
Niacin Inj.	S,M	A	
Niacinaimide Inj.	S,M	A	
Norepinephrine Bitartrate Inj.	S	A	LR
Nylidrin HCl Inj.	S,M	A	
Orphenadrine Citrate Inj.	S,M	A	L
Oxacillin Sodium for Inj.	I	D	RT
Sterile Oxacillin Sodium	I		
Oxymorphone HCl Inj.	S,M	A	L
Oxytetracycline Inj.	S,M		L
Sterile Oxytetracycline	I		L
Oxytetracycline HCl for Inj.	I	B	L
Sterile Oxytetracycline HCl	I		L
Papaverine HCl Inj.	S,M	A	
Sterile Paraldehyde	S	A,B	LR,RT
Parathyroid Inj.	S,M	A,B	R
Sterile Penicillin G Benzathine	I		
Sterile Penicillin G Benzathine Susp.	S,M	A,B	R
Sterile Penicillin G Benzathine and Penicillin G Procaine Susp.	S,M	A,C	
Penicillin G Potassium for Inj.	I	D	
Sterile Penicillin G Potassium	I	D	
Sterile Penicillin G Procaine	I		
Sterile Penicillin G Procaine for Susp.	S,M	A,C	
Penicillin G Sodium for Inj.	I		
Sterile Penicillin G Procaine Susp.	S,M	A,C	R
Sterile Penicillin G Procaine w/Aluminum Stearate Susp.	S,M	A,C	
Penicillin G Sodium for Inj.	I	D	
Sterile Penicillin G Sodium	I	D	
Pentazocine Lactate Inj.	S,M	A	

Drugs	Container	Glass Type	Storage Conditions
Pentobarbital Sodium Inj.	S,M	A	
Perphenazine Inj.	S,M	A	L
Pertussis Vaccine	U		R
Pertussis Vaccine Adsorbed	U		R
Phenobarbital Sodium Inj.	I	D	
Sterile Phenobarbital Sodium	I	D	
Phenolsulfonphthalein Inj.	S	A	
Phentolamine Mesylate for Inj.	I	B	
Phenylephrine HCl Inj.	S,M	A	L
Phenytoin Sodium Inj.	S,M	A	RT
Sterile Phenytoin Sodium	I	C	
Physostigmine Salicylate Inj.	S	A	L
Phytonadione Inj.	S,M	A	L
Pilocarpine Ocular System	S		R
Sterile Piperacillin Sodium	I		
Plicamycin for Inj.	I	D	L
Posterior Pituitary Inj.	S,M	A	
Poliovirus Vaccine Inactivated	U		R
Sterile Polymyxin B Sulfate	I	D	L
Potassium Acetate Inj.	S,M	A,B	
Potassium Chloride Inj.	S,M	A,B	
Potassium Chloride in Dextrose Inj.	S	A,B	
Chromic Phosphate P32 Susp.	S,M		
Potassium Phosphates Inj.	S,M	A	
Sterile Pralidoxone Chloride	I	B	
Sterile Prednisolone Acetate Susp.	S,M	A	
Prednisolone Sodium Phosphate Inj.	S,M	A	L
Prednisolone Sodium Succinate for Inj.	I	D	
Sterile Prednisolone Tebutate Susp.	S,M	A	
Prilocaine HCl Inj.	S,M	A	
Procainamide HCl Inj.	S,M	A	
Procaine HCl Inj.	S,M	A,B	
Sterile Procaine HCl	I	D	
Procaine HCl and Epinephrine Inj.	S,M	A,B	LR
Procaine and Phenylephrine HCls Inj.	S,M	A	
Procaine HCl, Tetracycline HCl and Levonordefrin Inj.	S,M	A	
Prochlorperazine Edisylate Inj.	S,M	A	L
Progesterone Inj.	S,M	A,C	
Sterile Progesterone Susp.	S,M	A	
Progesterone Intrauterine Contraceptive Sys.	S		
Promazine HCl Inj.	S,M	A	L
Promethazine HCl Inj.	S,M	A	L
Sterile Propantheline Bromide	S	D	
Propiomazine HCl Inj.	S	A	RT,L
Propoxycaine HCl, Procaine HCl and Levonordefrin Inj.	S	A	
Propoxycaine HCl, Procaine HCl and Norepinephrine Bitartrate Inj.	S,M	A	
Propranolol HCl Inj.	S	A	LR
Sterile Propyliodone Oil Susp.	S	D	LR
Protamine Sulfate Inj.	S	A	R
Protamine Sulfate for Inj.	I	D	
Protein Hydrolysate Inj.	S	A,B	H
Pyridostigmine Bromide Inj.	S	A	L
Pyridoxine HCl Inj.	S,M	A	L
Quinidine Gluconate Inj.	S,M	A	
Rabies Immune Globin	U		R

Drugs	Container	Glass Type	Storage Conditions
Rabies Vaccine	U		R
Reserpine Inj.	S	A	LR
Riboflavin Inj.	S,M	A	LR
Ringer's Inj.	S	A,B	
Lactated Ringer's Inj.	S	A,B	
Ritodrine HCl Inj.	S	A	RT
Rolitetracycline for Inj.	I	B	L
Sterile Rolitetracycline	I		L
Rubella Virus Vaccine Live	S,M		LR,R
Rubella and Mumps Virus Vaccine Live	S,M		LR,R
Scopolomine Hydrobromide Inj.	S,M	A	LR
Secobarbital Sodium Inj.	S,M	A	L,R
Sisomicin Sulfate Inj.	S,M	A	
Sterile Secobarbital Sodium	I	D	
Selenomethionine Se75 Inj.	U		R
Smallpox Vaccine	U		R
Sodium Acetate Inj.	S	A	
Sodium Bicarbonate Inj.	S	A	
Sodium Chloride Inj.	S	A,B	
Bacteriostatic Sodium Chloride Inj.	S,M	A,B	
Sodium Lactate Inj.	S	A,B	
Sodium Nitrate Inj.	S	A	
Sterile Sodium Nitroprusside	I	D	L
Sodium Phosphates Inj.	S,M	A	
Sodium Sulfate Inj.	S	A	
Sodium Thiosulfate Inj.	S	A	
Sterile Spectinomycin HCl	I	B	
Streptomycin Sulfate Inj.	S,M	A	
Sterile Streptomycin Sulfate	I	D	
Succinylcholine Chloride Inj.	S,M	A,B	R
Sterile Succinylcholine Chloride	I	D	
Sulfadiazine Sodium Inj.	S	A	LR
Sulfisoxazole Diolamine Inj.	S,M	A	L
Sulfobromophthalein Sodium Inj.	S	A	
Technetium Tc99m Albumin Inj.	S,M		R
Technetium Tc99m Albumin Aggregated Inj.	S,M		R
Technetium Tc99m Etiodonate Inj.	S,M		
Technetium Tc99m Ferpentate Inj.	S,M		R,L
Technetium Tc99m Gluceptate Inj.	S,M		R
Technetium Tc99m Medronate Inj.	S,M		
Technetium Tc99m Oxidronate Inj.	S,M		
Technetium Tc99m Penetate Inj.	S,M		R
Sodium Pertechnetate Tc99m Inj.	S,M		R
Technetium Tc99m Pyrophosphate Inj.	S,M		R
Technetium Tc99m (Pyro- and trimeta-) Phosphates Inj.	U	D	
Technetium Tc99m Succimer Inj.	S		RT,L
Technetium Tc99m Sulfur Colloid Inj.	S,M		
Terbutaline Sulfate Inj.	S	A	L,RT
Sterile Testolactone Susp.	S,M	A	
Sterile Testosterone Susp.	S,M	A	
Testosterone Cypionate Inj.	S,M	A	L
Testosterone Enanthate Inj.	S,M	A	
Testosterone Propionate Inj.	S,M	A	
Tetanus Antitoxin	U		R
Tetanus Immune Globulin	U		R
Tetanus Toxoid	U		R
Tetanus Toxoid Adsorbed	U		R

Drugs	Container	Glass Type	Storage Conditions
Tetanus and Diphtheria Toxoids Adsorbed (for adult use)	U		R
Tetracaine HCl Inj.	S,M	A	R,L
Sterile Tetracaine HCl	I	A	
Tetracycline HCl for Inj.	I	B	L
Sterile Tetracycline HCl	I		L
Tetracycline Phosphate Complex for Inj.	I		L
Tetracycline Phosphate Complex for Inj.	I	B	L
Sterile Tetracycline Phosphate Complex	I		L
Thallous Chloride Tl201 Inj.	S,M		
Thiamine HCl Inj.	S,M	A	L
Thiamylal Sodium for Inj.	I	C	
Thiethylperazine Malate Inj.	S	A	L
Thiopental Sodium for Inj.	I	C	
Thiotepa for Inj.	I	D	R,L
Thiothixene HCl Inj.	S	A	L
Thiothixene HCl for Inj.	I		LR
Sterile Ticarcillin Disodium	I	D	
Tobramycin Sulfate Inj.	S,M	A	
Sterile Tobramycin Sulfate	I		
Tolazoline HCl Inj.	S,M	A	
Sterile Tolbutamide Sodium	I	D	
Sterile Triamcinolone Diacetate Susp.	S,M	A	
Sterile Triamcinolone Hexacetonide Susp.	S,M	A	
Tridihexethyl Chloride Inj.	S	A	
Trifluoperazine HCl Inj.	M	A	L
Trifluopromazine HCl Inj.	S,M	A	L
Trimethaphan Camsylate Inj.	S,M	A	R
Trimethobenzamide HCl Inj.	S,M	A	
Tromethamine for Inj.	I	C	
Tubocurarine Chloride Inj.	S,M		R
Typhoid Vaccine	U		
Sterile Urea	I	D	
Vaccinia Immune Globulin	U		R
Sterile Vancomycin HCl	I	B	
Variccila-Zoster Immune Globulin	U		R
Vasopressin Inj.	S,M	A	
Vidarabine Concentrate for Inj.	S,M	A	
Sterile Vinblastine Sulfate	I	D	R
Vincristine Sulfate for Inj.	I	D	R
Warfarin Sodium for Inj.	I	D	LR
Bacteriostatic Water for Inj.	S,M	A,B	
Sterile Water for Inj.	S	A,B	
Sterile Water for Irrigation	S	A,B	
Xenon Xe133 Inj.	S (totally filled)		R
Yellow Fever Vaccine	U (nitrogen filled ampuls®)		
Ytterbium Yb169 Pentetate Inj.	S		RT
Zinc Chloride Inj.	S,M	A,B	
Zinc Sulfate Inj.	S,M		

LISTED IN NUMERICAL ORDER

0002
Lilly, Eli, & Co.

0003
Squibb Pharmaceutical Co.

0004
Roche Laboratories

0005
Lederle Laboratories,
Davis & Geck, American
Cyanamid Co.

0006
Merck Sharp & Dohme

0007
Smith Kline & French
Laboratories

0008
Wyeth Laboratories

0009
Upjohn Company, The

0011
Hynson, Westcott & Dunning
Inc.

0013
Warren-Teed Laboratories
Div. of Adria Laboratories, Inc.

0014
Searle & Co.

0015
Bristol Labs

0016
Pharmacia Laboratories

0017
Wampole Laboratories
Wallace Laboratories

0018
Pennwalt Corporation
Prescription Division

0021
Reed & Carnrick

0022
McKesson Laboratories

0023
Herbert Laboratories
Allergan Pharmaceuticals, Inc.

0024
Winthrop Laboratories

0025
Searle Laboratories

0026
Miles Pharmaceuticals

0028
Geigy Pharmaceuticals

0029
Beecham Laboratories

0031
Robins, A.H., Company

0032
Rowell Laboratories, Inc.

0033
Syntex Laboratories, Inc.

0034
Purdue Frederick Co., The

0035
Eaton Laboratories

0037
Wallace Laboratories

0038
Stuart Pharmaceuticals

0039
Hoechst-Roussel
Pharmaceuticals, Inc.

0041
Cooper Laboratories,
Inc.

0043
Dorsey Laboratories

0044
Knoll Pharmaceutical Co.

0045
McNeilab, Inc.

0046
Ayerst Laboratories

0047
Warner/Chilcott
Laboratories

0048
Flint Laboratories

0049
Roerig

0051
Unimed, Inc.

0052
Organon Inc.

0053
Armour Pharmaceutical
Co.

0054
Phillips Roxane Labs., Inc.

0055
Cole Pharmacal Co., Inc.

0056
Endo Labs., Inc.

0057
Breon Laboratories Inc.

0058
SMP, Div. CooperVision P.R.,
Inc.

0062
Ortho Pharmaceutical
Corporation

0063
Reid-Provident Labs., Inc.

0065
Alcon Laboratories, Inc.

0066
Dermik Laboratories, Inc.

0067
Rorer, William H., Inc.

0068
Merrell-National Labs.

0069
Pfizer Laboratories

0070
USV Laboratories Inc.

0071
Parke, Davis & Co.

0072
Westwood Pharmaceuticals,
Inc.

0073
Lakeside Laboratories

0074
Abbott Laboratories
Murine Company
Ross Laboratories

0075
USV Laboratories, Div.
USV Pharmaceutical Corp.

0076
Star Pharmaceuticals, Inc.

0078
Sandoz Pharmaceuticals

0081
Burroughs Wellcome Co.

0082
Ives Laboratories Inc.

0083
CIBA Pharmaceutical
Company

0084
American Pharmaceutical Co.
0085
Schering Corporation

0086
Carnrick Laboratories

0087
Mead Johnson & Company

0088
Marion Laboratories, Inc.
Derm-Arts Laboratories

0089
Riker Laboratories, Inc.

• The "Pharmaceutical Company Labeler Code Index" is presented to aid the practitioner in the identification of drug products. In this section the codes are listed in numerical order. Additionally, the pharmaceutical labeler codes are also listed with the alphabetical listing of Pharmaceutical Manufacturers and/or Drug Distributors.

0091
Kremers-Urban Co.

0093
Lemmon Company

0094
American Critical Care

0095
Poythress, Wm. P., & Co., Inc.

0096
Person & Covey, Inc.

0098
Kirkman Laboratories, Inc.

0105
USV (P.R.) Development Corp.

0107
Ortho Pharmaceuticals, Inc.

0109
Allergan Caribbean

0110
Tarmac Products, Inc.

0111
Emko Company, The

0112
Mitchum-Thayer, Inc.

0116
Xttrium Laboratories, Inc.

0118
Hollister-Stier Laboratories

0123
Stayner Corp.

0124
Reid-Provident Pharmaceuticals

0125
International Pharmaceutical
Corporation

0126
Hoyt Laboratories

0127
Ulmer Pharmacal Co.

0128
Calgon Consumer Products Co.,
Inc.

0131
The Central Pharmacal Co.

0132
Fleet, C. B., Co., Inc.

0133
Zemmer Co., The
Moore Kirk Labs.

0137
Johnson & Johnson
Dermatological Division

0138
Plough, Inc.

0139
Park Laboratories, Inc.

0141
Fuller Laboratories, Inc.

0142
Amfre-Grant
Ormont Drug & Chemical Co.,
Inc.

0143
West-ward, Inc.

0145
Stiefel Laboratories, Inc.

0147
Camall Company

0149
Norwich-Eaton Pharmaceuticals

0152
Gray Pharmaceutical Company

0154
Blair Laboratories, Inc.

0157
American Labs.
Towne, Paulsen & Co., Inc.

0158
Denver Chemical Mfg. Co., The

0159
Noyes, P.J. Co., The

0161
Cutter Laboratories, Inc.

0162
Arch Laboratories

0163
Elder, Paul B., Co.
Campbell Laboratories, Inc.

0165
Blaine Co., Inc.

0166
Mallard Inc.

0168
Fougera, E. & Co., Inc.

0171
Johnson, Matt, Co.

0172
Zenith Laboratories, Inc.

0173
Glaxo Incorporated

0175
Hartford Laboratories

0177
International Drug, Inc.

0178
Mission Pharmacal Co.

0179
Madland Laboratories, Inc.

0181
Vita Elixir Co., Inc.

0182
Generix Drug Sales Co., Inc.

0183
Dow Pharmaceuticals

0184
Medics Pharmaceutical Corp.

0185
Vitarine Co., Inc.
Laboratorios Gimenez, Inc.

0186
Astra Pharmaceutical Products,
Inc.

0187
ICN Pharmaceuticals

0191
Mahon, Thomas J., Inc.
Ortega Pharmaceutical Co.

0192
Miles Laboratories, Inc.

0193
Ames Company

0195
Wharton Laboratories, Inc.

0196
Rachelle Laboratories

0197
Ex-Lax Inc.

0198
North American Pharmacal

0212
Doyle Pharmaceutical Co.

0215
Medical Chemicals, Inc.
Medwick Laboratories, Inc.

0217
Dunhall Pharmaceuticals, Inc.

0219
Humphreys Pharmacal, Inc.

0221
Dooner Laboratories, Inc.

0222
Boyle & Co.

0223
Consolidated Midland Corp.

0225
Ascher, B.F., & Co., Inc.

0228
Purepac Pharmaceutical Co.

0233
Trent Pharmaceuticals, Inc.

0234
Schmid Laboratories

0235
Pharmacraft Division
Pennwalt Corporation

0237
Webber Pharmaceuticals, U.S.A.,
Inc.
Fellows Medical Division

0242
Stanlabs Pharmaceutical Co.

0244
Medicone Company

0245
Upsher-Smith Laboratories, Inc.

0247
Alcon/B. P.
Burton, Parsons & Company,
Inc.

0248
Brown Pharmaceutical Co., Inc.,
The

0249
Geriatric Pharmaceutical Corp.

0251
Spanner, G.O., Inc.

0252
Bowman Pharmaceuticals, Inc.
Bowman, Inc.

0253
Sutliff & Case Co., Inc.

0256
Fleming & Company

0258
Inwood Laboratories, Inc.

0259
Mayrand Incorporated

0261
Drug Industries Co., Inc.

0263
Rystan Co., Inc.

0267
Federal Pharmacal Corp.

0268
Center Laboratories, Inc.

0269
Roussel Corporation

0271
Palmedico, Inc.

0273
Lorvic Corp., The

0274
Scherer Laboratories, Inc.

0275
Arco Pharmaceuticals, Inc.

0276
Misemer Pharmaceuticals, Inc.

0277
Laser, Inc.

0279
Robinson Laboratory, Inc.

0281
Savage Laboratories

0282
Dalin Pharmaceuticals, Inc.

0283
Beutlich, Inc.

0284
Lexington Chemical Co., Inc.

0285
King Pharmaceutical Co., Inc.

0288
Fluoritab Corp.

0291
Westerfield

0292
Watson, T.E., Co.

0299
Owen Laboratories

0311
Almay Inc.

0314
Hyrex Pharmaceuticals
Matco Drug Company

0315
Len-Tag Co.

0316
Del-Ray Laboratories, Inc.

0317
Whorton Pharmaceuticals, Inc.
Yeager Specialty Co.

0318
Ormont Drug & Chemical Co.,
Inc.

0322
Merrick Medicine Co.

0323
Welty Corporation

0326
Calbio Pharmaceuticals

0327
Guardian Chemical Corp.

0329
Scruggs Pharmacal Company,
Inc.

0331
Premo Pharmaceutical Labs.,
Inc.

0341
Parker Laboratories, Inc.

0343
Youngs Drug Products Corp.

0346
Softcon Products

0348
Lambda Pharmacal Labs.,
Inc.

0349
Parmed Pharmaceuticals, Inc.

0351
Kay Pharmacal Co., Inc.

0352
Schuemann Laboratories, Inc.

0357
Cumberland Mfg. Co.
Arcum Pharmaceutical Corp.

0359
Columbia Medical Co.

0362
Novocol Chemical Mfg. Co., Inc.

0365
Progressive Enterprises

0368
Bell Pharmacal Corp.

0369
Key Pharmaceuticals, Inc.

0371
Layton Laboratories

0372
Hannaway, R. T., Inc.
Scot-Tussin Pharmacal Co., Inc.

0373
Baker, J.T., Chemical Company

0374
Lyne Laboratories

0375
Corvit Pharmaceuticals

0377
Vale Chemical Co., Inc., The

0381
Carter-Glogau Laboratories

0382
Northrup Pharmaceutical Co.

0383
Hoffman Laboratories, Inc.

0385
Coast Laboratories, Inc.

0386
Gebauer Chemical Co.

0391
Lardon Labs.

0393
Salem Pharmacal

0394
Mericon Industries, Inc.

0395
Humco Laboratory, Inc.

0396
Milex Products, Inc.

0397
Jenkins Laboratories, Inc.

0398
C & M Pharmacal, Inc.
Ries-Hamly, Inc.
0411
Forbes Pharmacal, Inc.

0414
Suppositoria Labs., Inc.

0417
Hall, Don, Laboratories

0418
Pasadena Research
Laboratories, Inc.

0419
Santa Pharmaceuticals, Inc.

0421
Fielding Pharmaceutical Co., The

0425
Day-Baldwin, Inc.

0427
Winston Pharmaceuticals, Inc.

0429
Merit Pharmaceutical Co., Inc.

0432
Rex Laboratory, Inc.

0436
Century Pharmaceuticals, Inc.

0444
Carr Drug Co.
Scrip, Inc.

0446
Leeds Pharmacal Corp.

0451
Muro Pharmacal Labs., Inc.

0452
Brunswick Laboratories

0454
Metro Med., Inc.

0456
O'Neal, Jones & Feldman, Inc.

0461
Yager Drug Co.

0463
Truxton, Inc.

0466
Macsil, Inc.

0467
Invenex Pharmaceuticals

0472
Barre Drug Co., Inc.

0473
Carbisulphoil Co.

0475
Berkeley Laboratories

0477
Obetrol Pharmaceuticals

0479
Burlington Pharmacal, Inc.

0482
Kenwood Laboratories, Inc.

0484
SK&F Co.

0485
Edwards Pharmacal Co.

0486
Beach Pharmaceuticals
    Hill Dermaceuticals

0487
Nephron Corporation

0491
Coastal Pharmaceutical Co., Inc.

0493
Amid Laboratories, Inc.

0494
Foy Laboratories, Inc.

0496
Ferndale Laboratories, Inc.

0511
Sandia Pharmaceuticals, Inc.

0512
Marsh-Emory Laboratories, Inc.

0514
Dow B. Hickam, Inc.

0516
Glenwood Laboratories, Inc.

0517
American Quinine

0518
Advance Biofactures Corp.

0523
Acid-Eze Company, Inc.

0524
Rucker Pharmacal Co., Inc.

0526
Carlton Corp., The

0527
Lannett Co., Inc.

0529
Blue Line Chemical Co., The

0534
Aeroceuticals, Inc.

0535
Gilbert Laboratories

0538
Landry Pharmaceuticals, Inc.

0539
American Urologicals, Inc.

0543
Mosso, C. A., Co.

0544
Eastwood Pharmacal Co., Inc.

0551
Seatrace Co., The

0552
Comatic Laboratories, Inc.

0553
Hydrosal Co.

0555
Barr Laboratories, Inc.

0556
Cenci, H.R., Laboratories, Inc.

0558
Tri-State Pharmaceutical Co.,
    Inc.

0563
Bock Pharmacal Company

0568
Baylor Laboratories, Inc.

0569
Rand Labs., Inc.

0571
Archer Pharmaceutical Co., Inc.

0572
Sheraton Laboratories, Inc.

0573
Whitehall Labs.

0574
Paddock Laboratories

0575
Cummins Pharmaceutical Co.,
    Inc.

0576
Medical Prods. Panamericana,
    Inc.

0578
Jones & Vaughan, Inc.

0585
Fisons Corporation

0587
Dermakon Laboratories Division,
    Preston Pharmaceutics, Inc.

0588
Keene Pharmaceuticals, Inc.

0592
Jones, Ed, Inc.

0596
Canright Corp.

0597
Boehringer Ingelheim Ltd.

0598
Approved Pharmaceutical Corp.
Pharmacy Associates

0611
Jalco Pharmaceuticals, Inc.

0614
Douglas Pharmacal Industries, Inc.

0615
Vangard Laboratories

0617
Dios Chemical Co.

0618
Luyties Pharmacal Co.

0619
Walker Pharmacal Co.

0621
Wise's K.C. Homeopathic
    Pharmacy

0633
Inland Alkaloid Company

0638
Fray Corp.

0639
Paraeusal Co.

0641
Elkins-Sinn, Inc.

0642
Everett Laboratories, Inc.

0645
Medi-Rx Pharmaceuticals, Inc.

0648
Truett Laboratories

0653
Nejo Pharmacal Co.

0655
Bomiseco Laboratories, Inc.

0656
Tennessee Pharmaceutical Co.,
    Inc.

0657
DDR Pharmaceutical Corp.

0659
Circle Pharmaceuticals, Inc.

0664
Bocan Drug Co.

0667
Fort David Laboratories, Inc.

0669
Lepler Laboratories, Inc.

0673
Sidal Pharmaceutical Co., Inc.

0674
General Pharmaceutical Prods.,
    Inc.

0689
Daniels Pharmaceuticals

0692
Martin-Phillips Laboratories,
    Inc.

0697
Delco Chemical Co., Inc.

0698
Grafton Pharmaceutical Co.

0711
Scott-Alison Pharmaceuticals,
    Inc.

0713
G & W Laboratories, Inc.

0716
Standex Laboratories, Inc.

0721
Eastern Research Labs., Inc.

0727
Park Plaza Pharmaceuticals,
    Inc.

0731
Alto Pharmaceuticals, Inc.

0733
Laboratorios Terrier, Inc.

0734
Tablicaps, Inc.

0737
Amazol Company, The
D'Franssia Corp.

0741
Walker Corp. & Co., Inc.

0749
Mill-Mark Pharmaceuticals, Inc.

0752
Norgine Laboratories, Inc.

0758
Moffet, Inc.

0759
Chrisman Co.

0762
Rhode, J. G., Co., The

0764
Medco Supply Co.

0766
Norcliff Thayer Inc.

0777
Dista Products Co.

0781
Geneva Generics

0785
UAD Laboratories, Inc.

0793
Rals Laboratories

0795
Brothers Pharmaceuticals, Inc.

0799
Perry Laboratories, Inc.

0814
Interstate Drug Exchange

0815
Reiss Williams Company

0816
Midway Medical Co., Inc.

0823
Sheryl Pharmaceuticals, Inc.

0827
Delta Drug Corp.

0832
Western Research Laboratories,
    Inc.

0834
Saron Pharmacal Corp.

0835
Geneva Drugs Ltd.

0836
Virtal Pharmacal Co., Inc.

0839
Moore, H. L., Drug Exchange,
    Inc.

0841
Haberle Drug Co.

0849
Ingram Pharmaceutical Co.

0875
Bio-Factor Labs.

0884
Pedinol Pharmacal, Inc.

0892
Bell Therapeutic Supplies,
    Inc.

0893
Barry Martin Pharmaceuticals,
    Inc.

0897
National Magnesia Co., Inc.

0917
Wesley Pharmacal Co., Inc.

0919
Werner Laboratories, Inc.

0923
Whitew001th, Inc.

0928
Wolins Pharmacal Corp.

0944
Hyland Laboratories

0971
Winthrop Products, Inc.

0991
Webcon Pharmaceuticals

0992
Kahlenberg Laboratories

0993
American Felsol Co.

0995
Pfipharmecs

1016
Bluco Incorporated

1097
Rilox Company, The

1212
Brown Medicine Co.

1215
Galen Pharmaceuticals, Inc.

1237
King's Specialty Co.

1246
Thera-Medic, Inc.

1277
Morton Pharmaceuticals,
    Inc.

10244
Otis Clapp & Son, Inc.
Buffington Division
Cross Division

10003
A.V.P. Pharmaceuticals, Inc.

10038
Velvet Pharmcal Co.

10040
Amco Drug Products Co.,
    Inc.

10125
Phoenix Pharmacal

10153
Bisleri Co., Inc.

10244
Otis Clapp & Son, Inc.

10310
Del Laboratories, Inc.
Commerce Drug Co., Inc.

10327
DeWitt International Corp.

10341
Doktors Laboratories, Inc.

10440
G. E. Laboratories, Inc.

10648
Larson Labs., Inc.

10651
Lavoptik Co., Inc.

10706
Manne, Kenneth A., Co.

10797
Natcon Chemical Co., Inc.

10824
Nortech Laboratories

10833
Spirt & Company
Hart Laboratories

10929
Pyro-Sana Laboratory

10945
Rasman Pharmacal Co., Inc.

10952
Recsei Laboratories

10956
Reese Chemical Co.

10973
Richards Pharmaceutical Co.

10989
ROR Pharmacal Co., Inc.

11086
Summers Laboratories, Inc.

11089
Superior Chemical International,
   Inc.
McGregor & Co.

11299
Torch Laboratories, Inc.

11311
Trimen Laboratories, Inc.

11312
Carbo-Fung Labs., Inc.

11365
Wade Chemical Company

11370
Warner-Lambert Company

11397
Western Pharmacal Co.

11414
Willen Drug Co.

11422
Winton, Ralph, Co.

11463
Barry Laboratories, Inc.

11489
Cunningham Distributors

11530
Stanback Co., Ltd.

11588
Jeffrey Martin, Inc.

11649
Press Chemical &
   Pharmaceutical Laboratories

11694
Key Company, The

11696
Dattel Pharmaceutical Co.,
   Inc.

11701
Sween Corp.

11808
Ion Laboratories, Inc.

11853
Gaddy, R. L., Company

11868
Monticello Drug Co.

11940
Medco Lab. Inc.

11980
Allergan America

12072
Temesco

12120
Wisconsin Pharmacal Co.,
   Inc.
Badger Pharmacal, Inc.

12126
Ivy Corp.

12136
Bird Corporation

12154
Allison Laboratories, Inc.

12336
Econo-Rx, Inc.

12359
Rawl Chemical Co., Inc.

12418
Culminal, Inc.

12434
Last, Alvin, Inc.

12620
Reaco Products, Inc.

12758
Mason Pharmaceuticals,
   Inc.

12766
Miller Laboratories

12805
International Chemical
   Laboratories

12814
Merchant, W. F., Pharmaceutical
   Co., Inc.

12843
Glenbrook Laboratories

12939
Marlop Pharmaceuticals,
   Inc.

14869
Lexalabs, Inc.

17021
Cameron Medical Corp.

17154
Danal Laboratories Inc.

17201
Leland Laboratories, Inc.

19041
Doshire, Inc.

19810
Bristol-Myers Products

21769
Reily Chemical Co.

23900
Vicks Health Care

35476
Vitacorp.

36969
Merrell-National Laboratories,
   Inc., (PR)

38242
Adria Laboratories Inc.
(Includes Warren-Teed Products)

41167
Chattem Laboratories

42021
Sclavo, Inc.

44081
Med-Corp, Inc.

44384
Biological Corp. of America

45800
Menley and James Laboratories

50419
Berlex Laboratories

50821
Springbrook Pharmaceuticals,
   Inc.

76660
Vicks Toiletry Products

0074
Abbott Laboratories
Abbott Park
North Chicago, IL 60064

0074
Abbott Consumer Products
Div. of Abbott Laboratories

0074
Abbott Diagnostic Products
Div. of Abbott Laboratories

0074
Abbott Hospital Products
Div. of Abbott Laboratories

0074
Abbott Pharmaceutical
Products
Div. of Abbott Laboratories

0523
Acid-Eze Company, Inc.
Triangle Shopping Center
Trion, GA 30753

38242
Adria Laboratories Inc.
P.O. Box 16529
Columbus, OH 43216

0518
Advance Biofactures Corp.
35 Wilbur St.
Lynbrook, NY 11563

0534
Aeroceuticals Health Care
Prods.
49 John Street
Southport, CT 06490

Alberto-Culver Co.
2525 W. Armitage Ave.
Melrose Park, IL 60160

0065
Alcon Labs., Inc.
6201 S. Freeway
Box 1959
Ft. Worth, TX 76101

0065
Alcon Labs., Inc.
Surgical Products Div.
P.O. Box 1959
Ft. Worth, TX 76101

Alconox, Incorporated
215 Park Avenue, S.
New York, NY 10003

Alkalol Co.
Box 964
Taunton, MA 02780

11980
Allergan America
See: Allergan Pharmaceuticals,
Inc.

0109
Allergan Caribbean
See: Allergan Pharmaceuticals,
Inc.

0023
Allergan Pharmaceuticals, Inc.
2525 duPont Drive
Irvine, CA 92713

Alpern Laboratories
Subs. Lesch Corp.
414 West Lenox Ave.
Oak Park, IL 60302

Alpha Pharmaceuticals,
Inc.
1336 N. Carolan St.
P.O. Box 1336
Burlingame, CA 94010

0731
Alto Pharmaceuticals, Inc.
P.O. Box 271369
Tampa, FL 33688

Alton Products Inc.
93 Border St.
W. Newton, MA 02165

10040
Amco Drug Prods. Co., Inc.
Box 10
North Olmsted, OH 44070

Amend Drug & Chemical Co.,
Inc.
83 Cordier St.
Irvington, NJ 07111

0094
American Critical Care
Div. American Hospital Supply
Corp.
1600 Waukegan Road
McGraw Park, IL 60085

0005
American Cyanamid Co.
Agriculture Division
P.O. Box 400
Princeton, NJ 08540

American Dermal Corp.
P.O. Box 427
Somerset, NJ 08873

0993
American Felsol Company
Div. T.E. Watson Co.
P.O. Box 3829
Sarasota, FL 33578

0157
American Labs. (Amlab)
Div. Towne, Paulsen & Co.,
Inc.

American Lecithin Co.,
Inc.
32–34 61st Street
Woodside, L.I., NY 11377

American McGaw
Div. Am. Hosp. Supply Corp.
2525 McGaw Ave.
Santa Ana, CA 92711

American Pharmaceutical
Products Co.

0517
American Quinine
Hosp. Div. Natcon Chemical Co.,
Inc.
1 Fairchild Court
Plainview, NY 11803

0539
American Urilogicals, Inc.

0193
Ames Company
Div. Miles Labs., Inc.
P.O. Box 70
1127 Myrtle Street
Elkhart, IN 46514

0142
Amfre-Grant, Inc.
See: U.S. Products, Inc.

0493
Amid Laboratories, Inc.
See: T. E. Williams
Pharmaceuticals, Inc.

0598
Approved Pharm. Corp.
1643 E. Genesee St.
Syracuse, NY 13202

Arbrook, Inc.
P.O. Box 130
Arlington, TX 76010

0162
Arch Laboratories
Div. of Norcliff Thayer Inc.
319 S. 4th Street
St. Louis, MO 63102

Archar Drug Co.
107 E. Markham St.
P.O. Box 2701
Little Rock, AR 72203

0275
Arco Pharmaceuticals, Inc.
105 Orville Drive
Bohemia, NY 11716

0357
Arcum Pharm. Corp.

Ar-Ex Products Co.
1036 W. Van Buren St.
Chicago, IL 60607

0053
Armour Pharm. Co.
Div. Revlon Health Care Group
303 South Broadway
Tarrytown, NY 10591

Arnar Stone Labs.
See: American Critical Care

0225
Ascher, B.F. & Co., Inc.
P.O. Box 827
Kansas City, MO 64141

Associated Concentrates
Div. American Lecithin Co., Inc.
P.O. Box 4056
Atlanta, GA 30302

---

* A Pharmaceutical Labeler Code appears prior to the address for each company. This code has been added as an aid in the identification of drug products.

0186
Astra Pharm. Products, Inc.
50 Otis street
Westboro, MA 01581

Atlas Chemical Co.
See: ICI United States Inc.

Aveeno Dermatologicals
See: Cooper Labs, Inc.

Avicon, Inc.
Div. of Alcon Labs., Inc.
6201 S. Freeway
P.O. Box 85
Fort Worth, TX 76101

10003
A.V.P. Pharmaceuticals, Inc.
9829 Main Street
Clarence, NY 14031

0046
Ayerst Labs.
Div. Amer. Home Products
   Corp.
685 Third Ave.
New York, NY 10017

12120
Badger Pharmacal, Inc.
P.O. Box 171
Cedarburg, WI 53012

Baker/Cummins
Div. of Key Pharmaceuticals, Inc.

Barnes-Hind Pharmaceuticals,
   Inc.
895 Kifer Rd.
Sunnyvale, CA 94086

0555
Barr Laboratories, Inc.
265 Livinston St.
Northvale, NJ 07647

0472
Barre Drug. Co., Inc.

11463
Barry Labs., Inc.
461 N.E. 27th St.
Pompano Beach, FL 33064

0893
Barry-Martin Pharmaceuticals, Inc.
5792 S. W. 8th St.
Miami, FL 33144

Barth Nutritional Supplements,
   Inc.
270 W. Merrick Rd.
Valley Stream, NY 11582

Bay Laboratories, Inc.
3654 West Jarvis
Skokie, IL 60076

Bausch & Lomb
Rochester, NY 14692

Baybank Drug Co., Inc.
See: Endo Labs.

0568
Baylor Laboratories Inc.
See: Norwich Eaton
   Pharmaceuticals

0486
Beach Pharmaceuticals
Div. of Beach Products, Inc.
P.O. Box 13447
Tampa, FL 33611

0029
Beecham Laboratories
Div. of Beecham, Inc.
501 Fifth St.
Bristol, TN 37620

Beecham Products
Div. of Beecham, Inc.
P.O. Box 1467
Pittsburgh, PA 15230

Beiersdorf, Inc.
P.O. Box 5529
South Norwalk, CT 06856

Bell & Co.
See: C. S. Dent & Co.

0368
Bell Pharmacal Corp.
P.O. Box 1968
Greenville, SC 29602

0892
Bell Therapeutic Supplies, Inc.
396 Rockaway Ave.
Valley Stream, NY 11581

Bellis' Santa Maria Drug
See: Anatox Co.

Bentex Pharmaceuticals
Div. ICN Corporation

Berkeley Biologicals
1831 Second Street
Berkeley, CA 94710

Berkeley Drug Co.
See: Alton Products Inc.

0475
Berkeley Laboratories
356 Warren Ave.
Stirling, NJ 07980

50419
Berlex Laboratories, Inc.
Subs. Schering AG
110 East Hanover Ave.
Cedar Knolls, NJ 07927

Beta Dyne Corp.
22 Park Place
New York City, NY 10007

0283
Beutlich, Inc.
7006 N. Western Ave.
Chicago, IL 60645

0875
Bio-Factor Labs.
103 South Elm St.
Marshville, NC 28103

Birchwood Laboratories, Inc.
7900 Fuller Road
Eden Prairie, MN 55344

12136
Bird Corp.
Subs. 3M Company
2800 East Alejo Road
Palm Springs, CA 92263

0165
Blaine Co.
2700 Dixie Highway
Fort Mitchell, KY 41017

0154
Blair Laboratories, Inc.
Subs. Purdue Fredrick Co.

Block Drug Co., Inc.
257 Cornelison Ave.
Jersey City, NJ 07302

1016
Bluco, Inc.
14849 W. McNichols
Detroit, MI 48235

Blue Cross
See: Halsey Drug Co., Inc.

0529
Blue Line Chemical Co., The
302 S. Broadway
St. Louis, MO 63102

0563
Bock Pharmacal Co.
5435 Highland Park Drive
St. Louis, MO 63110

0597
Boehringer Ingelheim
90 East Ridge
P.O. Box 368
Ridgefield, CT 06877

Boots Laboratories, Inc.
433 Commercial Ave.
Palisades Park, NJ 07650

11489
Boots Pharmaceuticals, Inc.
6540 Line Avenue
P.O. Box 6750
Shreveport, LA 71136

Borden Inc., Pharmaceutical
   Prod.
Div. Syntex Lab., Inc.
Stanford Industrial Park
Palo Alto, CA 94304

0252
Bowman Pharmaceuticals,
   Inc.
119 Schroyer Ave., S.W.
Canton, OH 44702

Boyd Pharmacal Co.
205 Mitchell St.
P.O. Box 552
Newland, NC 28657

0222
Boyle & Co.
13260 Moore Street
St. Cerritos, CA 90701

Breck, John H., Inc.
Berdan Ave.
P.O. Box 325
Wayne, NJ 07470

0057
Breon Laboratories Inc.
See: Winthop-Breon Labs.

Briar Pharmacal, Inc.
See: North American
   Pharmacal

0015
Bristol Laboratories
Div. Bristol-Myers Co.
P.O. Box 657
Syracuse, NY 13201

19810
Bristol-Myers Products
Div. Bristol-Myers Co.
345 Park Avenue
New York, NY 10154

Broemmel Pharmaceuticals
See: Riker Labs.

1212
Brown Medicine Co.
P.O. Box 3345
Knoxville, TN 37917

0248
Brown Pharmaceutical Co., The
2500 West 6th Street
Los Angeles, CA 90057

Buckley Pharmaceuticals
Subs. Schaffer Labs.

10244
Buffington
Div. of Otis Clapp & Son, Inc.

Burgin-Arden, Inc.
Portland, OR 97230

Burleson Ointment Co.
P.O. Box 6405
Grand Rapids, MI 49506

0479
Burlington Pharmacal, Inc.
274 N. Graham
Hopedale Road, Box 3311
Burlington, NC 27215

0081
Burroughs Wellcome Co.
3030 Cornwallis Road
Research Triangle Park, NC
27709

0247
Burton, Parsons & Co., Inc.
See: Alcon/ B. P.

Bush Labs.
4200 Laclede Ave.
St. Louis, MO 63108

0128
Calgon Consumer Prod. Co., Inc.
Sub. of Merck & Co.

Calvital Pharmaceutical Corp.
679 E. 138th Street
Bronx, NY 10454

17021
Cameron Medical Corp.
2716 E. Florence Ave.
Huntington Park, CA 90255

0163
Campbell Laboratories, Inc.
P.O. Box 812, FDR Station
New York, NY 10150

Campana Corp.
Campana Bldg.
Div. of Purex Corp.
Batavia, IL 60510

Campbell Pharmaceuticals, Inc.
See: Ayerst Laboratories

0398
C and M Pharmacal, Inc.
1519 E. Eight Mile Rd.
Hazel Park, MI 48030

0574
Canfield, C.R., & Co.
See: Paddock Labs.

11312
Carbo-Fung Labs., Inc.
798 No. Coney Ave.
Azusa, CA 91702

0526
Carlton Corp., The
See: Glenwood Labs. Inc.

Carnation Co.
5045 Wilshire Blvd.
Los Angeles, CA 90036

Carnation Research Labs.
8015 Van Nuys Blvd.
Van Nuys, CA 91412

Carnrick Laboratories
Div. of G. W. Carnrick Co.
65 Horse Hill Road
Cedar Knolls, NY 07927

0444
Carr Drug Co.
101 South St.
Peoria, IL 61602

Carrtone Labs., Inc.
See: Century Labs., Inc.

0381
Carter-Glogau Laboratories
Div. of Chromalloy
  Pharmaceuticals, Inc.
5160 W. Bethany Home Road
Glendale, AZ 85301

Carter Products
Div. Carter-Wallace, Inc.
Half Acre Rd.
Cranbury, NJ 08512

Celebre, Ernest P., R. Ph
4500 6th St.
Kenosha, WI 53140

0556
Cenci, H. R., Laboratories, Inc.
152 N. Broadway
Fresno, CA 93701

0268
Center Laboratories
35 Channel Drive
Port Washington, NY 11050

Centerchem Pharmaceuticals,
  Inc.
475 Park Avenue South
New York, NY 10016

0131
Central Pharmaceuticals, Inc.
110–128 E. Third St.
P.O. Box 328
Seymour, IN 47274

0436
Century Pharmaceuticals, Inc.
10377 Hague Road
Indianapolis, IN 46256

Cetylite Industries, Inc.
9051 River Road
Pennsauken, NJ 08110

41167
Chattem Laboratories
Div. of Chattem, Inc.
1715 W. 38th St.
Chattanooga, TN 37409

Chesebrough-Pond's Inc.
Div. Professional Prods.
40 Merritt Boulevard
Trumbull, CT 06611

Chicago Pharmacal Co.
See: Conal Pharmaceuticals

Chilton Laboratories, Inc.
See: Ivy Corporation

Chromalloy Pharmaceuticals,
  Inc.
See: Carter-Glogau Laboratories.

Churchill Pharmaceuticals, Inc.
P.O. Box 8581
Richmond, VA 23226

0083
Ciba Pharmaceutical Co.
Div. of Ciba-Geigy Corp.
556 Morris Ave.
Summit, NJ 07901

0659
Circle Pharmaceuticals,
  Inc.
10377 Hague Road
Indianapolis, IN 46256

Citroleum Co.
1054 North Ave.
Bridgeport, CT 06606

City Chemical Corp.
132 W. 22nd St.
New York, NY 10011

10244
Clapp, Otis & Son, Inc.
See: Otis Clapp

Clark-West
Div. of Syntex Labs.

0223
CMC Pharmaceuticals
Div. of Consolidated Midland

0385
Coast Laboratories, Inc.
521 W. 17th St.
Long Beach, CA 90813

30491
Coastal Pharmaceutical Co.,
  Inc.
2509 Granby St.
Norfolk, VA 23517

0055
Cole Pharmacal Co., Inc.
See: O'Neal, Jones and
  Feldman Pharmaceuticals

0359
Columbia Medical Co.
262 Route 59
Monsey, NY 10952

0552
Comatic Labs., Inc.

Combe Inc.
1101 Westchester Ave.
White Plains, NY 10604

10310
Commerce Drug Co., Inc.
Div. Del Labs, Inc.
565 Broad Hollow Rd.
Farmingdale, NY 11735

Conal Pharmaceuticals
Alcon—Specialty Products
  Division
P.O. Box 1959
Fort Worth, TX 76101

Connaught Laboratories, Inc.
Subs. E.R. Squibb Co.

0223
Consolidated Midland Corp.
195 E. Main St., Box 74
Brewster, NY 10509

C-D Consumer Products
P.O. Box 5716
Jacksonville, FL 32207

Continental Labs., Inc.
3106 Spring St.
P.O. Box 5242
Redwood City, CA 94063

ConvaTec
Subs. E.R. Squibb Co.
P.O. Box 4000
Princeton, NJ 08540

Cook-Waite Laboratories, Inc.
90 Park Avenue
New York, NY 10016

0058
CooperCare, Inc.
Mountain View Division
170 South Whisman Road
Mountain View, CA 94043

0041
Cooper Laboratories (P.R.), Inc.
P.O. Box 367
San German, PR 00753

0041
Cooper Laboratories, Inc.
Oral-B Division
305 Fairfield Avenue
Fairfield, NJ 07006

0041
Cooper Laboratories, Inc.
Dermatological Division
305 Fairfield Avenue
Fairfield, NJ 07006

0041
Cooper Laboratories, Inc.
Sparta Instrument Division
600 McCormick Street
San Leandro, CA 94577

0058
CooperVision, Inc.
Mountain View Division
455 E. Middlefield Road
Mountain View, CA 94043

0058
CooperVision Pharmaceuticals,
Inc.
P.O. Box 367
San German, PR 00753

Cord Pharmaceuticals
See: Geneva Generics

B.C. Cowley Co.
P.O. Box 185
Worcester, MA 01613

Crane-Hall Corp.
659 Lofstrand Lane
P.O. Box 1531
Rockville, MD 20850

Creighton Products Corp.
605 Third Avenue
New York, NY 10158

Creomulsion Co.
345 Glen Iris Dr., N.E.
Box 1214
Atlanta, GA 30301

10244
Cross
Div. of Otis Clapp & Son, Inc.

12418
Culminal, Inc.
Box 8
Union City, NJ 07087

0357
Cumberland Mfg. Co.
501 25th Avenue No.
Nashville, TN 37202

0575
Cummins Pharmaceutical Co.,
Inc.

0161
Cutter Laboratories, Inc.
Div., Miles Labs., Inc.
2200 Powell Street
Emeryville, CA 94608

Dairy House Inc.
105 W. Adams St.
Chicago, IL 60603

0282
Dalin Pharmaceuticals, Inc.

0689
Daniels Pharmaceuticals
2527 25th Ave. N.
St. Petersburg, FL 33713

11696
Dattel Pharmaceutical Co., Inc.
4300 Houma Blvd., Suite 101
Metairie, LA 70002

Davies, Rose-Hoyt
    Pharmaceutical
Hoyt Labs
633 Highland Ave.
Needham, MA 02194

Davis Labs., Inc.
P.O. Box 747
Cherry Hill, NJ 08034

0005
Davis and Geck
Div. of American Cyanamid Co.

0425
Day-Baldwin Inc.

Daywell Laboratories Corp.
78Unquowa Place
P.O. Box 490
Fairfield, CT 06430

0657
DDR Pharmaceutical Corp.
8 Ditomas Ct.
Copiague, NY 11726

Defco Pharmaceuticals
7223 Canoga Ave.
P.O. Box 627
Canoga Park, CA 91305

Dekens Products
Div. of J. H. Guild Co. Inc.
Rupert, VT 05678

Delbay Pharmaceuticals, Inc.
See: Schering Corporation

de Leon Labs.
P.O. Box 867
Douglasville, GA 30133

Delmont Laboratories, Inc.
P.O. Box AA
Swarthmore, PA 19081

10310
Del Laboratories, Inc.
See: Commerce Drug. Co.

0316
Del-Ray Laboratories, Inc.
27-Twentieth Avenue N.W.
Birmingham, AL 35215

0827
Delta Drug Corp.
1034 Hendricks Ave.
P.O. Box 10126
Jacksonville, FL 32207

DePree Co., The
See: Eckerd Drug Co.

0587
Dermakon Laboratories
Div. Preston Pharmaceutics, Inc.
P.O. Box 8
Butler, NJ 07405

0088
Derm-Arts Labs.
See: Marion Labs., Inc.

Dermatologicals, Inc.
Div. of Day-Baldwin, Inc.

0066
Dermik Laboratories, Inc.
1777 Walton Road, Dublin Hall
Blue Bell, PA 19422

Devlin Pharmaceuticals, Inc.
700 North Sepulveda Blvd.
El Segundo, CA 90245

DeWitt Drug & Beauty
    Products, Inc.
See: DeWitt International Corp.

10327
DeWitt International Corp.
P.O. Box 6827
Greenville, SC 29606

0737
D'Franssia Corp.
4505 W. First St.
Los Angeles, CA 90004

Dickey Drug Co.
1009 West State St.
Bristol, VA 24201

Dillard & Co., R. Yates
See: Hyrex Co.

0617
Dios Chem. Co.
4200 Laclede Ave.
St. Louis, MO 63108

0777
Dista Products Co.
Div. of Eli Lily Co.
P.O. Box 1407
Indianapolis, IN 46206

Doak Pharmacal Co., Inc.
700 Shames Drive
P.O. Box 1023
Westbury, L.I., NY 11590

Dolcin Corporation
381 Broadway
Westwood, NJ 07675

Dome Laboratories
See: Miles Pharmaceuticals

0221
Dooner Labs., Inc.
See: William H. Rorer, Inc.

0043
Dorsey Laboratories
Div. Sandoz Inc.
N.E., U.S. 6 & Interstate 80
P.O. Box 83288
Lincoln, NE 68501

19041
Doshire, Inc.
Superon Drug Division
3441 W. Montrose
Chicago, IL 60618

Douglas Pharmaceutical
Industries, Inc.
8906 Rosehill Road
Leneya, KS 66215

Dover Pharmaceutical, Inc.
Subs. Otis Clapp

0183
Dow Pharmaceuticals
See: Merrell Dow
Pharmaceuticals

0212
Doyle Pharmaceutical Co.
Div. Sandoz Inc.
5320 West 23 st.
Minneapolis, MN 55440

Drackett Products Co.
Div. Mead Johnson Nutritionals
201 East 4th Street
Cincinnati, OH 45201

Dram Pharmaceuticals, Inc.

0261
Drug Industries Co. Inc.
3237 Hilton Road
Ferndale, MI 48220

Drug Products Co., Inc.

Duke Labs, Inc.
See: Beiersdorf, Inc.

Dumas-Wilson & Co.
See: Mallinckrodt

0217
Dunhall Pharmaceuticals, Inc.
Highway 59 N
P.O. Box 100
Gravette, AR 72736

DuPont de Nemours, E.I.,
& Co., Inc.
Pharmaceutical Div.
1007 Market Street
Wilmington, DE 19898

Durst, S.F. & Co., Inc.
See: O'Neal, Jones & Feldman
Pharmaceuticals

Eastern Chemical Div.
Guardian Chemical Corp.
230 Marcus Blvd.
Hauppage, NY 11787

0721
Eastern Research Lab., Inc.
302 S. Central Ave.
Baltimore, MD 21202

0544
Eastwood Pharmacal Co., Inc.

0035
Eaton Laboratories
See: Norwich-Eaton
Pharmaceuticals

Eaton-Merz Laboratories
Div. Norwich-Eaton
Pharmaceuticals
17 Eaton Avenue
Norwich, NY 13815

Eckerd Drug Company
8333 Bryan Dairy Road
P.O. Box 4689
Clearwater, FL 33518

Economed Pharmaceuticals, Inc.
P.O. Box 3303
Burlington, NC 27215

12336
Econo-Rx, Inc.
2 Blue Ridge St.
Blairsville, GA 30512

0485
Edwards Pharmacal Co.
100 East Hale
P.O. Drawer 129
Osceola, AR 72370

0163
Elder Pharmaceuticals
705 E. Mulberry St.
P.O. Box 31
Bryan, OH 43506

0641
Elkins-Sinn, Inc.
Subs. A.H. Robins Co.
2 Esterbrook Lane
P.O. Box 5483
Cherry Hill, NJ 08034

Emerson Labs.
P.O. Box 1449
1407 San Jacinto
Dallas, TX 75221

0111
Emko Co.
Div. Schering Corp.
7912 Manchester Ave.
St. Louis, MO 63143

0056
Endo Labs., Inc.
See E.I. du Pont de Nemours &
Co., Inc.

Enzyme Process Co., Inc.
19727 Bahama St.
Northridge, CA 91324

Eric, Kirk & Gary, Inc.
9474 Crestfield
Westchester, OH 45069

Etherea Inc.
See: Revlon Inc.

Ever-Dry Corp.
Div. Scherer Labs., Inc.
P.O. Drawer 400009
Dallas, TX 75240

0642
Everett Laboratories, Inc.
76 Franklin Street
East Orange, NJ 07017

Ex-Lax Pharmaceutical Co., Inc
See: Creighton Products Corp.

Factor, Max, & Co.
Sales Div.
1655 N. McCadden
Pl.
P.O. Box 2323
Hollywood, CA 90028

Faraday Labs., Inc.
100 Hoffman Place
Hillside, NJ 07205

0267
Federal Pharmacal
Corp.,
See: U.S. Products, Inc.

0496
Ferndale Labs, Inc.
780 W. Eight Mile Rd.
Ferndale, MI 48220

Ferring Pharmaceuticals, Inc.
See: Centerchem Products, Inc.

Fidelity Prescriptions Labs., Inc.
42 Wyoming St.
Daytona, OH 45409

0421
Fielding Pharm. Co., Inc.
8181 Big Bend
P.O. Box 13017
St. Louis, MO 63119

0274
First Texas Pharmaceuticals,
Inc.
See: Scherer Labs., Inc.

0585
Fisons Corp.
Pharmaceutical Div.
Two Preston Court
Bedford, MA 01730

0132
Fleet, C.B., Co., Inc.
4615 Murray Pl.
P.O. Box 11349
Lynchburg, VA 24505

Fleming and Company
1600 Fenpark Drive
Fenton, MO 63026

0048
Flint Laboratories
Div. Travenol Labs. Inc.
One Baxter Parkway
Deerfield, IL 60015

Flow Pharmaceuticals
See: CooperVision
Pharmaceuticals

0288
Fluoritab Corp.
1927 Copeman Blvd., Box 381
Flint, MI 48501

0168
Fougera, E., & Co.
Div. of BYK-Gulden, Inc.
60 Baylis Road
Melville, NY 11747

0494
Foy Laboratories Div.
Foy Industries, Inc.
351 W. Penn Ave.
Wernersville, PA 19565

Freeport Drug Co., Inc.
4677 Stenstrom Road
Rockford, IL 61109

0141
Fuller Labs., Inc.
Div. of Parke, Davis & Company
7900 Fuller Rd.
Eden Prairie, MN 55343

0713
G & W Laboratories, Inc.
111 Coolidge Street
South Plainfield, NJ 07080

11853
Gaddy, R. L. Company
511 Hart St., P.O. Box 1076
Tallahassee, FL 32302

Galen Labs., Inc.
917 McGee St.
Kansas City, MO 64106

Garret Laboratories, Inc.
77 Brook E 23
Passiac, NJ 07055

0386
Gebauer Chemical Co.
9410 St. Catherine Ave.
Cleveland, OH 44104

0028
Geigy Pharmaceuticals
Div. of Ciba-Geigy Corp.
Ardsley, NY 10502

0674
General Pharmaceutical Prods.,
Inc.
3205 Johnson Rd.
Steubenville, OH 43952

General Drug Co.
200 N. Fairfield Ave.
Chicago, IL. 60612

0182
Generix Drug Sales Co., Inc.
3001 N. 29th Ave.
Hollywood, FL 33020

0835
Geneva Drugs Ltd.
P.O. Box 10
Pomona, NY 10970

Gerber Products Co.
445 State St.
Fremont, MI 49412

0249
Geriatric Pharm. Corp.
397 Jericho Turnpike
Floral Park, L.I., NY 11001

0535
Gilbert Laboratories
31 Fairmount Avenue
Chester, NJ 07930

0173
Glaxo Incorporated
P.O. Box 13960
Five Moore Drive
Research Triangle Park, NC
27709

12843
Glenbrook Labs.
Div. of Sterling Drug, Inc.
90 Park Ave.
New York City, NY 10016

0516
Glenwood Labs., Inc.
83 North Summit St.
Box 518
Tenafly, NJ 07670

Golden-West, Co.
135 S. Central Street
Knoxville, TN 37902

Good Samaritan Laboratories,
Inc.
P.O. Box 782
Norristown, PA 19404

Gordon Laboratories
State & Parkview Roads
Upper Darby, PA 19082

Gotham Pharm. Co., Inc.
See: Ormont Drug and
Chemical Co., Inc.

Graco Pharmaceutical Co.
172 West Main St.
Meriden, CT 06450

0698
Grafton Pharmaceutical Co.

Grant Labs.
6020 Adeline Street
Oakland, CA 94608

0152
Gray Pharmaceutical Co.
Subs. Purdue Fredrick Co.

Greco Pharmacal, Inc.
See: Doak Pharmacal Co.,
Inc.

Grove Lab., Inc.
See: Bristol-Myers Co.

0327
Guardian Chem. Corp.
See: United-Guardian, Inc.

Guild, J. H., Co., Inc.
10 Main Street
Rupert, VT 05768

Haack Labs., Inc.
See: Lemmon Pharmacal Co.

Haag Inc.
5 South 15th St.
Richmond, VA 23219

0841
Haberle Drug Co.
See:. Bowman Pharmaceuticals,
Inc.

Halsey Drug Co., Inc.
1827 Pacific St.
Brooklyn, NY 11233

Halsted Pharmaceuticals, Inc.
444 Bedford Rd.
P.O. Box 3
Pleasantville, NY 10570

Hanford, G. C., Mfr. Co.
304 Oneida St.
Post Office Box 1055
Syracuse, NY 13201

Hankscraft Co.
Div. of Gerber Products Co.
Booster Blvd.
P.O. Box 120
Reedsburg, WI 53959

Hanlon Drug Prods.
500 Church St.
Poughkeepsie, NY 12601

0372
Hannaway, R. T., Inc.
P.O. Box 8217, 50 Clemence St.
Cranston, RI 02920

Haskell, Charles C. & Co.,
Div. Arnar Stone Labs., Inc.

Hauck, W. E., Inc.
1207 Alpharetta St.
P.O. Box 1065
Roswell, GA 30075

Health Care Industries Inc.
2825 Middlebury St.
P.O. Box 878
Elkhart, IN 46515

0023
Herbert Laboratories
See: Allergan Pharmaceuticals,
Inc.

Herring, Louis C., & Co.
P.O. Box 2191
2501 S. Orange Ave.
Orlando, FL 32806

0514
Hickam, Dow B., Inc.
P.O. Box 2006
Sugar Land, TX 77478

High Chemical Company
1760 N. Howard St.
Philadelphia, PA 19122

Hill Dermaceuticals
Div. of Beach Products, Inc.
P.O. Box 19283
Orlando, FL 32814

Hobart Labs., Inc.
900 N. Franklin St.
Chicago, IL 60610

0039
Hoechst-Roussel
Pharmaceuticals Inc.
Div. American Hoechst
Corp.
Route 202–206 North
Somerville, NJ 08876

Holland-Rantos Co., Inc.
Enterprise Avenue
P.O. Box 5147
Trenton, NJ 08638

0118
Hollister-Stier Labs.
Div. Cutter Labs., Inc.
3525 N. Regal St.
Box 3145, Term. Annex
Spokane, WA 99220

Hope Co.
158 Saddleford Dr.
Chesterfield, MO 63017

0126
Hoyt Laboratories
Div. Colgate-Palmolive
Co.
633 Highland Ave.
Needham, MA 02194

0395
Humco Laboratory, Inc.
P.O. Drawer 2550
Texarkana, TX 75501

0219
Humphreys Pharmacal,
Inc.
63 Meadow Rd.
Rutherford, NJ 07070

0553
Hydrosal Co.
5927 St. Rt. 128
P.O. Box 8
Miamitown, OH 45041

Hygiene Research, Inc.
See Day-Baldwin

0944
Hyland Labs.
Div. Travenol Labs., Inc.
P.O. Box 1976
Glendale, CA 91202

0011
Hynson, Westcott & Dunning
Subs. Becton Dickinson
Charles & Chase Sts.
Baltimore, MD 21201

0314
Hyrex Pharmaceuticals
3494 Democrat Road
P.O. Box 18385
Memphis, TN 38118

ICI Americas, Inc.
3411 Silverside Road
P.O. Box 751
Wilmington, DE 19897

0187
ICN Pharmaceuticals
222 N. Vincent Ave.
Covina, CA 91722

Image Products, Inc.
See: U.S. Products, Inc.

Ingram Pharmaceuticals
See: Syntex Laboratories

0633
Inland Alkaloid Co.
4200 Laclede Ave.
St. Louis, MO 63108

Inolex Pharm.
Div. of Inolex Corp.
3 Science Rd.
Glenwood, IL 60425

12805
International Chem. Labs
185 Park Dr.
Eastchester, NY 10707

0177
International Drug, Inc.
See: C-D Consumer Products

0125
International Pharmaceutical
Corporation
See: Marion Labs., Inc.

0814
Interstate Drug Exchange,
Inc.
Engineers Hill
Plainview, L.I., NY 11803

0467
Invenex Laboratories
Div. Dexter Corp.
P.O. Box 200
Chagrin Falls, OH 44022

0258
Inwood Laboratories, Inc.
Div. of Forest Laboratories, Inc.
300 Prospect St.
Inwood, NY 11696

11808
Ion Labs, Inc.
112 Holder Dr.
Hurst, TX 76053

0082
Ives Labs., Inc.
685 Third Ave.
New York, NY 10017

12126
Ivy Corporation
23 Fairfield Pl.
West Caldwell, NJ 07006

Jackson-Mitchell
Pharmaceuticals, Inc.
P.O. Box 5425
Santa Barbara, CA 93108

Jalco
See: Misemer Pharm., Inc.

Jamieson-McKames, Inc.
3227 Morganford Road
St. Louis, MO 63116

Jamol Labs., Inc.
13 Ackerman Ave.
Emerson, NJ 07630

Janssen Pharmaceutica
Div. Johnson and Johnson
40 Kingsbridge Road
Piscataway, NJ 08854

11588
Jeffrey Martin, Inc.
410 Clermont Terrace
Union, NJ 07083

0397
Jenkins Labs., Inc.

0171
Johnson, Matt, Co.
1114 4th Street
Devils Lake, ND 58301

0137
Johnson & Johnson
Baby Products Co.
Grandview Rd.
Skillman, NJ 08558

0992
Kahlenberg Labs.
Div. T. E. Watson Co.
P.O. Box 3829
Sarasota, FL 33578

Kasdenol Corporation
50 Elm Street
Huntington, NY 11743

0351
Kay Pharmacal Co., Inc.
P.O. Box 50375
1312 N. Utica Ave.
Tulsa, OK 74150

Kedrin Pharmacals, Inc.
See: Dolcin Corp.

0588
Keene Pharmaceuticals Inc.
P.O. Box 7
333 S. Mockingbird
Keene, TX 76059

Kendall Co., The
Bauer & Black Div.
1 Federal St.
Boston, MA 02110

0482
Kenwood Labs., Inc.
490A Main Street
New Rochelle, NY 10801

Kenyon Drug Co.
Box 362
Mechanicsville, IA 52306

Kerr, Frank, Chemical Co.
43155 W. Nine Mile Rd.
Northville, MI 48167

Ketchum Labs., Inc.
See: Steri-Med, Inc.

0369
Key Pharmaceuticals, Inc.
50 N.W. 176 Street
P.O. Box 693670
Miami, FL 33169

0285
King Pharmaceutical Co., Inc.
26 N. 77th St.
Birmingham, AL 35206

Kinney & Co., Inc.
1307 12th St.
P.O. Box 307
Columbus, IN 47201

0098
Kirkman Labs., Inc.
934 N.E. 25th Avenue
Portland, OR 97232

Klug Labs., Inc.
See: Galen Labs.

Knickerbocker Biologics Div.
See: Charles Pfizer & Co., Inc.

0044
Knoll Pharm. Co.
30 North Jefferson Rd.
Whippany, NJ 07981

Kondon Mfg. Co.
Div. Wonderful Dream Salve
Corp.
P.O. Box 223
Croswell, MI 48422

0091
Kremers-Urban Co.
See: William H. Rorer

Laboratory Diagnostics Co., Inc.
Drawer 160
620 Route 520
Morganville, NJ 07751

La Cross
Div. Del Labs., Inc.

La Crosse Pharm. Co.
Div. Whittaker Corp.
1502 Miller Dr.
La Crosse, WI 54601

Lactona Prods.(Div.-
Warner-Lambert Pharm.)
201 Tabor Rd.
Morris Plains, NJ 07950

Lafayette Pharmacal, Inc.
4200 South Hulen Street
Fort Worth, TX 76109

0073
Lakeside Laboratories, Inc.
See: Richardson-Merrell Inc.

0348
Lambda Pharmacal Lab.
See: Medtech Laboratories, Inc.

0527
Lannett Co., Inc., The
9000 State Rd.
Philadelphia, PA 19136

10648
Larson Labs., Inc.
1320 Irwin Drive
Erie, PA 16505

La Salle Laboratories
Div. Del Labs., Inc.

0277
Laser, Inc.
2000 N. Main St.
P.O. Box 905
Crown Point, IN 46307

12434
Last, Alvin, Inc.
145 Palisades St.
Dobbs Ferry, NY 10522

10651
Lavoptik Co., Inc.
661 Western Av. N.
St. Paul, MN 55103

0005
Lederle Laboratories
Div. of American Cyanamid
  Co.
N. Middletown Rd.
P.O. Box 500
Pearl River, NY 10965

Lee-Colbert Div.
See: Daniels, Robert and Co.

Leeming Division
Pfizer, Incorporated
100 Jefferson Road
Parsippany, NJ 07054

Lehn & Fink Products Group
Div. Sterling Drug Inc.
225 Summit Ave.
Montvale, NJ 07645

Leicy's, Inc.
1531–33 W. Market St.
Steubenville, OH 43952

17201
Leland Laboratories, Inc.
West Wade Hampton Blvd.
Greer, SC 29651

0093
Lemmon Company
P.O. Box 30
Sellersville, PA 18960

0162
Lewis-Howe Co.
319 S. 4th St.
St. Louis, MO 63102

0284
Lexington Chemical Co., Inc.
27 Jones Road
Box 609
Waltham, MA 02154

14869
Lexalabs, Inc.
P.O. Box 5234
Lenexa, KS 66215

Lif-O-Gen, Div.
Allied Healthcare Prods., Inc,
1720 Sublette Ave.
St. Louis, MO 63110

0002
Lilly, Eli & Co.
740 S. Alabama St.
Box 618
Indianapolis, IN 46206

Lincoln Labs., Inc.
Hickory Point Rd.
Box 1139
Decatur, IL 62525

Lloyd Brothers, Inc.
See: Hoechst-Roussel

Loma Linda Food Co.
11503 Pierce St.
Riverside, CA 92515

0273
Lorvic Corp., The
8810 Frost Ave.
St. Louis, MO 63134

Luden's Inc.
200 North 8th St.
Reading, PA 19603

0618
Luyties Pharmacal Co.
4200 Laclede Ave.
St. Louis, MO 63108

0466
Macsil, Inc.
1326 Frankford Ave.
Philadelphia, PA 19125

Madison Labs.
380 North St.
Teterboro, NJ 07608

0179
Madland Laboratories,
  Inc.

0166
Mallard, Inc.
3021 Wabash Ave.
Detroit, MI 48216

Mallincrodt Pharmaceutics
  Div.
See: Wallace Laboratories

Maltbie Lab.
See: WTS-Pharmacraft
Div. Wallace and Tiernan

Mann Chemical Corp.
520 W. Main St.
Louisville, KY 40202

10706
Manne, Kenneth A. Co.
1522 Cleveland Ave., N.W.
P.O. Box 8649
Canton, OH 44711

Manola Company
4200 Laclede Ave.
St. Louis, MO 63108

Marin Pharmaceuticals
P.O. Box 174
Miami, FL 33144

0088
Marion Laboratories, Inc.
P.O. Box 9627
Kansas City, MO 64134

12939
Marlop Pharmaceuticals, Inc.
5752 Fieldston Road, Box 536
Bronx, NY 10471

Marlyn Company, Inc.
3071 S. Harbour Blvd.
Santa Ana, CA 92704

Marsh-Emory Laboratories, Inc.
600 Chama, N.E.
Albuquerque, NM 87108

0692
Martin-Phillips Labs.
8604 Verree Rd.
Philadelphia, PA 19115

12758
Mason Pharmaceuticals
P.O. Box 8330
1201 Dove Street, Suite 520
Newport Beach, CA 92660

Massengill, S.E., Co., The
See: Beecham Laboratories

0314
Matco Drug Company
See: Hyrex Pharmaceuticals

Maurry Biological Co., Inc.
6109 S. Western Avenue
Los Angeles, CA 90047

Mayer Lab., Inc.
701 Bridgeway Blvd.
P.O. Box 1336
Sausalito, CA 94965

0259
Mayrand, Inc.
1026 E. Lindsay St.
P.O. Box 20246
Greensboro, NC 27407

11089
McGregor & Co.
32580 Grand River Ave.
Farmington, MI 48024

0022
McKesson Laboratories
See: M.K. Laboratories, Inc.

0045
Mc Neil Consumer Products Co.
Subs. McNEILAB, Inc.
500 Office Center Drive
Fort Washington, PA 19034

Mc Neil Pharmaceutical
Subs. McNEILAB, Inc.
Spring House, PA 19477

0087
Mead Johnson & Company
2404 Pennsylvania St.
Evansville, IN 47721

11940
Medco Lab., Inc.
716 West Seventh St.
P.O. Box 864
Sioux City, IA 51102

0764
Medco Supply Co.
2410 Kilgore Ave.
Muncie, IN 47304

0244
Medicone Co.
225 Varick St.
New York, NY 10014

0184
Medics Pharmaceutical
See: U.S. Chemical Marketing
Group

0645
Medi-Rx Pharmaceuticals, Inc.
45 N. Palmer
Houston, TX 77003

Medtech Laboratories, Inc.
721 Sheridan Avenue
Cody, WY 82414

45800
Menley & James Labs.
Subs. SmithKline Corp.
P.O. Box 8082
1500 Spring Garden St.
Philadelphia, PA 19101

Mennen Co.
Hanover Ave.
P.O. Box 1000
Morristown, NJ 07960

Mentholatum Co., The
1360 Niagara St.
Buffalo, NY 14213

12814
Merchant Pharmaceutical Co.,
Inc.
4 South Third St., P.O. Box 527
Warrenton, VA 22186

0006
Merck Sharp & Dohme
Div. Merck & Co., Inc.
West Point, PA 19486

Merck Sharp & Dohme AGVET
Div. Merck & Co., Inc.
P.O. Box 2000
Rahway, NJ 07065

0394
Mericon Industries, Inc.
420 S. W. Washington St.
P.O. Box 5759
Peoria, IL 61601

Merieux Institute, Inc.
1200 N.W. 78th Ave.
Suite 109
Miami, FL 33126

0429
Merit Pharmaceutical Company,
Inc.
See: Scherer Labs., Inc.

0183
Merrell Dow Pharmaceuticals,
Inc.
Subs. Dow Chemical Company
2110 E. Galbraith Rd.
Cincinnati, OH 45215

36969
Merrell Dow Laboratories Inc.
(P.R.)
2110 E. Galbraith Rd.
Cincinnati, OH 45215

0322
Merrick Medicine Co.
P.O. Box 1489
Waco, TX 76703

Meyer Labs., Inc.
See: Glaxo Inc.

0816
Midway Medical Co., Inc.
103 Samson St.
Glasgow, KY 42141

0192
Miles Laboratories, Inc.
Consumer Products Div.
1127 Myrtle Street
Elkhart, IN 46514

0026
Miles Pharmaceuticals
Div. Miles Laboratories, Inc.
400 Morgan Lane
West Haven, CT 06516

0396
Milex Products
5915 Northwest Hwy.
Chicago, IL 60631

Miller Pharmacal Co.
P.O. Box 299
West Chicago, IL 60185

Mills Pharmaceuticals, Inc.

Mill-Mark Pharmaceuticals, Inc.
1090 Englewood Ave.
Buffalo, NY 14223

Milton Roy Company
Milroy Laboratories Division
P.O. Drawer 849
Sarasota, FL 33578

Minette Pharm. Corp.
3024 Genesee St.
P.O. Box 142
Buffalo, NY 14225

0276
Misemer Pharmaceuticals, Inc.
4553 South Campbell St.
P.O. Box 3177
Glenstone Sta.
Springfield, MO 65804

0178
Mission Pharmacal Co.
1325 E. Durango St.
P.O. Box 1676
San Antonio, TX 78296

M. J. Labs.
P.O. Box 432, Little River Sta.
Miami, FL 33138

M.K. Laboratories, Inc.
424Grasmere Ave.
Fairfield, CT 06430

Modern Products, Inc.
3015 W. Vera Ave.
P.O. Box 09398
Milwaukee, WI 53209

Monsanto Chemical Co.
800 North Lindbergh
Boulevard
St. Louis, MO 63167

11868
Monticello Drug Co.
45 Broad St. Viaduct
Jacksonville, FL 32202

Moore, Edward J., Sons, Inc.
46–44 11th St.
Long Island City, N.Y. 11101

0839
Moore, H. L., Drug Exchange,
Inc.
370 John Downey Dr.
New Britain, CT 06050

0133
Moore Kirk Labs., Inc.
Div. of the Zemmer Co.

01277
Morton Pharmaceuticals, Inc.
1625–39 N. Highland St.
P.O. Box 8037
Memphis, TN 38108

Moss Chemical Co. Inc.
183 St. Paul St.
Rochester, NY 14604

0543
Mosso, C. A. Co., Inc.
See: Health Care Industries
Inc.

Moyco Industries, Inc.
S.E. Cor 21st and Clearfield
Sts.
Philadelphia, PA 19132

M.P.L. Labs.
509 Washington Ave., S.
Minneapolis, MN 55401

Mulford Labs.
Div. Lemmon Pharmacal Co.
Sellersville, PA 18960

Murine Company
See: Abbott Labs., Consumer
Prods. Div.

0451
Muro Pharmacal Inc.
890 East Street
Tewksbury, MA 01876

0897
National Magnesia Co., Inc.
83rd Street & Cooper Avenue
Glendale, NY 11227

Neisler Labs., Inc.
See: Marion Labs., Inc.

Neoco Corp.
See: Nion Corp.

0487
Nephron Corporation
3319 Pacific Ave., P.O.
Box 1974
Tacoma, WA 98401

Neutrogena Corp.
5755 W. 96th St.
Los Angeles, CA 90045.

Nevin, J. R., Co., Inc.
183 Royal Parkway West
Williamsville, NY 14221

New England Pharmaceutical
Co.
14 Westerfield Rd.
Hamden, CT 06714

10797
New Skin Company
See: Medtech Laboratories,
Inc.

Nion Corporation
11581 Federal Drive
El Monte, CA 91731

0766
Norcliff Thayer Inc.
One Scarsdale Road
Tuckahoe, NY 10707

Nordisk-USA
6500 Rock Spring Drive
Bethesda, MD 20817

Norgine Laboratories, Inc.
2 Overhill Road
Scarsdale, NY 10583

Nortech Laboratories Inc.
4 Midland Avenue
Hicksville, NY 11801

0298
North American Pharm., Inc.
See: Vortech Pharm., Ltd.

0149
Norwich Eaton Pharmaceuticals
17 Eaton Ave.
Norwich, NY 13815

Novo Industries
Subs. E. R. Squibb Co.
120 Alexander St.
Princeton, NJ 08540

0362
Novocol Chemical Mfg. Co.,
   Inc.
2911 Atlantic Ave.
Brooklyn, NY 11207

Noxell Corp.
11050 York Rd.
P.O. Box 1799
Baltimore, MD 21203

0159
Noyes, P. J. & Co.
101 Main St.
Lancaster, NH 03584

Nutrition Control Products
Div. Pharmex Inc.
2113 Lincoln St.
P.O. Box 151
Hollywood, FL 33022

Nutritional Biochemicals Corp.
26201 Miles Ave.
Cleveland, OH 44128

0477
Obetrol Pharmaceuticals
Div. of Rexar Pharmacal
   Corp.
396 Rockway Ave.
Valley Stream, NY 11581

O'Connor Products Co.
24400 Capitol
Redford, MI 48239

O'Neal, Jones and Feldman
   Pharmaceuticals
2510 Metro Boulevard
St. Louis County, MO 63043

Orbar International Ltd.
711 S. Sleight St.
Naperville, IL 60540

Orbit Pharmaceutical Company
   Inc.
1304 N. 5th St.
Kansas City, KS 66101

0052
Organon Pharmaceuticals
375 Mt. Pleasant Ave.
West Orange, NJ 07052

0142
Ormont Drug & Chem. Co.
See: U.S. Products, Inc.

0191
Ortega Pharm. Co.
586 S. Edgewood Ave.
P.O. Box 6212
Jacksonville, FL 32205

0062
Ortho Diagnostic Systems Inc.
Div. Johnson and Johnson
Route 202
Raritan, NJ 08869

0062
Ortho Pharmaceutical Corp.
Route 202
Raritan, NJ 08869

0107
Ortho Pharmaceuticals, Inc.
P.O. Box 463
Manati, PR 00701

10244
Otis Clapp & Son, Inc.
143 Albany St.
Cambridge, MA 02139

0299
Owen Laboratories, Inc.
Div. of Alcon Labs., Specialty
   Prod. Div.
P.O. Box 1959
Ft. Worth, TX 76101

Oxford Laboratories Inc.
Dayton, VA 22821

0574
Paddock Laboratories, Inc.
3101 Louisiana Ave. North
Minneapolis, MN 55427

0271
Palmedico, Inc.
See: W. E. Hauck, Inc.

Pannett Products, Inc.
Div. of Dormin, Inc.
P.O. Box 723
Orleans, MA 02653

0318
Panray Pharmaceuticals
See: U.S. Products, Inc.

0638
Paraeusal Co.
1809 Belmont Ave.
Youngstown, OH 44504

0071
Parke-Davis
Div. Warner-Lambert Co.
201 Tabor Road
Morris Plains, NJ 07950

Parker Laboratories, Inc.
307 Washington Street
Orange, NJ 07050

0727
Park Plaza Pharmaceuticals,
   Inc.
11122 Walnut
Kansas City, MO 64114

0349
Parmed Pharmaceuticals
4220 Hyde Park Boulevard
Niagara Falls, NY 14305

0418
Pasadena Research Labs.,
   Inc.
2107 E. Villa St.
Pasadena, CA 91107

Pascal Company, Inc.
2929 N. E. Northrup Way
Bellevue, WA 98004

Paschall Labs., Inc.
4116 Rainier Ave., S.
Seattle, WA 98118

Paxton, F. H. & Sons, Inc.
P.O. Box 729
Evanston, IL 60204

0884
Pedinol Pharmacal Inc.
110 Bell Street
West Babylon, NY 11704

0018
Pennwalt Corporation
Prescription Division
P.O. Box 1710
Rochester, NY 14603

Penta Products, Inc.
425 2nd St.
San Francisco, CA 94107

Perfumeria Brisas, Inc.
P.O. Box 384
Forest Hills, NY 11375

0799
Perry Labs., Inc.
14713 Gratiot St.
Detroit, MI 48205

0096
Person & Covey, Inc.
616 Allen Ave.
Glendale, CA 91201

Peterson Ointment Co.
257 Franklin St.
Buffalo, NY 14202

Pfanstiehl Labs., Inc.
1219 Glen Rock Ave.
Waukegan, IL 60085

0995
Pfipharmecs
Div. of Pfizer, Inc.
235 E. 42nd St.
New York, NY 10017

0069
Pfizer Laboratories
Div. of Pfizer, Inc.
235 E. 42nd St.
New York, NY 10017

Pharmachem Corp.
Broad & Wood Sts.
Bethlehem, PA 18018

0016
Pharmacia Laboratories
Div. Pharmacia Inc.
800 Centennial Ave.
Piscataway, NJ 08854

0235
Pharmacraft Division
Pennwalt Corporation
P.O. Box 1710
Rochester, NY 14603

0598
Pharmacy Associates
1643 E. Genesee St.
Syracuse, NY 13201

Pharmex, Inc.
2113 Lincoln St., Box 151
Hollywood, FL 33022

Pharmics, Inc.
1878 S. Redwood Rd.
Salt Lake City, UT 84104

0054
Philips Roxane Labs.
See Roxane Laboratories,
Inc.

Pixacol Company
Dept. DB
P.O. Box 29277
Parma, OH 44129

Plessner, Paul, Co., The
2232 4th Street North
St. Petersburg, FL 33704

0138
Plough, Inc.
Subs: Schering-Plough Corp.
P.O. Box 377
Memphis, TN 38151

0095
Poythress, Wm. P. & Co.,
Inc.
16 N. 22nd Street
Box 26946
Richmond, VA 23261

0331
Premo Pharmaceutical Labs.,
Inc.
111 Leuning Street
South Hackensack, NJ 07606

11649
Press Chemical &
Pharmaceutical Labs.
P.O. Box 09103
584 East Whittler St.
Columbus, OH 43209

0587
Preston Pharmaceutics,
Inc.
Post Office Box #8
Butler, NJ 07405

Primedics Labs.
California Division
1123 Goodrich Blvd.
Los Angeles, CA 90022

Procter and Gamble
Professional Services
Division
P.O. Box 39175
Cincinnati, OH 45247

Professional Pharmacal Co.
See: Steri-Med, Inc.

Pruvo Pharmacal Co.
2018 W. Bender Rd.
Milwaukee, WI 53209

0034
Purdue Frederick Co.
50 Washington Street
Norwalk, CT 06856

0228
Purepac Pharmaceutical Co.
200 Elmora Ave.
Elizabeth, NJ 07207

Quinton, George, & Son, Inc.
Wantagh, NY 11793

0196
Rachelle Labs., Inc.
Sub. of International Rectifier
Corp.
700 Henry Ford Ave.
Long Beach, CA 90801

0793
Rals Laboratories
Div. Schuemann Labs.

Randob Labs., Ltd.
508 Franklin Ave.
Mt. Vernon, NY 10551

10952
Recsei Labs., The
330 S. Kellogg, Blvd. M.
Goleta, CA 93117

Redford Laboratories
See: Bay Laboratories, Inc.

0021
Reed & Carnrick
Pharmaceuticals
Piscataway, NJ 08854

10956
Reese Chemical Co.
10617 Frank Ave.
Cleveland, OH 44106

0063
Reid-Provident Labs, Inc.
640 Tenth Street, N.W.
Atlanta, GA 30318

21769
Reily Chemical Co.
P.O. Box 50372
New Orleans, LA 70150

0815
Reiss Williams Company
Blair Park
Port Reading, NJ 07064

Renalab
Div. of Ries Biologicals

Republic Drug Co., Inc.
175 Great Arrow Ave.
Buffalo, NY 14207

Requa Mfg. Co., Inc.
1 Seneca Pl., Box 4008
Greenwich, CT 06830

Research Industries Corp.
Pharm. Division
1847 W. 2300 South
Salt Lake City, UT 84119

Revlon Health Care
See: USV Laboratories

Rexall Drug Co.
P.O. Box 7189
3901 N. Kingshighway Blvd.
St. Louis, MO 63115

Rexar Pharmacal Corp.
396 Rockaway Ave.
Valley Stream, NY 11581

0762
Rhode, J.G., Co.
302 S. Central Ave.
Baltimore, MD 21202

10973
Richards Pharmaceutical Co.
P.O. Box 1129
Santa Monica, CA 90406

Richlyn Laboratories
3725 Castor Ave.
Philadelphia, PA 19124

0398
Ries-Hamly, Inc.
P.O. Box 83
Algonac, MI 48001

0089
Riker Labs., Inc.
Subs. 3M Company
19901 Nordhoff Street
Northridge, CA 91324

0031
Robins, A.H. Co.
1407 Cummings Drive
Richmond, VA 23220

0004
Roche Laboratories
Div. Hoffmann-LaRoche,
Inc.
Roche Park
Nutley, NJ 07110

0049
Roerig
Div. Pfizer Pharmaceuticals
235 E. 42nd Street
New York, NY 10017

Roger Pharmacal, Inc.
P.O. Box 011022
1654 N.W. 35th St.
Miami, FL 33142

Rohm & Haas Co.
Independence Mall West
Philadelphia, PA 19105

0067
Rorer, William H., Inc.
500 Virginia Drive
Ft. Washington, PA 19034

0074
Ross Laboratories
Div. Abbott Laboratories
585 Cleveland Ave.
Columbus, OH 43216

0269
Roussel Corp.
155 E. 44th St.
New York, NY 10017

0032
Rowell Laboratories, Inc.
210 Main Street, West
Baudette, MN 56623

0054
Roxanne Laboratories,
Inc.
330 Oak Street
P.O. Box 16532
Columbus, OH 43216

0524
Rucker Pharmacal Co.,
Inc.
6540 Line Avenue
Shreveport, LA 71106

Ruson Labs.
P.O. Box 42154
Portland, OR 97242

0263
Rystan Company, Inc.
47 Center Avenue
P.O. Box 214
Little Falls, NJ 07424

Salsbury Laboratories
2000 Rockford Road
Charles City, IA 50616

0511
Sandia Pharmaceuticals, Inc.

0078
Sandoz Pharmaceuticals
Div. of Sandoz Inc.
59 Route 10
E. Hanover, NJ 07936

Saron Pharmacal Corp
1640 Central Ave.
St. Petersburg, FL 33712

0281
Savage Labs., Inc.
Div. of Byk-Gulden, Inc.
60 Baylis Road
Melville, Long Island, NY 11747

Schaffer Laboratories
P.O. Box 539
Arcadia, CA 91006

0274
Scherer Laboratories, Inc.
14335 Gills Road
Dallas, TX 75240

0085
Schering Corp.
Div. Schering-Plough Corp.
2000 Galloping Hill Rd.
Kenilworth, NJ 07033

0234
Schmid, Julius, Inc.
Route 46 West
Little Falls, NJ 07424

Scholl, Inc.
See: Plough, Inc.

0352
Schuemann Laboratories, Inc.
480 W. Auroa Road
Northfield, OH 44067

42021
Sclavo, Incorporated
5 Mansard Court
Wayne, NJ 07470

0711
Scott-Allison Pharmaceuticals,
   Inc.
581 Sagamore Avenue
Teaneck, NJ 07666

0372
Scot-Tussin Pharmacal Co., Inc.
50 Clemence St., P.O. Box 8217
Cranston, RI 02920

0444
Scrip, Inc.
101 South St.
Peoria, IL 61602

0329
Scruggs Pharmacal Co., Inc.

0014
Searle & Co.
San Juan, PR 00936

0025
Searle Laboratories
Div. Searle Pharmaceuticals
   Inc.
P.O. Box 5110
Chicago, IL 60680

0551
Seatrace Co.
P.O. Box 363
Gadsden, AL 35902

SeMed Pharmaceuticals
See: Beecham-Massengill
   Co.

Serono Laboratories, Inc.
280 Pond Street
Randolph, MA 02368

Serums and Vaccines of
   America
Division of Murai Laboratories,
   Inc.

Shear-Kershman Labs., Inc.
14500 South Outer 40 Rd.
Chesterfield, MO 63017

Shepard Laboratories
500 Virginia Dr.
Ft. Washington, PA 19034

Sherwood Laboratories,
   Inc.
1601 E. 361st St.
Willoughby, OH 44094

0823
Sheryl Pharmaceuticals,
   Inc.

Shield Laboratories
99–101 Saw Mill River Rd.
Yonkers, NY 10701

Shulton, Inc.
697 Route 46
Clifton, NY 07011

Shuptrine Company
P.O. Box 22127
Savannah, GA 31403

Sig: Pharmaceuticals, Inc.
Div. International Chemical &
   Nuclear Corp.
185 Park Drive
Eastchester, NY 10707

Silver's Pharmaceuticals
P.O. Box 238
Neptune Beach, FL 32233

Smalley & Williams, Inc.
806 Lexington Ave.
New York, NY 10021

0007
Smith Kline & French Company
Subsidiary of SmithKline Corp.

0007
Smith Kline & French
   Laboratories
Division of SmithKline Corp.

0484
SmithKline Corporation
1500 Spring Garden St.
Philadelphia, PA 19101

0058
Smith, Miller & Patch
Div. of CooperVision
   Pharmaceuticals Inc.

0058
Smith, Miller & Patch
Div. of Berlex Laboratories

0346
Softcon Products
Div. Warner-Lambert Co.
201 Tabor Road
Morris Plains, NJ 07950

Southern Drug & Mfg. Co.
1639 N. Highland
Memphis, TN 38108

0251
Spanner, G.O., Inc.
20 Church St.
Monclair, NJ 07042

Spence McCord
Div. of General Medical
   Corp.
La Crosse, WI 54601

Spencer-Mead, Inc.
270 West Merrick Road
Valley Stream, NY 11582

Sperti Drug Products, Inc.
7 Sperti Dr.
Fort Mitchell, KY 41017

10833
Spirt & Company
Subs. Hyrex Pharmaceuticals

50821
Springbok Pharmaceuticals,
   Inc.
12502 South Garden Street
Houston, TX 77071

0003
Squibb, E.R.
P.O. Box 4000
Princeton, NJ 08540

Squibb-Connaught
Subs. E.R. Squibb Co.

11530
Stanback Co., Ltd.
1500 S. Main St.
P.O. Box 1669
Salisbury, NC 28144

Standard Process Laboratories,
   Inc.
2023 West Wisconsin Ave.
Milwaukee, WI 53201

0716
Standex Laboratories
585 W. Second Ave.
Columbus, OH 43215

0242
Stanlabs Pharmaceutical
   Co.
Subs. Simpak Corporation

Star Pharmaceuticals, Inc.
5064 Nadina Lane
Box 4161
Atlanta, GA 30302

Stecker Chemicals, Inc.
See: Pfister Chemical
   Inc.

0346
Steri-Med, Inc.
P.O. Box 459
Lindenhurst, NY 11757

Stewart-Jackson Pharmacal, Inc.
P.O. Box 28701
Memphis, TN 38128

0145
Stiefel Laboratories, Inc.
2801 Ponce de Leon
 Blvd.
Coral Gables, FL 33134

Stillman Co., The
323 East Galena Blvd.
Aurora, IL 60507

Strassenberg Labs.
See: Pennwalt Corp.

Strickland and Co.
1400 Ragan
Memphis, TN 38101

Strubel Drugs
4500 6th St.
Kenosha, WI 53142

0038
Stuart Pharmaceuticals
Div. of ICI Americas Inc.
P.O. Box 751
Wilmington, DE 19897

11086
Summers Labs., Inc.
Morris Road
Fort Washington, PA 19034

0414
Suppositoria Labs., Inc.
135 Florida St.
Farmingdale, L.I., NY 11735

Surgikos Co.
See: Johnson & Johnson

Surgitube Products Corp.
83 North Summit St.
Tenafly, NJ 07670

0253
Sutliff & Case Co., Inc.
P.O. Box 838
201 Spring St.
Peoria, IL 61603

11701
Sween Corp.

0033
Syntex Laboratories, Inc.
3401 Hillview Ave.
Stanford Industrial Park
Palo Alto, CA 94304

0033
Syntex Puerto Rico, Inc.
Humacao, PR 00661

0734
Tablicaps, Inc.

12072
Temesco
5135 Galaxy Dr., P.O. Box
 16328
Jackson, MS 39206

Tennessee Wholesale Drug
 Co.
200 Cumberland Bend.
Nashville, TN 37228

Texas Pharmacal
See: Alcon Laboratories or
 Parke-Davis

Thompson Medical Co., Inc.
919 Third Ave.
New York, NY 10022

3M Personal Care Products
Subs. 3M Company
19901 Nordhoff Street
Northridge, CA 91324

Three P Products Corp.
5 Cooper Street
Burlington, NJ 08018

Thurston Laboratories, Inc.
P.O. Box 8
Solana Beach, CA 92075

11299
Torch Laboratories, Inc.
P.O. Box 248
Reisterstown, MD 21136

Torigian Labs., Inc.
218–20 98th Ave.
Queens Village, NY 11429

0157
Towne, Paulsen & Co., Inc.
140 E. Duarte Rd.
Monrovia, CA 91016

Travenol Labs., Inc.
1425 Lake Cook Road
Deerfield, IL 60015

11311
Trimen Laboratories, Inc.

0558
Tri-State Pharm. Co., Inc.
See: Mismer Pharm., Inc.

0648
Truett Labs.
Div. Southwestern Drug Corp.
13450 Harry Hines Blvd.
P.O. Box 34029
Dallas, TX 75234

0463
Truxton, C.O. Inc.
1458–60 Haddon Ave.
Camden, NJ 08103

50023
Tunex Pharmaceuticals, Inc.
5909 Shelby Oaks Dr.
Suite 233
Memphis, TN 38134

0124
Tutag Pharmaceuticals
See: Reid-Provident

0785
UAD Laboratories, Inc.
1400 Commerce St.
Minden, LA 71055

0127
Ulmer Pharmacal
Div. Physicians & Hospital
 Supply Co.
2440 Fernbrook Lane
Plymouth, MN 55441

0051
Unimed, Inc.
35 Columbia Rd.
Somerville, NJ 08876

United-Guardian, Inc.
P.O. Box 2500
Smithtown, NY 11787

0009
Upjohn Company, The
7171 Portage Road
Kalamazoo, MI 49001

0245
Upsher-Smith Laboratories, Inc.
14905 23rd Ave. N.
Minneapolis, MN 55441

U.S. Chemical Marketing
 Group
203 Rio Circle
Decatur, GA 30030

U.S. Products, Inc.
16636 N.W. 54th Ave.
Miami Lakes, FL 33014

U.S. Ethicals
See: Wharton Labs., Inc.

0070
USV Laboratories Inc.
Manati, P.R. 00701

0075
USV Laboratories
Div. Revlon Health Care
 Group
303 South Broadway
Tarrytown, NY 10591

0105
USV (P.R.) Development Corp.
Manati, P.R. 00701

U-Tri Products, Inc.
P.O. Box 2152
Gardena, CA 90247

0377
Vale Chemical Co. Inc., The
1201 Liberty St.
Allentown, PA 18102

0615
Vangard Laboratories
Div. of M.W.M. Corp.
103 Samson St.
Glasgow, KY 42141

VanPelt & Brown, Inc.
See: Mallinckrodt Pharm.

10038
Velvet Pharmacal
See: Ambix Laboratories

Vernon Laboratories, Inc.
See: Ranbod Laboratories,
 Ltd.

25866
Vicks Health Care
Div. of Richardson-Vicks Inc.
One Far Mill Crossing
Shelton, CT 06484

23900
Vicks Pharmacy Products
Div. of Richardson-Vicks Inc.
10 Westport Road
Wilton, CT 06897

76660
Vicks Toiletry Products
Div. of Richardson-Vicks Inc.
One Far Mill Crossing
Shelton, CT 06484

Viobin Corporation
Subs: A.H. Robins Co.
226 W. Livingston
Monticello, IL 61856

0836
Virtal Pharmacal Co., Inc.
Brightwood Rd.
Woodbridge, CT 06525

0181
Vita Elixir Co., Inc.
P.O. Box 9026
Atlanta, GA 30314

Vitamins by Spirit, Inc.
39 Prospect St.
Waterbury, CT 06702

0185
Vitarine Co., Inc., The
227–15 N. Conduit Ave.
Springfield Gardens, NY 11413

0298
Vortech Pharmaceuticals,
   Ltd.
6851 Chase Rd.
Dearborn, MI 48126

Walgreen Laboratories, Inc.
3532 West 47th Place
Chicago, IL 60632

0741
Walker, Corp. & Co., Inc.
P.O. Drawer 1320
Syracuse, NY 13201

0619
Walker Pharmacal Co.
4200 Laclede Ave.
St. Louis, MO 63108

0037
Wallace Laboratories
Div. Carter-Wallace, Inc.
Half Acre Road
P.O. Box # 1
Cranbury, NJ 08512

0017
Wampole Laboratories
Div. Carter-Wallace, Inc.
Half Acre Road
Cranbury, NJ 08512

Wampole-Zeus
See: Wampole Labs.

0047
Warner/Chilcott Laboratories
See: Parke-Davis

11370
Warner-Lambert Company
201 Tabor Rd.
Morris Plains, NJ 07950

0013
Warren-Teed Laboratories
See: Adria Labs. Inc.

Wayne Medical Co.
111 N. Railroad St.
Pikeville, NC 27863

0991
Webcon Pharmaceuticals
Div. of Alcon Labs.
P.O. Box 1629
Fort Worth, TX 76101

Weber Pharmacenticals
105 Treehouse Lane
Zanesville, OH

Webster, William A. Co.,
   The
See: Webcon Pharm.

Weeks and Leo Co. Inc.
P.O. Box 3570
Des Moines, IA 50322

0917
Wesley Pharmacal Co., Inc.

0291
Westerfield Laboratories,
   Inc.
See: O'Neal, Jones & Feldman
   Pharmaceuticals

11397
Western Pharmacal Co.
1537 So. Main St.
Salt Lake City, UT 84115

Western Research Labs.,
   Inc.
P.O. Box 9327
301 S. Cherokee St.
Denver, CO 80223

0072
Westwood Pharmaceuticals
468 Dewitt St.
Buffalo, NY 14213

0195
Wharton Labs., Inc.
Div. U.S. Ethicals, Inc.
37–02 48th Ave.
Long Island City, NY 11101

0573
Whitehall Laboratories
Div. American Home Products
   Corp.
685 Third Ave.
New York, NY 10017

0923
Whiteworth, Inc.
14527 S. San Pedro St.
Gardena, CA 90248

Whittaker General Medical
See: La Crosse Pharm. Co.

0317
Whorton Pharmaceuticals, Inc.
4202 Gary Ave.
Fairfield, AL 35064

11414
Willen Drug Co.
18 N. High St.
Baltimore, MD 21202

Williams, J.B., Co., Inc.
See: Beecham Products

Williams, T. E.
Pharmaceuticals, Inc.
P.O. Box 1860
Edmond, OK 73034

0427
Winston Pharmaceuticals, Inc.
4706 Kirk Rd., P.O. Box 5275
Winston-Salem, NC 27103

Winthrop Laboratories
See: Winthrop-Breon Labs.

0024
Winthrop-Breon Laboratories
90 Park Avenue
New York, NY 10016

0971
Winthrop Products Inc.
See: Winthrop-Breon Labs.

11422
Winton, Ralph, Co.
18–20 No. High St.
Baltimore, MD 21202

12120
Wisconsin Pharmacal Co.
Div. Badger Pharmacal Inc.
2977 Hwy 60
P.O. Box 198
Jackson, WI 53037

0621
Wise's K.C. Homeopathic
   Pharmacy
4200 Laclede
St. Louis, MO 63108

0928
Wolins Pharmacal Corp.
Subsidiary of
Generics Corp. of America

0008
Wyeth Labs.
Div. American Home Prods.
   Corp.
P.O. Box 8299
Philadelphia, PA 19101

0116
Xttrium Lab. Inc.
415 W. Pershing Rd.
Chicago, IL 60609

0461
Yager Drug Co.
430 W. Mulberry St.
Baltimore, MD 21201

0317
Yeager Specialty Co.
Box 250
Blountsville, AL 35031

Young, W.F., Inc.
111 Lyman St.
Springfield, MA 01101

0343
Youngs Drug Products Corp.
See: Holland-Rantos

0133
Zemmer Co., Inc., The

0172
Zenith Laboratories, Inc.
140 LeGrand Ave.
Northvale, NJ 07647

Zeus Scientific, Inc.
Distributed by Wampole Labs.

Zitar Industries
P.O. Box 200
Fenton, MO 63026